Lippincott's

Nurses' Drug Manual

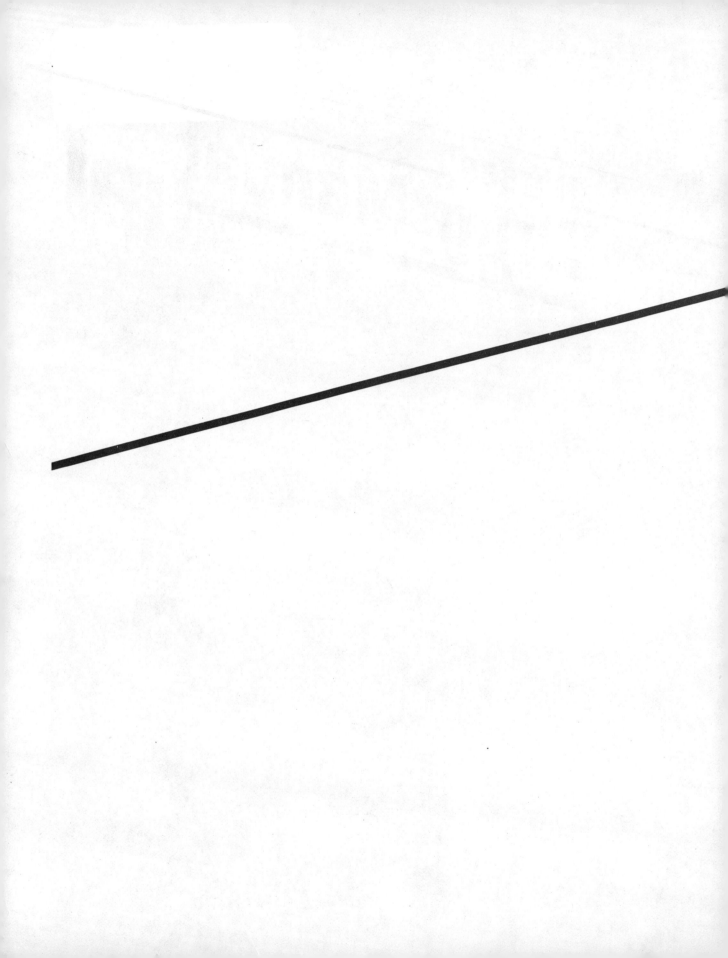

Lippincott's
Nurses'
Drug Manual

Jeanne C. Scherer, R.N., M.S.,
Editor and Nursing Author

Instructor, formerly Assistant Director

and Medical-Surgical Coordinator

Sisters of Charity Hospital

School of Nursing, Buffalo, New York

J. B. Lippincott Company

Philadelphia

London   Mexico City

New York   St. Louis

São Paulo   Sydney

Sponsoring Editor: David T. Miller/Joyce Mkitarian
Manuscript Editor: Barbara Farabaugh
Art Director: Tracy Baldwin
Design Coordinator: Charles W. Field

Designer: Arlene Putterman
Production Supervisor: J. Corey Gray
Production Coordinator: Charlene Catlett Squibb
Compositor: Tapsco Inc.
Printer/Binder: R. R. Donnelley & Sons Company

6 5 4 3 2 1

Library of Congress Cataloging in Publication Data

Main entry under title:

Lippincott's nurses' drug manual.

    Derived from: Drug facts and comparisons.
    Includes index.
    1. Pharmacology—Handbooks, manuals, etc.
2. Drugs—Handbooks, manuals, etc. 3. Nursing—
Handbooks, manuals, etc. I. Scherer, Jeanne C. II. Drug facts and comparisons. III. Title: Nurses' drug manual.
[DNLM: 1. Drugs—nurses' instruction. QV 55 L765]
RM301.L47 1985   615'.1   84-23331
ISBN 0-397-54435-9

The author and publisher have exerted every effort to ensure that drug selection and dosage set forth in this text are in accord with current recommendations and practice at the time of publication. However, in view of ongoing research, changes in government regulations, and the constant flow of information relating to drug therapy and drug reactions, the reader is urged to check the package insert for each drug for any change in indications and dosage and for added warnings and precautions. This is particularly important when the recommended agent is a new or infrequently employed drug.

This book is for Joey MacPeek

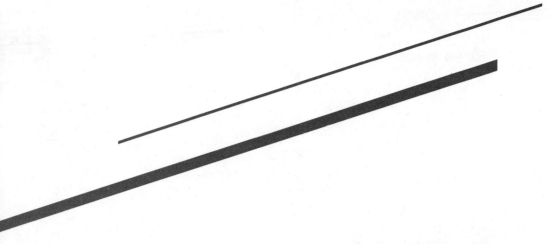

Drug Data Sources

The drug information in this book has been derived from *Facts and Comparisons,* Facts and Comparisons Division, J. B. Lippincott Company, St. Louis, Missouri.

EDITORIAL STAFF

Erwin K. Kastrup, B.S. Pharm.
Founding Editor

James R. Boyd, M.S. Pharm.
Editor-in-Chief

Bernie R. Olin, Pharm.D.
Managing Editor

Lois M. Hunsaker, Pharm.D.
Assistant Editor

Gene H. Schwach
Publisher

EDITORIAL PANEL

Timothy R. Covington, Pharm.D., M.S.
Professor and Chairman, Clinical Programs and
   Services
School of Pharmacy
West Virginia University Medical Center

Joseph R. DiPalma, M.D., D.Sc.
Professor of Pharmacology and Medicine
Hahnemann University School of Medicine
Philadelphia

Daniel A. Hussar, Ph.D.
Remington Professor of Pharmacy
Philadelphia College of Pharmacy and Science

Louis Lasagna, M.D.
Dean
Sackler School of Graduate Biomedical Sciences
Academic Dean
School of Medicine
Tufts University

David S. Tatro, Pharm.D.
Assistant Director of Pharmacy, Drug Information
   and Educational Services
Stanford University Hospital
Assistant Clinical Professor
University of California, San Francisco

Thomas L. Whitsett, M.D.
Professor of Medicine and Pharmacology
Director, Clinical Pharmacology Program
Health Sciences Center
University of Oklahoma

Consultants and Reviewers

The sections of this book that concern the nursing implications of drug therapy have been reviewed by the following consultants:

Anne Collins Abrams, R.N., B.S.N., M.S.N.
Assistant Professor, Department of Baccalaureate
  Nursing
College of Allied Health and Nursing
Eastern Kentucky University
Richmond, Kentucky

Virginia Poole Arcangelo, R.N., M.S.N.
Clinical Instructor
Helene Fuld School of Nursing
Camden, New Jersey

Sandra Beaumont, R.N., B.S.N., M.Ed.
Coordinator, Medical-Surgical Nursing
Sisters of Charity Hospital School of Nursing
Buffalo, New York

Alice Maus Blazeck, R.N., M.S.
Doctoral Candidate
University of Pennsylvania School of Nursing
Philadelphia, Pennsylvania

Marcia E. Blicharz, R.N., M.S.N., Ed.D. Candidate
Assistant Professor
Coordinator, Learning Resource Center
Trenton State College School of Nursing
Trenton, New Jersey

Stefana Campanella, R.N.
Adjunct Instructor
Sisters of Charity Hospital School of Nursing
Buffalo, New York

E. Dale Corbett, R.N., M.S.N.
Assistant Professor
University of Florida College of Nursing
Gainesville, Florida

Susan Dudek, R.D., B.S.
Instructor
Sisters of Charity Hospital School of Nursing
Buffalo, New York

Leslie Feinauer, Ph.D.
Associate Professor
University of Utah College of Nursing
Salt Lake City, Utah

Karine A. Guard, R.N., M.N.
Professor of Nursing
Shoreline Community College
Seattle, Washington

June Hastreiter, R.N., B.S.N., M.Ed.
Coordinator, Fundamentals of Nursing
Sisters of Charity Hospital School of Nursing
Buffalo, New York

Suzanne M. Kurtz, R.N., B.S.N., M.S.N.
Instructor
Sisters of Charity Hospital School of Nursing
Buffalo, New York

Patricia LaMancuso, R.N., M.Ed.
Associate Professor of Nursing
St. Petersburg Junior College
St. Petersburg, Florida

Bernadette Larson, R.N., B.S.
Instructor
Sisters of Charity Hospital School of Nursing
Buffalo, New York

Joanne Lejca, R.N., B.A., B.S.N.
Instructor
Sisters of Charity Hospital School of Nursing
Buffalo, New York

Donna Loughran, R.N., B.S.N., M.S.
Coordinator, Psychiatric Nursing
Sisters of Charity Hospital School of Nursing
Buffalo, New York

Euphemia Nowak, R.N., B.S.N., M.S.
Coordinator, Pediatric Nursing
Sisters of Charity Hospital School of Nursing
Buffalo, New York

*Sandy J. K. Oestreich, R.N.C., M.S., Doctoral
   Candidate*
Adult Health Nurse Practitioner
Associate Professor
Adelphi University
Garden City, New York

Christine S. Pakatar, M.S., R.N.C.
Assistant Professor
Russell Sage College
Troy, New York

Carol Porth, R.N., M.S.N., Ph.D.
Associate Professor
School of Nursing
University of Wisconsin-Milwaukee
Adjunct Assistant Professor
Department of Physiology
Medical College of Wisconsin
Milwaukee, Wisconsin

Margaret A. Reilly, M.S., Ph.D.
Research Scientist, The Nathan S. Kline Institute
   for Psychiatric Research
Orangeburg, New York
Adjunct Assistant Professor of Pharmacology
College of New Rochelle School of Nursing
New Rochelle, New York

Alberta A. Tedford, R.N., M.A.
Assistant Professor
Mount Mercy College
Cedar Rapids, Iowa

SPECIAL DRUG DATA REVIEWER:

Freddy Grimm, M.S., Pharm.D.
Director, Outpatient Pharmacy, Hospital of the
   University of Pennsylvania
Clinical Assistant Professor, Philadelphia College of
   Pharmacy and Science

Acknowledgments

The editor wishes to acknowledge the many individuals instrumental in the development and production of this book:

David T. Miller, John M. Connolly, and Barton H. Lippincott for their encouragement and commitment to this project from inception to completion.

James R. Boyd for creative ideas in developing the format for the drug monographs.

Joyce Mkitarian, whose close work with the editor during manuscript preparation is deeply appreciated.

Tracy Baldwin and Arlene Putterman for their expertise in book design.

Barbara Farabaugh for carefully editing the manuscript, and Charlene Squibb for coordinating its production.

Janet Lees, who ably handled many details of correspondence and record keeping.

Chris Ogden for easing the editor into word processing, and Ed MacPeek for his technical expertise when things went wrong.

The nursing consultants, who thoughtfully read the manuscript and offered many valuable suggestions.

Faculty members and students at Sisters of Charity Hospital School of Nursing, with whom discussions provided valuable input.

Contents

How to Use This Book

This manual is a joint effort between the editorial staff of *Facts and Comparisons* and the editor/nursing author. Its aim is to assemble and present the comprehensive, up-to-date drug information—both clinical pharmacology and nursing implications—required by today's nurses. The manual contains three main divisions: the product identification guide, the drug monographs, and the appendixes.

PRODUCT IDENTIFICATION GUIDE

This section depicts about 1000 selected dosage forms of approximately 500 of the most commonly prescribed drugs. Products have been photographed in full color, and markings such as product identification codes are indicated. This section is intended as a quick identification aid or for use in emergency situations to identify a drug not found in its original container. (Under no circumstances should it be used prior to drug administration to identify a drug in an unlabeled container.) This section can also be of value for patient teaching, especially for instruction regarding a multiple drug regimen, or for taking a patient history.

DRUG MONOGRAPHS

Drugs are presented in alphabetical order according to generic name. To avoid repetition, some drugs (*e.g.,* the narcotic analgesics and the cardiac glycosides) are presented as group monographs rather than individually, because their basic pharmacology and nursing implications are principally the same; individual variations are then indicated within the monograph.

Here is an example of a drug listing, along with an explanation of the information provided:

Methadone Hydrochloride   *Rx*   *C-II*
injection: 10 mg/ml   *Dolophine HCl*
tablets: 5 mg, 10 mg   *Dolophine HCl,* **Generic**
dispersible tablets: 40 mg   *Methadone HCl Diskets*
oral solution: 5 mg/5 ml,   **Generic**
  10 mg/5 ml

On the first line is the generic name of the drug and the notation of its availability on a prescription (*Rx*) or a nonprescription or over-the-counter (*otc*) basis. The *C* indicates that the manufacture, distribution, and dispensation of this drug are under the jurisdiction of the Controlled Substances Act of 1970, which concerns drugs that have potential for abuse; the Roman numeral identifies the Drug Enforcement Administration schedule under which the drug is categorized. (See Appendix 7 for a list of controlled substances and an explanation of each schedule.)

Below the generic drug name, the generally available dosage forms and strengths are listed; trade names for each form are given in the right-hand column. The term *Generic* indicates that the dosage form is available by generic name, manufactured and distributed by one or more pharmaceutical companies.

The monograph then continues with the drug's indications (including investigational uses), contraindications, actions, warnings, precautions, drug interactions, adverse reactions, overdosage symptoms and treatment, and dosage.*

The nursing implications are then presented sequentially. They have been structured in order to categorize the nursing assessments and interventions related to therapy with the specific drug and to facilitate their integration into the total nursing care plan.

History. A general format for the patient history is provided in Appendix 4. If necessary, additional data related to administration of the specific drug are noted in this section.

Physical Assessment. Relevant drug-specific physical assessments are noted under this heading. In some cases, the nurse may find it necessary to perform additional assessments based on patient symptoms, disease status, concurrent problems, or other factors. Also included here are the laboratory tests or diagnostic studies that may be performed or are recommended prior to initiation of drug therapy.

Administration. This section takes up such topics as preparation of solutions, timing of administration as related to food intake, and other techniques of administration related to the particular drug. Compatibility, storage, and stability data are also included here. For intravenous drugs, administration rates given in this manual are those recommended by the manufacturer. When used, terms such as *slowly* or *at a rapid rate* also refer to the manufacturer's guidelines. When no specific intravenous administration rate is given, it is because the manufacturer makes no recommendation and the administration rate must be based on factors such as age and weight of the patient; nature and severity of the disorder being treated; or cardiovascular, renal, and hepatic function or dysfunction. Whenever a drug is given by the intravenous route, the physician or hospital policy must establish written guidelines for its administration. Even when a manufacturer recommends an administration rate, the physician still exercises final judgment, because there may be instances when the recommended rate may need to be increased or decreased.

Ongoing Assessments and Nursing Management. This section describes the observations and nursing interventions necessary to help patients obtain optimal benefits from their drug regimens. Some attempt has been made to indicate priorities; however, this is not always practical or even possible, because each patient is a unique individual with varying potential responses to pharmacologic and other treatment modalities. Concurrent diseases or conditions and the severity of the problem being treated are among the factors that may require periodic reevaluations in the sequence of recommended assessments or interventions.

Patient and Family Information. Conveying and clarifying drug information for the patient and family are important nursing functions that can significantly influence patient compliance with a therapeutic drug regimen. The teaching points listed in this section are applicable to discharge teaching plans as well as to hospitalized patients and outpatients. Additionally, nursing assessment may indicate that other information, based on an individual patient's needs, may also be required. General points of patient and family information that apply to therapy with almost all drugs are given in Appendix 5.

APPENDIXES

Appendix 1 lists general principles for the safe and accurate administration of drugs. Special considerations for drug administration to geriatric and pediatric patients are taken up in Appendixes 2 and 3.

Points to be covered in the patient history at the time of admission to the hospital or a first visit to a clinic or physician's office are listed in Appendix 4. Appendix 5 covers general points of patient information, concerning purchase of prescription drugs, storage of drugs, drug labels and inserts, the dosage regimen, adverse drug effects, and drug use while traveling.

Appendix 6 gives signs and symptoms of various types of adverse reactions related to drug administration and also covers nursing management in anemia, leukopenia, stomatitis, and thrombocytopenia.

A general explanation of the Controlled Substances Act of 1970, the Drug Enforcement Administration schedules, and a list of the controlled substances covered in this book are given in Appendix 7.

Appendix 8 lists abbreviations used in this manual. Definitions of some of the terms used in the manual are found in Appendix 9.

Appendix 10 lists combination chemotherapeutic regimens currently used in the treatment of neoplastic diseases.

---

* All basic drug data in this book were derived from *Facts and Comparisons,* and updated information has been incorporated whenever possible up to the time of publication. If any drug information appearing herein is at variance with *Facts and Comparisons,* the responsibility for such changes is the editor/nursing author's.

COLOR LOCATOR

To identify a drug, use this Color Locator to find the pages
on which the product is most likely to appear.

The following pages illustrate approximately 1,000 dosage forms,
representing over 400 of the most commonly used products.

TABLETS

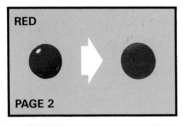

RED

PAGE 2

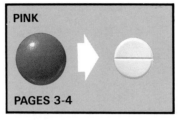

PINK

PAGES 3-4

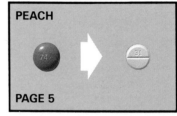

PEACH

PAGE 5

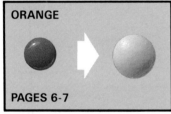

ORANGE

PAGES 6-7

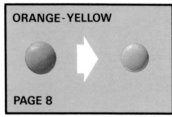

ORANGE-YELLOW

PAGE 8

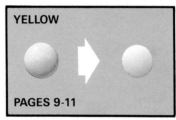

YELLOW

PAGES 9-11

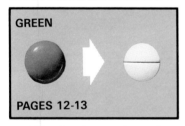

GREEN

PAGES 12-13

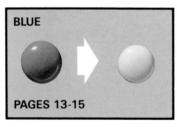

BLUE

PAGES 13-15

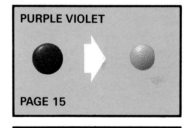

PURPLE VIOLET

PAGE 15

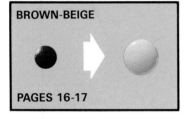

BROWN-BEIGE

PAGES 16-17

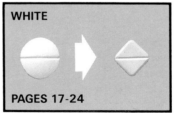

WHITE

PAGES 17-24

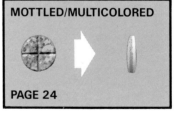

MOTTLED/MULTICOLORED

PAGE 24

CAPSULES

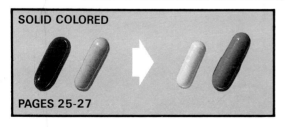

SOLID COLORED

PAGES 25-27

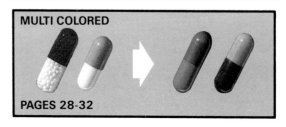

MULTI COLORED

PAGES 28-32

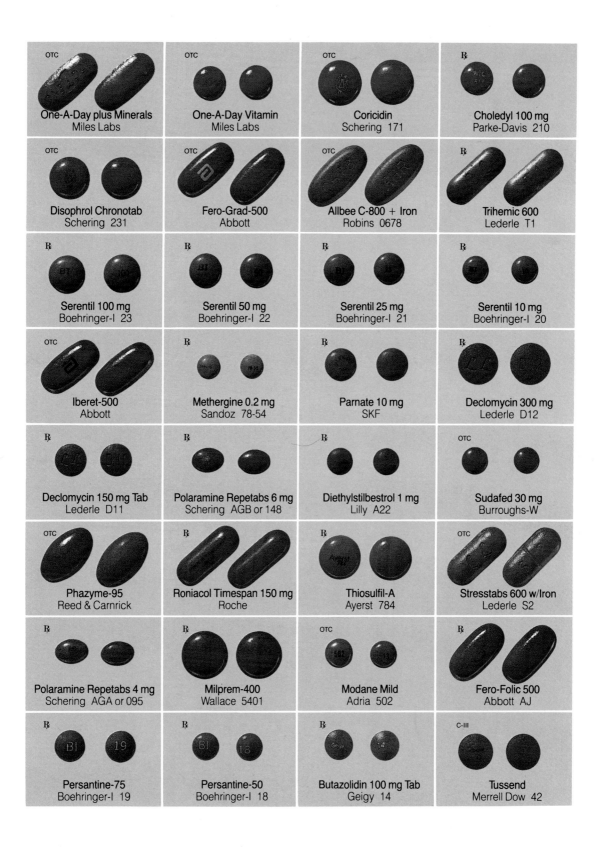

One-A-Day plus Minerals
Miles Labs

One-A-Day Vitamin
Miles Labs

Coricidin
Schering 171

Choledyl 100 mg
Parke-Davis 210

Disophrol Chronotab
Schering 231

Fero-Grad-500
Abbott

Allbee C-800 + Iron
Robins 0678

Trihemic 600
Lederle T1

Serentil 100 mg
Boehringer-I 23

Serentil 50 mg
Boehringer-I 22

Serentil 25 mg
Boehringer-I 21

Serentil 10 mg
Boehringer-I 20

Iberet-500
Abbott

Methergine 0.2 mg
Sandoz 78-54

Parnate 10 mg
SKF

Declomycin 300 mg
Lederle D12

Declomycin 150 mg Tab
Lederle D11

Polaramine Repetabs 6 mg
Schering AGB or 148

Diethylstilbestrol 1 mg
Lilly A22

Sudafed 30 mg
Burroughs-W

Phazyme-95
Reed & Carnrick

Roniacol Timespan 150 mg
Roche

Thiosulfil-A
Ayerst 784

Stresstabs 600 w/Iron
Lederle S2

Polaramine Repetabs 4 mg
Schering AGA or 095

Milprem-400
Wallace 5401

Modane Mild
Adria 502

Fero-Folic 500
Abbott AJ

Persantine-75
Boehringer-I 19

Persantine-50
Boehringer-I 18

Butazolidin 100 mg Tab
Geigy 14

Tussend
Merrell Dow 42

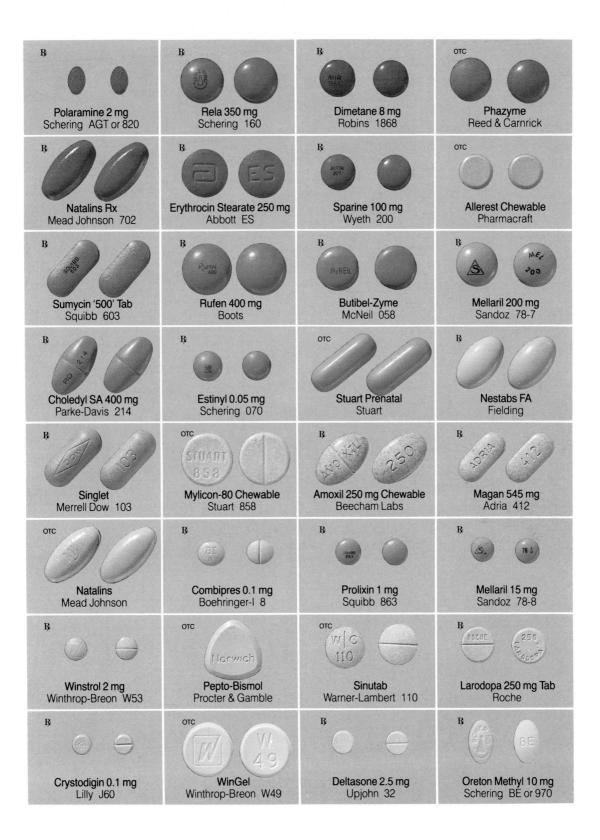

Polaramine 2 mg Schering AGT or 820	**Rela 350 mg** Schering 160	**Dimetane 8 mg** Robins 1868	**Phazyme** Reed & Carnrick
Natalins Rx Mead Johnson 702	**Erythrocin Stearate 250 mg** Abbott ES	**Sparine 100 mg** Wyeth 200	**Allerest Chewable** Pharmacraft
Sumycin '500' Tab Squibb 603	**Rufen 400 mg** Boots	**Butibel-Zyme** McNeil 058	**Mellaril 200 mg** Sandoz 78-7
Choledyl SA 400 mg Parke-Davis 214	**Estinyl 0.05 mg** Schering 070	**Stuart Prenatal** Stuart	**Nestabs FA** Fielding
Singlet Merrell Dow 103	**Mylicon-80 Chewable** Stuart 858	**Amoxil 250 mg Chewable** Beecham Labs	**Magan 545 mg** Adria 412
Natalins Mead Johnson	**Combipres 0.1 mg** Boehringer-I 8	**Prolixin 1 mg** Squibb 863	**Mellaril 15 mg** Sandoz 78-8
Winstrol 2 mg Winthrop-Breon W53	**Pepto-Bismol** Procter & Gamble	**Sinutab** Warner-Lambert 110	**Larodopa 250 mg Tab** Roche
Crystodigin 0.1 mg Lilly J60	**WinGel** Winthrop-Breon W49	**Deltasone 2.5 mg** Upjohn 32	**Oreton Methyl 10 mg** Schering BE or 970

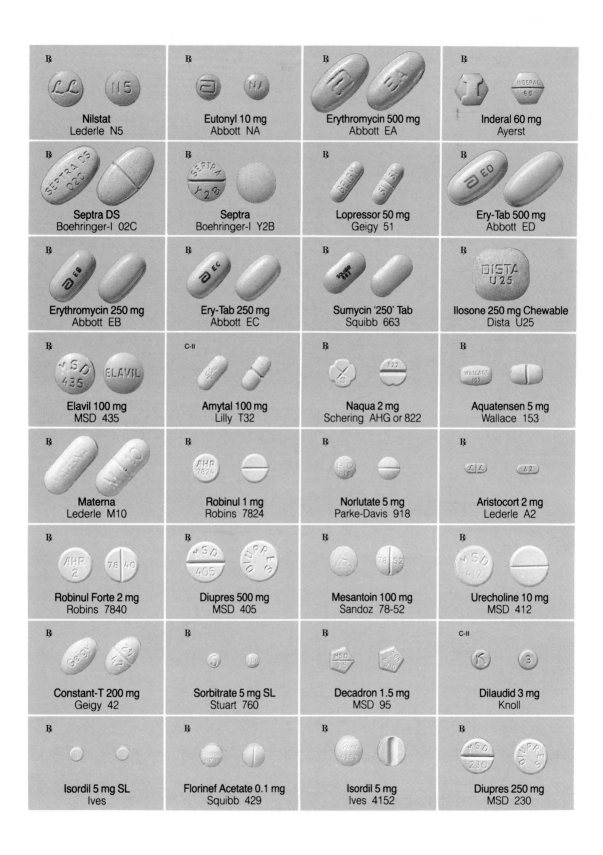

Nilstat Lederle N5	**Eutonyl 10 mg** Abbott NA	**Erythromycin 500 mg** Abbott EA	**Inderal 60 mg** Ayerst
Septra DS Boehringer-I 02C	**Septra** Boehringer-I Y2B	**Lopressor 50 mg** Geigy 51	**Ery-Tab 500 mg** Abbott ED
Erythromycin 250 mg Abbott EB	**Ery-Tab 250 mg** Abbott EC	**Sumycin '250' Tab** Squibb 663	**Ilosone 250 mg Chewable** Dista U25
Elavil 100 mg MSD 435	C-II **Amytal 100 mg** Lilly T32	**Naqua 2 mg** Schering AHG or 822	**Aquatensen 5 mg** Wallace 153
Materna Lederle M10	**Robinul 1 mg** Robins 7824	**Norlutate 5 mg** Parke-Davis 918	**Aristocort 2 mg** Lederle A2
Robinul Forte 2 mg Robins 7840	**Diupres 500 mg** MSD 405	**Mesantoin 100 mg** Sandoz 78-52	**Urecholine 10 mg** MSD 412
Constant-T 200 mg Geigy 42	**Sorbitrate 5 mg SL** Stuart 760	**Decadron 1.5 mg** MSD 95	C-II **Dilaudid 3 mg** Knoll
Isordil 5 mg SL Ives	**Florinef Acetate 0.1 mg** Squibb 429	**Isordil 5 mg** Ives 4152	**Diupres 250 mg** MSD 230

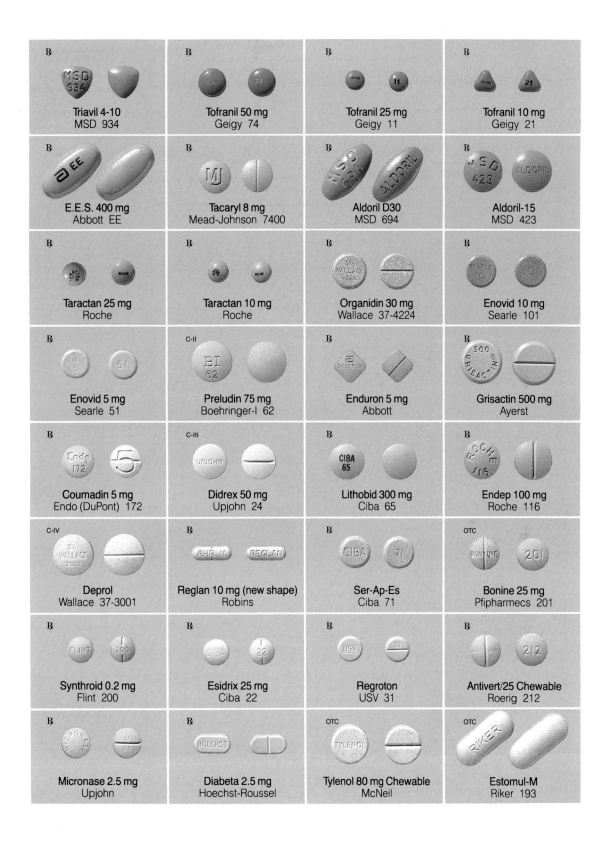

℞ Triavil 4-10
MSD 934

℞ Tofranil 50 mg
Geigy 74

℞ Tofranil 25 mg
Geigy 11

℞ Tofranil 10 mg
Geigy 21

℞ E.E.S. 400 mg
Abbott EE

℞ Tacaryl 8 mg
Mead-Johnson 7400

℞ Aldoril D30
MSD 694

℞ Aldoril-15
MSD 423

℞ Taractan 25 mg
Roche

℞ Taractan 10 mg
Roche

℞ Organidin 30 mg
Wallace 37-4224

℞ Enovid 10 mg
Searle 101

℞ Enovid 5 mg
Searle 51

C-II Preludin 75 mg
Boehringer-I 62

℞ Enduron 5 mg
Abbott

℞ Grisactin 500 mg
Ayerst

℞ Coumadin 5 mg
Endo (DuPont) 172

C-III Didrex 50 mg
Upjohn 24

℞ Lithobid 300 mg
Ciba 65

℞ Endep 100 mg
Roche 116

C-IV Deprol
Wallace 37-3001

℞ Reglan 10 mg (new shape)
Robins

℞ Ser-Ap-Es
Ciba 71

OTC Bonine 25 mg
Pfipharmecs 201

℞ Synthroid 0.2 mg
Flint 200

℞ Esidrix 25 mg
Ciba 22

℞ Regroton
USV 31

℞ Antivert/25 Chewable
Roerig 212

℞ Micronase 2.5 mg
Upjohn

℞ Diabeta 2.5 mg
Hoechst-Roussel

OTC Tylenol 80 mg Chewable
McNeil

OTC Estomul-M
Riker 193

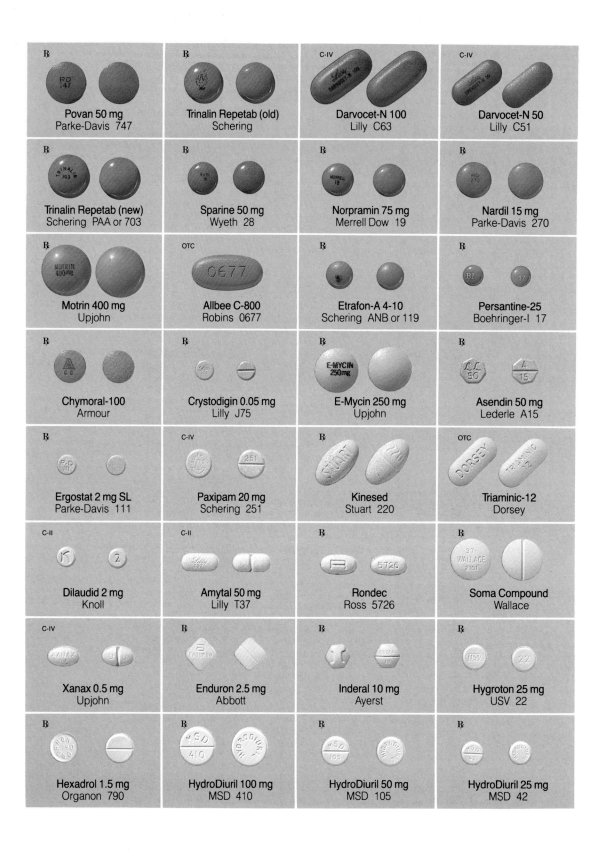

Povan 50 mg
Parke-Davis 747

Trinalin Repetab (old)
Schering

Darvocet-N 100
Lilly C63

Darvocet-N 50
Lilly C51

Trinalin Repetab (new)
Schering PAA or 703

Sparine 50 mg
Wyeth 28

Norpramin 75 mg
Merrell Dow 19

Nardil 15 mg
Parke-Davis 270

Motrin 400 mg
Upjohn

Allbee C-800
Robins 0677

Etrafon-A 4-10
Schering ANB or 119

Persantine-25
Boehringer-I 17

Chymoral-100
Armour

Crystodigin 0.05 mg
Lilly J75

E-Mycin 250 mg
Upjohn

Asendin 50 mg
Lederle A15

Ergostat 2 mg SL
Parke-Davis 111

Paxipam 20 mg
Schering 251

Kinesed
Stuart 220

Triaminic-12
Dorsey

Dilaudid 2 mg
Knoll

Amytal 50 mg
Lilly T37

Rondec
Ross 5726

Soma Compound
Wallace

Xanax 0.5 mg
Upjohn

Enduron 2.5 mg
Abbott

Inderal 10 mg
Ayerst

Hygroton 25 mg
USV 22

Hexadrol 1.5 mg
Organon 790

HydroDiuril 100 mg
MSD 410

HydroDiuril 50 mg
MSD 105

HydroDiuril 25 mg
MSD 42

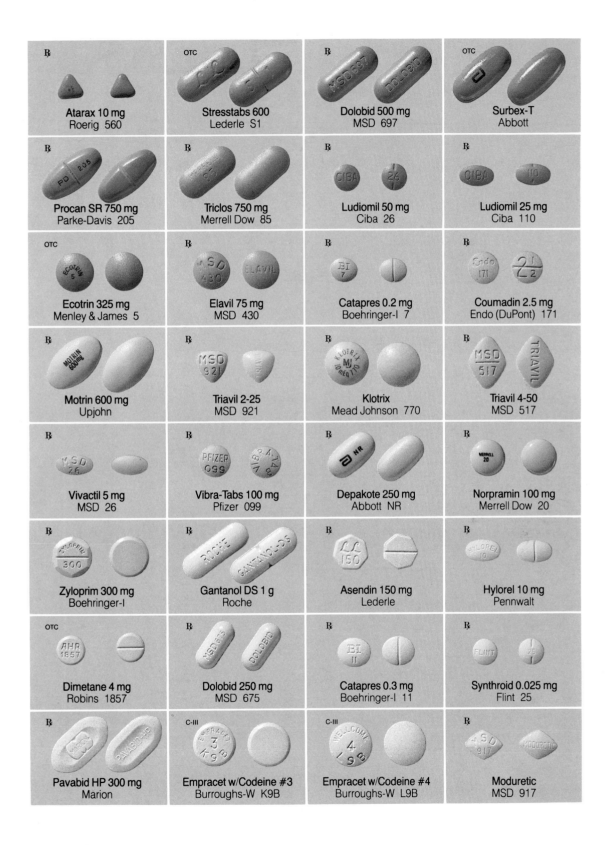

Atarax 10 mg Roerig 560	**Stresstabs 600** Lederle S1	**Dolobid 500 mg** MSD 697	**Surbex-T** Abbott
Procan SR 750 mg Parke-Davis 205	**Triclos 750 mg** Merrell Dow 85	**Ludiomil 50 mg** Ciba 26	**Ludiomil 25 mg** Ciba 110
Ecotrin 325 mg Menley & James 5	**Elavil 75 mg** MSD 430	**Catapres 0.2 mg** Boehringer-I 7	**Coumadin 2.5 mg** Endo (DuPont) 171
Motrin 600 mg Upjohn	**Triavil 2-25** MSD 921	**Klotrix** Mead Johnson 770	**Triavil 4-50** MSD 517
Vivactil 5 mg MSD 26	**Vibra-Tabs 100 mg** Pfizer 099	**Depakote 250 mg** Abbott NR	**Norpramin 100 mg** Merrell Dow 20
Zyloprim 300 mg Boehringer-I	**Gantanol DS 1 g** Roche	**Asendin 150 mg** Lederle	**Hylorel 10 mg** Pennwalt
Dimetane 4 mg Robins 1857	**Dolobid 250 mg** MSD 675	**Catapres 0.3 mg** Boehringer-I 11	**Synthroid 0.025 mg** Flint 25
Pavabid HP 300 mg Marion	**Empracet w/Codeine #3** Burroughs-W K9B	**Empracet w/Codeine #4** Burroughs-W L9B	**Moduretic** MSD 917

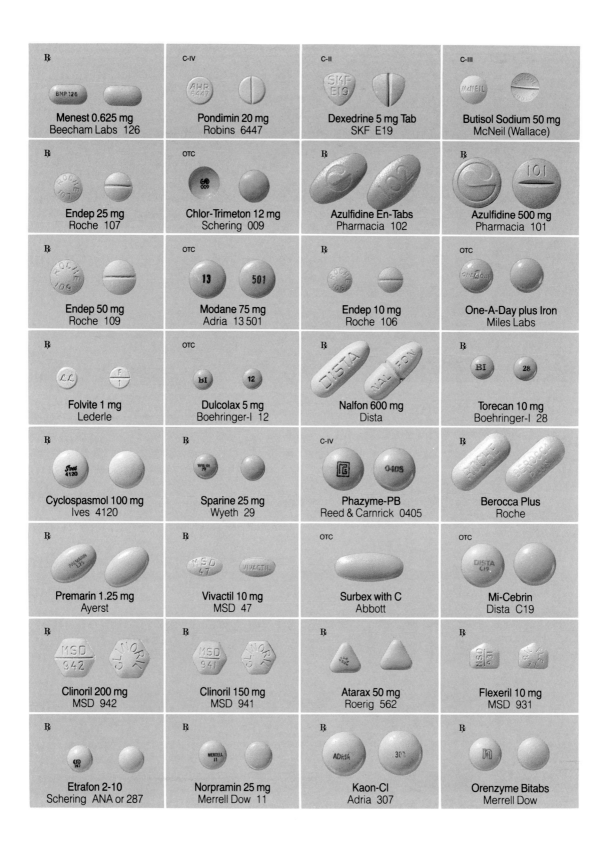

Menest 0.625 mg Beecham Labs 126	C-IV **Pondimin 20 mg** Robins 6447	C-II **Dexedrine 5 mg Tab** SKF E19	C-III **Butisol Sodium 50 mg** McNeil (Wallace)
Endep 25 mg Roche 107	OTC **Chlor-Trimeton 12 mg** Schering 009	**Azulfidine En-Tabs** Pharmacia 102	**Azulfidine 500 mg** Pharmacia 101
Endep 50 mg Roche 109	OTC **Modane 75 mg** Adria 13 501	**Endep 10 mg** Roche 106	OTC **One-A-Day plus Iron** Miles Labs
Folvite 1 mg Lederle	OTC **Dulcolax 5 mg** Boehringer-I 12	**Nalfon 600 mg** Dista	**Torecan 10 mg** Boehringer-I 28
Cyclospasmol 100 mg Ives 4120	**Sparine 25 mg** Wyeth 29	C-IV **Phazyme-PB** Reed & Carnrick 0405	**Berocca Plus** Roche
Premarin 1.25 mg Ayerst	**Vivactil 10 mg** MSD 47	OTC **Surbex with C** Abbott	OTC **Mi-Cebrin** Dista C19
Clinoril 200 mg MSD 942	**Clinoril 150 mg** MSD 941	**Atarax 50 mg** Roerig 562	**Flexeril 10 mg** MSD 931
Etrafon 2-10 Schering ANA or 287	**Norpramin 25 mg** Merrell Dow 11	**Kaon-Cl** Adria 307	**Orenzyme Bitabs** Merrell Dow

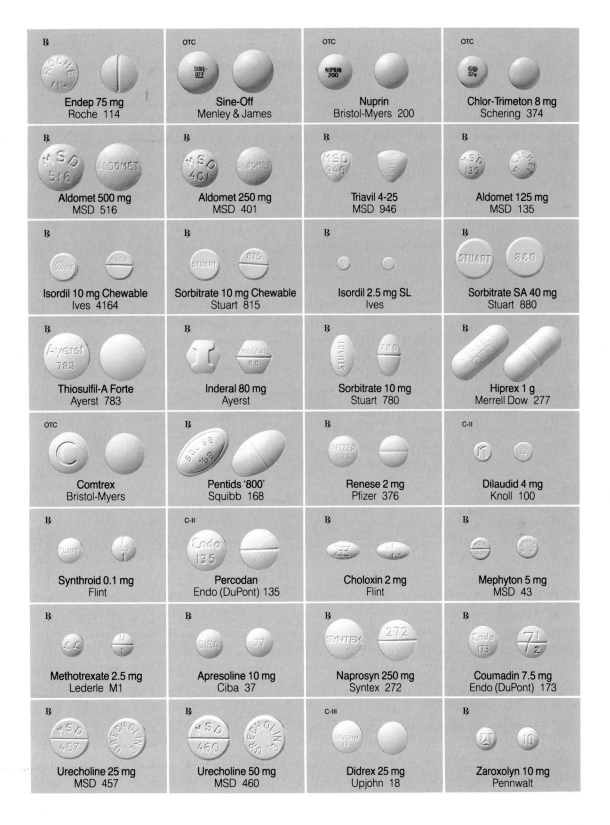

Endep 75 mg
Roche 114

Sine-Off
Menley & James

Nuprin
Bristol-Myers 200

Chlor-Trimeton 8 mg
Schering 374

Aldomet 500 mg
MSD 516

Aldomet 250 mg
MSD 401

Triavil 4-25
MSD 946

Aldomet 125 mg
MSD 135

Isordil 10 mg Chewable
Ives 4164

Sorbitrate 10 mg Chewable
Stuart 815

Isordil 2.5 mg SL
Ives

Sorbitrate SA 40 mg
Stuart 880

Thiosulfil-A Forte
Ayerst 783

Inderal 80 mg
Ayerst

Sorbitrate 10 mg
Stuart 780

Hiprex 1 g
Merrell Dow 277

Comtrex
Bristol-Myers

Pentids '800'
Squibb 168

Renese 2 mg
Pfizer 376

Dilaudid 4 mg
Knoll 100

Synthroid 0.1 mg
Flint

Percodan
Endo (DuPont) 135

Choloxin 2 mg
Flint

Mephyton 5 mg
MSD 43

Methotrexate 2.5 mg
Lederle M1

Apresoline 10 mg
Ciba 37

Naprosyn 250 mg
Syntex 272

Coumadin 7.5 mg
Endo (DuPont) 173

Urecholine 25 mg
MSD 457

Urecholine 50 mg
MSD 460

Didrex 25 mg
Upjohn 18

Zaroxolyn 10 mg
Pennwalt

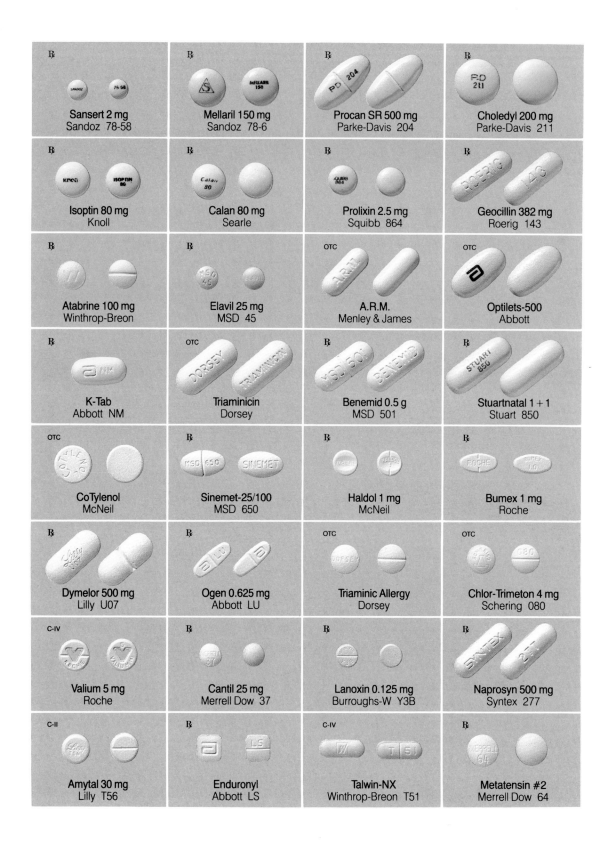

℞ Sansert 2 mg Sandoz 78-58	**℞** Mellaril 150 mg Sandoz 78-6	**℞** Procan SR 500 mg Parke-Davis 204	**℞** Choledyl 200 mg Parke-Davis 211
℞ Isoptin 80 mg Knoll	**℞** Calan 80 mg Searle	**℞** Prolixin 2.5 mg Squibb 864	**℞** Geocillin 382 mg Roerig 143
℞ Atabrine 100 mg Winthrop-Breon	**℞** Elavil 25 mg MSD 45	OTC A.R.M. Menley & James	OTC Optilets-500 Abbott
℞ K-Tab Abbott NM	OTC Triaminicin Dorsey	**℞** Benemid 0.5 g MSD 501	**℞** Stuartnatal 1 + 1 Stuart 850
OTC CoTylenol McNeil	**℞** Sinemet-25/100 MSD 650	**℞** Haldol 1 mg McNeil	**℞** Bumex 1 mg Roche
℞ Dymelor 500 mg Lilly U07	**℞** Ogen 0.625 mg Abbott LU	OTC Triaminic Allergy Dorsey	OTC Chlor-Trimeton 4 mg Schering 080
C-IV Valium 5 mg Roche	**℞** Cantil 25 mg Merrell Dow 37	**℞** Lanoxin 0.125 mg Burroughs-W Y3B	**℞** Naprosyn 500 mg Syntex 277
C-II Amytal 30 mg Lilly T56	**℞** Enduronyl Abbott LS	C-IV Talwin-NX Winthrop-Breon T51	**℞** Metatensin #2 Merrell Dow 64

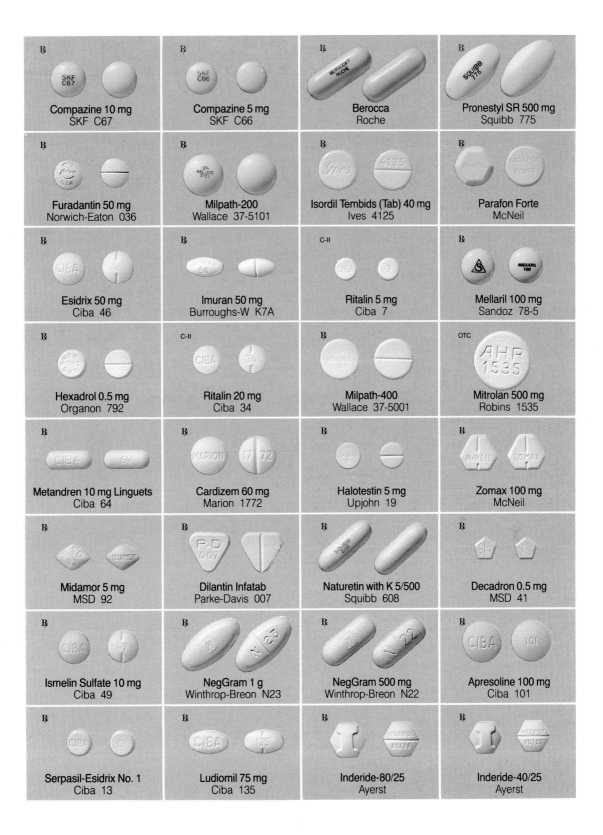

Compazine 10 mg
SKF C67

Compazine 5 mg
SKF C66

Berocca
Roche

Pronestyl SR 500 mg
Squibb 775

Furadantin 50 mg
Norwich-Eaton 036

Milpath-200
Wallace 37-5101

Isordil Tembids (Tab) 40 mg
Ives 4125

Parafon Forte
McNeil

Esidrix 50 mg
Ciba 46

Imuran 50 mg
Burroughs-W K7A

Ritalin 5 mg
Ciba 7

Mellaril 100 mg
Sandoz 78-5

Hexadrol 0.5 mg
Organon 792

Ritalin 20 mg
Ciba 34

Milpath-400
Wallace 37-5001

Mitrolan 500 mg
Robins 1535

Metandren 10 mg Linguets
Ciba 64

Cardizem 60 mg
Marion 1772

Halotestin 5 mg
Upjohn 19

Zomax 100 mg
McNeil

Midamor 5 mg
MSD 92

Dilantin Infatab
Parke-Davis 007

Naturetin with K 5/500
Squibb 608

Decadron 0.5 mg
MSD 41

Ismelin Sulfate 10 mg
Ciba 49

NegGram 1 g
Winthrop-Breon N23

NegGram 500 mg
Winthrop-Breon N22

Apresoline 100 mg
Ciba 101

Serpasil-Esidrix No. 1
Ciba 13

Ludiomil 75 mg
Ciba 135

Inderide-80/25
Ayerst

Inderide-40/25
Ayerst

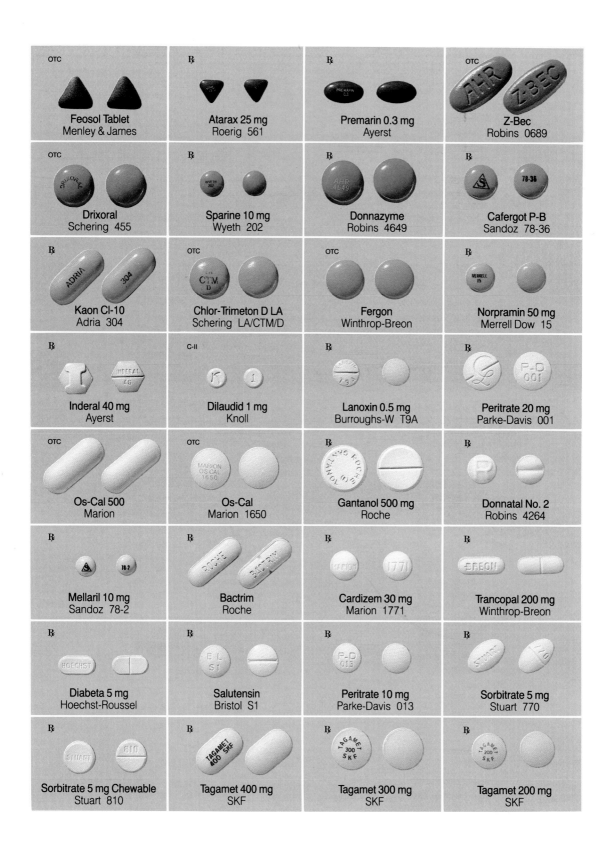

Feosol Tablet
Menley & James
OTC

Atarax 25 mg
Roerig 561
Rx

Premarin 0.3 mg
Ayerst
Rx

Z-Bec
Robins 0689
OTC

Drixoral
Schering 455
OTC

Sparine 10 mg
Wyeth 202
Rx

Donnazyme
Robins 4649
Rx

Cafergot P-B
Sandoz 78-36
Rx

Kaon Cl-10
Adria 304
Rx

Chlor-Trimeton D LA
Schering LA/CTM/D
OTC

Fergon
Winthrop-Breon
OTC

Norpramin 50 mg
Merrell Dow 15
Rx

Inderal 40 mg
Ayerst
Rx

Dilaudid 1 mg
Knoll
C-II

Lanoxin 0.5 mg
Burroughs-W T9A
Rx

Peritrate 20 mg
Parke-Davis 001
Rx

Os-Cal 500
Marion
OTC

Os-Cal
Marion 1650
OTC

Gantanol 500 mg
Roche
Rx

Donnatal No. 2
Robins 4264
Rx

Mellaril 10 mg
Sandoz 78-2
Rx

Bactrim
Roche
Rx

Cardizem 30 mg
Marion 1771
Rx

Trancopal 200 mg
Winthrop-Breon
Rx

Diabeta 5 mg
Hoechst-Roussel
Rx

Salutensin
Bristol S1
Rx

Peritrate 10 mg
Parke-Davis 013
Rx

Sorbitrate 5 mg
Stuart 770
Rx

Sorbitrate 5 mg Chewable
Stuart 810
Rx

Tagamet 400 mg
SKF
Rx

Tagamet 300 mg
SKF
Rx

Tagamet 200 mg
SKF
Rx

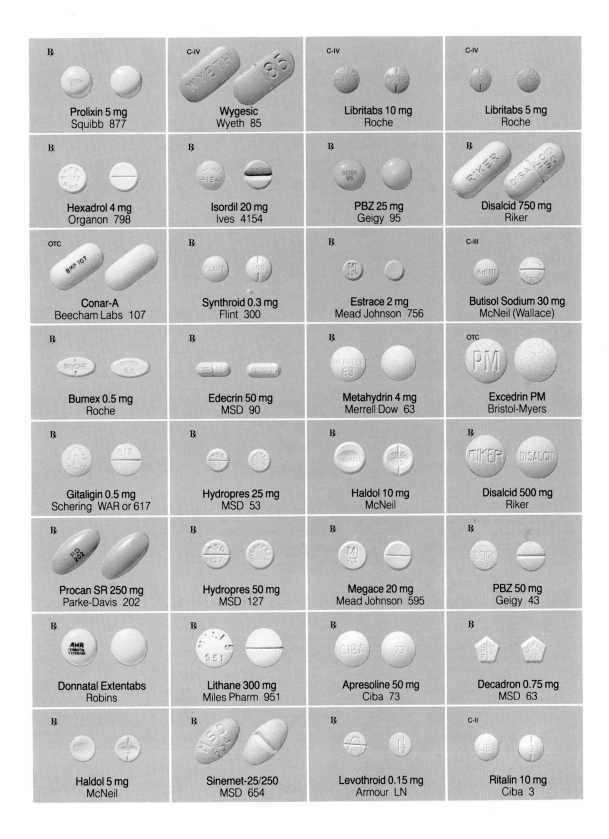

Prolixin 5 mg Squibb 877	**Wygesic** Wyeth 85	**Libritabs 10 mg** Roche	**Libritabs 5 mg** Roche
Hexadrol 4 mg Organon 798	**Isordil 20 mg** Ives 4154	**PBZ 25 mg** Geigy 95	**Disalcid 750 mg** Riker
Conar-A Beecham Labs 107	**Synthroid 0.3 mg** Flint 300	**Estrace 2 mg** Mead Johnson 756	**Butisol Sodium 30 mg** McNeil (Wallace)
Bumex 0.5 mg Roche	**Edecrin 50 mg** MSD 90	**Metahydrin 4 mg** Merrell Dow 63	**Excedrin PM** Bristol-Myers
Gitaligin 0.5 mg Schering WAR or 617	**Hydropres 25 mg** MSD 53	**Haldol 10 mg** McNeil	**Disalcid 500 mg** Riker
Procan SR 250 mg Parke-Davis 202	**Hydropres 50 mg** MSD 127	**Megace 20 mg** Mead Johnson 595	**PBZ 50 mg** Geigy 43
Donnatal Extentabs Robins	**Lithane 300 mg** Miles Pharm 951	**Apresoline 50 mg** Ciba 73	**Decadron 0.75 mg** MSD 63
Haldol 5 mg McNeil	**Sinemet-25/250** MSD 654	**Levothroid 0.15 mg** Armour LN	**Ritalin 10 mg** Ciba 3

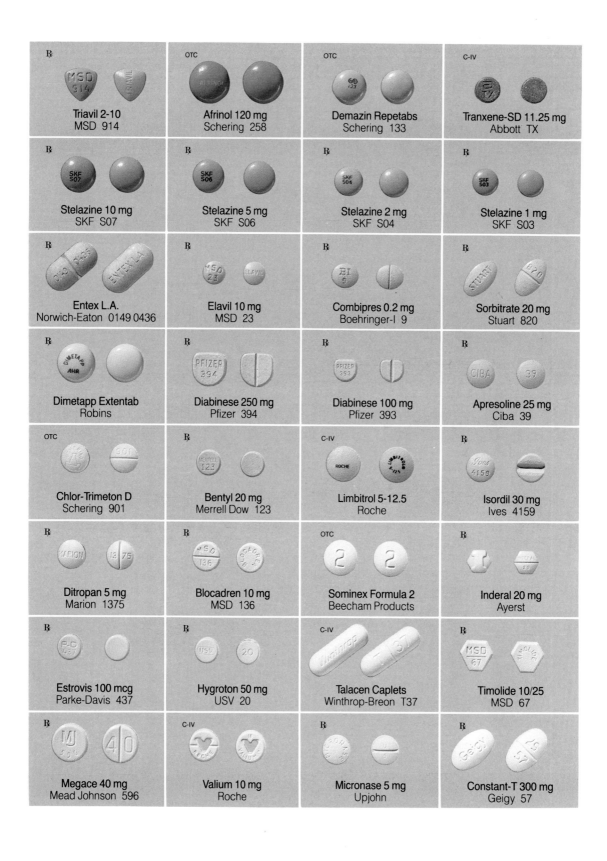

Rx Triavil 2-10 MSD 914	**OTC** Afrinol 120 mg Schering 258	**OTC** Demazin Repetabs Schering 133	**C-IV** Tranxene-SD 11.25 mg Abbott TX
Rx Stelazine 10 mg SKF S07	**Rx** Stelazine 5 mg SKF S06	**Rx** Stelazine 2 mg SKF S04	**Rx** Stelazine 1 mg SKF S03
Rx Entex L.A. Norwich-Eaton 0149 0436	**Rx** Elavil 10 mg MSD 23	**Rx** Combipres 0.2 mg Boehringer-I 9	**Rx** Sorbitrate 20 mg Stuart 820
Rx Dimetapp Extentab Robins	**Rx** Diabinese 250 mg Pfizer 394	**Rx** Diabinese 100 mg Pfizer 393	**Rx** Apresoline 25 mg Ciba 39
OTC Chlor-Trimeton D Schering 901	**Rx** Bentyl 20 mg Merrell Dow 123	**C-IV** Limbitrol 5-12.5 Roche	**Rx** Isordil 30 mg Ives 4159
Rx Ditropan 5 mg Marion 1375	**Rx** Blocadren 10 mg MSD 136	**OTC** Sominex Formula 2 Beecham Products	**Rx** Inderal 20 mg Ayerst
Rx Estrovis 100 mcg Parke-Davis 437	**Rx** Hygroton 50 mg USV 20	**C-IV** Talacen Caplets Winthrop-Breon T37	**Rx** Timolide 10/25 MSD 67
Rx Megace 40 mg Mead Johnson 596	**C-IV** Valium 10 mg Roche	**Rx** Micronase 5 mg Upjohn	**Rx** Constant-T 300 mg Geigy 57

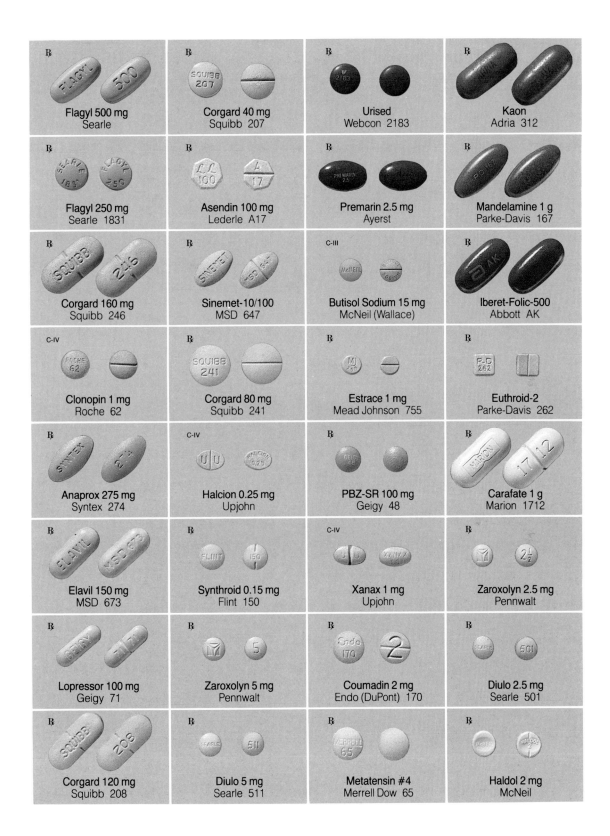

Flagyl 500 mg
Searle

Corgard 40 mg
Squibb 207

Urised
Webcon 2183

Kaon
Adria 312

Flagyl 250 mg
Searle 1831

Asendin 100 mg
Lederle A17

Premarin 2.5 mg
Ayerst

Mandelamine 1 g
Parke-Davis 167

Corgard 160 mg
Squibb 246

Sinemet-10/100
MSD 647

C-III

Butisol Sodium 15 mg
McNeil (Wallace)

Iberet-Folic-500
Abbott AK

C-IV

Clonopin 1 mg
Roche 62

Corgard 80 mg
Squibb 241

Estrace 1 mg
Mead Johnson 755

Euthroid-2
Parke-Davis 262

Anaprox 275 mg
Syntex 274

C-IV

Halcion 0.25 mg
Upjohn

PBZ-SR 100 mg
Geigy 48

Carafate 1 g
Marion 1712

Elavil 150 mg
MSD 673

Synthroid 0.15 mg
Flint 150

C-IV

Xanax 1 mg
Upjohn

Zaroxolyn 2.5 mg
Pennwalt

Lopressor 100 mg
Geigy 71

Zaroxolyn 5 mg
Pennwalt

Coumadin 2 mg
Endo (DuPont) 170

Diulo 2.5 mg
Searle 501

Corgard 120 mg
Squibb 208

Diulo 5 mg
Searle 511

Metatensin #4
Merrell Dow 65

Haldol 2 mg
McNeil

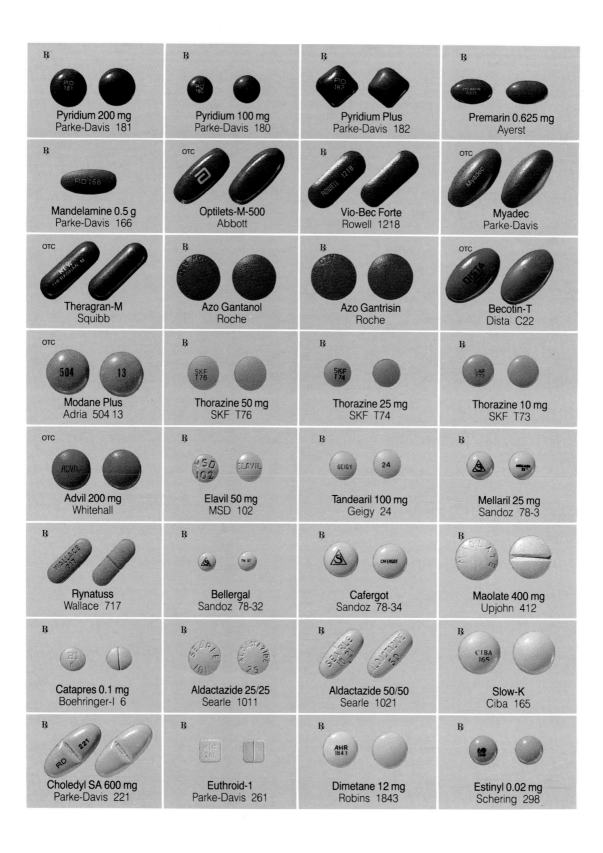

Pyridium 200 mg
Parke-Davis 181

Pyridium 100 mg
Parke-Davis 180

Pyridium Plus
Parke-Davis 182

Premarin 0.625 mg
Ayerst

Mandelamine 0.5 g
Parke-Davis 166

Optilets-M-500
Abbott

Vio-Bec Forte
Rowell 1218

Myadec
Parke-Davis

Theragran-M
Squibb

Azo Gantanol
Roche

Azo Gantrisin
Roche

Becotin-T
Dista C22

Modane Plus
Adria 504 13

Thorazine 50 mg
SKF T76

Thorazine 25 mg
SKF T74

Thorazine 10 mg
SKF T73

Advil 200 mg
Whitehall

Elavil 50 mg
MSD 102

Tandearil 100 mg
Geigy 24

Mellaril 25 mg
Sandoz 78-3

Rynatuss
Wallace 717

Bellergal
Sandoz 78-32

Cafergot
Sandoz 78-34

Maolate 400 mg
Upjohn 412

Catapres 0.1 mg
Boehringer-I 6

Aldactazide 25/25
Searle 1011

Aldactazide 50/50
Searle 1021

Slow-K
Ciba 165

Choledyl SA 600 mg
Parke-Davis 221

Euthroid-1
Parke-Davis 261

Dimetane 12 mg
Robins 1843

Estinyl 0.02 mg
Schering 298

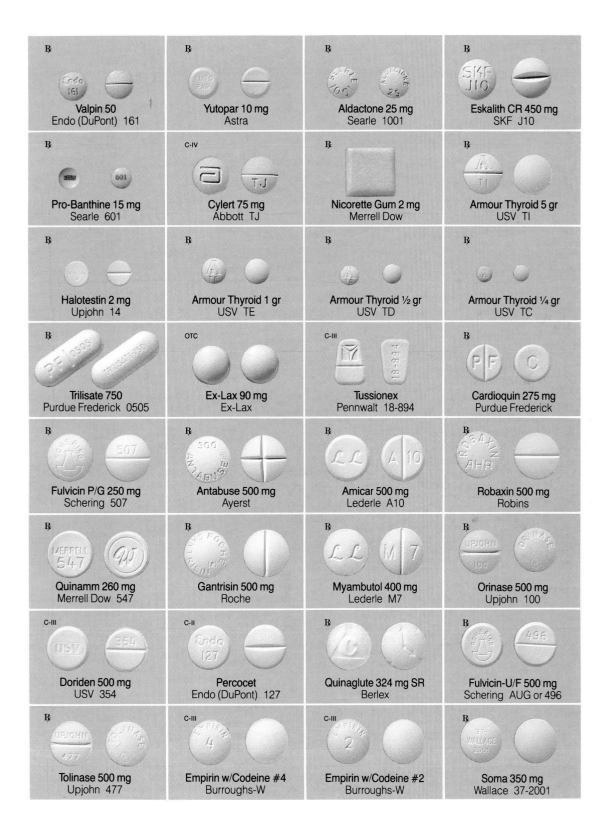

℞	℞	℞	℞
Valpin 50 Endo (DuPont) 161	**Yutopar 10 mg** Astra	**Aldactone 25 mg** Searle 1001	**Eskalith CR 450 mg** SKF J10
℞	C-IV	℞	℞
Pro-Banthine 15 mg Searle 601	**Cylert 75 mg** Abbott TJ	**Nicorette Gum 2 mg** Merrell Dow	**Armour Thyroid 5 gr** USV TI
℞	℞	℞	℞
Halotestin 2 mg Upjohn 14	**Armour Thyroid 1 gr** USV TE	**Armour Thyroid ½ gr** USV TD	**Armour Thyroid ¼ gr** USV TC
℞	OTC	C-III	℞
Trilisate 750 Purdue Frederick 0505	**Ex-Lax 90 mg** Ex-Lax	**Tussionex** Pennwalt 18-894	**Cardioquin 275 mg** Purdue Frederick
℞	℞	℞	℞
Fulvicin P/G 250 mg Schering 507	**Antabuse 500 mg** Ayerst	**Amicar 500 mg** Lederle A10	**Robaxin 500 mg** Robins
℞	℞	℞	℞
Quinamm 260 mg Merrell Dow 547	**Gantrisin 500 mg** Roche	**Myambutol 400 mg** Lederle M7	**Orinase 500 mg** Upjohn 100
C-III	C-II	℞	℞
Doriden 500 mg USV 354	**Percocet** Endo (DuPont) 127	**Quinaglute 324 mg SR** Berlex	**Fulvicin-U/F 500 mg** Schering AUG or 496
℞	C-III	C-III	℞
Tolinase 500 mg Upjohn 477	**Empirin w/Codeine #4** Burroughs-W	**Empirin w/Codeine #2** Burroughs-W	**Soma 350 mg** Wallace 37-2001

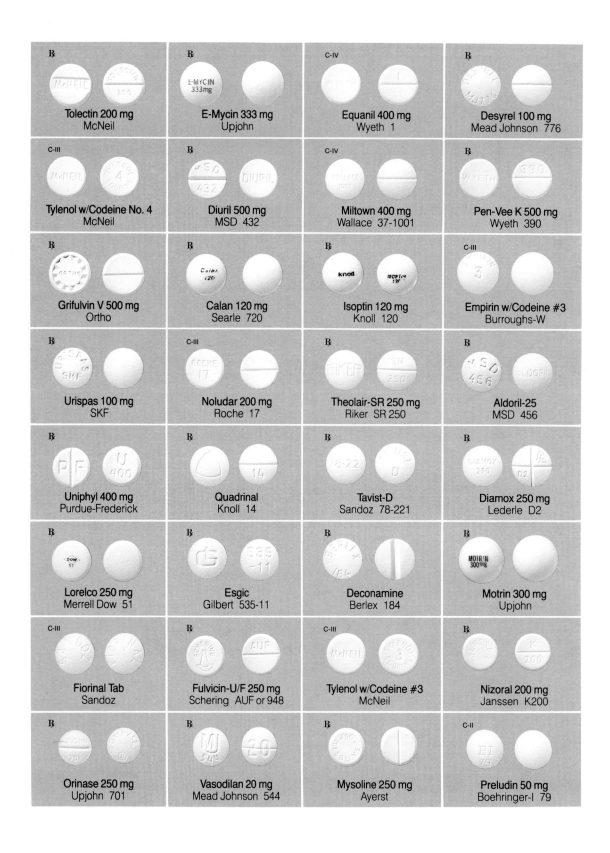

Tolectin 200 mg McNeil	**E-Mycin 333 mg** Upjohn	**Equanil 400 mg** Wyeth 1	**Desyril 100 mg** Mead Johnson 776
Tylenol w/Codeine No. 4 McNeil	**Diuril 500 mg** MSD 432	**Miltown 400 mg** Wallace 37-1001	**Pen-Vee K 500 mg** Wyeth 390
Grifulvin V 500 mg Ortho	**Calan 120 mg** Searle 720	**Isoptin 120 mg** Knoll 120	**Empirin w/Codeine #3** Burroughs-W
Urispas 100 mg SKF	**Noludar 200 mg** Roche 17	**Theolair-SR 250 mg** Riker SR 250	**Aldoril-25** MSD 456
Uniphyl 400 mg Purdue-Frederick	**Quadrinal** Knoll 14	**Tavist-D** Sandoz 78-221	**Diamox 250 mg** Lederle D2
Lorelco 250 mg Merrell Dow 51	**Esgic** Gilbert 535-11	**Deconamine** Berlex 184	**Motrin 300 mg** Upjohn
Fiorinal Tab Sandoz	**Fulvicin-U/F 250 mg** Schering AUF or 948	**Tylenol w/Codeine #3** McNeil	**Nizoral 200 mg** Janssen K200
Orinase 250 mg Upjohn 701	**Vasodilan 20 mg** Mead Johnson 544	**Mysoline 250 mg** Ayerst	**Preludin 50 mg** Boehringer-I 79

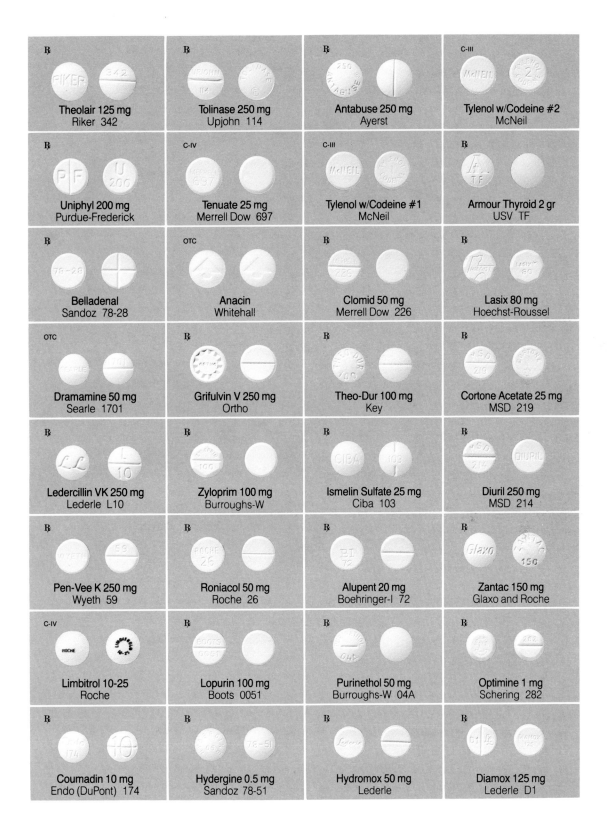

Theolair 125 mg Riker 342	**Tolinase 250 mg** Upjohn 114	**Antabuse 250 mg** Ayerst	**Tylenol w/Codeine #2** McNeil
Uniphyl 200 mg Purdue-Frederick	**Tenuate 25 mg** Merrell Dow 697	**Tylenol w/Codeine #1** McNeil	**Armour Thyroid 2 gr** USV TF
Belladenal Sandoz 78-28	**Anacin** Whitehall	**Clomid 50 mg** Merrell Dow 226	**Lasix 80 mg** Hoechst-Roussel
Dramamine 50 mg Searle 1701	**Grifulvin V 250 mg** Ortho	**Theo-Dur 100 mg** Key	**Cortone Acetate 25 mg** MSD 219
Ledercillin VK 250 mg Lederle L10	**Zyloprim 100 mg** Burroughs-W	**Ismelin Sulfate 25 mg** Ciba 103	**Diuril 250 mg** MSD 214
Pen-Vee K 250 mg Wyeth 59	**Roniacol 50 mg** Roche 26	**Alupent 20 mg** Boehringer-I 72	**Zantac 150 mg** Glaxo and Roche
Limbitrol 10-25 Roche	**Lopurin 100 mg** Boots 0051	**Purinethol 50 mg** Burroughs-W 04A	**Optimine 1 mg** Schering 282
Coumadin 10 mg Endo (DuPont) 174	**Hydergine 0.5 mg** Sandoz 78-51	**Hydromox 50 mg** Lederle	**Diamox 125 mg** Lederle D1

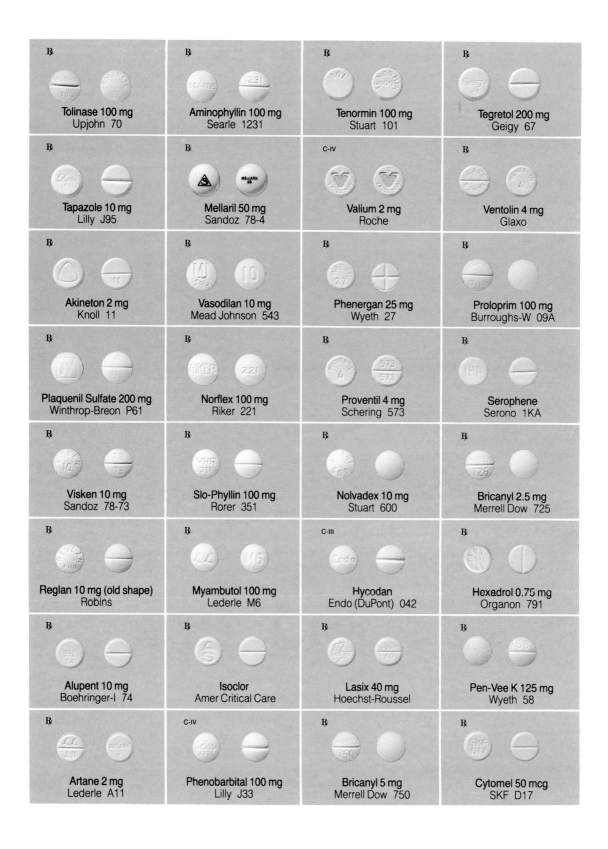

Tolinase 100 mg
Upjohn 70

Aminophyllin 100 mg
Searle 1231

Tenormin 100 mg
Stuart 101

Tegretol 200 mg
Geigy 67

Tapazole 10 mg
Lilly J95

Mellaril 50 mg
Sandoz 78-4

C-IV
Valium 2 mg
Roche

Ventolin 4 mg
Glaxo

Akineton 2 mg
Knoll 11

Vasodilan 10 mg
Mead Johnson 543

Phenergan 25 mg
Wyeth 27

Proloprim 100 mg
Burroughs-W 09A

Plaquenil Sulfate 200 mg
Winthrop-Breon P61

Norflex 100 mg
Riker 221

Proventil 4 mg
Schering 573

Serophene
Serono 1KA

Visken 10 mg
Sandoz 78-73

Slo-Phyllin 100 mg
Rorer 351

Nolvadex 10 mg
Stuart 600

Bricanyl 2.5 mg
Merrell Dow 725

Reglan 10 mg (old shape)
Robins

Myambutol 100 mg
Lederle M6

C-III
Hycodan
Endo (DuPont) 042

Hexadrol 0.75 mg
Organon 791

Alupent 10 mg
Boehringer-I 74

Isoclor
Amer Critical Care

Lasix 40 mg
Hoechst-Roussel

Pen-Vee K 125 mg
Wyeth 58

Artane 2 mg
Lederle A11

C-IV
Phenobarbital 100 mg
Lilly J33

Bricanyl 5 mg
Merrell Dow 750

Cytomel 50 mcg
SKF D17

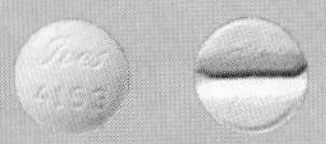

Isordil 10 mg Ives 4153	C-II **Demerol HCl 100 mg** Winthrop-Breon D37	C-IV **Paxipam 40 mg** Schering 538
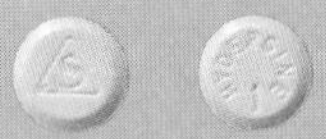 **Hydergine 1 mg** Sandoz	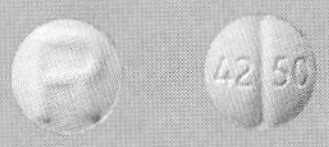 **Donnatal Tabs** Robins 4250	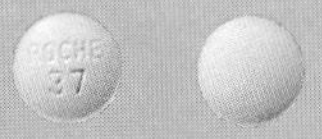 **Synkayvite 5 mg** Roché 37
Lanoxin 0.25 mg Burroughs-W X3A	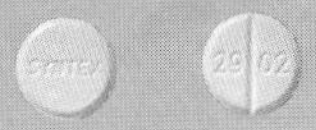 **Anadrol-50** Syntex 2902	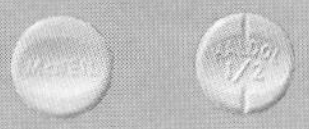 **Haldol 0.5 mg** McNeil
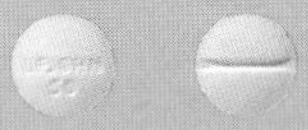 **Provera 10 mg** Upjohn 50	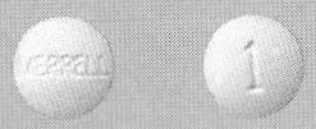 **Susadrin 1 mg** Merrell Dow	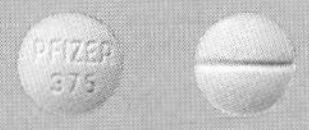 **Renese 1 mg** Pfizer 375
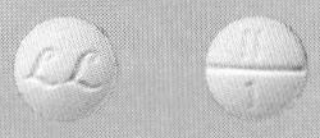 **Neptazane 50 mg** Lederle N1	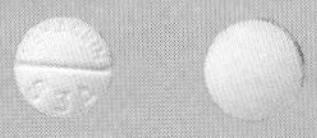 **Kemadrin 5 mg** Burroughs-W S3A	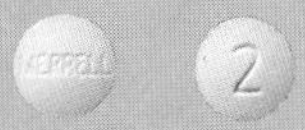 **Susadrin 2 mg** Merrell Dow
Mysoline 50 mg Ayerst	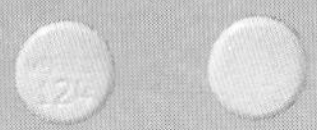 **Bentyl 20 mg w/Pb** Merrell Dow 124	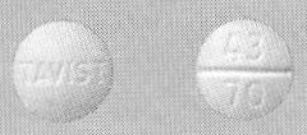 **Tavist** (Dorsey)
Periactin 4 mg MSD 62	C-IV **Cylert 18.75 mg** Abbott TH	**Lozol 2.5 mg** USV 82
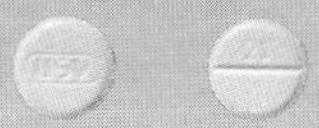 **Hygroton 100 mg** USV 21	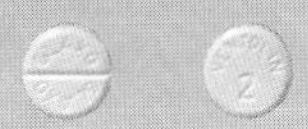 **Ventolin 2 mg** Glaxo	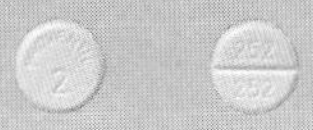 **Proventil 2 mg** Schering 252

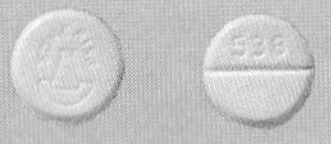

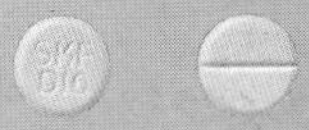

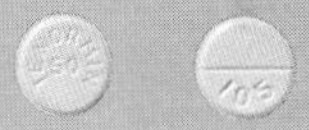

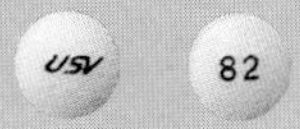

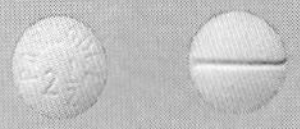

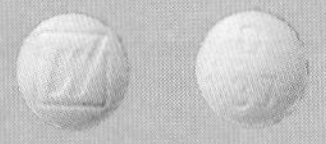

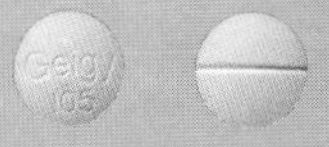

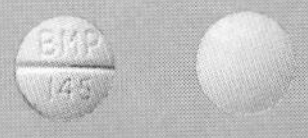

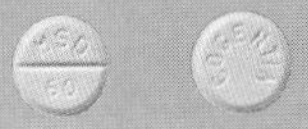

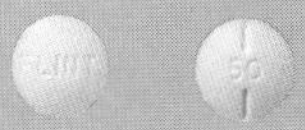

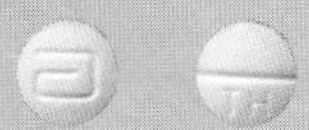

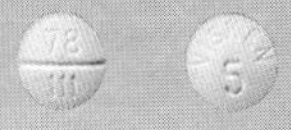

Brethine 5 mg
Geigy 105

Daricon 10 mg
Beecham Labs 145

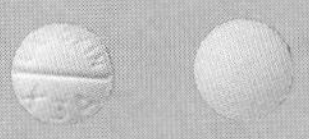

Cogentin 2 mg
MSD 60

Cytomel 25 mcg
SKF D16

Synthroid 0.05 mg
Flint 50

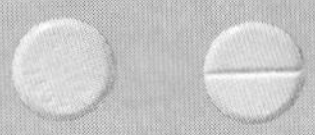

Tenormin 50 mg
Stuart 105

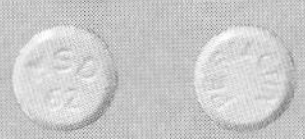

Parlodel 2.5 mg
Sandoz

Visken 5 mg
Sandoz 78-111

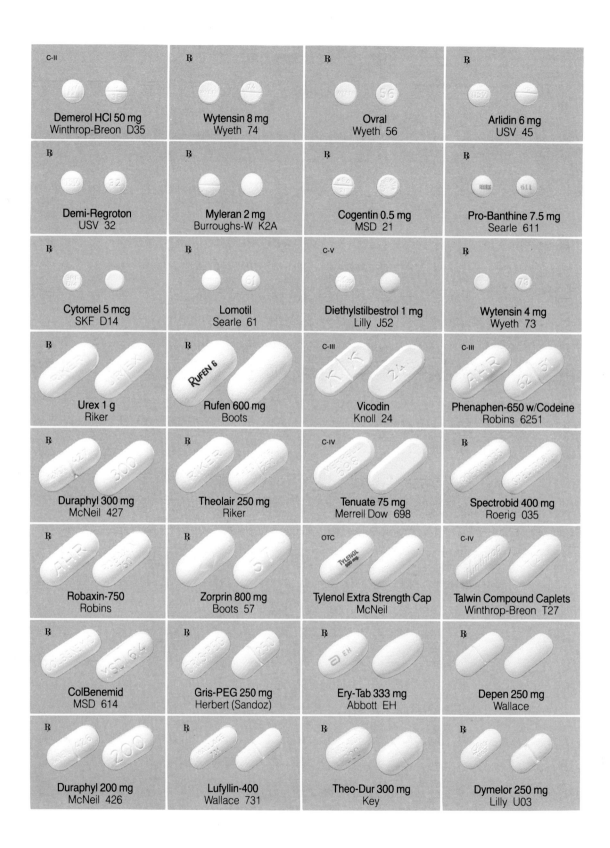

C-II Demerol HCl 50 mg Winthrop-Breon D35	**℞** Wytensin 8 mg Wyeth 74	**℞** Ovral Wyeth 56	**℞** Arlidin 6 mg USV 45
℞ Demi-Regroton USV 32	**℞** Myleran 2 mg Burroughs-W K2A	**℞** Cogentin 0.5 mg MSD 21	**℞** Pro-Banthine 7.5 mg Searle 611
℞ Cytomel 5 mcg SKF D14	**℞** Lomotil Searle 61	**C-V** Diethylstilbestrol 1 mg Lilly J52	**℞** Wytensin 4 mg Wyeth 73
℞ Urex 1 g Riker	**℞** Rufen 600 mg Boots	**C-III** Vicodin Knoll 24	**C-III** Phenaphen-650 w/Codeine Robins 6251
℞ Duraphyl 300 mg McNeil 427	**℞** Theolair 250 mg Riker	**C-IV** Tenuate 75 mg Merrell Dow 698	**℞** Spectrobid 400 mg Roerig 035
℞ Robaxin-750 Robins	**℞** Zorprin 800 mg Boots 57	**OTC** Tylenol Extra Strength Cap McNeil	**C-IV** Talwin Compound Caplets Winthrop-Breon T27
℞ ColBenemid MSD 614	**℞** Gris-PEG 250 mg Herbert (Sandoz)	**℞** Ery-Tab 333 mg Abbott EH	**℞** Depen 250 mg Wallace
℞ Duraphyl 200 mg McNeil 426	**℞** Lufyllin-400 Wallace 731	**℞** Theo-Dur 300 mg Key	**℞** Dymelor 250 mg Lilly U03

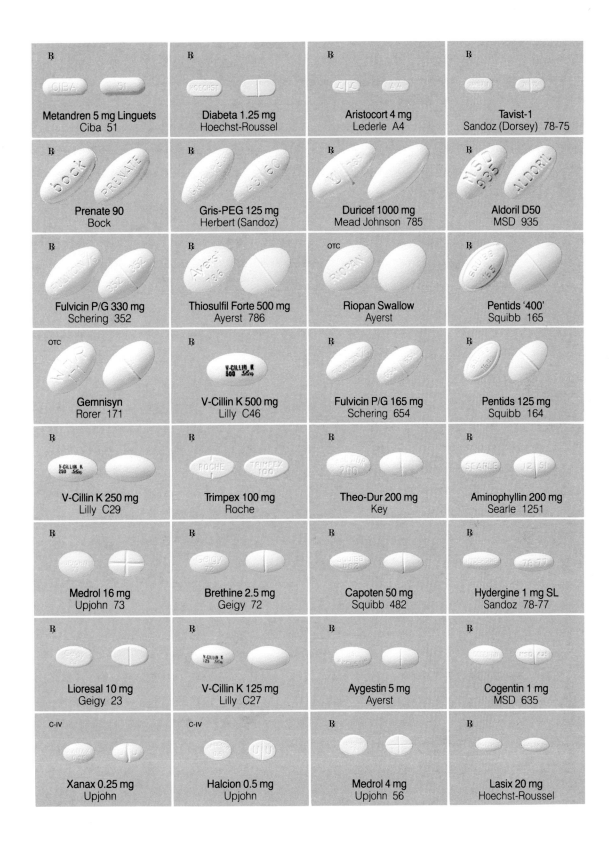

℞	℞	℞	℞
Metandren 5 mg Linguets Ciba 51	**Diabeta 1.25 mg** Hoechst-Roussel	**Aristocort 4 mg** Lederle A4	**Tavist-1** Sandoz (Dorsey) 78-75
℞	℞	℞	℞
Prenate 90 Bock	**Gris-PEG 125 mg** Herbert (Sandoz)	**Duricef 1000 mg** Mead Johnson 785	**Aldoril D50** MSD 935
℞	℞	OTC	℞
Fulvicin P/G 330 mg Schering 352	**Thiosulfil Forte 500 mg** Ayerst 786	**Riopan Swallow** Ayerst	**Pentids '400'** Squibb 165
OTC	℞	℞	℞
Gemnisyn Rorer 171	**V-Cillin K 500 mg** Lilly C46	**Fulvicin P/G 165 mg** Schering 654	**Pentids 125 mg** Squibb 164
℞	℞	℞	℞
V-Cillin K 250 mg Lilly C29	**Trimpex 100 mg** Roche	**Theo-Dur 200 mg** Key	**Aminophyllin 200 mg** Searle 1251
℞	℞	℞	℞
Medrol 16 mg Upjohn 73	**Brethine 2.5 mg** Geigy 72	**Capoten 50 mg** Squibb 482	**Hydergine 1 mg SL** Sandoz 78-77
℞	℞	℞	℞
Lioresal 10 mg Geigy 23	**V-Cillin K 125 mg** Lilly C27	**Aygestin 5 mg** Ayerst	**Cogentin 1 mg** MSD 635
C-IV	C-IV	℞	℞
Xanax 0.25 mg Upjohn	**Halcion 0.5 mg** Upjohn	**Medrol 4 mg** Upjohn 56	**Lasix 20 mg** Hoechst-Roussel

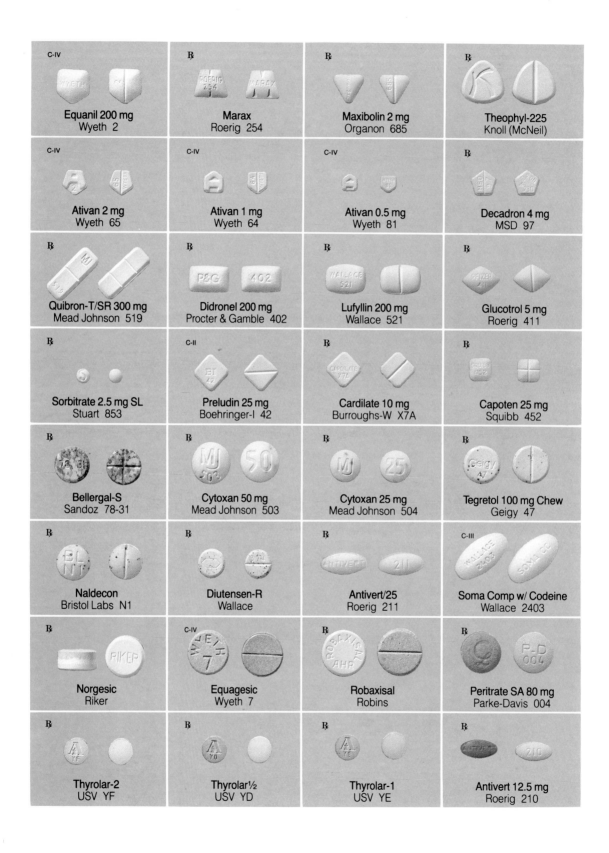

C-IV	Rx	Rx	Rx
Equanil 200 mg Wyeth 2	**Marax** Roerig 254	**Maxibolin 2 mg** Organon 685	**Theophyl-225** Knoll (McNeil)
C-IV	C-IV	C-IV	Rx
Ativan 2 mg Wyeth 65	**Ativan 1 mg** Wyeth 64	**Ativan 0.5 mg** Wyeth 81	**Decadron 4 mg** MSD 97
Rx	Rx	Rx	Rx
Quibron-T/SR 300 mg Mead Johnson 519	**Didronel 200 mg** Procter & Gamble 402	**Lufyllin 200 mg** Wallace 521	**Glucotrol 5 mg** Roerig 411
Rx	C-II	Rx	Rx
Sorbitrate 2.5 mg SL Stuart 853	**Preludin 25 mg** Boehringer-I 42	**Cardilate 10 mg** Burroughs-W X7A	**Capoten 25 mg** Squibb 452
Rx	Rx	Rx	Rx
Bellergal-S Sandoz 78-31	**Cytoxan 50 mg** Mead Johnson 503	**Cytoxan 25 mg** Mead Johnson 504	**Tegretol 100 mg Chew** Geigy 47
Rx	Rx	Rx	C-III
Naldecon Bristol Labs N1	**Diutensen-R** Wallace	**Antivert/25** Roerig 211	**Soma Comp w/ Codeine** Wallace 2403
Rx	C-IV	Rx	Rx
Norgesic Riker	**Equagesic** Wyeth 7	**Robaxisal** Robins	**Peritrate SA 80 mg** Parke-Davis 004
Rx	Rx	Rx	Rx
Thyrolar-2 USV YF	**Thyrolar½** USV YD	**Thyrolar-1** USV YE	**Antivert 12.5 mg** Roerig 210

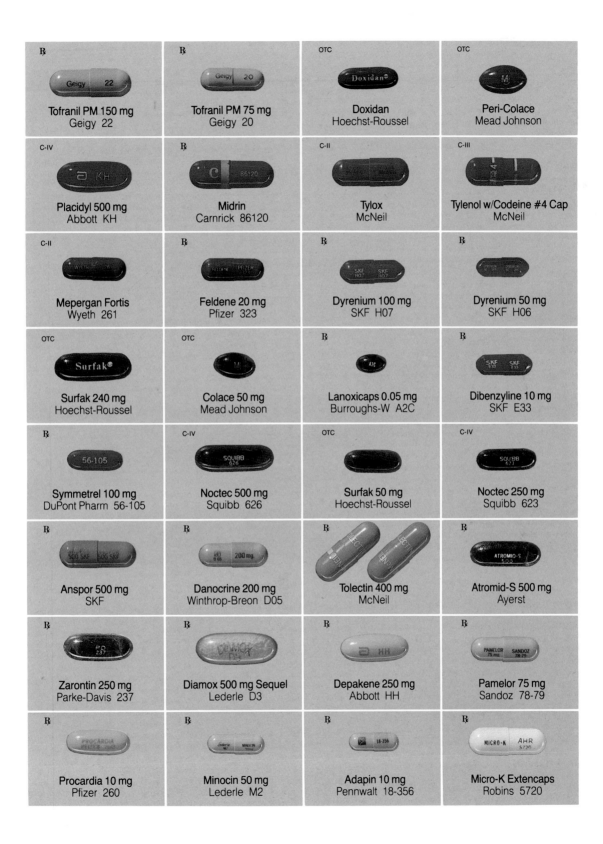

Rx Tofranil PM 150 mg Geigy 22	**Rx** Tofranil PM 75 mg Geigy 20
OTC Doxidan Hoechst-Roussel	**OTC** Peri-Colace Mead Johnson
C-IV Placidyl 500 mg Abbott KH	**Rx** Midrin Carnrick 86120
C-II Tylox McNeil	**C-III** Tylenol w/Codeine #4 Cap McNeil
C-II Mepergan Fortis Wyeth 261	**Rx** Feldene 20 mg Pfizer 323
Rx Dyrenium 100 mg SKF H07	**Rx** Dyrenium 50 mg SKF H06
OTC Surfak 240 mg Hoechst-Roussel	**OTC** Colace 50 mg Mead Johnson
Rx Lanoxicaps 0.05 mg Burroughs-W A2C	**Rx** Dibenzyline 10 mg SKF E33
Rx Symmetrel 100 mg DuPont Pharm 56-105	**C-IV** Noctec 500 mg Squibb 626
OTC Surfak 50 mg Hoechst-Roussel	**C-IV** Noctec 250 mg Squibb 623
Rx Anspor 500 mg SKF	**Rx** Danocrine 200 mg Winthrop-Breon D05
Rx Tolectin 400 mg McNeil	**Rx** Atromid-S 500 mg Ayerst
Rx Zarontin 250 mg Parke-Davis 237	**Rx** Diamox 500 mg Sequel Lederle D3
Rx Depakene 250 mg Abbott HH	**Rx** Pamelor 75 mg Sandoz 78-79
Rx Procardia 10 mg Pfizer 260	**Rx** Minocin 50 mg Lederle M2
Rx Adapin 10 mg Pennwalt 18-356	**Rx** Micro-K Extencaps Robins 5720

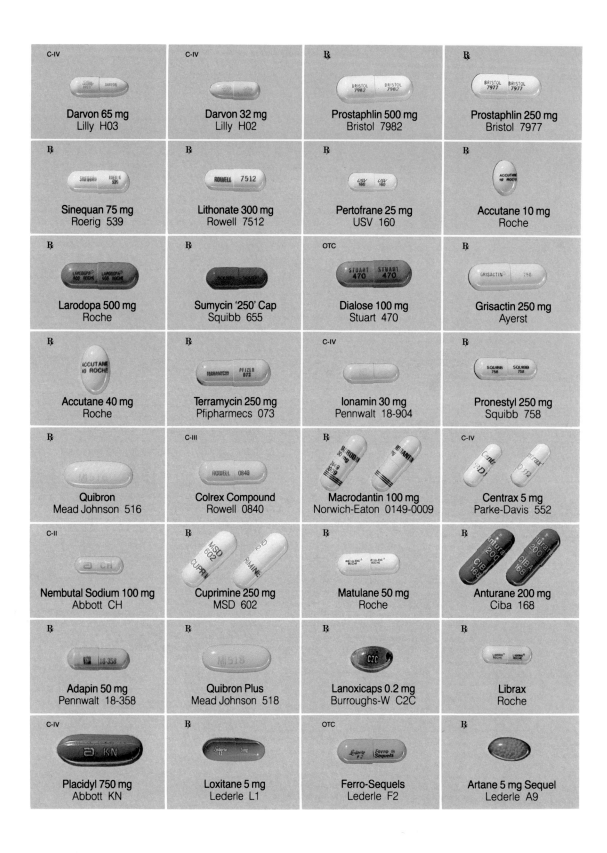

C-IV	C-IV	℞	℞
Darvon 65 mg Lilly H03	**Darvon 32 mg** Lilly H02	**Prostaphlin 500 mg** Bristol 7982	**Prostaphlin 250 mg** Bristol 7977
℞	℞	℞	℞
Sinequan 75 mg Roerig 539	**Lithonate 300 mg** Rowell 7512	**Pertofrane 25 mg** USV 160	**Accutane 10 mg** Roche
℞	℞	OTC	℞
Larodopa 500 mg Roche	**Sumycin '250' Cap** Squibb 655	**Dialose 100 mg** Stuart 470	**Grisactin 250 mg** Ayerst
℞	℞	C-IV	℞
Accutane 40 mg Roche	**Terramycin 250 mg** Pfipharmecs 073	**Ionamin 30 mg** Pennwalt 18-904	**Pronestyl 250 mg** Squibb 758
℞	C-III	℞	C-IV
Quibron Mead Johnson 516	**Colrex Compound** Rowell 0840	**Macrodantin 100 mg** Norwich-Eaton 0149-0009	**Centrax 5 mg** Parke-Davis 552
C-II	℞	℞	℞
Nembutal Sodium 100 mg Abbott CH	**Cuprimine 250 mg** MSD 602	**Matulane 50 mg** Roche	**Anturane 200 mg** Ciba 168
℞	℞	℞	℞
Adapin 50 mg Pennwalt 18-358	**Quibron Plus** Mead Johnson 518	**Lanoxicaps 0.2 mg** Burroughs-W C2C	**Librax** Roche
C-IV	℞	OTC	℞
Placidyl 750 mg Abbott KN	**Loxitane 5 mg** Lederle L1	**Ferro-Sequels** Lederle F2	**Artane 5 mg Sequel** Lederle A9

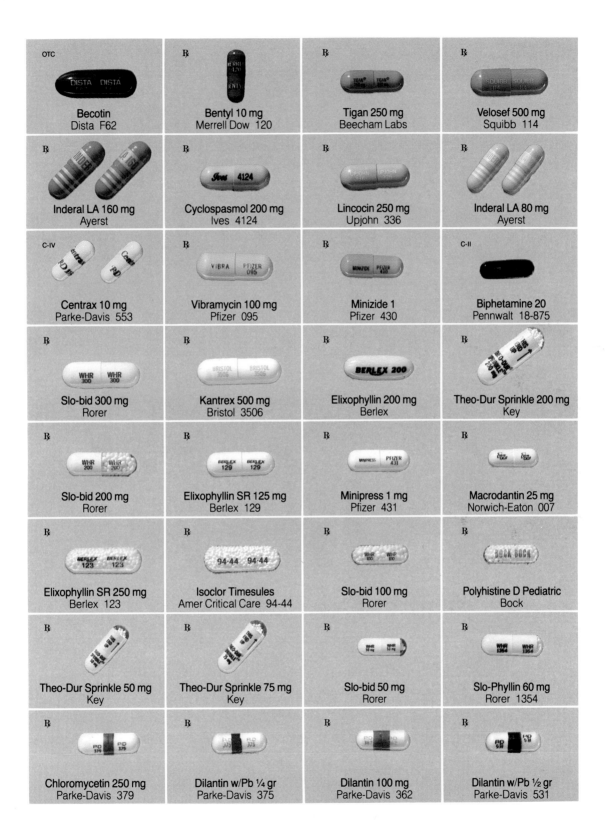

OTC **Becotin** Dista F62	℞ **Bentyl 10 mg** Merrell Dow 120	℞ **Tigan 250 mg** Beecham Labs	℞ **Velosef 500 mg** Squibb 114
℞ **Inderal LA 160 mg** Ayerst	℞ **Cyclospasmol 200 mg** Ives 4124	℞ **Lincocin 250 mg** Upjohn 336	℞ **Inderal LA 80 mg** Ayerst
C-IV **Centrax 10 mg** Parke-Davis 553	℞ **Vibramycin 100 mg** Pfizer 095	℞ **Minizide 1** Pfizer 430	C-II **Biphetamine 20** Pennwalt 18-875
℞ **Slo-bid 300 mg** Rorer	℞ **Kantrex 500 mg** Bristol 3506	℞ **Elixophyllin 200 mg** Berlex	℞ **Theo-Dur Sprinkle 200 mg** Key
℞ **Slo-bid 200 mg** Rorer	℞ **Elixophyllin SR 125 mg** Berlex 129	℞ **Minipress 1 mg** Pfizer 431	℞ **Macrodantin 25 mg** Norwich-Eaton 007
℞ **Elixophyllin SR 250 mg** Berlex 123	℞ **Isoclor Timesules** Amer Critical Care 94-44	℞ **Slo-bid 100 mg** Rorer	℞ **Polyhistine D Pediatric** Bock
℞ **Theo-Dur Sprinkle 50 mg** Key	℞ **Theo-Dur Sprinkle 75 mg** Key	℞ **Slo-bid 50 mg** Rorer	℞ **Slo-Phyllin 60 mg** Rorer 1354
℞ **Chloromycetin 250 mg** Parke-Davis 379	℞ **Dilantin w/Pb ¼ gr** Parke-Davis 375	℞ **Dilantin 100 mg** Parke-Davis 362	℞ **Dilantin w/Pb ½ gr** Parke-Davis 531

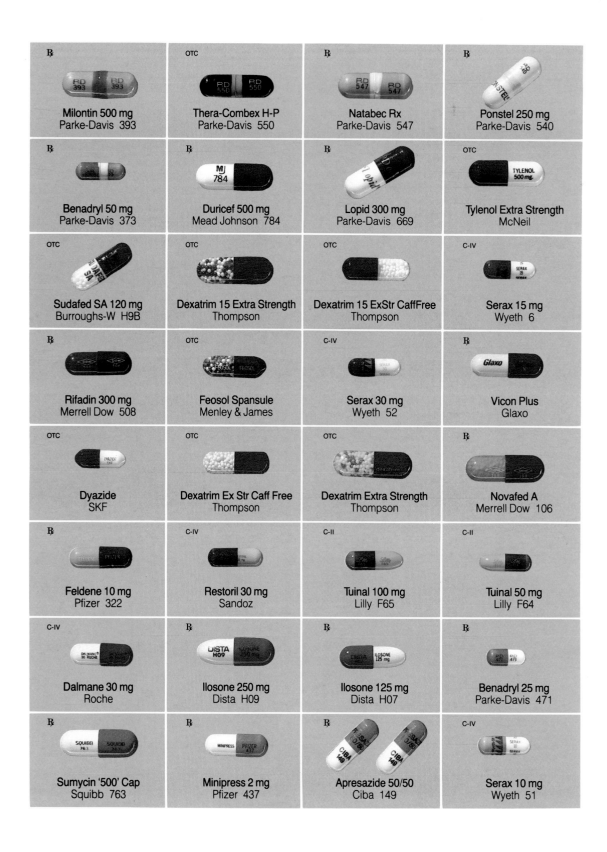

Rx	**OTC**	**Rx**	**Rx**
Milontin 500 mg Parke-Davis 393	Thera-Combex H-P Parke-Davis 550	Natabec Rx Parke-Davis 547	Ponstel 250 mg Parke-Davis 540
Rx	**Rx**	**Rx**	**OTC**
Benadryl 50 mg Parke-Davis 373	Duricef 500 mg Mead Johnson 784	Lopid 300 mg Parke-Davis 669	Tylenol Extra Strength McNeil
OTC	**OTC**	**OTC**	**C-IV**
Sudafed SA 120 mg Burroughs-W H9B	Dexatrim 15 Extra Strength Thompson	Dexatrim 15 ExStr CaffFree Thompson	Serax 15 mg Wyeth 6
Rx	**OTC**	**C-IV**	**Rx**
Rifadin 300 mg Merrell Dow 508	Feosol Spansule Menley & James	Serax 30 mg Wyeth 52	Vicon Plus Glaxo
OTC	**OTC**	**OTC**	**Rx**
Dyazide SKF	Dexatrim Ex Str Caff Free Thompson	Dexatrim Extra Strength Thompson	Novafed A Merrell Dow 106
Rx	**C-IV**	**C-II**	**C-II**
Feldene 10 mg Pfizer 322	Restoril 30 mg Sandoz	Tuinal 100 mg Lilly F65	Tuinal 50 mg Lilly F64
C-IV	**Rx**	**Rx**	**Rx**
Dalmane 30 mg Roche	Ilosone 250 mg Dista H09	Ilosone 125 mg Dista H07	Benadryl 25 mg Parke-Davis 471
Rx	**Rx**	**Rx**	**C-IV**
Sumycin '500' Cap Squibb 763	Minipress 2 mg Pfizer 437	Apresazide 50/50 Ciba 149	Serax 10 mg Wyeth 51

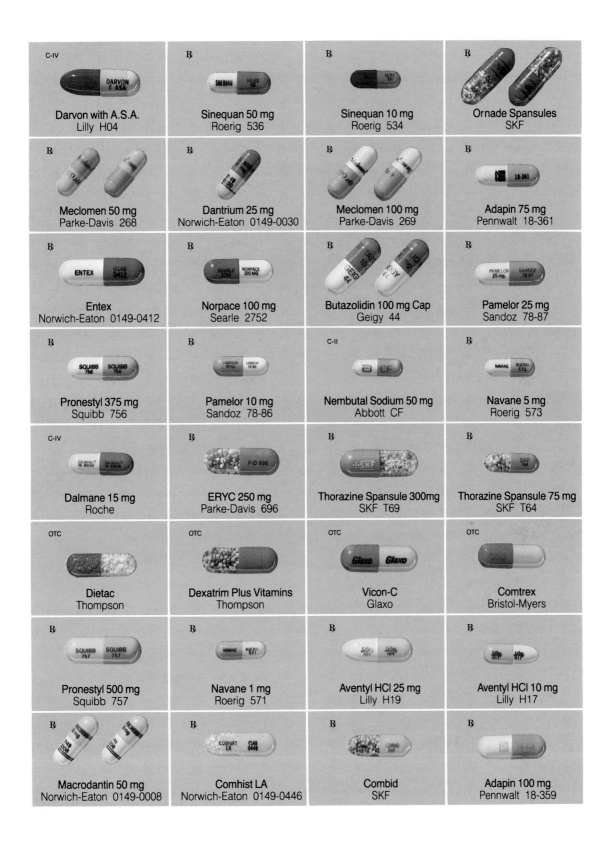

C-IV

Darvon with A.S.A.
Lilly H04

Rx

Sinequan 50 mg
Roerig 536

Rx

Sinequan 10 mg
Roerig 534

Rx

Ornade Spansules
SKF

Rx

Meclomen 50 mg
Parke-Davis 268

Rx

Dantrium 25 mg
Norwich-Eaton 0149-0030

Rx

Meclomen 100 mg
Parke-Davis 269

Rx

Adapin 75 mg
Pennwalt 18-361

Rx

Entex
Norwich-Eaton 0149-0412

Rx

Norpace 100 mg
Searle 2752

Rx

Butazolidin 100 mg Cap
Geigy 44

Rx

Pamelor 25 mg
Sandoz 78-87

Rx

Pronestyl 375 mg
Squibb 756

Rx

Pamelor 10 mg
Sandoz 78-86

C-II

Nembutal Sodium 50 mg
Abbott CF

Rx

Navane 5 mg
Roerig 573

C-IV

Dalmane 15 mg
Roche

Rx

ERYC 250 mg
Parke-Davis 696

Rx

Thorazine Spansule 300mg
SKF T69

Rx

Thorazine Spansule 75 mg
SKF T64

OTC

Dietac
Thompson

OTC

Dexatrim Plus Vitamins
Thompson

OTC

Vicon-C
Glaxo

OTC

Comtrex
Bristol-Myers

Rx

Pronestyl 500 mg
Squibb 757

Rx

Navane 1 mg
Roerig 571

Rx

Aventyl HCl 25 mg
Lilly H19

Rx

Aventyl HCl 10 mg
Lilly H17

Rx

Macrodantin 50 mg
Norwich-Eaton 0149-0008

Rx

Comhist LA
Norwich-Eaton 0149-0446

Rx

Combid
SKF

Rx

Adapin 100 mg
Pennwalt 18-359

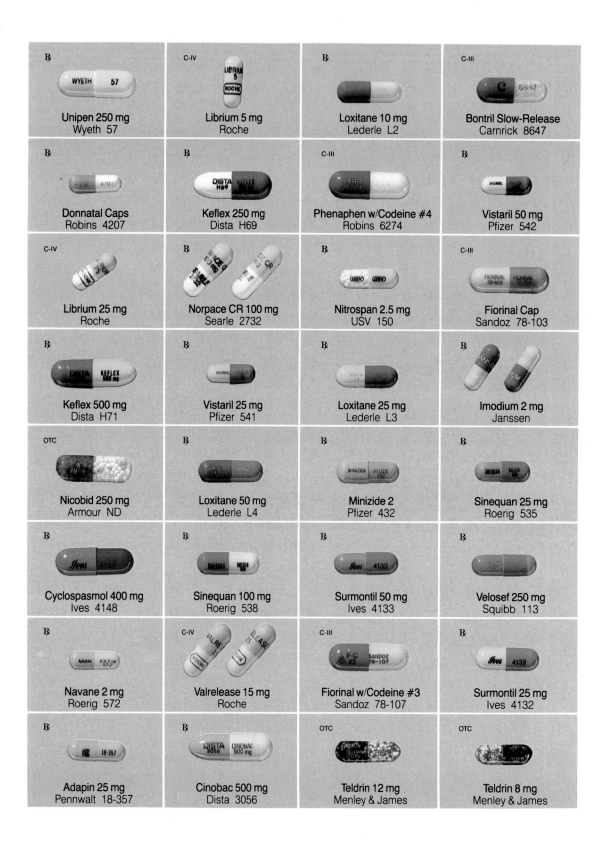

R̶	C-IV	R̶	C-III
Unipen 250 mg Wyeth 57	**Librium 5 mg** Roche	**Loxitane 10 mg** Lederle L2	**Bontril Slow-Release** Carnrick 8647
R̶	R̶	C-III	R̶
Donnatal Caps Robins 4207	**Keflex 250 mg** Dista H69	**Phenaphen w/Codeine #4** Robins 6274	**Vistaril 50 mg** Pfizer 542
C-IV	R̶	R̶	C-III
Librium 25 mg Roche	**Norpace CR 100 mg** Searle 2732	**Nitrospan 2.5 mg** USV 150	**Fiorinal Cap** Sandoz 78-103
R̶	R̶	R̶	R̶
Keflex 500 mg Dista H71	**Vistaril 25 mg** Pfizer 541	**Loxitane 25 mg** Lederle L3	**Imodium 2 mg** Janssen
OTC	R̶	R̶	R̶
Nicobid 250 mg Armour ND	**Loxitane 50 mg** Lederle L4	**Minizide 2** Pfizer 432	**Sinequan 25 mg** Roerig 535
R̶	R̶	R̶	R̶
Cyclospasmol 400 mg Ives 4148	**Sinequan 100 mg** Roerig 538	**Surmontil 50 mg** Ives 4133	**Velosef 250 mg** Squibb 113
R̶	C-IV	C-III	R̶
Navane 2 mg Roerig 572	**Valrelease 15 mg** Roche	**Fiorinal w/Codeine #3** Sandoz 78-107	**Surmontil 25 mg** Ives 4132
R̶	R̶	OTC	OTC
Adapin 25 mg Pennwalt 18-357	**Cinobac 500 mg** Dista 3056	**Teldrin 12 mg** Menley & James	**Teldrin 8 mg** Menley & James

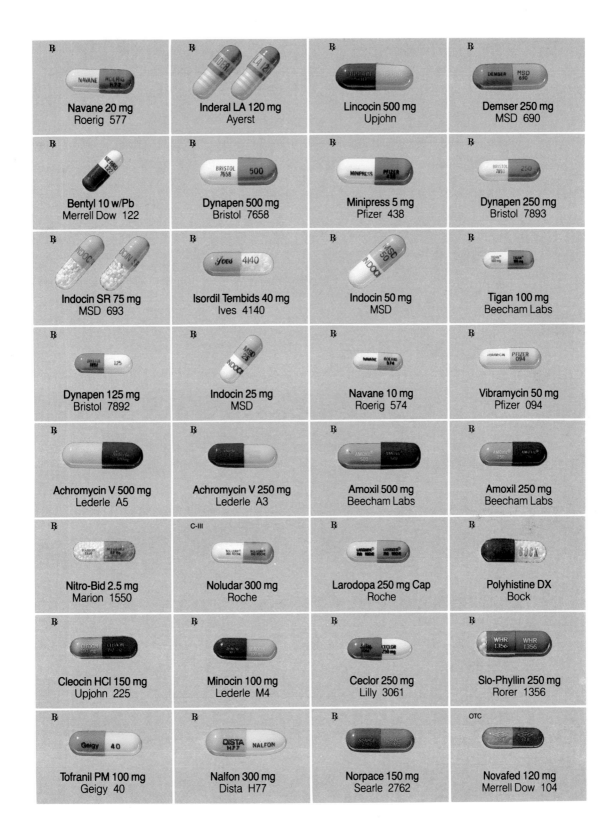

Navane 20 mg
Roerig 577

Inderal LA 120 mg
Ayerst

Lincocin 500 mg
Upjohn

Demser 250 mg
MSD 690

Bentyl 10 w/Pb
Merrell Dow 122

Dynapen 500 mg
Bristol 7658

Minipress 5 mg
Pfizer 438

Dynapen 250 mg
Bristol 7893

Indocin SR 75 mg
MSD 693

Isordil Tembids 40 mg
Ives 4140

Indocin 50 mg
MSD

Tigan 100 mg
Beecham Labs

Dynapen 125 mg
Bristol 7892

Indocin 25 mg
MSD

Navane 10 mg
Roerig 574

Vibramycin 50 mg
Pfizer 094

Achromycin V 500 mg
Lederle A5

Achromycin V 250 mg
Lederle A3

Amoxil 500 mg
Beecham Labs

Amoxil 250 mg
Beecham Labs

Nitro-Bid 2.5 mg
Marion 1550

C-III

Noludar 300 mg
Roche

Larodopa 250 mg Cap
Roche

Polyhistine DX
Bock

Cleocin HCl 150 mg
Upjohn 225

Minocin 100 mg
Lederle M4

Ceclor 250 mg
Lilly 3061

Slo-Phyllin 250 mg
Rorer 1356

Tofranil PM 100 mg
Geigy 40

Nalfon 300 mg
Dista H77

Norpace 150 mg
Searle 2762

OTC

Novafed 120 mg
Merrell Dow 104

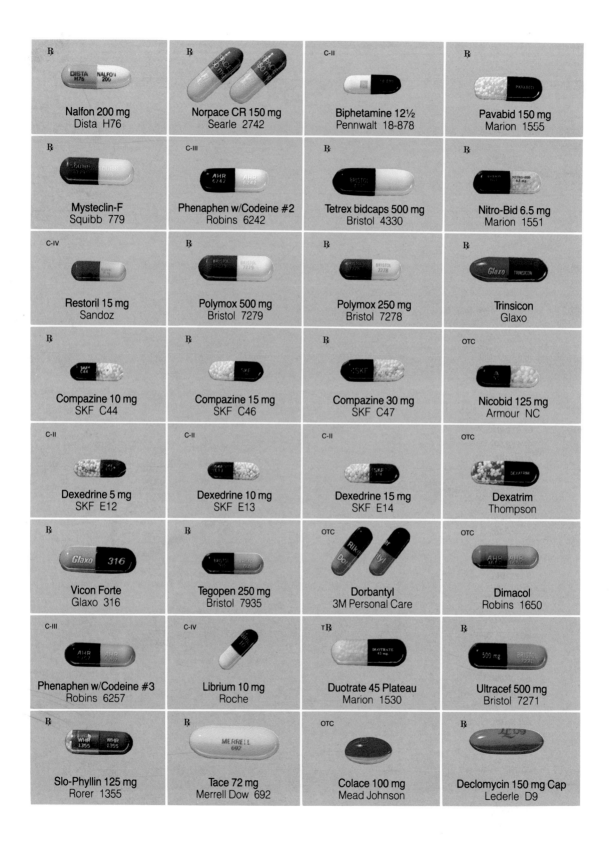

R̸

Nalfon 200 mg
Dista H76

R̸

Norpace CR 150 mg
Searle 2742

C-II

Biphetamine 12½
Pennwalt 18-878

R̸

Pavabid 150 mg
Marion 1555

R̸

Mysteclin-F
Squibb 779

C-III

Phenaphen w/Codeine #2
Robins 6242

R̸

Tetrex bidcaps 500 mg
Bristol 4330

R̸

Nitro-Bid 6.5 mg
Marion 1551

C-IV

Restoril 15 mg
Sandoz

R̸

Polymox 500 mg
Bristol 7279

R̸

Polymox 250 mg
Bristol 7278

R̸

Trinsicon
Glaxo

R̸

Compazine 10 mg
SKF C44

R̸

Compazine 15 mg
SKF C46

R̸

Compazine 30 mg
SKF C47

OTC

Nicobid 125 mg
Armour NC

C-II

Dexedrine 5 mg
SKF E12

C-II

Dexedrine 10 mg
SKF E13

C-II

Dexedrine 15 mg
SKF E14

OTC

Dexatrim
Thompson

R̸

Vicon Forte
Glaxo 316

R̸

Tegopen 250 mg
Bristol 7935

OTC

Dorbantyl
3M Personal Care

OTC

Dimacol
Robins 1650

C-III

Phenaphen w/Codeine #3
Robins 6257

C-IV

Librium 10 mg
Roche

TR̸

Duotrate 45 Plateau
Marion 1530

R̸

Ultracef 500 mg
Bristol 7271

R̸

Slo-Phyllin 125 mg
Rorer 1355

R̸

Tace 72 mg
Merrell Dow 692

OTC

Colace 100 mg
Mead Johnson

R̸

Declomycin 150 mg Cap
Lederle D9

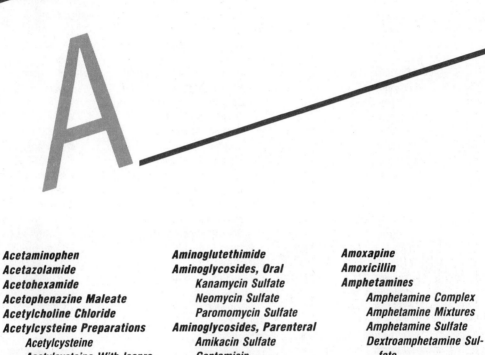

Testosterone
Testosterone Cypionate
Testosterone Enanthate
Testosterone Propionate
Anesthetics, General
Barbiturates
Methohexital Sodium
Thiamylal Sodium
Thiopental Sodium
Nonbarbiturates
Etomidate
Fentanyl Citrate and Droperidol
Ketamine Hydrochloride
Gases
Cyclopropane
Ethylene
Nitrous Oxide
Volatile Liquids
Enflurane
Halothane
Isoflurane
Methoxyflurane
Anesthetics, Local, Injectable
Bupivacaine Hydrochloride
Chloroprocaine Hydrochloride
Dibucaine Hydrochloride
Lidocaine Hydrochloride
Mepivacaine Hydrochloride
Prilocaine Hydrochloride
Procaine Hydrochloride, Injectable
Tetracaine Hydrochloride
Anesthetics, Local, Topical
Benzocaine
Butamben Picrate
Cocaine
Cyclomethycaine Sulfate
Dibucaine
Dyclonine Hydrochloride
Hexylcaine Hydrochloride
Lidocaine
Lidocaine Hydrochloride
Pramoxine Hydrochloride
Tetracaine
Tetracaine Hydrochloride
Anorectal Preparations
Anesthetics, Ophthalmic
Benoxinate Hydrochloride and Fluorescein Sodium
Proparacaine Hydrochloride
Tetracaine
Anisotropine Methylbromide

Anorexiants
Benzphetamine Hydrochloride
Diethylpropion Hydrochloride
Fenfluramine Hydrochloride
Mazindol
Phendimetrazine Tartrate
Phenmetrazine Hydrochloride
Phentermine Hydrochloride
Antacids
Aluminum Carbonate Gel, Basic
Aluminum Hydroxide Gel
Aluminum Phosphate Gel
Calcium Carbonate
Dihydroxyaluminum Sodium Carbonate
Magaldrate
Magnesia (Magnesium Hydroxide)
Magnesium Carbonate
Magnesium Oxide
Magnesium Trisilicate
Sodium Bicarbonate
Antacid Combinations
Anthralin
Antibiotics, Ophthalmic
Drops
Ointments
Antibiotics, Topical
Single Antibiotic Preparations
Multiple Antibiotic Preparations
Anticholinergic Antiparkinsonism Agents
Benztropine Mesylate
Biperiden
Diphenhydramine
Ethopropazine Hydrochloride
Orphenadrine Hydrochloride
Procyclidine
Trihexyphenidyl Hydrochloride
Anticonvulsants
Benzodiazepines
Clonazepam
Clorazepate Dipotassium
Diazepam
Hydantoins
Ethotoin
Mephenytoin

Phenytoin
Phenytoin Sodium, Extended
Phenytoin Sodium, Parenteral
Phenytoin Sodium, Prompt
Phenytoin Sodium With Phenobarbital
Oxazolidinediones
Paramethadione
Trimethadione
Succinimides
Ethosuximide
Methsuximide
Phensuximide
Antidepressants
Trazodone Hydrochloride
Tricyclic Compounds
Amitriptyline Hydrochloride
Amoxapine
Desipramine Hydrochloride
Doxepin Hydrochloride
Imipramine Hydrochloride
Imipramine Pamoate
Maprotiline Hydrochloride
Nortriptyline Hydrochloride
Protriptyline Hydrochloride
Trimipramine Maleate
Monoamine Oxidase Inhibitors
Isocarboxazid
Phenelzine Sulfate
Tranylcypromine Sulfate
Antiemetic/Antivertigo Agents
General Statement
Phenothiazines
Chlorpromazine Hydrochloride
Perphenazine
Prochlorperazine
Promethazine Hydrochloride
Thiethylperazine Maleate
Triflupromazine Hydrochloride
Antihistamines
Buclizine Hydrochloride
Cyclizine, Meclizine
Dimenhydrinate
Diphenhydramine Hydrochloride
Miscellaneous Preparations
Benzquinamide Hydrochloride

Diphenidol
Scopolamine Preparations
Trimethobenzamide Hydrochloride
Antiemetic/Antivertigo Combinations
Phosphorated Carbohydrate Solution
Combinations of Antihistamines, Pyridoxine HCl, Pentobarbital
Antihemophilic Factor
Antihistamines
Azatadine Maleate
Brompheniramine Maleate
Carbinoxamine Maleate
Chlorpheniramine Maleate
Clemastine Fumarate
Cyproheptadine Hydrochloride
Dexchlorpheniramine Maleate
Diphenhydramine Hydrochloride
Diphenylpyraline Hydrochloride
Methdilazine Hydrochloride
Phenindamine Tartrate
Promethazine Hydrochloride
Pyrilamine Maleate
Trimeprazine

Tripelennamine Hydrochloride
Triprolidine Hydrochloride
Anti-inhibitor Coagulant Complex
Antipsychotic Agents
Acetophenazine Maleate
Chlorpromazine Hydrochloride
Chlorprothixene
Fluphenazine Enanthate and Decanoate
Fluphenazine Hydrochloride
Haloperidol
Loxapine
Mesoridazine
Molindone Hydrochloride
Perphenazine
Piperacetazine
Prochlorperazine
Promazine Hydrochloride
Thioridazine Hydrochloride
Thiothixene
Trifluoperazine
Triflupromazine Hydrochloride
Antirabies Serum, Equine Origin
Antiseptics and Germicides
Benzalkonium Chloride
Chlorhexidine Gluconate

Hexachlorophene
Iodine
Povidone-Iodine
Merbromin
Thimerosal
Silver Nitrate
Silver Protein, Mild
Antithyroid Agents
Methimazole
Propylthiouracil
Antitoxins and Antivenins
Diphtheria Antitoxin
Tetanus Antitoxin
Antivenin (Crotalidae) Polyvalent
Antivenin (Micrurus Fulvius)
Antivenin (Latrodectus Mactans)
Apomorphine Hydrochloride
Aprobarbital
Aromatic Ammonia Spirit
Ascorbic Acid
Asparaginase
Aspirin
Atenolol
Atracurium Besylate
Atropine Sulfate
Aurothioglucose
Azatadine Maleate
Azathioprine
Azlocillin Sodium

Acetaminophen

(n-acetyl-P-aminophenol, APAP) otc

tablets, chewable: 80 mg	Children's Anacin-3, St. Joseph Aspirin-Free, Tylenol Pedric
wafers: 120 mg	
capsules: 325 mg	Phenaphen, Tylenol Regular Strength
tablets: 325 mg	A'Cenol, Aceta, Actamin, Anacin-3, Conacetol, Dapa, Febrinol, Panex, Sudoprin, Tapar, Tenol, Tylenol Regular Strength, Ty-tabs, Valadol, Valorin, *Generic*
capsules: 500 mg	A'Cenol, Anacin-3 Maximum Strength, Datril Extra Strength, Halenol Extra Strength, Panadol, Tylenol Extra Strength, *Generic*
tablets: 500 mg	Anacin-3 Maximum Strength, Banesin, Datril Extra Strength, Halenol Extra Strength, Panadol, Panex 500, St. Joseph Adult Maximum Strength, Tapanol Extra Strength, Tylenol Extra Strength, *Generic*
tablets: 650 mg	Acenol D.S., *Generic*
suppositories: 120 mg	Acetaminophen Uniserts, Acephen, Anuphen, Suppap-120, *Generic*
suppositories: 125 mg	Neopap Supprettes (*Rx*)
suppositories: 325 mg	Acetaminophen Uniserts, *Generic*
suppositories: 650 mg	Acephen, Acetaminophen Uniserts, Anuphen, Suppap-650, *Generic*
elixir: 120 mg/5 ml	Oraphen-PD, Pedric, Peedee Dose Aspirin Alternative, Valadol, *Generic*
elixir: 160 mg/5 ml	Aceta, Bayapap, Children's Anacin-3, Halenol, Tempra Syrup, Tenol, Tylenol, *Generic*
elixir: 325 mg/5 ml	Dolanex
liquid: 165 mg/5 ml	Tylenol Extra Strength
solution: 100 mg/ml	Bayapap Drops, Infant's Anacin-3 Drops, Tempra Drops, Tylenol Drops, *Generic*
solution: 120 mg/2.5 ml	Liquiprin Drops

INDICATIONS

Analgesic–antipyretic for use in presence of aspirin allergy, hemostatic disturbances (including anticoagulant therapy), bleeding disorders (*e.g.,* hemophilia), upper GI disease (*e.g.,* ulcer, gastritis, hiatus hernia), gouty arthritis, common cold, "flu," and other bacterial and viral infections. Analgesia in a wide variety of arthritic and rheumatic conditions as well as headache, toothache, abrasions, dysmenorrhea, myalgias, neuralgias, teething, immunization, and tonsillectomy.

CONTRAINDICATIONS

Hypersensitivity.

ACTIONS

Site and mechanism of analgesic effect unclear; reduces fever by direct action on hypothalamic heat-regulating centers resulting in increased dissipation of body heat via vasodilatation and sweating. Almost as potent as aspirin in inhibiting prostaglandin synthesis in CNS. Ability to inhibit prostaglandin synthesis peripherally is minimal, which may account for lack of significant anti-inflammatory and antirheumatic effects. Antipyretic and analgesic effects are comparable to those of aspirin; aspirin is clearly superior for treating pain of inflammatory origin. Acetaminophen does not inhibit platelet aggregation, affect prothrombin response or produce GI ulceration (see Acetylsalicylic Acid). Hepatotoxic effects noted with this drug have not been reported with aspirin.

Acetaminophen is rapidly and almost completely absorbed from the GI tract. Peak plasma concentrations occur within ½ to 2 hours; the rate and extent of absorption from suppositories is variable. Acetaminophen is extensively metabolized and excreted in the urine.

WARNINGS

Use with caution in those with impaired hepatic function. Hepatotoxicity and severe hepatic failure have been reported in chronic alcoholics following therapeutic doses.

PRECAUTIONS

If rare sensitivity occurs, discontinue use. Severe or recurrent pain or continued high fever may indicate serious illness. If pain persists more than 10 days, if redness is present, or if children under 12 are affected by arthritic or rheumatic conditions, consult physician immediately.

DRUG INTERACTIONS

In those treated with **prothrombin-reducing anti-coagulants,** acetaminophen is preferable to aspirin when antipyretic or analgesic action is desired. The hepatic metabolism of acetaminophen may be increased by **oral contraceptives,** decreasing elimination half-life by 20% to 30%. Drugs that may delay gastric emptying (*e.g.,* **anticholinergics, narcotics**) may decrease the rate of absorption of acetaminophen; the clinical significance is unknown. Chronic, excessive **ethanol** ingestion apparently increases the toxicity of larger therapeutic doses or overdoses of acetaminophen; evidence suggests that acute ethanol ingestion protects against overdose toxicity. **Activated charcoal** given immediately after acetaminophen ingestion reduces both the rate and extent of acetaminophen absorption. Studies indicate that **caffeine** enhances the analgesic activity of acetaminophen.

ADVERSE REACTIONS

Acetaminophen is free of severe toxicity or side-effects when used as directed. Adverse effects associated with use (usually chronic) have included the following:

Hematologic: Cyanosis, methemoglobinemia, sulfhemoglobinemia, hemolytic anemia, neutropenia, pancytopenia, thrombocytopenia.

Allergic: Skin eruptions, urticarial and erythematous skin reactions, fever.

Other: Hypoglycemia, CNS stimulation, jaundice, glossitis, drowsiness.

OVERDOSAGE

Acute poisoning may be manifested by cyanosis, tachycardia, anemia, pancytopenia, neutropenia, jaundice, leukopenia, skin eruptions, chills, fever, emesis, CNS stimulation, excitement, delirium followed by depression, coma, vascular collapse, convulsions, and death. Overdosage causes hepatotoxicity; minimal toxic dose is 10 g (140 mg/kg). Minimum lethal dose is 15 g (200 mg/kg). Children appear to be less susceptible than adults to toxicity. Initial signs of toxicity include nausea, vomiting, general malaise, diaphoresis, abdominal pain, and diarrhea. Clinical and laboratory evidence of toxicity usually is not apparent until after 48 to 72 hours and may be delayed up to 1 week. Serial hepatic enzyme determinations are recommended. Hepatic failure may be severe leading to encephalopathy, coma, and death. Plasma levels and plasma half-life of the drug may be used to determine need for treatment and predict degree of hepatic damage. Hepatic damage is unlikely if plasma levels at 4 hours are below 120 mcg/ml. If plasma half-life is greater than 4 hours, hepatic necrosis is probable. Chronic ingestion of 5 g to 8 g daily over several weeks or 2.9 g to 3.9 g daily for a year has resulted in liver damage.

Treatment: Gastric lavage if recently ingested. Activated charcoal may be used; lavage until clear. Magnesium or sodium sulfate may be instilled into stomach after lavage. Emesis, lavage, and activated charcoal should be instituted within 1 hour to be of significant value. Transfusion may be required for acute hemolytic anemia in severe poisoning. Early (0 to 10 hours after ingestion) administration of compounds supplying sulfhydryl groups may prevent or minimize hepatic damage. Oral and IV administration of acetylcysteine has been used (see Acetylcysteine).

DOSAGE

Adults: 300 mg to 650 mg q4h. Doses up to 1000 mg may be given qid for short-term therapy. Long-term therapy: Doses above 2.6 g/day are not recommended. Monitor hepatic function of those on long-term therapy.

Children: Doses may be repeated 4 or 5 times daily, not to exceed 5 doses in 24 hours.

0–3 months—40 mg
4–11 months—80 mg
12–24 months—120 mg
2–3 years—160 mg
4–5 years—240 mg
6–8 years—320 mg
9–10 years—400 mg
11–12 years—480 mg

A 10 mg/kg dose for children has also been recommended.

NURSING IMPLICATIONS

HISTORY

See Appendix 4. If relevant, obtain history of analgesic drug use and effectiveness of agent(s) used. Especially note recent or prolonged use of acetaminophen in normal or high doses and history of liver disease.

PHYSICAL ASSESSMENT

Evaluate pain—type, intensity, location, and duration; take temperature, pulse, respirations if drug is used as an antipyretic.

ADMINISTRATION

Instruct patient to chew the chewable tablet form thoroughly before swallowing (chewable tablets are flavored).

Evaluate analgesic effect of drug; notify physician if pain or discomfort is not relieved.

If drug is used as an antipyretic check temperature in 45 to 60 minutes. Profuse diaphoresis requires frequent changing of gown and bed linen.

Suppositories: Check in ½ hour to be sure product has not been expelled from the rectum. If it has been expelled, check with physician for instructions (*e.g.,* repeat of same or smaller dose).

Observe for adverse drug reactions.

PATIENT AND FAMILY INFORMATION

Do not exceed recommended dose, take for more than 10 days, or give to children under 3 without consulting physician.

Acetazolamide

See Carbonic Anhydrase Inhibitors.

Acetohexamide

See Sulfonylureas.

Acetophenazine Maleate

See Antipsychotic Agents.

Acetylcholine Chloride

See Miotics, Direct Acting.

Acetylcysteine Preparations

Acetylcysteine Rx

solution: 10%, 20%   Mucomyst

Acetylcysteine With Isoproterenol Rx

solution: 10% acetyl-   Mucomyst with Isoprotere-
cysteine, 0.05%   nol
isoproterenol

INDICATIONS
ACETYLCYSTEINE

Adjuvant therapy for abnormal, viscid, or inspissated mucous secretions in such conditions as chronic bronchopulmonary disease; acute pulmonary complications of cystic fibrosis; tracheostomy; pulmonary complications associated with surgery; anesthesia; posttraumatic chest conditions; atelectasis due to mucous obstruction; diagnostic bronchial studies.

Investigational uses: Acetylcysteine has been used successfully as an antidote to prevent or minimize hepatotoxicity in acute acetaminophen overdosage. Acetylcysteine is given orally as a 5% solution mixed with soda, water, or grapefruit juice. An initial dose of 140 mg/kg is followed by 17 maintenance doses of 70 mg/kg every 4 hours. Administer as early as possible after ingestion of potentially toxic doses of acetaminophen; however, preliminary evidence suggests that acetylcysteine may be effective as late as 18 hours after ingestion.

Acetylcysteine has also been used with some success as an ophthalmic solution, primarily to treat keratoconjunctivitis sicca (dry eye). It has been used successfully as an enema in a few neonates, children, and adults with bowel obstruction due to meconium ileus or meconium ileus equivalent.

ACETYLCYSTEINE WITH ISOPROTERENOL

For conditions listed under Acetylcysteine in those who might react to inhaled acetylcysteine aerosol with increased airway obstruction. The isoproterenol component is present only to decrease possible increased airway obstruction caused by acetylcysteine.

CONTRAINDICATIONS
Sensitivity to acetylcysteine.

ACTIONS
Mucolytic action is related to the sulfhydryl group in the molecule, which probably "opens" disulfide linkage in mucus, thus lowering viscosity.

WARNINGS
After administration, an increased volume of liquefied bronchial secretions may occur. If necessary, maintain an open airway by mechanical suction when coughing is inadequate. When there is a large mechanical block caused by a foreign body or local accumulation, the airway may be cleared by endotracheal aspiration with or without bronchoscopy. Watch asthmatics carefully; if bronchospasm progresses, discontinue treatment immediately. Drug should be used during pregnancy only if clearly needed. Exercise caution in administration to nursing mothers.

PRECAUTIONS
With administration, patient may notice a slight disagreeable odor, which is soon not noticeable. Un-

der certain conditions a color change may occur in the opened bottle. The light purple color is the result of a chemical reaction and does not impair safety or mucolytic drug activity. Continued nebulization with a dry gas results in increased concentration of the drug in the nebulizer because of evaporation. Extreme concentration may impede nebulization and efficient drug delivery; dilute the nebulizing solution with Sterile Water for Injection.

ADVERSE REACTIONS

Stomatitis, nausea, rhinorrhea. Sensitivity and sensitization reported rarely. A few susceptible patients, particularly asthmatics (see *Warnings*) may experience varying degrees of bronchospasm; most are quickly relieved by use of a bronchodilator given by nebulization. See also Isoproterenol.

DOSAGE
ACETYLCYSTEINE

Nebulization by face mask, mouthpiece, tracheostomy: 1 ml to 10 ml of the 20% solution or 2 ml to 20 ml of the 10% solution may be given q2h to q6h. The recommended dose for most patients is 3 ml to 5 ml of the 20% solution or 6 ml to 10 ml of the 10% solution tid to qid.

Nebulization by tent, croupette: Large volumes are required (as much as 300 ml during a single treatment period) to maintain a very heavy mist for the desired period. Administration for intermittent or continuous prolonged periods may be desirable.

Direct instillation: For routine management of a tracheostomy, 1 ml to 2 ml of a 10% to 20% solution may be instilled into the tracheostomy q1h to q4h. The drug may also be introduced directly into a particular segment of the bronchopulmonary tree by inserting (under local anesthesia and direct vision) a catheter into the trachea; 2 ml to 5 ml of the 20% solution may be instilled by means of a syringe attached to the catheter. Acetylcysteine may also be given through a percutaneous intratracheal catheter; 1 ml to 2 ml of the 20% solution may be instilled by a syringe attached to the catheter.

Diagnostic bronchograms: 2 to 3 administrations of 1 ml to 2 ml of the 20% solution given by nebulization prior to the procedure.

ACETYLCYSTEINE WITH ISOPROTERENOL

Adults: When nebulized into face mask or mouthpiece, 3 ml to 5 ml q3h to q6h up to 4 times/day. Recommended dose is 4 ml qid.

Children: Use with caution in children 6 years old and younger. Age two to six years: 2 ml to 3 ml bid. Ages 7 to 14 years: 2 ml to 3 ml bid or tid.

NURSING IMPLICATIONS

HISTORY
See Appendix 4.

PHYSICAL ASSESSMENT
Check respiratory rate, type (abdominal thoracic); visually inspect sputum raised; look for intercostal retractions or bulges during respiratory cycle; identify factors that may impede chest movement during inspiration, expiration (*e.g.,* ankylosing spondylitis, kyphosis, scoliosis, ascites, malignancies); auscultate lungs.

ADMINISTRATION
The 20% solution may be diluted to a lesser concentration by adding normal saline or Water for Injection; the 10% solution may be used undiluted.

Use compressed air for nebulization.

Nebulization equipment with parts made of certain metals (notably copper and iron) or rubber may interact with the drug. Parts made of glass, plastic, aluminum, chromed metal, tantalum, sterling silver, or stainless steel may be used. Silver may become tarnished; this is not harmful to drug action or to the patient.

Read label carefully. Two products are available: acetylcysteine and acetylcysteine with isoproterenol.

Do *not* mix this drug with antibiotics, iodized oil, or hydrogen peroxide.

Have the patient cough to clear airway prior to treatment. Explain the disagreeable odor that may be noted early in treatment.

Storage: If only a portion is used, the remainder should be refrigerated and used within 96 hours to minimize contamination. Write expiration date on container.

ONGOING ASSESSMENTS AND NURSING MANAGEMENT
During administration: Place tissues and paper bag for disposal within patient's reach.

Observe sputum raised (amount, color, consistency); observe patient's ability to participate in and tolerate treatment.

CLINICAL ALERT: The elderly and those with a history of asthma should be observed closely. If bronchospasm should occur, discontinue treatment immediately and notify physician.

Check nebulizing solution and dilute if it becomes concentrated (see *Precautions*).

When drug is instilled into a tracheostomy or through a percutaneous catheter, have suction equipment available for aspiration of secretions.

Duration of treatment will vary with type of nebulizing equipment and the capabilities and respiratory status of the patient. Usual time is 15 to 30 minutes.

Following administration: Auscultate lungs. If patient is unable to cough and raise sputum, suctioning may be necessary. Use of suctioning procedure should be discussed with and approved by physician prior to treatment.

A sticky residue is often deposited on the face. Following treatment, wash the patient's face with mild soap and water. Thoroughly wash and dry all equipment after use.

Evaluate and record respiratory status between treatments.

When applicable, encourage the patient to abstain from smoking between treatments.

Use a team approach to formulate short- and long-term goals for respiratory rehabilitation.

Acrisorcin Rx

cream   Akrinol

INDICATIONS
Treatment of tinea versicolor, a superficial fungal infection caused by *Malassezia furfur*.

ACTIONS
Possesses antifungal and mild antibacterial activity.

PRECAUTIONS
Do not use around the eyes. If irritation or sensitization develops, discontinue treatment.

ADVERSE REACTIONS
A few topical reactions have been reported (*e.g.,* blisters, erythematous vesicular eruptions, hives). Pruritus has occurred after exposure to ultraviolet light. With eczema, a burning sensation may occur.

DOSAGE
Apply a small quantity to affected areas bid, in A.M. and H.S. The H.S. application should follow a warm soapy bath and use of a stiff brush on the lesions. All soap must be removed by thorough rinsing, followed by thorough drying with a towel before the cream is applied. Treatment should continue for at least 6 weeks.

NURSING IMPLICATIONS

HISTORY
See Appendix 4.

PHYSICAL ASSESSMENT
Inspect lesions; record size, color, location.

ADMINISTRATION
See *Dosage* (above).

ONGOING ASSESSMENTS AND NURSING MANAGEMENT
Inspect affected areas weekly; note any change in size and appearance of lesions and record findings.

A Wood's light may be used to identify the lesions and monitor therapeutic drug response.

Notify physician if topical reactions occur.

PATIENT AND FAMILY INFORMATION
Area may be washed with warm water and soap; rinse well and dry thoroughly before cream is applied.

Do not use around the eyes.

Avoid prolonged exposure to sunlight; photosensitivity (manifested by pruritus) may occur.

If condition worsens or if irritation, blisters, or hives develop, discontinue use and notify physician.

Acyclovir (Acycloguanosine) Rx

ointment: 5%   Zovirax
powder for injection: Zovirax
  500 mg/vial

INDICATIONS
Ointment: Management of initial herpes genitalis and limited non-life-threatening mucocutaneous herpes simplex virus infections in immunocompromised patients. Clinical trials of acyclovir for treatment of initial herpes genitalis have shown a decrease in healing time and, in some cases, a decrease in duration of viral shedding and duration of pain. In some studies of immunocompromised patients, mainly with herpes labialis, there was a decrease in duration of viral shedding and a slight decrease in duration of pain. By contrast, in studies of recurrent herpes genitalis and of herpes labialis in nonimmunocompromised patients, there was no evidence of clinical benefit. There was some decrease in the duration of viral shedding. Positive cultures for herpes simplex virus offer a reliable means of confirming the diagnosis.

Parenteral: Treatment of initial and recurrent mucosal and cutaneous herpes simplex virus types 1 and 2 (HSV-1 and HSV-2) infections in immunocompromised adults and children and of severe initial clinical episodes of herpes genitalis in patients who are nonimmunocompromised.

CONTRAINDICATIONS
Hypersensitivity.

ACTIONS
Ointment: A synthetic acyclic purine nucleoside analogue with activity against HSV-1, HSV-2, varicella-zoster, Epstein-Barr virus, and cytomegalovirus. In clinical studies, no local tolerance, systemic toxicity, or contact dermatitis was observed.

Parenteral: A synthetic acyclic purine nucleoside analogues with activity the same as that of ointment. It is widely distributed in tissues and body fluids including brain, kidney, lung, liver, muscle, spleen, uterus, vaginal mucosa, vaginal secretions, CSF, and herpetic vesicular fluid. Renal excretion of unchanged drug by glomerular filtration and tubular secretion is major route of elimination. The half-life and total body clearance are dependent on renal function. Half-life and total body clearance in pediatric patients over 1 yr of age are similar to those in adults with normal renal function.

WARNINGS
Ointment: For cutaneous use only; do not use in the eye. Use in pregnancy only if potential benefit justifies the potential risk to the fetus. It is not known whether the drug is excreted in human milk; exercise caution when administering to nursing women.

Parenteral: For IV infusion only. Administered over a period of at least 1 hour to prevent renal tubular damage. Use in pregnancy only if potential benefit justifies the potential risk to the fetus. It is not known whether drug is excreted in human milk. Exercise caution when administering to nursing women.

PRECAUTIONS
Ointment: Do not exceed recommended dosage, frequency of application, or length of treatment. There are no available data demonstrating that use will either prevent transmission of infection to other persons or prevent recurrent infections when applied in the absence of signs and symptoms. Although clinically significant viral resistance has not been observed, the possibility exists.

Parenteral: Do not exceed recommended dosage, frequency, or length of treatment. Dosage based on creatinine clearance. Precipitation of acyclovir crystals in renal tubules can occur if the maximum solubility of free acyclovir (2.5 mg/ml at 37°C in water) is exceeded or if drug is administered by bolus injection. This complication can cause a rise in serum creatinine and BUN and a decrease in renal creatinine clearance.

Bolus administration leads to a 10% incidence of renal dysfunction; infusion of 5 mg/kg over 1 hour is associated with a lower frequency. Concomitant use of other nephrotoxic drugs, preexisting renal disease, and dehydration make further renal impairment with acyclovir more likely. In most instances, alterations of renal function are transient and resolve spontaneously or with improvement of water and electrolyte balance, adjustments in drug dosage, or discontinuation of administration. In some instances these changes may progress to acute renal failure.

Administration by IV infusion must be accompanied by adequate hydration. Because maximum urine concentration occurs within the first 2 hours following infusion, sufficient urine flow must be established during that period to prevent precipitation in renal tubules.

Approximately 1% of patients receiving drug IV have manifested encephalopathic changes characterized by lethargy, obtundation, tremors, confusion, hallucinations, agitation, seizures, or coma. Use with caution in those with serious renal, hepatic, or electrolyte abnormalities or significant hypoxia and in those who have manifested poor neurologic reactions to cytotoxic drugs.

DRUG INTERACTIONS
Ointment: None known.

Parenteral: Use with caution in those receiving concomitant intrathecal administration of **methotrexate** or **interferon. Probenecid** may decrease the mean urinary excretion of acyclovir.

ADVERSE REACTIONS
Ointment: Because ulcerated genital lesions are characteristically tender and sensitive to any contact, patient may experience discomfort upon application.

Parenteral: Most frequent adverse reactions are inflammation or phlebitis at injection site following extravasation of IV fluid, transient elevations of serum creatinine, rash, or hives. Approximately 1% of patients have manifested encephalopathic changes (see *Precautions*). Elevated serum creatinine, usually following rapid (over fewer than 10 minutes) IV infusion, thrombocytosis, and jitters also have been reported.

OVERDOSAGE (PARENTERAL)
Symptoms: No acute massive overdosage reported. Precipitation of free acyclovir in renal tu-

bules may occur when solubility in the intratubular fluid is exceeded.

Treatment: Is dialyzable. In the event of acute renal failure and anuria, the patient may benefit from hemodialysis until renal function is restored.

DOSAGE

Initiate therapy as early as possible following onset of signs and symptoms.

Ointment: Apply sufficient quantity to cover all lesions adequately, q3h, 6 times/day, for 7 days. The dose size per application will vary depending on total lesion area, but should approximate a half-inch ribbon of ointment per 4 sq in of surface area.

Parenteral: Avoid rapid or bolus IV, IM, or SC injection.

HSV-1 and HSV-2 in immunocompromised patients: Adults—Infuse 5 mg/kg at a constant rate over 1 hour, q8h (15 mg/kg/day) for 7 days. *Children under 12*—Infuse 250 mg/m² at a constant rate over 1 hour q8h (750 mg/m²/day) for 7 days.

Severe initial clinical episodes of herpes genitalis: Same dose as above, but administer for 5 days.

Acute or chronic renal impairment: Reduce dosage or increase intervals between doses.

Hemodialysis: Administer dose after hemodialysis.

NURSING IMPLICATIONS

HISTORY

Determine (if possible) whether symptoms are initial or recurrent.

PHYSICAL ASSESSMENT

Examination of affected areas and culture of lesions are usually performed by physician. Renal function studies are usually ordered prior to parenteral administration. If infection is severe and has caused other complications, additional assessments will be necessary.

ADMINISTRATION

Ointment

Whenever possible, drug is applied by patient. Provide fingercots or disposable gloves for application to prevent autoinoculation of other body sites and transmission of infection to others; dispose of application materials in the same manner as for isolation technique.

If nurse applies drug, gloves should be worn on both hands; dispose of application materials in same manner as for isolation technique.

In order to protect patients and personnel, hospitals, clinics, and physicians' offices should establish guidelines for examination and treatment of persons known to have or suspected of having an HSV-2 infection.

Storage: 15°C–25°C (59°F–78°F) in a dry place.

Parenteral

Dissolve contents of vial in 10 ml Sterile Water for Injection yielding a final concentration of 50 mg/ml. Shake well to assure complete dissolution before measuring and transferring individual doses.

Remove and add the calculated dose to any appropriate IV solution at a volume selected for administration during each 1-hour infusion. Physician must specify type and volume of IV solution.

Infusion concentrations of approximately 7 mg/ml or lower are recommended. An average 70-kg (154-lb) adult usually requires approximately 60 ml of fluid (IV solution + drug) per dose.

Calculate the drops-per-minute infusion rate necessary to infuse solution at a constant rate over a period of at least 1 hour.

Storage: Once drug is in solution in the vial (*i.e.,* reconstituted) at concentration of 50 mg/ml, use within 12 hours. Once it is diluted for administration in an IV fluid, use within 24 hours. Refrigeration of reconstituted solutions may result in formation of a precipitate that will redissolve at room temperature. Store at 15°C–30°C (59°F–86°F).

ONGOING ASSESSMENTS AND NURSING MANAGEMENT

Parenteral administration must be accompanied by adequate hydration because maximum urine concentration occurs within the first 2 hours following infusion.

Measure intake and output and total q8h. Because infusion is given q8h, schedule 8-hour intake/output measurements to conclude prior to time of next infusion. Notify physician if urinary output decreases, hydration does not appear adequate, or urine appears concentrated.

Physician may establish guidelines for establishing adequate hydration (*e.g.,* push oral fluids, continuous IV therapy, and minimal 8-hour urinary output) necessary for administration of drug. If guidelines for establishing adequate hydration are unclear, request clarification.

Monitor infusion rate q5m to q10m, especially if patient is restless, because movement may increase or decrease rate of infusion. Adjust infusion rate as necessary to complete infusion in no less than 1 hour.

CLINICAL ALERT: Incidence of renal tubular damage is increased if solution is infused in less than 1 hour or given by IV bolus injection. Do not administer next dose if hydration appears inadequate or does not meet prescribed guidelines, and notify physician immediately.

Monitor vital signs q4h; observe for adverse drug reactions. Additional assessments may be necessary if infection is severe or has resulted in complications.

Inspect injection site for evidence of inflammation or phlebitis daily. If either of these should occur, IV should be discontinued and another site selected, preferably in the opposite arm.

If extravasation of drug should occur, discontinue IV infusion and select new site. Pain, inflammation, or phlebitis may occur. Notify physician of problem as soon as possible; treatment of problem (_e.g.,_ cold compresses followed by warm moist packs) may be necessary.

Physician may order renal-function studies during therapy.

PATIENT AND FAMILY INFORMATION

Ointment must be applied q3h, 6 times/day for 1 week. Thoroughly cover all lesions. Use a fingercot or disposable glove to apply in order to prevent spread of infection; these materials are available at most pharmacies.

Ointment may cause transient burning, itching, rash; notify physician or nuse if these become pronounced.

Keep ointment in a cool, dry place.

Albumin, Human, 5%, 25%

See Plasma Protein Fractions.

Albuterol Sulfate

See Bronchodilators and Decongestants, Systemic.

Allopurinol Rx

tablets: 100 mg, 300 mg   Lopurin, Zyloprim, _Generic_

INDICATIONS

Treatment of gout, either primary or secondary to the hyperuricemia associated with blood dyscrasias and their therapy. Treatment of uric-acid nephropathy, primary or secondary, with or without symptoms of gout. Treatment of recurrent uric-acid stone formation. Prophylactic treatment: to prevent tissue urate deposition, renal calculi, or uric-acid nephropathy in those with leukemias, lymphomas, and malignancies who are receiving cancer chemotherapy.

This is not an innocuous drug; use in other hyperuricemic states is contraindicated.

CONTRAINDICATIONS

Do not use in children except those with hyperuricemia secondary to malignancy. Do not use in nursing mothers. Patients who have developed a severe reaction should not be restarted on the drug.

ACTIONS

A potent inhibitor of xanthine oxidase, the enzyme responsible for the conversion of hypoxanthine or xanthine to uric acid. Allopurinol acts on purine catabolism, reducing the production of uric acid without disrupting biosynthesis of vital purines. Administration generally results in a fall in both serum and urinary uric acid within 2 to 3 days. The magnitude of this decrease is dose dependent. A week or more of treatment may be required for manifestation of full effects. Uric acid may return slowly to pretreatment levels following cessation of therapy.

Hyperuricemia may be primary, as in gout, or secondary to diseases such as acute and chronic leukemia, polycythemia vera, multiple myeloma, and psoriasis. It may occur with the use of diuretic agents, during renal dialysis, in the presence of renal damage, during starvation or reducing diets, and in the treatment of neoplastic diseases in which rapid resolution of tissue masses may occur. The major manifestations in gout (kidney stones, tophi in soft tissues, deposits in joints and bones) result from the deposit of urates. If progressive deposition of urates is to be arrested or reversed, it is necessary to reduce the serum uric acid to a level below the saturation point to suppress urate precipitation. Allopurinol avoids the hazard of hyperuricosuria in those with gouty nephropathy or a predisposition to form uric-acid stones.

WARNINGS

Discontinue at first sign of a skin rash or any other adverse reaction. In some instances, skin rash may be followed by more severe hypersensitivity reactions such as exfoliative, urticarial, or purpuric lesions, the Stevens-Johnson syndrome (erythema multiforme), and (very rarely) generalized vasculitis, which may lead to irreversible hepatotoxicity and death. A few cases of hepatotoxicity have been noted and asymptomatic rises in serum alkaline phosphatase or serum transaminase levels have been observed.

Usage in pregnancy: Use only when clearly needed and potential benefits outweigh the unknown hazards to the fetus.

PRECAUTIONS

An increase in acute attacks of gout during early stages of therapy have been reported. A fluid intake sufficient to yield a daily urinary output of at least 2 liters and the maintenance of neutral or slightly alkaline urine are desirable to avoid the theoretic possibility of xanthine calculi formation and to help prevent renal precipitation of urates in those receiving concomitant uricosuric agent (*e.g.,* probenecid, sulfinpyrazone). A mild reticulocytosis has appeared in some patients; the significance of this is not known.

Usage in impaired renal function: A few patients have shown an increased BUN; decreased BUN levels have also been seen. Those with impaired renal function require less of the drug and require careful observation during early stages of treatment; discontinue drug if increased abnormalities in renal function occur.

Periodic determination of liver and kidney function and complete blood counts are performed, especially during first few months of therapy.

DRUG INTERACTIONS

Do not give **iron salts** simultaneously with allopurinol; do not administer allopurinol to immediate relatives of patients with idiopathic hemochromatosis. In patients receiving **mercaptopurine** or **azathioprine,** concomitant administration of 300 mg to 600 mg of allopurinol daily requires dose reduction to approximately one-third to one-fourth the usual dose of mercaptopurine or azathioprine. The half-life of **anticoagulants** is prolonged; this interaction requires reassessment of the coagulation time. Allopurinol has been reported to increase serum levels of **theophylline.** Hypersensitivity may occur in those with renal compromise receiving allopurinol and **thiazides** concurrently.

ADVERSE REACTIONS

Dermatologic: Skin rash, which in some instances has been followed by severe hypersensitive reactions (see *Warnings*).

Drug idiosyncrasy: Reported in a few patients and characterized by one or more of the following: fever, chills, leukopenia, leukocytosis, eosinophilia, arthralgias, skin rash, pruritus, nausea, and vomiting.

GI: Nausea, vomiting, diarrhea, intermittent abdominal pain.

Hematopoietic: Agranulocytosis, anemia, aplastic anemia, bone-marrow depression, leukopenia, pancytopenia, and thrombocytopenia have been reported.

Neurologic: Peripheral neuritis, drowsiness.

Ophthalmic: There have been a few reports of cataracts.

Vascular: Rare instances of generalized hypersensitivity vasculitis or necrotizing angiitis have led to irreversible hepatotoxicity and death.

DOSAGE

Control of gout, hyperuricemia: Dosage varies with severity of disease. The average is 200 mg/day to 300 mg/day for those with mild gout and 400 mg/day to 600 mg/day for those with moderately severe tophaceous gout. Dosage in excess of 300 mg should be given in divided doses. Children (6 to 10 years) with secondary hyperuricemia associated with malignancy are given 300 mg/day. Those under 6 years are generally given 150 mg/day.

Prevention of uric-acid nephropathy during therapy of neoplastic disease: 600 mg/day to 800 mg/day for 2 to 3 days together with a high fluid intake. Minimum effective dose is 100 mg/day to 200 mg/day. Maximum recommended dose is 800 mg/day.

Reduction of possibility of flare-up of acute gouty attacks: Start with 100 mg/day; increase at weekly intervals by 100 mg until serum uric acid level of 6 mg/100 ml or less is attained.

Renal impairment: Dose should be reduced.

Concomitant therapy: In patients treated with colchicine or anti-inflammatory agents, continue therapy and adjust dosage of allopurinol until normal serum acid level and freedom from acute attacks have been maintained for several months.

Replacement therapy: In transferring from a uricosuric agent to allopurinol, the dose of the uricosuric agent should be reduced gradually over a period of several weeks and the dose of allopurinol increased to the dose needed to maintain a normal serum uric acid level.

NURSING IMPLICATIONS

HISTORY
See Appendix 4.

PHYSICAL ASSESSMENT
Gout: examine involved joints for pain, tenderness, swelling, inflammation, limitation of motion; note appearance of skin over joints; when applicable, evaluate ability to carry out activities of daily living. Baseline laboratory tests may include CBC, serum uric acid, and renal- and hepatic-function tests.

ADMINISTRATION

Give with food or meals or immediately after meals to minimize GI side-effects. Give with full glass of water. For acute attacks of gout, maintenance doses of colchicine (0.5 mg bid) may be given prophylactically during initial therapy with allopurinol.

ONGOING ASSESSMENTS AND NURSING MANAGEMENT

Evaluate and record therapeutic drug response; assess involved joints; ask patient to compare present symptoms with those experienced prior to therapy.

Measure intake and output.

Encourage and provide a liberal fluid intake so that daily output is at least 2 liters. Consult physician before instituting a plan to increase fluid intake because extra fluids may be contraindicated in certain disorders such as congestive heart failure or syndrome of inappropriate ADH secretion (SIADH), which may occur in some malignancies or when patient is receiving certain antineoplastic agents. In those having recurrent uric-acid stones or receiving prophylactic agents during therapy for neoplastic disease, observe for signs of uric-acid stone formation (*e.g.,* pain, hematuria, pyuria, fever, abdominal distention).

If drowsiness occurs, assist with ambulation.

Sodium bicarbonate or potassium citrate may be prescribed to keep urine alkaline and prevent urinary calculi. Physician may request periodic check of urine *p*H with Nitrazine paper.

Laboratory: Serum uric acid levels usually return to normal in 1 to 3 weeks; physician may order periodic evaluation of renal, hematopoietic, and liver function and serum uric acid levels.

CLINICAL ALERT: Withhold next dose of drug and notify physician immediately if skin rash or other dermatologic manifestations occur.

PATIENT AND FAMILY INFORMATION

If GI upset occurs, drug may be taken with food. Take each dose with a full glass of water. Drink at least 10 to 12 8-oz glasses of fluid daily.

May produce drowsiness; observe caution while driving or performing other tasks requiring alertness.

Notify physician or nurse immediately if skin rash occurs.

Avoid taking vitamin C unless use has been approved by physician, because urinary acidification may increase the possibility of kidney stones.

Do not take iron or vitamin preparations containing iron unless approved by physician.

Keep a record of increase or decrease in pain or other symptoms; bring record to each office visit or clinic apointment.

Gout pain may persist for several weeks into drug therapy.

Alphaprodine Hydrochloride

See Narcotic Analgesics.

Alprazolam

See Benzodiazepines.

Alseroxylon

See Rauwolfia Derivatives.

Aluminum Acetate Solution

See Wet Dressings and Soaks.

Aluminum Carbonate Gel, Basic

See Antacids.

Aluminum Hydroxide Gel

See Antacids.

Aluminum Phosphate Gel

See Antacids.

Amantadine Hydrochloride Rx

capsules: 100 mg	Symmetrel
syrup: 50 mg/5 ml	Symmetrel

INDICATIONS

Parkinson's disease/syndrome and drug-induced extrapyramidal reactions: Treatment of idiopathic

Parkinson's disease (paralysis agitans), postencephalitic parkinsonism, drug-induced extrapyramidal reactions, and symptomatic parkinsonism following injury to the nervous system by carbon-monoxide intoxication. Indicated in elderly patients believed to develop parkinsonism in association with arteriosclerosis. Less effective than levodopa in treatment of Parkinson's disease.

Influenza A virus respiratory tract illness: For prophylaxis and symptomatic management, especially for high-risk patients, close household or hospital contacts of index cases, and patients with severe influenza A virus. In prophylaxis, early immunization is method of choice. When this is not feasible, or when vaccine is contraindicated or not available, amantadine can be used for prophylaxis. Because it does not appear to suppress antibody response, amantadine can be used in conjunction with inactivated influenza A virus vaccine until protective antibody responses develop.

CONTRAINDICATIONS
Known hypersensitivity to drug.

ACTIONS
Mechanism of action in Parkinson's disease and drug-induced extrapyramidal reactions is not known. Antiviral activity against influenza A virus is not completely understood but the mode of action appears to be prevention of release of infectious viral nucleic acid into the host cell. Amantadine is well absorbed after oral administration and readily crosses the blood–brain barrier. It passes the placental barrier and is excreted in breast milk. The drug may accumulate in those with impaired renal function.

WARNINGS
Those with epilepsy or other seizure disorders should be observed closely for possible increased seizure activity. Patients with a history of congestive heart failure or peripheral edema should be followed closely; patients have developed congestive heart failure while receiving amantadine.

Patients with Parkinson's disease improving on amantadine should resume normal activities gradually and cautiously, consistent with other medical considerations such as presence of osteoporosis or phlebothrombosis.

Usage in pregnancy and lactation: Use only when clearly needed and when potential benefits outweigh the unknown potential hazards to the fetus. Drug is excreted in breast milk; do not administer to nursing mothers.

DRUG INTERACTIONS
The dose of **anticholinergic drugs** or of amantadine should be reduced if atropinelike effects (pp 503–504) appear when the drugs are used concurrently. Careful observation is required when administered concurrently with **CNS stimulants.**

PRECAUTIONS
May cause blurring of vision or CNS effects.

Do not discontinue abruptly; patients with Parkinson's disease may experience a parkinsonian crisis (*i.e.,* sudden, marked clinical deterioration) when drug is suddenly stopped.

Dose may need careful adjustment in those with renal impairment, congestive heart failure, peripheral edema, or orthostatic hypotension.

Exercise care when administering to patients with liver disease, a history of recurrent eczemoid rash, or psychosis or severe psychoneurosis not controlled by chemotherapeutic agents.

ADVERSE REACTIONS
Most frequent serious reactions: Depression, congestive heart failure, orthostatic hypotensive episodes, psychosis, urinary retention, convulsions, leukopenia, neutropenia.

Less serious reactions: Hallucinations, confusion, anxiety, irritability, anorexia, nausea, constipation, ataxia, dizziness, livedo reticularis, peripheral edema.

Less frequent reactions: Vomiting, dry mouth, headache, dyspnea, fatigue, insomnia, sense of weakness.

Infrequent reactions: Skin rash, slurred speech, visual disturbances.

Rare reactions: Eczemoid dermatitis, oculogyric episodes; reversible loss of vision has been reported.

OVERDOSAGE
Symptoms: Nausea; vomiting; anorexia; CNS effects including hyperexcitability, tremors, ataxia, blurred vision, lethargy, depression, slurred speech, convulsions. CNS symptoms occur because of drug's ability to increase dopamine concentration in the brain.

Treatment: No specific antidote. Employ general supportive measures along with immediate gastric lavage or induction of emesis. Force fluids; if necessary give fluids IV. Physostigmine salicylate has been found to be of benefit in controlling neurologic manifestations. Urinary acidification may increase elimination from the body. Monitor blood pressure, pulse, respiration, temperature. Administer sedatives and anticonvulsants if required. Give appropriate antiarrhythmic and antihypotensive therapy should symptoms warrant. Monitor electrolytes, urine *p*H, urinary output. If there is no record of recent voiding, catheterize patient.

DOSAGE

Parkinsonism: Usual dose is 100 mg bid when used alone. Onset of action is usually within 48 hours. Initial dose is 100 mg/day for those with serious associated medical illness or those who are receiving high doses of other antiparkinsonian drugs. After 1 to several weeks at 100 mg/day, dose may be increased to 100 mg bid if necessary. If responses are not optimal at 200 mg/day, patient may benefit from a dosage increase up to a total dose of 400 mg/day in divided doses; supervise such patients closely. Patients initially deriving benefit may experience a fall-off of effectiveness after a few months. Benefit may be regained by increasing dose to 300 mg/day or by temporary discontinuation for several weeks followed by reinitiation of therapy. Other antiparkinsonian drugs may be necessary.

Concomitant therapy: Amantadine may be given with anticholinergic antiparkinsonian drugs. When amantadine and levodopa are initiated concurrently, there can be rapid therapeutic benefits. Hold constantly at 100 mg daily or bid while daily dose of levodopa is gradually increased to optimal benefit.

Drug-induced extrapyramidal reactions: Usual dose is 100 mg bid. If responses are not optimal, patient may benefit from 300 mg/day in divided doses.

Prophylaxis and symptomatic management of influenza A virus illness

Start drug in anticipation of contact or as soon as possible after contact with individuals with the illness. Continue daily for 10 days following known exposure. If used in conjunction with vaccine, give for 2 to 3 weeks after vaccine has been administered. When vaccine is contraindicated or unavailable, administer for up to 90 days.

Adults: 200 mg/day as single dose or 100 mg bid. If CNS effects develop on once-a-day dose, divided doses may be necessary.

Children: *1 to 9 years*—2 mg/lb/day to 4 mg/lb/day (not to exceed 150 mg/day) in 2 or 3 divided doses (as syrup); *9 to 12 years*—100 mg bid.

NURSING IMPLICATIONS

HISTORY
See Appendix 4.

PHYSICAL ASSESSMENT
Parkinson's disease/syndrome: Neurologic assessment of parkinsonism plus current diseases/ disorders identified during health history; evaluation of abilities or limitations in carrying out activities of daily living (ADL); when applicable, evaluate mental status; vital signs.

Drug-induced extrapyramidal symptoms: Identify and describe symptoms; determine whether symptoms interfere with ADL; when applicable, evaluate mental status; vital signs.

Influenza A virus illness: Base on type of illness (respiratory, cardiac), type and severity of complications; vital signs.

ADMINISTRATION
If patient with parkinsonism or drug-induced extrapyramidal reactions has difficulty swallowing capsule, check with physician about change to syrup.

If tremors are severe, assist in holding capsule or container with syrup and in holding water glass.

ONGOING ASSESSMENTS AND NURSING MANAGEMENT
Record vital signs (frequency depends on diagnosis, severity of disorder); evaluate mental status (see *Adverse Reactions*); evaluate drug response by comparing present data with data base; observe for adverse drug reactions.

CLINICAL ALERTS: Mental changes, especially depression, confusion, anxiety, and hallucinations, require notifying physician immediately along with *frequent* observation of patient's behavior. Nursing intervention will depend on the potential or actual dangers associated with these changes.

When administered for parkinsonism, drug must not be suddenly discontinued (see *Precautions*). Ensure continuity of therapy: inform all nursing personnel of therapeutic regimen; identify importance of continuity on Kardex and during team reports and conferences.

Orthostatic hypotension may occur. Caution patient to rise slowly from a sitting or lying position and to dangle legs for 5 to 10 minutes before getting out of bed. Assist with ambulation when necessary. Instruct patient to lie down immediately if lightheadedness or dizziness occurs.

Plan rehabilitation of those with parkinsonism using a team approach; revise short- and long-term goals according to drug response.

Anticholinergic side-effects: Dry mouth may be relieved by sips of cold water, ice chips, hard candy; if patient is elderly or urinary retention is suspected, measure intake and output. If visual disturbance occurs, patient may need assistance with ambulation, ADL.

Severe influenza A virus illness: Management based on needs and problems associated with the disease and its complications.

PATIENT AND FAMILY INFORMATION

Medication may impair ability to drive or perform other tasks requiring alertness.

If dizziness or lightheadedness (orthostatic hypotension) occurs, avoid sudden changes in position; notify physician or nurse of this problem.

Notify physician or nurse of mood or mental changes, swelling in the extremities, difficult urination, shortness of breath, failure of drug to relieve symptoms.

Do not discontinue drug or omit prescribed dose except on advice of physician.

If insomnia occurs, take last dose immediately after evening meal.

Do not use nonprescription drugs (especially cold remedies) without first checking with physician.

Ambenonium Chloride

See Muscle Stimulants, Anticholinesterase.

Amcinonide

See Corticosteroids, Topical.

Amikacin Sulfate

See Aminoglycosides, Parenteral.

Amiloride Hydrochloride   Rx

tablets: 5 mg   Midamor
tablets: 5 mg with 50   Moduretic
   mg hydrochloro-
   thiazide

INDICATIONS

Adjunctive treatment with thiazide diuretics or other kaliuretic–diuretic agents in patients with congestive heart failure or hypertension to help restore normal serum potassium levels in those developing hypokalemia on the kaliuretic–diuretic and to prevent hypokalemia in those at risk if hypokalemia were to develop (*e.g.,* digitalized patients or patients with significant cardiac arrhythmias). It is rarely used alone.

CONTRAINDICATIONS

Hypersensitivity to amiloride; presence of elevated serum potassium levels (>5.5 mEq/liter); those receiving other potassium-conserving drugs (triamterene, spironolactone); anuria; acute or chronic renal insufficiency; evidence of diabetic nephropathy.

ACTIONS

A potassium-conserving (antikaliuretic) drug possessing weak (compared with thiazide diuretics) natriuretic, diuretic, and antihypertensive activity. Amiloride has potassium-conserving ability in those receiving kaliuretic–diuretic agents. It is not an aldosterone antagonist.

Amiloride begins to act within 2 hours with a peak effect on electrolyte excretion between 6 and 10 hours; drug effects last about 24 hours. It is excreted unchanged by the kidneys and has little effect on the glomerular filtration rate or renal blood flow. It is not metabolized by the liver, and drug accumulation is not anticipated in those with hepatic dysfunction; however, accumulation can occur if the hepatorenal syndrome develops.

WARNINGS

Hyperkalemia: Serum levels above 5.5 mEq/liter, if uncorrected, may be potentially fatal. It is essential to monitor serum potassium levels, particularly when drug is first introduced at the time of diuretic dosage adjustments and during any illness affecting renal function.

Treatment of hyperkalemia: Discontinue drug immediately. If serum potassium level exceeds 6.5 mEq/liter, active measures must be taken to reduce it (*e.g.,* IV sodium bicarbonate, oral or parenteral glucose with a rapid-acting insulin preparation). If needed, a cation exchange resin (*e.g.,* sodium polystyrene sulfonate) may be given orally or by enema. Persistent hyperkalemia may require dialysis.

Potassium supplementation, in the form of medication or a potassium-rich diet, should not be used except in severe or refractory hypokalemia.

Diabetes mellitus: Use of amiloride is usually avoided in diabetic patients. If amiloride is used, monitor serum electrolytes and renal function closely.

Metabolic or respiratory acidosis: Cautiously institute therapy in severely ill patients in whom this may occur, such as those with cardiopulmonary disease and poorly controlled diabetes. If drug is given, frequently monitor acid–base balance because shifts alter the ratio of extracellular–intracellular potassium and the development of acidosis may cause a rapid increase in serum potassium levels.

Use in pregnancy: Safety not established; use only when clearly needed and potential benefits outweigh the unknown potential hazards to the fetus.

Use in children: Safety, efficacy not established.

PRECAUTIONS

Hyponatremia and hypochloremia may occur when amiloride is used with other diuretics. Increases in BUN levels have been reported and usually accompany vigorous fluid elimination, especially in seriously ill patients such as those with hepatic cirrhosis with ascites, metabolic acidosis, or resistant edema. Carefully monitor electrolytes and BUN levels when drug is given with other diuretics to these patients. In patients with preexisting severe liver disease, hepatic encephalopathy manifested by tremors, confusion, coma, and increased jaundice has been reported.

DRUG INTERACTIONS

Do not give **lithium** with diuretics because they reduce its renal clearance and add risk of lithium toxicity. Concomitant use of potassium-sparing agents (*e.g.*, **triamterene, spironolactone**) or **potassium supplements** can lead to hyperkalemia.

ADVERSE REACTIONS

Incidence greater than 1%:

CNS: Headache, dizziness, encephalopathy.

GI: Nausea, anorexia, diarrhea, vomiting, abdominal pain, gas, appetite changes, constipation.

Metabolic: Elevated serum potassium levels (>5.5 mEq/liter).

Musculoskeletal: Weakness, fatigability, muscle cramps.

Respiratory: Cough, dyspnea.

GU: Impotence.

Incidence less than 1%:

Angina; orthostatic hypotension; arrhythmia; palpitation; jaundice; GI bleeding; abdominal fullness; thirst; heartburn; dyspepsia; rash; dry mouth; pruritus; alopecia; joint pain; leg ache; back pain, neck/shoulder ache; pain of the extremities; paresthesias; tremors; vertigo; nervousness; mental confusion; insomnia; decreased libido; somnolence; visual disturbances; nasal congestion; increased intraocular pressure; polyuria; dysuria; urinary frequency; bladder spasms.

Causal relationship unknown: Activation of probable preexisting peptic ulcer, aplastic anemia, neutropenia, abnormal liver-function tests.

OVERDOSAGE

Symptoms: No data available; most likely signs are dehydration, electrolyte imbalance.

Treatment: No specific antidote; discontinue therapy and observe closely. Induce emesis or perform gastric lavage. Treatment is symptomatic and supportive. If hyperkalemia occurs, reduce serum potassium levels. It is not known whether amiloride is dialyzable.

DOSAGE

Concomitant therapy: Add amiloride 5 mg/day to usual antihypertensive or kaliuretic–diuretic dosage. Increase to 10 mg/day if necessary; more than 10 mg/day is usually not needed. If hypokalemia persists, dose can be increased to 15 mg, then 20 mg with careful monitoring of electrolytes. In treating patients with congestive heart failure, potassium loss may decrease after initial diuresis has been achieved; the need for amiloride should be reevaluated. Maintenance therapy may be on an intermittent basis.

Single drug therapy: Starting dose, 5 mg/day, if necessary increased to 10 mg/day. If persistent hypokalemia is documented, dose may be increased to 15 mg, then 20 mg, with careful monitoring of electrolytes.

Amiloride with hydrochlorothiazide: 1 to 2 tablets/day with meals.

NURSING IMPLICATIONS

HISTORY

See Appendix 4.

PHYSICAL ASSESSMENT

Monitor blood pressure with patient standing, sitting, and lying down (have patient rest 20–30 minutes before taking BP), pulse, respirations, weight; examine extremities for edema; look for symptoms of congestive heart failure (when applicable). Baseline laboratory/diagnostic tests may include serum electrolytes, renal and hepatic function tests, ECG.

ADMINISTRATION

Give immediately with or after meals or with food if drug and meal schedule are different.

ONGOING ASSESSMENTS AND NURSING MANAGEMENT

Daily, resting blood pressure (use same position and arm each time), pulse, respiratory rate; weigh at same time each day with approximately same clothing; record intake and output; evaluate clinical status if congestive heart failure is present by checking areas of edema, auscultating lungs; evaluate dietary intake (normal food intake is desirable); look for signs of hyperkalemia (see Appendix 6, section 6-15) and other adverse drug reactions.

Monitor serum electrolytes and other laboratory tests.

CLINICAL ALERT: Withhold next dose of drug and notify physician immediately if signs of hyperkalemia are apparent or serum potassium level exceeds normal range values.

When used with other diuretics, hyponatremia (see Appendix 6, section 6-17) and hypochloremia may occur; add observations for these imbalances to daily assessments.

Provide patient on bedrest with call light and, if necessary, a bedpan or urinal.

Have patient rise slowly from a sitting or lying position and dangle legs 5 to 10 minutes before getting out of bed. Ambulatory patients may require assistance, especially early in therapy.

Report excessive vomiting (due to any cause) to physician immediately because serum electrolyte determinations may be necessary.

Bring nausea or prolonged anorexia to the attention of the physician.

Diet adjustments (deletion of potassium-rich foods) may be necessary if serum potassium levels are elevated or in the high-normal range.

See Thiazide Diuretics if combination of amiloride and hydrochlorothiazide (Moduretic) or concomitant thiazide therapy is prescribed.

PATIENT AND FAMILY INFORMATION

Frequent urination may occur and diuresis will most probably begin in about 2 hours.

May cause GI upset; take with food or meals.

Notify physician or nurse if any of the following occurs: muscular weakness or cramps, fatigue, generalized weakness.

May cause dizziness, headache, visual disturbances; observe caution while driving or performing tasks requiring alertness.

Avoid large quantities of potassium-rich foods (*e.g.,* tea, coffee, bananas, chocolate, bran).

Aminocaproic Acid Rx

tablets: 500 mg	Amicar
solution for injection: 250 mg/ml	Amicar, *Generic*
syrup: 250 mg/ml	Amicar

INDICATIONS

Treatment of excessive bleeding that results from systemic hyperfibrinolysis and urinary fibrinolysis.

In life-threatening situations, fresh whole blood transfusions, fibrinogen infusions, and other emergency measures may be required.

Investigational use: Oral or IV aminocaproic acid, 36 g/day in 6 divided doses, has been used to prevent recurrence of subarachnoid hemorrhage. In the management of amegakaryocytic thrombocytopenia, the need for platelet transfusion may be decreased by administration of aminocaproic acid, 8 g/day to 24 g/day, for 3 days to 13 months.

CONTRAINDICATIONS

Evidence of active intravascular clotting process.

Disseminated intravascular coagulation (DIC): It is important to differentiate between hyperfibrinolysis and DIC, because this drug administered to a patient with DIC may produce potentially fatal thrombus formation. Criteria that may be useful to characterize hyperfibrinolysis include platelet count (normal), protamine paracoagulation (negative), and euglobulin clot lysis (reduced). Do not use drug in presence of DIC without concomitant heparin. Use should be accompanied by tests to determine amount of fibrinolysis present.

ACTIONS

Inhibits fibrinolysis via inhibition of plasminogen activator substances and, to a lesser degree, through antiplasmin activity. Drug is rapidly absorbed following oral administration; peak plasma levels occur in 2 hours. A single IV dose has a duration of under 3 hours. After prolonged administration, it distributes throughout both the extravascular and intravascular compartments and readily penetrates red blood cells and other tissue cells.

WARNINGS

Safety for use in pregnancy is not established. Use only when clearly needed and potential benefits outweigh unknown potential hazards to the fetus. In patients with upper urinary-tract bleeding, administration has been known to cause intrarenal obstruction in the form of glomerular capillary thrombosis or clots in the renal pelvis and ureters.

PRECAUTIONS

Hyperfibrinolysis: Do not administer without definite diagnosis or laboratory findings.

Use in cardiac, hepatic, renal disease: Use when the benefit outweighs the hazard. Avoid rapid IV administration because this may induce hypotension, bradycardia, or arrhythmia.

Clotting: Inhibition of fibrinolysis may theoretically result in clotting or thrombosis.

DRUG INTERACTIONS
An increase in clotting factors, leading to a hyper-coagulable state, may be produced by concomitant administration of **oral contraceptives** or **estrogens.**

Drug/lab tests: Serum potassium may be elevated, especially in impaired renal function.

ADVERSE REACTIONS
GI: Nausea, cramps, diarrhea.

Cardiovascular: Hypotension.

Muscular: Malaise. Myopathy characterized by symptomatic weakness, fatique, elevated CPK, serum aldolase and SGOT, and in some cases acute rhabdomyolysis with myoglobinuria and renal failure reported.

CNS: Dizziness; tinnitus; headache; delirium; auditory, visual, and kinesthetic hallucinations; psychotic reactions; weakness, dizziness, and headache preceding a grand mal seizure. A definite association between the seizures and the drug has not been established.

Miscellaneous: Conjunctival effusion; nasal congestion; skin rash; reversible acute renal failure; thrombophlebitis; prolongation of menstruation, in some cases with cramping.

DOSAGE
An initial dose of 5 g PO or IV, followed by 1 g/hour to 1.25 g/hour thereafter, should achieve and sustain drug plasma levels at 0.13 mg/ml; this is the concentration apparently necessary for inhibition of systemic fibrinolysis. Administration of more than 30 g/24 hours is not recommended.

IV: Administer by infusion. Administer 4 g to 5 g by infusion during the first hour, followed by a continuing infusion at the rate of 1 g/hour. Rapid IV injection of undiluted drug into a vein is not recommended, because hypotension, bradycardia, or arrhythmias may result. For treatment of acute bleeding syndromes, administer 4 g to 5 g in 250 ml of diluent by infusion during the first hour of treatment, followed by continuous infusion at a rate of 1 g/hour in 50 ml of diluent. Continue for 8 hours or until bleeding is controlled.

Oral: If patient is able to take oral medication, an identical dosage regimen may be followed.

NURSING IMPLICATIONS

HISTORY
See Appendix 4.

PHYSICAL ASSESSMENT
Depends on cause of hyperfibrinolysis (*e.g.,* open heart surgery, abruptio placentae, profound hem-orrhagic shock, hematologic disorders, cirrhosis, prostatectomy, neoplastic disorders). If an emergency exists, obtain blood pressure, pulse, and respirations and determine needs that have the highest priority; document any visible blood loss. *Nonemergency:* record vital signs; determine immediate needs and evaluate present signs and symptoms.

ADMINISTRATION
Initial dose is 5 g (10 tablets or 20 ml of syrup), followed by hourly administration. Provide ample water and time for taking large number of tablets. If there is difficulty swallowing tablets, contact physician because the liquid form may be necessary.

IV: Use Sterile Water for Injection, normal saline, 5% dextrose, Ringer's solution to dilute solution for injection.

Physician must specify infusion rate for first hour as well as continuing infusion rate.

Solution for injection is available in 20-ml vials and provides 5 g per vial.

An infusion pump may be used to ensure consistent delivery of the drug.

ONGOING ASSESSMENTS AND NURSING MANAGEMENT DURING ADMINISTRATION
Monitor rate of infusion and check needle site for signs of extravasation q10m to q15m.

Monitor BP, P, R q½h (more frequent determinations may be necessary if condition warrants); immediately notify physician of any change in vital signs.

Measure intake and output q1h or as ordered; notify physician immediately if a decrease in urinary output occurs.

Assess overt bleeding (when present) q15m to q30m. Keep physician informed of apparent response or lack of response to treatment.

Observe closely for thromboembolitic episodes (*e.g.,* chest or leg pain, dyspnea, blood-tinged sputum, hypotension) and notify physician immediately if symptoms are apparent.

Aminoglutethimide Rx

tablets: 250 mg   Cytadren

INDICATIONS
Suppression of adrenal function in selected patients with Cushing's syndrome.

Unlabeled uses: Has been used successfully in postmenopausal patients with advanced breast carcinoma and in patients with metastatic prostatic carcinoma.

CONTRAINDICATIONS
Hypersensitivity to glutethimide or aminoglutethimide.

ACTIONS
Inhibits enzymatic conversion of cholesterol to pregnenolone, thus reducing the synthesis of adrenal glucocorticoids, mineralocorticoids, and other steroids. The major portion is excreted unchanged in the urine within 24 hours. Because aminoglutethimide does not affect the underlying disease process, it has been used primarily during clinical investigations either as an interim measure until more definitive therapy such as surgery can be undertaken, or in cases in which such therapy is not appropriate.

WARNINGS
Cortical hypofunction: May occur especially under conditions of stress such as surgery, trauma, acute illness. Patient is monitored carefully and hydrocortisone and mineralocorticoid supplements given as needed.

Hypotension: May suppress aldosterone production and cause orthostatic or persistent hypotension.

Use in pregnancy: Can cause fetal harm; if drug must be taken during pregnancy or if patient becomes pregnant while taking drug, she should be apprised of the potential hazard to the fetus.

Use in children: Safety and efficacy not established.

PRECAUTIONS
Laboratory tests: Hypothyroidism may occur. Make appropriate clinical observations; thyroid-function studies may be necessary. Supplementary thyroid hormone may be required. Hematologic abnormalities have been reported; baseline hematologic studies should be followed by periodic hematologic checks. Elevation in SGOT, alkaline phosphatase, bilirubin have been reported. Tests of these levels, as well as of serum electrolytes, should be checked before and during therapy.

DRUG INTERACTIONS
Aminoglutethimide accelerates the metabolism of **dexamethasone.** If glucocorticoid replacement is needed, hydrocortisone should be prescribed.

ADVERSE REACTIONS
Untoward effects have been reported in 2 out of 3 patients treated solely with aminoglutethimide for 4 or more weeks. Most frequent effects are drowsiness, morbilliform rash, nausea, and anorexia.

These are reversible and often disappear within 1 to 2 weeks of continued therapy.

Hematologic abnormalities: Rare, but some have been reported.

Endocrine: Adrenal insufficiency has been reported during 4 or more weeks of therapy. Hypothyroidism, occasionally associated with thyroid enlargement, masculinization, and hirsutism in females and precocious sex development in males, has occurred.

CNS: Headache and dizziness, possibly caused by lowered vascular resistance or orthostasis.

Cardiovascular: Hypotension (occasionally orthostatic), tachycardia.

GI, hepatic: Vomiting, isolated instances of abnormal hepatic-function tests, hepatotoxicity (rare).

Dermatologic: Rash, pruritus, rarely urticaria.

Miscellaneous: Fever, myalgia.

OVERDOSAGE
Symptoms: Intentional overdosage has caused ataxia, sedation, deep coma with hypoventilation and hypotension. Extreme weakness has been reported with divided doses of 3 g/day. No deaths have been reported following doses estimated as high as 7 g.

Treatment: Gastric lavage, supportive treatment. Dialysis may be considered in severe intoxication. A parenteral glucocorticoid, preferably hydrocortisone, and/or a mineralocorticoid such as fludrocortisone, may be used in extreme adrenocortical hypofunction.

DOSAGE
Institute in hospital until stable dosage regimen is achieved. Administer 250 mg qid, preferably q6h. Response is monitored by measuring plasma cortisol. If cortisol suppression is inadequate, dosage may be increased in increments of 250 mg daily at 1- to 2-week intervals, to a total daily dose of 2 g.

Dose reduction or temporary discontinuation may be required in the event of adverse reactions (*e.g.,* extreme drowsiness, severe skin rash, excessively low cortisol levels). If rash persists for more than 5 to 8 days or becomes severe, discontinue drug. It may be possible to reinstate therapy at a lower dosage after rash disappears. If glucocorticoid replacement therapy is needed, 20 mg to 30 mg of hydrocortisone orally in the morning will replace endogenous secretion.

NURSING IMPLICATIONS

HISTORY
See Appendix 4.

PHYSICAL ASSESSMENT

Look for overt signs of Cushing's syndrome; vital signs; weight; evaluate mental status (Cushing's syndrome may produce emotional lability).

ADMINISTRATION

See *Dosage* above.

ONGOING ASSESSMENTS AND NURSING MANAGEMENT

Monitor blood pressure, pulse, and respirations q4h or as ordered; monitor temperature, weight; observe for adverse drug reactions; monitor dietary intake and report anorexia to physician; check for skin rash during morning care and report occurrence to physician.

Instruct patient to rise slowly from a sitting or lying position to minimize orthostatic hypotension. If orthostatic hypotension does occur, have patient dangle legs 5 to 10 minutes before getting out of bed and have him immediately lie down should weakness or dizziness occur.

Monitor laboratory studies during therapy; bring abnormal values to attention of physician.

Observe frequently (q½h–q1h) during periods of stress (surgery, trauma, acute illness); look for signs of cortical hypofunction (see adrenal insufficiency, Appendix 6, section 6-3); report evidence of adrenal insufficiency to physician immediately because hydrocortisone and mineralocorticoid replacement may be necessary.

PATIENT AND FAMILY INFORMATION

May produce drowsiness, dizziness; observe caution while driving or performing other tasks requiring alertness.

May cause rash, fainting, weakness, headache; notify physician or nurse if any of these becomes pronounced.

Nausea and loss of appetite may occur during first 2 weeks of therapy; notify physician or nurse if these become pronounced.

Aminoglycosides, Oral

Kanamycin Sulfate Rx

capsules: 500 mg   Kantrex

Neomycin Sulfate Rx

tablets: 500 mg   Mycifradin Sulfate, Neobiotic, *Generic*

oral solution: 125 mg/5 ml   Mycifradin Sulfate

Paromomycin Sulfate Rx

capsules: 250 mg   Humatin

INDICATIONS

KANAMYCIN SULFATE

Suppression of intestinal bacteria: When suppression of normal bacterial flora of the bowel is desirable for short-term adjunctive therapy.

Hepatic coma: Prolonged administration is effective adjunctive therapy because of the reduction of ammonia-forming bacteria in the intestine. This reduction results in neurologic improvement.

NEOMYCIN SULFATE

Preoperative suppression of intestinal bacteria: When suppression of normal bacterial flora is desirable for either short- or long-term adjunctive therapy.

Hepatic coma: Prolonged administration has shown to be effective adjunctive therapy by reduction of ammonia-forming bacteria in the intestine. Subsequent reduction in blood ammonia results in neurologic improvement.

Diarrhea due to enteropathic Escherichia coli: May be effectively treated with neomycin sulfate. When occurring in epidemic form, all patients and carriers should be treated concurrently.

PAROMOMYCIN SULFATE

Intestinal amebiasis (acute, chronic): Not effective in extraintestinal amebiasis.

Hepatic coma: Prolonged administration shown to be effective adjunctive therapy by reducing ammonia-forming bacteria in the intestine. Subsequent reduction in blood ammonia results in neurologic improvement.

CONTRAINDICATIONS

Intestinal obstruction; hypersensitivity to aminoglycosides.

ACTIONS

Oral aminoglycosides are not significantly absorbed and are used for suppression of GI bacterial flora. The small absorbed fraction is rapidly excreted with normal kidney function; the unabsorbed drug is eliminated unchanged in the feces. In rare instances, it is possible that systemic toxicity may result from unintended absorption. Growth of most intestinal bacteria is rapidly suppressed, with suppression persisting for 48 to 72 hours. Nonpathogenic yeasts and occasionally resistant strains of *Enterobacter aerogenes* replace intestinal bacteria. See also Aminoglycosides, Parenteral.

WARNINGS

Although negligible amounts are absorbed through intact mucosa, the possibility of increased absorption from ulcerated or denuded areas should be considered. In renal dysfunction, this could lead to accumulation and toxicity. Because of reported cases of deafness following oral use and the potential nephrotoxic effects, patients should be under close clinical supervision. Urine and blood examinations and audiometric tests should be performed before and during extended therapy, especially in those with hepatic or renal disease, to avoid nephrotoxicity and eighth-cranial-nerve damage from improper dosage. If renal insufficiency develops, reduce dosage or discontinue drug.

Use in pregnancy: Safety not established; use only when clearly needed and potential benefits outweigh potential hazards.

PRECAUTIONS

Use of antibiotics (especially prolonged or repeated therapy) may result in bacterial or fungal overgrowth of nonsusceptible organisms. Such overgrowth may lead to a secondary infection (superinfection).

DRUG INTERACTIONS

Concomitant use of **penicillin V potassium** and neomycin therapy should be avoided, because malabsorption of penicillin V potassium has been reported. Use caution in concurrent use of **other ototoxic** or **nephrotoxic antimicrobial agents.**

Decreased therapeutic effect of **digitalis glycosides** due to inhibition of absorption may occur with concurrent use of neomycin. Spacing doses between the two drugs may not be sufficient. Addition or withdrawal of oral neomycin in patients stabilized on **digoxin** may result in fluctuations in serum digoxin concentration.

Oral aminoglycosides may increase the effects of **oral anticoagulants** by causing malabsorption of vitamin K. It may be necessary to reduce the anticoagulant dose.

Neomycin and paromomycin may decrease the absorption of oral **methotrexate,** whereas kanamycin may have the opposite effect.

Avoid concurrent use of **potent diuretics** such as ethacrynic acid, furosemide, urea, and mannitol (particularly when they are given IV) because they may cause cumulative adverse effects on the kidney and auditory nerve.

ADVERSE REACTIONS

Nausea, vomiting, and diarrhea are most common reactions. The malabsorption syndrome characterized by increased fecal fat, decreased serum carotene, and a fall in xylose absorption has been reported with prolonged therapy. *Clostridium difficile*-associated colitis has been reported following prolonged, high-dose therapy in hepatic coma.

DOSAGE

KANAMYCIN SULFATE

Suppression of intestinal bacteria: As adjunct to mechanical cleansing of large bowel in short-term therapy—1.0 g hourly for 4 hours, followed by 1.0 g q6h for 36 to 72 hours.

Hepatic coma: 8 g/day to 12 g/day in divided doses.

NEOMYCIN SULFATE

Preoperative preparation in abdominal surgery: Used in conjunction with a low-residue diet and a cathartic for 24 hours and should not extend beyond 72 hours. *Regimen for 2- to 3-day preparation for children and adults:* Total daily dose calculated on basis of 40 mg/lb (88 mg/kg) and administered in 6 equally divided doses (1 dose q4h). First dose is given immediately after a saline cathartic. *Regimen for 24-hour preparation in adults:* 1 g q1h for 4 doses, followed by 1 g q4h for balance of 24 hours (*i.e.,* 5 doses).

Hepatic coma: Withdraw protein from diet; avoid use of diuretics. Use supportive therapy, including transfusions, as indicated. Give drug in doses of 4 g/day to 12 g/day in divided doses. In children, 50 mg/kg/day to 100 mg/kg/day in divided doses. Continue treatment for 5 to 6 days, during which time protein should be returned incrementally to the diet. Chronic hepatic insufficiency may require doses up to 4 g/day over an indefinite period.

Infectious diarrhea: May be administered to infants and children in doses of 50 mg/kg/day for 2 to 3 days in divided doses. In adults, a dose of 3 g/day is usually sufficient to obtain benefit in responsive cases.

PAROMOMYCIN SULFATE

Intestinal amebiasis: For adults and children, usual dose is 25 mg/kg/day to 35 mg/kg/day in 3 doses with meals, for 5 to 10 days.

Hepatic coma: For adults, usual dose is 4 g/day in divided doses given at regular intervals for 5 to 6 days.

NURSING IMPLICATIONS

HISTORY

Suppression of intestinal bacteria: Review chart for type of surgery, preoperative orders.

Hepatic coma: Review chart for current medical problems, present supportive therapy, current laboratory and diagnostic studies.

Intestinal amebiasis: Travel history and source of infection (if known); review laboratory tests supporting diagnosis.

Infectious diarrhea: Nonprescription drugs previously used to treat diarrhea (if any); review laboratory tests for evaluation of present status.

See also Appendix 4.

PHYSICAL ASSESSMENT

Suppression of intestinal bacteria: Routine preoperative assessments.

Hepatic coma: Assess present status, including the neurologic system, and document current symptoms; monitor vital signs; evaluate patient's ability to take oral medication and fluids without danger of aspiration.

Intestinal amebiasis (acute form): Monitor vital signs; evaluate state of hydration; palpate abdomen for tenderness; examine and describe stools; examine perianal area for excoriation if diarrhea is severe. Baseline laboratory tests may include serum electrolytes, CBC.

Infectious diarrhea: Monitor vital signs; evaluate state of hydration and general physical status; examine and describe stools; check perianal area for excoriation. Baseline laboratory tests may include culture and sensitivity, serum electrolytes.

ADMINISTRATION

Hepatic coma: Be sure patient is able to swallow capsules/tablets and water without danger of aspiration; give assistance in holding medicine cup, water glass when needed.

Administer paromomycin sulfate with meals.

Suppression of intestinal bacterial: Make sure medicine card and Kardex clearly state time of day drug is given, the number of doses, and the date and time of the last dose.

ONGOING ASSESSMENTS AND PATIENT MANAGEMENT

Patient should be well hydrated during therapy.

Suppression of intestinal bacteria (kanamycin sulfate, neomycin sulfate): Observe for nausea, vomiting, diarrhea; if these occur, withhold next dose of drug and contact physician immediately.

Contact physician if patient cannot (or will not) complete course of therapy or if adverse drug reactions occur.

Hepatic coma (kanamycin sulfate, neomycin sulfate, paromomycin sulfate): Monitor vital signs q4h; evaluate symptoms and compare to data base; examine each bowel movement; save stool and bring to attention of physician if appearance changes; record intake and output; contact physician if vomiting or diarrhea occurs, if patient is unable to take medication or protein-

restricted diet, or if clinical status changes rapidly.

PROLONGED THERAPY: Observe for signs of superinfection (Appendix 6, section 6-22), ototoxicity, nephrotoxicity, other adverse drug reactions.

Intestinal amebiasis (paromomycin sulfate): Monitor vital signs (q1h–q2h if condition is acute); observe for adverse drug reactions; record frequency and appearance of stools; observe for signs of superinfection.

Infectious diarrhea (neomycin sulfate): Monitor vital signs q1h–q2h; observe for adverse drug reactions; record frequency and appearance of stools; record intake and output; evaluate hydration (fluid and electrolyte replacement may be needed).

Notify physician if oral intake or urinary output decreases or if signs of dehydration are apparent.

Drug response (*i.e.,* decrease in frequency of bowel movements) may not be evident for 2 to 3 days; notify physician if condition worsens or appears unchanged.

PATIENT AND FAMILY INFORMATION

Take drug as prescribed; complete full course of therapy.

Notify physician or nurse if any of the following occurs: vaginal or perianal itching, sore mouth or tongue, fever, cough, sore throat, black furry tongue.

Intestinal amebiasis: Make every effort to control spread of infection (*e.g.,* wash hands before eating, preparing food, after defecation; ensure sanitary disposal of human wastes). Keep physician or clinic appointments for reexamination of stool. Repeated stool examinations will be necessary (weekly for 6 weeks, monthly for 2 years). Family and close personal contacts should have stool examined for amebae.

Infectious diarrhea: Contact physician if diarrhea becomes more severe or other symptoms appear, if diarrhea does not respond to therapy in 2 to 3 days, or if fluid intake is poor.

Aminoglycosides, Parenteral

Amikacin Sulfate Rx

solution for injection: Amikin
  100 mg/2-ml vial;
  500 mg/2-ml vial;
  500 mg/2-ml disposable syringe; 1
  g/4-ml vial

Gentamicin Rx

solution for injection: 100 mg/dose	IV Piggyback (*Generic*)
solution for injection: 60 mg/dose, 80 mg/dose	Apogen, Garamycin, Garamycin IV Piggyback, *Generic*
solution for injection: 40 mg/ml	Apogen, Garamycin, Jenamicin, *Generic*
solution for injection: 10 mg/ml	Apogen Pediatric, Garamycin Pediatric, *Generic* (labeled as pediatric)
solution for injection: 2 mg/ml	Garamycin Intrathecal

Kanamycin Sulfate Rx

injection: 500 mg, 1 g	Kantrex, Klebcil
injection, pediatric: 75 mg	Kantrex, Klebcil

Neomycin, Intramuscular Rx

powder for injection: 500-mg vials	Mycifradin Sulfate

Netilmicin Sulfate Rx

injection: 100 mg/ml	Netromycin
injection, pediatric: 25 mg/ml	Netromycin
injection, neonatal: 10 mg/ml	Netromycin

Streptomycin Sulfate Rx

solution for injection: 400 mg/ml, 500 mg/ml	*Generic*
powder for injection: 1-g, 5-g vials	*Generic*

Tobramycin Sulfate Rx

solution for injection: 40 mg/ml, 60 mg/dose, 80 mg/dose	Nebcin
powder for injection: 40 mg/ml	Nebcin
pediatric solution for injection: 10 mg/ml	Nebcin

INDICATIONS

See the following individual drug listings. It is recommended that these drugs be reserved for treatment of infections caused by organisms not sensitive to other, less toxic agents.

AMIKACIN SULFATE

Organisms: Short-term treatment of serious infections due to susceptible strains of gram-negative bacteria including: *Pseudomonas* species, *Escherichia coli, Proteus* species, *Providencia* species, *Klebsiella–Enterobacter–Serratia* species, *Acinetobacter* species.

Infections: Bacteremia and septicemia (including neonatal sepsis); in serious infections of respiratory tract, bones, joints, CNS (including meningitis); burns and postoperative infections (including postvascular surgery). Also effective in serious complicated and recurrent urinary-tract infection (UTI) due to these organisms. Not intended in uncomplicated initial episodes of UTI unless causative organism is not susceptible to antibiotics having less toxicity.

Suspected gram-negative infections: May be used in initial therapy before obtaining results of susceptibility testing. Decision to continue therapy is based on test results, severity of infection, response of patient, and concepts discussed in *Warnings.*

Staphylococcal infections: May be considered as initial therapy under certain conditions in treatment of known or suspected staphylococcal disease.

Neonatal sepsis: When susceptibility testing indicates other aminoglycosides cannot be used. In severe infections, concomitant therapy with a penicillin-type drug may be indicated.

GENTAMICIN

Treatment of serious infections caused by susceptible strains of *Pseudomonas aeruginosa, Proteus* species, *Escherichia coli, Klebsiella–Enterobacter–Serratia* species, *Citrobacter* species, *Staphylococcus* species (coagulase-positive, coagulase-negative). Effective in neonatal sepsis; septicemia; serious infections of CNS, of urinary, respiratory, and GI tract (including peritonitis), and of skin, bone, and soft tissue (including burns). Not indicated in uncomplicated initial episodes of UTI unless causative organisms are susceptible to this drug and are not susceptible to antibiotics with less potential for toxicity.

Gram-negative infections: Consider as initial therapy in suspected or confirmed infections; institute therapy before obtaining results of susceptibility tests. Decision to continue is based on test results, severity of the infection, and concepts listed under *Warnings.*

Unknown causative organisms: In serious infections, administered as initial therapy in conjunction with penicillin or cephalosporin before obtaining results of susceptibility tests. If anaerobic organism is suspected, other suitable antimicrobial therapy in conjunction with gentamicin may be used.

Combination therapy: Effective with carbenicillin for treatment of life-threatening infections caused by *P. aeruginosa.* Also effective when used with a penicillin for treatment of endocarditis caused by group D streptococci. In the neonate with suspected sepsis or staphylococcal pneumonia, a penicillin drug is usually indicated as concomitant therapy with gentamicin.

Staphylococcal infections: Effective in treatment of serious infections.

Intrathecal administration: Indicated as adjunctive therapy to systemically administered gentamicin in treatment of serious CNS infections (meningitis, ventriculitis) caused by susceptible *Pseudomonas* species.

KANAMYCIN SULFATE

Treatment of serious infections caused by susceptible organisms. Culture and sensitivity studies should be performed; therapy may be instituted before obtaining results. Kanamycin may be considered as initial therapy when one or more of the following are known or suspected pathogens: *E. coli, Proteus* species, *Enterobacter aerogenes, Klebsiella pneumoniae, Serratia marcescens, Acinetobacter.* In serious infections in which the organism is unknown, kanamycin may be administered as initial therapy with penicillin or cephalosporin before obtaining susceptibility-test results. If anaerobic organisms are suspected, suitable antimicrobial therapy with kanamycin may be used. Although not the drug of choice, kanamycin may be indicated under certain conditions for treatment of staphylococcal disease.

NEOMYCIN, INTRAMUSCULAR

Treatment of UTI due to susceptible strains of *P. aeruginosa, K. pneumoniae, Proteus vulgaris, E. coli, E. aerogenes.* Because of potential toxicity, use is reserved for hospitalized cases in which no other antimicrobial agent is effective.

NETILMICIN SULFATE

Short-term treatment of patients with serious or life-threatening bacterial infections caused by susceptible strains of the following: Complicated UTIs caused by *E. coli, K. pneumoniae, P. aeruginosa, Enterobacter* species, *Proteus mirabilis,* indole-positive *Proteus* species, *Serratia* and *Citrobacter* species, *Staphylococcus aureus.* Septicemia caused by *E. coli, K. pneumoniae, P. aeruginosa, Enterobacter* and *Serratia* species, *P. mirabilis.* Skin and skin structure infections caused by *E. coli, K. pneumoniae, P. aeruginosa, Enterobacter* and *Serratia* species, *S. aureus.* Intra-abdominal infections caused

by *E. coli, K. pneumoniae, P. aeruginosa, Enterobacter* species, *P. mirabilis,* indole-positive *Proteus* species, *S. aureus.* Lower respiratory-tract infections caused by *E. coli, K. pneumoniae, P. aeruginosa, Enterobacter* and *Serratia* species, *P. mirabilis, Proteus* species, *S. aureus.*

Although not the antibiotic of first choice, it may be considered for treatment of serious staphylococcal infections for which penicillins or other, less potentially toxic, drugs are contraindicated. May also be considered in mixed infections caused by susceptible strains of staphylococci and gram-negative organisms.

Netilmicin is indicated for those infections for which less potentially toxic antimicrobial agents are ineffective or contraindicated. Not indicated in treatment of uncomplicated initial episodes of UTI unless causative organisms are resistant to antimicrobial agents having less potential toxicity.

May be considered as initial therapy in suspected or confirmed gram-negative infections; therapy may be instituted before obtaining results of susceptibility testing. In serious infections, when causative organism unknown, netilmicin may be administered as initial therapy in conjunction with a penicillin-type or cephalosporin-type drug before results of susceptibility testing are obtained. In neonates with suspected sepsis, a penicillin-type drug is also usually indicated as concomitant therapy. If anaerobic organisms are suspected as etiologic agents, other suitable antimicrobial therapy should also be given. Following identifcation of the organism and its susceptibility, appropriate antibiotic therapy should be continued.

STREPTOMYCIN SULFATE

Mycobacterium tuberculosis, all forms, when infecting organisms are susceptible. Use only in combination with other antituberculosis drugs.

Nontuberculous infections: Use only in serious infections caused by organisms shown to be susceptible and when less potentially hazardous agents are ineffective or contraindicated. Organisms usually sensitive include *Yersinia pestis* (plague); *Francisella tularensis* (tularemia); *Brucella;* donovanosis (granuloma inguinale); *Hemophilus ducreyi* (chancroid); *H. influenzae* (concomitantly with another agent); *E. coli, Proteus, E. aerogenes, K. pneumoniae,* and *Streptococcus fecalis* in UTI; *S. viridans, S. fecalis* (in endocardial infections with penicillin); gram-negative bacilli (in bacteremia, concomitantly with another agent).

TOBRAMYCIN SULFATE

Treatment of serious infections caused by susceptible strains of *P. aeruginosa, E. coli, Proteus* species,

Providencia species, *Klebsiella–Enterobacter–Serratia* species, *Citrobacter* species, and staphylococci, including *S. aureus* (coagulase-positive and coagulase-negative). Indicated in treatment of septicemia; CNS infections including meningitis; neonatal sepsis; serious lower respiratory-tract infections; GI infections including peritonitis; serious skin, bone, and soft-tissue infections including burns; serious complicated and recurrent UTIs due to above organisms. In patients in whom gram-negative septicemia, neonatal sepsis, or meningitis is suspected, including those in whom concurrent therapy with a penicillin or cephalosporin and an aminoglycoside may be indicated, treatment with tobramycin is initiated before results of susceptibility tests are obtained. Decision to continue therapy is based on test results, severity of the infection, and concepts listed under *Warnings*.

CONTRAINDICATIONS

Do not use in those who have shown previous reactions to these agents. With the exception of the use of streptomycin in tuberculosis, these agents are *not* indicated in long-term therapy because of ototoxic hazards with extended administration.

ACTIONS

Absorption from the alimentary tract is negligible and systemic infections must be treated parenterally. Absorption from IM injection is rapid, with peaks blood levels achieved within 1 hour. The serum half-life of these agents is between 2 and 3 hours in those with normal renal function but is longer in young infants. Prolonged half-life may also occur in the elderly.

Aminoglycosides are widely distributed in extracellular fluids and cross the placental barrier. Serum concentrations in febrile patients may be lower than those in afebrile patients given the same dose. These agents do not achieve significant levels in CSF in normal patients, although penetration is enhanced in the presence of inflamed meninges. Excretion is by glomerular filtration.

Because of the narrow range between therapeutic and toxic serum levels, careful attention to dosage calculations, especially in those with renal impairment, is essential (Table 1). When possible, drug serum levels should be monitored.

Bactericidal activity is through inhibition of protein synthesis in the bacterial cell. These agents are more active in an alkaline media; alkalinization of the urine with sodium bicarbonate may be beneficial in the therapy of UTI. Culture and sensitivity testing is performed to determine appropriate antimicrobial therapy. Resistance to the aminoglycosides develops in a slow, stepwise manner, except

Table 1. Therapeutic and Toxic Serum Levels of Aminoglycosides

Drug	Therapeutic Serum Level (mcg/ml)	Toxic Serum Level (Peak) (mcg/ml)
Amikacin	8–16	>35
Gentamicin	4–10	>12
Kanamycin	8–16	>35
Neomycin	5–10	>10
Netilmicin	0.5–10	>16
Streptomycin	25	>50
Tobramycin	4–8	>12

with streptomycin, to which resistance may develop in single-step process.

WARNINGS

Use of these drugs may be associated with significant nephrotoxicity and ototoxicity, which may develop even with conventional doses, particularly in those with impaired renal function. These agents are excreted by glomerular filtration; serum half-life will be prolonged and significant accumulation will occur with impaired renal function. Those with impaired renal function or prerenal azotemia are especially likely to develop toxicity. Use with caution in such patients.

Patients should be under close observation. Monitoring of renal and eighth-cranial-nerve function is essential for those with known renal impairment. This testing is also recommended in those with normal renal function at the onset of therapy who develop evidence of nitrogen retention. Evidence of renal impairment or ototoxicity requires discontinuation of the drug or appropriate dosage adjustments. Concomitant use of other neurotoxic or nephrotoxic drugs should be avoided. Other factors that may increase risk of ototoxicity are advanced age and dehydration.

Ototoxicity (auditory and vestibular): Can occur in those treated at higher doses or for longer periods than recommended. The risk is greater in those with renal impairment and in those with preexisting hearing loss. High-frequency deafness usually occurs first and can be detected by audiometric testing. There may be no clinical symptoms to warn of developing cochlear damage. Tinnitus and vertigo may occur and are evidence of vestibular injury and impending bilateral *irreversible* deafness. Onset of deafness may occur several weeks after drug is discontinued and may progress to a complete loss of hearing. Vestibular deafness is more prominent with gentamicin and streptomycin; auditory toxicity may be more common with kanamycin and neomycin.

Renal toxicity: May be characterized by cylindruria, oliguria, proteinuria, or evidence of nitrogen retention (increasing BUN, nonprotein nitrogen, creatinine). Renal tubular damage is usually reversible.

Neuromuscular blockade: Neuromuscular blockade resulting in respiratory paralysis has occurred, especially when an aminoglycoside is administered simultaneously with or soon after the use of anesthesia or muscle relaxants or in patients with myasthenia gravis or parkinsonism. This effect is more pronounced with neomycin and streptomycin, but has also been reported with kanamycin.

Use in pregnancy and lactation: Safety not established. Aminoglycosides may be excreted in breast milk; breast-feeding should not be undertaken while using these agents.

PRECAUTIONS

Cross-allergenicity among the aminoglycosides has been demonstrated.

The possibility of acute toxicity increases in premature infants, neonates, and the elderly.

Hydration: Patients should be *well hydrated* to prevent chemical irritation of renal tubules. When patient is well hydrated and kidney function is normal, the risk of nephrotoxic reactions is low if dosage recommendations are not exceeded.

Assessment of renal function: Assess prior to therapy and periodically during course of treatment. If signs of renal irritation (casts, white or red cells, albumin in urine) appear, increase hydration. Reduction in dosage may be desirable if other evidence of renal dysfunction occurs (*e.g.,* increased BUN or creatinine, oliguria, decreased urine specific gravity). These findings usually disappear when treatment is completed; if azotemia or progressive decrease in urine output occurs, stop treatment.

Use in impaired renal function: If therapy is expected to last 5 or more days, obtain a pretreatment audiogram and repeat it during therapy. Therapy is stopped if tinnitus or subjective hearing loss develops or follow-up audiograms show significant loss of high-frequency perception.

Superinfection: Use of antibiotics (especially prolonged or repeated therapy) may result in bacterial or fungal overgrowth of nonsusceptible organisms and may lead to a secondary infection.

DRUG INTERACTIONS

Concurrent or sequential administration with other ototoxic, neurotoxic, or nephrotoxic agents may increase the potential for adverse effects. Avoid concurrent use with **other aminoglycosides, cisplatin, cephalothin** (and possibly other cephalosporins) **vancomycin,** or **methoxyflurane,** or with **potent diuretics** (ethacrynic acid, furosemide, mannitol). IV-admin-

istered diuretics enhance aminoglycoside toxicity by altering concentrations in serum and tissue.

Neuromuscular blockade and muscular paralysis have been reported with the use of several aminoglycosides. The risk should be considered when administered concomitantly or sequentially with **anesthetics, neuromuscular blocking drugs** (succinylcholine, tubocurarine, decamethonium) or in patients receiving massive transfusions of **citrate-anticoagulated blood.** If blockade occurs, calcium salts or neostigmine may reverse this phenomenon.

Aminoglycosides may exert a synergistic effect when used in combination with **carbenicillin** or **ticarcillin** for *Pseudomonas* infections.

ADVERSE REACTIONS

Nephrotoxic: Proteinuria; presence of red and white blood cells, granular casts; azotemia; oliguria.

Hepatic: Increased SGOT, SGPT, LDH, bilirubin; hepatomegaly; hepatic necrosis.

Hematologic: Increased and decreased reticulocyte count; transient agranulocytosis; leukopenia; thrombocytopenia; eosinophilia; pancytopenia; anemia; hemolytic anemia.

Ototoxic: Tinnitus, dizziness, vertigo, and partial to irreversible deafness have been reported, usually associated with higher than recommended dosage.

CNS: Confusion; depression; lethargy; respiratory depression; visual disturbances; amblyopia; headache; fever; pseudomotor cerebri; acute organic brain syndrome.

Hypersensitivity: Purpura; rash; urticaria; angioneurotic edema; pruritus; exfoliative dermatitis; generalized burning; alopecia; anaphylactoid reactions; laryngeal edema.

Neurotoxic: Numbness; skin tingling; circumoral or peripheral paresthesia; tremor; muscle twitching; convulsions; muscular weakness. Hypomagnesemia resulting in neuromuscular irritability and seizures has been reported in association with long-term *Gentamicin* therapy.

GI: Nausea; vomiting; decreased appetite; weight loss; increased salivation; stomatitis.

Other: Pulmonary fibrosis; myocarditis; splenomegaly; arthralgia; hypotension; hypertension; decreased serum calcium, sodium, potassium. Some local irritation or pain may follow IM injection.

OVERDOSAGE

In event of overdosage or toxic reaction, peritoneal dialysis or hemodialysis (preferred) will aid in removal from the blood.

DOSAGE

AMIKACIN SULFATE

Evidence of impairment in renal, vestibular, or auditory function requires discontinuation of drug or dosage adjustment. Obtain patient's ideal weight for calculation of correct dosage. Administer IM or IV.

Usual duration of treatment is 7 to 10 days. Do not exceed 15 mg/kg/day. In unusual circumstances in which treatment exceeds 10 days, monitor renal and auditory functions daily. Uncomplicated infections due to sensitive organisms should respond in 24 to 48 hours. If definite clinical response does not occur within 3 to 5 days, therapy should be stopped and antibiotic sensitivity pattern rechecked.

Adults, children, older infants: 15 mg/kg/day divided into 2 or 3 equal doses at equally divided intervals. Treatment of heavier patients should not exceed 1.5 g/day. In uncomplicated UTI, use 250 mg bid.

Neonates: Loading dose of 10 mg/kg recommended, followed by 7.5 mg/kg q12h.

IV: Dose same as IM dose. See *Administration.*

GENTAMICIN

Usually given IM. Serum level monitoring may be ordered.

Recommended dosage for serious infections and normal renal function is 3 mg/kg/day in 3 equal doses q8h. For life-threatening infections, administer up to 5 mg/kg/day in 3 or 4 equal doses, to be reduced to 3 mg/kg/day as soon as clinically indicated.

Children: 6 mg/kg/day to 7.5 mg/kg/day (2 mg/kg to 2.5 mg/kg q8h).

Infants and neonates: 7.5 mg/kg/day (2.5 mg/kg q8h).

Premature or full-term neonates (1 week of age or less): 5 mg/kg/day (2.5 mg/kg q12h).

Duration of therapy: Usually 7 to 10 days. In difficult or complicated cases, a longer course may be necessary. In such cases renal, auditory, and vestibular function is monitored.

Prevention of bacterial endocarditis in GI- or GU-tract surgery, instrumentation: 2 million units aqueous penicillin G or 1.0 g ampicillin IM or IV, plus gentamicin 1.5 mg/kg (not to exceed 80 mg) IM or IV ½ to 1 hour before procedure. Give 2 additional doses at 8-hour intervals. *Pediatric doses:* aqueous penicillin G 30,000 units/kg or ampicillin 50 mg/kg; gentamicin 2 mg/kg. Pediatric doses should not exceed recommended single dose or 24-hour dose for adults.

Impaired renal function: Adjust dosage; when possible, serum concentrations of gentamicin are monitored.

Hemodialysis: Amount removed from blood may vary. An 8-hour dialysis may reduce serum concentration by approximately 50%.

IV: Same as IM dose. IV administration is useful for treating patients with septicemia or in shock.

May also be preferred route for some patients with congestive heart failure, hematologic disorders, severe burns, or reduced muscle mass. See *Administration.*

Intrathecal: 2 mg/ml intrathecal preparation without preservatives is recommended. Dosage varies. Recommended dose for infants 3 months of age and older and children is 1 mg to 2 mg once a day. *Adults:* 4 mg to 8 mg once a day. See *Administration.*

KANAMYCIN SULFATE

Do not exceed 1.5 g/day by any route of administration.

IM

Recommended dose for adults, children: 7.5 mg/kg q12h for a total dose of 15 mg/kg/day. If continuously high blood levels are desired, give 15 mg/kg/day in equally divided doses q6h to q8h.

Usual duration of treatment: 7 to 10 days. Uncomplicated infections should respond in 24 to 48 hours. If definite clinical response does not occur within 3 to 5 days, therapy should be stopped and antibiotic susceptibility rechecked.

IV

Adults: Do not exceed 15 mg/kg/day. See *Administration.*

Children: See *Administration.*

Dosage in renal failure

Follow therapy by appropriate serum assays; if not feasible, reduce frequency of administration.

Intraperitoneal

500 mg diluted in 20 ml sterile distilled water instilled through a polyethylene catheter sutured into wound at closure.

Aerosol

250 mg 2 to 4 times/day. Withdraw 250 mg (1 ml) from 500-mg vial, dilute with 3 ml normal saline, and nebulize.

Other routes

Concentrations of 0.25% have been used in irrigating solutions in abscess cavities, pleural space, peritoneal and ventricular cavities.

NEOMYCIN, INTRAMUSCULAR

For IM use only. Injection of 300 mg q6h for 4 doses, followed by 300 mg q12h, yields blood concentrations of 12 mcg/ml to 30 mcg/ml in 48 to 72 hours. Therapy should not be continued beyond 10 days; total daily dose should not exceed 1 g.

Adults: 15 mg/kg/day in divided doses q6h. See *Administration.*

Children: Do not use in infants and children.

NETILMICIN SULFATE

Give IM or IV. Recommended dosage for both methods is identical. Obtain patient's pretreatment body weight for calculation of dosage. Dosage for obese patients is based on estimate of lean body mass. Status of renal function should be estimated by measurement of serum creatinine concentration or calculation of the endogenous creatinine clearance rate.

Burn patients: Extensive body-surface burns may result in reduced serum concentrations of aminoglycosides. Measurement of netilmicin serum concentrations is important as a basis for dosage adjustment.

Duration of treatment: Usual duration is 7 to 14 days. In complicated infections, a longer course may be necessary. Patient must be carefully monitored for changes in renal, auditory, and vestibular functions and dosage adjusted as indicated.

Periodically during therapy, measure serum concentrations to determine adequacy and safety of administration. The following dosages are guides for initial therapy.

Patients with normal renal function

Adults: For uncomplicated UTI, 1.5 mg/kg to 2 mg/kg q12h (3 mg/kg/day to 4 mg/kg/day). For serious systemic infections, 1.3 mg/kg to 2.2 mg/kg q8h or 2 mg/kg to 3.25 mg/kg q12h (4 mg/kg/day to 6.5 mg/kg/day).

Infants, children (6 weeks through 12 years): 1.8 mg/kg to 2.7 mg/kg q8h or 2.7 mg/kg to 4 mg/kg q12h (5.5 mg/kg/day to 8 mg/kg/day).

Neonates (under 6 weeks): 2 mg/kg to 3.25 mg/kg q12h (4 mg/kg/day to 6.5 mg/kg/day).

Patients with impaired renal function

Dosage is individualized and based on serum drug concentrations during treatment. Serum creatinine and creatinine clearance values may be used as a guide for dosage adjustment. In adults with renal failure undergoing hemodialysis, the amount of netilmicin removed from the body may vary. A dose of 2 mg/kg at the end of each dialysis period is recommended until results of tests measuring serum levels are available.

IV administration

See *Administration.*

STREPTOMYCIN SULFATE

Administer IM only.

Tuberculosis: 1 g streptomycin daily, along with one or more additional antitubercular agents. Give elderly smaller doses in accordance with age and renal and eighth-cranial-nerve function. Ultimately discontinue or reduce dosage to 1 g 2 or 3 times/week. Terminate therapy when toxic symptoms appear, toxicity is feared, organisms become resistant, or full therapeutic effect is obtained. Total treatment period is a minimum of 1 year.

Tularemia: 1 g to 2 g daily in divided doses for 7

to 10 days or until patient is afebrile for 5 to 7 days.

Plague: 2 g to 4 g daily in divided doses until patient is afebrile for 3 days.

Bacterial endocarditis due to penicillin-sensitive α-hemolytic and nonhemolytic streptococci: 1 g bid for 1 week and 0.5 g bid for second week. *In patients over 60 years:* 0.5 g bid for 2 weeks. Use penicillin concurrently.

Enterococcal endocarditis: 1 g bid for 2 weeks and 0.5 g bid for 4 weeks, in combination with penicillin.

Prevention of bacterial endocarditis in high-risk patients undergoing dental procedures or upper respiratory-tract surgery or instrumentation: 1 million units aqueous penicillin G mixed with 600,000 units procaine penicillin G IM, plus 1 g streptomycin ½ to 1 hour prior to procedure. Then, 500 mg penicillin V orally q6h for 8 doses. *Pediatric doses:* 30,000 units/kg aqueous penicillin G; 600,000 units procaine penicillin G; 20 mg/kg streptomycin. For children under 60 lb, the penicillin V dose is 250 mg q6h.

Prevention of bacterial endocarditis in GI- and GU-tract surgery or instrumentation: 2 million units aqueous penicillin G or 1 g ampicillin IM or IV, plus 1 g streptomycin IM. Administer ½ to 1 hour prior to procedure; give 2 additional doses q12h. *Pediatric doses:* 30,000 units/kg aqueous penicillin G or 50 mg/kg ampicillin; 20 mg/kg streptomycin. *For penicillin-allergic patients,* use 1 g vancomycin IV over 30 to 60 minutes, plus 1 g streptomycin IM. Repeat these doses in 12 hours for prolonged procedures or delayed healing. *Pediatric doses:* 20 mg/kg vancomycin; 20 mg/kg streptomycin. Pediatric doses should not exceed the recommended single or 24-hour dose for adults.

For use with other agents to which infecting organism is also sensitive (streptomycin is a secondary choice): Severe fulminating infections, 2 g/day to 4 g/day (children, 20 mg/kg/day to 40 mg/kg/day) in divided doses q6h to q12h; less severe infections and highly susceptible organisms, 1 g/day to 2 g/day.

TOBRAMYCIN SULFATE

Obtain patient's ideal body weight for calculation of correct dosage. Given IM or IV. Following IM dose of 1 mg/kg, maximum serum concentrations reach about 4 mcg/ml and measurable levels persist for as long as 8 hours. Serum concentrations of the drug administered by IV infusion over a 1-hour period are similar to those obtained by IM administration. Monitor serum concentrations when feasible.

Adults with serious infections: 3 mg/kg/day in 3 equal doses q8h. *Life-threatening infections:* Up to 5 mg/kg/day in 3 or 4 equal doses; reduce dosage to 3 mg/kg/day as soon as clinically indicated. Do not exceed 5 mg/kg/day unless serum levels are monitored.

Children: 6 to 7.5 mg/kg/day in 3 or 4 equally divided doses (2 mg/kg to 2.5 mg/kg q8h or 1.5 mg/kg to 1.9 mg/kg q6h).

Premature or full-term neonates (1 week of age or less): Up to 4 mg/kg/day in 2 equal doses q12h.

Usual duration of treatment: 7 to 10 days; a longer course of therapy may be necessary in complicated infections.

Impaired renal function: When possible, obtain serum levels. Following loading dose of 1 mg/kg, adjust subsequent dosage, either with reduced doses given q8h or normal doses given at prolonged intervals.

IV: Same as IM dose. See *Administration.*

NURSING IMPLICATIONS

HISTORY
See Appendix 4.

PHYSICAL ASSESSMENT
Base on location, type of infection; monitor vital signs; describe wound drainage (if present); weigh patient because dosage is usually calculated according to body weight (use bed scale if patient is acutely ill). Baseline laboratory tests may include urinalysis, renal- and hepatic-function tests, hematologic studies, culture and sensitivity studies. Pretreatment audiometric testing is recommended (some patients receiving these drugs are acutely ill and testing is not always practical).

ADMINISTRATION
Obtain culture and sensitivity *before* giving first dose of drug.

Check drug label carefully because the aminoglycosides are available in various dosage strengths.

Do not mix other drugs in same syringe or IV additive set without first checking with physician or pharmacist.

When administering with IV additive line, monitor infusion rate q5m to q15m.

When adding diluent for pediatric IV administration, check with physician about amount of diluent to be used and, when applicable, type of diluent.

Rotate IM injection sites and record site used. Warn patient that injection may cause discomfort or pain. Give slowly, deep IM.

Be sure drug is given at intervals stated because continuous therapeutic blood levels are necessary. When equal intervals are recommended, divide 24 hours by number of doses/day to obtain number of hours/interval (*e.g.,* for 3 doses/day, divide 24 by 3; drug should be given q8h).

AMIKACIN SULFATE, IV
Normal adults: Prepare solution for administration by adding contents of 500-mg vial to 200 ml of sterile diluent. Administer over a 30- to 60-minute period. Do not exceed 15 mg/kg/day, and divide into 2 or 3 equal doses at equal intervals.

Infants: In pediatric patients, the amount of fluid used for administration will depend on the amount ordered for patient, but it should be sufficient to infuse drug over a period of 30 to 60 minutes. Infants should receive a 1- to 2-hour infusion.

Stability of IV fluids: Stable for 24 hours at room temperature at concentrations of 0.25 mg/ml and 5.0 mg/ml in 5% Dextrose Injection, USP; 5% Dextrose and 0.2% Sodium Chloride Injection, USP; 5% Dextrose and 0.45% Sodium Chloride Injection, USP; 0.9% Sodium Chloride Injection, USP; Lactated Ringer's Injection, USP; Normosol M in 5% Dextrose Injection, USP (or Plasma-Lyte 56 Injection in 5% Dextrose in Water); Normosol R in 5% Dextrose Injection, USP (or Plasma-Lyte 148 Injection in 5% Dextrose in Water). Do not physically premix amikacin with other drugs.

GENTAMICIN, IV
For intermittent administration in adults, dilute single dose in 50 ml to 200 ml of sterile isotonic saline or in sterile solution of 5% Dextrose in Water (not to exceed 1 mg/ml). *Infants and children:* Volume of diluent should be less. Infuse over period of ½ to 2 hours. Do *not* physically premix gentamicin with other drugs.

GENTAMICIN, INTRATHECAL
Administered into lumbar area, usually by means of a lumbar puncture. May also be administered directly into the subdural space or directly into the ventricles, including administration by use of an implanted reservoir.

KANAMYCIN SULFATE, IM
Inject deep into upper outer quadrant of gluteal muscle.

KANAMYCIN SULFATE, IV
Do Not physically mix with other antibacterial agents; administer separately. Prepare solution by adding contents of 500-mg vial to 100 ml to 200

ml of sterile diluent or contents of 1-g vial to 200 ml to 400 ml of sterile diluent. Administer prescribed dose over 30 to 60 minutes.

Children: Use amount of diluent sufficient to infuse drug over 30 to 60 minutes.

Stability: Darkening of unopened vials during shelf life does not indicate loss of potency.

NEOMYCIN, IM

Preparation and storage: Add 2 ml sterile normal saline to vial to provide concentration of 250 mg/ml. Store and label prepared solutions in refrigerator at 2°C to 8°C (36°F to 46°F) and use as soon as possible, preferably within a week. Store unreconstituted product at room temperature.

NETILMICIN, IV

In adults, a single dose may be diluted in 50 ml to 200 ml of one of the parenteral solutions listed below. In infants and children, the volume of diluent should be less, according to the fluid requirements of the patient. Solutions may be infused over a period of ½ to 2 hours.

Netilmicin is stable in the following parenteral solutions for up to 72 hours when stored in glass containers, both when refrigerated and at room temperature. Do not use after this time period.

Sterile Water for Injection
0.9% Sodium Chloride
Sodium Chloride w/5% Dextrose
5% or 10% Dextrose Injection in Water
5% Dextrose in Polysal Injection
5% Dextrose w/Electrolyte #48 or #75
Ringer's and Lactated Ringer's
Lactated Ringer's w/5% Dextrose
10% Travert w/Electrolyte #2 or #3
Isolyte E, M, or P w/5% Dextrose
10% Dextran 40 or 6% Dextran 75 in 5% Dextrose
Plasma-Lyte 56 or 148 w/5% Dextrose
Plasma-Lyte M Injection w/5% Dextrose
Ionosol B in D5-W
Normosol R
Polysal (Plain)
Aminosol 5% Injection
Fre-Amine II 5% Injection
Plasma-Lyte 148
10% Fructose
Electrolyte #3 w/10% Inverted Sugar
Normosol M or R in D5-W
Isolyte H or S w/5% Dextrose
Polyonic R-148 or M-56 w/5% Dextrose
Polyonic R-148, Isolyte S, Plasma-Lyte 148 Injection in Water
Normosol R *p*H 7.4

Storage: Store between 2°C and 30°C (between 36°F and 86°F). Protect from freezing.

TOBRAMYCIN SULFATE, IV

Diluents: 0.9% Sodium Chloride Injection, 5% Dextrose Injection. Volume for adult doses is 50 ml to 100 ml; for children volume is proportionately less. Infuse diluted solution over a period of 20 to 30 minutes. *Do not* physically premix with other drugs.

ONGOING ASSESSMENTS AND NURSING MANAGEMENT

Check vital signs q4h (more often if warranted); accurately record intake and output; observe for adverse drug reactions and report occurrence immediately; check previous IM injection sites for irritation, swelling, induration.

If output measurement is assigned to nursing assistant, visually inspect urine for color changes, cloudiness, sediment (which may indicate presence of casts, red and white blood cells); notify physician if urine appears abnormal.

Observe for early manifestations of serious adverse drug effects by monitoring renal and eighth-cranial-nerve function (see *Adverse Reactions,* p 27).

Patient should be well hydrated (unless contraindicated) before and during therapy to prevent chemical irritation to the renal tubules and reduce risk of nephrotoxicity. For those allowed oral fluids, obtain physician's approval for increasing oral fluid intake.

CLINICAL ALERT: If oliguria or anuria develops or if patient complains of vertigo, dizziness, or tinnitus, withhold next dose of drug and notify physician immediately.

Monitor laboratory tests; report new abnormal values to physician immediately.

Observe for signs of superinfection (Appendix 6, section 6-22).

Culture and sensitivity studies are performed before, and sometimes during, therapy. It is important to use the correct procedure and obtain an adequate sample of infectious material. Take culture tubes to the laboratory *immediately.*

Neuromuscular blockade and respiratory paralysis can occur when an aminoglycoside is administered soon after use of anesthesia or muscle relaxants or in those with myasthenia gravis or parkinsonism (see *Warnings*). If blockade occurs, calcium salts or neostigmine may reverse this problem. These drugs, plus resuscitation equipment (including a respirator), should be available when the aminoglycosides are administered under these circumstances.

Streptomycin therapy for tuberculosis (usually given on outpatient basis): Keep clinic or physician appointments for periodic review of therapeutic regimen. Notify physician or nurse if dizziness, tinnitus, or hearing loss occurs.

Aminophylline

See Bronchodilators and Decongestants, Systemic.

4-Aminoquinoline Compounds

Chloroquine Hydrochloride Rx

injection: 50 mg/ml   Aralen HCl

Chloroquine Phosphate Rx

tablets: 250 mg   *Generic*
tablets: 500 mg   Aralen Phosphate

Hydroxychloroquine Sulfate Rx

tablets: 200 mg   Plaquenil Sulfate

INDICATIONS
CHLOROQUINE HYDROCHLORIDE
See Chloroquine Phosphate, below. Chloroquine hydrochloride is used when oral therapy is not feasible.

CHLOROQUINE PHOSPHATE
Suppression and treatment of acute attacks of malaria due to *Plasmodium vivax, P. malariae, P. ovale,* and susceptible strains of *P. falciparum.* (For radical cure of vivax and malariae malaria, concomitant therapy with primaquine is necessary.) Also used in the treatment of extraintestinal amebiasis.

HYDROXYCHLOROQUINE SULFATE
Antimalarial (see Chloroquine Phosphate, above). Also used for treatment of chronic discoid and systemic lupus erythematosus and acute or chronic rheumatoid arthritis.

CONTRAINDICATIONS
Presence of retinal or visual-field changes; known hypersensitivity to these agents; long-term therapy in children. Exception should be considered in specific circumstances such as treatment of acute malarial attacks caused by strains of plasmodia susceptible only to these compounds.

ACTIONS
Highly active against erythrocytic forms of *P. vivax* and *P. malariae* and most strains of *P. falciparum* (but not gametocytes of *P. falciparum*). Provides suppression without prevention of infection. These drugs do not prevent relapses of vivax or malariae malaria because they are not effective against exo-erythrocytic forms of the parasite, nor do they prevent vivax or malariae infection when administered prophylactically. Highly effective as suppressive agents in those with vivax or malariae malaria in terminating acute attacks and lengthening the interval between treatment and relapse. They abolish the acute attack of falciparum malaria and effect complete cure of the infection unless the infection is due to a resistant strain of *P. falciparum.* The precise mechanism of action of hydroxychloroquine sulfate in the treatment of collagen diseases is unknown.

These drugs are absorbed rapidly from the GI tract; peak plasma levels are reached in 1 to 3 hours. Blood levels fall off rapidly after treatment is stopped. Rapid excretion of the unchanged drug occurs in the urine; renal excretion is enhanced by urinary acidification.

WARNINGS
Certain strains of *P. falciparum* have become resistant to these compounds. Treatment with quinine or other forms of therapy are advised for those infected with a resistant strain.

Retinopathy: Irreversible retinal damage has been observed in some who have received long-term therapy or high doses. Initial and periodic ophthalmologic examinations should be performed. If there is any indication of ophthalmologic abnormality, therapy is discontinued. Retinal changes and visual disturbances may progress even after discontinuation of therapy.

Long-term therapy: Question and examine patients periodically; examine knee and ankle reflexes to detect muscular weakness and, if it occurs, discontinue therapy. These drugs may also precipitate a severe attack of psoriasis in those with this disorder. When used in those with porphyria, the condition may be exacerbated.

Use in pregnancy: Use only when clearly needed and potential benefits outweigh unknown potential hazards to the fetus.

Use in lactation: Safety not established; these agents are excreted in breast milk.

Use in children: Children are especially sensitive to these compounds; fatalities have been reported following accidental ingestion of relatively small doses.

PRECAUTIONS

Perform periodic CBCs during prolonged therapy. If any severe blood disorder is apparent, therapy may be discontinued. Measure glucose-6-phosphate dehydrogenase in American blacks or those of Mediterranean ancestry prior to therapy because these compounds may induce hemolysis in G6PD-deficient persons in presence of stress or infection.

DRUG INTERACTIONS

HYDROXYCHLOROQUINE SULFATE

May cause hepatotoxicity; use with caution with known **hepatotoxic drugs.** Concomitant use of **phenylbutazone, gold salts,** or other drugs known to cause sensitization or dermatitis may increase risk of severe skin reaction.

ADVERSE REACTIONS

Cardiovascular: Hypotension; ECG changes (particularly inversion or depression of the T wave, widening of QRS complex).

CNS: Mild, transient headache; psychic stimulation; rarely, psychotic episodes, convulsions.

GI: Anorexia; nausea; vomiting; diarrhea; abdominal cramps.

Otologic: A few cases of nerve-type deafness have been reported.

Ophthalmic: Blurred vision; difficulty in focusing or accommodation. *Other disturbances* (usually occurring when daily doses are used for long period of time): reversible corneal changes; generally irreversible and sometimes progressive or, rarely, delayed retinal changes that may be asymptomatic (especially early) or patient may complain of nyctalopia, scotomatous vision.

Other: Agranulocytosis; pruritus; neuropathy; blood dyscrasias; lichenlike skin eruptions; skin, mucosal pigmentary changes; pleomorphic skin eruptions.

OVERDOSAGE

Drugs are rapidly and completely absorbed; toxicity may occur within 30 minutes in overdosage (or, rarely, with lower doses in hypersensitive patients).

Symptoms: Headache, drowsiness, visual disturbances, cardiovascular collapse, convulsions followed by sudden and early cardiac and respiratory arrest. Respiratory depression, cardiovascular collapse, shock, convulsions, and death have been reported with overdose of parenteral **chloroquine HCl,** especially in infants and children. ECG may reveal atrial standstill, nodal rhythm, prolonged intraventricular conduction time, progressive bradycardia leading to ventricular fibrillation or arrest.

Treatment: Symptomatic, and must be prompt with immediate evacuation of stomach by emesis (at home) or gastric lavage until stomach is empty. After lavage, finely powdered activated charcoal (in a dose not less than 5 times the estimated ingested dose) may inhibit intestinal absorption when given by stomach tube within 30 minutes after ingestion. Control convulsions before attempting gastric lavage. If convulsions are due to cerebral stimulation, cautious administration of an anticonvulsant may be tried. Anoxia-induced convulsions should be controlled by oxygen, artificial respiration, or (in shock) with hypotension, by vasopressor therapy. Tracheal intubation or tracheostomy followed by gastric lavage may also be necessary. Peritoneal dialysis and exchange transfusions have also been suggested. An asymptomatic patient surviving the acute attack should be observed for 6 hours. Force fluids and administer ammonium chloride (8 g/day in divided doses of adults) for a few days to acidify the urine and promote excretion of drug.

DOSAGE

CHLOROQUINE HYDROCHLORIDE

Chloroquine HCl 50 mg is equivalent to 40 mg chloroquine base.

Extraintestinal amebiasis

Adults unable to tolerate oral therapy, 200 mg to 250 mg (160 mg to 200 mg base) injected daily for 10 to 12 days. Oral therapy begun as soon as possible.

Malaria

Adults: 4 ml or 5 ml IM initially; repeat in 6 hours if necessary. Total dose in first 24 hours not to exceed 800 mg (base). Begin oral therapy as soon as possible and continue for 3 days until approximately 1.5 g (base) are administered.

Children: Recommended dose for infants, children is 5 mg (base)/kg; repeat in 6 hours. Do not exceed 10 mg (base)/kg/day. (See also *Overdosage, symptoms*).

CHLOROQUINE PHOSPHATE

Chloroquine phosphate 500 mg is equivalent to 300 mg chloroquine base.

Extraintestinal amebiasis

1 g (600 mg base) daily for 2 days, followed by 500 mg (300 mg base) daily for at least 2 to 3 weeks. Treatment is usually combined with an effective intestinal amebicide.

Malaria

Suppression: 5 mg (base)/kg, not to exceed 300 mg (base) weekly, on *same day each week*. Begin 2 weeks prior to exposure; continue for 6 to 8 weeks after leaving endemic area. If suppressive therapy is not begun prior to exposure, double initial loading dose (adults—600 mg of base, children—10 mg of base/kg) and give in 2 divided doses 6 hours apart. *Children* (doses expressed in mg/kg but should not exceed recommended adult dose): 5 mg (base)/kg weekly.

Acute attack: Dosage expressed in mg of base. *Initial dose on day 1:* adults 600 mg, children 10 mg/kg. *Second dose, 6 hours later:* adults 300 mg, children 5 mg/kg. *Third dose, day 2:* adults 300 mg, children 5 mg/kg. *Fourth dose, day 3:* adults 300 mg, children 5 mg/kg.

HYDROXYCHLOROQUINE SULFATE

Hydroxychloroquine sulfate 200 mg is equivalent to 150 mg hydroxychloroquine base.

Malaria

Suppression: 5 mg (base)/kg, not to exceed 310 mg (base)/week, on *same day each week.* Begin 2 weeks prior to exposure; continue for 6 to 8 weeks after leaving endemic area. If suppressive therapy is not begun prior to exposure, double initial loading dose (adults, 620 mg of base; children, 10 mg of base/kg) and give in 2 doses, 6 hours apart. *Children* (dose expressed in mg/kg but should not exceed recommended adult dose): 5 mg (base)/kg/week.

Acute attack: Dosage in mg of base. *Initial dose on day 1:* adults 620 mg, children 10 mg/kg. *Second dose, 6 hours later:* adults 310 mg, children 5 mg/kg. *Third dose, day 2:* adults 310 mg, children 5 mg/kg. *Fourth dose, day 3:* adults 310 mg, children 5 mg/kg.

Rheumatoid arthritis: Initial adult dose 400 mg/day to 600 mg/day, with meal or glass of milk. Rarely, side-effects require temporary reduction. Later (usually 5–10 days), dose may be gradually increased to optimum response levels, often without return of side-effects. *Maintenance dose:* When good response is obtained (usually 4–12 weeks), reduce dosage 50% and continue at a level of 200 mg/day to 400 mg/day. Incidence of retinopathy is higher when this dose is exceeded. Drug is cumulative in action and requires several weeks to exert therapeutic effects. Minor side-effects may occur early. Several months may be required before maximum effects are obtained. If objective improvement (reduced joint swelling, increased mobility) does not occur in 6 months, discontinue drug. Safe use in juvenile rheumatoid arthritis is not established. Should relapse occur after medication is withdrawn, therapy may be resumed or continued on an intermittent schedule if there are no ocular contraindications. Corticosteroids and salicylates may be used with this drug; dose can be gradually decreased or eliminated after drug is used for several weeks.

When gradual reduction of steroid dosage is indicated, reduce cortisone dosage every 4 to 5 days by no more than from 5 mg to 15 mg; hydrocortisone by from 5 mg to 10 mg; prednisolone and prednisone by from 1 mg to 2.5 mg; methylprednisolone and triamcinolone by from 1 mg to 2 mg; dexamethasone by from 0.25 mg to 0.5 mg.

Lupus erythematosus: Initially, average adult dose is 400 mg/day or bid; may be continued for several weeks or months, depending on response. *Prolonged maintenance:* Smaller dose (200 mg to 400 mg daily) will frequently suffice. Incidence of retinopathy has been reported higher when maintenance dose exceeded.

NURSING IMPLICATIONS

HISTORY

See Appendix 4. In addition, obtain travel history from those with extraintestinal amebiasis or malaria; review laboratory tests supporting diagnosis. If travel history does not support diagnosis of malaria, inquire about recent blood transfusions or investigate possibility of drug abuse (IV self-administration with contaminated syringes).

PHYSICAL ASSESSMENT

Extraintestinal amebiasis: If patient is relatively asymptomatic, evaluate general health. If hospitalized, check vital signs; evaluate hydration, nutrition status; describe stools. Baseline laboratory tests may include serum electrolytes, CBC.

Malaria: Describe nature and duration of symptoms; check vital signs; check for myalgia, arthralgia; assess mental state (*e.g.,* confusion, disorientation); if pulmonary involvement is evident, note type and amount of sputum raised; assess hydration; look for jaundice (skin, sclera). Baseline laboratory tests may include blood smears for malaria, serum electrolytes, CBC, urinalysis.

Rheumatoid arthritis: Examine affected joints; describe joint deformities on patient's chart; evaluate ability to carry out activities of daily living.

ADMINISTRATION

Give with food or milk.

Those with arthritis may require assistance in removing tablet from medicine glass, holding glass of water.

Chloroquine HCl: Initial dose is 4 ml to 5 ml IM. Divide dose and give in two sites.

ONGOING ASSESSMENTS AND NURSING MANAGEMENT

Monitor drug response by comparing ongoing assessments with initial data.

Long-term therapy: Question and examine patient periodically at time of clinic/office appointments. Physician or nurse should examine knee and ankle reflexes to detect evidence of muscular weakness (which requires discontinuing therapy).

Periodic blood counts and ophthalmologic examinations are recommended during long-term therapy.

Acute attack of malaria: Record vital signs q4h or as ordered; administer antipyretics as ordered; record intake and output; observe q1h to q2h and record response to antimalarial therapy; observe for adverse drug reactions.

PATIENT AND FAMILY INFORMATION

May cause GI upset; take with food.

Complete full course of prescribed therapy.

Keep out of reach of children (overdose is especially dangerous to children).

Notify physician or nurse if any of the following occurs: blurring or other visual changes; ringing in the ears, difficulty hearing; fever; sore throat; unusual bleeding or bruising; unusual pigmentation (blue-black) of skin, inside mouth; skin rash or itching; unusual muscle weakness; bleaching or loss of hair; yellow discoloration of skin or eyes; mood or mental changes.

Drug may cause diarrhea, loss of appetite, nausea, stomach pain, vomiting. Notify physician or nurse if these become pronounced.

Suppression of malaria: Take drug on *same day each week.*

Aminosalicylate Sodium

(Para-aminosalicylate Sodium, PAS) Rx

tablets: 0.5 g	Teebacin, *Generic*
tablets: 1 g	*Generic*
powder: 4.18-g packets	*Generic*
powder: 1 lb	Teebacin, *Generic*

INDICATIONS

Treatment of tuberculosis with other antituberculous drugs when due to susceptible strains of tubercle bacilli.

Unlabeled uses: Has been shown to have serum lipid-lowering activity.

CONTRAINDICATIONS

Severe hypersensitivity.

ACTIONS

Has a bacteriostatic effect on the organism *Mycobacterium tuberculosis.* Mechanism of action similar to that of the sulfonamides; involves competition with bacterial enzyme systems for para-aminobenzoic acid (PABA) and inhibition of bacterial folic acid synthesis. Inhibits the onset of bacterial resistance to streptomycin and isoniazid. Drug is excreted in the urine.

PRECAUTIONS

If symptoms of hypersensitivity develop, *all* medications should be stopped. After symptoms have abated, medications may be restarted one at a time, in small and gradually increasing doses, to determine which drug is responsible for the symptoms. Use cautiously in patients with impaired renal or hepatic function or gastric ulcer. Crystalluria may be prevented by maintaining urine at a neutral or alkaline *p*H. Drug deteriorates rapidly in contact with water, heat, sunlight; brownish or purplish color of powder or tablets, especially of a solution made with them, indicates deterioration and drug should be discarded.

Use with caution in known or impending congestive heart failure and in other situations in which excess sodium is potentially harmful.

DRUG INTERACTIONS

Probenecid inhibits renal excretion of PAS, thus increasing PAS plasma levels. PAS toxicity may occur if dosage is not reduced. PAS may inhibit absorption of **rifampin;** dosage should be separated by 8 to 12 hours. The pharmacologic effects of oral **folic acid** may be decreased owing to decreased GI absorption: parenteral folic acid may be required. **Vitamin B_{12}** deficiency may be induced due to PAS interference of its GI absorption; parenteral vitamin B_{12} may be required.

ADVERSE REACTIONS

GI: Nausea, vomiting, diarrhea, abdominal pain.

Hypersensitivity: Fever, skin eruptions of various types, infectious mononucleosis–like syndrome, leukopenia, agranulocytosis, thrombocytopenia, hemolytic anemia, jaundice, hepatitis, encephalopathy, Löffler's syndrome, vasculitis.

Endocrine: Goiter with or without myxedema.

Metabolic: Hypokalemia, acidosis.

DOSAGE

Adults, 14 g/day to 16 g/day in 2 or 3 divided doses. Children, 275 mg/kg/day to 420 mg/kg/day in 3 to 4 divided doses.

NURSING IMPLICATIONS

HISTORY
See Appendix 4.

PHYSICAL ASSESSMENT
Identify present problems and needs (physical, psychological, social) related to diagnosis; evaluate general health, nutritional status.

ADMINISTRATION
Give orally with food or meals; powdered form may be added to juice or water, depending on patient preference.

Add powder to liquid *immediately prior to* administration.

Note color of (plain) tablets, powder each time drug is administered. If color change is noted, discard drug and obtain new supply.

Total daily dose of 14 g to 16 g requires administration of large number of tablets. Patient should be encouraged to take tablets at spaced intervals while eating.

ONGOING ASSESSMENTS AND NURSING MANAGEMENT
Monitor vital signs daily (sudden rise in temperature may indicate hypersensitivity; see *Adverse Reactions*); observe for adverse drug reactions.

If GI side-effects occur, discuss problem with physician; use of an antacid, a temporary decrease in dose, or temporary cessation of therapy may be necessary.

Monitor intake and output. Report decreased urinary output, hematuria, dysuria, or cloudy urine to physician.

Sour aftertaste may be relieved with hard candy, ice chips.

Physician will order periodic evaluation of treatment modalities (*e.g.,* smears, cultures, sensitivity testing, x-rays, urinalysis, CBC).

PATIENT AND FAMILY INFORMATION
May cause GI upset; take with food or meals.

Experiment with methods (*e.g.,* mouthwash, gum, juice) to alleviate sour aftertaste.

Do not use tablets or powders, or solutions made from them, that are brown or purple in color; obtain fresh supply of medication.

Do not use nonprescription drugs (especially aspirin or products containing aspirin) unless use is approved by physician.

Notify physician or nurse if fever, sore throat, unusual bleeding or bruising, or skin rash occurs.

Amitriptyline Hydrochloride

See Antidepressants, Tricyclic Compounds.

Ammonium Biphosphate, Sodium Biphosphate, and Sodium Acid Pyrophosphate Rx

tablets, plain, enteric   pHos-pHaid
    coated: 0.25 g,
    0.5 g

INDICATIONS
Increasing solubility of calcium in urine to assist in preventing formation of calculi in urinary tract. Can decrease urine pH to 5 to 5.5 in conjunction with acid ash diet.

PRECAUTIONS
Give with caution to patients with severe or extensive renal damage.

ADVERSE REACTIONS
Occasional hyperacidity, particularly when gastritis or ulceration exists; nausea with high dosage. This may be decreased or eliminated with use of enteric-coated tablets. Excessive doses may act as a saline cathartic and cause diarrhea. Dose is usually decreased until symptoms disappear.

DOSAGE
Usual dose is 1 g qid, in conjunction with acidifying diet. Occasionally, a higher dose is required.

NURSING IMPLICATIONS

HISTORY
See Appendix 4.

ADMINISTRATION
Drug is followed by a full glass of water.

ONGOING ASSESSMENTS AND NURSING MANAGEMENT
Observe for adverse drug reactions.

Physician may order daily monitoring of urine pH (test materials may include Nitrazine paper, Chemstrip).

PATIENT AND FAMILY INFORMATION
Take with a full glass of water.

Adhere to prescribed acid ash diet (if ordered).

Notify physician or nurse if nausea, diarrhea, or symptoms of hyperacidity occur.

Ammonium Chloride Rx, otc

tablets: 325 mg, 500 mg (otc) — Generic

tablets, enteric coated: 500 mg, 1 g (otc) — Generic

injection: 2.14% (0.4 mEq/ml), 26.75% (5 mEq/ml) (Rx) — Generic

INDICATIONS

Oral form used as a diuretic or systemic and urinary acidifying agent. Injectable form indicated in treatment of hypochloremic states and metabolic alkalosis (not accompanied by severe hepatic disease) to prevent tetany or renal damage due to persistent severe alkalemia, hypochloremia, and dehydration. Because metabolic alkalosis is frequently associated with hypokalemia, concomitant correction of potassium deficiency is often indicated. Severe metabolic alkalosis requiring parenteral ammonium chloride is most likely seen in infants with severe, protracted vomiting due to pyloric obstruction.

Oral form also used as an expectorant in combination with other respiratory agents (such as antihistamines and antitussives) in cough and cold preparations.

CONTRAINDICATIONS

Markedly impaired renal or hepatic function, respiratory acidosis. Ammonium chloride solutions should not be given subcutaneously, intraperitoneally, or rectally.

ACTIONS

When loss of hydrogen and chloride ions occurs, serum bicarbonate and pH rise; consequently, there is a fall in serum potassium owing to intracellular shift and increased urinary excretion of potassium. The ammonia ion is converted to urea in the liver. Liberated hydrogen and chloride ions in the blood and extracellular fluid result in a decreased pH and correction of alkalosis. As a result, serum bicarbonate and serum chloride rise and pH returns to normal.

PRECAUTIONS

Observe patient carefully for symptoms of ammonia toxicity. Monitor plasma electrolyte balance. If intracellular potassium depletion is cause of secondary alkalosis, sustained correction of hypochloremia cannot be achieved unless potassium chloride is given.

ADVERSE REACTIONS

A serious degree of metabolic acidosis may result (see *Overdosage*).

Rapid IV administration may be accompanied by pain or irritation at site of injection or along venous route.

Oral: Gastric irritation, nausea, vomiting, acidosis with large doses.

OVERDOSAGE

Symptoms: Headache, progressive drowsiness, mental confusion, local and general twitching, tonic convulsions, hyperventilation, jerky respirations with apneic periods; hyperchloremic acidosis, hypokalemia, bradycardia, cardiac arrhythmias, pallor, sweating, nausea, vomiting, thirst, coma, death.

Treatment: For acidosis and electrolyte loss, administer sodium lactate or sodium bicarbonate IV. Treat hypokalemia with an oral potassium product.

DOSAGE

Oral: Usual dose is 1 g to 3 g bid or qid.

IV: Administer by slow IV infusion. Potassium chloride is generally added to the ammonium chloride infusion to provide 20 mEq to 40 mEq potassium/liter. Dosage is dependent on condition and tolerance of the patient and should be monitored by repeat sodium chloride, pH, and bicarbonate determinations. In the absence of edema and hyponatremia, the required dose in milliequivalents may be estimated as the product of the extracellular fluid volume (20% of body weight in kilograms) times the serum chloride deficit in mEq/ml. Initially, one-half the calculated dose should be given slowly and pH rechecked.

NURSING IMPLICATIONS

HISTORY
See Appendix 4.

PHYSICAL ASSESSMENT
In metabolic alkalosis, hypochloremia: Check vital signs; identify symptoms; evaluate hydration; weigh patient for calculation of drug dosage.

As diuretic, urinary acidification: Check vital signs; identify symptoms; record weight; check urinary pH (if used for acidification). Baseline laboratory studies may include serum electrolytes, urinalysis.

ADMINISTRATION
Give tablets with or immediately after meals to minimize GI distress.

Give drug by *slow* IV infusion to avoid pain, local irritation at venipuncture site and along course of the vein, and toxic drug effects. Physician must order rate of infusion.

When exposed to low temperatures, concentrated solutions of ammonium chloride may crystallize. If crystals are observed, warm solution slowly to room temperature in a water bath. Recheck solution in strong light to be sure all crystals are dissolved.

Check physician's order *carefully*. Note that two different strengths are available: 2.14% and 26.75%. The 26.75% solution must be diluted before use. Physician will order diluent for IV administration of the 26.75% solution.

ONGOING ASSESSMENTS AND NURSING MANAGEMENT

Oral administration as diuretic: Weigh daily; record intake and output; assess areas of edema (if present); observe for signs of electrolyte imbalance, mainly hypokalemia (Appendix 6, section 6-15), hyponatremia (Appendix 6, section 6-17), adverse drug reactions.

Oral administration to acidify urine: Physician may order daily *p*H of urine (testing materials include Nitrazine paper, Combistix).

Intravenous administration: Monitor infusion rate q15m to q30m, adjusting as necessary; check needle site, vein for signs of local irritation; check blood pressure, pulse, respirations q1h (more often if warranted); observe for symptoms of ammonia toxicity (pallor, irregular breathing, vomiting, bradycardia, cardiac arrhythmias, local and generalized twitching, asterixis, tonic convulsions, coma) and metabolic acidosis (Appendix 6, section 6-1).

Frequent laboratory tests will be ordered to monitor therapy; do not perform venipuncture for blood samples on arm used for IV administration of drug.

PATIENT AND FAMILY INFORMATION

Take drug with or immediately after meal or with food.

Do not exceed recommended dosage.

Notify physician or nurse if nausea or vomiting occurs.

Amobarbital, Amobarbital Sodium

See Barbiturates.

Amoxapine

See Antidepressants, Tricyclic Compounds.

Amoxicillin

See Penicillins.

Amphetamines

Amphetamine Complex *Rx C–II*

capsules: dextroamphetamine 6.25 mg and amphetamine 6.25 mg	Biphetamine 12½
capsules: dextroamphetamine 10 mg and amphetamine 10 mg	Biphetamine 20

Amphetamine Mixtures *Rx C–II*

tablets, capsules: 1.25 mg each of dextroamphetamine sulfate, dextroamphetamine adipate, amphetamine sulfate, and amphetamine adipate	Delcobese-5 mg
tablets, capsules: 2.5 mg each of amphetamines in Delcobese-5 mg	Delcobese-10 mg
tablets, capsules: 3.75 mg each of amphetamines in Delcobese-5 mg	Delcobese-15 mg
tablets, capsules: 5 mg each of amphetamines in Delcobese-5 mg	Delcobese-20 mg
tablets: 2.5 mg each of dextroamphetamine saccharate, amphetamine aspartate, amphetamine sulfate, dextroamphetamine sulfate	Obetrol-10
tablets: 5 mg each of amphetamines in Obetrol-10	Obetrol-20

Amphetamine Sulfate
(Racemic Amphetamine Sulfate) *Rx C–II*

tablets: 5 mg, 10 mg	*Generic*

Dextroamphetamine Sulfate Rx C–II

tablets: 5 mg	Dexampex, Dexedrine, Ferndex, *Generic*
tablets: 10 mg	Dexampex, Oxydess II, *Generic*
elixir: 5 mg/5 ml	Dexedrine
capsules, sustained release: 5 mg, 10 mg	Dexedrine Spansules
capsules, sustained release: 15 mg	Dexedrine Spansules, Span-cap No. 1, *Generic*
capsules: 15 mg	Dexampex

Methamphetamine Hydrochloride
(Desoxyephedrine Hydrochloride) Rx C–II

tablets: 5 mg	Desoxyn
tablets, long acting: 5 mg, 10 mg, 15 mg (contains tartrazine)	Desoxyn Gradumets
tablets: 10 mg	Methampex

INDICATIONS

Exogenous obesity: As short-term adjunct in regimen of weight reduction based on calorie restriction for those refractory to alternative therapy (*e.g.,* repeated diets, group programs).

Abnormal behavioral syndrome in children: As integral part of total treatment program that includes other measures (psychological, educational, social) for stabilizing effect in children with a behavioral syndrome characterized by the following group of developmentally inappropriate symptoms: moderate to severe distractibility, short attention span, hyperactivity, emotional lability, impulsiveness.

Narcolepsy: Amphetamines are also indicated in narcolepsy.

CONTRAINDICATIONS

Advanced arteriosclerosis; symptomatic cardiovascular disease; moderate to severe hypertension; hyperthyroidism; known hypersensitivity or idiosyncrasy to sympathomimetic amines; glaucoma; agitated states; patients with a drug-abuse history; patients receiving MAO inhibitors.

ACTIONS

Amphetamines are sympathomimetic amines with CNS stimulant activity. Peripheral actions include elevation of systolic and diastolic blood pressures and weak bronchodilator and respiratory stimulant action. At therapeutic doses, cardiac output is not increased, cerebral blood flow is not affected, and heart rate may be reflexly slowed. Following oral administration, amphetamines are absorbed within 3 hours.

WARNINGS

Amphetamines have potential for drug abuse; administration for prolonged periods may lead to drug dependence. When tolerance to the anorectic effect develops, drug should be discontinued. These drugs may impair the ability to engage in potentially hazardous activity.

Amphetamines have been extensively abused. Tolerance, extreme psychological dependence, and severe social disability have occurred. Abrupt cessation following prolonged high dosage results in extreme fatigue, mental depression; EEG changes have been noted. Signs of chronic intoxication include severe dermatoses, marked insomnia, irritability, hyperactivity, and personality changes. The most severe sign is psychosis, which is often clinically indistinguishable from schizophrenia.

Use in pregnancy: Safety not established. Use in women who are or may become pregnant only when clearly needed and potential benefits outweigh unknown potential hazards to the fetus.

Use in children: Not recommended as anorectics in those under 12. In behavioral syndrome described under *Indications,* amphetamine and dextroamphetamine not recommended for children under 3. Experience suggests amphetamines may exacerbate symptoms of behavioral disturbance and thought disorder in psychotic children.

PRECAUTIONS

Behavioral syndrome: Drug treatment not necessary in all cases and should be considered in light of complete history and evaluation of child.

Tartrazine sensitivity: Some products contain tartrazine (see Appendix 6, section 6-23).

DRUG INTERACTIONS

Administration during or within 14 days following use of **MAO inhibitors** may result in hypertensive crisis.

Insulin requirements in diabetes mellitus may be altered in association with the use of amphetamines and concomitant dietary regimen.

Amphetamines may decrease the effects of **antihypertensive agents.**

ADVERSE REACTIONS

Cardiovascular: Palpitation, tachycardia, elevation of blood pressure.

CNS: Overstimulation, restlessness, dizziness, insomnia, dyskinesia, euphoria, dysphoria, tremor, headache; rarely, psychotic episodes at recommended doses.

GI: Dry mouth, unpleasant taste, diarrhea, constipation, other GI disturbances. Anorexia and weight loss may occur as undesirable effects when used for effect other than anorectic.

Allergic: Urticaria.

Endocrine: Impotence, changes in libido. Reversible elevations of serum T_4 have been reported with heavy use.

OVERDOSAGE

Symptoms: Restlessness, tremor, hyperreflexia, rapid respiration, confusion, assaultiveness, hallucinations, panic states. Fatigue and depression usually follow central stimulation. *Cardiovascular effects:* arrhythmias, hypertension or hypotension, circulatory collapse. *GI effects:* nausea, vomiting, diarrhea, abdominal cramps. Fatal poisoning is usually preceded by convulsions and coma.

Treatment: Largely symptomatic; includes gastric lavage and sedation with a barbiturate. Acidification of the urine increases amphetamine excretion. If acute hypertensive episode occurs, administration of IV phentolamine has been suggested; however, gradual drop in blood pressure will occur with sedation. *Long-acting form:* Therapy is directed at reversing drug effects and supporting patient as long as overdosage symptoms remain. Saline cathartics are useful for hastening evacuation of the pellets that have not already released medication.

DOSAGE
AMPHETAMINE COMPLEX

Obesity: 1 capsule/day, 10 to 14 hours before retiring.

Abnormal behavioral syndrome in children: Begin with dextroamphetamine to determine appropriate dose; once optimal response is obtained, amphetamine complex may be used for once-a-day dosage.

AMPHETAMINE MIXTURES

See Amphetamine Sulfate, below.

AMPHETAMINE SULFATE

Narcolepsy: 5 mg/day to 60 mg/day in divided doses, depending on response. *Children (age 6 to 12):* Narcolepsy seldom occurs under age 12. When it does, suggested initial dose is 5 mg/day; daily dose may be raised in increments of 5 mg at weekly intervals until optimal response is obtained. *Adults (12 years and older):* Start with 10 mg/day; dosage may be raised in increments of 10 mg/day at weekly intervals until optimal response is obtained. If bothersome effects (*e.g.,* insomnia, anorexia) appear, dose is reduced. Give first dose on awakening; additional doses (1 or 2) at 4- to 6-hour intervals.

Abnormal behavior syndrome in children: *Age 3 to 5:* Start with 2.5 mg/day; dosage may be raised in increments of 2.5 mg/day at weekly intervals until optimal response is obtained.

Age 6 and older: Start with 5 mg daily or bid; dosage may be raised in increments of 5 mg/day at weekly intervals until optimal response is obtained. Dosage will rarely exceed 40 mg/day.

Give first dose on patient's awakening; additional doses (1 or 2) at intervals of 4 to 6 hours. When possible, stop administration to determine if there is a recurrence of symptoms sufficient to require continued therapy.

Exogenous obesity: 5 mg to 30 mg daily in divided doses of 5 mg to 10 mg, 30 to 60 minutes A.C.

DEXTROAMPHETAMINE SULFATE

See Amphetamine Sulfate, above.

METHAMPHETAMINE HYDROCHLORIDE

Obesity: 5 mg 30 minutes before each meal. *Long-acting form:* 10 mg to 15 mg in A.M. Treatment should not exceed a few weeks' duration. Not recommended as anorectic for children under 12.

Abnormal behavioral syndrome: Recommended initial dose is 5 mg daily or bid. Daily dose may be raised in increments of 5 mg at weekly intervals until optimal response is obtained. Usual effective dose is 20 mg/day to 25 mg/day. Total daily dose may be given as tablets in 2 divided doses or once daily using the long-acting form.

NURSING IMPLICATIONS

HISTORY
See Appendix 4. In addition, in those being treated for abnormal behavioral syndrome, obtain description and pattern of abnormal behavior and review psychological evaluations and testing (if available).

PHYSICAL ASSESSMENT

Exogenous obesity: Record blood pressure, pulse, respirations, weight.

NOTE: Physician-supervised weight reduction programs usually perform a more extensive evaluation of obesity.

Abnormal behavioral syndrome: Record blood pressure, pulse, respirations, weight; height measurement may be of value to evaluate weight loss correctly (weight gain or loss is compared to increase in height) owing to anorectic effect of drug.

Narcolepsy: Check general health status; if history warrants, conduct additional assessments; record blood pressure, pulse, respirations, weight.

ADMINISTRATION
Avoid late-evening doses, particularly with long-acting form, because drug may cause insomnia; last dose given approximately 6 hours before retiring.

In management of obesity, drug is given 30 to 60 minutes A.C.; long-acting form is administered in early A.M.

ONGOING ASSESSMENTS AND NURSING MANAGEMENT
Record blood pressure, pulse, respirations daily or as ordered.

Observe for adverse reactions, especially CNS side-effects.

CLINICAL ALERT: Withdrawal from prolonged high dosages should be gradual because abrupt cessation results in extreme fatigue and mental depression. Observe for possible abuse potential of these drugs.

Exogenous obesity: Weigh at regular intervals (biweekly, weekly) or as ordered; explore patient's attitudes toward and acceptance of dietary management; look for development of tolerance (*e.g.,* failure of drug to decrease appetite; tolerance may develop in a few weeks, but time may vary).

Abnormal behavioral syndrome: Observe and record child's activities, interactions with others (peers, adults), emotional responses, attention span.

Narcolepsy: Observe as frequently as possible; record narcoleptic episodes.

PATIENT AND FAMILY INFORMATION
Take drug early in day (especially sustained-release forms) to avoid insomnia.

Do not chew or crush sustained-release or long-acting tablets, capsules.

Do not increase dosage except on advice of physician.

May impair ability to drive or perform other tasks requiring alertness; may mask extreme fatigue and cause dizziness.

May cause nervousness, restlessness, insomnia, dizziness, dry mouth, GI disturbances. Notify physician or nurse if these effects become bothersome.

Dry mouth may be relieved by frequent sips of water, chewing gum.

Avoid other CNS stimulants, including beverages containing caffeine (*e.g.,* coffee, some carbonated drinks).

Amphotericin B, Parenteral Rx

injection: 50-mg vial   Fungizone IV

INDICATIONS
Treatment of cryptococcosis (torulosis); North American blastomycosis; disseminated forms of moniliasis; coccidioidomycosis and histoplasmosis; mucormycosis caused by species of the genera *Mucor, Rhizopus, Absidia, Entomophthora, Basidiobolus;* sporotrichosis; aspergillosis. May be helpful in treatment of American mucocutaneous leishmaniasis, but is not drug of choice in primary therapy.

Administered primarily to those with progressive, potentially fatal infections. Not used to treat common inapparent forms of fungal disease that show only positive skin or serologic tests.

CONTRAINDICATIONS
Hypersensitivity, unless condition requiring treatment is life threatening and amenable only to amphotericin B therapy.

ACTIONS
An antibiotic with activity against many species of fungi, but without effect on bacteria, rickettsiae, and viruses. It is fungistatic or fungicidal depending on concentration in body fluids and susceptibility of the fungus. It probably acts by binding to sterols in the fungus cell membrane with a resultant change in membrane permeability, which allows leakage of a variety of small molecules. Amphotericin B potentiates antifungal effects of flucytosine and other antibiotics probably by allowing concentration of these drugs into the fungal cell. It also acts synergistically in combination with flucytosine, rifampin, or tetracycline. Plasma half-life is about 24 hours; the elimination half-life is 15 days and amphotericin B is very slowly excreted by the kidneys. It has been reported that amphotericin B is highly bound to plasma proteins and is poorly dialyzable. Penetration into inflamed pleural cavities and joints is good; penetration into the parotid gland, bronchial secretions, CSF, aqueous humor, pancreas, muscle, and bone is poor.

WARNINGS
Safety for use in pregnancy is not established. Use only when clearly needed and potential benefits outweigh the unknown potential hazards to the fetus.

DRUG INTERACTIONS

Corticosteroids should not be administered concurrently unless necessary to control drug reactions. Not administered concomitantly with other nephrotoxic antibiotics and antineoplastics (*e.g.,* nitrogen mustard) except with great caution. May potentiate the effects of **digitalis** and **skeletal muscle relaxants** because of its hypokalemic action; may also increase the therapeutic effect and toxicity of **5-fluorocytosine.**

PRECAUTIONS

Prolonged therapy is usually necessary; unpleasant reactions are common when drug is given parenterally at therapeutic dosage levels. Some of these reactions are potentially dangerous. BUN, serum creatinine or creatinine clearance test, hemograms, serum potassium should be performed weekly during therapy. If the BUN exceeds 40 mg/100 ml or serum creatinine exceeds 3 mg/100 ml, discontinue drug or reduce dosage until renal function improves. Discontinue therapy if hepatic-function tests are abnormal. Whenever medication is interrupted for longer than 7 days, resume therapy by starting at lowest possible dosage and increasing gradually.

Amphotericin B should be used parenterally only in hospitalized patients or in those under close supervision by trained personnel.

ADVERSE REACTIONS

Most patients will exhibit some intolerance, often at less than therapeutic dosage. Severe reactions may be lessened by giving aspirin, antihistamines, and/or antiemetics and by maintaining sodium balance. Administration on alternate days may decrease anorexia and phlebitis. IV administration of small doses of adrenal corticosteroids just prior to or during the infusion may decrease febrile reactions. Heparin may lessen thrombophlebitis. Extravasation of drug may cause chemical irritation.

Most frequent

General toxic reactions: Fever (sometimes with shaking chills); headache; anorexia; malaise; generalized pain including muscle and joint pains.

Renal: Abnormal renal function, including hypokalemia, azotemia, hyposthenuria, renal tubular acidosis, and nephrocalcinosis, is commonly observed and usually improves on interruption of therapy. Some permanent impairment often occurs, especially in those receiving large doses (over 5 g). Supplemental alkali medication may decrease renal tubular acidosis complications.

GI: Nausea and vomiting; dyspepsia; diarrhea; cramping; epigastric pain.

Hematologic: Normochromic, normocytic anemia.

Local: Venous pain at injection site with phlebitis and thrombophlebitis.

Miscellaneous: Weight loss.

Less frequent (or rare)

Cardiovascular: Arrhythmias; ventricular fibrillation; cardiac arrest; hypertension; hypotension.

Hematologic: Coagulation defects; thrombocytopenia; leukopenia; agranulocytosis; eosinophilia; leukocytosis.

CNS: Peripheral neuropathy; convulsions; other neurologic symptoms.

Senses: Hearing loss; tinnitus; transient vertigo; blurred vision; diplopia.

GI: Melena or hemorrhagic gastroenteritis.

Renal: Anuria; oliguria; permanent damage is usually related to a large total dose.

Hepatic: Acute liver failure.

Miscellaneous: Anaphylactoid reactions; flushing.

DOSAGE

For test dose, infuse 1 mg slowly to determine patient tolerance. Therapy usually instituted with daily dose of 0.25 mg/kg and gradually increased as tolerance permits. Optimal dose is unknown and total daily dose may range up to 1 mg/kg; alternate-day dosages range up to 1.5 mg/kg. Do not exceed 1.5 mg/kg/day. Several months of therapy are usually necessary.

NURSING IMPLICATIONS

HISTORY
See Appendix 4.

PHYSICAL ASSESSMENT
Patient is often acutely ill. Therefore, perform general assessment to determine present status and identify immediate needs; check vital signs; record weight (bed scale may be necessary) for calculation of drug dosage. Baseline laboratory tests may include renal-function tests, CBC, hematocrit, serum potassium, culture and sensitivity.

ADMINISTRATION

CLINICAL ALERT: Aseptic technique must be strictly observed in all handling, because no preservative or bacteriostatic agent is present in vial.

For initial concentration of 5 mg/ml: Rapidly express 10 ml of Sterile Water for Injection *without a bacteriostatic agent* directly into lyophilized cake (which may be partially reduced to a powder following manufacture) in the vial. Use a sterile 18- to 20-gauge needle.

CLINICAL ALERT: Read diluent label, including the fine print, _carefully;_ if in doubt, check with pharmacist. _Do Not_ reconstitute with saline solutions. The use of any diluent except water, or presence of a bacteriostatic agent in the diluent, may cause precipitation. _Do Not_ administer drug in which a precipitate has formed.

Shake vial _immediately_ after adding diluent until colloidal solution is clear.

The IV infusion solution, providing 0.1 mg/ml, is then obtained by further dilution (1:50) with 5% Dextrose Injection, USP of _p_H above 4.2.

An in-line membrane filter may be used for IV administration. To assure passage of the colloidal suspension, the filter's mean pore diameter should be greater than 1 micron.

Vials should be stored in a refrigerator protected from light. The concentrate (after reconstitution) may be stored in the dark at room temperature for 24 hours, or under refrigeration for 1 week, with minimal loss of potency and clarity. Any unused material should then be discarded. Label reconstituted stored solution with date of preparation.

Solutions prepared for IV infusion (_i.e.,_ diluted 1:50) should be used promptly after preparation.

Manufacturer recommends that solution be protected from light during administration. Although solutions are light sensitive, loss of drug activity is reported to be negligible when solution is exposed to light for 8 hours. Check with physician about need for protecting infusing solution. A brown paper bag or aluminum foil may be used to cover the container during administration.

Administer by slow IV infusion over 6 hours at a concentration of 0.1 mg/ml. Physician should specify IV infusion rate or total number of hours drug is to infuse. Apply timing label or use infusion pump.

Rotate venipuncture sites. Check vein to be used for signs of thrombophlebitis, phlebitis; do not use vein if these are apparent.

ONGOING ASSESSMENTS AND NURSING MANAGEMENT

Every 15 to 30 minutes, check IV infusion for rate, needle placement in vein, signs of extravasation; check patient for adverse reactions.

Monitor vital signs q1h to q2h; more frequent determinations may be necessary if patient is critically ill or there is a change in vital signs.

If severe adverse reactions occur, slow infusion to KVO (keep vein open) or discontinue infusion and contact physician immediately. Because repeated venipunctures may decrease the number of available venipuncture sites, check with physician for preferred intervention before infusion is started.

Monitor intake and output; in some instances hourly output measurements may be warranted. Immediately report any decrease in urinary output, change in appearance (sediment, cloudiness, hematuria), or other signs of abnormal renal function (anuria, signs of hypokalemia, low urine specific gravity).

Observe for signs of hypokalemia (Appendix 6, section 6-15), hearing loss, dizziness, or tinnitus.

Maintaining sodium balance may lessen severe reactions. Periodic serum electrolytes may be ordered and hyponatremia corrected by adding foods containing sodium to diet or by IV fluid therapy.

Periodic laboratory tests will be ordered to monitor possible toxic drug effects, response to therapy.

Amphotericin B, Topical Rx

cream, lotion, oint-   Fungizone
  ment: 3%

INDICATIONS
Treatment of cutaneous and mucocutaneous mycotic infections caused by _Candida (Monilia)_ species.

CONTRAINDICATIONS
Hypersensitivity.

ACTIONS
An antibiotic with antifungal activity.

PRECAUTIONS
Should hypersensitivity occur, discontinue treatment.

ADVERSE REACTIONS
Cream may have drying effect on some skin. Local irritation (erythema, pruritus, burning sensation) sometimes occurs, particularly in folds of the skin. With lotion, rare local intolerance has included increased pruritus, with or without other evidence of local irritation, or exacerbation of preexisting candidal lesions. Allergic contact dermatitis is rare. The ointment may occasionally irritate when applied to moist skin folds.

DOSAGE

Apply liberally to the candidal lesions 2 to 4 times/day. Duration of therapy depends on patient response.

NURSING IMPLICATIONS

HISTORY
See Appendix 4.

PHYSICAL ASSESSMENT
Examine lesions; record appearance, location, size.

ADMINISTRATION
Skin should be clean and dry before application. Apply liberally to lesions and rub in.

ONGOING ASSESSMENTS AND NURSING MANAGEMENT
Hospitalized patient may prefer to self-apply medication; supervise as needed.

Inspect lesions daily; chart size and location every other day. If condition worsens or improvement is not noted in 1 to 2 weeks, notify physician.

PATIENT AND FAMILY INFORMATION
Cleanse affected areas of skin prior to application (unless directed otherwise).

Apply liberally to lesions; rub in gently.

The cream may cause drying and slight discoloration of the skin. The lotion and ointment may cause staining of nail lesions. Redness, itching, or burning may also occur, particularly in skin folds; notify physician if these effects become bothersome, if skin rash develops, or if condition being treated worsens.

Discoloration of fabrics from cream or lotion may be removed by gently handwashing the fabric with soap and warm water. Discoloration from the ointment may be removed with cleaning fluid. Be sure room is well ventilated when using cleaning fluid because inhalation of fumes can be extremely dangerous.

Ampicillin Sodium

See Penicillins.

Ampicillin With Probenecid

See Penicillins.

Amyl Nitrite

See Nitrates.

Anabolic Hormones

Ethylestrenol Rx

tablets: 2 mg	Maxibolin
elixir: 2 mg/5 ml	Maxibolin

Methandriol Rx

injection (aqueous): 50 mg/ml	Andriol, Methydiol Aqueous
injection (in oil): 50 mg/ml	Andriol, Methydiol in Oil, *Generic*

Nandrolone Decanoate Rx

injection (in oil): 50 mg/ml	Analone-50, Androlone-D 50, Deca-Durabolin, Hybolin Decanoate, *Generic*
injection (in oil): 100 mg/ml	Anabolin LA 100, Analone-100, Androlone-D 100, Deca-Durabolin, Hybolin Decanoate, *Generic*
injection (in oil): 200 mg/ml	Deca-Durabolin

Nandrolone Phenpropionate Rx

injection (in oil): 25 mg/ml	Androlone, Durabolin, Hybolin Improved, Nandrobolic, Nandrolin, *Generic*
injection (in oil): 50 mg/ml	Anabolin I.M., Androlone 50, Durabolin, Hybolin Improved, *Generic*

Oxandrolone Rx

tablets: 2.5 mg	Anavar

Oxymetholone Rx

tablets: 50 mg	Anadrol-50

Stanozolol Rx

tablets: 2 mg	Winstrol

INDICATIONS
See below for approved indications of specific drugs.

Weight gain: In those who are underweight because of recent illness or constitutional factors contributing to a catabolic state.

Senile and postmenopausal osteoporosis: Probably effective—are without value as primary therapy, but may be of value as adjunctive therapy. Equal or greater consideration should be given to diet, calcium balance, physical therapy, good general health measures.

Corticosteroid catabolism: May reverse the profound nitrogen loss that occurs during administration of corticosteroids. If not corrected, such loss may lead to muscle wasting and osteoporosis, especially in postmenopausal women.

Anemia: Androgens stimulate erythropoiesis and may be of value in treating certain types of anemia.

ETHYLESTRENOL
Weight gain; adjunctive therapy in osteoporosis; corticosteroid catabolism; anemias.

METHANDRIOL
"Possibly effective" as adjunctive therapy in senile and postmenopausal osteoporosis.

NANDROLONE DECANOATE
"Probably effective" as adjunctive therapy in senile and postmenopausal osteoporosis; possibly effective for conditions in which potent tissue-building or protein-sparing action is desired (_e.g.,_ pre- and postsurgical care, burns), in control of metastatic breast cancer, as adjunctive therapy in certain types of refractory anemia.

NANDROLONE PHENPROPIONATE
Control of metastatic breast cancer.

OXANDROLONE
Weight gain; adjunctive therapy in osteoporosis; protein catabolism associated with prolonged administration of corticosteroids.

OXYMETHOLONE
Anemias caused by deficient red cell production; acquired aplastic anemia; congenital aplastic anemia; myelofibrosis and the hypoplastic anemias due to myelotoxic drugs.

STANOZOLOL
Aplastic anemia. Probably effective as adjunctive, but not primary, therapy in senile and postmenopausal osteoporosis.

CONTRAINDICATIONS
Hypersensitivity; men with carcinoma of the breast, prostate; carcinoma of the breast in some females; pregnancy (because of masculinization of fetus); pituitary insufficiency; those with history of myocardial infarction because of hypercholesterolemic effects; nephrosis or nephrotic stage of nephritis; hepatic dysfunction. Evidence of beneficial effects in prematures and newborns is lacking; use is not recommended.

ACTIONS
Promote body-tissue-building processes and reverse catabolic or tissue-depleting processes. Administer adequate amount of calories and protein to achieve positive nitrogen balance. Whether this positive nitrogen balance is of primary benefit in utilization of protein-building dietary substances has not been established. The androgenic properties of anabolic agents may cause serious disturbances of growth and sexual development if given to young children. These agents suppress the gonadotropic functions of the pituitary and may exert a direct effect on the testes.

Anabolic steroids have _not_ been proven to enhance athletic ability. Their serious health hazards minimize any potential gain they may confer.

These agents are derived from, or are closely related to, the androgen testosterone and have both androgenic and anabolic activity. Although claimed to possess a high-anabolic, low-androgenic activity ratio, the dissociation of anabolic from androgenic effects is incomplete and variable.

PRECAUTIONS
Hepatotoxicity: Hepatotoxic effects, including jaundice, are common with prescribed dosage. Clinical jaundice may be painless, with or without pruritus. It may also be associated with acute hepatic enlargement and right-upper-quadrant pain. Drug-induced jaundice is usually reversible when medication is discontinued. Continued therapy has been associated with hepatic coma and death. Prolonged administration of oxymetholone and other androgens to those with congenital and acquired aplastic anemia has resulted in hepatocellular carcinoma and peliosis hepatitis (blood-filled cysts in the liver).

Virilization: May occur in women. Amenorrhea usually occurs in the adult woman. Concomitant administration of large doses of progestational agents for menorrhagia is not recommended. Discontinue drug if menstrual irregularities occur until cause is determined.

Benign prostatic hypertrophy: Use with caution in such patients.

Iron deficiency: Has been observed. Periodic determinations of serum iron, iron-binding capacity recommended. Deficiency may be treated with supplementary iron.

Tartrazine sensitivity: Some of these products contain tartrazine (see Appendix 6, section 6-23).

Leukemia: Has been observed in those with aplastic anemia treated with oxymetholone.

Edema: Caution is required in administering to those with cardiac, renal, or hepatic disease. Edema, with or without congestive heart failure, may occur occasionally. Concomitant administration with adrenal steroid or ACTH may add to edema. This is generally controllable with diuretic and/or digitalis therapy.

Serum cholesterol levels: May increase or decrease during therapy; use caution in administering to those with a history of myocardial infarction or coronary artery disease.

Hypercalcemia: May develop both spontaneously and as result of hormonal therapy in women with disseminated breast carcinoma. If hypercalcemia develops, discontinue therapy.

Use in children: May accelerate epiphyseal maturation more rapidly than linear growth; effect may continue for 6 months after drug is stopped. Monitor patient by x-ray studies at 3- to 6-month intervals and discontinue drug well before bone age reaches the norm for chronological age to avoid risk of compromising adult height.

Benign prostatic hypertrophy: Use with caution in patients with benign prostatic hypertrophy.

DRUG INTERACTIONS

May potentiate **oral-anticoagulant** effects; dosage of anticoagulant may have to be decreased. Requirements for **insulin** or **oral hypoglycemic agent** may be decreased in insulin-dependent diabetics. *Methandrostenolone* may increase the therapeutic and toxic response to **corticosteroids. Oxyphenbutazone** plasma levels may be increased by concomitant administration of anabolic hormones.

Drug/lab tests

Interferences may occur in the following.

Glucose tests: Fasting blood sugar, glucose tolerance test.

Thyroid-function tests: Decrease in protein-bound iodine, T_4-binding capacity, radioactive-iodine uptake. Increase in T_3 uptake by red blood cells or resin.

Hepatic-function tests: SGOT; serum bilirubin; alkaline phosphatase.

Electrolytes: Retention of sodium, chloride, water, potassium, calcium, inorganic phosphates.

Blood coagulation tests: May alter clotting factors II, V, VII, X.

Miscellaneous: Creatinine; creatinine excretion; 17-ketosteroids; metyrapone test; serum cholesterol.

ADVERSE REACTIONS

Hepatotoxicity is the most serious reaction. Increase in serum bilirubin, with or without an increase in SGOT and SGPT, indicates a higher degree of excretory dysfunction. Reversible clinical jaundice may occur. Continued therapy may be associated with hepatic coma, death.

GI: Nausea; vomiting; diarrhea; abdominal fullness; loss of appetite; burning of tongue. Symptoms resembling those of peptic ulcer have been reported.

CNS: Excitation, insomnia, chills.

Virilization: Virilization is the most common undesirable side-effect; acne occurs frequently in all age groups. *Prepubertal males:* First signs are phallic enlargement, increase in frequency of erection; hirsutism and increased skin pigmentation may also occur. *Postpubertal males:* Inhibition of testicular function with oligospermia, decrease in seminal volume, change in libido, impotence (with prolonged therapy), gynecomastia, testicular atrophy. Chronic priapism, male-pattern baldness, epididymitis, and bladder irritability have been reported. *Females:* Hirsutism, hoarseness or deepening of voice, clitoral enlargement, change in libido, menstrual irregularities, male-pattern baldness. Voice change and clitoral enlargement are usually not reversible. Use of estrogens will not prevent virilization.

Fluid and electrolyte imbalance: Retention of sodium, chlorides, water, potassium, phosphates, and calcium has occurred.

Other: Muscle cramps, premature closure of epiphyses in children, habituation, toxic confusion, choreiform movement.

OVERDOSAGE

Symptoms: Those associated with the known effects of the drug.

Treatment: Symptomatic and supportive. Evacuate stomach by emesis and, if indicated, gastric lavage. Monitor liver function.

DOSAGE

ETHYLESTRENOL

Will produce an anabolic effect in daily doses that need not exceed 0.1 mg/kg. It is recommended that drug be given for 6 weeks. If, at the end of a 4-week rest period, indication for use continues, treatment may be resumed for an additional 6 weeks.

Adults: Average dose is 4 mg/day; higher doses of 6 mg/day or 8 mg/day for severe catabolic stress or other complicating factors may be required initially. Reduce higher doses following discernible response.

Children: Average dose is 2 mg/day; will vary according to age, size, and underlying disease. Satisfactory response is usually noted with 1 mg/day to 3 mg/day. After initial 6-week period, x-rays are usually taken to determine amount of bone maturation before reinstituting therapy.

METHANDRIOL
IM use only.

Adults: 10 mg/day to 40 mg/day of the aqueous preparation or 50 mg to 100 mg once or twice weekly of the preparation in oil.

Children: 5 mg/day to 10 mg/day, or less frequently, until susceptibility to androgenic effects has been ruled out.

NANDROLONE DECANOATE
If possible, therapy should be intermittent. Duration of therapy will depend on response and appearance of adverse reactions.

Adults: Average dose is 50 mg to 100 mg every 3 to 4 weeks.

Children (2–13 years): Average dose is 25 mg to 50 mg every 3 to 4 weeks.

Higher doses may be required for treatment of metastatic breast cancer, refractory anemias, and so on. Recommended dose is 100 mg/week to 200 mg/week.

NANDROLONE PHENPROPIONATE
Inject deep IM, preferably into gluteal muscle. If possible, therapy should be intermittent. Duration of therapy depends on response and appearance of adverse reactions.

Adults: Recommended dose is 25 mg/week to 50 mg/week.

Children (2–12 years): Recommended dose is 12.5 mg to 25 mg every 2 to 4 weeks.

Higher doses may be required for treatment of metastatic breast cancer, refractory anemias, and so on. Recommended dose is 50 mg/week to 100 mg/week based on therapeutic response and consideration of the benefit–risk ratio.

OXANDROLONE
Adults: Average dose is 2.5 mg 2 to 4 times/day. Response varies; a daily dosage of as little as 2.5 mg or up to 20 mg may be required. A 2- to 4-week course of therapy is usually adequate and may be repeated intermittently as needed.

Children: Total daily dose is 0.25 mg/kg, repeated intermittently as needed.

OXYMETHOLONE
Recommended dose for children and adults is 1 mg/kg/day to 5 mg/kg/day. Usual effective starting dose is 1 mg/kg/day to 2 mg/kg/day; higher doses may be required. Doses are individualized. Response is not always immediate; a minimum trial of 3 to 6 months should be given. Following remission, some patients may be maintained without the drug and others may be maintained with a lower daily dosage. Continuous maintenance is usually necessary in those with congenital aplastic anemia.

STANOZOLOL
Therapy should be intermittent. Duration of treatment depends on patient response and appearance of adverse reactions.

Adults: Suggested initial dose is 2 mg tid, just before or with meals. Higher doses have been employed in those with bone-marrow damage and patients on corticosteroid therapy. For young women who appear particularly susceptible to the androgenic effects of the drug, a dosage of 2 mg bid appears adequate for long-term administration. If this amount does not produce desired results, dosage may be raised to 2 mg tid.

Children: 6 to 12 years, 2 mg tid; under 6 years, 1 mg bid.

NURSING IMPLICATIONS

HISTORY
See Appendix 4.

PHYSICAL ASSESSMENT
Evaluate general physical and nutritional status; weight; blood pressure, pulse, respirations. Baseline laboratory studies may include serum cholesterol, hepatic-function tests, CBC.

ADMINISTRATION
Oral: Give immediately before or with meals.
Intramuscular: Preferred site is gluteal muscle.

ONGOING ASSESSMENTS AND NURSING MANAGEMENT
Observe for jaundice; check sclera, skin color (in natural rather than fluorescent or incandescent light). If jaundice is suspected or apparent, withhold next dose and notify physician.

When used for weight gain, weigh daily, weekly, or as ordered.

A good dietary regimen is necessary to promote weight gain; obtain dietitian consultation if diet is taken poorly.

Observe children and women for signs of virilization; inform physician of its appearance because drug may need to be withdrawn or dosage reduced. If continued drug therapy is necessary and virilization is allowed to develop, the female patient may be responsive to suggestions such as use of makeup to disguise acne, skin pigmentation, facial hair; change of hair style or use of wig to disguise male-pattern baldness.

Observe for signs of hypercalcemia (Appendix 6, section 6-13) in women with disseminated breast carcinoma; report observations to physician because drug may be discontinued.

Observe for evidence of edema, especially in lower extremities. If it is apparent, notify physician because a salt-restricted diet or diuretics may be necessary.

Periodic laboratory studies may be ordered, such as hepatic-function tests, CBC, serum cholesterol, fasting blood sugar (FBS), serum electrolytes. Periodic hand and wrist x-rays of children to monitor epiphyseal changes are recommended. Include name of drug and dose on all laboratory and x-ray request slips, because anabolic-steroid therapy may alter some test results.

Diabetic patient: Check urine for glucose, ketone bodies qid. Notify physician if percentage of urine glucose increases, ketonuria is present, or signs of hypoglycemia are noted because dosage of insulin or oral hypoglycemic agent may require adjustment.

PATIENT AND FAMILY INFORMATION

May cause nausea, GI upset; take with food or meals. Notify physician or nurse if jaundice occurs.

Keep scheduled physician or clinic appointments because close monitoring of therapy is essential.

Diabetic patients: Glucose tolerance may be altered; monitor urine glucose frequently and report abnormalities to physician.

Female patients: Notify physician or nurse if hoarseness, deepening of voice, male-pattern baldness, hirsutism, acne, clitoral enlargement, or menstrual irregularities occur.

Androgens

Fluoxymesterone Rx

tablets: 2 mg	Halotestin
tablets: 5 mg	Halotestin, Ora-Testryl
tablets: 10 mg	Android-F, Halotestin, *Generic*

Methyltestosterone Rx

tablets: 10 mg	Android-10, Metandren, Oreton Methyl, *Generic*
capsules: 10 mg	Testred, Virilon

tablets: 25 mg	Android-25, Metandren, Oreton Methyl, *Generic*
tablets, buccal: 5 mg	Android-5, Metandren Linguets
tablets, buccal: 10 mg	Metandren Linguets, Oreton Methyl, *Generic*

Testosterone (in Aqueous Suspension) Rx

injection: 25 mg/ml	*Generic*
injection: 50 mg/ml	Histerone 50, Testaqua, Testoject-50, *Generic*
injection: 100 mg/ml	Andro 100, Android-T, Histerone 100, Testaqua, *Generic*

Testosterone Cypionate (in Oil) Rx

injection: 50 mg/ml	Depo-Testosterone
injection: 100 mg/ml	Andro-Cyp 100, Andronate 100, depAndro 100, Depo-Testosterone, Duratest 100, Testoject-LA, *Generic*
injection: 200 mg/ml	Andro-Cyp 200, Andronate 200, Depo-Testosterone, Depotest, Duratest 200, depAndro 200, Testa-C, T-Ionate P.A., *Generic*

Testosterone Enanthate (in Oil) Rx

injection: 100 mg/ml	Android-T, Everone, Testate, Testone L.A., *Generic*
injection: 200 mg/ml	Andro-L.A. 200, Andryl 200, Anthatest, Delatestryl, Everone, Testone L.A. 200, Testostroval P.A., *Generic* Testoject-E.P.
injection: 200 mg testosterone enanthate, 25 mg testosterone propionate/ml	

Testosterone Propionate (in Oil) Rx

injection: 25 mg	*Generic*
injection: 50 mg, 100 mg	Testex, *Generic*

INDICATIONS

Males: Replacement therapy in hypogonadism associated with deficiency or absence of endogenous testosterone. Prior to puberty, androgen replacement will be needed during adolescent years for development of secondary sex characteristics. Prolonged androgen treatment is needed to maintain sexual characteristics in these and other men who develop testosterone deficiency after puberty. Androgens may be used to stimulate puberty in men in carefully selected cases of delayed puberty.

Females: May be used secondarily in women with advancing inoperable metastatic (skeletal) breast cancer who are 1 to 5 years past menopause. Primary goal of therapy is ablation of the ovaries. Other methods of counteracting estrogen activity are adrenalectomy, hypophysectomy, and antiestrogen therapy. This treatment has also been used in premenopausal women who have benefited from oophorectomy and are considered to have a hormone-responsive tumor. Methyltestosterone, fluoxymesterone, and testosterone propionate have been used in the management of postpartum breast pain and engorgement in the nonnursing mother.

CONTRAINDICATIONS

Men with carcinoma of the breast or known or suspected carcinoma of the prostate. Also contraindicated in women who are or may become pregnant because androgens cause virilization of the external genitalia of the female fetus. The degree of masculinization is related to the amount of drug given and age of the fetus, with masculinization most likely to occur when androgens are given in the first trimester. If the patient becomes pregnant while taking androgens, she should be apprised of the potential hazard to the fetus.

ACTIONS

Testosterone, produced by the Leydig cells of the testis, is the primary endogenous androgen. Fluoxymesterone and methyltestosterone are synthetic derivatives of testosterone that have predominant anabolic and minor androgenic activity. Endogenous hormones are responsible for normal growth and development of the male sex organs and for maintenance of secondary sex characteristics. These drugs also cause retention of nitrogen, sodium, potassium, and phosphorus and decreased urinary excretion of calcium. Androgens have been reported to increase protein anabolism and decrease protein catabolism. Oral testosterone is metabolized by the gut. Oral doses as high as 400 mg/day are needed to achieve clinically effective blood levels. Testosterone esters in oil are absorbed slowly; thus testosterone cypionate and enanthate can be given at 2- to 4-week intervals. Exogenous administration of androgens inhibits release of endogenous testosterone through feedback inhibition of pituitary LH. Large doses may suppress spermatogenesis through feedback inhibition of pituitary FSH.

WARNINGS

Patients with breast cancer: Androgen therapy may cause hypercalcemia by stimulating osteolysis. If this occurs, discontinue drug.

Hepatic effects: Prolonged use of high doses has been associated with peliosis hepatitis and hepatic neoplasms (see _Precautions, Anabolic Hormones)._ Cholestatic hepatitis and jaundice occur with fluoxymesterone and methyltestosterone at a relatively low dose. If cholestatic hepatitis with jaundice or abnormal hepatic-function studies occur, discontinue drug and determine etiology. Drug-induced jaundice is reversible when drug is discontinued.

Geriatric patients: May be at an increased risk of developing prostatic hypertrophy, prostatic carcinoma.

Edema: With or without congestive heart failure, edema may be a serious complication in those with preexisting cardiac, renal, or hepatic disease. In addition to discontinuation of drug, diuretic therapy may be required.

Gynecomastia: Frequently develops and occasionally persists in those treated for hypogonadism.

Bone maturation: Use androgens cautiously in healthy males with delayed puberty. Monitor bone maturation by assessing bone age of the wrist and hand every 6 months.

Use in lactation: It is not known whether androgens are excreted in human milk. Because of the potential for serious adverse reactions in breast-fed infants, a decision should be made whether to discontinue breast-feeding or discontinue drug.

Use in children: Use androgen therapy very cautiously in children; should be used only by specialists who are aware of the adverse effects on bone maturation.

PRECAUTIONS

General: Observe women for signs of virilization (deepening of voice, hirsutism, acne, enlarged clitoris, menstrual irregularities). Discontinuing drug when mild virilism is evident is necessary to prevent irreversible virilization. Some virilization will be tolerated during treatment of breast carcinoma.

Laboratory monitoring: Women with disseminated breast carcinoma should have frequent determination of urine and serum calcium levels during therapy. Because of hepatotoxicity associated with methyltestosterone and fluoxymesterone, periodic hepatic-function tests are obtained. X-ray examination of bone age should be made every 6 months during treatment of prepubertal males. Hemoglobin and hematocrit are checked periodically for polycythemia in patients who are receiving high doses of androgens.

Hypercholesterolemia: Serum cholesterol levels may increase or decrease during therapy. Periodic determinations of serum cholesterol are recommended.

Carcinogenesis: Hepatocellular carcinoma (rare) in those receiving long-term therapy in high doses.

Tartrazine sensitivity: Some products contain tartrazine (Appendix 6, section 6-23).

Others: If abnormal bleeding develops, discontinue drug until etiology is determined.

DRUG INTERACTIONS

Certain testosterone derivatives may decrease anticoagulant requirements in patients receiving **oral anticoagulants**. Anticoagulant dosage may need to be decreased in order to maintain the prothrombin time at desired therapeutic level. Close monitoring, especially when androgens are started or stopped, is essential. Concurrent administration of **oxyphenbutazone** may result in elevated serum levels of oxyphenbutazone. Androgens may decrease blood glucose and requirements for **insulin** or **oral hypoglycemic agents** in diabetic patients. Concomitant use of androgens with **adrenal steroids** or **ACTH** may potentiate edema resulting from androgen use.

Drug/lab tests

Alterations may occur in the following.

Glucose tests: Fasting blood sugar (FBS), glucose tolerance test.

Thyroid-function tests: May decrease levels of thyroxine-binding globulin, resulting in decreased T_4 serum levels and increased resin uptake of T_3 and T_4. Free thyroid hormones remain unchanged, and there is no clinical evidence of thyroid dysfunction.

Blood coagulation tests: Suppression of clotting factors II, V, VII, X.

Miscellaneous: Creatinine and creatine excretion lasting up to 2 weeks after discontinuing therapy; 17-ketosteroid excretion; metyrapone test.

ADVERSE REACTIONS

Female: Most common are amenorrhea and other menstrual irregularities; inhibition of gonadotropin secretion; virilization, including deepening of voice, clitoral enlargement (usually not reversible after drug is discontinued); virilization of external genitalia of the female fetus.

Male: Gynecomastia; excessive frequency and duration of penile erections; inhibition of testicular function; testicular atrophy; impotence; chronic priapism; decreased ejaculatory volume; epididymitis; bladder irritability; phallic enlargement. Oligospermia may occur at high dosages.

Skin, appendages: Hirsutism, male-pattern baldness, acne.

Fluid and electrolyte disturbances: Retention of sodium, chloride, water, potassium, calcium, inorganic phosphates. Hypercalcemia may occur, particularly in immobile patients and in those with metastatic breast carcinoma.

GI: Nausea; cholestatic jaundice; alterations in hepatic-function tests; rarely, hepatocellular neoplasms, peliosis hepatitis.

Hematologic: Suppression of clotting factors II, V, VII, X; bleeding in patients on concomitant anticoagulant therapy; polycythemia; leukopenia.

Nervous system: Increased or decreased libido; headache; anxiety; depression; generalized paresthesia.

Metabolic/endocrine: Increased serum cholesterol; menstrual irregularities; inhibition of gonadotropin; female virilization.

Miscellaneous: Inflammation, pain at site of IM injection or subcutaneous implantation of testosterone-containing pellets; stomatitis with buccal preparations; rarely, anaphylactoid reactions.

DOSAGE

Administer as oral or buccal tablets, IM. Do not administer IV. Dosage varies depending on age, sex, and diagnosis and is adjusted according to the patient's response and appearance of adverse reactions.

FLUOXYMESTERONE

Male: Hypogonadism; impotence due to testicular deficiency; male climacteric—2 mg/day to 10 mg/day; *delayed puberty*—2 mg/day and increase gradually.

Female: Inoperable carcinoma of breast—15 mg/day to 30 mg/day in divided doses; continue for 1 month for a subjective response and 2 to 3 months for an objective response; *postpartum breast engorgement*—2.5 mg when active labor starts; thereafter administer 5 mg to 10 mg daily in divided doses for 4 to 5 days.

METHYLTESTOSTERONE

Absorption through buccal mucosa into systemic circulation provides twice the bioavailability of oral tablets.

Male: Eunuchoidism; eunuchism; male climacteric; impotence resulting from androgen deficiency—10 mg/day to 40 mg/day (5 mg to 20 mg buccal); *postpubertal cryptorchidism*—30 mg/day (15 mg buccal).

Female: Postpartum breast pain, engorgement—80 mg/day (40 mg buccal) for 3 to 5 days; *breast cancer*—200 mg/day (100 mg buccal).

TESTOSTERONE (IN AQUEOUS SUSPENSION)

IM use only; do not inject IV. Shake well before use. These preparations are absorbed relatively slowly; frequent injections may cause overdosage.

Male: Eunuchoidism, eunuchism, male climacteric symptoms, impotence due to androgen deficiency: 10 mg to 25 mg 2 or 3 times/week.

Female: Postpartum breast engorgement—25 mg to 50 mg daily for 3 to 4 days, starting at time of delivery. *Carcinoma of the breast*—100 mg, 3 times/week as long as improvement is maintained. If response will occur, it will be apparent within 3 months of beginning therapy. When disease becomes progressive, discontinue therapy and observe patient for another period of improvement known as "rebound regression." These doses will likely have masculinizing effects, particularly in young women. There may be a disturbing increase in libido, for which sedation may be helpful. Acceleration of tumor growth may occur occasionally during androgen therapy, in which case immediate cessation of drug is indicated. In some of these cases the use of estrogen at this point causes regression.

TESTOSTERONE CYPIONATE (IN OIL)

IM injection only, deep into gluteal muscle.

Eunuchism, eunuchoidism, severe deficiency after castration, male climacteric when secondary to androgen deficiency—200 mg to 400 mg every 4 weeks; *oligospermia*—100 mg to 200 mg every 4 to 6 weeks; *suppression and rebound stimulation*—200 mg every week for 6 to 12 weeks; *palliation of inoperable mammary cancer in women*—200 mg to 400 mg every 2 to 4 weeks.

TESTOSTERONE ENANTHATE (IN OIL)

See Testosterone Cypionate, above.

TESTOSTERONE PROPIONATE (IN OIL)

See Testosterone (in aqueous suspension), above.

NURSING IMPLICATIONS

HISTORY
See Appendix 4.

PHYSICAL ASSESSMENT

Primary hypogonadism, hypogonadotropic hypogonadism, delayed puberty: Record height, weight. Baseline laboratory studies may include serum electrolytes, hepatic-function tests. X-ray examination of wrist and hand is obtained prior to therapy in prepubertal males.

Metastatic carcinoma of breast: Evaluate present status (physical, emotional, nutritional); identify problem areas such as pain, limitation of movement, ability to participate in activities of daily living. Baseline laboratory tests may in-clude CBC, hepatic-function tests, serum electrolytes, serum and urine calcium.

ADMINISTRATION

IM preparations given in gluteal muscle; warn patient that inflammation and pain may be noted at injection site.

Buccal tablets: Instruct patient in placement of tablet; warn not to swallow, but to allow tablet to dissolve; patient should not drink or smoke until tablet has dissolved.

Oral tablets: Give with meals.

ONGOING ASSESSMENTS AND NURSING MANAGEMENT

Breast carcinoma: Record weight (if on complete bedrest, weigh every 3 to 4 days using bed scale, or as ordered); record vital signs; evaluate mental status; observe for adverse effects, especially early signs of virilization (deepening or hoarseness of voice, hirsutism), signs of hypercalcemia (Appendix 6, section 6-13), hypernatremia (Appendix 6, section 6-17), hyperkalemia (Appendix 6, section 6-15), evidence of jaundice; check lower extremities for evidence of edema.

If virilization develops and must be tolerated, patient may be responsive to suggestions such as use of makeup to disguise acne, skin pigmentation, and facial hair or change of hairstyle or use of wig to disguise male-pattern baldness.

If androgen therapy is discontinued and additional treatment modalities are not possible, patient will need emotional support from all members of the health team.

Postpartum breast engorgement/pain: Check breasts for pain/discomfort when applying or reapplying breast binder or supportive brassiere; ask patient to describe any breast discomfort or pain. Notify physician if pain/discomfort remains unrelieved or becomes worse.

Hypogonadism: Physician usually discusses response to hormone therapy with patient; under certain conditions, nurse may assume this function.

Patient on complete bedrest, limited activity: Obtain physician's approval for ROM exercises bid or tid to prevent or decrease mobilization of calcium from the bone and consequent hypercalcemia.

Diabetic patient: Check urine qid for glucose, ketone bodies. Observe for signs of hypoglycemia (Appendix 6, section 6-14), especially during time of peak effect of antidiabetic agent. Contact physician if apparent hypoglycemic episode occurs because dosage adjustment of antidiabetic agent may be necessary.

Patient receiving oral anticoagulant ther-

apy: Check for petechiae, ecchymosis, hematuria, marked fluctuations in prothrombin time, partial thromboplastin time; immediately report bleeding tendencies, fluctuations in laboratory tests to physician.

General considerations: If abnormal vaginal bleeding develops, withhold next dose of drug and contact physician.

Periodic laboratory studies may be ordered, such as hepatic-function tests, CBC, serum cholesterol, fasting blood sugar (FBS), serum electrolytes, urine and serum calcium. Periodic hand, wrist x-rays of children to monitor epiphyseal changes are recommended. Include name and dose of drug on all laboratory and x-ray request slips because androgen therapy may alter some test results.

Fluid retention may be relieved by diuretics or dietary sodium restriction; in some instances, intake and output measurement may be indicated.

The anabolic effect of androgens (see Anabolic Hormones) is enhanced by adequate dietary intake of protein and calories. Some patients may have a poor dietary intake because of age, disease (*e.g.,* breast carcinoma), concurrent drug therapy (*e.g.,* narcotics). A dietary consultation may be warranted.

PATIENT AND FAMILY INFORMATION

Oral tablets: May cause GI upset; take with meals or snack.

Buccal tablets: Do not swallow; allow to dissolve between gum and cheek (preferred) or under tongue; avoid eating, drinking, smoking while tablet is in place. Change site where each tablet is dissolved.

General considerations: Notify physician or nurse if nausea, vomiting, swelling of extremities (edema), priapism, or jaundice occurs. Female patient should report hoarseness, deepening of voice, male-pattern baldness, acne, hirsutism, menstrual irregularities, enlarged clitoris, increase in libido.

Diabetic patient: If hypoglycemic episodes occur, contact physician; dosage adjustment of insulin or oral hypoglycemic agent may be necessary.

Anesthetics, General

Barbiturates

Methohexital Sodium Rx C–IV

powder for injection   Brevital Sodium

Thiamylal Sodium Rx C–III

injection   Surital

Thiopental Sodium Rx C–III

injection; rectal sus-   Pentothal
pension

INDICATIONS

Induction of anesthesia, supplementation of other anesthetic agents, IV anesthesia for short surgical procedures with minimal painful stimuli, or induction of a hypnotic state. Thiopental sodium for IV use is indicated for control of convulsive states, narcoanalysis, and narcosynthesis in psychiatric disorders. Thiopental sodium rectal suspension is recommended whenever preanesthetic sedation or basal narcosis by the rectal route is desired. It may be employed as a sole agent in selected brief minor procedures for which muscle relaxation and analgesia are not desired.

CONTRAINDICATIONS

Absolute: Latent or manifest porphyria; known hypersensitivity to barbiturates; absence of suitable veins for IV administration; status asthmaticus (thiopental).

Relative: Severe cardiovascular disease; hypotension or shock; conditions in which hypnotic effect may be prolonged or potentiated (excessive premedication, Addison's disease, hepatic or renal dysfunction, myxedema, increased blood urea, severe anemia); increased intracranial pressure; asthma; myasthenia gravis.

Rectal suspension is not used in severe respiratory embarrassment; inflammatory conditions of mouth, jaw, neck; in those who are to undergo rectal surgery; in the presence of inflammatory, ulcerative, bleeding, or neoplastic lesions of lower bowel.

ACTIONS

These ultra-short-acting barbiturates depress the CNS to produce hypnosis and anesthesia without analgesia. Administered IV, they produce anesthesia within 1 minute. Recovery after a small dose is rapid, with somnolence and retrograde amnesia. Muscle relaxation occurs about 30 seconds after unconsciousness is attained with thiopental. Methohexital does not possess muscle-relaxant properties. These drugs are frequently used to provide hypnosis during balanced anesthesia with other agents for muscle relaxation and analgesia. These drugs rapidly cross the blood–brain barrier but are rapidly redistributed from the brain to other body tissues. Duration of anesthetic activity following a single IV dose is 10 to 30 minutes for thiopental and thiamylal and 5 to 7 minutes for methohexital. Repeated doses or continuous infusion causes accumulation and slow release of the drug from lipoidal storage sites, resulting in prolonged anesthesia, somnolence, and respiratory and circulatory depression. Plasma half-life is 3 to 8 hours.

WARNINGS

May be habit forming. Resuscitative equipment and drugs should be immediately available. Repeated infusion may cause cumulative effects resulting in prolonged somnolence and respiratory and circulatory depression. Safety for use in pregnancy is not established. Use only when clearly needed and potential benefits outweigh unknown potential hazards to the fetus.

DRUG INTERACTIONS

CNS depressant effects may be additive to those of other **CNS depressants,** including **alcohol.**

PRECAUTIONS

Respiratory depression, apnea, hypotension may occur owing to individual variations in tolerance or to physical status of patient. Caution is exercised in debilitated patients or those with impaired function of respiratory, circulatory, renal, hepatic, or endocrine system.

ADVERSE REACTIONS

Circulatory depression; thrombophlebitis, pain, or nerve injury at injection site; respiratory depression including apnea; laryngospasm; bronchospasm; salivation; hiccups; emergence delirium; headache; skin rashes; nausea, vomiting; skeletal muscle hyperactivity; myocardial depression; cardiac arrhythmias; prolonged somnolence and recovery; sneezing; coughing; shivering. Acute allergic reactions include erythema, pruritus, urticaria, rhinitis, dyspnea, hypotension, restlessness, anxiety, abdominal pain, peripheral vascular collapse. Rectal irritation, diarrhea, cramping, and rectal bleeding have been reported following rectal instillation. If evacuation of drug occurs, effects of retained portion are assessed before repeat dose is administered.

DOSAGE

These drugs are administered by a physician or CRNA.

METHOHEXITAL SODIUM

Administered IV. Dosage is individualized according to patient response. A 1% solution is recommended for induction and maintenance by intermittent injection. Usual range is 5 ml to 12 ml of 1% solution (50 mg to 120 mg); this induction dose will provide anesthesia for 5 to 7 minutes. Continuous drip method uses a 0.2% solution with the rate of flow individualized.

THIAMYLAL SODIUM

Administered IV. Dosage is individualized according to patient response. A 2.5% solution is recommended for induction; a dilute solution (0.3%) may be administered by continuous drip.

THIOPENTAL SODIUM

Administered by IV or rectal route. Individual response is varied; therefore, there is no fixed dosage. _Anesthesia dose:_ Average adult injection is 50 mg to 75 mg (2 ml to 3 ml of 2.5% solution) at 20- to 40-second intervals. Once anesthesia is established, additional injections of 25 mg to 50 mg may be given. _When used for convulsive states:_ 75 mg to 125 mg (3 ml to 5 ml of 2.5% solution), given as soon as possible after convulsion begins. _Rectal suspension:_ Onset of action is usually 8 to 10 minutes. _Preanesthetic sedation:_ Average dose is 1 g/75 lb instilled rectally.

NURSING IMPLICATIONS
See p 56.

Nonbarbiturates

Etomidate Rx

injection: 2 mg/ml   Amidate

ACTIONS AND INDICATIONS

Etomidate is a hypnotic without analgesic activity for IV use in the induction of general anesthesia, supplementation of subpotent anesthetic agents (_e.g.,_ nitrous oxide), during maintenance of anesthesia for short operative procedures such as dilation and curretage, cervical conization.

ADVERSE REACTIONS

Most frequent are transient venous pain, transient skeletal muscle movements, averting movements, tonic movements, eye movements. Also seen are hyperventilation, hypoventilation, apnea of short duration (5–90 seconds with spontaneous recovery), laryngospasm, hiccups, snoring, hypertension, hypotension, tachycardia, bradycardia, other arrhythmias, and postoperative nausea and/or vomiting following induction of anesthesia.

DOSAGE

For adults and children above 10 years, dose will vary between 0.2 mg/kg and 0.6 mg/kg and is individualized. Usual induction is 0.3 mg/kg injected over a period of 30 to 60 seconds. Smaller increments may be administered to adults during short operative procedures to supplement subpotent anesthetic agents. Compatible with commonly used preanesthetic medication.

▌ NURSING IMPLICATIONS
See p 56.

Fentanyl Citrate and Droperidol Rx C–II

injection: 0.05 mg fentanyl (as citrate), 2.5 mg droperidol/ml Innovar

ACTIONS AND INDICATIONS
Combination drug containing a narcotic analgesic, fentanyl, and a neuroleptic (major tranquilizer), droperidol. The combined effect, sometimes referred to as neuroleptanalgesia, is characterized by general quiescence, reduced motor activity, and profound analgesia. Complete loss of consciousness usually does not occur from use of this combination alone. Indicated to produce tranquilization and analgesia for surgical and diagnostic procedures. May be used as an anesthetic premedication, for induction of anesthesia, and as an adjunct in the maintenance of general and regional anesthesia. Dosage is variable depending on response of patient.

ADVERSE REACTIONS
Respiratory depression; apnea; muscle rigidity; hypotension, which if untreated may lead to respiratory arrest; circulatory depression or cardiac arrest. Extrapyramidal reactions (dystonia, akathisia, oculogyric crisis) have been seen. Restlessness, hyperactivity and anxiety, elevated blood pressure, dizziness, chills and/or shivering, twitching, blurred vision, laryngospasm, bronchospasm, bradycardia, tachycardia, nausea, emesis, diaphoresis, emergence delirium, and postoperative hallucinatory episodes (sometimes associated with transient periods of mental depression) have been reported. See also *Fentanyl Citrate; Droperidol.*

ADMINISTRATION AND DOSAGE
Premedication for surgery, diagnostic procedures: 0.5 ml to 2 ml IM given 45 to 60 minutes prior to surgery, with or without atropine. Dosage is lower for elderly, debilitated patients or those who have received other depressant drugs. *Children:* 0.25 ml/20 lb body weight IM 45 to 60 minutes prior to surgery, with or without atropine.

Adjunct to general anesthesia: 1 ml/20–25 lb of body weight IV. Smaller doses may be given. *Children:* Total combined dose for induction and maintenance is 0.5 ml/20 lb body weight.

▌ NURSING IMPLICATIONS
See p 56.

Ketamine Hydrochloride Rx

injection: 50 mg/ml, 100 mg/ml Ketaject, Ketalar

ACTIONS AND INDICATIONS
Rapid-acting general anesthetic producing an anesthetic state characterized by profound analgesia, normal pharyngeal–laryngeal reflexes, normal or slightly enhanced skeletal muscle tone, cardiovascular and respiratory stimulation, and occasionally transient and minimal respiratory depression. Recommended for diagnostic and surgical procedures that do not require skeletal muscle relaxation; for induction of anesthesia prior to the administration of other general anesthetic agents; for supplementation of low-potency agents such as nitrous oxide.

ADVERSE REACTIONS
Blood pressure, pulse may be elevated but hypotension and bradycardia may also occur; respirations often stimulated but depression of respirations and apnea may be seen with too-rapid injection; diplopia; nystagmus; enhanced skeletal muscle tone manifested by tonic and clonic movements; anorexia; nausea, vomiting.

Emergence reactions have occurred in approximately 12% of patients and vary in severity and type. Reactions seen include dreamlike state, hallucinations, vivid imagery, and delirium. In some instances these have been accompanied by confusion, excitement, and irrational behavior, with some patients describing these as an unpleasant experience. Duration of emergence reactions is a few hours; a few patients have experienced recurrences of these effects up to 24 hours postoperatively. No permanent psychological effects have been reported. In order to terminate a severe emergence reaction, use of a small hypnotic dose of a short-acting or ultra-short-acting barbiturate may be required.

DOSAGE
Usual dose range is 1 mg/kg to 4.5 mg/kg IV or 6.5 mg/kg to 13 mg/kg IM for induction. Subsequent doses are titrated to response of patient.

▌ NURSING IMPLICATIONS
See p 56.

Gases

Cyclopropane

Supplied in orange cylinders. An anesthetic gas with a rapid onset of action. May be used for analgesia and induction and maintenance of anesthesia. Produces skeletal muscle relaxation in full anesthetic doses. Administered in a closed system with oxygen. Disadvantages include difficulty in detection of planes of anesthesia, occasional laryngospasm, and cardiac arrhythmias. Postanesthetic nausea, vomiting, and headache are frequent. _Caution:_ cyclopropane/oxygen mixtures are _explosive._

NURSING IMPLICATIONS
See p 56.

Ethylene

Supplied in red cylinders. An anesthetic gas with rapid onset and recovery. Provides adequate analgesia but has poor muscle-relaxant properties. Must be administered in high (80%) concentrations with oxygen (20%). Advantages include little bronchospasm and laryngospasm and little postanesthetic vomiting. Ethylene is nontoxic; hypoxia is the primary complication. _Caution:_ ethylene/oxygen mixtures are flammable and _explosive._

NURSING IMPLICATIONS
See p 56.

Nitrous Oxide

Supplied in blue cylinders. The most commonly used anesthetic gas. It is a weak anesthetic, usually used in combination with other anesthetics. Does not cause skeletal muscle relaxation. Chief danger in the use of nitrous oxide is hypoxemia; at least 20% oxygen should be used. A primary advantage over other anesthetic gases is that it is nonexplosive.

NURSING IMPLICATIONS
See p 56.

Volatile Liquids

Enflurane Rx

liquid: 125 ml, 250 ml   Ethrane

INDICATIONS AND ADMINISTRATION
An inhalation anesthetic. Induction and recovery from anesthesia are rapid. There is mild stimulus to salivation or tracheobronchial secretions when used alone. Pharyngeal and laryngeal reflexes are readily obtunded. The level of anesthesia changes rapidly. Reduces ventilation as depth of anesthesia increases. Provokes a sigh response reminiscent of that seen with diethyl ether. Progressive increases in depth of anesthesia produce corresponding increases in hypotension. Heart rate remains relatively constant without significant bradycardia. Cardiac rhythm remains stable. Elevation of carbon dioxide level in arterial blood does not alter cardiac rhythm. Muscle relaxation is adequate for intra-abdominal surgery at normal levels of anesthesia. Should greater relaxation be necessary, minimal doses of muscle relaxants may be used. Induction of anesthesia with enflurane 3.5% to 4.5% is in 7 to 10 minutes. Surgical levels of anesthesia may be attained with 1.5% to 3% concentrations.

NURSING IMPLICATIONS
See p 56.

Halothane Rx

liquid: 125 ml   Fluothane
liquid: 250 ml   Fluothane, _Generic_

INDICATIONS AND ADMINISTRATION
Inhalation anesthetic for induction and maintenance of general anesthesia. Induction and recovery are rapid and depth of anesthesia can be rapidly altered. Not an irritant to the respiratory tract and no increase in salivary or bronchial secretions ordinarily occurs. Pharyngeal and laryngeal reflexes are rapidly obtunded. Halothane causes bronchodilation. Hypoxia, acidosis, or apnea may develop during deep anesthesia. Sensitizes the myocardial conduction system to the action of epinephrine and norepinephrine; the combination may cause serious cardiac arrhythmias. Produces moderate muscle relaxation. Muscle relaxants are used as adjuncts in order to maintain lighter levels of anesthesia. The induction and maintenance doses vary. May be administered with oxygen or a mixture of oxygen and nitrous oxide.

NURSING IMPLICATIONS
See p 56.

Isoflurane Rx

liquid: 100 ml   Forane

INDICATIONS AND ADMINISTRATION
For induction and maintenance of general anesthesia. For induction, inspired concentrations of

1.5% to 3% usually produce surgical anesthesia in 7 to 10 minutes. Surgical anesthesia may be sustained with a 1% to 2.5% concentration when nitrous oxide is used concomitantly.

NURSING IMPLICATIONS

See below.

Methoxyflurane Rx

liquid: 15 ml, 125 ml   Penthrane

INDICATIONS AND ADMINISTRATION

Provides anesthesia or analgesia. Used (usually in combination with nitrous oxide) to provide anesthesia for surgical procedures in which the total duration of administration is anticipated to be 4 hours or less and when methoxyflurane is not to be used in concentrations that will provide skeletal muscle relaxation. May be used alone or in combination with oxygen and nitrous oxide for analgesia in obstetrics and minor surgical procedures. When used alone in safe concentration it will not produce appreciable skeletal muscle relaxation; a skeletal muscle relaxing agent is usually used as an adjunct. Bronchiolar constriction or laryngeal spasm is not ordinarily provoked.

NURSING IMPLICATIONS: ANESTHETICS, GENERAL

PREOPERATIVE

If laboratory or diagnostic tests are performed within 24 hours of surgery, review each test for abnormal results. If test results are not on chart, contact the appropriate laboratory or department for test results.

CLINICAL ALERTS: If *any* one or more recent laboratory or diagnostic tests are abnormal, contact the anesthesiologist or surgeon or attach a copy of the abnormal test results to the front of the patient's chart.

If the patient appears extremely apprehensive 20 to 30 minutes after receiving the preoperative medication, inform the anesthesiologist of this finding and enter observations on patient's chart.

Fentanyl citrate and droperidol may be administered by the nurse as a preoperative medication.

POSTOPERATIVE

Admit patient to recovery room according to department procedure; check airway for patency; position patient to prevent aspiration of vomitus, secretions; assess respiratory status and give oxygen if needed; check blood pressure, pulse, respirations; check IV lines; when appropriate, check Foley catheter, chest tubes, drainage tubes, casts, surgical dressing, and so on.

Review surgical and anesthesia records.

Monitor blood pressure, pulse, and respirations q5m to q15m.

Check for emergence from anesthesia q5m to q15m.

Suction prn.

Have resuscitative equipment readily available.

Exercise caution in administering narcotics; check respiratory rate before and 20 to 30 minutes after administration. Contact physician if respiratory rate is below 10/minute because a narcotic antagonist may be necessary. (Have a narcotic antagonist readily available.)

Ketamine: Keep visual, verbal, tactile stimuli to a minimum. Move patient to dimly lit area; do not talk to patient unless absolutely necessary; do not touch patient except when checking dressing, tubes, and so on or monitoring vital signs.

Anesthetics, Local, Injectable

Bupivacaine Hydrochloride Rx

injection: 0.25%, 0.5%, 0.75%	Marcaine HCl, Sensorcaine, *Generic*
injection: 0.25%, 0.5%, 0.75% with 1:200,000 epinephrine	Marcaine HCl

Chloroprocaine Hydrochloride Rx

injection: 1%, 2% (with preservatives)	Nesacaine
injection: 2%, 3% (without preservatives)	Nesacaine-CE

Dibucaine Hydrochloride Rx

injection: 1:200, 1:1500 solution	Nupercaine HCl
injection, heavy solution: 2.5 mg with 5% dextrose/ml	Nupercaine HCl

Lidocaine Hydrochloride _Rx_

injection: 0.5%	Xylocaine HCl
injection: 1%	Dilocaine, L-Caine, Lido-ject-1, Nervocaine, Nuli-caine, Ultracaine, Xylo-caine HCl, _Generic_
injection: 1.5%	Xylocaine HCl
injection: 2%	Dilocaine, Dolicaine, L-Caine, Lidoject-2, Nervo-caine, Nulicaine, Ultra-caine, Xylocaine HCl, _Generic_
injection: 4%	Duo-Trach Kit, Xylocaine HCl
injection: 1.5% w/ 7.5% dextrose, 5% w/7.5% glucose	Xylocaine HCl

With epinephrine (strength in parentheses)

injection: 0.5% (1:200,000)	Xylocaine HCl
injection: 1% (1:100,000)	Xylocaine HCl, _Generic_
injection: 1%, 1.5% (1:200,000)	Xylocaine HCl
injection: 2% (1:50,000)	Otocaine HCl, Xylocaine HCl
injection: 2% (1:100,000)	L-Caine E, Otocaine HCl, Xylocaine HCl, _Generic_
injection: 2% (1:200,000)	Xylocaine HCl

Mepivacaine Hydrochloride _Rx_

injection: 1%, 1.5%, 2%	Carbocaine
injection: 3%	Carbocaine, Isocaine HCl
injection: 2% with 1:20,000 levonor-defrin	Carbocaine with Neo-Cob-efrin, Isocaine

Prilocaine Hydrochloride _Rx_

injection: 1%, 2%, 3%	Citanest HCl
injection, plain: 4% (dental)	Citanest HCl
injection, Forte: 4% with 1:200,000 epinephrine (den-tal)	Citanest HCl

Procaine Hydrochloride, Injectable _Rx_

injection: 1%, 2%	Novocain, _Generic_
injection: 10%	Novocain

Tetracaine Hydrochloride _Rx_

injection: 1%; 0.2%, 0.3% with 6% dex-trose	Pontocaine HCl
powder for reconsti-tution	Pontocaine HCl

INDICATIONS

BUPIVACAINE HYDROCHLORIDE
Local infiltration 0.25%; epidural block 0.25%, 0.5%, 0.75%; caudal block 0.25%, 0.5%; peripheral nerve block 0.25%, 0.5%; sympathetic block 0.25%, retrobulbar block 0.75%.

CHLOROPROCAINE HYDROCHLORIDE
Infiltration and nerve block 1% to 2%; caudal and epidural block 2% or 3% (without preservative).

DIBUCAINE HYDROCHLORIDE
Isobaric spinal anesthesia 1:200, hypobaric spinal anesthesia 1:1500. For low spinal anesthesia, heavy solution is used.

LIDOCAINE HYDROCHLORIDE
Infiltration: Percutaneous 0.5%, 1%; IV regional 0.5%; oral dentistry 2%.
Peripheral nerve block: Brachial 1.5%; dental 2%; intercostal, paravertebral 1%; pudendal, paracervical obstetric 1%.
Sympathetic nerve block: Cervical (stellate gan-glion), lumbar 1%.
Central neural blocks: _Epidural_—thoracic 1%, lumbar analgesia 1%, lumbar anesthesia 1.5%, 2%.
Caudal: Obstetric analgesia 1%; surgical anes-thesia 1.5%.
Spinal anesthesia: 5% with glucose.
Low spinal or saddle block anesthesia: 1.5% with dextrose.
Retrobulbar or transtracheal: 4%.

MEPIVACAINE HYDROCHLORIDE
Nerve block 1%, 2%; transvaginal block 1%; para-cervical block in obstetrics 1%; caudal, epidural block 1%, 1.5%, 2%; infiltration 0.5%, 1%; therapeu-tic block (management of pain) 1%, 2%; dental pro-cedures 3%.

PRILOCAINE HYDROCHLORIDE
Infiltration: 1%, 2%.
Peripheral nerve block: Therapeutic (intercostal, paravertebral) 1%, 2%; brachial plexus, sciatic (femoral) 2%, 3%.
Central neural blocks: Epidural 1%, 2%, 3%; caudal obstetric analgesia 1%, caudal surgical anesthesia 2%, 3%.
Local dental anesthesia by nerve block, infiltration: 4%.

PROCAINE HYDROCHLORIDE, INJECTABLE
Infiltration, extensive field block 0.25% to 0.5%; nerve block 0.5% to 2%; spinal anesthesia 10%.

TETRACAINE HYDROCHLORIDE
Spinal anesthesia 0.2% to 1%.

CONTRAINDICATIONS
Hypersensitivity. Large doses should not be used in patients with heart block. Prilocaine should not be used in patients with methemoglobinemia.

ACTIONS
Stabilize the neuronal membrane so that the neuron is less permeable to ions. This prevents initiation and transmission of nerve impulses, thereby effecting local anesthetic action. The exact mechanism whereby local anesthetics influence permeability of the nerve-cell membrane is unknown.

The approximate duration of action is as follows:

Bupivacaine—4–8 hr
Chloroprocaine—1 hr
Dibucaine—3–4 hr
Lidocaine—1–1½ hr
Mepivacaine—2–2½ hr
Prilocaine—1–1½ hr
Procaine—1 hr
Tetracaine—3 hr

The use of vasoconstrictors (e.g., epinephrine) in conjunction with local anesthetics decreases systemic absorption and prolongs the duration of action.

WARNINGS
Resuscitative equipment and drugs should be immediately available when any local anesthetic is used. Preparations containing preservatives should *Not* be used for spinal or epidural anesthesia. When using preparations without preservatives, discard unused portion. Safety for use in pregnant women, other than those in labor, has not been established. Administration of bupivacaine to children under 12 is not recommended.

PRECAUTIONS
Care is taken to prevent intravascular injection. Debilitated or elderly patients, acutely ill patients, and children should be given reduced doses. Use with caution in patients with known drug allergies or sensitivities. Patients allergic to para-aminobenzoic acid (PABA) derivatives (e.g., procaine, tetracaine, benzocaine) have not shown cross-sensitivity to lidocaine. Use mepivacaine with caution in those with renal disease.

DRUG INTERACTIONS
Use solutions containing a vasoconstrictor with extreme caution in patients receiving drugs known to produce blood-pressure alterations (e.g., **MAO inhibitors, tricyclic antidepressants, phenothiazines**) because severe and sustained hypotension or hypertension may occur.

ADVERSE REACTIONS
May result from excessive dosage, rapid absorption, or inadvertent intravascular injection or from hypersensitivity, idiosyncrasy, or diminished tolerance on the part of the patient. CNS reactions are excitatory or depressant and may be characterized by nervousness, dizziness, blurred vision, and tremors followed by drowsiness, convulsions, unconsciousness, and possible respiratory arrest. Excitatory reactions may be brief or not occur at all, in which case the first manifestation of toxicity may be drowsiness, sometimes merging into unconsciousness and respiratory arrest. Other CNS effects may be nausea, vomiting, chills, pupil constriction, and tinnitus. Cardiovascular reactions include depression of the myocardium, hypotension or hypertension, bradycardia, and cardiac arrest. In obstetrics, fetal bradycardia has been reported.

Allergic reactions are characterized by cutaneous lesions of delayed onset, urticaria, edema, or anaphylactoid reactions.

Reactions following epidural or caudal anesthesia may include high or total spinal block; urinary retention; fecal incontinence; loss of perineal sensation and sexual function; persistent analgesia, paresthesia and paralysis of the lower extremities; headache and backache; slowing of labor and increased incidence of forceps delivery.

OVERDOSAGE
Treatment of toxic manifestations: Maintain a patent airway; support ventilation using oxygen and assisted or controlled respiration as required. Should circulatory depression occur, vasopressors and IV fluids may be used. Epinephrine should not be given in the presence of anoxia because of the risk

of causing ventricular fibrillation. Should a convulsion persist, small increments of anticonvulsant agents such as diazepam, an ultra-short-acting barbiturate (thiopental or thiamylal), or a short-acting barbiturate (pentobarbital or secobarbital) may be given IV.

DOSAGE

Dosage varies with area to be anesthetized, vascularity of the tissues, number of neuronal segments to be blocked, individual tolerance, and the technique of anesthesia.

NURSING IMPLICATIONS

HISTORY
See Appendix 4.

ADMINISTRATION
Prepare area (shave, cleanse) and position patient as directed by the physician.

Check entire label carefully: drug name, percentage, and contents (epinephrine, preservative) of solution.

Show label to physician while at same time stating drug name and percentage. If the drug contains **epinephrine,** include this information when giving drug name and percentage.

Be sure resuscitative equipment and drugs are available.

MANAGEMENT DURING ADMINISTRATION
Children, elderly, or uncooperative patients may require restraint while drug is injected. Restrain hands to prevent contamination of needle, injury to self or medical personnel; other types of restraint to prevent sudden movement may also be required.

Observe for adverse reactions (see _Adverse Reactions,_ above).

ONGOING ASSESSMENTS AND NURSING MANAGEMENT
Continue to observe for adverse reactions.

Nerve block: Protect extremity in which drug is given because sensory loss will occur. Pad siderail, insert pillows between siderail and extremity, place limb/body part in position of comfort. Assess affected extremity for color, temperature q15m to q30m or as ordered until sensation returns. Monitor blood pressure, pulse, and respirations q30m or as ordered.

Spinal anesthesia: Keep patient flat for length of time ordered; administer analgesics as ordered. Observe for adverse reactions, headache.

Note the times when sensation and lower-extremity movement begin to return and when all effects of anesthesia are reversed. Monitor blood pressure, pulse, and respirations q30m or as ordered.

Anesthetics, Local, Topical*

Benzocaine (Ethyl Aminobenzoate) _otc_

lotion: 0.5%	Solarcaine
lotion: 2%	Foille
cream: 1%	Soft 'N Soothe, Solarcaine
cream: 5%	Benzocol, _Generic_
cream: 6%	BiCOZENE
ointment: 2%	Foille
liquid: 2.1%	Chigger-Tox
liquid, gel: 20%	Hurricaine†
solution: 2%	Foille
solution: 3%	Unguentine
solution: 5%	Foille Plus
solution: 9.4%	Solarcaine
solution: 20%	Americaine Anesthetic, Dermoplast

Butamben Picrate _otc_

ointment: 1%	Butesin Picrate

Cocaine _Rx C-II_

soluble tablets: 135 mg	Cocaine HCl Solvets
powder	_Generic_
topical solution: 40 mg/ml, 100 mg/ml	_Generic_

Cyclomethycaine Sulfate _Rx, otc_

cream: 0.5% (_otc_)	Surfacaine
ointment: 1% (_otc_)	Surfacaine
jelly: 0.75% (_Rx_)	Surfacaine†

Dibucaine _otc_

ointment: 1%	Nupercainal, _Generic_
cream: 0.5%	Nupercainal

---

* Although some of the percentages/strengths of the products listed in this section are identical, products may differ because of additional ingredients (_e.g.,_ type of base, alcohol, benzethonium chloride, methylparaben).

† Products followed by a dagger are indicated for local anesthesia of mucous membranes; the other products are indicated for topical anesthesia in local skin disorders (see Indications).

Dyclonine Hydrochloride Rx

solution: 0.5%	Dyclone†

Hexylcaine Hydrochloride Rx

solution: 5%	Cyclaine†

Lidocaine Rx, otc

ointment: 2.5% (otc)	Xylocaine
ointment: 5% (Rx)	Generic
cream: 3% (Rx)	Lida-Mantle Creme

Lidocaine Hydrochloride Rx

solution: 2%	Anestacon†
solution: 2%	Baylocaine 2% Viscous,† Xylocaine Viscous†
solution: 4%	Baylocaine 4%,† Xylocain†
aerosol: 10%	Xylocaine 10% oral†
jelly: 2%	Xylocaine†
cream: 3%	Lida-Mantle†
ointment: 5%	Xylocaine†

Pramoxine Hydrochloride otc

cream: 1%	Proxine, Tronothane HCl
jelly: 1%	Tronothane HCl
lotion: 1%	Prax Anti-Itch

Tetracaine otc

ointment: 0.5%	Pontocaine
cream: 1%	Pontocaine

Tetracaine Hydrochloride Rx

solution: 2%	Pontocaine HCl†

Anorectal Preparations otc

ointment: 0.8% ben-zocaine	Pazo Hemorrhoid
ointment: 1% benzo-caine	Hemocaine, Tanurol
ointment: 1% pra-moxine HCl	Anusol
ointment: 2% benzo-caine	Rectal Medicone Unguent
ointment: 3.5% ben-zocaine	Rectagene Balm
ointment: 0.25% di-perodon HCl	A-Caine Rectal, Emeroid
cream: 1% pramox-ine HCl	Tronolane

suppositories: 130 mg benzocaine	Rectal Medicone
suppositories: 0.8% benzocaine	Pazo Hemorrhoid
suppositories: 70 mg benzocaine	Rectagene
suppositories: 2.5 mg dibucaine	Nupercainal
suppositories: 1% pramoxine HCl	Tronolane
aerosol foam: 1% pramoxine HCl	Perifoam

INDICATIONS

Skin disorders: For topical anesthesia in local skin disorders. These disorders include pruritus, pain, soreness, and discomfort due to minor burns, scalds, fungus infections, skin manifestations of systemic disease (e.g., chickenpox), prickly heat, diaper rash, wounds, bruises, abrasions, sunburn, plant poisoning, insect bites, eczema, and episiotomy.

Mucous membranes: For local anesthesia of accessible mucous membranes. These areas may include the oral, nasal, and gingival mucous membranes; the respiratory, upper GI, or urinary tracts. Also for the treatment of pruritus ani, pruritus vulvae, hemorrhoids, and fissures.

Anorectal preparations: Local-anesthetic-containing products are used to relieve symptoms of pain, itching, and irritation. To minimize the potential for systemic toxicity due to absorption from mucous membranes, use the lowest satisfactory dose. Used externally, these agents are effective for temporary discomfort. Their safety and efficacy when used intrarectally is currently under further study. The most frequent adverse effect is sensitization. Many of these products contain multiple ingredients such as vitamins A and D, ephedrine sulfate, tannic acid, or zinc oxide. Only the local-anesthetic content is included in the product list. All are available as nonprescription products.

CONTRAINDICATIONS

Hypersensitivity; use in the eyes; in secondary bacterial infection of the area.

ACTIONS

Inhibits conduction of nerve impulses from sensory nerves. This action results from an alteration of cell-membrane permeability to ions. These agents are poorly absorbed through intact epidermis but are readily absorbed through mucous membranes. When skin permeability has been increased by abrasions, ulcers, or blisters, the absorption and effectiveness are improved and incidence of side-effects increased.

WARNINGS

If extensive areas are treated, the possibility of systemic absorption exists. Exercise caution in persistent, severe, or extensive skin disorders or bleeding hemorrhoids. When there is a possibility of systemic involvement, resuscitative equipment and drugs should be available. Safety for use in pregnancy is not established. Use in women of childbearing potential, particularly in early pregnancy, only when potential benefits outweigh unknown potential hazards to the fetus.

PRECAUTIONS

Topical application may produce the same untoward effects as those following parenteral administration. Reactions and complications are best averted by employing the minimal effective dose. Acutely ill, debilitated, or elderly patients, as well as children, should be given dosages commensurate with their age, size, physical condition. Use cautiously in those with known sensitivity or in those with severely traumatized mucosa and sepsis in the region of application. If irritation or sensitivity occurs or infection appears, discontinue use. Use of oral topical anesthetics may interfere with the second (pharyngeal) stage of swallowing; exercise care, particularly in children, when food is ingested within 60 minutes following use of oral topical anesthetics, to prevent aspiration of food.

ADVERSE REACTIONS

Cutaneous lesions, urticaria, edema, contact dermatitis, burning, tenderness, swelling, tissue irritation, and in some patients sloughing and tissue necrosis. Urethritis has occurred rarely. Methemoglobinemia characterized by cyanosis has been reported following topical application of benzocaine or lidocaine for teething discomfort and as a laryngeal anesthetic spray.

OVERDOSAGE

Symptoms: Reactions due to high plasma levels are systemic and involve the CNS and/or cardiovascular system. _CNS:_ Reactions are excitatory or depressant and may be characterized by nervousness, dizziness, blurred vision, tremors, followed by drowsiness, convulsions, unconsciousness, and possibly respiratory arrest. Excitatory reactions may be brief or not occur at all, in which case the first sign of toxicity may be drowsiness, merging into unconsciousness and respiratory arrest. _Cardiovascular:_ Reactions are depressant and may be characterized by hypotension, myocardial depression, bradycardia, possibly cardiac arrest.

Treatment: Maintain patent airway, support ventilation using oxygen and assisted or controlled respiration as required, vasopressors (preferably those that stimulate the myocardium), IV fluids. Convulsions may be controlled by slow IV administration of 0.1 mg/kg diazepam or 10 mg to 50 mg succinylcholine, with continued oxygen administration.

NURSING IMPLICATIONS

HISTORY
See Appendix 4.

PHYSICAL ASSESSMENT
Check size and location of skin or rectal lesion (when applicable).

ADMINISTRATION
Apply in thin layer unless physician orders otherwise. Other methods of application may be ordered by physician (_e.g.,_ on tip of urethral catheter prior to insertion).

In some instances topical anesthetics are administered by the physician (_e.g.,_ anesthetic lubricant for endotracheal intubation).

Patient using Xylocaine Viscous should be instructed to hold the jellylike substance in his mouth for the time prescribed by the physician. The medication is not to be swallowed.

Insert rectal suppositories gently; apply creams, ointments gently.

ONGOING ASSESSMENTS AND NURSING MANAGEMENT
Evaluate relief from pain/discomfort; notify physician if drug is ineffective.

Notify physician if adverse reactions ocur.

Rectal medications: Notify physician of bleeding or increase in pain.

PATIENT AND FAMILY INFORMATION
Apply drug as directed by physician or on label; do not use on large areas of body.

If symptoms persist, or irritation or signs of infection occur, stop using preparation and see a physician.

Rectal medication: Notify physician or nurse if symptoms become worse or bleeding is noted.

Anesthetics, Ophthalmic

Benoxinate Hydrochloride and Fluorescein Sodium Rx

solution: 0.4% benoxinate HCl, 0.25% sodium fluorescein   Fluress

Proparacaine Hydrochloride Rx

solution: 0.5%   Ak-Taine, Alcaine, Ophthaine, Ophthetic, *Generic*

Tetracaine Rx

solution: 0.5%   Pontocaine HCl, *Generic*
ointment: 0.5%   Pontocaine Eye

INDICATIONS

BENOXINATE HYDROCHLORIDE AND FLUORESCEIN SODIUM

For procedures in which a topical ophthalmic anesthetic in conjunction with a disclosing agent is indicated: corneal anesthesia of short duration, removal of corneal foreign bodies, short corneal, conjunctival procedures.

PROPARACAINE HYDROCHLORIDE

Tonometry, gonioscopy, removal of foreign bodies and sutures, short corneal and conjunctival procedures, cataract surgery, conjunctival and corneal scraping for diagnostic purposes, paracentesis of anterior chamber.

TETRACAINE

See Proparacaine Hydrochloride, above.

CONTRAINDICATIONS

Hypersensitivity.

ACTIONS

Stabilizes the neuronal membrane so that the neuron is less permeable to ions, preventing initiation and transmission of nerve impulses, and thereby producing local anesthetic action. The exact mechanism whereby local anesthetics influence the permeability of the nerve-cell membrane is unknown.

WARNINGS

For topical use only. Prolonged use is not recommended.

PRECAUTIONS

Safety and effectiveness depend on proper dosage, correct technique, adequate precautions, readiness for emergencies. Use cautiously in those with known allergies, cardiac disease, hyperthyroidism.

ADVERSE REACTIONS

Occasional temporary stinging, burning, lacrimation, photophobia, chemosis, increased winking, conjunctival redness. Corneal epithelial erosions, retardation or prevention of healing of corneal erosions, and permanent corneal opacification and scarring have also been reported.

Proparacaine: Allergic contact dermatitis with drying and fissuring of fingertips, pupillary dilatation, cycloplegic effects, conjunctival congestion and hemorrhage, effuse stromal edema have been reported.

Tetracaine: Transient smarting of the eye may occur with concentrations greater than 0.5%. Systemic toxicity, usually manifested as CNS stimulation followed by CNS and cardiovascular depression, may occur.

DOSAGE

BENOXINATE HYDROCHLORIDE AND FLUORESCEIN SODIUM

Removal of foreign bodies, sutures and for tonometry: 1 to 2 drops (in single instillations) in each eye.

Deep ophthalmic anesthesia: 2 drops in each eye at 90-second intervals for 3 instillations.

PROPARACAINE HYDROCHLORIDE

Deep anesthesia as in cataract extraction: Instill 1 drop every 5 to 10 minutes for 5 to 7 doses.

Removal of sutures: 1 or 2 drops 2 or 3 minutes before removal.

Removal of foreign bodies: 1 or 2 drops prior to operating.

Tonometry: 1 or 2 drops immediately before measurement.

TETRACAINE

Solution: Instill 1 to 2 drops. Prolonged use, especially for at-home self-medication, is not recommended. Epinephrine 1:1000 may be added to produce vascular constriction.

Ointment: Apply ½ to 1 inch to lower conjunctival fornix. Prolonged use is not recommended.

NURSING IMPLICATIONS

HISTORY

See Appendix 4. If used in emergency treatment, determine whether patient is allergic to local anesthetics and whether there is a history of cardiac disease or hyperthyroidism; inform physician of findings.

NOTE: Patient may be in acute pain and unable to give accurate history. Family may be able to supply information.

PHYSICAL ASSESSMENT

Usually performed by physician.

ADMINISTRATION

If eye injury, physician may instill drug.

Check label carefully; drug must be labeled "ophthalmic."

Preoperative anesthesia: Drops must be instilled *Exactly* as ordered; failure to adhere to prescribed intervals or instill prescribed number of doses may result in inadequate anesthesia.

Eye injury, foreign body: Uncooperative patient may need to be restrained during and after instillation of drug.

NURSING MANAGEMENT

Protect eye from irritating chemicals, foreign bodies, and rubbing during period of anesthesia.

Thoroughly rinse tonometers with sterile distilled water prior to use.

Warn patient not to touch or rub eye until anesthesia has worn off because inadvertent damage may be done to anesthetized cornea, conjunctiva. The uncooperative patient may require restraints during this time.

The blink reflex is temporarily eliminated; physician may order eye patch following instillation of drug. Ask physician length of time covering is to remain in place.

PATIENT AND FAMILY INFORMATION

Do not rub eye or touch dropper tip to eyelids or surrounding area.

May retard healing: Use sparingly and *only as directed.*

Anisotropine Methylbromide

See Gastrointestinal Anticholinergics/Antispasmodics.

Anorexiants

Benzphetamine Hydrochloride   Rx C-III

tablets: 25 mg (contains tartrazine), 50 mg	Didrex

Diethylpropion Hydrochloride   Rx C-IV

tablets: 25 mg	Depletite-25, Tenuate, Tepanil, *Generic*
tablets, sustained release: 75 mg	Tenuate Dospan, Tepanil Ten-Tab

Fenfluramine Hydrochloride   Rx C-IV

tablets: 20 mg	Pondimin

Mazindol   Rx C-IV

tablets: 1 mg	Mazanor, Sanorex
tablets: 2 mg	Sanorex

Phendimetrazine Tartrate   Rx C-III

tablets: 35 mg	Adphen, Bacarate, Bontril PDM, Di-Ap-Trol, Limit, Melfiat, Metra, Obalan, Obeval, Obezine, PDM, Phenzine, Plegine, Sprx-1, Statobex, Statobex-G, Trimstat, Trimtabs, Weightrol, *Generic*
capsules: 35 mg	Sprx-3, Statobex, Wehless, *Generic*
capsules, sustained release: 105 mg	Melfiat-105 Unicelles, Prelu-2, Sprx-105, Wehless Timecelles-105, *Generic*

Phenmetrazine Hydrochloride   Rx C-II

tablets: 25 mg	Preludin
tablets, sustained release: 50 mg, 75 mg (contains tartrazine)	Preludin

Phentermine Hydrochloride   Rx C-IV

tablets: 8 mg	Phentrol, Tora, *Generic*
capsules: 15 mg	*Generic*
capsules: 30 mg	Fastin, Obephen, Obermine, Obestin-30, Phentrol 2, Unifast Unicelles, Wilpowr, *Generic*
capsules: 15 mg, 30 mg (as resin complex)	Ionamin
capsules, timed release: 30 mg	Parmine, Phentrol 4, Phentrol 5, *Generic*

INDICATIONS

Short-term (8–12-weeks) management of exogenous obesity as adjunct in a regimen of weight reduction based on caloric restriction. May be useful for obese persons who have inherited a tendency to gain weight easily and lose it with great difficulty, for those with metabolic changes resulting from long-standing obesity making weight reduction difficult, and those who have reached a 4- to 6-week plateau in their weight-loss program.

CONTRAINDICATIONS

Advanced arteriosclerosis; symptomatic heart disease; moderate to severe hypertension; hyperthyroidism; known hypersensitivity or idiosyncrasy to sympathomimetic amines; glaucoma; agitated states; history of drug abuse. Do not administer **fenfluramine** to alcoholics, because psychiatric symptoms (paranoia, depression, psychosis) have been reported.

ACTIONS

These nonamphetamine anorexiants, also called anorectics or anorexigenics, are indirectly acting sympathomimetic amines. Except for mazindol, phenmetrazine, and phendimetrazine, all are phenethylamine (amphetaminelike) analogues and possess pharmacologic activity similar to that of amphetamines. Although exact mechanism of action has not been established, it is thought that appetite suppression is produced by direct stimulant effect on the satiety center in the hypothalamic and limbic regions. Secondary actions include CNS stimulation and blood-pressure elevation. **Fenfluramine** produces CNS depression. The conventional dosage forms generally exert their effects for 4 to 6 hours, except for mazindol, which has an 8- to 15-hour duration.

WARNINGS

Tolerance: May develop within a few weeks; cross-tolerance among anorexiants is universal. The recommended dose should not be exceeded.

Drug dependence: These drugs have a potential for abuse. Intense psychological or physical dependence and severe social dysfunction may be associated with long-term therapy or abuse. If this occurs, dosage is gradually reduced to avoid withdrawal symptoms. Chronic intoxication is manifested by severe dermatoses, marked insomnia, irritability, hyperactivity, personality changes. Psychosis, often clinically indistinguishable from schizophrenia, is the most severe manifestation.

Use in pregnancy: Safety not established; use only when clearly needed and when potential benefits outweigh unknown potential hazards to the fetus.

Use in children: Not recommended in children under 12.

PRECAUTIONS

May impair ability to engage in potentially hazardous activities; patient should observe caution while driving or performing tasks requiring alertness. Use with caution in patients with mild hypertension, coronary or cardiovascular disease, hyperexcitability states, hyperthyroidism. **Diethylpropion** may increase convulsions in some epileptics. **Mazindol** and **fenfluramine** moderately lower blood glucose levels by increasing glucose uptake in skeletal muscle.

Tartrazine sensitivity: Some products contain tartrazine (see Appendix 6, section 6-23).

DRUG INTERACTIONS

Concomitant use of **CNS stimulants** is contraindicated. These drugs are contraindicated during or within 14 days following administration of **MAO inhibitors** (hypertensive crisis may result). Anorexiants may decrease the hypotensive effect of **guanethidine** and other **antihypertensive agents** and may markedly potentiate the pressor effect of **exogenous catecholamines.** If it is necessary to give a pressor amine agent to a patient in shock who has been taking anorexiants, monitor the blood pressure at frequent intervals.

Antidiabetic-drug requirements in diabetes mellitus may be altered in association with use of anorectics and concomitant dietary restrictions. Concurrent use of **general anesthetics** may result in cardiac arrhythmias. Fenfluramine may potentiate the effects of antihypertensive agents including **thiazide diuretics.** Use **alcohol, tricyclic antidepressants,** and other **CNS depressants** with caution in those taking fenfluramine, because effects may be additive.

ADVERSE REACTIONS

Cardiovascular: Palpitation; tachycardia; arrhythmia; hypertension or hypotension; fainting; dyspnea; precordial pain.

CNS: Overstimulation; nervousness, dizziness; jitters; insomnia; weakness or fatigue; anxiety; euphoria; depression; dysphoria; tremor; dyskinesia; agitation; dysarthria; confusion; incoordination; headache; rarely, psychotic episodes. An increase in convulsive episodes has been reported in a few epileptics; fenfluramine may cause drowsiness.

GI: Dry mouth; glossitis; stomatitis; unpleasant taste; nausea; vomiting; abdominal cramps; diarrhea; constipation.

Allergic: Urticaria; rash; ecchymosis; erythema; burning sensation.

Ocular: Mydriasis; eye irritation; blurred vision.

GU: Dysuria; difficulty in initiating micturition; diuresis; cystitis.

Endocrine: Impotence; changes in libido; menstrual upset; gynecomastia.

Hematopoietic: Bone marrow depression; agranulocytosis; leukopenia.

Miscellaneous: Hair loss; muscle pain; excessive sweating; chills; flushing; fever; clamminess.

OVERDOSAGE

Symptoms: Restlessness; tremor; hyperreflexia; rapid respiration; dizziness; confusion; assaultiveness; hallucinations and panic states may be manifestations of acute overdosage. Depression and fatigue usually follow stimulation. *Cardiovascular effects:* Arrhythmias (tachycardia); hypertension or hypotension, secondary to hypovolemia; circulatory collapse. _GI symptoms:_ Nausea; vomiting; diarrhea; abdominal cramps. Convulsions, coma, and death may result.

Fenfluramine: Agitation and drowsiness; confusion; flushing; tremor (or shivering); fever; sweating; abdominal pain; hyperventilation; dilated, nonreactive pupils are frequent. Reflexes may be exaggerated or depressed. Rotary nystagmus and continuous tremor of the lower jaw are specific characteristics of overdosage. Tachycardia may be present; blood pressure may be normal or slightly elevated. Convulsions, coma, and ventricular extrasystoles, culminating in ventricular fibrillation, may occur at higher dosage. Death has occurred.

Treatment: Symptomatic and supportive management includes lavage and sedation with a barbiturate and, if possible, cardiac monitoring. Chlorpromazine may be of value in antagonizing CNS stimulation effect. If acute severe hypertension occurs, a nitrate or rapidly acting alpha-adrenergic blocking agent (_e.g.,_ phentolamine) may be used. If hypotension occurs secondary to hypovolemia, attempt IV fluid administration prior to use of vasopressors. Acidification of urine should increase excretion.

Fenfluramine: Forced diuresis with acidification of the urine may be beneficial to hasten excretion.

DOSAGE

BENZPHETAMINE HYDROCHLORIDE

25 mg/day to 50 mg/day; increase according to response. Dosage range: 25 mg to 50 mg, 1 to 3 times/day.

DIETHYLPROPION HYDROCHLORIDE

25 mg tid, 1 hour A.C. and in midevening if needed to overcome night hunger. Sustained release: 75 mg/day in midmorning.

FENFLURAMINE HYDROCHLORIDE

Initial dose 20 mg tid. May be increased at weekly intervals by 20 mg daily to maximum of 40 mg tid. If initial dose is not well tolerated, dosage may be reduced to 40 mg/day and then gradually increased in order to minimize chance of side-effects.

MAZINDOL

Usual dose, 1 mg tid 1 hour A.C. or 2 mg once daily, 1 hour A.C. lunch. Therapy may be initiated at 1 mg/day and adjusted according to need and response. Taken with meals to avoid GI discomfort.

PHENDIMETRAZINE TARTRATE

Tablets, capsules: 35 mg bid or tid, 1 hour A.C.
Sustained release: 105 mg in A.M.

PHENMETRAZINE HYDROCHLORIDE

Maximum adult dose range is 50 mg to 75 mg.
Tablets: 25 mg bid or tid, 1 hour A.C.
Sustained release: 50 mg/day or 75 mg/day in A.M.

PHENTERMINE HYDROCHLORIDE

8 mg tid, A.C. or 15 mg to 37.5 mg as single daily dose in A.M.

NURSING IMPLICATIONS

HISTORY
See Appendix 4.

PHYSICAL ASSESSMENT
Record blood pressure, weight (Note: physician-supervised weight-reduction programs/clinics usually perform more extensive evaluation of obesity).

ADMINISTRATION
Give A.C.; see also _Dosage,_ above. Avoid late-evening doses because drug may cause insomnia.

ONGOING ASSESSMENTS AND NURSING MANAGEMENT
Monitor blood pressure, weight at time of clinic/office visits.

Encourage adherence to prescribed diet plan, exercise program.

These drugs are subject to abuse. Requests for new prescriptions or prescription renewals are entered on patient's record. Note especially date of last prescription and number of tablets/capsules prescribed.

Observe for adverse reactions, especially CNS effects (see _Adverse Reactions, Warnings_).

PATIENT AND FAMILY INFORMATION
May cause insomnia; avoid taking medication late in day.

Weight reduction requires strict adherence to dietary restrictions.

Do not take more frequently than prescribed.

Notify physician or nurse if palpitation, nervousness, or dizziness occurs.

May cause dryness of mouth, constipation; notify physician or nurse if these become pronounced or bothersome.

May produce dizziness, blurred vision; observe caution while driving or performing tasks requiring alertness.

Fenfluramine: May cause drowsiness.

Mazindol: May be taken with meals to reduce GI irritation.

Antacids*

Aluminum Carbonate Gel, Basic otc

	ANC (mEq)	
capsules: equivalent to 608 mg dried aluminum hydroxide gel or 500 mg aluminum hydroxide, 2.8 mg sodium	13	Basaljel
swallow tablets: same as capsules but with 2.1 mg sodium	14	Basaljel
suspension: equivalent to 400 mg aluminum hydroxide, 2.4 mg sodium per 5 ml	14	Basaljel
suspension, extra strength: equivalent to 1000 mg aluminum hydroxide, 23 mg sodium/5 ml	11	Basaljel

Aluminum Hydroxide Gel otc

	ANC (mEq)	
capsules: 475 mg		Alu-Cap
capsules: 500 mg (<1.2 mg sodium)	10	Dialume
tablets: 300 mg	9	Amphojel
tablets: 600 mg	18	Amphojel
tablets, chewable: 487.5 mg		Generic
suspension: 320 mg/5 ml (<0.3 mEq sodium)	6.5	Amphojel*
suspension: aluminum hydroxide equivalent to 4% aluminum oxide		Generic
liquid: 600 mg/5 ml, (<2 mg sodium)	12	Alternagel

Aluminum Phosphate Gel otc

	ANC (mEq)	
suspension: 233 mg (12.5 mg sodium)	1.5	Phosphaljel

* The acid-neutralizing capacity (ANC) is given per capsule, tablet, or 5 ml. Products that are starred (*) are flavored.

Calcium Carbonate otc

	ANC (mEq)	
tablets: 650 mg		Generic
tablets, chewable: 350 mg		Amitone
tablets, chewable: 420 mg		Mallamint*
tablets, chewable: 500 mg	10	Alka-2
	8.25	Dicarbosil*
	10	Tums (2.7 mg sodium)* Chooz,* Equilet

Dihydroxyaluminum Sodium Carbonate otc

	ANC (mEq)	
tablets, chewable: 334 mg (53 mg sodium)	7.5–8	Rolaids Antacid

Magaldrate otc

	ANC (mEq)	
swallow tablets, chewable tablets, suspension (5 ml): 480 mg (0.3 mg sodium)	13.5	Riopan

Magnesia (Magnesium Hydroxide) otc

tablets: 325 mg, 650 mg	Generic
liquid: approximately 7.75% magnesium hydroxide	Generic

Magnesium Carbonate otc

powder	Generic

Magnesium Oxide otc

capsules: 140 mg	Par-Mag, Uro-Mag
tablets: 400 mg	Mag-Ox 400
tablets: 420 mg	Maox
powder	Generic

Magnesium Trisilicate otc

tablets: 488 mg	Generic
powder	Generic

A

Sodium Bicarbonate

(Contains 27% sodium) otc

tablets: 325 mg	Soda Mint, _Generic_
tablets: 487.5 mg	Soda Mint
tablets: 520 mg	Bell/ans*
tablets: 650 mg	_Generic_
powder	_Generic_

Antacid Combinations*

	ANC (mEq)	Sodium (mg)
Alka-Seltzer w/o Aspirin, Effervescent Tablets: 958 mg sodium bicarbonate, 832 mg citric acid, 312 mg potassium bicarbonate	10.6	296
Alkets Tablets: 780 mg calcium carbonate, 130 mg magnesium carbonate, 65 mg magnesium oxide		
Aludrox Tablets: 233 mg aluminum hydroxide, 83 mg magnesium hydroxide	11.5	1.6
Aludrox Suspension: 307 mg aluminum hydroxide, 103 mg magnesium hydroxide	14	1.15
Bisodol Tablets: 178 mg magnesium hydroxide, 194 mg calcium carbonate		0.03
Bisodol Powder: 644 mg sodium bicarbonate, 475 mg magnesium carbonate		157/5 g
Bromo-Seltzer, Effervescent Granules: 0.325 g acetaminophen, 2.781 g sodium bicarbonate, 2.224 g citric acid		0.761 g/dose
Calcilac Tablets: 420 mg calcium carbonate, 180 mg glycine*		
Camalox Tablets: 225 mg aluminum hydroxide, 200 mg magnesium hydroxide, 250 mg calcium carbonate*	18	1.5
Camalox Suspension: 225 mg aluminum hydroxide, 200 mg magnesium hydroxide, 250 mg calcium carbonate*	18	2.5
Creamalin Tablets: 248 mg aluminum hydroxide, 75 mg magnesium hydroxide		<41

* These antacid preparations contain more than one ingredient. All are available as nonprescription products. Products that are starred (*) are flavored.

	ANC (mEq)	Sodium (mg)
Delcid Suspension: 600 mg aluminum hydroxide, 665 mg magnesium hydroxide	42	<15
Di-Gel Tablets: 85 mg magnesium hydroxide, 282 mg (aluminum hydroxide and magnesium carbonate), 25 mg simethicone*		10.6
Di-Gel Liquid: 282 mg aluminum hydroxide, 87 mg magnesium hydroxide, 25 mg simethicone*	10.5	8.5
ENO Powder: 2160 mg sodium tartrate, 495 mg sodium citrate		780/5 g
Estomul-M Tablets: 500 mg (aluminum hydroxide and magnesium carbonate), 45 mg magnesium oxide	8	16
Gaviscon Tablets: 80 mg aluminum hydroxide, 20 mg magnesium trisilicate, plus alginic acid, sodium bicarbonate		0.8
Gaviscon-2 Tablets: 160 mg aluminum hydroxide, 40 mg magnesium trisilicate, plus alginic acid, sodium bicarbonate		36.8
Gaviscon Liquid: 31.7 mg aluminum hydroxide, 137 mg magnesium carbonate*		39.1
Gelusil Tablets: 200 mg aluminum hydroxide, 200 mg magnesium hydroxide, 25 mg simethicone*	11	0.8
Gelusil-M Tablets: 300 mg aluminum hydroxide, 200 mg magnesium hydroxide, 25 mg simethicone*	12.5	1.3
Gelusil-II Tablets: 400 mg aluminum hydroxide, 400 mg magnesium hydroxide, 30 mg simethicone*	21	2.1
Gelusil Liquid: 200 mg aluminum hydroxide, 200 mg magnesium hydroxide, 25 mg simethicone*	12	0.7
Gelusil-M Liquid: 300 mg aluminum hydroxide, 200 mg magnesium hydroxide, 25 mg simethicone*	15	1.2
Gelusil-II Liquid: 400 mg aluminum hydroxide, 400 mg magnesium hydroxide, 30 mg simethicone*	24	1.3

Kolantyl Gel: 150 mg aluminum hydroxide, 150 mg magnesium hydroxide	10.5	
Kolantyl Wafers: 180 mg aluminum hydroxide, 170 mg magnesium hydroxide	10.8	
Maalox No. 1 Tablets: 200 mg aluminum hydroxide, 200 mg magnesium hydroxide	8.5	0.84
Maalox No. 2 Tablets: 400 mg aluminum hydroxide, 400 mg magnesium hydroxide	18	1.84
Maalox Plus Tablets: 200 mg aluminum hydroxide, 200 mg magnesium hydroxide, 25 mg simethicone*	11	0.8
Maalox Suspension: 225 mg aluminum hydroxide, 200 mg magnesium hydroxide*	13.5	1.35
Maalox Plus Suspension: 225 mg aluminum hydroxide, 200 mg magnesium hydroxide, 25 mg simethicone	13.5	1.3
Maalox Therapeutic Concentrate: 600 aluminum hydroxide, 300 mg magnesium hydroxide*	28.3	0.8
Magnagel Tablets: 325 mg (aluminum hydroxide and magnesium carbonate)		
Magnatril Tablet: 260 mg aluminum hydroxide, 130 mg magnesium hydroxide, 455 mg magnesium trisilicate		
Marblen Tablets: 520 mg calcium carbonate, 400 mg magnesium carbonate	18	3.2
Mylanta Tablets: 200 mg aluminum hydroxide, 200 mg magnesium hydroxide, 20 mg simethicone	11.5	0.77
Mylanta-II Tablets: 400 mg aluminum hydroxide, 400 mg magnesium hydroxide, 30 mg simethicone	23	1.3
Mylanta Liquid: 200 mg aluminum hydroxide, 200 mg magnesium hydroxide, 20 mg simethicone	12.7	0.68
Mylanta-II Liquid: 400 mg aluminum hydroxide, 400 mg magnesium hydroxide, 30 mg simethicone	25.4	1.14
Nephrox Suspension: 320 mg aluminum hydroxide, 10% mineral oil*	9	3.1
Ratio Tablets: 400 mg calcium carbonate, 50 mg magnesium carbonate*	9	
Riopan Plus Chew Tablets: 480 mg magaldrate, 20 mg simethicone	13.5	0.3
Riopan Plus Suspension: 480 mg magaldrate, 20 mg simethicone	13.5	<0.3
Silain-Gel Liquid: 282 mg aluminum hydroxide, 285 mg magnesium hydroxide, 25 mg simethicone*	15	4.8
Simeco Suspension: 365 mg aluminum hydroxide, 300 mg magnesium hydroxide, 30 mg simethicone*		6.9–13.8
Spastosed Tablets: 226 mg calcium carbonate, 162 mg magnesium carbonate		
WinGel Liquid: 180 mg aluminum hydroxide, 160 mg magnesium hydroxide*	11.6	
WinGel Tablets: 180 mg aluminum hydroxide, 160 mg magnesium hydroxide	12.3	

INDICATIONS

Symptomatic relief of upset stomach associated with hyperacidity (heartburn, acid indigestion, sour stomach) and hyperacidity associated with diagnosis of peptic ulcer, gastritis, peptic esophagitis, gastric hyperacidity, hiatal hernia. Although sufficient doses have been demonstrated to promote healing in peptic ulcer, their efficacy in relieving pain is not well documented. Antacids must be administered frequently owing to rapid emptying of gastric contents. Liquid dosage forms are usually preferred because of their rapid action and greater activity; tablets may be more acceptable and convenient for many patients.

Aluminum carbonate gel, basic, is also used with a low-phosphate diet to prevent formation of phosphatic urinary stones by reducing phosphates in the urine.

ACTIONS

Antacids are basic compounds that neutralize or reduce the acidity of gastric contents. Additionally, by increasing the pH to above 4, they inhibit the proteolytic activity of pepsin.

Acid-neutralizing capacity (ANC): The ANC is a primary consideration in the selection of an antacid. Sodium bicarbonate and calcium carbonate possess the greatest ANC but are not suitable for chronic therapy because of their systemic effects. The ANC of commercial antacid preparations varies and is dependent on the amount of antacid included as well as on other formulation factors. Suspensions have greater ANC than powders or tablets.

Phosphate binding: Aluminum-containing antacids are capable of binding with phosphate ions in the intestine to form insoluble aluminum phosphate, which is excreted in the feces. Large doses or prolonged therapy may result in hypophosphatemia. This effect is of therapeutic value in treating hyperphosphatemia in chronic renal failure. Aluminum carbonate gel exhibits the greatest phosphate-binding capacity and is indicated for prevention of phosphatic urinary stones. Only aluminum carbonate and aluminum hydroxide have clinically useful phosphate-binding capacity.

WARNINGS

Sodium content: Antacid products may contain significant amounts of sodium. Patients with hypertension, with congestive heart failure, or on restricted or low-sodium diets should use one of the low-sodium preparations.

Sodium bicarbonate is an absorbable antacid and may lead to systemic alkalosis if used chronically. **Magnesium-containing products** should be used with caution in patients with renal insufficiency, particularly when more than 50 mEq of magnesium are given daily. **Aluminum ions** inhibit spontaneous and induced smooth-muscle contraction, thus inhibiting gastric emptying. Aluminum-containing products should be used with caution in patients with gastric outlet obstruction.

DRUG INTERACTIONS

The physical and the chemical nature of antacids suggest a high potential for drug interaction by absorption and by alterations of the gastric pH. In general, it is best not to administer **other oral drugs** within 1 to 2 hours of antacid administration.

Calcium-, aluminum-, and magnesium-containing products may complex with **tetracycline derivatives** when given concomitantly, thus reducing absorption of these antibiotics. Antacids may impair the absorption of **digoxin, isoniazid, phenytoin, corticosteroids, quinidine,** and **warfarin.** Although the clinical significance of this interaction is uncertain, avoid concurrent use of antacids and drugs intended for systemic absorption. Antacids may inhibit the absorption of **oral iron** products when given concur-

rently, and may impair the absorption of **oral anticholinergics** and **phenothiazines.**

Systemic antacids may accelerate the excretion of **acidic drugs** like the salicylates by raising urine pH; urinary excretion of basic drugs such as **amphetamines** or **quinidine** may be inhibited and toxicity may occur.

ADVERSE REACTIONS

Magnesium-containing products have a laxative effect and may cause diarrhea. Aluminum- and calcium-containing products tend to cause constipation and may lead to intestinal obstruction. Mixtures of magnesium and aluminum antacids are frequently used in an attempt to avoid changes in bowel function.

Magnesium-containing antacids: In renal failure, chronic use may produce hypermagnesemia and toxicity. Chronic use may result in silicate renal stones. Ingestion of large amounts may result in acute renal failure.

Calcium carbonate and sodium bicarbonate: May cause rebound hyperacidity and milk alkali syndrome (hypercalcemia, metabolic acidosis, and possibly renal impairment).

Aluminum-containing products: May lead to decreased absorption of fluoride and accumulation of aluminum in serum, bone, and the CNS.

DOSAGE

ALUMINUM CARBONATE GEL, BASIC

Antacid: 2 capsules or tablets, 10 ml of regular suspension (in water, fruit juice), or 5 ml of extra-strength suspension as often as q2h, up to 12 times/day.

Prevention of phosphate stones: Capsules, tablets—2 to 6, 1 hour P.C. and at H.S.; *suspension*—10 ml to 30 ml 1 hour P.C. and H.S.; extra-strength suspension—5 ml to 15 ml in water or fruit juice, 1 hour P.C. and H.S.

ALUMINUM HYDROXIDE GEL
600 mg 3 to 6 times/day, between meals and H.S.

ALUMINUM PHOSPHATE GEL
15 ml to 30 ml undiluted q2h between meals and H.S.

CALCIUM CARBONATE
0.5 to 2 g as needed.

DIHYDROXYALUMINUM SODIUM CARBONATE
Chew 1 to 2 tablets prn.

MAGALDRATE
480 mg to 960 mg between meals and H.S.

MAGNESIA (MAGNESIUM HYDROXIDE)

Adults, children over 12: Antacid dose, 5 ml to 10 ml liquid or 600 mg tablet qid. Laxative dose, 15 ml to 30 ml liquid or 1.8 g to 3.6 g tablets daily with water.

Children: 2 to 6 years, laxative dose in 5 ml to 15 ml as single dose with water; 6 to 12 years, 15 ml to 30 ml liquid or 900 mg to 1.8 g tablets as single dose with water.

MAGNESIUM CARBONATE
0.5 g to 2 g with water.

MAGNESIUM OXIDE
250 mg to 1.5 g with water or milk qid.

MAGNESIUM TRISILICATE
1 g to 14 g qid with water.

SODIUM BICARBONATE
0.3 g to 2 g 1 to 4 times/day.

NURSING IMPLICATIONS

HISTORY
See Appendix 4.

ADMINISTRATION
Shake liquid preparations thoroughly before pouring.

Advise patient to chew tablets *thoroughly* before swallowing; tablets should not be broken into small pieces and swallowed.

Follow tablets with approximately 1 glass of water or milk unless physician orders a specific volume and type of liquid to follow each dose. In some instances the physician may allow juice to be substituted for milk or water.

Liquid antacids should be followed with a small amount of water or milk, usually 1 oz or 2 oz, unless the physician orders a specific volume and type of liquid to follow each dose.

If the physician orders drug to be left at bedside for self-administration, be sure patient has an adequate supply of ice water, juice, or milk that is refilled as needed; an adequate supply of measuring (medicine) cups; and a clock or watch.

If drug is self-administered, instruct patient in measurement of prescribed dose. Supervise as needed.

If milk is taken with or after medication, only a small amount should be left at the bedside, preferably in an insulated container. Check milk periodically to be sure it has not become warm.

Generally, it is best not to administer other oral drugs within 1 to 2 hours of antacid administration. Check times of other medications and adjust as needed.

If antacid is administered through a nasogastric tube, check to be sure tube is in stomach before administration; follow drug with water in sufficient amount to clear tube (approximately 30 ml to 60 ml) or as ordered by physician.

ONGOING ASSESSMENTS AND NURSING MANAGEMENT
If used for antacid effects, assess patient for relief of pain/discomfort daily; notify physician if pain is not relieved or becomes worse.

Note and record number and frequency of stools; report episodes of diarrhea or constipation to physician because medication change or laxative may be necessary. This is especially important if the patient is elderly, unable to participate in his own care (*e.g.*, brain damaged or retarded), on complete bedrest, or receiving drugs that decrease intestinal motility (*e.g.*, narcotics, antispasmodics, antidiarrheals).

If drug is self-administered, monitor patient to ensure compliance with medication schedule and dose.

If tablets are not chewed properly, if there is an expressed dislike for this form of the drug, or if the patient complains about the taste or aftertaste, discuss problem with physician because a liquid preparation or a flavored tablet or liquid may be ordered.

When used in acute peptic ulcer disease, antacids may be administered hourly during waking hours for the first 2 weeks; during the healing stage, they are usually administered 1 to 3 hours after meals and H.S. Other medication schedules may also be prescribed.

A nutritional diet plan with some restrictions (*e.g.*, coffee, strong spices, alcohol) is usually incorporated into the treatment of peptic-ulcer disease as well as gastritis, hiatal hernia, and peptic esophagitis. Meals may be 3 times/day or given in smaller portions with up to 6 feedings/day. Antacid administration is often scheduled between the 3 or more meals/day.

If aluminum carbonate gel, basic, is prescribed for prevention of phosphatic urinary stones, the physician may order a high fluid intake. Offer excess fluids between doses of antacid unless physician orders otherwise.

General considerations
Use of drugs containing alcohol (*e.g.*, elixirs) is usually avoided.

The neutralization of gastric acid by the ingestion and digestion of food is followed by increased gastric secretion; thus, the timing of administration of antacids (*e.g.,* 1–3 hours P.C.) is important. Prescribed dosage schedules must be adhered to strictly.

The physician should be notified if the prescribed diet is taken poorly or if the patient is found eating or drinking foods not on his diet.

PATIENT AND FAMILY INFORMATION

If pain/discomfort remains the same or becomes worse, if stools turn black, or if other symptoms occur, contact physician as soon as possible.

Chew tablets thoroughly before swallowing; follow with a glass of water or milk.

Adhere to prescribed dosage schedule; do not increase dose or frequency unless directed to do so by physician.

Follow prescribed diet. Omit foods as directed, eat well-balanced diet; make note of any foods that cause discomfort, pain, nausea, vomiting.

Follow suggestions made by physician (*e.g.,* sleeping with head of bed elevated for those with hiatal hernia, or eating smaller, more frequent meals).

Antacids impair the absorption of many drugs. It is best not to take other oral drugs within 1 to 2 hours before or after taking antacids.

Do not take any nonprescription drug without first checking with physician.

Magnesium-containing products have a laxative effect and may cause diarrhea; aluminum- and calcium-containing products may cause constipation. If either diarrhea or constipation becomes severe, contact physician.

Antacids may change the color of the stool (white, white streaks).

Anthralin *(Dithranol)* Rx

ointment: 0.1%, 0.25%, 0.5%, 1%	Anthra-Derm
ointment: 0.4%	Lasan Unguent
cream: 0.1%, 0.25%, 0.5%	Drithocreme

INDICATIONS
Psoriasis.

CONTRAINDICATIONS
Hypersensitivity. Used only on quiescent or chronic patches; not used on acute eruptions or where inflammation is present. Drug is absorbed through the skin; a part is excreted unchanged and can cause renal irritation, casts, proteinuria.

ACTIONS
Reduces the mitotic rate and proliferation of epidermal cells by inhibiting the synthesis of nucleic protein.

WARNINGS
Safety for use in pregnancy not established. Use only when clearly needed and when potential benefits outweigh unknown potential hazards to the fetus. It is not known whether drug is excreted in human milk.

PRECAUTIONS
Erythema occurring on normal skin adjacent to lesions is criterion of dosage form concentration. When redness is observed on adjacent skin, dosage or frequency is reduced or drug is discontinued. For external use only. Not to be used in or near eyes. Drug is an ocular irritant; if accidentally applied, severe conjunctivitis, keratitis, corneal opacity may result. Do not apply to face, genitalia, or intertriginous skin areas. Avoid excessive concentrations because excessive and harmful irritation may result. Wash hands thoroughly after using. May stain fabrics and temporarily discolor gray or white hair.

DOSAGE
Apply thin layer once or twice daily. Treatment is continued until scales are removed, lesions are flattened, and no palpable differences exist between the lesion site and normal surrounding skin.

Skin: Apply H.S. to plaque sites.

Scalp: Massage into affected areas; shampoo scalp in morning.

NURSING IMPLICATIONS

HISTORY
See Appendix 4.

PHYSICAL ASSESSMENT
Examine lesions; record appearance and size.

ADMINISTRATION
Wear plastic gloves to protect hands.

Explain to patient purpose of gloves (*i.e.,* effect of drug on normal skin of both patient and nurse).

A thin layer of petrolatum applied to the areas surrounding the plaques may be helpful in preventing drug action on normal skin.

Apply a thin layer. Do not apply to face, genitals, or intertriginous areas or allow ointment or cream to come into contact with unaffected areas.

If applied near hairline take extreme care to keep medication away from the eyes. Cover head with a plastic cap after scalp application.

Drug may stain fabrics; patient's clothing should not touch treated areas. Warn patient with gray or white hair that there may be a temporary discoloration.

Wash hands, forearms thoroughly after administration, even though plastic gloves are worn.

ONGOING ASSESSMENTS AND NURSING MANAGEMENT

In the morning, remove any remaining surplus with warm liquid petrolatum, followed by a bath. If drug is applied to the scalp, hair is shampooed the following morning.

Inspect skin before each application; compare appearance, size of lesions with data base.

Notify physician if sensitivity reaction is observed, especially normal skin surrounding the plaques, or if pustular folliculitis occurs.

The urine may appear red owing to absorption of drug.

Renal irritation may occur. Notify physician if urine appears cloudy (may be indication of casts), urinary output decreases, or patient offers complaints related to the GU tract.

PATIENT AND FAMILY INFORMATION

Patient instructions are available with product; read instructions thoroughly before use and direct any questions about application to physician, nurse, or pharmacist.

Apply petrolatum to areas around plaques.

Wear old clothing over lesions; use disposable plastic gloves to protect hands during application; wash hands, forearms thoroughly after application.

Do not get drug in or near eyes.

Contact physician or nurse if redness occurs on skin adjacent to plaques or if condition does not improve or becomes worse.

Antibiotics, Ophthalmic*

Drops

10 mg tetracycline HCl/ml	Achromycin Ophthalmic (suspension)
500,000 units polymyxin B sulfate	*Generic* (powder for solution)

* All of these are prescription drugs. Ointments with identical antibiotics may have additional ingredients or different bases (*e.g.,* mineral oil, petrolatum, anhydrous liquid lanolin). Drops with identical antibiotics may have additional ingredients such as preservatives or polyethylene glycol.

5 mg chloramphenicol/ml	Antibiopto Ophthalmic, Chloroptic Ophthalmic, Econochlor Ophthalmic Ophthochlor Ophthalmic, *Generic* (solutions)
25 mg chloramphenicol/vial (with 15 ml diluent)	Chloromycetin Ophthalmic (powder for solution)
3 mg gentamicin/ml	Garamycin Ophthalmic, Genoptic Ophthalmic, *Generic* (solutions)
10,000 units polymyxin B sulfate, 1.75 mg neomycin sulfate, 0.025 mg gramicidin/ml	Neosporin Ophthalmic, *Generic* (solutions)
16,250 units polymyxin B sulfate, 3.5 mg neomycin sulfate/ml	Statrol Ophthalmic (solution)
3 mg tobramycin/ml	Tobrex Ophthalmic

Ointments

10 mg tetracycline HCl/g	Achromycin Ophthalmic
10 mg chlortetracycline HCl/g	Aureomycin Ophthalmic
500 units bacitracin/g	Baciguent Ophthalmic, *Generic*
10 mg chloramphenicol/g	Chloromycetin Ophthalmic, Chloroptic S.O.P. Ophthalmic, Econochlor Ophthalmic
10 mg chloramphenicol, 10,000 units polymyxin B (as sulfate)/g	Chloromyxin Ophthalmic
5 mg erythromycin/g	Ilotycin Ophthalmic
3 mg gentamicin sulfate/g	Garamycin Ophthalmic, Genoptic S.O.P. Ophthalmic, *Generic*
10,000 units polymyxin B sulfate, 3.5 mg neomycin sulfate, 400 units bacitracin zinc/g	Neosporin Ophthalmic, AK-Sporin Ophthalmic
10,000 units polymyxin B sulfate, 500 units bacitracin zinc/g	Polysporin Ophthalmic
10,000 units polymyxin B sulfate, 3.5 mg neomycin sulfate/g	Statrol Ophthalmic

10,000 units poly-myxin B sulfate, 5 mg oxytetracycline HCl/g	Terramycin Ophthalmic
3 mg tobramycin/g	Tobrex Ophthalmic

INDICATIONS

Treatment of superficial ocular infections due to strains of microorganisms susceptible to the antibiotic contained in the product.

CONTRAINDICATIONS

Hypersensitivity.

WARNINGS

Because sensitization may contraindicate later use in serious infections, topical preparations containing antibiotics not ordinarily administered systemically are preferable. Prolonged or frequent intermittent use should be avoided because of the possibility of hypersensitivity reactions, including bone marrow hypoplasia (chloramphenicol). Ophthalmic ointments may retard corneal healing.

PRECAUTIONS

Use (especially prolonged use, repeated therapy) may result in bacterial or fungal overgrowth (superinfection) of nonsusceptible organisms, which may lead to a secondary infection. It is recommended that in all except very superficial infections, topical use be supplemented by appropriate systemic medication.

ADVERSE REACTIONS

Sensitivity reactions such as burning, stinging, itching, angioneurotic edema, urticaria, and vesicular and maculopapular dermatitis have occurred. Systemic **chloramphenicol** has been known to produce bone marrow hypoplasia, depression of erythropoiesis, aplastic anemia, visual disturbances. Bone marrow hypoplasia has been reported after prolonged (23 mo) use of opthalmic solution. Dermatitis and allied symptomatology have been reported with use of **tetracycline HCl.**

DOSAGE

Solutions: _Acute infections_—1 to 2 drops every 15 minutes to 1 hour; frequency reduced as infection is controlled. _Moderate infections_—1 to 2 drops 2 to 6 times/day or more often as needed. _Acute and chronic trachoma_—2 drops in each eye, 2 to 4 times/day. Continue for 1 to 2 months or longer. Concomitant oral tetracycline therapy is helpful.

Ointments: _Acute infections_—½ inch ribbon q3h to q4h until improvement is seen; reduce treatment prior to discontinuation. _Mild to moderate infections_—½ inch ribbon, 2 to 3 times/day.

NURSING IMPLICATIONS

HISTORY

Description and duration of symptoms; allergy history; previous prescription, nonprescription drugs used to treat current (and previous) ophthalmic infection.

PHYSICAL ASSESSMENT

Inspect periorbital area, external eye for redness, swelling, exudate, ulceration of lid margins, excessive tearing, hyperemia of the conjunctiva.

ADMINISTRATION

Place patient in upright position (when possible). Tilt head back.

Instill solution or ointment in lower conjunctival sac.

Drops: Apply light finger pressure on lacrimal sac for 1 minute following instillation.

Ointment: Have patient close eyes (without squeezing shut) for 1 to 2 minutes following instillation.

Advise patient that temporary blurring of vision or stinging may occur following administration.

ONGOING ASSESSMENTS AND NURSING MANAGEMENT

Withhold drug and contact physician if amount of exudate increases, pain/discomfort increases, or sensitivity reactions (severe burning, itching, stinging) occur.

Assess response to therapy each time drug is instilled; record observations.

Observe for signs of superinfection (_e.g.,_ increase in exudate or in signs of infection, redness). Notify physician if these are apparent.

PATIENT AND FAMILY INFORMATION

NOTE: If necessary, demonstrate instillation to patient or family member; if for child, demonstrate restraining methods.

Tilt head back and place amount of medication prescribed by physician into lower conjunctival sac of affected eye.

Do not increase amount of drug or frequency of dose, except on physician's order.

Wash hands thoroughly before and after instilling drug.

Do not contaminate dropper/tip of ointment tube by touching eye, eyelid, or surrounding area.

Keep bottle or tube tightly closed. Do not wash tip of tube or dropper. Do not lay dropper on table (or other surface); replace immediately in bottle after use. Replace cap on tube immediately after use.

May cause temporary blurring of vision or stinging following instillation. Notify physician if stinging, burning, or itching becomes prominent or if condition does not improve.

Use own towel and washcloth.

Do not attempt to drive or engage in potentially hazardous tasks while vision remains blurred.

Antibiotics, Topical

Single Antibiotic Preparations

ointment: 500 units bacitracin/g	Baciguent, *Generic* (*otc*)
ointment: 3% chlortetracycline HCl	Aureomycin (*otc*)
cream: 1% chloramphenicol	Chloromycetin (*Rx*)
ointment: 1% erythromycin	Ilotycin (*Rx*)
ointment: 0.1% gentamicin	Garamycin, *Generic* (*Rx*)
cream: 0.1% gentamicin	Garamycin, *Generic* (*Rx*)
ointment: 5 mg/g neomycin sulfate	Myciguent, *Generic* (*otc*)
cream: 5 mg/g neomycin sulfate	Myciguent (*otc*)
ointment: 3% tetracycline HCl	Achromycin (*otc*)

Multiple Antibiotic Preparations

ointment: 2.5 mg neomycin sulfate, 0.25 mg gramicidin/g	Spectrocin (*otc*)
ointment: 30 mg oxytetracycline, 10,000 units polymyxin B sulfate/g	Terramycin w/Polymyxin B Sulfate (*otc*)
aerosol: 100,000 units polymyxin B sulfate, 70 mg neomycin sulfate, 8000 units zinc bacitracin/90 g	Neosporin (*Rx*)
cream: 10,000 units polymyxin B sulfate, 3.5 mg neomycin sulfate, 0.25 mg gramicidin/g	Neosporin-G (*Rx*)
ointment: 10,000 units polymyxin B sulfate, 500 units zinc bacitracin/g	Biotres, Polysporin (*otc*)
ointment: 5000 units polymyxin B sulfate, 3.5 mg neomycin sulfate, 500 units bacitracin/g	BPN, Mycitracin (*otc*)
ointment: 5000 units polymyxin B sulfate, 3.5 mg neomycin sulfate, 400 units bacitracin/g	Clinicydin, N.B.P., Neo-Thrycex, Septa, Triple Antibiotic (*otc*)
ointment: 5000 units polymyxin B sulfate, 3.5 mg neomycin sulfate, 400 units bacitracin, 10 mg diperodon HCl/g	Epimycin "A," Mity-Mycin (*otc*)
ointment: 500 units zinc bacitracin, 3.5 mg neomycin sulfate/g	Bacimycin (*otc*)
ointment: 5000 units polymyxin B sulfate, 3.5 g neomycin sulfate, 400 units zinc bacitracin/g	Neomixin, Neo-Polycin, Neosporin (*otc*)
powder: 5000 units polymyxin B sulfate, 3.5 g neomycin sulfate, 400 units zinc bacitracin/g	Neosporin (*otc*)

INDICATIONS

Infection prophylaxis in minor skin abrasions; treatment of superficial skin infections due to susceptible organisms and amenable to local treatment.

CONTRAINDICATIONS

Prior sensitization to any of the ingredients; discontinue if sensitivity, irritation appears. Do not use in eyes or in external ear canal if eardrum is perforated.

ACTIONS

See individual (systemic) antibiotic monographs.

WARNINGS

For topical use only. Severe infection may require systemic therapy in addition to local treatment. Owing to potential nephrotoxicity and ototoxicity of **neomycin,** use products containing this drug with care in treating extensive burns, trophic ulceration, and other conditions in which absorption is possible. Do not apply more than once daily in burns when more than 20% of body surface is affected, especially if patient has impaired renal function or is receiving other aminoglycoside antibiotics concurrently. Avoid prolonged or frequent intermittent use of **chloramphenicol** because of possibility of hypersensitivity reactions including bone marrow hyperplasia.

PRECAUTIONS

Prolonged use may result in overgrowth (suprainfection) of nonsusceptible organisms, particularly fungi, which may lead to a secondary infection. Chronic application of **neomycin sulfate** to inflamed skin of those with contact dermatitis increases possibility of sensitization. Low-grade reddening with swelling, dry scaling, and itching or failure to heal is usually a manifestation of hypersensitivity.

During long-term use of neomycin-containing products, periodic examinations are recommended and drug should be discontinued if symptoms appear. Symptoms regress on withdrawal of medication. **Tetracycline** should be discontinued if redness, irritation, or swelling occurs or if pain or infection increases or persists.

Neurotoxic and nephrotoxic antibiotics (neomycin, polymyxin B sulfate, gentamicin) may be absorbed from body surfaces after local application.

ADVERSE REACTIONS

Itching, burning, angioneurotic edema, urticaria, and vesicular and maculopapular dermatitis have occurred in those sensitive to **chloramphenicol** and are causes for discontinuing drug. Bone marrow hyperplasia, including aplastic anemia and death, has been reported following local application of **chloramphenicol.** Allergic contact dermatitis has been reported with use of **bacitracin** ointment. Ototoxicity and nephrotoxicity have been reported with use of **neomycin.**

DOSAGE

Apply 1 to 5 times/day.

NURSING IMPLICATIONS

HISTORY

Record etiology of infection (if known); description and duration of symptoms; allergy history.

PHYSICAL ASSESSMENT

Assess area of superficial infection; record description.

ADMINISTRATION

Cleanse affected area (unless physician directs otherwise); apply as directed by physician.

Area may be covered with a sterile bandage, if needed.

ONGOING ASSESSMENTS AND NURSING MANAGEMENT

Inspect area each time drug is applied; withhold next application if adverse reaction noted. If **neomycin** is used, look for signs of hypersensitivity (_e.g.,_ redness, swelling, dry scaling or itching, failure to heal).

Notify physician if infection worsens or if rash or irritation develops.

PATIENT AND FAMILY INFORMATION

Cleanse affected area of skin prior to application (unless directed otherwise).

Area may be covered with a sterile dressing unless physician directs otherwise.

Notify physician or nurse if condition worsens or rash or irritation occurs.

Do not use other skin products (drugs) on area unless directed to do so by physician.

Tetracycline may stain clothing.

Anticholinergic Antiparkinsonism Agents*

Benztropine Mesylate Rx

tablets: 0.5 mg, 1 mg, 2 mg	Cogentin
injection: 1 mg/ml	Cogentin

Biperiden Rx

tablets: 2 mg	Akineton
injection: 5 mg/ml	Akineton

* For other agents used in the treatment of parkinsonism see Amantadine HCl, Carbidopa Preparations, and Levodopa. Also see Belladonna, Levorotatory Alkaloids of Belladonna, Hyoscyamine Hydrobromide, and Scopolamine HBr.

Diphenhydramine Rx

(See Antihistamines for product availability.)

Ethopropazine Hydrochloride Rx

tablets: 10 mg, 50 mg	Parsidol

Orphenadrine Hydrochloride Rx

tablets: 50 mg	Disipal

Procyclidine Rx

tablets: 5 mg	Kemadrin

Trihexyphenidyl Hydrochloride Rx

tablets: 2 mg	Artane, Tremin, Trihexane, Trihexidyl, Trihexy-2, *Generic*
tablets: 5 mg	Artane, Tremin, Trihexane, Trihexidyl, Trihexy-5, *Generic*
capsules, sustained release: 5 mg	Artane Sequels
elixir: 2 mg/5 ml	Artane

INDICATIONS

BENZTROPINE MESYLATE
Adjunct in therapy of all forms of parkinsonism. May also be used in control of extrapyramidal disorders (except tardive dyskinesia) due to neuroleptic drugs (*e.g.,* phenothiazines).

BIPERIDEN
Adjunct in therapy of all forms of parkinsonism. Useful in control of extrapyramidal disorders due to CNS drugs such as reserpine and phenothiazines.

DIPHENHYDRAMINE
Parkinsonism (including drug-induced extrapyramidal reactions) in the elderly unable to tolerate more potent agents; mild cases of parkinsonism (including drug-induced parkinsonism) in other age groups; in other cases of parkinsonism (including drug-induced parkinsonism) in combination with centrally acting anticholinergic agents.
Other indications: See Index.

ETHOPROPAZINE HYDROCHLORIDE
Adjunct in therapy of all forms of parkinsonism. Chemically a phenothiazine derivative but is distinct from other drugs in its class and is useful in control of extrapyramidal disorders due to CNS drugs such as reserpine and phenothiazines.

ORPHENADRINE HYDROCHLORIDE
Adjunct in therapy of all forms of parkinsonism.

PROCYCLIDINE
Treatment of all forms of parkinsonism. More efficacious in relief of rigidity than of tremor, but tremor, fatigue, weakness, and sluggishness are frequently influenced beneficially. Procyclidine can be substituted for all previous medications in mild and moderate cases. For severe cases, other drugs may be added to therapy. Relieves symptoms of extrapyramidal dysfunction that accompany therapy of mental disorders with phenothiazine and rauwolfia compounds.

TRIHEXYPHENIDYL HYDROCHLORIDE
Adjunct in treatment of all forms of parkinsonism. Useful as adjuvant therapy with levodopa; control of extrapyramidal disorders due to CNS drugs such as reserpine, dibenzoxazepines, phenothiazines, thioxanthenes, butyrophenones. The sustained-release form is indicated for maintenance therapy after patient is stabilized on tablets or elixir.

CONTRAINDICATIONS
Hypersensitivity; angle-closure glaucoma (simple-type glaucomas do not appear to be adversely affected); pyloric or duodenal obstruction, stenosing peptic ulcers, prostatic hypertrophy, or obstructions of bladder neck; achalasia; myasthenia gravis. **Benztropine** is contraindicated in children under 3 and used with caution in older children.

ACTIONS
Therapy of Parkinson's disease is directed at correcting a neurotransmitter imbalance within the CNS (a relative dopamine deficiency and acetylcholine excess in the corpus striatum). Use of levodopa or amantadine enhances dopaminergic activity. Centrally active anticholinergic agents are useful in inhibiting acetylcholine but are generally less effective than levodopa.

These agents are useful in treatment of all forms of parkinsonism: postencephalitic, arteriosclerotic, and idiopathic. They reduce the incidence and severity of akinesia, rigidity, and to a lesser extent, tremor; secondary symptoms such as drooling, hyperhidrosis, and depressed mood are also reduced. In addition to suppressing cholinergic activity in the CNS, these agents may also inhibit the re-uptake and storage of dopamine at central dopamine receptors, thereby prolonging the action of dopamine.

Peripheral anticholinergic side-effects (*e.g.,* urinary retention, tachycardia, constipation) frequently limit dosages that can be used. Antihistamines with central anticholinergic effects are also used and may have lower incidence of peripheral side-effects than belladonna alkaloids or synthetic derivatives; these agents are generally better tolerated by elderly patients. Antihistamines provide mild antiparkinsonian effects and are useful for initiating therapy in those with minimal symptoms. Benztropine has both anticholinergic and antihistaminic properties and a prolonged duration of activity. Ethopropazine is a phenothiazine with prominent anticholinergic effects and is reported to be less effective than synthetic anticholinergic agents. In spite of limited efficacy, the anticholinergic antiparkinsonism drugs are widely used and are useful in mild cases of Parkinson's disease in which the risks and demands of levodopa therapy are not warranted. These agents are also useful in therapy of drug-induced extrapyramidal symptoms.

WARNINGS

Intraocular pressure should be closely monitored at regular intervals. Safety for use in pregnancy is not established; use only when clearly needed and potential benefits outweigh unknown hazards to fetus. Safety and efficacy for use of **procyclidine** in children are not established. Patients, particularly over age 60, frequently develop increased sensitivity to these drugs and require strict dosage regulation.

PRECAUTIONS

Those with cardiac, liver, or kidney disease or hypertension should be under close observation. These drugs should be used with caution in elderly men with possible prostatic hypertrophy. Incipient glaucoma may be precipitated by these drugs. When used to treat extrapyramidal reactions due to phenothiazines or reserpine in patients with mental disorders, antiparkinsonism agents may exacerbate mental symptoms and precipitate a toxic psychosis. Tardive dyskinesia may appear in some on long-term therapy with phenothiazines or related agents, or it may occur after therapy has been discontinued. _Antiparkinsonism agents do not alleviate symptoms of tardive dyskinesia and, in some instances, may aggravate or unmask such symptoms._

Tolerance may develop and dosage may require adjustment. These drugs may produce anhidrosis and are given with caution in hot weather, especially to the elderly, the chronically ill, the alcoholic, those with CNS disease, and those who do manual labor in a hot environment. Dosage may need to be decreased so that ability to maintain body-heat equilibrium by perspiration is not impaired.

May impair mental and physical abilities required for performance of potentially hazardous tasks.

DRUG INTERACTIONS

When giving these agents with phenothiazines or other drugs with anticholinergic activity, advise patients to report gastrointestinal complaints promptly. Paralytic ileus (sometimes fatal) has occurred in those taking anticholinergic-type antiparkinsonism drugs in combination with **phenothiazines** or **tricyclic antidepressants.**

Use with caution in patients also taking **barbiturates,** or **alcohol.** There may be a possible interaction between **orphenadrine** and **propoxyphene,** resulting in mental confusion, anxiety, and tremors. By delaying gastric emptying, large doses of anticholinergic agents may increase gastric degradation of **levodopa** and decrease the amount of levodopa absorbed. Trihexyphenidyl has been associated with decreased plasma **chlorpromazine** levels.

ADVERSE REACTIONS

Frequently seen side-effects, such as dry mouth occasionally in conjunction with soreness of mouth and tongue, blurred vision, dizziness, mild nausea, or nervousness, tend to become less pronounced as treatment continues or may be controlled by careful adjustment of dose or interval between doses. If dry mouth is severe, with difficulty in swallowing or speaking, or anorexia with weight loss occurs, dosage may need to be reduced or drug temporarily discontinued.

There have been isolated instances of suppurative parotitis secondary to excessive dry mouth; skin rashes; dilatation of the colon; paralytic ileus; certain psychiatric manifestations such as delusions, hallucinations, paranoia, mental confusion, agitation, and disturbed behavior; nausea; and vomiting. If a severe reaction should occur, drug should be discontinued for a few days and resumed at a lower dose. Some patients may exhibit short periods of euphoria or disorientation. Psychiatric disturbances can result from indiscriminate use (leading to overdosage) to sustain euphoria. Other potential side-effects include constipation, drowsiness, urinary hesitancy or retention, tachycardia, palpitation, diplopia, increased ocular tension, mental dullness, weakness, epigastric distress, headache, giddiness, elevated temperature, flushing, decreased sweating, mydriasis, mild transient postural hypotension, listlessness, depression, memory loss, muscular cramping, paresthesia, a sensation of heaviness of the limbs, fullness of the stomach, and swelling of the feet. The occurrence of angle-closure glaucoma due to long-term treatment has been reported.

Because **ethopropazine** is a phenothiazine, the following side-effects may be possible: EEG slowing; seizures; ECG abnormalities (_e.g.,_ tachycardia); rare hematologic reactions (agranulocytosis, pancytopenia; purpura); certain endocrine disturbances; jaundice; pigmentation of cornea, lens, retina, skin; visual hallucinations.

OVERDOSAGE

Symptoms: Similar to those of atropine or antihistamine overdose. May include dry mucous membranes; dilatation of pupils; hot, dry, flushed skin; hyperpyrexia; tachycardia; glaucoma; constipation; nausea; vomiting; confusion; coma; convulsions; circulatory collapse; respiratory depression; CNS depression preceded or followed by stimulation, nervousness, listlessness, intensification of mental symptoms, or toxic psychosis in those with mental illness treated with neuroleptic drugs (*e.g.,* phenothiazines); hallucinations (especially visual); dizziness; muscle weakness; ataxia; blurred vision; palpitations; dysuria; numbness of fingers; dysphagia; allergic reactions (*e.g.,* skin rash); headache.

Treatment: Immediately following acute ingestion, remove drug from stomach by inducing emesis (contraindicated in precomatose, convulsive, and psychotic states) or by gavage. Active charcoal is an effective adsorbent. Treatment is symptomatic. To relieve peripheral effects, oral pilocarpine, 5 mg, may be given at repeated intervals. Physostigmine salicylate, 1 mg to 2 mg given subcutaneously or intravenously, will reverse symptoms of anticholinergic intoxication. A second injection may be given after 2 hours if needed. Artificial respiration and oxygen therapy may be needed for respiratory depression. A short-acting barbiturate may be used for CNS excitement, but is used with caution to avoid subsequent respiratory depression. Institute supportive care for depression (avoid convulsant stimulants such as pentylenetetrazol). Urinary retention may require catheterization. Hyperpyrexia may be treated with alcohol sponges, ice bags, other cold applications. To counteract mydriasis and cycloplegia, pilocarpine nitrate 0.5% may be used. Because of photophobia, the patient may be more comfortable in a darkened room. A vasopressor and fluids may be used for circulatory collapse.

DOSAGE

Administration and dosage depend on age of patient, etiology of disease, individual patient response. The dosage required for treatment of drug-induced extrapyramidal symptoms will depend on severity of side-effects associated with tranquilizer (neuroleptic) administration. Dosage must remain flexible to permit adjustment to individual tolerance and requirements. In general, younger and postencephalitic patients require somewhat higher doses than older patients and those with arteriosclerotic or idiopathic parkinsonism. See below for specific dosages.

BENZTROPINE MESYLATE

Tablets should be used when patient is able to take oral medication. Injectable form is useful for psychotic patients with acute dystonic or other reactions that make oral medication difficult or impossible, or when more rapid response is desired. There is no significant difference in onset of action after IV or IM injection. In emergency situations, when condition of patient is alarming, 1 mg to 2 mg will usually provide quick relief. If parkinsonism begins to return, dose may be repeated. Because of cumulative action, therapy is usually initiated with a low dose and increased gradually at 5 to 6 day intervals to the smallest amount necessary for optimal relief. Increases should be made in increments of 0.5 mg to a maximum of 6 mg or until optimal results are obtained without excessive side-effects.

Parkinsonism: Usual daily dose is 1 mg to 2 mg with range of 0.5 mg to 6 mg orally or parenterally. *Idiopathic parkinsonism:* Start with 0.5 mg to 1 mg H.S.; 4 mg/day to 6 mg/day may be required for some patients. For postencephalitic parkinsonism, start with 2 mg/day in 1 or more doses. In highly sensitive patients, begin therapy with 0.5 mg H.S.; increase as needed. Some patients experience greatest relief taking entire dose H.S.; others react more favorably to divided doses bid to qid. Do not terminate therapy with other antiparkinsonism drugs abruptly. Benztropine mesylate may be used concomitantly with a combination of carbidopa and levodopa or with levodopa. Periodic dosage adjustment may be necessary.

Drug-induced extrapyramidal disorders: 1 mg to 4 mg once or twice daily, orally or parenterally. *Acute dystonic reactions:* 1 mg to 2 mg (1 ml to 2 ml) of injection usually relieves condition quickly and may be followed by 1 mg to 2 mg orally bid. Extrapyramidal disorders that develop soon after treatment with neuroleptic drugs are likely to be transient. One milligram to two milligrams PO, two or three times/day usually gives relief in one to two days. Drug may be withdrawn after 1 to 2 weeks to determine need for it. Certain drug-induced extrapyramidal disorders that develop slowly may not respond to benztropine mesylate.

BIPERIDEN

Parkinsonism: 2 mg tid, qid orally.

Drug-induced extrapyramidal disorders: *Oral*—2 mg daily to tid; *parenteral*—average dose is 2 mg IM or IV. May be repeated q½h until symptoms are resolved but no more than 4 consecutive doses/24 hours.

DIPHENHYDRAMINE

Oral: _Adults_—25 mg to 50 mg tid, qid; _children over 20 lb_—12.5 mg to 25 mg tid, qid or 5 mg/kg/ 24 hours.

Parenteral: Administer IV or deep IM. _Adults_— 10 mg to 50 mg, 100 mg if required. Maximum daily dose, 400 mg. _Children_—5 mg/kg/24 hours divided into 4 doses. Maximum daily dose is 300 mg.

ETHOPROPAZINE HYDROCHLORIDE

Initially 50 mg daily or bid; increased gradually if necessary. _Mild to moderate symptoms_—100 mg to 400 mg/day. _Severe cases_—Increased to 500 mg or 600 mg or more/day.

ORPHENADRINE HYDROCHLORIDE

Usual dose 50 mg tid. In combination with other agents and in treatment of Parkinson's syndrome, smaller doses often suffice. Doses up to 250 mg/day have been used.

PROCYCLIDINE

Parkinsonism (for those who have received no other therapy): Initial dose 2.5 mg tid P.C. If tolerated, dose may be gradually increased to 4 mg to 5 mg tid and, if necessary, H.S. Smaller doses may also be used.

Transferring patients from other therapy: Substitute 2 mg to 2.5 mg tid for all or part of original drug. Dose is then increased as needed, while that of the other drug is omitted or reduced until complete replacement is achieved.

Drug-induced extrapyramidal symptoms: Initial dose 2.5 mg tid. May be increased by 2 mg to 2.5 mg daily increments until relief is obtained. Most cases respond with 10 mg to 20 mg/day.

TRIHEXYPHENIDYL HYDROCHLORIDE

Give A.C. or P.C. as determined by patient's reaction. Postencephalitic patients (more prone to salivation) may prefer P.C. administration and, in addition, require small amounts of atropine. If dry-mouth symptoms are severe, take A.C. unless nausea occurs.

Sustained release: Given as single dose P.C. breakfast or in 2 divided doses q12h.

Idiopathic parkinsonism: For initial therapy, give 1 mg to 2 mg first day; increase by 2 mg every 3 to 5 days until total of 6 mg to 10 mg is given daily. Some patients may require 12 mg/day to 15 mg/ day. Drug is tolerated best if given tid with meals. High doses may be divided into 4 doses with the fourth at H.S.

Drug-induced parkinsonism: Daily dose ranges between 5 mg and 15 mg. Initially, 1 mg; if reac-

tions are not controlled in a few hours, subsequent doses may be progressively increased until control is achieved. Control may be more rapidly achieved by temporarily reducing tranquilizer dose when instituting therapy with trihexyphenidyl HCl and then adjusting dose until desired effect is obtained.

Concomitant use with levodopa: Usual dose of each drug may need to be reduced. Dosage of 3 mg/day to 6 mg/day in divided doses is usually adequate.

Concomitant use with other anticholinergics: May be substituted, in whole or part, for other anticholinergics. Usual technique is partial substitution initially, with progressive reduction in other medication as dose of trihexyphenidyl HCl is increased.

NURSING IMPLICATIONS

HISTORY
See Appendix 4.
  NOTE: Because of memory impairment or alterations in thought processes in some patients with parkinsonism, history may be unreliable and should be obtained from family members or patient's chart.

PHYSICAL ASSESSMENT
Look for neurologic alterations (_e.g.,_ tremor [head, hands at rest], masklike facial expression, muscular rigidity with resistance to passive movement, shuffling gait, monotone speech, postural deformities, drooling). Evaluate mental status, thought processes, ability to participate in activities of daily living (ADL).

ADMINISTRATION
If GI upset occurs, give drug with meals or milk or immediately P.C. If severe dryness of mouth occurs, trihexyphenidyl HCl may be taken A.C. or P.C. Manufacturer recommends that procyclidine be administered P.C.

  If difficulty in swallowing oral tablet occurs because of parkinsonism or dry mouth caused by medication, have patient take a few sips of water before taking medication. If dysphagia persists, discuss problem with physician.

  Inspect oral cavity after patient swallows medication, especially if patient has dysphagia, is elderly, or is receiving psychotherapeutic drug.
  NOTE: Benztropine mesylate, injectable, is available as 1 mg/ml in 2-ml ampules (2 mg/ampule).

ONGOING ASSESSMENTS AND NURSING MANAGEMENT
Check vital signs daily. Observe for changes in pulse rate, rise in temperature.

Assess results of drug therapy by observing neurologic status and comparing to data base; observe changes in participation in ADL; observe for appearance of adverse effects, especially excessive dryness of mouth, urinary retention, paralytic ileus, visual and mental changes.

Patient should be assessed at more frequent intervals during initial therapy as well as each time dose is adjusted upward or downward.

Therapy should not be terminated abruptly unless serious adverse reactions occur. If the nurse, exercising clinical judgment, withholds the next dose of the drug and plans to contact the physician, this should be done as soon as possible.

Measure intake and output if urinary retention is suspected or patient has history of prostatic enlargement or nocturia.

Because some patients may communicate poorly, observe for overt symptoms of distress: apparent abdominal discomfort or pain (*e.g.,* urinary retention, paralytic ileus, constipation), changes in behavior (*e.g.,* hallucinations, depression, confusion), apparent visual difficulty (*e.g.,* diplopia, blurred vision, increased intraocular tension).

If postural hypotension or mental or physical impairment develops, assist with ambulation, ADL.

During hot weather, closely monitor patient for anhidrosis, hot dry skin, rise in body temperature. Should these occur, withhold next dose and contact physician immediately.

Dry mouth may be relieved by sips of water, ice chips, chewing gum (preferably sugarless), or hard candy. If dry mouth is severe, discuss problem with physician as well as observe for signs of parotitis (tenderness, swelling in front of ear, earache intensified by chewing, pain in gland when chewing or eating sour or acidic foods).

Accurate observations, document daily, assist the physician in adjusting dosage upward or downward to achieve desired therapeutic results.

When used to treat extrapyramidal reactions resulting from reserpine or the phenothiazines in patients with mental disorders, antiparkinsonism agents may exacerbate mental symptoms and precipitate a psychosis. Observe patient's behavior at frequent intervals; if behavioral changes are noted, withhold next dose of drug and contact physician.

Periodic ophthalmic examinations may be ordered.

See also Antihistamines.

PATIENT AND FAMILY INFORMATION

If GI upset occurs, take with food.

May cause drowsiness, dizziness, blurred vision; observe caution while driving, performing tasks requiring alertness; assistance with activities such as walking, dressing, and going up or down stairs may be required.

NOTE: If patient is elderly, family should be encouraged to remove objects or remedy situations that may cause falling (*e.g.,* small rugs, slippery floors).

Avoid alcohol, other CNS depressants.

May cause dry mouth, difficult urination, constipation; notify physician or nurse if these effects persist or become bothersome.

Notify physician or nurse if rapid or pounding heartbeat, confusion, eye pain, visual changes, or rash occurs.

Dry mouth may be relieved by sips of water, gum, hard candy. If it is persistent or uncomfortable, discuss problem with physician (saliva substitutes may be recommended).

Consult dentist if dry mouth interferes with wearing, inserting, or removing dentures.

Anticonvulsants*

WARNINGS

Recent reports strongly suggest an association between the use of anticonvulsant drugs by women with epilepsy and an elevated incidence of birth defects in children born to these women. The possibility exists that other factors may also contribute to the higher incidence of birth defects.

Anticonvulsant drugs are not discontinued in pregnant patients in whom the drug is administered to prevent major seizures because of the strong possibility of precipitating status epilepticus with attendant hypoxia and risk to both mother and unborn child. The physician may consider discontinuation of anticonvulsants prior to and during pregnancy when the nature, frequency, and severity of seizures do not pose a serious threat to the patient. It is not known whether even minor seizures constitute some risk to the developing embryo or fetus.

Reports suggest that maternal use of anticonvulsants, particularly barbiturates, is associated with a neonatal coagulation defect that may cause bleeding

---

* The barbiturates used as anticonvulsants are discussed in Barbiturates, and include *Amobarbital Sodium, Pentobarbital Sodium, Phenobarbital Sodium,* and *Secobarbital Sodium.* Also see the discussion of *Thiopental Sodium,* a barbiturate general anesthetic.

Miscellaneous agents used as anticonvulsants include *Acetazolamide, Carbamazepine, Magnesium Sulfate, Paraldehyde, Phenacemide, Primidone,* and *Valproic Acid.*

during the early (usually within 24 hours of birth) neonatal period. It has been suggested that prophylactic vitamin K be given to the mother 1 month prior to and during delivery, and to the infant, IV, immediately after birth.

Benzodiazepines

Clonazepam Rx C–IV

tablets: 0.5 mg,   Clonopin
   1 mg, 2 mg

INDICATIONS
Alone or as adjunct in treatment of Lennox-Gastaut syndrome (petit mal variant), akinetic and myoclonic seizures. May be useful in absence (petit mal) seizures not responding to succinimides.

CONTRAINDICATIONS
Hypersensitivity, clinical or biochemical evidence of significant liver disease. May be used in those with open-angle glaucoma receiving appropriate therapy, but not in acute narrow-angle glaucoma.

ACTIONS
Capable of depressing the spike and wave discharge in absence (petit mal) seizures and decreasing the frequency, amplitude, duration, and spread of discharge in motor seizures. Therapeutic serum concentrations: 20 ng/ml to 80 ng/ml.

WARNINGS
Withdrawal symptoms similar to those noted with barbiturates and alcohol have occurred following abrupt discontinuation. These symptoms include convulsions, tremor, abdominal and muscle cramps, vomiting, sweating. Keep addiction-prone persons under careful surveillance because of predisposition to habituation and dependence.

Abrupt withdrawal, particularly in patients on long-term, high-dose therapy, may precipitate status epilepticus. While clonazepam is being gradually withdrawn, simultaneous substitution of another anticonvulsant may be indicated.

Use in pregnancy, lactation: Effects are unknown. Use only when clearly needed and when potential benefits outweigh the unknown potential hazards to the fetus. Mothers receiving clonazepam should not breast-feed their infants. See also statement on page 80 regarding use of anticonvulsants.

Children: Because of the possibility that adverse effects on physical and mental development could become apparent only after many years, a benefit-to-risk consideration of long-term use is important.

PRECAUTIONS
Produces CNS depression; caution should be observed while driving or performing tasks requiring alertness. When used in those in whom several different types of seizure disorders coexist, clonazepam may increase incidence or precipitate onset of generalized tonic–clonic (grand mal) seizures. This may require the addition of other anticonvulsants or an increase in dosage. Periodic blood counts and hepatic-function tests are advisable during long-term therapy. Caution is exercised in patients with renal impairment because clonazepam metabolites are excreted by the kidney. May produce increase in salivation; exercise caution in giving to patients who have difficulty in handling secretions; use with caution in patients with chronic respiratory disease.

DRUG INTERACTIONS
The CNS depressant effect may be potentiated by **alcohol, narcotics, barbiturates, nonbarbiturate hypnotics, antianxiety agents, phenothiazines, thioxanthene, butyrophenone** classes of antipsychotic agents, **monoamine oxidase inhibitors, tricyclic antidepressants,** other **anticonvulsant drugs.** Concomitant use of **valproic acid** and **clonazepam** may produce absence (petit mal) status. **Phenobarbital** or **phenytoin** may decrease steady-state clonazepam serum levels.

ADVERSE REACTIONS
Most frequent are referable to CNS depression. Drowsiness has occurred in approximately 50% of patients, ataxia in approximately 30%. In some cases, these diminish with time. Behavioral problems have been noted in approximately 25%. Other adverse effects include the following.

Neurologic: Abnormal eye movements; aphonia; choreiform movements; coma; diplopia; dysarthria; glassy-eyed appearance; headache; hemiparesis; hypotonia; nystagmus; respiratory depression; slurred speech; tremor; vertigo.

Psychiatric: Confusion; depression; forgetfulness; hallucinations; hysteria; increased libido; insomnia; psychosis; suicidal attempts (behavioral effects are more likely to occur in those with a history of psychiatric disturbances).

Respiratory: Chest congestion; rhinorrhea; shortness of breath; hypersecretion in upper respiratory passages.

Cardiovascular: Palpitations.

Dermatologic: Hair loss; hirsutism; skin rash; ankle, facial edema.

_GI:_ Anorexia; coated tongue; constipation; diarrhea; dry mouth; fecal incontinence; gastritis; increased appetite; nausea; sore gums.

_GU:_ Dysuria; enuresis; nocturia; urinary retention.

Musculoskeletal: Muscle weakness, pains.

Hematopoietic: Anemia; leukopenia; thrombocytopenia; eosinophilia.

Hepatic: Hepatomegaly; transient elevations of serum transaminases, alkaline phosphatase.

Miscellaneous: Dehydration; general deterioration; fever; lymphadenopathy; weight loss, gain.

OVERDOSAGE

Symptoms: Somnolence, confusion, coma, diminished reflexes.

Treatment: Monitor respiration, pulse, blood pressure; take general supportive measures; perform immediate gastric lavage with activated charcoal; hypotension may be combated with vasopressors. Dialysis is of no known value.

DOSAGE

Adults: Initial dose should not exceed 1.5 mg/day, divided into 3 doses. Dosage may be increased by increments of 0.5 mg to 1 mg every 3 days until seizures are adequately controlled or side-effects preclude further increase. Maintenance dosage is individualized. Maximum recommended dosage is 20 mg/day.

Infants, children (up to 10 years): To minimize drowsiness, initial dose should be between 0.01 mg/kg/day and 0.03 mg/kg/day, not to exceed 0.05 mg/kg/day given in 2 or 3 divided doses. Dosage should be increased by not more than 0.25 mg to 0.5 mg every third day until a daily maintenance dose of 0.1 mg/kg to 0.2 mg/kg has been reached, unless seizures are controlled or side-effects preclude further increase. Whenever possible, daily dose should be divided into 3 equal doses; if not equally divided, largest dose should be given H.S.

Use of multiple anticonvulsants may result in an increase of depressant adverse effects.

▎ NURSING IMPLICATIONS
See p 89.

Clorazepate Dipotassium Rx C–IV

tablets, capsules: 3.75 mg, 7.5 mg, 15 mg	Tranxene
tablets: 11.25 mg	Tranxene-SD Half Strength
tablets: 22.5 mg	Tranxene-SD

INDICATIONS

Adjunctive therapy in management of partial seizures. Also indicated for anxiety (see Benzodiazepines).

CONTRAINDICATIONS, WARNINGS, PRECAUTIONS, DRUG INTERACTIONS, ADVERSE REACTIONS, OVERDOSAGE
See Benzodiazepines.

DOSAGE

To minimize drowsiness, recommended initial dosages and dosage increments should not be exceeded.

Adults: Maximum recommended initial dose is 7.5 mg tid. Dosage should be increased by no more than 7.5 mg every week and should not exceed 90 mg/day.

Children (9–12): Maximum recommended initial dose is 7.5 mg bid. Dosage should be increased by no more than 7.5 mg every week and should not exceed 60 mg/day. Not recommended in patients under 9 years of age.

▎ NURSING IMPLICATIONS
See p 89.

Diazepam Rx C–IV

tablets: 2 mg, 5 mg, 10 mg	Valium
capsules, sustained release: 15 mg	Valrelease
injection: 5 mg/ml	Valium

INDICATIONS

Oral: Adjunct in treatment of convulsive disorders; has not been proved useful as sole therapy. When used as an adjunct, the possibility of an increase in frequency or severity of grand mal seizures may require an increase in dosage of standard anticonvulsant medication. Abrupt withdrawal in such cases may also be associated with temporary increase in frequency or severity of seizures.

Parenteral: Adjunct in status epilepticus, severe recurrent convulsive seizures. Also used as an antianxiety agent, muscle relaxant, and in acute alcohol withdrawal (see Benzodiazepines).

CONTRAINDICATIONS, WARNINGS, PRECAUTIONS, DRUG INTERACTIONS, ADVERSE REACTIONS, OVERDOSAGE
See Benzodiazepines.

DOSAGE

Doses given below will meet the needs of most patients; some may require higher doses. Lower doses are used, and dose is increased slowly in elderly or debilitated patients or when other sedative drugs are administered.

Oral: Adults—2 mg to 10 mg bid to qid; geriatric or debilitated patients—2 mg to 2.5 mg daily or bid; increase gradually as needed. Children—1 mg to 2.5 mg tid, qid; increase gradually as needed. Not for children under 6 months.

Oral, sustained release: Adults—15 mg to 30 mg once daily.

Parenteral: *Adults*—5 mg to 10 mg initially (IV preferred); may be repeated if necessary at 10 to 15 minute intervals up to maximum dose of 30 mg. If necessary, may be repeated in 2 to 4 hours. *Children*—infants over 30 days and children under 5 years, 0.2 mg to 0.5 mg (IV preferred) every 5 minutes to a maximum of 5 mg. Children 5 and over, 1 mg every 2 to 5 minutes up to maximum of 10 mg. Repeat in 2 to 4 hours if needed. Efficacy and safety of parenteral diazepam in neonates (under 30 days) not established.

Hydantoins

Ethotoin Rx

tablets: 250 mg, 500 mg	Peganone

Mephenytoin Rx

tablets: 100 mg	Mesantoin

Phenytoin Rx

tablets: 50 mg	Dilantin Infatab
oral suspension: 30 mg/5 ml	Dilantin-30 Pediatric
oral suspension: 125 mg/5 ml	Dilantin-125

Phenytoin Sodium, Extended Rx

capsules: 30 mg, 100 mg	Dilantin Kapseals

Phenytoin Sodium, Parenteral Rx

injection: 50 mg/ml	Dilantin, *Generic*

Phenytoin Sodium, Prompt Rx

capsules: 30 mg	Diphenylan Sodium
capsules: 100 mg	Diphenylan Sodium, Ditan, *Generic*

Phenytoin Sodium With Phenobarbital Rx

capsules: 100 mg w/ phenobarbital 16 mg or 32 mg	Dilantin with Phenobarbital Kapseals

INDICATIONS

ETHOTOIN

Grand mal (tonic–clonic) and psychomotor (temporal lobe, complex partial) seizures.

MEPHENYTOIN

Grand mal (tonic–clonic), psychomotor (temporal lobe, complex partial), focal, and Jacksonian seizures in patients refractory to less toxic anticonvulsant drugs.

PHENYTOIN PREPARATIONS

Grand mal (tonic–clonic) and psychomotor (temporal lobe, complex partial) seizures.

Parenteral phenytoin is used for control of status epilepticus of the grand mal type and prevention and treatment of seizures occurring during neurosurgery.

Investigational: Although not FDA approved, IV phenytoin is useful as an antiarrhythmic agent, particularly in digitalis-induced arrhythmias.

CONTRAINDICATIONS

Hypersensitivity to hydantoins. **Ethotoin** is contraindicated in those with hepatic abnormalities or hematologic disorders. Because of its effect on ventricular automaticity, **IV phenytoin** is not used in sinus bradycardia, sinoatrial block, second- and third-degree heart block, Adams-Stokes syndrome.

ACTIONS

Primary site of action appears to be the motor cortex, where spread of seizure activity is inhibited. Possibly by promoting sodium efflux from neurons, hydantoins tend to stabilize the threshold against hyperexcitability caused by excessive stimulation or environmental changes capable of reducing membrane sodium gradient. This includes reduction of post-tetanic potentiation at synapses, which in turn prevents cortical seizure foci from detonating adjacent cortical areas. Hydantoins reduce the maximal activity of brain-stem centers responsible for the tonic phase of grand mal seizures.

Phenytoin is slowly absorbed from the small intestine. Oral phenytoin sodium, extended, dissolves slowly and reaches peak plasma levels in 5 to 6 hours; phenytoin sodium prompt achieves peak levels within 2 to 3 hours. Phenytoin is very slowly and erratically absorbed after IM administration. Phenytoin is metabolized in the liver and excreted in the urine. Individual variation in drug metabolism occurs; half-life ranges from 8 to 60 hours (average 20–30 hours). Steady-state therapeutic levels are achieved 7 to 10 days after initiation of therapy with recommended doses of 300 mg/day.

Serum levels: Therapeutic serum concentration for phenytoin is 10 mcg/ml to 20 mcg/ml; 5 mcg/ml to 10 mcg/ml may be therapeutic for some patients. Serum concentrations of less than 5 mcg/ml are not likely to be effective. Toxic concentrations are between 30 mcg/ml and 50 mcg/ml; lethal concentrations are approximately 100 mcg/ml. Serum level monitoring is essential. Therapeutic plasma concentrations of ethotoin range from 15 mcg/ml to 50 mcg/ml.

WARNINGS

Abrupt withdrawal in epileptic patients may precipitate status epilepticus. Reduce dosage, discontinue drug, or gradually substitute another anticonvulsant. Not indicated in seizures due to hypoglycemia or other causes that may be immediately identified and corrected. **Phenytoin** is used with caution in hypotension and severe myocardial insufficiency. See general warning, p 80, for use in pregnancy. These drugs are excreted in breast milk. Because of potential for serious adverse reactions in nursing infants, a decision should be made to discontinue nursing or discontinue drug.

PRECAUTIONS

Impaired hepatic function: Liver is chief site of biotransformation; patients with impaired liver function, the elderly, or those gravely ill may show early signs of toxicity. If hepatic dysfunction is suspected, hepatic-function tests should be made.

Hematologic effects: It is recommended that blood counts and urinalysis be performed when therapy is begun and at monthly intervals for several months thereafter. Blood dyscrasias have been reported, most commonly with *Mephenytoin.* Avoid use in combination with other drugs known to affect the hematopoietic system adversely. There is some evidence that hydantoinlike compounds may interfere with folic acid metabolism, precipitating a megaloblastic anemia. If this should occur during gestation, folic acid therapy may be considered.

Dermatologic effects: If rash appears, discontinue drug. If rash is exfoliative, purpuric, or bullous, use of drug should not be resumed. If rash is milder, therapy may be resumed after rash has completely disappeared. If rash recurs, further anticonvulsant medication is contraindicated.

Lymph node hyperplasia: These drugs have been associated with lymph node hyperplasia, which is usually reversible. Rarely, this may progress to malignant lymphoma. If hyperplasia occurs, an effort should be made to substitute another anticonvulsant.

Hypersensitivity: Allergic or hypersensitivity reactions may require rapid substitution of alternate therapy with a drug not of the hydantoin chemical class.

Hyperglycemia: Hyperglycemia, resulting from an inhibitory effect on insulin release, has been reported. Hydantoins may raise blood glucose levels in those with hyperglycemia.

Cardiovascular: Observe patient closely when drug is administered IV when possibility of sino-atrial node depression exists. Administer cautiously in presence of atrioventricular block.

Others: Drugs that control grand mal seizures are not effective for petit mal seizures; if both types of seizure are present, combined therapy is needed. Osteomalacia has been associated with hydantoin therapy. Hydantoins are administered cautiously to those with acute intermittent porphyria.

DRUG INTERACTIONS

The following have been reported with use of phenytoin but may occur with use of any of the hydantoins.

Agents that increase the effects of phenytoin: **Coumarin anticoagulants, disulfiram, phenylbutazone, isoniazid, chloramphenicol, cimetidine, sulfonamides** (sulfamethizole, sulfadiazine, sulfamethoxazole), co-trimoxazole, and Trimethoprim may inhibit phenytoin metabolism, resulting in prolonged half-life and increased phenytoin serum levels. Dicumarol inhibits phenytoin metabolism in the liver; concurrent administration of warfarin does not appear to impair phenytoin metabolism. Concomitant administration of **isoniazid** and phenytoin therapy may cause phenytoin intoxication. **Chloramphenicol** may cause a threefold to fourfold increase in phenytoin levels. Increased phenytoin levels have been reported during concomitant **dexamethasone** therapy. High doses of **salicylates** may displace phenytoin from protein binding, thereby increasing plasma concentration of free phenytoin.

Agents that decrease the effects of phenytoin: **Barbiturates** may enhance the rate of metabolism of phenytoin; this effect is variable and unpredictable. When there is difficulty establishing dosage levels when both drugs are used as anticonvulsants, this interaction may be a contributing factor. Administration of **folic acid** to folate-deficient patients receiving phenytoin may result in increased phenytoin metabolism and decreased phenytoin serum levels; increased frequency of seizures has been reported. Acute **alcohol** intoxication may increase the anticonvulsant effect; chronic **alcohol** abuse may result in a decreased anticonvulsant effect. Decreased GI absorption and bioavailability has been reported following **antacid** (aluminum hydroxide, magnesium hydroxide, calcium carbonate) administration, **calcium gluconate, oxacillin,** and **antineoplastic** therapy (vinblastine, cisplatin, bleomycin), and increased **dietary calcium** intake (either as nutritional supplement or in various antacids).

Phenytoin decreases the effects of the following drugs

Dicumarol—decreased anticoagulant effects.

Disopyramide, quinidine—decreased half-life, reduced antiarrhythmic effects. Larger doses may be required to maintain therapeutic antiarrhythmic effects of these agents.

Prednisolone, dexamethasone, possibly other **corticosteroids**—inhibition of effect; corticosteroid dosages may need to be increased.

Oral contraceptives—reduced efficacy, breakthrough bleeding. Risk of oral-contraceptive failure is higher with low-estrogen-component contraceptives.

Digitoxin—metabolism may be increased.

Furosemide—absorption may be impaired.

Miscellaneous drug interactions: Infusion of **dopamine** and phenytoin may lead to hypotension, bradycardia. Phenytoin increases the anticoagulant effects of **warfarin**. Concomitant administration of **valproic acid** and pheyntoin has been reported to produce breakthrough seizures. Paranoid symptoms have occurred with administration of **phenacemide** and phenytoin. **Tricyclic antidepressants** in high doses may precipitate seizures; dosage of phenytoin may need to be adjusted.

Drug/lab tests: Phenytoin may interfere with the **Metyrapone** and the 1-mg **dexamethasone** tests. It may also suppress protein-bound iodine and the unbound concentration of T_4.

ADVERSE REACTIONS

CNS: Most common manifestations involve the CNS and include nystagmus, ataxia, dysarthria, slurred speech, and mental confusion. Dizziness, insomnia, transient nervousness, motor twitchings (*i.e.,* choreiform movements), diplopia, fatigue, irritability, depression, tremor, headache may also be seen. These may disappear by continuing therapy at reduced dosage. Drowsiness is dose related. Transient hyperkinesia following IV phenytoin infusion has been reported.

The most notable signs of toxicity associated with IV phenytoin sodium are cardiovascular collapse and CNS depression. Hypotension occurs when drug is administered rapidly. Cardiac arrhythmias, including ventricular fibrillation or arrest, may occur. Rate of administration is *very important; do not exceed 50 mg/minute.* Drowsiness, nystagmus, circumoral tingling, nausea, and rarely vomiting may also be seen; however, these usually occur when plasma concentrations are above 20 mcg/ml.

GI: Nausea, vomiting, diarrhea, constipation.

Dermatologic: Manifestations have included scarlatiniform, morbilliform, maculopapular, urticarial, and nonspecific rashes, sometimes accompanied by fever. Rashes are more common in children and young adults. Other, more serious, forms that *may be fatal* include bullous, exfoliative, or purpuric dermatitis, lupus erythematosus, and Stevens-Johnson syndrome.

Hematopoietic: Thrombocytopenia, leukopenia, granulocytopenia, agranulocytosis, and pancytopenia have been reported; some have been fatal. Macrocytosis and megaloblastic anemia have occurred; these usually respond to folic acid therapy. Eosinophilia, monocytosis, and leukocytosis have occurred. *Rare:* Simple anemia, hemolytic anemia, aplastic anemia.

Lymphadenopathy, which simulates Hodgkin's disease, has been seen. The occurrence of Hodgkin's disease, monoclonal gammopathy, and multiple myeloma during prolonged therapy with **phenytoin sodium** have been reported.

Gingival hyperplasia: Occurs frequently with **phenytoin;** incidence is reduced by good oral hygiene.

Hepatic: Toxic hepatitis, liver damage, periarteritis nodosa may occur and can be fatal.

Miscellaneous: Polyarthropathy, hirsutism, alopecia, weight gain, numbness, chest pain, edema, fever, photophobia, conjunctivitis, pulmonary fibrosis, acute pneumonitis, lupus erythematosus syndrome.

OVERDOSAGE

Symptoms: Mean lethal dose is estimated to be 2 g to 5 g. Initial symptoms are nystagmus, ataxia, and dysarthria; the patient then becomes comatose, his pupils become unresponsive, and hypotension occurs. Death is due to respiratory depression, apnea.

Treatment: Nonspecific; no known antidote. Begin by inducing emesis; gastric lavage is an alternative. If gag reflex is absent, support airway. Oxygen, vasopressors, and assisted ventilation may be necessary. Hemodialysis can be considered. Total exchange transfusion has been used in treatment of severe intoxication in children.

DOSAGE
ETHOTOIN

Adults: Initial dose 1000 mg/day or less in 4 to 6 divided doses with subsequent gradual dosage increases over a period of several days. Optimum dosage determined by patient response. Usual maintenance dose, 2 g/day to 3 g/day.

Children: Dosage depends on age and weight; initial dose should not exceed 750 mg/day. Maintenance dose ranges from 500 mg/day to 1 g/day; occasionally 2 g/day or, rarely, 3 g/day may be needed.

Replacement therapy: Dosage of other drug is reduced gradually as that of ethotoin is increased.

Concomitant anticonvulsant therapy: Ethotoin is compatible with all anticonvulsant medications except phenacemide. In grand mal seizures, use of drug with metharbital or phenobarbital may be beneficial. It may be used with drugs such as trimethadione or paramethadione as an adjunct in patients with petit mal associated with grand mal.

MEPHENYTOIN

Maintenance dose is smallest amount necessary to suppress seizures completely or reduce their frequency. Optimum dosage is attained by starting with 50 mg/day or 100 mg/day for the first week and increasing daily dose by 50 mg or 100 mg at weekly intervals.

Adults: Average dose is 200 mg/day to 600 mg/day; up to 800 mg/day may be necessary.

Children: 100 mg/day to 400 mg/day depending on age and nature of seizures.

Replacement therapy: 5 mg to 100 mg mephenytoin first week; dose gradually increased at weekly intervals while dose of other drug is gradually reduced. If patient is also receiving phenobarbital, it is advisable to continue it until transition is completed, at which time phenobarbital can be gradually withdrawn.

PHENYTOIN

Oral

Serum level determinations may be necessary for optimal dosage adjustments.

Adults: Patients who have received no previous treatment—100 mg tid. For most, maintenance dose will be 300 mg/day to 400 mg/day; up to 600 mg/day may be needed by some patients.

Pediatric: Initially, 5 mg/kg/day in 2 or 3 equally divided doses; subsequent dosage is individualized to maximum of 300 mg/day. Daily maintenance dose is usually 4 mg/kg to 8 mg/kg. Children over 6 require the minimum adult dose (300 mg/day).

Phenytoin sodium, extended: May be used for once-a-day dosing as well as tid administration. Once seizure control is established with divided doses, total daily dose may be administered as a single daily dose.

NOTE: Because of potential bioavailability differences among products, brand interchange is not recommended. Dosage adjustments may be required when switching from the extended to the prompt products.

Parenteral

IM route should be avoided because of erratic absorption and pain and necrosis at injection site. When IM route is required for a patient previously stabilized orally, dosage adjustments are necessary. An IM dose 50% greater than the oral dose is necessary to maintain therapeutic plasma levels. When returning to oral administration, dose is reduced by 50% of original oral dose for 1 week. If more than 1 week of IM administration is required, alternate routes such as gastric intubation may be considered.

Status epilepticus: 150 mg to 250 mg IV administered *Slowly,* then 100 mg to 150 mg is administered 30 minutes later if necessary. Higher doses may be required. Dose for children is determined according to weight in proportion to dose for a 150-lb adult or calculated on a basis of 250 mg/m². If immobilization of an extremity is impossible because of convulsions, or if veins are inaccessible, give IM. If seizures are not terminated, other anticonvulsants, IV barbiturates, general anesthesia, or other measures may be tried.

Neurosurgery (prophylactic) dosage: 100 mg to 200 mg IM at approximately q4h intervals during surgery and the postoperative period. A total of 1000 mg should not usually be exceeded during first 24 hours of therapy; thereafter, maintenance-level dosages are usually sufficient.

NURSING IMPLICATIONS
See p 89.

Oxazolidinediones

Paramethadione Rx

capsules: 150 mg, 300 mg	Paradione (300 mg contains tartrazine)
solution: 300 mg/ml	Paradione

Trimethadione Rx

dulcets (tablets, chewable): 150 mg	Tridione
capsules: 300 mg	Tridione
solution: 40 mg/ml	Tridione

INDICATIONS
Control of absence (petit mal) seizures. Because of their potential to produce fetal malformations and serious side-effects, these agents should be used only when other, less toxic drugs, are ineffective.

CONTRAINDICATIONS
Hypersensitivity.

ACTIONS
Elevates seizure threshold in cerebral cortex and basal ganglia and reduces response to low-frequency repetitive stimulation. Readily absorbed from GI tract. Therapeutic serum levels (measured as active metabolite, dimethadione): 700 mcg/ml or above.

May cause serious side-effects; strict supervision of patient is mandatory, especially during initial therapy. See p 80 for statement on usage in pregnancy.

PRECAUTIONS
Abrupt withdrawal may precipitate absence (petit mal) status; withdraw gradually unless serious adverse effects dictate otherwise. Withdraw promptly if skin rash appears, because of grave possibility of occurrence of exfoliative dermatitis and severe forms of erythema multiforme. Even a minor rash should be allowed to clear before treatment is resumed.

Hepatic: Hepatic-function tests should be performed prior to therapy and monthly thereafter. Jaundice or other signs of liver dysfunction are indication for drug withdrawal. Rarely, hepatitis is associated with use of these drugs.

Renal: Perform urinalysis prior to therapy and monthly thereafter. Fatal nephrosis has been reported. Persistent or increasing proteinuria or development of significant renal abnormality is indication for drug withdrawal.

Ophthalmic: Diminished vision in bright light (hemeralopia), which can be reversed by dosage reduction. Scotomata are indication for drug withdrawal.

Lupus: Manifestations of systemic lupus erythematosus and lymphadenopathies simulating malignant lymphoma. Lupuslike manifestations, lymph node enlargement are indications for drug withdrawal.

Myasthenia gravis-like syndrome: This syndrome has been associated with use of these drugs; symptoms suggestive of this condition are indication for drug withdrawal.

Hematologic: A CBC should be taken prior to therapy and monthly thereafter. Marked depression of the blood count is indication for drug withdrawal.

Use **trimethadione** with caution in patients with acute intermittent porphyria.

Tartrazine sensitivity: Some of these products contain tartrazine (see Appendix 6, section 6-23).

DRUG INTERACTIONS
Drugs known to cause toxic effects similar to those of the oxazolidinediones should be avoided or used with extreme caution.

ADVERSE REACTIONS
Renal: Fatal nephrosis, proteinuria.

Hematologic: Fatal aplastic anemia, hypoplastic anemia, pancytopenia, agranulocytosis, leukopenia, neutropenia, thrombocytopenia, eosinophilia, retinal and petechial hemorrhages, vaginal bleeding, epistaxis, bleeding gums.

Hepatic: Hepatitis (rare).

Dermatologic: Acneiform or morbilliform rash that may progress to severe forms of erythema multiforme or exfoliative dermatitis; hair loss.

CNS/neurologic: Myasthenia gravis-like syndrome, precipitation of tonic–clonic (grand mal) seizures, vertigo, personality changes, increased irritability, drowsiness, headache, paresthesias, fatigue, malaise, insomnia. Drowsiness usually subsides with continued therapy; if it persists, dose reduction is indicated.

Ophthalmologic: Diplopia, hemeralopia, photophobia.

Cardiovascular: Changes in blood pressure.

GI: Vomiting, abdominal pain, gastric distress, nausea, anorexia, weight loss, hiccups.

Other: Lupus erythematosus and lymphadenopathies simulating malignant lymphoma. Pruritus associated with lymphadenopathy and hepatosplenomegaly has occurred in hypersensitive individuals.

OVERDOSAGE
Symptoms: Acute overdosage—nausea, drowsiness, dizziness, ataxia, visual disturbances. Coma may follow massive overdosage.

Treatment: Immediate gastric evacuation by induced emesis, lavage, or both. General supportive care including frequent monitoring of vital signs. Alkalinization of urine has been reported to increase renal excretion. A blood count and evaluation of hepatic and renal function should be done following recovery.

DOSAGE
PARAMETHADIONE AND TRIMETHADIONE

Adults: 900 mg to 2.4 g/day in 3 or 4 equally divided doses (300 mg to 600 mg tid, qid). Initially, 900 mg daily; increased by 300 mg at weekly intervals until therapeutic results are seen or toxic symptoms occur. Adjust maintenance dosage to minimum required to maintain control.

Children: Usually 300 mg/day to 900 mg/day, in 3 or 4 equally divided doses.

❚ NURSING IMPLICATIONS
See p 89.

Succinimides

Ethosuximide Rx

capsules: 250 mg	Zarontin
syrup: 250 mg/5 ml	Zarontin

Methsuximide Rx

| capsules, half strength: 150 mg | Celontin Kapseals (contains tartrazine) |
| capsules: 300 mg | Celontin Kapseals (contains tartrazine) |

Phensuximide Rx

| capsules: 500 mg | Milontin Kapseals |

INDICATIONS

ETHOSUXIMIDE
Absence (petit mal) seizures.

METHSUXIMIDE
Absence (petit mal) seizures. Recommended only for patients refractory to other drugs.

PHENSUXIMIDE
Absence (petit mal) seizures.

CONTRAINDICATIONS
Hypersensitivity.

ACTIONS
Suppression of the paroxysmal three cycle per second spike and wave activity, associated with lapses of consciousness, that is common in absence seizures. Frequency of attacks is reduced, apparently by depression of the motor cortex and elevation of the threshold of the CNS to convulsive stimuli. Therapeutic serum levels of ethosuximide: 40 mcg/ml to 100 mcg/ml.

WARNINGS
Blood dyscrasias, some fatal, have been reported; periodic blood counts should be performed. Administer with caution to those with known hepatic or renal disease. Periodic urinalysis, hepatic-function studies are advised. Cases of lupus erythematosus have been reported. See p 80 for statement regarding use in pregnancy.

PRECAUTIONS
These drugs, when used alone in mixed types of epilepsy, may increase grand mal seizures in some patients. Dosage should be increased or decreased slowly; abrupt withdrawal may precipitate absence (petit mal) status. It is recommended that these drugs be withdrawn slowly on appearance of unusual depression, aggressiveness, or other behavioral alterations. Use **phensuximide** with caution in patients with acute intermittent porphyria.

Tartrazine sensitivity: One product (methsuximide) contains tartrazine (see Appendix 6, section 6-23).

ADVERSE REACTIONS
The following have been reported with one or more of the succinimides.

GI: Symptoms occur frequently and include nausea or vomiting, vague gastric upset, cramps, anorexia, diarrhea, weight loss, epigastric and abdominal pain, constipation.

Hematopoietic: Eosinophilia, granulocytopenia, leukopenia, agranulocytosis, aplastic anemia, monocytosis, pancytopenia.

Psychiatric/psychological: Confusion, instability, mental slowness, depression, hypochondriacal behavior, sleep disturbances, night terrors, inability to concentrate, aggressiveness. These effects may be noted particularly in those who have previously exhibited psychological abnormalities. *Rare:* paranoid psychosis, suicidal behavior, auditory hallucinations, increased libido, increased state of depression.

Dermatologic: Pruritus, urticaria, Stevens-Johnson syndrome, pruritic erythematous rashes, skin eruptions, erythema multiforme, systemic lupus erythematosus.

GU: Urinary frequency, renal damage, hematuria reported with use of phensuximide.

Other: Periorbital edema, hyperemia, alopecia, muscular weakness, myopia, vaginal bleeding, swelling of tongue, gum hypertrophy, hirsutism.

DOSAGE

ETHOSUXIMIDE
Children 3–6 years: Initial dose is 250 mg/day.
Children over 6 and adults: 500 mg/day.
Maintenance: Individualized. One method is to increase daily dose by 250 mg every 4 to 7 days until control is achieved with minimal side-effects. Administer dosages exceeding 1.5 g/day in divided doses under strict supervision.

May be administered in combination with other anticonvulsants when other forms of epilepsy coexist.

METHSUXIMIDE
Suggested schedule is 300 mg/day first week; if required, increase at weekly intervals by 300 mg/day up to 1.2 g/day.

May be administered in combination with other anticonvulsants when other forms of epilepsy coexist.

PHENSUXIMIDE
500 mg to 1000 mg bid, tid. Total dosage may vary between 1 g/day and 3 g/day (average 1.5 g/day).

May be administered in combination with other anticonvulsants when other forms of epilepsy co-exist.

NURSING IMPLICATIONS

HISTORY
See Appendix 4; obtain from family, or review chart for, history of seizure disorder, including average length of seizure, aura (if any), degree of impairment of consciousness, motor and psychic activity, previous drug therapy.

PHYSICAL ASSESSMENT
Vital signs; if seizures are frequent, observe and enter accurate description in patient's chart. EEG, CT scan may be ordered. Laboratory tests may include CBC, hepatic- and renal-function tests, urinalysis, especially when drug is known to be toxic to specific body organs or systems.

ADMINISTRATION
To prevent GI distress, give with or immediately after meals.

Exercise caution in oral administration if patient appears drowsy; test swallowing ability by offering small sips of water before giving drug.

ETHOTOIN
Give in 4 to 6 divided doses daily, after food. Doses should be spaced as evenly as practicable.

PHENYTOIN
Oral suspension: Shake well to ensure uniform drug distribution.

IV administration: Addition of phenytoin to an IV infusion is not recommended owing to lack of solubility and resultant precipitation. Do not exceed an infusion rate of 50 mg/minute; there is a small margin between full therapeutic effect and minimally toxic doses. For status epilepticus, IV route is preferred because of delay in absorption when given IM. Each IV injection should be followed by an injection of sterile saline through the same needle or IV catheter to avoid local irritation (physician should write order for use and amount of saline). Continuous infusion should be avoided. Observe for possible cardiovascular collapse, CNS depression, cardiac arrhythmias or arrest; monitor blood pressure, pulse, respirations q5m to q10m or as ordered. If drug is used as antiarrhythmic, patient should be on a cardiac monitor during and after administration.

Storage: Solution is suitable for use as long as it remains free of haziness and precipitate. Upon refrigeration or freezing, a precipitate may form; this will dissolve after solution is allowed to stand at room temperature. The solution is still suitable for use. Use only a clear solution; a faint yellow coloration may develop but has no effect on potency. Store at room temperature: 15°C to 30°C (59°F–86°F).

PARAMETHADIONE ORAL SOLUTION
This product has a high alcohol content (65%); it may be desirable to dilute with water before administration to small children (obtain physician's approval for dilution). Solution is supplied as 300 mg/ml; dropper is supplied with drug and measures 0.5 ml and 1 ml.

DIAZEPAM, PARENTERAL
To reduce possibility of venous thrombosis, phlebitis, local irritation, swelling, and (rarely) vascular impairment, inject IV solution *slowly,* taking at least 1 minute for each 5 mg in adults (for children, see *Dosage*). Do not use small veins such as those on dorsum of hand or wrist; exercise care to void extravasation, intra-arterial administration. In the convulsing patient, IV route is preferred; if IV administration is impossible, IM route may be used; inject deep into muscle. *Do not mix or dilute parenteral preparation with other solutions or drugs in a syringe or infusion solution.* If it is not feasible to administer directly IV, inject slowly through the infusion tubing as closely as possible to the vein insertion.

Extreme care is used in administering parenteral diazepam to elderly, debilitated, or very ill patients because of possibility that apnea or cardiac arrest may occur.

Observe closely for apnea following IV administration.

ONGOING ASSESSMENTS AND NURSING MANAGEMENT
Monitor vital signs daily to qid or as ordered; observe for adverse drug effects (see individual drug monographs); observe patient at frequent intervals (q1h–q2h) for occurrence of seizures, especially early in therapy and in those with a history of frequent seizures. Inspect skin (trunk, extremities) for evidence of rash; contact physician immediately if skin rash is apparent.

CLINICAL ALERT: Do *not* abruptly withdraw any anticonvulsant drug unless ordered to do so by the physician because of the development of one or more serious adverse effects. Ensure continuity of prescribed therapy by notation on Kardex, informing health-team members responsible for drug administration.

Dosage of anticonvulsants is adjusted to individual needs and patient response to therapy. For those with frequent seizures, accurate observations and documentation assist physician in adjusting dosage.

Some pharmacologic agents may interact with anticonvulsant drugs. When any new drug is added to the therapeutic regimen, check with the hospital pharmacist about possible drug interactions. See also Drug Interactions in monographs.

Serum levels may be performed at periodic intervals.

Physician may order periodic renal-, hepatic-function tests, CBC.

Drowsiness is common, especially during early therapy. Assist with ambulation, activities of daily living as needed or if patient is elderly, debilitated, or chronically ill. Take precautions to prevent falls, other injuries.

Neonates: If mother had been or is taking any anticonvulsants, particularly a barbiturate, observe for bleeding (due to a coagulation defect), especially during first 24 hours after birth. If bleeding is noted, contact physician immediately.

HYDANTOINS, SUCCINIMIDES

Be alert for general malaise, sore throat, fever, mucous-membrane bleeding, glandular swelling, cutaneous reaction, other symptoms indicative of possible blood dyscrasia. If one or more of these occur, contact physician immediately, preferably before next dose of drug is due.

Hydantoins: Hyperglycemia has been reported during administration. During early therapy, check urine daily or every other day for glucose; report positive findings to physician. Check urine of diabetic patient qid; discuss with physician procedure to be followed if urine positive for glucose.

Gingival hyperplasia occurs frequently with phenytoin. Institute good oral-hygiene regimen as soon as drug therapy instituted.

Phenytoin may discolor urine pink, red, or red-brown.

Succinimides: Psychiatric/psychological abnormalities have been reported. Report any behavioral changes to physician and observe patient at frequent intervals until seen by physician. If aggressiveness occurs, safety of other patients and hospital personnel must be kept in mind.

Drugs may discolor urine pink, red, or red-brown.

PATIENT AND FAMILY INFORMATION

NOTE: Patient and family may need assistance in adjusting to diagnosis of epilepsy. Discuss with physician possibility of referral to discharge-planning coordinator or social-service worker prior to discharge from hospital. Formulate a teaching plan for family, including care of patient during and after seizure; importance of some restriction of activities until seizures are controlled by medication.

Do not discontinue medication abruptly or change dosage except on advice of physician.

May cause drowsiness, dizziness; observe caution while driving or performing other tasks requiring alertness.

Carry identification (such as Medic-Alert) indicating medication usage and epilepsy.

Avoid alcohol unless use is approved by physician.

Do not use *any* nonprescription drug unless use has been approved by physician.

Inform (other) physicians, dentists, other health-care professionals of health problem, medication regimen.

Keep record of all seizures (date, time, description of seizure) as well as minor problems (*e.g.,* mild drowsiness, photophobia, lethargy) and bring to each office or clinic visit; this helps physician adjust medication and dosage.

Contact local agencies (such as Epilepsy Foundation of America) for assistance with legal, insurance, driver's license, problems, low-cost prescription services, job training or retraining, and so on.

HYDANTOINS

Take (phenytoin) with food to enhance absorption and reduce GI upset.

Medication (phenytoin) may discolor urine pink, red, red-brown. This is not harmful.

Notify physician or nurse if any of following occurs: skin rash; severe nausea or vomiting; swollen glands; bleeding, swollen, or tender gums; yellowish discoloration of skin or eyes; joint pain; unexplained fever; sore throat; unusual bleeding (*e.g.,* epistaxis); unusual bruising; persistent headache; malaise; any indication of an infection or bleeding tendency; pregnancy or suspected pregnancy.

Do not take calcium supplements, antacids or *Any* nonprescription drug without first checking with physician.

Maintain good oral hygiene and frequent brushing, gum massage. Visit dentist as soon as possible to discuss plan of oral hygiene including type of toothbrush to use, use of dental floss. Follow-up dental appointments should be made every 6 months or as suggested by dentist. A dental consultation is also essential for young children as well as infants (even those who have not begun tooth eruption) because good oral hygiene is best carried out with guidance of a dentist.

Diabetic patient: Monitor urine for glucose daily or as ordered by physician; report any abnormalities.

SUCCINIMIDES

If GI upset occurs, take drug with food or milk.

Phensuximide may discolor urine pink, red or red-brown. This is not harmful.

Notify physician or nurse if any of the following occurs: skin rash; joint pain; unexplained fever; sore throat; unusual bleeding; unusual bruising; drowsiness; dizziness; blurred vision; pregnancy or suspected pregnancy.

OXAZOLIDINEDIONES

If GI upset occurs, may be taken with food.

Notify physician or nurse if any of following occurs: visual disturbances; excessive drowsiness or dizziness; sore throat; fever; unusual bleeding or bruising; skin rash; pregnancy or suspected pregnancy.

Parents of small children: Check with physician about dilution of paramethadione solution with water prior to administration.

Antidepressants

Trazodone Hydrochloride *Rx*

tablets: 50 mg,   Desyrel
  100 mg

INDICATIONS

Treatment of depression. Efficacy demonstrated in both inpatient and outpatient settings and for depressed patients with or without prominent anxiety. The depressive illness of patients studied corresponds to the Major Depressive Episode criteria of the American Psychiatric Association's Diagnostic and Statistical Manual, III. *Major Depressive Episode* implies a prominent and relatively persistent (nearly every day for at least 2 weeks) depressed or dysphoric mood that usually interferes with daily functioning and includes at least four of the following eight symptoms: change in appetite, change in sleep, psychomotor agitation or retardation, loss of interest in usual activities, increased fatigability, feelings of guilt or worthlessness, slowed thinking or impaired concentration, and suicidal ideation or attempts.

CONTRAINDICATIONS

Hypersensitivity.

ACTIONS

Mechanisms of antidepressant action are not fully understood; does not stimulate the CNS. Trazodone is well absorbed after oral administration. When taken shortly after ingestion of food, there may be a slight increase in amount of drug absorbed, a decrease in maximum concentration, and a lengthening in the time to maximum concentration. Peak plasma levels occur in approximately 1 hour. Patients who respond to trazodone have a significant therapeutic response by the end of the first or second week of treatment; a few may require 2 to 4 weeks for a significant therapeutic response.

WARNINGS

Not recommended for use during the initial recovery phase of myocardial infarction. Use during pregnancy only if potential benefit justifies the potential risk to the fetus. Exercise caution when administering to nursing women. Safety and efficacy for use in children not established. May be arrhythmogenic in some patients with preexisting cardiac disease.

PRECAUTIONS

The possibility of suicide in depressed patients is inherent in the illness and may persist until remission occurs. Hypotension (including orthostatic hypotension and syncope) and priapism have been reported.

Laboratory tests: Occasional low white blood cell and neutrophil counts have been noted but are not considered clinically significant and do not necessitate discontinuation of the drug. White blood cell and differential counts are recommended for patients developing fever, sore throat, or other signs of infection during therapy. Drug should be discontinued in any patient whose white blood cell or neutrophil count falls below normal levels.

Electroshock therapy: Administration concurrent with electroshock therapy avoided.

DRUG INTERACTIONS

Increased serum **digoxin** or **phenytoin** levels have been reported with concurrent trazodone therapy. May enhance response to **alcohol, barbiturates,** other **CNS depressants.** Because trazodone can cause hypotension, concomitant administration with **antihypertensives** may require reduction in dose of antihypertensive drug. However, hypotensive effects of **clonidine** may be inhibited by trazodone. It is not known whether interactions will occur between **monoamine oxidase (MAO) inhibitors** and trazodone; if MAO inhibitors are discontinued shortly before administration or are to be given concomitantly, therapy should be initiated cautiously with gradual increase in dosage until optimum response is achieved. Little is known about interaction between trazodone and **general anesthetics;** prior to elective surgery, trazodone should be discontinued for as long as clinically feasible.

ADVERSE REACTIONS

Allergic: *Greater than 1%*—skin conditions; edema. *Less than 1%*—allergic reaction.

Anticholinergic: *Greater than 1%*—blurred vision; constipation; dry mouth; nasal/sinus congestion.

Cardiovascular: *Greater than 1%*—hypertension; hypotension; shortness of breath; syncope; tachycardia; palpitations. *Less than 1%*—chest pain, myocardial infarction, ventricular ectopic activity. Occasionally, sinus bradycardia.

CNS: *Greater than 1%*—anger/hostility; nightmares/vivid dreams; confusion; decreased concentration; disorientation; dizziness; lightheadedness; drowsiness; malaise; excitement; fatigue; headache; insomnia; impaired memory; nervousness. *Less than 1%*—hallucinations; hypomania; impaired speech.

GI/GU: *Greater than 1%*—gastric disorder; bad taste in mouth; diarrhea; nausea; vomiting. *Less than 1%*—flatulence; hematuria; delayed urine flow; increased urinary frequency.

Musculoskeletal: *Greater than 1%*—aches, pains.

Neurologic: *Greater than 1%*—incoordination; paresthesia; tremors. *Less than 1%*—akathisia; muscle twitches; numbness.

Sexual function: *Greater than 1%*—decreased libido. *Less than 1%*—impotence; increased libido; retrograde ejaculation.

Other: *Greater than 1%*—decreased or increased appetite; red eyes (tired/itching); head full/heavy; sweating/clamminess; tinnitus; weight gain; weight loss; anemia; hypersalivation. *Less than 1%*—early menses; missed periods.

OVERDOSAGE

Symptoms: Overdosage may cause an increase in incidence or severity of adverse reactions.

Treatment: No specific antidote; treatment is symptomatic and supportive in case of hypotension or excessive sedation. Suspected cases of overdose should have stomach emptied by gastric lavage. Forced diuresis may be useful in facilitating elimination of the drug.

DOSAGE

Dosage initiated at low level and increased gradually. Occurrence of drowsiness may require administration of major portion of daily dose at H.S. or reduction in dosage. Give shortly after a meal or light snack. *Usual adult dosage:* Initially, 150 mg/day. Dose may be increased by 50 mg/day every 3 to 4 days. Maximum dose for outpatients usually should not exceed 400 mg/day in divided doses. Inpatients or the more severely depressed may be given up to, but not in excess of, 600 mg/day in divided doses. *Maintenance:* Once adequate response is achieved, dosage may be gradually reduced.

NURSING IMPLICATIONS
See p 102.

Tricyclic Compounds
(Tricyclic Antidepressants, TCAs)

Amitriptyline Hydrochloride Rx

tablets: 10 mg, 25 mg, 50 mg, 75 mg, 100 mg	Amitril, Elavil, Endep, SK-Amitriptyline, *Generic*
tablets: 150 mg	Amitril, Elavil, Endep, SK-Amitriptyline, *Generic*
injection: 10 mg/ml	Elavil, *Generic*

Amoxapine Rx

tablets: 25 mg, 50 mg, 100 mg, 150 mg	Asendin

Desipramine Hydrochloride Rx

tablets: 25 mg, 50 mg, 75 mg, 100 mg, 150 mg	Norpramin
capsules: 25 mg, 50 mg	Pertofrane

Doxepin Hydrochloride Rx

capsules: 10 mg, 25 mg, 50 mg, 75 mg, 100 mg	Adapin, Sinequan
capsules: 150 mg	Sinequan
oral concentrate: 10 mg/ml	Sinequan

Imipramine Hydrochloride Rx

tablets: 10 mg	Janimine (contains tartrazine), SK-Pramine, Tofranil (contains tartrazine), *Generic*
tablets: 25 mg	Janimine (contains tartrazine), SK-Pramine, Tofranil (contains tartrazine), *Generic*

| tablets: 50 mg | Janimine, SK-Pramine, Tofranil (contains tartrazine), *Generic* |
| injection: 25 mg/ 2 ml | Tofranil |

Imipramine Pamoate Rx

| capsules: 75 mg, 100 mg (contains tartrazine), 125 mg (contains tartrazine), 150 mg | Tofranil-PM |

Maprotiline Hydrochloride Rx

| tablets: 25 mg, 50 mg, 75 mg | Ludiomil |

Nortriptyline Hydrochloride Rx

capsules: 10 mg, 25 mg	Aventyl HCl, Pamelor
capsules: 75 mg	Pamelor
solution: 10 mg/5 ml	Aventyl HCl

Protriptyline Hydrochloride Rx

| tablets: 5 mg, 10 mg | Vivactil |

Trimipramine Maleate Rx

| capsules: 25 mg, 50 mg, 100 mg | Surmontil |

INDICATIONS

Relief of symptoms of depression; endogenous depression is most responsive to therapy with these agents. Specific indications for individual drugs are as follows.

AMITRIPTYLINE HYDROCHLORIDE

Relief of symptoms of depression. Endogenous depression more likely alleviated than other depressive states.

Investigational uses: Control of chronic pain (*e.g.,* intractable pain associated with cancer, peripheral neuropathies, postherpetic neuralgia, tic douloureux, central pain syndromes); prevention of cluster and migraine headaches.

AMOXAPINE

Relief of symptoms of depression in those with neurotic or reactive depressive disorders as well as in those with endogenous and psychotic depressions; for depression accompanied by anxiety or agitation.

DESIPRAMINE HYDROCHLORIDE

Relief of symptoms in various depressive syndromes, especially endogenous depression.

DOXEPIN HYDROCHLORIDE

Psychoneurotic anxiety and depressive reactions; mixed symptoms of anxiety and depression; anxiety or depression associated with alcoholism; anxiety associated with organic disease; psychotic depressive disorders including involutional depression and manic-depressive reactions. Target symptoms of psychoneurosis that respond to doxepin include anxiety, tension, depression, somatic symptoms and concerns, sleep disturbances, guilt, lack of energy, fear, apprehension, and worry.

IMIPRAMINE HYDROCHLORIDE

Relief of symptoms of depression; endogenous depression is more likely than other depressive states to be alleviated. One to three weeks of treatment may be needed before optimal therapeutic effects are evident.

Childhood enuresis: Temporary adjunctive therapy in children 6 years and older. Safety for long-term use not established. A dose of 2.5 mg/kg/day should not be exceeded.

Investigational uses: Control of chronic pain (*e.g.,* intractable pain associated with cancer, peripheral neuropathies, postherpetic neuralgia, tic douloureux, central pain syndromes).

IMIPRAMINE PAMOATE

See Imipramine hydrochloride, above.

MAPROTILINE HYDROCHLORIDE

Treatment of depressive illness in patients with depressive neurosis (dysthymic disorder) and manic-depressive illness, depressed type (major depressive disorder).

NORTRIPTYLINE HYDROCHLORIDE

Relief of symptoms of depression. Endogenous depression is more likely than other depressive states to be alleviated.

PROTRIPTYLINE HYDROCHLORIDE

Treatment of symptoms of depression in patients under close medical supervision. Its activating properties make it suitable for withdrawn, anergic patients.

TRIMIPRAMINE MALEATE

Relief of symptoms of depression. Endogenous depression is more likely than other depressive states to be alleviated.

CONTRAINDICATIONS

Prior sensitivity to any tricyclic drug. Not recommended for use during acute recovery phase following myocardial infarction. Concomitant use of MAO inhibiting compounds is generally contraindicated.

ACTIONS

Tricyclic antidepressants (TCAs) are structurally related to the phenothiazine antipsychotic agents and have similar secondary pharmacologic effects responsible for side-effects (anticholinergic effects, sedation). In contrast to phenothiazines, which act on dopamine receptors, tricyclic antidepressants block the re-uptake of norepinephrine and serotonin (5-hydroxytryptamine, 5-HT) by the presynaptic neuron in the CNS. Because re-uptake terminates amine activity, inhibition of re-uptake enhances activity at the receptor site (postsynaptic neuron). These effects appear to be directly related to the antidepressant effects.

Other pharmacologic effects: Inhibition of histamine and acetylcholine activity; increase in the pressor effect of norepinephrine, but blockage of the pressor response of phenylethylamine. Clinical effects, in addition to antidepressant effects, include sedation, anticholinergic effects, mild peripheral vasodilator effects. Because of their effects on the autonomic nervous system, which can cause adverse cardiovascular effects, these drugs are used cautiously in those with preexisting cardiovascular disorders. Amitriptyline, doxepin, amoxapine, maprotiline, and trimipramine have significant sedative action, which may be useful in depression associated with anxiety and sleep disturbances. Because of its activating properties, protriptyline may be useful for withdrawn and anergic patients.

The tricyclic antidepressants are well absorbed from the GI tract; highly bound to plasma proteins; widely distributed in tissues (including CNS); metabolized by the liver; and excreted primarily in the urine. These agents have a long serum half-life and require 4 to 6 days to establish steady-state plasma levels. Because of the long half-life, a single daily dose may be given; dosage adjustments should not be made more frequently than every 4 days. *Up to 2 to 4 weeks may be required to produce maximum clinical response.* Desipramine, amoxapine, and protriptyline may have a more rapid onset than imipramine, with initial clinical effects seen within 1 week. Protriptyline and amoxapine also show a more rapid onset than amitriptyline. Maprotiline may have an onset of therapeutic effects within 3 to 7 days, although 2 to 3 weeks are usually necessary.

Serum levels: Nortriptyline—50 ng/ml and 150 ng/ml; *protriptyline*— 70 ng/ml and 170 ng/ml.

Minimum effective plasma levels: Amitriptyline— >100 ng/ml; *imipramine*—>200 ng/ml; *doxepin*— >100 ng/ml; *desipramine*—>125 ng/ml.

WARNINGS

Seizure disorders: Because these drugs lower the convulsive threshold, use with caution in those with history of seizures. Seizures have occurred in patients both with and without past history of seizures.

Anticholinergic effects: Because of atropinelike action of these drugs, use with caution in those with history of urinary retention, angle-closure glaucoma, increased intraocular pressure. In occasional susceptible patients or those receiving anticholinergic drugs (including antiparkinsonism agents), the atropinelike effect may become more pronounced (e.g., paralytic ileus).

Cardiovascular disorders: Use with extreme caution in patients with cardiovascular disorders because these agents, especially in high doses, may produce arrhythmias, sinus tachycardia, prolongation of conduction time. Tachycardia may increase frequency and severity of anginal attacks in patients with coronary artery disease. Myocardial infarction and stroke have been reported.

Hyperthyroidism: Close supervision required when used in hyperthyroid patients or in those receiving a thyroid drug; these patients are more likely to develop cardiac arrhythmias.

Drowsiness: May impair mental or physical abilities.

Impaired renal or hepatic function: Use with caution and in reduced doses.

Use in psychiatric patients: Schizophrenic or paranoid patients may exhibit worsening of psychosis; manic-depressive patients, in depressed or normal phase, may experience shift to hypomanic or manic phase. In overactive or agitated patients, increased anxiety or agitation may occur. Reduction in dosage or concomitant antipsychotic therapy may be necessary. Troublesome patient hostility may be aroused by use of these drugs. Epileptiform seizures may accompany administration. The possibility of suicide in depressed patients remains during treatment and until significant remission occurs.

Use in pregnancy, lactation: These drugs cross the placental barrier slowly and may be secreted in breast milk. Safety for use during pregnancy and lactation is not established; use only when clearly needed and when potential benefits outweigh unknown potential hazards to the fetus.

Use in children: Not recommended for children under 12. Imipramine may be used for treatment of enuresis in children ages 6 to 12.

PRECAUTIONS

ECG recommended prior to initiation of larger than usual doses and at appropriate intervals thereafter until steady state is achieved. Patients with evidence of cardiovascular disease require cardiac surveillance at all dosage levels. Elderly patients and patients with cardiac disease or prior history of cardiac disease are at special risk of developing cardiac abnormalities associated with use of TCAs.

Therapy is discontinued for as long as possible before elective surgery.

Both elevation and lowering of blood sugar levels have been reported. Baseline and periodic leukocyte and differential counts and hepatic-function studies should be performed. Fever or sore throat may signal serious neutrophil depression, and therapy should be discontinued.

Imipramine has been reported to precipitate attacks of acute intermittent porphyria and is used with caution in susceptible patients.

Photosensitization may occur.

Tartrazine sensitivity: Some of these products contain tartrazine (see Appendix 6, section 6-23).

DRUG INTERACTIONS

TCAs generally are not given concomitantly with **MAO inhibitors** because hyperpyretic crisis, severe convulsions, hypertensive episodes, and deaths have occurred. In certain instances, combined therapy may be used with extreme caution (see _Administration_). When it is desired to replace an MAO inhibitor with a tricyclic drug, a minimum of 14 days should elapse after the former is discontinued.

These agents block the antihypertensive effect of **guanethidine, clonidine,** and similarly acting compounds. Exercise caution when TCAs are used with agents that lower blood pressure. If these drugs are given with **anticholinergic agents** or **sympathomimetic drugs** (including epinephrine combined with a local anesthetic), close supervision and careful adjustment of dosage are required. TCAs can potentiate the effects of **catecholamines.** In occasional susceptible patients or in those receiving anticholinergic drugs (including antiparkinsonism drugs), atropinelike effects may become more pronounced (_e.g.,_ paralytic ileus).

Tricyclic antidepressants may enhance the response to **alcohol** and the effects of **barbiturates, benzodiazepines,** and other **CNS depressants.** Barbiturates may stimulate the metabolism of TCAs and subsequently decrease their plasma levels.

Close supervision is required when these drugs are given to hyperthyroid patients or to those receiving **thyroid medication,** because tachycardia and cardiac arrhythmias may develop. Combined therapy may enhance the antidepressant response.

Administration of **reserpine** during therapy with these drugs has been shown to produce a "stimulating" effect in depressed patients. Reserpine should not be used because it may contribute to depression in long-term use.

Methylphenidate and **phenothiazines** inhibit the metabolism of tricyclic antidepressants and may increase their blood levels.

Caution is advised if patients receive large doses of **ethchlorvynol** concurrently; transient delirium has been reported in patients receiving 1 g of ethchlorvynol and 75 mg to 150 mg amitriptyline.

Smoking may increase the metabolic biotransformation of imipramine.

Concomitant administration of **quinidine** or **procainamide** with TCAs produces dangerous additive effects. The effects of **beta-adrenergic blocking agents** are antagonized by TCAs and excessive alpha stimulation may be produced. **oral contraceptives** may inhibit the effects of TCAs if given concomitantly.

ADVERSE REACTIONS

Sedation, anticholinergic effects reported most frequently. Tolerance develops but may be minimized by gradually increasing the dose.

Cardiovascular: Orthostatic hypotension; hypertension; syncope; tachycardia; palpitation; myocardial infarction; arrhythmias; heart block; ECG changes (occur most frequently with toxic doses but may occur at therapeutic levels); precipitation of congestive heart failure (CHF); stroke. Hypertensive episodes have been observed during surgery in patients taking desipramine.

CNS: Confusional states (especially in elderly); disturbed concentration; hallucinations, disorientation; decrease in memory; feelings of unreality; delusions; anxiety; excitement; nervousness; restlessness; agitation; panic; insomnia; nightmares; hypomania; mania; exacerbation of psychosis; drowsiness; dizziness; weakness; fatigue; headache.

Neurologic: Numbness; tingling; paresthesias of extremities; incoordination; motor hyperactivity; ataxia; tremors; peripheral neuropathy; tardive dyskinesia; extrapyramidal symptoms; seizures; speech blockage; alterations in EEG patterns; tinnitus.

Anticholinergic: Dry mouth and, rarely, associated sublingual adenitis; blurred vision, disturbance of accommodation, increased intraocular pressure, mydriasis; constipation; paralytic ileus; urinary retention; delayed micturition; dilation of urinary tract.

Allergic: Skin rash; pruritus; petechiae; urticaria; photosensitization (avoid excessive exposure to sunlight); edema (general or of face, tongue); drug fever; cross-sensitivity with other tricyclic drugs.

Hematologic: Bone-marrow depression, including agranulocytosis; eosinophilia; purpura; thrombocytopenia; leukopenia.

GI: Nausea; vomiting; anorexia; epigastric distress; flatulence; dysphagia; peculiar taste; increased salivation; stomatitis; glossitis; abdominal cramps; black tongue. Rarely, hepatitis, including altered liver function, jaundice.

Endocrine: Gynecomastia, testicular swelling in male; breast enlargement, menstrual irregularity, galactorrhea in female; increased or decreased libido; impotence; elevation or depression of blood sugar levels; inappropriate ADH secretion.

Other: Nasal congestion; excessive appetite; weight gain or loss; increased perspiration; flushing; chills; urinary frequency; nocturia; parotid swelling; alopecia; proneness to falling.

Withdrawal symptoms: Although not indicative of addiction, abrupt cessation after prolonged therapy may produce nausea, headache, vertigo, nightmares, malaise.

Enuretic children: All adverse reactions reported should be considered. Most common adverse reactions: nervousness, sleep disorders, tiredness, mild GI disturbances. These usually disappear with continued therapy or dose reduction. Other reactions include constipation; convulsions; anxiety; emotional instability; syncope; collapse. Children may have increased risk of cardiotoxicity. Do not exceed 2.5 mg/kg/day.

OVERDOSAGE

Children reportedly are more sensitive than adults to acute overdosage. Consider any overdose in infants or young children serious and potentially fatal.

Symptoms: High doses may cause temporary confusion, disturbed concentration, or transient visual hallucinations. Overdosage may cause drowsiness; ataxia; hypothermia; tachycardia or other arrhythmias such as bundle-branch block; ECG evidence of impaired conduction; CHF; dilated pupils; athetoid and choreiform movements; respiratory depression; cyanosis; convulsions; severe hypotension; stupor; shock; coma. Other symptoms may be agitation, hyperactive reflexes, muscle rigidity, vomiting, hyperpyrexia, or any of those listed under *Adverse Reactions.* Doses of 1.5 g to 2.5 g may be fatal.

Treatment: Hospitalization and close observation necessary even when amount ingested is thought to be small or initial degree of intoxication appears slight. Monitor for at least 72 hours if ECG abnormalities exist; observe closely until well after cardiac status returns to normal because relapses may occur.

Maintain adequate respiratory exchange; do not use respiratory stimulants. In the alert patient, induce emesis and follow with lavage. In the obtunded patient, secure airway with a cuffed endotracheal tube before beginning lavage (do not induce emesis). Continue lavage for 24 hours or longer and use normal or half-normal saline to avoid water intoxication, especially in children. Instillation of activated charcoal slurry may help to reduce absorption.

Direct slow IV administration of 1 mg to 3 mg physostigmine salicylate has been reported to reverse most cardiovascular and CNS effects of overdosage. In children, administer 0.5 mg physostigmine salicylate and repeat at 5-minute intervals to determine minimum effective dosage; do not exceed 2 mg. Because of short duration of action of physostigmine, repeat effective dose at 30- to 60-minute intervals as needed. Avoid rapid injection; give by slow IV push. Lidocaine, propranolol, and phenytoin have been used for life-threatening arrhythmias, but they may cause myocardial depression.

Shock and metabolic acidosis should be treated with supportive measures such as IV fluids, bicarbonate, oxygen, corticosteroids. If congestive heart failure requires rapid digitalization, care must be exercised. Minimize external stimulation (darken room) to prevent seizures. If an anticonvulsant is necessary, diazepam may be useful. Control hyperpyrexia by external means (*e.g.,* ice packs, hypothermia blanket) if necessary.

DOSAGE

If minor side-effects develop, dosage is usually reduced. Treatment is discontinued promptly if adverse effects of a serious nature or allergic manifestations occur.

Adolescent, elderly patients, outpatients: Lower dosages are recommended. Therapy is begun at lower dosage level and increased gradually at 4-day intervals; note carefully clinical response and any evidence of intolerance.

Single daily dose: May be used for maintenance therapy. A single daily dose at H.S. is more convenient for patient, will minimize daytime side-effects (sedation, anticholinergic effects), and may be beneficial in those with sleep disorders. The elderly may not tolerate single daily dose because of increased risk of cardiovascular and other complications.

Tricyclic antidepressant/MAO inhibitor combined use has been traditionally contraindicated because of potential for serious adverse reactions. Recent evidence indicates combination may offer significant advantages in those refractory to more conservative therapy.

Specific dosage guidelines for individual agents follow.

AMITRIPTYLINE HYDROCHLORIDE

Depression

Adults: _Outpatients_—75 mg/day in divided doses; if necessary, increase to a total of 150 mg/day. Increases are made preferably in late-afternoon or H.S. doses. A sedative effect may be apparent before antidepressant effect is noted. An adequate therapeutic effect may take as long as 30 days to develop. Alternately, therapy is initiated by beginning with 50 mg to 100 mg H.S. and increased by 25 mg to 50 mg as necessary, to a total of 150 mg/day. Hospitalized patients may require 100 mg/day initially. This may be increased gradually to 200 mg/day if needed. A small number of patients may require as much as 300 mg/day.

Adolescent, elderly patients: Lower doses are recommended; 10 mg tid with 20 mg H.S. may be satisfactory.

Maintenance: Usual dosage is 50 mg/day to 100 mg/day; in some patients, 40 mg/day is sufficient. Total daily dosage may be given as single dose, preferably H.S.

IM: Initially 20 mg to 30 mg IM qid. Effects may appear more rapidly with IM than with oral administration. Tablets should replace injection as soon as possible. Do not give IV.

Chronic pain (investigational)
75 mg/day to 150 mg/day.

Prevention of cluster and migraine headaches (investigational)
50 mg/day to 150 mg/day.

AMOXAPINE

Not recommended for those under 16. Effective dosage may vary. Usual effective dosage is 200 mg/day to 300 mg/day. Three weeks is adequate trial period if dosage has reached 300 mg/day for at least 2 weeks. If no response is seen, dosage may be increased up to 400 mg/day. Hospitalized patients who are refractory to antidepressant therapy and who have no history of seizures may have dosage cautiously increased up to 600 mg/day in divided doses. Once effective dosage is established, drug may be given in a single H.S. dose (not to exceed 300 mg). If total daily dose exceeds 300 mg, give in divided doses.

Adults: Usual starting dose is 50 mg tid. Depending on tolerance, this may be increased to 100 mg tid in third day of treatment. Lower doses are recommended in elderly. Recommended starting dose is 25 mg tid; if tolerated, this may be increased after 3 days to 50 mg tid. Although 150 mg/day may be adequate for most patients, some may require a higher dosage of up to 300 mg/day.

Maintenance: Use lowest dose that will maintain remission. For maintenance dose of 300 mg/day or less, a single dose at H.S. is recommended.

DESIPRAMINE HYDROCHLORIDE

Not recommended for children. Initial therapy may be given as single or divided dose. Maintenance therapy may be administered on a once-daily schedule.

Adults: Usual dose is 75 mg/day to 200 mg/day. In the more severely ill, dosage may be increased gradually to 300 mg/day. Dosages above 300 mg/day are not recommended. Treatment requiring as much as 300 mg/day should be initiated in hospitals, where regular visits by physician, skilled nursing care, and frequent ECGs are available. Continued therapy at optimal dosage level should be maintained during active phase of depression. It is recommended that a lower maintenance dosage be continued for at least 2 months after satisfactory response is achieved. Evidence of impending toxicity from very high doses is prolongation of the QRS or Q–T interval on the ECG. Prolongation of the P–R interval is also significant but is less closely correlated with plasma levels. Symptoms of intolerance (especially drowsiness, dizziness, postural hypotension) indicate need for reduction in dosage. Geriatric and adolescent patients usually can be managed on lower dosage; usual dose range is 25 mg/day to 100 mg/day. Dosages above 150 mg/day are not recommended.

DOXEPIN HYDROCHLORIDE

Not recommended for children under 12.

Mild to moderate anxiety and/or depression: 25 mg tid initially; adjust dosage at appropriate intervals according to patient response. Usual optimal dosage is 75 mg/day to 150 mg/day. _Alternate regimen:_ Total daily dose, up to 150 mg, given at H.S.

Mild symptomatology, emotional symptoms accompanying organic disease: Dosage as low as 25 mg/day to 50 mg/day is effective.

More severe anxiety and/or depression: 50 mg tid initially. If needed, may be gradually increased to 300 mg/day.

Optimal antidepressant response may not be evident for 2 to 3 weeks; antianxiety activity is readily apparent.

IMIPRAMINE HYDROCHLORIDE

Depression: Once-a-day maintenance dose can be given at H.S. In some patients it may be necessary to use a divided dose schedule. Parenteral route is used only for starting therapy in those unable or unwilling to take oral form. Do not administer IV. Initially up to 100 mg/day IM in divided doses. Oral form used as soon as possible.

Hospitalized patients: Initially, 100 mg/day to 150 mg/day orally in divided doses; gradually increased to 200 mg/day as required. If no response after 2 weeks, dosage may be increased to 250 mg/day to 300 mg/day. Total daily dose can be administered on once-a-day basis, preferably at H.S.

Outpatients: Initially, 75 mg/day orally, increased to 150 mg/day. Dosages over 200 mg/day not recommended. Total daily dosage can be administered on once-a-day basis, preferably at H.S. Maintenance dose is 50 mg/day to 150 mg/day.

Adolescent, geriatric patients: Initially, 30 mg/day to 40 mg/day orally; it is usually not necessary to exceed 100 mg/day.

Childhood enuresis: Initially, 25 mg/day, 1 hour before bedtime. If satisfactory response does not occur within 1 week, increase to 50 mg in children under 12, 75 mg in children over 12. Evidence suggests that in early-night bed wetters, drug is more effective given earlier and in divided amounts (*e.g.,* 25 mg midafternoon, repeated at bedtime).

Chronic pain (investigational): 50 mg/day to 200 mg/day.

IMIPRAMINE PAMOATE

See Imipramine hydrochloride, above.

MAPROTILINE HYDROCHLORIDE

Not recommended for those under 18. May be given as a single daily dose or in divided doses. Therapeutic effects sometimes seen within 3 to 7 days, although a period as long as 2 to 3 weeks is usually necesary.

Initial adult dosage: 75 mg/day for outpatients with mild to moderate depression; in some patients a lower dose may be used. Dosage may be increased as required and tolerated. Most patients respond to 150 mg/day, but doses as high as 225 mg/day may be required for some. *More severely depressed hospitalized patients:* 100 mg/day to 150 mg/day, which may be gradually increased as required and tolerated. Most patients with moderate to severe depression respond to 150 mg/day to 225 mg/day; dosages as high as 300 mg/day may be required. Dosage of 300 mg/day should not be exceeded.

Elderly patients: Lower doses are recommended for those over 60; 50 mg/day to 75 mg/day is satisfactory for those who do not tolerate higher amounts.

Maintenance: During prolonged maintenance therapy, dosage should be kept at lowest effective level and may be reduced to 75 mg/day to 150 mg/day, with subsequent adjustment depending on therapeutic response.

NORTRIPTYLINE HYDROCHLORIDE

Not recommended for children.

Usual adult dose: 25 mg tid, qid. Begin at a low level and increase as required. Doses above 100 mg/day not recommended.

Elderly, adolescent patients: 30 mg/day to 50 mg/day in divided doses.

PROTRIPTYLINE HYDROCHLORIDE

15 mg/day to 40 mg/day divided into 3 or 4 doses; may be increased to 60 mg/day if necessary. Dosages above 60 mg/day are not recommended. Increases should be made in the morning dose. Not recommended for children.

TRIMIPRAMINE MALEATE

Not recommended for children. Recommended dosage regimen may be modified by patient's age, chronicity, and severity of disease, patient's medical condition, degree of psychotherapeutic support.

Adult outpatients: 75 mg/day in divided doses; may be increased gradually in a few days to 200 mg/day. Dosages over 200 mg/day not recommended. *Maintenance therapy:* 50 mg/day to 150 mg/day. Total daily dosage may be given at H.S.

Adult hospitalized patients: Initially, 100 mg/day in divided doses; may be increased gradually in a few days to 200 mg/day. If improvement does not occur in 2 to 3 weeks, dose may be increased to maximum recommended dose of 250 mg/day to 300 mg/day.

Adolescent, elderly patients: Initially 50 mg/day with gradual increments up to 100 mg/day depending on patient response and tolerance.

Maintenance: Preferably administered as single dose at H.S. To minimize relapse, maintenance therapy may be continued for 3 months.

NURSING IMPLICATIONS
See p 102.

Monoamine Oxidase Inhibitors (MAOIs)

Isocarboxazid Rx

tablets: 10 mg	Marplan

Phenelzine Sulfate Rx

tablets: 15 mg	Nardil

Tranylcypromine Sulfate Rx

tablets: 10 mg	Parnate

INDICATIONS

ISOCARBOXAZID

Probably effective for treatment of depressed patients refractory to tricyclic antidepressants or electroconvulsive therapy (ECT) and depressed patients in whom tricyclic antidepressants are contraindicated.

PHENELZINE SULFATE

Effective in depressed patients clinically characterized as "atypical," "nonendogenous," or "neurotic." These patients often have mixed anxiety and depression and phobic or hypochondriacal features. Drug has been used in combination with dibenzazepine derivatives (imipramine, desipramine) in treatment-resistant patients without a significant incidence of serious side-effects.

TRANYLCYPROMINE SULFATE

Probably effective for symptomatic relief of severe reactive or endogenous depression in hospitalized or closely supervised patients not responding to other antidepressant therapy.

CONTRAINDICATIONS

Known hypersensitivity; pheochromocytoma; congestive heart failure; severe hepatic or renal impairment. Also, in confirmed or suspected cerebrovascular defect, cerebrovascular disease, hypertension, patients over 60 (because of possibility of existing cerebral sclerosis with damaged vessels).

ACTIONS

MAO is a complex enzyme system, widely distributed throughout the body, that is responsible for the metabolic decomposition of biogenic amines, thus terminating their activity. Drugs that inhibit this enzyme system (MAOIs) cause an increased concentration of endogenous epinephrine, norepinephrine, and serotonin (5-HT) in storage sites throughout the nervous system. It is believed that an increase in CNS concentration of monoamines is the basis for the antidepressant activity of these drugs. Drugs that have MAOI activity cause a wide range of clinical effects and have potential for serious interactions with other substances.

These agents are well absorbed orally. Tranylcypromine acts more rapidly (10 days) than do isocarboxazid and phenelzine (3–4 weeks). The clinical effects of the MAOIs may continue for up to 2 weeks after discontinuation of therapy.

WARNINGS

Because most serious reactions involve blood pressure, it is inadvisable to use these drugs in elderly or debilitated patients or in the presence of hypertension or cardiovascular or cerebrovascular disease. Not recommended for patients with frequent or severe headaches because headache may be first symptom of hypertensive reaction to the drug.

Hypertensive crisis: Usually occurs within several hours after ingestion of contraindicated substance; may be fatal. These crises are characterized by some or all of the following: occipital headache that may radiate frontally; palpitation; stiff or sore neck; nausea; vomiting; sweating (sometimes with fever, sometimes with cold clammy skin); dilated pupils; photophobia. Tachycardia or bradycardia may be present and can be associated with chest pain.

NOTE: Intracranial bleeding (sometimes fatal) has been reported in association with the paradoxical increase in blood pressure.

Treatment: Discontinue drug immediately. Institute therapy to lower blood pressure. Headaches tend to abate as blood pressure is lowered. Antihypertensive agents are administered slowly to avoid excessive hypotensive effect. Manage fever by external cooling (*e.g.,* hypothermia blanket, ice packs). Other supportive measures may be needed. Do not use parenteral reserpine.

In patients who may be suicidal risks, no single form of treatment such as MAOIs, ECT, or other therapy should be relied on as a sole therapeutic measure.

Patient warnings: Warn patient not to eat foods with high tyramine content (see list, below). Any high-protein food that is aged or undergoes breakdown by putrefaction to improve flavor is suspect of being able to produce hypertensive crisis in those taking MAOIs. Also give warnings about drinking alcoholic beverages, using nonprescription drugs, and consuming excessive amounts of caffeine.

Use in pregnancy, lactation: Safety not established. Use during pregnancy, lactation, or in women of childbearing age only when clearly needed and potential benefits outweigh the unknown hazards to the fetus.

Use in children: Not recommended for those under 16 years.

TYRAMINE-CONTAINING FOODS*

Cheese/Dairy Products

American, processed
Blue
*Boursault
Brick, natural
Brie
*Camembert

* Foods marked with an asterisk contain high to very high amounts of tyramine.

*Cheddar
*Emmenthaler
Gruyère
Mozzarella
Parmesan
Romano
Roquefort
*Stilton
Sour cream
Yogurt

Meat/Fish

Beef or chicken liver, other meats, fish (unrefriger-
   ated, fermented)
Meats prepared with tenderizer
Caviar
*Herring, pickled, spoiled
*Fermented sausages (bologna, pepperoni, salami,
   summer sausage)
Game meat
Dried fish (especially salted herring)

Alcoholic Beverages (undistilled)

Beer and ale (imports)
Red wine (especially Chianti)
Sherry

Fruit/Vegetables

Avocado (especially overripe)
*Yeast extracts (Marmite, etc.)
Bananas
Figs, canned (overripe)
Raisins
Soy sauce

Foods Containing Other Vasopressors

Fava beans (overripe)—dopamine
Chocolate—phenylethylamine
Coffee, tea, colas, etc.—caffeine

DRUG INTERACTIONS
Potentiation of sympathomimetic substances by
MAOIs may result in hypertensive crisis; patients
should not be given **sympathomimetic drugs** (including amphetamines, methyldopa, levodopa, dopamine, tryptophan, epinephrine, norepinephrine)
nor **foods with high concentrations of tryptophan**
(broad beans) or **tyramine** or other vasopressors (see
list, above). Excessive amounts of **caffeine, chocolate**
can also cause hypertensive reactions.

Do not use in combination with some **CNS depressants** such as alcohol, narcotics (*e.g.,* meperidine). Reduce doses of **barbiturates** if given concomitantly. MAOIs should not be administered together with or immediately following other **MAO
inhibitors** or **dibenzazepines** (imipramine, desipramine); such combinations may produce hypertensive crisis, severe convulsive seizures, fever, marked
sweating, excitation, delirium, tremor, twitching,
convulsions, coma, and circulatory collapse. At least
10 days should elapse between discontinuation of
MAOIs and institution of another antidepressant or
MAO inhibitor. Other **tricyclic antidepressants** have
been safely and successfully used in combination
with MAOIs.

Concomitant use of MAOIs and other **psychotropic agents** is not recommended because of possible potentiating effects and decreased margin of
safety.

Patients receiving MAOIs should not undergo
elective surgery requiring **general anesthesia** and
should not be given **cocaine** or **local anesthesia** containing sympathomimetic vasoconstrictors. The
combined hypotensive effects of MAOIs and **spinal
anesthesia** should be kept in mind. MAOIs should
be discontinued **at least 10 days** prior to elective
surgery.

Use caution in combination with **antihypertensive
drugs,** including **thiazide diuretics;** hypotension may
result. MAOIs are contraindicated in those receiving
guanethidine. Exercise caution when administering
rauwolfia concomitantly.

MAOIs have an additive hypoglycemic effect in
combination with **insulin** and **oral hypoglycemic
agents.** Monitor blood glucose and lower dosage of
hypoglycemic if necessary.

antiparkinsonism drugs are used cautiously in
those receiving **tranylcypromine;** severe reactions
have been reported.

MAOIs should not be used with **metrizamide.**

PRECAUTIONS
Follow patient closely for symptoms of postural hypotension, which may occur in hypertensive as well
as normal and hypotensive patients. Blood pressure
usually returns to pretreatment levels when drug is
discontinued or dosage reduced.

The effect of MAOIs on the convulsive threshold
may vary; take precaution when administering to
epileptic patients. Hypomania has been the most
common severe psychiatric side-effect and usually is
limited to those in whom disorders characterized by
hyperkinetic symptoms coexist with, but are obscured by, depressive affect; hypomania has usually
appeared as depression improves. If agitation is

present, it may be increased with the MAOIs. Hypomania, agitation have been reported at higher than recommended doses or following long-term therapy.

MAOIs may cause excessive stimulation in schizophrenic patients; in patients with manic-depressive states, this may result in a swing from a depressive to a manic phase. Brief discontinuation of the drug followed by resumption of therapy at a reduced dosage is advised.

Clinical evidence indicates a low incidence of altered hepatic function or jaundice. Watch for hepatic complications; periodic hepatic-function tests are recommended.

MAOIs may have the capacity to suppress anginal pain that would otherwise serve as a warning of myocardial ischemia. Use MAOIs cautiously in hyperthyroid patients because of their increased sensitivity to pressor amines.

ADVERSE REACTIONS

Common: Orthostatic hypotension, associated in some patients with falling; disturbances in cardiac rate, rhythm; dizziness, vertigo; constipation; headache; overactivity; hyperreflexia; tremors, muscle twitching; mania; hypomania; jitters, confusion, memory impairment; insomnia; peripheral edema; weakness; fatigue; drowsiness; dry mouth; blurred vision; hyperhidrosis; anorexia, body-weight changes; GI disturbances; minor sensitivity reactions such as skin rash.

Less common: Glaucoma; akathisia; ataxia; black tongue; coma; dysuria; euphoria; hematologic changes; incontinence; neuritis; photosensitivity; sexual disturbances; spider telangiectases; urinary retention; sweating; palilalia (repetitive use of words); nystagmus; hypernatremia; tachycardia; palpitation; chills. These side-effects sometimes require discontinuation of drug.

Rare: Edema of glottis; transient respiratory, cardiovascular depression following ECT; leukopenia; toxic delirium; reversible jaundice; convulsions; hepatitis; acute anxiety reaction and precipitation of schizophrenia. Fatal progressive necrotizing hepatocellular damage has been reported with high dosage but has disappeared when drug is discontinued or dosage reduced.

OVERDOSAGE

Symptoms: Depending on amount of overdosage, a mixed clinical picture may develop. Signs and symptoms may be absent or minimal during initial 12-hour period following ingestion and may develop slowly thereafter, reaching a maximum in 24 to 48 hours. Some symptoms may persist for 8 to 14

days. Immediate hospitalization, with continuous patient monitoring throughout the period, is essential. Early symptoms include excitement; irritability; anxiety; flushing; sweating; tachypnea; tachycardia; movement disorders, including grimacing, opisthotonos, clonic movements, muscular fasciculation. Tendon reflexes are often exaggerated; plantar responses may be extensor. In serious cases, coma, convulsions, hypertension and hypotension, acidosis, hyperpyrexia, cardiorespiratory arrest, and death may occur.

Treatment: Induce emesis or gastric lavage with instillation of charcoal slurry in early poisoning; protect airway against aspiration. Support respiration by appropriate measures, including management of the airway, use of supplemental oxygen, and mechanical ventilatory assistance, as required.

Cardiovascular complications include hypertension and hypotension; administer any cardiovascular agent cautiously and monitor blood pressure frequently. Severe hypotension may be treated with an alpha-adrenergic blocking agent (*e.g.*, phentolamine, phenoxybenzamine). Beta-adrenergic blocking agents may be useful for tachycardia, tachypnea, and hyperpyrexia. Treat hypotension and vascular collapse with IV fluids and, if necessary, titrate blood pressure with an IV infusion of dilute pressor agent. Adrenergic agents may produce a markedly increased pressor response.

CNS stimulation, including convulsions, may be treated with diazepam, given slowly IV. Avoid phenothiazine derivatives and CNS stimulants. Monitor temperature closely. Intensive management of hyperpyrexia may be required. Maintenance of fluid and electrolyte balance is essential. For serious hyperpyrexia, chlorpromazine has been effective.

ISOCARBOXAZID

Dosage is individualized. Usual starting dose is 30 mg/day in single or divided doses. A daily dose larger than 30 mg is not recommended. Many patients may show favorable response in a week or less but a beneficial effect may not be seen for 3 to 4 weeks.

PHENELZINE SULFATE

Initial dose, 15 mg tid; in early phase of treatment, increase dosage to at least 60 mg/day. It may be necessary to increase dosage up to 90 mg/day. Many patients do not show a clinical response until treatment at 60 mg is continued for at least 4 weeks. For maintenance, reduce dosage slowly over several weeks; dosage may be as low as 15 mg/day or every other day.

TRANYLCYPROMINE SULFATE

Dosage is individualized. Improvement should be seen within 48 hours to 3 weeks. Recommended starting dose is 20 mg/day (10 mg in A.M., 10 mg in afternoon). This may be continued for 2 weeks. If there is no response, dosage may be increased to 30 mg/day (20 mg in A.M., 10 mg in afternoon) and continued for 1 week. If there is no improvement, continued administration is unlikely to be beneficial. When satisfactory response is obtained, dosage may be reduced to maintenance level of 10 mg/day to 20 mg/day. When ECT is administered concurrently, 10 mg bid can usually be given during the series and reduced to 10 mg/day for maintenance.

Withdrawal: Reduction from peak to maintenance dosage is desirable before withdrawal. If drug is withdrawn prematurely, original symptoms will recur.

NURSING IMPLICATIONS: ANTIDEPRESSANTS

HISTORY

See Appendix 4.

PHYSICAL ASSESSMENT

Check blood pressure (in both arms with patient in sitting and/or lying position), pulse, respiratory rate; weight; observe and record overt symptoms—appearance, speech pattern, behavior, thought content, interest in surroundings, evidence of associated agitation, somatic (and other) complaints, affect (emotion).

ADMINISTRATION

Trazodone: Give with food or meals to enhance absorption.

Doxepin HCl: Dilute oral concentrate with approximately 120 ml of water, milk, or fruit juice just prior to administration. Carbonated beverages should *not* be used for dilution. Preparation and storage of bulk dilutions is not recommended. Drug is supplied with measuring dropper. For patients on methadone maintenance taking oral doxepin, mix concentrate with methadone and lemonade, orange juice, water, sugar water, or powdered fruit drink. *Do not* mix with grape juice.

Check oral cavity thoroughly if there is a suspicion that medication has not been swallowed.

Anergic or withdrawn patient: If medication is refused or not swallowed, discuss problem with physician as soon as possible. Physician may suggest crushing tablet and adding to a small amount of food or liquid or order drug to be given parenterally (if available in this form).

Tablets, when crushed, may dissolve poorly in liquids; check with pharmacist before using liquid medium to administer crushed tablets.

Amitriptyline HCl, Doxepin HCl: Two of the available strengths are 10 mg and 100 mg. Written order may be misinterpreted if not written clearly.

ONGOING ASSESSMENTS AND NURSING MANAGEMENT

Record vital signs (daily to qid or as ordered).

Observe for adverse reactions.

Monitor dietary intake (anorexia may be drug related or due to depression).

Observe and record behavior at frequent intervals, especially early in therapy, because dosage may be adjusted upward or downward according to patient response.

Daily behavioral assessments should include appearance, mood and affect, sensorium, speech and thought content, interest in surroundings, response to environment (other observations may also be appropriate).

The anergic or elderly patient may require assistance with ADL (*e.g.,* bathing, grooming, dressing, eating). The elderly patient may become confused and require supervision of all activities. Observe at frequent intervals during the day as well as in the nighttime hours.

Increased sweating may require clothing or bedding change, and sponge bath, especially in hot weather.

Keep a daily record of bowel movements; diarrhea or constipation is brought to the attention of the physician. Constipation may be relieved by addition of bulk foods to diet, increased fluid intake, or laxative.

Observe for shift to hypomania or manic phase, increased activity, agitation, anger. Hostility or agitation may require proper protection of staff members and other patients until physician examines patient.

The possibility of suicide, especially early in therapy as well as at time therapeutic response is noted, requires close patient observation.

Instruct patient to rise from a sitting or lying position slowly to prevent postural hypotension. Elderly and withdrawn patients (who may follow directions/instructions poorly) should be assisted with position changes and ambulation.

Carefully evaluate all behavior because the severely depressed patient may not communicate various physical problems (*e.g.,* pruritus, sore throat, constipation) that may indicate a drug side-effect.

Weigh 1 to 3 times/week (or as ordered) at approximately same time of day.

Dry mouth may be relieved by sips of water, hard candy, gum (sugarless). Inspect oral cavity daily, especially during early therapy; look for crusting, sore, or reddened areas. When applicable, have patient remove full or partial dentures prior to inspection of oral cavity.

Good oral care is essential, especially if dry mouth occurs. After each meal encourage thorough rinsing of the mouth and use of a soft toothbrush to brush teeth.

Daily physical and diversional therapies are geared to the patient's physical and emotional ability to participate.

Therapeutic response may vary. _Trazodone—_ end of first or second week and up to 4 weeks for some patients; _tricyclic compounds—_up to 2 to 4 weeks; _tranylcypromine_ (MAOI)—approximately 10 days; _isocarboxazid, phenelzine_—3 to 4 weeks.

The degree of psychotherapeutic support from all health-team members may influence therapeutic drug effect and therefore influence dosage.

TRICYCLIC COMPOUNDS

Observe for anticholinergic effects; monitor urinary output or check abdomen for evidence of bladder distention. Patient with blurred vision may require assistance with ambulation. If abdominal distention is noted, examine abdomen for tenderness and auscultate bowel sounds. Hyperactive, high-pitched sounds may indicate paralytic ileus; physician should be notified immediately.

These drugs have potential for bone-marrow depression (Appendix 6, section 6-8). Notify physician if one or more signs or symptoms occur.

CLINICAL ALERT: Abrupt cessation after prolonged therapy may produce withdrawal symptoms, which may include nausea, headache, vertigo, nightmares, and malaise. Ensure continuity of prescribed therapy by notation on Kardex, informing all health-team members responsible for drug administration. Termination of therapy requires gradual reduction of dosage.

Ambulatory patients who may be allowed outdoors must avoid exposure to sunlight.

These drugs lower the convulsive threshold. Seizure precautions should be carried out, especially in those with history of a seizure disorder.

Elevation and lowering of blood sugar has been reported. Check urine for glucose every 3 to 7 days or as ordered; check urine of diabetic patient qid.

Imipramine: Advise patient taking this drug not to smoke (smoking may increase metabolic biotransformation of drug).

See _Nursing Implications,_ Antianxiety Agents, if **doxepin HCl** is used to treat anxiety.

MONOAMINE OXIDASE INHIBITORS

Monitor blood pressure frequently (q2h–q4h), especially early in therapy, to detect evidence of a pressor response. If palpitation, headache, or rise in blood pressure occurs, notify physician immediately because these may be prodromal signs of hypertensive crisis.

CLINICAL ALERT: The most important reaction is hypertensive crisis, which can be fatal.

Hospitalized patient will receive a diet eliminating foods with high concentrations of tryptophan and tyramine. Visitors should be instructed not to send or bring in food for the patient.

The effect of MAOIs on the convulsive threshold may vary; institute seizure precautions when MAOIs are administered to the epileptic patient.

Observe patient for jaundice, signs of altered hepatic function.

Observe schizophrenic patient for excessive stimulation and manic-depressive patient for swing from depressive to manic phase. If these changes occur, notify physician immediately because discontinuation of drug may be necessary.

Diabetic patient: Observe for signs of hypoglycemia (Appendix 6, section 6-14); notify physician if these occur because dosage of the hypoglycemic agent may need to be reduced.

It is recommended that these drugs be discontinued _at least_ 10 days prior to elective surgery.

PATIENT AND FAMILY INFORMATION

NOTE: Patient and family cooperation with treatment modalities is essential. Give thorough explanation of dose and time of day drug is taken. Emphasize importance of physician or clinic follow-up. Because of possibility of suicide in depressed patients, physician may write outpatient prescriptions for the smallest number of tablets consistent with patient management.

Do not discontinue medication, increase or decrease dose, or take _any_ nonprescription drug without consent of physician.

Use caution when driving or performing tasks that require alertness.

Inform dentists and physicians consulted for other problems, as well as other health personnel (_e.g.,_ nurses, dietitians), of current therapy with these drugs.

To prevent postural hypotension, rise slowly from a sitting or lying position and avoid standing in one place for a prolonged period of time.

Avoid alcohol and other depressant drugs.

Dry mouth may be relieved by sips of water, hard candy, gum; good oral care is essential.

TRAZODONE

Take with food or meals to enhance absorption and decrease incidence of dizziness, lightheadedness.

Notify physician or nurse if dizziness, lightheadedness, fainting, or blood in urine occurs.

May cause dry mouth, irregular heartbeat, shortness of breath, nausea, vomiting; notify physician or nurse if any of these becomes pronounced.

If prolonged or inappropriate penile erection occurs, discontinue use immediately and consult physician.

TRICYCLIC COMPOUNDS

Avoid prolonged exposure to sunlight or sunlamps; photosensitivty may occur.

Notify physician or nurse if dry mouth persists or difficulty in urination or excessive sedation occurs.

Childhood enuresis: Give drug exactly as directed; report all adverse effects to physician or nurse as soon as possible. Keep record of bed wetting. Determine, if possible, whether enuresis occurs during the early or middle night or early morning hours. Bring records to physician at each office/clinic visit.

MONOAMINE OXIDASE INHIBITORS

Strict adherence to dietary restrictions is absolutely essential. Avoid ingestion of the following: alcohol; aged and natural cheeses; sour cream; pickled herring; broad beans; yeast extract; chicken livers; raisins; canned figs; chocolate; excessive amounts of caffeine (*e.g.*, coffee, cola beverages); soy sauce; yogurt; avocados; ripe bananas; pineapple; meat prepared with tenderizers. Check labels of frozen meat or packaged dinners containing meat for addition of a meat tenderizer (*e.g.*, papain); do not use if product contains a tenderizer.

Ask physician how many cups of coffee/tea are allowable each day.

Do not take *any* nonprescription drug unless its use has been approved by physician.

Notify physician or nurse if severe headache, skin rash, darkening of urine, pale stools, jaundice, or other unusual symptoms occur.

Antiemetic/Antivertigo Agents

General Statement

ACTIONS

Drug-induced vomiting (including drugs, radiation, metabolic disorders) is generally stimulated through the chemoreceptor trigger zone (CTZ), which in turn stimulates the vomiting center (VC) in the brain. The VC may also be stimulated directly by GI irritation, motion sickness, vestibular neuritis, and so on. Increased activity of central neurotransmitters, dopamine in the CTZ, or acetylcholine in the VC appear to be major mediators for induction of vomiting. Drugs shown to be effective as antiemetics are the antidopaminergic agents (phenothiazines, metoclopramide), which are especially effective for drug-induced emesis, and the anticholinergic agents (antihistamines, scopolamine, trimethobenzamide), which may be more appropriate in motion sickness, labyrinthine disorders, and so on. Other agents have been shown to be effective in various types of emesis; the mechanisms of these agents are not known or act differently (*e.g.*, hydroxyzine, cannabinoids, corticosteroids).

WARNINGS

Not recommended for uncomplicated vomiting in children; use should be limited to prolonged vomiting of known etiology for three principle reasons:

1. Although there is no confirming evidence, centrally acting antiemetics may contribute, in combination with viral illness (a possible cause of vomiting in children), to development of Reye's syndrome, a potentially fatal acute childhood encephalopathy. This syndrome is characterized by an abrupt onset, shortly following a nonspecific febrile illness, with persistent, severe vomiting, lethargy, irrational behavior, visceral fatty degeneration, especially involving the liver, progressive encephalopathy leading to coma, convulsions, and death.
2. Extrapyramidal symptoms secondary to some drugs may be confused with the CNS signs of an undiagnosed primary disease responsible for vomiting (*e.g.*, Reye's syndrome or other encephalopathy).
3. Drugs with hepatotoxic potential may unfavorably alter the course of Reye's syndrome. Avoid such drugs in children whose signs and symptoms (vomiting) could represent Reye's syndrome.

Severe emesis should not be treated with an antiemetic drug alone; when possible, establish cause of vomiting. Direct primary emphasis toward restoration of body fluids and electrolyte balance and toward relief of fever and causative disease process. Avoid overhydration, which may result in cerebral edema. Antiemetic effects may impede diagnosis of such conditions as brain tumors, intestinal obstruction, appendicitis, and obscure signs of toxicity from overdosage of other drugs.

Phenothiazines

Chlorpromazine Hydrochloride* Rx

See Antipsychotic Agents for complete listing of available products.

INDICATIONS
Control of nausea, vomiting; relief of intractable hiccups. See also Antipsychotic Agents for additional indications.

DOSAGE
Adults
Nausea, vomiting: _Oral_—10 mg to 25 mg q4h to q6h prn; dosage may be increased if necessary. _Rectal_—50 mg to 100 mg q6h to q8h prn. _IM_—25 mg; if no hypotension occurs, 25 mg to 50 mg q3h to q4h prn may be ordered until vomiting stops.
Intractable hiccups: _Oral_—25 mg to 50 mg tid or qid. If symptoms persist for 2 to 3 days, give 25 mg to 50 mg IM. Should symptoms persist, slow IV infusion may be used with patient flat in bed. Administer 25 mg to 50 mg in 500 ml to 1000 ml of saline. Follow blood pressure closely.
Children
Nausea, vomiting: Should not be used in children under 6 months. The duration of activity following IM administration may last 12 hours. _Oral_—0.25 mg/lb q4h to q6h. _Rectal_—0.5 mg/lb q6h to q8h prn. _IM_—0.25 mg/lb q6h to q8h prn. _Maximum IM dosage_—Children up to 5 years, 40 mg/day; 5 to 12 years, 75 mg/day except in severe cases.

NURSING IMPLICATIONS
See p 113.

Perphenazine* Rx

tablets: 2 mg, 4 mg,   Trilafon
  8 mg, 16 mg

* For _Actions, Contraindications, Warnings, Precautions, Drug Interactions, Adverse Reactions, Overdosage,_ and _Bioequivalence,_ see Antipsychotic Agents and General Statement, above.

repetabs (repeat-ac-   Trilafon
  tion tablets): 8 mg
concentrate: 16 mg/5   Trilafon
  ml
injection: 5 mg/ml   Trilafon

INDICATIONS
Control of severe nausea, vomiting; relief of intractable hiccups. See Antipsychotic Agents for additional indications.

DOSAGE
Oral—8 mg to 16 mg daily in divided doses; occasionally, 24 mg may be necessary.
_IM_—For rapid control of vomiting, 5 mg; increase to 10 mg only if necessary. Use higher doses only in hospitalized patients.
_IV_—Use only when necessary to control severe vomiting, intractable hiccups, or acute conditions such as violent retching during surgery. Limit use to recumbent hospitalized adults in doses not exceeding 5 mg. See _Administration,_ under Nursing Implications.

NURSING IMPLICATIONS
See p 113.

Prochlorperazine* Rx

See Antipsychotic Agents for complete listing of available products.

INDICATIONS
Control of severe nausea and vomiting. See Antipsychotic Agents for additional indications.

DOSAGE
Adults
Control of severe nausea and vomiting: _Oral_— usually 5 mg to 10 mg tid or qid; 15 mg sustained-release capsules on arising or 10 mg sustained-release capsules q12h. _Rectal_—25 mg bid. _IM_— initially 5 mg to 10 mg injected deeply into upper outer quadrant of buttock and repeated, if necessary, q3h to q4h. Total IM dosage should not exceed 40 mg/day.
Adult surgery (for severe nausea and vomiting): Total parenteral dose should not exceed 40 mg/day. Hypotension is a possibility if drug is given IV. _IM_—5 mg to 10 mg 1 to 2 hours before induction of anesthesia (may be repeated once in 30 minutes if needed) or to control acute symptoms during and after surgery. _IV injection_—5 mg to 10 mg 15 to 30 minutes before induction of anesthesia or to control acute symptoms during or after surgery; re-

peat once if necessary. *IV infusion*—20 mg/liter of isotonic solution; add to IV infusion 15 to 30 minutes before induction.

Children

Control of severe nausea and vomiting: Generally not used in children under 20 lb or 2 years of age.

Oral or *rectal*—20–29 lb: 2.5 mg daily or bid, not to exceed 7.5 mg/day; 30–39 lb: 2.5 mg bid or tid, not to exceed 10 mg/day; 40–85 lb: 2.5 mg tid or 5 mg bid, not to exceed 15 mg/day.

IM—0.06 mg/lb. Control is usually obtained with one dose. Duration of action may be 12 hours.

▌ NURSING IMPLICATIONS
See p 113.

Promethazine Hydrochloride* Rx

See Antihistamines for a complete list of available products.

INDICATIONS

Oral or *rectal*—active and prophylactic treatment of motion sickness; prevention and control of nausea and vomiting associated with certain types of anesthesia and surgery; antiemetic effect in postoperative patients. *Parenteral*—active treatment of motion sickness; prevention and control of nausea and vomiting associated with certain types of anesthesia and surgery. See Antihistamines for additional indications.

DOSAGE

Oral and rectal

Motion sickness: Average adult dose, 25 mg bid. Initial dose should be taken ½ to 1 hour before travel and repeated in 8 to 12 hours if needed. On succeeding days of travel, 25 mg should be taken on arising and again before the evening meal. *Children*—12.5 mg to 25 mg bid.

Nausea and vomiting: Average effective dose in children and adults is 25 mg. May be repeated as needed in doses of 12.5 mg to 25 mg q4h to q6h, or in children 0.25 mg to 0.5 mg/kg q4h to q6h IM or rectally as needed. Not used in premature or newborn infants.

Parenteral (IM, IV)

Motion sickness: Average adult dose, 25 mg. Doses of 12.5 mg to 25 mg may be repeated as needed q4h to q6h.

* For *Actions, Contraindications, Warnings, Precautions, Drug Interactions, Adverse Reactions, Overdosage,* and *Bioequivalence,* see Antipsychotic Agents and General Statement, above.

Nausea and vomiting: 12.5 mg to 25 mg, not repeated more frequently than q4h. When used for control of postoperative nausea and vomiting, administer IM or IV and reduce dosage of analgesics and barbiturates accordingly. In children under 12, dosage should not exceed one-half that of the suggested adult dose. As an adjunct to premedication, the suggested dose is 0.5 mg/lb in combination with an equal dose of narcotic or barbiturate and the appropriate dose of an atropinelike drug. Not used in premature or newborn infants.

See *Administration*.

▌ NURSING IMPLICATIONS
See p 113.

Thiethylperazine Maleate* Rx

tablets: 10 mg (contains tartrazine)	Torecan
suppositories: 10 mg	Torecan
injection: 5 mg/ml	Torecan

INDICATIONS

Effective for relief of nausea, vomiting.

DOSAGE

Do *not* administer IV (may cause severe hypotension). Not recommended for children under 12. When used in treatment of nausea or vomiting associated with anesthesia and surgery, administer by deep IM injection at, or shortly before, termination of anesthesia. *Adults*—10 mg to 30 mg daily in divided doses.

▌ NURSING IMPLICATIONS
See p 113.

Triflupromazine Hydrochloride* Rx

suspension: 50 mg/5 ml	Vesprin
injection: 10 mg/ml, 20 mg/ml	Vesprin

INDICATIONS

Control of severe nausea, vomiting. See Antipsychotic Agents for additional indications.

Adults: Recommended range is from 1 mg to a maximum total daily dose of 3 mg IV, or 5 mg to 15 mg IM repeated q4h to a maximum total daily dose of 60 mg. *Oral prophylaxis*—20 mg to a maximum total daily dose of 30 mg. For elderly or debilitated patients use 2.5 mg; maximum daily dose is 15 mg.

Children over 2½ years: 0.2 mg/kg to a maximum daily dose of 10 mg/day in 3 divided doses. *IM*—0.2 mg/kg to 0.25 mg/kg; maximum is 10 mg/day. Duration of activity following IM administration may be up to 12 hours.

▌*NURSING IMPLICATIONS*
See p 113.

Antihistamines

Buclizine Hydrochloride Rx

tablets: 50 mg (contains tartrazine)	Bucladin-S Softabs

INDICATIONS
Control of nausea, vomiting, and dizziness of motion sickness.

CONTRAINDICATIONS
Hypersensitivity, pregnancy.

ACTIONS
Acts centrally to suppress nausea, vomiting. See also General Statement, p 104.

WARNINGS
Safety and efficacy for use in children has not been established. See also General Statement, p 104.

PRECAUTIONS
Contains tartrazine. See Appendix 6, section 6-23.

ADVERSE REACTIONS
Drowsiness, dry mouth, headache, jitters.

DOSAGE
Adults: 50 mg usually relieves nausea. In severe cases 150 mg/day may be taken. Usual maintenance dose is 50 mg bid. In prevention of motion sickness, use 50 mg at least ½ hour before travel. For extended travel, a second 50 mg dose may be taken after 4 to 6 hours.

▌*NURSING IMPLICATIONS*
See p 113.

Cyclizine, Meclizine Rx, otc

CYCLIZINE

tablets: 50 mg (*otc*)	Marezine
injection: 50 mg/ml (*Rx*)	Marezine

MECLIZINE

tablets: 12.5 mg	Antivert (*Rx*), *Generic*
tablets: 25 mg	Antivert/25 (*Rx*), Wehvert (*otc*), *Generic*
tablets, chewable: 25 mg	Antivert/25 Chewable (*Rx*), Bonine (*otc*), Dizmiss (*otc*), Motion Cure (*otc*), *Generic*

INDICATIONS

CYCLIZINE
Prevention and treatment of nausea and vomiting of motion sickness.

MECLIZINE
Prevention and treatment of nausea and vomiting of motion sickness. Possibly effective for management of vertigo associated with diseases affecting the vestibular system.

CONTRAINDICATIONS
Hypersensitivity.

ACTIONS
Have antiemetic, anticholinergic, and antihistaminic properties. They reduce the sensitivity of the labyrinthine apparatus. Action may be mediated through nerve pathways to the vomiting center (VC) from the chemoreceptor trigger zone (CTZ), peripheral nerve pathways, the VC, or other CNS centers. Cyclizine and meclizine appear to have an onset of action of 30 minutes and 60 minutes respectively; their duration of action is 4 to 6 hours and 12 to 24 hours respectively. See also General Statement, p 104.

WARNINGS
Safety for use in children and the nursing mother has not been established. Use in pregnancy only when clearly needed and when potential benefits outweigh the unknown potential hazards to the fetus. See also General Statement, p 104.

PRECAUTIONS
May produce drowsiness. Because of their anticholinergic action, these drugs are used with caution in those with narrow-angle glaucoma or obstructive disease of the GI or GU tract as well as in elderly males with possible prostatic hypertrophy. Drugs may have hypotensive action; this may be confusing or dangerous in postoperative patients.

DRUG INTERACTIONS
May have additive effects with **alcohol** and other **CNS depressants** (*e.g.,* hypnotics, sedatives, tranquilizers, antianxiety agents).

ADVERSE REACTIONS

Urticaria; drug rash; dry mouth, nose, throat; drowsiness; restlessness; excitation; nervousness; insomnia; euphoria; anorexia; nausea; vomiting; diarrhea; constipation; hypotension; blurred vision; diplopia; vertigo; tinnitus; palpitation; tachycardia; urinary frequency; difficult urination; urinary retention; auditory and visual hallucinations (particularly when dosage recommendations are exceeded); cholestatic jaundice (cyclizine).

OVERDOSAGE

Symptoms: Moderate overdosage may cause hyperexcitability alternating with drowsiness. Massive overdosage may cause convulsions, hallucinations, respiratory paralysis.

Treatment: Appropriate supportive and symptomatic treatment. Consider dialysis. *Caution*—Do not use morphine or other respiratory depressants.

DOSAGE

Cyclizine

Oral: *Adults*—50 mg taken ½ hour before departure, to be repeated q4h to q6h, not to exceed 200 mg daily. *Children* (6–12 years)—½ adult dose up to 3 times/day.

IM: *Adults*—50 mg q4h to q6h.

Meclizine

Motion sickness: An initial dose of 25 mg to 50 mg 1 hour prior to travel; dose may be repeated every 24 hours for duration of journey.

Vertigo: 25 mg to 100 mg daily in divided doses.

NURSING IMPLICATIONS

See p 113.

Dimenhydrinate Rx, otc

tablets: 50 mg (*otc*)	Calm X, Dimentabs, Dramaban, Dramamine, Marmine (*Rx*), Motion-Aid, *Generic*
injection: 50 mg/ml (*Rx*)	Dinate, Dommanate, Dramamine, Dramilin, Dramoject, Dymenate, Hydrate, Marmine, Motion-Aid, Reidamine, Wehamine, *Generic*
liquid: 12.5 mg/4 ml (*otc*)	Dramamine, Motion-Aid Elixir, *Generic*

INDICATIONS

Prevention and treatment of nausea, vomiting, or vertigo of motion sickness.

ACTIONS

Dimenhydrinate consists of equal molar proportions of diphenhydramine and chlorotheophylline. It has a depressant action on hyperstimulated labyrinthine function. The precise mode of action is not known. Antiemetic effects are believed to be due to the diphenhydramine, an antihistamine also used as an antiemetic agent. See also General Statement, p 104.

WARNINGS

Safety for use in pregnancy has not been established. Use only when clearly needed and when potential benefits outweigh the unknown potential hazards to the fetus. See also General Statement, p 104.

PRECAUTIONS

May produce drowsiness, especially with high dosage. Use with caution in patients with conditions that might be aggravated by anticholinergic therapy (*e.g.,* prostatic hypertrophy, stenosing peptic ulcer, pyloroduodenal obstruction, bladder-neck obstruction, narrow-angle glaucoma, cardiac arrhythmias, asthma).

DRUG INTERACTIONS

Concomitant use of **alcohol** or other **CNS depressants** may have an additive effect. Use with caution in conjunction with certain antibiotics that may cause ototoxicity, because dimenhydrinate is capable of masking symptoms of ototoxicity and irreversible damage may result.

ADVERSE REACTIONS

CNS: *Most common*—Drowsiness; confusion; nervousness; restlessness; headache; insomnia; tingling, heaviness, and weakness of hands; vertigo.

GI: Nausea, vomiting, diarrhea, epigastric distress, constipation.

Ophthalmologic: Blurring of vision, diplopia.

Cardiovascular: Palpitation, hypotension.

Miscellaneous: Anaphylaxis; photosensitivity; urticaria; drug rash; hemolytic anemia; difficulty in urination; nasal congestion; tightness of chest; wheezing; thickening of bronchial secretions; dryness of mouth, nose, and throat.

DOSAGE

Adults

Oral: 50 mg to 100 mg q4h; do not exceed 400 mg in 24 hours.

IM: 50 mg as needed.

IV: 50 mg in 10 ml Sodium Chloride Injection USP given over a period of 2 minutes.

Children

Oral: *6 to 12 years of age*—25 mg to 50 mg q6h to q8h, not to exceed 150 mg in 24 hours; *2 to 6 years of age*—25 mg q6h to q8h, not to exceed 75 mg in 24 hours; *under 2 years of age*—give only on advice of physician.

IM: 1.25 mg/kg or 37.5 mg/m^2 4 times daily, up to 300 mg daily.

▌ NURSING IMPLICATIONS
See p 113.

Diphenhydramine Hydrochloride Rx

See Antihistamines for complete listing of available products.

INDICATIONS

Active and prophylactic treatment of motion sickness. See Antihistamines for additional indications.

CONTRAINDICATIONS, ACTIONS, WARNINGS, PRECAUTIONS, DRUG INTERACTIONS, ADVERSE REACTIONS, OVERDOSAGE

See Antihistamines, p 119, and General Statement, p 104.

DOSAGE

Oral

Adults: 25 mg to 50 mg tid or qid.

Children (over 20 lb): 12.5 mg to 25 mg tid or qid (5 mg/kg/24 hours). Do not exceed 300 mg. Give first dose 30 minutes before exposure to motion and repeat before meals and H.S. for duration of journey.

Parenteral

Adults: 10 mg to 50 mg IV or deep IM; 100 mg if required. *Maximum daily dose*—400 mg.

Children: 5 mg/kg/24 hours in 4 divided doses IV or deep IM. *Maximum daily dose*—300 mg.

▌ NURSING IMPLICATIONS
See p 113.

Miscellaneous Preparations

Benzquinamide Hydrochloride Rx

injection: 50 mg/vial   Emete-Con

INDICATIONS

Prevention and treatment of nausea and vomiting associated with anesthesia and surgery. Restrict prophylactic use to patients in whom emesis would endanger results of surgery or result in harm.

CONTRAINDICATIONS

Hypersensitivity.

ACTIONS

Mechanism of action is unknown. The onset of antiemetic activity usually occurs within 15 minutes; 5% to 10% of dose is excreted unchanged in the urine. The remaining drug undergoes metabolism in the liver. Plasma half-life is about 40 minutes and is 58% bound to plasma protein.

WARNINGS

Sudden increase in blood pressure and transient arrhythmias (premature ventricular and atrial contractions) have been reported following IV administration. IM route is preferable; restrict IV route to patients without cardiovascular disease who are receiving no preanesthetic or concomitant cardiovascular drugs. May mask signs of overdosage to toxic drugs or obscure diagnosis of such conditions as intestinal obstruction or brain tumor. Safety for use in pregnancy is not established; use in pregnancy is not recommended. Safety and efficacy for use in children is not established. See also General Statement, p 104.

DRUG INTERACTIONS

If patient is receiving **pressor agents** or **epinephrine-like drugs** and is also given benzquinamide, give in fractions of normal dose. Blood pressure should be monitored, particularly in hypertensive patients.

ADVERSE REACTIONS

Autonomic nervous system: Dry mouth, shivering, sweating, increased temperature, hiccups, flushing, salivation, blurred vision.

Cardiovascular: Hypertension, hypotension, dizziness, atrial fibrillation, premature atrial and ventricular contractions.

CNS: Drowsiness, insomnia, fatigue, restlessness, headache, excitement, nervousness.

GI: Anorexia, nausea.

Musculoskeletal: Twitching, shaking/tremors, weakness.

Skin: Hives/rash.

OVERDOSAGE

Symptoms: May be manifested as a combination of CNS stimulant and depressant effects.

Treatment: No specific antidote. Institute general supportive measures. Atropine may be helpful.

DOSAGE

IM: 50 mg (0.5 mg/kg to 1 mg/kg). First dose may be repeated in 1 hour with subsequent doses q3h to q4h as necessary. Inject well within mass of a large muscle; use the deltoid area *Only* if it is well developed.

IV: 25 mg (0.2 mg/kg to 0.4 mg/kg as a single dose) slowly (1 ml every 30 seconds to 1 minute). Subsequent doses should be given IM.

NURSING IMPLICATIONS
See p 113.

Diphenidol Rx

tablets: 25 mg (con-   Vontrol
    tains tartrazine)

INDICATIONS
Peripheral (labyrinthine) vertigo and associated nausea and vomiting seen in such conditions as Meniere's disease and middle- and inner-ear surgery (for labyrinthitis). For control of nausea and vomiting seen in such conditions as postoperative states, malignant neoplasms, and labyrinthine disturbances.

CONTRAINDICATIONS
Known hypersensitivity, anuria (approximately 90% of drug is excreted in urine).

ACTIONS
Exerts specific antivertigo effect on the vestibular apparatus to control vertigo and inhibits the chemoreceptor trigger zone (CTZ) to control nausea and vomiting.

WARNINGS
May cause hallucinations, disorientation, and confusion—for this reason, use is limited to hospitalized patients or to those under comparable continuous close professional supervision. Incidence of these reactions appears to be less than 0.5%; they usually occur within 3 days of starting drug therapy and subside spontaneously, usually within 3 days after drug is discontinued. Safety for use in pregnancy is not established. Safety for use in the breast-feeding mother is not established. See also General Statement, p 104.

PRECAUTIONS
Antiemetic action may mask signs of drug overdose (*e.g.,* digitalis) or may obscure diagnosis of such conditions as intestinal obstruction or brain tumor. Has a weak peripheral anticholinergic effect and is used with caution in those with glaucoma; obstructive lesions of the GI and GU tracts such as stenos-

ing peptic ulcer, prostatic hypertrophy, pyloric and duodenal obstruction; and organic cardiospasm. Contains tartrazine. See Appendix 6, section 6-23.

ADVERSE REACTIONS
Auditory and visual hallucinations, disorientation, and confusion have been reported. Drowsiness, overstimulation, depression, sleep disturbance, dry mouth, GI irritation (nausea, indigestion), or blurred vision may occur. Mild jaundice and slight lowering of blood pressure have been reported.

OVERDOSAGE
Treatment is supportive, with maintenance of blood pressure and respiration. Early gastric lavage may be indicated, depending on amount of overdose and symptoms.

DOSAGE
Adults, for vertigo or nausea and vomiting: Usual dose is 25 mg q4h; some may require 50 mg.
Children, for nausea and vomiting only: Usual dose is 0.4 mg/lb. Dosage for children 50 lb to 100 lb is 25 mg. Children's doses should usually not be given more often than q4h. However, if symptoms persist after first dose, repeat after 1 hour. Thereafter, doses may be given q4h, as needed. Total dose in 24 hours should not exceed 2.5 mg/lb. Not recommended for use in infants under 6 months or 25 lb.

NURSING IMPLICATIONS
See p 113.

Scopolamine Preparations Rx, otc

SCOPOLAMINE HYDROBROMIDE, ORAL
tablets: 0.4 mg, 0.6   *Generic*
    mg (*Rx*)
capsules: 0.25 mg   Triptone
    (*otc*)

SCOPOLAMINE, TRANSDERMAL
transdermal thera-   Transderm-Scōp
    peutic system: 1.5
    mg (delivering 0.5
    mg over 3 days)
    (*Rx*)

INDICATIONS
Prevention of nausea and vomiting associated with motion sickness in adults. See Gastrointestinal Anticholinergics/Antispasmodics for additional indications.

CONTRAINDICATIONS

Oral: Narrow-angle glaucoma, prostatic hypertrophy, pyloric obstruction. Do not give to those with impaired renal or hepatic function or those who have had an idiosyncratic reaction.

Transdermal: Hypersensitivity to scopolamine.

ACTIONS

In addition to having systemic anticholinergic effects, oral scopolamine is effective in motion sickness. See also Gastrointestinal Anticholinergics/Antispasmodics, p 500, and General Statement, p 104.

Transdermal system: This system is a 0.2-mm-thick film with 4 layers. It contains 1.5 mg of scopolamine, which is gradually released over 3 days from an adhesive matrix of mineral oil and polyisobutylene following application to the postauricular skin. An initial priming dose of scopolamine is released from the adhesive layer, saturates the skin binding site for scopolamine, and rapidly brings the plasma concentration to the required steady-state level. A continuous controlled release of scopolamine flows from the drug reservoir through the rate-controlling membrane to maintain a constant plasma level. Antiemetic protection is produced within several hours following application behind the ear.

WARNINGS

Potentially alarming idiosyncratic reactions may occur with therapeutic doses.

Administer during pregnancy only if clearly needed. It is not known whether drug is excreted in human breast milk. Safety and efficacy in children is not established. The transdermal system should not be used in children.

See also General Statement, p 104.

PRECAUTIONS

Use with caution in patients with cardiac disease and in the elderly. Use the transdermal system with caution in patients with glaucoma, pyloric obstruction, urinary-bladder-neck obstruction, and suspected intestinal obstruction. Use special caution in those with impaired metabolic, hepatic, or renal function because of increased likelihood of CNS effects.

ADVERSE REACTIONS

In comparison with transdermal administration, oral use requires larger total doses and is associated with a greater incidence of untoward systemic effects.

Most common: Dry mouth; drowsiness; transient impairment of eye accommodation, including

blurred vision and dilation of pupils. Unilateral fixed and dilated pupil has been reported, apparently from accidentally touching one eye after manipulation of the scopolamine patch.

Infrequent: Disorientation; memory disturbances; dizziness; restlessness; giddiness; hallucinations; confusion; difficult urination; rashes or erythema; dry, itchy, or red eyes. In susceptible patients, there may be dryness of the skin and other signs and symptoms typical of anticholinergic toxicity.

OVERDOSAGE

Oral form may cause delirium, fever, stupor, coma, respiratory failure, or death. Antidote is physostigmine, which may be given in repeated doses if patient lapses into coma again within 1 to 2 hours. Transdermal overdosage may cause disorientation, memory disturbances, restlessness, giddiness, hallucinations, or confusion. Should any of these occur, remove system immediately. Initiate appropriate parasympathomimetic therapy if symptoms are severe.

DOSAGE

Oral: 0.25 to 0.8 mg 1 hour before travel.

Transdermal: Initiation of therapy—apply one system to the postauricular skin several hours before antiemetic effect is required. Scopolamine 0.5 mg will be delivered over 3 days. If continued therapy is required, replace system every 3 days.

▌ NURSING IMPLICATIONS
See p 113.

Trimethobenzamide Hydrochloride Rx

capsules: 100 mg, 250 mg	Tigan
suppositories: 200 mg	Tegamide, Tigan, *Generic*
pediatric suppositories: 100 mg	Tegamide, Tigan, *Generic*
injection: 100 mg/ml	Tigan, *Generic*

INDICATIONS

Control of nausea, vomiting.

CONTRAINDICATIONS

Hypersensitivity to trimethobenzamide, benzocaine, or similar local anesthetics; parenteral administration to children; suppositories in premature or newborn infants.

ACTIONS

Mechanism is obscure, but drug may be mediated through the chemoreceptor trigger zone (CTZ); direct impulses to the vomiting center are not inhibited. See also General Statement, p 104.

WARNINGS

Safety for use in pregnancy and the nursing mother has not been established. See also General Statement, p 104.

PRECAUTIONS

May produce drowsiness. During acute febrile illness, encephalitides, gastroenteritis, dehydration, and electrolyte imbalance, especially in children and in the elderly or debilitated, CNS reactions (*e.g.,* opisthotonos, convulsions, coma, extrapyramidal symptoms) have been reported. Exercise caution in administering this drug, particularly with other CNS-acting agents such as phenothiazines, barbiturates, and belladonna derivatives.

ADVERSE REACTIONS

Hypersensitivity reactions; parkinsonlike symptoms; hypotension following parenteral administration; blood dyscrasias; blurred vision; coma; convulsions; depression of mood; diarrhea; disorientation; dizziness; drowsiness; headache; jaundice; muscle cramps; opisthotonos; allergic skin reactions. If any of these occurs, discontinue use. Intramuscular administration may cause pain, stinging, burning, redness, and swelling.

DOSAGE

Oral: *Adults*—250 mg tid or qid. *Children (30–90 lb)*—100 mg to 200 mg tid or qid.

Rectal: *Adults*—200 mg tid or qid. *Children (30–90 lb)*—100 mg to 200 mg tid or qid; *under 30 lb,* 100 mg tid or qid. Do not use in premature or newborn infants.

Injection: *Adults*—200 mg tid or qid, IM only, into upper outer quadrant of the gluteal region. *Children*—Use not recommended.

▌ NURSING IMPLICATIONS
See p 113.

Antiemetic/Antivertigo Combinations

Phosphorated Carbohydrate Solution otc

solution: fructose, dextrose, and orthophosphoric acid with controlled hydrogen ion concentration	Calm-X, Eazol, Emetrol, Nausetrol
solution: 33% dextrose, 33% fructose and phosphoric acid with controlled hydrogen ion concentration	Especol

INDICATIONS

Symptomatic relief of nausea, vomiting.

ACTIONS

These preparations are hyperosmolar carbohydrate solutions with phosphoric acid. They are claimed to relieve nausea and vomiting by direct local action on the wall of the GI tract, reducing smooth-muscle contraction and delaying gastric emptying time in direct proportion to the amount used. The data available do not appear sufficient to document effectiveness.

PRECAUTIONS

Nausea may be a sign of a serious condition. These preparations contain significant amounts of carbohydrates and therefore should be avoided by diabetic patients. Persons with hereditary fructose intolerance should not take preparations containing fructose.

DOSAGE

Epidemic and other functional vomiting or nausea; vomiting due to psychogenic factors: Infants, children—5 ml or 10 ml at 15-minute intervals until vomiting ceases. *Adults*—15 ml or 30 ml in same manner as for children. If emesis occurs after first dose, resume same dosage schedule in 5 minutes.

Regurgitation in infants: 5 ml or 10 ml, 10 to 15 minutes before each feeding; in refractory cases, 10 ml to 15 ml 30 minutes before feeding.

Morning sickness: 15 ml or 30 ml on arising; repeated q3h or when nausea occurs.

Motion sickness; nausea and vomiting due to drug therapy or inhalation anesthesia: 5-ml doses for young children; 15 ml for older children, adults.

▌ NURSING IMPLICATIONS
See p 113.

Combinations of Antihistamines, Pyridoxine HCl, Pentobarbital

capsules: 25 mg dimenhydrinate, 50 mg niacin. Dose: 1 or 2 capsules, 3 or 4 times/day. Not recommended for	Nico-Vert, Tega-Vert (*Rx*)

use in children under 12.

capsules: 12.5 mg pheniramine maleate, 50 mg nicotinic acid. Dose: 1 or 2 capsules tid, with meals or snacks. Not recommended for use in children under 12.   Vertex (*Rx*)

suppositories: 25 mg pyrilamine maleate, 30 mg pentobarbital sodium. Dose: Children 2–12, 1 suppository q6h–q8h; under 2, ½ suppository q6h–q8h. Not recommended for use in infants under 6 months. Do not exceed 3 doses in 24 hours.   Wans Children (*Rx, C–III*)

suppositories: 50 mg pyrilamine maleate, 50 mg pentobarbital sodium. Dose: 1 suppository initially; may be repeated in 4 to 6 hours. Do not exceed 4 doses in 24 hours.   Wans No. 1 (*Rx, C–III*)

suppositories: 50 mg pyrilamine maleate, 100 mg pentobarbital sodium. Dose: 1 suppository initially; may be repeated in 4 to 6 hours. Do not exceed 4 doses in 24 hours. (Contains tartrazine)   Wans No. 2 (*Rx, C–III*)

INDICATIONS
Symptomatic control of nausea, vomiting.

PRECAUTIONS
Some products contain tartrazine. See Appendix 6, section 6-23.

DOSAGE
See product listings, above.

NURSING IMPLICATIONS
See below.

NURSING IMPLICATIONS: ANTIEMETIC/ANTIVERTIGO AGENTS

HISTORY
See Appendix 4.

PHYSICAL ASSESSMENT
If vomiting is severe, monitor vital signs, weight; inspect mucous membranes; assess skin turgor; obtain urine sample and note color (pale yellow *vs* amber) to evaluate hydration. Baseline laboratory tests may include serum electrolytes, CBC, urinalysis.

ADMINISTRATION
If patient is unable to retain oral form of drug, contact physician because another route of administration may be necessary.

Liquid preparations may be diluted with a small amount of water or fruit juice immediately prior to administration. For use of other liquids, check with hospital pharmacist. Avoid using hot liquids (*e.g.,* soup) for dilution.

When administered IM, most of these drugs are injected deeply in the buttock (see also individual drug monographs).

TRADE NAME SIMILARITY
Wehamine (dimenhydrinate) and Wyamine (mephentermine sulfate), a drug used for shock.

PHENOTHIAZINES
Liquid concentrates: Avoid contact with the skin when pouring medication; contact dermatitis may result.

Parenteral administration: Administer with patient in a recumbent position. Keep patient recumbent for 30 or more minutes following administration because hypotension may occur.

Chlorpromazine HCl: If giving IV, place patient in a recumbent position. Monitor blood pressure, pulse q10m to q15m.

Perphenazine, IV administration: Place patient in a recumbent position; take blood pressure and pulse before drug is administered. Drug is given as a *diluted* solution by fractional injection (divided doses) or by slow IV drip infusion. Physician must specify diluent for fractional injection and specific dose administered with each injection (usually 1 mg/injection at 1- to 2-minute intervals). When administered in divided doses, dilute to 0.5 mg/ml and give not more than 1 mg per injection at not less than 1- to 2-minute intervals. Hypotensive and extrapyramidal side-effects may occur; monitor blood pressure and pulse continuously during and after administration. If hypotension occurs, slow IV infusion to KVO or withhold next dose of the fractional injection and contact physician immediately.

Prochlorperazine: Subcutaneous administration is not advisable because of local irritation; give deeply into upper outer quadrant of the buttock.

Promethazine, parenteral: Preferred route of administration is by deep IM injection. Proper IV administration is well tolerated but hazardous. When used IV, give in concentration no greater than 25 mg/ml, and at a rate not to exceed 25 mg/minute. It is preferable to inject through the tubing of an IV infusion set. Inadvertent intra-arterial injection can result in gangrene of the affected extremity. Subcutaneous injection is contraindicated because it may result in tissue necrosis.

ANTIHISTAMINES

Buclizine: Tablets may be taken whole without swallowing water; may be placed in mouth and allowed to dissolve, chewed, or swallowed whole.

Dimenhydrinate, IV administration: Dose (50 mg) diluted in 10 ml of Sodium Chloride Injection, USP and given over period of 2 minutes.

MISCELLANEOUS PREPARATIONS

Benzquinamide, IV administration: Must be reconstituted with 2.2 ml Sterile Water for Injection or Bacteriostatic Water for Injection with benzyl alcohol or methyl and propyl parabens. Dilution will yield 2 ml of solution with 25 mg/ml, which maintains potency for 14 days at room temperature.

Scopolamine, transdermal: Applied behind ear; directions supplied with product.

Trimethobenzamide, IM administration: Avoid escape of solution along IM route by using Z-track method of injection.

Phosphorated carbohydrate solution: Do not dilute solution for administration. Do not give oral fluids immediately before or for at least 15 minutes after dose.

ONGOING ASSESSMENTS AND NURSING MANAGEMENT

If nausea and vomiting are persistent or severe, monitor vital signs q2h to q4h or as ordered; weigh daily.

Measure intake and output (urine, emesis). If nausea and vomiting are temporary (*e.g.,* less than 1 day), measure intake and output until patient is taking oral fluids in sufficient quantity.

Observe for signs of dehydration (Appendix 6, section 6-10).

The parenteral route of administration may be ordered until emesis is controlled; the oral route is usually used as soon as emesis stops.

Antiemetic drugs may obscure signs of toxicity of other drugs or mask symptoms of disease (*e.g.,* brain tumor, intestinal obstruction, Reye's syndrome). Observe for *any* additional symptoms or complaints offered by the patient.

Observe for adverse drug reactions; if they occur, withhold next dose and notify physician immediately (see Antipsychotic Agents for complete list of adverse reactions for phenothiazine derivatives).

Administration of these drugs may also result in variable degrees of drowsiness. To prevent accidental falls or other injuries, instruct patient to request assistance with ambulation, including going to the bathroom, getting out of bed or into a chair, and so on.

PHENOTHIAZINES

Patients receiving phenothiazines by any route should be observed for hypotensive episodes. Monitor blood pressure and pulse q15m to q30m for 1 to 2 or more hours following administration. Keep patient recumbent for 30 or more minutes following parenteral administration.

CLINICAL ALERT: Phenothiazine derivatives may depress the cough reflex and aspiration of vomitus is possible. Observe patients, especially postoperative patients, at frequent intervals. A suction machine and suction catheters should be readily available.

The phenothiazine derivatives (with the exception of triethylperazine) may discolor urine pink or reddish brown. Inform patient of urine-color change. Mark laboratory slips for urinalysis with name of drug administered.

Children with acute illnesses or dehydration seem more susceptible to neuromuscular reactions, particularly dystonias. The elderly are more susceptible to parkinsonism and akathisia (these reactions are more likely to occur with prolonged therapy or high doses). If a neuromuscular reaction occurs, withhold next dose of drug and contact physician immediately.

The above adverse drug effects are distressing to the patient; if possible, have someone stay with the patient or check patient frequently until he is seen by the physician.

PATIENT AND FAMILY INFORMATION
Notify physician if problem is not relieved or becomes worse.

PHENOTHIAZINES
May cause drowsiness; observe caution while driving or performing other tasks requiring alertness.

Avoid alcohol and other depressants; do not use any nonprescription drug without first checking with physician.

May discolor urine pink or reddish brown (*exception*—triethylperazine).

Avoid prolonged exposure to sunlight; photosensitivity may occur. If exposure to sunlight is absolutely necessary, ask physician if a sunscreen lotion may be used and which product(s) provide reliable protection.

Notify physician or nurse if any of the following occurs: Weakness, lightheadness, dizziness, or fainting (signifying orthostatic hypotension, which can often be minimized by avoiding sudden changes in position); fever; sore throat; unusual bleeding, bruising; skin rash; weakness; tremors; impaired vision; darkly colored urine; pale stools; jaundice; extreme drowsiness.

Liquid (oral) preparations: Avoid contact with skin when pouring dose; skin rash may result.

ANTIHISTAMINES
May cause drowsiness; observe caution when driving or performing other tasks requiring alertness.

Avoid alcohol and other depressants; do not use any nonprescription drug without first checking with physician.

MISCELLANEOUS PREPARATIONS
Trimethobenzamide: May cause drowsiness; observe caution while driving or performing tasks requiring alertness.

Avoid alcohol and other depressants; do not take any nonprescription drug without first checking with physician.

Scopolamine hydrobromide: May cause dry mouth, blurred vision, drowsiness. Dry mouth may be relieved by hard candy or gum. Observe caution while driving or performing tasks requiring alertness.

Scopolamine, transdermal: Package insert available with product; read it carefully. (See also

discussion of Scopolamine Hydrobromide, above.)

Phosphorated carbohydrate solution: Nausea may be sign of a serious condition. If symptoms are not relieved or recur often, consult physician.

Do not dilute or take oral fluids immediately before or for at least 15 minutes after dose. Read package directions; follow manufacturer's recommendations.

COMBINATION ANTIEMETIC/ANTIVERTIGO AGENTS
Suppositories: Lubricate before insertion; purchase water-soluble lubricant, finger cot, or gloves from a pharmacy. Do *not* use Vaseline, mineral oil, or other lubricants except those marked "water soluble."

When inserting suppository in a small child, be sure suppository is well lubricated; use little finger (covered with lubricated finger cot) for insertion.

(See also discussion of Antihistamines, above.)

Antihemophilic Factor *(Factor VIII)* Rx

Stable lyophilized concentrate of Factor VIII in single-dose vials w/diluent	Factorate, Factorate Generation II
Stable dried preparation in concentrated form; contains trace amount of heparin and 3% dextrose; supplied w/diluent	Hemofil
Stable dried preparation in concentrated form; contains trace amount of heparin; in single-dose vials w/diluent	Hemofil T
Stable dried concentrate, contains 1% dextrose; w/diluent, sterile filter needle	Koāte
Stable freeze-dried concentrate in single-dose vials w/diluent	Profilate

INDICATIONS

Treatment of classical hemophilia (hemophilia A), in which there is demonstrated deficiency of plasma clotting factor, Factor VIII; no benefit may be expected from use in treating other causes of hemorrhage. Provides a means of temporarily replacing the missing clotting factor in order to correct or prevent bleeding episodes or perform emergency or elective surgery. Not effective in controlling bleeding associated with von Willebrand's disease.

ACTIONS

A plasma protein (Factor VIII), which corrects the coagulation defect of those with hemophilia A by accelerating the abnormally slow clotting time. It is needed for transformation of prothrombin (Factor II) to thrombin by the intrinsic pathway. Following administration, the half-disappearance time of Factor VIII from plasma is ordinarily about 8 hours. One antihemophilic factor (AHF) unit is defined as the activity present in 1 ml of human plasma pooled from at least 10 donors.

WARNINGS

Risk of transmitting hepatitis and acquired immune deficiency syndrome (AIDS) is present. Individual units of plasma used in preparation of these products and each lot of the final product have been found nonreactive when tested for hepatitis B surface antigen. Because present testing methods are not sensitive enough to detect potentially dangerous antigens, the risk of transmitting hepatitis still exists.

PRECAUTIONS

Approximately 5% to 8% of patients develop inhibitors to Factor VIII and require careful monitoring, especially if surgical procedures are indicated. In patients with inhibitors, the response to AHF may be less than expected and larger doses are often required. Patients with high inhibitor levels may not respond to AHF.

AHF contains naturally occurring blood-group-specific antibodies (Anti-A and Anti-B isoagglutinins). When large or frequently repeated doses are needed in those of blood group A, B, or AB, there is a possibility of intravascular hemolysis; the hematocrit and direct Coombs' test are monitored for signs of progressive anemia. Corrective therapy may include use of type-specific cryoprecipitate as an alternative source of AHF and, if red cell replacement is necessary, infusion of compatible group-O packed red cells.

ADVERSE REACTIONS

Allergic reactions: Mild reactions may result from administration. Bronchospasm, urticaria, chills, nausea, stinging at the infusion site, vomiting, headache, somnolence, and lethargy may also be seen. Rarely, massive doses have resulted in hemolytic anemia, increased bleeding tendency, or hyperfibrinogenemia. Acute reactions such as erythema, hives, fever, and backache may occur infrequently and ordinarily disappear in 15 to 20 minutes.

DOSAGE

Administer by IV route only. See *Administration.* Dosage is individualized according to the needs of the patient and is dependent on weight of patient, severity of deficiency, severity of hemorrhage, presence of inhibitors, and the Factor VIII level desired. Clinical effect on the patient is the most important factor in evaluation of therapy. It may be necessary to administer more AHF than estimated in order to obtain the desired result.

Prophylaxis of spontaneous hemorrhages: The level of Factor VIII required to prevent spontaneous hemorrhage is approximately 5% of normal; 30% of normal is the minimum required for hemostasis following trauma or surgery. Mild superficial or early hemorrhages may respond to a single dose of 10 AHF/IU/kg, leading to a rise of approximately 20% in the Factor VIII level. In those with early hemoarthrosis; smaller doses may be adequate.

Moderate hemorrhage and minor surgery: Requires the patient's plasma Factor VIII level to be 30% to 50% of normal for optimal clot formation. This usually requires an initial dose of 15 to 25 AHF/IU/kg; if further therapy is required, a maintenance dose of 10 to 15 AHF/IU/kg may be given every 8 to 12 hours.

Severe hemorrhage: For life-threatening bleeding or hemorrhage involving vital structures, the Factor VIII level is raised to 80% to 100% of normal. Administer an initial dose of 40 to 50 AHF/IU/kg and a maintenance dose of 20 to 25 AHF/IU/kg every 8 hours to 12 hours.

Major surgery: Requires a dose of AHF sufficient to achieve a level of 80% to 100% of normal, given an hour before the procedure. A second dose, half the size of the priming dose, is given about 5 hours after the first dose. The Factor VIII level is maintained at a daily minimum of at least 30% for a healing period of 10 to 14 days.

NURSING IMPLICATIONS

HISTORY

Obtain previous hospital records, if available, or obtain past history of bleeding episodes from patient or family; if bleeding has occurred, obtain description of trauma; if bleeding is external, attempt to determine approximate amount of blood loss; if bleeding is believed to be internal, obtain accurate description of symptoms (_e.g.,_ location and intensity of pain, other symptoms experienced).

PHYSICAL ASSESSMENT

Carefully examine external area(s) of bleeding and record findings. Baseline laboratory tests may include CBC, urinalysis, PTT, thromboplastin generation test, prothrombin generation test, type and cross-match.

ADMINISTRATION

Drug is administered by IV route only.

Actual number of AHF units is indicated on the vials. Check expiration data before using. Read enclosed directions carefully.

Use plastic syringes for preparation and administration.

Prior to reconstitution, warm diluent and the concentrate to room temperature.

Two needles are required to add diluent. One needle is used as an airway and a second needle (and plastic syringe) is used to add diluent.

Following addition of diluent, rotate vial gently (_do not shake_) until contents are dissolved (takes approximately 5 minutes).

Use a _plastic_ syringe to withdraw reconstituted solution because solutions may bind to the surface of ground glass.

After reconstitution, administer promptly (within 3 hours). Do not refrigerate after reconstitution.

Take vital signs prior to administration.

The solution must not be below room temperature during infusion.

Physician orders rate of administration. Preparations containing 34 or more AHF units/ml are given at a maximum rate of 2 ml/minute. Preparations containing less than 34 AHF units/ml are given at a rate of 10 ml to 20 ml over 3 minutes.

Monitor blood pressure and pulse during administration; contact physician immediately if pulse rate rises or acute reactions occur (see _Adverse Reactions_).

During and after administration, nausea, vomiting, chills, stinging sensation at needle site, headache, somnolence, or lethargy may occur. Use appropriate comfort measures.

After needle is removed from vein, prolonged pressure on venipuncture site is required. This may be followed by a pressure dressing. Check area carefully q5m to q15m to be sure there is no oozing from venipuncture site.

Discard unused portion of drug.

Diphenhydramine may be ordered before administration to prevent a reaction.

Storage: Store under normal refrigeration—2°C to 8°C (35°F to 46°F). _Do not freeze._ Factorate may be stored at room temperature. After reconstitution, administer promptly (within 3 hours) to avoid ill effects of any possible bacterial contamination occurring during reconstitution. Do not refrigerate after reconstitution.

ONGOING ASSESSMENTS AND NURSING MANAGEMENT

Assess frequently for signs of continued or further hemorrhage if reason for use was to control active hemorrhage. If used as prophylaxis, observe for signs of new bleeding.

Alert laboratory personnel to the fact that prolonged pressure and possibly a pressure dressing will be required following venipuncture.

Consider possibility of intravascular hemolysis, especially if large or repeated doses are given. Monitor urinary output, color of urine, and vital signs q1h to q2h or as ordered. Report cyanosis, hematuria (pink, red, or brown urine), or change in vital signs to physician immediately.

Protect patient from any injury that may result in further episodes of bleeding (_e.g.,_ pad siderails (if patient is restless), encourage use of electric shaver rather than safety razor, apply blood-pressure cuff carefully and avoid overinflation of cuff when monitoring vital signs, provide a soft toothbrush to prevent injury to gingiva, remove adhesive tape [use nonallergenic type when possible] from pressure dressing or IV infusion site slowly and carefully).

If intramuscular or subcutaneous administration of other drugs is ordered, apply prolonged pressure at injection site. In some cases it may be necessary to recheck injection site q15m for 1 to 2 hours to be sure no further oozing occurs.

Monitor coagulation studies before, during, and after administration.

PATIENT AND FAMILY INFORMATION

Patient and family must be thoroughly instructed in lifetime management of this disorder, including the importance of consistent medical management, ways to minimize trauma, how to manage bleeding emergencies, genetic counseling, and use of Medic-Alert or other identification.

Antihistamines

Azatadine Maleate Rx

tablets: 1 mg	Optimine

Brompheniramine Maleate Rx, otc

tablets: 4 mg	Bromamine (*Rx*), Bromphen (*Rx*), Dimetane (*otc*), Veltane (*Rx*), *Generic* (*Rx*)
tablets, timed release: 8 mg, 12 mg	Dimetane Extentabs (*otc*), *Generic* (*Rx*)
elixir: 2 mg/5 ml	Dimetane (*otc*), *Generic* (*Rx*)
injection: 10 mg/ml	Dimetane-Ten (*Rx*), *Generic* (*Rx*)

Carbinoxamine Maleate Rx

tablets: 4 mg	Clistin

Chlorpheniramine Maleate Rx, otc

tablets, chewable: 2 mg	Chlo-Amine (*otc*)
tablets: 4 mg	Alermine (*Rx*), Aller-Chlor (*otc*), Chlor-Niramine (*otc*), Chlortab 4 (*Rx*), Chlor-Trimeton (*otc*), Hal-Chlor (*Rx*), Histrey (*otc*), Phenetron (*Rx*), Trymegen (*Rx*), *Generic* (*Rx*)
tablets, timed release: 8 mg	Aller-Chlor (*otc*), Chlortab-8 (*Rx*), Chlor-Trimeton Repetabs (*otc*), Phenetron (*Rx*), *Generic* (*Rx*)
capsules, timed release: 8 mg	Aller-Chlor (*otc*), Allerid-O.D.-8 (*Rx*), Phenetron Lanacaps (*Rx*), T.D. Alermine (*Rx*), Teldrin (*otc*), *Generic* (*Rx*)
tablets, timed release: 12 mg	Aller-Chlor (*otc*), Chlor-Trimeton Repetabs (*otc*), Phenetron (*Rx*), *Generic* (*Rx*)
capsules, timed release: 12 mg	Aller-Chlor (*otc*), Allerid-O.D.-12 (*Rx*), Chlorspan 12 (*Rx*), Phenetron Lanacaps (*Rx*), T.D. Alermine (*Rx*), Teldrin (*otc*), *Generic* (*Rx*)
syrup: 2 mg/5 ml	Chlor-Mal (*Rx*), Chlor-Trimeton (*otc*), Phenetron (*Rx*), *Generic* (*Rx*)
injection: 10 mg/ml	Chlor-Pro (*Rx*), Chlor-Trimeton (*Rx*), *Generic* (*Rx*)
injection: 20 mg/ml	*Generic* (*Rx*)

Clemastine Fumarate Rx

tablets: 1.34 mg (equivalent to 1-mg clemastine base)	Tavist-1
tablets: 2.68 mg (equivalent to 2-mg clemastine base)	Tavist

Cyproheptadine Hydrochloride Rx

tablets: 4 mg	Periactin, *Generic*
syrup: 2 mg/5 ml	Periactin, *Generic*

Dexchlorpheniramine Maleate Rx

tablets: 2 mg	Polaramine
repetabs (repeat-action tablets): 4 mg, 6 mg	Polaramine
syrup: 2 mg/5 ml	Polaramine

Diphenhydramine Hydrochloride Rx, otc

capsules: 25 mg	Benadryl, Bendylate, Fenylhist, Nordryl, *Generic*
capsules: 50 mg	Benadryl Kapseals, Bendylate, Fenylhist, Nordryl, *Generic*
tablets: 50 mg	Valdrene
elixir: 12.5 mg/5 ml	Benadryl, Diahist, Noradryl, Phen-Amin, *Generic*
syrup: 12.5 mg/5 ml	Benylin Cough (*otc*), Diphen Cough, Noradryl Cough, *Generic*
syrup: 13.3 mg/5 ml	Valdrene (*otc*)
injection: 10 mg/ml	Bena-D 10, Benadryl, Benahist 10, Bendylate, Benoject-10, Nordryl, *Generic*
injection: 50 mg/ml	Bena-D 50, Benadryl, Benahist 50, Bendylate, Benoject-50, Dihydrex, Hyrexin-50, Nordryl, Wehdryl-50, *Generic*

Diphenylpyraline Hydrochloride Rx

capsules, timed release: 5 mg	Hispril Spansules

Methdilazine Hydrochloride Rx

tablets, chewable: 4 mg	Tacaryl
tablets: 8 mg	Tacaryl
syrup: 4 mg/5 ml	Tacaryl

Phenindamine Tartrate otc

tablets: 25 mg	Nolahist

Promethazine Hydrochloride Rx

tablets: 12.5 mg, 25 mg	Phenergan, *Generic*
tablets: 50 mg	Phenergan, Remsed, *Generic*
syrup: 6.25 mg/5 ml	Phenergan, *Generic*
syrup fortis: 25 mg/ml	Phenergan, *Generic*
suppositories: 12.5 mg	Phenergan
suppositories: 25 mg, 50 mg	Phenergan
injection: 25 mg/ml	Anergan 25, Phenazine 25, Phenergan, Prometh 25, Prorex, Prothazine, Provigan, V-Gan-25, Zipan-25, *Generic*
injection: 50 mg/ml	Anergan 50, Ganphen, K-Phen, Pentazine, Phenazine 50, Phencen-50, Phenergan, Phenoject-50, Prometh 50, Prorex, Prothazine, Provigan, V-Gan-50, Zipan-50, *Generic*

Pyrilamine Maleate otc

tablets: 25 mg	*Generic*

Trimeprazine Rx

tablets: 2.5 mg	Temaril
spansules (sustained release capsules): 5 mg	Temaril
syrup: 2.5 mg/5 mg	Temaril

Tripelennamine Hydrochloride Rx

tablets: 25 mg	PBZ
tablets: 50 mg	PBZ, *Generic*
tablets, sustained release: 100 mg	PBZ-SR
elixir: 37.5 mg tripelennamine citrate (equivalent to 25 mg tripelennamine HCl)/5 ml	PBZ

Triprolidine Hydrochloride Rx

tablets: 2.5 mg	Actidil
syrup: 1.25 mg/5 ml	Actidil, *Generic*

INDICATIONS

Oral: Symptomatic relief of symptoms associated with perennial and seasonal allergic rhinitis, vasomotor rhinitis, allergic conjunctivitis, mild uncomplicated urticaria and angioedema, and dermatographism; amelioration of allergic reactions to blood or plasma; adjunctive therapy in anaphylactic reactions.

Parenteral: Amelioration of allergic reactions to blood or plasma; in anaphylaxis as an adjunct to epinephrine and other measures; uncomplicated allergic conditions of the immediate type when oral therapy is not possible.

Cyproheptadine Hydrochloride, Diphenhydramine Hydrochloride, and *Promethazine Hydrochloride* have additional indications, as follows.

CYPROHEPTADINE HYDROCHLORIDE

In addition to uses listed above, this drug is also indicated for cold urticaria. *Investigational uses:* Drug has antihistaminic, antichlolinergic, antiserotonin, and appetite-stimulating properties. Dose of 4 mg tid has been used with variable success to stimulate appetite in underweight patients and in those with anorexia nervosa. Also has been used in doses of 4 mg tid or qid to treat vascular cluster headaches.

DIPHENHYDRAMINE HYDROCHLORIDE

In addition to uses given above, this drug is also used for active and prophylactic treatment of motion sickness (see Antiemetic/Antivertigo Agents) and for parkinsonism (see Anticholinergic Antiparkinsonism Agents). Diphenhydramine also has significant antitussive activity and is indicated as a nonnarcotic cough suppressant for the control of cough due to colds or allergy; only the syrup formulations are specifically labeled for this indication.

PROMETHAZINE HYDROCHLORIDE

Oral: In addition to general uses listed above, promethazine is also indicated for active and prophylactic treatment of motion sickness; preoperative, postoperative, or obstetric sedation; prevention and control of nausea and vomiting associated with certain types of anesthesia and surgery; as an adjunct to analgesics for control of postoperative pain; for sedation and relief of apprehension and to produce light sleep from which the patient can be easily aroused; as an antiemetic for postoperative patients (see Antiemetic/Antivertigo Agents).

Parenteral: Same as oral route. Intravenous administration may be used as an adjunct to anesthesia and analgesia in special surgical situations, such as repeated bronchoscopy, ophthalmic surgery, and poor-risk patients, with reduced amounts of meperidine or other narcotic analgesics.

CONTRAINDICATIONS

Hypersensitivity. Do not use in newborn or premature infants. Contraindicated in patients on monoamine oxidase (MAO) therapy.

Antihistamines should be avoided or used with caution in patients with the following: narrow-angle glaucoma, stenosing peptic ulcer, symptomatic protastic hypertrophy, asthmatic attack, bladder-neck obstruction, pyloroduodenal obstruction. Antihistamines may be excreted in breast milk. Owing to higher risk of adverse effects of antihistamines for infants generally and newborns and prematures in particular, antihistamines are contraindicated in nursing mothers. An inhibitory effect on lactation may also occur.

The **phenothiazine** antihistamines (see *Actions*) are contraindicated in comatose patients; in states of CNS depression from agents such as barbiturates, alcohol, narcotics, analgesics; in patients who have previously developed phenothiazine idiosyncrasy, jaundice, bone-marrow depression, hypersensitivity, or severe allergic reactions to these or other phenothiazines; and in acutely ill or debilitated children (there is greater susceptibility to dystonias). In patients who have previously developed phenothiazine-induced jaundice, phenothiazine antihistamines should be used only if essential for the patient's welfare.

ACTIONS

Antihistamines act by competitive antagonism of histamine at the H_1 histamine receptor. They do not block the release of histamine. They antagonize in varying degrees most, but not all, of the pharmacologic effects of histamine. Cyproheptadine and azatadine have also demonstrated antiserotonin activity. Antihistamines also have anticholinergic (drying), antipruritic, and sedative effects. Additionally, certain antihistamines have antiemetic effects and are useful in the management of nausea, vomiting, vertigo, and motion sickness.

Most antihistamines are metabolized by the liver. With few exceptions they are well absorbed after oral administration and have an onset of action within 30 to 60 minutes and a duration of 4 to 6 hours. The chemical classifications of the antihistamines are listed below.

Alkylamines: Brompheniramine, chlorpheniramine, dexchlorpheniramine, triprolidine.

Ethanolamines: Carbinoxamine, clemastine, diphenhydramine.

Ethylenediamines: Pyrilamine, tripelennamine.

Phenothiazines: Methdilazine, promethazine, trimeprazine.

Miscellaneous: Azatadine, cyproheptadine, diphenylpyraline.

WARNINGS

Hypersensitivity reactions including anaphylactic shock are more likely to occur following parenteral than oral administration.

Use in lower-respiratory-tract infections: Should not be used to treat lower-respiratory-tract infections including asthma because anticholinergic (drying) effects may cause thickening of secretions and impair expectoration.

Use in upper-respiratory-tract infections: Useful in allergic conditions affecting the upper respiratory tract, but drying effects may cause thickening of secretions and impair expectoration.

Use in elderly: Antihistamines are more likely to cause dizziness, sedation, syncope, toxic confusional states, and hypotension in elderly patients. Phenothiazine side-effects (extrapyramidal signs, especially parkinsonism; akathisia; persistent dyskinesia) are more prone to develop in this age group.

Use in pregnancy: Safety not established. Use only when clearly needed and when potential benefits outweigh the unknown potential hazards to the fetus. There are reports of jaundice and extrapyramidal symptoms in infants whose mothers received phenothiazines during pregnancy.

Use in children: In infants and children especially, antihistamine overdosage may cause hallucinations, convulsions, and death. Antihistamines may diminish mental alertness in children (young children particularly) and produce paradoxical excitation. Use *Phenothiazines* with caution in children with history of sleep apnea, a family history of sudden infant death syndrome (SIDS), or signs of Reye's syndrome.

PRECAUTIONS

May cause drowsiness. Antihistamines have atropine-like actions; use with caution in patients with predisposition to urinary retention, history of bronchial asthma, increased intravascular pressure, hyperthyroidism, cardiovascular disease, or hypertension. These drugs may thicken mucous secretions and inhibit expectoration and sinus drainage.

Tartrazine sensitivity: Some of these products contain tartrazine (Appendix 6, section 6-23).

Phenothiazine antihistamines: Should be used with caution in patients with cardiovascular disease, impairment of liver function, or history of ulcer disease. Use cautiously in persons with acute or chronic respiratory impairment, particularly children, because phenothiazines may suppress the cough reflex. If hypotension occurs, epinephrine is not recommended because phenothiazines may reverse its usual pressor effect and paradoxically cause a further lowering of blood pressure. Because these drugs have antiemetic action, they may obscure signs of intestinal obstruction, brain tumor, or overdosage of toxic drugs. Phenothiazines elevate prolactin levels; this elevation persists through chronic administration. This is of potential importance if drug is prescribed for a patient with previously detected breast cancer, because it is believed that some breast cancers may be prolactin dependent. Galactorrhea, amenorrhea, gynecomastia, and impotence have been reported; the clinical significance of elevated prolactin levels is unknown for most patients.

Others: Antihistamines should be used cautiously in patients with glucose-6-phosphate dehydrogenase deficiency; these drugs may induce hemolysis in such patients in the presence of infection or stress.

DRUG INTERACTIONS

Antihistamines may have additive depressant effects with **alcohol** and other **CNS depressants** (*e.g.,* hypnotics, sedatives, tranquilizers, antianxiety agents, depressant analgesics). Dosage adjustment of CNS depressants may be necessary.

The effects of **epinephrine** may be enhanced by certain antihistamines (*e.g.,* diphenhydramine, tripelennamine, or d-chlorpheniramine). MAO inhibitors may prolong and intensify the anticholinergic (drying) effects of antihistamines. See Antipsychotic Agents for complete discussion of **phenothiazine** drug interactions.

ADVERSE REACTIONS

General: Urticaria; drug rash; anaphylactic shock; photosensitivity; excessive perspiration; chills; dryness of mouth, nose, and throat.

Cardiovascular: Hypotension, headache, palpitations, tachycardia, extrasystoles.

Hematologic: Hemolytic anemia, thrombocytopenia, leukopenia, agranulocytosis, pancytopenia.

CNS: Most frequent—drowsiness, sedation, dizziness, disturbed coordination. *Other*—fatigue, confusion, restlessness, excitation, nervousness, tremor, irritability, insomnia, euphoria, paresthesias, blurred vision, diplopia, vertigo, tinnitus, acute labyrinthitis,

hysteria, neuritis, convulsions; paradoxical excitation, insomnia, euphoria, delusions (especially in children and the elderly).

GI: Most frequent—epigastric distress. *Other*—anorexia, increased appetite and weight gain, nausea, vomiting, diarrhea, constipation.

GU: Urinary frequency, difficulty in urinating, urinary retention, early menses, decreased libido, impotence.

Respiratory: Most frequent—thickening of bronchial secretions. *Other*—tightness of chest and wheezing, nasal congestion. Respiratory depression has been reported.

Phenothiazine Antihistamines infrequently cause typical phenothiazine adverse effects. See Antipsychotic Agents for discussion of phenothiazine adverse reactions. **Diphenhydramine** and **chlorpheniramine** have been reported to cause tingling, heaviness, and weakness of the hands.

OVERDOSAGE

Symptoms: May vary from CNS depression to stimulation, especially in children. Hallucinations have been reported following excessive tripelennamine dosage. Atropinelike signs and symptoms (*e.g.,* dry mouth, fixed dilated pupils, flushing), as well as GI symptoms, may occur. Marked cerebral irritation resulting in jerking of muscles and possible convulsions may be followed by deep stupor. Acute oral and facial dystonic reactions have been reported.

Treatment: If vomiting has not occurred spontaneously, induce emesis, except with *Phenothiazine Antihistamines* (see separate discussion, below). Syrup of ipecac is preferred. Precautions against aspiration must be taken, especially in infants and children. Following emesis, any drug remaining in the stomach may be absorbed by activated charcoal administered as a slurry with water. If vomiting is unsuccessful, gastric lavage is indicated within 3 hours after ingestion and even later if large amounts of milk or cream were given. Isotonic or 0.45% Sodium Chloride Solution is the lavage solution of choice. Saline laxatives such as milk of magnesia draw water into the bowel and are valuable for rapid dilution of bowel content. In the unconscious patient, secure the airway with cuffed endotracheal tube before emptying gastric contents. If breathing is significantly impaired, maintenance of an adequate airway and mechanical support of respiration are the safest and most effective means of providing oxygenation and preventing hypoxia (especially to the brain during convulsions).

Hypotension is early sign of impending cardiovascular collapse and is treated vigorously with IV infusion of a vasopressor (*e.g.,* dopamine) to maintain adequate blood pressure. Do not treat CNS depression with analeptics, which may precipitate convulsions; convulsions should be controlled by careful use of a short-acting barbiturate. Do not use CNS stimulants. Ice packs and cooling sponge baths can aid in reducing the fever commonly seen in children with antihistamine overdosage.

Management of phenothiazine overdosage: Early gastric lavage is helpful; treatment is essentially symptomatic and supportive. Keep patient under observation. Maintain open airway because involvement of extrapyramidal mechanism may produce dysphagia and respiratory difficulty in severe overdosage. Do *not* induce emesis, because a dystonic reaction of the head and neck may develop and result in aspiration of vomitus. Extrapyramidal symptoms may be treated with antiparkinsonism drugs, barbiturates, or diphenhydramine. Avoid analeptics, which may cause convulsions. If hypotension occurs, initiate standard measures for managing circulatory shock. If a vasopressor is needed, dopamine or norepinephrine is recommended. Other pressor agents, specifically epinephrine, are not recommended because phenothiazine derivatives may block the elevating action of these agents and paradoxically cause a further lowering of blood pressure.

DOSAGE

AZATADINE MALEATE
Individualized to needs of patient.
   Adults: 1 mg or 2 mg bid.
   Not for use in children under 12.

BROMPHENIRAMINE MALEATE
   Oral: *Adults (12 and older)*—4 mg q4h to q6h or 8 mg to 12 mg of sustained-release form q8h to q12h, not to exceed 24 mg/24 hours.
   Children—6 to 12 years, 2 mg q4h to q6h or 8 mg to 12 mg of sustained-release form q12h; 2 to 6 years, 1 mg q4h to q6h, not to exceed 6 mg/24 hours.
   Parenteral: See *Administration,* below.
   Adults—Usual dose is 10 mg; range is 5 mg to 20 mg. The period of protection is 3 to 12 hours; twice-daily administration is usually sufficient. Maximum recommended dose is 40 mg/24 hours.
   Children (under 12)—0.5 mg/kg/day or 15 mg/m²/day, divided into 3 or 4 doses.

CARBINOXAMINE MALEATE
Well tolerated in doses as high as 24 mg/day, in divided doses over prolonged periods. Some patients respond to as little as 4 mg/day.
   Adults: 4 mg to 8 mg tid or qid.
   Children: Approximately 0.2 mg to 0.4 mg/kg/day; *over 6 years*—4 mg to 6 mg tid or qid; *3 to 6*

years—2 mg to 4 mg tid or qid; *1 to 3 years*—2 mg tid or qid (**Note:** 4-mg tablets are scored).

CHLORPHENIRAMINE MALEATE
   Tablets or syrup: *Adults, children over 12*—4 mg, 3 to 6 times/day (for some patients 2 mg may be adequate); do not exceed 24 mg/24 hours. *Children (6–12)*—2 mg, 3 to 6 times/day; do not exceed 12 mg/24 hours. *Children under 6*—consult physician.
   Sustained release: *Adults (12 years and older)*—8 mg to 12 mg H.S. or q8h to q12h during the day.
   Not recommended for children under 12.
   Parenteral: See *Administration,* below.
   Allergic reactions to blood or plasma—10 mg to 20 mg as a single dose; maximum recommended dose is 40 mg/24 hours. *Anaphylaxis*—10 mg to 20 mg IV as single dose. *Uncomplicated allergic conditions*—5 mg to 20 mg as a single dose.

CLEMASTINE FUMARATE
Individualized according to needs and response of patient. *Adults, children over 12*—1.34 mg bid to 2.68 mg tid. Do not exceed 8.04 mg/day. For dermatologic conditions, only 2.68-mg dosage level is used. *Children under 12*—Safety, efficacy not established.

CYPROHEPTADINE HYDROCHLORIDE
Adults—Total daily dose should not exceed 0.5 mg/kg (0.23 mg/lb). Therapeutic range is 4 mg to 20 mg/day, with majority of patients requiring 12 mg to 16 mg/day. An occasional patient may require as much as 32 mg/day. Therapy is initiated with 4 mg tid and adjusted according to size and response of patient.
   Children—Total daily dosage may be calculated as approximately 0.25 mg/kg (0.11 mg/lb) or 8 mg/m². *Usual dose for children 2–6*—2 mg bid or tid; do not exceed 12 mg/day. *Usual dose for children 7–14*—4 mg bid or tid; do not exceed 16 mg/day.

DEXCHLORPHENIRAMINE MALEATE
Adults—2 mg q4h to q6h or 4 mg to 6 mg repeat-action tablets q8h to q10h. *Children (6–12)*—½ adult dose q4h to q6h or a 4-mg repeat-action tablet once daily at H.S. *Children (2–5)*—¼ adult dose q4h to q6h; do not use repeat-action form.

DIPHENHYDRAMINE HYDROCHLORIDE
   Oral: The basis for determining the most effective dose regimen is patient response and the condition under treatment. *Adults*—25 mg to 50 mg tid or qid.
   Children (over 10 kg)—12.5 mg to 25 mg tid or qid, or 5 mg/kg/day, or 150 mg/m²/day. Maximum daily dosage: 300 mg.
   Parenteral (IV or deep IM): *Adults*—10 mg to

50 mg; 100 mg if required. Maximum daily dosage is 400 mg.

Children—5 mg/kg/day or 150 mg/m²/day. Maximum daily dose: 300 mg divided into 4 doses.

For motion sickness, see p 109; for parkinsonism see p 76.

DIPHENYLPYRALINE HYDROCHLORIDE

Individualized to response and needs of patient.

Adults—5 mg q12h.

Children (6–12)—5 mg daily. Not recommended for children under 6.

METHDILAZINE HYDROCHLORIDE

Adults—8 mg, 2 to 4 times/day. _Children (over 3)_— 4 mg, 2 to 4 times/day.

PHENINDAMINE TARTRATE

Adults—25 mg q4h to q6h. Do not exceed 150 mg in 24 hours. _Children (6–12)_—12.5 mg q4h to q6h. Do not exceed 75 mg in 24 hours. _Children under 6_—As directed by physician.

PROMETHAZINE HYDROCHLORIDE

Oral

Allergy: Average dose is 25 mg H.S. or 12.5 mg A.C. and H.S. if necessary. _Children_—25 mg H.S. or 6.25 mg to 12.5 mg tid. When oral route is not feasible, suppositories in 25-mg doses may be used. Dose may be repeated in 2 hours if necessary. Promethazine in 25-mg doses will control minor transfusion reactions of an allergic nature.

Motion sickness, nausea, vomiting: See Antiemetic/Antivertigo Agents.

Sedation: _Adults_—25 mg to 50 mg. _Children_—12.5 mg to 25 mg, orally or rectally.

Preoperative use: _Adults_—50 mg. _Children_—12.5 mg to 25 mg, given night before surgery.

FOR PREOPERATIVE MEDICATION: Children, 0.5 mg/lb (1 mg/kg) in combination with an equal dose of meperidine and the appropriate dose of an atropinelike drug. Suppositories (25 mg in children up to 3 years, 50 mg in older children) may be used instead of oral or parenteral medication. Adults, 50 mg with an equal amount of meperidine and the required amount of belladonna alkaloid.

Postoperative sedation and adjunctive use with analgesics: 12.5 mg to 25 mg in children, 25 mg to 50 mg in adults.

Parenteral

See _Administration,_ below.

Adults

ALLERGY: Average dose is 25 mg IM or IV; repeat in 2 hours if necessary. Average adult dose for relief of allergic reactions to blood or plasma is 25 mg.

NAUSEA, VOMITING: See Antiemetic/Antivertigo Agents.

NIGHTTIME SEDATION: 25 mg to 50 mg.

PREOPERATIVE AND POSTOPERATIVE USE: 25 mg to 50 mg may be combined with appropriately reduced dosages of analgesics and anticholinergic drugs. Reduce dosage of concomitant analgesic or hypnotic accordingly.

OBSTETRICS: 50 mg in early stages of labor. When labor is definitely established, 25 mg to 75 mg IM or IV with appropriately reduced dose of any narcotic. Amnesic agents may be administered as needed. If necessary, 25-mg to 50-mg doses with a reduced dose of analgesic may be repeated once or twice at 4-hour intervals in the course of normal labor. Maximum total dose of 100 mg may be administered during 24-hour period to patients in labor.

Children (under 12): Dosage should not exceed half that of the suggested adult dose. As an adjunct to premedication, the suggested dose is 0.5 mg/lb (1 mg/kg) in combination with a narcotic or barbiturate and the appropriate dose of an anticholinergic drug. Antiemetics should not be used in vomiting of unknown etiology in children.

PYRILAMINE MALEATE

Adults—25 mg to 50 mg tid or qid. _Children (6 years and older)_—12.5 mg to 25 mg tid or qid.

TRIMEPRAZINE

Some side-effects appear to be dose related; lowest effective dose should be used.

Tablets, syrup: Adults—Usual dose is 2.5 mg qid. _Children (over 3)_—2.5 mg at H.S. or tid. _Children (6 months–3 years)_—1.25 mg at H.S. or tid if needed.

Sustained-release capsules: _Adults_—5 mg q12h. _Children (over 6)_—5 mg/day. _Children (6 and under)_—use tablets or syrup.

TRIPELENNAMINE HYDROCHLORIDE

Tablets, elixir: Adults—Usual dose is 25 mg to 50 mg q4h to q6h, but as little as 25 mg may control symptoms; as much as 600 mg/day may be given in divided doses. _Children, infants_—5 mg/kg/day or 150 mg/m²/day divided into 4 to 6 doses. Maximum total dose is 300 mg/day.

Long-acting, sustained-release forms: _Adults_—100 mg in the morning and evening; in difficult cases, 100 mg q8h may be required. _Children (over 5)_—50 mg in the morning and evening is usually sufficient; some may require 50 mg q8h. The 100-mg sustained-release form should not be used in children.

TRIPROLIDINE HYDROCHLORIDE
Adults—2.5 mg tid or qid. *Children*—6 to 12 years, ½ adult dose tid or qid; 4 to 6 years, 0.9 mg (syrup only) tid or qid; 2 to 4 years, 0.6 mg (syrup only) tid or qid; 4 months to 2 years, 0.3 mg (syrup only) tid or qid.

NURSING IMPLICATIONS

HISTORY
See Appendix 4.

PHYSICAL ASSESSMENT (will depend on reason for use)
For symptoms of allergy, assess involved areas (*e.g.*, eyes, skin, upper or lower respiratory tract). For parkinsonism see p 79; for nausea, vomiting, and vertigo see p 113. If promethazine is used with narcotic analgesic, obtain blood pressure, pulse, and respiratory rate; see also Narcotic Analgesics. If cyproheptadine is used as an appetite stimulant, weigh patient.

ADMINISTRATION
Oral form: Administer with food to prevent GI upset.
IM route: Give deep IM; alternate injection sites.
Suppositories: Insert beyond rectal sphincter; check patient in ½ hour to be sure suppository has been retained.
Amelioration of allergic reactions to blood or plasma: Monitor patient q15m to q30m following drug administration. If symptoms are not relieved or become worse, contact physician immediately. Follow hospital policy for blood transfusion, plasma reactions.

BROMPHENIRAMINE, PARENTERAL
May be administered without dilution IM or subcutaneously. May be administered IV either undiluted or diluted 1 to 10 with Sterile Saline for Injection. If given IV, drug is given slowly, preferably with the patient in a recumbent position. If desired, add to normal saline, 5% glucose, or whole blood for IV administration.

CHLORPHENIRAMINE, PARENTERAL
The 10-mg/ml injection is intended for IV, IM, and subcutaneous administration. The 20-mg/ml and 100-mg/ml injections are intended for IM or subcutaneous use *only*. Intradermal administration is not recommended.

PROMETHAZINE, PARENTERAL
Preferred route is deep IM injection. IV administration is well tolerated but not without hazard. Subcutaneous injection is contraindicated because it may result in tissue necrosis. Under no circumstances should this be given by intra-arterial injection, owing to the likelihood of severe angiospasm and possibility of resultant gangrene. Administer IV in a concentration no greater than 25 mg/ml and at a rate not to exceed 25 mg/minute. When given concomitantly with promethazine, dose of barbiturates should be reduced by at least one-half and the dose of narcotics (*e.g.*, morphine, meperidine) reduced by one-fourth to one-half. Injection available as 50 mg/ml is for IM use *only*.

GENERIC NAME SIMILARITY
Diphenhydramine, diphenylpyraline, dimenhydrinate.

TRADE NAME SIMILARITY
Benadryl and Bendylate (both diphenhydramine); Nordryl and Noradryl (both diphenhydramine); Valdrene (diphenhydramine) and Veltane (brompheniramine).

ONGOING ASSESSMENT AND NURSING MANAGEMENT
Record vital signs daily. Monitor blood pressure of elderly or those with known cardiovascular disease q4h to q8h because these patients are more likely to develop hypotensive episodes.

Assess response to therapy; notify physician if nausea, vomiting, vertigo, or symptoms of allergy are not relieved.

When used to ameliorate allergic reactions to blood or plasma, continue to observe patient for 24 hours or as ordered.

Antihistamines may thicken mucous secretions and inhibit expectoration and sinus drainage. Contact physician if patient complains of a headache (which may be due to inhibition of sinus drainage), experiences difficulty raising secretions, or has an elevated temperature.

Dry mouth may be relieved by sips of water, hard candy, gum. Contact physician if dry mouth is severe or not relieved by ordinary measures.

If drowsiness is severe, patient (especially the elderly) may require assistance with ambulation.

Observe infant, child for paradoxical excitement, other mental changes (see *Warnings*). Withhold next dose and contact physician if CNS changes occur.

Treatment of nausea, vomiting, vertigo: See Antiemetic/Antivertigo Agents. Contact physician if nausea or vomiting persists.

Treatment of parkinsonism: See Anticholinergic Antiparkinsonism Agents.

Cyproheptadine used as appetite stimulant: Weigh patient 1 to 2 times/week or as ordered; check daily food intake. Physician may request dietitian to record approximate daily caloric intake.

PATIENT AND FAMILY INFORMATION

May cause drowsiness or dizziness; observe caution while driving or performing other tasks requiring alertness.

Avoid alcohol, other CNS depressants (*e.g.,* sedatives, hypnotics, tranquilizers); check with physician regarding use of nonprescription drugs (especially cold, cough, and hay-fever preparations).

May cause dry mouth, which may be relieved by sips of water, hard candy, or gum.

May cause GI upset; take with food or meals.

If condition is not relieved, contact physician.

Anti-inhibitor Coagulant Complex Rx

dried form with maximum of 2 units heparin/ml reconstituted material; diluent supplied	Autoplex
freeze-dried anti-inhibitor coagulant complex; heparin free; diluent supplied	Feiba Immuno

INDICATIONS

For use in patients with Factor VIII inhibitors (see Antihemophilic Factor) who are bleeding or are to undergo surgery.

CONTRAINDICATIONS

Signs of fibrinolysis; disseminated intravascular coagulation (DIC).

ACTIONS

Product is prepared from pooled human plasma and contains, in concentrated form, variable amounts of activated and precursor clotting factors. Factors of the kinin generating system are also present. The product is standardized by its ability to correct the clotting time of hemophilic plasma, or hemophilic plasma that contains inhibitors to Factor VIII.

WARNINGS

Product prepared from large pools of human plasma; such plasma may contain the causative agent of viral hepatitis or acquired immune deficiency syndrome (AIDS). Although each unit of source plasma used in preparation of this product has been found to be nonreactive for hepatitis B surface antigen, the concentrate has not been subjected to any treatment known to diminish the risk of transmission of hepatitis and therefore should be used only when its expected effect outweighs the hepatitis and AIDS risks associated with its use.

PRECAUTIONS

If signs of DIC occur, the infusion should be stopped promptly and the patient monitored for DIC by appropriate laboratory tests. Identification of the clotting deficiency as that caused by the presence of Factor VIII inhibitors is essential before initiating administration of this drug. Special precaution and consideration should be given to use in newborns, in whom a higher morbidity and mortality may be associated with hepatitis, and in patients with preexisting liver disease.

ADVERSE REACTIONS

Reactions manifested by fever and chills, changes in blood pressure (vasoactive reactions), or indications of protein sensitivity may be seen. It is advisable that appropriate medications be available for treatment of acute allergic or vasoreactive reactions. A rapid infusion rate may cause headache, flushing, and changes in pulse rate and blood pressure. In such instances, stopping the infusion allows symptoms to disappear promptly. With all but the most reactive individuals, infusion may be resumed at a slower rate.

DOSAGE

See also *Administration.*

Administer IV only. Recommended dosage range is 25 to 100 Factor VIII correctional units/kg, depending on the severity of hemorrhage. If no hemostatic improvement is observed approximately 6 hours after administration, dosage may be repeated.

NURSING IMPLICATIONS

HISTORY AND PHYSICAL ASSESSMENT

See Antihemophilic Factor.

ADMINISTRATION

Administer IV only. Use Y-tubing or tubing with secondary port because infusion may need to be stopped.

Anti-inhibitor coagulant complex may be infused at rates as high as 10 ml/minute. (Physician prescribes rate of administration.) If headache, flushing, or changes in pulse rate or blood pressure appear, the infusion rate should be decreased. In such instances, it is advisable to stop the infusion initially until symptoms disappear, then reinitiate infusion at a rate of approximately 2 ml/minute. Physician should order IV solution to infuse to keep vein open (KVO) should infusion be temporarily discontinued.

It is advisable that appropriate medications be available for the treatment of acute allergic or vasoactive reactions. Discuss this potential problem with the physician and obtain recommended drugs.

Laboratory tests: Hemostatic improvement may occur without a reduction of partial thromboplastin time (PTT); however, the prothrombin time would be expected to be shortened. The prothrombin time should be monitored in all patients treated with this product. The postinfusion prothrombin time should be no less than two-thirds of the preinfusion value if the patient is to receive subsequent infusions. In children, fibrinogen levels should be determined prior to the initial infusion and monitored during the course of treatment.

Storage: Unreconstituted complex is stored under refrigeration (2°C–8°C). Avoid freezing.

ONGOING ASSESSMENTS AND NURSING MANAGEMENT

Monitor blood pressure, pulse, respirations, infusion rate (drops/minute) q15m or as ordered during infusion of drug.

Notify physician immediately if prescribed administration rate is slowed or stopped because of adverse reactions.

If infusion is stopped, switch to the prescribed IV solution and infuse at a rate to KVO.

Observe patient for signs of DIC (*e.g.,* chest pain; cough; changes in blood pressure, pulse rate). If these occur, stop drug infusion immediately, infuse prescribed IV solution at a rate to KVO, and notify physician. Laboratory indications of DIC include prolonged thrombin time, prothrombin time, and PTT. Other indications are decreased fibrinogen concentration, decreased platelet count, and the presence of fibrin split products.

In addition, see *Ongoing Assessments and Nursing Management* and *Patient and Family*

Information discussions under Antihemophilic Factor.

Antipsychotic Agents*

Acetophenazine Maleate Rx

| tablets: 20 mg | Tindal |

Chlorpromazine Hydrochloride Rx

tablets: 10 mg	Promapar, Thorazine, Thor-Prom, *Generic*
tablets: 25 mg, 50 mg, 100 mg, 200 mg	Promapar, Thorazine, Thor-Prom, *Generic*
capsules, timed release: 30 mg, 75 mg, 150 mg, 200 mg, 300 mg	Thorazine Spansules
syrup: 10 mg/5 ml	Thorazine
concentrate: 30 mg/ml	Thorazine, *Generic*
concentrate: 100 mg/ml	Thorazine, *Generic*
suppositories: 25 mg, 100 mg	Thorazine
injection: 25 mg/ml	BayClor, Clorazine, Ormazine, Promaz, Thorazine, *Generic*

Chlorprothixene Rx

tablets: 10 mg, 25 mg, 50 mg, 100 mg	Taractan
concentrate: 100 mg/ 5 ml	Taractan
injection: 12.5 mg/ml	Taractan

Fluphenazine Enanthate and Decanoate Rx

| injection: 25 mg/ml | Prolixin Enanthate, Prolixin Decanoate |

* The antipsychotic agents include the phenothiazines, the thioxanthenes, a butyrophenone, a dihydroindolone, and a dibenzoxazepine (see *Actions*). Although these are chemically distinct classes, pharmacologic and clinical effects are similar. The pharmacologic similarities between these agents suggest that all of this information should be considered when using any of these agents.

Fluphenazine Hydrochloride _Rx_

tablets: 0.25 mg	Permitil
tablets: 1 mg	Prolixin (contains tartrazine)
tablets: 2.5 mg, 5 mg, 10 mg	Permitil, Prolixin (contains tartrazine)
concentrate: 5 mg/ml	Permitil
elixir: 2.5 mg/5 ml	Prolixin
injection: 2.5 mg/ml	Prolixin

Haloperidol _Rx_

tablets: 0.5 mg, 1 mg (contains tartrazine), 2 mg, 5 mg (contains tartrazine), 10 mg (contains tartrazine), 20 mg	Haldol
concentrate: 2 mg/ml	Haldol
injection: 5 mg/ml	Haldol

Loxapine _Rx_

capsules: 5 mg, 10 mg, 25 mg, 50 mg	Loxitane
concentrate: 25 mg/ml	Loxitane C
injection: 50 mg/ml	Loxitane IM

Mesoridazine _Rx_

tablets: 10 mg, 25 mg, 50 mg, 100 mg	Serentil
concentrate: 25 mg/ml	Serentil
injection: 25 mg/ml	Serentil

Molindone Hydrochloride _Rx_

tablets: 5 mg, 10 mg, 25 mg, 50 mg, 100 mg	Moban
concentrate: 20 mg/ml	Moban

Perphenazine _Rx_

tablets: 2 mg, 4 mg, 8 mg, 16 mg	Trilafon
repetabs (repeat-action tablets): 8 mg	Trilafon
concentrate: 16 mg/5 ml	Trilafon
injection: 5 mg/ml	Trilafon

Piperacetazine _Rx_

tablets: 10 mg, 25 mg (both contain tartrazine)	Quide

Prochlorperazine _Rx_

tablets: 5 mg, 10 mg, 25 mg	Compazine, _Generic_
sustained release capsules: 10 mg, 15 mg, 30 mg	Compazine Spansules
syrup: 5 mg/5 ml	Compazine, _Generic_
concentrate: 10 mg/ml	_Generic_
suppositories: 2.5 mg, 5 mg, 25 mg	Compazine
injection: 5 mg/ml	Compazine, _Generic_

Promazine Hydrochloride _Rx_

tablets: 10 mg, 25 mg, 50 mg, 100 mg	Sparine
syrup: 10 mg/5 ml	Sparine
concentrate: 30 mg/ml	Sparine
injection: 25 mg/ml, 50 mg/ml	Sparine, _Generic_

Thioridazine Hydrochloride _Rx_

tablets: 10 mg, 15 mg, 25 mg, 50 mg, 100 mg, 150 mg, 200 mg	Mellaril, Millazine, _Generic_
concentrate: 30 mg/ml, 100 mg/ml	Mellaril
suspension: 25 mg/5 ml, 100 mg/5 ml	Mellaril-S

Thiothixene _Rx_

capsules: 1 mg, 2 mg, 5 mg, 10 mg, 20 mg	Navane
concentrate: 5 mg/ml	Navane
injection: 2 mg/ml or powder for injection 5 mg/ml	Navane

Trifluoperazine _Rx_

tablets: 1 mg, 2 mg, 5 mg, 10 mg	Stelazine, Suprazine, _Generic_
concentrate: 10 mg/ml	Stelazine, _Generic_
injection: 2 mg/ml	Stelazine

Triflupromazine Hydrochloride Rx

suspension: 50 mg/   Vesprin
   5 ml
injection: 10 mg/ml,   Vesprin
   20 mg/ml

INDICATIONS

Management of psychotic disorders. In addition to use as antipsychotics, some of these agents are used as antiemetics. Specific indications for individual drugs are as follows:

ACETOPHENAZINE MALEATE

Management of manifestations of psychotic disorders.

CHLORPROMAZINE HYDROCHLORIDE

Management of manifestations of psychotic disorders; control of manifestations of the manic type of manic-depressive illness; relief of intractable hiccups; relief of restlessness and apprehension prior to surgery; adjunct in treatment of tetanus; treatment of acute intermittent porphyria. Also, in treatment of severe behavioral problems in children marked by combativeness or explosive hyperexcitable behavior (out of proportion to immediate provocations). Short-term treatment of hyperactive children who show excessive motor activity with accompanying conduct disorders consisting of some or all of the following: impulsiveness, difficulty sustaining attention, aggression, mood lability, poor frustration tolerance. Also indicated for control of nausea and vomiting.

CHLORPROTHIXENE

Management of manifestations of psychotic disorders.

FLUPHENAZINE ENANTHATE AND DECANOATE

Management of manifestations of schizophrenia.

FLUPHENAZINE HYDROCHLORIDE

Management of manifestations of psychotic disorders.

HALOPERIDOL

Management of manifestations of psychotic disorders; control of tic and vocal utterances of Gilles de la Tourette's syndrome. Effective in treatment of severe behavioral problems in children with combative, explosive hyperexcitability (which cannot be accounted for by immediate provocation). Also effective in short-term treatment of hyperactive children who show excessive motor activity with accompanying conduct disorders consisting of impulsiveness, difficulty sustaining attention, aggression, mood lability, and/or poor frustration tolerance.

LOXAPINE

Manifestations of schizophrenia.

MESORIDAZINE

Schizophrenia: Reduces severity of emotional withdrawal, conceptual disorganization, anxiety, tension, hallucinatory behavior, suspiciousness, blunted affect.

Behavioral problems in mental deficiency and chronic brain syndrome: Reduces hyperactivity and uncooperativeness.

Alcoholism (acute and chronic): Ameliorates anxiety, tension, depression, nausea, and vomiting without producing hepatic dysfunction or hindering functional recovery of the impaired liver.

Psychoneurotic manifestations: Reduces symptoms of anxiety and tension, reduces prevalent symptoms often associated with neurotic components of many disorders, and benefits personality disorders in general.

MOLINDOME HYDROCHLORIDE

Management of manifestations of schizophrenia.

PERPHENAZINE

Management of manifestations of psychotic disorders. Also indicated for control of severe nausea and vomiting in adults.

PIPERACETAZINE

Management of manifestations of psychotic disorders.

PROCHLORPERAZINE

Management of manifestations of psychotic disorders, management of psychoneurotic patients displaying primarily symptoms of moderate to severe anxiety and tension. Also indicated for control of severe nausea and vomiting.

PROMAZINE HYDROCHLORIDE

Management of manifestations of psychotic disorders.

THIORIDAZINE HYDROCHLORIDE

Management of manifestations of psychotic disorders and short-term treatment of moderate to marked depression with variable degrees of anxiety in adult patients. Also effective in treatment of multiple symptoms such as agitation, anxiety, depressed mood, tension, sleep disturbances, and fears in geriatric patients. Treatment of severe behavioral problems in children marked by combativeness or explosive behavior out of proportion to immediate provocations. Also short-term treatment of hyperactive children showing excessive motor activity with accompanying conduct disorders consisting of some or all of the following: impulsiveness, difficulty in sustaining attention, aggression, mood lability, poor frustration tolerance.

THIOTHIXENE

Management of manifestations of psychotic disorders.

TRIFLUOPERAZINE

Management of psychotic disorders. "Possibly effective" in controlling excessive anxiety, tension, and agitation as seen in neurosis or associated with somatic disorders.

TRIFLUPROMAZINE HYDROCHLORIDE

Management of manifestations of psychotic disorders (excluding psychotic depressive reactions).

CONTRAINDICATIONS

Comatose or greatly depressed states; hypersensitivity (cross-sensitivity between phenothiazines may occur); presence of large amounts of CNS depressants; bone-marrow depression; preexisting thrombocytopenia; other blood dyscrasias; subcortical brain damage; Parkinson's disease; hepatic damage; jaundice; renal insufficiency; cerebral arteriosclerosis; coronary disease; severe hypotension or hypertension; mitral insufficiency; pheochromocytoma.

ACTIONS

The exact mode of antipsychotic action is not fully understood. The antipsychotics block postsynaptic dopamine receptors in the cerebral cortex, basal ganglia, hypothalamus, limbic system, brain stem, and medulla. The effects produced on the neuronal cells by antipsychotic agents include inhibition or alteration of dopamine release, an increased neuronal cell firing rate in the midbrain, and an increased turnover rate of dopamine in the forebrain. These actions appear to be directly related to the ability of these agents to suppress clinical manifestations of schizophrenia.

The chemical classifications of the antipsychotic agents are as follows:

Phenothiazines—Acetophenazine maleate, chlorpromazine hydrochloride, fluphenazine hydrochloride, fluphenazine enanthate and decanoate, mesoridazine, perphenazine, piperacetazine, prochlorperazine, promazine hydrochloride, thioridazine hydrochloride, trifluoperazine, triflupromazine hydrochloride.

Thioxanthenes—Chlorprothixene, thiothixene.
Butyrophenone—Haloperidol.
Dihydroindolone—Molindone hydrochloride.
Dibenzoxazepine—Loxapine.

The phenothiazine derivatives are believed to depress various components of the reticular activating system, which is involved in the control of basal metabolism and body temperature, wakefulness, vasomotor tone, emesis, and hormonal balance. In addition, the drugs exert peripheral autonomic effects (anticholinergic, alpha-adrenergic blocking effects).

These drugs may be administered, PO, IM, or IV. Oral administration is preferred for maintenance therapy but absorption tends to be erratic and variable. Peak plasma levels are seen 2 to 4 hours after oral administration; IM administration provides 4 to 10 times more active drug than do oral doses.

These agents are widely distributed in tissues and are found in the CNS in concentrations that exceed those in plasma. They are highly bound to plasma proteins. Because these agents are highly lipophilic, the antipsychotic agents and their metabolites accumulate in the brain, lung, and other tissues with high blood supply. They are stored in these tissues and may be found in the urine for up to 6 months after the last dose. Antipsychotic agents undergo biotransformation in the liver. Enzyme inducers, such as barbiturates and meprobamate, may enhance phenothiazine metabolism. Half of the excretion of these agents occurs via the kidneys; the other half occurs through enterohepatic circulation. These agents have plasma elimination half-lives ranging from 10 to 20 hours.

There is little evidence of clinical differences in efficacy among these agents when used in equitherapeutic dosages, but a patient who has failed to respond to one agent may respond to another. The principal differences between these agents are the type and severity of side-effects that accompany therapy. The predominant side-effects that differ in incidence among agents are sedation, extrapyramidal effects, anticholinergic effects, antiadrenergic effects (orthostatic hypotension). Changing from one agent to another may minimize undesirable or intolerable side-effects.

Oral liquid formulations are most predictably absorbed; conventional tablet forms are preferred over controlled-release preparations, which may have erratic absorption. In chronic therapy, full clinical effects may not be achieved for 4 to 8 weeks. Approximately 4 to 7 days are required to achieve steady-state plasma levels; therefore, in chronic therapy dosage adjustments should not be made more frequently than every week. Divided daily dosages are recommended for initiation of therapy; once-daily dosing may be used during chronic therapy. Administration at H.S. may be preferred to minimize sedation and orthostatic hypotension.

WARNINGS

CNS: May impair mental or physical abilities, especially during the first few days of therapy. Drowsiness, most often seen with chlorpromazine and thioridazine, may occur during the first or second week of therapy, after which it generally disappears. Nonsedating agents include trifluoperazine, haloperidol, and thiothixene. Use cautiously in patients with depression. When used in agitated states accompanying depression, precaution is indicated (particularly the recognition of a suicidal tendency).

Pulmonary: Bronchopneumonia (some fatal). It has been postulated that lethargy and decreased sensation of thirst due to central inhibition may lead to dehydration, hemoconcentration, and reduced pulmonary ventilation. If these signs appear, especially in the elderly, remedial therapy is instituted. Use with caution in respiratory impairment due to acute pulmonary infections or chronic respiratory disorders (*e.g.,* severe asthma, emphysema).

Ophthalmic: Use with caution in those with a history of glaucoma. During prolonged high-dose therapy, ocular changes may occur and include pigment deposition in the cornea and lens, progressing in more severe cases to lenticular opacities; epithelial keratopathies; pigmentary retinopathy. Ophthalmologic (slit-lamp) evaluation is recommended to detect corneal, lenticular deposits.

Use in seizure disorders: Can lower the convulsive threshold and induce seizures in those with or without history of seizure disorders. Petit mal and grand mal seizures have been reported, particularly in those with EEG abnormalities or history of such disorders. These drugs may be used concomitantly with anticonvulsants.

Use in impaired hepatic function: Use with caution. Because of possibility of liver damage, periodic hepatic-function tests are recommended.

Use in elderly: It has been reported that age lowers tolerance to the phenothiazines. The most common neurologic side-effects are parkinsonism and akathisia. There appears to be an increased risk of agranulocytosis and leukopenia.

Use in pregnancy, lactation: Safety is not established. Give only when potential benefits outweigh possible hazards. Hyperreflexia, jaundice, and extrapyramidal signs have been reported in the newborn when these drugs have been used during pregnancy. *Chlorpromazine* and *Haloperidol* have been detected in breast milk.

Use in children: Generally not recommended for children under 12 (see individual listings for those that may be used). Children with acute illnesses (*e.g.,* chickenpox, CNS infections, measles, gastroenteritis) or dehydration seem to be more susceptible to neuromuscular reactions, particularly dystonias.

PRECAUTIONS

Use with caution in patients with exposure to extreme heat or phosphorus insecticides; alcohol withdrawal; history of ulcer disease (aggravation of preexisting ulcer has occurred); cardiovascular disease; prostatic hypertrophy (because of anticholinergic activity of these drugs). Because myocardial hazards may be increased, concurrent electroshock treatment is reserved for patients for whom it is essential.

Renal: Monitor renal function during long-term therapy. If serum creatinine becomes elevated, therapy should be discontinued.

Hematologic: Monitor hematopoietic function periodically; appearance of blood dyscrasias requires immediate discontinuation of therapy.

Thyroid: Severe neurotoxicity (rigidity, inability to walk or talk) may occur in those with thyrotoxicosis.

Extrapyramidal reactions: If acute, may be relieved by dosage reduction or by anticholinergic antiparkinsonism agents. Antiparkinsonism agents should never be used prophylatically.

Tardive dyskinesia: Persistent and irreversible tardive dyskinesias may develop during or after discontinuation of phenothiazine therapy. Anticholinergic agents may worsen these effects (see *Adverse Reactions*).

Hypotension: If hypotension occurs, place patient in a recumbent position. Those with hypovolemia have increased sensitivity to the hypotensive effects of these agents.

Abrupt withdrawal: These drugs do not produce physical dependence; however, gastritis, nausea and vomiting, dizziness, and tremulousness have been reported with abrupt cessation of high-dosage therapy. These symptoms can be reduced by continuing antiparkinsonism agents for several weeks after the antipsychotic drug is withdrawn.

Antiemetic effects: Drugs that have antiemetic effects can obscure signs of toxicity of other drugs or mask symptoms of disease (*e.g.,* brain tumor, intestinal obstruction, Reye's syndrome). Because these drugs suppress the cough reflex, aspiration of vomitus is possible.

Tartrazine sensitivity: Some of these products contain tartrazine (see Appendix 6, section 6-23).

Cutaneous pigmentation changes/photosensitivity: Melanosis and blue-gray skin coloration have been reported. After prolonged administration of high doses, pigmentation has occurred chiefly in exposed areas, especially in women on large doses. Photosensitization may occur. These effects most commonly occur with chlorpromazine, prochlorperazine, and perphenazine.

DRUG INTERACTIONS
Use with caution in patients receiving **barbiturates, narcotics, anesthetics,** or **alcohol,** because of additive depressant effects, and in those receiving **atropine** or related drugs, because of additive anticholinergic effects. Concomitant administration of **antidiarrheal mixtures** and **antacids** may reduce phenothiazine absorption. Antipsychotic agents may inhibit the antihypertensive effect of **guanethidine.** Concomitant administration of phenothiazines with **propranolol** results in increased plasma levels of both drugs; **metoprolol** is similarly affected. **Lithium** may lower plasma levels of chlorpromazine. **Epinephrine** should not be used because phenothiazines block alpha-adrenergic receptors, permitting unopposed beta activity (vasodilatation, increased heart rate) to predominate. Concomitant administration of haloperidol and **methyldopa** may produce psychiatric symptoms (_i.e.,_ disorientation, irritability, aggressiveness, assaultiveness). **Caffeine-containing beverages** counteract the antipsychotic effects of these drugs.

Drug/lab tests: An increase in **cephalin flocculation,** sometimes accompanied by alterations in other **liver-function tests** has been reported in those receiving phenothiazines who have had no clinical evidence of liver damage. Phenothiazines may discolor the urine pink to red-brown. False-positive **pregnancy tests** have been reported but are less likely to occur when a serum test is used. An increase in **protein-bound iodine,** not attributable to an increase in T_4, has been noted.

ADVERSE REACTIONS
Sudden death: Has been reported. Previous brain damage or seizures may be predisposing factors; high doses should be avoided in known seizure patients. In some cases death was apparently due to cardiac arrest; others appeared to be due to asphyxia caused by failure of the cough reflex.

Hepatic: Incidence of jaundice is low. It usually occurs between the second and fourth weeks of therapy and is regarded as a hypersensitivity reaction. The clinical picture resembles hepatitis with laboratory features of extrahepatic obstructive jaundice. It is usually reversible, but chronic jaundice and biliary stasis have been reported.

Hematologic: Agranulocytosis; eosinophilia; leukopenia; leukocytosis; anemia; aplastic anemia; hemolytic anemia; thrombocytopenic or nonthrombocytopenic purpura; pancytopenia. Most cases of agranulocytosis occurred between the fourth and tenth weeks of therapy. If white cell count and differential show significant depression, drug is discontinued.

Cardiovascular: Postural hypotension; hypertension; tachycardia; bradycardia; cardiac arrest; faintness; dizziness. The hypotensive effect may produce a shocklike condition. ECG changes (increased Q–T interval, S–T depression, occasional atrioventricular block) may occur and are usually reversible.

Extrapyramidal: Usually dose related and takes three forms: pseudoparkinsonism, akathisia (motor restlessness), and dystonias. Dystonias include spasms of the neck muscles, extensor rigidity of back muscles, carpopedal spasm, rolled back eyes, convulsions, trismus, torticollis, opisthotonos, oculogyric crisis, and swallowing difficulties. These resemble serious neurologic disorders but usually subside within 48 hours. Management of extrapyramidal symptoms, depending on type and severity, includes antipsychotic dosage reduction and use of anticholinergic-type antiparkinsonism agents. Administration of parenteral diphenhydramine, 50 mg, will immediately reverse an acute dystonic reaction. Employ suitable measures, such as maintaining a clear airway and adequate hydration. In rare instances, persistent dyskinesias, usually involving the face, tongue, and jaw, have lasted months and even years, particularly in the elderly with previous brain damage.

Tardive dyskinesia: May appear in some patients on long-term therapy or may occur after drug therapy is discontinued. The risk appears greater in the elderly, especially those with previous brain damage. Symptoms are persistent and, in some patients, appear irreversible. Fine vermicular movements of the tongue may be an early sign; if medication is stopped at that time, the syndrome may not develop. The syndrome is characterized by rhythmic involuntary or semi-involuntary choreiform movements of the tongue, face, mouth, or jaw (_e.g.,_ protrusion of tongue, puffing of cheeks, puckering of mouth, chewing movements), sometimes accompanied by involuntary movements of the extremities. There is no effective treatment. It is suggested that all antipsychotic agents be discontinued if symptoms appear. Abrupt discontinuation may exacerbate symptoms, whereas gradual reduction of dosage may arrest the progression of symptoms.

Adverse behavioral effects: Paradoxical exacerbation of psychotic symptoms; catatoniclike states; paranoid reactions; lethargy; restlessness; hyperactivity; agitation; nocturnal confusion; toxic confusional states; bizarre dreams; insomnia; depression; despondency; euphoria; excitement.

Other CNS effects: Cerebral edema; headache; abnormality of CSF proteins; convulsive seizures; insomnia; vertigo; drowsiness; exacerbation of psychotic symptoms; hyperpyrexia; altered EEG tracings.

Allergic: Urticarial, maculopapular, petechial, or edematous hypersensitivity reactions; angioneurotic edema; itching; seborrhea; papillary hypertrophy of the tongue; erythema; photosensitivity; eczema; asthma; laryngeal edema; anaphylactoid reactions; acneiform skin rashes; loss of hair. Rarely, exfoliative dermatitis. Contact dermatitis appears in nursing personnel administering phenothiazine liquid concentrates.

Endocrine disorders: Lactation, moderate breast enlargement in women; galactorrhea; syndrome of inappropriate ADH secretion; mastalgia; gynecomastia in men on large doses; changes in libido; hyperglycemia or hypoglycemia; glycosuria; raised plasma cholesterol levels. Resumption of menses in previously amenorrheic women has been reported with **molindone.** Initially, heavy menses may occur. **chlorpromazine** blocks ovulation, suppresses the estrous cycle, causes infertility and pseudopregnancy, and reduces urinary levels of gonadotropins, estrogens, and progestins.

Autonomic: Dry mouth; nasal congestion; nausea; vomiting; anorexia; fever (including hyperpyrexia); pallor; salivation; perspiration; constipation; fecal impaction; diarrhea; adynamic ileus; urinary retention; urinary frequency; bladder paralysis; polyuria; enuresis; inhibition of ejaculation and impotence in men; urinary incontinence; increased libido in women.

Ocular: Aggravation of glaucoma; photophobia; blurred vision; myosis; mydriasis; ptosis. Star-shaped lenticular opacities, epithelial keratopathies, and pigmentary retinopathy may develop.

Respiratory: Laryngospasm; bronchospasm; dyspnea.

Other: Enlargement of parotid glands; increases in appetite and weight; dyspepsia; peripheral edema; fatigue; suppression of cough reflex; polydipsia. The occurrence of a systemic lupus erythematosus-like syndrome has been reported. Muscle necrosis has been reported following multiple IM injections of the acidic chlorpromazine HCl solution. Hirsutism has been reported during long-term therapy.

BIOEQUIVALENCE

Bioavailability differences between solid oral dosage forms and suppositories marketed by different manufacturers has been documented for various phenothiazines. Brand interchange is not recommended unless comparative bioavailability data is available.

OVERDOSAGE

Symptoms: CNS depression to the point of somnolence or coma that may persist for several days. Hypotension and extrapyramidal symptoms may occur. Other manifestations include agitation, restlessness, convulsions, fever, autonomic reactions, ECG changes, cardiac arrhythmias.

Treatment: Symptomatic and supportive. Early gastric lavage is helpful. Keep patient under observation and maintain open airway because involvement of the extrapyramidal mechanism may produce dysphagia and respiratory difficulty in severe overdosage. Do not induce emesis because dystonic reaction of the head or neck may develop, resulting in aspiration of vomitus. Extrapyramidal symptoms may be treated with antiparkinsonism drugs, barbiturates, or diphenhydramine. Stimulants that may cause convulsions are avoided. If hypotension occurs, the standard measures for managing circulatory shock, including volume replacement, should be initiated. If vasoconstrictor administration is desirable, levarterenol or dopamine is most suitable. Epinephrine is not recommended because phenothiazine derivatives may reverse the usual pressor action of this drug and cause a further lowering of blood pressure. Antipsychotic agents do not appear to be dialyzable.

DOSAGE

May be administered IM, IV, or PO (see individual drug dosages, below). Dosage is adjusted according to the individual and severity of the condition. Dosage should be increased gradually in elderly, debilitated, or emaciated patients. In continued therapy, gradually reduce dosage to the lowest effective maintenance level after symptoms are controlled. Increase parenteral dosage only if hypotension has not occurred. In combative patients or those with serious manifestations of acute psychosis, parenteral administration may be repeated q1h to q4h until desired effects are obtained or until cardiac rhythm, hypotension, or other disturbing side-effects emerge. Maintenance therapy can frequently be given as a single daily dose at H.S.

ACETOPHENAZINE MALEATE

Usual dosage is 20 mg tid. In patients having difficulty sleeping, the last tablet should be taken 1 hour before retiring. Total dosage may range from 40 mg/day to 80 mg/day. *Hospitalized patients:* Optimal dosage ranges from 80 mg/day to 120 mg/day in divided doses. Certain hospitalized patients with severe schizophrenia have received doses as high as 400 mg/day to 600 mg/day.

CHLORPROMAZINE HYDROCHLORIDE

Adults

Agitation, tension, apprehension or anxiety, and in psychiatric outpatients: For prompt control of severe symptoms, 25 mg IM. If needed, repeat in 1 hour. Subsequent doses are then given orally. Usual starting oral dose is 10 mg tid or qid or 25 mg bid or tid. Daily dosage may be increased by 20-mg to 50-mg increments until patient is calm and cooperative. Maximum improvement may not be seen for weeks or even months. Optimal dosage is continued for 2 weeks and then gradually reduced to maintenance level. Dosage of 200 mg/day is not unusual. Some patients require higher dosages (*e.g.,* 800 mg/day is not uncommon in discharged mental patients).

Preoperative: 25 mg to 50 mg orally 2 to 3 hours before surgery or 12.5 mg to 25 mg IM 1 to 2 hours before surgery.

Acute intermittent porphyria: 25 mg to 50 mg orally or 25 mg IM tid or qid until patient can take oral therapy.

Tetanus: 25 mg to 50 mg IM tid or qid, usually with barbiturates. For IV use, 25 mg to 50 mg IV. Dilute to at least 1 mg/ml and administer at a rate of 1 mg/minute.

Hospitalized psychiatric patients (acutely agitated, manic, or disturbed): 25 mg IM. If needed, give additional 25 mg to 50 mg in 1 hour. Increase gradually over several days (up to 400 mg q4h–q6h in exceptionally severe cases) until patient is controlled. Patient usually becomes quiet and cooperative within 24 to 48 hours and oral dosage may be substituted and increased until patient is calm; 500 mg/day is usually a sufficient dosage. Although gradual increases to 2000 mg or more/day may be necessary, there is little therapeutic gain from exceeding 1000 mg/day for extended periods.

Hospitalized psychiatric patients (less acutely agitated patients): *Oral*—25 mg tid. Increase gradually until effective dose is reached; usually 400 mg/day is sufficient dosage.

Nausea, vomiting (including postoperative administration), intractable hiccups: See Antiemetic/Antivertigo Agents.

Children

Psychiatric outpatients: *Oral*—0.25 mg/lb q4h to q6h as needed; *Rectal*—0.5 mg/lb q6h to q8h as needed. *IM*—0.25 mg/lb q6h to q8h as needed. Maximum IM dose: Up to 5 years, 40 mg/day; 5 to 12 years, 75 mg/day except in severe cases. Generally not used in children under 6 months.

Preoperative: 0.25 mg/lb orally 2 to 3 hours before surgery or 0.25 mg/lb IM 1 to 2 hours before surgery.

Nausea, vomiting: See Antiemetic/Antivertigo Agents.

Hospitalized psychiatric patients: *Oral*—Start with low dose and increase gradually. In severe behavioral disorders or psychotic conditions, higher doses of 50 mg/day to 100 mg/day or, in older children, 200 mg/day or more may be necessary. There is little evidence that behavioral improvement in severely disturbed mentally retarded patients is enhanced by doses above 500 mg/day.

IM—Up to 5 years, not over 40 mg/day; 5 to 12 years, not over 75 mg/day except in unmanageable cases.

Tetanus (IM or IV): 0.25 mg/lb q6h to q8h. When giving IV, dilute to at least 1 mg/ml and administer at rate of 1 mg/2 minutes. In children up to 50 lb, do not exceed 40 mg/day; 50 to 100 lb, do not exceed 75 mg/day except in severe cases.

CHLORPROTHIXENE

Not recommended for oral administration in children under 6 or for parenteral use in those under 12.

Oral: *Adults*—initially, 25 mg to 50 mg tid, qid; increase as needed. Dosages exceeding 600 mg/day are rarely required. For elderly or debilitated patients, initially use lower doses of 10 mg to 25 mg, tid, qid. *Children over 6 years*—10 mg to 25 mg tid, qid.

IM: *Adults, children over 12*—25 mg to 50 mg, up to 3 or 4 times daily. Pain or induration at site of injection is minimal. Administer with patient seated or recumbent because postural hypotension may occur.

FLUPHENAZINE ENANTHATE AND DECANOATE

Onset of action generally is 24 to 72 hours after injection; the effects on psychotic symptoms become significant within 48 to 96 hours. Duration of therapeutic effects ranges from 1 to 3 weeks or longer for the enanthate and up to 4 weeks or longer for the decanoate. Administer IM or subcutaneously. A dose of 12.5 mg to 25 mg may be given to initiate therapy. Subsequent injections and dosage intervals are determined by patient response. Dosage should not exceed 100 mg.

Severely agitated patients: May be treated initially with a rapid-acting phenothiazine such as fluphenazine HCl injection (see discussion above). When acute symptoms subside, 25 mg may be administered.

"Poor-risk" patients (those with known hypersensitivity to phenothiazines or with disorders that pre-

dispose them to undue reactions): Initiate therapy cautiously with oral or parenteral fluphenazine HCl. When pharmacologic effects and an appropriate dosage are apparent, an equivalent dose of fluphenazine enanthate or decanoate may be administered. Subsequent dosages are adjusted according to patient response.

FLUPHENAZINE HYDROCHLORIDE

Optimal dosage levels will vary. Oral dose has been found to be approximately 2 to 3 times the parenteral dose. Treatment is best instituted with low initial dosage, which may be increased until desired clinical effects are obtained. Therapeutic effect is often achieved with doses under 20 mg/day. Patients remaining severely disturbed or inadequately controlled may require up to 40 mg/day. Acutely ill patients may respond to lower doses and may require rapid increase of dosage. Elderly, debilitated, and adolescent patients may respond to low dosages. Outpatients should receive smaller doses. IM administration is useful when patient is unable or unwilling to take oral therapy. When symptoms are controlled, oral maintenance is generally instituted, often with single daily doses. Continued treatment, by the oral route if possible, is needed to produce maximum therapeutic benefits. Further adjustments in dosage may be necessary during course of therapy.

Oral: Dosage may range initially from 0.5 mg/day to 10 mg/day in divided doses administered q6h to q8h. In general, a daily dose in excess of 3 mg is rarely necessary. A dose in excess of 20 mg should be used with caution. When symptoms are controlled, dosage can be gradually reduced to daily maintenance doses of 1 mg to 5 mg, often given as a single daily dose. For geriatric patients, suggested starting dose is 1 mg/day to 2.5 mg/day, adjusted according to patient response.

IM: Average starting dose for adult patients is 1.25 mg IM. Depending on severity and duration of symptoms, initial total daily dosage may range from 2.5 mg to 10 mg and should be divided and given q6h to q8h. Dosages exceeding 10 mg/day IM are used with caution.

HALOPERIDOL

Initial dosage is based on patient's age, severity of illness, previous response to other neuroleptic drugs, and any concomitant medication or disease state.

Initial dose range: Moderate symptoms, 0.5 mg to 2 mg bid, tid; severe symptoms, 3 mg to 5 mg bid, tid; geriatric or debilitated patients, 0.5 mg to 2 mg bid, tid. Chronic or resistant patients, 3 mg to 5 mg bid, tid. Higher doses may be required in some cases. Patients who remain severely disturbed or inadequately controlled may require dosage adjustment. Daily doses above 100 mg have been used for severely resistant patients.

Maintenance dosage: After achieving a satisfactory therapeutic response, gradually reduce dosage to the lowest effective maintenance level.

IM: 2 mg to 5 mg (up to 10 mg to 30 mg) may be used for prompt control of acutely agitated patients with moderately severe to severe symptoms. Depending on response, subsequent doses may be administered as often as every hour, although 4- to 8-hour intervals may be satisfactory. Safety and efficacy of IM administration in children not established. The oral form should replace the injectable as soon as possible. The first oral dose should be given within 12 to 24 hours following the last parenteral dose.

Children 3 to 12 years or 15 to 40 kg (not intended for children under 3 years): Therapy should begin at the lowest possible dose (0.5 mg/day). Dosage can be increased in increments of 0.5 mg at 5- to 7-day intervals until desired therapeutic effect is obtained. The total dose may be divided and given bid or tid. *Psychotic disorders*—0.05 mg/kg/day to 0.15 mg/kg/day; *nonpsychotic behavioral disorders and Tourette's syndrome,* 0.05 mg/kg/day to 0.075 mg/kg/day. Severely disturbed psychotic children may require higher doses.

LOXAPINE

Drug is removed rapidly from plasma and distributed in tissues and is metabolized extensively and excreted in urine and feces. Signs of sedation are usually seen within 20 to 30 minutes after administration and are most pronounced within 1.5 to 3 hours and last through 12 hours.

Oral: Administer in divided doses, 2 to 4 times/day. Initial dosage of 10 mg bid is recommended, although in severely disturbed patients up to a total of 50 mg/day may be required. Dosage may be increased fairly rapidly over the first 7 to 10 days until there is effective control of psychotic symptoms. The usual range is 60 mg/day to 100 mg/day. Dosage higher than 250 mg/day is not recommended. *Maintenance therapy*—Reduce dosage to lowest level compatible with symptom control; many patients are maintained at dosages of 20 mg/day to 60 mg/day.

IM: Used for prompt symptomatic control in the acutely agitated patient and in patients whose symptoms render oral medication temporarily impractical. Administer 12.5 mg to 50 mg at intervals of 4 to 6 hours or longer. Many patients respond to bid administration. Not for IV use.

MESORIDAZINE

Schizophrenia: Starting oral dose of 50 mg tid is recommended. Usual optimal total dosage range is 100 mg/day to 400 mg/day.

Behavioral problems in mental deficiency and chronic brain syndrome: Recommended starting oral dose is 25 mg tid. Usual optimal total dosage range is 75 mg/day to 300 mg/day.

Alcoholism: Usual starting dose is 25 mg bid; optimal total dosage range is 50 mg/day to 200 mg/day.

Psychoneurotic manifestations: Usual starting oral dose is 10 mg tid; optimal total dosage range is 30 mg/day to 150 mg/day.

IM administration: Starting dose of 25 mg is recommended; may be repeated in 30 to 60 minutes, if necessary. Usual optimal dosage range is 25 mg/day to 200 mg/day.

MOLINDONE HYDROCHLORIDE

Usual starting dose is 50 mg/day to 75 mg/day, to be increased to 100 mg/day in 3 to 4 days. An increase to 225 mg/day may be required in some patients. Start elderly and debilitated patients on lower dosage.

Maintenance therapy: _Mild_—5 mg to 15 mg tid, qid; _moderate_—10 mg to 25 mg tid, qid; _severe_— up to 225 mg/day.

NOTE: Tablet form contains calcium sulfate, which may interfere with the absorption of some drugs such as **phenytoin sodium** or **tetracyclines.**

PERPHENAZINE

Children: Pediatric dosage not established; children over 12 may receive lowest limit of adult dosage.

Moderately disturbed nonhospitalized psychotic patients: 4 mg to 8 mg tid or 8 mg to 16 mg repeat-action form bid; reduce as soon as possible to minimum effective dosage.

Hospitalized psychotic patients: 8 mg/day to 16 mg/day in divided doses or 8 mg repeat-action form bid; occasionally, 24 mg may be necessary. Early dosage reduction is desirable; 16 mg repeat-action form may be used in acute cases.

IM: Use when rapid effect and prompt control of acute or intractable condition are required or when oral administration is not feasible. Therapeutic effect is usually evident in 10 minutes and is maximal in 1 to 2 hours. Average duration of effective action is 6 hours (occasionally 12–24 hours). Usual initial dose is 5 mg; this may be repeated in 6 hours. Ordinarily, the total daily dose should not exceed 15 mg in ambulatory patients or 30 mg in hospitalized patients. When required for control of severe conditions, an initial dose of 10 mg may be given. Patients should be placed on oral therapy as soon as possible. Equal or higher dosage should be used when patient is transferred to oral therapy.

Psychotic conditions: 5 mg IM will have a definite tranquilizing effect but it may be necessary to use 10 mg to initiate therapy in severely agitated states. Most patients will be controlled and amenable to oral therapy within 24 to 48 hours. Acute conditions (hysteria, panic reaction) often respond to a single dose whereas chronic conditions may require several injections.

Nausea, vomiting, and intractable hiccups: See Antiemetic/Antivertigo Agents.

IV: Use with caution and only when absolutely necessary for control of severe vomiting, intractable hiccups.

PIPERACETAZINE

Starting dose of 10 mg, 2 to 4 times/day; may be increased to 160 mg/day within a 3- to 5-day period. Reduce dosage or discontinue drug if side-effects occur.

Maintenance therapy: Up to 160 mg/day in divided doses.

PROCHLORPERAZINE

Adults

Subcutaneous administration is not advisable because of local irritation.

Elderly patients: Dosages in lower range usually sufficient.

Severe anxiety: _Oral_—5 mg or 10 mg tid, qid, or 15 mg of sustained-release form on arising, or 10 mg of sustained-release form q12h.

Rectal—25 mg bid.

IM—Initially 5 mg or 10 mg, repeated q3h to q4h if necessary. Total IM dosage should not exceed 40 mg/day.

Psychiatry: _Oral_—For relatively mild conditions 5 mg or 10 mg tid, qid. In moderate to severe conditions, starting dose is 10 mg tid, qid for hospitalized or adequately supervised patients. Increase dosage gradually until symptoms are controlled or side-effects are bothersome. Some patients respond to 50 mg/day to 75 mg/day; in more severe disturbances, optimal dosage is usually 100 mg/day to 150 mg/day.

_IM_—For immediate control of severely disturbed patients, 10 mg to 20 mg deep IM in upper outer quadrant of buttock. If necessary, repeat initial dose q2h to q4h (in resistant cases, every hour) to control patient. More than 3 or 4 doses seldom necessary. After control is achieved, patient is usually changed to oral form at same dosage level or higher. If parenteral therapy is needed for a prolonged period, 10 mg to 20 mg q4h to q6h is usually given.

Control of severe nausea, vomiting: See Antiemetic/Antivertigo Agents.

Children

Not recommended for children under 20 lb or 2 years. Occasionally patient may react to drug with restlessness and excitement; if this occurs, additional doses are not administered.

Child psychiatry: *Oral or rectal*—2 to 12 years, 2.5 mg bid or tid and not more than 10 mg on first day; 2 to 5 years, total daily dose usually does not exceed 20 mg; 6 to 12 years, total daily dose usually does not exceed 25 mg.

IM—Under 12 years, 0.06 mg/lb deep IM; after control is achieved, oral form at same dosage level or higher is usually administered.

PROMAZINE HYDROCHLORIDE

Parenteral administration should be reserved for bed patients, although acute states in ambulatory patients may be treated by IM injection. IV administration should be reserved for hospitalized patients. Use IV in concentrations no greater than 25 mg/ml; administer slowly in dilute solutions (25 mg/ml or less).

Adults: Recommended initial dose for severely agitated patients is 50 mg to 150 mg IM, depending on degree of excitation. If desired calming effect is not apparent in 30 minutes, additional doses up to a total of 300 mg may be given. Once desired control is obtained, administer drug orally. The oral or IM dose is 10 mg to 200 mg q4h to q6h. In less severe disturbances, dosage is adjusted downward. *Maintenance dosage*—10 mg to 200 mg q4h to q6h. When tablet medication is unsuitable or refused, the syrup or liquid concentrate may be used by diluting in citrus or chocolate-flavored drinks. It is recommended that the total daily dose not exceed 1000 mg. In the acute inebriated patient, the initial dose should not exceed 50 mg.

Children over 12: In acute episodes of chronic psychotic disease, 10 mg to 25 mg q4h to q6h.

THIORIDAZINE HYDROCHLORIDE

Psychotic manifestations: Usual initial dose is 50 mg to 100 mg tid, with a gradual dose increment to a maximum of 800 mg/day, if necessary. Once effective control of symptoms is achieved, dosage may be reduced gradually to determine minimum maintenance dose. The total daily dose ranges from 200 mg to 800 mg divided into 2 to 4 doses.

Short-term treatment of moderate to marked depression with variable degrees of anxiety; in geriatric patients, treatment of multiple symptoms such as agitation, anxiety, depressed mood, tension, sleep disturbances, fears: Usual starting dose is 25 mg tid. Dosage ranges from 10 mg bid, to 10 mg qid in milder cases, to 50 mg tid or qid for more severely disturbed patients. Total daily dosage range is from 20 mg to a maximum of 200 mg/day.

Children: Not recommended for children under 2 years. For ages 2 to 12 the dosage ranges from 0.5 mg/kg/day to 3 mg/kg/day. *Moderate disorders*—10 mg bid or tid is usual starting dose. *Hospitalized, severely disturbed, or psychotic children*—25 mg bid or tid. Dosage may be increased gradually until optimal therapeutic effect is obtained. The concentrate may be administered in distilled or acidified tap water or suitable juices.

THIOTHIXENE

Not recommended for children under 12.

Oral: In milder conditions, an initial dose of 2 mg tid; may be increased to 15 mg/day. In more severe conditions an initial dose of 5 mg bid is recommended. Usual optimal dose is 20 mg/day to 30 mg/day; if indicated, dosage may be increased to 60 mg/day. Dosages exceeding 60 mg/day rarely increase beneficial response.

IM: Used for more rapid control and treatment of acute behavior; also of benefit when nature of patient's symptoms renders oral administration impractical or impossible. Usual dose is 4 mg administered 2 to 4 times/day and increased or decreased depending on patient's response. Most patients are controlled on a total dosage of 16 mg/day to 20 mg/day.

Maximum recommended dosage: 30 mg/day. See *Administration.*

TRIFLUOPERAZINE

Adjusted to individual needs; dosage is increased more gradually in debilitated or emaciated patients. Because of inherent long action of the drug, patients may be controlled with twice-daily administration; some patients may be maintained on once-a-day administration.

Outpatients: 1 mg or 2 mg bid. It is seldom necessary to exceed 4 mg/day except in those with more severe conditions and in discharged mental patients.

Hospitalized patients or those under close supervision: Usual starting dosage is 2 mg to 5 mg bid. Most patients show optimal response with 15 mg/day or 20 mg/day, but some may require 40 mg/day or more. Optimal therapeutic dosage should be reached in 2 or 3 weeks.

IM: For prompt control of severe symptoms, usual dosage is 1 mg to 2 mg deep IM q4h to q6h as needed. More than 6 mg/24 hours is rarely necessary. Only in exceptional cases should the IM dosage exceed 10 mg/24 hours. Do not give at intervals less than 4 hours because of a possible cumulative effect. When administered IM, equivalent oral dosage may be substituted once symptoms are controlled.

Children: Adjust dosage to weight of child and severity of symptoms. The following dosages are for children ages 6 to 12 who are hospitalized or under close supervision.

Oral— Starting dose is 1 mg once or twice daily; dosage may be increased gradually until symptoms are controlled or side-effects become troublesome. Although it is not usually necessary to exceed 15 mg/day, some older children with severe symptoms may require higher doses.

IM— If necessary to achieve rapid control of symptoms, 1 mg may be administered once or twice daily.

Elderly: Usually dosages in the lower range are sufficient. Because the elderly are more susceptible to hypotension and neuromuscular reactions, observe closely.

TRIFLUPROMAZINE HYDROCHLORIDE

Psychotic disorders: Initially, 100 mg orally, up to a maximum total dose of 150 mg/day. After treatment is instituted, adjust daily dosage until desired clinical effect is obtained. Continued treatment is necessary to achieve maximum therapeutic benefits; in some, optimal improvement may occur only after prolonged treatment. When symptoms are controlled, dosage can gradually be reduced to maintenance levels. Recommended IM dose is 60 mg, up to a maximum of 150 mg/day. For maintenance therapy, recommended oral dose is 30 mg, up to a total of 150 mg/day.

Children: Recommended dosage schedule is 2 mg/kg up to a maximum of 150 mg/day in divided doses. For maintenance therapy, dosage is increased or decreased to meet individual requirements. When IM use is indicated, recommended range is 0.2 mg/kg to 0.25 mg/kg, up to a maximum total dose of 10 mg/day. Do not administer to children under 2½ years of age.

Nausea and vomiting: See Antiemetic/Antivertigo Agents.

NURSING IMPLICATIONS

HISTORY
See Appendix 4.

MENTAL AND PHYSICAL ASSESSMENT
Monitor blood pressure, (sitting and recumbent), pulse, respirations, temperature, weight. Observe overt symptoms—general appearance and behavior; response to immediate environment; level of consciousness; emotional status; intellectual responses to verbal questions; and thought content. Additional areas or limitation of assessment will depend on health history and severity of patient's illness. Perform baseline laboratory tests such as CBC, renal- and hepatic-function tests. An ophthalmologic evaluation may also be performed.

ADMINISTRATION
Oral
When diluting concentrated solutions, add diluent *immediately before* administering the drug. Some manufacturers supply a graduated dropper for measurement.

Use fruit juice for dilution of the oral concentrate unless patient is on a special diet or dislikes fruit juice. The manufacturers recommend the following vehicles for dilution of the concentrate.

Loxapin: Mix with orange or grapefruit juice.

Promazine: Dilute in citrus juice, chocolate-flavored drink, or other suitable vehicle. For best taste dilute 25 mg in 10 ml.

Thioridazine: Use distilled water, acidified tap water, or suitable juices. If water is used, check with pharmacist regarding water acidity.

Trifluoperazine: Add concentrate to 60 ml or more of diluent just prior to administration. Vehicles suggested are tomato or fruit juice, milk, simple syrup, orange syrup, carbonated beverages, coffee, tea, water, semisolid foods (*e.g.,* puddings).

Exercise caution in giving oral medication (liquid, capsule, tablet) to a resistant patient because aspiration can occur.

Oral liquid concentrates are sensitive to light and are dispensed in amber or opaque bottles and protected from light.

Check the oral cavity following oral administration, especially if patient is elderly, a child, debilitated, or resistant (mentally or physically) to treatment. If problems occur with administering drug in oral form, contact physician because another administration route may be necessary.

Phenothiazine liquid concentrates: Exercise care in preparing for administration, because contact dermatitis may occur. If drug is spilled on skin or clothing during preparation or administration, wash area immediately.

Suppositories
Insert beyond rectal sphincter; check patient in 30 minutes to be sure suppository is retained.
Parenteral
Thiothixene: The powder for injection is reconstituted with 2.2 ml of Sterile Water for Injection; each ml contains 5 mg.

Chlorpromazine, perphenazine: Slight yellow coloring does not alter potency; discard if markedly discolored.

Loxapine, fluphenazine, triflupromazine: May vary in color from colorless to light amber; if any darker than light amber or discolored in any other way, do not use.

General considerations

If drug is given IV, place patient in a recumbent position because postural hypotension may occur. Monitor blood pressure, pulse q15m to q30m. Notify physician if hypotension occurs. If a vasopressor is needed, levarterenol or dopamine is usually ordered.

If drug is administered IM, give with patient seated (deltoid) or recumbent (gluteus). Inject drug slowly. In some instances it may be advisable to have the patient remain seated or recumbent (if possible) for ½ hour after the injection.

Rotate IM injection sites.

Do *Not* mix these drugs with other pharmacologic agents without first consulting the pharmacist because they are incompatible with many other agents.

Chlorpromazine HCl: The recommended site of IM administration is the upper outer quadrant of the buttock. Drug may be irritating to tissues and cause pain on injection. If discomfort occurs, physician may order injection diluted with normal saline or 2% procaine.

Generic name similarity: Triflupromazine and trifluoperazine.

Dosage similarities: Prochlorperazine suppositories 2.5 mg, 25 mg.

ONGOING ASSESSMENTS AND NURSING MANAGEMENT
Monitor vital signs daily (monitor blood pressure, pulse, respirations more frequently during early therapy or as ordered).

Observe behavior and compare to data base.

Observe for side-effects, especially those related to the nervous system. Report any marked changes in behavior (*e.g.,* extreme sedation, withdrawal, hyperexcitability, aggressiveness) to physician immediately because dosage change or other changes in treatment may be necessary.

Drug dosage is adjusted upward or downward according to patient response. In chronic therapy, full clinical effects may not be seen for 4 to 8 weeks.

CLINICAL ALERT: Observe patients with known depression hourly (or more often if condition warrants). When antipsychotic agents are used in treatment of agitated states accompanying depression, precaution (particularly recognition of a suicidal tendency) is indicated.

Antipsychotic agents should not be suddenly discontinued (except by physician's order). Ensure continuity of prescribed therapy by notation on Kardex, informing health-team members responsible for drug administration.

If extrapyramidal reactions or tardive dyskinesia occurs, notify the physician immediately. Review *Adverse Reactions* for signs of both disorders.

The occurrence of extrapyramidal reactions is usually extremely upsetting and the patient will require emotional support and reassurance that the symptoms will subside (dosage reduction or an antiparkinsonism agent is usually ordered by the physician).

If hypotension occurs, place patient in a recumbent position.

To prevent orthostatic hypotension, advise patient to make position changes slowly and to dangle legs 5 to 10 minutes before getting out of bed.

Owing to a decreased sensation of thirst (see *Warnings*), a liberal liquid intake is essential, especially for the elderly or withdrawn patient. Provide easy access to fluids such as water and juice at the bedside, in the open ward or recreational setting, and at meals. If fluid intake is questionable, measure intake and output and offer fluids hourly while the patient is awake.

These drugs may impair mental or physical abilities. If drowsiness is severe, patient should remain in bed, with siderails raised, and ambulate only with assistance.

Autonomic side effects

Dry mouth: May be relieved by sips of water, hard candy, or gum. Encourage good oral hygiene; assist elderly, debilitated, and withdrawn patients and children with oral care as needed.

Constipation, fecal impaction, adynamic ileus: Record bowel movements daily. Palpate abdomen, auscultate bowel sounds if patient complains of discomfort or has not had a bowel movement for several days. Abdominal distention or change in bowel sounds may indicate adynamic ileus; notify physician of findings. Increase in fluid intake and addition of fiber to the diet may alleviate constipation. Some patients may require a laxative such as a stool softener.

Urinary retention: Record intake and output; palpate lower abdomen if urinary retention is suspected.

Blurred vision: Assist with ambulation, activities of daily living as needed.

Photophobia: Keep room semidark by drawing curtains or closing blinds or move patient to a dimly lit area.

Suppression of cough reflex: Closely observe

those with respiratory or pulmonary disorders for pooling of respiratory secretions, signs of pulmonary infection.

Concomitant administration of barbiturates, narcotics, or other CNS depressants may produce additive effects; dosages of these drugs should be *decreased* (see *Drug Interactions*).

Agranulocytosis may occur between the fourth and tenth weeks of therapy. Observe patient for sudden appearance of soreness of the mouth, gums, or throat or other signs of infection. Use a flashlight and tongue blade to inspect the oral cavity, especially if the patient is a child, elderly, debilitated, or withdrawn. If symptoms occur, notify the physician immediately. A WBC and differential are usually ordered.

Hepatic reactions may occur and include jaundice or fever with flulike symptoms; report occurrence to the physician. Hepatic-function tests are usually ordered.

Adverse behavioral effects (*e.g.,* paradoxical exacerbation of psychotic symptoms, catatonic-like states, paranoid reactions, lethargy, restlessness, hyperactivity, agitation, nocturnal confusion, toxic confusional states, insomnia, depression, despondency, euphoria, or excitement) may occur. Once behavioral change is identified, observations are reported to the physician and, when applicable, steps are taken to protect the patient, other patients, and health-team members.

Patients allowed out of doors or on sun-porches or roofs should avoid prolonged exposure to sunlight because photosensitivity and cutaneous skin pigmentation changes may occur. Patients who are relatively immobile should be placed in a shaded area that will not be in direct sunlight during the time they are out of doors.

When women are receiving these drugs during pregnancy, observe the newborn infants for hyperreflexia, jaundice, and prolonged extrapyramidal signs. If these should occur, notify physician immediately.

GI absorption of the phenothiazine derivatives may be reduced by concomitant administration of antacids or antidiarrheal mixtures. If an antacid or antidiarrheal mixture is prescribed, it should be given 1 to 2 hours before or after phenothiazine administration. Rapid-acting laxatives, such as saline laxatives, should not be administered if patient is receiving timed-release capsules or repeat-action tablets.

Note complaints of visual changes such as diminution of visual acuity, brownish coloring of vision, impairment of night vision; if these should occur, notify physician.

All behavior should be carefully evaluated because some patients may not communicate various physical problems (*e.g.,* pruritus, sore throat, constipation) that may indicate a drug side-effect.

Weigh patient weekly or as ordered. If patient exhibits a steady weight loss, discuss with physician.

Enter names of drugs currently administered on all laboratory and diagnostic request slips.

Daily physical and diversional therapies are geared to the patient's physical and emotional ability to participate.

The degree of psychotherapeutic support from all health-team members may influence therapeutic drug effect and infuence dosage.

PATIENT AND FAMILY INFORMATION

NOTE: Some patients may fail to comply with their therapeutic regimen. Whenever possible, one or more family members should receive full instruction and information about treatment modalities and should be encouraged to discuss noncompliance with the physician. If the patient neglects to take his medication or shows rapid deterioration in mental or physical status, the physician should be contacted or the patient taken to a designated psychiatric center.

May cause drowsiness; use caution while driving or performing tasks requiring alertness.

Do not increase, decrease, or omit doses without first checking with physician.

Avoid alcohol and other depressant drugs.

Do not use any nonprescription drug without first checking with physician. This includes laxatives, cold remedies, and tonics.

Keep all physician or clinic appointments because continued monitoring of drug regimen is an essential part of therapy.

Notify physician or nurse if sore throat, fever, unusual bleeding or bruising, skin rash, weakness, tremors, muscle twitching, impaired vision, darkly colored urine, pale stools, jaundice, lack of coordination occurs.

Phenothiazines

Avoid prolonged exposure to sunlight; photosensitivity (which in some cases resembles a severe sunburn) may occur. If exposure to sunlight is unavoidable, wear protective clothing and ask physician about use of a sunscreen lotion.

Drug may discolor urine pink or reddish brown.

If dizziness or fainting occurs, avoid sudden changes in position and use caution while climbing stairs. Rise slowly from a sitting or lying position.

Liquid concentrates: Avoid contact with skin because a rash may occur. If spilled on skin or clothing, wash area immediately.

Antirabies Serum, Equine Origin

See Rabies Prophylaxis Products.

Antiseptics and Germicides*

Benzalkonium Chloride (BAC) otc

concentrate: 17%	Zephiran, *Generic*
solution: 17%	Germicin
solution, aqueous: 1:750	Zephiran
tincture, tincture spray: 1:750	Zephiran
solution: 0.13%	Mercurochrome II
vaginal gel: 1:2000	Nonsul jelly

INDICATIONS

Antisepsis of skin, mucous membranes, wounds; preoperative preparation of skin; surgeon's hand, arm soaks; treatment of wounds; preservation of ophthalmic solutions; irrigations of the eye, body cavities, bladder, urethra; vaginal douching.

Vaginal gel: Combatting causative and associated organisms in trichomonal, monilial, and nonsporulating bacterial or nonspecific vaginal infections; after cauterizations or conizations to prevent secondary infections; and as an aid in proliferation and restoration of healthy, resistant vaginal epithelia.

CONTRAINDICATIONS

Use in occlusive dressings, casts, and anal or vaginal packs is inadvisable because irritation or chemical burns may result.

ACTIONS

Rapidly acting anti-infective with a moderately long duration of action. Active against bacteria and some viruses, fungi, and protozoa. Bacterial spores are resistant. Solutions are bacteriostatic or bactericidal according to their concentration. The exact mechanism of bactericidal action is unknown but is thought to be due to enzyme inactivation. Solutions have deodorant, wetting, detergent, keratolytic, and emulsifying activity.

---

* An antiseptic is an agent that stops, slows, or prevents the growth of microorganisms. A germicide is an agent that destroys microorganisms.

WARNINGS

Use Sterile Water for Injection as diluent for aqueous solutions intended for use on deep wounds or for irrigation of body cavities; otherwise use freshly distilled water.

Do not rely on antiseptic solutions to achieve complete sterilization because they do not destroy bacterial spores and certain viruses. The tinted tincture and spray contain flammable organic solvents; do not use near an open flame or electric cautery.

If solutions stronger than 1:3000 enter the eyes, irrigate immediately and repeatedly with water. Do not use concentrations greater than 1:5000 on mucous membranes except the vaginal mucosa (see recommended dilutions).

PRECAUTIONS

In preoperative antisepsis of the skin, do not permit solutions to remain in prolonged contact with patient's skin. Avoid pooling of solution on the operating room table. Solutions used on inflamed or irritated tissues must be more dilute than those used on normal tissues. Keep tinted tincture and spray away from eyes, other mucous membranes.

Vaginal gel: Patient must not scratch the vulva in the early stages of treatment. Itching is relieved by applying a washcloth containing cracked ice to the area of pruritus.

To reduce the possibility of marital reinfection, sexual relations are contraindicated during the first ten days of therapy. In cases of frequent recurrence, when all possible foci of infection have been ruled out, a urologic examination of the marital partner is indicated.

Discontinue use of applicators in those stages of pregnancy in which possible damage to amniotic sac of the fetus is possible.

ADVERSE REACTIONS

Rarely, hypersensitivity.

Vaginal gel: Occasionally, a local burning sensation may occur. Hypersensitivity reactions are rare; however, if encountered, discontinue use and flush vulvovaginal tissues with water.

ACCIDENTAL INGESTION

Symptoms: If solution (particularly a concentrated solution) is ingested, marked local irritation of the GI tract, manifested by nausea and vomiting, may occur. Signs of systemic toxicity are restlessness, apprehension, weakness, confusion, dyspnea, cyanosis, collapse, convulsions, and coma. Death occurs as a result of paralysis of the respiratory muscles.

Treatment: Immediate administration of several glasses of mild soap solution, milk, or egg whites beaten in water. This may be followed by gastric lavage with a mild soap solution. Avoid alcohol because it promotes absorption. To support respiration, clear airway, administer oxygen, and employ artifical ventilation if necessary. If convulsions occur, a short-acting barbiturate, given parenterally, may be ordered.

DOSAGE

Before use, thoroughly rinse anionic soaps and detergents from skin or other areas because they reduce antibacterial activity of BAC solutions. The following are incompatible with BAC solutions: iodine, silver nitrate, fluorescein, nitrates, peroxide, lanolin, potassium permanganate, aluminum, caramel, kaolin, pine oil, zinc sulfate, zinc oxide, and yellow oxide of mercury.

The following are recommended dilutions for specific applications of BAC solutions:

Preoperative disinfection of skin—1:750 tincture, aqueous solution, or spray
Surgeon's hand, arm soaks—1:750 aqueous solution
Minor wounds, lacerations—1:750 tincture or spray
Deep infected wounds—1:3000 to 1:20,000 aqueous solution
Denuded skin and mucous membranes—1:5000 to 1:10,000 aqueous solution
Vaginal douche and irrigation—1:2000 to 1:5000 aqueous solution
Postepisiotomy care—1:5000 to 1:10,000 aqueous solution
Breast and nipple hygiene—1:1000 to 1:2000 aqueous solution
Bladder and urethral irrigation—1:5000 to 1:20,000 aqueous solution
Bladder retention lavage—1:20,000 to 1:40,000 aqueous solution
Oozing and open infections—1:2000 to 1:5000 aqueous solution
Wet dressings—1:5000 or less aqueous solution
Eye irrigation—1:5000 to 1:10,000 aqueous solution

Vaginal gel: Fill applicator ½ its length (approximately 2½ inches) with 4 g jelly. Insert high into the vagina at bedtime for 24 days or twice daily for 12 days. Longer treatment may be required for resistant cases. Resume treatment during the last 3 days of the menstrual period and 2 days following menses for 3 or more menstrual cycles.

NURSING IMPLICATIONS

See p 145.

Chlorhexidine Gluconate   otc

cleanser: 4%	Hibiclens Antiseptic/Antimicrobial Skin
hand rinse: 0.5%, 70% isopropyl alcohol with emollients	Hibistat Germicidal Hand

INDICATIONS

Tincture: Preparation of skin at surgical site and prior to skin or vessel puncture.
Cleanser: Surgical scrub, handwash, skin-wound cleanser.
Hand rinse: Germicidal hand rinse.

CONTRAINDICATIONS

Hypersensitivity.

ACTIONS

Provides persistent antimicrobial effect against a wide range of microorganisms including gram-positive bacteria and gram-negative bacteria such as _Pseudomonas aeruginosa_.

PRECAUTIONS

Keep out of eyes, ears. If this accidentally occurs, rinse promptly with water and see a physician. For topical use only. Avoid excessive heat (45°C).

ADVERSE REACTIONS

Has been reported to cause deafness when instilled in middle ear. Take care in presence of perforated eardrum. Irritation or other adverse reactions such as dermatitis and photosensitivity are rare; if they occur, discontinue use.

DOSAGE

Tincture: Apply liberally to surgical site and swab for at least 2 minutes. Dry with sterile towel. Repeat procedure for an additional 2 minutes; allow skin to air-dry.
Cleanser: For surgical hand scrub, use 5 ml without adding water; scrub for 3 minutes using brush; rinse thoroughly; wash an additional 3 minutes with 5 ml and rinse under running water. For handwash, use 5 ml to wet hands, wash vigorously for 15 seconds, rinse thoroughly under running water. As skin-wound cleanser, rinse affected area with water; apply small amount, wash gently to remove dirt and debris; rinse thoroughly.
Hand rinse: Use 5 ml, rub hands vigorously until dry (about 15 seconds); pay particular attention to nails and interdigital spaces. Rinse dries rapidly; no water or towels are needed.

NURSING IMPLICATIONS

See p 145.

Hexachlorophene Rx

liquid: 3%	pHisoHex, Soy-Dome Cleanser
sponge: 3%	pHiso Scrub
liquid: 1%	Germa-Medica
liquid: 0.25%	Germa-Medica "MG," Septi-Soft
solution: 0.25%	Septisol
foam: 0.23%	Septisol

INDICATIONS

Surgical scrub, bacteriostatic skin cleanser. May also be used to control outbreak of gram-positive infection when other infection-control procedures have not been successful. Use only as long as necessary for infection control.

CONTRAINDICATIONS

Do not use on burned or denuded skin; as an occlusive dressing, wet pack, or lotion; routinely for prophylactic total-body bathing; as a vaginal pack or tampon, or on any mucous membranes.

ACTIONS

Bacteriostatic cleansing agent. Has bacteriostatic action against staphylococci, other gram-positive bacteria. Cumulative antibacterial action develops with repeated use. This antibacterial residue is resistant to removal by many solvents, soaps, detergents for several days.

WARNINGS

Rinse thoroughly after use, especially from sensitive areas such as the scrotum or perineum. Rapid absorption may occur with resultant toxic blood levels when applied to skin lesions such as ichthyosis congenita or other generalized dermatologic conditions. Application to burns has produced neurotoxicity and death. Discontinue promptly if signs of cerebral irritation occur.

Use in infants: Infants, especially premature infants or those with dermatoses, are susceptible to hexachlorophene absorption. Systemic toxicity may be manifested by signs of CNS irritation.

Use in pregnancy: Safety not established.

PRECAUTIONS

Suds entering eyes accidentally should be rinsed out promptly and thoroughly with water. Do not use in case of deep puncture wounds, serious burns. If redness, irritation, swelling, or pain persists or increases, or if infection occurs, discontinue use.

ADVERSE REACTIONS

Dermatitis, photosensitivity. In those with highly sensitive skin, use may produce a reaction characterized by redness and/or mild scaling or dryness.

ACCIDENTAL INGESTION

Symptoms: 30 ml to 120 ml has caused anorexia, vomiting, abdominal cramps, diarrhea, dehydration, convulsions, hypotension, shock; fatalities have been reported.

Treatment: If symptoms are seen early, evacuate stomach by emesis or lavage. Administer 60 ml of olive oil or vegetable oil to delay absorption, followed by a saline cathartic to hasten removal. Treatment is symptomatic and supportive. IV fluids (5% Dextrose in Normal Saline) may be given for dehydration. Correct electrolyte imbalance. If marked hypotension occurs, vasopressor therapy is indicated. Opiates may be used if GI symptoms are severe.

DOSAGE

Surgical wash or scrub: As indicated.

Bacteriostatic cleansing: Squeeze ½ tsp to 1 tsp into palm, add water, work up lather, apply to area to be cleansed. Rinse thoroughly after each washing.

Infant care: Do not use routinely for bathing. Use of baby skin products containing alcohol may decrease antibacterial action.

NURSING IMPLICATIONS

See p 145.

Iodine otc

solution: 2% iodine and 2.4% sodium iodide	Iodine Topical Solution
solution: 5% iodine and 10% potassium iodide	Strong Iodine Solution (Lugol's Solution)
tincture: 2% iodine and 2.4% sodium iodide in 50% alcohol	Iodine Tincture
tincture: 7% iodine and 5% potassium iodide in 85% alcohol	Strong Iodine Tincture

INDICATIONS

Externally for broad microbicidal spectrum against bacteria, fungi, viruses, protozoa, yeasts. Solution and tincture may be used to disinfect skin preoperatively.

DOSAGE
Apply to affected area.

CONTRAINDICATIONS
Hypersensitivity.

NURSING IMPLICATIONS
See p 145.

Povidone-Iodine _otc_

ointment; prep solution; skin cleanser; solution, swabsticks; solution, prep swabs	ACU-dyne
aerosol; gauze pads; lubricating gel; mouthwash/gargle; ointment; perineal wash concentrate; skin cleanser; skin cleanser foam; solution; solution, swab aid; solution, swabsticks; surgical scrub; surgi-prep sponge brush; whirlpool concentrate; vaginal gel	Betadine
aerosol; surgical scrub; ointment; perineal wash concentrate; scrub swabsticks; prep solution; solution, prep pads; solution, swabsticks; surgical scrub; whirlpool concentrate	Operand
ointment; perineal wash; skin cleanser; solution; solution, swabs; solution, swabsticks; spray; surgical scrub; surgical scrub sponge/brush; whirlpool concentrate	Pharmadine
cleansing bar; ointment; scrub; solution; solution, swabsticks; solution, wipes; whirlpool concentrate	Povadyne

ACTIONS
Water-soluble complex of iodine with povidone, which liberates approximately 10% free iodine. It retains the germicidal activity of iodine without irritation to skin and mucous membranes. Unlike iodine, treated areas may be bandaged or taped.

PRECAUTIONS
If irritation, redness, or swelling develops, discontinue use. Do not use, or use with caution, in those with history of iodine sensitivity.

DOSAGE
Apply as ordered.
  Vaginal gel: 1 applicator full nightly.

NURSING IMPLICATIONS
See p 145.

Merbromin _(25% Mercury, 20% Bromine)_ _otc_

solution: 2%	_Generic_ (as Mercurochrome)

INDICATIONS
General antiseptic; first-aid prophylactic.

PRECAUTIONS
Prolonged use or use on extensive areas should be under direction of physician.

ADMINISTRATION
Cleanse injury with soap and water; apply freely and continue to use until injury is healed.

NURSING IMPLICATIONS
See p 145.

Thimerosal _otc_

tincture: 1:1000	Mersol, Merthiolate, _Generic_
solution: 1:1000	Merthiolate, _Generic_
aerosol: 1:1000	Aeroaid Thimerosal, Merthiolate

INDICATIONS
  Aerosol: First aid; treatment of contaminated wounds after appropriate cleansing; antisepsis of intact skin; pustular dermatoses; dermatomycoses; preoperative, postoperative use.
  Solution: Use when tincture is contraindicated. A 1:5000 dilution may be used in the eye, nose, throat, or genitourinary tract.
  Tincture: Antisepsis of skin prior to surgery; first-aid treatment of contaminated wounds; antifungal agent in athlete's foot infection.

CONTRAINDICATIONS
Hypersensitivity.

ACTIONS
An organomercurial (49% mercury) antiseptic with sustained bacteriostatic and fungistatic activity.

PRECAUTIONS
Allow tincture to dry before covering with occlusive dressing. Avoid prolonged repeated application in mouths of infants. Thimerosal is incompatible with strong acids, salts of heavy metals, potassium permanganate, and iodine and should not be used in combination with or immediately following their application. Do not use when aluminum may come into contact with treated skin. May be used with or following soaps or sulfonamides.

OVERDOSAGE
Rare instances of mercury poisoning have been reported. After accidental ingestion of the tincture, account must be taken of alcohol and acetone content. After ingestion of the solution, account must be taken of the borate content. Treatment is supportive.

DOSAGE
Apply locally 1 to 3 times/day.

▎ NURSING IMPLICATIONS
See p 145.

Silver Nitrate (AgNO₃) Rx

ophthalmic solution: *Generic*
   1%
solution: 10%, 25%,   *Generic*
   50%

INDICATIONS
   1% solution: Prevention of gonorrheal ophthalmia neonatorum.
   10%, 25%, 50% solutions
   Use to treat indolent wounds, destroy exuberant granulations, touch the bases of vesicular, bullous, or aphthous lesions, and provide styptic action.
   10% solution: Impetigo vulgaris; pruritus. *Podiatry*—Helomas.
   25% solution: Pruritus.   *Podiatry*—Plantar warts.
   50% solution: Podiatry—Plantar warts; granulation tissue; papillomatous growths; granuloma pyogenicum.
   Unlabeled uses: Concentrations of 0.1% to 0.5% are used as wet dressings in burns and on lesions.

CONTRAINDICATIONS
Do not apply to wounds, cuts, or broken skin.

ACTIONS
1% solution is anti-infective. Silver nitrate is a strong caustic and escharotic providing antiseptic, astringent, germicidal, or caustic action externally. Germicidal action is due to precipitation of bacterial proteins by liberated silver ions.

WARNINGS
1% solution must be used with caution because cauterization of the cornea and blindness may result, especially with repeated applications. Is caustic and irritating to skin and mucous membranes.
   Prolonged or frequent use may result in permanent discoloration of the skin owing to deposition of reduced silver. However, topical silver nitrate for localized application as compresses on limited or extensive skin areas apparently does not produce argyria.
   Will stain clothing and linens.
   If wet dressings are used over extensive areas or prolonged periods, electrolyte abnormalities can result. Sodium and chloride leach into the dressing and hyponatremia or hypochloremia can occur. Absorbed nitrate can cause methemoglobinemia.

PRECAUTIONS
Handle solutions carefully because they stain skin, clothing, and utensils. Discontinue use if redness or irritation occurs.

ADVERSE REACTIONS
Mild chemical conjunctivitis should result from a properly performed Credé prophylaxis using silver nitrate. Chemical conjunctivitis occurs in 20% or fewer cases.

OVERDOSAGE
Highly toxic to GI tract and CNS when ingested. Swallowing can cause severe gastroenteritis that may be fatal. The fatal dose of silver nitrate may be as low as 2 g.
   Symptoms: The oral intake of silver nitrate causes a local corrosive effect including pain and burning of the mouth, salivation, vomiting, and diarrhea progressing to anuria, shock, coma, convulsions, and death. Blackening of the skin and mucous membranes occurs (sometimes permanent).
   Treatment: Administer sodium chloride in water, 10 g/liter; this causes precipitation of silver chloride. Follow with catharsis, including sodium chloride solution. Also attend to shock and methemoglobinemia if present.

If splashed in the eyes, wash copiously with water.

DOSAGE

1% solution: Immediately after birth, clean eyelids with sterile absorbent cotton or gauze and sterile water. Use a separate pledget for each eye; wash the unopened lids from the nose outward until free of all blood, mucus, or meconium. Separate the lids and instill 2 drops of 1% solution into eye. Separate the lids and elevate away from the eyeball so that a lake of silver nitrate may lie for 30 seconds or longer between them, coming into contact with every portion of the conjunctival sac. Irrigation of the eyes following instillation is *not* recommended.

10%, 25%, 50% solutions: Apply a cotton applicator dipped in solution on the affected area or lesion 2 or 3 times a week for 2 or 3 eeks as needed.

NURSING IMPLICATIONS
See this page.

Silver Protein, Mild *Rx, otc*

solution: 20%	Argyrol S.S. 20% (*Rx*)
solution: 10%	Argyrol S.S. 10% (*otc*)
powder for solution	*Generic (otc)*

INDICATIONS
20% solution used preoperatively in eye surgery and eye infections. *Other forms*—topical or local application in mild inflammatory conditions of eye, ear, nose, throat, rectum, urethra, vagina.

CONTRAINDICATIONS
Hypersensitivity.

ACTIONS
Has antimicrobial action against gram-positive and gram-negative organisms. When used prior to eye surgery, it stains and coagulates mucus.

WARNINGS
Safety and efficacy for use in children not established. Use in pregnant women only if clearly needed. It is not known whether drug is excreted in human milk.

PRECAUTIONS
Not for prolonged use.

ADVERSE REACTIONS
Prolonged or frequent use may result in permanent discoloration of skin, conjunctiva (argyria).

DOSAGE
Preoperatively, 2 to 3 drops of 20% solution in eye, rinsed out with sterile irrigating solution. *Eye infections*—1 to 3 drops q3h to q4h for several days. Other forms applied as directed on label or as directed by physician.

NURSING IMPLICATIONS: ANTISEPTICS AND GERMICIDES

ADMINISTRATION
Use, instill, or apply as directed by physician or on label of product. See also individual drug monographs.

Antiseptic or germicidal solutions kept at the bedside must be clearly labeled with name of drugs and strength. Replace hard-to-read or soiled, stained labels immediately.

CLINICAL ALERT: Caution is advised in keeping antiseptic or germicidal solutions at the bedsides of children, the elderly, or confused patients because the solution, even though labeled and colored, could be mistaken for water or another beverage and ingested.

Dilution of solutions or making solutions from powders: Usually prepared by hospital or dispensing pharmacist. Nurses preparing solutions from powders or diluting solutions must check calculations carefully; if there is any doubt, check with a pharmacist.

BENZALKONIUM CHLORIDE
Do not apply occlusive dressings following use.

IODINE TINCTURE OR SOLUTION
May impart a permanent stain to clothing; stains on the skin disappear with time. Protect patient's and own clothing. Do not apply occlusive dressings following use of iodine tincture or strong iodine solution.

POVIDONE-IODINE
Does not permanently stain skin or clothing; discoloration can be removed with soap and water.

SILVER COMPOUNDS
Impart a permanent stain to clothing, bedding, utensils, metal (including jewelry). Take precautions to protect patient's and own personal belongings and clothing when using these products. Remove rings, watches, articles of clothing that are near area of application. Staining of skin, although not permanent, must wear off; washing or rubbing area is usually ineffective.

Use only the ophthalmic solution of silver nitrate for eye instillation.

If silver is accidentally spilled on face of newborn infant following Credé prophylaxis, explain stain to parents (see above).

Storage (silver nitrate ophthalmic solution): Room temperature. Do not freeze. Do not use ampules when cold; protect from light. Supplied in wax ampules.

PATIENT AND FAMILY INFORMATION

Follow directions for use as stated on label or as directed by physician.

Do not use on areas other than those specified on the label or by the physician.

Keep away from eyes (unless product is recommended or prescribed for use in eye); wash eyes immediately with copious amounts of water if solution accidentaly enters them. Contact physician if burning, redness, discomfort, blurred vision, or pain persists for more than a few minutes.

See a physician if pain, redness, or signs of infection occur or, if product is used to treat an infection, the infection persists.

Discontinue use if itching, rash, or irritation occurs; if it persists even after use is discontinued, see a physician.

BAC vaginal gel: Complete full course of therapy. Notify physician if burning or irritation occurs. Avoid douches containing soap.

Antithyroid Agents*

Methimazole Rx

tablets: 5 mg, 10 mg   Tapazole

Propylthiouracil *(PTU)* Rx

tablets: 50 mg   *Generic*

INDICATIONS

Hyperthyroidism. Long-term therapy may lead to remission of the disease. May also be used to ameliorate hyperthyroidism in preparation for subtotal thyroidectomy or radioactive iodine therapy. Propylthiouracil (PTU) may be used when thyroidectomy is contraindicated.

CONTRAINDICATIONS

Hypersensitivity; nursing mothers.

---

* Antithyroid agents include methimazole, propylthiouracil, and sodium iodide I^{131}. This discussion concerns methimazole and propylthiouracil. Sodium iodide I^{131} is discussed separately.

ACTIONS

Inhibit the synthesis of thyroid hormones. They do not inactivate existing thyroxine (T_4) and triiodothyronine (T_3), which are stored in colloid or circulate in the blood, nor do they interfere with the effectiveness of exogenous thyroid hormones. PTU is reported to inhibit partially the conversion of T_4 to T_3.

WARNINGS

These drugs are effective in treatment of hyperthyroidism complicated by pregnancy. They readily cross placental membranes and can induce goiter and even cretinism in the developing fetus. It is important that a sufficient, but not excessive, dose be given. In many pregnant women, thyroid dysfunction diminishes as pregnancy proceeds, making dose reduction possible. In some instances, these drugs can be withdrawn 2 to 3 weeks before delivery. Concomitant administration of thyroid during antithyroid therapy of pregnant hyperthyroid women is recommended in order to prevent hypothyroidism in the mother and fetus. Administration should continue throughout pregnancy and delivery. Postpartum patients receiving antithyroid agents should not breast-feed their infants.

PRECAUTIONS

Patient should be under close surveillance and cautioned to report any evidence of illness, particularly sore throat, skin eruptions, fever, headache, or general malaise. If these occur, a WBC and differential are usually ordered to determine whether agranulocytosis has developed. Care is exercised with patients receiving additional drugs known to cause agranulocytosis.

Serious reactions are indications for permanently discontinuing the drug. Mild reactions may require dosage reduction or temporary discontinuation of the drug. PTU may cause hypoprothrombinemia and bleeding; the prothrombin time should be monitored during therapy, especially before surgical procedures.

DRUG INTERACTIONS

The activity of **anticoagulants** may be potentiated by anti-vitamin-K activity attributed to propylthiouracil.

ADVERSE REACTIONS

Agranulocytosis is the most serious effect. Rarely, exfoliative dermatitis, hepatitis, neuropathies, or CNS stimulation or depression are seen. Adverse reactions probably occur in fewer than 3% of patients.

Minor reactions: Skin rash; urticaria; abnormal

loss of hair; pruritus; skin pigmentation; nausea, vomiting; epigastric distress; loss of taste; jaundice; arthralgia; myalgia; paresthesia; neuritis; headache; vertigo; drowsiness; edema; sialadenopathy; lymphadenopathy.

Major reactions: Inhibition of myelopoiesis (agranulocytosis, granulocytopenia, thrombocytopenia); hypoprothrombinemia; bleeding; vasculitis; exfoliative dermatitis; lupuslike syndrome; periarteritis; drug fever; hepatitis, which has been fatal; nephrotic syndrome; nephritis.

OVERDOSAGE

Symptoms: Nausea, vomiting; epigastric distress; headache; fever; arthralgia; puritus; edema; pancytopenia. Prolonged therapy may result in hypothyroidism.

Treatment: Discontinue drug in presence of agranulocytosis, pancytopenia, hepatitis, fever, or exfoliative dermatitis. For bone-marrow depression, use antibiotic and transfusion of fresh whole blood. A corticosteroid may be prescribed. For hepatitis, rest and adequate diet and, in severe cases, corticosteroid therapy may be indicated. General management may consist of symptomatic and supportive therapy including rest, analgesics, gastric lavage, IV fluids, and mild sedation.

DOSAGE
METHIMAZOLE

Adults: Initial daily dose is 15 mg for mild hyperthyroidism, 30 mg to 40 mg for moderately severe hyperthyroidism, and 60 mg for severe hyperthyroidism, in 3 doses at 8-hour intervals. Maintenance dose is 5 mg/day to 15 mg/day.

Pediatric: Initially, daily dosage is 0.4 mg/kg divided into 3 doses at 8-hour intervals. Maintenance dose is approximately one-half the initial dose.

PROPYLTHIOURACIL (PTU)

Adults: Initial dose is 300 mg/day. In those with severe hyperthyroidism, very large goiters, or both, initial dose is usually 400 mg/day; an occasional patient may require 600 mg/day to 900 mg/day initially. Maintenance daily dose is usually 100 mg/day to 150 mg/day.

Children: *6 to 10 years*—initial dose is 50 mg/day to 150 mg/day; *10 or older*—initial dose is 150 mg/day to 300 mg/day. Maintenance dosage is determined by patient response.

NURSING IMPLICATIONS

HISTORY
See Appendix 4.

PHYSICAL ASSESSMENT
Hyperthyroidism: Record vital signs, weight; note presence of overt signs of hyperthyroidism (*e.g.,* nervousness, fine tremor of hands, visible enlargment in the thyroid area, skin changes [usually warm, moist, flushed], eyes [exophthalmos]); review previous laboratory, diagnostic tests (if available). Baseline laboratory tests may include T_3 and T_4 uptake, serum cholesterol, CBC. Baseline diagnostic tests may include radioactive iodine uptake, thyroid ultrasonography.

ADMINISTRATION
Drug is taken at 8-hour intervals around the clock.

Patient with an enlarged thyroid may have difficulty swallowing medication; if this occurs, discuss problem with physician before attempting to crush tablet or administer with food.

ONGOING ASSESSMENTS AND NURSING MANAGEMENT
Record vital signs q4h or as ordered (physician may order sleeping pulse rate).

Observe and record patient's overt symptoms because dosage may need to be adjusted upward or downward, according to clinical response.

Observe for adverse drug effects.

Weigh weekly or at time of each clinical or office visit. Weight gain may be seen several weeks after initiation of therapy.

Observe for inhibition of myelopoiesis; symptoms that may be noted are easy bruising, signs of infection (fever, cough, sore throat), malaise; report symptoms promptly.

Several months may be required for development of a euthyroid state. Therapy may be continued for up to 2 years.

If drug is administered preoperatively for thyroidectomy, Strong Iodine Solution (Lugol's Solution) may be added to the therapeutic regimen. Iodine reduces friability and vascularity of the thyroid and may decrease incidence of intraoperative and postoperative hemorrhage.

Long-term therapy: Physician will monitor drug effectiveness by periodic thyroid-function tests and evaluation of symptoms, weight, and blood pressure. The prothrombin time may also be monitored.

Once a euthyroid state is achieved, low doses of thyroid hormone may be prescribed to suppress thyroid-stimulating hormone (TSH) production and to prevent or treat hypothyroidism that may occur as a result of antithyroid therapy.

A hypothyroid state may develop insidiously during long-term antithyroid therapy.

Do not take drug in larger doses, more frequently, or for a longer time than specifically directed. Take at regular intervals around the clock (usually q8h) unless physician directs otherwise.

Notify physician or nurse promptly if fever, sore throat, unusual bleeding or bruising, headache, or general malaise occurs.

Record weight twice a week or as directed by physician. Take pulse daily (patient may need instruction) and record. Bring record of weight and pulse rate to each office or clinic visit.

Avoid use of nonprescription drugs unless approved by physician.

Antitoxins and Antivenins

These preparations contain antitoxic substances derived from the blood of horses immunized against specific toxins and are used for passive immunization. The following general information applies to all antitoxins and antivenins. For specific indications and dosage guidelines refer to individual drug monographs below.

WARNINGS

Parenteral administration of any biological product requires that every precaution be taken to prevent or arrest allergic or other untoward reactions. A careful history should review possible sensitivity to the type of protein injected.

PRECAUTIONS

Before administering any product containing horse serum, obtain a complete history of previous injections and any allergic manifestations that occurred. A test for sensitivity to horse serum is usually performed. When possible, both the conjunctival and intracutaneous scratch tests are performed in every patient prior to each administration of foreign serum, regardless of clinical history. Negative tests are usually reliable but do not completely rule out systemic sensitivity. Manufacturer's recommendations vary on sensitivity testing; package literature is consulted prior to use of a specific product.

ADVERSE REACTIONS

Systemic reactions: Acute anaphylaxis characterized by sudden onset of urticaria, respiratory distress, vascular collapse, and serum sickness (usually appearing 7 to 12 days after administration) with symptoms of lymphadenopathy, polyarthritis, arthralgias, skin rash, fever, and so on may develop. Serum sickness is largely related to the amount of

horse serum administered, hypersensitivity of the patient, and history of previous serum injection.

Location reactions: Local pain or local erythema and urticaria without constitutional disturbance may occur 7 to 10 days after administration and may last for 2 days.

Diphtheria Antitoxin Rx

injection: 20,000 units/vial	Diphtheria Antitoxin-Connaught
injection: 10,000 units/vial, 20,000 units/vial	*Generic*

INDICATIONS

Prevention and treatment of diphtheria; neutralizes the toxins produced by *Corynebacterium diphtheriae.*

DOSAGE

Administer IM or by slow IV infusion. Antitoxin may be warmed to 90°F to 95°F.

Therapeutic regimen: Any person with clinical symptoms of diphtheria should receive diphtheria antitoxin at once, without waiting for bacteriologic confirmation of diagnosis. Treatment should be continued until all local and general symptoms are controlled or some other etiologic agent is identified.

Sensitivity tests are performed.

Required antitoxin is given IM or IV, at once. Each hour's delay increases dosage requirement and decreases beneficial effects.

Suggested dosage ranges—Pharyngeal or laryngeal disease of 48 hours duration, 20,000 to 40,000 units; nasopharyngeal lesions, 40,000 to 60,000 units; extensive disease of 3 or more days' duration or in any patient with brawny swelling of the neck, 80,000 to 120,000 units.

Children are given same dose as adults.

Administration of antimicrobial agents is recommended.

Prophylactic regimen: All asymptomatic, unimmunized contacts of patients with diphtheria should receive prompt prophylaxis with appropriate antimicrobial therapy, with cultures before and after treatment. Immunize with diphtheria toxoid (p 567) and continue surveillance for 7 days. Close contacts not under surveillance should receive appropriate antimicrobial therapy and immunization with toxoid and diphtheria antitoxin. If sensitivity test is negative, administer 10,000 units IM. Dose also depends on length of time since exposure, extent of exposure, and medical condition of the patient.

NURSING IMPLICATIONS
See p 150.

Tetanus Antitoxin Rx

injection: 1500 units/   *Generic*
   vial, 20,000 units/
   vial

INDICATIONS
Tetanus immune globulin is preferred for the prevention and treatment of tetanus (see Immunizations). Tetanus antitoxin should be used only when tetanus immune globulin is not available. Antitoxin may be used for passive immunization and prevention of tetanus. Prophylactic doses should be given to those who have had fewer than two previous injections of tetanus toxoid if the wound is untended for more than 24 hours. Concomitant administration of tetanus antitoxin and tetanus toxoid adsorbed is indicated for those who must receive an immediate injection of tetanus antitoxin and for whom it is desirable to begin a process of active immunization.

DOSAGE
Prophylaxis: Usually 1500 to 5000 units IM or subcutaneously, according to body weight. Protection lasts about 15 days or less.

Treatment: Usually given as single dose of about 50,000 to 100,000 units. Preferably, part of the dose is given IV and the remainder IM.

NURSING IMPLICATIONS
See p 150.

Antivenin (Crotalidae) Polyvalent Rx

injection   *Generic*

INDICATIONS
Capable of neutralizing toxic effects of crotalids (pit vipers) native to North, Central, and South America, including rattlesnakes (*Crotalus, Sistrurus*); copperhead and cottonmouth moccasins (*Agkistrodon*), *A. halys* of Korea and Japan; the Fer-de-lance and other species of *Bothrops;* the tropical rattler (*C. durissus* and similar species); the Cantil (*A. bilineatus*); and the bushmaster (*Lachesis mutus*).

PIT VIPER BITES AND ENVENOMATION
Symptoms, signs, and severity of snake-venom poisoning depend on many factors including species; age and size of snake; number and location of bites; depth of venom deposit; condition of snake's fangs and venom glands; length of time snake "hangs on"; age, general health, and size of the victim; type of clothing around the bite area; type and efficacy of first treatment rendered and how soon treatment was applied.

Local signs and symptoms: Edema is usually seen around the bite area within 5 minutes. It may progress rapidly and involve the entire extremity within an hour. Generally, edema spreads more slowly, usually over a period of 8 or more hours. Ecchymosis and discoloration of the skin often appear in the bite area within a few hours. Vesicles may form in a few hours and are usually present in 24 hours. Hemorrhagic blebs and petechiae are common. Necrosis may develop, necessitating amputation. Pain frequently begins shortly after the bite (pain may be absent after bites by Mojave rattlers).

Systemic signs and symptoms: Weakness; faintness; nausea; sweating; numbness or tingling around the mouth, tongue, scalp, fingers, toes, bite area; muscle fasciculations; hypotension; prolongation of bleeding and clotting times; hemoconcentration followed by decrease in erythrocytes; thrombocytopenia; hematuria; proteinuria; vomiting, including hematemesis; melena; hemoptysis; epistaxis. In fatal poisoning, death is usually due to destruction of erythrocytes and changes in capillary permeability, especially in the pulmonary system, leading to pulmonary edema.

DOSAGE
IV administration is preferred; to be most effective, antivenin should be administered within 4 hours of bite.

Recommended initial doses: Minimal envenomation—2 to 4 vials; *moderate envenomation*—5 to 9 vials; *severe envenomation*—10 to 15 vials.

IM administration: Administer into large muscle mass, preferably the gluteal area.

Children: Dosage is not based on weight. Envenomation by large snakes in children or small adults requires larger doses of antivenin.

NURSING IMPLICATIONS
See p 150.

Antivenin (Micrurus Fulvius)
(North American Coral Snake Antivenin) Rx

injection   *Generic*

INDICATIONS
Neutralization of venom of *M. fulvius fulvius* (eastern coral snake) and *M. fulvius tenere* (Texas coral snake). Will *Not* neutralize venom of *M. euryxanthus* (Arizona or Sonoran coral snake).

ENVENOMATION

Coral-snake venom is chiefly neurotoxic (paralytic) and usually causes only minimal to moderate tissue reaction and pain. Symptoms begin 1 to 7 hours after the bite but may be delayed for as long as 18 hours. Symptoms may progress rapidly and precipitously. Paralysis has been observed 2½ hours after the bite and appears to be of a bulbar type, involving cranial motor nerves. Death from respiratory paralysis has occurred within 4 hours of the bite.

Systemic signs and symptoms: Euphoria, lethargy, weakness, nausea, vomiting, excessive salivation, ptosis of eyelids, dyspnea, abnormal reflexes, convulsions, and motor weakness or paralysis, including respiratory paralysis.

Local signs and symptoms: No edema to moderate edema, erythema, pain at the bite area, paresthesia in the bitten extremity.

Supportive therapy: Tetanus prophylaxis. Morphine or any narcotics that depress respiration are contraindicated; use sedatives with extreme caution.

DOSAGE

Given promptly by IV route. Start IV drip of 250 ml to 500 ml of Sodium Chloride Injection, USP immediately; then test for horse-serum sensitivity. If patient is not sensitive to horse serum, contents of 3 to 5 vials are administered by slow IV injection directly into tubing or by addition to the reservoir bottle of the IV drip. The first 1 ml or 2 ml are injected over 3 to 5 minutes. If no anaphylaxis occurs, injection is continued. Some patients may require 10 or more vials to neutralize the venom.

▌ NURSING IMPLICATIONS

See this page.

Antivenin (Latrodectus Mactans)

(Black Widow Spider Antivenin) Rx

injection   *Generic*

INDICATIONS

Treatment of symptoms of black-widow-spider bites. Early use is emphasized for prompt relief.

ENVENOMATION

Symptoms include muscle cramps, beginning from 15 minutes to several hours after the bite. Exact sequence of symptoms depends on location of bite. Venom acts on the myoneural junctions or nerve endings, causing ascending paralysis or destruction of peripheral nerve endings. Muscles most frequently affected are thigh, shoulder, and back muscles. Later, pain becomes more severe, spreading to

the abdomen; weakness and tremor usually develop. The abdominal muscles assume a boardlike rigidity, but tenderness is slight. Other symptoms include thoracic respirations, restlessness, feeble pulse, cold clammy skin, labored breathing and speech, light stupor, delirium, and convulsions. The temperature may be elevated. Urinary retention, shock, cyanosis, nausea, vomiting, insomnia, and cold sweats have been reported. Symptoms increase in severity for several hours up to a day and then slowly become less severe. Residual symptoms such as weakness, tingling, nervousness, and transient muscle spasms may persist for weeks or months.

Supportive therapy: Prolonged warm baths; IV injection of 10 ml of 10% solution of calcium gluconate repeated as necessary to control muscle pain. Morphine may be required and barbiturates used for extreme restlessness; neurotoxicity (respiratory paralysis) of venom must be considered when administering these drugs. Corticosteroids may be used. In healthy patients between the ages of 16 and 60, use of antivenin may be deferred and treatment with muscle relaxants considered.

DOSAGE

Adults and children—1 vial of antivenin. It may be given IM in the region of the anterolateral thigh, so that a tourniquet may be applied in case of a systemic reaction. Symptoms usually subside in 1 to 3 hours. A second dose may be necessary in some cases. Antivenin may also be given IV in 10 ml to 50 ml of saline solution over a 15-minute period. This route is preferred in severe cases, children under 12, and patients in shock.

▌ NURSING IMPLICATIONS: ANTITOXINS AND ANTIVENINS

HISTORY

Allergy history is important before antitoxin or antivenin is administered; however, because the situation often is an emergency, inquire whether the patient has *any* known allergies. The physician will decide on the relevance of information.

Snake or spider envenomation: Record symptoms, location of bite, time interval since bite, description of snake or spider (if seen), health history.

Injury requiring tetanus antitoxin: Record type and location of injury, where injury occurred, health history.

Diphtheria: Record description and duration of symptoms or history of exposure to diphtheria, health history.

PHYSICAL ASSESSMENT

Snake or spider envenomation: Record vital signs; assess neurologic, respiratory, and cardiovascular systems (see _Envenomation_). If bite is by _Crotalidae_ (rattlesnake), immediately draw sufficient blood (from uninvolved extremity) for laboratory studies; type and cross-match, CBC, hematocrit, platelet count, prothrombin time, clot retraction, bleeding and coagulation times, BUN, electrolytes, bilirubin recommended for baseline studies.

Injury requiring tetanus antitoxin: Record vital signs; examine wounds; note debris present in and around wound. If antitoxin will be used to treat tetanus, document symptoms.

Diphtheria: Record vital signs, assess for signs of upper respiratory obstruction. Examination of nasopharyngeal, laryngeal areas is usually performed by physician.

ADMINISTRATION

Read package inserts of drug carefully; follow manufacturer's directions about preparation, dilution, and administration of antitoxin or antivenin.

Have equipment available for respiratory support.

Sensitivity test will be performed prior to administration of antitoxin or antivenin.

Epinephrine injection 1:1000, a tourniquet, and needle and syringe should be immediately available when sensitivity test is performed and also when antitoxin or antivenin is administered.

Closely observe patient during and after administration of antivenin. Monitor blood pressure, pulse, and respirations q15m or as ordered; be alert to symptoms of shock, respiratory distress.

ONGOING ASSESSMENTS AND NURSING MANAGEMENT

Diphtheria antitoxin

Prophylaxis: Appropriate antimicrobial therapy, with bacterial cultures before and after prophylaxis, is recommended. Advise patient to take antimicrobial agent as directed by physician and return as requested for further surveillance.

Treatment of diphtheria: Record vital signs q2h to q4h or as ordered; observe patient for signs of respiratory obstruction. Tracheostomy is usually performed if respiratory distress is present.

Tetanus antitoxin

Prophylaxis: Observe patient for development of tetanus and sensitivity reactions to antitoxin. Monitor vital signs q4h or as ordered.

Treatment: Development of tetanus requires

intensive nursing care. Physician's orders usually include IV fluids, drug therapy (_e.g.,_ antibiotics, muscle relaxants), and observations and therapies based on the severity of the disease.

Antivenin (Crotalidae) polyvalent for rattlesnake envenomation

Monitor blood pressure, pulse, and respirations q5m to q15m or as ordered; obtain urine samples at frequent intervals for microscopic examination for erythrocytes (patient may require indwelling catheter); measure intake and output, IV fluids (use Y-tubing). Measure the circumference of the bitten extremity proximal to the bite and at one or more additional points, each several inches closer to the trunk; repeat measurements q15m to q30m to monitor progression of edema. Have available oxygen, resuscitation equipment, airway, tourniquet, epinephrine, parenteral antihistamines, and corticosteroids. Shock will be treated with whole blood, plasma, albumin, plasma expanders, and so on. Use one IV line for supportive therapy and the other for administration of antivenin and electrolytes.

Antivenin (Micrurus fulvius) for coral snake envenomation

If possible, immobilize victim completely to prevent spread of venom; IV fluids (use Y-tubing); monitor blood pressure, pulse, and respiration q30m or as ordered. Response to IV injection of antivenin may be rapid and dramatic. The patient is kept under observation as directed by physician.

Antivenin (Latrodectus mactans) for black widow spider envenomation

Monitor blood pressure, pulse, and respirations q30m or as ordered; observe for respiratory paralysis; may require IV fluids, analgesics, sedatives. Muscle relaxants may also be administered.

Apomorphine Hydrochloride Rx

tablets, soluble: 6 mg   _Generic_

INDICATIONS

Centrally acting emetic. Results are usually obtained within 10 to 15 minutes after parenteral administration.

CONTRAINDICATIONS AND PRECAUTIONS

Do not use in impending shock; corrosive-poisoning cases; narcosis due to opiates, barbiturates, alchol, or other CNS depressants; patients too inebriated to stand unaided; unconscious patients; those having ingested petroleum distillates (kerosene, paint thinner, cleaning fluid, gasoline). Use with caution in children, debilitated individuals, those with cardiac decompensation, and persons predisposed to nausea and vomiting.

ADVERSE REACTIONS
Therapeutic doses may cause CNS depression; at times, euphoria, tachypnea, restlessness, and tremors may be produced. Peripheral vascular collapse has been reported. Dangerous depression (even death) may occur when used in patients in shock (from corrosive poisons) or those narcotized from overdoses of opiates, barbiturates, alcohol, or other CNS depressants. Excessive doses may cause violent emesis, cardiac depression, and death.

DOSAGE
Adults—5 mg subcutaneously (dosage ranges between 2 mg and 10 mg). *Children*—70 mcg/kg to 100 mcg/kg subcutaneously. *Do not repeat.*

NURSING IMPLICATIONS

HISTORY
Obtain name and amount of substance(s) ingested. History (Appendix 4) is important but often unobtainable because of condition of patient and emergency situation.

PHYSICAL ASSESSMENT
Record blood pressure, pulse, and respirations; check for odor of alcohol on breath, clothes. When ingested substance is unknown, assess oral cavity for signs of corrosive-substance ingestion because emetic would be contraindicated. Evaluate CNS (*e.g.,* level of consciousness, pupil size and equality, reaction to light).

ADMINISTRATION
Physician may order administration of activated charcoal before or after administration of apomorphine.

Drug given subcutaneously only.

Administration of oral fluids immediately after administration facilitates emetic action of drug. *Recommended for adults*—200 ml to 300 ml of water or (preferably) evaporated milk; for children, use smaller amounts. Physician must give a specific order for amount and type of oral fluid to be administered.

Gently bouncing a small child may produce earlier emetic effects.

Position patient on his side before or immediately after administration of drug to prevent aspiration of vomitus.

Have available suction machine, emesis basin, towels, and laboratory specimen bottles (physician may request laboratory analysis of emesis).

Soluble (hypo) tablets are dissolved in 1 ml to 2 ml of 0.9% sodium chloride for injection or sterile water for injection. Because resulting solution should be sterilized by filtration (not by heat) prior to use, solution is usually prepared by a pharmacist. Prepared solutions are labeled and dated and are stable for 48 hours when protected from light and kept under refrigeration.

Check label of previously prepared solutions for expiration date and time (48 hours); do not use if expired or if solution is discolored or contains a precipitate.

Monitor blood pressure, pulse, and respirations every 5 minutes while waiting for evacuation of stomach by emesis.

Protect tablets from light; keep in tightly closed bottles. This preparation changes with age; discoloration may occur.

ONGOING ASSESSMENTS AND NURSING MANAGEMENT
Vomiting usually occurs 5 to 15 minutes after administration. Be prepared to suction patient prn to prevent aspiration of vomitus.

Obtain nasogastric tube and activated charcoal because further treatment may be necessary if drug fails to produce emesis sufficient to empty stomach.

Naloxone may be used to terminate violent, protracted vomiting or to counteract CNS and respiratory depression.

Save all emesis for physician's inspection or laboratory analysis.

Continue observations for signs of respiratory or CNS depression for 2 or more hours after emesis is produced.

Aprobarbital

See Barbiturates.

Aromatic Ammonia Spirit otc

inhalant: 0.33 ml	Aromatic Ammonia Vaporoles, *Generic*
inhalant: 0.4 ml	Aromatic Ammonia Aspirols
solution	*Generic*

INDICATIONS
To prevent or treat fainting.

ACTIONS
A respiratory and circulatory stimulant.

ADMINISTRATION AND DOSAGE
Inhale as needed.

NURSING IMPLICATIONS

ADMINISTRATION
Wrap glass vial in several layers of cloth or gauze
and crush with fingers. If solution is used, pour
on cloth or gauze.
 Place near patient's nose and have him inhale.
 Dispose of material used to wrap ampule.
 Stay with patient until cause of fainting has
been determined.

Ascorbic Acid

See Vitamin C Preparations.

Asparaginase Rx

powder for injection: Elspar
 10,000 IU

INDICATIONS
Therapy for acute lymphocytic leukemia. Useful in
combination with other chemotherapeutic agents in
induction of remissions of disease in children.
Should not be used as sole induction agent unless
combination chemotherapy is deemed inappropriate. The possibility of achieving therapeutic benefit is weighed against the risk of toxicity. Not recommended for maintenance therapy.

CONTRAINDICATIONS
Those who have had anaphylactic reactions to asparaginase or history of pancreatitis. Acute hemorrhagic pancreatitis, sometimes fatal, has occurred
following administration.

ACTIONS
Asparaginase contains the enzyme L-asparagine
amidohydrolase, type EC-2, derived from *Escherichia coli.* In a significant number of patients with
acute (particularly lymphocytic) leukemia, the malignant cells depend on exogenous asparagine for
survival. Normal cells are able to synthesize asparagine and thus are less affected by rapid depletion
produced by treatment with the enzyme asparaginase. This approach to therapy is based on a meta-

bolic defect of asparagine synthesis of some malignant cells. Plasma levels of asparaginase are dose
dependent and show a cumulative effect on repeated administration. Plasma half-life varies from
8 to 30 hours.

WARNINGS
Because of the unpredictability of adverse reactions,
drug is used only in a hospital setting. Hypersensitivity reactions are frequent and may occur during
primary course of therapy. Anaphylaxis and death
have occurred. Once a patient has received asparaginase, there is increased risk of hypersensitivity reactions with retreatment. In those found hypersensitive by skin testing and in any patient previously
under therapy with asparaginase, the drug is instituted or reinstituted only after successful desensitization.
 Hepatotoxicity: Has an adverse effect on hepatic
function. Therapy may increase preexisting hepatic
impairment caused by prior therapy or underlying
disease. Asparaginase may increase the toxicity of
other medications.
 Use in pregnancy and lactation: Use in women
who are or may become pregnant only when potential benefits outweigh the potential hazards to the
fetus.

PRECAUTIONS
The fall in circulating lymphoblasts is often
marked; normal or below-normal leukocyte counts
are noted frequently several days after therapy is instituted. This may be accompanied by a marked
rise in serum uric acid. The possible development
of uric-acid neuropathy is kept in mind and appropriate preventive measures taken (*e.g.,* allopurinol,
increased fluid intake, alkalinization of urine). Asparaginase toxicity is reported to be greater in
adults than in children.

DRUG INTERACTIONS
Administer concurrently with or immediately before
a course of **vincristine** and **prednisone** may be associated with increased toxicity. Asparaginase may diminish or abolish the effect of **methotrexate** on malignant cells, and use of methotrexate with or following asparaginase is not recommended. May also
interfere with enzyme detoxification of **other drugs,**
particularly in the liver.

ADVERSE REACTIONS
 Hypersensitivity: Allergic reactions including skin
rashes, urticaria, arthralgia, respiratory distress, and
acute anaphylaxis have been reported. Acute reactions have occurred in the absence of a positive skin

test and during continued maintenance of therapeutic levels of the drug.

Hyperglycemia: Hyperglycemia, along with glucosuria and polyuria, has been reported. Serum and urine acetone usually are absent or negligible; this syndrome resembles hyperosmolar, nonketotic hyperglycemia induced by a variety of other agents. This complication usually responds to discontinuation of drug and judicious use of IV fluids and insulin, but it may be fatal.

Bleeding: In addition to hypofibrinogenemia, depression of various other clotting factors may occur. Most marked has been a decrease in plasma levels of factors V and VIII with a variable decrease in factors VII and IX. A decrease in platelets has occurred. Fatal bleeding and increased fibrinolytic activity have been reported.

CNS: Depression, somnolence, fatigue, coma, confusion, agitation, hallucinations varying from mild to severe. Rarely, a parkinsonlike syndrome has occurred, with tremor and a progressive increase in muscle tone. These side-effects usually reverse spontaneously after treatment is stopped.

Renal: Azotemia, usually prerenal, occurs frequently. Acute renal shutdown and fatal renal insufficiency have been reported. Proteinuria may occur.

Hepatic: Elevation of SGOT, SGPT, alkaline phosphatase, bilirubin (direct and indirect); depression of serum albumin, cholesterol (total and esters), and plasma fibrinogen. Increases and decreases of total lipids have occurred. Marked hypoalbuminemia associated with peripheral edema has occurred. These abnormalities are usually reversible on discontinuation of therapy and some reversal may occur during the course of therapy. Fatty changes in the liver and the malabsorption syndrome have been reported.

Hematologic: Transient bone-marrow depression, marked leukopenia.

Miscellaneous: Chills, fever, nausea, vomiting, anorexia, abdominal cramps, weight loss, headache, irritability. Fatal hyperthermia has been reported. Pancreatitis, sometimes fulminant, has occurred during or following therapy.

DOSAGE
May be administered IM or IV.

Recommended induction regimens: One of the following combination regimens is recommended for acute lymphocytic leukemia in children. Day 1 is considered to be the first day of therapy.

Regimen I

Prednisone 40 mg/m^2/day PO in 3 divided doses for 15 days, followed by a tapering of dosage as follows: 20 mg/m^2 for 2 days, 10 mg/m^2 for 2 days, 5 mg/m^2 for 2 days, 2.5 mg/m^2 for 2 days, and then discontinue.

Vincristine sulfate 2 mg/m^2 IV once weekly on days 1, 8, and 15 of treatment period. The single maximum dose should not exceed 2 mg.

Asparaginase 1000 IU/kg/day IV for 10 successive days beginning on day 22.

Regimen II

Prednisone 40 mg/m^2/day PO in 3 divided doses for 28 days, followed by gradual discontinuation over a 14-day period.

Vincristine sulfate 1.5 mg/m^2 IV weekly for 4 doses, on days 1, 8, 15, and 22. Maximum single dose should not exceed 2 mg.

Asparaginase 6000 IU/m^2 IM on days 4, 7, 10, 13, 16, 19, 22, 25, and 28. When remission is obtained with either of above regimens, maintenance therapy is instituted.

Intradermal skin test: Because allergic reactions can occur, an intradermal skin test is performed prior to initial administration of asparaginase as well as when asparaginase is given after a week or more has elapsed between doses. An allergic reaction, even to the skin-test dose, in certain patients may occur rarely. A negative skin test does not preclude the possibility of development of an allergic reaction.

Desensitization: May be performed before giving first dose of asparaginase on initiating therapy in positive reactors and on retreatment of any patient in whom such therapy is deemed necessary. Physician will determine the number of injections and dose necesary for desensitization.

NURSING IMPLICATIONS

HISTORY
See Appendix 4.

PHYSICAL ASSESSMENT
Record vital signs; weight; general assessment of present physical status. Baseline laboratory and diagnostic studies may include bone-marrow aspiration, CBC, urinalysis, hepatic- and renal-function tests.

ADMINISTRATION

CLINICAL ALERT: Anaphylactic reactions require immediate use of epinephrine, oxygen, and IV steroids. Check with physician about the specific drugs to be made available and procedure to follow if anaphylaxis occurs. Depending on hospital policy or physician's order, emergency drugs may be prepared in advance and kept at bedside, in medicine room, or in another designated area.

An antiemetic may be administered prior to treatment to alleviate nausea, vomiting.

Record baseline temperature, pulse, respirations, and blood pressure immediately before administration of drug.

Intradermal skin test: Reconstitute 10,000-IU vial with 5 ml of diluent; this will result in 2000 IU/ml. Withdraw 0.1 ml and inject it into another vial containing 9.9 ml of diluent, which will yield 20 IU/ml. Withdraw 0.1 ml of this solution (about 2 IU) for the intradermal skin test. Observe skin-test site for 1 hour for appearance of a wheal or erythema (either indicates positive findings); chart observations.

Preparation of solutions

Visually inspect solution for particulate matter and discoloration prior to administration. Solution should be clear and colorless. If solution is cloudy, discard.

_IV:_ Reconstitute with Sterile Water for Injection or sodium chloride injection. Recommended volume for reconstitution is 5 ml/ 10,000-IU vial. Ordinary shaking during reconstitution does not inactivate the enzyme. As long as solution remains clear, it may be used for direct IV administration within 8 hours after reconstitution. For administration by infusion, solutions should be diluted with isotonic solutions, sodium chloride injection, or 5% dextrose injection. These solutions should be infused within 8 hours and only if clear.

Occasionally, a small number of gelatinous fiberlike particles may develop on standing. Filtration through a 5-micron filter during administration will remove these particles with no loss of potency. Some loss of potency has been seen with use of a 0.2-micron filter. If filter is necessary, check size (as stated on package) before using in IV line.

A running solution of sodium chloride injection or 5% dextrose is recommended. The asparaginase is added to the running solution, usually by piggyback method. Physician will order IV solution type and amount and exact administration procedure.

Drug is given over a period of not less than 30 minutes.

If drug is administered by IV infusion, compute rate of administration in gtt/min before drug is administered.

_IM:_ Reconstitute with 2 ml sodium chloride injection added to 10,000-IU vial. Use within 8 hours and only if clear.

An IV infusion may be ordered prior to IM administration to provide immediate administration of emergency medications, should they be required.

Volume of single injection site should be limited to 2 ml. If volume greater than 2 ml is to be given, two injection sites should be used. Use a separate needle and syringe for each injection.

Storage

Store powder below 8°C (46°F). Store unused reconstituted solution at 2°C to 8°C (36°F to 46°F) and discard after 8 hours, or sooner if cloudy.

Label reconstituted solution with date and time of reconstitution.

ONGOING ASSESSMENTS AND NURSING MANAGEMENT

CLINICAL ALERT: Patient is monitored continuously by physician and nurse during administration of drug. Observe for development of immediate adverse reactions, especially hypersensitivity reactions (_e.g.,_ skin rash, urticaria, arthralgia, respiratory distress, acute anaphylaxis). Monitor blood pressure, pulse, and respirations q10m to q15m or as directed.

Measure intake and output before treatment to establish data base as well as after treatment. Report any decrease in output to physician.

Record vital signs q4h or as ordered; test urine for glucose and ketone bodies qid and record on flow sheet; observe for adverse reactions q2h to q4h.

Assessments for adverse reactions should include observing patient for peripheral, sacral edema; evidence of a bleeding tendency (easy bruising, hematuria, petechiae, melena); decrease in urinary output (when compared with intake); development of sudden abdominal pain, discomfort, nausea, vomiting (may indicate pancreatitis); signs of infection (fever, sore throat, malaise); CNS changes (depression, somnolence, fatigue, coma, confusion, agitation); polydipsia, polyuria, glycosuria, ketonuria.

Document and report all adverse effects to physician immediately.

Encourage increased fluid intake to prevent uric-acid nephropathy; offer liquids q1h (or more often). If patients fails to increase fluid intake, consult physician and dietitian about possible methods of increasing fluid intake.

Allopurinol and alkalinization of the urine may be used to prevent uric-acid nephropathy.

Weigh weekly or as ordered.

Dietary changes may be necessary to prevent or treat uric-acid nephropathy, nausea, vomiting, anorexia, weight loss, edema, hyperglycemia, azotemia.

If bleeding tendencies are noted, apply prolonged pressure on parenteral administration sites, veins used for venipuncture. Inform laboratory personnel performing venipuncture of bleeding tendency.

CNS changes (see above) may require frequent supervision of activities. Extreme confusion or agitation may require restraining measures to protect patient. A physician's order is usually necessary for application of restraining devices.

Other drugs are given with caution because asparaginase may interfere with enzymatic detoxification, particularly in the liver.

Physician usually orders frequent laboratory monitoring of clinical status. Tests may include CBC, urinalysis, hepatic- and renal-function tests, blood ammonia, serum amylase, fasting blood sugar, serum uric acid, PT, PTT, and so on.

Alert the physician to patient or family problems that may require referral to community agencies such as public health, social service, or private support groups formed to help the patient with a malignant disease (and his family).

Emotional support for the patient and family is an integral part of nursing management.

PATIENT AND FAMILY INFORMATION

NOTE: Physician usually explains chemotherapeutic regimen to patient and family. Patient and family should receive full, detailed explanation of possible delayed adverse reactions and symptoms that may indicate pancreatitis (abdominal pain, nausea, vomiting); renal insufficiency (decreased urine output, edema); bone-marrow depression (signs of infection, bleeding tendencies); CNS toxicity; hyperglycemia (polyuria, polydipsia). The name and phone number of the persons to be contacted should adverse reactions occur should be given to patient or family.

Contact physician or nurse immediately if *Any* adverse drug reaction occurs (physician may limit extent of description of drug reactions or include all known adverse drug reactions).

Occurrence of CNS reactions may necessitate restriction of activities requiring alertness.

Frequent laboratory tests will be required for monitoring therapy.

Follow physician's recommendations regarding weight. Report anorexia, weight loss to physician or nurse.

Medication may be prescribed between treatments with asparaginase. The physician should be notified immediately if there is any problem with adhering to the prescribed therapeutic regimen.

The use of all other drugs, including nonprescription preparations, must be avoided unless drug is prescribed or approved by physician supervising chemotherapeutic regimen.

Drink at least 8 to 10 8-oz glasses of liquids per day.

Aspirin

See Salicylates.

Atenolol

See Beta-Adrenergic Blocking Agents.

Atracurium Besylate Rx

injection: 10 mg/ml   Tracrium

INDICATIONS
A muscle relaxant used as an adjunct to anesthesia to facilitate endotracheal intubation and to relax skeletal muscle during surgery or mechanical ventilation.

CONTRAINDICATIONS
Hypersensitivity.

ACTIONS
A nondepolarizing skeletal muscle relaxant that antagonizes the neurotransmitter action of acetylcholine by binding competitively with cholinergic receptor sites on the motor end-plate. It is a less potent histamine releaser than d-tubocurarine or metocurine.

WARNINGS
Atracurium should be used only by those skilled in airway management and respiratory support. Equipment and personnel must be immediately available for endotracheal intubation and support of ventilation (assisted or controlled), including administration of positive pressure oxygen. Anticholinesterase reversal agents should be immediately available.

Do not give by IM administration.

Has no known effects on consciousness, pain threshold, or cerebration.

Use only with adequate anesthesia.

Use in pregnancy: Use only if the potential benefit justifies the potential risk to the fetus.

Use in labor and delivery: Atracurium (0.3 mg/kg) has been administered during delivery by cesarean section. No harmful effects were attributable to the drug in any of the newborn infants, although small amounts crossed the placental barrier. Consider the possibility of respiratory depression in the newborn infant following cesarean section during which a neuromuscular blocking agent has been administered. The possibility of forceps delivery may increase. In patients receiving **magnesium sulfate,** the reversal of neuromuscular blockade may be unsatisfactory; lower the atracurium dose as indicated.

Use in lactation: Safety not established.

Use in children: Safety and efficacy for use in children below the age of 2 years have not been established.

PRECAUTIONS

Exercise special caution when substantial histamine release would be hazardous (*e.g.,* in patients with significant cardiovascular disease, severe anaphylactoid reactions, or asthma). The recommended initial dose is lower; administer slowly or in divided doses over 1 minute.

Bradycardia during anesthesia may be more common with atracurium than with other muscle relaxants because atracurium has no clinically significant effects on heart rate in recommended dosages.

Use in neuromuscular diseases in which potentiation of nondepolarizing agents has been noted (*e.g.,* myasthenia gravis, Eaton-Lambert syndrome) may cause atracurium to have profound effects. Use of a peripheral nerve stimulator is especially important. Take similar precautions in patients with severe electrolyte disorders or carcinomatosis. Safety has not been established in patients with bronchial asthma.

DRUG INTERACTIONS

Drugs that may enhance the neuromuscular blocking action of atracurium include **enflurane, isoflurane, halothane;** certain antibiotics, especially the **aminoglycosides** and **polymyxins; lithium; magnesium salts; procainamide;** and **quinidine.**

Prior administration of **succinylcholine** does not enhance the duration, but quickens the onset and increases the depth, of atracurium-induced blockade. Do not give atracurium until the patient has recovered from succinylcholine-induced neuromuscular blockade.

ADVERSE REACTIONS

Most adverse reactions suggest histamine release and may include skin flush, erythema, itching, wheezing/bronchial secretions, and hives. An increase or decrease in mean arterial pressure and an increase or decrease in heart rate may also be seen.

DOSAGE

To avoid patient distress do not administer drug until unconsciousness has been induced. Given by the IV route as IM administration, drug may result in tissue irritation. A peripheral nerve stimulator to monitor muscle twitch suppression and recovery is recommended to minimize the possibility of overdosage.

Recommended initial dose: 0.4 mg/kg to 0.5 mg/kg as IV bolus injection.

Maintaining neuromuscular blockade during prolonged surgical procedures: 0.08 mg/kg to 0.1 mg/kg. The first maintenance dose will usually be required 20 to 45 minutes after the initial injection. Maintenance doses may be given at relatively regular intervals.

Significant cardiovascular disease and history suggesting greater histamine release: 0.3 mg/kg to 0.4 mg/kg given slowly or in divided doses over 1 minute.

Following use of succinylcholine for intubation under balanced anesthesia: Initially, 0.3 mg/kg to 0.4 mg/kg. Further reductions may be desirable with use of potent inhalation anesthesia.

Dosage reductions may be used in those with neuromuscular disease, severe electrolyte disorders, or carcinomatosis.

NURSING IMPLICATIONS

HISTORY

Alert anesthesiologist to current drug therapy and history of allergies. Notification may be made by attaching note on cover of chart before transporting patient to surgery.

ADMINISTRATION TECHNIQUES

Drug administered by anesthesia department.

ONGOING ASSESSMENTS and NURSING MANAGEMENT

CLINICAL ALERT: Patient must not be left unattended until responding fully from anesthesia. This includes a partially awake patient with adequate respiratory exchange, movement in the extremities, return of swallowing and gag reflexes, and adequate circulation (arterial blood pressure returns to preanesthetic level).

Postanesthesia: Monitor blood pressure, pulse, and respirations q15m (or as ordered) until there is full recovery from anesthesia.

Maintain patent airway until patient is able to swallow or speak or until gag reflex returns.

Complete recovery from muscle relaxant effect may require several hours. Check for movement in the extremities, chest muscles (on inspiration and expiration), jaw and neck muscles, swallowing, and gag reflexes.

Notify anesthesia department immediately if any of the following occurs: Erythema, edema, flushing, tachycardia, hypotension, bronchospasm (all are signs of histamine release); prolonged muscle relaxation; choking, noisy respirations; cyanosis; prolonged apnea.

Additional nursing management is based on individual factors, such as type of surgery, condition of patient, complications during surgery (*e.g.*, prolonged procedure, hemorrhage, episodes of hypotension, development of a cardiac arrhythmia), additional medical problems present before surgery (*e.g.*, diabetes mellitus, COPD), patient's age.

Atropine Sulfate

See Gastrointestinal Anticholinergics/Antispasmodics; Mydriatics, Cycloplegic.

Aurothioglucose

See Gold Compounds.

Azatadine Maleate

See Antihistamines.

Azathioprine Rx

tablets: 50 mg   Imuran
injection: 100 mg/   Imuran
    vial

INDICATIONS
Adjunct for prevention of rejection in renal homotransplantation and rheumatoid arthritis. Indicated only for those patients meeting criteria for classic or definite rheumatoid arthritis. Use is restricted to those with severe, active, erosive disease not responsive to conventional management.

CONTRAINDICATIONS
Hypersensitivity. Not used to treat rheumatoid arthritis in pregnant women. Rheumatoid-arthritis patients previously treated with alkylating agents (cyclophosphamide, chlorambucil, melphalan, or others) may have risk of neoplasia if treated with azathioprine.

ACTIONS
An imidazolyl derivative of 6-mercaptopurine; many of its biological effects are similar to those of the parent compound.

Homograft survival: Mechanism of this action is somewhat obscure. Drug suppresses hypersensitivities of the cell-mediated type and causes variable alterations in antibody production. Suppression of T cells, including ablation of T-cell suppression, is dependent on the temporal relationship to antigenic stimulus or engraftment. Drug has little effect on established graft rejections or secondary responses. Transplant recipients on azathioprine also receive corticosteroids and may be given antilymphocyte globulin; there are no known hazards or toxicities due to interactions of these agents.

Immunoinflammatory response: Mechanisms whereby drug affects autoimmune diseases are not known. Azathioprine is considered a slow-acting drug; effects may persist after drug is discontinued.

Azathioprine is well absorbed following oral administration. Usual doses produce blood levels of azathioprine, and of mercaptopurine derived from it, that are low. Blood levels are of little predictive value for therapy. Azathioprine and mercaptopurine are moderately bound to serum proteins (30%) and are partially dialyzable. Azathioprine is cleaved *in vivo* to mercaptopurine. Both compounds are rapidly eliminated from blood and are oxidized or methylated in erythrocytes and liver. Neither compound is detectable in urine after 8 hours. Proportions of metabolites are different in individual patients, which may account for the variable magnitude and duration of drug effects.

WARNINGS
Severe leukopenia or thrombocytopenia may occur. Macrocytic anemia and severe bone-marrow depression may also occur. Hematologic toxicities are dose related and may be more severe in renal-transplant patients whose homograft is undergoing rejection. Serious infections are a constant hazard for patients on chronic immunosuppression, especially homograft recipients. Fungal, bacterial, and protozoal infections may be fatal and are treated vigorously.

Carcinogenicity: Azathioprine may increase the patient's risk of neoplasia. Renal-transplant patients are known to have an increased risk of malignancy, predominantly skin cancer and reticulum-cell or lymphomatous tumors. The risk is lower for patients with rheumatoid arthritis; however, acute myelogenous leukemia and solid tumors have been reported.

Use in pregnancy: Do not give during pregnancy without weighing risk *vs* benefit. Whenever possible, avoid use in pregnant patients.

DRUG INTERACTIONS

The principal pathway for detoxification of azathioprine is inhibited by **allopurinol;** therefore, during administration the dose of azathioprine is reduced to approximately one-third to one-fourth of the usual dose. Combined use of azathioprine with **gold, antimalarials,** or **penicillamine** has not been evaluated. Use of azathioprine with these agents is not recommended.

ADVERSE REACTIONS

The principle and potentially serious toxic effects are hematologic and gastrointestinal. Risks of secondary infection and neoplasia are also important. The frequency and severity of adverse reactions depend on the dose and duration as well as the patient's underlying disease or concomitant therapies.

Hematologic: Leukopenia and thrombocytopenia are dose dependent and may occur late in the course of therapy. Dose reduction or temporary withdrawal allows reversal of these toxicities. Infection may occur as a secondary manifestation of bone-marrow suppression or leukopenia, but incidence of infection in renal homotransplanation is 30 to 60 times that in rheumatoid arthritis.

GI: Nausea and vomiting may occur within the first few months of therapy. Frequency of gastric disturbance can be reduced by administration in divided doses or after meals. Vomiting with abdominal pain may occur rarely with a hypersensitivity pancreatitis. Hepatotoxicity with elevated serum alkaline phosphatase and bilirubin is known to occur in homograft recipients. It is generally reversible after interruption of azathioprine therapy. Hepatotoxicity is uncommon in rheumatoid-arthritis patients.

Others: Additional side-effects of low frequency include skin rashes, alopecia, fever, arthralgias, diarrhea, steatorrhea, and negative nitrogen balance.

DOSAGE

Renal homotransplantation: Dose required to prevent rejection and minimize toxicity will vary. *Initial dose*—3 mg/kg/day to 5 mg/kg/day, beginning at the time of transplant. Drug is usually given as a single daily dose on the day of, and in a minority of cases 1 to 3 days before, transplantation. Therapy is often initiated with IV administration, with subsequent use of tablets (at the same dose level) after the postoperative period. IV administration is indicated only in those unable to tolerate

oral medication. Dose reduction to maintenance levels of 1 mg/kg/day to 3 mg/kg/day is usually possible. The dose is not increased to toxic levels because of threatened rejection. Discontinuation may be necessary for severe hematologic or other toxicity, even if rejection of the homograft may be a consequence of drug withdrawal.

Rheumatoid arthritis: Drug is usually given on a daily basis; initial dose is approximately 1 mg/kg (50 mg to 100 mg) given as a single dose or bid. Dose may be increased beginning at 6 to 8 weeks, and thereafter by steps at 4-week intervals, if there are no serious toxicities and initial response is unsatisfactory. Dose increments should be 0.5 mg/kg/day, up to a maximum of 2.5 mg/kg/day. Therapeutic response occurs after several (6–8) weeks. Patients not improved after 12 weeks can be considered refractory. Drug may be continued long-term in those with clinical response, but patient is monitored closely and gradual dose reduction attempted to reduce risk of toxicities. Maintenance therapy should be at the lowest effective dose. Dose can be lowered incrementally with changes of 0.5 mg/kg (approximately 25 mg/day) every 4 weeks while other therapy is kept constant. Drug can be discontinued abruptly but delayed effects are possible.

Use in renal dysfunction: Relatively oliguric patients, especially those with tubular necrosis in the immediate postcadaveric transplant period may require lower doses.

Use with allopurinol: Patient receiving these drugs concomitantly should have a dose reduction of azathioprine to approximately one-third to one-fourth of the usual dose.

NURSING IMPLICATIONS

HISTORY
See Appendix 4.

PHYSICAL ASSESSMENT
CBC, differential, and platelet count are usually ordered; other laboratory tests may also be appropriate.

Renal homotransplantation: Assess general health status and problems identified in history.

Rheumatoid arthritis: Identify and describe joints involved; evaluate ability to participate in activities of daily living and list those activities requiring assistance.

ADMINISTRATION
Parenteral administration: Add 10 ml sterile water for injection; swirl until clear solution results. This solution is for IV use only and should

be used within 24 hours. Label if solution prepared in advance. Further dilution into sterile saline or dextrose is usually made for IV infusion. The final volume is ordered by the physician and depends on time for the infusion; this is usually 30 to 60 minutes, but as short a time as 5 minutes and as long a time as 8 hours may be ordered for daily administration.

Oral administration: Arthritic patient may require assistance removing drug from medicine container, holding water glass.

If GI upset occurs, administer with food or after meals.

ONGOING ASSESSMENTS AND NURSING MANAGEMENT

Renal homotransplantation: Physician writes detailed orders during pre- and postoperative period. Orders generally include vital signs; close monitoring of intake, output, urine specific gravity; observation for electrolyte imbalances; weight; evaluation of mental status; observation for signs and symptoms of graft rejection, infection.

Urinary output is usually measured at frequent intervals (q30m) during early postoperative period. Report any decrease in urinary output or change in intake–output ratio to physician *immediately.*

Drug therapy, as well as functioning of the graft, is monitored by frequent laboratory studies such as CBC, platelet counts, urinalysis, renal- and hepatic-function tests, serum electrolytes.

CLINICAL ALERT: Infection is a serious hazard. Observe closely for signs of infection: fever, chills, sore throat, malaise. Report any evidence of infection (*e.g.,* surgical wound, urinary, upper respiratory) to physician immediately.

If leukopenia occurs, dose reduction or drug withdrawal may be necessary to reverse this toxicity. Reverse isolation may be used until WBC returns to safe levels. Both patient and family should have full explanation of reason for and importance of reverse isolation.

Observe for signs of thrombocytopenia (ecchymoses, petechiae, hematuria, GI bleeding) and hepatotoxicity (jaundice, clay-colored stools, abdominal pain or discomfort, pruritus); report any occurrences immediately.

Rheumatoid arthritis: Record vital signs daily or as ordered.

Observe for adverse effects, especially signs of infection, thrombocytopenia, and hepatotoxicity (see above).

Monitor drug response by evaluation of general appearance, joint mobility, relief of joint pain or tenderness.

If nausea or vomiting persists despite giving drug with food or meals, notify physician; a bland diet or antiemetic drugs may be ordered.

Rest, physical therapy, and salicylates are usually continued while azathioprine is given; the dose of corticosteroids may be reduced.

PATIENT AND FAMILY INFORMATION

Close medical supervision is necessary. Frequent appointments and laboratory studies are necessary to monitor therapy.

If GI upset occurs, drug may be taken with food.

Notify physician or nurse if any of the following occurs: unusual bleeding or bruising, fever, sore throat, mouth sores, signs of infection, abdominal pain, pale stools, darkened urine, yellowing of skin.

May cause nausea, vomiting, rash, fever, aches, pains, diarrhea; notify physician or nurse if these persist or become bothersome.

All health-care personnel must be made aware of present drug therapy; this includes physicians consulted for other health problems, dentist, nurses, and so on.

Avoid use of any nonprescription drug unless use is approved by the physician prescribed azathioprine.

Vaccinations and other immunity-conferring agents (*e.g.,* "flu shots") are often avoided.

Avoid contact with persons with upper respiratory infection or another type of communicable disease and those recently exposed to a communicable disease.

Patient of childbearing age: Pregnancy is not recommended during therapy or for several months after therapy is terminated. Methods of contraception, if required, should be discussed.

Azlocillin Sodium

See Penicillins.

B

B

Bacampicillin Hydrochloride

See Penicillins.

Bacitracin, Intramuscular* Rx

injection: 10,000-   _Generic_
    unit, 50,000-unit
    vials

INDICATIONS
Use is limited to treatment of infants with pneumonia and empyema caused by staphylococci shown to be sensitive to the drug. See also Ophthamlic Anti-infectives; Topical Anti-infectives.

CONTRAINDICATIONS
Hypersensitivity or toxic reaction to bacitracin.

ACTIONS
Exerts profound antibacterial action against a variety of gram-positive and a few gram-negative organisms. Among systemic disease, only staphylococcal infections qualify for consideration of bacitracin therapy. Absorption following IM injection is rapid and complete. A dose of 200 units/kg or 300 units/kg q6h gives serum levels of 0.2 mcg/ml to 2 mcg/ml. Drug is excreted slowly by glomerular filtration and widely distributed in all body organs. It is demonstrable in ascitic and pleural fluids.

PRECAUTIONS
Parenteral use may cause renal failure due to tubular and glomerular necrosis. Adequate oral or parenteral fluid intake must be maintained. Use of antibiotics (especially prolonged or repeated therapy) may result in bacterial or fungal overgrowth of non-susceptible organisms (superinfection). Such overgrowth may lead to a secondary infection.

DRUG INTERACTIONS
Concurrent use of other **nephrotoxic drugs** (_e.g.,_ aminoglycosides) is avoided because toxic effects will be additive. Neuromuscular blockade and muscular paralysis may occur; these effects are additive when drug is administered concomitantly with **anesthetics, neuromuscular blocking agents, other drugs with neuromuscular blocking ability** (_e.g.,_ aminoglycosides).

ADVERSE REACTIONS
Proteinuria; cylindruria; azotemia; rising blood levels without any increase in dosage; nausea and vomiting; pain at injection site; skin rash.

* For ophthalmic preparations of bacitracin, see Antibiotics, ophthalmic. For topical preparations, see Antibiotics, topical.

DOSAGE
For IM use only.
   Infants under 2.5 kg: 900 units/kg/24 hours in 2 or 3 divided doses.
   Infants over 2.5 kg: 1000 units/kg/24 hours in 2 or 3 divided doses.

NURSING IMPLICATIONS

HISTORY
See Appendix 4. Obtain history of fluid intake (IV, bottle-feeding or breast-feeding).

PHYSICAL ASSESSMENT
Monitor vital signs, weight (exact weight will be necessary for calculation of dosage); assess hydration, respiratory status, general condition. Baseline laboratory studies may include renal-function tests, CBC, urinalysis, culture and sensitivity testing.

ADMINISTRATION
   Recommended reconstitution: Dissolve in Sodium Chloride Injection containing 2% procaine HCl.
   Concentration of the antibiotic should not be less than 5000 units/ml or more than 10,000 units/ml.
   Diluents containing parabens should not be used to reconstitute bacitracin; cloudy solutions and precipitate have occurred. Read label of diluent carefully before using.
   To the 10,000-unit vial add 2 ml of diluent. To the 50,000-unit vial add 9.8 ml of diluent. This will result in a concentration of 5000 units/ml.
   Label reconstituted solution with date and concentration/ml.
   Storage: _Unreconstituted vials_—store in refrigerator at 2°C to 8°C (36°F to 46°F). _Reconstituted solutions_—stable for 1 week when stored at 2°C to 8°C.
   Administer IM only; rotate injection sites. Record site used for each injection.

ONGOING ASSESSMENTS AND NURSING MANAGEMENT
Record vital signs q1h to q4h or as ordered.
   Record accurate intake and output; visually inspect urine for hematuria, cloudiness (may indicate cylindruria, infection).
   Examine oral cavity daily for evidence of _Candida_ (superinfection); check stool at time of diaper change and report diarrhea immediately.
   Assess hydration by checking oral mucous membranes, skin turgor.

Check urine *p*H daily or as ordered; record on flow sheet.

Evidence of superinfection must be reported immediately because appropriate measures must be instituted.

CLINICAL ALERT: Adequate oral or parenteral hydration must be maintained to avoid renal toxicity. If infant is maintained on oral fluids, notify physician immediately if prescribed intake decreases; parenteral fluids may be necessary. Report vomiting or diarrhea immediately because dehydration, which increases the risk of renal toxicity, can occur rapidly. Neuromuscular blockade resulting in respiratory paralysis may occur. Equipment for treating respiratory distress should always be immediately available. Report skin rash immediately because dermatologic manifestations may indicate hypersensitivity.

Urine should be kept at *p*H of 6 or greater to decrease renal irritation; physician may order sodium bicarbonate or other alkali to adjust urine *p*H.

Check previous injection sites for evidence of induration; notify physician if area becomes warm or red.

Baclofen Rx

| tablets: 10 mg | Lioresal |
| tablets: 20 mg | Lioresal DS |

INDICATIONS
Alleviation of signs and symptoms of spasticity resulting from multiple sclerosis, particularly for the relief of flexor spasms and concomitant pain, clonus and muscular rigidity. Patient should have reversible spasticity so that treatment will aid in restoring residual function. May also be of value in patients with spinal cord injuries and other spinal cord diseases. Not indicated in treatment of skeletal muscle spasm resulting from rheumatic disorders.

CONTRAINDICATIONS
Hypersensitivity.

ACTIONS
Precise mechanism of action is not fully known. Baclofen is capable of inhibiting both monosynaptic and polysynaptic reflexes at the spinal level, possibly by hyperpolarization of afferent terminals; actions at supraspinal sites may also occur and contribute to the clinical effect.

Baclofen is rapidly and extensively absorbed. Absorption may be dose dependent, being reduced with increasing doses. Peak serum levels are reached in approximately 2 hours; half-life is 3 to 4 hours. Drug is excreted primarily by the kidney in unchanged form.

WARNINGS
Hallucinations have occurred with abrupt withdrawal. Because drug is excreted primarily by the kidneys, it is given with caution to those with impaired renal function. Patients with stroke have shown poor tolerance to the drug. Use in pregnancy only when potential benefits outweigh the unknown potential hazards to the fetus. It is not known whether drug is excreted in breast milk. Safety for use in children under 12 has not been established.

PRECAUTIONS
In those with epilepsy, the clinical state and EEG should be monitored at regular intervals because deterioration of seizure control and EEG changes have been reported. Use drug with caution when spasticity is used to sustain upright posture and balance in locomotion or when spasticity is used to obtain increased function.

DRUG INTERACTIONS
The CNS effects of baclofen may be additive to those of **alcohol** and other **CNS depressants.**

ADVERSE REACTIONS
Most common: Transient drowsiness (10%–63%); dizziness (5%–15%); weakness (5%–15%); fatigue (2%–4%).

Neuropsychiatric: Confusion (1%–11%); headache (4%–8%); insomnia (2%–4%). *Rare*—euphoria, excitement, depression, hallucinations, paresthesia, muscle pain, tinnitus, slurred speech, coordination disorder, tremor, rigidity, dystonia, ataxia, blurred vision, nystagmus, miosis, mydriasis, diplopia, dysarthria, epileptic seizure.

Cardiovascular: Hypotension (0%–9%). *Rare*—dyspnea, palpitation, chest pain, syncope.

GI: Nausea (4%–12%); constipation (2%–6%). *Rare*—dry mouth, anorexia, taste disorder, abdominal pain, vomiting, diarrhea, positive test for occult blood in stool.

GU: Urinary frequency (2%–6%). *Rare*—enuresis, urinary retention, dysuria, impotence, inability to ejaculate, nocturia, hematuria.

Miscellaneous: Rash, pruritus, ankle edema, excessive perspiration, weight gain, nasal congestion.

Some of the CNS and GU symptoms may be related to the underlying disease rather than to drug therapy.

Abnormal laboratory tests: Increased SGOT; elevated alkaline phosphatase; elevated blood glucose.

OVERDOSAGE

Symptoms: Vomiting, muscular hypotonia, muscle twitching, drowsiness, accommodation disorders, respiratory depression, seizures.

Treatment: In the alert patient, promptly empty stomach by induced emesis followed by lavage. In the obtunded patient, secure airway with a cuffed endotracheal tube before beginning lavage (do not induce emesis). Maintain adequate respiratory exchange; respiratory stimulants are not recommended. Atropine has been used to improve ventilation, heart rate, blood pressure, core body temperature.

DOSAGE

Dosage is individualized. Start therapy at a low dosage and increase gradually until optimal effect is achieved (usually between 40 mg/day and 80 mg/day). The following dosage schedule is recommended: 5 mg tid for 3 days; 10 mg tid for 3 days; 15 mg tid for 3 days; 20 mg tid for 3 days. Thereafter, additional increases may be necessary but total daily dosage should not exceed 80 mg (20 mg qid).

NURSING IMPLICATIONS

HISTORY
See Appendix 4.

PHYSICAL ASSESSMENT
Evaluate and record description of symptoms (_e.g.,_ muscle rigidity, clonus, flexor spasms), ability to carry out activities of daily living (ADL). Monitor vital signs, weight.

ADMINISTRATION
If nausea occurs, check with physician whether drug may be given with food or meals.

Patient may require assistance in removing medication from dispensing container and in holding water glass.

ONGOING ASSESSMENTS AND NURSING MANAGEMENT
Record vital signs q4h to q8h or as ordered; observed for adverse drug reactions; evaluate drug response by assessing range of joint motion, increased ability to carry out ADL; look for flexor spasms, clonus and muscle rigidity and compare with data base; record observations.

Transient drowsiness, dizziness may occur. Supervise ambulatory activities. If patient is in a wheelchair, provide adequate body support or use restraining methods to prevent his falling from or tipping wheelchair.

If patient is diabetic, check urine for glucose, ketone bodies qid; record on flow sheet and report positive findings to physician.

Drug should not be withdrawn abruptly except in cases of serious adverse reactions. Ensure continuity of prescribed therapy by notation on Kardex, informing health-team members responsible for drug administration.

Fatigue may occur. Allow patient to perform ADL at own pace.

If constipation occurs, notify physician. An increase in fluid intake (unless contraindicated) or addition of bulk foods to the diet may correct problem. The physician may also order a laxative.

PATIENT AND FAMILY INFORMATION
May cause drowsiness, dizziness, fatigue. Observe caution while driving or performing other tasks requiring alertness.

Avoid alcohol, other CNS depressants.

Do not discontinue therapy except on advice of physician. Abrupt withdrawal may result in hallucinations.

May cause frequent urge to urinate or painful urination, constipation, nausea, headache, insomnia, or confusion. Notify physician or nurse if any of these effects persists.

Can be taken with food if there is GI distress.

Diabetic patient: Check urine daily or as recommended by physician. Keep record of urine tests and report any changes to physician immediately.

Barbiturates*

Amobarbital _Rx C–II_

tablets: 15 mg, 30 mg, 50 mg, 100 mg	Amytal
elixir: 44 mg/5 ml	Amytal

Amobarbital Sodium _Rx C–II_

capsules: 65 mg	Amytal Sodium Pulvules
capsules: 200 mg	Amytal Sodium Pulvules, _Generic_
powder for injection: 250-mg, 500-mg vials	Amytal Sodium

* For barbiturates used as general anesthetics (methohexital, thiamylal, and thiopental), see Anesthetics, general.

Aprobarbital *Rx C–III*

elixir: 40 mg/5 ml	Alurate

Butabarbital Sodium *Rx C–III*

tablets: 15 mg, 100 mg	Butisol Sodium, *Generic*
tablets: 30 mg	Butatran, Butisol Sodium (contains tartrazine), Sarisol No. 2 (contains tartrazine), *Generic*
tablets: 50 mg	Butisol Sodium (contains tartrazine)
capsules: 15 mg, 30 mg	Buticaps (30 mg contains tartrazine)
elixir: 30 mg/5 ml	Butisol Sodium (contains tartrazine), *Generic*
elixir: 33.3 mg/5 ml	Butalan

Mephobarbital *Rx C–IV*

tablets: 32 mg, 50 mg, 100 mg, 200 mg	Mebaral

Metharbital *Rx C–III*

tablets: 100 mg	Gemonil

Pentobarbital and Pentobarbital Sodium *Rx C–II*

capsules: 30 mg	Nembutal Sodium
capsules: 50 mg, 100 mg	Nembutal Sodium, *Generic*
elixir: 18.2 mg pentobarbital (equiv. to 20 mg pentobarbital sodium)/5 ml	Nembutal
suppositories: 30 mg, 60 mg, 120 mg, 200 mg	Nembutal Sodium (*C–III*)
injection: 50 mg/ml	Nembutal Sodium, *Generic*

Phenobarbital *Rx C–IV*

tablets: 8 mg, 65 mg, 100 mg	*Generic*
tablets: 15 mg, 30 mg	SK-Phenobarbital
tablets: 16 mg	Barbita, Luminal Ovoids, Solfoton, *Generic*
tablets: 32 mg	Luminol Ovoids, *Generic*
capsules: 16 mg	Solfoton
capsules, timed release: 65 mg	PBR/12

drops: 16 mg/ml	Sedadrops (contains tartrazine)
liquid: 15 mg/5 ml	*Generic*
elixir: 20 mg/5ml	*Generic*

Phenobarbital Sodium *Rx C–IV*

injection: 30 mg/ml, 60 mg/ml, 65 mg/ml, 130 mg/ml	*Generic*
powder for injection: 120 mg/ampule	*Generic*

Secobarbital and Secobarbital Sodium *Rx C–II*

capsules: 50 mg, 100 mg	Seconal Sodium Pulvules, *Generic*
tablets: 100 mg	*Generic*
elixir: 22 mg secobarbital/5 ml	Seconal
suppositories: 30 mg, 60 mg, 120 mg, 200 mg	Seconal Sodium (*C–III*)
injection: 50 mg/ml	Seconal Sodium, *Generic*

Talbutal *Rx C–III*

tablets: 120 mg	Lotusate Caplets

Oral Combinations *Rx*

25 mg amobarbital; 25 mg secobarbital	Tuinal 50 mg Pulvules (*C–II*)
50 mg amobarbital; 50 mg secobarbital	Tuinal 100 mg Pulvules (*C–II*)
100 mg amobarbital; 100 mg secobarbital	Tuinal 200 mg Pulvules (*C–II*)

INDICATIONS

AMOBARBITAL

Conditions requiring degrees of sedation ranging from minimum doses for relief of anxiety to hypnotic doses for preanesthetic medication.

AMOBARBITAL SODIUM

Sedation and relief of anxiety (at minimum doses); for hypnotic effects; as preanesthetic medication. Injectable form used for management of catatonic and negativistic reactions and for epileptiform seizures. Is also useful in narcoanalysis and narcotherapy and as a diagnostic aid in schizophrenia. Also indicated IV or IM for control of convulsive seizures such as those due to eclampsia, meningitis, tetanus, procaine or cocaine reactions, or poisoning from such drugs as strychnine or picrotoxin.

APROBARBITAL

Sedation and induction of sleep; on a short-term basis, in conditions requiring a sedative or hypnotic.

BUTABARBITAL SODIUM

Sedative and hypnotic.

MEPHOBARBITAL

As a sedative for relief of anxiety, tension, and apprehension. As an anticonvulsant for treatment of grand mal and petit mal epilepsy.

METHARBITAL

Control of grand mal, petit mal, myoclonic, and mixed types of seizures.

PENTOBARBITAL AND PENTOBARBITAL SODIUM

Sedative or hypnotic for short-term treatment of insomnia. May be used as preanesthetic medication. Use suppositories whenever oral or parenteral administration is undesirable. Injectable form may be used as a sedative, as a preanesthetic medication, as a hypnotic for short-term treatment of insomnia, and as an anticonvulsant. In anesthetic doses, for emergency control of acute convulsive episodes.

PHENOBARBITAL

As a preanesthetic and for sedation; as a hypnotic for short-term treatment of insomnia; as a long-term anticonvulsant for treatment of generalized tonic–clonic and cortical focal seizures. Also in the emergency control of certain acute convulsive episodes (*e.g.,* those associated with status epilepticus, eclampsia, meningitis, tetanus, and toxic reactions to strychnine or local anesthetics).

PHENOBARBITAL SODIUM

As a sedative in anxiety-tension states, hyperthyroidism, essential hypertension, nausea and vomiting of functional origin, motion sickness, acute labyrinthitis, pylorospasm in infants, cardiac failure, and in pediatrics as a preoperative and postoperative sedative. As an adjunct in treatment of hemorrhage from the respiratory and GI tract. Also used for symptomatic control of acute convulsions (*e.g.,* in tetanus, eclampsia, status epilepticus, cerebral hemorrhage). For pediatric patients as an anticonvulsant.

SECOBARBITAL AND SECOBARBITAL SODIUM

Intermittent use as a sedative or hypnotic. Use rectal form when indicated. Parenteral form may be used as a sedative or hypnotic as well as in anesthetic doses for emergency control of certain acute convulsive conditions.

TALBUTAL

Hypnotic for short-term treatment of insomnia.

ORAL COMBINATIONS

Hypnotic.

CONTRAINDICATIONS

Hypersensitivity; those with a history of manifest or latent porphyria; marked impairment of hepatic function. Large doses contraindicated in nephritic patients. Contraindicated in those with severe respiratory distress and respiratory disease if dyspnea, obstruction, or cor pulmonale is present. Not given to those with known previous addiction; ordinary doses may be ineffectual and may contribute to further addiction. Do not give *Secobarbital Sodium* in the presence of acute or chronic pain. Parenteral *Secobarbital* is contraindicated in obstetric delivery.

ACTIONS

Barbiturates are capable of producing all levels of CNS mood alteration from excitation to mild sedation, hypnosis, and deep coma. In sufficiently high therapeutic doses, barbiturates induce anesthesia. These agents depress the sensory cortex, decrease motor activity, alter cerebellar function, and produce drowsiness, sedation, and hypnosis. They appear to act at the level of the thalamus, where they inhibit ascending conduction in the reticular formation, thereby interfering with impulse transmission to the cortex.

Barbiturates have little analgesic action at subanesthetic doses and may increase the reaction to painful stimuli. All barbiturates exhibit anticonvulsant activity in anesthetic doses, but only phenobarbital, mephobarbital, and metharbital are effective as oral anticonvulsants in subhypnotic doses.

Barbiturates are respiratory depressants; the degree of respiratory depression is dose dependent. With hypnotic doses, respiratory depression is similar to that occurring during physiologic sleep.

Barbiturates are absorbed in varying degrees following oral, rectal, or parenteral administration. The salts are more rapidly absorbed than are acids. The rate of absorption is increased if the sodium salt is ingested as a dilute solution or taken on an empty stomach. The onset of action for oral or rectal administration varies from 20 to 60 minutes; for IM administration, onset of action is slightly faster. Following IV administration, onset of action ranges from almost immediately for pentobarbital sodium to 5 minutes for phenobarbital. Maximum CNS depression may not occur for 15 or more minutes after IV administration of phenobarbital. Duration of action is related to dose and to the rate at which the drug is redistributed throughout the body and varies among persons and in the same person from time to time. Classification of barbiturates according to duration of action is:

Long-acting—mephobarbital, metharbital, phenobarbital
Intermediate-acting—amobarbital, aprobarbital, butabarbital, talbutal
Short-acting—pentobarbital, secobarbital

Barbiturates are bound to plasma and tissue proteins in varying degrees. They are metabolized primarily by the hepatic microsomal enzyme system and the metabolic products are excreted in urine and, less commonly, in feces.

Barbiturate-induced sleep reduces the amount of time spent in the rapid eye movement (REM) phase of sleep or dreaming stage. Also, stages III and IV sleep are decreased. Following abrupt cessation of barbiturates that have been used regularly, patients may experience markedly increased dreaming, nightmares, or insomnia.

Secobarbital and pentobarbital lose most of their effectiveness for inducing and maintaining sleep by the end of 2 weeks of continued administration, even with use of multiple doses. Other barbiturates might also be expected to lose their effectiveness after about 2 weeks. However, definitions of tolerance vary, and these two barbiturates have been given for weeks to months for chronic sedation with little development of tolerance. The short-acting agents may be preferred for those with difficulty in falling asleep, whereas long-acting agents are preferred in those with the problem of awakening during sleep.

WARNINGS

Barbiturates may be habit forming. Tolerance and psychological or physical dependence may occur with continued use. Administer with caution, if at all, to those who are mentally depressed or who have suicidal tendencies or history of drug abuse.

Too-rapid IV administration may cause respiratory depression, apnea, laryngospasm, or vasodilatation with fall in blood pressure. Exercise caution when administering to those with acute or chronic pain, because paradoxical excitement could be induced or important symptoms could be masked. However, use of these drugs as sedatives in postoperative surgery or as adjuncts to cancer chemotherapy is well established.

Barbiturates that are excreted either partially or completely unchanged in urine (*i.e.,* phenobarbital, mephobarbital, aprobarbital, talbutal) are contraindicated in patients with impaired renal function.

Status epilepticus may result from abrupt discontinuation, even when barbiturates have been administered in small daily doses in treatment of epilepsy.

Barbiturates may increase vitamin D requirements, possibly by increasing the metabolism of vitamin D via enzyme induction. Rickets and osteomalacia have been reported rarely following prolonged use.

Barbiturates may produce marked excitement, depression, and confusion in elderly or debilitated patients. In some, barbiturates repeatedly produce excitement rather than depression.

In those with hepatic damage, give these drugs with caution and, initially, in reduced doses; do not give to those showing premonitory signs of hepatic coma.

Use in pregnancy: Barbiturates can cause fetal damage when administered to pregnant women. If drug is used during pregnancy or if the patient becomes pregnant while using this drug, she should be apprised of the potential hazards to the fetus. Barbiturates readily cross the placental barrier and are distributed throughout fetal tissues. Fetal blood levels approach maternal blood levels following parenteral administration. Withdrawal symptoms occur in infants born to mothers who receive barbiturates throughout the last trimester of pregnancy. Maternal ingestion of anticonvulsant drugs, particularly barbiturates, may be associated with a neonatal coagulation defect that may cause bleeding during the early (usually within 24 hours) neonatal period. This defect is characterized by decreased levels of vitamin-K-dependent clotting factors and prolongation of prothrombin time, partial thromboplastin time, or both.

Hypnotic doses of barbiturates do not appear to impair uterine activity significantly during labor. Full anesthetic doses decrease the force and frequency of uterine contractions. Administration of barbiturates to the mother during labor may result in respiratory depression in the newborn; premature infants are particularly susceptible to the depressant effects of barbiturates. A delayed interest in breastfeeding and a depressed response to auditory and visual stimuli have been noted in neonates.

Exercise caution when administering barbiturates to nursing women because small amounts are excreted in breast milk. Drowsiness in the nursing infant has been seen.

Use in children: Barbiturates may produce irritability, excitability, inappropriate tearfulness, and aggression. Hyperkinetic states may also be induced or aggravated and are primarily related to a specific drug sensitivity.

Untoward effects may occur in the presence of fever, hyperthyroidism, diabetes mellitus, or severe anemia. Use extreme caution in cases of great debility, severely impaired liver function, pulmonary or cardiac disease, status asthmaticus, shock, or uremia. Administer with caution to those with border-line hypoadrenal function.

Tartrazine sensitivity: Some of these products contain tartrazine. See Appendix 6, Section 6-23.

DRUG INTERACTIONS

Most reports of clinically significant drug interactions occurring with barbiturates have involved phenobarbital.

Agents that increase the effects of barbiturates:
Valproic acid appears to decrease barbiturate metabolism; monitoring of barbiturate levels is recommended. Concomitant use of **ether** or **curarelike drugs** may produce additive respiratory depressant effects. Concomitant use of other **CNS depressants,** including other sedatives and hypnotics, antihistamines, tranquilizers, phenothiazines, and alcohol, may produce additive depressant effects. **Monoamine oxidase inhibitors** (MAOIs) prolong the effects of barbiturates, probably because metabolism of the barbiturate is inhibited. **Chloramphenicol** may inhibit the metabolism of **phenobarbital.**

Barbiturates decrease the effects of the following drugs: Barbiturates do not impair normal hepatic function but can induce hepatic microsomal enzymes resulting in increased metabolism and decreased anticoagulant response of **oral anticoagulants.** Patients stabilized on anticoagulant therapy may require dosage adjustments if barbiturates are added or withdrawn from the dosage regimen. Barbiturates increase metabolism of **digitoxin** and **tricyclic antidepressants.** They also enhance the metabolism of exogenous **corticosteroids.** Patients stabilized on corticosteroid therapy may require dosage adjustments if barbiturates are added to or withdrawn from the dosage regimen. **Phenobarbital** shortens the half-life of **doxycycline** for as long as 2 weeks after barbiturate therapy is discontinued. If these drugs are administered concurrently, clinical response to doxycycline is closely monitored. Pretreatment with or concurrent administration of **phenobarbital** may decrease the effect of **estradiol** by increasing metabolism. There have been reports of patients treated with antiepileptic drugs (*e.g.,* phenobarbital) who have become pregnant while taking **oral contraceptives.** Concurrent administration of **phenobarbital** may significantly reduce the serum half-life of **quinidine.**

Miscellaneous drug interactions: The effect of barbiturates on the metabolism of **phenytoin** is variable and unpredicatable; monitoring of phenytoin and barbiturate levels is recommended when these drugs are given concurrently. **Phenobarbital** appears to interfere with absorption of orally administered **griseofulvin,** thus decreasing its blood level, but the effect on therapeutic response has not been estab-

lished. Concomitant administration of these drugs is avoided.

Concomitant administration of **furosemide** and barbiturates may produce or aggravate orthostatic hypotension.

ADVERSE REACTIONS

CNS: Somnolence is the most common adverse reaction. Others include agitation, confusion, hypokinesia, ataxia, CNS depression, nightmares, lethargy, residual sedation (hangover effect), paradoxical excitement, nervousness, psychiatric disturbance, hallucinations, insomnia, anxiety, dizziness, thinking abnormality.

Respiratory: Hypoventilation, apnea, respiratory depression, laryngospasm, bronchospasm, circulatory collapse.

Cardiovascular: Bradycardia, hypotension, syncope.

GI: Nausea, vomiting, constipation, diarrhea, epigastric pain.

Hypersensitivity: Skin rashes, angioneurotic edema, fever, serum sickness, morbilliform rash, and urticaria are most likely with in those with asthma, urticaria, or angioneurotic edema. Exfoliative dermatitis and Stevens-Johnson syndrome are rare and may prove fatal.

Local reactions: Inadvertant intra-arterial injection may produce arterial spasm with resulting thrombosis and gangrene of an extremity. Reactions range from transient pain to severe tissue necrosis and neurologic tissue deficit. Subcutaneous injection may produce tissue necrosis, pain, tenderness, and redness. Injection into or near peripheral nerves may result in permanent neurologic deficit. Thrombophlebitis after IV use and pain at IM injection site have been reported.

Other: Headache, fever, liver damage, megaloblastic anemia following chronic phenobarbital use. Blood dyscrasias (*e.g.,* agranulocytosis, thrombocytopenia) are extremely rare. Rarely, barbiturates may produce a pain syndrome suggestive of myalgic, neuralgic, or arthritic pain. Rickets and osteomalacia have also been rarely reported following prolonged use.

OVERDOSAGE

The toxic dose of barbiturates varies considerably. In general, an oral dose of 1 g produces serious poisoning in an adult. Death commonly occurs after 2 g to 10 g.

Symptoms: Acute overdosage is manifested by CNS and respiratory depression, which may progress to Cheyne-Stokes respiration, areflexia, constriction of the pupils to a slight degree (in severe poisoning pupils may show paralytic dilation), oliguria, tachycardia, hypotension, lowered body temperature, and coma. Typical shock syndrome (apnea, circulatory collapse, respiratory arrest, and death) may occur.

In extreme overdose, all electrical activity in the brain may cease, in which case a "flat" EEG, normally equated with clinical death, cannot be accepted. This effect is fully reversible unless hypoxic damage occurs. Complications such as pneumonia, pulmonary edema, cardiac arrhythmias, congestive heart failure, and renal failure may occur. Uremia may increase CNS sensitivity to barbiturates if renal function is impaired.

Treatment: Is mainly supportive. Maintain an adequate airway, with assisted respiration and oxygen administration as necessary. Monitor vital signs and fluid balance. If patient is conscious and has not lost the gag reflex, emesis may be induced with ipecac. Care should be taken to prevent pulmonary aspiration of vomitus. After patient has completed vomiting, give him 30 g activated charcoal in a glass of water. Nasogastric administration of multiple doses of activated charcoal has been used to accelerate elimination of phenobarbital from the body. If emesis is contraindicated, gastric lavage may be performed with a cuffed endotracheal tube in place with the patient in the face-down position. Activated charcoal may be left in the emptied stomach and a saline cathartic given.

Administer fluid and other standard treatment for shock, if needed. If renal function is normal, forced diuresis may aid in elimination of the barbiturate. Alkalinization of the urine increases renal excretion of some barbiturates, especially phenobarbital, aprobarbital, and mephobarbital. Hemodialysis may be used in severe intoxication if patient is anuric or in shock. Patient should be rolled from side to side every 30 minutes.

DRUG ABUSE AND DEPENDENCE

Barbiturates may be habit forming. Tolerance and psychological and physical dependence may occur, especially following prolonged use and high doses. Doses of pentobarbital or secobarbital in excess of 400 mg/day for approximately 90 days are likely to produce some degree of physical dependence. A dose of 600 mg to 800 mg taken for at least 35 days may be sufficient to produce withdrawal seizures. As tolerance develops, the amount needed to maintain the same level of intoxication increases; tolerance to a fatal dosage does not increase more than twofold. As this occurs, the margin between an intoxicating dosage and fatal dosage becomes smaller.

Symptoms of acute intoxication include unsteady gait, slurred speech, and sustained nystagmus. Mental signs of chronic intoxication include confusion, poor judgment, irritability, insomnia, and somatic complaints.

Symptoms of dependence: Are similar to those of chronic alcoholism and include a strong desire or need to continue taking the drug; tendency to increase the dose; psychic dependence on the effects of the drug related to subjective and individual appreciation of these effects; and physical dependence on the effects of the drug requiring its presence for maintenance of homeostasis resulting in a definite, characteristic, and self-limited abstinence syndrome when drug is withdrawn.

Symptoms of withdrawal: Can be severe and may cause death.

Minor symptoms—May appear 8 to 12 hours after last dose of a barbiturate. Symptoms usually appear in the following order: anxiety, muscle twitching, tremor of hands and fingers, progressive weakness, dizziness, distortion in visual perception, nausea, vomiting, insomnia, orthostatic hypotension.

Major symptoms (convulsions and delirium)— May occur within 16 hours and last up to 5 days after abrupt cessation of these drugs. Intensity of symptoms gradually declines over a period of approximately 15 days.

Treatment of dependence: Cautious and gradual withdrawal of the drug. Patients can be withdrawn by using a number of different withdrawal regimens over an extended period of time.

DOSAGE

Must be individualized. Factors considered are patient's age, weight, and condition. Parenteral routes are used only when oral administration is impossible or impractical. Dosage is reduced in the elderly or debilitated because these patients may be more sensitive to barbiturates. Dosage is reduced in impaired hepatic or renal function.

AMOBARBITAL

Daytime sedation: Adult dosage range may be from 15 mg to 120 mg PO 2 to 4 times/day, but usual adult dosage for daytime sedation is 30 mg to 50 mg PO 2 or 3 times/day.

Hypnotic: Usual adult dose is 100 mg to 200 mg PO. On occasion a larger dose may be necessary to produce the desired degree of hypnosis.

AMOBARBITAL SODIUM

Insomnia: 65 mg to 200 mg PO at H.S.

Preanesthetic sedation: 200 mg PO 1 to 2 hours before surgery.

Labor: Initial dose is 200 mg to 400 mg PO; additional quantities of 200 mg to 400 mg PO may be given at 1- to 3-hour intervals to a total dose of not more than 1 g.

APROBARBITAL

Sedative: 40 mg PO tid.
Mild insomnia: 40 mg to 80 mg PO H.S.
Pronounced insomnia: 80 mg to 160 mg PO H.S.

BUTABARBITAL SODIUM

Adults: _Daytime sedation_—15 mg to 30 mg PO tid or qid. _Hypnotic_—50 mg to 100 mg PO H.S.

Children: _Daytime sedation_—7.5 mg to 30 mg PO depending on age, weight, and degree of sedation desired. _Hypnotic_— Dosage based on age and weight.

MEPHOBARBITAL

Sedative: _Adults_—32 mg to 100 mg PO tid or qid. Optimum dose is 50 mg PO tid or qid. _Children_—16 mg to 32 mg PO tid or qid.

Epilepsy: _Adults_—Average dose is 400 mg to 600 mg PO/day. _Children (under 5)_—16 mg to 32 mg PO tid or qid. _Children over 5_—32 mg to 64 mg PO tid or qid. Taken at H.S. if seizures generally occur at night and during the day if attacks are diurnal. Initiate treatment with a small dose and gradually increase it over 4 to 5 days until optimum dosage is determined.

Replacement therapy: If patient is taking some other antiepileptic drug, it should be tapered off as the doses of mephobarbital are increased; this will guard against temporary marked attacks that may occur when any treatment for epilepsy is changed abruptly. Similarly, when the dose is to be lowered to a maintenance level or discontinued, the amount is reduced gradually over 4 to 5 days.

Combination drug therapy: May be used in combination with phenobarbital, in alternating courses or concurrently. When the two are used at the same time, the dose should be about one-half the amount of each used alone. _Average daily dose for adults_— 50 mg to 100 mg PO phenobarbital and 200 mg to 300 mg PO mephobarbital. Drug may also be used with phenytoin; in some cases, combined therapy appears to give better results than either agent used alone. When used concurrently, a reduced dose of phenytoin is advised, but full dose of mephobarbital may be used. Satisfactory results have been obtained with an average daily dose of 230 mg phenytoin plus about 600 mg mephobarbital.

METHARBITAL

Usual adult starting dose is 100 mg PO, 1 to 3 times/day. A dose of 5 mg/kg/day to 15 mg/kg/day has been recommended for children. According to the patient's tolerance, this dosage may be gradually increased to the level required to control seizures. In some cases, very small doses may be effective; in others, as much as 600 mg/day to 800 mg/day may

be required. May be used alone or with other antiepileptic drugs. When added to an established regimen to replace or supplement other anticonvulsant therapy, gradually reduce dosage of other medication while increasing that of metharbital.

PENTOBARBITAL, PENTOBARBITAL SODIUM

Adults: _Daytime sedation_—30 mg PO 3 or 4 times/day. _Hypnotic_—100 mg PO. _Suppositories_— 120 mg to 200 mg.

Children: _Daytime sedation_—2 mg/kg/day to 6 mg/kg/day PO (maximum 100 mg), depending on age, weight, and desired degree of sedation. _Hypnotic_—Judged on individual age and weight. _Suppositories_—Children 12 to 14 years (80–110 lb), 60 mg or 120 mg; 5 to 12 years (40–80 lb), 60 mg; 1 to 4 years (20–40 lb), 30 mg or 60 mg; 2 months to 1 year (10–20 lb), 30 mg.

IV: Restricted to conditions in which other routes are not feasible. There is no average IV dose. An initial dose of 100 mg in the 70-kg adult may be used. Reduce dosage for pediatric or debilitated patients. Rate of injection should not exceed 50 mg/minute. At least 1 minute is necessary to determine the full effect. If needed, additional small increments may be given, up to a total of 200 mg to 500 mg for normal adults.

IM: Dosage is calculated on basis of patient's age, weight, and condition. Usual adult dose is 150 mg to 200 mg; children's dosage frequently ranges from 25 mg to 80 mg or 2 mg/kg to 6 mg/kg as a single IM injection, not to exceed 100 mg.

PHENOBARBITAL

Adults: _Daytime sedation_—30 mg/day to 120 mg/day PO in 2 to 3 divided doses. _Hypnotic_—100 mg to 320 mg PO. _Anticonvulsant_—50 mg to 100 mg PO 2 to 3 times/day. _Timed-release form_—65 mg PO in the morning and 1 hour before H.S.

Children: _Preoperative sedation_—1 mg/kg to 3 mg/kg PO. _Anticonvulsant_—4 mg/kg/day to 6 mg/kg/day PO for 7 to 10 days to blood level of 10 mcg/ml to 15 mcg/ml or 10 mg/kg/day to 15 mg/kg/day PO. Adjusted to blood levels. Timed-release form not recommended for use in children under 12.

PHENOBARBITAL SODIUM

Sedation: _Adults_—100 mg to 130 mg IM or IV. _Infants and children_—2 mg/kg IM tid.

Convulsions, status epilepticus, eclampsia: _Adults_—200 mg to 300 mg IV or IM, repeated if necessary after 6 hours. _Infants and children_—3 mg/kg to 5 mg/kg/dose IM.

Vomiting of pregnancy: 100 mg to 300 mg IM q6h.

Preoperative: Adults—130 mg to 200 mg IM. *Children*—16 mg to 100 mg IM.

Postoperative sedation: Adults—32 mg to 100 mg IM. *Children*—8 mg to 30 mg IM.

SECOBARBITAL, SECOBARBITAL SODIUM

Adults: Insomnia—100 mg PO at H.S. *Preoperative sedation*—200 mg to 300 mg PO 1 to 2 hours before surgery. *Sedative*—30 mg to 50 mg PO. *Hypnotic*—100 mg to 200 mg PO. *Suppositories*—120 mg to 200 mg.

Children: Preoperative sedation—50 mg to 100 mg PO. *Sedative*—6 mg/kg/day PO divided into 3 equal doses. *Suppositories*—Up to 6 months, 15 mg to 60 mg; 6 months to 3 years, 60 mg; over 3 years, 60 mg to 120 mg. *Injectable solution*—For rectal administration of the solution to children prior to ear, nose, and throat procedures, solution is usually diluted to a concentration of 1% to 1.5% and administered after a cleansing enema. Children weighing under 40 kg may receive 5 mg/kg. Atropine may be given for its drying effect on respiratory-tract secretions.

Parenteral

Hypnotic: Adults—Usual dose is 100 mg to 200 mg IM. *Children*—3 mg/kg to 5 mg/kg or 125 mg/m² IM (maximum 100 mg).

Anesthetic procedures: To provide basal hypnosis for general, spinal, or regional anesthesia or to facilitate intubation, give secobarbital IV at a rate not exceeding 50 mg/15-second period and discontinue as soon as desired response is obtained. Total dosage in excess of 250 mg not recommended.

Dentistry: Adults and children, 2.2 mg/kg (maximum 100 mg) or 1.1 mg/kg to 1.6 mg/kg for light sedation. IM rather than IV administration, 10 to 15 minutes before procedure is started, is recommended. Sedative effects persist 3 to 4 hours. For nerve blocks, 100 mg to 150 mg IV may be used.

Convulsions in tetanus: Initial dose of 5.5 mg/kg may be used and repeated q3h to q4h as needed. The rate of IV injections should not exceed 50 mg/15 seconds.

TALBUTAL

Adults: 120 mg 15 to 30 minutes before retiring.

ORAL COMBINATIONS

Tuinal: 50 mg to 200 mg H.S. or 1 hour preoperatively.

NURSING IMPLICATIONS

HISTORY
See Appendix 4.

PHYSICAL ASSESSMENT
Record blood pressure, pulse, and respirations. Determine whether specific factors that may be controlled or eliminated are interfering with sedation or sleep. Such factors may include noise, bright lights, pain, and discomfort.

ADMINISTRATION
Do not administer a barbiturate if the patient has pain that should be controlled with an analgesic. Barbiturates have little analgesic action at subanesthetic doses and may increase reaction to painful stimuli.

Do not administer a barbiturate shortly before or after administration of a narcotic analgesic or other CNS depressant. If patient has an order for a narcotic analgesic (or other CNS depressant) and a hypnotic, check with physician regarding time interval between administration of these agents. Usually 2 or more hours should elapse between administration of a barbiturate and another CNS depressant, but this interval may vary with a specific CNS and the dose administered.

Dosage should be reduced in the elderly or debilitated because these patients may be more sensitive to barbiturates.

The rate of absorption is increased if the sodium salts are ingested in a dilute solution or taken on an empty stomach.

Do not use parenteral solutions if they are not absolutely clear or if they contain a precipitate.

Obtain blood pressure, pulse, and respirations before administration, especially if patient is elderly or baseline vital signs are low normal.

CLINICAL ALERT: Parenteral solutions of barbiturates are highly alkaline. When barbiturates are given IV, use extreme care to avoid perivascular extravasation, which may cause local tissue damage with subsequent necrosis. When barbiturates are given IM, exercise care to avoid intra-arterial injection (aspirate the syringe before injection). Consequences of accidental intra-arterial injection may vary from transient pain to gangrene of the limb. Any complaint of pain in the limb warrants stopping the injection immediately.

IM
Give deep into a large muscle such as gluteus maximus or vastus lateralis or other areas where there is little risk of encountering a nerve trunk or major artery. Injection into or near peripheral nerves may result in permanent neurologic deficit. Do not exceed 5 ml at any one site.

Amobarbital sodium: Do not exceed 500 mg per IM dose. Superficial IM or subcutaneous injection may be painful and may produce sterile abscesses or sloughs. Twenty-percent solutions may be used. Add Sterile Water for Injection to vial (1.25 ml to 250-mg vial or 2.5 ml to 500-mg vial) to make a 20% solution.

IV

Use a larger vein to minimize possibility of thrombosis and perivascular extravasation. Slow injection of these drugs is essential.

Keep an oropharyngeal airway at bedside for use (if needed) to maintain a patent airway.

Amobarbital sodium: To make a 10% solution, add 2.5 ml to the 250-mg vial or 5 ml to the 500-mg vial. Rotate to facilitate solution of the powder. Do *Not* shake the vial.

RECOMMENDED RATES OF INJECTION: *Amobarbital Sodium*—Do not exceed 1 ml/minute; *Secobarbital Sodium*—Do not exceed 50 mg/15-second period; *Pentobarbital Sodium*—Do not exceed 50 mg/minute.

Stability of parenteral solutions

Amobarbital sodium: Under no circumstances should a solution be used that is not absolutely clear after 5 minutes. Solution hydrolyzes upon exposure to air; no more than 30 minutes should elapse from time vial is opened until contents are injected.

Secobarbital sodium: Store in refrigerator; protect from light.

Rectal administration

Secobarbital sodium (children): Cleansing enema recommended prior to administration. Using secobarbital sodium injection (50 mg/ml), dilute with lukewarm tap water to a concentration of 1% to 1.5%. Three milliliters of tap water added to the 1-ml (50-mg) solution will equal a 1.25% solution. A different concentration may also be ordered.

Do not divide suppositories.

ONGOING ASSESSMENT AND NURSING MANAGEMENT

Following administration of barbiturates as a hypnotic, raise the siderails and advise patient to remain in bed and call for assistance if it is necessary to get out of bed. Those receiving a barbiturate as a sedative may require assistance with ambulatory activities if drowsiness occurs.

When barbiturates are administered IV, patient must be under continuous observation. Maintain a patent airway; use an oropharyngeal airway if necessary. Monitor blood pressure, pulse, and respirations q15m or as ordered. Inform physician immediately if respiratory depression occurs.

Expected onset and peak following oral administration are shown in Table 2.

Observe patient for 1 to 2 hours after administration to evaluate effect of the drug.

Table 2. Onset and Peak of Effects of Oral Barbiturates

Barbiturate	Onset (minutes)	Peak (hours)
Mephobarbital, metharbital, phenobarbital	≥60	10–12
Amobarbital, aprobarbital, butabarbital, talbutal	45–60	6–8
Secobarbital, pentobarbital	10–15	3–4

In some instances, supplemental doses may be ordered if patient wakes during the night. If no order for a supplemental dose has been written and patient wakes during the night, record length of sleep from H.S. dose and discuss with physician.

Observe for adverse reactions.

Elderly and debilitated patients are observed for marked excitement, depression, and confusion. If excitement or confusion occurs, observe at freqent intervals (as often as every 5 to 10 minutes may be necessary) for duration of these adverse effects. Inform physician of problem because a different drug may be necessary.

CLINICAL ALERT: Abrupt discontinuation of barbiturates in those on prolonged therapy may result in withdrawal symptoms, which may include anxiety, muscle twitching, tremor of hands and fingers, progressive weakness, dizziness, distortion of visual perception, nausea, vomiting, insomnia, and orthostatic hypotension, within 8 to 12 hours after the last dose. Convulsions and delirium may occur within 16 hours. When barbiturates used for control of epilepsy, status epilepticus may also occur.

Infants born of mothers given barbiturates throughout the last trimester of pregnancy may experience the acute withdrawal syndrome of seizures and hyperirritability from birth to a delayed onset of up to 14 days.

Periodic laboratory evaluation of the hematopoietic, renal, and hepatic systems is recommended during prolonged therapy.

Concomitant administration of a barbiturate and an oral anticoagulant may result in decreased anticoagulant response. Patients stabilized on anticoagulant therapy may require dosage adjustment if a barbiturate is added to or withdrawn from the dosage regimen.

Maternal use of anticonvulsants, particularly barbiturates, may be associated with a neonatal coagulant defect. It has been suggested that prophylactic vitamin K be given to the mother 1 month prior to, and during, delivery and to the infant, IV, immediately after birth.

If barbiturates are used during labor and delivery, resuscitation equipment should be available for treatment of neonatal respiratory depression.

Barbiturates may increase vitamin D requirements. Patients, especially children, may receive supplemental vitamin D when on long-term barbiturate therapy for convulsive disorders.

If used as an anticonvulsant, see p 89.

PATIENT AND FAMILY INFORMATION

Do *Not* increase or decrease the dose unless a change in dosage is recommended by the physician.

May impair mental or physical abilities required for performance of potentially hazardous tasks (*e.g.,* driving, operating machinery).

Alcohol must not be consumed by patients taking this drug. Concurrent use of barbiturates with other CNS depressants (alcohol, narcotics, tranquilizers, antihistamines) may result in additive depressant effects.

Do not use cold, cough, or allergy preparations unless use has been approved by the physician. (These preparations may contain antihistamines or other drugs that may cause drowsiness or sympathomimetics, which are CNS stimulants and may defeat the purpose of the barbiturate.)

Notify physician or nurse if any of the following occurs: fever, sore throat, mouth sores, easy bruising or bleeding, nosebleed, petechiae.

Pregnancy should be avoided while taking these drugs because fetal abnormalities have occurred.

Use of oral contraceptives while on phenobarbital therapy may result in decreased effectiveness of the oral contraceptive and possible pregnancy. An alternative method of contraception is advisable.

Accidental overdose may occur when a patient awakens during the night and forgets that a pill has been ingested only a short time earlier. To avoid accidental overdose, keep these medications in an area other than the bedroom or bathroom.

Children: Supervision of activities including playtime may be required. Some activities such as sports or riding a bicycle may be potentially hazardous if drowsiness occurs.

Barley Malt Extract

See Laxatives.

BCG Vaccine

See Immunizations, Active.

Beclomethasone Dipropionate

See Corticosteroids, Intranasal; Corticosteroid, Respiratory Inhalants.

Belladonna

See Gastrointestinal Anticholinergics/Antispasmodics.

Bendroflumethiazide

See Thiazides and Related Diuretics.

Benoxinate HCl and Fluorescein Sodium

See Anesthetics, Ophthalmic.

Benzalkonium Chloride (BAC)

See Antiseptics and Germicides.

Benzocaine

See Anesthetics, Local, Topical.

Benzodiazepines*

Alprazolam Rx C–IV

tablets: 0.25 mg, 0.5 mg, 1 mg	Xanax

Chlordiazepoxide Rx C–IV

tablets: 5 mg, 10 mg, 25 mg	Libritabs
capsules: 5 mg	A-poxide, Librium, SK-Lygen, *Generic*
capsules: 10 mg	A-poxide, Librium, Murcil, Reposans-10, Sereen, SK-Lygen, *Generic*

* This monograph covers benzodiazepines used for management of anxiety. Benzodiazepines discussed elsewhere include clonazepam (see Anticonvulsants), flurazepam, and temazepam.

| capsules: 25 mg | A-poxide, Librium, SK-Lygen, _Generic_ |
| powder for injection: 100 mg | Librium |

Clorazepate Dipotassium Rx C–IV

capsules: 3.75 mg, 7.5 mg, 15 mg	Tranxene
tablets: 3.75 mg, 7.5 mg, 15 mg	Tranxene
tablets: 11.25 mg	Tranxene-SD Half Strength
tablets: 22.5 mg	Tranxene-SD

Diazepam Rx C–IV

tablets: 2 mg, 5 mg, 10 mg	Valium
capsules, sustained release: 15 mg	Valrelease
injection: 5 mg/ml	Valium

Halazepam Rx C–IV

| tablets: 20 mg, 40 mg | Paxipam |

Lorazepam Rx C–IV

| tablets: 0.5 mg, 1 mg, 2 mg | Ativan |
| injection: 2 mg/ml, 4 mg/ml | Ativan |

Oxazepam Rx C–IV

| capsules: 10 mg, 15 mg, 30 mg | Serax |
| tablets: 15 mg | Serax (contains tartrazine) |

Prazepam Rx C–IV

| capsules: 5 mg, 10 mg, 20 mg | Centrax |
| tablets: 10 mg | Centrax |

INDICATIONS
ALPRAZOLAM

Management of anxiety disorders; short-term relief of symptoms of anxiety, anxiety associated with depression.

CHLORDIAZEPOXIDE

Management of anxiety disorders: short-term relief of symptoms of anxiety, symptoms of acute alcohol withdrawal, preoperative apprehension, anxiety.

CLORAZEPATE DIPOTASSIUM

Management of anxiety disorders; short-term relief of symptoms of anxiety; symptomatic relief of acute alcohol withdrawal. Also indicated in management of partial seizures (see Anticonvulsants, Benzodiazepines).

DIAZEPAM

Anxiety: Management of anxiety disorders; short-term relief of symptoms of anxiety.

Acute alcohol withdrawal: May be useful in symptomatic relief of acute agitation, tremor, impending or acute delirium tremens, hallucinosis.

Muscle relaxant: Adjunct for relief of skeletal-muscle spasm due to reflex spasm to local pathology (_i.e.,_ inflammation of muscles or joints or secondary to trauma); spasticity caused by upper motor neuron disorders (_i.e.,_ cerebral palsy, paraplegia); athetosis; stiff-man syndrome. Useful in treatment of tetanus.

Anticonvulsant: Adjunct in status epilepticus, severe recurrent convulsive seizures (see Anticonvulsants, Benzodiazepines).

Preoperative: Used parenterally for relief of anxiety and tension in those about to undergo surgical procedures; IV prior to cardioversion for relief of anxiety, tension; adjunct to endoscopic procedures for apprehension, anxiety, and acute stress reactions and to diminish patient's recall.

HALAZEPAM

Management of anxiety disorders; short-term relief of symptoms of anxiety.

LORAZEPAM

Management of anxiety disorders; short-term relief of symptoms of anxiety, anxiety associated with depressive symptoms. Also used for insomnia due to anxiety or transient situational stress. Parenteral route used in adults for preanesthetic medication producing sedation, relief of anxiety, and a decreased ability to recall events related to the day of surgery.

OXAZEPAM

Management of anxiety disorders; short-term relief of symptoms of anxiety, anxiety associated with depression; management of anxiety, tension, agitation, irritability in older patients; management of acute tremulousness or inebriation in alcoholics or of anxiety associated with alcohol withdrawal.

PRAZEPAM

Management of anxiety disorders; short-term relief of symptoms of anxiety.

CONTRAINDICATIONS

Hypersensitivity; psychoses; acute narrow-angle glaucoma (may be used in those with open-angle glaucoma receiving appropriate therapy).

ACTIONS

Have a depressant effect on subcortical levels of the CNS. Although exact mechanisms are not fully understood, calming effect appears to be due to actions on the limbic system and reticular formation. The cortex is relatively unaffected compared with the effects of barbiturates upon it. There is a wide margin of safety between therapeutic and toxic doses. Ataxia and sedation occur only at doses beyond dose needed for antianxiety effects. These drugs are readily absorbed following oral administration; IM administration of chlordiazepoxide and diazepam is painful, results in slow erratic absorption, and produces lower peak plasma levels than do oral and IV administration. These drugs are highly lipid soluble, widely distributed in body tissues, and highly bound to plasma proteins.

Oxazepam, lorazepam, and alprazolam are metabolized to inactive compounds and therefore have relatively short half-lives and duration of activity. The other benzodiazepines have active metabolites with very long half-lives; cumulative effects occur with chronic administration. Oxazepam or lorazepam may be preferred in patients with liver disease and in the elderly.

WARNINGS

These agents *not* intended for patients with a primary depressive disorder or psychosis or for those psychiatric disorders in which anxiety is not a prominent feature.

Dependence: Withdrawal symptoms similar to those with barbiturates and alcohol have occurred following abrupt discontinuation of therapy and have been reported in those receiving excessive doses over extended periods of time. These effects can range from mild dysphoria and insomnia to convulsions, tremor, abdominal and muscle cramps, vomiting, and sweating. Withdrawal psychosis with agitation, confusion, and disorientation has occurred. Symptoms of nervousness, anxiety, agitation, insomnia, irritability, diarrhea, muscle aches, occasional convulsions, and memory impairment have followed abrupt withdrawal after long-term use of high dosage. Addiction-prone patients should be kept under close surveillance. When discontinuing therapy after prolonged use, decrease dosage gradually to avoid possibility of withdrawal symptoms.

Parenteral administration: Administer parenterally (particularly IV) with extreme care to the elderly or very ill and to those with limited pulmonary reserve because of possibility of apnea or cardiac arrest. Resuscitative facilities should be available. When used with a narcotic analgesic, reduce narcotic dosage by at least one-third and administer in small increments. In some cases, use of a narcotic may not be necessary. Not recommended for obstetric use. Do not administer to patients in shock, coma, or acute alcoholic intoxication with depression of vital signs. Tonic status epilepticus has been precipitated in those treated with IV diazepam for petit mal status or petit mal variant status.

Parenteral therapy is indicated primarily in acute states and patient should be kept under observation, preferably in bed, for up to 3 hours. Ambulatory patients should not be permitted to operate a motor vehicle following an injection. Laryngospams, increased cough reflex, depressed respiration, dyspnea, hyperventilation, and pain in the throat or chest have been reported during peroral endoscopic procedures; topical anesthetics should be used and necessary countermeasures available. Hypotension and muscular weakness are possible, particularly when these drugs are used with narcotics, barbiturates, or alcohol.

Usage in pregnancy, lactation: An increased risk of congenital malformations associated with use of minor tranquilizers during the first trimester has been suggested. The child born of a mother taking these drugs may be at some risk for withdrawal symptoms during the postnatal period. Neonatal flaccidity has occurred. These drugs are excreted in breast milk. Neonates metabolize these drugs more slowly than do adults, and accumulation to toxic levels is possible; therefore, these drugs are not administered to nursing mothers. Chronic administration of diazepam to nursing mothers has been reported to cause infants to become lethargic and lose weight.

PRECAUTIONS

In those in whom a degree of depression accompanies anxiety, suicidal tendencies may be present; protective measures may be required. In elderly or debilitated patients or children, the initial dose should be small and increments made gradually to prevent ataxia or excessive sedation. Although hypotension rarely occurs, administer with caution when drop in blood pressure might lead to cardiac complications. Observe caution in those with impaired renal or hepatic function to avoid accumulation of drug. **Chlordiazepoxide** has been reported to precipitate attacks of acute intermittent porphyria. Some of these products contain tartrazine (see Appendix 6, section 6-23).

Long-term therapy: Because of isolated reports of neutropenia and jaundice, periodic blood counts and hepatic-function tests are recommended.

DRUG INTERACTIONS

Avoid simultaneous use of **alcohol** and other **CNS depressants.** If combined with other **psychotropics** or **anticonvulsants,** individual pharmacologic effects, particularly of compounds which may potentiate action of benzodiazepines (*e.g.,* **phenothiazines, antihistamines, narcotics, barbiturates, MAO inhibitors, tricyclic antidepressants**), must be considered. **Disulfiram** may inhibit plasma clearance of benzodiazepines with pharmacologically active metabolites. Oxazepam and lorazepam should be unaffected by concurrent administration with disulfiram. Variable effects on blood coagulation have been reported in those receiving **oral anticoagulants** and chlordiazepoxide. **Cigarette smoking** may alter clinical effects of benzodiazepines. The rate of absorption of diazepam and chlordiazepoxide is delayed by concomitant administration of **antacids** or **food.** The half-life of some benzodiazepines has been reported to be increased in those taking **cimetidine.** The elimination half-lives of lorazepam and oxazepam are not affected. **Isoniazid** impairs the clearance and increases the half-life of **diazepam; rifampin** increases clearance and decreases half-life.

ADVERSE REACTIONS

Transient mild drowsiness is commonly seen in the first few days of therapy. Drowsiness, ataxia, and confusion have been reported, especially in the elderly and debilitated. If these are persistent, dosage may be reduced. Other adverse effects less frequently reported include the following.

CNS: Sedation, sleepiness, depression, lethargy, apathy, fatigue, lightheadedness, disorientation, headache, agitation, stimulation, slurred speech, dysarthria, stupor, syncope, tremor, dystonia, vertigo, dizziness, euphoria, insomnia, sleep disturbances, nervousness, irritability, difficulty in concentration, akathisia, weakness, auditory disturbances, vivid dreams, psychomotor retardation, extrapyramidal symptoms.

GI: Constipation, diarrhea, dry mouth, nausea, anorexia, change in appetite, vomiting, difficulty in swallowing, increased salivation, gastric disorders.

GU: Incontinence, changes in libido, urinary retention, menstrual irregularities.

Cardiovascular: Bradycardia, cardiovascular collapse, hypotension, tachycardia, palpitations, edema.

Eye-ear-nose-throat: Visual disturbances, blurred vision, diplopia, nystagmus.

Dermatologic: Urticaria, pruritus, skin rash, dermatitis, allergy.

Other: Hiccups; fever; diaphoresis; paresthesias; muscular disturbance; respiratory disturbances; congestion; leukopenia; elevations of lactate dehydrogenase, alkaline phosphatase, SGOT, and SGPT; hepatic dysfunction including jaundice; blood dyscrasias including agranulocytosis; increase or decrease in weight; joint pain. Phlebitis and thrombosis at IV sites and pain following IM injection have occurred. Lactic acidosis has been reported with high IV dosage of diazepam.

Paradoxical reactions: Mild paradoxical reactions (excitement, stimulation) have been reported in psychiatric patients; these reactions may be secondary to relief of anxiety and usually appear during first two weeks of therapy. Drug should be discontinued if reactions such as acute hyperexcited states, anxiety, hallucinations, increased muscle spasticity, insomnia, rage, and sleep disturbances occur.

OVERDOSAGE

Symptoms: *Mild cases*—Drowsiness, mental confusion, lethargy; *more serious*—Ataxia, hypotonia, hypotension, hypnosis, coma, and (rarely) death.

Treatment: If vomiting has not occurred spontaneously, it should be induced. Monitor blood pressure, pulse, and respirations. General supportive measures, along with immediate gastric lavage, may be used. Administer IV fluids and maintain an adequate airway. Norepinephrine or metaraminol may be used for hypotension. Dialysis is of limited value. There have been reports of excitation following overdosage; if this occurs, barbiturates should not be used.

DOSAGE
ALPRAZOLAM

Usual starting dose is 0.25 mg to 0.5 mg tid. This may be titrated according to needs to a maximum total dose of 4 mg/day, given in divided doses. If side-effects occur with the starting dose, the dose should be lowered. *For elderly or debilitated patients*— Usual starting dose is 0.25 mg bid or tid. This may be gradually increased if needed or tolerated.

CHLORDIAZEPOXIDE

Optimum dose varies with diagnosis and response of patient and is individualized for maximum benefit.

Oral

Mild to moderate anxiety and tension: 5 mg or 10 mg tid or qid.

Severe anxiety and tension: 20 mg to 25 mg tid or qid.

Geriatric patients or those with debilitating disease: 5 mg bid to qid.

Preoperative apprehension and anxiety: On days preceding surgery, 5 mg to 10 mg tid or qid.

Acute alcohol withdrawal: Parenteral form usually used initially. If oral, initial dose is 50 mg to 100 mg followed by repeated doses as needed (up to 300 mg/day). Then reduce to maintenance levels.

Children: Initiate therapy with lowest dose; increase as required. Initially, 5 mg bid to qid. (May be increased in some children to 10 mg bid or tid). Not recommended for children under 6 years.

Parenteral

Lower doses (usually 25 mg to 50 mg) should be used for elderly or debilitated patients and for older children. In most cases, acute symptoms may be rapidly controlled by parenteral administration so that further treatment, if needed, may be given orally. Although 300 mg may be given in a 6-hour period, this dose should not be exceeded in any 24-hour period. Not recommended for children under 12 years.

Acute alcohol withdrawal: 50 mg to 100 mg IM or IV initially; repeat in 2 to 4 hours if necessary.

Acute or severe anxiety and tension: 50 mg to 100 mg IM or IV initially; then 25 mg to 50 mg tid or qid if necessary.

Preoperative apprehension and anxiety: 50 mg to 100 mg IM 1 hour prior to surgery.

CLORAZEPATE DIPOTASSIUM

Symptomatic relief of anxiety: May be given in divided doses tid. Usual dose is 30 mg/day. Adjusted gradually within range of 15 mg/day to 60 mg/day according to patient response. In elderly or debilitated patients, suggested initial dose is 7.5 mg/day to 15 mg/day. May be administered as single daily dose H.S.; recommended initial dose is 15 mg. Patient response may require adjustment. Lower doses may be indicated in the elderly. Drowsiness may occur at initiation of treatment and with dosage increments.

Maintenance therapy: 22.5 mg may be administered as single dose as an alternate dosage form for those stabilized with 7.5 mg tid. Not used to initiate therapy.

Symptomatic relief of acute alcohol withdrawal: *Day 1*—30 mg initially; followed by 30 mg to 60 mg in divided doses. *Day 2*—45 mg to 90 mg in divided doses. *Day 3*—22.5 mg to 45 mg in divided doses. *Day 4*—15 mg to 30 mg in divided doses. Thereafter, gradually reduce daily dose to 7.5 mg to 15 mg; discontinued as soon as patient's condition is stable. Maximum recommended total daily dose is 90 mg.

Management of seizures: See Anticonvulsants.

DIAZEPAM

Oral: Dose is individualized. Doses listed below will meet the needs of most patients; some may require higher doses, which are increased cautiously to avoid adverse effects.

Anxiety disorders, anxiety symptoms: 2 mg to 10 mg bid to qid. *Sustained-release capsules*—15 mg/day to 30 mg/day.

Acute alcohol withdrawal: 10 mg tid or qid during first 24 hours; reduce to 5 mg tid or qid as needed. *Sustained-release capsules*—30 mg first 24 hours, then 15 mg/day as needed.

Skeletal muscle spasm: 2 mg to 10 mg tid or qid. *Sustained-release capsules*—15 mg/day to 30 mg/day.

Geriatric or debilitated patients: Initially 2 mg to 2.5 mg daily or bid; increase gradually as needed and tolerated.

Management of seizures: See Anticonvulsants.

Children: Initially 1 mg to 2.5 mg tid or qid; increase gradually as needed and tolerated. Not for use in children under 6 months.

Parenteral (see also Administration): Dose is individualized. *Recommended dose in older children, adults*—2 mg to 20 mg IM, or IV. In some conditions (*e.g.,* tetanus), larger doses may be required. In acute conditions, injection may be repeated within 1 hour. Lower doses (usually 2 mg to 5 mg) and slow increase in dosage should be used for elderly or debilitated patients and when other sedative drugs are administered.

Moderate anxiety disorders, anxiety symptoms: 2 mg to 5 mg IM or IV; repeat in 3 to 4 hours if necessary.

Severe anxiety disorders, anxiety symptoms: 5 mg to 10 mg IM or IV; repeat in 3 to 4 hours if necessary.

Acute alcohol withdrawal: 10 mg IM or IV initially; then 5 mg to 10 mg in 3 to 4 hours if necessary.

Endoscopic procedures: *IV*—dose is titrated to desired response, such as slurring of speech. Administer slowly just prior to procedure. Reduce dosage of narcotics by at least one-third or omit narcotics. Ten milligrams or less is usually an adequate dose; up to 20 mg may be used. *IM*—5 mg to 10 mg 30 minutes prior to procedure if IV route cannot be used.

Muscle spasm: 5 mg to 10 mg IM or IV initially, then 5 mg to 10 mg in 3 or 4 hours if needed.

Preoperative: 10 mg IM before surgery. If atropine, scopolamine, or other premedication is desired, administer in *separate syringes.*

Cardioversion: 5 mg to 15 mg IV, 5 to 10 minutes prior to procedure.

Management of seizures: See Anticonvulsants.

Children: Administer slowly over 3-minute period to reduce risk of apnea, prolonged periods of somnolence. Dosage should not exceed 0.25 mg/kg. After 15 to 30 minutes, initial dose may be safely repeated. Facilities for respiratory assistance should be available.

Tetanus: *Infants over 30 days of age*—1 mg to 2 mg IM or IV slowly; repeat q3h to q4h as necessary. *Children 5 years or older*—5 mg to 10 mg repeated q3h to q4h may be required. Use IM route only when IV is impossible.

HALAZEPAM

Dose is individualized; some may require dosages higher than those listed. Administer in divided doses. Recommended dose is 20 mg to 40 mg tid or qid. Optimal dosage ranges from 80 mg/day to 160 mg/day. *Elderly or debilitated patients*—Initial recommended dosage is 20 mg daily or bid.

LORAZEPAM

Dose is individualized and increased gradually to minimize adverse effects. When higher dose is indicated, evening dose is increased before the daytime dose.

Oral: Usual range is 2 mg/day to 6 mg/day in divided doses, the largest dose being taken H.S. Dosage may vary from 1 mg/day to 10 mg/day.

Anxiety: Most patients require initial dose of 2 mg/day to 3 mg/day given bid or tid.

Insomnia due to anxiety, transient situational stress: Single daily dose of 2 mg to 4 mg, usually H.S.

Elderly or debilitated patient: Initial dose of 1 mg/day to 2 mg/day in divided doses.

Parenteral

IM: *Premedication*—usual dose is 0.05 mg/kg up to maximum of 4 mg. For optimum effect give at least 2 hours before surgery. Inject undiluted deep into the muscle mass.

IV: *Sedation, relief of anxiety*—usual dose is 2 mg total or 0.02 mg/lb (0.044 mg/kg), whichever is smaller. Larger doses of 0.05 mg/kg up to a total of 4 mg may be given. For optimum effect give 15 to 20 minutes before procedure.

Children (under 18): Not recommended.

OXAZEPAM

Dose is individualized.

Mild to moderate anxiety with associated tension, irritability, agitation, or related symptoms of functional origin or secondary to organic disease: 10 mg to 15 mg tid or qid.

Severe anxiety syndromes, agitation, or anxiety associated with depression: 15 mg to 30 mg tid or qid.

Older patients with anxiety, tension, irritability, agitation: 10 mg tid. If needed, increase cautiously to 15 mg tid or qid.

Alcoholics with acute inebriation, tremulousness, anxiety on withdrawal: 15 mg to 30 mg tid or qid.

Children (6 to 12 years): Dose not established.

PRAZEPAM

Usual dose is 30 mg/day in divided doses, adjusted gradually within range of 20 mg/day to 60 mg/day. In elderly or debilitated patients, it is advisable to initiate treatment at 10 mg/day to 15 mg/day in divided doses. May be given as single daily dose H.S.; recommended starting dose is 20 mg/night. Optimum dose ranges from 20 mg to 40 mg.

NURSING IMPLICATIONS

HISTORY

Note duration of symptoms; mental health history; drug history (because of potential for abuse of benzodiazepines, history of drug abuse may or may not be reliable). When applicable, inquire of woman patient possibility of current pregnancy or planned pregnancy in the immediate future. See also Appendix 4.

PHYSICAL ASSESSMENT

Record vital signs. Observe overt symptoms: motor responses (*e.g.,* trembling, tense, restless, tremors, unable to relax, agitated); autonomic responses (*e.g.,* cold clammy hands, sweating, tachycardia). Those in alcohol withdrawal should also be evaluated for memory impairment, disorientation, hallucinosis, depression, irritability, thinking and behavioral patterns. Baseline laboratory tests may include hepatic- and renal-function tests, CBC.

ADMINISTRATION

When used with a narcotic analgesic, narcotic dose should be reduced by at least one-third and administered in small increments.

May be given with food or meals if GI upset occurs.

Following administration, check oral cavity to be sure tablet/capsule has been swallowed if patient is in psychiatric setting, elderly, debilitated, uncooperative, addiction prone, or suspected of drug abuse.

Patients receiving drug by the parenteral route should be kept in bed and under observation for at least 3 hours.

Withhold drug and contact physician if there is suspicion that patient has recently consumed alcohol.

LORAZEPAM, IV

Immediately prior to use, drug must be diluted with an equal volume of compatible solution (Sterile Water for Injection, Sodium Chloride Injection, 5% Dextrose Injection). Drug is injected directly in vein or tubing of existing IV infusion; rate of infusion should not exceed 2 mg/minute. Equipment necessary to maintain a patent airway should be immediately available.

Storage, stability: Do not use if solution is discolored or contains a precipitate. Diluted solution should be refrigerated.

CHLORDIAZEPOXIDE

Prepare solution immediately before administration.

IV: Add 5 ml of sterile physiological saline or Sterile Water for Injection to ampule; agitate gently until *thoroughly* dissolved. Discard unused portion. Give slowly over 1-minute period.

IM: Reconstitute with special diluent provided in package; do not use diluent if opalescent or hazy. Discard unused solution. Give deep IM (slowly) into upper outer quadrant of gluteus muscle.

DIAZEPAM

IV: To reduce possibility of venous thrombosis, phlebitis, local irritation, swelling, and (rarely) vascular impairment, inject *Slowly.* Take at least 1 minute for each 5 mg (1 ml); do not use small veins (*e.g.,* dorsum of hand or wrist); avoid intra-arterial administration or extravasation. *Do not* mix or dilute with other solutions or drugs in syringe or IV infusion solutions. If not feasible to administer directly IV, it may be injected slowly through the infusion tubing as closely as possible to the vein insertion. Because of possibility of precipitation in IV fluids and adsorption of drug to the plastic of IV containers and tubing, IV infusion is not recommended.

IM: *Do Not* mix with other drugs in same syringe.

ONGOING ASSESSMENTS AND NURSING MANAGEMENT

Record vital signs daily or as ordered.

Observe behavior and compare to data base. Accurate observation of patient's response to drug is important because dose may need to be adjusted upward or downward to obtain desired effect.

If used as skeletal-muscle relaxant, evaluate relief of pain, discomfort.

When used to relieve preoperative anxiety and tension, notify physician if patient's anxiety remains the same or increases despite drug therapy.

CLINICAL ALERT: Suicidal tendencies may be present in some anxiety states; special precautions may be necessary. Notify physician and observe patient hourly (or more often) if depression is noted.

Abrupt discontinuation of long-term therapy may precipitate withdrawal symptoms (see *Warnings*). Ensure continuity of prescribed therapy by notation on Kardex, informing health-team members responsible for drug administration. When therapy is discontinued, dosage is reduced gradually.

Child born of mother taking benzodiazepines may be at risk for withdrawal symptoms. Observe neonate closely; report any apparent withdrawal symptoms to physician immediately.

Caution patient that drowsiness may occur. Assist with ambulation if drowsiness is noted. Elderly or debilitated patients may require supervision with ambulation and activities of daily living, especially early in therapy.

Observe q4h to q6h for adverse effects, paradoxical reactions; withhold drug and contact physician if adverse effects or paradoxical reactions are noted.

When applicable, encourage patient to stop smoking, because smoking reduces drug effectiveness. Patient who continues to smoke should be supervised if drowsiness is present.

Physician may order periodic hepatic- and renal-function tests, CBC during long-term therapy.

PATIENT AND FAMILY INFORMATION

May cause drowsiness; avoid driving or other tasks requiring alertness.

Avoid alcohol or other CNS depressants. Do *Not* exceed recommended dosage. May be taken with food or water if stomach upset occurs.

Do not discontinue drug abruptly without first checking with physician.

Concomitant use of antacids is to be avoided; absorption of drug may be impaired. Check with physician before using any nonprescription preparation.

Take drug as prescribed. Do not increase or decrease dose or dose intervals.

Benzoin Preparations *otc*

Benzoin: tincture	*Generic*
Benzoin compound: tincture	*Generic*

INDICATIONS
Protection of skin against irritants and coating of minor sores.

CONTRAINDICATIONS
Hypersensitivity. Do not use near eyes.

ADVERSE REACTIONS
Contact dermatitis.

NURSING IMPLICATIONS

ADMINISTRATION
Wash and dry area thoroughly before applying. Previous applications of this or other skin products must be removed prior to application of benzoin.

Apply as directed by physician or by manufacturer's directions.

Do not apply to acutely inflamed areas.

If an occlusive dressing will be applied, allow preparation to dry thoroughly; then place dressing lightly over area.

Remove an occlusive dressing carefully to be sure dressing has not adhered to skin. If dressing adheres to the area, soaking usually facilitates removal.

If area is to be left uncovered, do not allow bedding to come into contact with area until area is thoroughly dry.

CLINICAL ALERT: Never force removal of a dressing that has adhered to the skin following application of benzoin because skin can be removed along with the dressing.

Benzonatate Rx

capsules: 100 mg   Tessalon Perles

INDICATIONS
Symptomatic relief of nonproductive cough.

CONTRAINDICATIONS
Hypersensitivity.

ACTIONS
Acts peripherally by anesthetizing stretch receptors located in the respiratory passages, lungs, and pleura, dampening their activity and thereby reducing the cough reflex at its source. Has no inhibitory effect on the respiratory center in recommended dosage. Onset of action occurs in 15 to 20 minutes; effects last for 3 to 8 hours.

WARNINGS
Safety for use in pregnancy or in the nursing mother not established. Use only when clearly needed and when potential benefits outweigh the unknown hazards to the fetus.

PRECAUTIONS
Release of benzonatate in the mouth can produce temporary local anesthesia of oral mucosa.

ADVERSE REACTIONS
Sedation, headache, mild dizziness, pruritus and skin eruptions, nasal congestion, constipation, nausea, GI upset, sensation of burning in the eyes, a vague "chilly" sensation, numbness in the chest, hypersensitivity.

OVERDOSAGE
Symptoms: Drug is chemically related to tetracaine and other topical anesthetics. If capsules are chewed or dissolved in the mouth, oropharyngeal anesthesia develops rapidly. CNS stimulation may cause restlessness and tremors, which may proceed to clonic convulsions followed by profound CNS depression.

Treatment: Evacuate gastric contents and administer copious amounts of activated charcoal slurry. Even in the conscious patient, cough and gag reflexes may be so depressed as to necessitate special attention to protection against aspiration of gastric contents. Treat convulsions with a short-acting barbiturate given IV and carefully titrated for the smallest effective dosage. Intensive support of respiration and cardiovascular–renal function is essential in treatment of severe intoxication from overdosage. CNS stimulants are avoided.

DOSAGE
Usual dose for adults and children over 10 years is 100 mg tid, as required. If necessary, up to 600 mg/day may be given.

NURSING IMPLICATIONS

HISTORY
See Appendix 4. Inquire whether cough is nonproductive (drug not recommended for productive cough) and whether coughing is more prevalent at a certain time of day.

PHYSICAL ASSESSMENT
Monitor vital signs; auscultate chest; note character of respirations (rate, depth).

ADMINISTRATION

Instruct patient to swallow capsules whole; provide sufficient amount of water to ensure swallowing of capsules.

ONGOING ASSESSMENT AND NURSING MANAGEMENT

Assess response to drug; if cough becomes productive (see *Indications*) note amount and appearance of sputum and inform physician.

Additional measures to relieve coughing include increasing fluid intake; humidifying immediate environment (vaporizer, nebulizer); barring smoking (by patient, visitors).

Moisture delivered by vaporizer or nebulizer may result in increased water absorption and overhydration. In certain patients this could result in increased cardiac workload or pulmonary edema.

Frequent linen and clothing changes may be necessary if surrounding air receives extra humidification.

PATIENT AND FAMILY INFORMATION

Do not chew or break capsules; swallow whole.

Contact physician if cough is not relieved or becomes productive, or if chills, fever, or chest pain occurs.

Benzphetamine Hydrochloride

See Anorexiants.

Benzquinamide Hydrochloride

See Antiemetic/Antivertigo Agents.

Benzthiazide

See Thiazides and Related Diuretics.

Benztropine Mesylate

See Anticholinergic Antiparkinsonism Agents.

Beta-Adrenergic Blocking Agents

Atenolol Rx

tablets: 50 mg,   Tenormin
  100 mg

Metoprolol Tartrate Rx

tablets: 50 mg,   Lopressor
  100 mg

Nadolol Rx

tablets: 40 mg, 80   Corgard
  mg, 120 mg,
  160 mg

Pindolol Rx

tablets: 5 mg, 10 mg   Visken

Propranolol Hydrochloride Rx

tablets: 10 mg, 20   Inderal
  mg, 40 mg, 60 mg,
  80 mg, 90 mg
capsules, sustained   Inderal LA
  release: 80 mg,
  120 mg, 160 mg
injection: 1 mg/ml   Inderal

Timolol Maleate Rx

tablets: 5 mg, 10 mg, Blocadren
  20 mg

INDICATIONS

See below for specific indications for individual drugs.

Hypertension: Generally used in combination with other drugs, particularly a thiazide diuretic. Not indicated for treatment of hypertensive emergencies.

Angina pectoris due to coronary atherosclerosis: For selected patients with moderate to severe angina not responding to conventional measures. Not used in those with angina that occurs only with considerable effort or infrequent precipitating factors. These drugs exert both favorable and unfavorable effects, the preponderance of which may be beneficial. Use is not continued unless there is reduced pain or increased work capacity. Because of potential for adverse results, treatment is monitored closely and patient evaluated periodically because dosage requirement and need to continue treatment may be altered by clinical exacerbation or remission.

Hypertrophic subaortic stenosis: Useful in treatment of exertional or other stress-induced angina, palpitations, and syncope. Improves exercise performance. Effectiveness appears to be due to reduction of elevated outflow pressure gradient, which is exacerbated by beta-receptor stimulation. Clinical improvement may be temporary.

Cardiac arrhythmias

Supraventricular arrhythmias: PAROXYSMAL ATRIAL TACHYCARDIA, particularly those induced by catecholamines or digitalis or associated with the Wolff-Parkinson-White syndrome.

PERSISTENT SINUS TACHYCARDIA that is noncompensatory and impairs well-being.

TACHYCARDIAS AND ARRHYTHMIAS due to thyrotoxicosis when they cause distress or increased hazard and when immediate effect is necessary as adjunctive short-term (2–4 weeks) therapy. May be used with, but not in place of, specific therapy.

PERSISTENT ATRIAL EXTRASYSTOLES that impair well-being and do not respond to conventional measures.

ATRIAL FLUTTER AND FIBRILLATION when the ventricular rate cannot be controlled by digitalis alone or when digitalis is contraindicated.

Ventricular tachycardias: In ventricular tachycardias, with exception of those induced by catecholamines or digitalis, propanolol is not the drug of first choice. Drug may be considered in critical situations when cardioversion techniques or other drugs are not indicated or not effective. Also may be used in persistent premature ventricular extrasystoles that do not respond to conventional measures and impair well-being.

Tachyarrhythmias of digitalis intoxication: If tachyarrhythmias persist following discontinuation of digitalis and correction of electrolyte abnormalities, they are usually reversible with oral propanolol. IV propanolol is reserved for life-threatening arrhythmias.

Resistant tachyarrhythmias during anesthesia: Tachyarrhythmias may occur because of release of endogenous catecholamines or administration of catecholamines during anesthesia. When usual measures fail, IV propanolol may be given. All general anesthetics produce some degree of myocardial depression. Use propanolol with caution when treating arrhythmias during anesthesia; the ECG and CVP are monitored constantly.

Myocardial infarction: Indicated to reduce cardiovascular mortality and risk of reinfarction in clinically stable patients who have survived the acute phase. Initiation of treatment recommended within 1 to 4 weeks after infarction.

Pheochromocytoma: After primary treatment with an alpha-adrenergic blocking agent has been instituted, propanolol may be used as adjunctive therapy if control of tachycardia becomes necessary before or during surgery. It is hazardous to use propanolol unless alpha-adrenergic blocking drugs are already in use, because this would predispose the patient to serious blood-pressure elevation. With inoperable or metastatic pheochromocytoma, drug may be useful as an adjunct in management of symptoms due to excessive beta-receptor stimulation.

Migraine: Prophylaxis of common migraine headache. Efficacy in the treatment of a migraine attack that has already started has not been established.

ATENOLOL
Management of hypertension.

METOPROLOL TARTRATE
Management of hypertension.

Investigational use: Metoprolol has been used investigationally in acute myocardial infarction.

NADOLOL
Management of angina pectoris, hypertension.

PINDOLOL
Management of hypertension.

PROPRANOLOL HYDROCHLORIDE
Arrhythmias, hypertrophic subaortic stenosis, pheochromocytoma, hypertension, migraine, angina pectoris due to atherosclerosis, myocardial infarction.

Investigational uses: Propranolol has been evaluated for use in recurrent GI bleeding in cirrhotic patients, schizophrenia, tardive dyskinesia, acute panic reactions (_e.g.,_ stage fright).

TIMOLOL MALEATE
Hypertension, myocardial infarction. Also available as an ophthalmic solution for use in glaucoma (see Index).

CONTRAINDICATIONS
Allergic rhinitis during the pollen season; sinus bradycardia and greater than first-degree block; cardiogenic shock; right ventricular failure secondary to pulmonary hypertension; congestive heart failure (CHF), unless secondary to beta blockers; patients on adrenergic-augmenting psychotropic drugs including MAO inhibitors (and during 2-week withdrawal from such drugs); hypersensitivity.

Propranolol, nadolol, timolol, and **pindolol** are contraindicated in those with bronchial asthma or bronchospasm, including severe chronic obstructive pulmonary disease.

ACTIONS
Beta-adrenergic blocking agents compete with beta-adrenergic agonists for available beta-receptor sites.

Propranolol, nadolol, timolol, and pindolol inhibit both the beta$_1$ receptors, located chiefly in cardiac muscle, and beta$_2$ receptors, located chiefly in bronchial and vascular musculature, inhibiting the chronotropic, inotropic, and vasodilator responses to beta-adrenergic stimulation. Metoprolol and atenolol are cardioselective and preferentially inhibit beta$_1$ adrenoreceptors.

In dosages greater than those required for beta blockade, propranolol and, to a lesser extent, metoprolol exert a quinidinelike or anestheticlike membrane action that affects the cardiac action potential and depresses cardiac function. Nadolol, atenolol, and timolol do not have any membrane-stabilizing effects and have little direct myocardial depressant activity. Only pindolol has intrinsic sympathomimetic activity in therapeutic dosages; it does not have quinidinelike membrane stabilizing activity.

Clinical response to beta blockade includes slowing of sinus rate (heart rate), depression of AV conduction, decreased cardiac output at rest and on exercise, reduction of systolic blood pressure on exercise, general reduction of blood pressure in both supine and standing positions, inhibition of isoproterenol-induced tachycardia, and reduction of reflex orthostatic tachycardia.

Systemic bioavailability following oral administration of propranolol, metoprolol, and timolol is low because of significant first-pass hepatic metabolism. Pindolol has no significant first-pass effect. Ingestion with food enhances bioavailability of propranolol and metoprolol. Atenolol is approximately 50% absorbed; pindolol is rapidly absorbed and achieves peak plasma concentrations within 1 hour of administration. Only propranolol is significantly bound to plasma proteins. Metoprolol and propranolol readily enter the CNS. Because of their high water solubility, nadolol and atenolol do not pass the blood–brain barrier and may therefore have a lower incidence of CNS side-effects.

Metabolism/excretion: Propranolol and metoprolol are extensively metabolized by the liver; nadolol and atenolol are excreted unchanged by the kidneys. Timolol is partially metabolized by the liver; timolol and its metabolites are excreted by the kidneys. Pindolol undergoes extensive metabolism; 35% to 40% is excreted unchanged in the urine and 60% to 65% is metabolized and excreted as glucuronides and ethereal sulfate.

Antihypertensive actions: Beta blockers decrease standing and supine blood pressure and are effective when used alone or with other antihypertensives. Possible pharmacologic mechanisms include competitive antagonism of catecholamines at peripheral (nonCNS) adrenergic neuron sites (especially cardiac) leading to decreased cardiac output; a central effect leading to reduced sympathetic outflow to the periphery, and blockade of the beta-adrenergic receptors responsible for renin release from the kidneys.

Antianginal actions: Propranolol and nadolol may reduce oxygen requirement of the heart at any given level by blocking catecholamine-induced increases in heart rate, systolic blood pressure, and the velocity and extent of myocardial contraction. These agents may increase oxygen requirements by increasing left ventricular fiber length, end-diastolic pressure, and systolic ejection period, particularly in heart failure.

Antiarrhythmic action: Propranolol exerts antiarrhythmic effects in concentrations associated with beta-adrenergic blockade; this appears to be its principal antiarrhythmic mechanism of action. The membrane effect also plays a role, particularly in digitalis-induced arrhythmias. Beta-adrenergic blockade is of importance in management of arrhythmias due to increased levels of circulating catecholamines or enhanced sensitivity of the heart to catecholamines (arrhythmias associated with pheochromocytoma, thyrotoxicosis, exercise). Propranolol prolongs the refractory period, depresses automaticity, and slows AV conduction.

Myocardial infarction: Timolol and propranolol are the only beta-adrenergic blocking agents approved for use in prevention of reinfarction. The effectiveness of other beta blockers in the reduction of reinfarction and mortality in those surviving an acute MI has been demonstrated. The mechanism is unknown.

Antimigraine actions: Mechanism of propranolol's antimigraine effect has not been established. It may be due to inhibition of vasodilation or the fact that beta-adrenergic receptors have been demonstrated in the pial vessels of the brain and the arteriolar spasms over the cortex can be inhibited.

WARNINGS

Cardiac failure: Sympathetic stimulation is a vital component supporting circulatory function in CHF and beta blockade carries the potential of further depressing myocardial contractility and precipitating more severe failure. Administer these drugs cautiously in hypertensive patients who have CHF controlled by digitalis and diuretics. Beta-adrenergic blocking agents do not abolish the inotropic action of digitalis on heart muscle but, in those receiving digitalis, the positive inotropic action of digitalis may be reduced by the negative inotropic effect of beta blockade. The effects of beta blockers and digitalis are additive in depressing AV conduction.

In patients without a history of cardiac failure, continued depression of the myocardium over a period of time can, in some cases, lead to cardiac failure. At first sign of cardiac failure, the patient should be fully digitalized and/or treated with diuretics and the response observed closely.

In patients with Wolff-Parkinson-White syndrome there have been reports of tachycardia replaced by severe bradycardia after administration of propranolol.

Abrupt withdrawal: Hypersensitivity to catecholamines has been observed in those withdrawn from beta-blocker therapy. Exacerbation of angina, myocardial infarction, and ventricular arrhythmias have occurred after abrupt discontinuation of therapy. When discontinuing chronically administered beta-adrenergic blocking agents, reduce dosage gradually over 1 to 2 weeks and monitor patient closely. Because coronary artery disease may be unrecognized, therapy may not be abruptly discontinued in those treated for hypertension because abrupt withdrawal has resulted in transient symptoms, including tremulousness, sweating, palpitations, headache, and malaise.

Diabetes and hypoglycemia: Beta-adrenergic blockade may prevent the appearance of premonitory signs and symptoms (*e.g.,* pulse rate, blood-pressure changes) of acute hypoglycemia. Nonselective beta blockers may potentiate insulin-induced hypoglycemia. **Atenolol** does not potentiate insulin-induced hypoglycemia and, unlike nonselective beta blockers, does not delay recovery of blood glucose to normal levels. Hypoglycemic attacks may be accompanied by a precipitous elevation of blood pressure. These drugs are used with caution in diabetics, especially those with labile diabetes. Beta blockade also reduces release of insulin in response to hyperglycemia; it may be necessary to adjust the dose of antidiabetic drugs.

Thyrotoxicosis: May potentially aggravate CHF and mask clinical signs (*e.g.,* tachycardia) of developing or continuing hyperthyroidism or complications and give false impression of improvement. Abrupt withdrawal may be followed by exacerbation of symptoms of hyperthyroidism, including thyroid storm.

Nonallergenic bronchospasm (*e.g.,* chronic bronchitis, emphysema): Patients with these diseases should generally not receive beta blockers. Administer nadolol, propranolol, timolol, and pindolol with caution because they may block bronchodilation produced by endogenous or exogenous catecholamine stimulation of beta$_2$ receptors. Low doses of metoprolol and atenolol may be used with caution in those who do not respond to, or cannot tolerate, other antihypertensive treatment. Metoprolol may be administered tid in smaller doses to avoid higher plasma levels.

Major surgery: Beta blockade impairs ability of the heart to respond to reflex stimuli and may increase risk of general anesthesia and surgical procedures, resulting in protracted hypotension and low cardiac output. Therapy may be withdrawn several days prior to surgery, except in pheochromocytoma. In emergency surgery, effects of beta blockers can be reversed by administration of beta receptor agonists (*e.g.,* isoproterenol, dopamine, dobutamine, norepinephrine).

Use in impaired hepatic or renal function: Use beta blockers with caution. Renal function does not appear to affect elimination or clinical effect of metoprolol. Timolol's half-life is essentially unchanged in those with moderate renal insufficiency; marked hypotensive responses have been seen in those with marked renal impairment undergoing dialysis after 20 mg of timolol. Because nadolol and atenolol are eliminated primarily by the kidneys, half-life increases in renal failure. Propranolol, metoprolol, and timolol are not significantly dialyzable. Poor renal function has only minor effects on pindolol clearance, but poor hepatic function may cause blood levels to increase substantially.

Use in pregnancy: Safety not established.

Use in lactation: In general, nursing should not be undertaken by mothers receiving these drugs.

Use in children: Safety and efficacy not established.

DRUG INTERACTIONS

Catecholamine-depleting drugs (*e.g.,* reserpine): May have an additive effect. Patients receiving a beta-adrenergic blocking agent plus a catecholamine-depleting drug are monitored closely for excessive reduction in sympathetic tone (hypotension or excessive bradycardia), which may produce vertigo, syncope, postural hypotension.

MAO inhibitors: Contraindicated in patients on these drugs and during 2-week withdrawal period from such drugs.

Digitalis: Inotropic action may be reduced by the beta-adrenergic blocking agents' negative inotropic effects. Effects are additive in depressing AV conduction.

Verapamil: *Oral*—use may be beneficial in those with chronic stable angina, but the combination can have adverse effects on cardiac function. If combined therapy is used, closely monitor vital signs, evaluate patient's clinical status. *IV*—concomitant administration with beta blockers has, on rare occasions, resulted in serious adverse reactions, especially in those with severe cardiomyopathy, CHF, or recent myocardial infarction.

Nifedipine: Rarely, increase in likelihood of CHF, severe hypotension, exacerbation of angina.

Lidocaine: Clearance may be impaired with concomitant use of propranolol.

Anesthesia: During anesthesia with agents that require catecholamine release for maintenance of adequate cardiac function, beta blockade will impair the desired inotropic effect.

Isoproterenol, norepinephrine, dopamine, dobutamine: Effects of beta-adrenergic blocking agents can be reversed by these drugs, but patient can be subject to severe protracted hypotension.

Aminophylline: Concomitant use of beta blockers may have antagonistic effects. **Theophylline** clearance may decrease.

Insulin: Hypoglycemic effects may be prolonged by beta blockade.

Clonidine: During concomitant administration with beta blockers, rapid withdrawal of clonidine prior to discontinuation of the beta-adrenergic blocking agent may produce hypertension due to increase in circulating catecholamines.

Prazosin: Beta-adrenergic blocking agents may increase the "first-dose response" (acute postural hypotension) that often occurs following initiation of prazosin therapy.

Indomethacin: May inhibit antihypertensive response of propranolol.

Chlorpromazine, cimetidine, furosemide, hydralazine: An increase in propranolol plasma levels and increase in beta blockade may occur with concomitant administration with these drugs.

IV phenytoin: May produce additive cardiac depressant effects. May decrease propranolol levels.

Phenobarbital: May decrease propranolol plasma levels.

Smoking: May reduce serum levels and increase clearance of propranolol.

Drug/lab tests: Beta-adrenergic blocking agents may produce hypoglycemia and interfere with **glucose**- or **insulin**-tolerance tests.

ADVERSE REACTIONS

Most adverse effects are mild and transient and rarely require withdrawal of drug.

Allergic: Pharyngitis; erythematous rash; fever with aching, sore throat; laryngospasm; respiratory distress.

Cardiovascular: Bradycardia; chest pain; worsening of angina; shortness of breath; symptoms of peripheral vascular insufficiency (cold extremities, paresthesia of hands) usually of Raynaud type; cardiac failure; sinoatrial block; cerebral vascular accident; edema; pulmonary edema; vasodilatation; syncope; hypotension; tachycardia; arrhythmia; rhythm/conduction disturbances; palpitations; worsening of atrial insufficiency; first-degree and third-degree heart block; intensification of AV block.

CNS/Psychiatric: Dizziness; vertigo; fatigue; mental depression (insomnia, lassitude, weakness, fatigue); paresthesias; local weakness; lethargy; claudication; sedation and change in behavior; anxiety; nervousness; diminished concentration; somnolence; sleep disturbances; bizarre or many dreams; reversible mental depression progressing to catatonia; hallucinations; an acute reversible syndrome characterized by disorientation of time, place; short-term memory loss; emotional lability; slightly clouded sensorium; decreased performance on neuropsychometrics; lightheadedness. Headache, nightmares, insomnia also reported. Acute mental changes (paranoia, disorientation, combativeness) in elderly have occurred.

Endocrine: Hyperglycemia, hypoglycemia.

GI/GU: Gastric pain; flatulence; heartburn; nausea; diarrhea; dry mouth; dyspepsia; abdominal discomfort; vomiting; indigestion; anorexia; bloating; abdominal cramping; mesenteric arterial thrombosis; ischemic colitis; retroperitoneal fibrosis; hepatomegaly; urination difficulties; pollakiuria; impotence or decreased libido.

Hematologic: Agranulocytosis; nonthrombocytopenic or thrombocytopenic purpura.

Integumentary: Rash; pruritus; skin irritation; increased pigmentation; sweating; dry skin. Peripheral skin necrosis and psoriasiform lesions have occurred with propranolol.

Ophthalmologic: Eye irritation; visual disturbances; dry eyes; blurred vision.

Respiratory: Bronchospasm; dyspnea; cough; bronchial obstruction; rales; nasal congestion.

Musculoskeletal: Chest pain; joint pain; muscle cramps and pain.

Miscellaneous: Reversible alopecia; acute pancreatitis; facial swelling; weight gain, loss; body pain; slurred speech; tinnitus; arthralgia; decreased exercise tolerance; hyperhydrosis; Peyronie's disease.

Clinical laboratory test findings: Propranolol may elevate blood urea levels in those with severe heart disease, elevate serum transaminase, alkaline phosphatase, and lactate dehydrogenase (LDH). Timolol may produce slight increases in BUN, serum potassium, and serum uric acid and slight decreases in hemoglobin and hematocrit. Minor persistent elevations in SGOT and SGPT have occurred in some patients given pindolol. Rarely, alkaline phosphatase, LDH, and uric acid may be elevated.

OVERDOSAGE

In addition to gastric lavage, the following treatments should be employed as appropriate for the reactions listed.

Bradycardia: IV atropine (0.25 mg to 2 mg); if no response to vagal blockade, IV isoproterenol. In

AV block, transvenous cardiac pacing may be needed.

Bronchospasm: A beta$_2$ stimulating agent and/or theophylline may be administered.

Cardiac failure: A digitalis glycoside, a diuretic, and oxygen are administered immediately. In refractory cases, IV aminophylline is suggested. Glucagon may also be used. In shock resulting from inadequate cardiac contractility, dobutamine may be considered.

Hypotension: Vasopressors (*e.g.,* dopamine, dobutamine, norepinephrine) may be administered; blood pressure is monitored frequently. There is evidence that epinephrine may be the drug of choice. Glucagon may be used in refractory cases.

Heart block (second or third degree): Isoproterenol or transvenous cardiac pacemaker.

Dialysis: Nadolol and atenolol can be removed by hemodialysis. Propranolol, metoprolol, and timolol are not significantly dialyzable.

DOSAGE

ATENOLOL

Initially, 50 mg/day as one tablet/day either alone or added to diuretic therapy. Full effect of this dose usually seen in 1 to 2 weeks. If optimal response is not achieved, dosage may be increased to 100 mg given as one tablet/day. Dosage above 100 mg/day is unlikely to produce further benefit.

Renal failure: Dosage adjusted in cases of severe renal impairment. Recommended dosages are 50 mg daily if creatinine clearance is 15 ml/minute to 35 ml/minute; 50 mg every other day if creatinine clearance is less than 15 ml/minute. Patients on hemodialysis should be given 50 mg after each dialysis; this should be done under hospital supervision because marked falls in blood pressure can occur.

METOPROLOL TARTRATE

Initially, 100 mg/day in single or divided doses, whether used alone or added to a diuretic. Dosage may be increased at weekly or longer intervals until optimum response is achieved. Generally, the maximum effect of any given dosage level will be apparent after 1 week of therapy.

Maintenance dose: Effective dosage range is 100 mg/day to 450 mg/day. Dosages above 450 mg/day presently not recommended. Although once-daily dosing is effective and can maintain reduction in blood pressure throughout the day, lower doses (especially 100 mg) may not maintain a full effect at the end of a 24-hour period; larger or more frequent daily doses may be required. Blood pressure should be measured at the end of the dosing interval to determine whether satisfactory control is being maintained throughout the day.

NADOLOL

Drug may be given without regard to meals.

Angina pectoris: Usual initial dose is 40 mg once daily. Dosage is gradually increased in 40-mg to 80-mg increments at 3- to 7-day intervals until optimum response is obtained or there is pronounced slowing of the pulse. Usual maintenance dosage range is 80 mg to 240 mg administered once daily. Most patients respond to 160 mg or less daily. Usefulness and safety of dosages above 240 mg/day not established.

Hypertension: Usual initial dose is 40 mg once daily whether used alone or in addition to diuretic therapy. Dosage may be gradually increased in 40-mg to 80-mg increments until optimum blood-pressure reduction is achieved. Usual maintenance dose is 80 mg to 320 mg once daily. In rare instances, doses up to 640 mg/day may be needed.

Renal failure: Recommended dosage intervals are listed in Table 3.

PINDOLOL

Recommended initial dose is 10 mg bid, alone or in combination with other antihypertensive agents. Many respond to 15 mg/day (5 mg tid). Antihypertensive response usually occurs within first week. If a satisfactory reduction in blood pressure does not occur within 2 to 3 weeks, adjust dosage in increments of 10 mg/day at 2- to 3-week intervals to a maximum of 60 mg/day.

PROPRANOLOL HYDROCHLORIDE

Lower dosages may be required in patients with renal or hepatic dysfunction.

Oral

Arrhythmias: 10 mg to 30 mg tid or qid, A.C. and H.S.

Hypertension: Dosage individualized. Usual initial dose is 40 mg bid whether used alone or added to a diuretic. Increase gradually until optimum response is achieved. Usual dosage is 160 mg/day to 480 mg/day; up to 640 mg/day may be required.

Table 3. Recommended Nadolol Dosage Intervals in Renal Failure

Creatinine Clearance (ml/minute)	Dosage Interval (hours)
>50	24
31–50	24–36
10–30	24–48
<10	40–60

Time of response is variable and may range from a few days to several weeks. Although bid dosing is effective and can maintain reduction in blood pressure throughout the day, some patients, especially when lower doses are used, may experience a modest rise in blood pressure toward the end of the 12-hour dosing interval. If control is not adequate, a larger dose or tid therapy may achieve better control.

Angina pectoris: Dosage is individualized. Usual initial dose is 10 mg to 20 mg tid or qid, A.C. and H.S. May be gradually increased at 3- to 7-day intervals until optimum response is obtained. Average optimum dosage is 160 mg/day. Value and safety of dosage exceeding 320 mg/day not established.

Myocardial infarction: 180 mg/day to 240 mg/day in divided doses in a tid or qid regimen. The effectiveness and safety of daily dosages above 240 mg for prevention of cardiac mortality not established. Higher dosages may be needed to treat coexisting diseases (*e.g.,* angina or hypertension) effectively.

Hypertrophic subaortic stenosis: 20 mg to 40 mg tid or qid, A.C. and H.S.

Pheochromocytoma: Preoperatively, 60 mg/day in divided doses for 3 days prior to surgery, concomitantly given with an alpha-adrenergic blocking agent. *Management of inoperable tumor*—30 mg/day in divided doses.

Migraine: Dosage is individualized. Initial dose is 80 mg/day in divided doses. Usual effective dosage range is 160 mg/day to 240 mg/day. Dosage may be increased gradually to achieve optimum prophylaxis. If satisfactory response is not obtained within 4 to 6 weeks after reaching maximum dose, discontinue therapy. Withdraw drug gradually over a 2-week period.

Parenteral

IV administration reserved for life-threatening arrhythmias or arrhythmias occurring under anesthesia. Usual dose is from 1 mg to 3 mg administered under careful monitoring (CVP, ECG). Do not exceed 1 mg/minute to avoid lowering blood pressure and causing cardiac standstill. If necessary, a second dose may be administered after 2 minutes. Thereafter, drug not administered prior to 4 hours later. Additional propranolol not given after the desired alteration in rate or rhythm is achieved. Oral therapy started as soon as possible.

TIMOLOL MALEATE

Hypertension: Usual initial dosage is 10 mg bid whether used alone or added to a diuretic. Usual total maintenance dosage is 20 mg/day to 40 mg/day. May be increased to 60 mg/day divided into 2 doses, if necessary. There should be an interval of at least 7 days between dosage increases.

Myocardial infarction (long-term prophylactic use in those who have survived the acute phase of a myocardial infarction): 10 mg bid.

NURSING IMPLICATIONS

HISTORY
See Appendix 4.

PHYSICAL ASSESSMENT
Take blood pressure on both arms with patient in sitting and lying positions; take pulse (obtain apical and radial rate if patient has an arrhythmia); record respiratory rate, temperature, weight; auscultate lungs. Baseline laboratory and diagnostic tests/studies may include renal- and hepatic-function studies, serum electrolytes, fasting blood sugar, CBC, ECG.

ADMINISTRATION
Metoprolol: Give with food. Usual dose schedule is bid at 12-hour intervals. If patient is diabetic, request dietitian to provide H.S. snack if one is not currently included in diet regimen.

Propranolol, oral: Give before meals.

Propranolol, IV: Available in 1-ml ampules, 1 mg/ml. Do *not* exceed 1 mg/minute. It is recommended that patient be on cardiac monitor and have CVP line, both of which are monitored closely during and immediately following administration of drug.

ONGOING ASSESSMENTS AND NURSING MANAGEMENT
Nursing observations are essential determinants in achieving optimal drug response.

Record blood pressure, pulse, and respirations q2h to q4h or as ordered; monitor temperature, intake and output; observe for adverse effects (see *Adverse Reactions*); observe for beneficial drug response (*e.g.,* relief from angina, decrease in blood pressure, abolishment of arrhythmia). Notify physician if any adverse reaction occurs. If reaction appears serious, withhold next dose of drug and notify physician immediately.

During initial therapy, obtain additional blood pressure and pulse rate immediately before drug is administered. Withhold medication and notify physician immediately if there is a pronounced decrease or increase in blood pressure or change in heart rate, rhythm, or amplitude from baseline values. An apical or apical–radial pulse should be taken if patient has an arrhythmia and is not on a cardiac monitor. Changes in blood pressure or pulse rate may require dosage adjustment.

CLINICAL ALERT: Pronounced bradycardia may require emergency intervention; IV atropine or isoproterenol may be administered to produce vagal blockade. These emergency drugs should always be immediately available if patient is receiving a beta-adrenergic blocking agent.

Weigh daily or as ordered. Increase in weight and decrease in urinary output may indicate development of CHF.

Check extremities daily for evidence of vascular insufficiency (cold extremities, paresthesia of hands).

Drug is not discontinued abruptly (except in emergency situations); ensure continuity of prescribed therapy by notation on Kardex, informing health-team members responsible for drug administration. _Symptoms of abrupt withdrawal_—tremulousness, sweating, palpitations, headache, malaise.

Observe for signs of CHF (_e.g.,_ dyspnea on exertion, orthopnea, edema of extremities, night cough, distended neck veins); notify physician should one or more of these occur. If symptoms are severe, administer oxygen and notify physician immediately because emergency intervention (digitalis glycoside, diuretic, IV aminophylline) may be necessary.

May produce drowsiness, dizziness, lightheadedness, blurred vision. Patient should be assisted with ambulatory activities, especially early in therapy.

Diabetic patient may require dosage adjustment of antidiabetic agent. Monitor patient closely; administration of these drugs may prevent appearance of signs and symptoms of acute hypoglycemia (_e.g.,_ changes in pulse rate or blood pressure). Check urine for glucose, ketones qid; observe patient for other signs of hypoglycemia (_e.g.,_ fatigue, hunger, sweating, personality changes).

NOTE: Fatigue, sweating, personality changes may also be adverse drug reactions.

Hypoglycemic attacks may be accompanied by a precipitous rise in blood pressure. If hypoglycemia should occur, monitor blood pressure q30m until condition is stabilized.

Notify physician if diabetic patient has anorexia because dosage of antidiabetic drug or diabetic diet may require adjustment.

When therapy is discontinued, monitor patient closely during dosage-reduction period. Check blood pressure, pulse, and respirations q2h to q4h or as ordered; observe for recurrence of original symptoms. If angina markedly worsens or acute coronary insufficiency develops, notify physician immediately because therapy may need to be reinstituted.

If major surgery is scheduled, drug therapy is usually withdrawn several days prior to surgery (_exception_—pheochromocytoma). If scheduled or emergency surgery is necessary, always notify anesthetist of current drug therapy and tape notice on front of the patient's chart.

Hemodialysis patients: Atenolol administered after dialysis. Monitor blood pressure, pulse, and respirations q1h to q2h or as ordered because marked falls in blood pressure can occur.

PATIENT AND FAMILY INFORMATION

Do not discontinue medication abruptly except on advice of physician. Sudden cessation of therapy may precipitate or exacerbate angina.

Notify physician or nurse if any of the following occurs: difficulty breathing, especially on exertion or when lying down; night cough; swelling of extremities; dizziness; lightheadedness; confusion or depression; skin rash; fever; sore throat; unusual bleeding or bruising.

Take pulse before each dose; report any increase or decrease to physician. If drug is prescribed as antihypertensive, take pulse and blood pressure daily. (Physician approval should be obtained to include these in teaching plan. Patient or family member will also require instruction in taking pulse, blood pressure).

May produce drowsiness, dizziness, lightheadedness, blurred vision; observe caution while driving or performing tasks requiring alertness.

Keep all physician/clinic appointments because close monitoring of therapy is essential. Physician may order periodic laboratory tests, diagnostic studies to monitor progress.

Do not use any nonprescription drugs without consent of physician.

Inform dentists, other physicians of current therapy with this drug.

Propranolol: Avoid smoking because it may decrease drug's effect.

Propranolol and metoprolol: Take with food to enhance absorption.

Metoprolol, nadolol, timolol: May be taken without regard to meals.

Atenolol: Available in calendar pack 28s (50 mg), which may be of value for those having difficulty remembering dosage schedule.

Diabetics: These agents may mask signs of hypoglycemia or alter blood glucose levels. Adhere to prescribed diet; check urine one to two times a day (or as recommended by physician). Report positive urine glucose, ketones to physician.

Betamethasone Preparations

For systemic preparations, see Glucocorticoids. For topical preparations, see Corticosteroids, Topical.

Betazole Hydrochloride Rx

injection: 50 mg/ml   Histalog

INDICATIONS

For clinical testing of gastric secretion. In recommended dosage, will produce stimulation of gastric secretion equal to the usual dosage of histamine but has minimal effects on other organs and produces less severe side-effects. Not recommended for use in other conditions in which histamine is used clinically.

Testing of gastric secretion is usually performed to determine whether achlorhydria is present, as in those suspected of having pernicious anemia, or to measure the secretory capacity of the gastric glands, as in patients suspected of having a gastric carcinoma or peptic ulcer.

ACTIONS

Similar to histamine in respect to its effect on blood pressure, gastric-acid secretion, and smooth muscle. Unlike histamine, it is selective in action. Primary effect is to stimulate production of gastric acid. This is much more prominent than its other histamine-like actions. Antihistaminic drugs do not effect the stimulation of gastric secretion produced by betazole or histamine.

WARNINGS

Those with an allergic diathesis may react severely. Use with caution in patients with moderate to severe allergic disease. Safety for use in pregnancy not established.

PRECAUTIONS

Weakness, syncope may occur.

ADVERSE REACTIONS

Most common is flushing of the face accompanied by a sense of warmth; headache, urticaria may also occur.

OVERDOSAGE

If hypotension or acute asthma follows accidental overdosage, epinephrine is recommended. Urticaria has been improved with the use of antihistamines.

DOSAGE

Administer IM or subcutaneously. The 0.5-mg/kg dose is comparable to the usually employed dose of histamine in fractional gastric analysis. If a simplified procedure is desired, a fixed amount of 50 mg may be given to adult patients of average weight. There is a wide margin of safety in dosage; amounts of 200 mg have been given without apparent harm but have been associated with higher incidence and increased severity of side-effects.

Technique of fractional gastric analysis: Various methods are used; one procedure is described below:

The fasting patient is intubated with a Levin tube. Stomach contents are aspirated by continuous suction. The aspirate is fractionated into 15-minute specimens. After the first 15 minutes, betazole is injected and fractional specimens collected for 1 hour. Specimens are sent to the laboratory.

Interpretation of test results: Response varies according to age and general health. In general, the fasting specimen may normally contain 0 mEq to 2 mEq of free HCl and an additional 1 mEq of total HCl in a volume up to 50 ml of gastric juice. Maximum secretory response begins 45 minutes after administration of betazole and lasts approximately 2.5 hours. The secretory volume and acidity are usually increased 100% to 200% in normal patients.

High values are often associated with duodenal ulcer and pyloric obstruction. Low values may be found with gastric ulcer, carcinoma of the stomach, and chronic gastritis and in chronic diseases and debilitated states. Absence of free HCl is always found in patients with pernicious anemia. Normal patients may also have achlorhydria but normal amounts of mucus and pepsin are found; mucus and pepsin are absent or nearly absent in those with pernicious anemia.

NURSING IMPLICATIONS

HISTORY

See Appendix 4.

NOTE: Drug is contraindicated or used with caution in those with moderate to severe allergic disease.

PHYSICAL ASSESSMENT

Check blood pressure, pulse, and respirations; weigh patient (dosage may be based on weight);

inspect nares to see if deviation of septum will interfere with passage of nasogastric tube.

ADMINISTRATION
Explain general purpose and techniques of test and what side-effects might be experienced. Inform patient about fasting from midnight.

Physician may order a fixed dose of 50 mg or calculate dose according to weight. Drug may be administered IM or subcutaneously (physician will specify).

Review hospital manual for technique of fractional gastric analysis, insertion of nasogastric tube.

Epinephrine and an antihistamine should be immediately available. Epinephrine may be used if hypotension or acute asthma occurs; antihistamine is used for urticaria. Hospital's procedure policy may include dosage of epinephrine and antihistamine. If guidelines for administration of these drugs are not included in hospital procedure, discuss with physician.

Patient is kept fasting, usually from midnight throughout test. Usually smoking is not allowed. Certain drugs (_e.g.,_ anticholinergic agents) may affect gastric secretion and are withheld until the test is completed. The physician must specify drugs to be withheld.

Obtain required materials: gastric analysis tray or separate materials including nasogastric tube, aspiration/irrigation syringe, gastric decompression machine (_e.g.,_ Gomco Thermotic machine, Air Shields suction machine), water-soluble lubricant, stethoscope, clamp, emesis basin, bath towel.

Obtain baseline blood pressure, pulse, and respirations before procedure.

Restraints will be required for pediatric patient.

Obtain gastric aspirate samples according to hospital procedure; label each specimen with patient's name, time and date, sample number.

ONGOING ASSESSMENTS AND NURSING MANAGEMENT
Monitor blood pressure, pulse, and respirations during and for 1 hour after test. Hypotension and acute asthma require immediate intervention.

Send labeled aspirate to laboratory.

Bethanecol Chloride Rx

tablets: 5 mg	Urecholine, _Generic_
tablets: 10 mg, 25 mg	Duvoid, Myotonachol, Urecholine, _Generic_
tablets: 50 mg	Duvoid, Urecholine, _Generic_
injection: 5 mg/ml	Urecholine

INDICATIONS
Acute postoperative and postpartum nonobstructive (functional) urinary retention and neurogenic atony of the urinary bladder with retention.

**Investigational uses:** Reflux esophagitis.

CONTRAINDICATIONS
Hypersensitivity; hyperthyroidism; peptic ulcer; latent or active asthma; pronounced bradycardia; vasomotor instability; coronary artery disease; epilepsy; parkinsonism; coronary occlusion; atrioventricular conduction defects; hypertension; hypotension. Not used when strength or integrity of the GI or bladder wall is in question or in presence of mechanical obstruction; when increased muscular activity of the GI tract or urinary bladder might prove harmful (as following recent bladder surgery, GI resection, and anastomosis), or when there is a possible GI obstruction; in bladder-neck obstruction, spastic GI disturbances, acute inflammatory lesions of the GI tract, peritonitis; in marked vagotonia. Contraindicated in pregnancy.

ACTIONS
A synthetic choline ester that acts principally by producing the effects of stimulation of the parasympathetic nervous system. It increases the tone of the detrusor urinae muscle, usually producing contraction sufficiently strong to initiate micturition and empty the bladder. It stimulates gastric motility, increases gastric tone, and often restores impaired rhythmic peristalsis. When spontaneous stimulation of the parasympathomimetic system is reduced and therapeutic intervention is required, acetylcholine can be given, but it is rapidly hydrolyzed by cholinesterase and its effects are transient. Bethanechol is not destroyed by cholinesterase and its effects are more prolonged than those of acetylcholine. It has predominate muscarinic action and only slight nicotinic action. Doses that stimulate micturition and defecation and increase peristalsis do not ordinarily stimulate ganglia or voluntary muscles. Therapeutic doses have little effect on heart rate, blood pressure, peripheral circulation.

Drug effects appear within 30 to 90 minutes after oral administration and persist for up to 6 hours. Subcutaneous administration is usually effective in 5 to 15 minutes. In general, the onset of subcutaneous dosage activity is more rapid and of shorter duration.

WARNINGS

Parenteral form for subcutaneous use only. It should *never* be given IM or IV. Violent symptoms of cholinergic overstimulation, such as circulatory collapse, fall in blood pressure, abdominal cramps, bloody diarrhea, shock, or sudden cardiac arrest, are likely to occur if drug is given IM or IV. Although rare, these symptoms have occurred after subcutaneous injection and may occur in cases of hypersensitivity or overdosage.

PRECAUTIONS

In urinary retention, if sphincter fails to relax as bethanechol contracts the bladder, urine may be forced up the ureter into the kidney pelvis. If there is bacteriuria, this may cause reflux infection.

DRUG INTERACTIONS

Special care is required if given to patients receiving **quinidine** or **procainamide,** which may antagonize cholinergic effects; **cholinergic drugs,** particularly cholinesterase inhibitors, because additive effects may occur; **ganglionic blocking compounds** because there may be a critical fall in blood pressure, which is usually preceded by severe abdominal symptoms.

ADVERSE REACTIONS

Untoward effects usually due to overdosage and pharmacologic extension, but may occur infrequently with oral administration. Abdominal discomfort, salivation, flushing of skin ("hot feeling"), sweating, nausea, vomiting are early signs of overdosage. Involuntary defecation and urinary urgency may occur after large doses. Other effects include malaise, headache, colicky pain, abdominal cramps, diarrhea, belching, borborygmi. Asthmatic attacks, especially in asthmatics, may be precipitated. Substernal pressure or pain may occur; it is uncertain whether this is due to bronchoconstriction or spasm of the esophagus.

Transient syncope with cardiac arrest, transient complete heart block, dyspnea, and orthostatic hypotension may be associated with large doses. Myocardial hypoxia must be considered if a marked fall in blood pressure occurs. Patients with hypertension may react with a precipitous fall in blood pressure. Short periods of atrial fibrillation have been observed in hyperthyroid patients following administration of cholinergic drugs.

OVERDOSAGE

Symptoms: See *Adverse Reactions* (above).

Treatment: Atropine is a specific antidote. When using bethanechol parenterally, a syringe containing atropine sulfate, 0.6 mg to 1.2 mg (for adults),
should always be available. For children, use proportionately smaller amounts (*i.e.,* 0.01 mg/kg q2h, as necessary). See Atropine Sulfate for recommended pediatric dosage by weight. Maximum single dose should not exceed 0.4 mg. Subcutaneous injection is recommended, except in emergencies, when IV route may be used.

DOSAGE

Dose is individualized.

Oral: Usual adult dose is 10 mg to 50 mg two to four times/day; maximum, 120 mg. Minimum effective dose is determined by giving 5 mg or 10 mg initially and repeating the same amount at hourly intervals to a maximum of 30 mg until satisfactory response occurs. Alternatively, 10 mg may be given initially and administration repeated with 25 mg, then 50 mg, at 6-hour intervals until desired response is obtained.

Subcutaneous: Usual dose is 5 mg; some patients respond to as little as 2.5 mg. Minimum effective dose is determined by injecting 2.5 mg initially and repeating same amount at 15- to 30-minute intervals to a maximum of four doses until satisfactory response is obtained, unless disturbing reactions appear. Minimum effective dose is repeated thereafter three to four times/day as needed. Rarely, single doses up to 10 mg may be required. Such doses may cause severe reactions and are used only after adequate trial of single doses of 2.5 mg to 5 mg has established that smaller doses are not sufficient. If necessary, the effects of the drug can be abolished promptly by atropine.

NURSING IMPLICATIONS

HISTORY

See Appendix 4.

PHYSICAL ASSESSMENT

Palpate bladder to determine size; check blood pressure, pulse.

ADMINISTRATION

Oral: Administer 1 hour before meals or 2 hours after meals; if taken soon after eating, nausea and vomiting may occur.

CLINICAL ALERT: Parenteral form is for subcutaneous use only. It should *never* be given IM or IV (see *Warnings*).

Use correct technique for subcutaneous injection and aspirate syringe before injecting drug to avoid administration into a blood vessel.

Obtain blood pressure and pulse before administration, especially when drug is given subcutaneously.

Atropine sulfate should be immediately available for abolishing severe side-effects when drug is administered parenterally. Discuss with physician dose to be used and circumstances required for administration of antidote. Prepare syringe filled with prescribed dose and keep available. Atropine is usually administered subcutaneously, but in an emergency may be administered IV.

If drug is administered orally, be sure atropine is readily available and stocked in the clinical area.

ONGOING ASSESSMENTS AND NURSING MANAGEMENT

Physician usually titrates dosage to determine minimum effective dose (see *Dosage*). It is essential that each voiding be measured; record the amount and time on the patient's chart.

Measure total daily intake and output, as well as each voiding.

In some instances physician may order catheterization for residual urine after each voiding.

Patients with hypertension may react to drug with a precipitous fall in blood pressure; monitor such patients more frequently.

If patient is on bedrest, have call light, bedpan, or urinal within easy reach because voiding may occur rapidly and with little warning.

Drug may not always produce desired results. Keep physician informed of response or lack of response to therapy.

Oral: Drug effects usually appear within 30 to 90 minutes.

Observe for adverse drug effects. Monitor blood pressure, pulse, and respirations q1h to q2h when drug therapy is initiated. Check for early signs of overdosage: abdominal discomfort, salivation, flushing of skin, nausea, vomiting. If these should occur, contact physician immediately.

Subcutaneous: Drug effects usually appear within 5 to 15 minutes.

Observe patient frequently during initial therapy; monitor blood pressure, pulse, and respirations q15m to q30m. The serious adverse effects seen with incorrect administration (IM, IV), although rare, can occur with subcutaneous administration (review *Warnings*).

PATIENT AND FAMILY INFORMATION

To avoid nausea and vomiting, take on empty stomach 1 hour before or at least 2 hours after meals.

May cause abdominal discomfort, salivation, sweating, or flushing; notify physician or nurse if these effects are pronounced.

Do not take any nonprescription drug unless use is approved by physician.

Bile Acid Sequestrants

Cholestyramine Rx

powder: 4 g resin/9 g   Questran
   powder

Colestipol Hydrochloride Rx

water-insoluble beads   Colestid

INDICATIONS

Hyperlipoproteinemia: Adjunctive therapy to diet management in those with elevated cholesterol levels due to primary type II hyperlipoproteinemia (pure hypercholesterolemia). These agents have been shown to increase or have no effect on triglyceride levels.

Biliary obstruction: **Cholestyramine** also indicated for relief of pruritus associated with partial biliary obstruction.

Investigational uses: Cholestyramine has been used in treatment of pseudomembranous colitis, poisoning by the pesticide chlordecone (Kepone).

CONTRAINDICATIONS

Hypersensitivity; complete biliary obstruction.

ACTIONS

Cholesterol is the major (and probably the sole) precursor of bile acids. During normal digestion, bile acids are secreted via the bile from the liver and gallbladder into the intestines. Bile acids emulsify the fatty and lipid materials present in food, thus facilitating absorption. A major portion of the bile acids secreted is reabsorbed from the intestines and returned via the portal circulation to the liver, thus completing the enterohepatic cycle. Only very small amounts of bile acids are found in normal serum. Bile acid sequestering resins (cholestyramine, colestipol) combine with bile acids in the intestine to form an insoluble complex that is excreted in the feces. This results in a continuous, although partial, removal of bile acids from the enterohepatic circulation by preventing their reabsorption. The increased loss of bile acids leads to an increased oxidation of cholesterol to bile acids, a decrease in beta-lipoprotein or low-density lipoprotein plasma levels and a decrease in serum cholesterol levels. Bile acid sequestrants produce an increase in hepatic synthesis of cholesterol, but plasma cholesterol levels fall. There is evidence that this fall in cholesterol is secondary to an increased rate of clearance of cholesterol-rich lipoproteins from plasma. Serum triglyceride levels may increase or remain unchanged. The decline in serum cholesterol levels is usually evident in 1 month. When these drugs are discontinued, serum cholesterol levels usually return to baseline levels within 1 month.

When secretion of bile is partially blocked, the concentration of bile acids in the serum rises. In patients with partial biliary obstruction, reduction of serum bile acid levels by cholestyramine resin is thought to reduce excess bile acids deposited in dermal tissues, with resulting decrease in pruritus.

WARNINGS

Not taken in dry form, but mixed with water or other fluid. Safety for use in pregnancy and lactation not established. Use only when clearly needed and potential benefits outweigh the unknown potential hazards to the fetus. A practical dosage schedule for children has not been established and effects of long-term administration and effectiveness in maintaining lowered cholesterol levels are unknown.

DRUG INTERACTIONS

These resins are anion-exchange resins and have a strong affinity for anions other than the bile acids and may delay or reduce absorption of concomitant oral medication by binding the drugs in the gut. The intervals between administration of these resins and any other medication should be as long as possible.

These agents have been reported to delay or reduce absorption of concomitant oral medication such as **phenylbutazone, warfarin, chlorothiazide, digitalis preparations, penicillin G, tetracycline, phenobarbital, folic acid, iron, thyroid preparations, cephalexin, clindamycin, trimethoprim.** The absorption of chlorothiazide is markedly decreased even when administered 1 hour before colestipol. There are conflicting reports for the effect of these resins on the availability of digoxin and digitoxin. Malabsorption of **fat-soluble vitamins** may occur with doses greater than 24 g/day.

Discontinuance of these resins could pose a potential hazard if a potentially toxic drug (such as digitalis) that is significantly bound to the resin has been titrated to a maintenance level while the patient has been taking the resin.

PRECAUTIONS

Before therapy is instituted, an attempt is made to control serum cholesterol by appropriate dietary regimen and weight reduction, and any underlying disorder that may contribute to the hypercholesterolemia is treated.

These resins may interfere with normal fat absorption and may thus prevent absorption of fat-soluble vitamins such as A, D, and K. If given for long periods of time, supplemental vitamin A and D may be given daily in a water-miscible form or parenterally.

Chronic use of resins may be associated with increased bleeding tendency due to hypoprothrombinemia associated with vitamin K deficiency. This usually responds to parenteral vitamin K; recurrences can be prevented by oral administration of vitamin K.

There is a possibility that chronic use may produce hyperchloremic acidosis. These agents may produce or severely worsen preexisting constipation. Decreased dosages may be necessary in those with constipation because fecal impaction may occur. Particular effort should be made to avoid constipation in those with symptomatic coronary artery disease. Constipation associated with these drugs may aggravate hemorrhoids. A laxative, rather than a decrease in dose, may be prescribed if drug is effective and needed. The theoretical possibility of hypothyroidism exists, particularly in those with limited thyroid reserve.

ADVERSE REACTIONS

Most common adverse reactions are related to the GI tract. Constipation is the major single complaint and at times is severe and occasionally accompanied by fecal impaction and/or hemorrhoids, with or without severe bleeding. Most instances of constipation are mild, transient, and controlled with standard treatment. Some patients may require decrease in dosage or discontinuation of therapy.

Less frequent GI complaints: Abdominal discomfort (pain, distention), belching, flatulence, nausea, vomiting, diarrhea, heartburn, anorexia, feeling of indigestion, steatorrhea.

Other reactions: Bleeding tendencies due to hypoprothrombinemia (vitamin K deficiency) as well as vitamin A and D deficiencies; rash, irritation of skin, tongue, perianal area; hypochloremic acidosis in children; osteoporosis. Occasionally calcified material has been seen in the biliary tree, including calcification of the gall bladder. This may be a manifestation of the liver disease and not drug related.

Other reactions (not necessarily drug related)

GI: Rectal bleeding, black stools, hemorrhoidal bleeding, bleeding from known duodenal ulcer, dysphagia, hiccups, ulcer attack, sour taste, pancreatitis, rectal pain, diverticulitis, peptic ulceration, cholecystitis, cholelithiasis.

Hematologic: Decreased prothrombin time, ecchymosis, anemia.

Cardiovascular: Claudication, arteritis, thrombophlebitis, myocardial ischemia, angina, myocardial infarction.

Hypersensitivity: Urticaria and dermatitis.

Musculoskeletal: Backache, muscle and joint pains, arthritis.

Neurologic: Headache, anxiety, vertigo, dizziness, fatigue, tinnitus, syncope, drowsiness, femoral nerve pain, paresthesia.

Ophthalmologic: Arcus juvenilis, uveitis.

Renal: Hematuria, dysuria, burnt odor of urine, diuresis.

Miscellaneous: Xanthomas of hands and fingers, weight loss or gain, increased libido, swollen glands, edema, gingival bleeding, fatigue, weakness, shortness of breath. Transient and modest elevations of SGOT and alkaline phosphatase observed in those given colestipol HCl. Some patients have shown an increase in serum phosphorus and chloride with a decrease in sodium and potassium.

ADMINISTRATION

Although generally given three to four times/day, there appears to be no advantage to dosing more frequently than twice daily.

DOSAGE

CHOLESTYRAMINE

Adults: Initial dose is 4 g tid or qid A.C. and is adjusted to meet patient's needs.

Infants, children: Dosage not established. Initiated with small doses; subsequent adjustment depends on clinical response and benefit–risk ratio.

COLESTIPOL HYDROCHLORIDE

Adults: 15 g/day to 30 g/day in divided doses two to four times/day.

NURSING IMPLICATIONS

HISTORY
See Appendix 4.

PHYSICAL ASSESSMENT
Inspect areas identified during history. Baseline laboratory studies (cholesterol, triglyceride levels, total plasma lipids, phospholipids) are normally obtained prior to therapy.

ADMINISTRATION
These drugs must *never* be given in dry form; always mix with liquids (see below).

The interval between administration of these resins and any other medication should be as long as possible. Other drugs should be administered at least 1 hour before or 4 to 6 hours after administration of these resins to avoid impeding their absorption.

When other medications are included in the daily therapeutic regimen, there may be difficulty scheduling administration of these resins. Do not change the dosage time of other medications without first consulting with the physician.

CHOLESTYRAMINE

Place contents of one packet or one level scoopful on the surface of 120 ml to 180 ml of preferred beverage (water, milk, fruit juice).

Allow to stand without stirring for 1 to 2 minutes; twirl glass occasionally.

Product absorbs moisture; lumping can be avoided by permitting it to hydrate for approximately 1 minute before stirring. Stir to obtain uniform suspension.

Rinse glass with additional fluid to make sure all medication is taken.

May also be mixed with highly fluid soups (tomato, chicken noodle), pulpy fruits with high moisture content (*e.g.,* applesauce, crushed pineapple). Carbonated beverages may be used, with care because excessive foaming may result. Use a large glass; stir mixture slowly.

Different batches may vary in color.

COLESTIPOL HYDROCHLORIDE

Add prescribed amount to glassful (90 ml or more) of water, milk, flavored drink, carbonated beverages (use a large glass and stir slowly), fruit juice, hot or regular breakfast cereal, soups that have a high fluid content, pulpy fruits such as crushed pineapple, pears, peaches, fruit cocktail.

Stir until completely mixed (drug will not dissolve).

Rinse glass with small amount of additional beverage.

ONGOING ASSESSMENTS AND NURSING MANAGEMENT
Observe for adverse drug reactions daily; check for bleeding tendencies (*e.g.,* ecchymosis, petechiae, nose bleeds, tarry stools); rash; irritation of skin, tongue, perianal area.

Severe constipation may lead to fecal impaction. Keep record of bowel movements and inform physician if constipation is apparent.

Physician may manage constipation with laxatives, dose reduction, dietary changes (addition of bulk foods to diet), exercise, increase in water intake.

Concomitant dietary management (*e.g.,* weight reduction, cholesterol restricted) is usually necessary. Consult with dietitian if patient expresses dislike for diet or for some foods offered in diet.

Serum triglyceride, cholesterol levels are monitored periodically.

Failure of fall in cholesterol or a significant rise in triglyceride level may be indication to discontinue medication.

PATIENT AND FAMILY INFORMATION

Restriction of dietary intake of cholesterol and saturated fats and adherence to dietary regimen are important in controlling elevated serum cholesterol level. (*Note:* Have dietitian discuss diet plan if patient has questions about diet or fails to understand dietary restrictions.)

Medication is usually taken before meals. Follow physician's specific directions in taking this and other medications currently being taken. Failure to follow the timed dosage schedule may interfere with action of other medications.

Other drugs should be taken 1 hour before or 4 to 6 hours after this drug. If there is any difficulty in scheduling other drugs, discuss problem with physician.

Do not use nonprescription drugs or alcohol unless use has been approved by physician.

Never take in dry powder form. May be mixed with beverages, highly fluid soups, cereals, pulpy fruits.

Gastrointestinal upset (constipation, flatulence, nausea, heartburn) may occur and may disappear with continued therapy. Notify physician or nurse if these become bothersome of if unusual bleeding (*e.g.,* from gums, nose, or rectum) occurs.

Keep drug container tightly closed. Do not open single-dose packets until ready for use.

Biperiden

See Anticholinergic Antiparkinsonism Agents.

Bisacodyl

See Laxatives.

Bleomycin Sulfate (BLM) Rx

injection: 15 units/ ampule   Blenoxane

INDICATIONS

Should be considered as a palliative treatment. Shown useful in management of the following as ei-

ther a single agent or in combination with other chemotherapeutic agents.

Squamous cell carcinoma: Head and neck including mouth, tongue, tonsil, nasopharynx, oropharynx, sinus, palate, lip, buccal mucosa, gingiva, epiglottis, skin, and larynx. Also indicated in carcinoma of the penis, cervix, and vulva. Response poorer in those with head and neck cancer previously radiated.

Lymphomas: Hodgkin's, reticulum cell sarcoma, lymphosarcoma.

Testicular carcinoma: Embryonal cell, choriocarcinoma, teratocarcinoma.

CONTRAINDICATIONS

Hypersensitivity, idiosyncrasy.

ACTIONS

Bleomycin sulfate is a mixture of cytotoxic glycopeptide antibiotics isolated from a strain of *Streptomyces verticillus*. Although exact mechanism of action is unknown, evidence indicates that the main mode of action is the inhibition of DNA synthesis with evidence of lesser inhibition of RNA and protein synthesis. See also Antineoplastic Agents.

In patients with a creatinine clearance greater than 35 ml/min, plasma half-life is approximately 2 hours. In those with a creatinine clearance under 35 ml/min, plasma elimination half-life increases exponentially as the creatinine clearance decreases. Sixty percent to seventy percent of an administered dose is recovered in the urine as active bleomycin.

WARNINGS

Observe patients carefully and frequently during and after therapy. Use with extreme caution in those who have impaired renal function or compromised pulmonary function.

Pulmonary fibrosis is the most severe toxicity. It is most frequently seen as pneumonitis, which occasionally progresses to pulmonary fibrosis. Its occurrence is higher in the elderly and in those receiving over 400 units as a total dose, but pulmonary toxicity has been observed in young patients treated with lower doses. Pulmonary toxicities occur in 10% of treated patients. In approximately 1%, the nonspecific pneumonitis induced by the drug progresses to pulmonary fibrosis and death. Although age and dose related, the toxicity is unpredictable. Frequent x-rays are recommended. Total doses over 400 units are given with great caution. When bleomycin is used with other antineoplastic agents, pulmonary toxicities may occur at lower doses.

Idiosyncratic reactions similar to anaphylaxis have been reported in 1% of lymphoma patients.

Because these usually occur after the first or second dose, careful monitoring is essential.

Renal or hepatic toxicity, beginning as a deterioration in renal- or hepatic-function tests, has been reported infrequently. These toxicities may occur any time after initiation of therapy.

Safety for use in pregnancy not established.

ADVERSE REACTIONS

Pulmonary: Most frequent is pneumonitis, occasionally progressing to pulmonary fibrosis. Approximately 1% of patients treated have died of pulmonary fibrosis. Because of lack of specificity of the clinical syndrome, identifying pulmonary toxicity is extremely difficult. The earliest symptom is dyspnea and the earliest sign is fine rales. Radiographically, bleomycin-induced pneumonitis produces nonspecific patchy opacities, usually of the lower lung field. The most common changes in pulmonary-function tests are a decrease in lung volume and a decrease in vital capacity. These changes are not predictive of the development of pulmonary fibrosis. Chest x-rays should be taken every 1 to 2 weeks. If changes are noted, treatment should be discontinued until it is determined whether they are drug related. Sequential measurements of the pulmonary diffusion capacity for carbon monoxide may indicate subclinical pulmonary toxicities.

Idiosyncratic reactions: In approximately 1% of patients, an idiosyncratic reaction similar to anaphylaxis has been reported. This reaction may be immediate or delayed for several hours and usually occurs after the first or second dose. It consists of hypotension, confusion, fever, chills, and wheezing. Treatment is symptomatic and includes volume expansion, pressor agents, and steroids.

Integument and mucous membranes: These are the most frequent side-effects and are reported in 50% of patients. They consist of erythema, rash, striae, vesiculation, hyperpigmentation, and tenderness of the skin. Hyperkeratosis, nail changes, alopecia, pruritus, and stomatitis also have been reported. It was necessary to discontinue the drug in 2% of these patients because of these toxicities. Skin toxicity is a relatively late manifestation, usually developing in the second and third week of treatment after 150 units to 200 units have been administered.

Other: Fever, chills, and vomiting are frequently seen. Anorexia and weight loss are common and may persist long after termination of the drug. Pain at the tumor site, phlebitis, and other local reactions have been reported infrequently.

Combination therapy: There have been isolated reports of Raynaud's phenomenon occurring in patients with testicular carcinomas treated with bleomycin and vinblastine sulfate.

DOSAGE

Because of possibility of anaphylactoid reaction, lymphoma patients should be treated with 2 units or less for the first 2 doses. If no acute reaction occurs, the regular dosage schedule may be followed.

Squamous cell carcinoma, lymphosarcoma, reticulum cell sarcoma, testicular carcinoma: 0.25 units/kg to 0.5 units/kg (10 units/m^2 to 20 units/m^2) IV, IM, or subcutaneously, once or twice weekly.

Hodgkin's disease: 0.25 units/kg to 0.5 units/kg (10 units/m^2 to 20 units/m^2) IV, IM, or subcutaneously once or twice weekly. After a 50% response, a maintenance dose of 1 unit daily or 5 units weekly IV or IM.

Improvement in Hodgkin's disease or testicular tumors is prompt and noted within 2 weeks. If no improvement is seen by this time, it is unlikely to occur. Squamous cell carcinomas respond more slowly, sometimes requiring as long as 3 weeks before any improvement is noted.

NOTE: Some oncologists may employ a different dosage or frequency schedule than those stated above.

NURSING IMPLICATIONS

HISTORY
See Appendix 4.

PHYSICAL ASSESSMENT
Monitor physical, emotional status; vital signs; weight. Baseline laboratory tests and diagnostic studies may include chest x-ray, pulmonary diffusion capacity for carbon monoxide, pulmonary-function studies, BUN, creatinine.

ADMINISTRATION

Preparation of IM or subcutaneous solutions: Dissolve contents of ampule in 1 ml to 5 ml of Sterile Water for Injection, Sodium Chloride for Injection, 5% Dextrose for Injection, or Bacteriostatic Water for Injection (physician specifies diluent and amount).

Preparation of IV solution: Dissolve content of ampule in 5 ml or more of physiologic saline or glucose (physician specifies diluent and amount).

Obtain baseline temperature.

Physician may prescribe an antiemetic or antipyretic prior to administration of bleomycin to prevent vomiting, fever.

A Kold Kap or scalp tourniquet may be used to prevent alopecia. Outpatients may have purchased their own cap, which is brought to the physician's office or clinic each treatment in a cold state (placing the cap in a small foam cooler keeps it cold). The cap is put into place just prior to injection of the drug and may be left in place approximately 1 hour, or as directed by the physician, after the drug is injected. The outpatient may wear his cap while returning home.

IV: Administer slowly over period of 10 minutes.

IM: Give by deep intramuscular injection.

Rotate IV, IM, subcutaneous injection sites; record site used on patient's chart.

Stability: Stable for 24 hours at room temperature in Sodium Chloride, 5% Dextrose solution, and 5% Dextrose containing heparin 100 units/ml or 1000 units/ml.

ONGOING ASSESSMENTS AND NURSING MANAGEMENT

Prior to initial therapy, physician explains and discusses number and frequency of treatments, adverse reactions that may be experienced, possible physical changes (*e.g.,* skin pigmentation, stomatitis, alopecia), and tests required to monitor drug response.

Check vital signs q4h or as ordered for first 24 hours after administration. Report chills, fever to physician. If patient is receiving first or second dose, monitor more frequently (see *Clinical Alert*).

An antiemetic or antipyretic may be ordered q4h for 24 hours after administration.

If nausea or vomiting occurs, patient may be given a liquid diet. Foods or fluids that may relieve nausea include dry toast, unsalted crackers, and carbonated beverages. Patient may need to experiment to find suitable liquid or solid food that relieves hunger and thirst but does not increase nausea.

CLINICAL ALERT: An idiosyncratic reaction may occur immediately or be delayed for several hours and usually occurs after the first or second dose. Symptoms are hypotension, confusion, fever, chills, and wheezing. Monitor blood pressure, pulse, and general status immediately after drug is given and q15m for 1 to 2 hours, q1h for 3 to 4 hours, and then q4h. Notify physician immediately should symptoms of drug idiosyncrasy occur because volume expansion, pressor agents, antihistamines, and steroids may be necessary.

Observe for signs and symptoms of pulmonary toxicity. Earliest symptom is dyspnea; earliest sign is fine rales. Auscultate lungs q4h. Notify physician immediately if patient becomes dyspneic or fine rales are noted on auscultation of lungs.

When patient is receiving first or second dose, emergency intervention for an idiosyncratic reaction may be necessary. Check with physician about drug preference for treating this reaction. Drugs that may be used include diphenhydramine HCl, epinephrine or other pressor agent, and a steroid. The requested drugs, as well as an intravenous fluid and administration set, should be immediately available.

If an idiosyncratic reaction occurs and patient does not have an IV line, start an IV with the recommended fluid (see above), run to KVO, stay with patient, and monitor blood pressure, pulse, and respirations until physician arrives.

Inspect skin daily for erythema, rash, striae, vesiculation, hyperpigmentation, tenderness, hyperkeratosis, and nail changes. Note whether hair loss has begun to occur or patient complains of pruritus. Report these reactions to the physician.

If pain develops at IM or subcutaneous injection site, inform physician. Hot compresses may be ordered to relieve discomfort.

Stomatitis may develop, usually 10 to 14 days after therapy is instituted. Inspect oral cavity daily for erythema, ulcerations. Report reaction to physician. When stomatitis develops, begin stomatitis care (Appendix 6, section 6-21) q4h (around the clock).

Xylocaine Viscous 15 ml q3h to q4h prn may be prescribed for pain due to stomatitis. Instruct patient to swish Xylocaine Viscous around in mouth. Drug may be swallowed if pharynx is also sore. A topical local anesthetic ointment or spray may also be prescribed.

Physician or nurse should discuss with patient the purchase and use of a wig or scarf should alopecia occur. Patient may wish to purchase a wig before treatment or wait to see the degree of alopecia. Patient should be told that hair loss may be complete or partial and may involve scalp, eyebrows, eyelashes, and the underarm and pubic areas. Hair will grow back (possibly while the patient is still receiving drug) but may be a different texture or color.

Hair loss, other skin changes are often distressing; patient will require understanding from both family and medical team.

Weigh weekly or as ordered. Report weight loss to physician.

Notify physician if anorexia persists for more than 2 days because a dietary change may be necessary. Food intake may improve if food is given in small, frequent amounts. A high-protein, high-calorie diet may be ordered.

Pain at tumor site may occur. Patient should be told that this is not abnormal. Inform physician of this reaction, because an analgesic may be required.

Frequent pulmonary-function tests and chest x-rays are recommended. Periodic renal- and liver-function tests may also be ordered to detect early renal or hepatic toxicity.

Observe patient receiving bleomycin and vinblastine for Raynaud's phenomena (*e.g.,* changes in fingers, toes; numbness; tingling; blanching, which later becomes cyanotic and then red when exposed to cold).

PATIENT AND FAMILY INFORMATION

NOTE: The patient should receive a full explanation of all possible adverse reactions, what can be done to control or alleviate these reactions, and what specific reactions should be reported immediately to the physician or nurse. This information may be given by the physician or by the nurse with physician approval.

Keep all physician and clinic appointments for administration of drug and tests necessary to monitor therapy.

Inform physician or nurse if the following occur: chills, fever, anorexia (more than 2 to 3 days), nausea and vomiting for more than 12 hours, pronounced weight loss, sores or ulcerations in the mouth, skin tenderness. If shortness of breath occurs, contact physician immediately.

If drug is to be administered on outpatient basis, physician may prescribe one or more medications (an antiemetic or antipyretic) to be taken prior to administration of bleomycin. Be sure to take drugs at specified time intervals.

Physician may also prescribe or suggest other drugs (*e.g.,* antiemetic, antipyretic, Xylocaine Viscous) to be taken or used between treatments. Take or use these drugs exactly as directed.

Avoid use of nonprescription drugs unless use has been approved by physician.

A liquid diet, dry toast, unsalted crackers, and carbonated beverages may be taken if nausea or vomiting occurs.

Good oral care is essential. Use a soft toothbrush and rinse mouth thoroughly after taking food or beverages. Avoid use of mouthwashes or other oral products unless use approved by physician.

NOTE: Information about detection (examination of oral cavity daily) and treatment of stomatitis and diet for prolonged anorexia (see *Ongoing Assessments and Nursing Management*) may be given after initial or subsequent treatments. Discussion of use of wig or scarf for alopecia may be given during initial treatment or reserved for subsequent treatments.

Boric Acid otc

ointment: 5%	Borofax (topical), *Generic* (ophthalmic)
ointment: 10%	*Generic* (topical, ophthalmic)

INDICATIONS
Temporary relief of chapped skin, diaper rash, dry skin, abrasions, minor burns, sunburn, windburn, insect bites, other skin irritations. Ophthalmic ointment used in treatment of irritated and inflamed eyelids. A boric acid solution may be prepared by pharmacist for use as a topical solution or soak. The 5% solution is labeled "saturated" or SSBA (saturated solution of boric acid).

ACTIONS
Has fungistatic and weak bacteriostatic activity.

PRECAUTIONS
Do not apply to badly broken or raw skin or to large areas of the body. Do not use in eye unless labeled for ophthalmic use. For external use only.

DOSAGE
Ointment: Applied three or four times daily.
Ophthalmic ointment: 1 to 2 times/day or as directed by physician.

NURSING IMPLICATIONS

HISTORY
When applicable, determine cause of skin or eye irritation.

PHYSICAL ASSESSMENT
When applicable, examine and record appearance of skin or eye.

ADMINISTRATION
Ointment: Apply directly to affected area or on a dressing; cover with sterile gauze unless physician directs otherwise.
Ophthalmic ointment: Apply to the inner surface at the lower eyelid.
Solution: Apply as directed by physician.

ONGOING ASSESSMENTS AND NURSING MANAGEMENT
If problem persists, notify physician because other therapy may be indicated.
Solution: Not used on newborn infants. If solution is left at bedside, label clearly. Solution should not be left at bedside of the elderly,

young children, or the confused patient (may be mistaken for water).

PATIENT AND FAMILY INFORMATION

Read label carefully; only product labeled "for ophthalmic use" may be used in eye.

Follow label directions or physician's recommendations for use.

Boric acid is for external use only; do not apply to open skin lesions.

If condition does not improve, contact physician.

Bretylium Tosylate Rx

injection: 50 mg/ml   Bretylol

INDICATIONS

Prophylaxis and therapy of ventricular fibrillation. Treatment of life-threatening ventricular arrhythmias, such as ventricular tachycardia, that have failed to respond to adequate doses of a first-line antiarrhythmic agent such as lidocaine.

CONTRAINDICATIONS

There are no contraindications to use in treatment of ventricular fibrillation or life-threatening refractory ventricular arrhythmias.

ACTIONS

Inhibits norepinephrine release by depressing adrenergic nerve-terminal excitability. It induces a chemical sympathectomylike state that resembles a surgical sympathectomy. Catecholamine stores are not depleted but drug causes an early release of norepinephrine from the adrenergic postganglionic nerve terminals. Therefore, transient catecholamine effects on the myocardium (tachycardia) and on peripheral vascular resistance (rise in blood pressure) are often seen shortly after administration. Subsequently, bretylium blocks the release of norepinephrine in response to neuron stimulation. Peripheral adrenergic blockade regularly causes orthostatic hypotension but has less effect on supine blood pressure. The relationship of adrenergic blockade to the antifibrillatory and antiarrhythmic actions of the drug are not clear. It has a positive inotropic effect on the myocardium.

Following IV administration to patients with acute myocardial infarction, there is a mild increase in arterial pressure, followed by a modest decrease, remaining within normal limits throughout. Pulmonary artery pressure, pulmonary capillary wedge pressure, right atrial pressure, cardiac index, stroke volume index, and stroke work index are not significantly changed. There is sometimes an initial small increase in heart rate after administration, but this is an inconsistent and transient occurrence.

Peak plasma concentration and peak hypotensive effects are seen within 1 hour of IM administration. Suppression of premature ventricular beats is not maximal until 6 to 9 hours after dosing. Antifibrillatory effects can be seen within minutes of IV injection. Suppression of ventricular tachycardia and other ventricular arrhythmias develops more slowly, usually 20 minutes to 2 hours after parenteral administration. The drug is excreted primarily by the kidneys.

WARNINGS

Use should be limited to intensive care units, coronary care units, or other facilities where equipment and personnel for constant monitoring of cardiac arrhythmias and blood pressure are available.

Hypotension: Administration results in postural hypotension, subjectively recognized by dizziness, lightheadedness, vertigo, or faintness. Some degree of hypotension is present in about 50% of patients while they are supine. Hypotension may occur at doses lower than those needed to suppress arrhythmias. Patient should be kept supine until tolerance to the hypotensive effect develops. Tolerance occurs unpredictably but may be present after several days. Hypotension with supine systolic pressure greater than 75 mm Hg need not be treated unless there are associated symptoms. If supine systolic pressure falls below 75 mm Hg, an infusion of dopamine or norepinephrine may be used to raise the blood pressure. When catecholamines are administered, use a dilute solution and monitor blood pressure closely because the pressor effects of catecholamines should be given promptly if severe hypotension occurs.

Impaired renal function: Drug is excreted primarily by the kidneys and the dosage interval is increased in those with impaired renal function.

Use in pregnancy: Safety for use during pregnancy not established. Because drug is intended for use only in life-threatening situations, it may be used in pregnant women when potential benefits outweigh the unknown potential hazards to the fetus.

Use in children: Safety and efficacy not established.

DRUG INTERACTIONS

Initial release of norepinephrine caused by the drug may aggravate digitalis toxicity. When a life-threatening arrhythmia occurs in a digitalized patient, bretylium should be used only if the etiology of the arrhythmia does not appear to be digitalis toxicity and other antiarrhythmic drugs are not effective. Simultaneous initiation of therapy with **digitalis glycosides** is avoided.

ADVERSE REACTIONS

Hypotension and postural hypotension are most frequently reported. Nausea and vomiting may occur in about 3% of patients, primarily after rapid IV administration. Vertigo, dizziness, lightheadedness, and syncope, which sometimes accompany postural hypotension, may occasionally be seen.

The following have been reported in a small number of patients: bradycardia, increased frequency of PVCs, transitory hypertension, initial increase in arrhythmias, precipitation of anginal attacks, sensation of substernal pressure, renal dysfunction, diarrhea, abdominal pain, hiccups, erythematous macular rash, flushing, hyperthermia, confusion, paranoid psychosis, emotional lability, lethargy, generalized tenderness, anxiety, shortness of breath, diaphoresis, nasal congestion, mild conjunctivitis.

DOSAGE

Used only for short-term treatment of life-threatening ventricular arrhythmias. Optimal dosage schedule has not been determined. The following dosage schedule is suggested.

For immediately life-threatening ventricular arrhythmias (*e.g.,* ventricular fibrillation or hemodynamically unstable ventricular tachycardia): Administer undiluted at dosage of 5 mg/kg by rapid IV injection. Other usual cardiopulmonary resuscitative procedures, including electrical cardioversion, should be employed prior to and following the injection. If ventricular fibrillation persists, dosage may be increased to 10 mg/kg and repeated as necessary.

For continuous suppression: Administer the diluted solution as a constant infusion of 1 mg/minute to 2 mg/minute. As an alternative maintenance schedule, infuse the diluted solution at a dosage of 5 mg/kg to 10 mg/kg over 10 to 30 minutes, q6h. More rapid infusion may cause nausea and vomiting.

Other ventricular arrhythmias

IV: Must be diluted before IV administration as described under *Administration.* Administer the diluted solution at a dosage of 5 mg/kg to 10 mg/kg by IV infusion over a period of 10 to 30 minutes. More rapid infusion may cause nausea and vomiting. Subsequent doses may be given at 1- to 2-hour intervals if the arrhythmia persists.

IM: Do not dilute prior to IM injection. Inject 5 mg/kg to 10 mg/kg. Subsequent doses may be given at 1- to 2-hour intervals if arrhythmia persists.

Thereafter, maintain same dosage q6h to q8h. (See *Administration.*)

NURSING IMPLICATIONS

HISTORY

See Appendix 4. Immediate problem is identified by detection and identification of arrhythmia.

PHYSICAL ASSESSMENT

Baseline data provided by assessments made prior to the arrhythmia requiring emergency intervention. Weight should be obtained on admission to unit, when possible, using a standing or bed scale. If weight is obtained in pounds, convert to kilograms and record on Kardex or other area for immediate retrieval.

ADMINISTRATION

Dosage may be determined by weight in kilograms. If patient has not been weighed on admission, physician may need to approximate dose.

Drug is administered with patient under constant ECG monitoring.

Place patient in supine position (to lessen postural hypotension) unless physician orders otherwise.

Monitor blood pressure, pulse, respirations, and ECG during and after administration.

Have suction apparatus available because nausea and vomiting may occur and patient may be in danger of aspiration owing to clinical status and supine position.

A pressor agent such as dopamine or norepinephrine should be immediately available to treat hypotension (usually when systolic blood pressure falls below 75 mm Hg).

Life-threatening arrhythmias: Drug given undiluted by rapid IV injection. If patient has IV line, insert needle into the injection port, close the clamp on the IV line, draw back on the syringe to check integrity of IV line (look for blood backflow), and then administer drug. Following administration, open clamp on IV line.

Other ventricular arrhythmias

Drug is given IM or by IV infusion.

IV: Drug must be diluted before administration. Dilute contents of 1 ampule (500 mg/10 ml) to a minimum of 50 ml with 5% Dextrose Injection, USP, or Sodium Chloride Injection, USP. Administer diluted solution by IV infusion over 10 to 30 minutes. A volume control set on the primary IV line may be used to administer the solution.

Bretylium tosylate is compatible with the following IV solutions and additives:

5% Dextrose Injection
5% Dextrose in 0.45% Sodium Chloride
5% Dextrose in 0.9% Sodium Chloride
5% Dextrose in Lactated Ringer's
0.9% Sodium Chloride
5% Sodium Bicarbonate
20% Mannitol
$\frac{1}{6}$ M Sodium Lactate
Lactated Ringer's
Calcium Chloride (54.5 mEq/liter) in 5% Dextrose
Potassium Chloride (40 mEq/liter) in 5% Dextrose

IM: Do not dilute prior to injection. Inject deep IM, administering no more than 5 ml in any one site. Avoid injecting into or near a major nerve.

Rotate injection sites because repeated injection into same site may cause atrophy and necrosis of muscle tissue, fibrosis, vascular degeneration, and inflammatory changes. Record site used.

ONGOING ASSESSMENT AND NURSING MANAGEMENT

CLINICAL ALERT: The patient must be monitored closely during and after administration of this drug. Be alert to drug's adverse effects, which include hypotension, bradycardia, PVCs, transitory hypertension, initial increase in arrhythmias, precipitation of angina.

Monitor blood pressure, pulse, respirations, and ECG q5m or as ordered by physician. Pulse may be obtained from cardiac monitor; blood pressure may be monitored by an arterial line or ultrasonic blood-pressure monitor (set monitor to desired intervals between reading; preset high- and low-level alarms).

Patient should be kept in supine position until tolerance to hypotensive effect develops. If a position change is necessary because of respiratory difficulty, raise the head of the bed slowly and only to the point at which respirations improve.

If the supine systolic pressure falls below 75 mm Hg, an infusion of dopamine or norepinephrine may be ordered. A dilute solution is used and the blood pressure monitored closely because the pressor effects of these drugs are enhanced by bretylium.

Following treatment for a life-threatening ventricular arrhythmia, cardiopulmonary resuscitative efforts may be continued.

Patient is monitored closely (*i.e.,* q5m–q15m)

until arrhythmia is corrected or prophylaxis is no longer necessary.

Monitor intake and output; decrease in urinary output may indicate impairment in renal function.

As soon as possible, and when indicated, patient is changed to an oral antiarrhythmic agent for maintenance therapy.

Bromocriptine Mesylate *Rx*

| tablets: 2.5 mg | Parlodel |
| capsules: 5 mg | Parlodel |

INDICATIONS

Short-term treatment of amenorrhea/galactorrhea associated with hyperprolactinemia due to varied etiologies excluding demonstrable pituitary tumors. Not indicated in those with normal prolactin levels.

Treatment of female infertility associated with hyperprolactinemia in absence of a demonstrable pituitary tumor.

Prevention of physiologic lactation (secretion, congestion, engorgement) after parturition when mother elects not to breast-feed or breast-feeding is contraindicated. After stillbirth or abortion.

Treatment of signs and symptoms of idiopathic or postencephalitic Parkinson's disease. As adjunct to levodopa, bromocriptine may provide additional therapeutic benefits in those currently maintained on optimal dosages of levodopa, those beginning to deteriorate (develop tolerance to levodopa therapy), and those experiencing "end-dose failure" on levodopa therapy. May permit a reduction of the maintenance dose of levodopa and thus ameliorate the occurrence or severity of adverse reactions associated with long-term levodopa therapy such as abnormal involuntary movements (dyskinesias) and marked swings in motor function ("on–off" phenomenon). Continued efficacy during treatment of more than 2 years not established.

Investigational uses: Lowers plasma growth-hormone levels in those with acromegaly. In doses of 10 mg to 20 mg tid it may be a useful adjunct to radiotherapy or surgery. When bromocriptine is used alone, complete remission occurs in only a minority of patients.

CONTRAINDICATIONS

Sensitivity to any ergot alkaloids; patients with severe ischemic heart disease; pregnancy.

ACTIONS

A nonhormonal, nonestrogenic ergot derivative that inhibits secretion of prolactin with little or no effect on other pituitary hormones, except in acromegaly, in which it lowers elevated blood levels of growth hormone.

Has been shown to be a dopamine-receptor agonist in that it activates postsynaptic dopamine receptors. The dopaminergic neurons in the tuberoinfundibular process modulate the secretion of prolactin from the anterior pituitary by secreting prolactin inhibitory factor (thought to be dopamine). In the corpus striatum, the dopaminergic neurons are involved in the control of motor function. Drug has been shown to significantly reduce plasma levels of prolactin in patients with hyperprolactinemia.

In many cases of galactorrhea associated with amenorrhea, bromocriptine suppresses galactorrhea completely, or almost completely, and reinstates normal ovulatory menstrual cycles. Menses usually is reinitiated prior to complete suppression of galactorrhea; average time is 6 to 8 weeks, but some patients may respond in a few days. Galactorrhea may take longer to control, depending on the degree of stimulation of mammary tissue prior to therapy. At least 75% reduction in secretion is usually observed after 8 to 12 weeks. Some may fail to respond even after 24 weeks of therapy. Bromocriptine acts to prevent physiologic lactation when therapy is started after delivery and continued for 2 to 3 weeks.

Parkinson's disease: Produces therapeutic effect by directly stimulating the dopamine receptors in the corpus striatum.

Drug is absorbed from the GI tract and completely metabolized prior to excretion. Major route of excretion is via bile; only a small amount is excreted in urine. Almost all of the administered dose is excreted in feces in 120 hours.

WARNINGS

Because hyperprolactinemia with amenorrhea/galactorrhea and infertility has been found in those with pituitary tumors, complete evaluation of the sella turcica is recommended before treatment. Although drug will effectively lower plasma levels of prolactin in those with pituitary tumors, this does not obviate the necessity of radiotherapy or surgical procedures when appropriate.

Hypotension: Symptomatic hypotension can occur. Periodic monitoring of blood pressure, particularly during first few days of therapy, is advisable. Care is exercised when drug is administered concomitantly with other medications known to lower blood pressure.

Pulmonary effects: Long-term treatment (6–36 months) in doses ranging from 20 mg/day to 100 mg/day has been associated with pulmonary infiltrates, pleural effusion, and thickening of the pleura

in a few patients. When treatment was terminated, the changes slowly reverted toward normal.

Use in pregnancy: Safe use has not been demonstrated. If pregnancy occurs, drug is discontinued immediately and careful observation of patient throughout pregnancy is mandatory.

Use in lactation: Not administered to mothers who wish to breast-feed.

Use in children: Safety and efficacy for children under 15 not established.

PRECAUTIONS

Amenorrhea/galactorrhea: Treatment may result in restoration of fertility; patient is advised to use contraceptive measures during treatment.

Female infertility: Therapy is discontinued as soon as diagnosis of pregnancy established. Patient is monitored throughout pregnancy for signs and symptoms that may develop if a previously undetected prolactin-secreting tumor enlarges.

Parkinson's disease: Safety for use longer than 2 years not established. Periodic evaluation of hepatic, hematopoietic, cardiovascular, and renal function recommended. Symptomatic hypotension can occur; caution is advised in administering to those receiving antihypertensive agents. High doses may be associated with confusion or mental disturbances. May cause hallucinations (visual or auditory), which usually resolve with dose reduction. Exercise caution when administering to patients with a history of myocardial infarction who have a residual arrhythmia.

Use in impaired hepatic or renal function: Safety not established but, because very little drug is excreted in the urine, impaired renal function should not significantly influence plasma profile or elimination of the drug. Use with caution in those with hepatic dysfunction.

DRUG INTERACTIONS

Exercise care when administering concomitantly with **other drugs known to lower blood pressure. Phenothiazines** should be avoided.

ADVERSE REACTIONS

Amenorrhea/galactorrhea: Nausea, headache, dizziness, fatigue, abdominal cramps, lightheadedness, vomiting, nasal congestion, constipation, diarrhea.

Physiologic lactation: Transient decreases in blood pressure during first three postpartum days, headache, dizziness, nausea, vomiting, fatigue, syncope, diarrhea, cramps.

Parkinson's disease: Nausea, abnormal involuntary movements, hallucinations, confusion, on–off phenomenon, dizziness, drowsiness, faintness/fainting, vomiting, asthenia, abdominal discomfort, visual disturbances, ataxia, insomnia, depression, hypotension, shortness of breath, constipation, vertigo. *Less common*—Anorexia; anxiety; blepharospasm; dry mouth; dysphagia; edema of feet, ankles; erythromelalgia; epileptiform seizure; fatigue; headache; lethargy; mottling of skin; nasal congestion; nervousness; nightmares; paresthesia; skin rash; urinary frequency, incontinence, or retention; rarely, signs of ergotism such as tingling of fingers, cold feet, numbness, muscle cramps of feet and legs, or exacerbation of Raynaud's syndrome.

Laboratory test abnormalities: Elevations in BUN, SGOT, SGPT, GPT, CPK, alkaline phosphatase, and uric acid, which are usually transient and not of clinical significance.

DOSAGE

Amenorrhea/galactorrhea: 2.5 mg bid or tid with meals. Duration of treatment should not exceed 6 months. It is recommended that treatment be started with 2.5 mg/day and increased within the first week to reduce possibility of adverse reactions.

Female infertility: 2.5 mg bid or tid with meals. It is recommended that treatment be started with 2.5 mg/day and increased within the first week to reduce possibility of adverse reactions. A mechanical contraceptive should be used until normal ovulatory menstrual cycles have been restored; contraception should then be discontinued. If menstruation does not occur within 3 days of expected date, therapy should be discontinued and a pregnancy test performed.

Prevention of physiologic lactation: Start therapy only after patient's vital signs have been stabilized and no sooner than 4 hours after delivery. Recommended dosage is 2.5 mg bid with meals. Usual dosage range is from 2.5 mg/day to 2.5 mg tid. Continue therapy for 14 days; may be given up to 21 days if needed.

Parkinson's disease: Initial dose is one-half tablet (1.25 mg) bid with meals. Assessments are advised at 2-week intervals during dosage titration to ensure that the lowest dosage producing optimal effects is not exceeded. If needed, dosage may be increased every 14 to 28 days by 2.5 mg/day. Safety has not been demonstrated for dosages exceeding 100 mg/day.

NURSING IMPLICATIONS

HISTORY
See Appendix 4.

PHYSICAL ASSESSMENT
Monitor vital signs.

Amenorrhea/galactorrhea, infertility, prevention of physiologic lactation: Review patient's chart for physical examination performed by physician.

Parkinson's disease: See Anticholinergic Antiparkinsonism Agents.

ADMINISTRATION
Initiate therapy in postpartum patient only after vital signs have stabilized and no sooner than 4 hours after delivery.

First dose is best given with patient in a recumbent position because dizziness or fainting may occur, particularly following the first dose.

Give with meals or food.

Tablets are scored (one-half tablet may be ordered for patient with parkinsonism).

Patient with parkinsonism may require assistance in removing tablet from dispensing cup, holding water glass.

ONGOING ASSESSMENTS AND NURSING MANAGEMENT
Monitor blood pressure, pulse, and respirations q4h (first 3–4 days of therapy).

Observe for adverse reactions.

Monitor drug response. In the postpartum patient, there should be a decrease in breast engorgement, congestion, and secretion. In the patient with parkinsonism there should be a decrease in symptoms of the disorder; compare daily findings with data base.

If hypotension occurs, instruct patient to make position changes slowly and dangle legs 5 to 10 minutes before getting out of bed.

Increase dosage for parkinsonism slowly until maximum response is obtained. Patient is observed closely for adverse reactions, drug response. If levodopa (see p 619) is administered concomitantly, observe for adverse reactions of both drugs. Once maximum response is obtained, dosage for parkinsonism may be higher than dosages for other uses.

Observe for mental changes and other adverse reactions reported to occur in those with parkinsonism because close supervision and/or assistance with activities of daily living may be required. See also Anticholinergic Antiparkinsonism Agents.

PATIENT AND FAMILY INFORMATION
Take with meals or food.

Dizziness or fainting may occur, particularly after the first dose. The first dose is best taken while lying down. Avoid sudden changes in posture such as suddenly rising from a sitting position. Observe caution while driving or performing other tasks requiring alertness.

Infertility, amenorrhea/galactorrhea:
Contraceptive measures (other than oral contraceptives) should be employed during treatment. If pregnancy is suspected, do not take next dose but contact the physician immediately because drug will most likely be discontinued.

Brompheniramine Maleate

See Antihistamines.

Bronchodilators and Decongestants, Systemic

Sympathomimetics

Albuterol Sulfate _Rx_

tablets: 2 mg, 4 mg	Proventil, Ventolin

Ephedrine Sulfate _Rx, otc_

capsules: 25 mg (_otc_), 50 mg (_Rx_)	_Generic_
syrup: 11 mg/5 ml (_otc_), 20 mg/5 ml (_otc_)	_Generic_
injection: 25 mg/ml (_Rx_), 50 mg/ml (_Rx_)	_Generic_

Epinephrine _Rx_

injection: 1:1000 solution	Adrenalin Chloride Solution, _Generic_
injection: 1:200 suspension	Sus-Phrine

Ethylnorepinephrine Hydrochloride _Rx_

injection: 2 mg/ml	Bronkephrine

Isoproterenol Hydrochloride _Rx_

injection: (1:5000 solution) 0.2 mg/ml	Isuprel
tablets, sublingual: 10 mg, 15 mg	Isuprel Glossets

Metaproterenol Sulfate _Rx_

tablets: 10 mg, 20 mg	Alupent, Metaprel
syrup: 10 mg/5 ml	Alupent, Metaprel

Phenylpropanolamine Hydrochloride _Rx, otc_

tablets, 25 mg, 50 mg	_Generic_ (_otc_)
capsules: 25 mg, 50 mg	Propadrine (_otc_)
capsules, timed release: 75 mg	Rhindecon (_Rx_), _Generic_ (_otc_)

Pseudoephedrine HCl _(d-Isoephedrine HCl)_ _otc_

tablets: 30 mg	Sudafed, Sudrin, _Generic_
tablets: 60 mg	Cenafed, NeoFed, Sudafed, _Generic_
capsules, timed release: 120 mg	Neo-Synephrinol Day Relief, Novafed, Sudafed S.A.
liquid: 30 mg/5 ml	Cenafed Syrup, Novafed, Sudafed Syrup, _Generic_

Pseudoephedrine Sulfate _otc_

tablets, repeat action: 120 mg	Afrinol Repetabs

Terbutaline Sulfate _Rx_

tablets: 2.5 mg, 5 mg	Brethine, Bricanyl
injection: 1 mg/ml	Brethine, Bricanyl Subcutaneous

INDICATIONS
ALBUTEROL SULFATE
Relief of bronchospasm in patients with reversible obstructive airway disease.

EPHEDRINE SULFATE
Treatment of allergic disorders, such as bronchial asthma.

EPINEPHRINE
Relief of respiratory distress in bronchial asthma or during acute attacks and for bronchospasm in those with chronic bronchitis, emphysema, and other obstructive pulmonary diseases. In treatment of hypersensitivity reactions to drugs, sera, insect stings, or other allergens, including such symptoms as bronchospasm, urticaria, pruritus, angioneurotic edema, itching, hives, or swelling of the lips, eyelids, tongue, and nasal mucosa.

Epinephrine solutions have a rapid but short duration of effect. The suspensions provide both prompt and prolonged effects (up to 8 hours) owing to slow absorption of crystalline epinephrine.

ETHYLNOREPINEPHRINE HYDROCHLORIDE
Relief of bronchospasm in bronchial asthma.

ISOPROTERENOL HYDROCHLORIDE

Management of bronchospasm during anesthesia. Sublingual tablets used as bronchodilators in management of bronchopulmonary diseases.

METAPROTERENOL SULFATE

Bronchial asthma; reversible bronchospasm that may occur in association with bronchitis and emphysema.

PHENYLPROPANOLAMINE HYDROCHLORIDE

Nasal congestion associated with the common cold, rhinitis, sinusitis, nasopharyngitis, or allergic conditions such as hay fever and allergic rhinitis.

PSEUDOEPHEDRINE HCl (d-ISOEPHEDRINE HCl)

Symptomatic relief of nasal congestion or eustachian-tube congestion. Has fewer CNS and pressor effects than ephedrine, but is not effective as a bronchodilator.

PSEUDOEPHEDRINE SULFATE

Relief of nasal congestion.

TERBUTALINE SULFATE

Bronchodilator for relief of bronchial asthma and reversible bronchospasm that may occur in association with bronchitis and emphysema.

Investigational use: Oral and IV have been used successfully to inhibit premature labor. IV administration titrated at 10 mcg/minute, titrated upward to a maximum dose of 80 mcg/minute. IV dosage maintained at the minimum effective dose for 4 hours. Oral doses of 2.5 mg q4h to q6h have been used as maintenance therapy until term.

CONTRAINDICATIONS

Hypersensitivity to any component (allergic reactions are rare); severe hypertension; severe coronary artery disease; arrhythmias; tachycardia caused by digitalis intoxication; monoamine oxidase inhibitor therapy; angle-closure glaucoma; during general anesthesia with halogenated hydrocarbons or cyclopropane, which sensitize the myocardium.

ACTIONS

Pharmacologic actions of these agents include alpha-adrenergic stimulation (vasoconstriction, nasal decongestion, pressor effects) and beta$_2$-adrenergic stimulation (bronchial dilatation and vasodilatation). The relative selectivity of action of sympathomimetic agents is the primary determinant of their clinical usefulness and can be used to predict side-effects most likely to be encountered.

WARNINGS

Administer with caution to those with angina, stroke, hypertension, diabetes, hyperthyroidism, prostatic hypertrophy, a history of seizures, or glaucoma. Patients with atrial fibrillation will show an exaggerated increase in heart-rate response.

A sharp rise in blood pressure may result in cerebral or other hemorrhage. Sympathomimetics may produce CNS stimulation. Fatalities may result from pulmonary edema due to peripheral constriction and cardiac stimulation. Rapidly acting vasodilators, such as nitrites or alpha-adrenergic blocking agents, may counteract epinephrine's marked pressor effects.

Use in pregnancy, lactation: Safety not established. Use only when clearly needed and potential benefits outweigh unknown potential hazards to the fetus. Because of higher than usual risk for infants, breast-feeding should not be undertaken while mother is using these agents.

Use in elderly: Patients over 60 are more likely to have adverse reactions. Overdosage may cause hallucinations, convulsions, CNS depression, and death. Safe use of a short-acting agent should be demonstrated before using sustained-action form.

PRECAUTIONS

May cause toxic symptoms through idiosyncratic response or overdosage.

DRUG INTERACTIONS

Contraindicated in those taking **monoamine oxidase inhibitors** and **beta-adrenergic blockers,** because they potentiate alpha-sympathomimetic substances. Effects of sympathomimetics may be potentiated by **tricylic antidepressants,** certain **antihistamines,** and **sodium levothyroxine.** Sympathomimetics may reduce the effects of **antihypertensive agents** (guanethidine or reserpine).

Use of epinephrine and **general anesthetics** or with excessive doses of **digitalis, mercurial diuretics,** or other drugs that sensitize the heart to arrhythmias is not recommended. Anginal pain may be induced when coronary insufficiency is present.

Concomitant use of one sympathomimetic agent with another is not recommended; their combined effects may be deleterious. Sufficient time should elapse after discontinuing one agent before substituting another. This does not preclude use of an aerosol bronchodilator for relief of acute bronchospasm in patients receiving chronic therapy.

ADVERSE REACTIONS

CNS: Restlessness, anxiety, fear, tension, insomnia, tremor, convulsions, weakness, vertigo, dizziness, headache, flushing, pallor, sweating, nausea, vomiting, anorexia, muscle cramps, polyuria, dysuria.

Cardiovascular: Hypertension, palpitations, tachycardia, arrhythmias, anginal pain, precordial distress, cardiorespiratory arrest, cardiovascular collapse with hypotension.

Other: Vesicle sphincter spasm may result in difficult and painful urination. Urinary retention may develop in males with prostatism. Acute interstitial nephritis has been reported with phenylpropanolamine.

OVERDOSAGE

Symptoms: Palpitation, tachycardia, bradycardia, extrasystoles, heart block, chest pain, elevated blood pressure, fever, chills, cold perspiration, blanching of skin, nausea, vomiting, mydriasis. Central actions produce insomnia, anxiety, tremor; delirium, convulsions, collapse, and coma may occur.

Treatment: Discontinue drug or reduce dosage. If toxicity is pronounced, a beta blocker (propranolol) may be used to block effects of the beta-adrenergic agents, but the possibility of aggravation of airway obstruction is considered. Phentolamine (alpha blocker) may be used to block strong alpha-adrenergic actions.

DOSAGE

ALBUTEROL SULFATE

Adults, children over 12: Usual starting dosage is 2 mg or 4 mg tid or qid. Total daily dose should not exceed 32 mg. Doses above 4 mg qid are used only when patient fails to respond. If a favorable response does not occur with 4 mg, increase dosage cautiously, to a maximum of 8 mg qid, as tolerated.

Elderly patients, those sensitive to beta-adrenergic stimulators: An initial dose of 2 mg tid or qid. If adequate bronchodilatation is not obtained, increase dosage gradually to as much as 8 mg tid or qid.

Children under 12: Not recommended.

EPHEDRINE SULFATE

Adults: Usual parenteral dose is 25 mg to 50 mg subcutaneously, IM, or slow IV. Usual oral dose is 25 mg to 50 mg repeated q3h to q4h as necessary.

Children: 3 mg/kg/day divided into 4 to 6 doses.

EPINEPHRINE

1:1000 solution: *Adults*—0.3 mg to 0.5 mg subcutaneously or IM. *Children*—For bronchial asthma 0.01 mg/kg or 0.3 mg/m^2 subcutaneously.

1:200 suspension: *Adults*—0.1 ml to 0.3 ml subcutaneously. *Children*—0.025 mg/kg subcutaneously.

Epinephrine is readily destroyed by alkalies and oxidizing agents such as oxygen, chlorine, bromine, iodine, permanganates, chromates, nitrites, and salts of easily reducible metals, especially iron.

ETHYLNOREPINEPHRINE HYDROCHLORIDE

Adults: Usual dose by subcutaneous or IM injection is 0.5 ml to 1 ml. Depending on severity of the asthma attack, smaller doses (0.3 ml to 0.5 ml) may suffice.

Children: Dosage varies according to age, weight; usually 0.1 ml to 0.5 ml is sufficient.

ISOPROTERENOL HYDROCHLORIDE

Parenteral (management of bronchospasm during anesthesia): 1 ml of a 1:5000 solution diluted to 10 ml with Sodium Chloride Injection or 5% Dextrose Injection. An initial dose of 0.01 mg to 0.02 mg is administered IV and repeated as necessary.

Sublingual: Average adult dose is 10 mg (15 mg to 20 mg may be required) depending on patient's response. A dose of 15 mg qid or 20 mg tid should not be exceeded. *Children*—5 mg to 10 mg, not exceeding a total of 30 mg/day.

Tablets are allowed to disintegrate under the tongue. Treatment should not be repeated more often than q3h to q4h or more than three times daily.

METAPROTERENOL SULFATE

Adults, children over 9 years or over 60 lb: 20 mg tid or qid.

Children 6–9 years or less than 60 lb: 10 mg tid or qid.

Not recommended for children under 6.

PHENYLPROPANOLAMINE HYDROCHLORIDE

Adults: 25 mg q3h to q4h or 50 mg q6h to q8h, not to exceed 150 mg/day (or 75 mg sustained release q12h).

Children 6–12 years: 12.5 mg q4h or 25 mg q8h.

Children 2–6 years: 6.25 mg q4h or 12.5 mg q8h.

PSEUDOEPHEDRINE HCl

Adults: 60 mg q6h (120 mg sustained release q12h).

Children 6–12 years: 30 mg q6h.

Children 2–5 years: 15 mg q6h (as syrup).

PSEUDOEPHEDRINE SULFATE

120 mg q12h for adults and children over 12.

TERBUTALINE SULFATE

Oral: *Adults*—5 mg at 6-hour intervals tid, during waking hours. If side-effects are pronounced, dose may be reduced to 2.5 mg tid. Do not exceed 15 mg in 24 hours. *Children 12–15 years*—2.5 mg tid. Do not exceed 7.5 mg in 24 hours. Not recommended for children under 12.

Parenteral: Usual subcutaneous dose is 0.25 mg injected into the lateral deltoid area. If significant improvement does not occur in 15 to 30 minutes, a second dose of 0.25 mg may be administered. Do not exceed a total dose of 0.5 mg in a 4-hour period. If patient fails to respond, to a second 0.25 mg dose within 15 to 30 minutes and other therapeutic measures may be employed.

NURSING IMPLICATIONS
See p 213.

Xanthine Derivatives

Aminophylline *(Theophylline Ethylenediamine)*— *79% Theophylline* Rx

tablets: 100 mg (equivalent to 79 mg theophylline)	Amoline, *Generic*
tablets: 200 mg (equivalent to 158 mg theophylline)	Amoline, *Generic*
tablets, timed release (12 hours) 225 mg (equivalent to 182 mg theophylline)	Phyllocontin
tablets, sustained release (8–12 hours) 300 mg (equivalent to 236 mg theophylline)	Aminodur Dura-tabs
elixir: 250 mg/15 ml (equivalent to 215 mg theophylline)	Lixaminol
oral liquid: 105 mg/5 ml (equivalent to 90 mg theophylline)	Somophyllin, Somophyllin-DF, *Generic*
suppositories: 250 mg (equivalent to 198 mg theophylline)	Truphylline, *Generic*
suppositories: 500 mg (equivalent to 395 mg theophylline)	Truphylline, *Generic*
rectal solution: 300 mg/5 ml (equivalent to 255 mg theophylline)	Somophyllin

injection: 250 mg/10 ml (equivalent to 198 mg theophylline)	*Generic*
injection: 500 mg/20 ml (equivalent to 394 mg theophylline)	*Generic*
injection: 500 mg/2 ml (equivalent to 395 ml theophylline) (IM only)	*Generic*

Dyphylline *(Dihydroxypropyl Theophylline)* Rx

tablets: 200 mg	Dilor, Dyflex, Lufyllin, Neothylline, *Generic*
tablets: 400 mg	Dilor, Dyflex, Lufyllin-400, Neothylline, *Generic*
tablets, long acting: 400 mg	Droxine L.A.
liquid: 100 mg/5 ml	Droxine, Droxine S.F.
elixir: 100 mg/15 ml	Lufyllin
elixir: 160 mg/15 ml	Dilor
injection: 250 mg/ml	Asminyl, Dilin, Dilor, Lufyllin, Oxystat, *Generic*

Oxtriphylline
(Choline Theophyllinate)—64% Theophylline Rx

tablets: 100 mg, 200 mg (equivalent to 64 mg or 128 mg theophylline)	Choledyl
elixir: 100 mg/5 ml (equivalent to 64 mg theophylline)	Choledyl, *Generic*
syrup, pediatric: 50 mg/5 ml (equivalent to 32 mg theophylline)	Choledyl
tablets, sustained action: 400 mg, 600 mg (equivalent to 256 mg or 384 mg theophylline)	Choledyl SA

Theophylline Rx

capsules: 50 mg	Aquaphyllin, Somophyllin-T
capsules: 100 mg, 200 mg	Bronkodyl, Elixophyllin, Somophyllin-T
capsules: 250 mg	Somophyllin-T
tablets: 100 mg	Slo-Phyllin, *Generic*

tablets: 125 mg, 250 mg   Theolair

tablets: 200 mg   Slo-Phyllin, *Generic*

tablets: 225 mg   Theophyl-225

tablets: 300 mg   Quibron-T Dividose, *Generic*

elixir: 80 mg/15 ml   Asmalix, Bronkodyl, Elixophyllin, Lanophyllin, Liquophylline, Theo-Lix, Theolixir, *Generic*

elixir: 150 mg/15 ml   Theon

liquid: 80 mg/15 ml   Theolair

liquid: 150 mg/15 ml   Accurbron

liquid: 160 mg/15 ml   Aerolate

syrup: 80 mg/15 ml   Aquaphyllin, Slo-Phyllin 80, Theoclear-80, Theostat 80

suspension: 300 mg/15 ml   Elixicon

capsules, timed release (12 hours): 65 mg, 130 mg, 260 mg   Aerolate III, Aerolate JR., Aerolate SR.

capsules, timed release (12 hours): 125 mg, 250 mg   Elixophyllin SR

capsules, timed release (12 hours): 100 mg, 200 mg, 300 mg   Slo-bid Gyrocaps

capsules, timed release (8–12 hours): 60 mg, 125 mg, 250 mg   Slo-Phyllin Gyrocaps

capsules, timed release (12 hours): 130 mg   Theobid Jr. Duracaps

capsules, timed release (12 hours): 260 mg   Theobid Duracaps

capsules, timed release (6–8 hours): 130 mg, 260 mg   Theoclear L.A. Cenules

capsules, sustained release (12 hours): 300 mg   Bronkodyl S-R

capsules, sustained release (12 hours): 130 mg, 260 mg   Theospan SR

capsules, sustained release (12 hours): 125 mg, 250 mg   Theobron SR

capsules, controlled release (12 hours): 50 mg, 100 mg, 250 mg   Somophyllin-CRT

capsules, long acting (12 hours): 125 mg, 250 mg   Theovent

tablets, sustained action (12 hours): 200 mg, 300 mg   Constant-T

tablets, sustained release (12 hours) 300 mg   Quibron-T/SR Dividose

tablets, sustained release (6–8 hours): 250 mg, 500 mg   Respbid

tablets, timed release (12 hours): 100 mg, 300 mg   Sustaire

tablets, timed release (12 hours): 100 mg, 200 mg, 300 mg   Theo-Dur

tablets, timed release (8–12 hours): 250 mg, 500 mg   Theolair-SR

Theophylline Sodium Glycinate—
49% Theophylline   Rx

elixir: 330 mg/15 ml (equivalent to 165 mg theophylline/ 15 ml)   Synophylate

INDICATIONS
Symptomatic relief or prevention of bronchial asthma and treatment of reversible bronchospasm associated with chronic bronchitis and emphysema.

Investigational uses: Have been used in treatment of apnea and bradycardia of prematurity. Maintenance doses of 2 mg/kg/day have been used to maintain serum concentrations between 3 mcg/ml and 5 mcg/ml.

CONTRAINDICATIONS
Hypersensitivity to any xanthine. May be contraindicated in peptic ulcer and active gastritis. Aminophylline rectal suppositories are contraindicated in presence of irritation or infection of rectum or lower colon. Do not inject aminophylline through a central venous catheter.

ACTIONS
The methylxanthines (theophylline and its soluble salts and derivatives) directly relax smooth muscle of the bronchi and pulmonary blood vessels, stimulate the central nervous system, induce diuresis, and have weak positive chronotropic and inotropic effects. Theophylline is also a respiratory stimulant.

Xanthines competitively inhibit phosphodiesterase, which results in an increase of cyclic adenosine monophosphate (AMP). This action increases the release of endogenous epinephrine. Additionally, there is evidence that the increase in cyclic AMP may inhibit the release of the slow-reacting substance of anaphylaxis (SRS-A) and histamine.

Theophylline is well absorbed after oral administration; food has little effect on bioavailability. Absorption may be slower in the presence of food and more rapid in the presence of large volumes of fluid and high-protein meals. Rectal absorption is slow and unreliable; the oral route is generally preferred. Oral liquids and uncoated tablets are well absorbed; maximum concentrations are produced in the plasma in 2 hours. Enteric-coated tablets and sustained-release dosage forms may be unreliably absorbed; however, certain continuous-release formulations have demonstrated excellent drug serum level profiles.

Therapeutic serum levels range from 10 mcg/ml to 20 mcg/ml. Ideally, serum levels should be monitored. Levels above 20 mcg/ml may produce toxic effects. Once patient is stabilized, serum levels tend to remain constant with same dosage. When blood is difficult to obtain, theophylline saliva levels (approximately 60% of plasma levels) may be used for dosage adjustments.

Xanthines are eliminated through biotransformation in the liver and excreted by the kidneys. Plasma elimination half-life averages about 7 to 9 hours in adult nonsmokers, 4 to 5 hours in adult smokers, and 3.5 hours in children. Decreased plasma clearance in patients with heart failure, liver dysfunction, alcoholism, reduced renal function, pulmonary edema, chronic obstructive pulmonary disease, or respiratory infections, in premature infants, and in patients receiving certain antibiotics may result in a significantly prolonged plasma half-life.

WARNINGS

Toxicity: Excessive doses may cause severe toxicity. There are often no early signs of less serious theophylline toxicity, such as nausea and restlessness, which may appear in up to 50% of patients prior to onset of convulsions. Ventricular arrhythmias, tachycardia, or seizures may be the first signs of toxicity. Grand mal seizures may occur, particularly if serum level is above 50 mcg/ml.

Cardiac effects: May worsen preexisting arrhythmias. Overdosage may cause cardiac arrhythmias including sinus tachycardia, premature ventricular contractions, ventricular fibrillation, and ultimately cardiovascular collapse.

Use morphine and curare with caution in those with airflow obstruction; these agents may stimulate histamine release and can induce acute asthma. They may also depress respiration, leading to respiratory failure.

Rectal administration: Occasionally may be irritating. Although absorption from suppositories may be variable and unpredictable, administration by enema may result in blood levels comparable to those obtained by IV injection; retention enemas are more reliable than suppositories.

Use in pregnancy: Safety not established. Aminophylline administered to a pregnant asthmatic shortly before delivery has resulted in fetal tachycardia during labor and delivery and the appearance of "jitters" in the newborn. Apnea has been associated with theophylline withdrawal in the neonate. Use only when clearly needed and when potential benefits outweigh the unknown potential hazards to the fetus.

Use in lactation: It has been reported that theophylline distributes readily into breast milk. Use with caution in nursing women.

Use in children: Use with caution in children because they have marked sensitivity to the CNS stimulant action of theophylline. Xanthines are not generally well tolerated by small children because of CNS stimulation.

PRECAUTIONS

Use with caution in severe cardiac disease, severe hypoxemia, severe renal and hepatic disease, severe hypertension, acute myocardial injury, hyperthyroidism, cor pulmonale, congestive heart failure (CHF), and in elderly, particularly males, and neonates. In patients with CHF, theophylline may have a markedly prolonged half-life.

GI effects: Use cautiously in those with peptic ulcer. Local irritation may occur; centrally mediated GI effects may occur with serum levels over 20 mcg/ml.

Parenteral administration: Aminophylline must be injected slowly, not more than 25 mg/min when given IV. Rapid infusion has been associated with marked hypotension, syncope, and death. Hydration must be maintained. IM route not recommended; injection may cause severe, persistent pain. When switching from oral to IV dosing, amount of drug given previously must be considered. When switching from continuous IV infusions to oral therapy, wait at least 4 to 6 hours before giving first dose.

The addition of **alcohol** in liquid formulations is not necessary for absorption and may be potentially harmful, especially to the pediatric patient. Ethylenediamine in aminophylline may cause sensitivity reactions and dermatitis.

DRUG INTERACTIONS

Agents that decrease the effects of theophylline: **Cigarette** and **marijuana smoking, phenobarbital, charcoal-broiled foods** with a high polycyclic carbon content.

Agents that increase the effects of theophylline: **Troleandomycin, erythromycin, cimetidine, influenza vaccine,** and possibly **allopurinol** and **thiabendazole.**

Theophylline increases the effects of the following: **Furosemide, sympathomimetic drugs.** Enhances sensitivity to and toxicity of **digitalis.** Higher than usual doses may increase the effects of **oral anticoagulants.**

Theophylline decreases the levels of **phenytoin,** resulting in increased seizure activity. Aminophylline may increase excretion of **lithium carbonate.**

Miscellaneous: Concomitant administration of aminophylline and **beta-adrenergic blocking agents** may cause antagonistic effects. Beta-adrenergic blocking agents may decrease theophylline clearance, especially in those with increased theophylline clearance due to cigarette smoking. Concomitant administration of theophylline and **tetracycline** may increase incidence of GI side-effects. Administration of theophylline with **reserpine** can cause tachycardia; theophylline with **chlordiazepoxide** can cause fatty-acid mobilization. Coadministration with a **magnesium–aluminum hydroxide antacid** is reported to decrease rate, but not extent, of theophylline absorption.

Drug/lab test interferences: Theophylline may interfere with the assay of **uric acid** and increase test results for **urinary catecholamines, plasma free fatty acids, sedimentary rate.** Theophylline may decrease the results of ^{131}I **uptake tests.** Spectrophotometric methods for measuring theophylline in serum are affected by **furosemide, phenylbutazone, probenecid, theobromine.**

ADVERSE REACTIONS

GI: Nausea, vomiting, loss of appetite, gastric irritation, burning substernal or epigastric pain, hematemesis, diarrhea, rectal irritation or bleeding (aminophylline suppositories), reactivation of peptic ulcer, intestinal bleeding. Therapeutic doses of theophylline have been shown to induce GI reflux during sleep or while recumbent, thus increasing the opportunity for aspiration, which can aggravate bronchospasm.

CNS: Irritability (especially in children), restlessness, dizziness, nervousness, headache, insomnia, reflex hyperexcitability, muscle twitching, clonic and tonic generalized convulsions. Isolated cases of severe depression and stammering speech have been reported. Abnormal behavior manifested by withdrawal, mutism, and unresponsiveness alternating with periods of hyperexcitability (flailing of limbs, posturing on all four extremities, intense emotional lability).

Cardiovascular: Palpitations, ECG changes, sinus tachycardia, ventricular tachycardia, extrasystoles, flushing, decreased pulmonary vascular resistance, peripheral vascular collapse, hypotension, life-threatening ventricular arrhythmias, circulatory failure.

Respiratory: Tachypnea, respiratory arrest.

Renal: Proteinuria, increased excretion of renal tubular cells and red blood cells, diuresis (dehydration). Urinary retention has been reported in males with prostatic enlargement.

Other: Fever, hyperglycemia, inappropriate antidiuretic hormone (ADH) syndrome, rash, increased SGOT, shortened prothrombin and clotting times, leukocytosis. May cause presence of benign breast tumors. Rapid IV injection of aminophylline may produce headache, flushing, palpitations, dizziness, hyperventilation, fall in blood pressure, or precordial pain.

OVERDOSAGE

Symptoms: Early symptoms include anorexia, nausea, occasional vomiting, vertigo, agitation, wakefulness, restlessness, irritability, headache. Convulsions or ventricular arrhythmias may be first signs of toxicity. Other symptoms of intoxication include confusion, respiratory paralysis, hematemesis, dizziness, drowsiness, tremors, hyperactivity, coma, precordial pain, tachycardia, other arrhythmias, varying degrees of hypotension (including, in extreme cases, severe shock, cardiovascular collapse, and death). Agitated maniacal behavior and frequent vomiting accompanied by extreme thirst develop later, and lead to delirium, convulsions, hyperthermia, and vasomotor collapse. Gross overdosage, especially in children, may lead to seizures and death without preceding symptoms of toxicity. Serious toxicity can occur without earlier signs of less toxicity and are generally seen only with IV administration.

Treatment if overdose is established and seizure has not occurred: Induce vomiting, even if emesis has occurred spontaneously; administration of syrup of ipecac is preferred method. *Do not* induce emesis in those with impaired consciousness; take precautions against aspiration, especially in infants, children. If vomiting is unsuccessful or contraindicated, perform gastric lavage. Administer a cathartic (important if sustained-release preparation has been taken). Administer activated charcoal.

If patient is having a seizure: Establish airway and administer oxygen. Treat seizure with IV diazepam 0.1 mg/kg to 0.3 mg/kg, up to 10 mg. Monitor vital signs, maintain blood pressure, and provide adequate hydration.

Postseizure coma: Maintain airway and oxygenation. Follow above recommendations to prevent absorption of drug, but perform intubation and lavage instead of producing emesis. Introduce cathartic and charcoal via large-bore gastric tube. Continue to provide full supportive care and adequate hydration while waiting for drug to be metabolized. This generally occurs rapidly enough that dialysis is not warranted.

Supportive care: Do not use stimulants (analeptic agents); IV fluids may be required to overcome dehydration, acid–base imbalance, and hypotension. The latter may also be treated with vasopressors. Apnea will require ventilatory support. Treat hyperpyrexia, especially in children, with tepid-water sponge baths or a hypothermic blanket. Monitor theophylline serum levels until they fall below 20 mcg/ml. Forced diuresis is of no value.

DOSAGE

Dosage is individualized; adjustments may be based on clinical response with careful monitoring for manifestations of toxicity. If possible, serum levels are monitored to maintain serum levels in the therapeutic range of 10 mcg/ml to 20 mcg/ml. Levels above 20 mcg/ml may produce toxicity; toxicity may be seen with serum levels between 15 mcg/ml and 20 mcg/ml, particularly during initial therapy. Once stabilized, serum levels tend to remain constant. Dosages calculated on lean body weight because theophylline does not distribute into fatty tissue.

Frequency of dosing: When immediate-release products are used, dosing to maintain therapeutic serum levels usually requires administration q6h, particularly in children, but dosing intervals up to 8 hours may be satisfactory for adults.

Acute symptoms requiring rapid theophyllinization in those not receiving theophylline: To achieve a rapid effect, an initial loading dose is required. Dosage recommendations for theophylline anhydrous are given in Table 4.

Acute symptoms requiring rapid theophyllinzation in those currently receiving theophylline: Ideally, the loading dose should be deferred if a serum theophylline level can be obtained rapidly.

Chronic therapy: Initial dose—16 mg/kg/24 hours or 400 mg/24 hours of anhydrous theophylline in divided doses q6h to q8h. Dosage may be increased in approximately 25% increments at 2- to 3-day intervals.

Maximum dose when serum concentration is not measured: 9 years—24 mg/kg/day; *9–12 years*—20 mg/kg/day; *12–16 years*—18 mg/kg/day; *over 16 years*—13 mg/kg/day or 900 mg.

Maintenance of serum theophylline concentrations during chronic therapy: Serum levels obtained at time of peak absorption, 1 to 2 hours after administration of immediate-release products and 4 hours for most sustained-release products. Dosage is adjusted according to serum levels.

AMINOPHYLLINE (THEOPHYLLINE ETHYLENEDIAMINE)

For oral and rectal dosage, see above.

IM: Adults—500 mg as required. Preparations of 250 mg/ml are available for IM use. IM injection is painful; this route of administration is *not* recommended.

IV: Use only diluted (25 mg/ml) preparations; may be further diluted with IV solutions. Do not exceed 25 mg/min infusion rate.

Loading dose: In those not currently receiving theophylline products, a loading dose of 6 mg/kg is infused at rate not to exceed 25 mg/minute. Reduce loading dose in those receiving any theophylline-containing product.

Maintenance infusions: Monitoring of serum theophylline concentration is recommended for continuous IV infusion. The recommended dosage is given in Table 5.

DYPHYLLINE (DIHYDROCYPROPYL THEOPHYLLINE)

Is a derivative of theophylline; it is not a theophylline salt. Specific dyphylline serum levels may be used to monitor therapy; serum theophylline levels will *Not* measure dyphylline.

Table 4. Dosage Recommendations for Theophylline Anhydrous

Patients	Oral Loading Dose	Following Dosage	Maintenance Dosage
Children 6 months to 9 years	6 mg/kg	4 mg/kg q4h × 3 doses	4 mg/kg q6h
Children 9–16 years, young adult smokers	6 mg/kg	3 mg/kg q4h × 3 doses	3 mg/kg q6h
Otherwise healthy nonsmoking adults	6 mg/kg	3 mg/kg q6h × 2 doses	3 mg/kg q8h
Older patients or those with cor pulmonale	6 mg/kg	2 mg/kg q6h × 2 doses	2 mg/kg q8h
Those with CHF	6 mg/kg	2 mg/kg q8h × 2 doses	1–2 mg/kg q12

Table 5. Maintenance Infusion Rates for Aminophylline (mg/kg/hr)

Patients	First 12 Hours	Beyond 12 Hours
Neonates	—	0.2
Infants under 1 year	—	0.2–0.9
Children 1–9 years	1.2	1.0
Children 9–16 years, young adult smokers	1.0	0.8
Otherwise healthy nonsmoking adults	0.7	0.5
Older patients, those with cor pulmonale	0.6	0.3
Patients with CHF or liver disease	0.5	0.1–0.2

Oral: _Adults_—Up to 15 mg/kg q6h. Dosage is individualized.

IM (_Not_ for IV administration): _Adults_—250 mg to 500 mg, injected slowly. _Children_—2 mg/lb to 3 mg/lb (4.4 mg/kg to 6.6 mg/kg) daily in divided doses.

OXTRIPHYLLINE (CHOLINE THEOPHYLLINATE)

Adults: 200 mg qid.

Children (2–12 years): 100 mg/60 lb (3.7 mg/kg) qid.

Sustained action: 400 mg to 600 mg q12h.

THEOPHYLLINE SODIUM GLYCINATE

Adults: 330 to 660 mg q6h to q8h (P.C.).

Children (6–12 years): 220 mg to 330 mg q6h to q8h (P.C.).

Children (under 6 years): 55 mg to 165 mg q6h to q8h (P.C.).

NURSING IMPLICATIONS: BRONCHODILATORS AND DECONGESTANTS, SYSTEMIC

HISTORY
See Appendix 4.

PHYSICAL ASSESSMENT
Record blood pressure, pulse, and respirations; auscultate lungs.

Sympathomimetics: If a hypersensitivity reaction is apparent, auscultate lungs and examine affected areas (skin for urticaria, pruritus; edema of lips, eyelids, tongue, nasal mucosa; area of insect bite); emergency administration of epinephrine may be necessary.

Xanthine derivatives: Examine sputum raised (if any); assess additional problems identified in health history. Baseline studies may include ECG, pulmonary-function studies. Serum levels may be drawn if patient has been receiving a xanthine derivative.

ADMINISTRATION
SYMPATHOMIMETICS
Oral preparations may be given with food to avoid GI upset.

Insomnia may occur when these drugs are administered routinely. Last dose should be scheduled several hours before H.S.

If drug is given parenterally to relieve acute bronchospasm, obtain blood pressure, pulse, and respirations before drug is administered.

Epinephrine
Repeated local injections can result in necrosis at sites of injection from vascular constriction. If repeated injections are necessary, rotate sites and record site used.

Parenteral epinephrine 1:1000: Subcutaneous route preferred; if ordered IM, avoid use of buttocks; when possible use the deltoid muscle.

CLINICAL ALERT: Carefully check product label, physician's order (dosage, route) before administration. Epinephrine intended for inhalation is available as a 1:100 solution and is not used for injection. _Epinephrine 1:1000:_ Dose may be ordered in mg or ml. Dose range is 0.2 mg (0.2 ml or 3 minims) to 1 mg (1 ml). To determine patient's response, physician usually orders smallest dose when drug is first administered. If physician's written order is unclear, or decimal point is difficult to read (for dose less than 1 ml), request clarification.

Use a tuberculin syringe to ensure accuracy, especially when dosage is less than 1 ml. Aspirate syringe before injection to avoid IV injection.

Do not remove parenteral epinephrine from package until ready for use, because solution should be protected from exposure to light. Do not use if solution is brown in color or contains a precipitate.

Suspension: Shake vial or ampule thoroughly before withdrawing drug.

Isoproterenol, sublingual
Instruct patient to place tablet under tongue and allow to disintegrate; instruct patient not to swallow saliva until absorption has taken place.

Terbutaline
Subcutaneous injection given into the lateral deltoid area.

XANTHINE DERIVATIVES
Dosages for some liquid formulations are given in mg/15 ml.

There are two doses expressed for aminophylline, oxtriphylline, and theophylline sodium glycinate: the dosage stated on the product label and the dosage equivalent, in mg, to theophylline. If the physician's written dosage does not correspond to the dosage stated on the drug container, compare the written order to dosage equivalents or check with the hospital pharmacist.

IV aminophylline
Only aminophylline is administered IV.

Drug should always be well diluted (25 mg/ml) and warmed to room temperature prior to administration. Drug may also be further diluted with (added to) IV solutions. Do not use drug if crystals are present or solution appears cloudy or discolored.

CLINICAL ALERT: Do not exceed an infusion rate of 25 mg/minute. Rapid infusion has been associated with marked hypotension, syncope, and death. Rapid IV injection may produce headache, flushing, palpitations, dizziness, hyperventilation, fall in blood pressure, or precordial pain. *Do not* inject aminophylline through a central venous catheter.

Maintenance infusion dosages are normally lower than the loading dose.

IM administration of aminophylline is *not* recommended, because injection is painful.

The recommended IV loading dose or oral dose of aminophylline for acute asthmatic attacks may be reduced if patient has recently received any xanthine derivative. Notify physician before giving initial dose if history identified use or administration of a xanthine derivative in past 24 hours.

Compatibility: Do *not* mix the following solutions with aminophylline in IV fluids: Strong acid solutions, ascorbic acid, chlorpromazine, corticotropin, dimenhydrinate, erythromycin gluceptate, hydralazine, insulin, meperidine, methadone, methicillin, morphine sulfate, oxytetracycline, penicillin G potassium, phenobarbital, phenytoin, prochlorperazine, promethazine, tetracycline, vancomycin, vitamin B complex with C.

Insert lubricated aminophylline rectal suppository past the rectal sphincter. Only the pediatric suppository (125 mg) should be used on children. Do not break an adult suppository to obtain the pediatric dosage.

Aminophylline suppositories should be kept under refrigeration until use (unless manufacturer's label directs otherwise).

Rectal solution of aminophylline: Administer when patient is unable to take oral medication. Available solution is 300 mg/5 ml. Solution is best absorbed when rectum is free of feces. Keep patient recumbent 20 to 30 minutes or until defecation reflex subsides. If respiratory distress occurs or increases when patient is recumbent, slowly elevate the head of the bed until patient is comfortable.

If patient is unable to retain rectal solution or suppository, *Do not repeat dose;* notify physician, because another route of administration is usually necessary.

Oral preparations are best given q6h around the clock (exception is long-acting forms).

If GI upset occurs, drug may be given with food or meals. Theophylline sodium glycinate is given after meals (P.C.).

Warn patient not to chew timed-release capsules or tablets but to swallow whole.

ONGOING ASSESSMENTS AND NURSING MANAGEMENT
Parenteral administration for acute bronchospasm: Monitor blood pressure, pulse, respirations, and drug response q15m to q30m until bronchospasms are relieved or condition stabilized.

Notify the physician immediately if condition is not relieved, bronchospasms become worse, or adverse reactions occur.

Measure intake and output.

Other therapies such as oxygen, steroids, and intravenous fluids may be employed.

Patient may be diaphoretic and require frequent changes of gown and bed linen; avoid exposure to drafts, cool air.

Relief of mild bronchospasm: Monitor blood pressure, pulse, and respirations q4h to q8h; assess drug response q2h to q4h.

Observe for adverse reactions; report occurrence to the physician because dosage or frequency of administration may be changed.

SYMPATHOMIMETICS
Observe for hypertension, hypotension, palpitations, tachycardia, arrhythmias, chest pain, or precordial distress.

Difficulty breathing, as well as sympathomimetic activity of drug, may produce severe anxiety. Patient may require frequent reassurance until condition is relieved.

Observe for adverse reactions; report occurrence to physician because dosage or frequency may need to be reduced.

If difficult or painful urination occurs, or urinary retention is suspected, notify physician and measure intake and output.

XANTHINE DERIVATIVES
Morphine is administered with caution to patients receiving xanthine derivatives, because re-

spiratory suppression leading to respiratory failure may occur.

Occasionally, rectal administration may be irritating. If patient complains of rectal burning or discomfort, notify physician because another route of administration may be necessary.

Observe children for CNS adverse reactions, particularly irritability.

If dizziness occurs, the ambulatory patient may require assistance.

Early symptoms of toxicity include anorexia, nausea, occasional vomiting, vertigo, agitation, wakefulness, restlessness, irritability, and headache.

Observe for adverse reactions and signs of overdose (toxicity). Withhold the next dose and notify the physician if adverse reactions or signs of toxicity are apparent.

Serum levels may be monitored during titration period (exception: dyphylline) and periodically thereafter.

When switching from IV to oral route, wait at least 4 to 6 hours before giving first oral dose.

Rectal suppository: Check patient q15m to q30m after insertion to be sure suppository is retained. If patient is unable to retain suppository, contact physician.

PATIENT AND FAMILY INFORMATION

XANTHINE DERIVATIVES
If GI upset occurs, take with food or meals.

Do _Not_ chew or crush enteric-coated or sustained-release tablets.

Take every 6 hours around the clock (exception: time-release dosage forms) unless directed otherwise by physician.

Notify physician if nausea, vomiting, GI pain, or restlessness occurs or condition becomes worse.

Do not use nonprescription drugs, especially those for colds, cough, or asthma, unless use is approved by physician.

Avoid smoking cigarettes because this may interfere with proper dosage adjustment as well as contribute to the original problem.

Avoid excessive amounts of coffee, tea, and cola because these products contain varied amounts of xanthine derivatives.

SYMPATHOMIMETICS
Do not exceed prescribed or manufacturer's recommended dose; if drug fails to produce response, contact physician.

If GI upset occurs, take with food.

Do not use other nonprescription drugs, especially cold and cough remedies or nasal sprays or drops, unless use is approved by physician.

May cause nervousness, restlessness, insomnia (especially ephedrine), or anorexia (phenylpropanolamine); if these effects occur, notify physician because dosage or schedule may need to be changed.

Notify physician if palpitations, tachycardia, chest pain, muscle tremors (especially with terbutaline), dizziness, headache, flushing, or difficult urination (with ephedrine) occurs, or if breathing difficulty persists.

Buclizine Hydrochloride

See Antiemetic/Antivertigo Agents.

Bumetanide

See Loop Diuretics.

Bupivacaine Hydrochloride

See Anesthetics, Local, Injectable.

Busulfan Rx

tablets: 2 mg   Myleran

INDICATIONS
Palliative treatment of chronic myelogenous leukemia (myeloid, myelocytic, granulocytic). Although not curative, busulfan reduces total granulocyte mass, relieves symptoms, and improves clinical state of patient. Approximately 90% of adults with previously untreated chronic myelogenous leukemia will obtain hematologic remission. It has been shown to be superior to splenic irradiation with respect to survival times and maintenance of hemoglobin levels, and equivalent to irradiation in controlling splenomegaly. Busulfan is less effective in those with chronic myelogenous leukemia who lack the Philadelphia (Ph[1]) chromosome. Juvenile chronic myelogenous leukemia, typically occurring in young children and associated with the absence of a Ph[1] chromosome, responds poorly to busulfan. Drug is of no benefit in patients whose chronic myelogenous leukemia has entered a "blastic" phase. See also Antineoplastic Agents, Combination Chemotherapy.

CONTRAINDICATIONS
Should not be used unless a diagnosis of chronic myelogenous leukemia has been established; should not be used in patients whose disease has demon-

strated prior resistance to the drug. Busulfan is of no value in chronic lymphocytic leukemia, acute leukemia, or in "blastic crisis" of chronic myelogenous leukemia.

ACTIONS

Busulfan is an alkylating agent that undergoes a wide range of nucleophilic substitution reactions. Although chemical reactivity is relatively nonspecific, alkylation of deoxyribonucleic acid (DNA) is felt to be an important biological mechanism for its cytotoxic effect. See also Antineoplastic Agents.

WARNINGS

Hematopoietic toxicity: Most frequent and serious side-effect of treatment is the induction of bone-marrow failure, resulting in severe pancytopenia, which may be more pronounced than that induced with other alkylating agents. It is generally felt that the usual cause of pancytopenia is failure to stop the drug soon enough; individual idiosyncrasy to the drug does not seem to be an important factor. Use with extreme caution in those whose bone-marrow reserve may have been compromised by prior irradiation or chemotherapy or whose marrow is recovering from previous cytotoxic therapy. Although recovery from pancytopenia may take from 1 month to 2 years, this complication is potentially reversible and the patient is vigorously supported through any period of severe pancytopenia.

Pulmonary: A rare complication of therapy is development of bronchopulmonary dysplasia with pulmonary fibrosis. Symptoms have been reported to occur within 8 months to 10 years after initiation of therapy. Clinically, patients have reported the insidious onset of cough, dyspnea, and low-grade fever. Pulmonary-function studies have revealed diminished diffusion capacity and decreased pulmonary compliance. If measures such as sputum cultures, virologic studies, and exfoliative cytology fail to establish an etiology for the pulmonary infiltrates, lung biopsy may be necessary to establish the diagnosis. Treatment is unsatisfactory; in most cases patients died within 6 months after the diagnosis was established. There is no specific therapy for this complication other than immediate discontinuation of busulfan. Busulfan may cause cellular dysplasia in many organs in addition to the lung.

Chromosome aberrations: Chromosome aberrations have been reported. Also, busulfan is possibly mutagenic.

Carcinogenicity: Malignant tumors have been reported in patients receiving busulfan; drug may be a carcinogen.

Fertility: Ovarian suppression and amenorrhea with menopausal symptoms commonly occur during therapy in premenopausal patients. There have been reports of sterility, azoospermia, and testicular atrophy in male patients.

Use in pregnancy: Busulfan is potentially teratogenic and embryotoxic. The use of the drug during pregnancy should be avoided, if possible, particularly during the first trimester. The potential benefits to the mother must be weighed against the risk to the fetus.

PRECAUTIONS

Most consistent dose-related toxicity is bone-marrow suppression. This may be manifested by anemia, leukopenia, thrombocytopenia, or any combination of these. Patients must be instructed to report promptly the development of fever, sore throat, signs of local infection, bleeding from any site, symptoms suggestive of anemia. Any of these may indicate busulfan toxicity; however, they may also indicate transformation of the disease to the acute blastic form. Because drug may have a delayed effect, medication is usually withdrawn temporarily at first sign of an abnormally large or exceptionally rapid fall in any of the formed elements of the blood. It is recommended that evaluation of hemoglobin or hematocrit, total white blood cell count, and quantitative platelet count be obtained weekly during therapy. Bone-marrow examination may be useful for evaluation of marrow status when cause of fluctuation in the formed element of peripheral blood is obscure.

Dosage may need to be reduced if busulfan is combined with other drugs whose primary toxicity is myelosuppression. Occasionally, patients may be unusually sensitive to standard doses and suffer neutropenia or thrombocytopenia after relatively short exposure to the drug.

DRUG INTERACTIONS

Drug/lab tests: **Uric acid levels** in blood and urine may be increased.

ADVERSE REACTIONS

Hematologic: Most frequent, serious toxic effect is myelosuppression resulting in leukopenia, thrombocytopenia, and anemia.

Pulmonary: Interstitial pulmonary fibrosis reported rarely, but is a clinically significant adverse effect when observed, and calls for immediate discontinuation of drug.

Ocular: Drug capable of inducing cataracts; in cases reported, these have occurred after prolonged administration of the drug.

Dermatologic: Hyperpigmentation is most common (5%–10%) adverse reaction, particularly in those with a dark complexion.

Metabolic: In a few cases, a syndrome closely resembling adrenal insufficiency has developed after prolonged therapy and is characterized by weakness, severe fatigue, anorexia, weight loss, nausea and vomiting, and melanoderma. Hyperuricemia and hyperuricosuria are common in patients with chronic myelogenous leukemia. Additional rapid destruction of granulocytes may accompany the initiation of therapy and increase the urate pool.

DOSAGE

Remission induction: Usual dose range is 4 mg to 8 mg total dose daily. Because rate at which the leukocyte count falls is dose related, daily doses exceeding 4 mg/day should be reserved for patients with the most compelling symptoms. The greater the total daily dose, the greater the possibility of inducing bone-marrow aplasia.

A decrease in the leukocyte count is not usually seen during the first 10 to 15 days of treatment; the leukocyte count may actually increase during this period. Because the leukocyte count may continue to fall for more than 1 month after drug is discontinued, busulfan is discontinued prior to the total leukocyte count's falling into the normal range. When the total leukocyte count has declined to approximately 15,000/cu mm, the drug is usually withdrawn. With recommended doses, a normal leukocyte count is usually achieved in 12 to 20 weeks.

Maintenance therapy: During remission, patient is examined at monthly intervals and treatment resumed with the induction dosage when the total leukocyte count reaches approximately 50,000/cu mm. When remission is shorter than 3 months, maintenance therapy of 1 mg/day to 3 mg/day may be used to keep the hematologic status under control and prevent rapid relapse.

NURSING IMPLICATIONS

HISTORY
See Appendix 4.

PHYSICAL ASSESSMENT:
Monitor general physical and emotional status; vital signs; weight. Baseline laboratory tests may include CBC, differential platelet count, hematocrit, hemoglobin, serum uric acid, BUN, creatinine. Pulmonary-function studies and bone-marrow aspiration may also be performed.

ADMINISTRATION
Administer at same time each day. Encourage patient to drink 10 to 12 glasses (8 oz each) of water per day.

ONGOING ASSESSMENTS AND NURSING MANAGEMENT
Depending on clinical status, patient may require hospitalization at time of initiation of therapy. Maintenance therapy is almost always on an outpatient basis, unless complications of disease or therapy require hospitalization.

Monitor vital signs q4h or as ordered.

Observe for adverse reactions.

Measure intake and output; inform physician if intake is under 2500 ml/day.

A decrease in the leukocyte count is not usually seen in the first 10 to 15 days (leukocyte count may actually increase during this period).

CLINICAL ALERT: Observe for signs of myelodepression (see Appendix 6, section 6-8). Bronchopulmonary pulmonary dysplasia, a rare but extremely serious complication of therapy, may occur. Observe for an insidious onset of cough, dyspnea, low-grade fever. Inform physician immediately of findings.

Weigh weekly; report weight changes to physician.

Physician may order urine alkalinization or the prophylactic administration of a xanthine oxidase inhibitor such as allopurinol to minimize hyperuricemia or hyperuricosuria. Increased intake of oral fluids is also necessary.

IM administration of other pharmacologic agents is avoided, when possible, if thrombocytopenia occurs. When this route is necessary, prolonged pressure on the injection site is necessary.

Physician will order weekly hemoglobin or hematocrit, WBC, differential count, quantitative platelet count while patient is on busulfan therapy.

PATIENT AND FAMILY INFORMATION
NOTE: Patient should receive a full explanation of all possible adverse reactions and what specific reactions should be reported immediately to the physician, the length of therapy, and the results expected.

Notify physician or nurse immediately if unusual bleeding or bruising, fever, cough, shortness of breath, or flank, stomach, or joint pain occurs.

Medication may cause darkening of skin, diarrhea, dizziness, fatigue, loss of appetite, mental confusion, nausea, and vomiting; notify physician if these become pronounced.

Take medication at same time each day.

Drink at least 10 to 12 glasses (8 oz each) of fluid daily; this is an important part of therapy.

If additional drugs are prescribed, take them at the time specified.

Do not use any nonprescription drug, including aspirin, without obtaining prior approval of the physician.

Inform other physicians and dentists seen concurrently of therapy with busulfan.

Female patients: Contraceptive measures are recommended during therapy.

Butabarbital Sodium

See Barbiturates.

Butamben Picrate

See Anesthetics, Local, Topical.

Butorphanol Tartrate Rx

injection: 1 mg/ml, 2   Stadol
    mg/ml

INDICATIONS
Relief of moderate to severe pain. Also used for preoperative or preanesthetic medication, as a supplement to balanced anesthesia, and for relief of prepartum pain.

CONTRAINDICATIONS
Hypersensitivity.

ACTIONS
Is a potent analgesic with both narcotic agonist and antagonist effects. Exact mechanism of action is unknown.

Narcotic antagonist activity: Is approximately 30 times that of pentazocine and $\frac{1}{40}$ that of naloxone.

Effect on respiration: At the dose of 2 mg to 3 mg, butorphanol produces analgesia and respiratory depression approximately equal to those produced by 10 mg of morphine or 80 mg of meperidine. Respiratory depression is reversible by naloxone.

Cardiovascular effects: Hemodynamic changes after IV administration are similar to those seen after administration of pentazocine and include increased pulmonary artery pressure, pulmonary wedge pressure, left ventricular end-diastolic pressure, systemic arterial pressure, pulmonary vascular resistance, and cardiac workload.

Onset: The onset of analgesia is within 10 minutes following IM administration; peak analgesic activity is obtained in 30 to 60 minutes. Rapid effects occur with IV administration. Duration of analgesia is 3 to 4 hours. Butorphanol is metabolized by the liver and is excreted primarily in the urine.

On a weight basis, analgesic potency appears to be 3.5 to 7 times that of morphine, 30 to 40 times that of meperidine, and 15 to 20 times that of pentazocine.

WARNINGS
Patients physically dependent on narcotics: These patients should not receive butorphanol because its antagonist properties; it may precipitate withdrawal symptoms. Detoxification in such patients is required prior to use.

Drug dependence: Has low physical-dependence liability but care is exercised in administration to emotionally unstable patients and those prone to drug misuse and abuse.

Head injury and increased intracranial pressure: Butorphanol, like other potent analgesics, may elevate CSF pressure. Use in cases of head injury can produce effects (*e.g.,* miosis) that may obscure the clinical course of these patients. Use with extreme caution and only if essential.

Cardiovascular disease: Increases cardiac workload. Limit use in acute myocardial infarction or in ventricular dysfunction or coronary insufficiency to patients hypersensitive to morphine sulfate or meperidine. Use with caution in the hypertensive patient.

Use in labor and delivery: Safety to mother and fetus have been established, but use with caution in women delivering premature infants.

Use in pregnancy and lactation: Safety for use prior to labor not established. Use only when clearly needed and when potential benefits outweigh the unknown potential hazards to the fetus. Not recommended in nursing mothers. Butorphanol has been used safely for labor pain in mothers who subsequently nursed their infants.

Use in children: Not recommended for children under 18.

PRECAUTIONS
Respiratory conditions: Butorphanol causes some respiratory depression. Administer with caution and in low dosage to those with respiratory depression (*e.g.,* from other medication, uremia, or severe infection), severely limited respiratory reserve, bronchial asthma, obstructive respiratory conditions, or cyanosis.

Use in impaired renal or hepatic function: Drug is metabolized by liver and excreted by kidneys. Administer with caution to patient with renal or hepatic impairment. Extensive liver disease may predispose patient to side-effects and increased activity from the usual clinical dose, possibly the result of decreased drug metabolism.

Biliary surgery: Safety not established for administration to patients undergoing surgery of the biliary tract.

DRUG INTERACTIONS

Concomitant administration of **pancuronium** may cause an increase in conjunctival changes. Dose of butorphanol should be reduced when administered concomitantly with **phenothiazines, droperidol, other tranquilizers,** and **barbiturate anesthetics,** which may potentiate the action of butorphanol. Butorphanol will precipitate withdrawal reactions in patients physically dependent on **narcotics.**

ADVERSE REACTIONS

Most frequent

Sedation (40%); nausea, clamminess, sweating (6%); headache, vertigo, floating feeling (3%); dizziness, lethargy (2%); confusion, lightheadedness (1%).

Other adverse reactions, with incidence of less than 1%

CNS: Nervousness, unusual dreams, agitation, euphoria, hallucinations.

Autonomic: Flushing, warmth, dry mouth, sensitivity to cold.

Cardiovascular: Palpitation, increase or decrease in blood pressure.

GI: Vomiting.

Respiratory: Slowing of respiration, shallow breathing.

Dermatologic: Rash, hives, or pruritus.

Ophthalmic: Diplopia or blurred vision.

OVERDOSAGE

Symptoms: Overdosage could produce some degree of respiratory depression and variable cardiovascular and CNS effects.

Treatment: Immediate treatment of suspected overdosage is IV naloxone. Constantly evaluate the respiratory and cardiac status. Institute appropriate supportive measures (*e.g.,* oxygen, IV fluids, vasopressors, assisted or controlled respiration).

DOSAGE

Not recommended in children under 18 years.

IM: Usual single dose is 2 mg. May be repeated q3h to q4h as needed. Dosage range is 1 mg to 4 mg, repeated q3h to q4h. Do not exceed single doses of 4 mg.

IV: Usual single dose is 1 mg. May be repeated q3h to q4h as necessary. Dosage range is 0.5 mg to 2 mg, repeated q3h to q4h.

NURSING IMPLICATIONS

HISTORY

See Appendix 4. When applicable, review chart for etiology of pain, length of time drug has been given, time of last administration, therapeutic effect of analgesic, date of drug order.

PHYSICAL ASSESSMENT

At time patient requests analgesic, determine exact location of pain, type of pain (sharp, dull, stabbing), when pain began. In addition, look for controllable factors (*e.g.,* uncomfortable position, thirst, noise, bright lights, cold) that may decrease patient's tolerance to pain.

ADMINISTRATION

Obtain blood pressure, pulse, and respirations immediately before preparing drug for administration. If these vital signs are significantly increased or decreased from average baseline values, withhold drug and notify physician immediately.

ONGOING ASSESSMENTS AND NURSING MANAGEMENT

Onset of analgesia is with 10 minutes following IM administration and rapid following IV administration.

Assess patient 20 to 30 minutes following administration for relief of pain. Check blood pressure, pulse, and respirations. Because symptoms of overdosage can occur with normal doses, observe for some degree of respiratory depression and variable cardiovascular and CNS effects. Contact physician immediately if symptoms of overdosage are suspected.

Continue to monitor patient q30m to q60m following administration for analgesic effect, development of adverse reactions.

If drug fails to produce sufficient analgesia, discuss problem with physician because a different analgesic may be necessary.

If sedation occurs, patient should remain in bed or, when necessary, ambulate with assistance.

If patient is to be assisted out of bed at scheduled times during the day, attempt to schedule ambulatory activity 30 to 60 minutes after administration of drug because peak analgesic activity occurs at this time.

Although safety for use during labor and delivery has been established, observe neonate for signs of respiratory depression if mother received drug within 4 hours before delivery.

A patient history may not reveal dependence on narcotics. When initial dose of drug is administered, observe for development of narcotic withdrawal symptoms: yawning, perspiration, sneezing, tearing, restlessness. These can progress to more severe symptoms such as anxiety, vomiting, abdominal cramps, diarrhea, fever, chills, tremors, and so on.

C

Caffeine
Calcifediol
Calcitonin-Salmon
Calcitriol
Calcium Pantothenate
Calcium Preparations
    Calcium Carbonate
    Calcium Chloride
    Calcium Glubionate
    Calcium Gluceptate
    Calcium Gluconate
    Calcium Lactate
    Dibasic Calcium Phosphate
     Dihydrate
Capreomycin Sulfate
Captopril
Carbachol
Carbamazepine
Carbamide Peroxide
Carbarsone
Carbenicillin Disodium
Carbenicillin Indanyl Sodium
Carbidopa Preparations
    Carbidopa
    Carbidopa/Levodopa
Carbinoxamine Maleate
Carbonic Anhydrase Inhibitors
    Acetazolamide

Dichlorphenamide
Methazolamide
Carboprost Tromethamine
Cardiac Glycosides
    Deslanoside
    Digitalis
    Digitalis Glycoside Mixture
    Digitoxin
    Digoxin
    Gitalin
Carisoprodol
Carmustine
Cascara Sagrada
Castor Oil
Cephalosporins and Related
     Antibiotics
    Cefaclor
    Cefadroxil
    Cefamandole Nafate
    Cefazolin Sodium
    Cefoperazone Sodium
    Cefotaxime Sodium
    Cefoxitin Sodium
    Ceftizoxime Sodium
    Cefuroxime Sodium
    Cephalexin
    Cephalothin Sodium
    Cephapirin Sodium

    Cephradine
    Moxalactam Disodium
Charcoal, Activated
Chenodiol
Chloral Derivatives
    Chloral Hydrate
    Triclofos Sodium
Chlorambucil
Chloramphenicol
Chlordiazepoxide
Chlorhexidine Gluconate
Chlormezanone
Chloroprocaine Hydrochloride
Chloroquine Hydrochloride
Chloroquine Phosphate
Chlorothiazide
Chlorotrianisene
Chlorphenesin Carbamate
Chlorpheniramine Maleate
Chlorpromazine Hydrochloride
Chlorpropamide
Chlorprothixene
Chlortetracycline
Chlorthalidone
Chlorzoxazone
Cholera Vaccine
Cholestyramine
Choline Salicylate

221

Chorionic Gonadotropin
Chromic Phosphate P 32
Ciclopirox Olamine
Cimetidine
Cinoxacin
Cisplatin
Citrate of Magnesia
Clemastine Fumarate
Clidinium Bromide
Clindamycin
Clocortolone Pivalate
Clofibrate
Clomiphene Citrate
Clonazepam
Clonidine Hydrochloride
Clorazepate Dipotassium
Clotrimazole
Cloxacillin Sodium
Cocaine
Codeine
Colchicine
Colestipol Hydrochloride
Colistimethate Sodium
Colistin Sulfate
Collagenase
Combined Estrogens, Aqueous
Conjugated Estrogens
Contraceptives, Oral
  Combination Products
  Progestin-Only Products
Corticosteroid Respiratory In-
  halants
    Beclomethasone Dipro-
      pionate
    Dexamethasone Sodium
      Phosphate
Corticosteroids, Intranasal
    Beclomethasone Dipro-
      pionate

Dexamethasone Sodium
  Phosphate
Flunisolide
Corticosteroids, Ophthalmic
  Ointments
  Solutions
  Suspensions
Corticosteroids, Topical
  Amcinonide
  Betamethasone
  Betamethasone Benzoate
  Betamethasone Dipropion-
    ate
  Betamethasone Valerate
  Clocortolone Pivalate
  Desonide
  Desoximetasone
  Dexamethasone
  Dexamethasone Sodium
    Phosphate
  Diflorasone Diacetate
  Flumethasone Pivalate
  Fluocinolone Acetonide
  Fluocinonide
  Flurandrenolide
  Halcinonide
  Hydrocortisone
  Hydrocortisone Acetate
  Hydrocortisone Valerate
  Methylprednisolone Ace-
    tate
  Prednisolone
  Triamcinolone Acetonide
  Anorectal Preparations
Corticotropin (ACTH) Prepara-
  tions

Corticotropin Injection
Corticotropin Zinc Hydrox-
  ide
Repository Corticotropin
  Injection
Cortisone Acetate
Cosyntropin
Coumarin and Indandione De-
  rivatives
  Dicumarol
  Phenprocoumon
  Warfarin Potassium
  Warfarin Sodium
Cromolyn Sodium
Crotamiton
Curare Preparations
  Metocurine Iodide
  Tubocurarine Chloride
Cyanocobalamin
Cyclacillin
Cyclandelate
Cyclizine
Cyclobenzaprine Hydrochlo-
  ride
Cyclomethycaine Sulfate
Cyclopentolate Hydrochloride
Cyclophosphamide
Cyclopropane
Cycloserine
Cyclosporine
Cyclothiazide
Cyproheptadine Hydrochloride
Cytarabine

Caffeine _Rx, otc_

tablets: 100 mg (_otc_)	NōDōz, Tirend, _Generic_
tablets: 200 mg (_otc_)	Vivarin
tablets: 65 mg caffeine, 65 mg citric acid (_otc_)	Citrated Caffeine
tablets: 150 mg caffeine, 300 mg dextrose (_otc_)	Quick Pep
capsules, timed release: 200 mg (_otc_)	Caffedrine, _Generic_
capsules, timed release: 250 mg (_otc_)	_Generic_
injection: 250 mg/ml (equal parts caffeine and sodium benzoate) (_Rx_)	Caffeine and Sodium Benzoate (_Generic_)

INDICATIONS

Oral: As an aid in staying awake and restoring mental alertness.

Parenteral: Has been used by IM injection as an analeptic in treatment of poisoning, as a stimulant in acute circulatory failure, and as a diuretic. IV injection of 500 mg has been recommended to alleviate headaches following spinal puncture. Has also been used for treatment of excited or comatose alcoholic patients. Not recommended as a respiratory stimulant.

ACTIONS

Stimulates the CNS at all levels including the cerebral cortex, medulla, and spinal cord. Other actions include cardiac stimulation, dilatation of coronary and peripheral blood vessels, constriction of cerebral blood vessels, skeletal muscle stimulation, augmented gastric secretion, and diuretic activity. Small decreases in heart rate may be produced by low concentrations of caffeine; higher concentrations may produce tachycardia or premature ventricular contractions. Caffeine is contained in coffee (100 mg/cup to 150 mg/cup brewed, 86 mg/cup to 99 mg/cup instant), tea (60 mg/cup to 75 mg/cup), and cola drinks (40 mg/12 oz to 60 mg/12 oz). Excessive use may lead to toxicity, which is manifested as an exaggeration of pharmacologic effects. Tolerance to the cardiovascular, CNS, and diuretic effects of caffeine may develop.

Caffeine is well absorbed following oral administration. It readily crosses the blood–brain barrier and is transported across the placenta. Biological half-life is about 3.5 hours in adults; in newborn and premature infants, it is between 4 and 6 days. Caffeine is metabolized in the liver; about 10% is excreted unchanged by the kidneys.

Sodium benzoate or citric acid increases the solubility of caffeine in aqueous solutions.

WARNINGS

Lower dosage or avoid use if other agents are being used to treat cardiovascular, psychological, or renal disorders. Consumption of large quantities of caffeine-containing products may reactivate preexisting duodenal ulcers. Safety for use in pregnancy and lactation is not established; pregnant women should avoid, or consume sparingly, caffeine-containing food and drugs. Excessive caffeine intake has been associated with increased fetal loss and premature delivery. Caffeine appears in the breast milk of nursing mothers.

PRECAUTIONS

Because too-vigorous treatment with parenteral caffeine can produce further depression in the already depressed patient, a single dose of caffeine and sodium benzoate should not exceed 1 g. High blood glucose levels may result from caffeine use.

DRUG INTERACTIONS

Oral contraceptives may impair elimination of caffeine.

ADVERSE REACTIONS

Nausea, vomiting, insomnia, restlessness, excitement, nervousness, tinnitus, scintillating scotoma, muscular tremor, tachycardia, extrasystoles, diuresis.

Large doses may produce symptoms mimicking anxiety neurosis (_e.g.,_ tremulousness, muscle twitching, sensory disturbances, irritability, flushing, tachypnea, palpitations, arrhythmias, GI disturbances, diuresis). Withdrawal from caffeine may produce headache, anxiety, muscle tension.

OVERDOSAGE

Convulsions may occur if caffeine is consumed in doses larger than 10 g. Induce emesis to empty stomach. Caffeine overdosage has been reported in newborns given a single dose of caffeine, 36 mg/kg to 94 mg/kg, at birth. Symptoms included hypertonicity alternating with hypotonicity, opisthotonic posturing, coarse tremors, bradycardia, hypotension, and severe acidosis. Intracranial hemorrhage has also been reported.

DOSAGE

Oral: 100 mg to 200 mg q4h, as needed. Not recommended for children.

Parenteral: Usual adult dose is 500 mg IM, with a dosage range of 200 mg to 500 mg. May be given IV in emergency situations. _Infants and children_—8 mg/kg. Maximum dose in any case is 500 mg. Dose may be repeated q4h if necessary.

NURSING IMPLICATIONS

PHYSICAL ASSESSMENT
When caffeine is used in treatment of poisoning or as stimulant in acute circulatory failure obtain blood pressure, pulse, and respirations; record presenting symptoms.

ADMINISTRATION
Parenteral form administered IM; IV route may be used in emergencies.

ONGOING ASSESSMENTS AND NURSING MANAGEMENT
When caffeine is administered in treatment of poisoning or as stimulant in acute circulatory failure, monitor blood pressure, pulse, and respirations q15m until condition is stabilized; record response to drug.

If caffeine is used as a diuretic, monitor intake and output; observe patient for adverse reactions. If side-effects occur, notify physician because dosage may need to be decreased or drug discontinued.

PATIENT INFORMATION
Do not exceed recommended dosage. Discontinue use if rapid pulse, dizziness, or palpitations occur.

If fatigue persists or recurs, consult physician.

Caffeine use is not intended as a substitute for normal sleep.

Use during pregnancy, lactation should be avoided.

Use only with physician approval if there is a history of heart disease or ulcer.

Read labels of carbonated beverages, foods; avoid consumption of products containing caffeine if use is restricted.

Calcifediol

See Vitamin D.

Calcitonin-Salmon Rx

injection: 200 MRC Calcimar
   units/ml*

INDICATIONS
Treatment of symptomatic Paget's disease (osteitis deformans) of bone; treatment of hypercalcemia.

* MRC = Medical Research Council; 1 MRC unit is equivalent to 1 international unit (IU).

Paget's disease: Effectiveness demonstrated principally in those with moderate to severe disease. Bone pain and biochemical abnormalities have been substantially improved.

Hypercalcemia: Early treatment of hypercalcemic emergencies, along with other appropriate agents, when a rapid decrease in serum calcium is required (until more specific treatment of the underlying disease can be accomplished). Calcitonin-salmon may also be added to existing therapeutic regimens for hypercalcemia such as IV fluids and furosemide, oral phosphate, or corticosteroids.

CONTRAINDICATIONS
Hypersensitivity to synthetic salmon calcitonin.

ACTIONS
A polypeptide hormone secreted by the parafollicular cells of the thyroid. Calcitonin acts primarily on the bone, but direct renal effects and actions on the GI tract are also seen.

Bone: Single injections cause a marked transient inhibition of bone resorption process. With prolonged use, there is a persistent, smaller decrease in rate of bone resorption. Endogenous calcitonin participates with parathyroid hormone in the homeostatic regulation of blood calcium. High blood calcium levels cause increased secretion of calcitonin, which in turn inhibits bone resorption. This reduces transfer of calcium from bone to blood and tends to return blood calcium to the normal level.

Paget's disease of bone: Paget's disease is a disorder characterized by abnormal and accelerated bone formation and resorption in one or more bones. Salmon calcitonin, presumably by an initial blocking effect on bone resorption, causes a decreased rate of bone turnover with a resultant fall in serum alkaline phosphatase and urinary hydroxyproline excretion in approximately two-thirds of patients treated. These biochemical changes appear to correspond to changes toward more normal bone, as evidenced by (1) radiologic regression of lesions, (2) improvement of impaired auditory-nerve and other neurologic function, and (3) decreases in abnormally elevated cardiac output. Circulating antibodies to calcitonin have been reported in about half of those with Paget's disease, but calcitonin treatment remained effective in many cases. Occasionally, patients with high antibody titers are found; they usually have suffered a biochemical relapse and are unresponsive to the acute hypocalcemic effects of calcitonin.

Hypercalcemia: Has been shown to lower elevated serum calcium in patients with carcinoma (with or without metastases), multiple myeloma, or primary hyperparathyroidism (lesser response). Patients with higher serum calcium levels tend to show greater reduction. Decrease in calcium occurs about 2 hours after injection and lasts 6 to 8 hours. Given q12h, drug maintains a calcium-lowering effect for 5 to 8 days.

Kidney: Increases the excretion of filtered phosphate, calcium, and sodium by decreasing their tubular reabsorption. In some, the inhibition of bone resorption is of such magnitude that the consequent reduction of filtered calcium load more than compensates for the decrease in tubular resorption of calcium. The result is a decrease rather than an increase in urinary calcium. Transient increases in sodium and water excretion may occur after the initial injection; in most, these changes return to pretreatment levels with continued therapy.

Gastrointestinal tract: Short-term administration results in marked transient decreases in the volume and acidity of gastric juice and in the volume and trypsin and amylase content of pancreatic juice.

WARNINGS

Use in pregnancy and lactation: Use only when clearly needed in women who are or may become pregnant. Safety for use in the nursing mother not established.

Use in children: There are no adequate data to support use in children.

PRECAUTIONS

Because calcitonin is a protein, the possibility of a systemic allergic reaction cannot be overlooked. Skin testing may be performed prior to use of drug, particularly for those with suspected sensitivity.

Periodic examinations of urine sediment of patients on chronic therapy are recommended.

ADVERSE REACTIONS

Nausea, with or without vomiting (10% of patients), which is most evident when treatment is initiated and tends to decrease or disappear with continued administration. Local inflammatory reactions at the site of subcutaneous or IM injection (10%); flushing of face or hands (2%–5%); occasionally skin rashes.

OVERDOSAGE

A dose of 1000 MRC units subcutaneously may produce nausea and vomiting as the only adverse effect. Doses of 32 units/kg/day for 1 or 2 days demonstrate no other adverse effects.

DOSAGE

Paget's disease: Recommended starting dose is 100 MRC units (0.5 ml) per day subcutaneously or IM. In many patients, doses of 50 MRC units (0.25 ml) per day or every other day are sufficient.

Hypercalcemia: Recommended starting dose is 4 MRC units/kg/12 hours by subcutaneous or IM in-

jection. If response is not satisfactory after 1 or 2 days, dose may be increased to 8 MRC units/kg/12 hours. If response still remains unsatisfactory after 2 more days, dose may be increased to 8 MRC units/kg/6 hours.

NURSING IMPLICATIONS

HISTORY
See Appendix 4.

PHYSICAL ASSESSMENT
Base on present signs and record findings. Baseline laboratory and diagnostic studies (*e.g.,* serum alkaline phosphatase, 24-hour urinary hydroxyproline, serum calcium, CBC, urinalysis, bone scan or other bone x-rays) will depend on cause of hypercalcemia.

ADMINISTRATION
Skin testing may be performed prior to treatment, particularly for patients with suspected sensitivity. *Procedure for skin testing*—Prepare a dilution at 10 MRC units/ml. Mix well and discard 0.9 ml; 0.1 ml (approximately 1 MRC unit) is injected intracutaneously on inner aspect of forearm. Observe site 15 minutes after injection. Appearance of more than mild erythema or wheal constitutes a positive response.

May be administered IM or subcutaneously. Subcutaneous route preferred for outpatient self-administration.

Allow vial to stand 20 to 30 minutes at room temperature to facilitate withdrawal.

If volume to be injected exceeds 2 ml, IM route is preferred; rotate injection sites and record site used.

Provision for parenteral calcium (p 227) administration should be available during first several doses. Check with physician for drug preferred.

The possibility of a systemic allergic reaction must be considered. Check with physician about steps to be taken and emergency drugs (*e.g.,* epinephrine, antihistamine) to be administered should an allergic reaction occur.

Storage: Keep refrigerated.

ONGOING ASSESSMENTS AND NURSING MANAGEMENT
During initial therapy observe patient for 1 to 2 hours after injection for signs of an allergic reaction (rash or urticaria, difficulty breathing, itching, fever) or evidence of hypocalcemia (twitching, carpopedal spasm, positive Chvostek's sign, Trousseau's sign, cardiac arrhythmias, tetany).

Observe for therapeutic drug response:

Paget's disease: Decrease in bone pain and tenderness over affected bones, which may take one or more months, and improvement in neurologic symptoms, which may require more than a year.

Hypercalcemia: Decrease in symptoms (Appendix 6, section 6-13).

NOTE: In some instances, symptoms may be vague and nonspecific.

Drug effects are monitored by periodic serum calcium and alkaline phosphatase determinations, 24-hour urinary hydroxyproline, and examination of urinary specimens for sediments.

If patient has a good response and later relapses, either clinically or biochemically, the possibility of antibody formation may be explored. Patient compliance with treatment modalities should also be assessed.

Test for high antibody titer: Patient fasts from midnight, serum calcium is determined, and 100 MRC units are given IM. Patient is then permitted to eat his usual breakfast; 3- and 6-hour postinjection serum calcium values are compared. A decrease of 0.5 mg/dl or more from fasting level at 3 and 6 hours is usually seen in the responsive patient. Decreases of 0.3 mg/dl or less constitute an inadequate response and further therapy will not be effective.

A moderately reduced calcium diet or avoidance of foods high in calcium may be prescribed. A list of foods high in calcium or a moderately reduced calcium diet is given to the patient.

Foods high in calcium include milk and milk products; some leafy and green vegetables (kale, mustard and turnip greens, broccoli); some cereals and breads.

PATIENT AND FAMILY INFORMATION

NOTE: Patient or family member will require instruction in techniques of subcutaneous drug administration.

In order to attain optimal results, it will be necessary to adhere to the dosage schedule and dietary regimen (if prescribed).

Avoid use of nonprescription preparations, especially multivitamin preparations and antacids, unless use has been approved by the physician, because some of these drugs contain calcium.

Read labels of all food products (if dietary restrictions are prescribed). If calcium is listed on the label, check with the physician about advisability of eating the food.

Although symptoms may be controlled, drug must be continued. Do not increase or decrease the dose or stop taking the medication unless directed to do so by the physician.

Rotate injection sites; keep a daily record of sites used.

NOTE: An outline of a standing figure may be given to patient to record injection sites.

Contact physician or nurse if tenderness, swelling, or redness persists at an injection site.

Calcitriol

See Vitamin D.

Calcium Carbonate

See Calcium Preparations; Antacids.

Calcium Chloride

See Calcium Preparations.

Calcium Glubionate

See Calcium Preparations.

Calcium Gluceptate

See Calcium Preparations.

Calcium Gluconate

See Calcium Preparations.

Calcium Lactate

See Calcium Preparations.

Calcium Pantothenate

See Vitamin B_5.

Calcium Preparations

Calcium Carbonate* otc

tablets: 650 mg (260 mg calcium)	Generic
tablets: 1.25 g (500 mg calcium)	Os-Cal 500
powder	Generic

* See also Antacids for other indications for calcium carbonate.

Calcium Chloride Rx

injection: 10% solu-   *Generic*
tion (272 mg cal-
cium)

Calcium Glubionate otc

syrup: 1.8 g/5 ml   Neo-Calglucon
(115 mg calcium)

Calcium Gluceptate Rx

injection: 1.1 g/5 ml   *Generic*
(90 mg calcium)

Calcium Gluconate otc (oral) Rx (parenteral)

tablets: 500 mg (45   *Generic*
mg calcium), 650
mg (58.5 mg cal-
cium), 1 g (90 mg
calcium)
powder   *Generic*
injection: 10% solu-   Kalcinate, *Generic*
tion (90 mg cal-
cium)

Calcium Lactate otc

tablets: 325 mg   *Generic*
(42.25 mg cal-
cium), 650 mg
(84.5 mg calcium)
powder   *Generic*

Dibasic Calcium Phosphate Dihydrate otc

tablets: 500 mg (115   *Generic*
mg calcium)
powder   *Generic*

INDICATIONS

Oral: Dietary supplement when calcium intake may be inadequate (*e.g.,* childhood and adolescence, pregnancy, lactation, postmenopause, and old age). Also, in treatment of calcium-deficiency states that may occur in diseases such as tetany of newborn (as a supplement to parenteral calcium); hypoparathyroidism, acute and chronic; pseudohypoparathyroidism; postmenopausal and senile osteoporosis; rickets and osteomalacia.

Parenteral: Treatment of hypocalcemia in conditions requiring prompt increase in plasma calcium levels (*e.g.,* neonatal tetany and tetany due to parathyroid deficiency, vitamin D deficiency, and alkalosis); prevention of hypocalcemia during exchange transfusions. Also used as adjunctive therapy in management of acute symptoms in lead colic. Calcium is used in cardiac resuscitation, particularly after open heart surgery, epinephrine fails to improve weak or ineffective myocardial contractions. Calcium chloride is used to combat the deleterious effects of hyperkalemia as measured by ECG, pending correction of increased potassium in the extracellular fluid.

CONTRAINDICATIONS

Oral calcium is contraindicated in patients with renal calculi. Parenteral calcium chloride is contraindicated in the presence of ventricular fibrillation during cardiac resuscitation and in those with the risk of existing digitalis toxicity.

DESCRIPTION

Calcium is the fifth most abundant element in the body; the major fraction is in bony structure. Calcium plays important physiological roles, many of which are poorly understood. It is essential for the functional integrity of the nervous and muscular systems, and for normal cardiac function, and is one of the factors involved in blood coagulation. Calcium may be given by the oral or parenteral route.

ACTIONS

Adequate calcium intake is particularly important during periods of bone growth in childhood and adolescence and during pregnancy and lactation. An adequate supply of calcium is considered necessary in adults, especially those over 40, to prevent a negative calcium balance, which may contribute to the development of osteoporosis. The different calcium salts contain varying amounts of calcium (Table 6).

PRECAUTIONS

Oral: Avoid use when calcium levels are excessively high or when conditions favor kidney stones. When calcium is administered in therapeutic amounts for prolonged periods, hypercalcemia and hypercalciuria may result. These are most likely to occur in patients with hypoparathyroidism receiving

Table 6. Calcium Contents of Different Calcium Salts

Calcium Salt	% Calcium	mEq Ca/g
Calcium carbonate	40.0	20.0
Calcium chloride	27.2	13.6
Calcium glubionate	6.5	3.3
Calcium gluceptate	9.0	4.5
Calcium gluconate	9.0	4.5
Calcium lactate	13.0	6.5
Dibasic calcium phosphate dihydrate	23.0	11.5

high doses of vitamin D, and can be avoided by frequent checks of plasma and urine calcium levels. Urine calcium levels may rise before a rise is seen in plasma calcium levels. The former may be checked by determining 24-hour calcium excretion or by the Sulkowitch test.

Parenteral: Calcium gluconate and calcium gluceptate may be administered either IM or IV; calcium chloride is administered only by the IV route.

DRUG INTERACTIONS

Oral: Certain dietary substances interfere with the absorption of calcium. These include **oxalic acid** (found in large quantities in rhubarb and spinach), **phytic acid** (found in bran, whole cereals), and **phosphorus** (found in milk and dairy products). Administration of **corticosteroids** may interfere with calcium absorption. Oral calcium compounds reduce serum levels of **oral tetracyclines;** the drugs should not be taken within 1 hour of each other. Because of the potential for antagonism of the beneficial effects of **verapamil,** calcium administration should be avoided or used with caution to avoid significant increases in calcium levels.

Parenteral: Because of its additive effect, administer calcium cautiously to a **digitalized** patient. Calcium salts should not generally be mixed with **carbonates, phosphates, sulfates,** or **tartrates** in parenteral admixtures.

ADVERSE REACTIONS

Oral: Gastrointestinal disturbances are rare. Symptoms of hypercalcemia (Appendix 6, section 6-13) may occur.

Parenteral: Following IM administration, mild local reactions may occur. Rapid IV administration may cause patient to complain of tingling sensations, a calcium taste, or "heat waves."

DOSAGE: ORAL PREPARATIONS

Recommended dietary allowances (RDAs): *Adults*—800 mg.

Dietary supplement: Usual daily dose is 500 mg to 2 g, 2 to 4 times/day.

DOSAGE: PARENTERAL PREPARATIONS
CALCIUM CHLORIDE

IV Only; administration is not to exceed 1 ml/minute. 10 ml is equivalent to 1 g and contains 272 mg calcium.

Hypocalcemic disorders: 500 mg to 1 g at intervals of 1 to 3 days, depending on response of patient and results of serum calcium determination. Several injections may be required because of rapid excretion of calcium.

Magnesium intoxication: 500 mg promptly. Observe for signs of recovery before additional doses are given.

Hyperkalemic ECG disturbances of cardiac function: Adjust dosage by constant monitoring of ECG changes during administration.

Cardiac resuscitation: 200 mg to 800 mg injected into the ventricular cavity or 500 mg to 1 g IV.

CALCIUM GLUCEPTATE

5 ml = 1.1 g and contains 90 mg calcium.

IM: 2 ml to 5 ml. Inject 5-ml doses into the gluteal region or, in infants, into the lateral thigh.

IV: 5 ml to 20 ml.

Exchange transfusions in newborns: 0.5 ml after every 100 ml of blood is exchanged.

CALCIUM GLUCONATE

IV infusion preferred; administer at rate not to exceed 0.5 ml/minute. IM use not recommended, especially in infants and children. 10 ml = 1 g and contains 90 mg calcium.

Adults: 0.5 g to 2 g (5 ml to 20 ml), as required. Dosage range is 1 g to 15 g daily.

Children: 500 mg/kg/day given in divided doses.

NURSING IMPLICATIONS

HISTORY
See Appendix 4.

PHYSICAL ASSESSMENT
When applicable, document presenting symptoms of hypocalcemia (Appendix 6, section 6-13).

ADMINISTRATION
IV

Warm solutions to body temperature.

If calcium chloride is administered for hyperkalemic ECG disturbances, patient must be on cardiac monitor during administration of drug because dosage is adjusted according to ECG response.

Place patient in a recumbent position.

Administration should not exceed the following:

0.5 ml/minute calcium gluconate
1 ml/minute calcium chloride
2 ml/minute calcium gluceptate

CLINICAL ALERT: Stop administration if patient complains of tingling sensations, heat waves, a metallic taste, or any other discomfort; administration may be resumed when symptoms disappear.

Calcium chloride should be administered only by IV. This drug is irritating to veins and must _not_ be injected into tissues because severe necrosis and sloughing may occur. Take care to avoid extravasation or accidental injection into perivascular tissue.

Keep patient recumbent for 5 to 10 minutes following administration. Depending on response, patient should remain in bed 30 to 60 minutes after administration.

IM

Calcium gluconate and calcium gluceptate may be administered IM; however, this route is usually used for very young patients in emergencies when technical difficulty makes IV injection impossible. Calcium gluconate IM is not recommended for infants and children.

Calcium gluceptate: Inject 5-ml doses into the gluteal region; for infants, use lateral thigh.

ONGOING ASSESSMENTS AND NURSING MANAGEMENT

Once symptoms of hypocalcemia are identified, patient should be protected against injury that may occur if hypocalcemic tetany develops. Pad siderails, have airway and suction immediately available, and remove any objects that may cause injury (_e.g.,_ over-the-bed stands).

IV

Observe patient q5m to q15m until condition is stabilized. Look for decrease in symptoms, which may have included muscle spasms, paresthesias, twitching, cardiac arrhythmias, laryngospasm, carpopedal spasm, positive Chvostek's sign, and muscle cramps.

Monitor blood pressure, pulse, and respirations q30m until condition stabilized.

If symptoms are not relieved or recur, notify physician immediately.

Frequent serum calcium determinations may be ordered until hypocalcemia is controlled.

If calcium is administered for hyperkalemic ECG disturbances of cardiac function, continue to monitor ECG. If periodic ECG tracings are done, label each tracing with date and time and insert on patient's chart.

IM

Mild local reactions may occur following administration. Notify physician if reaction is severe.

Oral

Certain dietary substances interfere with the absorption of calcium. Physician may prescribe diet restricting intake of foods containing high amounts of oxalic acid, phytic acid, and phosphorus.

PATIENT AND FAMILY INFORMATION (ORAL CALCIUM)

Notify physician or nurse if any of the following occurs: anorexia, nausea, vomiting, constipation, abdominal pain, dry mouth, thirst, polyuria (symptoms of hypercalcemia).

Follow prescribed dosage recommendations.

Capreomycin Sulfate Rx

powder for injection: Capastat Sulfate
  1 g/5-ml vial

INDICATIONS

Used concomitantly with other antituberculosis agents in pulmonary infections caused by capreomycin-susceptible strains of _Mycobacterium tuberculosis_ when primary agents (isoniazid, ethambutol, and streptomycin) have been ineffective or cannot be used because of toxicity or presence of resistant tubercle bacilli. Susceptibility studies should be performed to determine presence of capreomycin-susceptible strain of _M. tuberculosis._

CONTRAINDICATIONS

Hypersensitivity.

ACTIONS

A polypeptide antibiotic isolated from _Streptomyces capreolus._ Drug is not absorbed in significant quantities from GI tract and must be administered parenterally. Peak serum concentrations following IM administration achieved in 1 to 2 hours. Capreomycin is excreted essentially unaltered; 52% is excreted in urine within 12 hours.

Varying degrees of cross-resistance between capreomycin and kanamycin and neomycin have been reported. No cross-resistance has been observed between capreomycin and isoniazid, aminosalicylic acid, cycloserine, streptomycin, ethionamide, or ethambutol.

PRECAUTIONS

Audiometric measurements and assessment of vestibular function may be performed prior to initiation of therapy and at regular intervals during treatment. Regular tests of renal function should be made throughout treatment; reduced dosage is recommended for those with renal impairment. Renal injury with tubular necrosis, elevation of BUN, and abnormal sediment have been noted. Slight elevation of BUN may be seen in some patients receiving prolonged therapy; the appearance of casts, red cells, and white cells in the urine has been noted in a high percentage of these cases.

Elevation of BUN above 30 mg/100 ml, or any

other evidence of decreasing renal function with or without a rise in BUN levels, usually requires careful patient evaluation.

Hypokalemia may occur during therapy; serum potassium levels may be determined frequently.

WARNINGS

Use of capreomycin in patients with renal insufficiency or preexisting auditory impairment is undertaken with great caution. The risk of additional eighth-nerve impairment or renal injury is weighed against benefits derived from therapy. Because other antituberculosis agents also have similar and sometimes irreversible toxic effects, particularly on eighth-cranial-nerve and renal function, simultaneous administration of these agents with capreomycin is not recommended. Use with nonantituberculosis drugs (polymyxin, colistin sulfate, gentamicin, tobramycin, vancomycin, kanamycin, neomycin) having ototoxic or nephrotoxic potential is undertaken with great caution.

Safety for use during pregnancy and for use in infants and children not established.

ADVERSE REACTIONS

Nephrotoxic: Elevation of BUN and nonprotein nitrogen (NPN), a depression of phenolsulfonphthalein (PSP) excretion, and abnormal urine sediment have been observed.

Ototoxic: Subclinical auditory loss noted in approximately 11% of patients. Clinically apparent hearing loss has occurred in 3%. Some audiometric changes were reversible. Other cases with permanent loss were not progressive following withdrawal of drug. Tinnitus and vertigo have occurred.

Hepatic: Serial tests of hepatic function have demonstrated a decrease in Bromsulphalein (BSP) excretion without change in SGOT or SGPT in the presence of preexisting liver disease. Abnormal results in hepatic-function tests have occurred in many receiving capreomycin in combination with other antituberculosis agents also known to cause changes in hepatic function.

Hematologic: Leukocytosis and leukopenia have been observed. Pain, induration, and excessive bleeding at injection sites have been reported. Sterile abscesses have been noted.

Hypersensitivity: Urticaria and maculopapular skin rashes, associated in some cases with febrile reactions, have been reported when capreomycin and other antituberculosis drugs were given concomitantly.

DOSAGE

Administer in combination with at least one other antituberculosis agent to which patient's strain of

tubercle bacilli is susceptible. Usual dose is 1 g daily (not to exceed 20 mg/kg/day, given IM for 60 to 120 days, followed by 1 g two to three times weekly.

NOTE: Therapy for tuberculosis should be maintained for 18 to 24 months. If facilities for administering injectable medication are not available, a change to oral therapy is indicated upon patient's release from the hospital.

NURSING IMPLICATIONS

HISTORY
See Appendix 4.

PHYSICAL ASSESSMENT
Record general physical and emotional status, vital signs, weight. Baseline laboratory tests and diagnostic studies may include audiometric testing, renal- and hepatic-function tests, CBC, serum potassium.

ADMINISTRATION

Preparation of solution: Dissolve in 2 ml of 0.9% Sodium Chloride Injection or Sterile Water for Injection. Allow 2 or 3 minutes for complete solution. For administration of 1-g dose, entire contents of vial are given. For dosages less than 1 g, see Table 7.

Administer by deep IM injection into large muscle mass; superficial injections may be associated with increased pain and sterile abscesses. Rotate injection sites; record site used.

At initiation of therapy, develop a plan of rotation of injection sites because drug may be given over a long period of time.

If excessive bleeding at injection site occurs, apply prolonged pressure to area and report findings to physician.

Storage: After reconstitution, solutions may be stored for 48 hours at room temperature and up to 14 days under refrigeration. Solution may acquire a pale straw color and darken with time; this is not associated with loss of potency or development of toxicity.

Table 7. Dilutions for Capreomycin Doses Under 1 g

Concentration (Approximate)	Diluent Added to 1-g Vial	Volume of Capreomycin Sulfate Solution
350 mg/ml	2.15 ml	2.85 ml
300 mg/ml	2.63 ml	3.33 ml
250 mg/ml	3.3 ml	4.0 ml
200 mg/ml	4.3 ml	5.0 ml

ONGOING ASSESSMENT AND NURSING MANAGEMENT

Daily: Check vital signs; check previous injection sites for evidence of inflammation, induration, pain, formation of sterile abscess; monitor intake and output, especially during early therapy or if nephrotoxicity is suspected.

Observe for development of adverse reactions. Instruct patient to inform physician or nurse if tinnitus or vertigo occurs (early signs of ototoxicity). Development of these symptoms may require withdrawal of drug.

Assess for signs of hypokalemia (Appendix 6, section 6-15).

Report to physician if any change in intake–output ratio occurs or appearance of urine changes (cloudy, pink-tinged, concentrated, contains sediment).

Weigh weekly or as ordered.

Periodic laboratory and diagnostic tests are performed during therapy and may include sputum culture and sensitivity; audiometric evaluation; renal- and hepatic-function tests; CBC; urinalysis; serum potassium.

PATIENT AND FAMILY INFORMATION

Injections must be given on a scheduled basis for therapy to be effective. Appointments for injections must not be missed. If illness or other problem prevents keeping an appointment, contact the physician (or clinic).

Keep all appointments for laboratory and diagnostic studies because therapy must be monitored closely.

Report any hearing changes, dizziness, or problem with balance to physician or nurse immediately.

Report any symptoms or changes (*e.g.,* change in urine output, cloudy urine, muscle weakness or cramping, diarrhea, abdominal discomfort, sore throat) to physician or nurse promptly.

Captopril Rx

tablets: 25 mg, 50   Capoten
   mg, 100 mg

INDICATIONS

Hypertension: Because of potential for serious side-effects, drug is reserved for treatment of hypertensive patients who have developed unacceptable side-effects or have failed to respond satisfactorily to multidrug antihypertensive regimens. Although captopril is effective alone, it usually is used in combination with a thiazide-type diuretic because the blood-pressure-lowering effects of captopril and thiazides appear to be additive.

Heart failure: For those who have not responded adequately to, or cannot be controlled by, conventional diuretic and digitalis therapy. Used with diuretics and digitalis.

ACTIONS

Mechanism of action not fully elucidated. It appears to act as an antihypertensive and as an adjunct in therapy for heart failure primarily through suppression of the renin–angiotensin–aldosterone system.

Renin is synthesized by the kidneys and released into the circulation to produce angiotensin I, which is then converted by angiotensin-converting enzyme (ACE) to angiotensin II, a potent endogenous vasoconstrictor. Angiotension II also stimulates aldosterone secretion from the adrenal cortex, contributing to sodium and fluid retention. Captopril prevents conversion of angiotensin I to angiotensin II by inhibition of ACE.

Inhibition of ACE results in decreased plasma angiotensin II and increased plasma renin activity, the latter resulting from loss of negative feedback on renin release caused by reduction in angiotensin II. The reduction in angiotensin II leads to decreased aldosterone secretion and, as a result, to small increases in serum potassium.

After oral administration, rapid absorption occurs with peak blood levels in about 1 hour. The presence of food reduces absorption by 30% to 40%.

Administration results in reduction of peripheral arterial resistance in hypertensive patients and either no change or an increase in cardiac output. Renal blood flow increases, but glomerular filtration rate is usually unchanged. Decreased peripheral resistance, reduced pulmonary capillary wedge pressure, and increased cardiac output have been observed in patients with heart failure.

Blood-pressure reduction is often maximal 60 to 90 minutes after administration. Duration of effect appears to be dose related. Reduction in blood pressure may be progressive; several weeks of therapy may be required to achieve maximal therapeutic effects. Blood pressure is lowered to about the same extent in both standing and supine positions. Orthostatic effects and tachycardia are infrequent but may occur in volume-depleted patients. Abrupt withdrawal has not been associated with a rapid increase in blood pressure.

In those with heart failure, significant decreased peripheral resistance, reduced pulmonary capillary wedge pressure and pulmonary vascular resistance, increased cardiac output, and increased exercise tolerance time have been seen. These effects occur after the first dose and appear to persist for the duration of therapy.

WARNINGS

Proteinuria: Total urinary protein greater than 1 g/day has been seen in 1.2% patients; nephrotic syndrome has occurred in about one-fourth of these cases. Existence of prior renal disease increases the likelihood of development of proteinuria. Because most cases of proteinuria occur by the eighth month of therapy, patient should have urinary protein estimates at monthly intervals during the first 9 months of therapy and periodically thereafter.

Neutropenia/agranulocytosis: Neutropenia has been observed in about 0.3% of patients and appears 3 to 12 weeks after initiation of therapy. WBC counts are recommended every 2 weeks for the first three months of therapy and periodically thereafter.

Hypotension: Excessive hypotension is seen rarely but is a possible consequence in severely salt/volume-depleted persons, such as those treated vigorously with diuretics (*e.g.,* patients with severe congestive heart failure).

Use in pregnancy: Use only if potential benefit justifies the potential risk to the fetus.

Use in lactation: Exercise caution when administering to a nursing mother; interruption of nursing is recommended.

Use in children: Safety and efficacy in children not established. Use only if other measures have been ineffective.

Impaired renal function: Some patients, particularly those with severe renal artery stenosis, have developed increases in BUN and serum creatinine after reduction of blood pressure with captopril. Dosage reduction of captopril and discontinuation of diuretic may be required. For some, it may not be possible to normalize blood pressure and maintain adequate renal perfusion.

Surgery/anesthesia: In patients undergoing major surgery, or during anesthesia with agents that produce hypotension, captopril will block angiotensin II formation secondary to compensatory renin release. If hypotension occurs, it can be corrected by volume expansion.

DRUG INTERACTIONS

Hypotension: Concomitant administration of **diuretic therapy** occasionally causes precipitous reduction in blood pressure within 3 hours after administration of the initial dose of captopril. This is especially true in those recently begun on diuretic therapy and those on severe dietary salt restriction or dialysis. The possibility of hypotensive effects can be minimized by either discontinuing the diuretic or increasing salt intake approximately 1 week prior to

treatment with captopril or by supervising patient for at least 3 hours after the initial dose.

Agents causing renin release: **Other antihypertensive agents** that cause renin release will augment the effect of captopril.

Agents affecting sympathetic activity: **Ganglionic blocking agents** or **adrenergic neuron blocking agents** should be used with caution. **Beta-adrenergic blocking agents** add some further antihypertensive effect to captopril.

Agents increasing serum potassium: Elevation of serum potassium may occur. **Potassium-sparing diuretics** or **potassium supplements** are given only for documented hypokalemia. If patient has received **spironolactone** at any time up to several months prior to captopril therapy, serum potassium levels should be determined frequently because the effects of spironolactone persist.

Drug/lab tests: May cause false-positive test for **urine acetone.**

ADVERSE REACTIONS

Renal: Proteinuria (1%–2%). Renal insufficiency, renal failure, polyuria, oliguria, urinary frequency (0.1%–0.2%).

Hematologic: Neutropenia/agranulocytosis (0.3%).

Dermatologic: Rash (usually maculopapular, rarely urticarial), often with pruritus, and sometimes fever and eosinophilia occur in about 10% of patients, usually during first 4 weeks of therapy. Rash is usually mild and disappears with dosage reduction, treatment with antihistamines, or discontinuation of therapy. Remission may occur even if captopril is continued. Angioedema of the face, mucous membranes of the mouth, or extremities, which is reversible on discontinuation of therapy, has been seen in approximately 1% of patients.

Cardiovascular: Hypotension (2%). Tachycardia, chest pain, palpitations (approximately 1%). Angina pectoris, myocardial infarction, Raynaud's syndrome, congestive heart failure (0.2%–0.3%).

Dysgeusia: Approximately 7% have developed diminution or loss of taste perception. Taste impairment is reversible and usually self-limited, even with continued therapy (2–3 months). Weight loss may be associated with loss of taste.

Miscellaneous: The following have been reported in about 0.5% to 2% of patients: gastric irritation, abdominal pain, nausea, vomiting, diarrhea, anorexia, constipation, aphthous ulcers, peptic ulcer, dizziness, headache, malaise, fatigue, insomnia, dry mouth, dyspnea, paresthesias.

Altered lab findings: Elevation of liver enzymes (few patients) with no causal relationship established. A transient elevation of BUN and creatinine may occur, especially in those with volume depletion or renovascular hypertension. Rapid reduction of longstanding or severely elevated blood pressure may transiently decrease the glomerular filtration rate, resulting in rises in creatinine and BUN. Small increases in serum potassium frequently occur, especially in those with renal impairment.

OVERDOSAGE

Correction of hypotension is the primary concern. Volume expansion with an IV infusion of normal saline is treatment of choice to restore blood pressure. Captopril may be removed by hemodialysis.

DOSAGE

Initiation of therapy requires consideration of recent antihypertensive drug therapy, extent of blood-pressure elevation, salt restriction, and other clinical considerations. If possible, previous antihypertensive drug regimen is discontinued 1 week before captopril is started.

Initial therapy: 25 mg tid. If reduction of blood pressure is not achieved after 1 to 2 weeks, dose may be increased to 50 mg tid. If blood pressure is not satisfactorily controlled after another 1 to 2 weeks, a thiazide diuretic may be added. The diuretic dose may be increased at 1- to 2-week intervals. If further blood-pressure reduction is required, dose of captopril may be increased to 100 mg tid and then, if necessary, to 150 mg tid (while continuing the diuretic). *Maximum dose—450 mg/day.*

Malignant hypertension: For accelerated or malignant hypertension, when temporary discontinuation of current antihypertensive therapy is not practical or when prompt titration of blood pressure is indicated, current medication may be stopped and captopril initiated at 25 mg tid. Dose may be increased every 24 hours until satisfactory response is obtained or maximum dose is reached. Addition of a more potent diuretic (*e.g.,* furosemide) may also be indicated. Beta blockers may be used, but the effects are less than additive.

Heart failure: In patients with either normal or low blood pressure who have been treated with diuretics and who may be hyponatremic or hypovolemic, a starting dose of 6.25 mg or 12.5 mg tid may minimize the magnitude or duration of the hypotensive effect; titration to the usual daily dosage can then occur within several days. Usual daily dosage is 25 mg tid. After a dose of 50 mg tid is reached, further increases in dosage should be delayed, when possible, for at least 2 weeks to determine whether satisfactory response occurs. Most patients have a satisfactory improvement at 50 mg or 100 mg tid. *Maximum dose—450 mg/day.* Used in conjunction with a diuretic and digitalis.

Use in renal impairment: Excretion is reduced in those with impaired renal function. These patients will take longer to reach steady-state levels and will reach higher steady-state levels for a given daily dose. Therefore, these patients may respond to smaller or less frequent doses. With significant renal impairment, initial dosage should be reduced and smaller increments used for titration, which should be slow (1–2 week intervals). After desired therapeutic effect is achieved, dosage should be titrated back to the minimal effective dose. When diuretic therapy is required, a loop diuretic (*e.g.,* furosemide) is recommended in those with severe renal impairment.

NURSING IMPLICATIONS

HISTORY
See Appendix 4.

PHYSICAL ASSESSMENT
Take blood pressure both arms with patient in standing, sitting, and supine positions after he has rested for approximately 10 minutes; record pulse, respirations, weight. For those with heart failure, also include auscultation of lungs and examination of extremities for edema. Baseline laboratory tests may include serum potassium, CBC, urinalysis, renal-function tests.

ADMINISTRATION
Drug is administered 1 hour before meals.

Withhold dose and contact physician if blood pressure has significantly decreased or hypotension has occurred.

Obtain blood pressure and pulse prior to administration; record arm used and position of patient (standing, sitting, supine). During initial therapy, patient should be at rest for approximately 10 minutes before vital signs are obtained.

Hypertension: Current antihypertensive agents may be discontinued up to 1 week prior to initiation of therapy with captopril. Blood pressure should be monitored closely during this interval and physician contacted if rise in blood pressure occurs.

Initial dose in patient receiving concomitant diuretic therapy: Hypotension may occur. Monitor blood pressure, pulse for at least 3 hours following initial dose. If hypotension occurs, place patient in a supine position and contact physician immediately. An IV infusion of normal saline may be required. Further doses may be given without difficulty once blood pressure has increased after volume expansion.

Storage: Do not store above 30°C (86°F). Keep bottles tightly closed; protect from moisture.

ONGOING ASSESSMENTS AND NURSING MANAGEMENT

If significant decrease in blood pressure is noted, withhold next dose and notify physician.

If dizziness occurs, patient should be assisted with ambulation.

Weigh weekly or as ordered. If patient is on concomitant diuretic therapy, obtain weight daily.

Observe for adverse drug effects daily. Contact physician if aphthous ulcers, sore throat, fever, edema of hands or feet, arrhythmia, chest pains, or other adverse effects are noted.

Rash, often with pruritus, may occur during first 4 weeks of therapy. Inspect skin daily and contact physician if rash is noted; treatment with an antihistamine, reduction in dosage, or discontinuation of therapy may be necessary.

If anorexia occurs because of loss of taste perception, discuss problem with physician. Small, frequent meals may increase dietary intake.

Periodic renal-function tests, CBC, and serum potassium may be ordered (see *Warnings*). Notify physician before next dose is due if laboratory tests are abnormal.

Urine samples sent to the laboratory should indicate drug therapy, because captopril may cause a false-positive test for acetone.

Hypertension: Blood pressure reduction is often maximal 60 to 90 minutes after administration. During initial therapy or until optimal therapeutic effect is achieved, monitor blood pressure (on same arm and with patient in same position as for preadministration assessment) and pulse 60 to 90 minutes after drug is administered.

Physician may order blood pressure to be monitored at intervals other than before and after drug administration.

Heart failure: Obtain vital signs q4h. In addition, obtain blood pressure and pulse 60 to 90 minutes after drug is administered. If blood pressure is markedly decreased, contact physician. Examine extremities for edema; auscultate lungs. Other assessments, based on original symptoms of heart failure, may also be appropriate.

Concomitant therapy with a diuretic and digitalis is recommended. Be familiar with adverse reactions and nursing management for these drugs.

PATIENT AND FAMILY INFORMATION

NOTE: If drug is administered for hypertension, physician may wish patient or family member to monitor blood pressure and pulse; instruction in obtaining blood-pressure measurements and taking pulse will be necessary.

Take drug 1 hour before meals.

Do not interrupt or discontinue medication without consulting physician.

Notify physician or nurse if any of the following occurs: mouth sores, sore throat, fever, swelling of hands or feet, irregular heartbeat, chest pains.

Excessive perspiration, dehydration, vomiting, and diarrhea may lead to a fall in blood pressure; consult physician or nurse if any of these should occur.

May cause dizziness or fainting; avoid sudden changes in posture.

May also cause skin rash or impaired taste perception. Notify physician or nurse if these persist.

Avoid cough, cold, or allergy medications, except those approved by physician.

Carbachol

See Miotics, Direct Acting.

Carbamazepine Rx

tablets, chewable: 100 mg	Tegretol
tablets: 200 mg	Tegretol

INDICATIONS

Refractory seizure disorders: For the following conditions in patients not responding satisfactorily to other agents such as phenytoin, phenobarbital, or primidone:

Partial seizures with complex symptoms (psychomotor, temporal lobe)
Generalized tonic–clonic seizures (grand mal)
Mixed seizure patterns, including those mentioned, or other partial or generalized seizures

Not recommended as drug of choice in seizure disorders. It is reserved for those whose seizures are difficult to control and for patients experiencing marked side-effects (*e.g.,* excessive sedation). Absence seizures (petit mal) do not appear to be controlled by this drug.

Trigeminal neuralgia: Treatment of pain associated with true trigeminal neuralgia. Beneficial results also reported in glossopharyngeal neuralgia.

CONTRAINDICATIONS

Previous bone-marrow depression; hypersensitivity to carbamazepine; known sensitivity to any of the tricyclic antidepressants.

ACTIONS

Has demonstrated anticonvulsant properties with convulsions induced by electrical and chemical methods. Is chemically unrelated to other anticonvulsants or other agents used to control severe pain. Absorption from the GI tract is slow and fairly complete. Food appears to increase peak concentrations. The parent drug is 75% bound to plasma protein and the metabolite 50% bound. Carbamazepine concentrations are found in the brain and cerebrospinal fluid.

Monitoring blood levels has increased the efficacy and safety of anticonvulsants. Plasma levels are variable and may range from 0.5 mcg/ml to 25 mcg/ml with no apparent relationship to daily drug intake. Therapeutic plasma levels in the adult range should be between 4 mcg/ml and 12 mcg/ml. Drug is metabolized in the liver. Because carbamazepine may induce its own metabolism, the half-life is also variable. Initial half-life values have been reported to range from 25 to 65 hours, with 12 to 17 hours on repeated doses. The drug and its metabolites are excreted in the urine and feces.

WARNINGS

Serious and sometimes fatal blood cell abnormalities (aplastic anemia, agranulocytosis, thrombocytopenia, leukopenia) have been reported following treatment with carbamazepine. Early detection of hematologic change is important because, in some patients, aplastic anemia is reversible. Complete pretreatment blood counts are recommended; any significant abnormalities should rule out use of this drug. Hematologic retests are recommended every week during the first 3 months of therapy and monthly thereafter for at least 2 to 3 years. Discontinue drug if evidence of bone-marrow depression develops.

Drug is not used as simple analgesic for relief of trivial aches and pains.

Use in glaucoma: Has shown mild anticholinergic activity; closely observe patients with increased intraocular pressure.

CNS effects: Because of relationship to other tricyclic compounds, the possibility of activating latent psychosis, or confusion or agitation in elderly patients, should be kept in mind.

Potentially hazardous tasks: May produce drowsiness, dizziness, or blurred vision.

Use in pregnancy and lactation: Effects in human pregnancy and lactation unknown. Use only when the clinical situation warrants the risk.

PRECAUTIONS

Carbamazepine prescribed only after critical benefit-to-risk appraisal in patients with a history of cardiac, hepatic, or renal damage, history of adverse hematologic reactions to other drugs, or previously interrupted courses of therapy with the drug. Baseline hepatic-function evaluation and eye examination (including slit lamp, fundoscopy, tonometry) recommended.

DRUG INTERACTIONS

Use with **MAO inhibitors** not recommended. **Troleandomycin** and **erythromycin** have been reported to increase serum levels of carbamazepine, causing manifestations of toxicity. Breakthrough bleeding has been reported in women receiving concomitant **oral contraceptives,** whose reliability may be adversely affected. Carbamazepine increases **warfarin** metabolism, thus decreasing oral-anticoagulant half-life and activity. **Phenytoin, ethosuximide,** and **valproic acid** may be potentially affected in the same way during concomitant therapy. The simultaneous administration of **phenobarbital, phenytoin,** or **primidone,** or a combination, produces a marked lowering of serum levels of carbamazepine.

The half-life of **doxycycline** was significantly shortened when administered concurrently with carbamazepine.

Cimetidine may elevate serum carbamazepine levels.

Isoniazid and **propoxyphene** may inhibit the metabolism of carbamazepine, which may result in carbamazepine CNS toxicity. Conversely, carbamazepine may increase risk of isoniazid-induced hepatotoxicity.

ADVERSE REACTIONS

If adverse reactions are so severe that drug must be discontinued, abrupt discontinuation in a responsive patient may lead to seizures or even status epilepticus.

Most frequent: Dizziness, drowsiness, unsteadiness, nausea, vomiting. To minimize such reactions, therapy may be started at low doses.

Hematopoietic: Aplastic anemia, leukopenia, agranulocytosis, eosinophilia, leukocytosis, thrombocytopenia, purpura.

Hepatic: Abnormal hepatic function, cholestatic and hepatocellular jaundice.

GU: Urinary frequency, acute urinary retention, oliguria with hypertension, renal failure, azotemia, impotence, albuminuria, glycosuria, elevated BUN, microscopic deposits in urine.

CNS: Dizziness, drowsiness, disturbances of coordination, confusion, headache, fatigue, blurred vision, visual hallucinations, transient diplopia and oculomotor disturbances, speech disturbances, abnormal involuntary movements, peripheral neuritis and paresthesias, depression with agitation, nystagmus, tinnitus, hyperacusis. There have been reports of associated paralysis and other symptoms of cerebral arterial insufficiency.

Pulmonary: Hypersensitivity pneumonitis.

Dermatologic: Pruritic and erythematous rashes, urticaria, Stevens-Johnson syndrome, photosensitivity reactions, alterations in pigmentation, exfoliative dermatitis, alopecia, diaphoresis, erythema multiforme and nodosum, aggravation of lupus erythematosus. Discontinuation of therapy may be necessary in certain cases.

Digestive: Nausea, vomiting, gastric distress, diarrhea, constipation, anorexia, dryness of mouth or pharynx, glossitis and stomatitis.

Cardiovascular: Congestive heart failure, aggravation of hypertension, hypotension, syncope and collapse, edema, primary thrombophlebitis, recurrence of thrombophlebitis, aggravation of coronary artery disease, adenopathy or lymphadenopathy. Some cardiac complications have resulted in fatalities. Arrhythmias and AV block have been reported. Myocardial infarction has been associated with other tricyclics.

Ophthalmologic: Scattered, punctate cortical lens opacities; conjunctivitis.

Musculoskeletal: Aching joints and muscles, leg cramps.

Metabolic: Fever and chills, inappropriate antidiuretic hormone syndrome. Alterations in thyroid function have been reported in combination with other anticonvulsant medications. Thyroid-function tests have been reported to have decreased values.

OVERDOSAGE

Symptoms: Dizziness, ataxia, drowsiness, stupor, nausea, vomiting, restlessness, agitation, disorientation, tremor, involuntary movements, opisthotonos, abnormal reflexes (slowed or hyperactive), mydriasis, nystagmus, flushing, cyanosis, urinary retention. Encephalopathy has been associated with acute overdosage. Hypotension or hypertension may develop followed by coma. ECG may show dysrhythmias.

Treatment: There is no specific antidote. Induced emesis and gastric lavage are recommended. Monitor vital signs; administer symptomatic treatment. Parenteral barbiturates may be used to treat hyperirritability (do not use if MAO inhibitors have also been taken, either in overdosage or within 1 week). Barbiturates may induce respiratory depression, particularly in children; equipment for artificial ventilation and resuscitation should be available. Paraldehyde may be used in children to counteract muscular hypertonus without producing respiratory depression. Treat shock with supportive measures such as IV fluids, oxygen, and corticosteroids. Because of carbamazepine's relationship to tricyclic antidepressants, monitor ECG, particularly in children.

TREATMENT OF BLOOD COUNT ABNORMALITIES: If evidence of bone-marrow depression develops, the following is recommended: Discontinue drug; obtain daily CBC, platelet, and reticulocyte counts; perform bone-marrow aspiration and trephine biopsy immediately and repeat to monitor therapy.

DOSAGE

Epilepsy

Adults, Children over 12: *Initial*—200 mg bid first day; increase gradually by 200 mg/day, in divided doses at 6- to 8-hour intervals, until best response is obtained. Do not exceed 1000 mg/day in children 12 to 15 years or 1200 mg/day in patients over 15. Doses up to 1600 mg/day have been used in rare instances.

Maintenance: Adjust to minimum effective level; usually 800 mg/day to 1200 mg/day.

Children 6 to 12: Initial dose 100 mg bid first day. Increase gradually by 100 mg/day at 6- to 8-hour intervals until best response is obtained. Do not exceed 1000 mg/day. Adjust maintenance dose to minimum effective level; usually 400 mg/day to 800 mg/day.

Combination therapy: May be used alone or with other anticonvulsants. When added to existing therapy, carbamazepine is added gradually while other anticonvulsants are maintained or gradually decreased.

Trigeminal neuralgia

Initial dose: 100 mg bid first day. This may be increased by up to 200 mg/day, using increments of 100 mg q12h as needed, not to exceed 1200 mg/day.

Maintenance: Control of pain is usually maintained with 400 mg/day to 800 mg/day. Some may be maintained on 200 mg/day; others may require 1200 mg/day. Reduce dosage to minimal effective level or discontinue drug at least once every 3 months.

NURSING IMPLICATIONS

HISTORY
See Appendix 4.

PHYSICAL ASSESSMENT

Refractory seizure disorder: Obtain vital signs; if seizures are frequent, observe and enter accurate description in patient's chart. Prior to initial therapy, recommended laboratory tests include CBC, serum iron, reticulocyte and platelet counts, hepatic- and renal-function tests. Ophthalmologic examination and evaluation of the cardiovascular system may also be performed.

Trigeminal neuralgia: Obtain vital signs, general health status, weight. See above for recommended tests.

ADMINISTRATION
Administer drug with food or meals.

When chewable tablet is administered, instruct patient to chew tablet before swallowing.

Patient with trigeminal neuralgia may not tolerate hot, warm, or cold food or liquids; offer water or other liquid at room temperature when administering drug.

ONGOING ASSESSMENTS AND NURSING MANAGEMENT
Drowsiness, dizziness, or unsteadiness may occur. Assist patient with ambulation, especially early in therapy.

The possibility of activating latent psychosis, or confusion or agitation in the elderly, should be kept in mind. Any change in mental status should be brought to the attention of the physician. If an elderly patient becomes confused or agitated, notify physician immediately and take necessary steps to prevent injury (*e.g.*, falling) until patient can be seen by a physician.

Notify physician if any change in blood pressure or pulse rate or rhythm is noted.

Periodic eye examinations, renal- and hepatic-function tests, and evaluation of the hematopoietic system are ordered.

CLINICAL ALERT: Observe for signs and symptoms of hematologic, renal, and hepatic reactions. Notify the physician immediately if any of the following occurs: fever, chills, sore throat, sores in the mouth, malaise, fatigue, easy bruising, oliguria, cloudy or dark urine, swelling of the hands or feet, jaundice, pale stools.

Refractory seizure disorder: Record vital signs q4h; measure intake and output (during initial therapy); observe for adverse effects; assess patient response to drug. If seizures are frequent, observe q1h until therapeutic drug response is attained.

Accurate documentation of patient response assists the physician in adjusting dosage.

CLINICAL ALERT: Do *not* abruptly discontinue an anticonvulsant drug unless ordered to do so by the physician. Ensure continuity of prescribed therapy by notation on Kardex, informing health-team members responsible for drug administration. Abrupt discontinuation may lead to seizures and even status epilepticus.

Trigeminal neuralgia: Obtain vital signs; measure intake and output (during initial therapy); observe for adverse drug effects; assess patient's response to drug. When attacks of pain occur, record factors that may have triggered the attack, time of attack, whether pain of attack appears to be decreasing with medication.

The pain of trigeminal neuralgia is severe. A narcotic analgesic may be ordered until drug response is obtained.

Observe patient for signs of depression or suicidal tendencies.

PATIENT AND FAMILY INFORMATION
Do not discontinue use except on advice of a physician.

May produce drowsiness, dizziness, blurred vision; observe caution while driving or performing tasks requiring alertness.

Notify physician or nurse immediately if any of the following occurs: unusual bleeding or bruising, jaundice, abdominal pain, pale stools, darkened urine, impotence, CNS disturbances, swelling of hands or feet, fever, chills, sore throat, ulcers in the mouth.

May cause GI upset; take with food.

Close medical supervision is necessary during therapy with this drug. Keep all physician, clinic, and laboratory appointments.

Carbamide Peroxide (Urea Peroxide) otc

solution: 10% in anhydrous glycerol	Cankaid, Gly-Oxide Liquid, Periolav
gel: 11% in water-free gel base	Proxigel

INDICATIONS
Relief of minor inflammation of gums and other mucosal surfaces of the mouth and lips. Also helpful against canker and denture irritation, post-dental-procedure irritation, irritation related to inflamed gums, and as an aid to oral hygiene when normal cleansing measures are inadequate. Used for debridement and cleansing of accessible oral lesions.

ACTIONS
Releases oxygen on contact with mouth tissues to provide cleansing effects. Helps reduce inflammation, relieve pain, and inhibit odor-forming bacteria.

WARNINGS
Discontinue use and consult physician or dentist promptly if irritation persists or if inflammation, fever, and infection develop.

DOSAGE
Solution: Apply undiluted four times daily and at bedtime, or as directed. Place several drops on affected area and expectorate after 1 to 3 minutes, or place 10 drops on tongue, mix with saliva, swish for several minutes, and expectorate. Do not rinse. Solution foams on contact with saliva.

Gel: Do not dilute. Use four times daily or as directed. Gently massage onto affected area. Do not drink or rinse for 5 minutes after use.

NURSING IMPLICATIONS

PHYSICAL ASSESSMENT
Inspect oral cavity with tongue blade, flashlight. Record observations.

ADMINISTRATION
Patient may be able to self-administer. Give instructions for use (see *Dosage,* above). Supervise patient as required.

If patient is unable to self-administer drug, apply as directed (see above).

If possible, have patient rinse mouth with warm water prior to use of solution or gel.

Best given after meals and H.S.

Explain foaming effects of drug. Warn patient not to swallow solution.

ONGOING ASSESSMENTS AND NURSING MANAGEMENT
Inspect oral cavity daily or before each treatment. Notify physician if oral problem does not improve or becomes worse.

PATIENT AND FAMILY INFORMATION
Severe or persistent oral inflammation or denture irritation may be serious. If these or unexpected effects occur, consult physician or dentist promptly.

Discontinue use if fever develops or condition persists or becomes worse.

Do not use for more than 7 days.

Do not use in children under 3 years unless directed by physician or dentist.

Carbarsone Rx

capsules: 250 mg   Carbarsone Pulvules

INDICATIONS
Treatment of intestinal amebiasis without hepatic involvement. Effective against the trophozoite form of *Entamoeba histolytica* in the lumen and shallow ulcers of the colon.

CONTRAINDICATIONS
Not used as initial agent when amebic hepatitis of any degree may be present; in the presence of contracted visual or color fields; when patient is hypersensitive or intolerant to organic or inorganic arsenic given systemically or applied topically; or in cases of hepatic or renal disease.

ACTIONS
An organic arsenic derivative containing 28.5% arsenic, with amebicidal activity in intestinal amebiasis. Excretion via the kidneys is slow.

WARNINGS
Safety for use in pregnancy not established. Use only when clearly needed and when potential benefits outweigh the unknown potential hazards to the fetus. Safety for use in lactation not established.

Use in children: Carbarsone is one of the most innocuous of the organic arsenicals. However, skin rashes may occur, but these are usually mild. Nausea, vomiting, abdominal pain, and diarrhea may also occur.

PRECAUTIONS
Because drug is absorbed readily from GI tract and eliminated slowly by the kidneys, accumulation may result. If prolonged treatment is indicated or contemplated, it is mandatory that the recommended daily dose not be exceeded, a course of treatment should last no more than 10 days, and rest intervals of at least 10 days should be allowed before beginning another treatment. Discontinue drug immediately if there is any evidence of intolerance or toxicity.

ADVERSE REACTIONS
Sore throat, splenomegaly, icterus, pruritus, skin eruption, GI irritation, hepatitis, neuritis, visual disturbances. Fatalities have occurred from exfoliative dermatitis, liver necrosis, and hemorrhagic encephalitis.

OVERDOSAGE
Symptoms: Nausea, vomiting, abdominal pain, diarrhea, shock, coma, convulsions, ulcerations of mucous membranes and skin, and kidney and liver damage.

Treatment: Dimercaprol, 3 mg/kg to 4 mg/kg q6h for first 2 days and then bid for a total of 10 days. General management is symptomatic and supportive and may include gastric lavage, oxygen, IV fluids, and maintenance of body temperature. Unexplained fatalities have occurred with usual doses.

DOSAGE
Discontinue therapy immediately if signs of toxicity occur.

Adults: 250 mg bid or tid for 10 days. Give additional courses of treatment as indicated following a rest period of 10 to 14 days.

Children: Average daily dose is 75 mg/kg over 10 days, given in divided doses tid.

NURSING IMPLICATIONS

HISTORY

See Appendix 4. Local health department regulations may require investigation into recent travel to foreign countries. If patient has not traveled, further investigation of local travel, use of restaurants, water source, and so on may be necessary.

PHYSICAL ASSESSMENT

Obtain vital signs, weight, general physical status. Look for signs of dehydration (see Appendix 6, section 6-10). Record appearance and consistency of stools.

ADMINISTRATION

To administer to children: Divide contents of capsule and administer tid in food, jelly, or liquid (*e.g.,* ½ glass of milk or orange juice or small volume of sodium bicarbonate solution). Taste is not objectionable, but solutions will not be clear.

Dose for child will be approximate, because only one dose (250-mg capsule) is available.

Alternative to dividing contents of capsule: Calculate percentage of 250-mg dose patient is to receive; convert percentage to nearest fraction. Using a graduated container, add contents of capsule to a given amount of fluid. When drug is dissolved, pour off unneeded fluid and give the remainder. *Example*—Dose ordered is 66 mg, which is approximately 26% (or ¼) of 250 mg. Amount of fluid used is 8 oz; ¼ × 8 = 2 ounces. Pour out 6 oz and give 2 oz. The hospital pharmacist should also be consulted for other ways to prepare a divided dose.

Drug may be administered by retention enema if ulcers of colon are present. Dissolve dose ordered in amount and type of fluid ordered. Usually 50 ml or 100 ml of tap water or normal saline is used. Check in 20 to 30 minutes to be sure fluid has been retained. Physician may order cleansing enema prior to administration by retention enema.

ONGOING ASSESSMENTS AND NURSING MANAGEMENT

Record number, character, color of each stool; assess for signs of dehydration; measure intake and output; record vital signs q4h or as ordered. Daily stool specimens may be examined for amebic cysts.

If an enema is administered to obtain stool specimen, contact the laboratory for proper procedure. Usually only tap water or normal saline is used.

Isolation is usually not necessary. Follow hospital procedure for disposal of feces (stool precautions). Wash hands thoroughly after attending to patient following bowel movement, linen changes, anal care, obtainment of stool specimen.

Deliver all stool specimens to the laboratory immediately because specimen must be kept warm until examined.

Observe for signs of toxicity or intolerance: increase in severity of GI symptoms already present; nausea, vomiting, abdominal pain or cramps, or diarrhea not previously present; urinary symptoms; dermatitis or other skin lesions suggesting sensitivity to arsenic; any CNS changes; any signs or symptoms listed under *Adverse Reactions.* Notify physician if one or more of these occur because therapy may need to be discontinued.

Special diet (*e.g.,* low-residue, high-calorie) may be prescribed.

Examination of stool specimens from all household members may be necessary.

PATIENT AND FAMILY INFORMATION

Take drug exactly as prescribed; complete full course of therapy.

Notify physician or nurse if GI upset, skin lesions, visual disturbances, or sore throat occurs.

Stool specimens will be required at periodic intervals, usually 3 times after therapy is completed and monthly for 3 months (physician usually informs patient of number and times of specimen).

It is important to wash hands thoroughly after each bowel movement and when preparing or eating food. Thoroughly wash raw foods before eating them.

NOTE: Food handlers must not return to employment until course of treatment has been completed and all stool samples are negative.

Carbenicillin Disodium

See Penicillins.

Carbenicillin Indanyl Sodium

See Penicillins.

Carbidopa Preparations

Carbidopa Rx

tablets: 25 mg   Lodosyn*

* Lodosyn is available only to physicians upon request from the manufacturer for use in patients requiring individual titration of carbidopa and levodopa.

Carbidopa/Levodopa Rx

tablets: 10 mg carbidopa, 100 mg levodopa	Sinemet-10/100
tablets: 25 mg carbidopa, 100 mg levodopa	Sinemet-25/100
tablets: 25 mg carbidopa, 250 mg levodopa	Sinemet-25/250

INDICATIONS

Carbidopa is for use with levodopa in treatment of symptoms of idiopathic Parkinson's disease (paralysis agitans), postencephalitic parkinsonism, and symptomatic parkinsonism that may follow injury to the nervous system by carbon monoxide or manganese intoxication.

Is used to permit administration of lower doses of levodopa with reduced nausea and vomiting, more rapid dosage titration, and a somewhat smoother response. Patients with markedly irregular ("on–off") response to levodopa have not been shown to benefit from the addition of carbidopa.

Carbidopa is for use with carbidopa/levodopa combinations in those who do not have adequate reduction in nausea and vomiting when the combination provides under 70 mg/day of carbidopa; it is also for use with levodopa in the occasional patient whose dosage requirement of carbidopa and levodopa requires separate titration of each drug. Carbidopa has not been shown to enhance the intrinsic efficacy of levodopa in parkinsonian syndromes.

CONTRAINDICATIONS

Hypersensitivity to carbidopa or levodopa.

ACTIONS

Inhibits decarboxylation of peripheral levodopa. It does not cross the blood–brain barrier and does not affect metabolism of levodopa within the nervous system. Administration of carbidopa with levodopa makes more levodopa available for transport to the brain and reduces the amount of levodopa required by about 75% to 80%. When administered with levodopa, carbidopa increases both plasma levels and plasma half-life of levodopa and decreases plasma and urinary dopamine and homovanillic acid. Pyridoxine HCl (vitamin B_6) in oral doses of 10 mg to 25 mg may reverse the effects of levodopa. Carbidopa inhibits this action of pyridoxine HCl, and this vitamin may be given to those receiving carbidopa and levodopa concomitantly.

WARNINGS

Carbidopa has *no effect* when given alone; it is indicated for use only with levodopa. Levodopa must be discontinued at least 8 hours before concomitant therapy with carbidopa and levodopa is started. Because carbidopa permits more levodopa to reach the brain and more dopamine to be formed, dyskinesias may occur at lower doses and sooner with concomitant administration than with levodopa alone. Occurrence of dyskinesias may require dosage reduction.

Use in pregnancy and lactation: Use only when clearly needed and potential benefits outweigh the unknown potential hazards to the fetus.

ADVERSE REACTIONS

Carbidopa has not been demonstrated to have any pharmacodynamic actions in recommended doses. The only adverse reactions observed have been with concomitant use of carbidopa and levodopa. Levels of BUN, creatinine, and uric acid are lower during concomitant administration of carbidopa and levodopa than during administration of levodopa alone.

DOSAGE

Optimal daily dose must be determined by individual titration.

Patients not presently receiving levodopa: Dosage may be initiated with one tablet of 10 mg carbidopa/100 mg levodopa or 25 mg carbidopa/100 mg levodopa tid and increased by 1 tablet every day or every other day until a dosage of 6 tablets/day is reached. When nausea and vomiting occur on low daily dosages of 10 mg carbidopa/100 mg levodopa, 1 tablet of the 25 mg/100 mg product may be substituted for 1 tablet of the 10 mg/100 mg product. When it is evident that more levodopa is needed, 25 mg carbidopa/250 mg levodopa at a dosage of 1 tablet tid or qid may be given. If further titration is necessary, dosage with 25 mg carbidopa/250 mg levodopa may be increased by ½ or 1 tablet every day or every other day to a maximum of 8 tablets/day. Alternately, dosage may be titrated to 6 tablets of 25 mg carbidopa/250 mg levodopa/day and further adjusted with increments of levodopa or carbidopa.

Patients receiving levodopa: Levodopa is discontinued before combination is started. May be started with a morning dose after a night (8 hours) when patient has not received any levodopa. A daily dose is chosen that will provide approximately 25% of the previous daily levodopa dosage. Suggested starting dose is 1 tablet of 25 mg carbidopa/250 mg levodopa tid or qid. Adjustment is made as necessary by adding or omitting ½ or 1 tablet/day.

Patients receiving carbidopa/levodopa who require additional carbidopa: When patient is taking 10 mg carbidopa/100 mg levodopa, 25 mg of carbidopa may be given with the first dose each day. When patient is taking 25 mg carbidopa/250 mg levodopa, 25 mg carbidopa may be given with any dose as required for optimum therapeutic response.

Dosage adjustment: Dosage may be adjusted by adding or omitting ½ to 1 tablet/day. Because therapeutic and adverse responses occur more rapidly with combined therapy than with levodopa alone, monitor patient closely.

NOTE: Other standard antiparkinsonism agents may be continued while carbidopa and levodopa are administered; the dosage of such drugs may require adjustment. If general anesthesia is required, therapy may be continued as long as patient is allowed to take fluids and medication by mouth. When therapy is interrupted temporarily, usual daily dosage may be resumed as soon as patient is able to take oral medication.

NURSING IMPLICATIONS

HISTORY
See Appendix 4.

PHYSICAL ASSESSMENT
Look for neurologic alterations (*e.g.,* tremor [head, hands at rest], masklike facial expression, muscular rigidity with resistance to passive movement, shuffling gait, monotone speech, postural deformities, drooling). Evaluate mental status, thought process, ability to participate in activities of daily living. If patient is presently receiving an antiparkinsonism agent, symptoms may be diminished.

ADMINISTRATION
Administer with food or meals.

Carbidopa is *not given alone* but rather in combination with levodopa. Combination may be 2 separate tablets or both drugs in one tablet.

Early in therapy, titration of dosage may be necessary (*e.g.,* ½ or 1 tablet may be added to or omitted from one of the doses).

Patient may require assistance in removing medicine from dispensing container and holding water glass.

ONGOING ASSESSMENTS AND NURSING MANAGEMENT
Dosage adjustments, when necessary, are based on patient response. Assess neurologic deficits identified during physical assessment during titration period; record observations.

Dyskinesia (difficulty in movement) may occur sooner with combined therapy than with levodopa alone. Observe patient for difficulty in movement, especially during titration period. In some patients, blepharospasm may be a useful early sign of excess dosage. Contact physician if

dyskinesia, blepharospasm, or adverse reactions to **levodopa** occur.

See also Levodopa for additional assessments and nursing management.

PATIENT AND FAMILY INFORMATION
NOTE: Detailed explanation may be necessary, especially when addition or omission of a tablet from the dosage schedule is required. In some instances it may be necessary to have a responsible family member administer the medication until dosage is stabilized.

Frequent office or clinic appointments may be necessary during the dosage adjustment period.

Contact physician if difficulty in movement or twitching of the eyelids occurs.

See also Levodopa.

Carbinoxamine Maleate

See Antihistamines.

Carbonic Anhydrase Inhibitors

Acetazolamide *Rx*

tablets: 125 mg	Diamox
tablets: 250 mg	Ak-Zol, Dazamide, Diamox, *Generic*
capsules, sustained release: 500 mg	Diamox Sequels
injection: 500 mg/vial	Diamox

Dichlorphenamide *Rx*

tablets: 50 mg	Daranide

Methazolamide *Rx*

tablets: 50 mg	Neptazane

INDICATIONS
Adjunctive treatment of simple (open-angle) glaucoma and secondary glaucoma and used preoperatively in acute angle-closure glaucoma when delay of surgery is desired in order to lower intraocular pressure (IOP).

Tablet and parenteral forms of **acetazolamide** are also used for adjunctive treatment of edema due to congestive heart failure, drug-induced edema, and centrencephalic epilepsy (petit mal, unlocalized seizures).

Investigational uses: Acetazolamide 500 mg/day for prophylactic treatment of acute mountain sickness produced at high altitudes. It reduces renal bicarbonate reabsorption and causes metabolic acidosis; as a result, sleep hypoxia and symptoms of acute mountain sickness are decreased.

CONTRAINDICATIONS

Situations in which serum sodium or potassium levels are depressed; marked kidney or liver disease or dysfunction; hyperchloremic acidosis; electrolyte imbalance; adrenocortical insufficiency; known hypersensitivity to these drugs.

Long-term use is contraindicated in patients with chronic noncongestive angle-closure glaucoma because it may permit organic closure of the angle to occur while the worsening glaucoma is masked by lowered IOP. These agents are of doubtful use in glaucoma due to severe peripheral anterior synechiae or hemorrhagic glaucoma. Not used in patients with severe pulmonary obstruction who are unable to increase their ventilation because acidosis may be increased.

ACTIONS

Are nonbacteriostatic sulfonamides. They inhibit the action of the enzyme carbonic anhydrase. This action decreases the secretion of aqueous humor and results in a decrease in IOP. Carbonic anhydrase inhibitors cause some decrease in renal blood flow and glomerular filtration rate. The effect in the kidney results in increased excretion of sodium, potassium, bicarbonate, and water, producing alkaline diuresis. The effects of these drugs are summarized in Table 8.

WARNINGS

Not used during pregnancy, especially during first trimester, unless potential benefits outweigh the potential hazards.

PRECAUTIONS

Increase in dose does not increase diuresis and may cause drowsiness or paresthesia; it often results in a decrease in diuresis. Under certain circumstances, very large doses have been given in conjunction with other diuretics to promote diuresis in complete refractory failure.

Table 8. IOP Lowering Effects

Carbonic Anhydrase Inhibitor	Onset	Peak Effect	Duration
Acetazolamide			
Tablets	1–1½ hr	2–4 hr	8–12 hr
Sustained release	2 hr	8–12 hr	18–24 hr
IV injection	2 min	15 min	4–5 hr
Dichlorphenamide	Within 1 hr	2–4 hr	6–12 hr
Methazolamide	2–4 hr	6–8 hr	10–18 hr

Hypokalemia: Potassium excretion is increased; hypokalemia may develop with brisk diuresis, when severe cirrhosis is present, or during concomitant use of **steroids** or **ACTH.** Interference with oral electrolyte intake will also contribute to hypokalemia. Hypokalemia can sensitize or exaggerate response of the heart to the toxic effects of **digitalis** (*e.g.,* increased ventricular irritability). Hypokalemia may be avoided or treated by use of potassium supplements such as foods with high potassium content.

Use in impaired hepatic function: Hepatic coma could be precipitated in those with hepatic cirrhosis or insufficiency.

Electrolyte imbalance: Adequate and balanced electrolyte intake is essential in those whose clinical condition may cause electrolyte imbalance.

Use in respiratory acidosis: Use with caution.

Periodic blood counts are recommended to determine possibility of agranulocytosis or thrombocytopenia.

DRUG INTERACTIONS

Quinidine, a weak base, may have its half-life prolonged by concomitant administration of carbonic anhydrase inhibitors, which alkalinize the urine. Concomitant use with **corticosteroids** or **ACTH** will enhance potassium depletion. Carbonic anhydrase inhibitors may induce hypokalemia, which sensitizes the patient to **digitalis** toxicity.

ADVERSE REACTIONS

Adverse reactions common to all sulfonamide derivatives may occur. These include fever, rash, crystalluria, renal calculi, bone-marrow depression, thrombocytopenic purpura, hemolytic anemia, leukopenia, pancytopenia, and agranulocytosis. Precaution is advised for early detection of such reactions.

Short-term therapy: Side-effects are minimal and include paresthesias, particularly a tingling feeling in the extremities or at the mucocutaneous junction of the lips, mouth, or anus; some loss of appetite; polyuria; occasionally drowsiness and confusion.

Long-term therapy: An acidotic state may occasionally supervene, which can usually be corrected by administration of bicarbonate.

Occasional reactions

GI/GU: Melena, anorexia, nausea, vomiting, constipation, hematuria, glycosuria, hepatic insufficiency, urinary frequency, renal colic and calculi, pancreatitis.

CNS: Convulsions, weakness, fatigue, nervousness, sedation, lassitude, depression, dizziness, disorientation, ataxia, tremor, tinnitus, globus hystericus, headache, malaise, vertigo.

Dermatologic: Urticaria, pruritus, skin eruptions. Photosensitivity reactions may occur.

Miscellaneous: Flaccid paralysis, weight loss. Transient myopia also has been reported and subsides upon dose reduction or discontinuation of therapy. Cross-sensitivity between antibacterial sulfonamides and sulfonamide-derivative diuretics, including acetazolamide and various thiazides, has been reported.

DOSAGE

ACETAZOLAMIDE

Chronic simple (open-angle) glaucoma: 250 mg to 1 g/24 hours, usually in divided doses for amounts over 250 mg. Adjust dosage to symptoms and ocular tension. Dosage in excess of 1 g daily does not usually produce an increased effect.

Secondary glaucoma and preoperative treatment of some cases of acute congestive (closed-angle) glaucoma: 250 mg q4h or 250 mg bid in short-term therapy. In some acute cases, 500 mg followed by 125 mg or 250 mg q4h. IV therapy may be used for rapid relief of increased intraocular pressure in acute cases. A complementary effect is noted when drug is used in conjunction with miotics or mydriatics.

Congestive heart failure: For diuresis, starting dose is usually 250 mg to 375 mg (5 mg/kg) once daily in A.M. If, after an initial response, patient fails to lose edema fluid, dose is not increased but kidney is allowed to recover by having the patient skip medication for a day. Yields best diuretic results when given on alternate days or for 2 days alternating with a day of rest.

Drug-induced edema: Recommended dosage is 250 mg to 375 mg once daily for 1 to 2 days, alternating with a day of rest.

Epilepsy: Suggested total daily dose is 8 mg/kg to 30 mg/kg in divided doses. Although some patients respond to a low dose, the optimum range appears to be 375 mg/day to 1000 mg/day. When given in combination with other anticonvulsants, suggested starting dose is 250 mg once daily, in addition to existing medication.

Sustained release: May be used twice daily. Not recommended for use as an anticonvulsant.

Bioavailability: Bioequivalence problems have been documented for products marketed by different manufacturers. Brand interchange is not recommended unless comparative bioavailability data are consulted.

DICHLORPHENAMIDE

Most successful when given with miotics. In acute angle-closure glaucoma, may be used with miotics and osmotic agents in an attempt to reduce intraocular tension rapidly. Dosage is adjusted carefully to meet individual requirements. A priming dose of 100 mg to 200 mg is suggested for adults, followed by 100 mg q12h until desired response is obtained. Recommended maintenance dosage is 25 mg to 50 mg 1 to 3 times/day.

METHAZOLAMIDE

50 mg to 100 mg bid or tid. May be used concomitantly with miotic and osmotic agents.

NURSING IMPLICATIONS

HISTORY
See Appendix 4.

PHYSICAL ASSESSMENT

Chronic simple (open-angle) glaucoma: Assess general visual deficiency (*e.g.,* peripheral vision; visual acuity, especially in darkened room); review physician's admission notes for results of ophthalmic examination; obtain vital signs.

Acute closed-angle glaucoma: Same as above; check pupil of affected eye for dilation, response to light.

Edema due to congestive heart failure: Obtain vital signs, cardiac rate (apical–radial) and rhythm; auscultate lungs; note location and extent of edema; record weight.

Drug-induced edema: Note location and extent of edema; record weight.

Epilepsy: See Anticonvulsants.

ADMINISTRATION

If GI upset occurs, give drug with food.

Patient with glaucoma may have limited vision and may require assistance in removing medication from dispensing container.

Parenteral (acetazolamide): Reconstitute 500-mg vial with at least 5 ml of Sterile Water for Injection prior to use. Label container with date of reconstitution, amount of diluent used, and mg/ml.

Parenteral acetazolamide is given by direct IV. IM administration may be employed but is painful.

Storage: Reconstituted solutions retain potency for 1 week if refrigerated. Because product contains no preservative, use within 24 hours is strongly recommended.

ONGOING ASSESSMENTS AND NURSING MANAGEMENT

Observe daily for adverse reactions.

Adequate and balanced electrolyte intake is essential in all whose clinical condition may cause electrolyte imbalance. If dietary intake is poor, discuss problem with physician.

Observe for signs of electrolyte imbalance, especially hypokalemia (Appendix 6, section 6-15). Hypokalemia may be avoided or treated by use of potassium supplements or foods high in potassium.

If patient is receiving a cardiac glycoside (*e.g.,* digitalis, digoxin), hypokalemia can sensitize and exaggerate the response of the heart to the toxic effects of digitalis. Observe for development of arrhythmias; contact physician immediately if an arrhythmia is noted.

If patient is ambulatory and has reduced visual acuity, keep room dimly lit at night.

If drowsiness occurs or visual acuity is reduced, assist with ambulation.

Long-term therapy may result in an acidotic state with early signs of headache and lethargy. If uncorrected, this may progress to drowsiness, CNS depression, and Kussmaul's respirations. Anorexia, nausea, vomiting, and diarrhea (which may lead to dehydration) may also occur. Administration of sodium bicarbonate usually corrects problem.

Physician usually orders periodic CBCs to determine the possibility of agranulocytosis or thrombocytopenia.

Glaucoma: Monitor drug response (*i.e.,* relief of symptoms). In acute closed-angle glaucoma, check pupil of affected eye for dilation and response to light. Notify physician immediately if ocular pain increases or pain is not relieved.

Edema due to congestive heart failure or drugs: Weigh daily at same time each day with approximately same clothing; monitor intake and output; evaluate symptoms and compare with baseline data; obtain blood pressure, pulse (rate and rhythm), and respirations daily to q4h depending on patient's condition.

Epilepsy: See Anticonvulsants.

PATIENT AND FAMILY INFORMATION

If GI upset occurs, drug may be taken with food.

May cause drowsiness; observe caution while driving or performing other tasks requiring alertness.

Notify physician or nurse if sore throat, fever, unusual bleeding or bruising, tingling or tremors in the hands or feet, flank or loin pain, skin rash, fatigue, muscle weakness, or leg cramps occur.

Avoid exposure to ultraviolet light and prolonged exposure to sunlight. If prolonged exposure to sunlight is unavoidable, discuss problem with physician.

Epilepsy: See Anticonvulsants.

Carboprost Tromethamine Rx

injection: 250 mcg   Prostin/15 M
   carboprost, 83 mcg
   tromethamine/ml

INDICATIONS

For aborting pregnancy between the 13th and 20th weeks of gestation as calculated from the first day of the last regular menstrual period (LMP).

CONTRAINDICATIONS

Hypersensitivity; acute pelvic inflammatory disease; known active cardiac, pulmonary, renal, or hepatic disease.

ACTIONS

Stimulates myometrial contractions, similar to labor contractions at the end of a full term of pregnancy, in the gravid uterus. In most instances, the products of conception are evacuated from the uterus. Carboprost also stimulates smooth muscle of the GI tract. This activity may produce the vomiting and diarrhea that are common when drug is used to terminate pregnancy. Large doses can raise blood pressure, probably by contracting the vascular smooth muscle. Body-temperature elevation may be seen in some patients.

WARNINGS

Like other oxytocics, should be used only with strict adherence to recommended dosages and in a hospital providing immediate intensive care and acute surgical facilities.

Carboprost does not appear to affect the fetoplacental unit directly. A live birth may occur, particularly as gestational age approaches the end of the second trimester.

Any failed attempts at pregnancy termination with carboprost should be completed by some other means.

PRECAUTIONS

Carboprost-induced abortion may be expected to be incomplete in about 20% of cases. Although incidence of cervical trauma is small, the cervix is carefully examined immediately postabortion.

Use of carboprost is associated with transient pyrexia that may be due to hypothalamic thermoregulation.

Use cautiously in patients with history of asthma; hypotension or hypertension; cardiovascular, adrenal, or hepatic disease; anemia; jaundice; diabetes; or epilepsy. Also use cautiously in those with previously compromised (scarred) uteri.

ADVERSE REACTIONS

Adverse effects are generally transient and are reversible when therapy ends. Adverse effects observed during use for abortion (not all of which are clearly drug related), in decreasing order of frequency, include vomiting, diarrhea, nausea, flushing or hot flashes, chills or shivering, coughing, headache, endometritis, hiccups, dysmenorrhealike pain, paresthesia, backache, muscular pain, breast tenderness, eye pain, drowsiness, dystonia, asthma, injection-site pain, tinnitus, vertigo, vasovagal syndrome, dry mouth, hyperventilation, respiratory distress, hematemesis, taste alterations, urinary-tract infection, septic shock, torticollis, lethargy, hypertension, tachycardia, perforated uterus, endometritis from intrauterine contraceptive devices, nervousness, nosebleed, sleep disorders, dyspnea, tightness in chest, wheezing, posterior cervical perforation, weakness, diaphoresis, dizziness, blurred vision, epigastric pain, excessive thirst, twitching eyelids, gagging, retching, dry throat, choking sensation, thyroid storm, syncope, palpitations, rash, upper respiratory infection, leg cramps, anxiety, chest pain, retained placental fragments, shortness of breath, fullness of throat, uterine sacculation, faintness, lightheadedness, and uterine rupture. The most common complications requiring additional treatment after discharge from the hospital are endometritis, retained placental fragments, and excessive uterine bleeding, occurring in about 1 out of 50 patients.

DOSAGE

For IM use only. Administer initial dose of 250 mcg (1 ml) deep into the muscle with a tuberculin syringe. Subsequent doses of 250 mcg should be administered at 1½- to 3½-hour intervals depending on uterine response.

An optional test dose of 100 mcg (0.4 ml) may be administered initially. Dose may be increased to 500 mcg (2 ml) if uterine contractibility is judged to be inadequate after several doses of 250 mcg.

The total dose administered should not exceed 12 mg.

NURSING IMPLICATIONS

HISTORY
See Appendix 4.

PHYSICAL ASSESSMENT
Obtain vital signs, general mental and physical status; review physical examination performed by physician.

ADMINISTRATION

Physician may prescribe antiemetic and antidiarrheal drugs prior to administration of abortifacient.

Use tuberculin syringe; administer deep IM.

Rotate injection sites when more than 1 dose is required.

Storage: Refrigerate at 2°C to 4°C (36°F to 39°F).

ONGOING ASSESSMENTS AND NURSING MANAGEMENT

Patient should be given a complete explanation of the procedure and should be told that some adverse drug effects may be noted after abortifacient is administered.

Emotional support is necessary before, during, and after the procedure; most patients require reassurance and understanding.

Monitor uterine response (contractions) q½h to q1h or as ordered. Note and record onset of labor as well as time between contractions and intensity and duration of contractions.

Monitor blood pressure, pulse, and respirations q½h, temperature q4h or as ordered.

Notify physician if any of the following occurs: fever; increase or decrease in blood pressure or pulse; vaginal bleeding; cessation or decrease in intensity, duration, or frequency of contractions; nausea, vomiting, or diarrhea.

Fluids should be forced in patients with drug-induced fever.

Save all tissue expelled for physician to inspect and/or for laboratory identification of the fetus and placenta.

After products of conception are expelled, continue to monitor vital signs q1h to q2h and observe patient for evidence of continued bleeding. Contact physician immediately if further bleeding is apparent.

If drug fails to terminate pregnancy, other methods may be employed.

PATIENT INFORMATION

Contact physician if any of the following occurs: fever, vaginal bleeding (other than normal lochia), abdominal cramps or pain, passage of clots or pieces of tissue, foul-smelling lochia.

Discuss with physician when sexual activity, use of douches or tampons may be resumed (usually in 2 weeks).

Reexamination will be necessary (usually in 2–4 weeks).

NOTE: Following an abortion, depression may occur. Advise patient to discuss problem with her physician.

Cardiac Glycosides (Digitalis Glycosides)*

Deslanoside (Desacetyl-Lanatoside C) Rx

injection: 0.2 mg/ml   Cedilanid-D

Digitalis Rx

tablets: 100 mg	*Generic*
capsules: 100 mg	Digifortis Kapseals, Digitalis Pulvules

Digitalis Glycoside Mixture Rx

tablets: 1 unit	Digiglusin

Digitoxin Rx

tablets: 0.05 mg, 0.15 mg	Crystodigin
tablets: 0.1 mg	Crystodigin, Purodigin, *Generic*
tablets: 0.2 mg	Crystodigin, Purodigin, *Generic*
injection: 0.2 mg/ml	Crystodigin

Digoxin Rx

tablets: 0.125 mg, 0.5 mg	Lanoxin
tablets: 0.25 mg	Lanoxin, *Generic*
capsules: 0.05 mg, 0.1 mg, 0.2 mg	Lanoxicaps
elixir, pediatric: 0.05 mg/ml	Lanoxin
injection: 0.25 mg/ml	Lanoxin, *Generic*
injection, pediatric: 0.1 mg/ml	Lanoxin

Gitalin Rx

tablets: 0.5 mg	Gitaligin (contains tartrazine)

INDICATIONS

Congestive heart failure (CHF) (all degrees): Increased cardiac output results in diuresis and general amelioration of disturbances characteristic of right heart failure (venous congestion, edema) and left heart failure (dyspnea, orthopnea, cardiac asthma).

Atrial fibrillation: Especially indicated when ventricular rate is elevated. Rapidly reduces ventricular rates and eliminates the pulse deficit. Palpitation, precordial distress or weakness are relieved and concomitant congestive failure ameliorated.

Atrial flutter: Slows the heart; regular sinus rhythm may appear. Frequently, the flutter is converted to atrial fibrillation with a slow ventricular rate. Stopping therapy at this point may result in restoration of sinus rhythm, especially if the flutter was of paroxysmal type. It is preferable to continue therapy if failure ensues or atrial flutter is a frequent occurrence.

Paroxysmal atrial tachycardia: Oral therapy may be used, especially if the tachycardia is resistant to lesser measures. Depending on the urgency, a parenteral preparation may be preferred to initiate digitalization. Not indicated in sinus tachycardia or premature systoles in the absence of heart failure.

Cardiogenic shock: Value has not been established; however, cardiac glycosides may be employed when the condition is accompanied by pulmonary edema.

CONTRAINDICATIONS

Ventricular fibrillation; ventricular tachycardia, unless CHF supervenes after a protracted episode not due to these drugs; presence of toxic effects (see *Overdosage*) induced by any digitalis preparation. Allergy, although rare, does occur. It may not extend to all cardiac glycosides and another may be tried. Contraindicated in beriberi heart disease and some instances of hypersensitive carotid sinus syndrome.

ACTIONS

Direct effects include an increase in the force of myocardial contraction (positive inotropic effect), an increase in the refractory period of the atrioventricular (AV) node, and an increase in total peripheral resistance. These drugs also depress the sinoatrial (SA) node and prolong conduction to the AV node via vagal stimulation. The cellular basis for the inotropic effects is probably enhancement of excitation–contraction coupling, triggered by membrane depolarization. Most evidence relates this process to the entry of calcium ions into the cell during depolarization of the membrane and/or to the release of calcium from intracellular binding sites on the sarcoplasmic reticulum. The free calcium ion mediates the interaction of actin and myosin. At high doses, the glycosides enhance automaticity and may increase atrial or ventricular rate.

---

* The cardiac glycosides include glycoside mixtures (digitalis leaf and the refined glycoside mixtures gitalin and digitalis glycoside mixture) and digitoxin, derived from *Digitalis purpurea,* and deslanoside and digoxin, derived from *D. lanata.* Although these glycosides differ pharmacokinetically, they have qualitatively the same therapeutic effects on the heart.

Digitalis leaf, Digiglusin, and gitalin are glycoside mixtures that may elicit a variable response. Digitoxin is the major glycoside of digitalis leaf and digitalis glycoside mixtures (Digiglusin). Gitalin appears to have a more rapid onset of action and a shorter half-life than digitalis.

Absorption: Only digitoxin is highly lipid soluble and almost completely absorbed.

Distribution: Widely distributed in tissues; high concentrations are found in the myocardium, intestine, liver, and kidneys. Digitalis glycosides are bound to plasma albumin in varying degrees.

Elimination: Digitoxin is inactivated by hepatic degradation with the metabolites excreted by the kidney. The other cardiac glycosides are excreted by the kidneys. In patients with impaired renal function, significant accumulation may occur, except with digitoxin.

Glycoside serum levels: Serum digitoxin and digoxin levels are of limited value in establishing therapeutic serum levels but are valuable as an indicator of toxicity (Table 9).

WARNINGS

Obesity: Digitalis alone or with other drugs has been promoted for use in treatment of obesity. This use is unwarranted; potentially fatal arrhythmias and other adverse effects make use dangerous.

Digitalis toxicity: Many of the arrhythmias for which these drugs are prescribed closely resemble those reflecting digitalis intoxication. If the possibility of digitalis intoxication cannot be excluded, and if clinical situation permits, cardiac glycosides may be temporarily withheld.

The patient with CHF may complain of nausea and vomiting. Because these symptoms may also be associated with digitalis intoxication, a determination of their cause is necessary. When risk of digitalis intoxication is great, use of a short-acting, rapidly eliminated glycoside, such as digoxin, is recommended.

Cardiovascular disease: Electrical conversion of arrhythmias may require reduction of dosage. Exercise caution when giving one of these drugs to a patient still under influence of a previously administered cardiac glycoside. Exercise caution in the presence of multiple ventricular extrasystoles or heart block. Patients with incomplete AV block, especially those subject to Stokes-Adams attacks, may develop advanced or complete heart block if cardiac glycosides are given.

Patients with acute myocardial infarction, severe pulmonary disease, rheumatic carditis, or far advanced heart failure may be more sensitive to cardiac glycosides and more prone to disturbances of rhythm. If heart failure develops, digitalization may be tried with relatively low doses and cautiously increased until beneficial effects are obtained. Patients with chronic constrictive pericarditis may respond unfavorably to these drugs.

Idiopathic hypertrophic subaortic stenosis is managed with extreme care. These drugs are used only when absolutely necessary in those with Wolff-Parkinson-White syndrome because of the possibility of fatal ventricular arrhythmias.

Impaired renal function: Renal insufficiency delays excretion of all glycosides except digitoxin. Adjust dosage in patients with renal disease. Digitoxin may be given in usual doses. The presence of acute glomerulonephritis accompanied by CHF requires extreme care in digitalization; constant ECG monitoring is essential.

Impaired hepatic function: May necessitate reduction of dosage.

Use in pregnancy and lactation: Use only when clearly needed.

Use in children: Newborn infants display considerable variability in tolerance, depending on their degree of maturity. Premature and immature infants are particularly sensitive; dosage must be reduced and digitalization individualized. ECG monitoring may be necessary to avoid intoxication.

Use in elderly: Exercise special care in the elderly because body mass tends to be small and renal clearance is likely to be reduced.

PRECAUTIONS

Electrolyte balance: Hypokalemia sensitizes the myocardium to the cardiac glycosides and may alter the rate of onset and intensity of positive inotropic drug effects. Toxicity may develop, even with usual doses. It is desirable to maintain normal serum potassium levels. Potassium loss may result from diuretic or corticosteroid therapy, hemodialysis, or suction of gastrointestinal secretions. It may accompany malnutrition, diarrhea, prolonged vomiting, diarrhea, old age, or long-standing CHF. Rapid changes in serum potassium or other electrolytes should be avoided. IV calcium should not be given to patients receiving these drugs. Elevated serum calcium increases the effect of cardiac glycosides and may produce serious arrhythmias in digitalized patients.

Thyroid dysfunction: The plasma half-life of cardiac glycosides is inversely related to the functional status of the thyroid. In patients with myxedema, drug requirements are lower because excretion rate is decreased. In thyrotoxic patients with heart failure, larger doses may be necessary.

Atrial arrhythmias associated with hypermeta-

Table 9. Therapeutic and Toxic Serum Digitoxin and Digoxin Levels

Glycoside	Therapeutic Serum Level	Toxic Serum Level
Digitoxin	14–26 ng/ml	>35 ng/ml
Digoxin	0.5–2.0 ng/ml	>2.5 ng/ml

bolic states are resistant to these drugs and care must be taken to avoid toxicity.

Tartrazine sensitivity: Some of these products contain tartrazine. See Appendix 6, section 6-23.

DRUG INTERACTIONS

Microsomal enzymes that metabolize digitoxin in the liver are stimulated by a number of drugs such as **barbiturates, hydantoins, hypoglycemic agents, phenylbutazone, rifampin,** and others. Drugs that are microsomal enzyme inducers should not be used concomitantly.

Decreased GI absorption and enterohepatic recycling of digitoxin and digoxin may occur when taken with **cholestyramine** or **colestipol.**

Hypokalemia may increase the effects and toxicity of digitalis. This is most frequently seen in those receiving concomitant diuretic therapy. The most widely used and most effective diuretics (*i.e.,* **thiazides, furosemide**) increase urinary loss of potassium. Administering a potassium-sparing agent (amiloride, spironolactone, triamterene) with the potassium-wasting diuretic is a means of maintaining serum potassium levels. Potassium chloride may also be prescribed. In digitalized patients with severe or complete heart block, concurrent use of **potassium salts** is not recommended. **Mineralocorticoids** (*e.g.,* prednisone) and, rarely, certain **antibiotics** (*e.g.,* amphotericin B) may cause increased potassium excretion.

Spironolactone may increase or decrease the toxic effects of digitalis.

Serum digoxin levels are two to three times higher in digitalized patients receiving **quinidine. Quinine** may have an effect similar to that of quinidine.

The effects of the cardiac glycosides may be additive with those of **quinidine, procainamide,** or **beta-adrenergic blocking agents.**

Administration of **thyroid hormones** or **thioamines** (methimazole, propylthiouracil) would likely change a stabilized, digitalized patient's dose of glycoside. (See *Precautions.*)

The glycosides are synergistic with **parenteral calcium salts, rauwolfia alkaloids, ephedrine, epinephrine,** and possibly other **adrenergic agents.** Pharmacologic toxicity may be increased with concomitant use of **succinylcholine.**

Decreased therapeutic effect, probably due to inhibition of absorption, may occur with concurrent use of **antacids** (aluminum or magnesium salts) and **kaolin-pectin** antidiarrheal suspensions, **oral aminoglycosides, aminosalicylic acid,** and **sulfasalazine. Metoclopramide** may decrease absorption of slowly dissolving digoxin preparations. **Combination chemotherapy** regimens have decreased digoxin absorp-

tion (bleomycin, cyclophosphamide, cytarabine, doxorubicin, procarbazine, *Vinca* alkaloids).

Exercise caution when administering **insulin** concurrently with cardiac glycosides.

Drugs shown to increase serum digoxin levels are **anticholinergic agents; erythromycin** and **tetracycline** in a small number of patients susceptible to their changes in bowel flora; **hydroxychloroquine; verapamil** and **nifedipine.**

Serum digoxin levels may be decreased by **penicillamine.**

ADVERSE REACTIONS

Because of the cumulative effect of cardiac glycosides, adverse reactions may ultimately develop in response to chronic use of doses that were initially well tolerated (see *Digitalis Toxicity*). When toxicity occurs, symptoms are typically those resulting from overdosage. Anorexia, nausea, and vomiting have been reported. These effects are central in origin, but following large oral doses there is also a local emetic action. Abdominal discomfort or pain and diarrhea may also occur. Gynecomastia, skin rash, and eosinophilia can occur. Rarely, allergy may occur.

DIGITALIS TOXICITY

GI: Most common early symptoms are anorexia, salivation, nausea, vomiting, and diarrhea. Abdominal discomfort or pain often accompanies GI symptoms.

CNS: Headache, weakness, apathy, drowsiness, visual disturbances (blurred, yellow, or green vision, halo effect). Mental depression may be an early symptom; confusion, disorientation, seizures, EEG abnormalities, and delirium may also be seen with more severe intoxication. Aphasia, hallucinations, psychosis, bad dreams, and neurologic pain stimulating trigeminal neuralgia, possibly with paresthesias, may occur.

Muscular: Weakness.

Cardiac disturbances: Major cardiac effects include either an enhancement of automaticity, a depression of conductivity, or a combination of these. Unifocal or multiform premature ventricular contractions (PVCs), especially in bigeminal or trigeminal patterns, are the most common toxic arrhythmias. Paroxysmal and nonparoxysmal nodal rhythms, AV dissociation, accelerated junctional (nodal) rhythm, paroxysmal atrial tachycardia with block, and coupled beat are most common. Excessive slowing of the pulse is a clinical sign of overdosage. AV block of increasing degree may proceed to complete heart block. Ventricular fibrillation is the most common cause of death from digitalis poisoning. The ECG is fundamental in determining presence and nature of these arrhythmias.

Children: Vomiting, diarrhea, neurologic and visual disturbances are rarely seen as initial signs of toxicity; cardiac arrhythmias are more frequent and reliable signs of toxicity. Common manifestations of digitalis toxicity include atrial arrhythmias (atrial ectopic rhythms and paroxysmal atrial tachycardia with AV block). Ventricular arrhythmias (premature ventricular systoles) are rarely seen.

TREATMENT OF TOXICITY

Adults: Discontinue drug until all signs of toxicity are abolished. This may be all that is necessary if manifestations are not severe and appear after peak effect of drug. Potassium salts may be used if renal function is adequate. When correction of arrhythmia is urgent and serum potassium level is low to normal, IV potassium (40 mEq to 100 mEq at a rate of 20 mEq/hour to 40 mEq/hour) may be given. Additional amounts may be given if arrhythmia is uncontrolled and potassium is well tolerated. ECG monitoring (_i.e.,_ for peaking T waves) is indicated to avoid potassium toxicity and to observe effect on the arrhythmia so that infusion may be stopped when desired effect is achieved. Potassium should not be used when severe or complete heart block is due to digitalis and not related to tachycardia.

Severe sinus bradycardia or a slow ventricular rate due to secondary AV block may be symptomatically treated with atropine 0.01 mg/kg IV. Insertion of a transvenous pacemaker may be necessary.

For atrial and ventricular arrhythmias that are unresponsive to potassium, phenytoin 0.5 mg/kg IV may be given at a rate not exceeding 50 mg/minute, at 1- to 2-hour intervals; the maximum dose should not exceed 10 mg/kg/24 hours. Alternately, lidocaine, 1 mg/kg IV over 5 minutes, followed by an infusion of 15 mcg/kg/minute to 50 mcg/kg/minute to maintain normal cardiac rhythm, may be used.

Cholestyramine, colestipol, or activated charcoal may be useful.

Fab (fragments, antigen-binding): A new and investigational treatment of digitalis intoxication is a specific, antigen-binding globulin fragment (Fab). Given in approximate equimolar quantities as the digitalis, it has rapidly and completely reversed all signs and symptoms and has led to total recovery in 80% of patients.

Children: Potassium preparations may be given orally in divided doses totaling 1 mEq/kg to 1.5 mEq/kg. When correction of arrhythmia is urgent, approximately 0.5 mEq/kg/hour of potassium may be given, with careful ECG monitoring, as a solution of 20 mEq or less per 500 ml. Total dose should not exceed 2 mEq/kg.

ADMINISTRATION

Loading doses: Large loading doses, administered initially, rapidly establish effective plasma levels; small daily doses are then given to replace daily losses due to metabolism and excretion. Loading doses are recommended with digitalis leaf and digitoxin because of the prolonged time necessary to achieve steady-state blood levels and clinical response. Without a loading dose, slow digitalization with digoxin may be achieved in 1 week. For a rapid effect in acutely ill patients, parenteral administration of digitoxin, deslanoside, or digoxin can be used. Use parenterally only when drug cannot be taken orally or rapid digitalization is urgent. Full loading doses should not be used in those who have taken a cardiac glycoside during the preceding 3 weeks; dosages are reduced for partially digitalized patients.

Maintenance therapy: Determined by amount necessary to sustain the desired therapeutic effect. Recommended dosages are average figures that may require modification. Diminished renal function is the most important factor requiring modification of recommended doses.

DOSAGE

DESLANOSIDE
When given IV, onset of action occurs in 10 to 30 minutes; peak effect is seen in 2 to 3 hours.

Loading dose: Rapid results are obtained in 12 hours by giving 1.6 mg IM or IV. _IV_—May be given as one injection or in portions of 0.8 mg each. _IM_—Inject 0.8-mg (4-ml) portions at each of two sites.

Maintenance: May be accomplished by starting administration of an oral preparation within 12 hours.

DIGITALIS
Loading dose: If patient has not received a long-acting cardiac glycoside within the previous 3 weeks or digoxin within the previous week, digitalization is carried out with a total average dose of 1.2 g in several equal parts, administered q6h.

Maintenance: Average dose is 100 mg/day to 200 mg/day. Individual requirements may vary widely, ranging from 30 mg/day to 400 mg/day. Determination of optimum daily dose depends on close and careful observations of patient, whose need for digitalis may vary from time to time.

DIGITALIS GLYCOSIDE MIXTURE
1 unit is equal to 1 USP unit.

Loading dose: For rapid digitalization, 6 units

initially, followed by 4 units 4 to 6 hours later and 2 units q4h to q6h thereafter until full therapeutic effect is obtained. *Slow*—In adult who has not received a cardiac glycoside during the preceding 3 weeks, 2 units, bid, for 4 days.

Maintenance: Ranges from 0.5 units/day to 3 units/day.

DIGITOXIN

Parenteral loading dose: Average digitalizing dose by IV route is 1.2 mg to 1.6 mg. Digitalization may be accomplished by slow IV injection of an initial dose of 0.6 mg followed by 0.4 mg 4 to 6 hours later and 0.2 mg q4h to q6h thereafter until full therapeutic effect is apparent (8–12 hours). Administration of the average digitalization dose in a single injection is not recommended. Patients with extensive myocardial damage or conduction defects may require smaller doses.

Oral loading dose: *Rapid*—0.6 mg initially, followed by 0.4 mg, then 0.2 mg q4h to q6h. *Slow*—0.2 mg bid for 4 days, followed by maintenance dose.

Maintenance: Dose ranges from 0.05 mg/day to 0.3 mg/day, with the most common dose being 0.15 mg/day. Larger or smaller doses may be required in some cases. Elderly patients with coronary artery disease may require less medication.

Children

Loading dose: Must be individualized. IV doses are given slowly, with continuous ECG monitoring. Generally, premature and immature infants are particularly sensitive and require reduced dosage, which must be determined by careful adjustment. Normal newborn infants, from birth to 1 month, require adult proportions by body weight. Infants 1 month to 2 years require approximately 50% more, by body weight, than adult proportions. Total dose should be divided into three, four, or more proportions, with 6 hours or more between doses. The following digitalizing doses are recommended:

Premature and newborn and in reduced renal function or myocarditis—0.022 mg/kg (0.3 mg/m^2–0.35 mg/m^2)
Under 1 year—0.045 mg/kg
1 to 2 years—0.04 mg/kg
Over 2 years—0.03 mg/kg (0.75 mg/m^2)

Maintenance dose: Patient should be given one-tenth of the digitalizing dose.

DIGOXIN

The IV dose is 20% to 30% less than the oral dose. The onset of action is 5 to 30 minutes IV and 30 to 120 minutes PO.

Lanoxicaps (gelatin capsules) have greater bioavailability than standard tablets. The 0.2-mg cap-

sule is equivalent to an 0.25-mg tablet, the 0.1-mg capsule is equivalent to an 0.125-mg tablet, and the 0.05-mg capsule is equivalent to an 0.0625-mg tablet.

Bioequivalence: Bioavailability differences have been documented. Current requirements for FDA-approved products should minimize problems; however, patients being changed from one product to another should be monitored for any changes in clinical response.

Adults

Rapid digitalization with a loading dose: Peak body digoxin stores of 8 mcg/kg to 12 mcg/kg should provide therapeutic effect; larger stores (10 mcg/kg–15 mcg/kg) are often required for control of ventricular rate in those with atrial flutter or fibrillation. In renal insufficiency, projected peak body stores are lower (*i.e.*, 6 mcg/kg to 10 mcg/kg). Loading dose is based on projected peak body stores and given in several portions, with roughly half the total given as the first dose and additional fractions at 4- to 8-hour intervals IV or PO, with careful assessment of clinical response before each additional dose.

In undigitalized patients, a single IV dose of 400 mcg to 600 mcg (0.4 mg to 0.6 mg) usually produces a detectable effect in 5 to 30 minutes, becoming maximal in 1 to 4 hours. The usual parenteral amount for a 70-kg patient to achieve peak body stores of 8 mcg/kg to 15 mcg/kg is 600 mcg to 1000 mcg (0.6 mg to 1 mg). A single initial oral dose of 500 mcg to 750 mcg (0.5 mg to 0.75 mg) usually produces a detectable effect in ½ to 2 hours, becoming maximal in 2 to 6 hours. Usual oral amount for a 70-kg patient to achieve peak body stores of 8 mcg/kg to 15 mcg/kg is 750 mcg to 1250 mcg (0.75 mg to 1.25 mg).

Maintenance dose: Based on the percentage of the peak body stores lost each day through elimination. The following formula may be used:

Maintenance dose

$$= \text{Peak body stores (i.e., loading dose)}$$
$$\times \frac{\% \text{ Daily loss}}{100} \text{ (i.e., } 14 + \text{Ccr/5)}$$

CCr is creatinine clearance, converted to 70 kg body weight or 1.73 m^2 body surface area.

GRADUAL DIGITALIZATION WITH A MAINTENANCE DOSE: Based on body weight and creatinine clearance (Ccr) to maintain peak body stores of 10 mcg/kg.

Infants and children

Divided daily dosing is recommended for infants and children under 10 years. Children over 10 require adult dosing in proportion to their body weight.

Table 10. Normal Digitalizing and Maintenance Dosages of Digoxin for Infants and Children With Normal Renal Function, Based on Lean Body Weight

Age	Digitalizing Dose*† (mcg/kg)		Daily Maintenance Dose
	Oral	IV	
Premature	20–30	15–25	20%–30% of the loading dose
Full term	25–35	20–30	
1–24 months	35–60	30–50	25%–35% of the loading dose
2–5 years	30–40	25–35	
5–10 years	20–35	15–30	
Over 10 years	10–15	8–12	

* IV digitalizing doses are 80% of oral digitalizing doses.

† Projected or actual digitalizing dose providing desired clinical response.

Rapid digitalization with a loading dose: Loading dose is given in several portions, with roughly half the total given as the first dose and additional fractions of the total dose at 6- to 8-hour intervals (PO) or 4- to 8-hour intervals (parenteral). See Table 10.

Elderly patients with impaired renal function
Daily dose based on creatinine clearance.

GITALIN

Loading dose: *Rapid*—Initially 2.5 mg, followed by 0.75 mg q6h until therapeutic effect or toxicity develops. Most patients respond to a total dose of approximately 6 mg. Digitalization is usually complete within 24 hours. *Slow*—A single daily dose of 1.5 mg for 4 to 6 days.

Maintenance: 0.5 mg, preferably administered in the morning. Dosage may be as low as 0.?5 mg or as high as 1.25 mg/day.

NURSING IMPLICATIONS

HISTORY

See Appendix 4. If patient has taken a cardiac glycoside with in the past 3 weeks, inform physician because a reduction in dosage may be necessary.

PHYSICAL ASSESSMENT

Obtain blood pressure, pulse (obtain apical–radial rate; note cardiac rhythm); auscultate lungs; obtain respiratory rate; inspect extremities and presacral area for evidence of edema; check jugular veins for distention; describe sputum raised (if any); record weight; look for evidence of cyanosis. Baseline laboratory tests and diagnostic studies may include ECG, renal- and hepatic-function tests, serum electrolytes.

ADMINISTRATION

Parenteral: Check label to be sure preparation can be administered by the prescribed route.

Pulse should be taken for 60 seconds prior to administration (30 seconds may suffice if patient is receiving maintenance therapy). Withhold drug and contact physician if adult patient's pulse is 60 or below or child's pulse is 70 or below, unless written order gives different guidelines for withholding drug.

When drug is given IV, inject slowly; patient should be on cardiac monitor and observed closely during and for 1 to 2 hours after drug is administered by this route. Observe for development of bradycardia, ventricular premature beats, or a new cardiac arrhythmia; report occurrence to physician immediately.

Alternate IM injection sites; chart site used. *IM injection sites for children*—either lateral aspect of thigh or buttocks.

Do not administer IM in gluteus muscle if edema is extensive and involves the upper legs or presacral area; administer in the deltoid unless physician directs otherwise.

Read label of disposable syringe for digoxin carefully. Drug is available in 1-ml or 2-ml disposable syringe or tubex. The 2-ml syringe contains a total of 0.5 mg (0.25 mg/ml).

DIGOXIN

Oral pediatric elixir is available as 0.05 mg/ml. If dose ordered is written in mcg, 0.05 mg = 50 mcg. Note similarity between mg and mcg. If written order is unclear or there is doubt concerning dose, check with physician.

When administering these drugs to infants and children, check written order for clarity; check dose with approved references to avoid possible misinterpretation of a written order.

If child is unable to swallow entire dose of pediatric elixir, or if part of drug is lost by spitting or drooling, notify physician. Avoid mixing elixir with food or beverages to encourage patient to take medication, because dose is critical.

Check oral cavity of elderly or incompetent patient if there is suspicion that the tablet has not been swallowed.

ONGOING ASSESSMENTS AND NURSING MANAGEMENT

Check blood pressure, pulse, and respirations q2h to q4h or as ordered, using same arm each time to measure blood pressure with patient in same position (*e.g.*, sitting, lying down); take temperature q4h while patient is awake or as ordered; monitor intake and output. Check for signs of toxicity or adverse drug effects q2h to q4h during digitalization and daily when patient is on maintenance dose.

CLINICAL ALERT: Toxicity can occur even when normal doses are given. These drugs have a narrow margin of safety. Assess patient for signs of toxicity q2h to q4h (review *Digitalis Toxicity*) while he is being digitalized and daily when he is receiving maintenance dose. Withhold drug and contact physician immediately if toxicity is suspected.

Cardiac arrhythmias (especially atrial arrhythmias) are the most common sign of digitalis toxicity in children. Frequent monitoring of the apical–radial rate, or ECG monitoring, aids in early detection of toxicity. Premonitory signs of toxicity in the newborn are undue slowing of the sinus rate, SA arrest, and prolongation of the P–R interval.

Hypokalemia sensitizes the myocardium to the cardiac glycosides and may alter the rate of onset and intensity of the positive inotropic effects of the drug. Potassium loss may result from diuretic or corticosteroid therapy, hemodialysis, suction of gastrointestinal secretions, malnutrition, diarrhea, prolonged vomiting, old age, or long-standing CHF.

Weigh daily or as ordered and record on flow sheet. Daily weight for infant or child usually is necessary because drug dose is usually based on weight.

Take apical–radial pulse for 60 seconds before administration of cardiac glycoside during period of digitalization. Taking a radial pulse for 30 to 60 seconds may suffice if patient is receiving maintenance dose.

Withhold next dose of drug and notify physician if one or more of the following occur: a pulse rate below 60 in adults or below 70 in children (unless written order states otherwise); a significant increase or decrease in the resting pulse rate; the development of an arrhythmia or, if an arrhythmia was present, the development of a new arrhythmia; a change in the patient's clinical condition; appearance of adverse effects or signs of digitalis toxicity.

Electrical conversion (cardioversion) of arrhythmias may require reduction of dosage. If elective arrhythmia conversion is scheduled, the physician usually orders a decrease in dosage or omission of drug.

Digitalization may be rapid or slow (see *Dosage*), depending on the dose used and the interval between doses. Check dosages carefully if rapid digitalization is used; dose and interval are decreased once digitalization is achieved. Be sure medication cards for rapid digitalization are destroyed once the prescribed rapid digitalization dose schedule is completed.

Digitoxin may be administered to those with impaired renal function.

Periodic determination of electrolytes, ECG, and renal- and hepatic-function tests may be ordered. Serum drug levels (of digoxin and digitoxin) may also be determined, especially if toxicity is suspected.

Review recent laboratory data. Check with physician before next dose is due if hypokalemia or abnormal hepatic or renal function is apparent.

PATIENT AND FAMILY INFORMATION

NOTE: Physician may wish patient to monitor own pulse rate while taking drug. Patient or family member will need instruction in proper technique.

Do not discontinue drug without first checking with physician.

Avoid use of antacids and of nonprescription cough, cold, allergy, antidiarrheal, and diet medications, except on physician's advice.

Notify physician if loss of appetite, lower-stomach pain, vomiting, diarrhea, unusual fatigue, weakness, blurred or yellow vision, or mental depression occurs.

Physician will closely monitor therapy. Periodic laboratory tests and diagnostic studies such as ECG are usually necessary.

Adhere to dietary restrictions recommended by physician.

Carisoprodol Rx

| tablets: 350 mg | Rela (contains tartrazine), Soma, Soprodol, *Generic* |

INDICATIONS

Adjunct to rest, physical therapy, and other measures for relief of discomfort associated with acute, painful musculoskeletal conditions.

CONTRAINDICATIONS

Acute intermittent prophyria; suspected porphyria; allergic or idiosyncratic reactions to carisoprodol or related compounds such as meprobamate or tybamate.

ACTIONS

Mode of action is not clearly identified but may be related to its sedative properties. Does not directly relax skeletal muscles.

Following administration, onset of action is in 30 minutes and duration is 4 to 6 hours. Peak plasma concentrations occur 4 hours after administration of 350 mg; half-life is 8 hours. Drug is metabolized in the liver and trace amounts are excreted unchanged in the urine.

WARNINGS

Idiosyncratic reactions: Rarely, first dose is followed by idiosyncratic symptoms appearing within minutes or hours. Symptoms reported include extreme weakness, transient quadriplegia, dizziness, ataxia, temporary loss of vision, diplopia, mydriasis, dysarthria, agitation, euphoria, confusion, disorientation. Symptoms usually subside over next several hours. Supportive and symptomatic therapy, including hospitalization, may be necessary.

Drug dependence: Abrupt cessation of large doses (100 mg/kg/day) may be followed by mild withdrawal symptoms (abdominal cramps, insomnia, chilliness, headache, nausea) in some patients. Psychological dependence and abuse have been rare, but drug is used with caution in addiction-prone individuals.

Use in pregnancy: Safety not established. Drug crosses the placenta. Use only when clearly needed and potential benefits outweigh the unknown potential hazards to the fetus.

Use in lactation: Drug is present in the breast milk of lactating mothers at concentrations 2 to 4 times that of maternal plasma.

Use in children: Not recommended for children under 12.

PRECAUTIONS

Use in impaired renal function: Exercise caution.

Tartrazine sensitivity: Some products contain tartrazine (see Appendix 6, section 6-23).

DRUG INTERACTIONS

Effects of carisoprodol and **alcohol,** other **CNS depressants,** and **psychotropic drugs** may be additive; exercise caution with patients who take more than one of these agents simultaneously.

ADVERSE REACTIONS

CNS: CNS effects may require dosage reduction. Reactions include dizziness, drowsiness, vertigo, ataxia, tremor, agitation, irritability, headache, depressive reactions, syncope, and insomnia.

Allergic or idiosyncratic: Reactions occasionally develop and are usually seen within first to fourth dose in those having no previous contact with the drug. Skin rash, erythema, pruritus, eosinophilia, and fixed drug eruption with cross-reaction to meprobamate have been reported. Severe reactions are manifested by asthmatic episodes, fever, weakness, dizziness, angioneurotic edema, smarting eyes, hypotension, and anaphylactoid shock. If such reactions occur, discontinue drug and institute appropriate symptomatic therapy, epinephrine, antihistamines, and possibly corticosteroids.

Cardiovascular: Tachycardia, postural hypotension, facial flushing.

GI: Nausea, vomiting, hiccups, epigastric distress.

OVERDOSAGE

Symptoms: Stupor, coma, shock, respiratory depression; rarely, death. Effects of carisoprodol and alcohol or other CNS depressants or psychotropic agents can be additive, even when one of the drugs has been taken in normal dosage.

Treatment: Any drug remaining in the stomach should be removed and symptomatic therapy given. Should respiration or blood pressure become compromised, respiratory assistance or pressor agents may be administered. Diuresis, osmotic diuresis, peritoneal dialysis, or hemodialysis may also be considered. Careful monitoring of urinary output is necessary and caution is used to prevent overhydration. Observe patient for possible relapse due to incomplete gastric emptying and delayed absorption.

DOSAGE

350 mg qid; last dose taken H.S.

NURSING IMPLICATIONS

HISTORY
See Appendix 4.

PHYSICAL ASSESSMENT
Evaluate limitations imposed by musculoskeletal disorder (*e.g.,* walking, sitting, movement or use of a limb).

ADMINISTRATION
May be given with meals or food if GI upset occurs. Last dose should be administered H.S.

TRADE NAME SIMILARITY
Soprodol and Sopronol (antifungal agent).

ONGOING ASSESSMENTS AND NURSING MANAGEMENT
Rest, physical therapy, and other measures may be part of therapeutic regimen.

If drowsiness or dizziness occurs, assist patient with ambulation.

Notify physician before next dose is due if excessive drowsiness or dizziness occurs.

PATIENT AND FAMILY INFORMATION
Follow physician's recommendations about rest and other therapy, because these are a necessary part of treatment.

Drug may be taken with food or meals if GI upset occurs.

May cause drowsiness, dizziness; observe caution while driving or performing other tasks requiring alertness.

Avoid alcohol and other CNS depressants. Do not use nonprescription preparations (*e.g.,* liquid cough medications) that contain alcohol. If there is doubt about whether a product contains alcohol, check with a pharmacist.

If dizziness (postural hypotension) occurs, avoid sudden changes in posture; use caution when climbing stairs and so on.

Contact physician if condition persists.

Carmustine (BCNU) Rx

injection: 100   BiCNU
mg/vial

INDICATIONS
Palliative therapy as single agent or in combination with other chemotherapeutic agents in the following.

Brain tumors: Glioblastoma, brainstem glioma, medulloblastoma, astrocytoma, ependymoma, metastatic brain tumors.

Multiple myeloma: In combination with prednisone.

Hodgkin's disease, Non-Hodgkin's lymphomas: As secondary therapy in combination with other drugs in patients who relapse with primary therapy or fail to respond to primary therapy.

CONTRAINDICATIONS
Previous hypersensitivity; patients with decreased circulating platelets, leukocytes, or erythrocytes from either previous chemotherapy or other causes.

ACTIONS
Is a nitrosurea alkylating agent. Carmustine alkylates deoxyribonucleic acid (DNA) and ribonucleic acid (RNA) and also has been shown to inhibit several enzymes by carbamoylation of amino acids in proteins. It is thought that its antineoplastic and toxic activities may be due to metabolites. Carmustine is rapidly degraded, with no drug detectable after 15 minutes. Crosses the blood–brain barrier effectively. Approximately 60% to 70% of total dose is excreted in the urine in 96 hours and 10% is excreted as respiratory CO_2. The fate of the remainder is undetermined.

See also Antineoplastic Agents.

WARNINGS
Therapy has carcinogenic potential. Acute leukemia and bone-marrow dysplasias have occurred. Safe use in pregnancy not established.

ADVERSE REACTIONS
Hematopoietic: Most frequent and serious adverse reaction is delayed myelosuppression, which usually occurs 4 to 6 weeks after administration and is dose related. Platelet nadirs usually occur at 4 to 5 weeks and leukocyte nadirs at 5 to 6 weeks after therapy. Thrombocytopenia is generally more severe than is leukopenia; however, both may be dose-limiting toxicities. Anemia is generally less severe.

GI: Nausea and vomiting frequently are noted and usually appear within 2 hours of dosing, last 4 to 6 hours, and are dose related. Prior administration of antiemetics is effective in diminishing or preventing these side-effects.

Renal: Decrease in kidney size, progressive azotemia, and renal failure have been reported in those receiving large cumulative doses after prolonged therapy with carmustine and related nitrosureas. Kidney damage has been reported occasionally in those receiving lower total doses.

Hepatic: When high doses are employed, a reversible type of hepatic toxicity, manifested by increased transaminase, alkaline phosphatase, and bilirubin levels, has been reported.

Local: Burning at site of injection is common, but true thrombosis is rare. Accidental contact of reconstituted carmustine with skin has caused transient burning and hyperpigmentation of affected areas.

Pulmonary: Toxicity characterized by pulmonary infiltrate and/or fibrosis has been reported in some patients receiving prolonged therapy.

Other: Rapid IV infusion may produce intensive flushing of the skin and suffusion of the conjunctiva within 2 hours, lasting about 4 hours.

DOSAGE
Recommended dose as a single agent in previously untreated patients is 200 mg/m^2 IV every 6 weeks. This may be given as a single dose or divided into daily injections, such as 100 mg/m^2, on 2 successive days. When used in combination with other myelosuppressive drugs or in patients whose bone-marrow reserve is depleted, doses are adjusted accordingly.

A repeat course should not be given until circulating blood elements have returned to acceptable levels (platelets above 100,000/mm^3; leukocytes above 4000/mm^3). Repeat courses are not given before 6 weeks because of delayed toxicity.

NURSING IMPLICATIONS

HISTORY
See Appendix 4.

PHYSICAL ASSESSMENT
Record physical and emotional status; vital signs; weight. Review recent laboratory and diagnostic

studies. Baseline hematologic studies, renal- and hepatic-function studies are usually ordered.

ADMINISTRATION

Drug may be administered in an inpatient or outpatient setting.

Physician may prescribe antiemetic prior to administration of carmustine.

Drug is prepared immediately before administration.

Preparation and handling of solutions:
Accidental contact of reconstituted solution with skin has caused transient burning and hyperpigmentation. Plastic disposal gloves may be worn to protect personnel preparing the solution.

Dissolve with 3 ml of the supplied sterile diluent. Do _not_ use other diluents for this first step of preparation.

Next, aseptically add 27 ml of Sterile Water for Injection, USP, to the alcohol solution.

Resulting solution will contain 3.3 mg/ml of carmustine in 10% ethanol having a _p_H of 5.6 to 6.0.

Reconstitution as recommended results in a clear, colorless solution.

Solution may be further diluted with Sodium Chloride for Injection, USP, or 5% Dextrose for Injection, USP (physician must specify which solution and amount to be used).

The recommended solution should be used IV only and administered by IV drip over a 1- to 2-hour period. Injection over shorter periods of time may produce intense pain and burning at site of injection.

Drug contains no preservatives and is not intended as a multidose vial; after dosage is removed, discard remainder of drug.

Avoid use of small veins because movement during infusion may displace needle. Secure arm on a board or other support device to protect IV injection site.

Inform patient that burning may occur at site of injection.

IV may be started with a separate IV solution that is the same as that used for further dilution (_e.g.,_ Sodium Chloride or 5% Dextrose). This prevents any drug contact with the skin when starting the intravenous line. Then add IV solution containing carmustine to IV line (piggyback or Y-tubing) immediately after preparation.

Stability: Refrigeration (2°C to 8°C) of unopened vials is required and prevents significant decomposition for at least 2 years. Decomposition of reconstituted solutions is linear with time; refrigeration of the reconstituted solution significantly increases stability. After 24 hours, when protected from light, there is only 4% decomposition. Further dilution of the reconstituted solution with 500 ml of Sodium Chloride for Injection, USP, or 5% Dextrose for Injection, USP, results in a solution that is stable for 48 hours when protected from light and refrigerated. Carmustine has a low melting point (approximately 30.5°C–32°C); exposure to this temperature or above will cause it to liquefy and appear as an oily film in the bottom of the vial. This is a sign of decomposition and the vial should be discarded.

ONGOING ASSESSMENTS AND NURSING MANAGEMENT

Solution must infuse within 2 hours of preparation because drug has tendency to decompose after that time. Calculate infusion rate in drops per minute; timing label may be applied to side of bottle.

Monitor IV infusion rate q15m.

Advise patient that flushing of skin and suffusion of conjunctiva may occur; this usually lasts about 4 hours.

If patient complains of burning at injection site or pain along pathway of vein (caused by venospasm), slow infusion rate. However, the infusion must be completed in 2 hours, and it may be necessary to increase rate of infusion at a later time.

If burning is not relieved, check with physician about further dilution of IV fluid.

Nausea and vomiting may occur within 2 hours of dosing. In some, vomiting may occur a few minutes after infusion is started.

Stay with patient and monitor IV infusion if vomiting occurs because retching and movement may result in displacement of the needle and extravasation of IV fluid.

If extravasation occurs or there is question of patency of the IV line, restart IV immediately, preferably in the opposite extremity.

If extravasation occurs, contact physician. Cold compresses may be applied to area.

Monitor vital signs q4h. Notify physician if temperature elevation occurs.

Nausea may be controlled with an antiemetic before and q4h after administration of drug. A liquid diet or dry toast, unsalted crackers, cola syrup in water, or carbonated beverages may relieve nausea. Patient may have to experiment with food or fluid that best relieves problem.

Advise patient that skin pigmentation may occur along vein pathway of injection site and is not permanent.

At time of future clinic or office visits, weigh patient; obtain blood pressure, pulse, and respirations; auscultate lungs; look for signs of jaundice, difficulty breathing, thrombocytopenia, infection, swelling of extremities.

PATIENT AND FAMILY INFORMATION

NOTE: Drug may be given in an outpatient setting or patient may be hospitalized and then discharged several days after drug is administered.

Promptly report any of the following to physician or nurse: chills, fever, sore throat, weakness, infections of any kind (including common cold, abscess formation, infections in cuts), easy bruising, blood in urine or stool, petechiae, bleeding gums, nosebleeds, foul-smelling urine, pain on urination, extended episodes of vomiting, jaundice, dark urine, light-colored stools, itching, swelling of extremities, nonproductive cough, dyspnea.

If dyspnea develops, contact physician immediately, regardless of time of day or night. If physician cannot be contacted, go to hospital emergency room for examination and possible treatment.

Physician will periodically order laboratory tests to monitor therapy. In some instances it may be necessary to avoid persons with infections; if this becomes necessary, physician will explain necessary precautions.

Inform other physicians and dentist of therapy with carmustine if medical/surgical or dental treatment is required.

Cascara Sagrada

See Laxatives.

Castor Oil

See Laxatives.

Cefaclor

See Cephalosporins and Related Antibiotics.

Cefadroxil

See Cephalosporins and Related Antibiotics.

Cefamandole Nafate

See Cephalosporins and Related Antibiotics.

Cefazolin Sodium

See Cephalosporins and Related Antibiotics.

Cefoperazone Sodium

See Cephalosporins and Related Antibiotics.

Cefotaxime Sodium

See Cephalosporins and Related Antibiotics.

Cefoxitin Sodium

See Cephalosporins and Related Antibiotics.

Ceftizoxime Sodium

See Cephalosporins and Related Antibiotics.

Cefuroxime Sodium

See Cephalosporins and Related Antibiotics.

Cephalexin

See Cephalosporins and Related Antibiotics.

Cephalosporins and Related Antibiotics

Cefaclor Rx

capsules: 250 mg, 500 mg	Ceclor
oral suspension: 125 mg/5 ml, 250 mg/5 ml	Ceclor

Cefadroxil Rx

capsules: 500 mg	Duricef, Ultracef
tablets: 1 g	Duricef, Ultracef
oral suspension: 125 mg/5 ml, 250 mg/5 ml	Duricef, Ultracef
oral suspension: 500 mg/5 ml	Duricef

Cefamandole Nafate Rx

injection: 500-mg, 1-g, 2-g vials	Mandol

Cefazolin Sodium Rx

| powder for injection:
250-mg, 500-mg,
1-g vials; 500-mg
or 1-g/100 ml pig-
gyback units; 5-g
or 10-g/100 ml
bulk vial | Ancef |
| powder for injection:
250-mg, 500-mg,
1-g, 10-g vials;
500-mg, 1-g Redi
vials; 10-g/100 ml
vials | Kefzol |

Cefoperazone Sodium Rx

| powder for injection:
1-g, 2-g vials | Cefobid |

Cefotaxime Sodium Rx

| powder for injection:
500-mg, 1-g, 2-g
vials; 1-g, 2-g infu-
sion bottles | Claforan |

Cefoxitin Sodium Rx

| powder for injection:
1-g/10 ml vial;
2-g/20 ml vial; 1-g
and 2-g/100 ml in-
fusion bottles | Mefoxin |

Ceftizoxime Sodium Rx

| powder for injection:
1-g, 2-g vials, pig-
gyback vials | Cefizox |

Cefuroxime Sodium Rx

| powder for injection:
750-mg vials, 1.5-g
vials, infusion bot-
tles | Zinacef |

Cephalexin Rx

capsules: 250 mg, 500 mg	Keflex
tablets: 1 g	Keflex
oral suspension: 125 mg/5 ml, 250 mg/5 ml	Keflex
pediatric oral suspen- sion: 100 mg/ml	Keflex

Cephalothin Sodium Rx

| powder for injection:
1-g, 2-g, 4-g, 20-g
vials | Keflin, Neutral |

Cephapirin Sodium Rx

| injection: 500-mg,
1-g, 2-g vials; 1-g,
2-g, 4-g piggyback
vials; 20-g bulk
package | Cefadyl |

Cephradine Rx

capsules: 250 mg, 500 mg	Anspor, Velosef
tablets: 1 g	Velosef
oral suspension: 125 mg/5 ml, 250 mg/ 5 ml	Anspor, Velosef
powder for injection: 250-mg, 500-mg, 1-g vials; 2-g and 4-g/100 ml infu- sion containers; 2-g/200 ml infu- sion container	Velosef

Moxalactam Disodium Rx

| powder for injection:
1-g, 2-g vials | Moxam |

INDICATIONS
See Table 11.

CEFACLOR
Lower respiratory-tract infections including pneumonia; upper respiratory-tract infections including pharyngitis and tonsillitis; otitis media; skin and skin-structure infections; urinary-tract infections (UTIs) including pyelonephritis and cystitis caused by susceptible organisms.

Unlabeled use: Single 2-g dose may be effective for uncomplicated UTI in selected populations.

CEFADROXIL
Treatment of UTI; skin and skin-structure infections; pharyngitis and tonsillitis caused by susceptible organisms.

CEFAMANDOLE NAFATE
Lower respiratory-tract infections including pneumonia; UTI; peritonitis; septicemia; skin and skin-structure infections; nongonococcal pelvic inflammatory disease caused by susceptible organisms in

Table 11. Organisms That Are Generally Susceptable to Various Cephalosporins

✓ = generally susceptible
‡ = demonstrated in vitro activity

		First Generation						Second Generation				Third Generation			
	Organism	Cefadroxil	Cephalexin	Cephradine	Cephapirin	Cephalothin	Cefazolin	Cefaclor	Cefamandole	Cefoxitin	Cefuroxime	Cefotaxime	Ceftizoxime	Cefoperazone	Moxalactam
Gram-positive	Staphylococci[1]	✓	✓[2]	✓	✓	✓	✓	✓	✓	✓	✓	✓[3]	✓	✓	✓
	Streptococcus pneumoniae	✓	✓	✓	✓	✓	✓	✓	✓	✓	✓	✓	✓	✓	✓
	Beta-hemolytic streptococci	✓	✓	✓	✓	✓	✓	✓	✓	✓	✓	✓	✓	✓	✓
	Streptococcus faecalis			✓[4]										✓	
Gram-negative	Escherichia coli	✓	✓	✓	✓	✓	✓	✓	✓	✓	✓	✓	✓	✓	✓
	Hemophilus influenzae	✓	✓	✓	✓	✓	✓	✓	✓	✓	✓	✓	✓	✓[2]	✓
	Klebsiella species	✓	✓	✓	✓	✓	✓	✓	✓	✓	✓	✓	✓	✓	✓
	Neisseria gonorrhoeae	✓	✓	✓	✓	✓	✓	✓	✓	✓	✓	✓	✓	✓[2]	
	Neisseria meningitidis	✓	✓	✓	✓	✓	✓	✓	✓	✓	✓	✓	‡	‡	‡
	Proteus mirabilis	✓	✓	✓	✓	✓	✓	✓	✓	✓	✓	✓	✓	✓	
	Salmonella species	✓	✓	✓	✓	✓	✓	✓	✓	✓	✓	‡	‡	‡	‡
	Shigella species	✓	✓	✓	✓	✓	✓	✓	✓	✓	✓	‡	‡	‡	‡
	Morganella morganii (Proteus morganii)								✓	✓	✓[2•]	✓	✓	✓	✓
	Proteus vulgaris								✓[2]	✓		✓	✓	✓	✓
	Providencia species								✓	✓	✓	‡	‡		‡
	Providencia rettgeri								✓	✓	✓	✓	✓	✓	✓
	Enterobacter species								✓		✓	✓	✓	✓	✓
	Citrobacter species										✓[2]	✓	‡	✓	✓
	Pseudomonas aeruginosa											✓[2]	✓	✓[2]	✓[2]
	Serratia species											✓	✓	✓	✓
	Salmonella typhi											‡	‡		‡
	Acinetobacter species													✓	✓[2]
Anaerobic	Clostridium species	✓	✓	✓	✓	✓	✓	✓	✓	✓	✓	✓	‡	✓	✓
	Peptococcus species	✓	✓	✓	✓	✓	✓	✓	✓	✓	✓	✓	✓	✓	✓
	Peptostreptococcus species	✓	✓	✓	✓	✓	✓	✓	✓	✓	✓	✓	✓	✓	✓
	Bacteroides fragilis									✓		✓	✓	✓	✓
	Fusobacterium species								✓		✓		‡	‡	✓
	Eubacterium species												‡	‡	✓
	Clostridium difficile													‡	

[1] Coagulase-positive, coagulase-negative, and penicillinase producing

[2] Some strains are resistant

[3] Including some beta-lactamase producing strains

[4] For urinary-tract infections only

women. Antibiotic therapy for beta-hemolytic streptococcal infections should continue for at least 10 days.

Aminoglycoside therapy: In certain cases of confirmed or suspected gram-positive or gram-negative sepsis, or in those with serious infections in which the causative organism has not been identified, drug may be used concomitantly with an aminoglycoside. Dosage recommended in the labeling of both may be given and depends on the severity of the infection and the patient's condition.

Perioperative prophylaxis: May reduce incidence of certain postoperative infections.

CEFAZOLIN SODIUM

Respiratory-tract infections; genitourinary-tract infections; skin and soft-tissue infections; biliary-tract infections; bone and joint infections; septicemia; endocarditis caused by susceptible organisms.

Prophylaxis: Preoperative, intraoperative, and postoperative administration may reduce incidence of certain postoperative infections in patients undergoing contaminated or potentially contaminated procedures. May also be effective in surgical patients in whom infection at the operative site would present a serious risk (*e.g.,* open heart surgery, prosthetic arthroplasty).

CEFOPERAZONE SODIUM

Respiratory-tract infections; peritonitis, other intra-abdominal infections; bacterial septicemia; infections of skin, skin structures; pelvic inflammatory disease, endometritis, and other infections in the female genital tract caused by susceptible organisms.

C

CEFOTAXIME SODIUM

Lower respiratory-tract infections, including pneumonia; genitourinary infections and uncomplicated gonorrhea caused by *Neisseria gonorrhoeae,* including penicillinase-producing strains; gynecologic infections including pelvic inflammatory disease, endometritis, and pelvic cellulitis; bacteremia/septicemia; skin and skin-structure infections; intra-abdominal infections; bone or joint infections caused by susceptible organisms.

Perioperative prophylaxis: Administration may reduce incidence of certain postoperative infections in those undergoing surgical procedures that are classified as contaminated or potentially contaminated. In patients undergoing cesarean section, intraoperative (after clamping the umbilical cord) and postoperative use may reduce incidence of certain postoperative infections.

Concomitant aminoglycoside therapy: See statement in Cefamandole Nafate, above.

CEFOXITIN SODIUM

Lower respiratory-tract infections; UTI including uncomplicated gonorrhea due to *N. gonorrhoeae;* intra-abdominal infections; gynecologic infections; septicemia; bone and joint infections; skin and skin-structure infections caused by susceptible organisms.

Perioperative prophylaxis: Prophylactic administration may reduce incidence of certain postoperative infections. In cesarean section, intraoperative use may reduce incidence of postoperative infections.

CEFTIZOXIME SODIUM

Lower respiratory-tract infections; genitourinary infections; gonorrhea (uncomplicated cervical and urethral); intra-abdominal infections; septicemia; skin and skin-structure infections; bone and joint infections caused by susceptible organisms.

CEFUROXIME SODIUM

Lower respiratory-tract infections; genitourinary infections; skin and skin-structure infections; septicemia; meningitis; gonorrhea caused by susceptible organisms.

Perioperative prophylaxis: May reduce incidence of certain postoperative infections in those undergoing surgical procedures classified as clean-contaminated or potentially contaminated.

CEPHALEXIN

Respiratory-tract infections; otitis media; skin and soft-tissue infections; bone infections; genitourinary-tract infections caused by susceptible organisms.

CEPHALOTHIN SODIUM

Respiratory-tract infections; skin and soft-tissue infections (including peritonitis); genitourinary-tract

infections; septicemia, including endocarditis; GI infections; meningitis; bone and joint infections caused by susceptible organisms. Also for prophylactic administration perioperatively to reduce incidence of certain postoperative infections in those undergoing surgical procedures classified as contaminated or potentially contaminated.

CEPHAPIRIN SODIUM

Respiratory-tract infections; skin and soft-tissue infections; genitourinary infections; septicemia; endocarditis; osteomyelitis caused by susceptible organisms.

Perioperative prophylaxis: May reduce incidence of certain postoperative infections in those undergoing surgical procedures classified as contaminated or potentially contaminated. Also may be effective in surgical patients in whom infection at operative site would be a serious risk.

CEPHRADINE

Oral: Infections of respiratory tract; otitis media; infections of skin and skin structures; infections of the urinary tract caused by susceptible organisms.

Parenteral: Respiratory-tract infections; genitourinary infections; infections of the skin and skin structures; bone infections; septicemia caused by susceptible organisms.

Perioperative prophylaxis: May reduce incidence of certain postoperative infections in those undergoing surgical procedures classified as contaminated or potentially contaminated. In cesarean section (after clamping of umbilical cord) and postoperatively to reduce incidence of certain postoperative infections.

MOXALACTAM DISODIUM

Lower respiratory-tract infections; genitourinary infections; intra-abdominal infections; septicemia; CNS infections; skin and skin-structure infections; bone and joint infections caused by susceptible organisms.

Concomitant aminoglycoside therapy: See statement in Cefamandole Nafate, above.

CONTRAINDICATIONS

Hypersensitivity to cephalosporins or related antibiotics.

ACTIONS

Are structurally and pharmacologically related to the penicillins. Cefoxitin (a cephamycin) and moxalactam (a beta-lactam) are included in this group because of their similarity to the cephalosporins.

Antibacterial activity is by inhibition of mucopeptide synthesis in the bacterial cell wall. The result is a defective wall that is osmotically unstable. Cephalosporins may be bactericidal or bacteriostatic depending on factors such as organism susceptibility, dose, tissue concentrations, and the rate at which the organisms are multiplying. They are more effective against rapidly growing organisms in the process of cell-wall formation.

Cephalexin, cephradine, cefaclor, and cefadroxil are well absorbed from the GI tract; oral absorption may be delayed by presence of food, but amount of drug absorbed is not affected. These drugs are widely distributed to most body tissues and fluids, with maximum concentrations being achieved in the liver and kidneys. First- and second-generation cephalosporins (except cefuroxime) do not readily enter cerebrospinal fluid (CSF); however, third-generation cephalosporins (moxalactam, cefotaxime, ceftizoxime, and cefoperazone) readily diffuse into the CSF. Therapeutic blood levels are reached in bone tissue following usual doses of cephradine, cefamandole, and cefoperazone, cefuroxime, and ceftizoxime. Cefazolin penetrates into acutely inflamed bone at considerably higher concentrations than it penetrates into normal bone tissue. Concentrations of cephalothin and cephapirin are low in normal and infected bone.

Cephalosporins and their metabolites are excreted primarily by the renal route. Oral probenecid will block cephalosporin excretion and produce higher and more prolonged serum levels, especially with those cephalosporins excreted primarily by tubular secretion; probenecid does not significantly affect elimination of moxalactam.

WARNINGS

Bleeding abnormalities: **Moxalactam, Cefamandole,** and **Cefoperazone** can interfere with hemostasis through hypoprothrombinemia (due to destruction of intestinal bacteria, altering vitamin K availability and/or a molecular attachment that prevents activation of prothrombin), platelet destruction, and, very rarely, immune-mediated thrombocytopenia. Bleeding associated with hypoprothrombinemia can be prevented with vitamin K. Bleeding may also be related to complications of underlying diseases (*e.g.,* sepsis, malignancy). Predisposing factors include hepatic and renal dysfunction, thrombocytopenia, the concomitant use of more than 20,000 units of heparin/day, oral anticoagulants, other drugs affecting hemostasis (*e.g.,* aspirin), and elderly, malnourished, or debilitated patients. "Normal" patients have also experienced bleeding problems.

Hypersensitivity: Before therapy is instituted, inquiry is made about previous hypersensitivity to cephalosporins and penicillin. If a hypersensitivity reaction occurs, drug is discontinued and patient treated with usual agents (*i.e.,* epinephrine or other pressor amines, antihistamines, or corticosteroids).

Administer oxygen, IV steroids, and airway management, including intubation, as indicated, for treatment of serious reactions.

Cross-allergenicity with penicillin: There is evidence of partial cross-allergenicity between penicillins and the cephalosporins. Cephalosporins are administered cautiously to penicillin-sensitive patients.

Pseudomembranous colitis: Has been reported with use of cephalosporins. Treatment alters normal flora of the colon and may permit overgrowth of clostridia. Mild cases of colitis may respond to drug discontinuance alone. Moderate to severe cases can be managed with fluid, electrolyte, and protein supplementation, as indicated. When colitis not relieved by discontinuing drug or when it is severe, oral vancomycin is the treatment of choice.

Use in pregnancy and lactation: Safety not established. Use only when clearly needed and when potential benefits outweigh the potential hazards to the fetus. Cephalosporins are secreted in breast milk during lactation.

Use in infants and children: The relative benefit–risk ratio is considered. In newborns, accumulation of cephalosporin antibiotics (with resulting prolongation of drug half-life) has been reported.

PRECAUTIONS

Superinfection: Use of antibiotics (especially prolonged or repeated therapy) may result in bacterial or fungal overgrowth of nonsusceptible organisms, which may lead to a secondary infection.

Impaired renal function: May be nephrotoxic; use with caution in the presence of markedly impaired renal function. In the elderly and in those with known or suspected renal impairment, laboratory studies should be made prior to and during therapy.

Impaired hepatic function: Cefoperazone is extensively excreted in bile. Serum half-life is increased in those with hepatic disease or biliary obstruction. If higher doses are used, serum concentrations are monitored.

Hypoprothrombinemia: Has been reported rarely with cefamandole, cefoperazone, and moxalactam; it is promptly reversed by administration of vitamin K. Such episodes usually have occurred in elderly, debilitated, or otherwise compromised patients with deficient stores of vitamin K. Treatment of such patients with antibiotics possessing significant gram-negative or anaerobic activity is thought to alter intestinal flora, with consequent reduction in vitamin K synthesis. In addition, prolonged bleeding times with bleeding diathesis and platelet dysfunction have been reported. Inhibition of platelet function has been reported with high doses of moxalactam.

Parenteral use: Inflammatory reactions to parenteral cephalosporins are common. IM preparations are injected deep into the musculature; IV preparations should be properly diluted and administered over an appropriate time interval. Prolonged or high-dosage IV may be associated with phlebitis and thrombophlebitis.

Gonorrhea: Patients with suspected concomitant syphilis should have darkfield examinations of all suspect lesions before treatment, as well as monthly serologic tests for a minimum of 3 months.

Urinary tract infections: Frequent bacteriologic and clinical appraisals are necessary during therapy and may be necessary for several months after.

Electrolyte imbalance: Sodium content of cefoperazone, cephapirin, cephalothin, cefazolin, cefoxitin, and cefotaxime ranges from 1.5 mEq/g to 2.8 mEq/g. Cefamandol and moxalactam contain 3.3 mEq/g and 3.8 mEq/g respectively; cephradine contains 6 mEq/g but is also available in sodium-free form.

DRUG INTERACTIONS

Bacteriostatic agents may interfere with bacterial activity of cephalosporins, particularly in acute infections in which organisms are proliferating rapidly.

Probenecid administered concurrently with cephalosporins increases and prolongs plasma levels. Probenecid does not significantly affect elimination of moxalactam.

Concomitant use of nephrotoxic agents (*e.g.,* **colistin, vancomycin, polymyxin B, aminoglycosides**) increases probability of nephrotoxicity. Cephalosporins can be administered with aminoglycosides but solutions should not be combined because of physical incompatibility. Potent "loop" diuretics may enhance the possibility of renal toxicity.

Alcoholic beverages consumed concurrently with **cefamandole, cefoperazone,** or **moxalactam** may produce alcohol intolerance (disulfiram reaction).

Drug/lab tests: A false-positive reaction for **urine glucose** may occur with Benedict's solution, Fehling's solution, or Clinitest tablets but not with enzyme-based tests such as Clinistix and Tes-Tape. There may be a false-positive for **proteinuria.** A false-positive direct **Coombs' test** has been reported. Cephalosporins have been implicated in the production of falsely elevated **urinary 17-ketosteroid** values. High concentrations of **cephalothin** or **cefoxitin** may interfere with measurement of *creatinine levels* (by the Jaffe reaction).

ADVERSE REACTIONS

Most common are GI disturbances and hypersensitivity phenomena. The latter are most likely to occur in patients previously demonstrating hypersensitivity and in those with history of allergy, asthma, hay fever, or urticaria.

Hypersensitivity: Severity of reactions ranges from mild to life threatening. Most common reactions are mild and appear as urticaria, pruritus, exfoliative dermatitis, or morbilliform eruptions. Reactions resembling serum sickness (erythema multiforme or the above skin manifestations accompanied by arthritis/arthralgia and, frequently, fever) have been reported. Anaphylactic reactions are rare but some fatalities have resulted. Allergic reaction in the recipient following passive transfer of **cephalothin** antibodies from the donor during a blood transfusion has been reported.

GI: Adverse effects most frequently noted with oral administration include nausea, vomiting, and diarrhea. Other effects include glossitis, abdominal pain, dyspepsia, heartburn, and tenesmus. Colitis, including rare instances of pseudomembranous colitis, has been reported with cephalosporin therapy. GI adverse effects occur rarely after parenteral administration of some cephalosporins.

Hematologic: Eosinophilia, transient neutropenia (more common with prolonged, high-dose therapy), leukopenia, thrombocytopenia, agranulocytosis, hemolytic anemia. Disturbances in vitamin-K-dependent clotting functions have been reported. A positive direct Coombs' test may develop in some patients, especially those with azotemia.

Hepatic: Elevated SGOT and SGPT and a few cases of elevated total bilirubin, alkaline phosphatase, and LDH have been seen. Values tend to return to normal after therapy.

Renal: Mild elevations in BUN have been seen; the frequency increases in patients who are over 50 years or under 3 years. Pyuria, dysuria, and hematuria have been reported.

CNS: Headache, malaise, dizziness, and vertigo have been reported. Neurotoxicity manifested by generalized tonic-clonic seizures, mild hemiparesis, and extreme confusion have been reported following large doses of cefazolin in renal failure.

Other: Fever; dyspnea; candidal overgrowth consisting of oral candidiasis, monilial vaginitis with vaginal discharge, and genitoanal pruritus. IM administration of cephalosporins, particularly **cephalothin and cefoxitin,** commonly results in pain, induration, fever, tenderness, and tissue sloughs. Sterile abscesses have been reported following accidental subcutaneous injection. IV administration has produced phlebitis and thrombophlebitis. IV cephalothin seems to produce a higher incidence of inflammatory reactions.

ADMINISTRATION

Administration is continued for minimum of 48 to 72 hours after fever abates or evidence of bacterial eradication is obtained.

Perioperative prophylaxis: Administration is usually discontinued within 24-hour period after surgical procedure. In certain surgeries in which occurrence of infection may be particularly devastating (*e.g.,* open heart surgery, prosthetic arthroplasty), prophylactic administration may be continued for 3 to 5 days following surgery.

DOSAGE

CEFACLOR

Adults: Usual dosage is 250 mg q8h. In severe infections or those caused by less susceptible organisms, dosage may be doubled. Do not exceed 4 g/day.

Children: 20 mg/kg/day in divided doses q8h. In more serious infections, otitis media, and infections caused by less susceptible organisms, 40 mg/kg/day with maximum dosage of 1 g/day.

CEFADROXIL

UTI: Usual dosage for uncomplicated infections is 1 g or 2 g/day in single or divided doses. For all other UTIs, usual dose is 2 g/day in divided doses.

Skin and skin-structure infections: Usual dosage is 1 g/day in single or divided doses.

Group A beta-hemolytic streptococcal pharyngitis or tonsillitis: 1 g/day in 2 divided doses for 10 days.

Renal impairment: Adjust dosage to prevent drug accumulation. Initial dose is 1 g; maintenance doses are based on creatinine clearance rate.

Children: Recommended daily dosage is 30 mg/kg/day in divided doses q12h.

CEFAMANDOLE NAFATE

Adults: Usual dose range is 500 mg to 1 g q4h to q8h. Dosage of 500 mg q6h is adequate in uncomplicated pneumonia and infections of skin structures. In uncomplicated UTIs, a dosage of 500 mg q8h is sufficient; in more serious infections, dose may be increased to 1 g q8h; in severe infections, dose may be increased to 1 g q4h to q6h. In life-threatening infections or infections due to less susceptible organisms, doses up to 2 g q4h may be needed.

Infants and children: 50 mg/kg/day to 100 mg/kg/day in equally divided doses q4h to q8h. May be increased to 150 mg/kg/day for severe infections.

Perioperative prophylaxis

Adults: 1 g or 2 g IM or IV ½ to 1 hour prior to the surgical incision, followed by 1 g or 2 g q6h for 24 to 48 hours.

Children (3 months and older)*:* 50 mg/kg/day to 100 mg/kg/day in equally divided doses IM or IV.

Patients undergoing prothestic arthroplasty: Administration is recommended for as long as 72 hours.

Patients undergoing cesarean section: Initial dose may be administered just prior to surgery or immediately after cord is clamped.

Impaired renal function

Reduced dosage is employed and serum levels closely monitored. After an initial dose of 1 g to 2 g, a maintenance dosage schedule is followed and is based on degree of renal impairment, severity of infection, and susceptibility of organism.

CEFAZOLIN SODIUM

Total daily dosages are the same for IV and IM administration.

Mild infections caused by susceptible gram-positive cocci: 250 mg to 500 mg q8h.

Moderate to severe infections: 500 mg to 1 g q6h to q8h.

Severe, life-threatening infections: 1 g to 1.5 g q6h; in rare instances, dosages of 12 g/day have been used.

Acute uncomplicated UTI: 1 g q12h.

Perioperative prophylaxis: *Preoperative*—1 g IV or IM ½ to 1 hour prior to surgery. *Intraoperative*—0.5 g to 1 g IV or IM during surgery. *Postoperative*—0.5 g to 1 g IV or IM q6h to q8h for 24 hours. May be continued for 3 to 5 days when occurrence of infection would be especially serious.

Impaired renal function: After a 500-mg loading dose, maintenance doses are based on BUN and creatinine clearance.

Children: *Mild to moderately severe infections*— 25 mg/kg/day to 50 mg/kg/day (approximately 10 mg/lb to 20 mg/lb) in 3 or 4 equal doses. *Severe infections*—Total daily dosage may be increased to 100 mg/kg (45 mg/lb). *Impaired renal function*— Dosage is adjusted according to creatinine clearance.

Premature infants (under 1 month): Safety for use not determined.

CEFOPERAZONE SODIUM

May be given IM or IV. Usual adult dose is 2 g/day to 4 g/day in equally divided doses q12h. In severe infections or infections caused by less sensitive organisms, total daily dose and/or frequency may be increased. Patients have been treated with total daily dosage of 6 g to 12 g divided into 2, 3, or 4 administrations ranging from 1.5 g/dose to 4 g/dose.

Hepatic disease and/or biliary obstruction: Drug is extensively excreted in bile. Serum half-life is increased in those with hepatic disease and/or biliary obstruction. In general, total daily dosage above 4 g is not necessary in these patients.

Impaired renal function: Patient usually does not require dosage adjustment unless high dosages are used. Half-life is reduced slightly during hemodialysis. Dosage is scheduled to follow a dialysis period.

CEFOTAXIME

May be administered IM or IV. Usual adult dose is 1 g q6h to q8h. Maximum daily dose should not exceed 12 g. Dosage guidelines are as follows.

Gonorrhea: 1 g IM (single dose).

Uncomplicated infections: 1 g q12h IM or IV.

Moderate to severe infections: 1 g to 2 g q6h to q8h IM or IV.

Infections commonly needing higher dosage (*e.g.,* septicemia): 2 g q6h to q8h IV.

Life-threatening infections: 2 g q4h IV.

Perioperative prophylaxis: 1 g IV or IM 30 to 90 minutes prior to surgery; 1 g IV or IM 30 to 120 minutes following first dose; 1 g IV or IM within 2 hours after surgery.

Cesarean section: 1 g IV as soon as umbilical cord is clamped; second and third doses of 1 g IV or IM at 6- and 12-hour intervals after first dose.

Pediatric: The following may serve as a guideline:

Age 0–1 week—50 mg/kg q12h IV

Age 1–4 weeks—50 mg/kg q8h IV

Age 1 month–12 years and <50 kg weight—50 mg/kg/day to 180 mg/kg/day in 4 to 6 divided doses IM or IV

Children ≥ 50 kg—Use adult dosage

Use in impaired renal function: Dosage determined by degree of renal impairment, severity of infection, and susceptibility of causative organism.

CDC-recommended treatment schedules for gonorrhea

Penicillinase-producing N. gonorrhoeae (PPNG): For positive cultures after spectinomycin therapy, 1 g IM as single injection.

Disseminated gonococcal infection: 500 mg IV qid for at least 7 days.

Gonococcal ophthalmia in adults: PPNG, give 500 mg IV qid.

CEFOXITIN SODIUM

Usual adult dose range is 1 g to 2 g q6h to q8h. Dosage guidelines are as follows.

Uncomplicated infection: 1 g q6h to q8h IV or IM.

Moderately severe or severe infections: 1 g q4h or 2 g q6h to q8h IV.

Infections needing higher dosage: 2 g q4h or 3 g q8h IV.

Uncomplicated gonorrhea: 2 g IM with 1 g oral probenecid given at same time or up to 30 minutes before cefoxitin.

Prophylactic use, surgery: 2 g IV or IM 30 to 60 minutes prior to surgery followed by 2 g q6h after

first dose for no more than 24 hours (72 hours after prosthetic arthroplasty).

Prophylactic use, cesarean section: 2 g IV as soon as umbilical cord is clamped; second and third 2-g dose IV or IM 4 and 8 hours after first dose. Give subsequent doses q6h for no more than 24 hours.

Impaired renal function: In adults, an initial loading dose of 1 g to 2 g followed by reduced maintenance doses based on creatinine clearance.

Hemodialysis: 1-g to 2-g loading dose after each hemodialysis. Maintenance doses based on renal function.

Infants and children: Recommended dosage in children 3 months and older is 80 mg/kg/day to 160 mg/kg/day in divided doses q4h to q6h. Higher doses are used for more serious infections. Total daily dosage should not exceed 12 g/day. *Prophylactic use (3 months and older)*—30 mg/kg/dose to 40 mg/kg/dose q6h. *Impaired renal function*—Dosage adjusted according to degree of renal impairment.

CDC-recommended treatment schedules for gonorrhea and acute pelvic inflammatory disease.

Penicillinase-producing N. gonorrhoeae (PPNG): A PPNG isolate resistant to spectinomycin may be treated with 2 g IM and 1 g probenecid PO.

Disseminated gonoccocal infection: 1 g IV qid for at least 7 days.

Gonococcal ophthalmia in adults: For PPNG, use 1 g IV qid.

Acute pelvic inflammatory disease: For hospitalized patients, 100 mg doxycycline IV bid plus 2 g cefoxitin IV qid. Continue for at least 4 days and at least 48 hours after patient defervesces. Continue 100 mg doxycycline PO bid after discharge to complete 10 to 14 days of therapy. For nonhospitalized patient, give 2 g cefoxitin IM with 1 g oral probenecid, followed by 100 mg doxycycline bid for 10 to 14 days.

CEFTIZOXIME SODIUM

Usual adult dosage is 1 g to 2 g q8h to q12h. Dosage is individualized.

Genitourinary infections: Higher dosage is recommended; other therapy is instituted if response is not prompt.

Gonorrhea, uncomplicated: A single 1-g IM injection is usual dose.

Life-threatening infections: IV route may be preferable. In those with normal renal function, IV dose is 2 g/day to 12 g/day. In conditions such as bacterial septicemia, 6 g/day to 12 g/day IV may be given initially for several days and dosage gradually reduced according to clinical response and laboratory findings.

Impaired renal function: Following an initial loading dose of 500 mg to 1 g IM or IV, the maintenance dose is based on the serum creatinine or creatinine clearance.

CEFUROXIME SODIUM

Adults: May be given IM or IV. Usual dosage range is 750 mg to 1.5 g q8h, usually for 5 to 10 days.

Perioperative prophylaxis: 1.5 g IV just prior to surgery (approximately ½ to 1 hour before initial incision). Thereafter, 750 mg IV or IM q8h when procedure is prolonged. For preventive use during open heart surgery, 1.5 g IV at the induction of anesthesia and q12h thereafter for a total of 6 g.

Impaired renal function: Dosage is reduced and based on degree of renal impairment and susceptibility of the causative organism.

Infants and children over 3 months: 50 mg/kg/day to 100 mg/kg/day in equally divided doses, q6h to q8h. The higher dose is used for more severe or serious infections (not to exceed the maximum adult dose). *Bacterial meningitis*—Larger doses initially of 200 mg/kg/day to 240 mg/kg/day IV in divided doses q6h to q8h. Dosage may be reduced to 100 mg/kg/day IV upon clinical improvement. In children with renal insufficiency, the frequency of dosage is modified as for adults.

CEPHALEXIN

Adults: 1 g to 4 g/day in divided doses. *Usual dose*—250 mg q6h. *For skin and skin-structure infections*—500 mg q12h. For more severe infections or those caused by less susceptible organisms, larger doses may be used. If doses larger than 4 g/day are required, a parenteral cephalosporin is used.

Children: 25 mg/kg/day to 50 mg/kg/day in 4 doses. For skin and skin-structure infections, total daily dose is divided and given q12h. In severe infections, dosage may be doubled. *Otitis media*—75 mg/kg/day to 100 mg/kg/day in 4 divided doses.

CEPHALOTHIN SODIUM

May be given IV or deep IM.

Adults: Range is 500 mg to 1 g q4h to q6h. *Severe infections*—500 mg q4h or dosage raised to 1 g. *Life-threatening infections*—Doses up to 2 g q4h may be needed.

Infants and children: 100 mg/kg/day in divided doses usually effective for most infections, but range may be 80 mg/kg/day to 160 mg/kg/day in divided doses.

Perioperative prophylaxis: 1 g to 2 g 30 to 60 minutes prior to initial incision; 1 g to 2 g during surgery and 1 g to 2 g q6h after surgery and discontinued within 24 hours after surgery. *Children*—20 mg/kg to 30 mg/kg given at same times before, during, and after surgery.

Peritoneal dialysis: Added to peritoneal dialysis fluid in concentrations up to 6 mg/100 ml and instilled into the peritoneal cavity throughout entire dialysis (16–30 hours).

Intraperitoneal administration: 0.1% to 4% solution in saline for treating peritonitis or contaminated peritoneal cavities.

CEPHAPIRIN SODIUM

Adults: Usual dose is 500 mg to 1 g q4h to q6h IM or IV. Very serious life-threatening infections may require doses up to 12 g daily. IV route is preferred when high doses are administered. Patients with reduced renal function may be treated with lower doses.

Perioperative prophylaxis: Recommended doses are 1 g to 2 g IM or IV administered ½ to 1 hour prior to surgery, 1 g or 2 g during surgery, and 1 g or 2 g IV or IM q6h for 24 hours postoperatively.

Children: Recommended total daily dose is 40 mg/kg to 80 mg/kg (20 mg/lb to 40 mg/lb) administered in 4 equally divided doses.

CEPHRADINE

Oral: May be given without regard to meals.

Adults: Infections of skin, skin structures, respiratory tract (other than lobar pneumonia)—250 mg q6h or 500 mg q12h. *Lobar pneumonia*—500 mg q6h or 1 g q12h. *Uncomplicated UTI*—Usual dose is 500 mg q12h. In more serious infections, 500 mg q6h or 1 g q12h. Severe or chronic infections may require larger doses.

Children (over 9 months): Usual dose is 25 mg/kg/day to 50 mg/kg/day, in equally divided doses q6h to q12h. For otitis media due to *Hemophilus influenzae,* 75 mg/kg/day to 100 mg/kg/day in equally divided doses q6h to q12h. Do not exceed 4 g/day.

All patients: Larger doses (up to 1 g qid) may be given for severe or chronic infections.

Parenteral: May be given IV or deep IM.

Adults: 2 g to 4 g in equally divided doses qid IM or IV. In bone infections, usual dosage is 1 g qid IV. *Uncomplicated pneumonia, skin and skin-structure infections, and UTI*—500 mg qid. *Severe infections*—Dose may be increased by giving q4h or by increasing dose up to maximum of 8 g/day.

Perioperative prophylaxis: Recommended doses are 1 g IM or IV 30 to 90 minutes prior to surgery, followed by 1 g q4h to q6h after first dose for 1 to 2 doses, or up to 24 hours postoperatively. *Cesarean section*—1 g IV when umbilical cord is clamped. Give second and third doses as 1 g IM or IV at 6 and 12 hours after first dose.

Infants, children: Usual range is 50 to 100 mg/kg/day in equally divided doses qid.

Renal impairment: Dosage is reduced and based on creatinine clearance.

MOXALACTAM DISODIUM

Adults: Usual dose is 2 g/day to 6 g/day in divided doses q8h for 5 to 10 days or up to 14 days. Most mild to moderate infections respond to 500 mg to 2 g q12h. *Mild skin and skin-structure infections and uncomplicated pneumonia*—500 mg q8h. *Mild uncomplicated UTI*—250 mg q12h. *Persistent UTI*—500 mg q12h; in serious UTIs, dosage may be increased to q8h. *Life-threatening infections, infections due to less susceptible organisms*—Up to 4 g q8h.

Neonates, infants, children: Dosage guidelines are as follows:

Age 0–1 week—50 mg/kg q12h
Age 1–4 weeks—50 mg/kg q8h
Infants—50 mg/kg q6h
Children—50 mg/kg q6h to q8h

The dosage for children may be increased to a total daily dosage of 200 mg/kg (not to exceed maximum adult dose) for serious infections. In pediatric gram-negative meningitis, an initial loading dose of 100 mg/kg is recommended prior to use of the above dosage schedule.

Use in impaired renal function: Dose is reduced; after initial dose of 1 g to 2 g, maintenance dosage is determined by degree of renal impairment, severity of infection, and susceptibility of organism. Maintenance doses should be repeated following regular hemodialysis.

NURSING IMPLICATIONS

HISTORY
See Appendix 4. If patient history reveals an allergy to penicillin, inform physician immediately.

PHYSICAL ASSESSMENT
Obtain vital signs; when applicable, assess area of infection (*e.g.,* respiratory tract, skin, genitourinary tract). Culture and sensitivity tests should be performed prior to institution of therapy, but therapy may be instituted before results are obtained. Other assessments, such as weight (pediatric dosage may be based on weight), may also be appropriate. Baseline laboratory tests may include renal- and hepatic-function studies and CBC prior to initiation of therapy.

ADMINISTRATION
Return oral suspensions to refrigerator immediately after measuring dose.

See *Stability and Storage,* below, or package insert regarding storage and length of time drug retains potency under refrigeration or room temperature. Discard all outdated preparations.

Oral administration may result in nausea, vomiting, or diarrhea. If nausea occurs, drug may be given with meals or food.

When reconstituting powder form for more than one dose, label vial with date, amount of diluent used, and dose/ml.

IM administration: Inject into large muscle mass such as the gluteus or lateral part of the thigh. Aspiration is necessary to avoid injection into a large blood vessel. Rotate injection sites; record site used.

IM injections are usually painful; patient should be informed that pain or discomfort will occur.

Do not administer these drugs subcutaneously; sterile abscesses may result.

If a cephalosporin and an aminoglycoside are given concomitantly by the IM route, administer in two different sites.

When drug is administered IV, physician's order must state method used (*e.g.,* direct IV infusion [directly into vein or through IV tubing injection port], use of a volume control set or Y-tubing infusion set). If order is unclear as to which method is to be used, request clarification.

When infusing with Y-tubing, it is desirable to discontinue the other solution. Pay careful attention to the volume of the drug solution so that the calculated dose is infused.

Prolonged or high-dosage IV administration may be associated with phlebitis and thrombophlebitis; using small IV needles and larger veins and alternating infusion sites may minimize phlebitis.

CEFAMANDOLE NAFATE
During storage of reconstituted drug at room temperature, carbon dioxide develops inside the vial. This pressure may be dissipated prior to withdrawal of contents or may be used to aid withdrawal if the vial is inverted *over* the syringe needle and contents are allowed to flow into the syringe. *Do not* place the vial upright on a surface and push needle down into the vial; the carbon dioxide may exert enough pressure to force the plunger out of the syringe and cause injury to the user.

IM: Dilute each gram with 3 ml of one of the following: Sterile Water for Injection, Bacteriostatic Water for Injection, 0.9% Sodium Chloride for Injection, or Bacteriostatic Sodium Chloride for Injection. Shake well until dissolved. Give deep IM.

Intermittent IV administration: Reconstitute each gram with 10 ml of Sterile Water for Injection, 5% Dextrose Injection, or 0.9% Sodium Chloride Injection. May be administered by slowly injecting directly into vein over period of 3 to 5 minutes or through tubing of an IV administration set while patient is receiving one of the following IV fluids: 0.9% Sodium Chloride Injection, 5% or 10% Dextrose Injection, 5% Dextrose and 0.9% Sodium Chloride Injection, 5% Dextrose and 0.2% Sodium Chloride Injection, or Sodium Lactate Injection (M/6).

Intermittent IV infusion with Y-type administration set or volume control set: May also be used with any of the IV fluids mentioned above. When a Y-tube hookup is used, add 100 ml of appropriate diluent to the 1-g or 2-g 100-ml piggyback vial. If Sterile Water for Injection is used as a diluent, reconstitute with approximately 20 ml/g to avoid a hypotonic solution.

Continuous IV infusion: Dilute each gram with 10 ml of Sterile Water for Injection. An appropriate quantity of the resulting solution may be added to an IV container of one of the fluids listed under intermittent IV administration.

CEFADROXIL MONOHYDRATE

Can be given without regard to meals.

CEFAZOLIN SODIUM

Reconstitute with Sterile Water for Injection, Bacteriostatic Water for Injection, or 0.9% Sodium Chloride Injection (Table 12). Shake well until dissolved. Dilute further as required for IV use.

Intermittent IV infusion: Administer along with primary IV fluid management programs in a volume control set or in a separate secondary IV container. Reconstituted 500 mg or 1 g of drug may be diluted in 50 ml to 100 ml of 0.9% Sodium Chloride Injection, 5% or 10% Dextrose Injection, 5% Dextrose in Lactated Ringer's Injection, 5% Dextrose and 0.2, 0.45, or 0.9% Sodium Chloride Injection, Lactated Ringer's Injection, 5% or 10% Invert Sugar in Sterile Water for Injection, 5% Sodium Bicarbonate in Sterile Water for Injection, or Ringer's Injection.

Direct IV injection: Dilute reconstituted 500 mg or 1 g of drug in minimum of 10 ml Sterile Water for Injection. Inject slowly over 3 to 5 minutes. Administer directly into a vein or through IV tubing.

CEFOPERAZONE SODIUM

If reconstituted powder for injection has been stored in freezer, thaw to room temperature before use. After thawing, discard unused portion; do not refreeze.

IV: Concentrations of between 2 mg/ml and 50 mg/ml are recommended. Reconstitute powder with 5% Dextrose Injection, 5% Dextrose and Lactated Ringer's Injection, 5% Dextrose and 0.2% or 0.9% Sodium Chloride Injection, 10% Dextrose Injection, Lactated Ringer's Injection, 0.9% Sodium Chloride Injection, Normosol M and 5% Dextrose Injection, or Normosol R. Vials may be reconstituted with 2.8 ml/g; the use of 5 ml/g for reconstitution is recommended.

The entire quantity of the resulting solution is then withdrawn for further dilution and administration as follows:

Intermittent infusion—Further dilute reconstituted drug in 20 ml to 40 ml of diluent per gram; administer over period of 15 to 30 minutes.

Continuous infusion—Dilute to a final concentration of between 2 mg/ml and 25 mg/ml.

IM: Reconstitute with Bacteriostatic Water for Injection (benzyl alcohol or parabens), 0.5% Lidocaine HCl Injection; or Sterile Water for Injection. When concentrations above 250 mg/ml are to be given, solutions should be prepared using 0.5% Lidocaine HCl injection. Do not use preparations containing benzyl alcohol in neonates. See Table 13.

Following reconstitution of IM or IV solution, let stand to allow any foaming to dissipate to permit visual inspection for complete stabilization. Vigorous and prolonged agitation may be necessary to solubilize higher concentrations (above 333 mg/ml).

CEFOTAXIME SODIUM

See Table 14.

Shake to dissolve; inspect for particulate matter and discoloration prior to use. Solutions range from light yellow to amber.

IV: Reconstitute with at least 10 ml of Sterile Water for Injection. Infusion bottles may be re-

Table 12. Guidelines for Preparing Solution of Cefazolin Sodium

Vial Size	Volume of Diluent to Be Added	Approximate Final Volume	Approximate Concentration
250 mg	2 ml	2 ml	125 mg/ml
500 mg	2 ml	2.2 ml	225 mg/ml
1 g	2.5 ml	3 ml	330 mg/ml

Table 13. Volumes and Concentrations of Cefoperazone

Package Size	Concentration	Volume of Diluent to Be Added	Withdrawable Volume
1-g vial	333 mg/ml	2.8 ml	3 ml
	250 mg/ml	3.8 ml	4 ml
2-g vial	333 mg/ml	5.6 ml	6 ml
	250 mg/ml	7.8 ml	8 ml

constituted with 50 ml or 100 ml of 0.9% Sodium Chloride Injection or 5% Dextrose Injection.

Intermittent IV administration: 1 g or 2 g in 10 ml of Sterile Water can be injected over a period of 3 to 5 minutes but may also be given for a longer period through the tubing system by which patient is receiving other IV solutions.

Continuous IV infusion: May be added to IV bottles of the following: 0.9% Sodium Chloride; 5% or 10% Dextrose; 5% Dextrose and 0.9%, 0.45%, or 0.2% Sodium Chloride; Lactated Ringer's Solution; Sodium Lactate Injection (M/6); 10% Invert Sugar.

_IM:_ Reconstitute with Sterile Water or Bacteriostatic Water for Injection. Individual IM doses of 2 g may be given if the dose is divided and administered in 2 different sites.

CEFOXITIN SODIUM

For preparation of solution, see Table 15.

_IV:_ Reconstitute each gram with at least 10 ml of Sterile Water for Injection. May be reconstituted with 50 ml or 100 ml of 0.9% Sodium Chloride Injection or 5% or 10% Dextrose Injection. These primary solutions may be further diluted in 50 ml to 1000 ml of the above mentioned solutions or any of the following injections: 5% Dextrose and 0.9% Sodium Chloride,

Table 14. Volumes and Concentrations of Cefotaxime Sodium After Reconstitution

Package Size	Volume of Diluent to Be Added (ml)	Approximate Withdrawable Volume (ml)	Approximate Concentration (mg/ml)
500-mg vial	2 (IM)	2.2	230
	10 (IV)	10.2	50
1-g vial	3 (IM)	3.4	300
	10 (IV)	10.4	95
2-g vial	5 (IM)	6.0	330
	10 (IV)	11.0	180

Table 15. Volumes and Concentrations of Cefoxitin Sodium After Reconstitution

Package Size	Volume of Diluent to Be Added (ml)	Approximate Withdrawable Volume (ml)	Approximate Concentration (mg/ml)
1-g vial	2 (IM)	2.5	400
	10 (IV)	10.5	95
2-g vial	4 (IM)	5	400
	10 or 20 (IV)	11.1 or 21.0	180 or 95
1-g infusion bottle	50–100 (IV)	50–100	20–10
2-g infusion bottle	50–100 (IV)	50–100	40–20

5% Dextrose with 0.02% Sodium Bicarbonate, 5% Dextrose with 0.2% or 0.45% Saline, Ringer's, Lactated Ringer's, 5% Dextrose in Lactated Ringer's, 5% or 10% Invert Sugar in Water, 10% Invert Sugar in Saline, 5% Sodium Bicarbonate, M/6 Sodium Lactate, 5% Aminosol, Polyonic M56 in 5% Dextrose, 2.5% and 5% Mannitol, Isolyte E, or Isolyte E with 5% Dextrose. When reconstituted with these solutions, drug's potency is maintained for 24 hours at room temperature or 48 hours under refrigeration. When reconstituted with Neut (sodium bicarbonate), Normosol-M in D5-W, Ionosol B with 5% Dextrose, or 10% Mannitol, drug is stable for 1 week under refrigeration.

Intermittent IV administration: Inject 1 g or 2 g in 10 ml Sterile Water for Injection over 3 to 5 minutes. May also be given for longer periods through system by which other IV solutions are administered.

Continuous IV infusion: May be added to IV container of 5% Dextrose Injection, 0.9% Sodium Chloride Injection, 5% Dextrose and 0.9% Sodium Chloride Injection, or 5% Dextrose with 0.02% Sodium Bicarbonate Solution.

_IM:_ Reconstitute each gram with 2 ml Sterile Water for Injection, or use 2 ml of 0.5% lidocaine HCl solution (without epinephrine) to minimize discomfort of IM injection. Physician must order lidocaine solution.

CEFTIZOXIME SODIUM

Preparation of Solution: Reconstitute with Sterile Water for Injection; shake well. Table 16 may be used as a guide.

Piggyback vials: Reconstitute with 50 ml to 100 ml of Sodium Chloride Injection or any other IV solution listed under IV administration, below. Shake well. Administer as a single dose with primary IV fluids.

Table 16. Volumes and Concentrations of Ceftizoxime Sodium After Reconstitution

Package Size	Volume of Diluent to Be Added (ml)	Approximate Withdrawable Volume (ml)	Approximate Concentration (mg/ml)
1-g vial	3 (IM)	3.7	270
	10 (IV)	10.7	95
2-g vial	6 (IM)	7.4	270
	20 (IV)	21.4	95

IV administration: Direct bolus injection, injected slowly over 3 to 5 minutes, directly or through IV tubing of running parenteral fluid.

Intermittent or continuous infusion: Dilute reconstituted drug in 50 ml to 100 ml of one of the following: Sodium Chloride Injection; 5% or 10% Dextrose Injection; 5% Dextrose and 0.9%, 0.45%, or 0.2% Sodium Chloride Injection; Ringer's Injection; Invert Sugar 10% in Sterile Water for Injection; 5% Sodium Bicarbonate in Sterile Water for Injection; 5% Dextrose in Lactated Ringer's Injection (only when reconstituted with 4% Sodium Bicarbonate Injection).

IM administration: Divide the 2-g doses and give in different large muscle masses.

CEFUROXIME SODIUM

For preparation of solution and suspension (drug is a suspension at IM concentrations), see Table 17. Use Sterile Water for Injection, 5% Dextrose in Water, 0.9% Sodium Chloride, or any solutions listed under IV.

IV: When the 750-mg and 1.5-g vials are reconstituted with Sterile Water for Injection, they maintain potency for 24 hours at room temperature and 48 hours when refrigerated. More dilute solutions, such as 1.5 g plus 50 ml of Sterile Water for Injection, 5% Dextrose Injection, or 0.9% Sodium Chloride Injection, maintain potency for

Table 17. Volumes and Concentrations of Cefuroxime Sodium After Reconstitution

Package Size	Volume of Diluent to Be Added (ml)	Approximate Withdrawable Volume (ml)	Approximate Concentration (mg/ml)
750 mg vial	3.6 (IM)	3.6	200
	9.0 (IV)	8.0	100
1.5-g vial	16.0 (IV)	Total	100
1.5-g infusion pack	50.0 (IV)	—	30

24 hours at room temperature or for 1 week under refrigeration.

These solutions may be further diluted to concentrations between 1 mg/ml and 30 mg/ml in the following and will not lose more than 10% activity for 24 hours at room temperature or for at least 7 days under refrigeration: 0.9% Sodium Chloride Injection, M/6 Sodium Lactate Injection, Ringer's Injection, Lactated Ringer's Injection, 5% Dextrose and 0.9%, 0.45%, or 0.225% Sodium Chloride Injection, 5% or 10% Dextrose Injection, and 10% Invert Sugar in Water for Injection.

Cefuroxime is compatible for 24 hours at room temperature when admixed in IV infusion with heparin (10 units/ml to 50 units/ml) or potassium chloride (10 mEq and 40 mEq) in 0.9% Sodium Chloride Injection.

IM: When reconstituted with Sterile Water for Injection, suspensions retain potency for 24 hours at room temperature and for 48 hours under refrigeration. Do not add to solutions of aminoglycoside antibiotics because of potential interaction. If concurrent therapy is indicated, each of these antibiotics may be given separately.

Administration

IV administration: May be preferable in those with bacterial septicemia or other severe or life-threatening infections, or in those who may be poor risks because of lowered resistance, particularly if shock is present or impending.

Direct intermittent IV administration: Inject slowly into a vein over 3 to 5 minutes or give through the tubing system by which the patient is receiving other IV solutions.

Intermittent IV administration with a Y-type administration set: Dosing is accomplished through the tubing system by which patient is receiving other IV solutions. During infusion, temporarily discontinue administration of any other IV solutions at the same site.

Continuous IV infusion: A solution may be added to an IV bottle containing one of the following: 0.9% Sodium Chloride Injection, 5% or 10% Dextrose Injection, 5% Dextrose and 0.9% or 0.45% Sodium Chloride Injection, or M/6 Sodium Lactate Injection.

IM administration: Give deep IM into a large muscle mass (such as the gluteus or lateral part of the thigh).

CEPHALOTHIN SODIUM

Intermittent IV administration: Slowly inject a solution of 1 g in 10 ml diluent directly into vein over 3 to 5 minutes, or give through IV tubing.

Intermittent infusion with Y-type administration set: Can be accomplished while bulk IV solutions are being infused.

Continuous IV infusion: 1 g or 2 g reconstituted and well mixed with 10 ml of Sterile Water for Injection may be added to an IV container of any of the following: Acetated Ringer's Injection, 5% Dextrose Injection, 5% Dextrose in Lactated Ringer's Injection, Lactated Ringer's Injection, Ringer's Injection, or 0.9% Sodium Chloride Injection.

Continuous IV infusion must be completed within 24 hours; for prolonged infusion, replace freshly prepared solution at least every 24 hours.

CEPHAPIRIN SODIUM

IM: Reconstitute 1-g vial with 2 ml of Sterile Water for Injection or Bacteriostatic Water for Injection (with parabens or benzyl alcohol). Each 1.2 ml contains 500 mg of drug.

Intermittent IV injection: Dilute 1-g or 2-g vial with 10 ml or more diluent and give slowly over 3 to 5 minutes, or give with IV infusions. The 2-g piggyback vial should be diluted with Dextrose Injection, USP, Sodium Chloride Injection, USP, or Bacteriostatic Water for Injection, USP.

Intermittent IV infusion with Y-tube: Can be accomplished while bulk IV solutions are being infused. When Y-tube hookup is used, dilute 4-g vial with 40 ml Bacteriostatic Water for Injection, USP, Dextrose Injection, USP, or Sodium Chloride Injection, USP.

Compatibility: Stable and compatible for 24 hours at room temperature at concentrations between 2 mg/ml and 30 mg/ml in any of the following: Sodium Chloride Injection; 10% Invert Sugar in NS or Water; Dextrose in Water; Sodium Lactate Injection; Lactated Ringer's; Dextrose plus Sodium Chloride; Ringer's Injection; Lactated Ringer's w/ 5% Dextrose; Sterile Water for Injection; 5% Dextrose in Ringer's Injection; Normosol R; Normosol R in 5% Dextrose; Ionosol D-CM; or Ionosol G in 10% Dextrose.

CEPHRADINE

IM: Add Sterile Water for Injection or Bacteriostatic Water for Injection as per Table 18.

IV: A 3 mcg/ml serum concentration can be maintained for each mg of cephradine/kg/hour of infusion. Diluents for direct IV injection are Sterile Water for Injection; 5% Dextrose Injection; Sodium Chloride Injection. IV infusion solutions include 5% and 10% Dextrose Injection; Sodium Chloride Injection; M/6 Sodium Lactate; Dextrose and Sodium Chloride Injection;

Table 18. Volume and Concentrations of Cephradine After Reconstitution

Package Size	Volume of Diluent to Be Added (ml)	Approximate Withdrawable Volume (ml)	Approximate Concentration (mg/ml)
250 mg	1.2	1.2	200
500 mg	2.0	2.2	227
1 g	4.0	4.5	222

10% Invert Sugar in Water; Normosol-R; Ionosol B with 5% Dextrose. Use Sterile Water for Injection to dilute to a final concentration of 30 mg/ml to 50 mg/ml.

Direct IV administration: Add 5 ml Sterile Water for Injection, 5% Dextrose for Injection, or Sodium Chloride for Injection or other suitable infusion fluid to the 250-mg or 500-mg vial, 10 ml to the 1-g vial, or 20 ml to the 2-g bottle. Inject directly into a vein over 3 to 5 minutes or give through IV tubing when the IV fluid is compatible with cephradine.

Continuous or intermittent IV infusion
IV infusion container: Add 10 ml, 20 ml, or 40 ml of Sterile Water for Injection or a suitable infusion fluid, respectively, to the 1-g vial, 2-g bottle, or 4-g bottle to prepare solution. Promptly withdraw entire contents of resulting solution and transfer to an IV infusion container.

2-g or 4-g IV bottle: Reconstitute 2-g bottle with 40 ml and 4-g bottle with 80 ml of a suitable infusion solution; attach an IV administration set directly to the IV bottle.

Use IM or direct IV solutions within 2 hours at room temperature. If stored under refrigeration, solutions retain potency for 24 hours. Continuous or intermittent IV infusion solutions retain full potency for 10 hours at room temperature. For prolonged infusions, replace infusions every 10 hours.

MOXALACTAM DISODIUM

IM: Dilute each gram with 3 ml Sterile Water, Bacteriostatic Water, 0.9% Sodium Chloride, Bacteriostatic Sodium Chloride, or 0.5% lidocaine. Shake well until dissolved.

Direct IV administration: Add 10 ml Sterile Water for Injection, 5% Dextrose Injection, or 0.9% Sodium Chloride Injection per gram. Slowly inject into vein over period of 3 to 5 minutes or give through IV tubing of administration set while patient is also receiving one of the following: 0.9% Sodium Chloride, 5% Dextrose,

5% Dextrose and 0.9%, 0.45%, or 0.2% Sodium Chloride, 5% Dextrose and 0.15% Potassium Chloride, 5% Osmitrol in Water, Sodium Lactate (M/6), Normosol-M in D5-W, Ionosol B in 5% Dextrose, Plasma-Lyte-M in 5% Dextrose, Ringer's Injection, Acetated Ringer's Injection, or Lactated Ringer's in 5% Dextrose. Avoid IV solutions containing alcohol.

Continuous IV infusion: Dilute each gram with 10 ml of Sterile Water for injection; add appropriate quantity to IV bottle containing one of the compatible fluids listed above.

STABILITY AND STORAGE

CEFACLOR, CEPHALEXIN

Refrigerate oral suspension. May be kept for 14 days after reconstitution without loss of potency.

CEFAMANDOLE NAFATE, CEFZOLIN SODIUM

Reconstituted solution stable for 24 hours at room temperature and 96 hours if stored under refrigeration.

CEFOPERAZONE SODIUM

Reconstituted drug may be stored at room temperature, under refrigeration (2°C to 8°C), or in a freezer. See package insert for manufacturer's recommended storage times for specific diluents at various temperatures. Protect from light; refrigerate sterile powder at 2°C to 8°C prior to reconstitution. After reconstitution, protection from light is not necessary.

CEFOTAXIME

Solutions in 0.9% Sodium Chloride Injection and 5% Dextrose Injection in IV bags are stable for 24 hours at room temperature, 5 days under refrigeration, and 13 weeks frozen. Thaw frozen samples at room temperature before use. After periods mentioned above, discard unused solutions or frozen material. Do not refreeze. Store in a dry state below 30°C. The dry material as well as solutions tend to darken depending on storage conditions; protect from elevated temperatures and excessive light.

CEPHALOTHIN SODIUM

Concentrated solutions will darken, especially at room temperature; slight discoloration is permissible.

Room temperature storage: Give solutions for IM injection within 12 hours after reconstitution. Start IV infusions within 12 hours and complete within 24 hours.

CEPHAPIRIN SODIUM

Utility time varies with diluent used, concentration, and storage temperature. See manufacturer's package insert.

CEPHRADRINE SODIUM

IM or IV solutions should be used within 2 hours at room temperature. If stored under refrigeration at 5°C, solutions retain potency for 24 hours. Reconstituted solutions may vary in color from light straw to yellow; this does not affect potency. Continuous or intermittent IV infusion solutions retain full potency for 10 hours at room temperature or 48 hours at 5°C. Mixture with other antibiotics is not recommended.

CEFTIZOXIME SODIUM

Protect unreconstituted drug from excessive light and store at controlled room temperature (15°C to 30°C) in the original package until used. After reconstitution or dilution with recommended diluents, these solutions are stable 8 hours at room temperature and 48 hours if refrigerated.

CEFUROXIME

Discard unused solutions or suspensions after the time periods mentioned in *Dosage* section. Store in a dry state at controlled room temperature; protect from light. Visually inspect for particulate matter and discoloration prior to administration. Powder solutions and suspensions tend to darken, depending on storage conditions, without adversely affecting product potency.

MOXALACTAM DISODIUM

Solutions are stable for 96 hours if stored under refrigeration and 24 hours at room temperature.

ONGOING ASSESSMENTS AND NURSING MANAGEMENT

Record vital signs q4h or as ordered (more frequent measurements may be necessary if patient is critically ill); assess for adverse drug reactions, especially hypersensitivity reactions; measure intake and output of children, elderly, acutely ill patients, or those suspected or known to have renal impairment. Look for signs of improvement (*e.g.,* response to antibiotic therapy); record all observations accurately, (*e.g.,* amount and type of drainage when present, general appearance of patient).

CLINICAL ALERT: Patient should be observed frequently, especially early in therapy, for hypersensitivity reactions (*e.g.,* rash, urticaria, difficulty breathing, hypotension, angioedema). If hypersensitivity occurs, discontinue drug (even when it is given IV) and contact physician immediately. Epinephrine or other pressor amines, antihistamines, or corticosteroids, oxygen, and airway management may be required.

Patient receiving moxalactam, cefamandole or cefoperazone—Observe for bleeding, which can be serious. Withhold the next dose and notify the physician immediately if bleeding (*e.g.,* GI, GU, ecchymosis, easy bleeding from cuts or injections, gums) is noted.

If drug is given IV, check injection site and vein pathway for evidence of phlebitis or thrombophlebitis (*e.g.,* redness, heat, tenderness over vein). If symptoms are apparent, IV should be restarted in opposite extremity and physician notified of problem.

If drug is given IM, check previous injection sites for evidence of induration, tenderness, tissue sloughing. If tissue sloughing or persistent induration, pain, or redness is apparent, notify physician.

If diarrhea occurs, contact physician before next dose is due. Colitis, which at times may be extremely serious, has been associated with use of these drugs.

Be alert to signs of superinfection (see Appendix 6, section 6-22).

Physician may order periodic evaluation of renal function. Impaired renal function during treatment may be indicated by appearance of casts in the urine, proteinuria, falling urinary output, rising BUN or serum creatinine. Bring changes in laboratory values, fall in urinary output, or development of cloudy urine to attention of physician.

Culture and sensitivity tests may be performed during therapy to determine continued organism susceptibility. Take samples to laboratory immediately because sample material must not be allowed to dry.

Probenecid may be administered concurrently to increase and prolong plasma levels of a cephalosporin.

If hypoprothrombinemia occurs, physician may order vitamin K.

Diabetics: Test urine with Tes-Tape, Clinistix, or other enzyme-based tests. False-positive reactions may occur with Benedict's or Fehling's solution, Clinitest tablets.

Label all laboratory request slips with the name of drug being administered. Patients receiving **cefoxitin** should not have blood drawn for serum creatinine within 2 hours of drug administration.

PATIENT AND FAMILY INFORMATION

If nausea occurs, take with food or meals.

Complete full course of therapy; do not stop taking drug even though symptoms have disappeared.

Notify physician if condition is not improved or becomes worse or if nausea, vomiting, diarrhea, rash, hives, or easy bruising occurs.

Oral suspensions: Keep refrigerated at all times and remove from refrigerator only to pour medication. Do not allow to stand at room temperature.

CEFAMANDOLE, MOXALACTAM

Avoid all alcoholic beverages; a severe reaction (nausea, vomiting, severe headache) may occur.

Diabetics: To test urine, use Tes-Tape, Clinistix, or other test materials recommended by physician while taking this drug.

Cephalothin Sodium

See Cephalosporins and Related Antibiotics.

Cephapirin Sodium

See Cephalosporins and Related Antibiotics.

Cephradine

See Cephalosporins and Related Antibiotics.

Charcoal, Activated otc

powder	CharcolantiDote, *Generic*
liquid: 12.5 g in 60-ml bottle; 25 g in 120-ml bottle	*Generic*
liquid: 40 g in 200-ml suspension	Liquid-Antidose

INDICATIONS

As emergency antidote for poisoning by most drugs and chemicals.

CONTRAINDICATIONS

Ineffective for poisoning or overdosage of cyanide, mineral acids, or alkalies. It is not particularly effective in poisonings of ethanol, methanol, and iron salts.

ACTIONS

Is a carbon residue derived from heating organic material in the absence of oxygen. Activation of the charcoal surface to increase absorptive properties occurs by treatment at high temperatures with steam and carbon dioxide or sulfuric acid, phosphoric acid, zinc chloride, or a combination of these. Is insoluble in water and not absorbed from the GI tract. It is a potent adsorbent; when given in overdosage or poisoning it rapidly inactivates and retains the absorbed material throughout GI transport.

WARNINGS

Induce emesis prior to administration. Administer to conscious persons only.

DRUG INTERACTIONS

Do not administer concomitantly with **syrup of ipecac** or **laxatives;** activated charcoal will absorb and inactivate these substances. The effectiveness of other medication may be decreased when used concurrently because of the adsorption by activated charcoal. Do not mix charcoal with **milk, ice cream** or **sherbet** because it will decrease the adsorptive capacity of activated charcoal.

ADVERSE REACTIONS

Rapid ingestion of high doses may cause vomiting. Constipation or diarrhea may occur; stools will be black.

DOSAGE

Dose should be approximately five to ten times amount of poison ingested. The initial dose in adults for acute intoxications is 30 g to 100 g as a suspension in 6 to 8 oz of water.

For maximum effect, give within 30 minutes after ingestion of poison.

Gastric dialysis: Multiple administration (*e.g.,* 20 g to 40 g q6h for 1–2 days) may be used in severe poisonings to prevent desorption from the charcoal; also promoted to increase GI clearance and rate of elimination of drugs that undergo an external recirculation pattern. Five to six tsp is approximately equal to 1 oz of activated charcoal.

NURSING IMPLICATIONS

HISTORY

When possible, obtain name and amount of drug or chemical ingested and approximate time of ingestion.

PHYSICAL ASSESSMENT

Obtain vital signs; look for toxic symptoms related to the respiratory, cardiac, and central nervous systems.

ADMINISTRATION

If there is question about type of treatment to be instituted, call the nearest poison control center for accurate information. Antidotes printed on the labels of some products are not always reliable.

Do not attempt to administer to an unconscious patient.

Patient should be cooperative; do not give to a resisting patient because aspiration may result.

Emesis should be induced prior to administration of charcoal.

To make a charcoal slurry, add powdered activated charcoal to tap water to form a thick soupy mixture. In an emergency, accurate measurements are not important.

If patient is not cooperative, a nasogastric (NG) tube may be inserted and the charcoal administered. If a slurry has been prepared, it will have to be thinned with water before administration via NG tube. Check to be sure tube is in the stomach before introducing any liquid.

Do not administer too rapidly because vomiting may occur.

Storage: Activated charcoal adsorbs gases from the air. Store in closed containers. Sealed aqueous suspensions can be stored for at least 1 year without loss of activity.

ONGOING ASSESSMENTS AND NURSING MANAGEMENT

Further assessments and management will depend on the type of poison ingested, as well as on the speed, effectiveness, and results of treatment.

Observe patient for signs and symptoms of drug overdose; notify physician if symptoms of overdose are not relieved or become worse.

If charcoal is used as chemical-poisoning antidote, consult appropriate references for symptoms.

PATIENT AND FAMILY INFORMATION

In cases of drug or chemical poisoning, call the nearest poison control center or a physician for directions for treatment. Post the telephone number of the nearest poison control center, your personal physician, and the nearest hospital in a visible place in the home, especially if there are young children in the household.

Do not use activated charcoal unless directed to do so by poison control center personnel or a physician. This is not an antidote for all poison ingestions.

When hospitalization is necessary, take the drug or chemical container with its remaining contents to the hospital. Identification of the ingested substance is vitally important.

Chenodiol *(Chenodeoxycholic Acid)* Rx

tablets: 250 mg   Chenix

INDICATIONS
For those with radiolucent stones in well-opacifying gallbladders, in whom elective surgery would be undertaken except for the presence of increased surgical risk due to systemic disease or age. The likelihood of successful dissolution is greater if the stones are floatable or small.

CONTRAINDICATIONS
Known hepatic dysfunction or bile-duct abnormalities; a gallbladder confirmed as nonvisualizing after two consecutive single doses of dye; radiopaque or radiolucent bile pigment stones; or gallstone complications or compelling reasons for gallbladder surgery.

Use in pregnancy: May cause fetal harm when administered to a pregnant woman. If drug is used during pregnancy or if pregnancy occurs while patient is taking this drug, apprise the patient of the potential harm to the fetus.

ACTIONS
A naturally occurring human bile acid. It suppresses hepatic synthesis of cholesterol and cholic acid, gradually replacing the latter and its metabolite, deoxycholic acid, in an expanded bile pool. These actions contribute to biliary cholesterol desaturation and gradual dissolution of radiolucent cholesterol gallstones. It has no effect on radiopaque (calcified) gallstones or on radiolucent bile pigment stones. Chenodiol is well absorbed from the small intestine and taken up by the liver, where it is conjugated and secreted in bile. It is ultimately converted to lithocholic acid, of which 80% is excreted in the feces.

WARNINGS
Hepatic effects: Lithocholic acid is a known hepatotoxin. Safe use depends on selection of patients without preexisting liver disease and monitoring of serum aminotransferase levels.

Colon cancer: The possibility that chenodiol might contribute to colon cancer cannot be ruled out.

Use in pregnancy, lactation, and children: See *Warnings* about use in pregnancy. Safety for use in the nursing mother is not established. Safety and efficacy for use in children are not established.

DRUG INTERACTIONS
Bile-sequestering agents (*e.g.,* cholestyramine, colestipol) may interfere with the action of chenodiol by reducing absorption. **Aluminum-based antacids** may interfere with chenodiol in the same manner as bile-sequestering agents. **Estrogens, oral contraceptives, clofibrate,** and perhaps other lipid-lowering drugs increase biliary cholesterol secretion and the incidence of cholesterol gallstones; as a result, these drugs may counteract the effectiveness of chenodiol.

ADVERSE REACTIONS
Hepatobiliary: Dose-related serum aminotransferase (mainly SGPT) elevations, usually not accompanied by rises in alkaline phosphatase or bilirubin, may occur.

GI: Dose-related diarrhea may occur at any time during treatment, but most commonly occurs when treatment is initiated. Usually it is mild and transient and does not interfere with therapy. Other, less frequent, effects include cramps, heartburn, constipation, nausea, vomiting, anorexia, epigastric distress, dyspepsia, flatulence, and nonspecific abdominal pain.

Serum lipids: Serum total cholesterol and low-density lipoprotein (LDL) cholesterol may rise 10% or more. No change has been seen in the high-density lipoprotein (HDL) fraction. Average decreases of 14% in serum triglyceride levels have been reported.

Hematologic: Decreases in WBC count (never below 3000) have been seen.

DOSAGE
Recommended dosage range is 13 mg/kg/day to 16 mg/kg/day in two divided doses, morning and night, starting with 250 mg bid the first 2 weeks and increasing by 250 mg/day each week thereafter until the recommended or maximum tolerated dose is reached.

NURSING IMPLICATIONS

HISTORY
See Appendix 4.

PHYSICAL ASSESSMENT
Obtain vital signs, weight. Baseline laboratory tests and diagnostic studies may include serum aminotransferase levels (SGOT, SGPT), serum bilirubin, serum and total cholesterol, serum triglycerides, lipoprotein-cholesterol fractions, lipoprotein phenotyping, oral cholecystogram, ultrasonogram. A pregnancy test may also be indicated.

ADMINISTRATION

Chenodiol is given in divided doses in the morning and evening.

ONGOING ASSESSMENTS AND NURSING MANAGEMENT

Instruct patient to report, or observe for, diarrhea. Notify the physician immediately if diarrhea occurs because dose reduction or discontinuation of the drug may be necessary.

CLINICAL ALERT: Notify the physician immediately if the patient experiences symptoms of gallstones (*i.e.*, nausea; vomiting; right upper quadrant pain, which may or may not radiate to the back between the shoulder blades or front of the chest; abdominal pain, chills; fever; diaphoresis; or jaundice). Surgical intervention may be necessary.

Weigh weekly or as ordered. Maintenance of reduced weight is recommended to forestall stone recurrence. Notify the physician if a weight gain is noted.

Dietary measures may include a low-cholesterol or low-carbohydrate diet and dietary bran (which have been reported to reduce biliary cholesterol). A weight-reduction diet (when appropriate) may also be ordered.

The following laboratory tests are recommended:

Serum aminotransferase levels monthly for the first 3 months and every 3 months during therapy. Elevations over three times the upper limit of normal require immediate discontinuation of therapy.

Serum cholesterol levels every 6 months. Therapy may be discontinued if levels rise above the accepted age-adjusted limit for a given patient.

Oral cholecystograms or ultrasonograms at 6- to 9-month intervals. Complete dissolution is confirmed by a repeat test after 1 to 3 months of continued administration of chenodiol. If partial dissolution is not seen by 9 to 12 months, the likelihood of success of continued treatment is greatly reduced. Drug is discontinued if there is no response by 18 months.

Stone recurrence can be expected within 5 years in 50% of cases.

Once dissolution of the gallstones is confirmed, drug is discontinued. A prophylactic dose has not been established.

PATIENT AND FAMILY INFORMATION

Notify the physician immediately if nausea; vomiting; right upper quadrant pain, which may or may not radiate; abdominal pain; chills; fever; diaphoresis; or jaundice (symptoms of gallstone complications) occurs.

If diarrhea occurs, notify the physician. A temporary dose reduction may be necessary.

It is important that the prescribed dosage regimen be followed. Do not omit, increase, or decrease the dose unless advised to do so by the physician Take the drug in the morning and at night.

Periodic laboratory tests and diagnostic studies are extremely important and will be necessary to monitor the results of therapy.

Chloral Derivatives

Chloral Hydrate Rx C–IV

capsules: 250 mg	Noctec, *Generic*
capsules: 500 mg	Noctec, Oradrate, SK-Chloral Hydrate, *Generic*
syrup: 250 mg/5 ml	*Generic*
syrup: 500 mg/5 ml	Noctec, *Generic*
elixir: 500 mg/5 ml	*Generic*
suppositories: 325 mg, 650 mg	Aquachloral Supprettes (325 mg contains tartrazine)
suppositories: 500 mg	*Generic*

Triclofos Sodium Rx

tablets: 750 mg	Triclos
liquid: 1.5 g/15 ml	Triclos

INDICATIONS

CHLORAL HYDRATE

Nocturnal sedation. As preoperative sedative to allay anxiety and induce sleep without depressing respiration or cough reflex. In postoperative care and control of pain as adjunct to opiates and analgesics.

TRICLOFOS SODIUM

Treatment of insomnia characterized by difficulty in falling asleep, frequent nocturnal awakenings, or early morning awakening. Also has been used as a premedication for obtaining sleep records in electroencephalography.

CONTRAINDICATIONS

Marked hepatic or renal impairment; severe cardiac disease; gastritis; hypersensitivity or idiosyncrasy to chloral derivatives. Because chloral hydrate passes the placental barrier and appears in breast milk, it is contraindicated in nursing mothers. See also *Warnings,* below.

ACTIONS

Hypnotic dosage produces mild cerebral depression and quiet, deep sleep with little or no "hangover." Blood pressure and respiration are depressed only slightly more than in normal sleep; reflexes are not significantly depressed, so that patient can be awakened and completely aroused. These agents do not depress REM sleep. Both chloral hydrate and tricoflos are metabolized to trichloroethanol, the principally active metabolite. Trichloroethanol has a half-life of 8 to 10 hours and is inactivated by conversion to trichloroacetic acid, which is excreted in the urine.

WARNINGS

Drug dependency: May be habit forming. Exercise caution in giving to those known to be addiction prone. Many patients take higher doses of hypnotics than they admit, and slurred speech, incoordination, tremulousness, and nystagmus should arouse suspicion of this. Drowsiness, lethargy, and hangover are frequently observed from excessive drug intake. Prolonged use of larger than usual therapeutic doses may result in psychic and physical dependence. Tolerance and psychological dependence may develop by the second week of continued administration. Chloral-hydrate addicts may take huge doses of the drug. Abuse is similar to alcohol addiction and sudden withdrawal may result in CNS excitation, with tremor, anxiety, hallucinations, or even delirium, which may be fatal. In those suffering from chronic chloral-hydrate intoxication, gastritis is common and skin eruptions may develop. Parenchymatous renal injury may also occur. Withdrawal should be undertaken in a hospital and supportive treatment similar to that used during barbiturate withdrawal is recommended.

Use in pregnancy: Safety not established. Chronic use during pregnancy may cause withdrawal symptoms in the neonate. It is not known whether these agents can affect reproductive capacity. Use only when clearly needed.

PRECAUTIONS

Continued use of therapeutic doses of **chloral hydrate** has been shown to be without deleterious effect on the heart. Large doses should not be used in those with severe cardiac disease. Use **triclofos** with caution in those with cardiac arrhythmias and with severe cardiac disease.

Most insomnias are of brief duration; long-term administration is not recommended. Chloral derivatives have been reported to precipitate attacks of acute intermittent porphyria; use with caution in susceptible patients.

Tartrazine sensitivity: Some of these products contain tartrazine. See Appendix 6, section 6-23.

DRUG INTERACTIONS

In those taking **oral anticoagulants,** chloral hydrate may cause an increased hypoprothrombinemic effect by displacement from protein binding sites. Monitor prothrombin levels and adjust coumarin dose accordingly. Administration of chloral hydrate followed by **IV furosemide** may result in sweating, hot flashes, and variable blood pressure including hypertension due to a hypermetabolic state caused by displacement of thyroid hormone from its bound state. Caution is recommended in combining chloral hydrate with other **CNS depressants** such as alcohol, barbiturates, and tranquilizers.

Drug/lab test interactions: Chloral hydrate may interfere with the **copper sulfate test** for glycosuria, **fluorometric tests** for urine catecholamines, or **urinary 17-hydroxycorticosteroid determinations.**

ADVERSE REACTIONS

CNS: Occasionally a patient becomes somnambulistic, disoriented, and incoherent and shows paranoid behavior. Rarely, excitement, tolerance, addiction, delirium, drowsiness, staggering gait, ataxia, lightheadedness, vertigo, dizziness, nightmares, malaise, mental confusion, and hallucinations are reported.

Hematologic: Leukopenia and eosinophilia occasionally occur.

Dermatologic: Allergic skin rashes including hives, erythema, eczematoid dermatitis, urticaria, and scarlatiniform exanthema are occasionally seen.

GI: Gastric irritation or GI upset, nausea, vomiting, flatulence, diarrhea, unpleasant or bad taste.

Other: *Rarely*—headache, hangover, idiosyncratic syndrome, ketonuria.

OVERDOSAGE

Symptoms: Symptoms resemble those of barbiturate overdosage and especially affect the CNS and cardiovascular systems. They may include hypothermia; pinpoint pupils; hypotension; comatose state; and slow, rapid, shallow breathing. Gastric irritation may result in vomiting and even gastric necrosis. If patient survives, icterus due to hepatic damage and albuminuria from renal irritation may appear. Toxic oral dose of chloral hydrate for adults is approximately 10 g but death has been reported from a dose of 4 g. Some patients have survived after taking as much as 30 g.

Treatment: Perform gastric lavage or induce vomiting to empty stomach. Supportive measures may be used. Hemodialysis has been reported to be effective.

DOSAGE

CHLORAL HYDRATE

Adults: Single or daily dose should not exceed 2 g. *Hypnotic*—500 mg to 1 g 15 to 30 minutes before retiring. *Sedative*—250 mg tid after meals.

Children: *Hypnotic*—50 mg/kg, up to 1 g per single dose. May be given in divided doses. *Sedative*—½ the hypnotic dose.

TRICLOFOS SODIUM

Hypnotic dose: 1500 mg 15 to 30 minutes before retiring.

Sleep induction in electroencephalography (children under 12): 0.22 ml/kg (0.1 ml/lb). Except for sleep induction in electroencephalography, use is not recommended in children.

NURSING IMPLICATIONS

HISTORY

See Appendix 4.

PHYSICAL ASSESSMENT

Determine whether specific factors that may be controlled or eliminated are interfering with sleep. Such factors may include noise, bright lights, pain, and discomfort.

ADMINISTRATION

Patient's immediate area should be free from disturbance (*e.g.,* noise, lights) before drug is given.

Do not administer if patient has pain, which should be controlled by administration of an analgesic. *Exception*—Use of chloral hydrate as an adjunct to opiates and analgesics.

Chloral hydrate capsules are taken with a full glass of water, swallowed whole, and not chewed or bitten. The syrup or elixir may be administered in a half glass of water, fruit juice, or ginger ale.

Chloral hydrate suppositories: Check patient ½ hour after suppository is inserted to be sure suppository has been retained.

When drug is used as a hypnotic, raise siderails and advise patient to remain in bed and call for assistance if it is necessary to get out of bed during the night.

ONGOING ASSESSMENTS AND NURSING MANAGEMENT

Observe patient in approximately 1 hour for effect of drug (hypnosis or sedation). If drug fails to produce sleep or sedation (depending on reason for use), inform physician. Another drug may be necessary.

If paradoxical excitement occurs, observe patient closely until effect of drug has worn off. In some instances, restraints may be necessary to protect patient from injury. Inform physician of occurrence because a different drug or lower dosage may be necessary.

If extreme morning sedation (after H.S. hypnotic dose) is noted, inform physician.

Observe for adverse reactions.

Patient receiving oral (coumarin, coumarin-related) anticoagulants and chloral hydrate may require adjustment of anticoagulant dosage (see *Warnings*). Upon withdrawal of chloral hydrate, observe for bleeding tendency and hemorrhage.

PATIENT AND FAMILY INFORMATION

Chlorate hydrate may cause GI upset. Take capsules with a full glass of water. Swallow capsules whole; do not chew or bite the capsule. Dilute syrup or elixir with ½ glass of water, fruit juice, or ginger ale. Inform physician if gastric irritation or upset occurs.

May cause drowsiness. Do not drive or engage in hazardous tasks after taking drug. Hypnotic use: It is advisable to remain in bed once drug is taken for sleep.

Do not drink alcohol before or after taking this drug because the combination can be dangerous.

Avoid use of CNS depressants.

May be habit forming. Take only as prescribed. Do not increase dose except on advice of a physician.

Notify physician or nurse if excessive morning drowsiness, headache, or skin rash occurs or if drug is ineffective in producing sleep.

Chloral Hydrate

See Chloral Derivatives.

Chlorambucil Rx

tablets: 2 mg   Leukeran

INDICATIONS

Treatment of chronic lymphocytic leukemia, malignant lymphomas including lymphosarcoma, giant follicular lymphoma, and Hodgkin's disease. Produces remission in a substantial proportion of patients.

CONTRAINDICATIONS

Not given within 4 weeks of a full course of radiation therapy or chemotherapy because of vulnerability of bone marrow to damage under these conditions. Small doses of palliative radiation over iso-

C

lated foci remote from bone marrow will not usually depress the neutrophil and platelet counts; in these cases chlorambucil may be given. Full dosage is not given when bone marrow is infiltrated with lymphomatous tissue or is hypoplastic as a result of long-standing and extensively treated disease.

ACTIONS

A derivative of nitrogen mustard; a potent drug. It is easier than nitrogen mustard and some related drugs to handle because it produces fewer side-effects and is not damaging to the hematopoietic system in therapeutic doses. Appears to be relatively free from GI effects or other evidence of toxicity apart from the bone-marrow depressant action.

Chlorambucil is a cell-cycle nonspecific drug that interacts with cellular DNA to produce a cytotoxic cross-linkage. It is absorbed following oral administration. Plasma half-life is approximately 90 minutes. In 24 hours after administration, 60% of drug is excreted in the urine; approximately 40% is tissue bound. Fat storage may occur due to drug's lipophilic properties.

See also Appendix 10.

WARNINGS

Excessive or prolonged dosage will produce severe bone-marrow depression. Blood counts are recommended once or twice weekly. Discontinue drug or reduce dosage upon evidence of abnormal depression of the bone marrow.

Use in pregnancy: May be mutagenic and embryotoxic. Avoid use during first trimester, if at all possible.

PRECAUTIONS

Bone-marrow damage: Patients must be followed carefully to avoid irreversible damage to the bone marrow. Weekly examination of blood is recommended to determine hemoglobin levels and total and differential leukocyte counts. During the first 3 to 6 weeks of therapy, it is recommended that white blood cell counts (WBCs) be taken 3 to 4 days after each weekly complete blood count (CBC). Many patients develop a slowly progressive lymphopenia during treatment. The lymphocyte count usually returns rapidly to normal levels on completion of therapy. Most patients have some neutropenia after the third week of therapy, which may continue for up to 10 days after the last dose; the neutrophil count usually rapidly returns to normal. Severe neutropenia appears to be dose related. Drug is not discontinued at the first sign of a fall in the neutrophil count; decreases may continue for 10 days after the last dose is given.

DRUG INTERACTIONS

Drug/lab tests: **Serum** and **urine uric acid** levels may be increased during therapy.

ADVERSE REACTIONS

Bone-marrow depression (see *Precautions*) and hyperuricemia are the major adverse effects.

DOSAGE

Initial and short courses of therapy: Usual dose is 0.1 mg/kg/day to 0.2 mg/kg/day for 3 to 6 weeks as required (4 mg/day to 10 mg/day for average patient). Entire daily dose may be given at one time. Adjust dosage to response of patient and reduce it immediately if there is an abrupt fall in the WBC. Patients with Hodgkin's disease usually require 0.2 mg/kg/day, whereas those with lymphomas or chronic lymphocytic leukemia usually require 0.1 mg/kg/day. When lymphocytic infiltration of bone marrow is present or bone marrow is hypoplastic, do not exceed 0.1 mg/kg/day (about 6 mg for average patient).

Short courses of treatment are safer than continuous maintenance therapy, although both methods have been effective.

Maintenance therapy: If maintenance dosage is used, 0.1 mg/kg/day should not be exceeded. Dose may be as low as 0.03 mg/kg/day (usually 2 mg/day to 4 mg/day or less).

NURSING IMPLICATIONS

HISTORY
See Appendix 4.

PHYSICAL ASSESSMENT
Obtain vital signs, weight, general physical and emotional status. Baseline laboratory studies usually include CBC, serum uric acid, liver-function tests. Other studies may be performed, depending on diagnosis.

ADMINISTRATION
Entire daily dose may be given at one time; give at same time each day.

ONGOING ASSESSMENTS AND NURSING MANAGEMENT
Obtain vital signs q4h; obtain weight; observe for signs of hepatic toxicity (jaundice, dark urine). Observe for signs of bone-marrow depression (Appendix 6, section 6-8). If one or more signs occur, notify physician immediately.

Place on intake and output. Have patient drink at least 10 to 12 glasses (8 oz each) of fluid each day. Provide water as well as other fluids (*e.g.,* gelatin, juices, carbonated beverages) according to patient's preference. If fluid intake is not sufficient, remind patient hourly to drink fluids.

Rarely, nausea and vomiting may occur. A liquid diet, cola syrup, dry crackers, or carbonated beverages may be used. If nausea persists, contact physician because an antiemetic may be necessary.

Periodic blood counts (see *Precautions*) are made to avoid irreversible bone-marrow damage.

Physician may chart blood counts on a chart or graph and at the same time record body weight, temperature, spleen size. A summary of patient's present status may also be included.

PATIENT AND FAMILY INFORMATION

NOTE: Therapy is often on an outpatient basis. Strict patient compliance is necessary. Physician should explain expected results, possible adverse effects of therapy and tests necessary to monitor therapy.

Take drug as directed by physician; follow instructions carefully.

Notify physician or nurse if unusual bleeding or bruising, fever, chills, sore throat, cough, shortness of breath, flank or stomach pain, joint pain, sores in the mouth or on the lips, or yellow discoloration of skin or eyes occurs.

Medication may cause nausea, vomiting, skin rash, aching, or hair loss. Notify physician or nurse if these become pronounced.

Drink at least 10 to 12 glasses (8 oz each) of fluid each day. Gelatin, ice cream, and carbonated beverages as well as water count as fluid.

Contraceptive measures are recommended during therapy. Discuss method of contraception with physician.

Frequent monitoring of therapy is necessary. Physician will order laboratory tests and possibly other diagnostic studies during as well as after therapy.

Inform other physicians and dentist of therapy with this drug.

Vaccinations, flu shots, and immunizations are not recommended during therapy.

Chloramphenicol* Rx

capsules: 250 mg	Chloromycetin Kapseals, Mychel, *Generic*
capsules: 500 mg	*Generic*
oral suspension: 150 mg/5 ml	Chloromycetin Palmitate

* For other preparations of chloramphenicol, see Antibiotics, ophthalmic; Antibiotics, topical; Otic preparations.

powder for injection: 100 mg/ml	Chloromycetin Sodium Succinate, Mychel-S, *Generic*

INDICATIONS

Use only in serious infections for which less potentially dangerous drugs are ineffective or contraindicated. May be chosen to initiate antibiotic therapy if one or more of the conditions listed below is believed present. Sensitivity tests are performed concurrently so that drug may be discontinued as soon as possible if less potentially dangerous agents are indicated.

May be prescribed for acute infections caused by *Salmonella typhi* and is drug of choice. Not recommended for routine treatment of typhoid "carrier state." Also may be prescribed for acute infections caused by susceptible strains of *Salmonella* species; *Hemophilus influenzae,* specifically meningeal infections; rickettsia; lymphogranuloma-psittacosis group; various gram-negative bacteria causing bacteremia, meningitis, or other serious gram-negative infection; other susceptible organisms that have demonstrated to be resistant to all other appropriate antimicrobial agents. May also be included in cystic fibrosis regimens.

CONTRAINDICATIONS

History of hypersensitivity or toxicity to chloramphenicol. Must not be used in treatment of trivial infections or infections other than those indicated or as a prophylactic agent to prevent bacterial infections.

ACTIONS

Mode of action is interference or inhibition of protein synthesis. Exerts mainly a bacteriostatic effect on a wide range of gram-negative and gram-positive bacteria and is active against rickettsias, the lymphogranuloma-psittacosis group, and *Vibrio cholerae.* It is particularly active against *S. typhi* and *H. influenzae.*

Is absorbed rapidly from intestinal tract. Recommended therapeutic range is 5 mcg/ml to 20 mcg/ml (may be lower in neonates). Drug is approximately 50% bound to plasma proteins. Chloramphenicol diffuses rapidly, but distribution is not uniform. Highest concentrations are found in liver and kidney, lowest in brain and CSF. Measurable levels are also found in pleural and ascitic fluids, saliva, milk, and aqueous and vitreous humors. Transport across placental barrier occurs. Drug is excreted in the urine.

WARNINGS

Serious and fatal blood dyscrasias (aplastic anemia, hypoplastic anemia, thrombocytopenia, granulocytopenia) are known to occur after administration of chloramphenicol. There have been reports of aplastic anemia, which later terminated in leukemia, attributed to this drug. Blood dyscrasias have occurred after both short-term and prolonged therapy. This drug must not be used when less potentially dangerous agents are effective. It is essential that adequate blood studies be made during treatment. Although blood studies may detect early peripheral blood changes (_e.g.,_ leukopenia, reticulocytopenia, granulocytopenia) before they become irreversible, such studies cannot be relied on to detect bone-marrow depression prior to development of aplastic anemia. To facilitate appropriate studies and observation during therapy, it is desirable that patients be hospitalized.

Use in pregnancy and lactation: Safety not established. Drug readily crosses placental barrier; use cautiously during pregnancy at term or during labor because of potential toxic effects on fetus (gray syndrome). Chloramphenicol is secreted in breast milk; use caution during lactation because of possible toxic effects in the nursing infant.

Use in infants: Use with caution in premature and full-term infants to avoid gray syndrome toxicity (see _Adverse Reactions_). Drug serum levels should be carefully followed.

PRECAUTIONS

Hematology: Baseline blood studies should be followed by periodic blood studies approximately every 2 days during therapy. Discontinue drug upon appearance of reticulocytopenia, leukopenia, thrombocytopenia, anemia, or any other blood-study findings. Concurrent therapy with other drugs that may cause bone-marrow depression is avoided. Repeated courses are avoided if at all possible. Treatment is not continued longer than required.

Use in impaired hepatic or renal function: Excessive blood levels may result from use of recommended dosages in those with impaired liver or kidney function. Adjust dosage accordingly in these patients.

Use with caution in those with acute intermittent porphyria or glucose-6-phosphate dehydrogenase deficiency.

Superinfection: Use of antibiotics (especially prolonged or repeated therapy) may result in bacterial or fungal overgrowth of nonsusceptible organisms. Such overgrowth may lead to a secondary infection.

DRUG INTERACTIONS

Chloramphenicol inhibits metabolism of **dicumarol, phenytoin, phenobarbital, tolbutamide, chlorpropamide, cyclophosphamide.** The half-life of these drugs may be prolonged and their pharmacologic effects enhanced. Because cyclophosphamide's activity

may be mediated through active metabolites, its therapeutic value may be theoretically reduced. Elevated serum levels may occur with concurrent administration of **acetaminophen;** the dosage of chloramphenicol may need to be reduced. Hematologic response to **iron salts** and **vitamin B$_{12}$** may be decreased. Concurrent administration with **penicillin** may decrease penicillin's effect and increase the half-life of chloramphenicol.

ADVERSE REACTIONS

Blood dyscrasias: Most serious adverse effect is bone-marrow depression (see _Warnings_). An irreversible type of marrow depression leading to aplastic anemia with a high rate of mortality is characterized by appearance of bone-marrow aplasia or hypoplasia weeks or months after therapy. Peripherally, pancytopenia is most often observed. A dose-related reversible type of bone-marrow depression may occur.

_GI:_ Nausea, vomiting, glossitis and stomatitis, diarrhea, or enterocolitis may occur in low incidence.

CNS: Headache, mild depression, mental confusion, and delirium. Optic and peripheral neuritis have been reported, usually following long-term use.

Hypersensitivity: Fever, macular and vesicular rashes, angioedema, urticaria, or anaphylaxis may occur.

Gray syndrome: Toxic reactions including fatalities have occurred in the premature and newborn; signs and symptoms associated with these reactions are referred to as the _gray syndrome._ In most cases, therapy was instituted within the first 48 hours of life; symptoms first appeared after 3 to 4 days of treatment with high doses. Symptoms appear in the following order: abdominal distention with or without emesis; progressive pallid cyanosis; vasomotor collapse frequently accompanied by irregular respiration; death within a few hours of onset of symptoms. The progression of symptoms was accelerated with higher doses. Termination of therapy upon early evidence of the associated symptoms frequently reversed the process with complete recovery.

DOSAGE

Majority of organisms susceptible to chloramphenicol will respond to a concentration between 5 mcg/ml and 20 mcg/ml.

Adults: 50 mg/kg/day in divided doses q6h. Exceptional infections due to moderately resistant organisms may require up to 100 mg/kg/day.

Impaired hepatic or renal function: Dosages adjusted and based on drug concentrations in blood.

Children: 50 mg/kg/day in divided doses q6h; severe infections may require up to 100 mg/kg/day.

Newborn infants (see *Gray syndrome* under *Adverse Reactions*): 25 mg/kg/day in divided doses q12h usually produces therapeutic concentrations. After first 2 weeks of life, full-term infants ordinarily may receive 50 mg/kg/day in divided doses q12h. These dosage recommendations are extremely important because blood concentration in all premature and full-term infants under 2 weeks differs from that of other infants, owing to variations in maturity of the metabolic functions of the liver and kidneys.

Infants and children with immature metabolic processes: 25 mg/kg/day. In this group, the concentration of the drug in the blood should be carefully followed.

IV administration: Chloramphenicol sodium succinate is intended for IV use *only;* it is ineffective if given IM. Dosage same as for oral form.

NURSING IMPLICATIONS

HISTORY
See Appendix 4. If patient has salmonellal infection, inquiry is usually necessary to determine possible source of infection.

PHYSICAL ASSESSMENT
Record vital signs, weight; review recent laboratory and diagnostic studies. Additional assessments should be based on diagnosis and patient's symptoms. Baseline studies may include CBC (including differential) and platelet count. Heptic- and renal-function studies may also be ordered.

ADMINISTRATION
Culture and sensitivity studies performed prior to institution of therapy.

Oral: Give on empty stomach at least 1 hour before or 2 hours after meals. Drug usually given q6h; therefore, select administration times according to meal schedule.

If GI upset occurs, drug may be taken with food.

Parenteral: Administered *IV only* as a 10% solution injected over at least 1 minute (in infants and small children a slower rate of injection may be preferred by physician). Prepare by adding 10 ml of aqueous diluent (*e.g.,* Water for Injection or 5% Dextrose Injection), giving a dose of 100 mg/ml.

ONGOING ASSESSMENTS AND PATIENT MANAGEMENT
Record vital signs q4h; measure intake and output; observe for adverse reactions. Look for signs of improvement (*e.g.,* response to antibiotic therapy); record observations.

Laboratory monitoring of serum levels is recommended; a concentration between 5 mcg/ml and 20 mcg/ml is desirable.

Blood studies every 2 days are recommended during therapy; notify physician immediately if recent blood studies are abnormal.

CLINICAL ALERT: Observe for signs of bone-marrow depression (Appendix 6, section 6-8). If one or more signs or symptoms occur, contact physician immediately.

Observe premature and newborn infants receiving this drug for symptoms of gray syndrome (see *Adverse Reactions*); if any of these should occur, contact physician immediately.

Observe for signs of superinfection (Appendix 6, section 6-22); notify physician immediately if one or more signs or symptoms occur.

Notify physician if there is any change in the intake–output ratio.

Diabetics receiving tolbutamide, chlorpropamide: Pharmacologic effects of these drugs may be enhanced. Physician may decrease dose and monitor blood glucose during therapy with chloramphenicol. Report any changes in urine test results (glucose, ketone bodies) to physician.

PATIENT AND FAMILY INFORMATION
NOTE: Occasionally drug may be prescribed for short-term therapy following hospitalization.

Preferably, take on empty stomach at least 1 hour before or 2 hours after meals. Take with food only if GI upset occurs.

Take at evenly paced intervals (every 6 hours) around the clock, or as ordered by the physician.

Notify physician or nurse immediately if fever, sore throat, tiredness, or unusual bleeding or bruising occurs.

Physician may order follow-up laboratory tests at frequent intervals to monitor therapy.

Food handlers with salmonellal infection may not return to work until physician is sure infection has cleared and is not transmittable to others.

Chlordiazepoxide

See Benzodiazepines.

Chlorhexidine Gluconate

See Antiseptics and Germicides.

Chlormezanone Rx

| tablets: 100 mg | Trancopal Caplets |
| tablets: 200 mg | Trancopal Caplets, *Generic* |

INDICATIONS
Treatment of mild anxiety and tension states.

CONTRAINDICATIONS
Hypersensitivity.

ACTIONS
Improves emotional state by allaying mild anxiety, usually without impairing clarity of consciousness. Mechanism of action is unknown. Relief of symptoms often apparent 15 to 30 minutes after administration; may last up to 6 or more hours.

WARNINGS
Should drowsiness occur, dosage may be reduced. Safety for use in pregnancy and lactation not established. Use only when clearly needed and potential benefits outweigh the unknown potential hazards to the fetus.

DRUG INTERACTIONS
Possible additive effects may occur when taken with **alcohol** or other **CNS depressants.**

ADVERSE REACTIONS
Drug rash, dizziness, flushing, nausea, drowsiness, depression, edema, inability to void, dry mouth, weakness, excitement, tremor, confusion, headache. Chlolestatic jaundice has occurred rarely but was reversible on discontinuance.

DOSAGE
Adults: Usual dose is 200 mg tid or qid; in some, 100 mg may suffice.

Children (5–12 years): 50 mg to 100 mg tid or qid. Because the effect of CNS drugs varies, treatment, particularly in children, should begin with the lowest dosage possible; this may then be increased as needed.

NURSING IMPLICATIONS

HISTORY
See Appendix 4.

PHYSICAL ASSESSMENT
Monitor vital signs, weight; observe overt symptoms (if present).

ADMINISTRATION
If nausea occurs, check with physician as to whether drug can be administered with food.

ONGOING ASSESSMENTS AND NURSING MANAGEMENT
Assess patient's response to drug; if anxiety appears to persist or become more intense, notify the physician.

Observe for adverse drug effects; some adverse effects may require decrease in dosage or discontinuance of drug.

If drowsiness occurs, patient may require assistance with ambulation; if excessive drowsiness, slurred speech, or lethargy occurs, contact physician.

Weigh weekly because anxiety may cause an increase or decrease in appetite.

If drug is administered over a long period of time, dose should be tapered and patient observed for return of symptoms of anxiety.

Should not be administered to those with a history of drug abuse.

PATIENT AND FAMILY INFORMATION
Drug may impair mental or physical abilities required for performance of potentially hazardous tasks such as driving or operating machinery.

Avoid alcohol while taking drug.

Some nonprescription drugs (*e.g.,* cough medications) may contain alcohol. Check with a pharmacist about alcohol content before purchasing nonprescription drugs.

Dry mouth may be relieved by frequent sips of water, ice chips, gum.

Notify physician or nurse if skin rash, sore throat, or fever occurs, or if there is difficulty in voiding.

Do not increase prescribed dose. If symptoms are not relieved, discuss problem with physician.

Chloroprocaine Hydrochloride

See Anesthetics, Local, Injectable.

Chloroquine Hydrochloride

See 4-Aminoquinoline Compounds.

Chloroquine Phosphate

See 4-Aminoquinoline Compounds.

Chlorothiazide

See Thiazides and Related Diuretics.

Chlorotrianisene

See Estrogens.

Chlorphenesin Carbamate Rx

tablets: 400 mg (contains tartrazine)   Maolate

INDICATIONS

Adjunct to rest, physical therapy, and other measures for relief of discomfort associated with acute, painful musculoskeletal conditions.

CONTRAINDICATIONS

Hypersensitivity.

ACTIONS

Mode of action not identified but may be related to drug's sedative properties. Has no direct action on striated muscle, the motor endplate, or the nerve fiber. Readily absorbed from GI tract. Maximum serum concentration attained 1 to 3 hours after administration. Biological half-life is approximately 3.5 hours; is rapidly excreted in the urine.

WARNINGS

May impair mental or physical alertness. Safety for use in pregnancy not established. Use during pregnancy, in the nursing mother, or in women who may become pregnant only when clearly needed and when potential benefits outweigh the potential hazards. Safety and efficacy for use in children not established.

PRECAUTIONS

Safe use for periods exceeding 8 weeks not established. Use with caution in those with preexisting liver disease or impaired liver funtion. Liver-function studies as well as blood counts should be considered for patients receiving this drug.

This product contains tartrazine (see Appendix 6, section 6-23).

ADVERSE REACTIONS

Hematopoietic: Rarely, leukopenia, thrombocytopenia, agranulocytosis, pancytopenia.

Hypersensitivity: Anaphylactoid reactions and drug fever have been observed occasionally. Such reactions are an indication for discontinuing medication.

Miscellaneous: Drowsiness, dizziness, confusion, nausea, epigastric distress. Occasionally, paradoxical excitation, insomnia, increased nervousness, and headache have been reported. Dose reduction usually controls these symptoms.

OVERDOSAGE

Dangerous side-effects from accidental overdosage appear unlikely.

Treatment: Vomiting may be induced or gastric lavage or saline catharsis employed. Supportive therapy should suffice in most instances.

DOSAGE

Initially, 800 mg tid until desired effect is obtained. May be reduced to 400 mg qid, or less, as required for maintenance.

NURSING IMPLICATIONS

HISTORY
See Appendix 4.

PHYSICAL ASSESSMENT
Evaluate limitations imposed by musculoskeletal disorder (*e.g.,* walking, sitting, movement or use of limb). Baseline laboratory tests may include liver-function studies, CBC.

ADMINISTRATION
If nausea occurs, check with physician as to whether drug can be given with food or meals.

ONGOING ASSESSMENTS AND NURSING MANAGEMENT
Rest, physical therapy, and other measures may also be part of therapeutic regimen.

If drowsiness or dizziness occurs, assist with ambulation. Notify physician before next dose is due if drowsiness is excessive.

PATIENT AND FAMILY INFORMATION
May cause drowsiness or dizziness. Observe caution while driving or performing other tasks requiring alertness.

Avoid alcohol and other CNS depressants. Do not use nonprescription preparations (*e.g.,* liquid cough medications) that contain alcohol. If there is doubt about whether a product contains alcohol, check with a pharmacist.

Notify physician or nurse if any of the following occurs: easy bruising, unusual bleeding, fever, chills, sore throat, sores in the mouth or on lips.

Contact physician if condition persists.

Chlorpheniramine Maleate

See Antihistamines.

Chlorpromazine Hydrochloride

See Antiemetic/Antivertigo Agents; Antipsychotic Agents.

Chlorpropamide

See Sulfonylureas.

Chlorprothixene

See Antipsychotic Agents.

Chlortetracycline

See Antibiotics, Topical.

Chlorthalidone

See Thiazides and Related Diuretics.

Chlorzoxazone Rx

tablets: 250 mg   Paraflex, *Generic*

INDICATIONS
Adjunct to rest, physical therapy, and other measures for the relief of discomfort associated with acute, painful musculoskeletal conditions.

CONTRAINDICATIONS
Intolerance to chlorzoxazone.

ACTIONS
A centrally acting skeletal muscle relaxant. Mode of action may be related to its sedative properties. Acts primarily at the level of the spinal cord and subcortical areas of the brain by inhibiting multisynaptic reflex arcs involved in producing and maintaining skeletal muscle spasm of varied etiology. Skeletal muscle spasm is reduced with relief of pain and increased mobility of the involved muscles. Drug does not directly relax tense skeletal muscles. Serum levels can be detected during the first hour after administration and peak in 3 to 4 hours. Half-life is approximately 60 minutes. It is rapidly metabolized and excreted in the urine.

WARNINGS
Safety for use in pregnancy not established. Use only when clearly needed and when potential benefits outweigh the unknown potential hazards.

PRECAUTIONS
Use with caution in patients with known allergies or a history of allergic drug reactions. If a sensitivity reaction occurs, such as urticaria, redness, or itching, discontinue use.

Hepatic effects: If signs and symptoms of liver dysfunction are observed, discontinue drug.

DRUG INTERACTIONS
Concomitant use of **alcohol** or other **CNS depressants** may have an additive effect.

ADVERSE REACTIONS
GI: GI disturbances; rarely, GI bleeding.

CNS: Drowsiness, dizziness, lightheadedness, malaise, overstimulation.

Dermatologic: Allergic-type skin rashes; petechiae or ecchymosis occurs rarely.

Hypersensitivity: Skin rashes, angioneurotic edema, and anaphylaxis are very rare.

Hepatic: Is suspected to have caused liver damage in a few patients.

Miscellaneous: Urine discoloration.

OVERDOSAGE
Symptoms: Initially, GI disturbances such as nausea, vomiting, or diarrhea together with drowsiness, dizziness, lightheadedness, or headache may occur. Early there may be malaise or sluggishness followed by marked loss of muscle tone, making voluntary movement impossible. Deep tendon reflexes may be decreased or absent. The sensorium remains intact and there is no peripheral loss of sensation. Respiratory depression may occur with rapid, irregular respiration and intercostal and substernal retraction. The blood pressure is lowered, but shock has not been observed.

Treatment: Employ gastric lavage or induce emesis, followed by activated charcoal. Thereafter, treatment is supportive. If respirations are depressed, employ oxygen and artificial respiration and assure a patent airway. Hypotension may be counteracted by use of plasma volume expanders or vasopressors. Cholinergic drugs or analeptic drugs are of no value and should not be used.

DOSAGE
Adults: 250 mg tid or qid. Initial dosage for painful musculoskeletal conditions is 500 mg tid or qid. If adequate response is not obtained, dosage may be increased to 750 mg tid or qid. As improvement occurs, dosage may be reduced.

Children: 125 mg to 500 mg tid or qid, according to age and weight.

NURSING IMPLICATIONS

HISTORY
See Appendix 4.

CLINICAL ALERT: If patient has known allergies or a history of allergic drug reactions, discuss this fact with the physician (see *Precautions*) before first dose is administered.

PHYSICAL ASSESSMENT
Evaluate limitations imposed by musculoskeletal disorder (*e.g.,* walking, sitting, movement or use of a limb).

ADMINISTRATION
May be given with food or meals if GI upset occurs.

Paraflex and Parafon (chlorzoxazone with acetaminophen).

ONGOING ASSESSMENTS AND NURSING MANAGEMENT
Evaluate response to drug daily; observe for allergic-type skin reactions, hypersensitivity reactions. Withhold next dose of drug and notify physician if these should occur.

Rest, physical therapy, and other measures may also be part of therapeutic regimen.

If drowsiness or dizziness occurs, assist with ambulation. Notify physician before next dose is due if drowsiness is excessive.

Although rare, liver damage has occurred. Observe for signs of hepatitis (*e.g.,* fever, malaise, jaundice [skin, sclera], pruritus, dark urine).

PATIENT AND FAMILY INFORMATION
Drug may be taken with food or meals if GI upset occurs. Notify physician or nurse if skin rash or itching occurs.

May cause drowsiness, dizziness, lightheadedness; observe caution while driving or performing other tasks requiring alertness. Avoid alcohol and other CNS depressants.

May discolor urine orange or purple-red.

Contact physician if condition persists.

Cholera Vaccine

See Immunizations, Active.

Cholestyramine

See Bile Acid Sequestrants.

Choline Salicylate

See Salicylates.

Chorionic Gonadotropin

(Human Chorionic Gonadotropin, HCG) Rx

powder for injection: 200 units/ml	Glukor
powder for injection: 5000 units/ml	A.P.L. Secules, Chorex, Corgonject-5, Profasi HP, *Generic*
powder for injection: 10,000 units/ml	Android-HCG, A.P.L. Secules, Chorex, Follutein, Gonic, Libigen, Pregnyl, Profasi HP, *Generic*
powder for injection: 20,000 units/ml	A.P.L. Secules, *Generic*

INDICATIONS
Prepubertal cryptorchidism not due to anatomic obstruction. HCG is thought to induce testicular descent in situations when descent would have occurred at puberty. HCG may help predict whether orchiopexy will be needed in the future. In some cases, descent following HCG administration is permanent, but in most cases, response is temporary. Therapy is usually instituted between the ages of 4 and 9.

Selected cases of hypogonadotropic hypogonadism (hypogonadism secondary to a pituitary deficiency) in males.

Induction of ovulation and pregnancy in the anovulatory woman when cause of anovulation is secondary and not due to primary ovarian failure and when woman has been appropriately pretreated with human menotropins.

HCG has *not* been demonstrated to be effective adjunctive therapy in treatment of obesity.

CONTRAINDICATIONS
Precocious puberty, prostatic carcinoma, or other androgen-dependent neoplasm; prior allergic reaction to HCG.

ACTIONS
HCG, a polypeptide hormone produced by the human placenta, is composed of an alpha and beta subunit. The alpha subunit is essentially identical to the alpha subunits of the human pituitary gonadotropins, luteinizing hormone (LH) and follicle-stimulating hormone (FSH), as well as the alpha subunit of human thyroid-stimulating hormone (TSH). The action of HCG is virtually identical to that of pituitary LH, although HCG appears to have a small degree of FSH activity as well. It stimulates production of gonadal steroid hormones by stimulating the interstitial cells (Leydig cells) of the testes to produce androgens and the corpus luteum of the ovary to produce progesterone. Androgen stimulation in the male leads to the development of secondary sex characteristics and may stimulate testicular descent when no anatomic impediment to descent is present. The descent is usually reversible when HCG is discontinued. During the normal menstrual cycle, LH participates with FSH in the development and maturation of the normal ovarian follicle, and the midcycle LH surge triggers ovulation. HCG can substantially substitute for LH in this function. During a normal pregnancy, HCG secreted by the

placenta maintains the corpus luteum after LH secretion decreases, supporting continued secretion of estrogen and progesterone and preventing menstruation.

WARNINGS
Use with caution in conjunction with human menopausal gonadotropins. The principal serious adverse reactions experienced with this indication are ovarian hyperstimulation, a syndrome of sudden ovarian enlargement, ascites with or without pain and pleural effusion, rupture of ovarian cysts with resultant hemoperitoneum, multiple births, and arterial thromboembolism.

PRECAUTIONS
May induce precocious puberty in those treated for cryptorchidism; discontinue use if this occurs. May cause fluid retention and should be used with caution in patients with epilepsy, migraine, or cardiac or renal disease. Not recommended for hypogonadism of testicular origin.

ADVERSE REACTIONS
Headache, irritability, restlessness, fatigue, edema, precocious puberty, gynecomastia, pain at site of injection.

DOSAGE
For IM use only. Dosage regimens may vary but the following have been recommended.

Prepubertal cryptorchidism not due to anatomical obstruction: (1) 4000 units 3 times weekly for 3 weeks; (2) 5000 units every second day for 4 injections; (3) 15 injections of 500 to 1000 units over a period of 6 weeks; (4) 500 units 3 times weekly for 4 to 6 weeks and, if not successful, another course 1 month later giving 1000 units per injection.

Selected cases of hypogonadotropic hypogonadism in males: (1) 500 to 1000 units 3 times a week for 3 weeks, followed by same dose twice a week for 3 weeks; (2) 4000 units 3 times weekly for 6 to 9 months; dosage reduced to 2000 units 3 times weekly for an additional 3 months.

Use with menotropins: After pretreatment with HCG, menotropins may be administered to stimulate spermatogenesis (see Menotropins). Recommended HCG dosage is 5000 units 3 times weekly for 4 to 6 months. With beginning of menotropin therapy, HCG dose is continued at 2000 units twice weekly.

Induction of ovulation and pregnancy: After pretreatment with menotropins, 5000 to 10,000 units 1 day following last dose of menotropins.

NURSING IMPLICATIONS

HISTORY AND PHYSICAL ASSESSMENT
Performed by physician; review patient's chart. Obtain weight, blood pressure.

ADMINISTRATION
Diluent may be supplied by manufacturer. Refer to package insert for preparation and storage of drug.

For IM use only. Advise patient of pain at injection site.

Rotate injection sites; record site used.

ONGOING ASSESSMENTS AND NURSING MANAGEMENT
Drug usually administered in outpatient setting.

Weigh patient and obtain blood pressure before drug is administered. Inform physician if weight gain or edema is noted.

Inspect previous injection sites for signs of redness, induration.

PATIENT AND FAMILY INFORMATION
NOTE: Treatment regimen, results expected, and possible adverse effects are explained by physician prior to institution of therapy.

Headache, irritability, depression, or fatigue may be noted. If these become pronounced, discuss with physician.

If swelling of extremities or weight gain is noted, inform physician.

When prescribed for induction of ovulation and pregnancy: Follow physician's recommendations about timing of intercourse. Following course of treatment, contact physician if thought to be pregnant or if vaginal bleeding or abdominal pain or distention occurs.

When prescribed for cryptorchidism: Physician will examine child for evidence of precocious puberty during treatment. Inform physician if acne; growth of facial, axillary, and pubic hair; or penile enlargement is apparent.

Chromic Phosphate P 32 Rx

suspension: 10 mCi   Phosphocol P 32
or 15 mCi

INDICATIONS
Intracavity instillation for treatment of peritoneal or pleural effusions caused by metastatic disease. Interstitial injection for treatment of cancer.

CONTRAINDICATIONS
Not used in presence of ulcerative tumors or administered in exposed cavities or where there is evi-

dence of loculation (division into small cavities) unless extent of loculation is determined.

ACTIONS
Local irradiation by beta emission.

WARNINGS
Not for intravascular use. Use in pregnancy and lactation only when clearly needed and when potential benefits outweigh the potential hazards to the fetus.

PRECAUTIONS
Radioactive material. Care must be taken to ensure minimum radiation exposure to patient and medical personnel.

ADVERSE REACTIONS
Transitory radiation sickness, bone-marrow depression, pleuritis, peritonitis, nausea, abdominal cramping.

DOSAGE
Dosage determined by radioactivity calibration system immediately prior to administration.

Interstitial use: Dosage based on estimated gram weight of tumor.

PHYSICAL CHARACTERISTICS
Phosphorus 32 (P 32) decays by beta emission with a physical half-life of 14.3 days.

NURSING IMPLICATIONS

HISTORY
See Appendix 4.

PHYSICAL ASSESSMENT
Evaluate physical and mental status; identify immediate patient needs.

ADMINISTRATION
Administered by a physician.

ONGOING ASSESSMENTS AND NURSING MANAGEMENT
Hospital protocol for management of patient receiving radiopharmaceuticals is developed by department of radiology or nuclear medicine. Protocol usually includes type of isolation necessary; disposal of linens, drainage, food, excreta, and other body fluids; time allowed at bedside per day; monitoring of radioactivity.

Patient management is planned so that each member of the health team receives minimum exposure. Radiation badges must be worn.

Observe for adverse reactions; report to physician if nausea or abdominal cramping occurs.

Observe for signs of bone-marrow depression (Appendix 6, section 6-8), other signs of infection. These may occur after treatment.

Monitor vital signs q4h or as ordered by physician. Notify physician of respiratory distress or acute abdominal pain; these may indicate development of pleuritis or peritonitis.

Other assessments and management are based on patient's diagnosis, present physical status, and individual needs.

Ciclopirox Olamine Rx

cream: 1%   Loprox

INDICATIONS
Tinea pedis, tinea cruris, and tinea corporis due to *Trichophyton rubrum, T. mentagrophytes, Epidermophyton floccosum,* and *Microsporum canis;* candidiasis (moniliasis) due to *Candida albicans;* tinea versicolor due to *Malassezia furfur.*

CONTRAINDICATIONS
Hypersensitivity.

ACTIONS
A broad-spectrum, antifungal agent that inhibits growth of pathogenic dermatophytes, yeasts, and *M. furfur.* Exhibits activity against *T. rubrum, T. mentagrophytes, E. floccosum, M. canis, C. albicans.*

WARNINGS
No adequate or well-controlled studies in pregnant women. It is not known whether drug is excreted in human milk. Safety and effectiveness in children under 10 not established.

PRECAUTIONS
If sensitivity or chemical irritation occurs, discontinue treatment.

ADVERSE REACTIONS
Rarely, pruritus.

DOSAGE
Gently massage cream into affected and surrounding areas bid, morning and evening.

NURSING IMPLICATIONS

HISTORY
See Appendix 4.

PHYSICAL ASSESSMENT

Examine and describe lesions; record in patient's chart.

ADMINISTRATION

Prior to application, cleanse with soap and warm water, rinse thoroughly, and gently pat dry, unless directed otherwise by physician.

Gently massage cream into affected and surrounding skin.

Do not use an occlusive dressing unless directed by physician.

ONGOING ASSESSMENTS AND NURSING MANAGEMENT

Inspect lesions at time of each application. If redness, blistering, swelling, or oozing is noted or if patient complains of itching or burning, do not apply next dose and contact physician.

Record appearance of lesions daily. Compare with data base.

Clinical improvement usually occurs within first week of treatment. If no clinical improvement is noted after 4 weeks, physician reevaluates diagnosis. Patients with tinea versicolor usually exhibit clinical and mycologic clearing 2 weeks after treatment.

PATIENT AND FAMILY INFORMATION

Use medication for the full treatment time, even though symptoms may have improved. Notify physician if there is no improvement after 4 weeks.

Inform physician if area of application shows signs of increased irritation (redness, itching, burning, blistering, swelling, oozing) indicative of possible sensitization.

Clean area with soap and warm water, rinse thoroughly, and gently pat dry, unless directed otherwise by physician.

Do not apply dressing or wrapping over the area.

Tinea infections

Keep towels, face cloths, and bedding separate from those of other family members. Launder clothing, linens daily; use hot water and detergent. Do not wash clothes or bedding used by other family members at same time.

Tinea corporis, tinea cruris: Change clothing contacting infected area after each application.

Tinea pedis: Keep feet dry; change socks daily or whenever damp or wet; expose feet to air as much as possible. Follow directions of physician about shoes and care of feet until infection is cleared.

Cimetidine Rx

tablets: 200 mg, 300 mg	Tagamet
liquid: 300 mg/5 ml	Tagamet
injection: 300 mg/2 ml	Tagamet

INDICATIONS

Active duodenal ulcer: Short-term (6–8 weeks) treatment.

Active benign gastric ulcer: Short-term (up to 8 weeks) treatment.

Prophylactic use in duodenal ulcer patients: At reduced dosage, to prevent ulcer recurrence in those likely to need surgical treatment (history of recurrence or complications) and in patients with concomitant illness in whom surgery would constitute a greater than usual risk.

Pathologic hypersecretory conditions: Zollinger-Ellison syndrome, systemic mastocytosis, multiple endocrine adenomas.

Unlabeled uses: 400 mg to 600 mg PO and/or 300 mg IV 60 to 90 minutes before anesthesia induction for prophylaxis of aspiration pneumonitis. Doses of 1 g/day used with variable success for treatment of primary hyperparathyroidism and to control secondary hyperparathyroidism in chronic hemodialysis patients. May have promise in the prophylaxis of acute upper GI bleeding. Has been evaluated for use in reflux esophagitis, tinea capitis, herpesvirus infection, and hirsutism in women.

CONTRAINDICATIONS

None known.

ACTIONS

Competitively inhibits action of histamine at histamine H_2 receptors of parietal cells. Inhibits both daytime and nocturnal basal gastric acid secretion, and gastric acid secretion stimulated by food, histamine, pentagastrin, caffeine, and insulin.

Is rapidly absorbed after oral administration; peak levels occur in 45 to 90 minutes. Half-life is approximately 2 hours in those with normal renal function; in renal impairment, half-life is prolonged. Both oral and parenteral administration provide comparable periods of therapeutically effective serum levels; blood concentrations remain above those required to provide 80% inhibition of basal gastric acid secretion for 4 to 5 hours following a 300-mg dose. Principal route of excretion is in the urine, mainly as unchanged drug.

WARNINGS

Safety for use in pregnancy not established. Use only when clearly needed and potential benefits outweigh the unknown potential hazards to the fetus. Cimetidine is secreted in human milk; breast-feeding should not be undertaken. Not recommended for children under 16 years unless anticipated benefits outweigh the potential risks.

PRECAUTIONS

Has demonstrated a weak antiandrogenic effect. Cases of gynecomastia in those treated for 1 month or longer may be related to this effect. A few cases of reversible confusional states have been reported, usually in the elderly or severely ill, such as those with renal insufficiency or organic brain syndrome; overdosage may have played a role in some cases. Symptomatic response to therapy does not preclude the presence of a gastric malignancy.

DRUG INTERACTIONS

Has an apparent effect on certain microsomal enzyme systems and reduces hepatic metabolism of **Warfarin-type anticoagulants, phenytoin, beta-adrenergic blocking agents** (propranolol, metoprolol), **lidocaine,** and **theophylline,** thereby delaying elimination and increasing plasma levels of these drugs. The half-life of **benzodiazepine** derivatives (chlordiazepoxide and diazepam) has been reported to be increased. Dosage adjustment of these drugs may be required to maintain optimal therapeutic blood levels when starting or stopping concomitantly administered cimetidine. Clinically significant effects have been reported with warfarin anticoagulants. The prothrombin time is closely monitored and dosage adjusted if necessary. Interaction with phenytoin, lidocaine, and theophylline has been reported to produce adverse clinical effects.

Decreased white blood cell counts, including agranulocytosis, have been reported in cimetidine-treated patients who also received **antimetabolites, alkylating agents,** or other drugs or treatment known to produce neutropenia.

Although commonly used with **antacids,** it may be advisable to administer cimetidine between doses of the antacid to avoid possible inhibition of cimetidine absorption.

Concurrent administration of cimetidine and **morphine** has been reported to precipitate apnea, confusion, and muscle twitching. Increase in gastric *p*H by cimetidine may cause decreased absorption of **ketoconazole;** administer at least 2 hours apart. **Cigarette smoking** reverses the inhibition of nocturnal gastric secretion produced by cimetidine. Concurrent administration of **Carbamazepine** and cimetidine may increase carbamazepine's pharmacologic effects and toxicity. A decrease in serum digoxin concentrations may occur during concomitant administration of **digoxin** and cimetidine.

ADVERSE REACTIONS

Mild and transient diarrhea, muscular pain, dizziness, and rash have been reported in approximately 1%. Severe diarrhea occasionally reported. Mild gynecomastia has been reported in a few patients treated for 1 month or longer.

A few cases of neutropenia have been reported in those with serious concomitant illness or receiving drugs or treatment known to produce neutropenia; therefore, a cause-and-effect relationship cannot be established. Isolated cases of granulocytopenia, thrombocytopenia, and autoimmune hemolytic anemia or aplastic anemia have been reported.

Regularly observed small increases in serum creatinine have been reported. These did not progress with continued therapy and disappeared at the end of therapy. Some increases in serum transaminase and rare cases of fever and interstitial nephritis and hepatitis, which cleared on withdrawal of drug, have been reported.

Other adverse effects include galactorrhea, bradycardia, impotence, alopecia, and CNS effects including hallucinations and delirium (particularly in the elderly), symptoms of brainstem dysfunction (*e.g.*, dysarthria, ataxic gate, diplopia). Cardiac arrhythmias and arrest have been reported following IV administration.

OVERDOSAGE

Symptoms: Experience with gross overdosage is limited. In cases reported, dosages up to 10 g have not been associated with any untoward effects.

Treatment: Usual measures to remove unabsorbed material from the GI tract, clinical monitoring, and supportive therapy should be employed.

DOSAGE

Active duodenal ulcer: 300 mg qid, with meals and H.S. Antacids may be given concomitantly for relief of pain.

Prophylaxis of recurrent ulcer: 400 mg H.S.; prophylactic treatment with higher doses does not improve effectiveness.

Pathologic hypersecretory conditions: 300 mg qid, with meals and H.S. In some patients it may be necessary to administer 300 mg more frequently. Maximum daily dose: 2400 mg/day.

Active benign gastric ulcer: Recommended dose is 300 mg qid with meals and H.S.

Severely impaired renal function: 300 mg q12h PO or IV recommended. An increase in frequency to q8h may be made. Whether hemodialysis reduces level of cimetidine is controversial; dosage schedule should be adjusted so that dose is given at the end of hemodialysis.

Parenteral: Usual dose is 300 mg q6h. In some,

dosage may be increased by more frequent administration not exceeding 2400 mg/day.

NURSING IMPLICATIONS

HISTORY
See Appendix 4.

PHYSICAL ASSESSMENT
Monitor vital signs, weight. If ulcer is active and bleeding, observe color of stool. Baseline studies include CBC, gastrointestinal x-rays. Additional diagnostic tests may be ordered for pathologic hypersecretory conditions.

ADMINISTRATION
If patient is concomitantly receiving an antacid, it may be advisable to administer cimetidine between doses of antacid. Clarify with physician times when antacid and cimetidine are to be administered.

Administer oral form with or immediately after meals.

Transient pain at IM injection site has been reported. Rotate injection sites; record site used.

IV injection: Dilute with 0.9% Sodium Chloride Injection or other compatible IV solution to a total volume of 20 ml and inject over period of not less than 2 minutes.

Intermittent IV infusion: Dilute 300 mg in 100 ml of 5% Dextrose Injection or other compatible IV solution. Add the solution to a volume-control set and infuse over 15 to 20 minutes.

Cardiac arrhythmias and arrest have been reported following rapid IV (bolus) administration. Observe patient frequently during and for 1 to 2 hours after IV injection.

Stability: Stable for 48 hours at room temperature when added to most commonly used IV solutions (_i.e.,_ 0.9% Sodium Chloride Injection, 5% or 10% Dextrose Injection, Lactated Ringer's Solution, or 5% Sodium Bicarbonate Injection).

Incompatibility: Incompatible with aminophylline and barbiturates in IV solutions.

ONGOING ASSESSMENTS AND NURSING MANAGEMENT
Record vital signs q4h or as ordered (more frequent monitoring may be necessary in those with a bleeding ulcer); observe for signs and symptoms of hemorrhage (hematemesis, frequent tarry stools, signs of shock); observe for adverse drug reactions; observe response to therapy (_e.g.,_ decrease in symptoms, control of bleeding).

If blood loss is severe, other therapies such as blood transfusion and treatment of shock may be necessary.

Confusional states may occur in the elderly or severely ill patient. Observe q1h to q2h and contact physician if confusion is apparent; drug may need to be discontinued. Adequate support (and possibly restraint) of the IV arm may be necessary to maintain integrity of the IV line.

Hematologic studies may be performed frequently if patient has active bleeding ulcer.

Parenteral therapy is discontinued and oral therapy instituted once bleeding is controlled.

PATIENT AND FAMILY INFORMATION
Take with meals.

Keep physician informed of response to therapy (_e.g.,_ decrease in symptoms of ulcer, if present).

If dizziness occurs, avoid tasks requiring alertness.

When applicable, caution patient that cigarette smoking may interfere with drug's therapeutic effect.

Cinoxacin Rx

capsules: 250 mg, 500 mg   Cinobac Pulvules

INDICATIONS
Treatment of initial and recurrent urinary tract infections in adults caused by the following susceptible organisms: _Escherichia coli, Proteus mirabilis, P. vulgaris, Klebsiella pneumoniae, Klebsiella_ and _Enterobacter_ species.

CONTRAINDICATIONS
Hypersensitivity.

ACTIONS
Is bactericidal; acts by inhibiting DNA replication. Drug is active within range of urinary _p_H. Is rapidly absorbed after oral administration with 97% excreted in the urine within 24 hours. Presence of food does not affect total absorption.

WARNINGS
Use in prepubertal children not recommended. Use in pregnancy not recommended. Because of the potential for serious adverse reactions in nursing infants, a decision must be made to discontinue nursing or discontinue drug.

PRECAUTIONS
Because drug is eliminated primarily by the kidney, dosage should be decreased in patients with reduced

renal function. Administration not recommended for anuric patients. Use with caution in those with hepatic disease.

ADVERSE REACTIONS

GI: Most common (5%) are nausea, abdominal cramps. Less frequent are anorexia, vomiting, diarrhea, and perineal burning.

CNS: Most frequent (1%–2%) are headache, dizziness. Less frequent (fewer than 1%) are insomnia, nervousness, confusion, tingling sensation, photophobia, blurred vision, tinnitus.

Hypersensitivity (less than 3%): Rash, urticaria, pruritus, edema.

Laboratory tests: Laboratory values reported to be abnormal were, in order of frequency, BUN (1%) and SGOT, SGPT, serum creatinine, alkaline phosphatase (fewer than 1%).

DOSAGE

Usual adult dosage is 1 g/day in 2 to 4 divided doses for 7 to 14 days. Although susceptible organisms may be eradicated within a few days after therapy is begun, a full course of treatment is recommended.

When renal function is impaired, reduced dosage is employed. The following is recommended: Mild impairment, 250 mg tid; moderate impairment, 250 mg bid; marked impairment, 250 mg daily.

NURSING IMPLICATIONS

HISTORY
See Appendix 4.

PHYSICAL ASSESSMENT
Urine for culture and sensitivity obtained before institution of therapy.

ADMINISTRATION
May be taken with food.

Dosage intervals should be evenly spaced to provide adequate urinary concentration of drug.

ONGOING ASSESSMENTS AND NURSING MANAGEMENT
Obtain vital signs q4h; observe for adverse drug reactions; observe for response to therapy (*i.e.,* decrease in symptoms of urinary tract infection). Monitor intake and output if renal function is impaired.

Culture and sensitivity tests may be repeated during therapy.

If dizziness occurs, patient may need assistance with ambulation.

Contact physician if symptoms are not relieved after several days of therapy.

If symptoms become more severe or a sudden rise in temperature is noted, contact physician immediately.

PATIENT AND FAMILY INFORMATION
May be taken with or without food. Take with food if nausea occurs.

The full course of therapy must be completed; do *not* stop taking drug if symptoms are relieved.

Contact physician if symptoms are not relieved within a few days after therapy is begun or if symptoms become worse.

If dizziness occurs, avoid tasks (such as driving) that require alertness.

If rash or hives occur, contact physician as soon as possible.

Cisplatin Rx

powder for injection: Platinol
   10 mg, 50 mg/vial

INDICATIONS

Metastatic testicular and ovarian tumors: In combination therapy with other chemotherapeutic agents with metastatic testicular or ovarian tumors in patients who have received appropriate surgical or radiotherapeutic procedures.

Advanced bladder cancer: As single agent for patients with transitional-cell bladder cancer that is no longer amenable to local treatments such as surgery or radiotherapy.

CONTRAINDICATIONS

Preexisting renal impairment; myelosuppressed patients; patients with hearing impairment; history of allergic reactions to cisplatin or other platinum-containing compounds.

ACTIONS

Has biochemical properties similar to those of bifunctional alkylating agents, producing interstrand cross-links in DNA. It is apparently cell-cycle nonspecific. Following a single dose, drug concentrates in the liver, kidneys, and large and small intestines. It has poor penetration into the CNS. Initial plasma half-life is 25 to 49 minutes and postdistribution plasma half-life is 58–73 hours. Cisplatin is excreted primarily in the urine.

WARNINGS

Nephrotoxicity: Cumulative renal toxicity is severe. At recommended dosage, do not give more frequently than once every 3 to 4 weeks.

Hypersensitivity: Anaphylacticlike reactions have been reported. These have occurred within minutes of administration to patients with prior exposure to drug and have been alleviated by administration of epinephrine, corticosteroids, and antihistamines.

Ototoxicity: Is cumulative. Audiometric testing, performed prior to initiating therapy and prior to each subsequent dose, is recommended.

Use in pregnancy: Safety not established.

PRECAUTIONS

Monitor peripheral blood counts weekly and liver function periodically. Neurologic examination should also be performed regularly.

ADVERSE REACTIONS

Nephrotoxicity: Dose-related and cumulative renal insufficiency is the major dose-limiting toxicity. Renal toxicity has been noted in 28% to 36% of patients treated with a single dose of 50 mg/m^2. It is first noted during second week after a dose and manifested by elevations in BUN, creatinine, and serum uric acid and/or a decrease in creatinine clearance. Renal toxicity becomes more pronounced and severe with repeated courses. Renal function must return to normal before another dose can be given. Impairment of renal function has been associated with renal tubular damage. Administration using a 6- to 8-hour infusion with IV hydration and mannitol has been used to reduce nephrotoxicity; renal damage can still occur after use of these procedures.

Ototoxicity: Has been observed in 31% of patients treated with a single dose of 50 mg/m^2 and is manifested by tinnitus or hearing loss in the high-frequency range. Decreased ability to hear normal conversational tones may occur. Ototoxic effects are more severe in children. Hearing loss can be unilateral or bilateral and tends to become more frequent and severe with repeated doses. It is unclear whether ototoxicity is reversible. Vestibular toxicity, manifested by transient dizziness, has been reported.

Hematologic: Myelosuppression occurs in 25% to 30% of patients. The nadirs of circulating platelets and leukocytes occur between days 18 and 23 (range 7.5 to 45), with most patients recovering by day 39 (range 13 to 62). Leukopenia and thrombocytopenia are more pronounced at higher doses. Anemia occurs at approximately the same frequency and with the same timing as leukopenia and thrombocytopenia.

GI: Marked nausea and vomiting occur in almost all patients and are occasionally so severe that drug must be discontinued. Nausea and vomiting usually begin 1 to 4 hours after treatment and last up to 24 hours. Various degrees of nausea and anorexia may persist for up to 1 week after treatment.

Hyperuricemia: Has been reported to occur at approximately the same frequency as increases in BUN and serum creatinine. It is more pronounced after doses greater than 50 mg/m^2; peak levels of uric acid generally occur 3 to 5 days after the dose. Allopurinol therapy effectively reduces uric-acid levels.

Neurotoxicity: Usually characterized by peripheral neuropathies; has occurred in some patients. Seizures and loss of taste also reported. Neuropathies resulting from treatment may occur after prolonged therapy (4–7 months) but neurologic symptoms have been reported after a single dose. Discontinue therapy when symptoms are first observed. There is some evidence that peripheral neuropathy may be irreversible in some patients.

Anaphylacticlike reactions: Have occasionally been reported in patients previously treated with cisplatin. These include facial edema, wheezing, tachycardia, and hypotension and appear within a few minutes of administration. Reactions may be controlled by IV epinephrine, corticosteroids, or antihistamines.

Other: Infrequently reported are cardiac abnormalities, anorexia, elevated SGOT, hypomagnesemia, hypocalcemia, and persistent systemic hypertension.

DOSAGE

Metastatic testicular tumors: The following combination may be used: Cisplatin 20 mg/m^2 day IV for 5 days every 3 weeks for 3 courses; bleomycin 30 units IV weekly (day 2 of each week) for 12 consecutive weeks; vinblastine 0.15 mg/kg to 0.2 mg/kg IV twice weekly (days 1 and 2) every 3 weeks for 4 courses. Maintenance therapy for those who respond to this regimen consists of vinblastine 0.3 mg/kg IV every 4 weeks for a total of 2 years.

Metastatic ovarian tumors: The following combination may be used: Cisplatin 50 mg/m^2 IV once every 3 weeks (day 1); doxorubicin 50 mg/m^2 IV once every 3 weeks (day 1). In combination therapy, cisplatin and doxorubicin are administered sequentially. As a single agent, cisplatin 100 mg/m^2 IV every 4 weeks.

Advanced bladder cancer: Administered as single agent; 50 mg/m^2 to 70 mg/m^2 IV once every 3 to 4 weeks, depending on extent of prior exposure to radiation therapy or prior chemotherapy. For heavily pretreated patients, an initial dose of 50 mg/m^2 repeated every 4 weeks is recommended.

Repeat courses: Should not be given until the serum creatinine level is below 1.5 mg/ml or the BUN is below 25 mg/100 ml or until circulating blood elements are at acceptable levels. Subsequent doses should not be given until an audiometric analysis indicates auditory acuity within normal limits.

NURSING IMPLICATIONS

HISTORY
See Appendix 4.

PHYSICAL ASSESSMENT
Monitor physical and emotional status, vital signs, weight. Other assessments may also be applicable. Laboratory tests and diagnostic studies include renal-function tests, CBC, differential, platelet count, serum uric acid, serum enzymes, serum bilirubin, alkaline phosphatase, ECG, audiometric testing.

ADMINISTRATION
Needles or IV sets containing aluminum parts that may come into contact with drug should not be used for preparation or administration. Aluminum reacts with cisplatin, causing precipitate formation and loss of potency.

CLINICAL ALERT: Caution should be exercised in handling the powder and preparing the solution. Skin reactions associated with accidental exposure may occur. Plastic gloves are recommended. If powder or solution contacts the skin or mucosa, wash immediately with soap and water.

Hydration: Pretreatment hydration with 1 to 2 liters of fluid infused for 8 to 12 hours prior to dose is recommended. The drug is then diluted in 2 liters of 5% Dextrose in ½ or ⅓ Normal Saline containing 37.5 g of mannitol, and infused over a 6- to 8-hour period. Adequate hydration and urinary output must be maintained during the following 24 hours.

Physician may order a diuretic such as furosemide to be administered instead of mannitol.

Preparation of solution: Dissolve the 10-mg and 50-mg vials with 10 ml or 50 ml of Sterile Water for Injection, USP, respectively. Resulting solutions will contain 1 mg/ml of cisplatin. Reconstitution as recommended results in a clear, colorless solution. Use the reconstituted solution IV *only* and administer over a 6- to 8-hour period.

An infusion pump may be used to administer the IV solution containing cisplatin. If an infusion pump is not used, apply a timing label.

Do not refrigerate the reconstituted solution; a precipitate will form. The reconstituted solution is stable for 20 hours at room temperature.

Physician may order an antiemetic to be ad-ministered ½ to 1 hour before cisplatin is administered.

Have immediately available (preferably at patient's bedside) drugs to be used if an anaphylacticlike reaction occurs. Physician orders drugs and dosage to be administered.

Obtain vital signs before treatment is started.

Stability: Unopened vials of dry powder must be stored in a refrigerator (2°C to 8°C); product is stable for 2 years.

ONGOING ASSESSMENTS AND NURSING MANAGEMENT
If drug is administered on an outpatient basis, patient usually is hospitalized in a short-term care unit for 24, 48, or more hours. Pretreatment hydration may be started the evening before with the cisplatin administered early in the morning or may be started early in the morning with cisplatin administered in the late afternoon. Pretreatment hydration requires an 8- to 12-hour infusion of IV fluids.

The hospital or physician usually establishes guidelines about time of pretreatment hydration and cisplatin infusion and specific events requiring immediate notification of the physician (*e.g.*, vomitus exceeding 750 ml/8 hours, urinary output less than 100 ml/hour).

CLINICAL ALERT: If patient has previously received cisplatin, observe closely for possible anaphylacticlike reaction. Symptoms may include facial edema, wheezing, tachycardia, and hypotension, which may appear within a few minutes of administration.

Monitor intake and output q1h to q2h starting with pretreatment hydration and continue for 48 hours after cisplatin therapy. Measurement of urine specific gravity may also be ordered q1h to q2h.

Notify physician immediately if urinary output decreases.

Monitor blood pressure, pulse, and respirations q1h to q2h (or as ordered); take temperature q4h.

Nausea and vomiting occur in most all patients and usually begin 1 to 4 hours after treatment. Measure all vomitus. Notify physician if vomitus exceeds guideline limit because proper hydration must be maintained to prevent nephrotoxicity.

A parenteral antiemetic may be ordered q3h to q4h during and after treatment and until nausea and vomiting subside.

Assess patient for signs of dehydration (Appendix 6, section 6-10).

Cola syrup, carbonated beverages, dry toast, and unsalted crackers may be used to relieve nausea.

Serum electrolytes may be determined if vomiting is severe. Observe for signs of hypokalemia and hyponatremia (Appendix 6, sections 6-15 and 6-17). Notify physician if laboratory results are abnormal.

Neurotoxicity may occur after prolonged therapy but may be seen after a single dose. Observe patient for motor or sensory changes; note any patient complaints of numbness, tingling, or difficulty in moving the extremities.

If combination chemotherapy is administered, the adverse reactions and nursing management of each drug must be considered.

In combination therapy, cisplatin and doxorubicin are administered sequentially.

Unless complications develop or disease process is severe, patient may be discharged approximately 24 hours after treatment is completed. Toxic drug effects may not be noted until after discharge.

Toxic drug effects occur at different intervals as follows:

1. Nausea and vomiting may persist up to 24 hours after treatment. Various degrees of nausea and anorexia may persist for up to 1 week after treatment. Physician usually prescribes an antiemetic (oral or suppository form) q4h to q6h prn.
2. Nephrotoxicity usually is first noted in the second week after dosing and is manifested by elevations in renal-function tests. Physician monitors renal function at periodic intervals. Renal function must return to normal before another dose can be given.
3. Ototoxicity is manifested by tinnitus or hearing loss. Physician orders audiometric testing prior to initial dose as well as subsequent doses. Hearing loss tends to become more frequent and severe with repeated doses. Vestibular toxicity is manifested by transient dizziness. If hearing loss is severe, a decision will be made about further treatment.
4. Leukopenia, thrombocytopenia, and anemia (myelosuppression, Appendix 6, section 6-8) may occur between days 18 and 23 (range 7.5 to 45). Peripheral blood counts are recommended weekly after therapy.
5. Serum uric acid may be elevated; peak uric-acid levels generally occur 3 to 5 days after dosing. Physician may prescribe allopurinol.

6. Occasionally, cardiac abnormalities may occur. Periodic ECGs are recommended.
7. Neurotoxicity may occur after a single dose or after prolonged therapy. Periodic neurologic examinations are recommended.
8. Persistent systemic hypertension may occur, which may require drug therapy.
9. Hypocalcemia and hypomagnesemia (Appendix 6, sections 6-13 and 6-16) have been reported.
10. Abnormal liver function may be seen; periodic liver-function tests are recommended.

PATIENT AND FAMILY INFORMATION

NOTE: When cisplatin is administered on an outpatient basis, patient will be instructed to report for laboratory tests at periodic intervals. Complete detailed instruction about possible adverse effects and describe the symptoms of these effects to the patient.

An antiemetic may be prescribed for nausea and vomiting. If nausea and vomiting continue for more than a week, contact physician.

Sips of liquids such as water, carbonated beverages, or tea may relieve nausea. Dry toast and unsalted crackers may also be of value. Experiment with the foods and liquids that help the most.

Anorexia may occur. If it persists for more than 2 to 3 days, contact physician. Eating small portions 4 to 6 times a day may provide adequate nutritional intake until anorexia subsides.

Notify physician or nurse if any of the following is noted: fatigue; easy bruising or bleeding in small cuts, nose, or gums; blood in the urine or stool; sore throat; common cold; cough; fever; pain on urination; abscesses, infections in small cuts; ringing or buzzing in the ears; hearing loss; loss of taste; numbness or tingling in the extremities; loss of balance; constipation; diarrhea; muscle cramps or spasms; any other changes or symptoms experienced.

Inform other physicians or dentist of therapy with cisplatin.

Keep all appointments for follow-up tests and monitoring of therapy.

Citrate of Magnesia

See Laxatives.

Clemastine Fumarate

See Antihistamines.

Clidinium Bromide

See Gastrointestinal Anticholinergics/Antispasmodics.

Clindamycin Rx

capsules: 75 mg, 150 mg (contains tartrazine)	Cleocin HCl
granules, flavored: 75 mg (as palmitate)/ 5 ml when reconstituted	Cleocin Pediatric
injection: 300 mg/2 ml, 600 mg/4 ml	Cleocin Phosphate
topical solution: 10 mg/ml	Cleocin T

INDICATIONS

Oral, parenteral

Treatment of serious infections caused by susceptible anaerobic bacteria. Also for treatment of serious infections due to susceptible strains of streptococci, pneumococci, and staphylococci. Reserved for penicillin-allergic patients or for others when penicillin is inappropriate.

Anaerobes: Serious respiratory infections such as empyema, anaerobic pneumonitis, and lung abscess; serious skin infections; septicemia; intra-abdominal infections and abscess; infections in the female pelvis and genital tract such as endometritis, nongonococcal tubo-ovarian abscess, pelvic cellulitis, and postsurgical vaginal cuff infection. *Streptococci and staphylococci*—Serious respiratory-tract infections; serious skin and soft-tissue infections. *Pneumococci*—Serious respiratory-tract infections. Injectable clindamycin is indicated in septicemia caused by streptococci or staphylococci, acute hematogenous osteomyelitis due to staphylococci, and as adjunctive therapy in the surgical treatment of chronic bone and joint infections due to susceptible organisms.

Topical: Treatment of acne vulgaris. Because of the potential for diarrhea, bloody diarrhea, and pseudomembranous colitis, consider whether other agents are more appropriate.

CONTRAINDICATIONS

History of hypersensitivity to preparations containing clindamycin or lincomycin. Topical solution is also contraindicated in patients with a history of regional enteritis or ulcerative colitis or a history of antibiotic-associated colitis.

ACTIONS

Oral, parenteral: Binds to the 50 S subunit of bacterial ribosomes and suppresses protein synthesis. Is rapidly absorbed after oral administration. Oral doses are 90% absorbed; concomitant administration of food does not appreciably modify serum concentrations. Serum concentrations increase linearly with dose. Is widely distributed in body fluids and tissues (including bones). Significant levels are not attained in cerebrospinal fluid. Serum half-life is increased slightly in patients with markedly reduced renal or hepatic function. Approximately 10% of the bioactivity is excreted in the urine and 3.6% in the feces; the remainder is excreted as inactive metabolites. Hemodialysis and peritoneal dialysis are not effective in removing clindamycin from serum.

Cross-resistance has been demonstrated between clindamycin and lincomycin.

Topical: Clindamycin has been shown to have *in vitro* activity against isolates of *Propionibacterium acnes,* which may account for its usefulness in acne. Approximately 10% of the dose is absorbed into human skin.

WARNINGS

Colitis: Can cause severe colitis that may be fatal. Mild cases may respond to drug discontinuation alone. Moderate to severe cases should be managed with fluid, electrolyte, and protein supplementation as indicated. Systemic corticoids and corticoid-retention enemas may help relieve colitis.

Antiperistaltic agents such as opiates and diphenoxylate with atropine may prolong or aggravate the condition. Diarrhea, colitis, and pseudomembranous colitis can begin up to several weeks following cessation of therapy.

Vancomycin is effective in the treatment of antibiotic-associated pseudomembranous colitis produced by *Clostridium difficile.*

Anaphylactoid reactions: Require immediate emergency treatment with epinephrine. Oxygen and IV corticosteroids may also be used.

Use in pregnancy and lactation: Safety not established.

Use in newborns and infants: Monitor organ system functions.

PRECAUTIONS

Oral, parenteral

Use in the elderly: Monitor carefully for change in bowel frequency; older patients with associated severe illness may tolerate diarrhea less well. Give with caution to those with history of GI disease, particularly colitis, and to atopic individuals.

Superinfection: Use of antibiotics (especially prolonged and repeated therapy) may result in bacterial and fungal overgrowth of nonsusceptible organisms. Such overgrowth may lead to a secondary infection.

Tartrazine sensitivity: Capsules contain tartrazine (see Appendix 6, section 6-23).

Patients with very severe renal disease or very severe hepatic disease accompanied by severe metabolic aberrations should be given drug with caution and serum levels should be monitored during high-dose therapy.

Topical

Solution has an alcohol base, which will cause burning and irritation of the eye. In case of accidental contact with eye, abraded skin, or mucous membranes, bathe with copious amounts of cool tap water. Use caution when applying medication around the mouth. Prescribe with caution in atopic individuals.

DRUG INTERACTIONS

Antagonism has been demonstrated between clindamycin and **erythromycin.** Concomitant administration may produce cross-interference because both drugs have an affinity for the 50 S ribosomal unit of the bacterial cell. These two drugs are not administered concurrently.

Clindamycin has been shown to have neuromuscular blocking properties that may enhance the action of other **neuromuscular blocking agents;** use with caution in patients receiving such agents.

Simultaneous administration of **kaolin** reduces GI absorption.

ADVERSE REACTIONS

_GI:_ Abdominal pain, esophagitis, nausea, vomiting, diarrhea, pseudomembranous colitis.

Hypersensitivity reactions: Maculopapular rash and urticaria have been seen. Generalized mild to moderate morbilliformlike skin rashes are the most frequently reported adverse reactions. _Rarely_—Erythema multiforme, sometimes resembling Stevens-Johnson syndrome. A few cases of anaphylactic reactions have been reported. If a hypersensitivity reaction occurs, discontinue drug. The usual agents (epinephrine, corticosteroids, antihistamines) should be available for emergency treatment of serious reactions.

Hepatic: Jaundice and abnormalities in hepatic-function tests.

Hematopoietic: Transient leukopenia, eosinophilia, agranulocytosis, and thrombocytopenia have been seen. No direct relationship has been shown.

Musculoskeletal: Rarely, polyarthritis.

Injectable clindamycin: Pain, induration, and sterile abscesses after IM injection and thrombo-

phlebitis after IV infusion. Reactions can be minimized or avoided by giving deep IM injections and avoiding prolonged use of indwelling IV catheters.

Topical: See GI, above. _Other_—Contact dermatitis; dryness; fatigue; gram-negative folliculitis; headache; irritation; oily skin; sensitization; sore throat; stinging of the eye; swelling of the face; pain; urinary frequency; vaginitis.

DOSAGE

In treatment of anaerobic infections, parenteral clindamycin may be used initially followed by oral therapy. In beta-hemolytic infections, continue treatment for at least 10 days.

Oral

Adults: _Serious infections_—150 mg to 300 mg q6h. _More severe infections_—300 mg to 450 mg q6h.

Children: _Clindamycin HCl_—Serious infections, 8 mg/kg/day to 16 mg/kg/day divided into 3 to 4 equal doses; more severe infections, 16 mg/kg/day to 20 mg/kg/day divided into 3 to 4 equal doses.

Clindamycin palmitate—Serious infections, 8 mg/kg/day to 12 mg/kg/day divided into 3 to 4 equal doses; _severe infections_—13 mg/kg/day to 16 mg/kg/day divided into 3 to 4 equal doses; _more severe infections_—17 mg/kg/day to 25 mg/kg/day divided into 3 to 4 equal doses. _Children weighing 10 kg or less_—37.5 mg tid should be considered the minimum recommended dose.

Parenteral

Adults: _Serious infections due to aerobic gram-positive cocci and the more sensitive anaerobes_—600 mg/day to 1200 mg/day in 2, 3, or 4 equal doses. _More severe infections_—1200 mg/day to 2700 mg/day in 2, 3, or 4 equal doses. _More serious infections_—These doses may need to be increased. In life-threatening situations, doses of as much as 4.8 g/day have been given. Alternatively, may be administered in the form of a single rapid infusion of the first dose followed by continuous IV infusion (Table 19).

Children (over 1 month): _Serious infections_—15 mg/kg/day to 25 mg/kg/day in 3 to 4 equal doses.

Table 19. Infusion Rates to Maintain Prescribed Serum Levels of Clindamycin

Serum Clindamycin Level to Be Maintained	Rapid Infusion Rate	Maintenance Infusion Rate
>4 mcg/ml	10 mg/min for 30 min	0.75 mg/min
>5 mcg/ml	15 mg/min for 30 min	1.00 mg/min
>6 mcg/ml	20 mg/min for 30 min	1.25 mg/min

More severe infections—25 mg/kg/day to 40 mg/kg/day in 3 to 4 equal doses. Dose may also be determined on basis of square meters of body surface: 350 mg/m²/day for serious infections and 450 mg/m²/day for more severe infections. In severe infections it is recommended that children be given no less than 300 mg/day regardless of body weight.

Topical solution
Apply a thin film to affected area twice daily.

NURSING IMPLICATIONS

HISTORY
See Appendix 4. Careful inquiry should be made about previous sensitivities to drug and other allergens. Inform physician if patient has an allergy history.

PHYSICAL ASSESSMENT
Monitor vital signs, weight (if dosage is to be determined by weight). Additional assessments are based on patient's symptoms. Order culture and sensitivity tests prior to therapy. Other laboratory tests may include CBC, hepatic- and renal-function tests.

ADMINISTRATION
Parenteral administration
Single IM injections greater than 600 mg are not recommended. Administer deep IM; rotate injection sites and chart site used.

Injection form is available as 300 mg/2 ml or 600 mg/4 ml with each milliliter containing 150 mg.

Clindamycin must be diluted prior to IV administration to a dilution of 300 mg/50 ml or more of diluent. For infusion rates, see Table 20.

Do *not* inject as IV bolus; infuse over at least 10 to 60 minutes. A volume control set may be used to administer IV. Time infusion rate as stated in Table 20.

Compatibility: Compatible with IV solutions containing sodium chloride, glucose, calcium, or potassium; solutions containing vitamin B complex in concentrations used clinically; the antibiotics cephalothin, kanamycin, gentamicin, penicillin, and carbenicillin. Physically incompatible with ampicillin, phenytoin, barbiturates, aminophylline, calcium gluconate, magnesium sulfate.

Oral administration
Have patient take capsule with a full glass (8 oz) of water. Food does not appreciably modify serum levels.

Cleocin Pediatric (granules) is reconstituted by the pharmacist. The solution is *not* refrigerated; chilled solution may thicken and be difficult to pour. Solution is stable for 2 weeks at room temperature. Note expiration date; discard outdated drug.

ONGOING ASSESSMENTS AND NURSING MANAGEMENT
Record vital signs q4h; record *each* bowel movement; observe for adverse drug effects, particularly hypersensitivity reactions and diarrhea; check previous IM injection sites for induration, development of sterile abscess; check IV infusion sites for evidence of thrombophlebitis (*e.g.,* pain or tenderness, redness at injection site or along pathway of vein); observe patient's general drug response (*e.g.,* improvement in clinical condition).

CLINICAL ALERT: Because of danger of pseudomembranous colitis, drug must be discontinued when significant diarrhea occurs. If necessary, administration may be continued with patient under close observation. Record frequency as well as appearance and consistency of bowel movements. Note if blood, pus, or mucus is present. Withhold next dose of drug and contact physician if abdominal cramping or diarrhea occurs.

Rarely, anaphylactoid reactions may occur. Observe for hypotension, facial edema, dyspnea, restlessness; contact physician immediately if these should occur because emergency intervention may be necessary.

If severe diarrhea occurs, the physician may order an endoscopic examination of the large bowel.

To minimize phlebitis, avoid prolonged use of indwelling IV catheters.

Observe for signs of superinfection (Appendix 6, section 6-22). If signs or symptoms occur, withhold next dose and notify physician.

During prolonged therapy, periodic hepatic- and renal-function tests and blood counts may be performed.

Culture and sensitivity tests may be repeated during therapy.

Table 20. Dilution and Infusion Rates for Clindamycin

Dose (mg)	Diluent (ml)	Infusion Time (minutes)
300	50	10
600	100	20
900	150	30
1200	200	45

PATIENT AND FAMILY INFORMATION

Complete full course of therapy; take entire prescription unless advised to do otherwise by physician.

Take each dose with a full (8 oz) glass of water.

May cause diarrhea; notify physician or nurse immediately should this occur. Do not use nonprescription antidiarrheal agents to treat diarrhea unless advised to do so by physician.

Notify physician or nurse if any of the following occurs: fever; ulcerations of the mouth; anogenital itching; vaginal itching and discharge; rash; yellowing of skin or eye whites; nausea; vomiting.

Topical solution: Notify physician if swelling of the face, abdominal pain, or diarrhea occurs. Avoid contact with eyes, abraded skin, or mucous membranes; clindamycin may cause burning and irritation.

Clocortolone Pivalate

See Corticosteroids, Topical.

Clofibrate Rx

capsules: 500 mg   Atromid-S

INDICATIONS

Adjunctive therapy in patients with significant hyperlipidemia and a high risk of coronary artery disease who do not respond to diet and weight loss. Is drug of first choice for primary dysbetalipoproteinemia (type III hyperlipidemia). In other types of hyperlipidemia other antilipidemic drugs may prove more effective in individual patients, particularly when cholesterol is the lipid of greatest concern. May be useful in patients individually selected for recognized disorders of fat metabolism that may predispose them to an increased risk of heart disease. Response to drug is variable.

CONTRAINDICATIONS

Clinically significant hepatic or renal dysfunction; primary biliary cirrhosis because clofibrate may raise the already elevated cholesterol in these cases. Pregnancy and lactation.

ACTIONS

An antihyperlipidemic agent that predominantly lowers serum triglycerides and very low-density lipoprotein (VLDL) levels; serum cholesterol and low-density lipoprotein (LDL) levels are lowered less predictably and effectively. Mechanism of action is not established; the triglyceride-lowering effect appears to be due to accelerated catabolism of VLDL to LDL and decreased hepatic synthesis of VLDL. Cholesterol formation is inhibited early in the biosynthetic chain, and excretion of natural sterols is increased. Clofibrate also has a platelet-inhibiting effect. The plasma elimination half-life ranges from 6 hours to 25 hours.

WARNINGS

Because of possible increased risk of malignancy associated with clofibrate, as well as increased risk of cholelithiasis, drug is used only for patients described under *Indications* and should be discontinued if significant lipid response is not obtained. Strict birth control procedures must be exercised by women of childbearing potential. In patients who plan to become pregnant, drug should be withdrawn several months before conception. Because of the possibility of occurrence of pregnancy despite birth control precautions, potential benefits of the drug are weighed against potential hazards to the fetus.

DRUG INTERACTIONS

Caution should be exercised when **oral anticoagulants** are given concomitantly; dosage of anticoagulant should be reduced, usually by one-half (depending on individual case), to maintain desired prothrombin time level to prevent bleeding complications. Frequent prothrombin time determinations are advised until level is stabilized.

PRECAUTIONS

Baseline studies and frequent determinations of serum lipid levels are recommended during the first few months of therapy and periodically thereafter. Drug may be withdrawn after 3 months if response is inadequate.

Subsequent serum lipid determinations should be done to detect a paradoxical rise in serum cholesterol or triglyceride levels. Clofibrate will not alter seasonal variations of serum cholesterol: peak elevations are in midwinter and late summer and decreases are in fall and spring. If drug is discontinued, serum lipids may be monitored until stabilized because a rise in these values to or above original baseline may occur.

During therapy, frequent serum transaminase determinations and other hepatic-function tests should be performed, because drug may produce abnormalities in these parameters. These effects are usually reversible after drug is withdrawn. Withdraw drug if hepatic-function tests steadily rise or show excessive abnormalities. Use with caution in those with history of jaundice or hepatic disease.

Because cholelithiasis is possible side-effect, appropriate diagnostic procedures should be performed if signs and symptoms related to disease of the biliary tract should occur. Use with caution in those with peptic ulcer because reactivation has been reported. Complete blood counts should be done periodically because anemia and, more frequently, leukopenia have occurred. Various cardiac arrhythmias have been reported.

ADVERSE REACTIONS
Most common is nausea. Less frequent GI reactions are vomiting, loose stools, dyspepsia, flatulence, and abdominal distress. Reactions reported less often are headache, dizziness, and fatigue; muscle cramping, aching, and weakness; skin rash, urticaria, and pruritus; dry brittle hair and alopecia.

Cardiovascular: Increased or decreased angina, cardiac arrhythmias, both swelling and phlebitis at site of xanthomas. An increased incidence of thrombophlebitis and pulmonary emboli has been reported.

Dermatologic: Skin rash; alopecia; allergic reaction including urticaria, dry skin, dry brittle hair, and pruritus.

GI: Nausea, diarrhea, GI upset (bloating, flatulence, abdominal distress), hepatomegaly (not associated with hepatotoxicity), gallstones, vomiting, stomatitis, gastritis.

GU: Impotence and decreased libido; findings consistent with renal dysfunction as evidenced by dysuria, hematuria, proteinuria, decreased urine output.

Musculoskeletal: Myalgia (muscle cramping, aching, weakness), flulike symptoms, arthralgia.

Neurologic: Fatigue, weakness, drowsiness, dizziness, headache.

Miscellaneous: Weight gain, polyphagia.

Laboratory findings: Abnormal hepatic-function tests as evidenced by increased serum transaminase (SGOT, SGPT), Bromsulphalein retention; increased creatine phosphokinase.

Reported adverse reactions whose direct relationship to drug is not established: Peptic ulcer, GI hemorrhage, rheumatoid arthritis, tremors, increased perspiration, systemic lupus erythematosus, blurred vision, gynecomastia, thrombocytopenic purpura.

OVERDOSAGE
None reported. Should it occur, symptomatic supportive measures should be taken.

DOSAGE
Initially 2 g daily in divided doses. Some patients may respond to lower dosage. *Maintenance*—Same as initial dosage.

Insufficient data for efficacy and safety in children.

NURSING IMPLICATIONS

HISTORY
See Appendix 4. Note family history of coronary artery disease, hyperlipidemia, dietary history, methods previously used to reduce serum triglycerides. Inquire about use of tobacco, alcohol.

PHYSICAL ASSESSMENT
Obtain vital signs, weight; examine skin for xanthomas, especially over elbows, knees, palms, and fingertips. Review laboratory tests identifying type of hyperlipidemia. Hepatic- and renal-function studies, CBC, and ECG may also be ordered.

ADMINISTRATION
If GI upset occurs, give with meals, food, or skim milk.

ONGOING ASSESSMENTS AND NURSING MANAGEMENT
Record vital signs daily; observe for adverse reactions.

Physician will order a fat-controlled diet; if patient has difficulty accepting foods on this diet, contact the dietitian.

Weigh weekly or as ordered by physician. Weight should also be obtained at time of each clinic or office visit.

Periodic monitoring of hepatic-function tests, CBC, serum triglycerides, and serum cholesterol is recommended.

PATIENT AND FAMILY INFORMATION
NOTE: A copy of a fat-controlled diet is given to the patient; intake of saturated fats, sugars, and cholesterol is usually restricted. Review diet and sample meal plans with patient and family. Books or pamphlets on fat-controlled meal planning may be recommended. Strict birth control procedures must be exercised by women of childbearing potential; this should be discussed with the patient by the physician.

Patient package insert available with product.

If GI upset occurs, drug may be taken with food or skim milk.

Do not stop taking drug or increase or decrease the dose unless advised to do so by physician.

Inform other physicians of therapy with this drug.

Adherence to prescribed diet is an important part of therapy.

Alcohol intake should be limited. Discuss with physician how much alcohol is allowed.

Notify physician or nurse if any of the following occurs: chest pain, shortness of breath; irregular heartbeat; severe stomach pain with nausea and vomiting; fever and chills or sore throat; blood in the urine or unusually low urine output; swelling of the lower extremities; weight gain; flulike symptoms.

Clomiphene Citrate Rx

tablets: 50 mg   Clomid, Serophene

INDICATIONS

Treatment of ovulatory failure in patients who desire pregnancy and whose partners are fertile and potent. Indicated only when ovulatory dysfunction is demonstrated. Good levels of endogenous estrogen provide favorable prognosis for treatment. A reduced estrogen level, although less favorable, does not preclude successful therapy. Therapy is ineffective in patients in whom primary pituitary or ovarian failure precludes possibility of stimulating normal function.

Investigational use: Treatment of male infertility. Has been administered in doses of 25 mg/day for 25 days with 5 days of rest and at doses of 100 mg every Monday, Wednesday, and Friday.

CONTRAINDICATIONS

Liver disease, history of liver dysfunction, abnormal bleeding of undetermined origin; pregnancy.

ACTIONS

A nonsteroidal agent that may induce ovulation in anovulatory women in appropriately selected cases.

Ovulatory response to cyclic therapy appears to be mediated through increased output of pituitary gonadotropins, which in turn stimulates maturation and endocrine activity of the ovarian follicle and the subsequent development and function of the corpus luteum. Clomiphene binds to estrogenic receptors in the cytoplasmin and decreases the number of available estrogenic receptors. The hypothalamus and pituitary interpret the false signal that estrogen levels are low and respond by increasing secretion of luteinizing hormone, follicle-stimulating

hormone, and gonadotropins. This results in ovarian stimulation. Clomiphene is readily absorbed orally and excreted principally in the feces.

WARNINGS

If visual symptoms occur, treatment may be discontinued and an ophthalmologic examination performed. Evaluation of hepatic function is recommended before therapy. Patients with abnormal bleeding should be evaluated prior to therapy to assure that neoplastic lesions are not present. Not given in presence of ovarian cyst; further enlargement of the ovary may occur.

To minimize hazard associated with occasional abnormal ovarian enlargement, employ lowest dose consistent with expectation of good results.

PRECAUTIONS

Not given in presence of ovarian cyst; further enlargement may occur. Some patients with polycystic ovary syndrome who are unusually sensitive to gonadotropin may have an exaggerated response to usual doses. Maximal enlargement of the ovary, whether physiologic or abnormal, does not occur until several days after discontinuation of the drug. Patients complaining of pelvic pain after receiving clomiphene should be examined. If enlargement of the ovary occurs, additional doses are not given until the ovaries have returned to pretreatment size. The incidence of multiple pregnancies increases when conception takes place during clomiphene therapy.

DRUG INTERACTIONS

Drug/lab tests: May increase levels of serum **thyroxine** and **thyroxine-binding globulin (TBG)**.

ADVERSE REACTIONS

At recommended doses, side-effects are not prominent, interfere with treatment infrequently, and tend to be dose related. Common side-effects include vasomotor flushes, abdominal discomfort (distention, bloating, pain, soreness), ovarian enlargement, and visual blurring.

Vasomotor: Resemble menopausal hot flashes, are usually not severe, and disappear promptly after treatment is discontinued.

Abdominal: May be most often related to ovulatory (mittelschmerz) or premenstrual phenomena or to ovarian enlargement. Nausea and (rarely) vomiting, constipation, and diarrhea have been reported.

Miscellaneous: Nausea, vomiting; nervousness, insomnia; headache; dizziness, lightheadedness; increased urination; depression, fatigue; urticaria, allergic dermatitis; weight gain; reversible hair loss.

Abnormal ovarian enlargement: Infrequent at recommended dosage but usual cyclic variation in ovarian size may be exaggerated. Cyclic ovarian pain may also be accentuated. With higher or prolonged dosage, more frequent ovarian enlargement and cyst formation may occur.

Ophthalmologic: Usually described as "blurring" or spots or flashes; increase in incidence with increasing total dose and disappear within a few days or weeks after discontinuation. Symptoms most often appear with or are accentuated by exposure to a more brightly lit environment.

Birth defects: Have been reported.

DOSAGE

Many patients respond to 50 mg/day for 5 days. Ovulation and pregnancy are slightly more attainable on 100 mg/day for 5 days. The recommended initial dose for the first course is 50 mg/day for 5 days. Therapy may be started at any time in those who have had no recent uterine bleeding. If ovulation has not occurred after the first course, a second course of 100 mg/day for 5 days is started as early as 30 days after the previous course. The majority of patients who respond will respond to the first course of therapy; three courses should be an adequate therapeutic trial. Further treatment is not recommended. Properly timed coitus is necessary.

NURSING IMPLICATIONS

HISTORY AND PHYSICAL ASSESSMENT

Physician obtains health and gynecologic history and performs a physical examination. Evaluation of hepatic function is recommended prior to initiating treatment. A complete pelvic examination and endometrial biopsy are also recommended.

PATIENT INFORMATION

Take the drug for 5 days.

Physician will discuss the timing of sexual intercourse.

Notify physician or nurse if bloating, stomach or pelvic pain, blurred vision, jaundice, hot flashes, breast discomfort, headache, nausea, or vomiting occurs.

May cause dizziness, lightheadedness, and visual disturbances; observe caution while driving or performing other tasks requiring alertness.

Clonazepam

See Anticonvulsants, Benzodiazepines.

Clonidine Hydrochloride Rx

tablets: 0.1 mg, 0.2   Catapres
mg, 0.3 mg

INDICATIONS

Treatment of hypertension. Is mild to moderate in potency and may be employed in a general treatment program with a diuretic or other antihypertensive agent, as needed.

Investigational uses: Treatment of Gilles de la Tourette syndrome (0.05 mg to 0.6 mg/day) and to decrease the severity and frequency of migraine attacks and episodes of menopausal flushing. Also used to detoxify patients from chronic methadone administration and may be a useful alternative to methadone in rapid opiate detoxification. Relief from withdrawal symptoms has been reported with an average dose of 0.8 mg/day; doses up to 17 mcg/kg/day have been administered in divided doses.

ACTIONS

Mechanism of action appears to be central alpha-adrenergic stimulation. This results in inhibition of bulbar sympathetic cardioaccelerator and sympathetic vasoconstriction centers, thereby causing a decrease in sympathetic outflow from the brain. Initially, clonidine stimulates peripheral alpha-adrenergic receptors producing transient vasoconstriction. Orthostatic effects are mild and infrequent because supine blood pressure is reduced essentially to the same extent as standing pressure. Does not alter hemodynamic responses to exercise. Renal blood flow and glomerular filtration rate remain essentially unchanged. During long-term therapy, cardiac output tends to return to normal control values, while peripheral resistance remains decreased. Slowing of the pulse rate has been observed in most patients. Concomitant administration of a diuretic has been shown to enhance antihypertensive efficacy. Acts fairly rapidly; blood pressure declines within 30 to 60 minutes after dose, the maximum decrease occurring within 2 to 4 hours. The antihypertensive effect lasts approximately 12 to 24 hours. Peak plasma level occurs in approximately 3 to 5 hours, with a plasma half-life of 12 to 16 hours. In those with impaired renal function, half-life increases to 25 to 40 hours. Clonidine and its metabolites are excreted mainly in the urine.

WARNINGS

Use with caution in those with severe coronary insufficiency, recent myocardial infarction, cerebrovascular disease, or chronic renal failure. Tolerance may develop, necessitating reevaluation of therapy.

Not recommended in women who are or may become pregnant, unless potential benefits outweigh the unknown potential hazards to the mother and infant. Safety and efficacy for use in children not established.

PRECAUTIONS

Rebound hypertension: Discontinue therapy by reducing dose gradually over 2 to 4 days to avoid a rapid rise in blood pressure and associated subjective symptoms (*e.g.,* nervousness, agitation, headache). Rare instances of hypertensive encephalopathy and death have been reported after abrupt cessation of therapy, but a causal relationship has not been established. If an excessive rise in blood pressure should occur, it can be reversed by resumption of therapy or by IV phentolamine.

Ophthalmologic effects: Periodic eye examination is recommended because retinal degeneration has been noted in animal studies.

DRUG INTERACTIONS

May enhance CNS effects of **alcohol, barbiturates,** and other sedatives. **Tolazoline** and **tricyclic antidepressants** may block the antihypertensive effects of clonidine.

ADVERSE REACTIONS

Most common are dry mouth (40%), drowsiness (35%), and sedation (8%). Constipation, dizziness, headache, and fatigue have also been reported. Generally, these effects tend to diminish with continued therapy within 4 to 6 weeks. The following have been associated with the drug, some of them rarely. In some instances, exact causal relationship has not been established.

GI: Anorexia, malaise, nausea and vomiting, parotid pain, mild transient abnormalities in hepatic-function tests.

Metabolic: Weight gain, transient elevation in blood glucose or serum creatine phosphokinase, gynecomastia.

Cardiac: Congestive heart failure, Raynaud's phenomenon, ECG abnormalities manifested as Wenckebach period or ventricular trigeminy.

CNS: Vivid dreams or nightmares, insomnia, delirium, other behavioral changes, nervousness, restlessness, anxiety, mental depression.

Dermatologic: Rash, angioneurotic edema, hives, urticaria, thinning of hair; pruritus not associated with rash.

GU: Impotence, urinary retention.

Other: Increased sensitivity to alcohol; dryness, itching, burning of eyes; dryness of nasal mucosa; pallor; weakly positive Coombs' test.

OVERDOSAGE

Symptoms: Bradycardia, CNS depression, respiratory depression, apnea, hypothermia, miosis, seizures, lethargy, agitation, irritability, diarrhea, and arrhythmias have been reported. Profound hypotension, weakness, somnolence, diminished or absent reflexes, and vomiting have followed accidental ingestion by children 19 months to 5 years.

Treatment: Establish respiration if necessary, perform gastric lavage, administer activated charcoal. A saline cathartic (magnesium sulfate) will increase rate of transport through the GI tract. Dopamine, 200 mg in 500 ml of 5% Dextrose in Water, infused at a rate of 10 mcg/kg/minute may be used. Atropine sulfate (0.6 mg for adults; 0.01 mg/kg in children) IV may be used to treat persistent bradycardia. Tolazoline IV, in doses of 10 mg at 30-minute intervals, may be used in those failing to respond to dopamine and IV fluids.

DOSAGE

Adjusted to patient's blood-pressure response. Initial dose is 0.1 mg bid. *Maintenance dose*—Increments of 0.1 mg/day to 0.2 mg/day may be made until desired response is obtained. Therapeutic doses most commonly used range from 0.2 mg/day to 0.8 mg/day in divided doses. Maximum dose is 2.4 mg/day. Sedative effects can be minimized by slowly increasing daily dosage and giving majority of daily dose H.S.

NURSING IMPLICATIONS

HISTORY
See Appendix 4.

PHYSICAL ASSESSMENT
Take blood pressure in both arms with patient in sitting and lying positions; take pulse rhythm and rate; record weight. Eye examination, pregnancy test (see *Warnings*), ECG, fasting blood sugar (FBS) may be ordered.

ADMINISTRATION
Majority of daily dose may be ordered H.S. to minimize sedative effects.

During initial therapy monitor blood pressure and pulse before each dose.

ONGOING ASSESSMENTS AND NURSING MANAGEMENT
Record blood pressure and pulse q4h as well as before each dose is administered; observe for adverse effects.

Weigh daily if patient is receiving concomitant diuretic therapy; otherwise, weigh weekly.

CLINICAL ALERT: Drug should not be suddenly discontinued because rebound hypertension as well as hypertensive encephalopathy may occur. Ensure continuity of prescribed therapy by notation on Kardex, informing health-team members responsible for drug administration.

Use same arm and same patient position for each blood-pressure reading; chart position, arm used.

If blood pressure markedly increases or decreases from baseline values, withhold next dose of drug and notify physician.

If drowsiness, dizziness, or lightheadedness occurs, patient may require assistance with ambulation.

Diabetic patients: FBS may be monitored more frequently because transient elevation in blood glucose may occur.

If drug is gradually being withdrawn, monitor blood pressure and pulse at more frequent intervals; notify physician immediately if a rise in blood pressure or nervousness, agitation, and headache occur.

Periodic eye examinations may be performed during long-term therapy.

PATIENT AND FAMILY INFORMATION

Do not discontinue drug unless directed by physician. Abrupt withdrawal may cause a rapid rise in blood pressure.

Avoid cough, cold, or allergy medications (some may contain sympathomimetics) unless use of a specific product is approved by physician.

May have sedative effect; observe caution while driving or performing other tasks requiring alertness. Drowsiness and dry mouth are common, especially during first days of therapy.

Dry mouth may be relieved by sips of water, ice chips, hard candy, or gum.

If dizziness (orthostatic hypotension) occurs, avoid sudden changes in posture.

Clorazepate Dipotassium

See Benzodiazepines; Anticonvulsants, Benzodiazepines.

Clotrimazole Rx

vaginal tablets: 100 mg	Gyne-Lotrimin, Mycelex-G
vaginal cream: 1%	Gyne-Lotrimin, Mycelex-G
topical cream: 1%	Lotrimin, Mycelex
topical solution: 1%	Lotrimin, Mycelex
troche, oral: 10 mg	Mycelex

INDICATIONS

Vaginal cream and tablets: Treatment of vulvovaginal candidiasis (moniliasis).

Topical cream or solution: Treatment of tinea pedis, tinea cruris, or tinea corporis due to *Trichophyton rubrum, T. mentagrophytes, Epidermophyton floccosum, Microsporum canis;* candidiasis due to *Candida albicans;* tinea versicolor due to *Malassezia furfur.*

Troche: Oropharyngeal candidiasis.

CONTRAINDICATIONS

Hypersensitivity.

ACTIONS

Vaginal: A broad-spectrum antifungal agent that inhibits growth of pathogenic yeasts. Application has shown negligible absorption after insertion of cream or tablets.

Topical: A broad-spectrum antifungal agent that inhibits growth of dermatophytes, yeasts, *M. furfur.*

WARNINGS

Topical cream and solution for dermatologic use only. Not for ophthalmic use.

PRECAUTIONS

Vaginal: Intractable candidiasis may be presenting symptom of diabetes mellitus. Perform urine and blood glucose studies on those not responding to treatment. A persistently resistant infection may be evidence of reinfection.

Topical: If irritation or sensitivity develops, discontinue use. Use during only first trimester of pregnancy when considered essential to welfare of patient.

ADVERSE REACTIONS

Vaginal tablets, cream: Adverse effects uncommon. Mild burning may occasionally occur. Skin rash, itching, vulval irritation, lower abdominal cramps and bloating, slight urinary frequency, slight cramping, erythema, and burning or irritation in the sexual partner occur rarely.

Topical: Erythema, stinging, blistering, peeling, pruritus, urticaria, general irritation of skin.

DOSAGE

Vaginal tablets: Insert 1 daily for 7 consecutive days, preferably H.S. An alternate regimen of 2 tablets daily for 3 consecutive days is similarly effective in nonpregnant patients.

Vaginal cream: Effective when used for 7 to 14 days. Recommended dose is 1 applicatorful/day for 7 to 14 days. Insert intravaginally, preferably H.S.

Topical: Gently massage into affected and surrounding skin areas twice daily, in morning and evening.

Troche: 1 troche, 5 times daily, for 14 days.

NURSING IMPLICATIONS

HISTORY
Obtain description and duration of symptoms.

PHYSICAL ASSESSMENT
Vaginal: Physician confirms diagnosis by potassium hydroxide (KOH) smears or cultures.

Topical: Inspect areas of infection and describe in patient's record.

ADMINISTRATION
Vaginal tablets: Applicator is supplied with drug. Insert prescribed dose (1 or 2 tablets) high into vagina.

Vaginal cream: Applicator supplied with drug. Insert 1 applicatorful.

Topical cream or solution: Cleanse affected area with tap water or other solution as directed by physician. Rinse thoroughly if soap or other cleanser is used. Gently massage cream or lotion into affected area. If applying to head area, avoid contact with eyes. Wear disposable gloves when cleaning skin, applying drug.

ONGOING ASSESSMENTS AND NURSING MANAGEMENT
Vaginal tablets, cream: Provide patient with sanitary napkins to prevent staining of clothing, bedding.

Notify physician before next dose is due if patient complains of itching or burning.

If improvement is not noted in 1 week or infection becomes worse, inform physician.

Topical cream, solution: If condition worsens or irritation occurs, notify physician.

PATIENT AND FAMILY INFORMATION
Vaginal tablets, cream: Directions for use and applicator are supplied with drug.

Insert high into vagina with applicator provided.

Full course of therapy must be completed; do not stop use because condition appears to improve.

Notify physician or nurse if burning or irritation occurs.

Use sanitary napkin to prevent staining of clothing, bedding.

Topical solution, cream: Apply after cleansing area (unless directed otherwise); use method of cleansing recommended by physician.

Change clothing (socks, underwear) contacting infected area(s) after each application.

If condition persists or becomes worse, or if irritation occurs, discontinue use and notify physician.

If diagnosis is ringworm—Keep towels, facecloths, bedding separate from those of other family members. Launder clothing, linens daily; use hot water and detergent. Do not wash clothes or bedding used by other family members at same time. Follow instructions of physician about type of clothes or shoes (if feet are infected) to be worn. Keep infected areas clean and dry.

Cloxacillin Sodium

See Penicillins.

Cocaine

See Anesthetics, Local, Topical.

Codeine

See Narcotic Analgesics.

Colchicine ℞

tablets: 0.6 mg, 0.5 mg	*Generic*
tablets: 0.432 mg	Colsalide
granules: 0.5 mg	*Generic*
injection: 1 mg/2 ml	*Generic*

INDICATIONS
Treatment of gout. Is effective in relieving pain of acute attacks, especially if therapy is begun early and adequate doses are given. May be used as interval therapy to prevent acute attacks. Has no effect on nongouty arthritis or on uric-acid metabolism. IV use is advantageous when a rapid response is desired or when GI side-effects interfere with oral administration. Occasionally IV is effective when oral preparation is not. After acute attack subsides, patient is usually given oral form.

CONTRAINDICATIONS
Hypersensitivity; serious GI, renal, hepatic or cardiac disorders; blood dyscrasias.

ACTIONS
Exact mechanism of action in gout unknown. It is involved in leukocyte migration inhibition; reduc-

tion of lactic acid production by leukocytes, which results in decreased deposition of uric acid; interference with kinin formation; and reduction of phagocytosis with inflammatory response abatement. It apparently exerts its effect by reducing the inflammatory response to the deposited crystals and also by diminishing phagocytosis. Colchicine diminishes lactic acid production by leukocytosis directly and by diminishing phagocytosis, and thereby interrupts the cycle of urate crystal deposition and inflammatory response that sustains the acute attack. The oxidation of glucose in phagocytizing as well as in nonphagocytizing leukocytes is suppressed.

Colchicine is not an analgesic, although it relieves pain in acute attacks. It is not a uricosuric agent and will not prevent progression of gout to chronic gouty arthritis. It has a prophylactic, suppressive effect that helps reduce incidence of acute attacks and relieves occasional residual pain and mild discomfort.

Colchicine is rapidly absorbed after oral administration. Large amounts of the drug and metabolites enter the intestinal tract in bile and intestinal secretions. High concentrations are found in the kidney, liver, and spleen. It does not appear to be tightly bound to serum protein; the drug rapidly leaves the bloodstream; excretion occurs primarily by biliary and renal routes.

WARNINGS

Use in impaired hepatic function: Possibility of increased colchicine toxicity is considered.

Fertility: Has adversely affected spermatogenesis.

Use in elderly: Administer with caution to aged and debilitated patients, especially those with renal, GI, or heart disease. Reduction of dosage is recommended if weakness, anorexia, nausea, vomiting, or diarrhea occurs.

Use in pregnancy: Can cause fetal harm when administered to a pregnant woman. Use only when clearly needed and when potential benefits outweigh the unknown potential hazards to the fetus.

Use in lactation: Not known if drug is excreted in human milk.

Use in children: Safety, efficacy not established.

PRECAUTIONS

Rarely, thrombophlebitis occurs at site of IV injection. Periodic blood counts are recommended during long-term therapy.

DRUG INTERACTIONS

Has been shown to induce reversible malabsorption of **vitamin B$_{12}$,** apparently by altering the function of ileal mucosa. Colchicine is inhibited by **acidifying agents.** Action of colchicine is potentiated by **alkalinizing agents.** May increase sensitivity to **CNS de-**

pressants. Response to **sympathomimetic agents** may be enhanced by colchicine.

Drug/lab tests: May cause elevated **alkaline phosphatase** and **SGOT** values; decreased **thrombocyte** values may be seen. May cause false-positive results when testing **urine** for **RBC** or **hemoglobin.**

ADVERSE REACTIONS

In decreasing order of severity: Bone-marrow depression with aplastic anemia, agranulocytosis, or thrombocytopenia may occur during long-term therapy. Peripheral neuritis, purpura, myopathy, loss of hair, and reversible azoospermia also have been reported.

Vomiting, diarrhea, abdominal pain, and nausea may occur, especially when maximum doses are necessary for therapeutic effect. These may be particularly troublesome in the presence of peptic ulcer or spastic colon. At toxic doses may cause severe diarrhea, generalized vascular damage, and renal damage with hematuria and oliguria. GI symptoms may occur even with IV therapy, usually with large doses. To avoid more serious toxicity, discontinue use when these symptoms appear, regardless of whether joint pain has been relieved. Dermatoses have been reported. Hypersensitivity reactions occur infrequently.

ACUTE OVERDOSAGE

Symptoms: There is usually a latent period between overdosage and onset of symptoms, regardless of route of administration. Lethal dose has been estimated to be 65 mg; deaths have been reported with as little as 7 mg. First symptoms are gastrointestinal (nausea, vomiting, abdominal pain, diarrhea). Diarrhea may be severe and bloody, owing to hemorrhagic gastroenteritis. Burning sensations in the throat, stomach, and skin may also occur. Extensive vascular damage may result in shock. Kidneys may show evidence of damage by hematuria and oliguria. Severe dehydration and hypotension may develop. Muscular weakness is marked, and ascending paralysis of the CNS may develop. The patient usually remains conscious, but delirium and convulsions may occur. Death is usually the result of respiratory depression.

Treatment: Begin with gastric lavage and measures to prevent shock. Recent studies support use of hemodialysis or peritoneal dialysis as part of treatment in addition to gastric lavage. Respiratory assistance may be needed. Paregoric may be administered to control diarrhea and cramps.

DOSAGE

Parenteral

Must be given IV. Severe local irritation occurs if administered subcutaneously or IM.

**Acute gouty arthritis:** Average initial dose is 2 mg. May be followed by 0.5 mg q6h until satisfactory response is obtained. In general, total dosage for 24-hour period should not exceed 4 mg. A single IV dose of 1 mg or 3 mg may also be administered initially, followed by 0.5 mg once or twice daily, if needed. If pain recurs, a daily dose of 1 mg or 2 mg may be administered for several days. Patient may be transferred to oral therapy, with a dose similar to IV dose.

**Prophylaxis or maintenance therapy of recurrent or chronic gouty arthritis:** Dosage of 0.5 mg to 1 mg once or twice daily. Oral administration is preferable, usually in conjunction with a uricosuric agent.

**Oral**

**Treatment of acute gouty arthritis:** Usual dose to relieve or abort attack is 1 mg to 1.2 mg. May be followed by 0.5 mg to 1.2 mg q1h to q2h until pain is relieved. Drug should be stopped if there is GI discomfort or diarrhea. Total amount needed to control pain and inflammation during an acute attack usually ranges from 4 mg to 8 mg. If a second course is required, an interval of 3 days between courses is advised to minimize possibility of toxic effects. If corticotropin (ACTH) is administered for treatment of an acute attack of gouty arthritis, it is recommended colchicine also be given in doses of at least 1 mg/day and be continued for a few days after ACTH is withdrawn.

**Prophylaxis during intercritical attacks:** To reduce frequency of paroxysms and lessen their severity, colchicine may be administered continuously. In those who have fewer than one attack per year, usual dose is 0.5 mg or 0.6 mg daily for 3 to 4 days per week. In cases involving more than one attack per year, usual dose is 0.5 mg to 0.6 mg daily; severe cases may require 1 mg to 1.8 mg daily.

**Prophylaxis against attacks of gout in patients undergoing surgery:** In patients with gout, an attack may be precipitated by even minor surgical procedures; 0.5 mg or 0.6 mg may be administered tid for 3 days before and 3 days after surgery.

NURSING IMPLICATIONS

HISTORY
See Appendix 4.

PHYSICAL ASSESSMENT
Monitor vital signs; note appearance of joints involved and record observations. Baseline serum uric acid, CBC usually ordered. If renal or hepatic disease is suspected, function studies may be ordered.

ADMINISTRATION
Physician may order dose in milligrams (mg) or grains (gr). The following are the equivalents: 0.432 mg = gr 1/140; 0.5 mg = gr 1/120; 0.6 mg = gr 1/100; 1 mg = gr 1/69.

**Oral:** Usually can be given with food or milk. Check with physician about administration with food when drug is given q1h to q2h to abort an acute attack.

**Parenteral:** Administer _IV only_ over period of 2 to 5 minutes. Do not dilute with 5% Dextrose in Water if a decrease in concentration is ordered. Use 0.9% Sodium Chloride Injection, which does not contain a bacteriostatic agent. Do not use solutions that have become turbid.

In IV administration, needle must be properly positioned in the vein and good blood return seen before drug is injected. Extravasation into surrounding tissues results in extreme irritation.

If extravasation does occur, local application of heat or cold may relieve discomfort. Analgesics may also be given.

ONGOING ASSESSMENTS AND NURSING MANAGEMENT
Oral form is administered q1h to q2h until pain is relieved _or_ there is GI discomfort (nausea, vomiting, abdominal pain) or diarrhea. Drug is discontinued as soon as these symptoms appear. Physician will then decide when to begin daily dosages.

CLINICAL ALERT: It is imperative that drug be stopped when GI symptoms occur, because continued administration will result in overdosage (see _Acute Overdosage_).

During initial therapy to relieve an acute attack, assess drug response q½h to q1h; either adverse reactions or lack of pain relief requires discontinuing drug. Chart all subjective and objective symptoms on a flow chart because these aid physician in evaluating present and future therapy. Measure intake and output during the acute attack.

If the patient has had repeated acute attacks, he may be able to judge his drug requirement accurately enough to stop short of his "diarrheal dose" and request that medication be stopped.

Articular pain and swelling typically abate within 12 hours and are usually gone in 24 to 48 hours. Analgesics may be ordered for pain relief until acute attack subsides.

An increased fluid intake and a urinary output of approximately 2000 ml/day is necessary to promote urate excretion and prevent formation of urate stones. Alkalinization of the urine with sodium bicarbonate or other agents may be prescribed.

IV administration: Check site of injection for signs of thrombophlebitis (*e.g.,* pain or tenderness, redness, warmth).

An antidiarrheal agent, such as the opiate paregoric, may be needed to control diarrhea.

Periodic blood counts are recommended for patients on long-term therapy.

Serum uric-acid levels may be monitored frequently during initial therapy; periodic serum uric-acid determinations are usually performed during long-term therapy.

A uricosuric agent such as probenecid may be added to the therapeutic regimen after the acute attack has subsided.

Restriction of foods containing purine is usually not necessary; foods very high in purine (*e.g.,* liver, kidney) may be eliminated from diet or eaten in limited amounts.

PATIENT AND FAMILY INFORMATION

Notify physician or nurse if skin rash, sore throat, fever, unusual bleeding or bruising, fatigue or weakness, or numbness or tingling occurs.

Discontinue medication as soon as gout pain is relieved or at first sign of nausea, vomiting, stomach pain, or diarrhea. If symptoms persist, notify physician.

Contact physician if an attack recurs or present drug therapy fails to control symptoms.

Follow physician's recommendation regarding weight loss, diet.

Alcohol should be avoided or taken in small amounts.

Do not fast to lose weight because this may precipitate an acute attack; weight loss (when necessary) should be gradual.

If a minor surgical or dental procedure is necessary, notify physician in advance because a dosage change may be necessary 3 days before and after the procedure.

Periodic laboratory tests will be prescribed to monitor drug therapy.

Always keep drug on hand so that therapy can be started or increased as recommended by physician. When traveling, have an adequate supply available.

Colestipol Hydrochloride

See Bile Acid Sequestrants.

Colistimethate Sodium Rx

powder for injection: Coly-Mycin M
150 mg

INDICATIONS

Treatment of acute and chronic infections due to sensitive strains of certain gram-negative bacilli. Particularly indicated when infection is caused by sensitive strains of *Pseudomonas aeruginosa.* Also proven effective in treatment of infections due to *Enterobacter aerogenes, Escherichia coli, Klebsiella pneumoniae.* Pending results of culture and sensitivity tests, may be used to initiate therapy in serious infections suspected to be due to gram-negative organisms.

CONTRAINDICATIONS

Hypersensitivity.

ACTIONS

Has bactericidal activity against gram-negative organisms listed above. Administered IM or IV; higher blood levels obtained after IV administration. Serum half-life is 2 to 3 hours. Blood levels peak at over 5 mcg/ml between 1 to 2 hours after IM administration. Is transferred across the placental barrier.

WARNINGS

Do not exceed 5 mg/kg/day in patients with normal renal function. Transient neurologic disturbances may occur and include circumoral paresthesias or numbness, tingling of extremities, generalized pruritus, vertigo, dizziness, and slurred speech. Reduction of dosage may relieve symptoms. Therapy may not be discontinued but patient is observed closely. Overdosage can result in renal insufficiency, muscle weakness, or apnea. Safety for use in pregnancy is not established. Use only when potential benefits outweigh the potential risks.

PRECAUTIONS

Drug is eliminated mainly by renal excretion. Use with caution when possibility of impaired renal function exists. The decline in renal function with advanced age is considered. When renal impairment exists, modify dosage in proportion to the extent of impairment. Administration of amounts in excess of renal excretory capacity will lead to high serum levels, resulting in further impairment of renal function. If not recognized, this can lead to acute renal insufficiency, renal shutdown, and further concentration of the antibiotic to toxic levels. At this point, interference with nerve transmission at neuromuscular junctions may occur and result in muscular weakness and apnea.

Early signs indicating development of impaired renal function are diminishing urine output and rising BUN and serum creatinine. If these are present, discontinue drug immediately. If a life-threatening situation exists, therapy may be reinstated at lower dosages after blood levels have fallen. If apnea occurs, it is treated with assisted respiration, oxygen, and calcium chloride injections.

DRUG INTERACTIONS

Concurrent use with other **nephrotoxic** drugs (*e.g.,* aminoglycosides) is avoided; these toxic effects will be additive. Neuromuscular blockade and muscular paralysis may occur; these effects are additive when drug is administered concurrently with **anesthetics, neuromuscular blocking agents,** or **other drugs with neuromuscular blocking activity.**

ADVERSE REACTIONS

Respiratory arrest has been reported following IM administration. Impaired renal function increases the possibility of apnea and neuromuscular blockade, generally because of failure to follow recommended guidelines, overdosage, failure to reduce dose commensurate with the degree of renal impairment, or concomitant use of other antibiotics or drugs with neuromuscular blocking potential.

Renal: A decrease in urine output or an increase in BUN or serum creatinine can mean nephrotoxicity, which is probably a dose-dependent effect. Values usually return to normal following cessation of therapy.

Miscellaneous: Paresthesia, tingling of the extremities, or tingling of the tongue and generalized itching or urticaria have been reported with IV and IM use. In addition, the following have been reported: drug fever, GI upset, vertigo, and slurring of speech.

DOSAGE

For IM or IV use.

Adults and children: 2.5 mg/kg/day to 5 mg/kg/day in 2 to 4 divided doses for those with normal renal function, depending on the severity of the infection. Reduce dosage in presence of any renal impairment.

Direct intermittent IV administration: One-half of total daily dose over period of 3 to 5 minutes q12h.

Continuous IV infusion: Inject one-half of total daily dose over period of 3 to 5 minutes. Add remaining half of daily dose to IV solution and administer starting 1 to 2 hours after the initial dose at rate of 5 mg/hour to 6 mg/hour.

❙ NURSING IMPLICATIONS

HISTORY

See Appendix 4.

PHYSICAL ASSESSMENT

Monitor vital signs, weight (if needed to determine drug dose). Other areas of assessment depend on symptoms. Renal-function tests, CBC, urinalysis may be ordered. Culture and sensitivity tests are obtained before first dose is administered.

ADMINISTRATION

Reconstitute vial with 2 ml Sterile Water for Injection, USP. Swirl gently to prevent frothing. Dilution yields 75 mg/ml.

IM: Inject deeply into upper outer quadrant of buttock. Rotate injection sites; record site used.

Warn patient that IM injection may produce discomfort or pain.

Respiratory arrest has been reported following IM administration. Oxygen, calcium chloride, and respiratory resuscitative equipment should be immediately available.

Direct intermittent IV administration: Inject one-half of total daily dose over a period of 3 to 5 minutes. Administer drug q12h.

Continuous IV infusion: Freshly prepare infusion solution.

Slowly inject one-half of total daily dose over period of 3 to 5 minutes.

The remaining half of the daily dose is added to one of the following IV solutions: 0.9% Sodium Chloride; 5% Dextrose in Water, 5% Dextrose with 0.9% Sodium Chloride, 5% Dextrose with 0.45% Sodium Chloride, 5% Dextrose with 0.225% Sodium Chloride, Lactated Ringer's solution, or 10% Invert Sugar. Swirl gently to prevent frothing. Type and volume of IV solution ordered by physician.

Starting 1 to 2 hours after administration of one-half of the daily dose, the remaining half, diluted in one of the above solutions, is added to the IV line and infused at a rate of 5 mg/hour to 6 mg/hour. If renal function is impaired, infusion rate is reduced according to physician's directions.

Apply timing label. Label infusion bottle with date and time, drug and dose added.

Stability: Freshly prepare infusion solutions and use for no longer than 24 hours.

BRAND NAME SIMILARITY

Coly-Mycin M and Coly-Mycin S (colistin sulfate).

ONGOING ASSESSMENTS AND NURSING MANAGEMENT

Record vital signs q4h; measure intake and output; assess patient for adverse reactions, response to drug (*e.g.,* signs of clinical improvement).

Following IM administration, observe patient approximately q15m to q30m for first 2 hours, especially during initial therapy. Observe for restlessness, respiratory distress, apnea. If these occur, contact physician immediately.

Observe patient for signs of respiratory distress; this is especially important in the elderly, infants, and those with renal impairment.

If renal output decreases, notify physician immediately because decrease may be indicative of renal impairment. Drug may need to be discontinued or dosage reduced.

Transient neurologic disturbances (see *Warnings, Adverse Reactions*) may occur. Because these symptoms are subjective, they may not be manifest in infants or young children. If these occur, notify physician because a reduction in dosage may be ordered.

If ambulatory and neurologic disturbances occur, assistance with ambulatory activities is usually necessary.

Repeat culture and sensitivity and renal-function tests may be performed during therapy.

Colistin Sulfate *(Polymyxin E)* Rx

oral suspension: 25 mg/5 ml   Coly-Mycin S

INDICATIONS
Diarrhea in infants and children caused by susceptible strains of enteropathogenic *Escherichia coli*. Gastroenteritis due to *Shigella* organisms. Clinical response may vary owing to absence of tissue levels in the bowel wall.

CONTRAINDICATIONS
Hypersensitivity.

ACTIONS
Bactericidal against most gram-negative enteric pathogens, especially enteropathogenic *E. coli* and *Shigella* species. In infants and children, has effectively controlled acute infections of the intestinal tract due to these pathogens. Susceptible strains rarely develop resistance. Cross-resistance to polymyxin B sulfate does exist; cross-resistance to broad-spectrum antibiotics has not been encountered.

WARNINGS
Although not absorbed systemically in measurable amounts, it is assumed that slight absorption may occur. A potential for possible renal toxicity exists in the presence of azotemia or if dosages above recommended range are used.

Superinfection: Use of antibiotics (especially prolonged or repeated therapy) may result in bacterial

or fungal overgrowth of nonsusceptible organisms. Such organisms may lead to secondary infection.

PRECAUTIONS
Assessment of renal function prior to therapy is recommended.

ADVERSE REACTIONS
None reported when recommended doses are used.

DOSAGE
Usual dose is 5 mg/kg/day to 15 mg/kg/day in 3 divided doses. Higher doses may be necessary.

NURSING IMPLICATIONS

HISTORY
See Appendix 4.

PHYSICAL ASSESSMENT
Record vital signs; examine abdomen for distention, tenderness; auscultate bowel sounds; look for signs of dehydration. Culture and sensitivity studies, renal-function studies, and serum electrolytes are usually obtained before therapy.

ADMINISTRATION
Normally comes from pharmacy reconstituted. Expiration date (2 weeks) should be on bottle.

Reconstitution directions are as follows: Measure 37 ml distilled water. Slowly add one-half this amount, replace cap, and shake well. Add remaining amount and shake well.

If child is unable to swallow entire dose or if part of dose is lost by spitting or drooling, notify physician.

Stability: After reconstitution, stable for 2 weeks when kept below 15°C (59°F).

BRAND NAME SIMILARITY
Coly-Mycin S and Coly-Mycin M (colistimethate sodium).

ONGOING ASSESSMENTS AND NURSING MANAGEMENT
Obtain vital signs q4h; note frequency and consistency of bowel movements and enter data on chart; observe for signs of dehydration, electrolyte imbalance.

If diarrhea is not improved or becomes worse, notify physician.

Note urinary output. If patient is an infant, determine adequacy of output by inspection of diaper during changes.

Observe for signs of superinfection (Appendix 6, section 6-22). Notify physician if signs and symptoms occur.

Isolation may be necessary. Good handwashing technique is essential to prevent transmission to other patients.

PATIENT AND FAMILY INFORMATION

Complete prescribed course of therapy. Do not discontinue without first checking with physician, even if bowel movements are normal.

If teaspoon is used to measure dose, use same type each time. Preferably, purchase calibrated measuring spoon available in most pharmacies.

Keep drug refrigerated.

If child does not swallow all of each dose, contact physician; do not repeat part of dose that is lost unless advised to do so by physician.

If problem is not relieved, diarrhea becomes more frequent, or white patches are seen in the mouth, contact physician.

Wash hands thoroughly after changing diapers or clothing or handling infant or child.

Collagenase Rx

ointment: 250 units/g   Biozyme-C, Santyl

INDICATIONS

For debriding dermal ulcers and severely burned areas.

CONTRAINDICATIONS

Local or systemic hypersensitivity.

ACTIONS

Collagen accounts for 75% of the dry weight of tissue. The ability of collagenase to digest collagen in the physiologic pH range and temperature makes it effective in removal of detritus. Collagenase contributes to the formation of granulation tissues and subsequent epithelialization of dermal ulcers and severely burned areas. Collagen in healthy tissue or in newly formed granulation tissue is not attacked.

PRECAUTIONS

Enzyme's optimal pH range is 6 to 8; higher or lower pH conditions decrease enzymatic activity. Monitor debilitated patients for systemic bacterial infections because debriding enzymes may increase risk of bacteremia. Slight transient erythema has been noted occasionally in surrounding tissue, particularly when ointment was not confined to the lesion.

DRUG INTERACTIONS

Enzymatic activity is adversely affected by **detergents, hexachlorophene,** and **heavy metal ions** such

as **mercury** and **silver,** which are used in some antiseptics. When it is suspected that such materials have been used, carefully cleanse site by repeated washings with normal saline before ointment is applied. Avoid soaks containing metal ions or acid solutions such as **Burow's solution** because of metal ion and low pH. Cleansing materials, such as hydrogen peroxide and Dakin's solution, do not interfere with enzyme activity.

ADVERSE REACTIONS

No allergic sensitivity or toxic reactions reported.

OVERDOSAGE

Action of enzyme may be stopped by application of Burow's solution (pH 3.6–4.4) to the lesion.

DOSAGE

Apply once daily (more frequently if dressing becomes soiled). When infection is present, as evidenced by positive cultures, pus, inflammation, or odor, an appropriate topical antibacterial agent may be prescribed. Neomycin-Bacitracin-Polymyxin B is compatible with collagenase ointment and should be applied to lesion in powder form or solution before application of collagenase ointment.

NURSING IMPLICATIONS

HISTORY

Review patient's chart for etiology, extent of lesions, health history, and previous treatment modalities (if any).

PHYSICAL ASSESSMENT

Describe location, extent, and appearance of lesions.

ADMINISTRATION

Burns: Physician may crosshatch thick eschar with a #10 blade to allow collagenase more surface contact with necrotic debris, and as much loosened detritus as possible is removed with sterile forceps and scissors.

Before application of ointment, lesion should be cleansed of debris and digested material. Physician orders preapplication treatment. _Recommended_—Gently rub with gauze pad saturated with hydrogen peroxide or Dakin's solution followed by sterile normal saline solution.

If antibiotic ointment is used, it is applied prior to application of collagenase ointment.

Use a wooden tongue depressor or spatula to apply ointment. Apply carefully within area of lesion. Physician may order dressing to be applied over treated area.

When dealing with shallow wounds, use sterile gauze pad: apply to wound and secure properly.

All excess ointment should be removed each time dressing is changed.

If dressing becomes soiled, ointment may be reapplied.

ONGOING ASSESSMENTS AND NURSING MANAGEMENT

Note response of drug application to ulcer or burned area; chart observations daily.

If lesion shows evidence of increased inflammation, pus formation, or odor, contact physician.

Burow's solution can be used to stop drug action.

Use of ointment is usually terminated when debridement of necrotic tissue is complete and granulation tissue is well established.

Combined Estrogens, Aqueous

See Estrogens.

Conjugated Estrogens

See Estrogens.

Contraceptives, Oral

Combination Products* Rx

2.5 mg norethynodrel, 100 mcg mestranol	Enovid-E (*20*), Enovid-E 21 (*21*)
2 mg norethindrone, 100 mcg mestranol	Norinyl 2 mg (*20*), Ortho-Novum 2 mg 21 (*21*)
1 mg ethynodiol diacetate, 100 mcg mestranol	Ovulen (*20*), Ovulen-21 (*21*), Ovulen-28 (*21 + 7 inert*)
1 mg norethindrone, 80 mcg mestranol	Norinyl 1 + 80 21-Day (*21*), Norinyl 1 + 80 28-Day (*21 + 7 inert*), Ortho-Novum 1/80 21 (*21*), Ortho-Novum 1/80 28 (*21 + 7 inert*)
5 mg norethynodrel, 75 mcg mestranol	Enovid 5 mg (*20*)
1 mg norethindrone, 50 mcg mestranol	Norinyl 1 + 50 21-Day (*21*), Norinyl 1 + 50 28-Day (*21 + 7 inert*), Ortho-Novum 1/50 21 (*21*), Or-
	tho-Novum 1/50 28 (*21 + 7 inert*)
1 mg norethindrone, 50 mcg ethinyl estradiol	Ovcon-50 (*21 or 28 + 7 inert*)
1 mg norethindrone acetate, 50 mcg ethinyl estradiol	Norlestrin 21 1/50 (*21*), Norlestrin 28 1/50 (*21 + 7 inert*), Norlestrin Fe 1/50 (*21 + 7 ferrous fumarate 75 mg*)
1 mg ethynodiol diacetate, 50 mcg ethinyl estradiol	Demulen (*21*), Demulen-28 (*21 + 7 inert*)
2.5 mg norethindrone acetate, 50 mcg ethinyl estradiol	Norlestrin 21 2.5/50 (*21*), Norlestrin Fe 2.5/50 (*21 + 7 ferrous fumarate 75 mg*)
0.5 mg norgestrel, 50 mcg ethinyl estradiol	Ovral (*21*), Ovral-28 (*21 + 7 inert*)
1 mg norethindrone, 35 mcg ethinyl estradiol	Norinyl 1 + 35 21-day (*21*), Norinyl 1 + 35 28-Day (*21 + 7 inert*), Ortho-Novum 1/35 21 (*21*), Ortho-Novum 1/35 28 (*21 + 7 inert*)
0.5 mg norethindrone, 35 mcg ethinyl estradiol	Brevicon 21-Day (*21*), Brevicon 28-Day (*21 + 7 inert*), Modicon (*21*), Modicon 28 (*21 + 7 inert*)
0.4 mg norethindrone, 35 mcg ethinyl estradiol	Ovcon-35 (*21*)
1 mg ethynodiol diacetate, 35 mcg ethinyl estradiol	Demulen 1/35 (*21*), Demulen 1/35 28 (*21 + 7 inert*)
0.5 mg norethindrone, 35 mcg ethinyl estradiol (10 tablets) followed by 1 mg norethindrone, 35 mcg ethinyl estradiol (11 tablets)	Ortho-Novum 10/11-21 (*21*), Ortho-Novum 10/11-28 (*21 + 7 inert*)
1.5 mg norethindrone, 30 mcg ethinyl estradiol	Loestrin 21 1.5/30 (*21*), Loestrin Fe 1.5/30 (*21 + 7 ferrous fumarate 75 mg*)
0.3 mg norgestrel, 30 mcg ethinyl estradiol	Lo/Ovral (*21*), Lo/Ovral-28 (*21 + 7 inert*)
0.15 mg levonorgestrel, 30 mcg ethinyl estradiol	Nordette (*21*), Nordette-28 (*21 + 7 inert*)
1 mg norethindrone acetate, 20 mcg ethinyl estradiol	Loestrin 21 1/20 (*21*), Loestrin Fe 1/20 (*21 + 7 ferrous fumarate 75 mg*)

* Combination products are listed in order of decreasing estrogen (mestranol or ethinyl estradiol) content. The number of tablets per dispenser is listed in parentheses.

Progestin-Only Products Rx

0.35 mg norethin- drone	Micronor, Nor-Q.D.
0.075 mg norgestrel	Ovrette (contains tartra- zine)

INDICATIONS

Prevention of pregnancy. Because of the positive association between the dose of estrogens and risk of thrombophlebitis, minimize exposure to estrogens by prescribing a product with the least estrogen activity compatible with an acceptable pregnancy rate and patient acceptance. New users of oral contraceptives (OCs) should generally be started on preparations that contain 50 mcg or less of estrogen.

CONTRAINDICATIONS

Thrombophlebitis; thromboembolic disorders; history of deep vein thrombosis; cerebral vascular disease; myocardial infarction (MI); coronary artery disease; known or suspected carcinoma of the breast or estrogen-dependent neoplasia; undiagnosed abnormal genital bleeding; known or suspected pregnancy (see _Warnings_); past or present benign or malignant liver tumors (see _Warnings_).

ACTIONS

Progestin-only: Mechanism by which progestin-only contraceptives prevent conception is not known, but they alter cervical mucus, exert a progestational effect on the endometrium (interfering with implantation), and in some patients suppress ovulation.

Combination OCs: Inhibit ovulation by suppression of the gonadotropins follicle-stimulating hormone (FSH) and luteinizing hormone (LH). Additionally, alterations in the genital tract, including alterations in cervical mucus (which inhibits sperm penetration) and the endometrium (which inhibits implantation) may also contribute to their effectiveness.

These products differ both in potency of the components and in the relative predominance of estrogenic or progestational activity. Two estrogens, mestranol and ethinyl estradiol, are generally considered to be equivalent in activity; 50 mcg of ethinyl estradiol is equivalent in ovulation suppression to 80 mcg of mestranol.

Progestins may modify the effects of estrogens; these effects are dependent on the type and amount of progestin present and the ratio of progestin to estrogen. Dosage, potency, length of administration, and concomitant administration with estrogen are factors that contribute to total progestational potency. Total estrogenic potency of an OC is based on the combined effects of the estrogen and the estrogenic/antiestrogenic effect of the progestin component.

WARNINGS

Cigarette smoking increases the risk of cardiovascular side-effects. This risk increases with age and with heavy smoking (15 or more cigarettes/day) and is quite marked in women over 36 years of age.

The use of OCs is associated with increased risk of venous and arterial thromboembolism, thrombotic and hemorrhagic stroke, MI, visual disorders, hepatic adenomas and tumors, gallbladder disease, hypertension, and fetal abnormalities.

Mortality associated with all methods of birth control is low compared with the risk of childbirth, with the exception of OC use in women over 40 who smoke.

Drug is discontinued at earliest symptoms of thromboembolic and thrombotic disorders. The incidence of thromboembolism is lower in those with type O blood.

An increased risk of MI has been reported. The greater the number of underlying risk factors (smoking, hypertension, hypercholesterolemia, obesity, diabetes, history of preeclamptic toxemia), the higher the risk of developing MI, regardless of OC use, although OCs are considered an additional risk factor. It is estimated that OC users are about twice as likely to have a fatal MI.

Preliminary data suggest that the increased risk of MI persists after discontinuation of long-term use of OCs; the highest-risk group includes women ages 40 to 49 who used OCs for more than 10 years.

Smoking: OC users who also smoke have about a fivefold increased risk of fatal infarction as compared with nonsmoking users.

Dose: Risk of thromboembolism, including coronary thrombosis, is directly related to the dose of estrogen (and in some cases, progestogen) used; however, this may not be the sole factor involved.

Age: Risk of thromboembolic and thrombotic disease associated with OCs increases after approximately age 30 and increases substantially at age 40 and over, especially in those with other risk factors (smoking). Use in women over 40 is not recommended.

Postsurgical thromboembolism: Risk is increased; if possible, discontinue OCs at least 4 weeks before surgery of a type associated with an increased risk of thromboembolism or prolonged immobilization.

Varicose veins: Presence substantially increases risk of superficial venous thrombosis of the leg, depending on severity of the varicosities. This has been correlated to the progestogen dose. Varicose veins seem to have little effect on deep vein thrombosis.

Factor XII deficiency: Patients with Factor XII deficiency are at increased risk of developing thromboembolism.

Progestin-only products: Thromboembolic risk associated with progestin-only products has not been studied. Thromboembolic disease has been reported; these products should not be assumed to be free of risk.

NOTE: The association between OCs and cardiovascular disease are based on a number of studies. These conclusions have been criticized for a number of reasons: national trends of cardiovascular mortality are incompatible with these risk estimates; excess deaths may not be attributable entirely to smoking; the clinical diagnosis of thromboembolism is often unreliable. New data about risks to ex-users of OCs have further confounded these analyses.

Ocular lesions: Neuro-ocular lesions (*e.g.,* optic neuritis, retinal thrombosis) have been reported. Discontinue drug if there is an unexplained loss of vision, onset of proptosis or diplopia, papilledema, or retinal vascular lesions.

Carcinoma: No evidence has been reported suggesting an increased risk of endometrial cancer in users of OCs. OCs may, in fact, have a protective effect; users appear about half as likely to develop ovarian and endometrial cancer as those who have never taken OCs.

Hepatic lesions (*e.g.,* adenomas, hepatomas, hamartomas, regenerating nodules, focal nodular hyperplasia, hemangiomas, hepatocellular carcinoma): Benign and malignant hepatic adenomas have been associated with use of OCs. High hormonal potency may be associated with higher risk than low-potency formulations.

Birth defects and malignancy in offspring: Use of female sex hormones during early pregnancy may seriously damage offspring.

Use during pregnancy: Safety not demonstrated. If pregnancy is confirmed in patient taking OCs, she should be apprised of potential risks to the fetus, and the advisability of continuing pregnancy should be discussed in light of these risks.

Progestin use: Administration of progestin-only OCs or progestin-estrogen combinations to induce withdrawal bleeding should not be used as a test for pregnancy.

Gallbladder disease: Studies indicate an increased risk of gallbladder disease in users of OCs or estrogens.

Carbohydrate and lipid metabolism: Glucose tolerance may decrease; triglycerides and total phospholipids may increase.

Elevated blood pressure: Blood pressure may increase; hypertension may occur within a few months of beginning use. Prevalence increases with duration of use. Age is also strongly correlated with development of hypertension. Women with a history of hypertension, preexisting renal disease, toxemia or elevated blood pressure during pregnancy, familial tendency toward hypertension or its consequences, or a history of excessive weight gain or fluid retention during the menstrual cycle may be more likely to develop elevation of blood pressure.

Headaches: Onset or exacerbation of migraine or development of headache of a new pattern that is recurrent, persistent, or severe requires discontinuation of OCs and evaluation of cause.

Bleeding irregularities: Breakthrough bleeding, spotting, and amenorrhea are frequent reasons for discontinuing OCs. In breakthrough bleeding, nonfunctional causes are considered. In undiagnosed persistent or recurrent abnormal vaginal bleeding, pregnancy or malignancy is ruled out. If pathology is excluded, time or formulation change may resolve problem.

Women with history of oligomenorrhea or secondary amenorrhea and young women without regular cycles have a tendency to remain anovulatory or become amenorrheic after discontinuation of OCs. Post-use anovulation, possibly prolonged, may occur in women with previous irregularities. A higher incidence of galactorrhea and of pituitary tumors has been associated with amenorrhea in former users as compared with nonusers. With progestin-only products, an alteration in menstrual patterns is likely to occur; amount and duration of flow, cycle length, breakthrough bleeding, spotting, and amenorrhea will be variable. Bleeding irregularities occur more frequently with progestin-only products than with combination products.

Ectopic pregnancy: Ectopic as well as uterine pregnancy may occur in contraceptive failures.

Use in lactation: OCs interfere with lactation, decreasing both quantity and quality. Use should be deferred until infant is weaned.

Infertility: There is evidence of fertility impairment in women discontinuing OCs in comparison with those discontinuing other methods of contraception. Impairment appears to be independent of the duration of use of the preparation and diminishes with time.

Treatment with OCs may mask onset of the climacteric.

PRECAUTIONS

Fibroids: Under influence of estrogen-progestin preparations, fibroids may increase in size.

Depression: In those with history of psychic depression, use is discontinued if depression recurs to a serious degree.

Fluid retention: May cause fluid retention. Prescribe with caution for patient with conditions that may be aggravated by fluid retention (_e.g.,_ convulsive disorders, migraine syndrome, asthma, or cardiac, hepatic, or renal dysfunction).

Hepatic function: Those with history of jaundice during pregnancy have an increased risk of recurrence of jaundice; if jaundice develops, discontinue use. Steroid hormones may be poorly metabolized in those with impaired hepatic function; administer OCs with caution.

Pyridoxine deficiency: OC users may have disturbances in normal tryptophan metabolism, resulting in a relative pyridoxine deficiency; clinical significance is unknown, although megaloblastic anemia has been reported.

Serum folate levels: May be depressed during therapy. Because a pregnant woman is predisposed to folate deficiency and its incidence increases with lengthening gestation, a woman who becomes pregnant shortly after stopping therapy may have a greater chance of developing folate deficiency and its attendant complications.

Acute intermittent porphyria: Estrogens are reported to precipitate attacks of acute intermittent porphyria and should be used with caution in susceptible patients.

Tartrazine sensitivity: See Appendix 6, section 6-23.

Photosensitivity: Photosensitization (photoallergy or phototoxicity) may occur.

DRUG INTERACTIONS

Reduced efficacy and increased incidence of breakthrough bleeding have been reported in users treated with **rifampin** and may occur with **barbiturates, phenylbutazone, phenytoin, carbamazepine, isoniazid, neomycin, penicillin V, tetracycline, chloramphenicol, sulfonamides, nitrofurantoin, analgesics, tranquilizers, and antimigraine preparations.** The broad-spectrum antibiotics may cause failure of OCs by inhibiting bacteria in the gut.

May decrease hypoprothrombinemic effects of **oral anticoagulants** and decrease effectiveness of **anticonvulsants, tricyclic antidepressants, antihypertensive agents** (_e.g.,_ **guanethidine**), **vitamins, hypoglycemic agents (tolbutamide).** Concomitant administration of OCs and **troleandomycin** may cause jaundice.

OCs may possibly impair elimination of **caffeine, diazepam, chlordiazepoxide, metoprolol** (and perhaps **propranolol**), **corticosteroids, imipramine, phenytoin,** and **phenybutazone** and increase metabolism of **lorazepam** and **oxazepam.**

Drug/lab tests: Estrogen-containing OCs may cause the following alterations in serum, plasma, or blood unless specified otherwise:

Increased—Factors II (prothrombin), VII, VIII, IX, X; plasminogen, fibrinogen; norepinephrine-induced platelet aggregation; thyroid-binding globulin (TBG), leading to increased total thyroid hormone (as measured by protein-bound iodine or T_4 by column or radioimmunoassay); transcortin; corticosteroid levels; triglycerides and phospholipids; ceruloplasmin; aldosterone; amylase; gamma-glutamyltranspeptidase; iron-binding capacity; transferrin; renin activity; vitamin A.

Decreased—Antithrombin III; free T_3 resin uptake; pregnanediol excretion; response to metyrapone test; folate; glucose tolerance; albumin; cholinesterase; haptoglobin; vitamin B_{12}; zinc.

ADVERSE REACTIONS

Serious: Thrombophlebitis and thrombosis; pulmonary embolism; coronary thrombosis; MI; cerebral thrombosis; renal artery thrombosis; cerebral hemorrhage; hypertension; gallbladder disease; congenital anomalies; liver tumors and other hepatic lesions with or without abdominal bleeding. There is evidence of an association between use of OCs and mesenteric thrombosis, Budd-Chiari syndrome, and neuro-ocular lesions. See also _Warnings._

The following adverse reactions are believed to be drug related.

Most common: Nausea and vomiting, occurring in approximately 10% during the first cycle.

_GI:_ Abdominal cramps, bloating.

Gynecologic: Breakthrough bleeding; spotting; change in menstrual flow; missed menses during treatment; dysmenorrhea; amenorrhea during and after treatment; temporary infertility after discontinuation; change in cervical erosion and secretions; increased size of uterine leiomyomata; vaginal candidiasis.

Breast changes: Tenderness; enlargement; secretion; possible diminution in lactation when OCs are given immediately postpartum.

Dermatologic: Melasma; rash (allergic).

CNS: Migraine; mental depression.

Ophthalmic: Changes in corneal curvature; intolerance to contact lenses.

Miscellaneous: Edema; weight change (increase, decrease); cholestatic jaundice; reduced tolerance to carbohydrate.

The following have been reported in users of OCs, but the association has been neither confirmed nor refuted: Premenstrual-like syndrome; cataracts; changes in libido; chorea; changes in appetite; cystitislike syndrome; headache; nervousness; dizziness; hirsutism; loss of scalp hair; erythema multiforme; erythema nodosum; hemorrhagic eruption; vaginitis; impaired renal function; porphyria; paresthesia; auditory disturbances; rhinitis; fatigue; backache; itching; anemia; pancreatitis; hepatitis; colitis; gingivitis; lupus erythematosus; rheumatoid arthritis; prolactin-secreting pituitary tumors with amenorrhea or galactorrhea after use; endometrial, cervical, and breast cancer.

OVERDOSAGE
Serious effects not reported following acute overdosage in young children. Overdosage may cause nausea. Withdrawal bleeding may occur in women.

DOSAGE
COMBINATION PRODUCTS
20–21-Day regimen: Day 1 of cycle is the first day of menstrual bleeding. Take one tablet daily for 20 or 21 days, according to the number of tablets supplied for one cycle, beginning on day 5 of cycle. If flow has not begun within 7 days after cessation of medication, resume next course. Withdrawal flow will normally occur 2 or 3 days after last tablet is taken. Schedule should be followed whether or not flow occurs as expected and whether or not the woman experiences spotting or breakthrough bleeding during her cycle.

28-Day regimen: To eliminate need to count days between cycles, some products are supplied in packages containing 7 inert or iron-containing tablets to permit continuous daily dosage during entire 28-day cycle.

Missed dose: There is little likelihood that ovulation will occur if only one tablet is missed, but the possibility of spotting or bleeding is increased. This is likely to occur if two or more consecutive tablets are missed. If patient forgets to take one or more tablets, the following is suggested:

One tablet missed—Take it as soon as remembered, or the next day take two tablets.

Two consecutive tablets missed—Take two tablets daily for next 2 days, then resume regular schedule.

Three consecutive tablets missed—Begin new compact of tablets, starting 7 days after the last tablet was taken. Use an additional form of birth control for 7 days (after two missed doses) or 14 days (after three missed doses). The possibility of ovulation increases with each successive day that scheduled tablets are missed.

Bleeding: In rare cases of bleeding that resembles menstruation, patient should discontinue drug and begin taking tablets from a new compact on the fifth day (day 5). Persistent bleeding requires reexamination of patient.

Missed menstrual period: If patient has not adhered to prescribed dosage, pregnancy is considered. If patient has adhered to prescribed dosage regimen and misses two consecutive menstrual periods, pregnancy is considered.

Postpartum administration: May be prescribed at first postpartum examination, regardless of whether patient has experienced spontaneous menstruation. In nonnursing mothers, administration may begin immediately after delivery if desired.

Dosage adjustments: A product with 50 mcg or less of estrogen is generally used for initial therapy. Side-effects noted may be transient; if they continue, adjustment may be necessary.

PROGESTIN-ONLY PRODUCTS
Starting on the first day of menstruation, take one tablet daily, at the same time each day, every day of the year. A nonhormonal method of contraception should be used for first 14 days with norgestrel. May be initiated postpartum to nonnursing mother. When administered during postpartum period, increased risk of thromboembolic disease is considered.

Missed dose: If one tablet is missed, take as soon as remembered, then take next tablet at regular time. If two tablets are missed, take one of the missed tablets, discard the other, and take daily tablet at usual time. If more than two tablets are missed, discontinue immediately. Use an additional method of contraception if two or more tablets are missed until menses appears or pregnancy is ruled out. If menses does not occur in 45 days, regardless of circumstances, discontinue drug and use nonhormonal method of contraception. Test for pregnancy is recommended. Because of slightly higher failure rate of progestin-only products, regimen may be discontinued if only one tablet is missed and alternate methods of contraception used until menses occurs or pregnancy is ruled out.

NURSING IMPLICATIONS

HISTORY
See Appendix 4. A *thorough* health history (including pregnancies, if any) and family history of breast cancer or other malignancies are important. Before taking history, review *Warnings*.

PHYSICAL ASSESSMENT
Obtain blood pressure, weight; physician performs physical examination including Pap smear, gynecologic examination. Laboratory tests may include hepatic-function tests, pregnancy test, and others as appropriate.

ONGOING ASSESSMENTS AND NURSING MANAGEMENT
Patients receiving OCs should discontinue drug at least 4 weeks prior to surgery, if possible.

Hepatic adenoma should be considered in women presenting symptoms of an "acute abdomen" (abdominal pain and tenderness, abdominal mass, shock).

Prediabetic and diabetic patients should be observed carefully while receiving oral contraceptives because glucose tolerance may decrease.

Patient status should be reevaluated by physician at periodic intervals. Periodic examination should include blood pressure; examination of breasts, abdomen, pelvic organs; Pap smear. Yearly examinations are recommended but more frequent examinations may be indicated for some patients.

Pap smear specimens are labeled indicating OC therapy.

Severe depression usually requires discontinuing drug to determine if symptoms are drug related.

PATIENT INFORMATION

NOTE: Physician or nurse should review therapeutic regimen with patient, including adverse effects and procedure to follow if dosage is missed. Using the patient package insert and highlighting appropriate areas may be of value.

Patient package insert is available with product.

To achieve maximum contraceptive effectiveness, take exactly as directed at intervals not exceeding 24 hours. Should be taken regularly with a meal or at bedtime. The efficacy of medication depends on strict adherence to dosage schedule.

May cause spotting or breakthrough bleeding during first months of therapy. If this continues past the second month, notify physician.

Use an additional method of birth control (as recommended by physician) until after first week of administration in the initial cycle.

Corticosteroid Respiratory Inhalants

Beclomethasone Dipropionate Rx

aerosol   Beclovent, Vanceril

INDICATIONS

Control of bronchial asthma in those requiring chronic treatment with corticosteroids in conjunction with other therapy, including those receiving systemic corticosteroids and those inadequately controlled on a nonsteroid regimen in whom steroid therapy has been withheld because of concern over potential adverse effects. *Not* indicated for relief of asthma controlled by bronchodilators and other nonsteroid drugs, in those who require systemic corticosteroid treatment infrequently, or in treatment of nonasthmatic bronchitis.

CONTRAINDICATIONS

Primary treatment of status asthmaticus or other acute episodes of asthma in which intensive measures are required; hypersensitivity to any ingredient.

ACTIONS

Has potent anti-inflammatory activity, but mechanism responsible for this action is not well understood. Systemic absorption occurs rapidly. The principal route of excretion is the feces.

WARNINGS

Adrenal insufficiency: Deaths due to adrenal insufficiency have occurred in asthmatic patients during and after transfer from systemic corticosteroids to this drug. After withdrawal from systemic corticosteroids, several months are required for recovery of hypothalamic-pituitary-adrenal (HPA) function. During this period, patients may exhibit symptoms of adrenal insufficiency when exposed to trauma, surgery, or infections, particularly gastroenteritis. Although this aerosol may provide control of asthmatic symptoms during these episodes, it does *not* provide the systemic steroid necessary for coping with these emergencies.

Stress/severe asthmatic attack: During periods of stress or severe asthmatic attack, patients withdrawn from systemic corticosteroids should resume them (in large doses) immediately and contact their physicians.

Infections: Localized infections with *Candida albicans* or *Aspergillus niger* have occurred frequently in the mouth and pharynx and occasionally the larynx and may require antifungal therapy or discontinuance of aerosol steroid treatment.

Replacement therapy: Transfer from systemic steroid therapy may unmask allergic conditions previously suppressed. During withdrawal from oral steroids, some patients may experience symptoms of active steroid withdrawal (*e.g.,* joint or muscular pain, lassitude, depression) despite maintenance or even improvement of respiratory function.

Use in pregnancy and lactation: Drug is used during pregnancy, in the nursing mother, or in women of childbearing potential only when clearly needed and when potential benefits outweigh the unknown potential hazards to the fetus or nursing infant.

PRECAUTIONS

In responsive patients, inhaled beclomethasone may permit control of asthmatic symptoms without suppression of HPA function. Because it is absorbed into the circulation and can be systemically active, its effects in minimizing or preventing HPA dysfunction may be expected only when recommended dosages are not exceeded. Long-term effects, particularly local effects on developmental or immunologic processes in the mouth, pharynx, trachea, and lung, are unknown.

ADVERSE REACTIONS

Deaths due to adrenal insufficiency have occurred during and after transfer from systemic corticosteroids to aerosol beclomethasone. Suppression of HPA function (reduction in early morning plasma cortisol levels) has been reported in those receiving over 1600 mcg/day for 1 month. A few patients have complained of hoarseness or dry mouth. Bronchospasm and rash have been reported rarely.

DOSAGE

50 mcg released at the valve delivers 42 mcg to the patient.

Adults: Usual dosage is two inhalations tid or qid. In those with severe asthma, start with 12 to 16 inhalations/day; dosage is then adjusted downward according to response. Do not exceed 20 inhalations/day.

Children 6–12 years: Usual dose is one or two inhalations tid or qid according to response. Do not exceed 10 inhalations/day.

Use in patients receiving concomitant systemic therapy: Patient's asthma should be stable before treatment is started. Initially, aerosol is used concurrently with usual maintenance dose of systemic steroid. After approximately 1 week, gradual withdrawal of the systemic steroid is started. A slow rate of withdrawal is essential.

NURSING IMPLICATIONS
See below.

Dexamethasone Sodium Phosphate Rx

aerosol   Decadron Phosphate
                           Respihaler

INDICATIONS

Bronchial asthma and related bronchospastic states intractable to adequate trial of conventional therapy. *Not* indicated for occasional mild and isolated attacks of asthma that are readily responsive to epinephrine, isoproterenol aminophylline, and so on. Not employed for treatment of severe status asthmaticus when intensive measures are required. Dexamethasone should be considered only for patients not on corticosteroid therapy who have not

responded to other treatment or for patients on systemic corticosteroid therapy, in an attempt to reduce or eliminate systemic administration.

CONTRAINDICATIONS

Systemic fungal infections; hypersensitivity to any component; persistently positive sputum cultures for *Candida albicans.*

ACTIONS

Has potent anti-inflammatory effects. When given by inhalation, it may decrease the need for systemically administered corticosteroids. Systemic glucocorticoids are potent antiasthmatic agents but are generally reserved for severe acute asthmatics. Following stabilization with parenteral agents, patients may be transferred to oral, then to inhalational respiratory products. The exact mode of action is unknown. The aerosolized particles dissolve readily in secretions of the bronchial and bronchiolar mucous membrane.

WARNINGS, PRECAUTIONS, AND DRUG INTERACTIONS

See Glucocorticoids.

ADVERSE REACTIONS

Rare: Laryngeal and pharyngeal fungal infections. These have responded promptly to cessation of therapy and institution of antifungal treatment.

Miscellaneous: Throat irritation, hoarseness, coughing.

For information on the systemic effects of glucocorticoids, see p 517.

DOSAGE

Recommended initial dosage: Adults—3 inhalations tid or qid. *Children*—2 inhalations tid or qid.

Maximum dosage: Adults—3 inhalations/dose; 12 inhalations/day. *Children*—2 inhalations/dose; 8 inhalations/day.

Concomitant systemic corticosteroid therapy: When a favorable response is obtained, gradually reduce dose. In those on systemic corticosteroids, reduce or eliminate systemic therapy before reducing aerosol dosage. Gradual reduction of systemic corticosteroid therapy is essential to avoid withdrawal symptoms.

NURSING IMPLICATIONS

HISTORY
See Appendix 4.

PHYSICAL ASSESSMENT
Auscultate lungs.

Drug is almost always self-administered. Remain with patient while drug is administered.

Auscultate lungs before each treatment; record findings.

If more than one inhalation prescribed, instruct patient to allow at least 1 minute between inhalations.

Beclomethasone dipropionate: If concomitant inhalation bronchodilator therapy is prescribed, the bronchodilator is used _before_ beclomethasone aerosol in order to enhance penetration of beclomethasone into the bronchial tree. After use of the bronchodilator, several minutes should elapse before use of beclomethasone aerosol to reduce potential toxicity from the inhaled fluorocarbon propellants.

Instruct patient to rinse mouth with water after inhalation to prevent candidiasis, hoarseness, and excessive drying of oral mucous membranes.

Clean inhaler daily by removing the canister and rinsing the inhaler with warm water; dry thoroughly.

ONGOING ASSESSMENTS AND NURSING MANAGEMENT

CLINICAL ALERT: If patient is receiving concomitant systemic steroids and gradual withdrawal of the systemic steroids is prescribed, observe patient for symptoms of steroid withdrawal (_e.g.,_ joint or muscular pain, lassitude, and depression) and signs of adrenal insufficiency (Appendix 6, section 6-3). Monitor blood pressure, pulse, and respirations q4h or as ordered during this period.

During periods of emotional or physical stress or severe asthma attack, patient being withdrawn from systemic steroid therapy will require supplementary treatment with systemic steroids.

Auscultate lungs between inhalations; record findings.

Inspect oral cavity daily for signs of _Candida_ infection (_e.g.,_ cream-colored or bluish white spots/patches on the tongue or mucous membranes). Inform physician of occurrence because therapy may be discontinued and appropriate antifungal treatment instituted.

PATIENT AND FAMILY INFORMATION

NOTE: Instructions for use are provided with these products. Review instructions with patient.

Medication is for preventive therapy only and should _not_ be used to abort an acute asthmatic attack. Follow physician's directions if an acute asthmatic attack occurs.

Use at prescribed intervals. _Do not_ increase the dose (_i.e.,_ number of inhalations) or frequency of use.

Allow at least 1 minute between inhalations.

Rinse mouth with warm water after use to reduce dry mouth and hoarseness.

Notify physician immediately if soreness of throat or mouth occurs or white patches or spots are seen in the mouth or on the tongue.

Patient receiving bronchodilator by inhalation concurrently: Use bronchodilator several minutes _before_ use of beclomethasone inhaler to enhance penetration of the steroid into the bronchial tree.

Clean inhalator daily (instructions for cleaning are included in patient instruction sheet available with these products).

Beclomethasone contains 200 doses per canister. Dexamethasone contains 170 doses per canister. Divide these figures by the number of inhalations prescribed per day to estimate the number of days a canister will last. Write the date of first use and the (probable) date the canister will be empty on the label. Purchase a refill canister 3 to 5 days before you expect the canister to be empty.

Inform other physicians and dentist of therapy with this drug.

If emotional stress, illness (even minor), or an asthmatic attack occurs, notify physician immediately.

Wear identification, such as Medic-Alert, to inform medical personnel of therapy with this drug.

Corticosteroids, Intranasal

Beclomethasone Dipropionate _Rx_

| aerosol | Beconase Nasal Inhaler, Vancenase Nasal Inhaler |

Dexamethasone Sodium Phosphate _Rx_

| aerosol | Turbinaire Decadron Phosphate |

Flunisolide _Rx_

| spray | Nasalide |

INDICATIONS

BECLOMETHASONE DIPROPIONATE

Relief of symptoms of seasonal or perennial rhinitis in cases poorly controlled with conventional methods. Although systemic effect is minimal at recommended doses, drug should not be continued beyond 3 weeks in absence of significant symptomatic improvement. Not used in presence of untreated localized infections involving the nasal mucosa.

DEXAMETHASONE SODIUM PHOSPHATE
Allergic or inflammatory nasal conditions; nasal polyps (excluding polyps originating within the sinuses).

FLUNISOLIDE
Relief of symptoms of seasonal or perennial rhinitis when effectiveness of or tolerance to conventional treatment is unsatisfactory. Although systemic effects are minimal at recommended doses, drug should not be continued beyond 3 weeks in absence of significant symptomatic improvement. Not used in presence of untreated localized infections involving the nasal mucosa.

CONTRAINDICATIONS
Hypersensitivity.

ACTIONS
Have potent glucocorticoid and weak mineralocorticoid activity. Mechanism responsible for anti-inflammatory action on nasal mucosa is unknown. When administered topically in recommended doses, these agents exert local anti-inflammatory effects with minimal systemic effects. Exceeding recommended dose may result in systemic effects, including suppression of endogenous cortisol production. See Glucocorticoids for discussion of physiological and pharmacologic effects of glucocorticoids.

WARNINGS
Combined administration of alternate systemic prednisone treatment with these products may increase likelihood of hypothalamic-pituitary-adrenal (HPA) suppression as compared with a therapeutic dose of either alone. During withdrawal from oral steroids, some patients may experience symptoms of withdrawal (*e.g.,* joint or muscular pain, lassitude, depression). Patients previously treated with systemic corticosteroids and transferred to intranasal steroids should be carefully monitored. This is particularly important in those with associated asthma or other clinical conditions, in whom too rapid a decrease in systemic corticosteroids may cause a severe exacerbation of symptoms.

Use in pregnancy: Topical administration of recommended doses is unlikely to achieve significant systemic levels; however, these drugs should be used during pregnancy only if potential benefits outweigh potential hazards to the fetus.

Use in lactation: Infants born to mothers who have received substantial doses during pregnancy should be monitored for signs of hypoadrenalism. Dexamethasone appears in breast milk and could suppress growth, interfere with endogenous corticosteroid production, or cause other unwanted effects. Use these drugs with caution in nursing women.

Use in children: Safety and efficacy of beclomethasone in children under 12 not established. Dexamethasone and flunisolide not recommended for children under 6.

PRECAUTIONS
Nasal infections: When steroids are used in presence of infection, proper adjunctive anti-infective therapy is employed. *Beclomethasone and flunisolide*—Rarely, localized infections of the nose and nasopharynx with *Candida albicans* has occurred. Nasal steroids are used with caution, if at all, in those with recent nasal septal ulcers, nasal surgery, or trauma.

Systemic effects: Systemic absorption is low when used as recommended. Adrenal suppression may occur, especially with excessive doses. Use with caution, if at all, in those with active or quiescent tuberculosis infections of the respiratory tract or with untreated fungal, bacterial, or systemic viral infections or ocular herpes simplex.

ADVERSE REACTIONS
Nasal irritation and dryness are the most common side-effects. The following have also been reported: Headache, lightheadedness, urticaria, nausea, epistaxis, rebound congestion, bronchial asthma, occasional sneezing attacks, transient episodes of bloody discharge from nose, perforation of nasal septum, anosmia. Ulceration of nasal mucosa, watery eyes, sore throat, and vomiting occur rarely. Signs of hypercorticism (*i.e.,* Cushing's syndrome) may occur in some patients, especially with overdosage.

DOSAGE
BECLOMETHASONE DIPROPIONATE
Each actuation delivers 42 mcg. Usual dosage for adults and children over 12 is one inhalation (42 mcg) in each nostril 2 to 4 times/day (total dose 168 mcg/day to 336 mcg/day). May be maintained on a maximum dose of one inhalation in each nostril tid (252 mcg/day).

DEXAMETHASONE SODIUM PHOSPHATE
Each metered spray delivers 0.084 mg. Adult dosage is two sprays in each nostril bid or tid. In children 6 to 12 years, use one or two sprays in each nostril, bid, depending on age. Some patients will be symptom free on one spray in each nostril bid. Maxi-

mum daily dose for adults is 12 sprays and for children 8 sprays. Discontinue therapy as soon as feasible; therapy may be reinstituted if symptoms recur.

FLUNISOLIDE

Each actuation delivers approximately 25 mcg.

Adults: Starting dose is two sprays (50 mcg) in each nostril bid. May be increased to two sprays in each nostril tid (total dose 300 mcg/day).

Children 6–14 years: Starting dose is one spray (25 mcg) in each nostril tid or two sprays (50 mcg) in each nostril bid (total dose 150 mcg/day to 200 mcg/day).

Maximum total daily dose should not exceed eight sprays in each nostril for adults (total dose 400 mcg/day) or four sprays in each nostril for children under 14 (total dose 200 mcg/day).

Maintenance dose: After desired clinical effects are obtained, reduce dosage to smallest amount necessary to control symptoms. Some patients may be maintained on as little as one spray in each nostril daily.

NURSING IMPLICATIONS

HISTORY

Record description and duration of symptoms; health history; complete allergy history; previous treatments for allergy symptoms; prescription and nonprescription drug history.

PHYSICAL ASSESSMENT

Using nasal speculum, check nares for signs of excessive nasal mucosa secretions, edema of nasal mucosa. If nasal speculum is not available, attempt to determine patency by having patient inhale through each nostril while pinching opposite side.

ADMINISTRATION

Drug is self-administered; children may require assistance with actuation of inhaler.

Have patient clear nasal passages of secretions before use. Instruct patient to blow nose without pinching off one nares and to keep mouth open.

Seat patient upright with head tilted slightly back.

If nasal passages appear edematous or secretions are excessive, do not give drug; inform physician. Excessive secretions or edema may prevent drug from reaching site of intended action. Physician may order a nasal vasoconstrictor instilled before use of drug.

Advise patient not to inhale forcefully through nose immediately following application because drug will not have time to come into contact with nasal mucosa.

If more than one application per nostril is prescribed, instruct patient to allow approximately 1 minute between sprays. Nose should not be blown during this time.

Clean inhaler as per directions in patient instruction sheet provided with drug. Rinse thoroughly and dry.

ONGOING ASSESSMENTS AND NURSING MANAGEMENT

Advise patient that effects are not immediate; several days of use are usually required.

Sensations of irritation or burning may follow use; if severe, inform physician.

Sneezing attacks may follow use. If drug appears to have been lost, do not repeat dose but contact physician.

Patients previously treated for prolonged periods with systemic corticosteroids and transferred to intranasal steroids should be carefully monitored for symptoms of acute adrenal insufficiency (Appendix 6, section 6-3). Monitor blood pressure, pulse, and respirations q4h. Notify physician immediately if signs of adrenal insufficiency are apparent.

Patients with history of asthma: Transfer from systemic to intranasal corticosteroids may result in an exacerbation of asthma symptoms. If this should occur, contact physician immediately because appropriate therapy will be necessary.

PATIENT AND FAMILY INFORMATION

NOTE: Patient package insert is provided with product. Review directions for use and care of spray, if needed.

Do not exceed recommended dosage. Effects are not immediate; full benefit requires regular use and is usually evident within a few days.

May cause irritation and drying of nasal mucosa. If severe, contact physician.

If nasal passages are blocked, use decongestant recommended by physician just before administration to ensure adequate penetration of spray.

Clear nasal passage of secretions prior to use. Do not forcefully blow nose with mouth closed and one nostril compressed. Blow nose with both nostrils open while keeping mouth open.

If bloody or purulent discharge from nose is noted, or sneezing occurs and drug is apparently lost, contact physician.

When container is empty, discard it. Do not incinerate.

Corticosteroids, Ophthalmic* Rx

Ointments

dexamethasone sodium phosphate 0.05%	Decadron Phosphate Ophthalmic, Maxidex Ophthalmic, *Generic*

Solutions (Drops)

dexamethasone sodium phosphate 0.1%	Ak-Dex Ophthalmic, Decadron Phosphate Ophthalmic
prednisolone sodium phosphate 0.125%	Ak-Pred Ophthalmic, Inflamase Ophthalmic, *Generic*
prednisolone sodium phosphate 0.5%	Metreton Ophthalmic
prednisolone sodium phosphate 1%	Ak-Pred Ophthalmic, Inflamase Forte Ophthalmic, *Generic*

Suspensions (Drops)

dexamethasone 0.1%	Maxidex Ophthalmic
fluorometholone 0.1%	FML Liquifilm Ophthalmic
medrysone 1%	HMS Liquifilm Ophthalmic
prednisolone acetate 0.12%	Pred Mild Ophthalmic
prednisolone acetate 0.125%	Econopred Ophthalmic
prednisolone acetate 0.25%	Predulose Ophthalmic
prednisolone acetate 1%	Ak-Tate Ophthalmic, Econopred Plus Ophthalmic, Pred Forte Ophthalmic, *Generic*

INDICATIONS

Treatment of responsive inflammatory conditions of the palpebral and bulbar conjunctiva, lid, cornea, and anterior segment of the globe, such as allergic conjunctivitis; episcleritis; epinephrine sensitivity reactions; acne rosacea; superficial punctate keratitis; nonpurulent blepharitis; nonpurulent phlyctenular keratoconjunctivitis; herpes zoster keratitis; iritis; cyclitis; and selective infective conjunctivitis when inherent hazard of steroid use is acceptable to obtain advisable diminution in edema and inflammation. Also used for corneal injury from chemical irritation, thermal burns, and penetration of foreign bodies.

*All of these are prescription drugs. Brand names may contain same percentage of the corticosteroid, but additional ingredients in suspensions (*e.g.*, glycerin, benzalkonium chloride, polysorbate 80, boric acid) may vary from product to product.

CONTRAINDICATIONS

Acute superficial herpes simplex keratitis; fungal diseases of ocular structures; vaccinia, varicella and most other viral diseases of cornea and conjunctiva; ocular tuberculosis; hypersensitivity.

ACTIONS

Exert anti-inflammatory action. Local application often gives rapid relief from pain and photophobia, particularly in corneal lesions. Effect is believed to be due to anti-inflammatory actions of hormones rather than to any specific analgesic effect. Other aspects of inflammatory process such as hyperemia, cellular infiltration, vascularization, and fibroblastic proliferation are also suppressed.

By inhibiting fibroblastic proliferation, may prevent symblepharon formation in chemical and thermal burns. Decreased scarring with clearer corneas is result of inhibiting fibroblastic proliferation and vascularization. Steroids cause inhibition of inflammatory response to inciting agents of mechanical, chemical, or immunologic nature. Chronic conditions respond less rapidly and relapses are more frequent. In traumatic conditions following intraocular surgery, inflammatory reaction may be effectively inhibited.

WARNINGS

Use with caution in treatment of stromal herpes simplex keratitis; frequent slit-lamp microscopy is required.

Ocular damage: Prolonged use may result in glaucoma, damage to optic nerve, defects in visual acuity and fields of vision, or posterior cataract formation or may aid in establishment of secondary ocular infections from pathogens liberated from ocular tissues. In diseases causing thinning of cornea or sclera, perforation has been known to occur. Acute purulent untreated infections of eye may be masked or activity enhanced by presence of steroid medication. Ophthalmic ointments may retard corneal healing.

Fungal infections: Have been reported with long-term use.

Use in pregnancy: Safety of intensive or protracted use not established. Expected benefit to mother should outweigh the risk to the fetus.

Use in children: Safety and efficacy in children under 2 not demonstrated.

ADVERSE REACTIONS

Occasional burning or stinging may occur. See also *Warnings,* above. Systemic side-effects may occur with extensive use. Rarely, filtering blebs have been reported with use following cataract surgery.

DOSAGE

Duration of treatment will vary and may extend from a few days to several weeks.

Ointments: Apply thin coating in lower conjunctival sac tid or qid. When favorable response is achieved, number of applications is usually reduced to two, and later one, per day.

Solutions: Instill one or two drops into conjunctival sac every hour during the day and every 2 hours during the night as initial therapy. When favorable response is achieved, dosage is usually reduced to 1 drop q4h. Later, further dosage reduction to 1 drop tid may be used.

NURSING IMPLICATIONS

HISTORY

See Appendix 4. If problem is due to chemical irritation, thermal burns, or penetration of foreign body, obtain circumstances of injury (from patient, family, or co-workers).

PHYSICAL ASSESSMENT

Performed by physician. Record general description of eye and surrounding area.

ADMINISTRATION

Check label carefully for percentage of solution and labeling of "ophthalmic," either in brand name of drug or printed on label. *Only* drugs labeled as ophthalmic may be used in the eye.

Some brand-name products may have same percentage of corticosteroid, but other ingredients may vary. Do not interchange these products without physician's approval.

Shake suspension gently immediately before instillation.

Physician may order cleansing or removal of ointment from lids and eyelashes prior to instillation. If purulent drainage is noted, withhold instillation and notify physician.

Place patient in sitting position with head tilted back.

Solutions, suspensions: Instill prescribed amount into conjunctival sac.

Ointment: Apply thin coating in lower conjunctival sac.

Take care to prevent contamination of tip of dropper or ointment tube.

Following instillation of drops, have patient close eye. Apply light finger pressure on lacrimal sac for 1 minute following instillation.

Physician may order application of eye pad following instillation of drug. Change eye pad with each application, unless ordered otherwise.

ONGOING ASSESSMENTS AND NURSING MANAGEMENT

Inspect eye each time drug is applied. Compare present symptoms with baseline data and record observations.

Occasional stinging or burning may occur on instillation. If symptoms are severe, if patient complains of itching, or if purulent drainage is noted, contact physician before next dose is due.

In some patients, physician may monitor intraocular pressure and perform slit-lamp microscopy at frequent intervals during therapy.

If child is uncooperative during instillation of medication, removes eye dressing (if one is used), or persists in rubbing or touching eyes, discuss with physician.

PATIENT AND FAMILY INFORMATION

NOTE: Patient or family member may require demonstration of drop or ointment instillation.

Shake suspension gently immediately before instillation of drug.

Tilt head back, place medication in conjunctival sac, and close eyes. When drops are used, apply light finger pressure on lacrimal sac for 1 minute following instillation.

May cause temporary blurring of vision or stinging following administration. Notify physician or nurse if stinging, burning, or itching becomes pronounced.

Use of ointment may impair vision, especially when medication is instilled in both eyes. Seek assistance in ambulatory activities when vision is impaired.

Avoid rubbing or touching eyes.

Do not exceed recommended dosage or instill more often than prescribed.

Do *not* add additional liquid to medication.

Do not contaminate dropper or tip of ointment tube by touching eye, eyelids, or surrounding area.

Solution/suspension: Amount dispensed is small, usually 5 ml to 15 ml. Take care not to spill contents of container. If contents are spilled, obtain additional medication.

Corticosteroids, Topical

Amcinonide Rx

cream, ointment: Cyclocort
0.1%

Betamethasone *Rx*

cream: 0.2%	Celestone

Betamethasone Benzoate *Rx*

ointment, lotion: 0.025%	Benisone, Uticort
cream: 0.025%	Benisone, Uticort
gel: 0.025%	Benisone, Uticort

Betamethasone Dipropionate *Rx*

ointment, cream, lotion: 0.05%	Diprosone
aerosol: 0.1%	Diprosone

Betamethasone Valerate *Rx*

ointment, cream, lotion: 0.1%	Valisone
cream: 0.01%	Valisone Reduced Strength

Clocortolone Pivalate *Rx*

cream: 0.1%	Cloderm

Desonide *Rx*

ointment, cream: 0.05%	Tridesilon

Desoximetasone *Rx*

cream, gel: 0.05%	Topicort Gel, Topicort LP
cream: 0.25%	Topicort

Dexamethasone *Rx*

cream: 0.04%	Hexadrol
gel: 0.1%	Decaderm
aerosol: 0.01%	Aeroseb-Dex, Decaspray

Dexamethasone Sodium Phosphate *Rx*

cream: 0.1%	Decadron Phosphate

Diflorasone Diacetate *Rx*

ointment, cream: 0.05%	Florone, Maxiflor

Flumethasone Pivalate *Rx*

cream: 0.03%	Locorten

Fluocinolone Acetonide *Rx*

ointment: 0.025%	Fluonid, Flurosyn, Synalar
cream: 0.01%	Fluonid, Flurosyn, Synalar, *Generic*
cream: 0.025%	Fluonid, Flurosyn, Synalar, Synemol, *Generic*
cream: 0.2%	Synalar-HP
solution: 0.01%	Fluonid, Synalar, *Generic*

Fluocinonide *Rx*

ointment: 0.05%	Lidex
cream: 0.05%	Lidex, Lidex-E
gel: 0.05%	Topsyn

Flurandrenolide *Rx*

ointment: 0.025%, 0.05%	Cordran
cream: 0.025%, 0.05%	Cordran SP
lotion: 0.05%	Cordran, *Generic*
tape: 4 mcg/cm^2	Cordran

Halcinonide *Rx*

ointment: 0.1%	Halog
cream: 0.025%	Halog
cream: 0.1%	Halog, Halog-E
solution: 0.1%	Halog

Hydrocortisone *Rx, otc*

ointment: 0.5% (*Rx, otc*)	Hytone (*otc*), *Generic* (*Rx, otc*)
ointment: 1% (*Rx*)	Cortril, Hytone, *Generic*
ointment: 2.5% (*Rx*)	Hytone, *Generic*
cream: 0.125%, 0.25% (*Rx*)	Cort-Dome
cream: 0.5% (*Rx, otc*)	*otc preparations:* Bactine Hydrocortisone, Cortril, DermiCort, Dermolate Anti-Itch, Pro-Cort, *Generic; Rx preparations:* Cort-Dome, Hydro-tex, Hytone, *Generic*
cream: 1% (*Rx*)	Cort-Dome, Dermacort, Eldecort, Hi-Cor, Hydro-tex, Hytone, nutracort, Synacort, Ulcort, *Generic*
cream: 2.5% (*Rx*)	Eldecort, Hi-Cor-2.5, Hytone, Synacort, *Generic*
gel: 1% (*Rx*)	nutracort
lotion: 0.125% (*Rx*)	Cort-Dome
lotion: 0.25% (*Rx*)	Cetacort, Cort-Dome, nutracort
lotion: 0.5% (*Rx, otc*)	*otc preparations:* Delacort, Dermolate Scalp-Itch, *Generic; Rx preparations:* Cetacort, Cort-Dome, Dermacort, My Cort, nutracort, Ulcort, *Generic*
lotion: 1% (*Rx*)	Acticort 100, Cetacort,

	Cort-Dome, Dermacort, Hytone, nutracort, Texacort Scalp Lotion, Ulcort, *Generic*
lotion: 2.5% (*Rx*)	Hytone
spray: 0.5% (*Rx, otc*)	Aeroseb-HC (*Rx*), Calde-Cort Anti-Itch (*otc*), Dermolate Anti-Itch (*otc*), Sensacort (*otc*)

Hydrocortisone Acetate *Rx, otc*

ointment: 0.5% (*otc*)	Cortaid
ointment: 1%, 2.5% (*Rx*)	Cortef Acetate
cream: 0.5% (*Rx, otc*)	*otc preparations:* Caladryl Hydrocortisone, Gynecort, Lanacort, Pharma-Cort, Resicort; *Rx preparations: Generic*
cream: 0.5% hydrocortisone equivalent (*otc*)	CaldeCort, Cortaid, Rhulicort
cream: 1% (*Rx*)	Carmol HC, *Generic*
lotion: 0.5% (*otc*)	Cortaid, Rhulicort
foam (aerosol): 1% (*Rx*)	Epifoam

Hydrocortisone Valerate *Rx*

cream: 0.2%	Westcort
ointment: 0.2%	Westcort

Methylprednisolone Acetate *Rx*

ointment: 0.25%, 1%	Medrol Acetate

Prednisolone *Rx*

cream: 0.5%	Meti-Derm

Triamcinolone Acetonide *Rx*

ointment: 0.025%	Kenalog, Trymex, *Generic*
ointment: 0.1%	Aristocort, Aristocort A, Kenac, Kenalog, Trymex
ointment: 0.5%	Aristocort, Aristocort A, Kenalog
cream: 0.025%	Aristocort, Aristocort A, Kenac, Kenalog, Trymex, *Generic*
cream: 0.1%	Aristocort, Aristocort A, Flutex, Kenac, Kenalog, Kenalog-H, Trymex, *Generic*
cream: 0.5%	Aristocort, Aristocort A, Flutex, Kenalog, Trymex, *Generic*
lotion: 0.025%, 0.1%	Kenalog, *Generic*

aerosol: 2-second spray delivers approximately 0.2 mg	Kenalog

Anorectal Preparations *Rx, otc*

cream: 0.5% hydrocortisone	Dermolate Anal-Itch (*otc*), Anusol-HC (*Rx*)
cream: 1% hydrocortisone	Proctocort (*Rx*)
ointment: 0.5% hydrocortisone	Cortef Rectal Itch (*otc*)
aerosol foam: 1% hydrocortisone	Proctofoam-HC (*Rx*)
suppositories: 10 mg hydrocortisone	Anugard-HC (*Rx*), Anusol-HC (*Rx*), Corticaine (*Rx*), Hemorrhoidal HC (*Rx*), Hemusol HC (*Rx*), Rectacort (*Rx*), Rectal Medicone-HC, (*Rx*) Wyanoids HC (*Rx*)
suppositories: 15 mg hydrocortisone	Cort-Dome Regular (*Rx*)
suppositories: 25 mg hydrocortisone	Cort-Dome High Potency (*Rx*)

INDICATIONS

Relief of inflammatory and pruritic manifestations of corticosteroid-responsive dermatoses. Nonprescription products indicated for temporary relief of minor skin irritations, itching, and rashes due to eczema; dermatitis; insect bites; poison ivy, oak, or sumac; soaps, detergents, cosmetics, or jewelry; and itchy genital and anal areas.

Anorectal products are used to reduce and control severe inflammation and swelling. They are contraindicated in tuberculosis and in fungal and most viral lesions of the skin, including herpes, vaccinia, and varicella. Many of these products contain additional ingredients such as extract of belladonna, zinc oxide, benzocaine, or ephedrine sulfate. Only the steroid content is included in the above product list.

CONTRAINDICATIONS

Fungal infections; when tuberculosis of skin is present; in vaccinia and varicella; in the ear if drum is perforated; hypersensitivity. These preparations are not for ophthalmic use. When applied to eyelids or skin near eyes, drug may enter eyes. Prolonged ocular exposure may cause steroid-induced glaucoma. Topical steroids should not be used when circulation is markedly impaired.

ACTIONS

Have anti-inflammatory, antipruritic, and vasoconstrictive actions when applied topically. Clinical efficacy is dependent on extent of percutaneous absorption or penetration of active drug through the skin. Factors influencing absorption include agent used; concentration of drug; vehicle used; anatomic site of application; and integrity of epidermal barrier. Occlusive dressings or transparent plastic wrap will enhance absorption. Increased absorption can cause adverse systemic steroid effects; this may occur in those with altered skin, as in atopic dermatitis.

Vehicles: Greasy ointment bases are generally more occlusive and preferred for dry scaly lesions; greasy creams may be equally effective. Gels are less occlusive. Aerosols, lotions, and solutions are preferred for hairy areas. Urea enhances hydration and may enhance absorption. Steroid-impregnated tapes are useful for occlusive therapy of small areas.

WARNINGS
Safety for use in pregnancy not established. Should not be used extensively, in large amounts, or for prolonged periods on pregnant patients.

PRECAUTIONS
Systemic effects: Systemic absorption of topical corticosteroid has produced reversible hypothalamic-pituitary-adrenal (HPA) axis suppression, manifestations of Cushing's syndrome, and glycosuria in some patients. Conditions augmenting systemic absorption include application of more potent steroids, use over large areas, prolonged use, and addition of occlusive dressing. Recovery of HPA axis function is generally prompt and complete when use is discontinued. Infrequently, signs of steroid withdrawal may occur.

Local irritation: Discontinue use if irritation develops. When applied to intertriginous areas, oleaginous ointments may be irritating and are not recommended. Medications containing alcohol may produce burning sensations in open lesions or drying skin. Ulceration has been reported with use in skin conditions involving impaired circulation. Care should be taken when used periorbitally, or in the scrotal, vulvar, or perineal areas, because of burning sensation.

Infections: In presence of infection, therapy with appropriate antifungal or antibacterial agents is instituted. If a favorable response does not occur, corticosteroid therapy is discontinued. Due to anti-inflammatory action, all topical corticosteroids may mask signs of and enhance dissemination of infection.

Occlusive therapy: Generally, occlusive dressing should not be used on weeping or exudative lesions. Inspect lesions between dressings for development of infection. When large areas of body are covered, thermal homeostasis may be impaired.

Pediatric use: Children may show greater susceptibility to topical steroid-induced HPA axis suppression and Cushing's syndrome. Administration should be limited to the least amount possible.

ADVERSE REACTIONS
The following have been reported, especially under occlusive dressings: burning sensations; itching; irritation; dryness; folliculitis; hypertrichosis; acneiform eruptions; hypopigmentation; perioral dermatitis; allergic contact dermatitis; maceration of skin; secondary infection; skin atrophy; striae; miliaria. Following prolonged contact around eyes, cataracts and glaucoma may develop. In diffusely atrophied skin, blood vessels may become visible on skin surface and purpura may occur at site of trauma.

Systemic effects: Excessive or prolonged application can produce systemic effects, including adrenal suppression. This is more likely to occur when drug is used on broken skin or with occlusive dressings and with more potent fluorinated steroid derivatives. Prolonged application has produced growth retardation in children. Benign intracranial hypertension, the development of cushingoid features, and edema have also been reported.

DOSAGE
See *Administration.*

NURSING IMPLICATIONS

HISTORY
See Appendix 4.

PHYSICAL ASSESSMENT
Examine and describe involved areas.

ADMINISTRATION
Avoid contact with eyes.

Apply sparingly in a light film and rub in lightly unless ordered otherwise by physician. Cover involved area only.

Cover application with an occlusive dressing only if ordered by physician. Use prescribed type of dressing.

Aerosols: Avoid inhalation when applying. If applied near patient's face, prevent inhalation by having patient hold small folded towel or several thicknesses of facial tissue in front of nose and mouth.

ONGOING ASSESSMENTS AND NURSING MANAGEMENT
Inspect area each time drug is applied. Note changes as compared with baseline data. If problem does not improve or worsens, infection is apparent, or sensitivity to drug (burning, irrita-

tion) or occlusive material (rash, itching, redness) is apparent, notify physician.

When large areas of body are covered with occlusive dressings, thermal homeostasis may be impaired. Check temperature q4h; if elevation occurs, notify physician immediately.

Patient may develop sensitivity reaction to a particular occlusive dressing material or adhesive. If this occurs, a substitute material may be necessary.

Avoid fire hazard from plastic occlusive material. Advise patient not to smoke unless supervised.

HPA suppression has been noted in children and adults. When drug is applied to large area or is used for a prolonged period of time, or occlusive dressing is used, physician may order urinary free cortisol or ACTH stimulation test. Patients (especially children) should be observed for Cushing's syndrome, intracranial hypertension (bulging fontanelles, headaches).

PATIENT AND FAMILY INFORMATION

Apply sparingly in a light film; rub in lightly. Apply only to involved areas; do not use more often than recommended.

Avoid getting drug in eyes.

Notify physician or nurse if condition persists or worsens, if burning or irritation occurs, or if infection develops.

Rectal medication: Notify physician or nurse if symptoms become worse or bleeding is noted.

Corticotropin (ACTH) Preparations

Corticotropin Injection *Rx*

injection: 40 units/ ml, 80 units/ml	*Generic*
for injection: 25 units/vial	Acthar
for injection: 40 units/vial	Acthar, *Generic*

Corticotropin Zinc Hydroxide *Rx*

repository injection: 40 units corticotropin, 2 mg zinc/ml	Cortrophin-Zinc

Repository Corticotropin Injection *Rx*

repository injection: 40 units/ml	Cortigel-40, Cortrophin Gel, Cotropic Gel 40, H.P. Acthar Gel, *Generic*
repository injection: 80 units/ml	Cortigel-80, Cortrophin Gel, Cotropic Gel 80, H.P. Acthar Gel, *Generic*

INDICATIONS

Diagnostic testing of adrenocortical function. Has limited therapeutic value in conditions responsive to corticosteroid therapy. May be employed in the following: nonsuppurative thyroiditis; hypercalcemia associated with cancer; acute exacerbations of multiple sclerosis; tuberculous meningitis with subarachnoid block or impending block (when accompanied by appropriate antituberculosis chemotherapy); trichinosis with neurologic or myocardial involvement. Also indicated in same manner as the glucocorticoids (p 514).

CONTRAINDICATIONS

Scleroderma, osteoporosis, systemic fungal infections, ocular herpes simplex, recent surgery, congestive heart failure (CHF), hypertension, sensitivity to proteins of porcine origin. IV administration is contraindicated (except in treatment of idiopathic thrombocytopenic purpura, in which only IV route is recommended). IV route may be used for diagnostic testing of adrenocortical function. Contraindicated in treatment of conditions accompanied by primary adrenocortical insufficiency or adrenocortical hyperfunction.

ACTION

Corticotropin is a secretion of the anterior pituitary that stimulates the adrenal cortex to produce and secrete adrenocortical hormones. Adequate adrenal function is necessary for corticotropin to elicit a pharmacologic response. ACTH secretion is regulated by a negative feedback mechanism whereby elevated plasma corticosteroid levels suppress ACTH stores and induce morphologic changes in the pituitary. In absence of ACTH stimulation, the adrenal cortex may atrophy. Injection has a rapid onset and a duration of activity of approximately 2 hours. Repository cortricototropin and corticotropin zinc hydroxide have a slower onset but may sustain effects for up to 3 days.

WARNINGS

Not administered until adrenal responsiveness is verified with route of administration to be used during treatment. A rise in urinary and plasma corticosteroid levels provides evidence of a stimulatory effect.

Chronic administration: May lead to irreversible adverse effects. May suppress signs and symptoms of chronic disease without altering natural course of the disease. Prolonged use increases risk of hypersensitivity and may also produce posterior subcapsular cataracts and glaucoma with possible damage to the optic nerve.

Stress: Although action is similar to that of endogenous adrenocortical steroids, the quantity of adrenocorticoid may be variable. In those receiving prolonged corticotropin therapy, additional use of rapidly acting corticosteroids before, during, and after an unusually stressful situation is indicated.

Infection: May mask signs of infection, and new infections, including those of the eye due to fungi or viruses, may appear during use. There may be decreased resistance and inability to localize infection. Patients with latent tuberculosis are observed for reactivation of the disease.

Electrolytes: Can cause elevation of blood pressure, salt and water retention, and increased potassium excretion. Dietary salt restriction and potassium supplementation may be necessary. Calcium excretion may be increased.

Immunosuppression: While on corticotropin therapy, patients should *not* be vaccinated against smallpox; other immunization procedures should be undertaken with caution, especially when high doses are administered, because of possible hazards of neurologic complications and lack of antibody response. Immunization with live vaccines is usually contraindicated.

Use in pregnancy: Use in pregnancy, lactation, or women of childbearing potential only when clearly needed and when potential benefits outweigh the unknown potential hazards to the fetus. Infants born to mothers who have received substantial doses during pregnancy should be observed for hypoadrenalism.

PRECAUTIONS

Maximal corticotropin stimulation of the adrenals may be limited during the first few days of treatment; other drugs (hydrocortisone) may be administered when immediate effect is desirable. Lowest possible dose is used; when reduction in dosage is possible, it should be gradual.

Skin testing is recommended before treatment of patients with suspected sensitivity to proteins of porcine origin.

Relative adrenocortical insufficiency induced by prolonged therapy may be minimized by gradual dosage reduction. This type of insufficiency may persist for months after therapy is discontinued; in situations of stress, hormone therapy may be instituted.

Hypothyroidism and cirrhosis: There is an enhanced corticotropin effect.

Acute gouty arthritis: Limit treatment to a few days. Because rebound attacks may occur when drug is discontinued, conventional concomitant

therapy is instituted during corticotropin treatment and for a few days after treatment is discontinued.

Mental disturbances: May appear during therapy and range from euphoria, insomnia, mood swings, personality changes, and depression to frank psychotic manifestations. Existing emotional instability or psychotic tendencies may be aggravated by corticotropin.

Others: Use with caution in patients with diabetes, abscess, pyogenic infections, diverticulitis, renal insufficiency, or myasthenia gravis.

ADVERSE REACTIONS

Fluid and electrolyte disturbances: Sodium retention; potassium loss; calcium loss; fluid retention; hypokalemic alkalosis.

Musculoskeletal: Muscle weakness; osteoporosis; vertebral compression fractures; pathologic fracture of long bones; steroid myopathy; loss of muscle mass; aseptic necrosis of femoral and humeral heads.

GI: Pancreatitis; ulcerative esophagitis; abdominal distention; peptic ulcer with possible perforation and hemorrhage has been reported but disputed in the literature.

Dermatologic: Impaired wound healing; petechiae and ecchymosis; increased sweating; hyperpigmentation; thin, fragile skin; facial erythema; acne; suppression of skin-test reactions.

Cardiovascular: Hypertension; CHF; necrotizing angiitis.

Neurologic: Convulsions; vertigo; headache; increased intracranial pressure with papilledema, usually after treatment. Isolated cases of intracerebral hemorrhage and reversible cerebral atrophy have been reported in infants.

Infections: Pneumonia; abscess and septic infection. Gastrointestinal and GU infections reported more frequently with higher doses.

Endocrine: Menstrual irregularities; suppression of growth in children; hirsutism; development of cushingoid state; manifestations of latent diabetes mellitus; decreased carbohydrate tolerance; increased requirements for insulin or oral hypoglycemic agents in diabetics; secondary adrenocortical and pituitary unresponsiveness, especially in times of stress.

Ophthalmic: Posterior subcapsular cataracts; increased intraocular pressure; glaucoma with possible damage to optic nerve; exophthalmos.

Metabolic: Negative nitrogen balance due to protein catabolism.

Allergic reactions: Especially in those with allergic responses to proteins manifesting as dizziness, nausea and vomiting, shock, skin reactions.

Miscellaneous: Prolonged use may result in antibody production and subsequent loss of stimulatory effect of ACTH.

DOSAGE

Standard tests for verification of adrenal responsiveness may utilize as much as 80 units/injection or one or more injections of a lesser dosage. Verification tests are performed prior to treatment, using the routes of administration proposed for treatment. Following verification, dosage is individualized according to disease under treatment and general medical condition of patient. Only gradual changes in dosage schedules are attempted after full drug effects are apparent.

CORTICOTROPIN INJECTION

May be given IM or subcutaneously. May be given IV for diagnostic purposes.

Usual IM or subcutaneous dose is 20 units qid; chronic administration of more than 40 units/day may be associated with uncontrollable adverse effects.

Acute exacerbations of multiple sclerosis: 80 units to 120 units/day IM for 2 to 3 weeks.

For diagnostic purposes: 10 units to 25 units dissolved in 500 ml of 5% Dextrose infused IV over an 8-hour period.

CORTICOTROPIN ZINC HYDROXIDE

For IM use only. 40 units to 80 units IM every 24 to 72 hours.

REPOSITORY CORTICOTROPIN INJECTION

May be given IM or subcutaneously. *Not* for IV use. 40 units to 80 units IM or subcutaneously every 24 to 72 hours.

NURSING IMPLICATIONS

HISTORY

See Appendix 4. If patient has a history of allergy to pork or other proteins, inform physician.

PHYSICAL ASSESSMENT

Based on symptoms. Baseline urinary and plasma corticosteroid levels may be obtained prior to therapy.

ADMINISTRATION

Skin testing may be performed by physician prior to treatment of patient with suspected sensitivity to proteins of porcine origin.

Reconstitute powder by dissolving in Sterile Water for Injection or Sodium Chloride Injection so that individual dose will be contained in 1 ml to 2 ml of solution. Label vial with date, units/ml.

CORTICOTROPIN ZINC

Gently swirl suspension before withdrawing dose.

REPOSITORY CORTICOTROPIN INJECTION

Use large needle (20 gauge, 21 gauge) for withdrawing and administering.

CORTICOTROPIN ZINC AND REPOSITORY CORTICOTROPIN

Give deep IM in the gluteus muscle. *Do not* give subcutaneously.

Storage: Refrigerate reconstituted solution.

ONGOING ASSESSMENTS AND NURSING MANAGEMENT

During IV administration or immediately after IM or subcutaneous administration, observe for hypersensitivity reactions. Patient may experience rash, urticaria, hypotension, tachycardia, difficulty breathing, or angioedema. If these symptoms occur, notify physician immediately. In some instances, an order for administration of epinephrine for a hypersensitivity reaction may be written before drug is administered.

Obtain vital signs q4h to q8h or as ordered; observe for adverse drug effects; observe symptoms and compare with baseline data.

Verification of drug effectiveness may be determined by urinary or plasma corticosteroid values. Collect urine or blood sample as directed by hospital or laboratory procedure manual or directions supplied with test containers. Adherence to collection-procedure directions is important because dosage and ongoing therapy are dependent on accurate laboratory results.

CLINICAL ALERT: Corticotropin must not be abruptly discontinued (*exception*—when used for diagnostic purposes). Dosage reduction is gradual. Ensure continuity of prescribed therapy by notation on Kardex, informing health-team members responsible for drug administration.

Observe for signs of infection, which may occur in any body system, including infections of the eye due to fungi or viruses. Report any evidence or suspicion of infection to the physician immediately.

Dietary management of hypokalemia and hypernatremia may be prescribed. If diet is taken poorly, request consultation by dietitian.

Periodic ophthalmic examinations are usually performed during prolonged therapy.

PATIENT AND FAMILY INFORMATION

Vaccinations and immunizations are avoided except when deemed necessary by physician.

Inform other physicians and dentist of therapy with this drug.

Cortisone Acetate

See Glucocorticoids.

Cosyntropin Rx

for injection: 0.25   Cortrosyn
    mg/vial

INDICATIONS
Diagnostic agent in screening patients presumed to have adrenocortical insufficiency. When presumptive adrenal insufficiency is diagnosed, further studies are indicated to determine whether it is primary or secondary.

CONTRAINDICATIONS
History of previous adverse reaction to cosyntropin.

ACTIONS
A synthetic derivative subunit of ACTH that exhibits full corticosteroidogenic activity of natural ACTH. Cosyntropin 0.25 mg stimulates the adrenal cortex maximally and to the same effect as 25 units of natural ACTH. The extra-adrenal effects that natural ACTH and cosyntropin have in common include increased melanotropic activity, increased growth hormone secretion, and an adipokinetic effect.

PRECAUTIONS
Exhibits slight immunologic activity, does not contain foreign animal protein, and is therefore less risky to use than natural ACTH. Most patients with a history of previous sensitivity to natural ACTH or a preexisting allergic disease will tolerate cosyntropin; however, hypersensitivity reactions are possible.

ADVERSE REACTIONS
Rare, because drug is used for diagnostic and not therapeutic purposes. Adverse reactions other than a rare hypersensitivity reaction are not anticipated.

DOSAGE
May be administered IM or IV as a rapid screening test for adrenal function. May also be given as an IV infusion over 4 to 8 hours to provide greater stimulus to the adrenals. Doses of 0.25 mg to 0.75 mg have been used. Suggested dose is 0.25 mg. In children 2 years old or younger, a dose of 0.125 mg will often suffice. When given as an IV infusion, 0.25 mg may be used.

NURSING IMPLICATIONS

HISTORY
See Appendix 4. Obtain smoking history (smoking may alter test results). If *any* drugs have been used or administered within 1 week prior to the test, check with physician and laboratory personnel because some drugs may interfere with test results.

ADMINISTRATION
Medications that interfere with test results are discontinued before test and resumed following last blood sample.

Fasting for 10 to 12 hours prior to test is usually required.

Patient should rest quietly in bed for approximately 30 minutes before test is started.

IM: Diluent is provided with product. Sterile Saline for Injection may also be used. Administer deep IM.

IV infusion: Dose is added to dextrose or saline intravenous solution (physician specifies type and volume); administration of approximately 40 mcg/hour over 6 hours is recommended. Physician may order different infusion rate and time. Label infusion with date, time started. Apply timing label.

Test may be listed as cosyntropin test or rapid ACTH test in hospital or laboratory procedure manual.

ONGOING ASSESSMENTS AND NURSING MANAGEMENT
Explain test procedure; number of blood samples (usually three); restrictions required before, during, and after test. Advise patient not to smoke.

Normally, plasma cortisol levels rise 7 or more mcg/dl above baseline values (laboratory values may vary slightly in some hospitals).

PATIENT AND FAMILY INFORMATION
NOTE: If test is given on outpatient basis, an instruction sheet explaining what is required is given to the patient and further explained as needed.

Coumarin and Indandione Derivatives

Dicumarol (Bishydroxycoumarin) Rx

tablets: 25 mg, 50   *Generic*
    mg, 100 mg
pulvules: 25 mg,   *Generic*
    50 mg

Phenprocoumon Rx

| tablets: 3 mg | Liquamar |

Warfarin Potassium Rx

| tablets: 5 mg | Athrombin-K |

Warfarin Sodium Rx

| tablets: 2 mg, 2.5 mg, 5 mg, 7.5 mg, 10 mg | Coufarin, Coumadin Sodium, Panwarfin (7.5 mg contains tartrazine) |
| injection: 50-mg vial | Coumadin Sodium |

INDICATIONS

These drugs are anticoagulants used for prophylaxis and treatment of venous thrombosis and its extension, for treatment of atrial fibrillation with embolization, for prophylaxis and treatment of pulmonary embolism, and as adjuncts in treatment of coronary occlusion. Although all these agents provide adequate anticoagulant effects, warfarin is generally considered the drug of choice.

Investigational uses: Oral anticoagulant therapy has been used to reduce the risk of recurrent myocardial infarction, but data are conflicting. There may be some benefit in elderly persons. Warfarin has shown potential benefit as an adjunct in treatment of small-cell carcinoma of the lung when given concomitantly with combination chemotherapy and radiation treatments.

CONTRAINDICATIONS

Any hemorrhagic diathesis due to reduction in plasma coagulation factors, platelet numbers or platelet function (_e.g.,_ hemorrhagic tendencies, hemophilia, thrombocytopenic purpura, leukemia with pronounced bleeding tendencies); recent or contemplated surgery of eye or CNS (brain, spinal cord); or surgery resulting in large open surfaces. Should not be given to those with bleeding from GI, GU, or respiratory tract or to those with lesions likely to cause bleeding from these parts. _Other contraindications_—abortion (threatened), aneurysm (cerebral, dissecting aorta), clinical ascorbic acid deficiency, acute nephritis, suspicion of cerebral hemorrhage, bleeding granuloma, diverticulitis, eclampsia, preeclampsia, blood dyscrasias, uncontrolled hypertension, hepatic insufficiency, pericardial effusion, polyarthritis, polycythemia vera, ulcerative lesions (somatic, surgical wounds), ulcerative colitis, and visceral carcinoma.

Do not use anticoagulants following spinal puncture or other diagnostic or therapeutic procedures (_e.g.,_ IUD insertion) with potential for uncontrollable bleeding. Contraindicated in patients with continuous GI drainage or regional block anesthesia. Anticoagulation use may be associated with increased risks in severe trauma, infectious diseases, antibiotic therapy that alters intestinal flora and interferes with vitamin K formation, moderate to severe renal or hepatic insufficiencies, prolonged dietary insufficiencies, menometrorrhagia, moderate to severe hypertension, vasculitis, allergic disorders, anaphylactic states, indwelling catheters, severe diabetes, and major surgery.

Use in pregnancy, lactation: Contraindicated in pregnancy because drug passes the placental barrier; fetal hemorrhage and death have occurred. There have been reports of congenital malformations in children born to mothers who received these drugs during pregnancy. If a patient becomes pregnant during therapy, she should be apprised of potential risks to the fetus, and the possibility of termination of pregnancy should be discussed. Because these drugs appear in breast milk, breast-feeding is contraindicated during therapy; if anticoagulant therapy is desired, heparin may be considered.

ACTIONS

Act by interfering with hepatic synthesis of vitamin-K-dependent clotting factors. This results in depletion of clotting factors VII, IX, X, and II (prothrombin). Although factor VII is depleted in a short time and initial prolongation of the prothrombin time is seen in 8 to 12 hours, maximum anticoagulation is not approached for 3 to 5 days, as the other factors are depleted and the drug achieves steady-state (Table 21).

Oral anticoagulants are generally rapidly and completely absorbed; dicumarol, with erratic bioavailability, is the exception. Dicumarol also exhibits a dose-dependent half-life, which increases with increasing doses; both of these facts make dosing difficult. Although serum levels are easily attained for most of these agents, their therapeutic effect is more dependent on depletion of clotting factors; their du-

Table 21. Half-Life, Time to Achieve Peak Coagulation Effect, and Duration of Hypoprothrombinemia Following Discontinuation of Coumarin and Indandione Derivatives

Drug	Half-life (days)	Peak Activity (days)	Duration (days)
Coumarin Derivatives			
Dicumarol	1–2	3–5	2–10
Phenprocoumon	4–9	2–3	up to 7
Warfarin	1.5–2	1.5–3	2–5
Indandione Derivative			
Phenindione	5 hours	1–2	1–2

ration of effect may vary more in relation to their half-lives. Oral anticoagulants are highly bound to plasma proteins, primarily albumin; therefore a potential exists for interaction with other drugs capable of displacing these agents from binding sites. These agents are metabolized by hepatic microsomal enzymes and excreted primarily in the urine and feces.

Oral anticoagulants have no direct effect on an established thrombus, nor do they reverse ischemic tissue damage. Once the thrombus has occurred, anticoagulant treatment aims to prevent further extension of the formed clot and prevent secondary thromboembolic complications.

WARNINGS

Treatment is highly individualized. Dosage is controlled by periodic determination of prothrombin time, which should be monitored daily during initiation of therapy and when any other drug that may alter patient's response to anticoagulants is added to or discontinued from therapy. Once the patient is stabilized on therapy, prothrombin times may be monitored every 4 to 6 weeks. Determination of whole blood clotting and bleeding times are not effective measures for control of therapy.

Caution is used when drug is administered in any condition in which added risk of hemorrhage is present. At earliest sign of bleeding or if prothrombin time is prolonged, drug is discontinued. When hemorrhage occurs during therapy, the possibility of an organic lesion, such as a silent neoplasm, is considered.

Delayed hypersensitivity reactions: Agranulocytosis and hepatitis have been rarely associated with use of oral anticoagulants (most frequently phenindione). Periodic blood studies and hepatic-function tests are performed periodically. Hypersensitivity reactions are rare and occur within 1 to 3 months following start of indandione medication; 10% of cases that develop are fatal. Discontinue medication at first sign of hypersensitivity reactions. Symptoms include dermatitis, erythematomacular or eczematous rash, fatal exfoliative dermatitis, exudative erythema multiforme, alopecia, eosinophilia, leukopenia, thrombocytopenia, agranulocytosis, pancytopenia, neutropenia, nephropathy, nephritis, acute tubular necrosis, nephrotic azotemia, oliguria, anuria, and albuminuria. Also, enanthema with diarrhea, severe stomatitis, ulcerative colitis, paralytic ileus, mixed hepatocellular damage, hepatitis, jaundice, microadenopathy, fever, cholestasis.

PRECAUTIONS

Uncooperative, alcoholic, senile, and emotionally unstable patients are usually not suitable for therapy on outpatient basis.

Endogenous factors that will result in an increased response to oral anticoagulants or an increased prothrombin time include carcinoma, hepatic disorders, vitamin K deficiency (due to obstructive jaundice, steatorrhea, or infectious hepatitis), congestive heart failure (CHF), diarrhea, poor nutritional state, collagen disease, disorders of the pancreas, fever, cachexia, renal insufficiency, x-ray therapy, and thyrotoxicosis.

Endogenous factors reducing response to oral anticoagulants and decreasing the prothrombin time include edema, hyperlipidemia, diabetes mellitus, hypercholesterolemia, visceral carcinoma, hypothyroidism, and hereditary resistance to oral anticoagulants. Decreased sensitivity has been reported in myxedema; treatment with triiodothyronine and thyroxine will restore sensitivity to oral anticoagulants. An increase in activity of the intrinsic clotting system has been observed when edematous patients with CHF are treated with diuretics.

Some patients exhibit a genetic resistance to oral anticoagulants; these patients also have an increased need for vitamin K.

Tartrazine sensitivity: see Appendix 6, section 6-23.

DRUG INTERACTIONS

As a group, oral anticoagulants have a greater potential for clinically significant drug interactions than any other group of drugs. Although concomitant administration of some drugs with oral anticoagulants may be contraindicated, careful monitoring and appropriate dosage adjustments usually permit safe administration of combined therapy. Critical times during therapy are when an interacting drug is being added to or discontinued from the regimen of a patient stabilized on anticoagulants.

Enhanced anticoagulant effects: The drugs listed in Table 22 may increase the hypoprothrombinemic effect of oral anticoagulants when administered concurrently. The mechanisms of these interactions include inhibition of vitamin K production or absorption; displacement of the anticoagulant from protein-binding sites; inhibition of microsomal enzymes; or other mechanisms not fully understood.

Increased bleeding tendency: Use of the agents listed in Table 23 with oral anticoagulants may increase the chances of hemorrhage by inhibition of platelet aggregation, inhibition of procoagulant factor production, or ulcerogenic effects.

Decreased anticoagulant effects: The drugs listed in Table 24 may decrease the hypoprothrombinemic effect of oral anticoagulants when administered concurrently by inducing hepatic microsomal metabolism of the anticoagulant, enhancing production of procoagulant factors, or decreasing anticoagulant absorption.

Table 22. Drugs That Enhance Anticoagulant Effects, Listed by Mechanism of Enhancement

Decrease in Vitamin K	Displacement of Anticoagulant	Inhibition of Metabolism	Other
Oral antibiotics	Chloral hydrate	Alcohol (acute) ingestion)	Anabolic steroids
	Clofibrate	Allopurinol	Clofibrate
	Phenylbutazone	Chloramphenicol	Danazol
	Salicylates	Cimetidine	Glucagon
	Sulfonamides	Co-trimoxazole	Quinidine
	Sulfonylureas	Disulfiram	Sulindac
	Triclofos	Metronidazole	Thyroid drugs
		Phenylbutazone	
		Sulfinpyrazone	
		Sulfonamides	

In patients in whom the anticoagulant dosage has been established while on therapy with enzyme reducers, discontinuation of the enzyme-inducing drug may lead to increased anticoagulant response, requiring dosage reduction. Diuretic-induced hemoconcentration with subsequent concentration of clotting factors has been reported to decrease the effects of oral anticoagulants.

Other drug interactions: Anticoagulants may increase the activity and toxicity of **sulfonylurea oral hypoglycemic agents** (chlorpropamide, tolbutamide) and **phenytoin.** The concomitant use of **alcohol** or other drugs or changes in life habits (especially diet, environment) could either increase or decrease the prothrombin-time response to oral anticoagulants.

Drug/lab test interactions: Because heparin prolongs the one-stage prothrombin time, a period of 4 to 5 hours after the last IV dose or 12 to 24 hours after the last subcutaneous dose of heparin should elapse before blood is drawn for testing prothrombin time.

ADVERSE REACTIONS

Hemorrhage: Is the principal adverse effect. Significant GI bleeding during therapy may indicate the presence of an underlying occult lesion. Excessive uterine bleeding may occur, but menstrual flow is usually normal. Reports indicate that women receiving short-term or long-term therapy with warfarin sodium may be at risk of developing ovarian hemorrhage at the time of ovulation. Ovarian and luteal hemorrhage have been reported. Hemorrhagic infarction, vasculitis, and necrosis of skin of the female breast have been reported rarely, as have hepatic hemorrhage and rupture resulting in death. Adrenal hemorrhage with resultant acute adrenal insufficiency has occurred rarely. Therapy is discontinued in those developing signs and symptoms characteristic of acute adrenal hemorrhage or insufficiency. Plasma cortisol levels should be measured and therapy with IV corticosteroids instituted promptly. Delay in recognition and institution of therapy in an acute situation may result in the patient's death.

Overdosage may cause hematuria, hemorrhage from wounds and ulcerative lesions, bleeding from mucous membranes, widespread petechiae, and ecchymotic hemorrhages. Paralytic ileus and intestinal obstruction from submucosal or intramural hemorrhage may occur.

Table 23. Drugs That Interact With Anticoagulants to Increase Bleeding Tendency, Listed by Mechanism of Effect

Inhibition of Platelet Aggregation	Inhibition of Procoagulant Factors	Ulcerogenic Effects
Dipyridamole	Alkylating agents	Adrenal corticosteroids
Indomethacin	Antimetabolites	Indomethacin
Oxyphenbutazone	Quinidine	Oxyphenbutazone
Phenylbutazone	Quinine	Phenylbutazone
Salicylates	Salicylates	Potassium products
Sulfinpyrazone		Salicylates
		Sulfinpyrazone

Table 24. Drugs That Decrease Anticoagulant Effects, Listed by Mechanism of the Decrease

Induction of Enzymes	Increase in Procoagulant Factors	Decrease in Drug Absorption
Barbiturates	Estrogens	Cholestyramine
Carbamazepine	Oral contraceptives	Colestipol
Chlorinated insecticides	Vitamin K	
Ethchlorvynol		
Glutethimide		
Griseofulvin		
Phenytoin		
Rifampin		

Coumarin derivatives: Side-effects other than hemorrhage are infrequent. Reported effects include alopecia, urticaria, dermatitis, skin necrosis, nausea, vomiting, anorexia, abdominal cramping, diarrhea, retroperitoneal hematoma, hepatitis, jaundice, fever, "purple toes" syndrome, hypersensitivity reactions, agranulocytosis, leukopenia, priapism, mouth ulcers, and nephropathy.

Other adverse effects including the following.

Hematopoietic: Aplastic anemia, leukopenia, red cell aplasia, leukocytosis, anemia, thrombocytopenia, atypical mononuclear cells, myeloid immaturity, presence of leukocyte agglutinins.

Cutaneous: Rash, which may progress to exfoliative dermatitis.

Hepatic: Hepatitis, jaundice.

Renal: Renal damage with tuberlar necrosis, proteinuria with massive edema.

Other: Steatorrhea; paralysis of accommodation, blurred vision; sore mouth, throat; pyrexia.

OVERDOSAGE

Symptoms: May cause hematuria, hemorrhage from wounds and ulcerative lesions, bleeding from mucous membranes, widespread petechiae, ecchymotic hemorrhages; paralytic ileus and intestinal obstruction from submucosal or intramural hemorrhage.

Treatment: If minor bleeding or excessive hypoprothrombinemia (excessive prolongation of prothrombin time) occurs, one or more doses should be omitted until prothrombin time returns to a therapeutic range or bleeding stops. If minor bleeding persists or progresses, oral vitamin K_1 (phytonadione) in doses of 1 mg to 10 mg may be given. If frank bleeding occurs, 5 mg to 50 mg of parenteral vitamin K_1 may be given. Use of vitamin K complicates subsequent anticoagulant therapy; therefore, use caution in determining need. A hypercoagulable state may occur following rapid reversal of a prolonged prothrombin time. Recent studies suggest that large doses of vitamin K are unnecessary and undesirable because of prolonged effects on further anticoagulation. Smaller doses (1 mg to 15 mg) of vitamin K may be sufficient except in cases of severe hemorrhage. In emergency situations, clotting factors can be returned to normal by administration of 250 ml to 500 ml fresh frozen plasma or commercial Factor IX complex.

DOSAGE

Adjust dosage to achieve and maintain a prothrombin time from 1.5 to 2.5 times the control value or prothrombin activity of 20% to 30% of normal. A prothrombin time that is twice the control value should provide adequate anticoagulation with less risk of hemorrhage. Although an initial loading dose has previously been recommended, use of heparin is preferred if rapid anticoagulation is necessary. Oral anticoagulants are started at anticipated maintenance levels, with the daily dosage adjusted based on prothrombin time determinations. Lower doses are recommended for the elderly.

Treatment during dentistry and surgery (warfarin): If anticoagulants are administered before, during, or immediately following dental or surgical procedures, it is recommended that dosage be adjusted to maintain the prothrombin time at approximately 1.5 to 2.5 times the control level.

DICUMAROL

200 mg to 300 mg first day; 25 mg to 200 mg on subsequent days if prothrombin activity is 25% or more of normal.

PHENPROCOUMON

Induction, 24 mg; maintenance, 0.75 mg/day to 6 mg/day.

WARFARIN POTASSIUM

Initial daily range 40 mg to 60 mg; 20 mg to 30 mg for elderly or debilitated patients.

Maintenance: 2.5 mg/day to 10 mg/day when prothrombin falls to 25 seconds. Interval between initial dose and first maintenance dose may vary from 2 to 6 days, depending on prothrombin time response.

WARFARIN SODIUM

Initiate with 10 mg/day to 15 mg/day PO, and thereafter (usually 2 or 3 days) adjust according to prothrombin time response. Alternatively, give 40 mg to 60 mg for average adults or 20 mg to 30 mg for elderly or debilitated patients for one dose only IM.

Maintenance: 2 mg/day to 10 mg/day.

NURSING IMPLICATIONS

HISTORY

See Appendix 4. The activity of oral anticoagulants is affected by many drugs; an accurate, detailed drug history from a newly admitted patient or a review of current drug therapy is essential.

PHYSICAL ASSESSMENT

Obtain vital signs, weight (if patient is to receive phenindione). Other assessments based on symptoms or diagnosis. Prothrombin time is ordered as baseline. If heparin is given concomitantly, a partial thromboplastin time and white blood cell count are ordered. Additional laboratory studies and diagnostic tests pertinent to diagnosis or clinical findings may also be ordered.

ADMINISTRATION
Baseline prothrombin time must be drawn and results obtained before administration of initial dose; in some instances physician may order drug to be given before test results are obtained.

A flow sheet is used to record anticoagulant administration as well as prothrombin time results. *Always* check this flow sheet before drug is administered and enter required data immediately after administration of an oral anticoagulant.

CLINICAL ALERT: If most recent prothrombin time is above 2.5 times control value (or 30% of normal) or exceeds limits set by the physician's written order or hospital policy, withhold next dose of drug and contact physician immediately.

Administer drug at approximately the same time each day.

Bioequivalence: Bioequivalence problems have been documented for warfarin sodium products marketed by different manufacturers. Brand interchange is not recommended.

Injection (warfarin sodium): Administered IM or IV. Reconstitute with diluent (2 ml Sterile Water for Injection) supplied with product. Each ml equals 25 mg. Use immediately after reconstitution; discard unused portion.

Injectable warfarin sodium may be given in same syringe as heparin when administered in emergency situations.

Trade name similarity: Liquamar (**phenprocoumon,** oral anticoagulant) and Liquaemin (**heparin**).

ONGOING ASSESSMENTS AND NURSING MANAGEMENT
In emergency situations, heparin may be administered along with an oral anticoagulant or injectable warfarin sodium.

Record vital signs q4h to q8h or as ordered; observe for adverse reactions and check for evidence of early bleeding tendencies q2h to q6h (see *Overdosage*); if noted, contact physician immediately.

Blood for prothrombin time is drawn daily during initial therapy and whenever any other drug is added to or discontinued from therapy.

Check the following for evidence of bleeding: urine (hematuria), stool (melena), mouth rinses after oral care (pink discoloration), gums (exces-

sive bleeding after brushing teeth, eating), skin (petechiae, bruising), emesis (hematemesis). In addition observe for unexplained nosebleeds and excessive bleeding from minor cuts or scratches. Areas of assessment should be noted on the Kardex and personnel made aware of the necessity of routinely checking these areas.

Oral anticoagulants may cause red-orange discoloration of alkaline urine; this may interfere with some laboratory tests as well as with visual detection of hematuria.

Label all laboratory request slips with notation of anticoagulant therapy.

When patient is receiving both heparin and an oral or injectable anticoagulant, the blood sample for prothrombin time should be drawn *just prior to* the next dose of heparin, at least 5 hours after the last IV dose or 24 hours after the last subcutaneous dose of heparin. It usually is the nurse's responsibility to inform laboratory personnel of the timing necessary when the patient is receiving both anticoagulants.

Apply prolonged pressure to the needle or catheter site following venipuncture, removal of central or peripheral IV lines, IM and subcutaneous injections. In some instances a pressure dressing may be required. Laboratory personnel should be made aware of anticoagulant therapy.

Provide patient with soft toothbrush; male patient should be encouraged to use an electric razor. Avoid use of red mouthwash, when possible, because color can interfere with evaluation of oral bleeding.

A well-balanced diet is important. Observe dietary intake; if diet is taken poorly, discuss problem with the physician.

Vitamin K_1 should be readily available on clinical units where oral anticoagulants are administered.

Nursing infants should be observed for evidence of unexpected bleeding because oral anticoagulants cross the placental barrier. If maternal anticoagulant therapy is necessary, physician usually suggests change to formula feeding.

If emergency surgery is necessary, physician may order vitamin K. Tape note on front of patient's chart about anticoagulant therapy, time and dose of vitamin K administration. Be sure all recent laboratory reports are on chart before patient is transported to surgery.

If future surgery is anticipated, anticoagulant therapy is usually discontinued several days before procedure (length of time depends on anticoagulant used).

Observe for adrenal hemorrhage resulting in signs of adrenal insufficiency (Appendix 6, section 6-3). If suspected, contact physician immediately because condition may become life threatening. See also *Adverse Reactions.*

Diuretic-induced hemoconcentration with subsequent concentration of clotting factors has been reported to decrease the effects of oral anticoagulants. Observe for erratic prothrombin times when patient is receiving a diuretic and taking insufficient oral fluids to compensate for diuresis.

Tapering the dose on discontinuation of oral anticoagulant therapy does not appear necessary.

Warfarin sodium administration: If female patient develops sudden abdominal pain or discomfort, notify physician. Ovarian hemorrhage at the time of ovulation has been reported.

Delayed hypersensitivity reactions: Seen most frequently with phenindione. Observe for complaints of marked fatigue, chills, sore throat, and fever. See *Warnings* for additional symptoms of hypersensitivity reactions. Contact physician immediately if any is noted. Periodic blood studies and hepatic-function tests are recommended.

PATIENT AND FAMILY INFORMATION

Strict adherence to prescribed dosage schedule and laboratory monitoring of drug's effect is necessary.

Do *not* take or discontinue *any* other medication except on advice of physician or pharmacist. This includes *all* nonprescription drugs.

Inform dentist and other physicians of anticoagulant therapy *before* any treatment is instituted or medications are prescribed.

Take drug at same time each day.

Avoid alcohol (unless use is approved by physician) and large amounts of green leafy vegetables. Avoid any changes in life habits such as drastic change in diet or alcohol consumption.

If unusual bleeding or bruising, red or dark brown urine (blood), red or black stools, or diarrhea occurs do not take next dose of drug and notify physician immediately. (Note: Additional adverse reactions can be discussed with patient if physician approves.)

Follow physician's advice about additional treatment or prophylactic measures such as avoiding prolonged periods of standing or sitting, tight garments (pants, garters, girdles, knee-high stockings), injury to legs, weight gain; exercising; wearing support or antiembolitic stockings; and elevating legs while sitting.

Use a soft toothbrush; men should use electric razor if possible. Consult dentist about oral-hygiene measures, including use of dental floss.

Keep all physician and laboratory appointments because therapy must be closely monitored.

Wear Medic-Alert tag or bracelet or other identification that will alert others to anticoagulant therapy.

Cromolyn Sodium

(Disodium Cromoglycate) Rx

capsules (inhalation): 20 mg	Intal
solution (nebulizer): 20 mg/ampule	Intal
solution (nasal): 40 mg/ml	Nasalcrom Nasal

INDICATIONS

Capsules (inhalation), ***solution*** (nebulizer): Adjunct in management of severe bronchial asthma when frequency, intensity, and predictability of episodes indicate continued use of symptomatic medication. Patients must have a significant bronchodilator-reversible component to their airway obstruction as demonstrated by a generally accepted pulmonary-function test of airway mechanics. The decision to continue therapy on a long-term basis is justified if use of drug produces a significant reduction in severity of symptoms of asthma; permits a significant reduction in, or elimination of, steroids or permits better management of patients who have intolerable side-effects to sympathomimetic agents or methylxanthines.

Nasal solution: Allergic rhinitis.

Investigational uses: Oral use is being evaluated for use in those with food allergies.

CONTRAINDICATIONS

Hypersensitivity.

ACTIONS

Studies show cromolyn inhibits degranulation of sensitized mast cells, which occurs after exposure to specific antigens. It inhibits the release of histamine and slow reacting substance of anaphylaxis (SRS-A). Bronchial asthma that is induced by inhalation of antigens can be inhibited to varying degrees with treatment. Drug has no intrinsic bronchodilator, antihistaminic, or anti-inflammatory activity. Because of prophylactic mechanism of action, it has no role in treatment of an acute asthma attack. Is poorly absorbed from the GI tract. After inhalation, about 8% of total dose is absorbed from the lung and rapidly excreted unchanged in bile and urine. Remainder of dose is either exhaled or deposited in the oropharynx, swallowed, and excreted via the alimentary tract.

WARNINGS

Has no role in treatment of acute asthma, especially status asthmaticus.

Because of biliary and renal routes of excretion, consideration is given to decreasing dosage or discontinuing administration in those with impaired renal or hepatic function. If eosinophilic pneumonia occurs during course of therapy, drug should be discontinued.

Use in pregnancy: Safety not established.

Use in children: Not recommended for children under 5 because of necessity to administer by inhalation. Because of possibility that adverse effects could become apparent only after many years, a benefit–risk consideration of long-term use is particularly important in pediatric patients.

PRECAUTIONS

Occasionally, patient experiences cough or bronchospasm following inhalation and at times may not be able to continue treatment. Symptoms of asthma may recur if cromolyn is reduced below the recommended dosage or discontinued.

ADVERSE REACTIONS

Most frequent involve the respiratory tract and include bronchospasm, cough, laryngeal edema (rare), nasal congestion, pharyngeal irritation, and wheezing.

Other adverse reactions are angioedema, dizziness, dysuria and urinary frequency, joint swelling and pain, lacrimation, nausea and headache, rash, swollen parotid gland, and urticaria.

The following are reported as rare and it is unclear whether they are attributable to cromolyn: anaphylaxis, anemia, exfoliative dermatitis, hemoptysis, hoarseness, myalgia, nephrosis, periarteric vasculitis, pericarditis, peripheral neuritis, polymyositis, pulmonary infiltrates with eosinophilia, and vertigo.

Adverse effects that have occurred in relation to the cromolyn delivery system are inhalation of gelatin particles and inhalation of mouthpiece or propeller.

DOSAGE

Capsules (inhalation), nebulizer solution: Usual starting dosage for adults and children 5 and over is 20 mg inhaled qid at regular intervals. Effect of therapy depends on administration at regular intervals.

Cromolyn is introduced into the patient's therapeutic regimen when the acute episode has been controlled, the airway has been cleared, and patient is able to inhale adequately. Once the patient is stabilized on cromolyn, and if there is no need for steroids, frequency of administration is adjusted downward to the least frequent level consistent with the desired effect. Usual decrease is from four to three capsules a day. Reduce dosage slowly to avoid exacerbation of asthma. In those using fewer than four capsules a day, an increase in dosage may be needed if clinical condition worsens.

Corticosteroid treatment and its relation to cromolyn use: An attempt may be made to decrease corticosteroid administration and to institute an alternate-day regimen. Concomitant corticosteroids as well as bronchodilators should be continued following introduction of cromolyn. If patient improves, an attempt to decrease corticosteroids may be made. Even if steroid-dependent patient fails to improve following cromolyn administration, gradual tapering of steroid dosage may be attempted. When inhalation of cromolyn is impaired, as may occur in severe exacerbation of asthma, a temporary increase in dosage of corticosteroids or other medications may be required.

Nasal solution: One spray in each nostril three or four times daily.

NURSING IMPLICATIONS

HISTORY

See Appendix 4.

PHYSICAL ASSESSMENT

Obtain vital signs; auscultate lungs (listen for expiratory wheezing, hyperresonance, decreased voice sounds, distant breath sounds); examine and describe sputum raised (if any). Pulmonary-function studies, renal- or hepatic-function tests (if impairment is suspected) may be ordered before institution of therapy.

ADMINISTRATION

Stay with patient during early therapy with inhaler to be sure device is used correctly.

Inhalation capsules

Patient must be cooperative in use of inhaler.

The capsules are for use in the inhaler and are *not* for oral administration.

Graphic instructions are supplied with the inhaler unit.

Patient should have demonstration of inhaler use before initial treatment. Use the inhaler (without capsule) and the instruction sheet. Go through use step by step. Then have patient practice use of inhaler, as needed.

Following patient's proficiency in use of inhaler, demonstrate insertion of capsule, preparation of inhaler for use, and cleaning of inhaler.

Preparation for use: Inhaler is held upright with mouthpiece at bottom. Open mouthpiece and insert colored end of capsule into center of propeller. Screw device back together, slide the sleeve down (to puncture capsule), then slide up. Inhaler is now ready for use.

Avoid overhandling capsule because it may soften.

Have patient clear air passages by coughing.

To use: Instruct patient to exhale as much air as possible, then tilt head back, place the mouthpiece in mouth, close lips around it, quickly inhale once, hold breath for several seconds, remove mouthpiece from mouth, and then exhale.

Inhalation solution

Administer cromolyn nebulizer solution from a power-operated nebulizer having an adequate flow rate and equipped with a suitable face mask. Hand-operated nebulizers are not suitable for administration of cromolyn solution.

Have patient clear air passages by coughing.

Place face mask over mouth and nose. Instruct patient to inhale deeply through the mouth as nebulization is administered.

Cleaning

Inhaler: Will be for patient's own use. Remove empty capsule. Daily, take apart and rinse thoroughly under warm running water. Allow to dry before reassembling unit. Rinse more frequently if needed.

Mask: Wipe off mask with warm water. Clean or soak in solution, as per hospital policy, because mask is used by others (unless disposable mask is used). Wash patient's face with warm water; dry thoroughly.

ONGOING ASSESSMENTS AND NURSING MANAGEMENT

If improvement occurs, it will ordinarily occur within the first 4 weeks of therapy, as manifested by a decrease in severity of clinical symptoms of asthma or decrease in the need for concomitant therapy.

During initial therapy, auscultate lungs following drug administration; record findings.

If cough, wheezing, or symptoms of asthma occur, notify physician.

If bronchospasm, severe coughing, or other respiratory adverse drug effects occur during administration, stop use and notify physician.

Physician may prescribe bronchodilator to be administered before administration of cromolyn.

Pharyngeal irritation, hoarseness may occur. Encourage patient to take sips of water following each treatment and prn. If condition persists or becomes uncomfortable, discuss problem with physician.

If the patient is unable to inhale adequately, is uncooperative, or is unable to follow directions for administration, discuss problem with physician.

CLINICAL ALERT: An attempt to decrease corticosteroid dosage may be made. Dose *must be* reduced *gradually.* Observe for exacerbation of asthma and signs of adrenal insufficiency (Appendix 6, section 6-3).

Adrenal insufficiency may persist asymptomatically for some time after gradual discontinuation of adrenocortical steroids. If patient is subjected to significant stress (asthma attack, trauma, severe illness, emotional stress) while being treated or within 1 year (and occasionally 2 years) after corticosteroid treatment is terminated, steroid treatment may need to be reinstituted.

If inhalation of cromolyn is impaired, as may occur in severe exacerbation of asthma, a temporary increase in dosage of corticosteroids or other medications may be required.

If cromolyn therapy is discontinued in those in whom its use has permitted reduction in the maintenance dose of steroids, observe patient for sudden appearance of severe manifestations of asthma. If this should occur, notify physician immediately because therapy, such as possible reintroduction of corticosteroids, may be necessary.

PATIENT AND FAMILY INFORMATION

Do not discontinue therapy with this or other prescribed drugs abruptly except on advice of physician.

Notify physician if cough or wheezing occurs.

For inhalation use *only;* capsule is *not* for oral use. Use with Spinhaler only; capsule cannot be used with other types of inhalers.

Patient instructions for use of Spinhaler are supplied with product.

Crotamiton Rx

cream or lotion: 10%   Eurax

INDICATIONS

For eradication of scabies (*Sarcoptes scabiei*) and for symptomatic treatment of pruritic skin.

CONTRAINDICATIONS

Do not administer to patients who are allergic to crotamiton or who manifest a primary irritation response.

ACTIONS

Scabicidal and antipruritic; mechanisms of these actions are not known.

WARNINGS

Do not apply to acutely inflamed skin or raw weeping surfaces or apply in the eyes or mouth. Defer use until acute inflammation subsides. If severe irritation or sensitization develops, discontinue use.

ADVERSE REACTIONS

Allergic sensitivity or primary irritation reactions may occur.

DOSAGE

See *Administration.*

NURSING IMPLICATIONS

HISTORY

Scabies: Record description, duration, and location of symptoms; inquire whether other household members have same symptoms.

Pruritus: Record description, duration, and location of pruritus, as well as cause (if known).

PHYSICAL ASSESSMENT

Scabies: Examine and described lesions. Note if lesions are excoriated or appear infected. Even if symptoms are not present, examine areas most likely affected: between fingers, toes; flexor surface of wrists; waist; axilla; genitalia (males); nipples (females); scalp and neck folds (infants). Look for brown/black threadlike lesions approximately ½ inch long. Because of intense itching (especially at night) and scratching, areas become excoriated. Physician may attempt superficial skin scraping and examine contents expressed from burrow under microscope. A drop of mineral oil may be placed over a burrow before scraping.

Pruritus: Examine and describe affected areas.

ADMINISTRATION

Scabies: Wearing gloves, thoroughly massage into skin of whole body from chin down, paying particular attention to all skin folds and creases.

Clothing and bed linen should be changed the next morning.

A second application is advisable 24 hours later.

Pruritus: Massage gently into affected areas until medication is completely absorbed. Repeat as necessary.

ONGOING ASSESSMENTS AND NURSING MANAGEMENT

Scabies: A cleansing bath should be taken 48 hours after last application.

Hospitalized patient should be isolated from others (when possible) to prevent transmission. Wash hands thoroughly after patient contact. Bed linens, hospital gown are placed in isolation linen bag and laundered separately. Keep infected personal clothing in sealed plastic bag; clothing should not be worn until thoroughly laundered with soap and hot water and then dry cleaned or pressed with a steam iron. Preferably, clothes should be discarded.

Following treatment, inspect skin areas and compare with pretreatment data. Itching should be relieved.

Pruritus: Note result of application. If condition does not improve or worsens, contact physician.

PATIENT AND FAMILY INFORMATION

NOTE: Patient instructions are available with product. Review instructions for use, if necessary.

Keep away from eyes and mouth; do not apply to inflamed skin.

Discontinue use and notify physician if irritation or skin rash occurs.

Scabies: Have household members or other contacts examined for scabies.

Thoroughly launder *all* infected clothing and bed linens with soap and hot water followed by dry cleaning or pressing with a steam iron. If possible, discard infected clothes and bed linens.

Pruritus: If condition is not relieved, contact physician.

Curare Preparations

Metocurine Iodide Rx

| injection: 2 mg/ml | Metubine Iodide |

Tubocurarine Chloride Rx

| injection: 3 mg (20 units)/ml | *Generic* |

INDICATIONS

Muscle relaxants used as adjunct to anesthesia to induce skeletal muscle relaxation. May be employed to reduce intensity of muscle contractions in pharmacologically or electrically induced convulsions. Also used to facilitate management of patients undergoing mechanical ventilation. **Tubocurarine** may be used as a diagnostic test for myasthenia gravis when results of tests with neostigmine or edrophonium are inconclusive.

CONTRAINDICATIONS
Hypersensitivity or allergic reaction to these drugs. **Tubocurarine** is contraindicated in those in whom histamine release is a definite hazard. **Metocurine iodide** is contraindicated in those sensitive to iodide.

ACTIONS
Curare preparations block nerve impulses to skeletal muscles at the myoneural junction. This is a nondepolarizing (competitive) neuromuscular blockade. Studies suggest that metocurine does not produce autonomic ganglionic blockade seen with other nondepolarizing muscle relaxants. Clinical findings suggest metocurine iodide reaches the neuromuscular junction more rapidly than does tubocurarine and is approximately twice as potent.

Use of repeated doses may be accompanied by a cumulative effect. Duration of action and degree of muscle relaxation may be altered by dehydration, body-temperature changes, hypocalcemia, excess magnesium, or acid-base imbalance. Because these drugs are excreted by the kidneys, severe renal disease or conditions associated with poor renal perfusion (shock) or hypotension may result in more prolonged action. Concurrently administered general anesthetics, certain antibiotics, abnormal states (*e.g.,* acidosis), electrolyte imbalance, and neuromuscular disease are reported to potentiate activity of these drugs. These preparations do not affect consciousness or cerebration and do not relieve pain. A patient in severe pain may not be able to communicate this to the anesthesiologist.

Following IV infusion, onset of flaccid paralysis occurs within a few minutes. Maximal effects persist for 35 to 60 minutes; effective muscle paralysis may persist for 25 to 90 minutes. Complete recovery may require several hours.

WARNINGS
Respiratory effects: These are potent drugs that may cause respiratory depression. Prolonged apnea, with its attendant hazards, due to hypoxia may result from overdosage.

Myasthenia gravis: Employ with extreme caution in these patients.

Use in pregnancy, lactation: Safety not established. Use in women of childbearing potential, especially during early pregnancy, only when clearly needed and when potential benefits outweigh the unknown potential hazards to the fetus. Metocurine is known to pass the placental barrier. It is not known whether these drugs are excreted in human milk. Exercise caution in administering to nursing women.

Use in labor and delivery: It is not known whether use of these drugs has immediate or delayed adverse effects on the fetus, prolongs duration of labor, or increases likelihood that forceps delivery, obstetric intervention, or resuscitation of newborn will be necessary.

Use in children: Metocurine appears to be twice as potent as tubocurarine in children, but rate of recovery is the same. There may be a slight increase in heart rate, but no change occurs in blood pressure or ECG. Doses calculated on basis of body weight or surface area may be applicable.

PRECAUTIONS
Use with caution in those with respiratory depression or impaired cardiovascular, renal, hepatic, pulmonary, or endocrine function. Hypotension may follow large doses. Rapid injection may produce increased release of histamine with resultant decreased respiratory capacity due to bronchospasm and paralysis of respiratory muscles. Hypotension may occur due to ganglionic blockade or may be a complication of positive pressure respiration. Histamine release occurs less frequently with metocurine and is related to dosage and rapidity of administration.

Tubocurarine accumulates and may be present in some quantity for several hours after the effects are not clinically apparent.

DRUG INTERACTIONS
Intensity of blockade and duration of action are increased in those receiving potent **volatile inhalation anesthetics** (halothane, diethyl ether, methoxyflurane, enflurane). Parenteral use of **aminoglycoside antibiotics, bacitracin, polymyxin B, colistin, sodium colistimethate,** and **tetracyclines** may intensify or resemble the action of curare. If muscle relaxants and antibiotics must be administered simultaneously, observe patient closely for prolongation of respiratory depression. Potassium depletion produced by **thiazide diuretics** may cause increased sensitivity to neuromuscular blocking agents. Adequate serum potassium levels should be assured or thiazide diuretic discontinued at least 4 days before elective surgery. Prior administration of **succinylcholine** may enhance relaxant effect of these drugs. Tubocurarine is antagonized by **acetylcholine** and **anticolinesterases.** Action is potentiated by **quinine, quinidine, calcium** and **magnesium salts, trimethaphan, diazepam,** and **propranolol.** Synergistic or antagonistic effects may result when **depolarizing** or

nondepolarizing muscle relaxants are administered simultaneously or sequentially.

ADVERSE REACTIONS

Most frequently noted is prolongation of drug's action. Profound and prolonged muscle relaxation may occur, with consequent respiratory depression to point of apnea. Hypersensitivity may exist in rare instances. Idiosyncrasy, interference with physical signs of anesthesia, circulatory depression, ganglionic blockade, and release of histamine can occur. Possible reactions to metocurine include allergic or hypersensitivity reactions to drug or its iodide content and histamine release when large doses are administered rapidly.

OVERDOSAGE

May be avoided by careful monitoring of response by means of a peripheral nerve stimulator.

Symptoms: May result in prolonged apnea, cardiovascular collapse, and sudden release of histamine. Massive doses are not reversible by the antagonists edrophonium or neostigmine and atropine.

Treatment: Maintain airway; administer manual or mechanical ventilation. Accompanying derangements of blood pressure, electrolyte balance, or circulating blood volume are determined and corrected by appropriate therapy. If hypotension occurs, determine etiology; hypotension may be treated with fluid and vasopressors. Edrophonium or neostigmine may antagonize skeletal muscle relaxant action; neostigmine should be accompanied or preceded by injection of atropine sulfate or its equivalent.

DOSAGE

Metocurine iodide: Give IV. Dosage is dependent on nature of surgical procedure. Initial dose range is 0.2 mg/kg to 0.4 mg/kg for endotracheal intubation. Supplemental doses average 0.5 mg to 1 mg. For electroshock therapy, doses range from 1.75 mg to 5.5 mg.

Tubocurarine chloride: Give IV or IM. *Surgery*—40 units to 60 units at time of skin incision and 20 units to 30 units in 3 to 5 minutes if required. Supplemental doses of 20 units are given as required. *Electroshock therapy*—0.5 units/lb given slowly IV as a sustained 1 to 1½ minute injection. The initial dose is 20 units less than this. **Diagnosis of myasthenia gravis**—When small doses are given, a profound exaggeration of this syndrome occurs. Dosage is $\frac{1}{15}$ to $\frac{1}{5}$ the average adult electroshock therapy dose administered IV.

NURSING IMPLICATIONS

HISTORY

Alert anesthesiologist to current drug therapy and history of allergies, especially to iodine, iodides, and seafoods. Notification may be made by attaching note on cover of chart before transporting patient to surgery.

ADMINISTRATION TECHNIQUES

Drug is administered by anesthesia department or by physician when testing for myasthenia gravis.

ONGOING ASSESSMENTS AND NURSING MANAGEMENT

CLINICAL ALERT: Patient must not be left unattended until fully recovered from anesthesia. This includes a partially awake patient with adequate respiratory exchange, movement in the extremities, return of swallowing and gag reflexes, and adequate circulation (arterial blood pressure returns to preanesthetic level).

Postanesthesia: Monitor blood pressure, pulse, and respirations q15m (or as ordered) until patient has full recovery from anesthesia.

Maintian patent airway until patient is able to swallow or speak or until gag reflex returns.

Complete recovery from muscle relaxant effect may require several hours. Check for movement in the extremities, chest muscles (on inspiration and expiration), jaw and neck muscles, swallowing and gag reflexes.

Notify anesthesia department immediately if any of the following occurs: erythema, edema, flushing, tachycardia, hypotension, bronchospasm (all are signs of histamine release); prolonged muscle relaxation; choking, noisy respirations; cyanosis; prolonged apnea.

Additional nursing management is based on individual factors, such as type of surgery, condition of patient, complications during surgery (*e.g.,* prolonged procedure, hemorrhage, episodes of hypotension, development of a cardiac arrhythmia), additional medical problems present before surgery (*e.g.,* diabetes mellitus, chronic obstructive pulmonary disease), patient's age.

Diagnosis of myasthenia gravis (tubocurarine): Have available edrophonium or neostigmine and atropine, suction equipment, oral airway, equipment for assisted or controlled ventilation, oxygen.

A peripheral nerve stimulator may be used to assess effects of administration.

Test is positive when a profound exaggeration of this syndrome occurs.

Electroshock therapy: Have available same equipment as listed for diagnosis of myasthenia gravis.

Cyanocobalamin

See Vitamin B_{12}.

Cyclacillin

See Penicillins.

Cyclandelate Rx

tablets: 100 mg	Cyclospasmol
capsules: 200 mg	Cyclospasmol, Cydel, *Generic*
capsules: 400 mg	Cyclospasmol, *Generic*

INDICATIONS
"Possibly effective" for adjunctive therapy in intermittent claudication; arteriosclerosis obliterans; thrombophlebitis (to control associated vasospasm and muscular ischemia); nocturnal leg cramps; Raynaud's phenomenon; selected cases of ischemic cerebral vascular disease. Not intended as substitute for other appropriate medical or surgical programs in treatment of peripheral or cerebral vascular disease.

CONTRAINDICATIONS
Hypersensitivity.

ACTIONS
An oral vasodilator. Activity exceeds that of papaverine. It is musculotropic, acting directly on vascular smooth muscle; has no significant adrenergic stimulating or blocking actions.

WARNINGS
Use with extreme caution in patients with severe obliterative coronary artery or cerebral vascular disease because there is a possibility that these diseased areas may be compromised by vasodilatory effects of the drug elsewhere. The hazard of prolonged bleeding time is considered when administering to patient with active bleeding or a bleeding tendency.

Use in pregnancy, lactation: Safety not established. Use only when clearly needed and when potential benefits outweigh unknown potential hazards to the fetus.

PRECAUTIONS
Use with caution in patients with glaucoma.

ADVERSE REACTIONS
GI: GI distress (pyrosis, pain, eructation) occur infrequently and are usually mild.

Miscellaneous: Mild flush, headache, dizziness, feeling of weakness, and tachycardia may occur, especially during first weeks of administration.

DOSAGE
Therapy initiated at high dosage (*e.g.,* 1200 mg/day to 1600 mg/day) given in divided doses A.C. and H.S. When clinical response is noted, decrease dosage in 200-mg increments until maintenance dose is reached.

Maintenance therapy: Usual dosage is between 400 mg/day and 800 mg/day given in two to four divided doses.

NURSING IMPLICATIONS

HISTORY
See Appendix 4.

PHYSICAL ASSESSMENT
Obtain vital signs.

Peripheral vascular disease: Check peripheral pulses; look for changes in affected extremities such as dry scaly skin, ulcerations, discoloration, temperature of extremities, and so on. If legs are affected, note color in supine and sitting position.

Cerebral vascular disease: Evaluate mental status.

ADMINISTRATION
If GI upset occurs, give with meals. Physician may prescribe concomitant antacid administration if giving with food does not relieve GI distress.

ONGOING ASSESSMENTS AND NURSING MANAGEMENT
Objective signs of therapeutic benefit may be rapid, but improvement usually occurs gradually over weeks of therapy. Anticipated therapeutic results for peripheral vascular disease include decrease in pain/discomfort/cramping in extremity, increased skin warmth, and increased amplitude of peripheral pulses. For cerebral vascular disease, improvement in mental status.

Obtain vital signs bid; observe for adverse reactions; repeat pretreatment physical assessments (daily to every 2–3 days).

If flushing, headache, and weakness are severe, inform physician; a dosage reduction may be necessary.

If dizziness occurs, assist patient with ambulatory activities.

Remove or move objects (*e.g.,* footstools, stands) that may result in falls or other injuries.

PATIENT AND FAMILY INFORMATION

Improvement usually occurs gradually over several weeks of therapy, although some rapid benefit may be noted. Prolonged use of drug may be necessary.

May cause GI distress; taking with meals or antacids (if physician approves) may help reduce these symptoms.

May cause flushing, headache, weakness.

If dizziness occurs, avoid sudden changes in posture; dangling legs for a few minutes before arising may eliminate dizziness.

Use caution when going up or down stairs or walking on ice, snow, slick pavement, or slippery floors. (Encourage family of elderly patient to remove small rugs, other objects that could cause falls.)

Stop smoking (if applicable).

For peripheral vascular disease: Follow physician's recommendations (*e.g.,* avoiding exposure to cold, keeping extremities warm, taking care of the feet) because these are an important part of treatment.

Cyclizine

See Antiemetic/Antivertigo Agents.

Cyclobenzaprine Hydrochloride ℞

tablets: 10 mg   Flexeril

INDICATIONS

Adjunct to rest and physical therapy for relief of muscle spasm associated with acute painful musculoskeletal conditions. Use only for short periods (2–3 weeks) because evidence for effectiveness for more prolonged use is not available. Not effective in treatment of spasticity associated with cerebral or spinal cord disease or in children with cerebral palsy.

CONTRAINDICATIONS

Hypersensitivity; concomitant use of monoamine oxidase (MAO) inhibitors or within 14 days after their discontinuation; acute recovery phase of myocardial infarction; arrhythmias, heart block, conduction disturbances, congestive heart failure; hyperthyroidism.

ACTIONS

Relieves skeletal muscle spasm of local origin without interfering with muscle function. Studies indicate drug reduces or abolishes muscle hyperactivity and does not act at the neuromuscular junction or directly on skeletal muscle. It acts primarily within the CNS at brain stem as opposed to spinal cord levels, although action on the latter may contribute to overall skeletal muscle relaxant activity. Evidence suggests that the net effect is a reduction of tonic somatic motor activity, influencing both gamma and alpha motor systems.

Is well absorbed after oral administration. Onset of action is 1 hour; duration of action is 12 to 24 hours and it is eliminated quite slowly, with a half-life as long as 1 to 3 days. It is highly bound to plasma proteins, extensively metabolized primarily to glucuronidelike conjugates, and excreted primarily via the kidneys.

WARNINGS

Use for longer than 2 to 3 weeks is not recommended. Is closely related to tricyclic antidepressants. Safety for use in pregnancy not established. Use only when clearly needed and when potential benefits outweigh the unknown potential hazards to the fetus. Because it is likely that drug is excreted in breast milk, it should not be given to nursing mothers. Safety and efficacy for use in children under 15 not established.

PRECAUTIONS

Hazardous tasks: May impair mental or physical abilities required for performance of hazardous tasks.

Ophthalmologic effects: Because of atropinelike action, use with caution in those with history of urinary retention, angle-closure glaucoma, or increased intraocular pressure.

DRUG INTERACTIONS

May enhance effects of **alcohol, barbiturates,** and other **CNS depressants.** Because of atropinelike action, use with caution in those taking **anticholinergic medication.** Because of structural and pharmacologic similarities to the **tricyclic antidepressants,** all interactions listed on p 65 should be considered.

ADVERSE REACTIONS

Most frequent: Drowsiness (40%); dry mouth (28%); dizziness (11%).

Less frequent: Increased heart rate; weakness; fatigue; dyspepsia; nausea; paresthesias; unpleasant taste; blurred vision; insomnia.

Rare: Sweating; myalgia; dyspnea; abdominal pain; constipation; coated tongue; tremors; dysarthria; euphoria; nervousness; disorientation; confusion; headache; urinary retention; decreased bladder tonus; ataxia; depressed mood; hallucinations; allergic reactions including skin rash, urticaria, edema of face and tongue.

Because of structural and pharmacologic similarities to the tricyclic antidepressants, all adverse reactions listed on p 65 should be considered.

OVERDOSAGE

Symptoms: High doses may cause temporary confusion, disturbed concentration, transient visual hallucinations, agitation, hyperactive reflexes, muscle rigidity, vomiting, or hyperpyrexia, in addition to effects listed under adverse reactions. Overdosage may cause drowsiness, hypothermia, tachycardia, and other cardiac rhythm abnormalities such as bundle branch block, ECG evidence of impaired conduction and congestive heart failure. Other manifestations may include dilated pupils, convulsions, severe hypotension, stupor, and coma.

Treatment: Is symptomatic and supportive. Empty stomach as quickly as possible by emesis, followed by gastric lavage. After lavage, give 20 g to 30 g activated charcoal q4h to q6h during first 24 to 48 hours after ingestion. An ECG should be taken and close monitoring of cardiac function instituted if there is any evidence of dysrhythmia. Maintenance of an open airway, adequate fluid intake, and regulation of body temperature are necessary. IV administration of 1 mg to 3 mg physostigmine salicylate is reported to reverse symptoms of anticholinergic poisoning; dosage may be repeated as often as required when life-threatening signs such as arrhythmias, convulsions, and deep coma recur or persist. Standard medical measures should be used to manage circulatory shock and metabolic acidosis. Cardiac arrhythmias may be treated with neostigmine, pyridostigmine, physostigmine, or propranolol. When signs of cardiac failure occur, use of short-acting digitalis preparation is considered. Close monitoring of cardiac function for not less than 5 days is advised. Dialysis is probably of no value.

Because overdosage is often deliberate, patient may attempt suicide by other means during the recovery phase. Deaths by deliberate or accidental overdosage have occurred with this drug.

DOSAGE

Usual dose is 10 mg tid with range of 20 mg/day to 40 mg/day in divided doses. Dosage should not exceed 60 mg/day. Use for periods longer than 2 to 3 weeks not recommended.

NURSING IMPLICATIONS

HISTORY
See Appendix 4.

PHYSICAL ASSESSMENT
Evaluate physical limitations imposed by musculoskeletal disorder (*e.g.,* walking, sitting, movement or use of limb).

TRADE NAME SIMILARITIES
Flexeril and Flaxedil (gallamine triethiodide).

ONGOING ASSESSMENTS AND NURSING MANAGEMENT
Assess response to drug. Improvement is manifested by relief of muscle spasm and its associated signs and symptoms.

Rest, physical therapy, and other measures may also be part of therapeutic regimen.

If drowsiness or dizziness occurs, assist with ambulation. Notify physician before next dose if drowsiness is excessive.

If patient has history of urinary retention, measure intake and output during early therapy. If urinary retention is suspected, notify physician.

PATIENT AND FAMILY INFORMATION
May cause drowsiness, dizziness, or blurred vision. Observe caution while driving or performing other tasks requiring alertness.

Avoid use of alcohol, other CNS depressants, and nonprescription drugs (especially cold and cough medications) unless use has been approved by physician.

May cause dry mouth, which may be relieved by sips of water, ice chips, chewing gum, or hard candy.

If drug fails to produce relief in a few days or becomes worse, contact physician.

Cyclomethycaine Sulfate

See Anesthetics, Local, Topical.

Cyclopentolate Hydrochloride

See Mydriatics, Cyclopegic.

Cyclophosphamide Rx

tablets: 25 mg, 50 mg	Cytoxan (contains tartrazine)
injection: 100 mg, 200 mg, 500 mg	Cytoxan, Neosar
injection: 1 g, 2 g	Cytoxan

INDICATIONS
Cyclophosphamide, although effective alone in susceptible malignancies, is more frequently used con-

currently or sequentially with other antineoplastic drugs. The following malignancies are often susceptible to cyclophosphamide treatment: malignant lymphomas (stages III and IV, Ann Arbor Staging System); Hodgkin's disease; lymphoma (nodular or diffuse); mixed-cell type lymphoma; histiocytic lymphoma; Burkitt's lymphoma; multiple myeloma; leukemias (chronic lymphocytic, chronic granulocytic [ineffective in acute blastic crisis], acute myelogenous and monocytic, acute lymphoblastic [stem cell] in children [given during remission, drug is effective in prolonging its duration]); mycosis fungoides (advanced disease); neuroblastoma (disseminated disease); adenocarcinoma of the ovary; retinoblastoma; carcinoma of the breast.

Unlabeled uses: Has been used in a wide variety of severe rheumatologic conditions. Benefit demonstrated in Wegener granulomatosis, other steroid-resistant vasculidities, and in some cases of severe progressive rheumatoid arthritis and systemic lupus erythematosus. Toxicity is limiting.

ACTIONS

Although generally classified as an alkylating agent, cyclophosphamide is not an alkylating agent but interferes with the growth of susceptible neoplasms and, to some extent, certain normal tissues. Mechanism of action not known. It is absorbed from the GI tract and parenteral sites. Details of metabolism are not fully known; the drug and its metabolites are distributed throughout the body, including the brain. After IV administration, serum half-life is about 4 hours; however, the drug and its metabolites may be detected in plasma for up to 72 hours. It is excreted by the kidneys; the extent by which it is excreted by other routes is not known. See also Antineoplastic Agents.

WARNINGS

Adjustment of doses of both replacement steroids and cyclophosphamide may be necessary in the adrenalectomized patient. Cyclophosphamide may interfere with wound healing.

Use in pregnancy and lactation: Use in pregnancy, particularly in the first trimester, only when clearly needed and when potential benefits outweigh the potential hazards to the fetus. Is excreted in breast milk; breast-feeding should be terminated prior to institution of therapy. Contraceptive measures are recommended during therapy for both men and women.

PRECAUTIONS

Give cautiously to patients with leukopenia; thrombocytopenia; tumor cell infiltration of bone marrow; previous x-ray therapy; previous therapy with other cytotoxic agents; impaired hepatic function; impaired renal function.

Immunosuppression: Because drug may exert a suppressive action on immune mechanisms, interrupting or modifying dosage may be considered for those who develop bacterial, viral, or fungal infections. This is especially true for patients receiving concomitant steroid therapy or who have recently received steroid therapy, because infections may be fatal. Varicella-zoster infections appear to be particularly dangerous under these circumstances.

Tartrazine sensitivity: Tablets contain tartrazine (see Appendix 6, section 6-23).

DRUG INTERACTIONS

Rate of metabolism and leukopenic activity of this drug are increased by chronic administration of high doses of **phenobarbital. Allopurinol** and **chloramphenicol** administered concurrently may enhance the effects and bone-marrow toxicity of cyclophosphamide. Cyclophosphamide may decrease pseudocholinesterase levels in plasma, thus inhibiting **succinylcholine** metabolism and resulting in prolonged apnea.

Drug/lab tests: May suppress positive reactions to the following skin tests: *Candida,* **mumps,** *Trichophyton,* **tuberculin PPD. Serum pseudocholinesterase** may be decreased; blood and urine **uric-acid levels** may be increased. Cyclophosphamide may produce false-positive **Papanicolaou test.**

ADVERSE REACTIONS

Secondary neoplasia: Has developed in some patients treated with this drug alone or with other antineoplastic drugs or radiation therapy. Most frequent have been urinary bladder, myeloproliferative, and lymphoproliferative malignancies. Secondary malignancies have developed most frequently in patients with primary myeloproliferative and lymphoproliferative malignancies and primary nonmalignant diseases in which immune processes are believed to be pathologically involved. In some cases, the secondary malignancy was detected up to several years after discontinuing cyclophosphamide. Secondary urinary bladder malignancies generally have occurred in those who previously developed hemorrhagic cystitis. Although no cause-and-effect relationship has been established between cyclophosphamide and the development of malignancy, the possibility of secondary malignancy is considered in any benefit-to-risk assessment for use of the drug.

Hematopoietic: Leukopenia is an expected effect and ordinarily is used as a guide to dosage. Thrombocytopenia or anemia may occur rarely. These effects are usually reversible when therapy is interrupted.

GI: Anorexia, nausea, vomiting, and diarrhea are common and related to dose as well as individual susceptibility. There are isolated reports of hemorrhagic colitis, oral mucosal ulceration, and hepatic dysfunction with jaundice.

GU: Urinary tract complications occur in about 25% of patients, and acute hemorrhagic cystitis occurs in 7% to 12%. These can be severe, or even fatal, and are probably due to metabolites in the urine. Nonhemorrhagic cystitis and fibrosis of the bladder have been reported. Atypical epithelial cells may be found in the urinary sediment. When cystitis occurs, it is usually necessary to interrupt therapy. Hematuria usually resolves spontaneously within a few days but may persist for several months. In severe cases, replacement of blood loss may be required. Application of electrocautery to telangiectatic areas of the bladder and diversion of urine flow have been used in protracted cases. Cryosurgery has also been used. Nephrotoxicity, including hemorrhage and clot formation in the renal pelvis, has been reported.

Gonadal suppression, resulting in amenorrhea or azoospermia, is related to dosage and duration of therapy. It may be irreversible and should be anticipated. It is not known to what extent this drug may affect prepubertal gonads. Ovarian fibrosis has been reported.

Integumentary: Alopecia is frequent; regrowth of hair can be expected, although it may be a different color and texture. Skin and fingernails may become darker. Nonspecific dermatitis has been reported.

Pulmonary: Interstitial pulmonary fibrosis with prolonged high dosage has been reported.

DOSAGE

Induction therapy: Initial IV loading dose for those with no hematologic deficiency is 40 mg/kg to 50 mg/kg, usually given in divided doses over a period of 2 to 5 days. A ⅓ to ½ reduction in the initial loading doses may be necessary for those who have previously received treatment that might have compromised the functional capacity of bone marrow (such as x-rays or cytotoxic drugs) and for patients with tumor infiltration of the bone marrow. Although marked leukopenia has been associated with these loading doses, recovery usually begins in 7 to 10 days. Initial therapy may be given orally in a dose of 1 mg/kg/day to 5 mg/kg/day, depending on patient response.

Maintenance therapy: To suppress or retard neoplastic growth, a variety of schedules have been used: 1 mg/kg/day to 5 mg/kg/day PO; 10 mg/kg to 15 mg/kg IV every 7 to 10 days; 3 mg/kg to 5 mg/kg IV twice weekly. Unless disease is unusually sensitive to cyclophosphamide, the largest maintenance dose that can be tolerated is given. The total leukocyte count is a guide for regulating maintenance doses. Ordinarily a leukopenia of 3000 to 4000 cells/cu mm can be maintained without undue risk of serious infection or other complications.

NURSING IMPLICATIONS

HISTORY
See Appendix 4.

PHYSICAL ASSESSMENT
Record physical, emotional status; vital signs; weight. Baseline laboratory studies include CBC, hepatic- and renal-function tests.

ADMINISTRATION
Antiemetic may be ordered prior to administration of drug.

Parenteral: Prepare solution by adding Sterile Water for Injection, USP, or Bacteriostatic Water for Injection, USP (paraben preserved only) to vial; shake to dissolve. Use 5 ml for the 100-mg vial, 10 ml for the 200-mg vial, or 25 ml for the 500-mg vial.

Prepared solutions may be injected IV, IM, intraperitoneally, or intrapleurally or may be infused IV in 5% Dextrose or 5% Dextrose and 0.9% Sodium Chloride (physician orders type and amount of IV solution, length of time for infusion).

IV infusion is best started in the morning.

A Kold Kap or scalp tourniquet may be used to prevent alopecia. The scalp tourniquet remains in place during and approximately 15 minutes after IV injection; the Kold Kap remains in place during and for approximately 1 hour after injection.

Storage: Use solutions within 24 hours if stored at room temperature or within 6 days if stored under refrigeration. Cyclophosphamide does not contain an antimicrobial agent; care must be taken to ensure sterility of prepared solutions.

Oral solution (prepared by pharmacist): Prepare by dissolving drug in Aromatic Elixir, USP. Store under refrigeration and use within 14 days. Preparation and expiration dates should be on container.

Tablets: Best given on empty stomach. If GI upset severe, may be given with food.

ONGOING ASSESSMENTS AND NURSING MANAGEMENT
Drug (tablets) may be prescribed for outpatient use. Parenteral administration of induction therapy usually requires hospitalization, although

maintenance therapy may be administered in a physician's office or outpatient clinic.

Obtain vital signs q4h or as ordered; measure intake and output for at least 24 hours after drug is administered; inspect each voided sample for hematuria (physician may also order use of chemical reagent sticks such as Hema-Combistix or Labstix for detecting occult blood in urine); push fluids to 2 to 3 liters on the day drug is administered as well as 1 to 2 days after administration or as ordered by physician; observe for adverse drug reactions.

CLINICAL ALERT: Hemorrhagic cystitis, which can be severe or even fatal, requires temporary discontinuation of therapy. If hematuria is apparent, contact physician immediately. Ensuring ample fluid intake and encouraging patient to void frequently help to prevent hemorrhagic cystitis.

Observe for signs of bone-marrow depression (Appendix 6, section 6-8). Contact physician immediately if one or more signs should occur.

Nausea and vomiting may begin 4 to 6 hours after drug is administered, especially when it is administered by parenteral route. Physician may order an antiemetic to be given parenterally or as a suppository q4h prn.

If patient is unable to take sufficient fluids orally because of nausea or vomiting, notify physician because parenteral fluid administration may be necessary.

A liquid diet, sips of carbonated beverage or cola syrup in water, dry toast, or crackers (preferably unsalted) may relieve nausea.

If vomiting persists despite antiemetic therapy, observe for signs of dehydration (Appendix 6, section 6-10). Report findings to physician.

WBC is monitored closely. Contact physician immediately if most recent laboratory report indicates leukopenia or a decided decrease from last sample.

Interstitial pulmonary fibrosis has been reported. Observe for dyspnea, nonproductive cough, basilar rales; notify the physician if these symptoms occur.

Weigh weekly (or as ordered) or at time of each office or clinic visit. Inform physician if a steady weight loss occurs. Nutritional supplements and a high-calorie diet offered in frequent, small amounts may prevent steady weight loss due to anorexia.

Hepatic dysfunction may occur. Observe for jaundice, dark urine, pruritus, and light-colored stools, and report occurrence to the physician. Hepatic-function studies may also be ordered.

Alopecia is a frequent complication. Physician or nurse should discuss purchase and use of a wig or scarf. Patient may wish to purchase wig before treatment or wait to see degree of alopecia. Patient should be told hair loss may be complete or partial and may involve scalp, eyebrows and lashes, and the underarm and pubic hair. Hair will grow back but may be different texture or color.

Oral mucosal ulceration may occur. Examine patient's mouth every 1 to 2 days. If noted, inform physician and begin stomatitis care (Appendix 6, section 6-21).

PATIENT AND FAMILY INFORMATION

NOTE: Diagnosis, chemotherapeutic regimen, anticipated adverse effects, and contraceptive measures should be discussed with the patient.

Preferably take drug on an empty stomach. If GI upset is severe, take with food.

Take medication exactly as directed. Do not omit, increase, or decrease the prescribed doses. If unable to take drug for *any* reason, contact physician.

Maintain a good fluid intake. Drink 8 to 10 glasses (8 oz) of water per day.

Notify physician if fever; chills; sore throat; missed menstrual period; blood in urine; painful urination; cough; shortness of breath; unusually rapid heartbeat; swelling of feet or lower legs; or joint, flank, or stomach pain occurs.

Medication may cause darkening of skin and fingernails, loss of appetite, loss of hair, nausea, or vomiting; notify physician if these become pronounced.

Contraceptive measures are recommended during therapy.

Blood tests will be performed frequently to monitor therapy.

Eat nutritious food. If anorexia occurs, try eating smaller quantities of food at more frequent intervals.

Cyclopropane

See Anesthetics, General, Gases.

Cycloserine Rx

capsules: 250 mg   Seromycin Pulvules

INDICATIONS

Treatment of active tuberculosis (including extrapulmonary) when organisms are susceptible, after failure of adequate treatment with the primary medications. Administered in conjunction with other effective chemotherapy. May be effective in treatment of acute urinary-tract infections caused by susceptible strains of bacteria, especially *Enterobacter* and *Escherichia coli.* Usually less effective than other antimicrobial agents in treatment of urinary-tract infections caused by bacteria other than mycobacteria. Use is considered only when more conventional therapy has failed and when organism has demonstrated sensitivity.

CONTRAINDICATIONS

Hypersensitivity to cycloserine; epilepsy; depression, severe anxiety, or psychosis; severe renal insufficiency; excessive concurrent use of alcohol.

ACTIONS

Inhibits cell wall synthesis in susceptible strains of gram-positive and gram-negative bacteria and *Mycobacterium tuberculosis.*

WARNINGS

Discontinue drug or reduce dosage if patient develops allergic dermatitis or symptoms of CNS toxicity such as convulsions, psychosis, somnolence, depression, confusion, hyperreflexia, headache, tremor, vertigo, paresis, or dysarthria. Risk of convulsions is increased in chronic alcoholics.

Toxicity is closely related to excessive blood levels (above 30 mcg/ml). The ratio of toxic dose to effective dose is small.

Use in pregnancy: Safety not established.

Use in children: Safety and dosage not established.

PRECAUTIONS

Blood levels should be determined weekly for patients with reduced renal function, for those taking more than 500 mg/day, and for those with symptoms of toxicity. Adjust dosage to keep blood level below 30 mcg/ml.

Anticonvulsant drugs or sedatives may be effective in controlling symptoms of CNS toxicity, such as convulsions, anxiety, and tremor. The value of pyridoxine in preventing CNS toxicity has not been proved.

Administration has been associated in a few instances with vitamin B_{12} or folic acid deficiency, megaloblastic anemia, and sideroblastic anemia. If evidence of anemia develops, appropriate studies and therapy are instituted.

DRUG INTERACTIONS

The CNS toxicity of cycloserine may be increased when it is administered concomitantly with **isoniazid.** Cycloserine discontinuation may be necessary.

ADVERSE REACTIONS

CNS (related to dosages over 500 mg/day): Convulsions, drowsiness, and somnolence; head-ache; tremor; dysarthria; vertigo; confusion and disorientation with loss of memory; psychoses, possibly with suicidal tendencies, character changes; hyperirritability; aggression; paresis; hyperreflexia; paresthesias; major and minor (localized) clonic seizures; coma.

Allergic (not related to dosage): Skin rash.

Miscellaneous: Elevated transaminase, especially in those with hepatic disease.

OVERDOSAGE

Symptoms: CNS depression with drowsiness, somnolence, dizziness, hyperreflexia, mental confusion, convulsions, and allergic dermatitis.

Treatment: Pyridoxine, 300 mg or more daily, and anticonvulsants to relieve convulsions. Management includes symptomatic and supportive therapy, such as gastric lavage, oxygen, artificial respiration, IV fluids, management of circulatory shock, and maintenance of body temperature.

DOSAGE

500 mg to 1 g daily in divided doses monitored by blood levels. Initial dosage most frequently given is 250 mg bid at 12-hour intervals for first 2 weeks. Daily dosage of 1 g should not be exceeded.

NURSING IMPLICATIONS

HISTORY

See Appendix 4. Warn patient that response to inquiry about alcohol consumption must be accurate because alcohol use could cause problem with administration of this drug.

PHYSICAL ASSESSMENT

Record vital signs. Culture and sensitivity tests are performed before institution of therapy. CBC, renal- and hepatic-function tests may also be ordered.

ADMINISTRATION

Initial dosage may be given q12h for first 2 weeks.

ONGOING ASSESSMENTS AND NURSING MANAGEMENT

Obtain vital signs daily; observe for adverse reactions, especially of overdosage (ratio of toxic dose to effective dose is small).

CLINICAL ALERT: Observe for allergic dermatitis or symptoms of CNS toxicity, such as convulsions, psychosis, somnolence, depression, confusion, hyperreflexia, headache, tremor, vertigo, paresis, or dysarthria. If any of these occurs, notify physician immediately. Dosage may be reduced or drug discontinued; an anticonvulsant drug or sedative may also be prescribed to control more serious CNS symptoms.

Weigh weekly or as ordered.

Periodic hematologic, renal-excretion, and liver-function studies, cycloserine blood levels, and culture and sensitivity studies are performed during therapy. Blood levels are recommended weekly for those with reduced renal function.

If drowsiness occurs, assist with ambulatory activities. If drowsiness is severe, inform physician.

PATIENT AND FAMILY INFORMATION

Take drug exactly as directed. Do not omit doses unless directed to do so by physician. Keep all physician and clinical appointments because monitoring of drug therapy is essential.

May cause drowsiness. Observe caution while driving or performing tasks requiring alertness.

Alcohol may be allowed, but discuss amount considered safe with physician. Excessive alcohol consumption may pose serious problems and must be avoided.

Notify physician or nurse if skin rash, somnolence, mental confusion, dizziness, headache, or tremors should occur.

Cyclosporine Rx

oral solution: Sandimmune
    100 mg/ml
IV solution: Sandimmune
    50 mg/ml

INDICATIONS

Prophylaxis of organ rejection in kidney, liver, and heart allogenic transplants in conjunction with adrenal corticosteroids; treatment of chronic rejection in those previously treated with other immunosuppressive agents.

Unlabeled uses: Has had limited but successful use in other procedures including transplantation of pancreas, bone-marrow, and heart/lung.

CONTRAINDICATIONS

Hypersensitivity to cyclosporine or polyoxyethylated castor oil.

ACTIONS

Is a potent immunosuppressant. The exact mechanism of action is unknown. Excretion is primarily biliary with only 6% of the dose excreted in the urine.

WARNINGS

Nephrotoxicity: Has been noted in 25% of renal, 38% of cardiac, and 37% of liver transplantations. Mild nephrotoxicity was generally noted 2 to 3

months after transplant and consisted of an arrest in the fall of preoperative elevations of BUN and creatinine. These elevations were often responsive to dosage reduction. More overt nephrotoxicity was seen early after transplantation and was characterized by a rapidly rising BUN and serum creatinine. Because these events are similar to rejection episodes, differentiation must be made between them. This form of nephrotoxicity is usually responsive to dosage reduction.

Impaired renal function: Requires close monitoring and possibly frequent dosage adjustment. In those with persistent high elevations of BUN and serum creatinine who are unresponsive to dosage adjustments, other immunosuppressive drugs may be tried.

Hepatotoxicity: Has been seen in 4% of renal, 7% of cardiac, and 4% of liver transplantations. This usually occurred during the first month of therapy when high doses were used and consisted of elevations of hepatic enzymes and bilirubin, which usually decreased with a reduction in dosage.

Lymphomas have developed in patients receiving cyclosporine and other forms of immunosuppressive therapy after transplantation. No causal relationship has been established.

Use in pregnancy, lactation: Safety not established. Use drug only when clearly needed and when potential benefits outweigh the unknown potential hazards to the fetus. Breast-feeding is avoided because drug is excreted in breast milk.

Use in children: Safety and efficacy not established. Patients as young as 6 months have received the drug with no unusual adverse effects.

PRECAUTIONS

Patients with malabsorption may have difficulty in achieving therapeutic levels with oral form.

Hypertension is a fairly common side-effect in some patients with cardiac transplants; antihypertensive therapy may be required.

DRUG INTERACTIONS

Use drug carefully with **nephrotoxic** drugs because potential synergies of nephrotoxicity may occur. **Ketoconazole** and **amphotericin B** have increased the plasma concentration of cyclosporine. Cyclosporine is not used with other **immunosuppressive agents** except adrenal corticosteroids. Immunosuppression can lead to increased susceptibility to infection and possible development of lymphoma.

ADVERSE REACTIONS

Principal adverse reactions: Renal dysfunction, tremor, hirsutism, hypertension, gum hyperplasia.
Other adverse reactions
GU: Hematuria.

Cardiovascular: Cramps, myocardial infarction.

Dermatologic: Acne, brittle fingernails, hair breaking, pruritus.

CNS: Convulsions, headache, confusion, anxiety, depression, lethargy, weakness.

GI: Diarrhea, nausea/vomiting, hepatotoxicity, abdominal discomfort, anorexia, gastritis, peptic ulcer, hiccups, mouth sores, swallowing difficulty, upper GI bleeding, pancreatitis, constipation.

Autonomic nervous system: Paresthesia, flushing, night sweats.

Hematopoietic: Leukopenia, lymphoma, anemia, thrombocytopenia.

Respiratory: Sinusitis.

Miscellaneous: Gynecomastia, allergic reactions, conjunctivitis, edema, fever, hearing loss, tinnitus, hyperglycemia, muscle pain, chest pain, joint pain, visual disturbances, weight loss.

Infectious complications developed in approximately 74% of patients receiving cyclosporine compared with 94% receiving standard therapy.

Discontinuation of cyclosporine occurred in 10% to 11.3%, primarily because of renal toxicity, infection, acute tubular necrosis, and lack of efficacy.

OVERDOSAGE

There is minimal experience with overdosage. Because of slow absorption, forced emesis would be of value up to 2 hours after oral administration. Transient hepatotoxicity and nephrotoxicity may occur, which should resolve following drug withdrawal. General supportive measures and symptomatic treatment should be followed. Drug is not dialyzable to any great extent nor is it cleared by charcoal hemoperfusion.

DOSAGE

Oral: 15 mg/kg/day initially, given 4 to 12 hours prior to transplantation. Dose continued postoperatively for 1 to 2 weeks, then tapered by 5% per week to a maintenance level of 5 mg/kg/day to 10 mg/kg/day. Lower initial doses after a 20 mg/kg preoperative dose may also be used.

Parenteral: Patients unable to take oral form preoperatively or postoperatively may be given drug IV. *Initial dose*—5 mg/kg/day to 6 mg/kg/day given 4 to 12 hours prior to transplantation as single IV dose as a slow infusion over 2 to 6 hours. This daily dose is continued postoperatively until patient can tolerate the oral solution.

NURSING IMPLICATIONS

HISTORY
See Appendix 4.

PHYSICAL ASSESSMENT

Obtain vital signs; weight. Baseline laboratory studies may include CBC, differential, platelet count, serum bilirubin, creatinine, hepatic enzymes. Other laboratory tests and diagnostic studies pertinent to the transplantation procedure are performed.

ADMINISTRATION

Oral solution: Use only a glass container to measure the dose and dispense the drug.

A graduated pipette is provided with the oral solution.

Drug may be mixed with milk, chocolate milk, or orange juice, preferably at room temperature.

Add drug to one of the above (according to patient preference) immediately before administration; stir to mix well.

Instruct patient to drink the solution immediately. Do not allow the solution to stand before drinking.

To ensure the total dose is taken, rinse the container used to measure the dose with a small amount of water or the solution used to mix the drug. Pour this liquid into the container used to dispense the drug, swirl, and again have patient drink immediately.

Parenteral solution: Immediately before use, dilute each 1 ml of the 50 mg/ml IV solution in 20 ml to 100 ml of 0.9% Sodium Chloride or 5% Dextrose Injection. Physician orders diluent and amount of diluent per milliliter of concentrate.

Give by slow IV infusion over 2 to 6 hours (physician orders time of infusion).

Storage: Store at less than 30°C. Protect IV solution from light. Do not store oral solution in the refrigerator; use contents within 2 months once opened.

ONGOING ASSESSMENTS AND NURSING MANAGEMENT

The protocol for pre- and postoperative nursing management pertaining to an allograft transplant varies according to the hospital or surgeon.

Record vital signs q1h to q4h or as ordered. Notify physician immediately of any change in vital signs because changes may be associated with adverse drug reactions, organ rejection, or infection.

Monitor intake and output at intervals ordered. Notify physician immediately of any change in the intake and output ratio.

CLINICAL ALERT: Nephrotoxicity and hepatotoxicity may occur with high doses of cyclosporine. Overt nephrotoxicity is noted by rapid increases in BUN and serum creatinine. Hepatotoxicity consists of elevations of hepatic enzymes and bilirubin.

BUN, serum creatinine, serum bilirubin, and hepatic enzymes are ordered to monitor the effect of cyclosporine on the hepatic and renal systems. Keep physician informed of all changes in laboratory tests as soon as they are reported because dosage adjustment may be necessary.

Keep physician informed of all adverse reactions. Although some may have to be tolerated (_e.g._, hirsutism, gynecomastia), others may require dosage adjustment or other methods of treatment.

Because absorption from the GI tract is incomplete and variable, blood level monitoring of cyclosporine may be useful in patient management. Although no fixed relationships have been established, 24-hour trough values of 250 ng/ml to 500 ng/ml (whole blood RIA) or 50 ng/ml to 300 ng/ml (plasma RIA) appear to minimize side-effects and rejection events.

PATIENT AND FAMILY INFORMATION

NOTE: Before discharge from the hospital, the patient and his family members require a thorough explanation of lifetime follow-up care including diet, prevention of infection, activities of daily living, fluid intake, measurement of blood pressure, daily weights, measurement of intake and output, signs of graft rejection, and so on. Included in this teaching plan is drug therapy, including demonstrations on measurement of the drug, all adverse reactions that may occur, and which adverse reactions require immediate notification of the physician. When applicable, advise the patient of potential risks of pregnancy during use of this drug.

Use a glass container to measure and take (or administer) the drug. Use the provided pipette to measure the dose.

For a more palatable solution, dilute the drug with milk, chocolate milk, or orange juice, preferably at room temperature.

Stir the mixture well and drink (or give) at once. _Do not_ allow the solution to stand before drinking.

To ensure the entire dose is taken, rinse the container used to measure the dose with a small amount of water or the solution used to dilute the drug. Pour this liquid into the glass used to take the drug mixed in milk or orange juice, swirl, and then again drink immediately.

Notify the physician immediately if fever, sore throat, tiredness, or unusual bleeding occurs.

Do not discontinue the medication or change the dosage unless advised to do so by the physician.

Inform other physicians and dentist of therapy with this drug.

Frequent follow-up visits and laboratory tests will be necessary to monitor the effect of therapy with cyclosporine.

Cyclothiazide

See Thiazides and Related Diuretics.

Cyproheptadine Hydrochloride

See Antihistamines.

Cytarabine _(Cytosine Arabinoside, ARA-C)_ Rx

powder for injection: Cytosar-U
  20 mg/ml in 100-
  mg vial, 50 mg/ml
  in 500-mg vial

INDICATIONS

Primarily indicated for induction and maintenance of remission in acute myelocytic leukemia (AML) of adults and children. Also found useful in treatment of other leukemias, such as acute lymphocytic leukemia, chronic myelocytic leukemia (blast phase), and erythroleukemia. May be used alone or in combination with other neoplastic agents; best results are often obtained with combination chemotherapy. Remissions not followed by maintenance treatment have been brief. Maintenance therapy has extended these and provided useful and comfortable remissions with relatively little toxicity.

Acute myelocytic leukemia: Responsiveness and course of childhood AML appear different from those of adults. Response rates are higher in children than in adults with similar treatment schedules.

Acute lymphocytic leukemia: Treatment of both adults and children. Used singly, or in combination with other agents, cytarabine has also been effective in treating patients relapsed on other therapy.

May also be injected intrathecally to treat meningeal leukemia.

CONTRAINDICATIONS

Hypersensitivity.

ACTIONS

Is cytotoxic and inhibits cell phase specificity, primarily killing cells undergoing DNA synthesis and under certain conditions blocking the progression of cells from the G_1 phase to the S-phase. Although mechanism of action is not completely understood, it appears drug acts through inhibition of DNA polymerase. Cytarabine is rapidly metabolized and is not effective orally. Relatively constant plasma levels can be achieved by continuous IV infusion. See also Antineoplastic Agents.

WARNINGS

Myelosuppression: This is a potent bone-marrow suppressant. Start therapy cautiously in those with preexisting drug-induced bone-marrow suppression. Suspend or modify therapy when drug-induced bone-marrow depression has resulted in a platelet count under 50,000 or a polymorphonuclear granulocyte count under 1000/mm³. Counts of formed elements in peripheral blood may continue to fall after drug is stopped and reach lowest values after drug-free intervals of 12 to 24 days. If indicated, therapy is restarted when definite signs of bone-marrow recovery appear (on successive bone-marrow studies). Patients whose drug is withheld until "normal" peripheral blood values are attained may escape from control.

Use in pregnancy: Use in women who are or may become pregnant only when clearly needed and when potential benefits outweigh potential hazards to the fetus. The potential for fetal abnormalities exists, particularly during the first trimester. A patient who becomes pregnant while taking cytarabine should be apprised of the potential risk to the fetus. There is a definite, but considerably lesser risk if therapy is initiated during the second or third trimester. Normal infants have been delivered to patients treated after the first trimester; however, follow-up of such infants is advisable.

PRECAUTIONS

When large IV doses are given quickly, patients are frequently nauseated and may vomit for several hours. This tends to be less severe when drug is infused slowly.

Impaired hepatic function: Liver apparently detoxifies a substantial fraction of an administered dose. Use with caution and at reduced dose in those with poor hepatic function.

Hyperuricemia: May induce hyperuricemia secondary to lysis of neoplastic cells.

When given intrathecally may cause systemic toxicity. Careful monitoring of the hematopoietic system is indicated; modification of other antileukemic therapy may be necessary. Major toxicity is rare. Most frequently reported reactions are nausea, vomiting, and fever and are mild and self-limiting.

ADVERSE REACTIONS

Because drug is a bone-marrow suppressant, anemia, leukopenia, thrombocytopenia, megaloblastosis, and reduced reticulocytes can be expected. Severity of these reactions is dose and schedule dependent. Cellular changes in the morphology of bone marrow and peripheral smears can be expected.

Most frequent: Anorexia, nausea, vomiting, diarrhea, oral and anal inflammation or ulceration, hepatic dysfunction, fever, rash, thrombophlebitis, and bleeding (all sites). Nausea and vomiting are most frequent following rapid IV injection.

Less frequent: Sepsis, pneumonia, cellulitis at injection site, skin ulceration, urinary retention, renal dysfunction, neuritis or neural toxicity, sore throat, esophageal ulceration, esophagitis, chest pain, abdominal pain, freckling, jaundice, conjunctivitis (may occur with rash), dizziness, alopecia, and anaphylaxis.

DOSAGE

Schedule and method of administration vary; may be given by IV infusion or injection or subcutaneously. Thrombophlebitis has occurred at IV site in some patients; pain and inflammation have been noted at subcutaneous injection sites. Higher doses are tolerated when drug is given by rapid IV injection as compared with slow infusion because of drug's rapid inactivation and brief exposure of susceptible normal and neoplastic cells to significant levels after rapid injection.

Success appears to be more dependent on adeptness in modifying day-to-day dosage to obtain maximum leukemic cell kill with tolerable toxicity than on the basic treatment schedule chosen at the onset of therapy. Toxicity necessitating dosage alteration almost always occurs. Use in combination therapy with other cytotoxic drugs may necessitate changes and dose alterations.

AML—induction, remission, and maintenance, adults: 200 mg/m²/day by continuous infusion for 5 days (120 hours) for total dose of 1000 mg/m² repeated approximately every 2 weeks. Modifications are made based on hematologic response. See Appendix 10.

Induction and maintenance in AML, children: When specified amounts of drug are indicated for adult dosage, these should be adjusted for children on the basis of factors such as age, body weight, and body surface area.

Acute lymphocytic leukemia: In general, dosage schedules similar to those used in AML.

Intrathecal use in meningeal leukemia: Dosage schedule is usually governed by type and severity of

CNS manifestations and response to previous therapy.

NURSING IMPLICATIONS

HISTORY
See Appendix 4.

PHYSICAL ASSESSMENT
Record physical, emotional status; vital signs; weight. Review most recent blood and bone-marrow studies. Baseline hematologic studies, renal- and hepatic-function tests, serum uric acid, and other tests as appropriate are obtained before institution of therapy.

ADMINISTRATION
100-mg vial: Reconstitute with 5 ml of Bacteriostatic Water for Injection with Benzyl Alcohol 0.9% to result in a solution containing 20 mg/ml.

500-mg vial: Reconstitute with 10 ml of Bacteriostatic Water for Injection with Benzyl Alcohol 0.9% to result in a solution containing 50 mg/ml.

Physician may order a special diluent for intrathecal use.

Drug may be administered by subcutaneous injection, IV infusion, or rapid IV injection.

Physician orders length of time for administration and IV fluid to be used when IV infusion is selected as method of administration.

An antiemetic may be ordered before administration of cytarabine.

Small children may require arm restraint when drug is given by infusion.

Storage: Solutions may be stored at controlled room temperature, 15°C to 30°C (59°F to 86°F) for 48 hours. Discard any solution in which a haze develops.

ONGOING ASSESSMENTS AND NURSING MANAGEMENT
Obtain vital signs q4h or as ordered; measure intake and output before, during, and for 24 to 48 hours after drug is administered; check IV infusion site for evidence of thrombophlebitis and notify physician if apparent.

CLINICAL ALERT: Cytarabine is a bone-marrow depressant. Observe for signs and symptoms of bone-marrow depression (Appendix 6, section 6-8) and report findings to physician immediately.

Following 5 days of infusion or acute injections of 50 mg/m^2 to 600 mg/m^2, white cell depression follows a biphasic course. WBC starts to fall the first 24 hours, with the nadir at days 7 to 9, followed by a brief rise, which peaks around the 12th day. A second and deeper fall reaches nadir at days 15 to 24. Then there is a rapid rise to above baseline in the next 10 days. Platelet depression is noticeable at 5 days, with a peak depression occurring between days 12 and 15. A rapid rise to above baseline occurs in the next 10 days.

At times of anticipated falls in the WBC and platelet count, patient should be closely observed for signs of bone-marrow depression. CBC, differential, and platelet count are usually drawn daily.

Protective (or reverse) isolation may be necessary if WBC is less than 2000/mm^3 or polymorphonuclear granulocyte count is under 1000/mm^3.

If the platelet count falls below 50,000, precautions will be necessary to minimize risk of bleeding or hemorrhage. Assess for evidence of bleeding q2h to q4h. Check oral cavity, nose, urine, stools, rectum, and vagina for bleeding and skin surfaces for petechiae and ecchymosis. Monitor blood pressure, pulse, and respirations q2h to q4h or as ordered. If signs of bleeding are apparent, notify physician immediately.

Inform laboratory personnel or those performing venipuncture of decreased platelet count. Prolonged pressure on venipuncture site will be necessary.

If IM or subcutaneous injections are given, apply prolonged pressure on site until bleeding or oozing has ceased.

If vomiting occurs, observe for signs of dehydration: poor skin turgor, dry mucous membranes, concentrated urine, decreased urinary output, restlessness, irritability, rapid respirations. Report findings to physician.

Antiemetic may be ordered q4h prn for nausea and vomiting after administration of cytarabine. Antiemetic is best given IM or by suppository if patient is vomiting. A liquid diet may be given until nausea and vomiting cease.

Check oral cavity for signs of inflammation or ulceration. Stomatitis care (Appendix 6, section 6-21) should be instituted as soon as oral changes are noted.

Xylocaine viscous 15 ml q3h to q4h prn may also be ordered for pain due to stomatitis. Instruct patient to swish solution around in mouth. Drug may be swallowed if pharynx is sore. A topical local anesthetic ointment or spray may also be ordered.

Force fluids to 2 to 3 liters per day to prevent urate stone formation.

Check anal area for inflammation and ulceration daily. If noted, contact physician. A topical anesthetic spray or ointment may be prescribed. Wash and dry area carefully after each bowel movement.

If diarrhea occurs, it is usually controlled by antidiarrheal agents.

Serum uric acid levels are monitored periodically during therapy. If serum level rises, physician may order push of fluids. Other treatment may also be instituted for hyperuricemia.

Periodic checks of bone marrow, liver function, and kidney function are performed during therapy.

If a rash develops, notify physician. If rash is severe, topical or systemic therapy may be ordered.

PATIENT AND FAMILY INFORMATION

NOTE: Explanation of expected side-effects that may occur following discharge from the hospital is given by the physician or nurse (with physician approval).

Notify the physician or nurse immediately if any of the following occurs: fever, chills, sore throat, fatigue, sores in mouth or on lips, other signs of infection, easy bruising or bleeding, petechiae.

Inform dentist or other physicians of therapy with this drug before any treatment is started or prescriptions are written.

If anorexia occurs, eat small meals at more frequent intervals. If it persists, discuss with physician.

D

Dacarbazine
Dactinomycin
Danazol
Danthron
Dantrolene Sodium
Dapsone
Daunorubicin Hydrochloride
Decongestants, Nasal, Topical
  Ephedrine
  Epinephrine Hydrochloride
  Naphazoline Hydrochloride
  Oxymetazoline Hydrochloride
  Phenylephrine Hydrochloride
  Tetrahydrozoline Hydrochloride
  Xylomethazoline Hydrochloride
Deferoxamine Mesylate
Dehydrocholic Acid
Demecarium Bromide
Demeclocycline Hydrochloride
Deserpidine
Desipramine Hydrochloride
Deslanoside
Desmopressin Acetate

Desonide
Desoximetasone
Desoxycorticosterone Preparations
  Desoxycorticosterone Acetate
  Desoxycorticosterone Pivalate
Dexamethasone Preparations
Dexchlorpheniramine Maleate
Dexpanthenol Preparations
  Dexpanthenol
  Dexpanthenol With Choline Bitartrate
Dextran, Low Molecular Weight
Dextran, High Molecular Weight
Dextranomer
Dextroamphetamine Sulfate
Dextromethorphan Hydrobromide
Dextrothyroxine Sodium
Diazepam
Diazoxide, Oral
Diazoxide, Parenteral

Dibasic Calcium Phosphate Dihydrate
Dibucaine
Dichlorphenamide
Dicloxacillin Sodium
Dicumarol
Dicyclomine Hydrochloride
Dienestrol
Diethylpropion Hydrochloride
Diethylstilbestrol
Diethylstilbestrol Diphosphate
Diflorasone Diacetate
Diflunisal
Digestive Enzymes
  Pancreatin
  Pancrelipase
Digitalis
Digitalis Glycoside Mixture
Digitoxin
Digoxin
Dihydroergotamine Mesylate
Dihydrotachysterol
Dihydroxyaluminum Sodium Carbonate
Diltiazem Hydrochloride
Dimenhydrinate
Dimercaprol

Dimethyl Sulfoxide
Dinoprost Tromethamine
Dinoprostone
Diphenhydramine Hydrochloride
Diphenidol
Diphenoxylate Hydrochloride With Atropine Sulfate
Diphenylpyraline Hydrochloride
Diphtheria Antitoxin
Diphtheria Toxoid, Adsorbed
Diphtheria and Tetanus Toxoids, Combined
Diphtheria and Tetanus Toxoids and Pertussis Vaccine, Adsorbed

Dipivefrin Hydrochloride
Dipyridamole
Disopyramide
Disulfiram
Dobutamine
Docusate Calcium, Sodium, Potassium
Dopamine Hydrochloride
Doxapram Hydrochloride
Doxepin Hydrochloride
Doxorubicin Hydrochloride
Doxycycline
Dromostanolone Propionate
Droperidol
Dyclonine Hydrochloride
Dyphylline

Dacarbazine

(DTIC, Imidazole Carboxamide)   Rx

injection: 100 mg/10-   DTIC-Dome
  ml vial, 200 mg/
  20-ml vial

INDICATIONS

Treatment of metastatic malignant melanoma; in Hodgkin's disease as a second-line therapy when used in combination with other effective agents (see Appendix 10).

CONTRAINDICATIONS

Hypersensitivity.

ACTIONS

Exact mechanism unknown. It is thought that it inhibits deoxyribonucleic acid (DNA) by acting as a purine analog, acts as an alkylating agent, and interacts with sulfhydryl (SH) groups. After IV administration, the volume of distribution exceeds total body water content, suggesting localization in some body tissue, probably the liver. At therapeutic concentrations, it is not appreciably bound to plasma protein. Disappearance from the plasma is biphasic with initial half-life of 19 minutes and a terminal half-life of 5 hours. The average cumulative excretion of unchanged dacarbazine in the urine is 40% of the injected dose in 6 hours. Drug is subject to renal tubular secretion rather than glomerular filtration.

WARNINGS

Hematopoietic toxicity: Hematopoietic depression is the most serious toxicity and involves primarily leukocytes and platelets, although anemia sometimes occurs. Leukopenia and thrombocytopenia may be severe enough to cause death. Possible bone-marrow depression requires careful monitoring of WBC, RBC, and platelet levels. Hematopoietic toxicity may warrant temporary suspension or cessation of therapy.

Hepatotoxicity: Hepatic toxicity, accompanied by hepatic-vein thrombosis and hepatocellular necrosis, resulting in death has been reported; the incidence of such reactions is low.

Anaphylaxis: Can occur following administration.

Use in pregnancy, lactation: Use in pregnancy only when potential benefit justifies the potential risk to the fetus. It is not known whether drug is excreted in breast milk. Because of a potential for tumorigenicity, a decision should be made whether to discontinue nursing or discontinue the drug, taking into account the importance of the drug to the mother.

PRECAUTIONS

Extravasation of drug during IV administration may result in tissue damage and severe pain.

ADVERSE REACTIONS

GI: Symptoms of anorexia, nausea, and vomiting were most frequently noted, with over 90% of patients affected with the initial few doses. Vomiting lasts 1 to 12 hours and is incompletely and unpredictably palliated with phenobarbital or prochlorperazine. Rarely, intractable nausea and vomiting have necessitated discontinuation of therapy. Diarrhea is rare. Rapid tolerance to these symptoms suggests that a CNS mechanism may be involved; symptoms usually subside after the first 1 to 2 days.

Flulike syndrome: An influenzalike syndrome of fever to 39°C, myalgias, and malaise may be experienced. Symptoms usually occur after large single doses, may last for several days, and may occur with successive treatments.

Clinical laboratory findings: There have been a few reports of significant liver- or renal-function test abnormalities.

Dermatologic: Erythematous and urticarial rashes have been observed infrequently; photosensitivity reactions occur rarely.

Miscellaneous: Alopecia, facial flushing, and facial paresthesias have been noted.

OVERDOSAGE

Give supportive treatment and monitor blood cell counts.

DOSAGE

Administer IV only.

Malignant melanoma: 2 mg/kg/day to 4.5 mg/kg/day IV for 10 days. Treatment may be repeated at 4-week intervals. An alternative dosage is 250 mg/m^2/day IV for 5 days. Treatment may be repeated every 3 weeks.

Hodgkin's disease: Recommended dosage is 150 mg/m^2/day for 5 days, in combination with other effective drugs. Treatment may be repeated every 4 weeks. An alternative recommended dosage is 375 mg/m^2 on day 1, in combination with other effective drugs, to be repeated every 15 days.

NURSING IMPLICATIONS

HISTORY

See Appendix 4.

PHYSICAL ASSESSMENT

Monitor physical, emotional status; vital signs; weight. Baseline laboratory studies include CBC, differential, platelet count, renal- and hepatic-function studies.

ADMINISTRATION

Physician may order restriction of oral intake of food and fluids for 4 to 6 hours before the administration of dacarbazine to reduce nausea and vomiting.

Physician usually orders antiemetic given before administration of dacarbazine.

Reconstitute 100-mg vial with 9.9 ml of Sterile Water for Injection, USP.

Reconstitute 200-mg vial with 19.7 ml of Sterile Water for Injection, USP.

The resulting solution of either vial contains 10 mg/ml.

The reconstituted solution may be further diluted with 5% Dextrose Injection, USP or Sodium Chloride Injection, USP and administered by IV infusion, usually over a period of 15 to 30 minutes.

Physician will order type, amount (usually 50 ml to 100 ml) of IV fluid and length of time for infusion. Physician may also administer by IV push over a period of 1 to 2 minutes. In preparing drug for administration by IV push, check with physician about further dilution once dose is removed from the vial.

Warn patient that drug may cause localized pain or a burning sensation as it is being administered.

Extravasation of drug during IV administration may result in tissue damage and severe pain.

If extravasation should occur, *immediately* stop and remove the intravenous infusion. Apply an ice pack to the infusion site and notify physician immediately.

Anaphylaxis can occur. Drugs used to treat anaphylaxis include epinephrine, oxygen, and an antihistamine.

Should anaphylaxis occur, stop infusion of dacarbazine by removing the IV infusion containing dacarbazine and immediately replace it with an IV infusion of 0.9% Sodium Chloride for Injection (other IV fluids may be hospital policy or physician preference). The IV line *must remain patent.* Have another member of the health team contact the physician immediately. Stay with the patient and monitor the blood pressure and pulse.

Stability: After reconstitution and prior to use, solution may be stored in the vial at 4°C for up to 72 hours or under normal room conditions (light and temperature) for up to 8 hours. If the reconstituted solution is further diluted in 5% Dextrose Injection, USP or Sodium Chloride Injection, USP, the resulting solution may be stored at 4°C for up to 24 hours or under normal room conditions for up to 8 hours.

ONGOING ASSESSMENTS AND NURSING MANAGEMENT

Hospitalization is not always necessary but adequate laboratory study capability must be available.

Obtain vital signs q4h; measure intake and output starting before drug is administered and continuing until vomiting stops.

Nausea and vomiting may begin 1 to 6 hours after drug is administered and may last up to 12 hours. They may or may not be controlled by administration of an antiemetic.

Notify physician if vomiting persists and total amount exceeds approximately 700 ml to 800 ml in 8 hours. Observe patient for electrolyte imbalance, especially hypokalemia (Appendix 6, section 6-15) and hyponatremia (Appendix 6, section 6-17) as well as evidence of dehydration (Appendix 6, section 6-10). Report findings to physician.

A liquid diet or sips of water or carbonated beverage may be tolerated in small amounts until nausea and vomiting cease.

CLINICAL ALERT: Hematopoietic toxicity is the most common toxicity and usually occurs in approximately 10 to 14 days. Observe for signs of bone-marrow depression (Appendix 6, section 6-8). Notify physician immediately if one or more should occur.

If bone-marrow depression is severe, protective (reverse) isolation may be necessary.

Local pain, burning sensation, and irritation at the site of injection may be relieved by locally applied hot packs.

PATIENT AND FAMILY INFORMATION

NOTE: If dacarbazine is given on outpatient basis, complete instructions should be given during an office or clinic visit before the day drug administration is scheduled. Instructions may include directions for taking an antiemetic, fasting from food or liquids for 4 to 6 hours, and so on. Patient should also be told of possible alopecia, the necessity for frequent blood tests, and the possibility of hospitalization should bone-marrow depression become severe.

Notify physician or nurse if any of the following occurs: fever, chills, sore throat, sores in the mouth or on the lips, other signs of infection, easy bleeding, or bruising.

A flulike syndrome may occur, with malaise, muscle aches, fever, and headache. (NOTE: Because fever may also be a sign of hematopoietic toxicity, patient should be encouraged to contact the physician and describe his symptoms.)

Inform dentist or other physicians of therapy with this drug before treatment is started or drugs are prescribed.

Do not take any nonprescription drugs unless use has been approved by the physician.

If anorexia is severe or weight loss is noted, discuss this with physician. Eating small meals at more frequent intervals may be of value.

Avoid exposure to ultraviolet light and prolonged exposure to sunlight.

Dactinomycin (Actinomycin D, ACT) Rx

injection: 0.5 mg/vial   Cosmegen

INDICATIONS

Wilms' tumor: With low doses of both dactinomycin and radiotherapy, temporary objective improvement may be as good as and last longer than with higher doses of each given alone. Combination therapy with vincristine, together with surgery and radiotherapy, significantly improves the prognosis of patients in groups II and III.

Rhabdomyosarcoma: Temporary regression and subjective results have occurred. Combination chemotherapy may also be used.

Carcinoma of the testes and uterus: Sequential use of dactinomycin and methotrexate, along with monitoring of human chorionic gonadotropin levels until normal, has resulted in survival of the majority of women with metastatic choriocarcinoma. Has been beneficial as a single agent in treatment of metastatic nonseminomatous testicular carcinoma.

Other neoplasms: Has been given IV or by regional perfusion, either alone or with other antineoplastic agents or x-ray therapy, in the palliative treatment of Ewing's sarcoma and sarcoma botryoides.

Radiation therapy: Evidence suggests that dactinomycin potentiates the effects of x-ray therapy; the converse also appears likely. This potentiation of radiation effect represents a special problem when irradiation includes the mucous membrane. Because of this potentiating effect, dactinomycin may be tried in radiosensitive tumors not responding to x-ray therapy.

Perfusion technique: Given alone or with other antineoplastic agents by isolation-perfusion, either as palliative treatment or as an adjunct to resection of a tumor. Some tumors considered resistant to chemotherapy and radiation therapy may respond when drug is given by the perfusion technique. Neoplasms in which this technique has been tried include various types of sarcoma, carcinoma, and adenocarcinoma. Isolation-perfusion technique offers advantages provided leakage of the drug into general circulation is minimal. By this technique the drug is in continuous contact with the tumor for the duration of treatment. The dose may be increased over that used by the systemic route, usually without danger of toxic effects. If the agent is confined to an isolated part, it should not interfere with the patient's defense mechanism. Systemic absorption of toxic products from neoplastic tissue can be minimized by removing the perfusate when procedure is finished.

CONTRAINDICATIONS

If given at or about the time of infection with chickenpox or herpes zoster, a severe generalized disease may occur, which could result in death.

ACTIONS

Is the principal component of the mixture of actinomycins produced by *Streptomyces parvullus.* Generally, actinomycins exert an inhibitory effect on gram-positive and gram-negative bacteria and some fungi. However, toxic properties of the actinomycins (including dactinomycin) in relation to antibacterial activity are such as to preclude their use as antibiotics in treatment of infectious disease. Actinomycins are cytotoxic and thus have an antineoplastic effect, which is the basis for their use. Dactinomycin is minimally metabolized. Plasma half-life is 36 hours. Drug tends to concentrate in nucleated cells and does not cross the blood–brain barrier. See also Antineoplastic Agents.

WARNINGS

Use in pregnancy, lactation: Danger to the fetus should be taken into consideration. Breast-feeding should be stopped before beginning treatment.

Use in infants: Should not be given to infants under 6 months because of greater frequency of toxic effects.

PRECAUTIONS

Dactinomycin is a toxic drug. Reactions may involve any body tissue; anaphylactoid reactions may occur. A variety of abnormalities of renal, hepatic and bone-marrow function have been reported. Increased incidence of GI toxicity and marrow suppression has been reported when given with x-ray therapy. Caution used in the first 2 months after irradiation for the treatment of right-sided Wilms' tumor, because hepatomegaly and elevated SGOT levels have been noted. Reports indicate an increased incidence of second primary tumors following treatment with radiation and antineoplastic agents such as dactinomycin. Multimodal therapy creates need for long-term observation of cancer survivors.

Nausea and vomiting may make it necessary to give dactinomycin intermittently. If stomatitis, diarrhea, or severe hematopoietic depression appears during therapy, treatment is discontinued until patient has recovered.

ADVERSE REACTIONS

Adverse reactions are usually reversible with discontinuation of therapy.

Miscellaneous: Malaise, fatigue, lethargy, fever, myalgia, proctitis, hypocalcemia.

Oral: Cheilitis, dysphagia, esophagitis, ulcerative stomatitis, pharyngitis.

GI: Anorexia, nausea, vomiting, abdominal pain, diarrhea, GI ulceration.

Hematologic: Anemia, including aplastic anemia, agranulocytosis, leukopenia, thrombocytopenia, pancytopenia, and reticulopenia. Platelet and WBC counts performed daily to detect severe hematopoietic depression. If either markedly decreases, drug is withheld until recovery occurs. This often takes up to 3 weeks.

Dermatologic: Alopecia, skin eruptions, acne, flare-up of erythema, or increased pigmentation of previously irradiated skin.

Soft tissues: Dactinomycin is extremely corrosive. Extravasation during IV administration causes severe damage to soft tissues.

Toxic reactions: Toxic reactions are frequent and may be severe, limiting the amount of drug that may be given. Severe toxicity varies and is only partly dependent on dose. Drug must be given in short courses.

DOSAGE

IV

Dosage varies depending on tolerance of patient, size and location of neoplasm, and use of other therapy. Dosage for adults and children should not exceed 15 mcg/kg or 400 mcg/m^2 to 600 mcg/m^2 daily IV for 5 days. Dosage is calculated for obese or edematous patients on basis of body surface area.

Adults: 0.5 mg/day IV for maximum of 5 days.

Children: 0.015 mg/kg/day IV for 5 days. An alternative schedule is a total dosage of 2.5 mg/m^2 IV over 1 week.

In both adults and children, a second course may be given after at least 3 weeks have elapsed, provided all signs of toxicity have disappeared.

Isolation-perfusion technique: 0.05 mg/kg for lower extremity or pelvis; 0.035 mg/kg for upper extremity. Lower doses are used in obese patients or when previous therapy has been employed.

NURSING IMPLICATIONS

HISTORY
See Appendix 4.

PHYSICAL ASSESSMENT
Record physical, emotional status; vital signs; weight. Baseline studies include CBC, differential, platelet count, renal- and hepatic-function tests. Other laboratory or diagnostic studies may also be appropriate.

ADMINISTRATION
An antiemetic is usually ordered before administration of drug.

Preparation of solution: Reconstitute by adding 1.1 ml Sterile Water for Injection (without preservative). Resulting solution will contain approximately 0.5 mg/ml. Use of Water for Injection with a preservative results in formation of a precipitate and drug cannot be used.

After removal of dose from vial, discard unused portion.

Drug can be added directly to infusion solutions of 5% Dextrose or Sodium Chloride Injection or to the tubing of a running IV infusion. May also be administered by IV push.

Physician must order exact method of administration and IV solution.

Adding to an IV infusion: Drug withdrawn from vial is further diluted with 30 ml to 50 ml of 5% Dextrose or Sodium Chloride Injection (*e.g.,* same as the IV infusion solution) and added to a volume-control set, used as a secondary IV line inserted into the injection port of the primary line. After drug is administered, run the IV solution in the primary line for a few minutes to clear the line of the drug. The primary line may then be removed, unless orders state otherwise.

Always use the type of IV set specified by physician or hospital policy because partial removal of dactinomycin from IV solutions by cellulose ester membrane filters (used in some IV in-line filters) has been reported.

To give through a running IV infusion, the primary line is run wide open and the drug is slowly injected into the IV injection port. The primary line is then run for a few minutes to clear the line of the drug. The primary line may then be removed, unless orders state otherwise.

CLINICAL ALERT: Determine patency of IV line and correct placement of needle in vein before attempting to administer dactinomycin. _Do not administer drug if there is any question regarding correct placement of the IV needle because this drug is extremely corrosive to tissue._ If extravasation does occur, discontinue IV immediately.

Remain with patient during administration of drug. Continue to monitor the IV site until drug is completely infused. If extravasation should occur during administration, stop IV immediately and contact the physician.

Instruct patient to mention immediately if burning is felt at the injection site (may be sign of extravasation). Stop administration to see if burning persists. If burning persists, treat as extravasation.

IV push (given directly into vein without use of an infusion): Use "two-needle technique." Reconstitute and withdraw drug with one sterile needle. Use another needle for direct injection into vein. A butterfly needle may also be inserted, then approximately 5 ml of Sodium Chloride is injected to be sure needle is correctly placed in the vein. The syringe is then removed and replaced with the syringe containing dactinomycin, which is injected slowly. Following administration, Sodium Chloride (approximately 15–20 ml) is then injected to clear the needle and flush the vein.

NOTE: Hospital or unit policies or the physician's order may vary on the exact technique of administration.

Isolation-perfusion technique: An intra-arterial catheter is inserted surgically or threaded through a peripheral artery to the tumor. An infusion pump or pressure cuff is used to deliver the solution. Consult hospital procedure manual for equipment needed and specific directions for administration.

ONGOING ASSESSMENTS AND NURSING MANAGEMENT

If extravasation of drug has occurred, follow procedure outlined by physician for treatment. Usually ice packs are applied immediately after needle is removed; area may also be treated with injections of a steroid. Any drugs used to treat extravasation should be immediately available and the physician should write specific orders for administration of agents used to decrease tissue necrosis.

Monitor vital signs q4h.

Measure intake and output, starting before

drug is administered and continuing for 48 hours after administration.

Severe nausea and vomiting usually begin 1 to 4 or more hours after administration of drug. An antiemetic is usually ordered q4h prn. If vomiting is severe, an antiemetic should be given by the parenteral route or as a suppository.

A liquid diet, sips of water, or carbonated beverages may be offered.

Evaluate hydration during period of severe vomiting. Signs of dehydration include poor skin turgor, dry mucous membranes, concentrated urine, decreased urinary output, restlessness, and rapid respirations. If these should occur, report findings to the physician.

If vomitus exceeds approximately 700 ml to 800 ml in 8 hours, notify physician.

Toxic effects (except nausea and vomiting) usually do not become apparent until 2 to 4 days after a course of therapy is stopped and may not be maximal before 1 to 2 weeks have elapsed. Deaths have been reported.

Careful and frequent observation of patient for adverse reactions is necessary. Begin to observe patient 2 days after course of therapy is stopped. Review section on _Adverse Reactions._ Generally, inspect skin surfaces for dermatologic reactions; examine mouth for ulcerative stomatitis; check all bowel movements for diarrhea, occult blood (physician may request testing each stool for blood using Hematest, Hemoccult, etc.); look for signs of bone-marrow depression (Appendix 6, section 6-8); monitor vital signs; observe for signs of hypocalcemia (Appendix 6, section 6-13); listen to and evaluate all patient complaints (_e.g.,_ fatigue, lethargy, dysphagia).

Bone-marrow depression may be seen within the first week after therapy is stopped. Platelet and WBC counts are usually performed daily to detect severe hematopoietic depression. Notify physician immediately if signs of bone-marrow depression (Appendix 6, section 6-8) are apparent or most recent laboratory report shows marked decrease in WBC or platelet count.

Anorexia may occur. Physician may order high-calorie, high-protein diet (in small servings, 4–6 times/day). A dietitian consult should also be obtained.

Erythema from previous x-ray therapy may be reactivated, even when radiation occurred months earlier.

With combined dactinomycin-radiation therapy, normal skin and the buccal and pharyngeal mucosa show early erythema. A smaller than usual x-ray dose given with dactinomycin causes erythema and vesiculation, which progress more rapidly through stages of tanning and desquamation. Healing may occur in 4 to 6 weeks rather than 2 to 3 months.

PATIENT AND FAMILY INFORMATION

NOTE: When drug is given on outpatient basis, complete instructions about therapy and anticipated adverse reactions are necessary and should include possibility of alopecia and severe bone-marrow toxicity that may require hospitalization.

Take antiemetic (if prescribed) before reporting for therapy. Continue to take this drug after therapy, as needed.

If antiemetic does not (partially) relieve nausea and vomiting, or if vomiting persists for longer than 8 hours, notify physician.

Anorexia may occur. If this persists for more than 2 to 3 days, notify physician. Try to eat small meals at more frequent intervals.

Notify physician or nurse if any of the following should occur: fever, chills, sore throat, sores in the mouth or on the lips, signs of infection, fatigue, easy bruising or bleeding, rectal pain, diarrhea, blood in the stool, black stools, abdominal pain, changes in color of skin, acne, difficulty swallowing or pain on swallowing, myalgia.

Frequent blood tests will be necessary to monitor results of therapy.

Danazol Rx

capsules: 50 mg, 100   Danocrine
  mg, 200 mg

INDICATIONS

Endometriosis: When amenable to hormonal management and only for those who cannot tolerate other drug therapy, those in whom other drugs are contraindicated, or those who fail to respond to other drug therapy. Not indicated when surgery alone is treatment of choice.

Fibrocystic breast disease: Most cases can be treated by simple measures (*e.g.,* analgesics). In some patients, symptoms of pain and tenderness may be severe enough to warrant treatment by suppression of ovarian function. Usually effective in decreasing nodularity, pain, and tenderness. This treatment involves considerable alterations in hormone levels, and recurrence of symptoms is common after cessation of therapy.

Hereditary angioedema: For prevention of attacks of angioedema of all types (cutaneous, abdominal, laryngeal) in males and females.

Investigational uses: Treatment of gynecomastia, infertility, menorrhagia.

CONTRAINDICATIONS

Undiagnosed abnormal genital bleeding; markedly impaired hepatic, renal, or cardiac function. Contraindicated during pregnancy and lactation.

ACTIONS

A synthetic androgen derived from ethisterone, which suppresses the pituitary–ovarian axis by inhibiting the output of pituitary gonadotropins. Also has weak, dose-related androgenic activity. Drug is not estrogenic or progestational. It depresses output of both follicle-stimulating hormone (FSH) and luteinizing hormone (LH), decreasing ovarian estrogen production. Generally, the pituitary suppressive action is reversible. Ovulation and cyclic bleeding usually return within 60 to 90 days after therapy is discontinued.

Endometriosis: Danazol alters normal and ectopic endometrial tissue so that it becomes inactive and atrophic. Complete resolution of endometrial lesions occurs in a majority of cases. Regression is due to suppression of ovarian function, resulting in anovulation with amenorrhea. Changes in vaginal cytology and cervical mucus reflect suppressive effect of drug on the pituitary–ovarian axis.

Fibrocystic breast disease: Usually produces partial to complete disappearance of nodularity and complete relief of pain and tenderness. Changes in the menstrual pattern may occur.

Hereditary angioedema: At effective doses, prevents attacks of the disease characterized by episodic edema of the abdominal viscera, extremities, face, and airway, which may be disabling and even fatal if the airway is involved.

Has a half-life of approximately 29 hours and is excreted primarily in the urine.

WARNINGS

Carcinoma of breast: Should be excluded before therapy is instituted for fibrocystic disease. Nodularity, pain, and tenderness due to fibrocystic disease may prevent recognition of underlying carcinoma before treatment is begun. If any nodule persists or enlarges during treatment, carcinoma should be considered and ruled out.

Androgenic effects: Patient is observed for signs of virilization. Some androgenic effects may not be reversible even when drug is discontinued.

PRECAUTIONS

May cause some degree of fluid retention; conditions influenced by edema (*e.g.,* epilepsy, cardiac or renal dysfunction) require careful observation. Because hepatic dysfunction has been reported, periodic hepatic-function tests are recommended. Semen is checked for volume, viscosity, sperm count, and motility every 3 to 4 months, especially in adolescents.

DRUG INTERACTIONS

Prolongation of prothrombin time in patients stabilized on **warfarin** has been reported. Abnormal **glucose tolerance** test and increased **insulin** requirements in diabetics have occurred.

ADVERSE REACTIONS

Androgenic: Acne, edema, mild hirsutism, decrease in breast size, deepening of voice, oiliness of skin or hair, weight gain, and (rarely) clitoral hypertrophy or testicular atrophy.

Hypoestrogenic: Flushing, sweating, vaginitis (itching, dryness, burning, vaginal bleeding), nervousness, emotional lability.

Hepatic: Dysfunction, evidenced by elevated serum enzymes or jaundice, has been reported in those receiving dosage of 400 mg/day or more.

Other: The following have been reported, but no causal relationship has been confirmed: skin rashes, nasal congestion (rare), dizziness, headache, sleep disorders, fatigue, tremor; rarely, paresthesia in extremities, visual disturbances, anxiety, depression, changes in appetite; muscle cramps or spasms; joint lock-up, joint swelling; pain in back, neck, legs; rarely, hematuria; loss of hair; changes in libido; elevated blood pressure; chills; rarely, pelvic pain.

DOSAGE

Endometriosis: Therapy is begun during menstruation, if possible; otherwise pregnancy test is done. *Dosage*—800 mg/day in 2 divided doses. Therapy is continued uninterrupted for 3 to 6 months; may be extended to 9 months. If symptoms recur after termination, treatment can be instituted.

Fibrocystic breast disease: Therapy is begun during menstruation, if possible; otherwise pregnancy test is done. Dosage ranges from 100 mg/day to 400 mg/day in two divided doses depending on patient response. A nonhormonal method of contraception is recommended when drug is administered at this dose because ovulation may not be suppressed. Elimination of nodularity usually requires 4 to 6 months. If symptoms recur after termination, treatment may be reinstated.

Hereditary angioedema: Dosage is individualized on basis of response. Recommended starting dose is 200 mg bid or tid. After favorable response is obtained, dosage may be decreased at intervals of 1 to 3 months or longer. If an attack occurs, dosage may be increased by up to 200 mg/day. During dose-adjusting phase patient is monitored closely, particularly if there is a history of airway involvement.

NURSING IMPLICATIONS

HISTORY
See Appendix 4.

PHYSICAL ASSESSMENT
Review chart or record for physician's physical examination, laboratory tests. Pregnancy test, hepatic-function tests may be performed before therapy is initiated.

ONGOING ASSESSMENTS AND NURSING MANAGEMENT
Record weight, blood pressure, and pulse rate at time of each clinic/office visit.

Periodic liver-function tests are recommended.

Physician performs periodic physical assessments to evaluate drug response.

PATIENT INFORMATION
May cause masculinization (*e.g.,* abnormal growth of facial or other fine body hair, deepening of voice). Notify physician or nurse if these occur.

Treatment of endometriosis: If menstrual period is missed, notify physician. A pregnancy test may be necessary.

Nonhormonal contraceptive measures are recommended during therapy; follow physician's recommendations in this matter.

If pregnancy is suspected, discontinue therapy immediately and make an appointment to see physician.

Flushing, sweating, vaginitis, or nervousness may occur. If these become uncomfortable, discuss with physician.

Fibrocystic breast disease: Symptoms may be relieved by first month and eliminated in 2 to 3 months. Menses may be regular or irregular. If symptoms do not appear to be relieved, contact physician.

Danthron

See Laxatives.

Dantrolene Sodium Rx

| capsules: 25 mg, 50 mg, 100 mg | Dantrium |
| powder for injection: 0.32 mg/ml | Dantrium Intravenous |

INDICATIONS

Spasticity: Oral form is indicated for controlling clinical spasticity resulting from upper motor neuron disorders such as spinal cord injury, stroke, cerebral palsy, or multiple sclerosis. Is of particular benefit to patient whose functional rehabilitation has been retarded by the sequelae of spasticity.

Malignant hyperthermia: Intravenous form indicated, along with appropriate supportive measures, for management of the fulminant hypermetabolism of skeletal muscle characteristic of malignant hyperthermic crisis as soon as it is recognized. Oral form is indicated to prevent or attenuate development of signs of malignant hyperthermia in known, or strongly suspected, susceptible patients requiring anesthesia or surgery. Oral form also administered following a malignant hyperthermic crisis to prevent recurrence of the signs of malignant hyperthermia.

Investigational: Used in exercise-induced muscle pain.

CONTRAINDICATIONS

Oral form is contraindicated in active hepatic disease such as hepatitis and cirrhosis, in which spasticity is used to sustain upright posture and balance in locomotion or whenever spasticity is used to obtain or maintain increased function.

ACTIONS

Has been shown to produce relaxation by affecting contractile response in skeletal muscle at site beyond the myoneural junction and directly on the muscle itself. Does not affect neuromuscular transmission. In skeletal muscle, it dissociates the excitation–contraction coupling, probably by interfering with the release of calcium from sarcoplasmic reticulum. This effect appears more pronounced in fast muscle fibers as compared to slow ones, but it generally affects both. A CNS effect occurs, with drowsiness, dizziness, and generalized weakness occasionally present.

Absorption after oral administration is incomplete and slow but consistent. Dose-related blood levels are obtained with duration and intensity of skeletal muscle relaxation related to dosage and blood levels. The mean biological half-life in adults is 9 hours after a 100-mg oral dose and 5 hours after IV administration. Significant amounts of drug are bound to plasma proteins, mostly albumin. The parent compound is found in significant amounts in blood and urine. It is probably metabolized by hepatic microsomal enzymes.

WARNINGS

Hepatic effects: Fatal and nonfatal liver disorders, of an idiosyncratic or hypersensitivity type, may occur. Use with particular caution in females and patients over 35 in view of greater likelihood of drug-induced, potentially fatal, hepatocellular disease in these groups.

Long-term use: Safety and efficacy not established.

Carcinogenicity: Cannot be fully excluded; this possible risk of chronic administration must be weighed against benefits of the drug for the individual patient.

Malignant hyperthermia (hyperpyrexia): IV use of this drug is not a substitute for previously known supportive measures. These measures must be individualized, but it will usually be necessary to discontinue the suspected triggering agents, attend to increased oxygen requirements, manage metabolic acidosis, institute cooling when necessary, attend to urinary output, and monitor for electrolyte imbalance.

Use in pregnancy and lactation: Safety for use in women who are or who may become pregnant not established. Do not use in nursing mothers.

Use in children: Safety for use in children under 5 not established.

PRECAUTIONS

Use with caution in patients with impaired pulmonary function, particularly those with obstructive pulmonary disease; severely impaired cardiac function due to myocardial disease; a history of previous liver disease or dysfunction.

DRUG INTERACTIONS

Although a definite drug interaction with **estrogen** therapy is not yet established, caution should be observed if the two drugs are given concomitantly. Hepatotoxicity has occurred more often in women over 35 years receiving concomitant estrogen therapy. Exercise caution in concomitant administration of **tranquilizing agents.**

ADVERSE REACTIONS

The following apply to oral therapy. None of the reactions reported in patients on oral therapy have been reported in patients treated with short-term IV therapy for malignant hyperthermia.

Most frequent: Drowsiness, dizziness, weakness, general malaise, fatigue, diarrhea. These effects are generally transient, occurring early in treatment, and can often be obviated by beginning with a low dose and increasing gradually until optimal regimen is established. Diarrhea may be severe and necessitate temporary withdrawal of therapy; if it recurs upon readministration, therapy is discontinued.

GI: Constipation, GI bleeding, anorexia, swallowing difficulty, gastric irritation, abdominal cramps.

Hepatobiliary: Hepatitis (see *Warnings*).

Neurologic: Speech disturbance, seizure, headache, lightheadedness, visual disturbance, diplopia, alteration of taste, insomnia.

Cardiovascular: Tachycardia, erratic blood pressure, phlebitis.

Psychiatric: Mental depression and confusion, increased nervousness.

GU: Increased urinary frequency, hematuria, crystalluria, difficult erection, urinary incontinence or nocturia, difficult urination or urinary retention.

Musculoskeletal: Myalgia, backache.

Hypersensitivity: Pleural effusion with pericarditis.

Other: Chills, fever, feeling of suffocation, excessive tearing.

OVERDOSAGE

General supportive measures are employed along with gastric lavage. IV fluids should be administered in fairly large quantities to avert possibility of crystalluria. Maintain adequate airway; artificial resuscitation equipment should be available. Monitor ECG; observe patient carefully. No experience reported with dialysis.

DOSAGE

Chronic spasticity

Dosage is increased until maximum performance compatible with dysfunction due to underlying disease is achieved. No further increase in dosage is then indicated. Dosage is titrated and individualized.

Adults: Therapy is usually begun with 25 mg once daily; increase to 25 mg bid to qid, then by increments of 25 mg up to as high as 100 mg bid to qid, if needed. Most patients will respond to 400 mg/day or less; higher doses are rarely needed. Each dosage level is maintained 4 to 7 days to determine patient's response.

Children: Usually 0.5 mg/kg bid, increased to 0.5 mg/kg tid or qid, then by increments of 0.5 mg/kg up to 3 mg/kg bid to qid, if needed. Doses higher than 100 mg qid should not be used.

Malignant hyperthermia

Preoperative prophylaxis: 4 mg/kg/day to 8 mg/kg/day PO in three or four divided doses for 1 to 2 days before surgery, with last dose being given approximately 3 to 4 hours before scheduled surgery with a minimum of water.

Treatment: As soon as malignant hyperthermia is recognized, all anesthetic agents are discontinued. Dantrolene is administered by rapid IV push beginning at a minimum dose of 1 mg/kg and continuing until all symptoms subside or maximum cumulative dose of 10 mg/kg is reached. Treatment may be repeated. Dose for children is same as for adults.

Postcrisis follow-up: 4 mg/kg/day to 8 mg/kg/day PO in four divided doses for 1 to 3 days to prevent recurrence.

NURSING IMPLICATIONS

HISTORY

Chronic spasticity: Review patient's chart or record for symptoms, etiology of spasticity, current treatment modalities.

Malignant hyperthermia: Question all surgical patients about previous exposure to anesthetics; personal or family history of muscle disorders; unexplained death of a family member during or shortly after surgery. If any answer is positive, notify surgeon and anesthesiologist.

PHYSICAL ASSESSMENT

Chronic spasticity: Evaluate neuromuscular function (*e.g.,* gait, muscle coordination and strength, areas of spasticity, posture, ability to carry out activities of daily living [ADL]). Review assessments of physician and physical and occupational therapists. Hepatic-function studies are recommended before institution of therapy.

Malignant hyperthermia: Early recognition is important. Signs include slow rise in heart rate, body temperature; cyanosis; muscle rigidity; hypotension. Respiratory and metabolic acidosis also present.

ADMINISTRATION

If child has difficulty swallowing capsule, discuss with physician or contact pharmacist about advisability of opening capsule and pouring contents into proper vehicle.

Parenteral: Add 60 ml of Sterile Water for Injection, USP (without bacteriostatic agent) to each vial; shake until solution is clear. Protect contents of vial from direct light and temperatures above 30°C (86°F) and below 15°C (59°F). Use within 6 hours after reconstitution.

Because of high *p*H of IV formulation, care must be taken to prevent extravasation into surrounding tissues.

ONGOING ASSESSMENTS AND NURSING MANAGEMENT

Chronic spasticity: It is important to establish a therapeutic goal (*e.g.,* regain and maintain a specific function such as therapeutic exercise program, use of braces, transfer maneuvers) before beginning therapy. These goals should be developed as a team effort (*i.e.,* by the physician, physical and occupational therapists, nursing personnel).

Evaluate response to drug by comparing daily neuromuscular assessments to baseline data; monitor vital signs; observe for adverse drug effects, especially signs of hepatotoxicity (rash, itching, jaundice).

When evaluating drug response look for reduction in painful or disabling spasticity such as clonus, reduction in the intensity or degree of nursing care required, and decrease in annoying manifestations of spasticity considered important by the patient.

Subtle but meaningful improvement may occur with therapy. Information about improvement should be solicited from the patient as well as documented in daily nursing summaries.

Drowsiness, dizziness, weakness, general malaise, and fatigue may be seen during early therapy. Patient may require assistance with ambulation, ADL. Physical and occupational therapies may prove tiring and time in therapy may need to be shortened until these transient effects disappear.

Diarrhea may occur. If severe, contact physician because therapy may be temporarily discontinued. If diarrhea occurs upon readministration, drug will be discontinued.

Hepatic-function tests are performed at periodic intervals during therapy. Abnormal values require discontinuation of therapy.

Therapy is usually discontinued if benefits are not evident within 45 days.

Malignant hyperthermia: Preoperative prophylaxis dosage is usually associated with skeletal muscle weakness and sedation (sleepiness, drowsiness). Notify physician if these become excessive because dosage adjustment may be made to avoid incapacitation or excessive GI irritation (nausea, vomiting).

Intraoperative and postoperative management of malignant hyperthermia include reduction of body temperature, correction of acidosis and other electrolyte imbalances, monitoring of intake and output and vital signs, and other appropriate measures depending on patient's condition.

PATIENT AND FAMILY INFORMATION

May cause drowsiness or dizziness; exercise caution while driving or performing other tasks requiring alertness.

Avoid alcohol and other CNS depressants.

Avoid prolonged exposure to sunlight; photosensitivity may occur.

May cause weakness, fatigue, nausea, diarrhea; notify physician or nurse if these effects persist.

Notify physician if skin rash, itching, bloody or black tarry stools, or yellowish discoloration of skin or eyes occurs.

Malignant hyperthermia: Wear Medic-Alert or other identification of problem. Always inform other physicians, dentists, and medical personnel of problem before any therapy that may require use of an anesthetic.

Dapsone (DDS) Rx

tablets: 25 mg,   *Generic*
    100 mg

INDICATIONS

All forms of leprosy (Hansen's disease) except for cases of proven dapsone resistance; dermatitis herpetiformis.

Unlabeled uses: Treatment of relapsing polychondritis and prophylaxis of malaria.

CONTRAINDICATIONS

Hypersensitivity.

ACTIONS

Is bactericidal as well as bacteriostatic against *Mycobacterium leprae.* The mechanism of action in dermatitis herpetiformis has not been established. It is slowly and nearly completely absorbed from the GI tract; peak plasma concentrations are reached in 4 to 8 hours. About 70% is excreted in the urine as conjugates and unidentified metabolites. Excretion of the drug is slow and a constant blood level can be maintained with the usual dosage.

WARNINGS

Deaths associated with dapsone administration have been reported from agranulocytosis, aplastic anemia, and other blood dyscrasias. Sore throat, fever, pallor, purpura, or jaundice may occur.

Anemia: Treat prior to initiation of therapy. Hemolysis and methemoglobin may be poorly tolerated by those with severe cardiopulmonary disease.

Hypersensitivity: Cutaneous reactions (especially bullous) include exfoliative dermatitis, toxic erythema, erythema multiforme, toxic epidermal necrolysis, morbilliform and scarlatiniform reactions, urticaria, and erythema nodosum. These are some of the most serious and rare complications of dapsone therapy and are directly related to drug sensitization. If new or toxic dermatologic reactions occur, promptly discontinue dapsone therapy and institute appropriate therapy.

Leprosy reactional states, including those that are cutaneous, are not hypersensitivity reactions and do not require discontinuation of therapy (see *Precautions*).

Use in pregnancy: Studies have not shown that dapsone increases the risk of fetal abnormalities if given during all trimesters. Because studies cannot rule out the possibility of harm, use drug during

D

pregnancy only if necessary. In general, for leprosy, the U.S. Public Health Service (USPHS) at Carville, Louisiana recommends maintenance of dapsone. Dapsone has been important for the management of some pregnant dermatitis herpetiformis patients. Dapsone is generally not considered to have an effect on the later growth, development, and functional maturation of the child.

Use in lactation: Because of potential tumorigenicity shown in animal studies, discontinue nursing or the drug.

PRECAUTIONS

Hemolysis and Heinz body formation may be exaggerated in those with G6PD deficiency, methemoglobin reductase deficiency, or hemoglobin M. This reaction is frequently dose related. Give dapsone with caution to these patients or if the patient is exposed to other agents or conditions such as infection or diabetic ketosis capable of producing hemolysis.

Toxic hepatitis and cholestatic jaundice have been reported early in therapy. Hyperbilirubinemia may occur more often in G6PD-deficient patients.

Leprosy reactional states are abrupt changes in clinical activity occurring in leprosy with any effective treatment and are classified into two groups.

Type 1: May occur in borderline or tuberculoid leprosy patients soon after chemotherapy is begun. The patient has enhanced delayed hypersensitivity response to residual infection leading to swelling of existing skin and nerve lesions. If severe, or if neuritis is present, use large doses of steroids and hospitalize the patient. In general, continue antileprosy treatment and therapy to suppress the reaction (*e.g.,* analgesics, steroids, or surgical decompression of swollen nerve trunks).

Type 2: Occurs mainly in lepromatous patients and small numbers of borderline patients. Principal clinical features are fever and tender erythematous skin nodules, sometimes associated with malaise, neuritis, orchitis, albuminuria, joint swelling, iritis, epistaxis, or depression. Skin lesions can become pustular or ulcerate. If severe, patient is hospitalized. In general, antileprosy treatment is continued. Analgesics, steroids, and other agents (available from the USPHS) are used to suppress the reaction.

DRUG INTERACTIONS

Rifampin lowers dapsone levels by accelerating plasma clearance. **Para-aminobenzoic acid** may antagonize the effect of dapsone by interfering with the primary mechanism of action. **Activated charcoal** may decrease GI absorption and enterohepatic recycling of dapsone.

ADVERSE REACTIONS

Hematologic: Hemolysis of varying degrees is most common toxic effect, including hemolytic anemia (in patients with or without G6PD deficiency). Hemolysis develops in almost every person given 200 mg to 300 mg dapsone/day. Doses of 100 mg or less in healthy individuals or 50 mg in those with G6PD deficiency do not cause hemolysis. Almost all patients demonstrate the interrelated changes of a loss of 1 g to 2 g hemoglobin, an increase in reticulocytes, a shortened red cell life span, and a rise in methemoglobin. G6PD-deficient patients have greater responses. Hypoalbuminemia without proteinuria has been seen.

Dermatologic: Hyperpigmented macules, drug-induced lupus erythematosus, phototoxicity.

CNS: Peripheral neuropathy is an unusual complication in nonleprosy patients. Motor loss is predominant. If muscle weakness appears, withdraw drug. Recovery on withdrawal is usually substantially complete. This complication is not reported in leprosy. Other CNS reactions include headache, psychosis, insomnia, vertigo, and paresthesia.

GI: Nausea, vomiting, abdominal pain, anorexia.

Renal: Albuminuria, the nephrotic syndrome, renal papillary necrosis.

Other: Blurred vision, tinnitus, fever, male infertility.

OVERDOSAGE

Symptoms: Nausea, vomiting, and hyperexcitability can appear within a few minutes up to 24 hours after ingestion of an overdose. Methemoglobin-induced depression, convulsions, and severe cyanosis require prompt treatment. Headache, hemolysis, and permanent retinal damage have occurred.

Treatment: Empty the stomach by aspiration and lavage. In normal and methemoglobin reductase–deficient patients, methylene blue, 1 mg/kg to 2 mg/kg, given slowly IV, is treatment of choice. The effect is complete in 30 minutes but may be repeated if methemoglobin reaccumulates. For nonemergencies, if treatment is needed, methylene blue may be given orally in doses of 3 mg/kg to 5 mg/kg q4h to q6h. Methylene blue reduction depends on G6PD; do not give to fully expressed G6PD-deficient patients. Hemolysis may be treated by blood transfusions. Other supportive measures include oxygen and IV fluids to maintain renal flow.

DOSAGE

Dermatitis herpetiformis: Dosage is individualized. Start with 50 mg/day in adults and correspondingly smaller doses in children. If full control is not achieved within range of 50 mg/day to 300 mg/day, higher doses may be tried. Reduce dosage to minimum maintenance level as soon as possible. In responsive patients, there is a prompt reduction in pruritus followed by clearance of the lesions. There is no effect on the GI component of the disease.

Maintenance dosage can often be reduced (approximately 50%) after 6 months on a gluten-free diet.

Leprosy: It is recommended that therapy be commenced and maintained at full dosage without interruption.

Recommended dosage—6 mg/kg/week to 10 mg/kg/week. The schedule amounts to 50 mg/day to 100 mg/day in adults, with correspondingly smaller doses in children.

In bacteriologically negative tuberculoid and indeterminate type leprosy, an adult dosage of 50 mg/day is usually sufficient. After all signs of clinical activity are controlled, continue therapy a minimum of 3 years for tuberculoid and indeterminate patients.

In lepromatous and borderline patients, administration for at least 10 years after patient is bacteriologically negative is recommended. More than 5 years of continuous therapy is required to render most patients with lepromatous leprosy bacteriologically negative.

Secondary dapsone resistance is suspected whenever a lepromatous or borderline lepromatous patient receiving dapsone treatment relapses clinically and bacteriologically. If such cases show no response to regular and supervised dapsone therapy within 3 to 6 months, consider dapsone resistance and confirm clinically. Patient with proven dapsone resistance is treated with other drugs.

NURSING IMPLICATIONS

HISTORY
Record description and duration of symptoms; location of cutaneous lesions (if present); health history; allergy history; prescription, nonprescription drug history.

PHYSICAL ASSESSMENT
Examine and describe superficial lesions (if present). CBC, hepatic-function tests may be ordered.

ADMINISTRATION
Administer with food to prevent GI distress.

ONGOING ASSESSMENTS AND NURSING MANAGEMENT
A U.S. citizen found to have leprosy may be admitted to Carville Hospital (Baton Rouge, La.)

for treatment. All costs of hospitalization are paid for by the federal government.

Nursing management is focused on (1) psychological support, (2) control of acute infection, (3) prevention of deformities and other complications, (4) rehabilitation, (5) preparation for treatment on an outpatient basis, and (6) patient and family education.

Record vital signs daily. Observe for adverse reactions and evaluate patient's physical and emotional status.

CLINICAL ALERT: Inspect skin daily for rash or other dermatologic manifestations. Notify physician immediately if any dermatologic reactions are noted because drug may need to be discontinued immediately and appropriate therapy instituted.

Weekly blood counts are recommended for the first month of therapy. Notify physician immediately of any reduction in the leukocyte or platelet count or if any change in CBC values occurs, because therapy may need to be discontinued.

Weigh weekly or as ordered; notify physician if weight loss occurs.

If nausea, vomiting, or anorexia occurs, notify physician. Hepatic-function tests may be ordered to detect hepatic involvement.

Dermatitis herpetiformis: In responsive patients there is a prompt reduction in pruritus followed by a clearance of skin lesions. Inspect skin daily and record findings.

PATIENT AND FAMILY INFORMATION
May cause GI upset; take with food.

Notify physician immediately if any of the following occurs: rash or any dermatologic symptoms, nausea, vomiting, weight loss, loss of appetite.

Do not discontinue drug except on advice of physician.

Long-term follow-up care will be necessary.

Daunorubicin Hydrochloride

(DNR) Rx

powder for injection: Cerubidine
    20 mg

INDICATIONS
Remission induction in acute nonlymphocytic leukemia (myelogenous, monocytic, erythroid) in adults. Used as a single agent, it has produced com-

plete remission rates of 40% to 50%; in combination with cytarabine, it has produced complete remission rates of 53% to 65%.

ACTIONS
An anthracycline antibiotic produced by *Streptomyces coeruleorubidus.* It inhibits synthesis of nucleic acids; its effect on DNA is particularly rapid and marked. Has antimitotic and cytotoxic activity, although precise mechanism of activity is unknown. Following IV injection, plasma levels decline rapidly, indicating tissue uptake and concentration. Thereafter, plasma levels decline slowly, with a half-life of 18.5 hours. There is no evidence that drug crosses the blood–brain barrier.

WARNINGS
Bone marrow: Is a potent bone-marrow suppressant. Suppression will occur in all patients given a therapeutic dose. Therapy is not started in those with preexisting drug-induced bone-marrow depression unless benefit from such treatment warrants the risk.

Cardiac toxicity: Preexisting heart disease and previous therapy with doxorubicin are cofactors of increased risk of daunorubicin-induced cardiac toxicity. The benefit-to-risk ratio in such patients is weighed before therapy is started. At total cumulative doses exceeding 550 mg/m^2, there is an increased incidence of drug-induced congestive heart failure (CHF). There is no reliable method for predicting which patients will develop acute CHF; however, certain changes in the ECG and a decrease in the systolic ejection fraction from pretreatment baseline may aid in recognizing patients at greatest risk. Early clinical diagnosis of drug-induced CHF appears to be essential for successful treatment with digitalis, diuretics, sodium restriction, and bedrest.

Evaluation of hepatic and renal function: Significant hepatic or renal impairment can enhance toxicity.

Use in pregnancy: Due to its teratogenic potential, drug can cause fetal harm when administered to a pregnant woman. If drug is used during pregnancy or if patient becomes pregnant while taking drug, she should be apprised of the potential hazard to the fetus.

PRECAUTIONS
Therapy requires close patient observation and extensive chemical and laboratory monitoring. May induce hyperuricemia secondary to rapid lysis of leukemic cells. Serum uric acid levels should be monitored and therapy initiated if hyperuricemia

develops. Measures must be taken to control any systemic infection before beginning therapy. Drug may impart a red coloration to urine.

ADVERSE REACTIONS
Dose-limiting toxicity includes myelosuppression and cardiotoxicity (see *Warnings*); other reactions include the following.

Cutaneous: Reversible alopecia occurs in most patients.

GI: Acute nausea and vomiting occur; antiemetic therapy may be of some help. Mucositis may occur 3 to 7 days after administration. Diarrhea has occasionally been reported.

Local: Extravasation during administration may result in tissue necrosis.

Acute reactions: Fever, chills, skin rash occur rarely.

DOSAGE
To eradicate leukemic cells and induce complete remission, a profound suppression of bone marrow is usually required. Appropriate maintenance therapy should be instituted following successful induction of complete remission.

As a single agent: 60 mg/m^2/day IV on days 1, 2, and 3 every 3 to 4 weeks.

In combination: 45 mg/m^2/day IV on days 1, 2, and 3 of the first course and on days 1 and 2 of subsequent courses with 100 mg/m^2/day cytosine arabinoside by IV infusion daily for 7 days for the first course and for 5 days for subsequent courses.

Attainment of bone marrow that appears normal may require up to three courses of induction therapy. Evaluation of bone marrow following recovery from the previous course of induction therapy determines whether a further course of induction treatment is required. Dosage may be reduced in hepatic or renal impairment.

NURSING IMPLICATIONS

HISTORY
See Appendix 4.

PHYSICAL ASSESSMENT
Record general physical and emotional status; vital signs; weight. Baseline studies such as bone marrow and peripheral blood samples, serum uric acid, hepatic- and renal-function tests, ECG and/or determination of systolic ejection fraction are performed prior to therapy.

ADMINISTRATION
Daunorubicin must be given by IV route. It is *never* given subcutaneously or IM.

Do not administer mixed with other drugs or heparin.

Antiemetic may be ordered prior to administration of daunorubicin.

A Kold Kap or scalp tourniquet may be used to prevent alopecia. The cap or tourniquet is put into place just before administration of drug. The tourniquet is removed in approximately 15 minutes after injection of the drug; the Kold Kap may be left on for as long as 1 hour after drug is injected. Check with physician about length of time either is to remain in place after injection of the drug.

Vial contents are reconstituted with 4 ml of Sterile Water for Injection, USP, which will provide 5 mg/ml.

Withdraw desired dose into a syringe containing 10 ml to 15 ml of normal saline.

IV of 5% glucose or normal saline solution is started (physician will order type and amount of IV solution). Use a large vein; avoid small veins, such as on back of hand, unless absolutely necessary.

Drug is injected slowly, a few milliliters at a time, into injection port or sidearm of *rapidly flowing* IV infusion.

CLINICAL ALERT: Extravasation can cause severe tissue necrosis. Be sure needle is positioned correctly in vein before as well as during injection of drug. *Do not administer drug if there is any question regarding correct placement of the IV needle because extravasation may result in severe tissue necrosis.* If extravasation does occur, discontinue IV immediately.

Instruct patient to mention immediately if burning is felt at the injection site (may be sign of extravasation). Stop administration to see if burning persists. If burning persists, treat as extravasation.

After drug is injected, allow IV solution to continue to run through the line for 1 to 2 minutes; then discontinue IV infusion (unless physician orders otherwise).

Storage: The reconstituted solution is stable for 24 hours at room temperature and for 48 hours under refrigeration. Protect from exposure to sunlight.

ONGOING ASSESSMENTS AND NURSING MANAGEMENT

If extravasation of drug has occurred, follow procedure outlined by physician for treatment. Usually ice packs are applied immediately after needle is removed; area may also be treated with injections of a steroid. Any drug used to treat extravasation should be immediately available and the physician should write specific orders for administration of agents used to decrease tissue necrosis.

Antiemetic is usually ordered q4h prn for nausea and vomiting. If vomiting occurs, antiemetic should be administered by parenteral or rectal route.

Measure intake and output, starting measurements before drug is administered as well as for 48 or more hours after drug is administered. Notify physician if output decreases or vomiting exceeds 700 ml to 800 ml/8 hours.

Monitor vital signs q4h.

Leukocyte and platelet nadirs usually occur 10 to 14 days following administration. Peripheral blood samples are usually obtained frequently to monitor bone-marrow depression.

CLINICAL ALERT: Drug causes severe myelosuppression when used in therapeutic doses. Observe for signs of bone-marrow depression (Appendix 6, section 6-8). If signs of bone-marrow depression are apparent, notify physician immediately.

Observe for early signs of CHF (Appendix 6, section 6-9). If CHF is apparent, notify physician immediately, because early recognition and treatment are essential.

Mucositis (stomatitis) may occur 3 to 7 days after therapy. Patient may first complain of a burning sensation; the oral mucosa may appear inflamed. This is usually followed in several days by ulceration of the oral mucosa. Examine patient's mouth daily for erythema and small white ulcerations and notify physician immediately if these are apparent. Stomatitis care should be instituted immediately (Appendix 6, section 6-21).

Xylocaine Viscous 15 ml q3h to q4h prn may be prescribed for pain due to stomatitis. Instruct patient to swish solution around in mouth. Drug may be swallowed if pharynx is also sore. A topical local anesthetic ointment or spray may also be prescribed.

Drug may transiently impart a red color to urine.

Periodic laboratory tests are usually performed during therapy. Physician may order CBC, serum electrolytes, renal- and hepatic-function tests, serum uric acid. Bone-marrow aspirations and ECG may also be performed.

If hyperuricemia occurs, physician may order increase of fluid intake as well as drug therapy such as with allopurinol. Increased fluid intake may also begin immediately after nausea and vomiting has stopped as a prophylactic measure.

Protective (reverse) isolation may be necessary for severe myelosuppression.

PATIENT AND FAMILY INFORMATION

NOTE: Drug may be given on outpatient basis or patient may be discharged from hospital after completion of course of therapy. Before institution of therapy, patient should have full explanation of all possible adverse reactions, what can be done to control or alleviate these reactions, and what specific reactions should be reported immediately to the physician. Patient should be told that alopecia may occur and what can be done (*e.g.*, purchase of wig, wearing scarves or knit cap) until hair grows back. This information should be given by the physician or by the nurse with physician approval.

Take antiemetic (if prescribed) as directed. If antiemetic does not (partially) relieve nausea and vomiting, or if vomiting persists for more than 8 hours, notify physician.

Notify physician or nurse immediately if any of the following occurs: fever, chills, sore throat or other signs of infection, easy bruising or bleeding, petechiae, shortness of breath on exertion, difficulty breathing while lying down.

Drug may impart a red color to the urine; this is not abnormal.

Reversible alopecia will most likely occur. The onset may be sudden. Hair will grow back, but it may be a different color or texture.

Inform other physicians and dentist of therapy with this drug.

Decongestants, Nasal, Topical

Ephedrine otc

drops: 0.5%	Vatronol
drops: 1%	Ephedsol-1%
drops: 3%	*Generic*
jelly: 0.6%	Efedron Nasal

Epinephrine Hydrochloride otc

drops: 0.1%	Adrenalin Chloride

Naphazoline Hydrochloride otc

drops, spray: 0.05%	Privine

Oxymetazoline Hydrochloride otc

pediatric drops: 0.025%	Afrin Pediatric Nose Drops, Neo-Synephrine 12 Hour Children's Drops
spray: 0.05%	Afrin, Bayfrin, Dristan Long Lasting, Duramist Plus, Duration, Neo-Synephrine 12 Hour, Nostrilla, *Generic*
drops: 0.05%	Afrin, Duration, Neo-Synephrine 12 Hour
vapor spray, mentholated: 0.05%	Afrin, Dristan Long Lasting, Duration, Neo-Synephrine 12 Hour

Phenylephrine Hydrochloride otc

drops: 0.125%	Neo-Synephrine
drops: 0.16%	Alconefrin 12
drops: 0.2%	Rhinall-10, Vacon
drops: 0.25%	Alconefrin 25, doktors Nose Drops, Neo-Synephrine, Newphrine, Nōstril, Rhinall
spray: 0.25%	Alconefrin 25, Neo-Synephrine, Rhinall, Super Anahist, Vacon Nasal
drops: 0.5%	Alconefrin 50, Neo-Synephrine
spray: 0.5%	Allerest Nasal, Coricidin Nasal Mist, Duration Mild, Neo-Synephrine, Sinarest Nasal, Sinex
jelly: 0.5%	Neo-Synephrine
drops: 1%	Neo-Synephrine, Newphrine, Sinophen Intranasal

Tetrahydrozoline Hydrochloride Rx

spray, drops: 0.1%	Tyzine
drops, pediatric: 0.05%	Tyzine Pediatric Drops

Xylomethazoline Hydrochloride otc

drops, pediatric: 0.05%	Neo-Synephrine II Long Acting Children's Nose Drops, Otrivin Pediatric Nasal Drops
drops: 0.1%	Neo-Synephrine II Long Acting, Otrivin
spray: 0.1%	Chlorohist-LA, 4-Way Long Acting, Dristan Long Acting, Neo-Synephrine II Long Acting, Otrivin, Sinex Long Acting

INDICATIONS

Symptomatic relief of nasal and nasopharyngeal mucosal congestion due to common cold, sinusitis, hay fever, or other upper respiratory allergies.

May also be useful in the adjunctive therapy of middle ear infections by decreasing congestion around the eustachian ostia. Nasal inhalers may be useful for the relief of ear block and pressure pain in air travel.

CONTRAINDICATIONS

Monoamine oxidase (MAO) inhibitor therapy; hypersensitivity or idiosyncrasy to sympathomimetic amines, which may be manifested by insomnia, dizziness, weakness, tremor, or arrhythmias.

Although systemic effects are less likely from topical administration, these agents should be used with caution in severe hypertension and severe coronary artery disease. Contraindicated in nursing mothers because of the higher than usual risk to infants from sympathomimetic amines. Adverse reactions are more likely to occur with excessive use, and in the elderly and children.

ACTION

Decongestants are sympathomimetic amines that are administered directly to the swollen membrane (*e.g.,* by spray, drops) or systemically via the oral route.

These decongestants act principally through stimulation of the alpha-adrenergic receptors of vascular smooth muscle (vasoconstriction, pressor effects, nasal decongestion), although some retain beta-adrenergic properties (*e.g.,* ephedrine, pseudoephedrine). The alpha-adrenergic effects cause intense vasoconstriction when applied directly to mucous membranes. Constriction in the mucous membranes results in their shrinkage, promoting drainage and improving ventilation and the stuffy feeling.

WARNINGS

Administer with caution to patients with hypertension, hyperthyroidism, diabetes mellitus, cardiovascular disease, ischemic heart disease, angina, advanced arteriosclerotic conditions, increased intraocular pressure, or prostatic hypertrophy. Sympathomimetics may cause CNS stimulation and convulsions or cardiovascular collapse with accompanying hypotension.

Excessive use: Systemic effects from excessive use of topical decongestants may occur owing to GI absorption or rapid absorption through nasal mucous membranes. Such reactions are more likely to occur in infants and the elderly. Habituation and toxic psychosis have been reported following long-term high-dose therapy.

Rebound congestion: Recurrence or exacerbation of symptoms may occur after the vasoconstrictor action wears off. As a result, patients may increase the amount of drug used and frequency of administration, thereby producing overdosage and toxicity. Frequent and continued use of the topical agents may cause rebound congestion.

Use in the elderly: Patients 60 years and older are more likely to experience adverse reactions to sympathomimetics. Overdosage of sympathomimetics in this age group may cause hallucinations, convulsions, CNS depression, and death. Therefore, safe use of a short-acting sympathomimetic should be demonstrated in the elderly patient before considering the use of a sustained-action formulation.

Use in pregnancy: Safety for use during pregnancy has not been established.

PRECAUTIONS

Use topical decongestants only in acute states and not longer than 3 to 5 days. Use sparingly in all patients, particularly infants, children, and patients with cardiovascular disease.

Some hypersensitive individuals may experience a mild, transient stinging sensation after topical application. This often disappears after a few applications.

DRUG INTERACTIONS

Beta-adrenergic blocking agents and **MAO inhibitors** increase the effects of sympathomimetics. Severe hypertensive reactions may occur when sympathomimetics are given to patients receiving MAO inhibitors.

The antihypertensive effects of **methyldopa, mecamylamine,** and **reserpine,** may be reduced by sympathomimetics.

Isoproterenol and epinephrine should not be administered simultaneously because both drugs are direct cardiac stimulants; their combined effects may induce serious arrhythmia.

ADVERSE REACTIONS

CNS: Fear; anxiety; tenseness; restlessness; headache; lightheadedness; dizziness; drowsiness; tremor; insomnia; hallucinations; psychological disturbances; prolonged psychosis (paranoia, terror, delusions); convulsions; CNS depression.

Cardiovascular: Arrhythmias and cardiovascular collapse with hypotension. Palpitations, sweating, tachycardia, precordial pain, and cardiac arrhythmias have been reported with ephedrine.

Ocular: Blepharospasm (ocular irritation, tearing, photophobia).

Ephedrinelike reactions: Hyperreactive individuals may display ephedrinelike reactions such as palpitations, tachycardia, hypertension, headache, dizziness, or nausea.

GI: Nausea, vomiting, and anorexia (ephedrine).

GU: Vesical sphincter spasm and urinary retention in males with prostatism have been reported with ephedrine.

D

Miscellaneous: Weakness, pallor, respiratory difficulty, orofacial dystonia, dysuria.

Topical use: Burning, stinging, sneezing, dryness, contact dermatitis (ephedrine).

OVERDOSAGE

Symptoms: Depending on the severity of overdosage, somnolence, sedation, or deep coma may occur. Overdosage may produce profound CNS depression and sedation in children, possibly requiring intensive supportive treatment. Sedation may be accompanied by profuse sweating. With marked overdosage, CNS depression is accompanied by hypertension, bradycardia, and decreased cardiac output, which may be followed by rebound hypotension and cardiovascular collapse. Respiration is centrally depressed in severe cases.

Treatment: Because these preparations are rapidly absorbed, evacuation of gastric contents following oral ingestion is useful if done very early. Intensive supportive care is required to sustain respiratory and cardiovascular function, especially following marked overdosage.

DOSAGE

EPHEDRINE

Adults, children 6 and over: 2 to 3 drops or small amount of jelly in each nostril q3h to q4h. Do not use for more than 3 or 4 consecutive days. Not used in children under 6 unless directed by physician.

EPINEPHRINE HCl

Adults, children 6 and over: 1 to 2 drops in each nostril q4h to q6h.

NAPHAZOLINE HCl

Adults, children 6 and over: 2 drops in each nostril as needed, no more often than q3h. Not used in children under 6 unless directed by physician.

OXYMETHAZOLINE HCl

Adults, children 6 and over: 2 or 3 drops or sprays of 0.05% solution in each nostril bid, morning and evening.

Children 2 to 6: 2 or 3 drops of 0.025% solution in each nostril bid, morning and evening.

PHENYLEPHRINE HCl

Adults: 0.25% to 0.5% in each nostril q3h to q4h.

Children over 6: 0.25% in each nostril q3h to q4h.

Infants: 0.125% to 0.2% in each nostril q2h to q4h.

TETRAHYDROZOLINE HCl

Adults and children over 6: 2 to 4 drops of 0.1% solution in each nostril as needed, no more often than q3h.

Children 2 to 6: 2 to 3 drops of 0.05% solution in each nostril as needed, no more often than q3h.

XYLOMETAZOLINE HCl

Adults: 2 or 3 drops or sprays of 0.1% solution in each nostril q8h to q10h.

Children under 12: 2 or 3 drops or sprays of 0.05% solution in each nostril q8h to q10h.

NURSING IMPLICATIONS

HISTORY
See Appendix 4.

PHYSICAL ASSESSMENT
Use nasal speculum to inspect nares. Note type of secretions (*e.g.,* clear and watery, profuse, purulent, blood tinged).

ONGOING ASSESSMENTS AND NURSING MANAGEMENT
Note results of use. Notify physician if condition is not improved, if patient resists instillation of drug, if appearance of drainage changes, or if side-effects occur.

Observe for symptoms of overdosage in children and the elderly.

PATIENT AND FAMILY INFORMATION
Notify physician or nurse if insomnia, dizziness, weakness, tremor, or irregular heartbeat occurs.

Do not exceed recommended dosage.

Because rebound congestion may occur, do not use longer than 3 to 5 days unless directed otherwise by physician.

Stinging, burning, or drying of the nasal mucosa may occur.

To help prevent contamination from nasal secretions, rinse dropper or spray tip in hot water after each use.

Deferoxamine Mesylate Rx

powder for injection: Desferal Mesylate
500 mg/vial

INDICATIONS

Acute iron intoxication: As adjunct to standard treatment measures such as induction of emesis, gastric lavage, maintenance of clear airway, control of shock, correction of acidosis.

Chronic iron overload: Promotes iron excretion

in patients who have secondary iron overload from multiple transfusions. Slows accumulation of hepatic iron and retards or eliminates progression of hepatic fibrosis. Not indicated for treatment of primary hemochromatosis.

CONTRAINDICATIONS

Severe renal disease or anuria.

ACTIONS

Chelates iron and therefore prevents iron from entering into chemical reactions. Is metabolized by plasma enzymes and excreted in urine. Some is excreted in the feces via bile.

WARNINGS

Rarely, cataracts have been observed in those treated for prolonged periods. Not administered to women of childbearing potential (particularly during pregnancy) unless clearly needed.

ADVERSE REACTIONS

Occasionally, pain and induration at injection site. Side-effects reported in acute therapy of iron intoxication include generalized erythema, urticaria, and hypotension, which have occurred with rapid IV injection. Adverse effects in long-term therapy include allergic-type reactions (cutaneous wheal formation, generalized itching, rash, anaphylactic reaction), blurring of vision, dysuria, abdominal discomfort, diarrhea, leg cramps, tachycardia, and fever. Effects reported with subcutaneous therapy include localized pain, pruritus, erythema, skin irritation, and swelling. These might also occur in patients treated for acute intoxication.

DOSAGE

May be administered IM, by continuous subcutaneous mini-infusion, or by slow IV infusion. Net iron excretion with subcutaneous use is greater than with equal doses given IM because the labile (chelatable) intracellular iron pool is constantly exposed to the drug.

Acute iron intoxication

IM: Initially, 1 g, followed by 0.5 g q4h for 2 doses. Depending on response, give subsequent doses of 0.5 g q4h to q12h, not to exceed 6 g daily.

IV: Dosage same as for IM use, given at rate not to exceed 15 mg/kg/hour. As soon as clinical condition permits, discontinue IV and administer drug IM.

Chronic iron overload

Administration is individualized.

IM: 0.5 g to 1 g daily. Give 2 g IV with, but separately from, each unit of blood. Rate of infusion must not exceed 15 mg/kg/hour.

Subcutaneous: 1 g to 2 g (20 mg/kg/day to 40 mg/kg/day) administered daily over 8 to 24 hours using a continuous mini-infusion pump. In some, iron excretion will be as great after a short infusion of 8 to 12 hours as it is if the same dose is given over 24 hours.

Children: 50 mg/kg/dose IM or IV q6h or up to 15 mg/kg/hr by continuous IV infusion, to maximum of 6 g/24 hour: or 2 g/dose.

NURSING IMPLICATIONS

HISTORY

Acute iron intoxication (history obtained from family, others): Amount and name of substance ingested (*e.g.,* iron tablets, capsules, suspension; preparations such as multivitamins containing iron); time product was ingested; general health history (especially history of renal disease).

Chronic iron overload: Review chart for general information (*e.g.,* diagnosis, number of transfusions, other treatment modalities, laboratory studies).

PHYSICAL ASSESSMENT

Acute iron intoxication: Clinical effects begin in 30 minutes to 2 hours and include lethargy, restlessness, bloody diarrhea, hematemesis, and abdominal pain. These may be followed by period of apparent recovery and then shock, cyanosis, fever, and respiratory acidosis develop. Several days later, hepatic necrosis may be seen. Record vital signs; perform general assessment and record symptoms; obtain weight.

Chronic iron overload: Obtain vital signs, weight; record symptoms. Renal-function tests may be performed before administration.

ADMINISTRATION

Reconstitute each vial with 2 ml Sterile Water for Injection. IV infusion or IM administration is used for acute iron intoxication. IM or subcutaneous route is used for chronic iron intoxication; may be given IV when blood is administered.

When given at same time as blood transfusion, do not add to blood container; give separately. Rate of infusion must not exceed 15 mg/kg/hour.

For IV use add to saline, glucose in water, or Ringer's solution (physician orders amount and type of solution). This route is used only for patients in cardiovascular collapse. Administer slowly.

If vein is not obtainable from IV administration, a cutdown may be performed by physician.

Subcutaneous: Use mini-infusion pump. Physician will designate site for injection and rate of infusion. Infusion time varies from 8 to 24 hours.

IM: Administer deep IM in gluteus muscle unless physician orders otherwise. This is the preferred route and should be used for all patients not in shock.

Storage: Store solutions reconstituted with sterile water for no longer than 1 week. Protect from light.

ONGOING ASSESSMENTS AND NURSING MANAGEMENT

Monitor vital signs q1h to q4h (depending on patient's condition); measure intake and output.

As iron is chelated and passes through the kidneys, it will impart a reddish color to urine.

Laboratory monitoring of therapy (serum iron) is usually performed at frequent intervals.

Cardiovascular collapse may be treated with additional drugs such as vasopressors, IV fluids, and oxygen.

Keep physician informed of any change in patient's general condition, vital signs, urinary output. Observe for adverse reactions; report allergic-type reactions immediately.

Inspect injection sites daily. If pain is reported or induration is noted, contact physician.

Patients treated for chronic iron overload: Periodic slit-lamp examinations may be performed to detect ophthalmologic effects of drug.

Dehydrocholic Acid otc

tablets: 244 mg	Hepahydrin, *Generic*
tablets: 250 mg	Cholan-DH, Decholin, Neocholan (contains tartrazine)

INDICATIONS

Temporary relief of constipation. As adjunct in clinical conditions involving the biliary tract, including recent surgery of the biliary tract, repeated surgery for biliary calculi or strictures, noncalculous cholecystitis, ascending cholangitis, recurring noncalculous cholangitis, biliary dyskinesia, chronic partial obstruction of common bile duct, prolonged drainage from biliary fistulas or T-tube drainage of an infected common bile duct, sclerosing choledochitis.

CONTRAINDICATIONS

Cholelithiasis; jaundice; marked hepatic insufficiency (severe hepatitis, suppurative cholangitis, advanced cirrhosis); partial or complete obstruction of the common or hepatic bile ducts (with or without jaundice) or of the GI or GU tracts due to any cause. Not used as a diuretic or as an adjunct to diuretics. Do not use when abdominal pain, nausea, or vomiting is present.

ACTIONS

Is a derivative of cholic acid and is a hydrocholeretic agent. Has no effect on production of bile salts. Administration leads to an increase in the amount of high-water-content, low-viscosity bile produced.

Is less effective than natural bile salts in lowering surface tension and in causing emulsification. Also less effective than bile salts in promoting absorption.

PRECAUTIONS

Increases bile volume and flow by hydrocholeretic action. There is no evidence that these products improve liver function or accelerate the rate of clearance of jaundice. Use cautiously in those with prostatic hypertrophy, acute hepatitis, or acute yellow atrophy of the liver. Use cautiously in children under 6, elderly patients, or those with partial GI or GU tract obstructions.

Tartrazine sensitivity: See Appendix 6, section 6-23.

OVERDOSAGE

Principal symptom is diarrhea associated with weakness. There is no specific antidote. Gastric lavage may be indicated, but treatment is directed principally toward relief of diarrhea. Laxatives and other hydrocholeretics may potentiate diarrhea produced by an overdose. Treatment consists of replenishment of fluid and electrolyte losses.

DOSAGE

Usual dose is 244 mg to 500 mg tid after meals. Simultaneous administration of bile salts may be indicated in order to ensure adequate digestion and absorption of nutrients in the presence of biliary fistula or other condition in which bile is draining away from the intestinal tract and during prolonged administration.

NURSING IMPLICATIONS

HISTORY

Obtain history of constipation including possible causes (*e.g.,* diet, lack of exercise, decreased fluid intake).

NOTE: Bowel changes may also be indicative of lower GI malignancy.

ADMINISTRATION
Give after meals. Bile salts may also be ordered.

ONGOING ASSESSMENTS AND NURSING MANAGEMENT
If constipation is not relieved, inform physician.

Other methods of relieving constipation such as increased fluid intake, exercise, and inclusion of roughage in diet may also be employed.

PATIENT AND FAMILY INFORMATION
Frequent use may result in laxative dependence.

Increasing fluid intake, eating fresh and cooked fruit and vegetables and whole-grain cereals and bread, and drinking prune juice may be of value in relieving constipation.

If problem is not relieved, see a physician.

Demecarium Bromide

See Miotics, Cholinesterase Inhibitors.

Demeclocycline Hydrochloride

See Tetracyclines, Oral.

Deserpidine

See Rauwolfia Derivatives.

Desipramine Hydrochloride

See Antidepressants, Tricyclic Compounds.

Deslanoside

See Cardiac Glycosides.

Desmopressin Acetate Rx

nasal solution: 0.1 mg/ml   DDAVP

INDICATIONS
Antidiuretic replacement therapy in management of cranial diabetes insipidus, for temporary polyuria and polydipsia associated with trauma to, or surgery in, the pituitary region. Ineffective for treatment of nephrogenic diabetes insipidus.

CONTRAINDICATIONS
Hypersensitivity.

ACTIONS
A synthetic analog of arginine vasopressin, the naturally occurring human antidiuretic hormone (ADH). Provides prompt onset of antidiuretic action with a long duration. Antidiuretic action is more specific and more prolonged than that of the natural hormone or lypressin. A single dose produces an antidiuretic effect that persists for 8 to 20 hours. Urine volume is reduced and urine osmolarity increased. Vasopressor and oxytocic activity are not noted at normal therapeutic dosages. Has been used successfully in patients with long-standing central diabetes insipidus when other antidiuretic agents were ineffective or not tolerated. Also has been used as a diagnostic agent to evaluate renal concentrating ability.

WARNINGS
For intranasal use only.

PRECAUTIONS
At high dosage has infrequently produced a slight elevation in blood pressure, which disappeared with reduction in dosage. Use with caution in those with coronary artery insufficiency or hypertensive cardiovascular disease.

DRUG INTERACTIONS
Other drugs that are known to potentiate endogenous ADH, such as **chlorpropamide, clofibrate** and **carbamazepine,** may potentiate the antidiuretic effects of desmopressin.

ADVERSE REACTIONS
Infrequent: High dosages have produced transient headache, nausea, and slight elevation of blood pressure.

Occasional: Nasal congestion, rhinitis, flushing, mild abdominal cramps, vulval pain. These symptoms disappear with dosage reduction.

OVERDOSAGE
In case of overdosage, frequency of administration is reduced or drug is withdrawn, according to severity of the condition. There is no known specific antidote. If considerable fluid retention causes concern, a saluretic such as furosemide may induce diuresis.

DOSAGE
Adults: Usual dosage range is 0.1 ml/day to 0.4 ml/day, either as single dose or divided into two or three doses. Most adults require 0.2 ml/day in two

divided doses. Morning and evening doses are adjusted separately for an adequate diurnal rhythm of water turnover.

Children (3 months to 12 years): Usual dosage range is 0.05 ml/day to 0.3 ml/day, either as a single dose or divided into two doses.

About one-fourth to one-third of cases can be controlled by a single daily dose.

NURSING IMPLICATIONS

HISTORY
See Appendix 4.

PHYSICAL ASSESSMENT
Review recent intake and output and ratio of output to intake; check for signs of dehydration; obtain vital signs, weight.

ADMINISTRATION
Medication is self-administered when patient is alert, cooperative, and old enough to understand administration. Patient will need instructions for filling the plastic tube and administering solution intranasally.

Desmopressin is supplied as a solution in 2.5-ml vials. A measured quantity of solution is drawn into a flexible calibrated plastic tube supplied with the product.

The calibrations on the applicator tube measure 0.2 ml, 0.15 ml, 0.1 ml, and 0.05 ml. Physician may order drug in milligrams or milliliters (1 ml = 0.1 mg). Usual (adult) dose is 0.1 ml/day to 0.4 ml/day, which is 0.01 mg/day to 0.04 mg/day. If written order is unclear, request clarification.

One end of the tube is inserted into the nose, and the patient blows on the other end to deposit the solution deep into the nasal cavity, where it is absorbed through the nasal mucosa.

Drug may be administered to infants, young children, or obtunded patients by using an air-filled syringe attached to the plastic tube.

Rinse plastic administration tube thoroughly under warm water.

Storage: Keep refrigerated at about 4°C.

ONGOING ASSESSMENTS AND NURSING MANAGEMENT
Obtain vital signs q4h or as ordered; monitor weight; measure intake and output; observe for adverse effects and signs of water retention (weight gain, edema), and notify physician if water retention is apparent.

Total of intake and output may be every 8 hours but physician may also order measurement of each voided sample as well as time of voiding during adjustment period. Use separate flow sheet to record time and amount of each voiding. Determination of specific gravity of each sample may also be ordered.

Dosage must be determined for each patient and is adjusted according to the diurnal (daytime) pattern of response. Accurate measurement of intake and output is important in determining individualized dosage.

Objective of therapy is to provide adequate duration of sleep (*i.e.,* without nocturia) and adequate, not excessive, water turnover.

Morning and evening doses are adjusted separately, so that urinary output is similar to that of normal diurnal pattern.

Physician may place limit on water intake, especially in the elderly or very young patient, to decrease potential occurrence of water intoxication (Appendix 6, section 6-12) and hyponatremia (Appendix 6, section 6-17). Plan fluid intake at intervals spaced throughout waking hours; explain importance of spacing fluid intake to patient.

Periodic laboratory determinations of electrolytes may be ordered.

Although manufacturer states that patients with nasal congestion and blockage respond well to drug, patient should be observed for a marked increase in urinary output, which may indicate drug is not being effectively absorbed by the nasal mucosa.

PATIENT AND FAMILY INFORMATION
NOTE: Administration technique must be explained to patient. A return demonstration of measuring and administering the drug assures proper self-administration.

Do not increase or decrease the dose or frequency unless directed by physician.

Notify physician or nurse if drowsiness, listlessness, headache, shortness of breath, heartburn, nausea, abdominal cramps, vulval pain, or severe nasal congestion or irritation occurs.

Desonide

See Corticosteroids, Topical.

Desoximetasone

See Corticosteroids, Topical.

Desoxycorticosterone Preparations

Desoxycorticosterone Acetate Rx

injection: 5 mg/ml   Doca Acetate
pellets: 125 mg   Percorten Acetate

Desoxycorticosterone Pivalate Rx

respository injection: Percorten Pivalate
   25 mg/ml

INDICATIONS

Partial replacement therapy for primary and secondary adrenocortical insufficiency in Addison's disease and treatment of salt-losing adrenogenital syndrome.

CONTRAINDICATIONS

Hypersensitivity; hypertension; congestive heart failure; cardiac disease.

ACTIONS

Has potent mineralocorticoid activity and is devoid of glucocorticoid effects. Single doses enhance sodium reabsorption and potassium excretion. After several days of administration, intact or adrenalectomized subjects may "escape" from the sodium-retaining action and come into sodium balance. However, potassium continues to be excreted despite developing hypokalemia.

Desoxycorticosterone acetate (DOCA) is available only in parenteral form and is used primarily in those unable to take oral medication.

WARNINGS

Mineralocorticoids should be accompanied by adequate glucocorticoid therapy. Safety for use in pregnancy is not established. Use only when clearly needed and when potential benefits outweigh the unknown potential hazards to the fetus. If necessary to give steroids during pregnancy, watch newborn infant closely for signs of hypoadrenalism and institute appropriate therapy if such signs are apparent.

PRECAUTIONS

Those with Addison's disease are more sensitive to the action of the hormone and may exhibit side-effects in an exaggerated degree. Patients should be closely monitored and treatment stopped if a significant increase in weight or blood pressure, edema, or cardiac enlargement occurs.

Sodium retention and loss of potassium are accelerated by a high intake of sodium. If edema occurs, dietary sodium restriction may be required. Glucose tolerance tests (particularly IV) should be performed only if absolutely necessary, as addisonian patients, with or without desoxycorticosterone therapy, have a tendency to react with severe hypoglycemia within 3 hours.

Patients should be watched for evidence of infection; should this occur, appropriate therapy is instituted.

Mineralocorticoid therapy may not be necessary if patient's disease can be controlled with an adequate salt intake and glucocorticoid therapy.

ADVERSE REACTIONS

Severe side-effects may occur if dosage is too high or prolonged.

Cardiac: Increased blood volume; edema; hypertension; cardiac arrhythmias and enlargement of cardiac shadow, especially if hypertension was present before onset of adrenal insufficiency. In those with essential hypertension or a tendency toward its development, a marked rise in blood pressure may follow use of this drug.

CNS: Frontal or occipital headaches.

Musculoskeletal: Arthralgia and tendon contractures; extreme weakness of extremities with ascending paralysis secondary to low serum potassium.

Other: Hypersensitivity reactions. Rarely, irritation at site of injection or pellet implantation.

DOSAGE

Mineralocorticoid therapy must be accompanied by adequate amounts of glucocorticoid; usual dose of glucocorticoid is 10 mg to 30 mg hydrocortisone or 10 mg to 37.5 mg cortisone/day.

DESOXYCORTICOSTERONE ACETATE

Injection: Average maintenance dose is 2 mg/day to 5 mg/day IM.

Pellets: Implant only after optimal daily maintenance dose is determined. Pellets are surgically implanted into subcutaneous tissue, most commonly in the infrascapular region. Several weeks are required to determine the ultimate optimal maintenance dose. Patient is usually maintained on injection therapy for at least 2 to 3 months prior to pellet implantation to eliminate possibility of overdosage. On the average, pellets last for 8 to 12 months. In case of infection, disease, or other stress, supplementary desoxycorticosterone may be necessary.

DESOXYCORTICOSTERONE PIVALATE

Repository injection: Average dose is 25 mg to 100 mg IM every 4 weeks. Not administered more frequently than once a month.

▌NURSING IMPLICATIONS

▌HISTORY
See Appendix 4.

List symptoms of disorder.

ADMINISTRATION
A 19-gauge needle may be used to withdraw drug from vial; use a 20- or 21-gauge needle for administration.

Give deep IM into upper outer quadrant of gluteal region. Avoid use of the deltoid muscle.

ONGOING ASSESSMENTS AND NURSING MANAGEMENT
Addison's disease: Record vital signs q4h or as ordered; monitor weight; monitor closely for appearance of adverse reactions because these patients are more susceptible to action of hormone; check extremities for edema; record intake and output; observe for signs of hypokalemia (Appendix 6, section 6-15) and hypernatremia (Appendix 6, section 6-17).

Patient may require dietary restriction of sodium.

Salt-losing adrenogenital syndrome: Record vital signs q2h to q4h or as ordered; monitor weight; record number and type of stools; assess for signs of dehydration (Appendix 6, section 6-10), hyponatremia (Appendix 6, section 6-17), hyperkalemia (Appendix 6, section 6-15), signs of adrenal crisis (Appendix 6, section 6-3).

Infants with salt-losing adrenogenital syndrome may require IV sodium chloride and dextrose until condition is stabilized.

General considerations: Develop a daily plan of care based on patient's symptoms. Those with extreme weakness or fatigue may require assistance with activities of daily living.

Observe for evidence of infection (*e.g.*, fever, chills, sore throat, abscess formation) and notify physician.

Dosage is individualized according to severity of disease and response of patient. Accurate documentation of assessments is essential.

Patient may be receiving a glucocorticoid concomitantly.

CLINICAL ALERT: Adrenal cortical steroids (desoxycorticosterone, a mineralocorticoid, and glucocorticoids) are essential to life. Ensure continuity of prescribed therapy by notation on Kardex, informing health-team members responsible for drug administration.

Monitor electrolyte studies. Notify physician if most recent studies are abnormal.

If drug is given during pregnancy, newborn infant is watched closely for signs of hypoadrenalism (Appendix 6, section 6-3).

Pellets (implanted surgically): Check incision for signs of infection, wound separation, delayed healing; observe for signs of overdosage (*e.g.*, edema, excessive weight gain, rise in blood pressure).

The effect of implanted pellets fades after approximately 8 to 12 months. A gradual decrease in blood pressure and weight, increased fatigue, and anorexia are usually the first indications of a decrease in hormonal supply.

Infection, disease, or other stress may require supplementary injections of DOCA until patient has returned to condition established when pellets were implanted.

PATIENT AND FAMILY INFORMATION
Keep all physician or clinic appointments because close supervision is imperative.

If placed on a sodium-restricted diet, do not use a salt substitute except on physician's approval of a specific brand.

Contact physician if stress, excessive exercise, infection or exposure to infection, increased fatigue, weight loss, or anorexia occurs.

NOTE: Physician may also approve of including signs of electrolyte imbalance in teaching plan.

Dexamethasone Preparations

See Corticosteroids, Intranasal; Corticosteroids, Ophthalmic; Corticosteroids, Topical; Corticosteroid Respiratory Inhalants; Glucocorticoids.

Dexchlorpheniramine Maleate

See Antihistamines.

Dexpanthenol Preparations

Dexpanthenol (Dextro Pantothenyl Alcohol) Rx

injection: 250 mg/ml   Ilopan, Panol, *Generic*

Dexpanthenol With Choline Bitartrate Rx

tablets: 50 mg with   Ilopan-Choline
25 mg choline bi-
tartrate

INDICATIONS
DEXPANTHENOL
Prophylactic use immediately after major abdominal surgery to minimize possibility of adynamic (paralytic) ileus; intestinal atony causing abdominal

distention; postoperative or postpartum retention of flatus or postoperative delay in resumption of intestinal motility; adynamic ileus.

DEXPANTHENOL WITH CHOLINE BITARTRATE

Relief of gas retention associated with splenic flexure syndrome, cholecystitis, gastritis, gastric hyperacidity, irritable colon, regional ileitis, postantibiotic and postoperative gas retention, or during laxative withdrawal.

CONTRAINDICATIONS

Hemophilia.

ACTIONS

Pantothenic acid is a precursor of coenzyme A, which serves as a cofactor for a variety of enzyme-catalyzed reactions involving transfer of acetyl groups. The final step in synthesis of acetylcholine is the choline acetylase transfer of an acetyl group form acetylcoenzyme A to choline. Acetylcholine is the neurohormonal transmitter in the parasympathetic nervous system and maintains normal functions of the intestine. Decrease in acetylcholine content would result in decreased peristalsis and, in extreme cases, adynamic ileus. The pharmacologic mode of action is unknown.

Choline: In addition to being a precursor for acetylcholine, choline is essential for normal transport of fat, as a constituent of the phospholipid lecithin. It can also serve as a methyl donor in intermediary metabolism. Choline has same pharmacologic actions as acetylcholine but is much less active.

WARNINGS

Do not administer within 1 hour of succinylcholine. Safety for use in pregnancy is not established. Use only when clearly needed and potential benefits outweigh the unknown potential hazards to the fetus. It is not known if drug is excreted in breast milk. Exercise caution when administering to nursing women. Safety and effectiveness in children not established.

PRECAUTIONS

If signs of hypersensitivity appear, discontinue drug. If ileus is a secondary consequence of mechanical obstruction, primary attention should be directed toward the obstruction.

DRUG INTERACTIONS

There have been rare instances of allergic reaction of unknown cause during use of this drug with other drugs such as **antibiotics, narcotics,** and **barbiturates.** Temporary respiratory difficulty was experienced following administration 5 minutes after **suc-cinylcholine** was discontinued; the effects of succinylcholine appeared to have been prolonged.

ADVERSE REACTIONS

The following have been reported and the causal relationship is uncertain: itching, tingling, difficulty in breathing, red patches of skin, generalized dermatitis, urticaria, slight drop in blood pressure, intestinal colic, vomiting, and diarrhea.

DOSAGE
DEXPANTHENOL

Prevention of postoperative adynamic ileus: 250 mg or 500 mg IM. Repeat in 2 hours, followed by doses q6h, or until all danger of adynamic ileus has passed.

Treatment of adynamic ileus: 500 mg IM. Repeat in 2 hours, followed by doses q6h as needed.

IV: 500 mg by IV infusion.

DEXPANTHENOL WITH CHOLINE BITARTRATE

2 to 3 tablets tid.

NURSING IMPLICATIONS

HISTORY

See Appendix 4.

PHYSICAL ASSESSMENT
DEXPANTHENOL

Monitor vital signs; palpate abdomen (rigid, soft, distented, tender); auscultate abdomen, note bowel sounds (present or absent, frequency/minute, pitch) and record description; measure abdominal girth with tape measure if distention is noted.

DEXPANTHENOL WITH CHOLINE TARTRATE

Palpate abdomen; auscultate abdomen and note bowel sounds.

ADMINISTRATION

Do not administer dexpanthenol directly into a vein.

IV administration: May be added to IV solutions such as glucose or Lactated Ringer's and infused slowly. Physician orders rate of infusion.

Storage: Protect from freezing, excessive heat.

ONGOING ASSESSMENTS AND NURSING MANAGEMENT

Adynamic (paralytic) ileus: Assess q1h to q2h; auscultate abdomen for bowel sounds and compare with baseline data; measure abdominal girth; note if flatus or stool is being passed; palpate abdomen and compare with baseline data;

measure intake and output; keep physician informed of observations.

If condition persists physician may order rectal tube, nasogastric decompression, other treatment modalities.

Prevention of adynamic ileus: Observe for development of adynamic ileus (*e.g.,* colicky abdominal pain, nausea, vomiting, abdominal distention, abnormal or absent bowel sounds).

Gas retention (treated with dexpanthenol with choline bitartrate): Assess daily for relief of symptoms; notify physician if symptoms persist.

PATIENT AND FAMILY INFORMATION (DEXPANTHENOL WITH CHOLINE TARTRATE)

Take as directed. Notify physician if symptoms persist.

Dextran, Low Molecular Weight

(Dextran 40) Rx

injection: 10% dextran 40 in 0.9% sodium chloride or 5% dextrose	Gentran 40, 10% LMD, Rheomacrodex, *Generic*

INDICATIONS

Adjunctive treatment of shock or impending shock due to hemorrhage, burns, surgery, or other trauma. Does not replace other forms of therapy known to be of value in treatment of shock.

Also used for use as priming fluid, either as sole primer or as an additive in pump oxygenators during extracorporeal circulation. Also used in prophylaxis therapy against venous thrombosis and pulmonary embolism (PE) in patients undergoing procedures known to be associated with a high incidence of thromboembolic complications, such as hip surgery.

CONTRAINDICATIONS

Known hypersensitivity; marked hemostatic defects of all types (*e.g.,* thrombocytopenia, hypofibrinogenemia), including those caused by drugs (*e.g.,* heparin, warfarin); marked cardiac decompensation; renal disease with severe oliguria or anuria.

ACTIONS

Has an average molecular weight of 40,000 (range 10,000 to 80,000). Approximately 50% administered to normovolemic subject is excreted in urine within 3 hours, 60% within 6 hours, and 75% within 24 hours. The remaining 25% is partly hydrolyzed and excreted in the urine, partly excreted in the feces, and partly oxidized. Dextran 40 10% solution is osmotically equivalent to approximately two times the volume of plasma.

Shock: Enhances blood flow, particularly in the microcirculation, by increasing blood volume, venous return, and cardiac output; decreasing blood viscosity and peripheral vascular resistance; reducing aggregation of erythrocytes and other cellular elements by coating them and maintaining their electronegative charges. Administration usually increases blood volume, arterial blood pressure, capillary perfusion, venous return, central venous pressure, and urinary output.

Extracorporeal circulation: As priming solution has advantages over homologous blood and other priming solutions. Advantages are decreased destruction of erythrocytes and platelets; reduced intravascular hemagglutination; maintenance of electronegativity of erythrocytes and platelets; reduced dangers attendant on use of homologous blood (*i.e.,* serum hepatitis, transfusion reactions).

Prophylaxis against venous thrombosis, thromboembolism: Reduces incidence of deep venous thrombosis (DVT) and PE. Acts by simultaneously inhibiting other mechanisms essential to thrombus formation, such as vascular stasis and platelet adhesiveness, and by altering the structure and thereby the lysability of fibrin clots.

WARNINGS

Infrequently, severe and fatal anaphylactoid reactions reported. Symptoms are marked hypotension and/or cardiac and respiratory arrest. Most occurred early in the infusion period, in those not previously exposed to IV dextran.

Product is a colloid hypertonic solution and will attract water from the extravascular space. This fluid shift is considered when drug is used for poorly hydrated patients where additional fluid therapy will be needed.

In patients with diminished urine flow, urine viscosity and specific gravity can be markedly increased.

Renal failure, sometimes irreversible, has been reported. Occasional abnormal renal- and hepatic-function values have been reported.

Caution is used when drug is given to patients with active hemorrhage because resulting increase in perfusion pressure and improved microcirculatory flow may result in additional blood loss.

Recommended doses should not be exceeded because a dose-related increase in the incidence of wound hematoma, wound seroma, wound bleeding, distant bleeding (hematuria, melena), and pulmonary edema have been reported. Recommended doses should never be exceeded in patients with advanced renal disease because excessive doses may precipitate renal failure.

Dextran may interfere to some extent with platelet function; use with caution in cases of thrombocytopenia. Transient prolongation of bleeding time and/or slightly increased bleeding tendency may occur with administration of doses greater than 1000 ml. Solutions containing sodium ions are used with care, if at all, in patients with congestive heart failure (CHF), severe renal insufficiency, and clinical states in which there exists edema with sodium retention.

Administration can cause fluid and/or solute overloading, resulting in dilution of serum electrolyte concentrations, overhydration, congested states, or pulmonary edema.

Safety for use in pregnancy not established. Use only when clearly needed and when potential benefits outweigh the unknown potential hazards to the fetus.

PRECAUTIONS

In individuals with normal hemostasis, dosages up to 15 ml/kg may prolong bleeding time and depress platelet function. Some of the changes induced by dextran may be reversed by infusion of factor VIII concentrate.

When the risk of pulmonary edema or CHF may be increased, dextran is used with caution.

DRUG INTERACTIONS

Drug/lab tests: Falsely elevated **glucose assays** may be reported. In other laboratory tests, presence of dextran may result in development of turbidity, which can interfere with the assay. This has been observed in some bilirubin assays, some **total protein** assays, and some **blood glucose** determinations (depending on laboratory methods used). **Blood typing** and **cross-matching** procedures employing enzyme techniques may give unreliable readings if samples are taken after infusion.

ADVERSE REACTIONS

Hypersensitivity reactions have been reported. Reactions that may occur because of the solution or technique of administration include febrile response, infection at site of injection, extravasation, and hypervolemia.

DOSAGE

Adjunctive therapy in shock: Total dosage during first 24 hours should not exceed 20 ml/kg. The first 10 ml/kg is infused rapidly while remaining dose is given slowly. Should therapy continue beyond 24 hours, total daily dosage should not exceed 10 ml/kg and therapy should not continue beyond 5 days.

Hemodiluent in extracorporeal circulation: Dosage varies. Generally, 10 ml/kg to 20 ml/kg is added.

Prophylactic therapy of venous thrombosis, thromboembolism: Treatment usually initiated during surgery—500 ml to 1000 ml (approximately 10 ml/kg) on day of surgery. Treatment continued at dose of 500 ml daily for additional 2 to 3 days. Thereafter, 500 ml may be given every second or third day during period of risk up to 2 weeks.

Supplied in 500-ml units.

NURSING IMPLICATIONS

HISTORY

Review chart for history, most recent vital signs, other monitoring parameters, and laboratory or diagnostic tests. In an emergency, review most recent vital signs, if possible.

PHYSICAL ASSESSMENT

Monitor blood pressure, pulse, respirations; weight (usually estimated if patient is in shock). Additional assessments based on reason for dextran use, patient's symptoms. When used for prophylaxis, baseline laboratory tests such as hemoglobin, hematocrit, renal-function studies, and urine or serum osmolarity may be ordered. Other laboratory tests may also be appropriate.

ADMINISTRATION

Blood samples (when necessary) should be drawn before dextran is administered. If necessary to start immediate IV infusion because of patient's condition, perform venipuncture, obtain blood samples, and then attach IV line to same needle.

Administered by IV infusion.

CVP line and monitoring of CVP recommended during initial infusion.

Physician will order rate of infusion. In shock, first infusion usually administered rapidly.

GENERIC NAME SIMILARITY

Dextran 40 and dextran 70 or 75.

TRADE NAME SIMILARITY

Gentran 40 and Gentran 75.

CLINICAL ALERT: Hypersensitivity reactions have been reported in those not previously exposed to dextran. Observe for generalized urticaria, hypotension, nausea, vomiting, headache, tightness of the chest, wheezing. Anaphylactoid reactions (Appendix 6, section 6-6) may also occur. If either hypersensitivity or anaphylaxis occurs, stop infusion immediately, remove dextran, and add 5% Dextrose in Water (or other IV solution ordered by physician) to IV

D

line. *Do not* discontinue IV because accessible vein is necessary for possible administration of emergency medications.

Drugs for treatment of hypersensitivity (epinephrine, steroids, antihistamines) should always be available when dextran is first administered.

ONGOING ASSESSMENTS AND NURSING MANAGEMENT

Monitor blood pressure, pulse, and respirations q5m to q30m (frequency also depends on patient's condition, reason for use of dextran); check IV infusion site q15m to q30m.

Monitor CVP (if line inserted) q30m or as ordered. *Normal CVP*—5 cm to 15 cm H_2O. Readings are relative; therefore compare with baseline value. Because CVP may be low at time of initiation of therapy, a rise is closely watched. Keep physician informed of CVP readings.

Monitor patient for signs of fluid overload (Appendix 6, section 6-12). A CVP above 15 cm H_2O is indicative of fluid overload.

Measure intake and output q15m to q30m or as ordered; urine specific gravity may also be ordered. Usually, an increase in urine output occurs in oliguric patients after administration of dextran. If no increase is observed after 500 ml is given, notify physician because drug may be discontinued until adequate diuresis develops spontaneously or is provoked by other means.

An osmotic diuretic such as mannitol may be ordered to maintain adequate urine flow.

State of hydration assessed by determination of urine or serum osmolarity, CVP, intake-output ratio.

Dextran, High Molecular Weight

(Dextran 70) Rx

injection: 6% dextran 75 in 0.9% sodium chloride	Gentran 75, *Generic*
injection: 6% dextran 70 in 0.9% sodium chloride	Macrodex, *Generic*
injection: 6% dextran 75 in 5% dextrose	*Generic*
injection: 6% dextran 70 in 5% dextrose	Macrodex

INDICATIONS

Treatment of shock or impending shock due to surgery or other trauma, hemorrhage or burns. Intended primarily for emergency treatment; not regarded as substitute for whole blood or plasma.

CONTRAINDICATIONS

See *Contraindications* for Dextran 40.

ACTIONS

Dextran 70 has molecular weight of 70,000 (range 25,000 to 125,000). IV infusion results in expansion of plasma volume slightly in excess of the volume infused and decreases from this maximum over the succeeding 24 hours. This expansion of plasma volume improves the hemodynamic status for 24 hours or longer. Dextran molecules over 50,000 molecular weight are eliminated in renal excretion with approximately 40% appearing in urine in 24 hours. The remaining drug is enzymatically degraded to glucose.

WARNINGS

Anaphylactoid reactions: See *Warnings* for Dextran 40.

Interference with platelet function: See *Warnings* for Dextran 40.

Use of solutions containing sodium ions: See *Warnings* for Dextran 40.

Fluid and/or solute overloading: See *Warnings* for Dextran 40.

Use in renal impairment: See *Warnings* for Dextran 40.

PRECAUTIONS

Prolonged bleeding time and depression of platelet function: See *Precautions* for Dextran 40.

Circulatory overload: See *Precautions* for Dextran 40.

Exercise caution in administration of parenteral fluids, especially those containing sodium ions, to patients receiving corticosteroids or corticotropin.

DRUG INTERACTIONS

See *Drug Interactions* for Dextran 40.

ADVERSE REACTIONS

Allergic reactions include urticaria, nasal congestion, wheezing, tightness of chest, and mild hypotension. Antihistamines may be effective in relieving these symptoms. Other adverse reactions include nausea, vomiting, fever, and joint pains. If a reaction develops, discontinue use and treat accordingly. Reactions that may occur because of the solution or technique of administration include febrile response, infection at site of injection, venous thrombosis or phlebitis extending from the site of injection, extravasation, and hypervolemia.

DOSAGE

It is suggested that total dosage not exceed 20 ml/kg during the first 24 hours. In adults, the amount usually administered is 500 ml, which may be given at a rate from 20 ml/minute to 40 ml/minute in an emergency.

In children, best guide to dosage is body weight or surface area of patient. Total dosage should not exceed 20 ml/kg.

NURSING IMPLICATIONS

HISTORY
If possible, review most recent vital signs.

PHYSICAL ASSESSMENT
Monitor blood pressure, pulse, and respirations. Obtain most recent weight because dosage is based on weight. If weight is not available, estimate will need to be made.

ADMINISTRATION
Administered by IV infusion.
  Drawing blood samples: See *Administration* for Dextran 40.
  CVP line may be inserted to monitor therapy. Physician will order rate of infusion.
  Hypersensitivity reactions: See *Clinical Alert* for Dextran 40.
  Drugs for treatment of hypersensitivity reaction: See Dextran 40.
  Solution contains no bacteriostat; discard partially used containers.

GENERIC NAME SIMILARITY
Dextran 70 or 75 and dextran 40.

TRADE NAME SIMILARITY
Gentran 75 and Gentran 40.

ONGOING ASSESSMENTS AND NURSING MANAGEMENT
See Dextran 40.

Dextranomer Rx

beads, paste   Debrisan

INDICATIONS
Used in cleansing secreting wounds such as venous stasis ulcers, decubitus ulcers, infected traumatic and surgical wounds, infected burns.

ACTIONS
Dextranomer's ability to remove exudates rapidly and continuously from the surface of a wound results in reduction of inflammation and edema. Evidence suggests that suction forces created by the drug may remove bacteria and bacterial toxins from the wound surface. The hydrophilic beads absorb approximately 4 ml of fluid per 1 g of beads. The beads swell to approximately four times their original size.

When applied to surface of secreting wounds, it removes exudates and particles that tend to impede tissue repair. Low molecular weight components of wound exudates are drawn within the beads or paste, while higher molecular weight components (plasma proteins, fibrinogen) are found between the swollen beads. Removal of these latter components (particularly fibrin and fibrinogen) retards eschar formation.

PRECAUTIONS
Wounds may appear larger during first few days of treatment because of reduction of edema. Drug is not effective in cleansing nonsecreting wounds. Not all wounds require treatment to complete healing. When wound is no longer secreting and healthy granulation tissue is established, use should be discontinued because the natural healing process usually leads to complete closure of the wound.

Drug is not used in sinus tracts, deep fistulas, or any cavity where complete removal would be difficult.

Treatment of the underlying condition (*e.g.,* venous or arterial flow, pressure) should proceed concurrently with use of dextranomer.

ADVERSE REACTIONS
Upon application or removal of beads, transitory pain, bleeding, blistering, and erythema have been reported.

ADMINISTRATION AND DOSAGE
See *Nursing Implications, Administration.*

NURSING IMPLICATIONS

HISTORY
See Appendix 4. Review chart for cause of secreting wound and previous treatment modalities, including nursing interventions.

PHYSICAL ASSESSMENT
Examine wound; record size, location, appearance of secretions, general wound appearance.

ADMINISTRATION
Beads or paste usually applied q12h; more frequent application may be necessary. Number of applications is diminished as exudate from wound diminishes.

Wash hands thoroughly before and after application of drug.

Cleanse wound using sterile water, saline, or other cleansing solution. Physician orders solution to be used.

Leave area moist and apply sufficient amount of beads or paste to cover area to a thickness of ¼ inch.

When treating decubitus ulcers, do not pack wound tightly. Allow for expansion of beads. Maceration of surrounding skin may result if occlusive dressings are used.

Cover area with a dry sterile dressing and close all sides using nonallergenic adhesive tape. Apply dressing so that beads are held in place but still have enough room to expand.

To apply to irregular body surfaces or hard to reach places: Pour small amount of glycerine on a dry, sterile dressing. Add beads in sufficient amount to make ¼-inch layer and apply to wound. Fasten all four sides of dressing.

Glycerin (1 part) and beads (3 parts) may be mixed in a receptacle and applied directly to the wound with a tongue depressor. Cover wound with a dry, sterile dressing and fasten on all four sides. Discard unused paste.

If beads or paste spills on floor, remove immediately because a slippery surface will result.

ONGOING ASSESSMENTS AND NURSING MANAGEMENT

Inspect dressing q2h to q4h. Dressings usually require changing once or twice daily. If wound is draining profusely, more frequent changes may be required.

Dressing should be changed before it becomes fully saturated to prevent drying and to make removal easier.

When saturated, beads and paste change color and should be removed.

Removal of beads or paste must be as complete as possible and is best achieved by rinsing with same solution ordered by physician to clean area. Vigorous irrigation may be required to remove patches of beads or paste that adhere to wound surface. Soaking or whirlpool may also be used to remove drug.

Never remove a dried dressing that has adhered firmly to the wound. Liberally apply solution used for cleansing to loosen dressing.

If treated area is on hip or other bony prominence, develop an orderly plan for q2h position changes and enter in Kardex. Avoid position change that requires full pressure on the treated area.

If wound is infected, dispose of contaminated dressings according to hospital policy.

PATIENT AND FAMILY INFORMATION

If drug is prescribed for home use, patient or family member will require complete instruction on application and removal of drug. Physician should be kept informed of wound's appearance.

Dextroamphetamine Sulfate

See Amphetamines.

Dextromethorphan Hydrobromide

otc

lozenges: 7.5 mg	Hold 4 Hour (Adult), Sucrets Cough Control
lozenges: 10 mg	Chloraseptic Cough Control
syrup: 2.5 mg/5 ml	Romilar Children's Cough
syrup: 5 mg/5 ml	Congespirin
syrup: 10 mg/5 ml	Benylin DM Cough, DM Cough
syrup: 15 mg/5 ml	Pertussin 8 hour Cough Formula, Romilar CF 8 hour Cough Formula
liquid: 30 mg/5 ml	Delsym Pennkinetic

INDICATIONS

Control of productive cough.

CONTRAINDICATIONS

Hypersensitivity.

ACTIONS

Controls cough spasms by depressing cough center in medulla.

WARNINGS

Do not use for persistent cough such as occurs with smoking, asthma, or emphysema, or when cough is accompanied by excessive secretions. Persons with high fever, persistent headache, nausea, or vomiting should not use these preparations except under medical supervision.

DRUG INTERACTIONS

Do not give to patients taking **MAO inhibitors.**

DOSAGE

Increasing dose will increase duration of action.
Lozenges and syrup
Adults, children over 12: 10 mg to 30 mg q4h to q8h. Do not exceed 60 mg to 120 mg in 24 hours.
Children 6–12: 2.5 mg to 5 mg q4h or 7.5 mg to

15 mg q6h to q8h. Do not exceed 40 mg to 60 mg in 24 hours.

Children 2–6: 1.25 mg to 2.5 mg q4h or 3.75 mg to 7.5 mg q6h to q8h. Do not exceed 30 mg in 24 hours.

Children under 2: Not recommended unless directed by physician.

Controlled-release liquid
Adults: 60 mg bid.
Children 6–12: 30 mg bid.
Children 2–5: 15 mg bid.

NURSING IMPLICATIONS

HISTORY
See Appendix 4. Also note duration of cough; type of cough (productive, nonproductive).

PHYSICAL ASSESSMENT
Record temperature; auscultate lungs.

ADMINISTRATION
Administer undiluted unless physician orders otherwise.

ONGOING ASSESSMENTS AND NURSING MANAGEMENT
If cough is not relieved or patient develops a productive cough, fever, or chest pain, contact physician.

PATIENT AND FAMILY INFORMATION
Use as directed by physician or directions on label.

Avoid irritants such as dust, smoking, fumes, other air pollutants.

Frequent sips of water, hard candy, or humidification of air may help relieve dry throat.

If cough persists more than 10 days or if fever, chest pain, or productive cough occurs, see a physician.

Dextrothyroxine Sodium Rx

tablets: 1 mg, 2 mg,   Choloxin (2-mg, 6-mg tab-
    4 mg, 6 mg   lets contain tartrazine)

INDICATIONS
Adjunct to diet and other measures for reduction of elevated serum cholesterol in euthyroid patients with no known organic heart disease. Also indicated in treatment of hypothyroidism in those with cardiac disease who cannot tolerate other types of thyroid medication.

CONTRAINDICATIONS
Administration to euthyroid patients with one or more of the following: known organic heart disease, including angina; history of myocardial infarction (MI); cardiac arrhythmia, including tachycardia, either active or in patients with demonstrated propensity for arrhythmias; rheumatic heart disease; history of congestive heart failure (CHF); decompensated or borderline compensated cardiac status; hypertensive states (other than mild, labile systolic hypertension); advanced liver or kidney disease; history of iodism.

Contraindicated in pregnancy and nursing mothers.

ACTIONS
Predominant effect is reduction of serum cholesterol and low-density lipoprotein (LDL) levels in hyperlipidemic patients. Beta-lipoprotein and triglyceride fractions may also be reduced from previously elevated levels. Evidence indicates dextrothyroxine stimulates the liver to increase catabolism and excretion of cholesterol and its degradation products via the biliary route into the feces. Cholesterol synthesis is increased, and abnormal metabolic end-products do not accumulate in the blood.

WARNINGS
Drugs with thyroid hormone activity have been used for obesity. Large doses may produce serious or even life-threatening manifestations of toxicity; low doses are ineffective for weight reduction.

When used as thyroid replacement in hypothyroid patients with concomitant coronary artery disease or other cardiac disease, treatment is initiated with care and special consideration of dosage schedule required. Drug may increase oxygen requirements of the myocardium, especially at high dosage levels.

Because possibility of precipitating cardiac arrhythmias during surgery exists, drug should be discontinued at least 2 weeks prior to elective surgery. During emergency surgery in euthyroid patients and in surgery in hypothyroid patients in whom it may not be advisable to withdraw therapy, observe patient closely.

When impaired liver function, impaired kidney function, or both are present, advantages of therapy are weighed against possibility of deleterious results.

Use in pregnancy: Women of childbearing age with familial hypercholesterolemia or hyperlipemia should not be deprived of use of this drug. It can be given to those exercising strict birth control procedures. Because pregnancy may occur despite strict birth control procedures, undertake administration only after weighing the possible risk to the fetus against possible benefits to the mother.

DRUG INTERACTIONS
There may be an additive effect when drug is administered to a patient receiving a **digitalis prepara-**

tion; the additive effect may possibly stimulate the myocardium excessively in those with significant myocardial impairment. Dosage of dextrothyroxine should not exceed 4 mg/day when patient is receiving a digitalis preparation.

May potentiate the effects of **oral coumarin anticoagulants** (such as warfarin and dicumarol) on prothrombin time. Reductions in anticoagulant dosage by as much as 30% may be required and the prothrombin time monitored closely. In the surgical patient, dextrothyroxine should be withdrawn 2 weeks before surgery if use of anticoagulants is contemplated.

Special consideration is given to dosage of other **thyroid** medications used concomitantly; hypothyroid patients are more sensitive to a given dose of dextrothyroxine than are euthyroid patients.

Epinephrine injection in those with coronary artery disease may precipitate an episode of coronary insufficiency. This condition may be enhanced in those receiving thyroid analogues.

It has been reported that dextrothyroxine may be capable of increasing blood sugar levels, with a resultant decrease in requirements of **insulin** or **oral hypoglycemic agents.**

PRECAUTIONS

Serum protein-bound iodine (PBI) levels will be increased, but this increased level is not indicative of hypermetabolism. It is also recommended that children with familial hypercholesterolemia receive this drug only if a significant serum cholesterol-lowering effect is seen.

Tartrazine sensitivity: See Appendix 6, section 6-23.

ADVERSE REACTIONS

Side-effects are mainly due to increased metabolism. Adverse effects are least commonly seen in euthyroid patients with no signs or symptoms of organic heart disease. Incidence of adverse effects is increased in hypothyroid patients and highest in those with organic heart disease superimposed on the hypothyroid state.

In the absence of known organic heart disease, some cardiac changes may occur during therapy. In addition to angina pectoris, arrhythmias consisting of extrasystoles, ectopic beats, or supraventricular tachycardia, ECG evidence of ischemic myocardial changes, and increase in heart size have been reported. MI has occurred; it is not known if this is drug related.

Changes in clinical status that may be related to the metabolic action of the drug include insomnia, nervousness, palpitations, tremors, weight loss, lid lag, sweating, flushing, hyperthermia, hair loss, diuresis, and menstrual irregularities. GI complaints include dyspepsia, nausea and vomiting, constipation, diarrhea, and increase in appetite. Other side-effects include headache, changes in libido, hoarseness, tinnitus, dizziness, peripheral edema, malaise, tiredness, visual disturbances, psychic changes, paresthesia, muscle pain, and various bizarre complaints. Skin rashes, including a few that appeared to be due to iodism, and itching have been noted. Occasionally, gallstones have occurred.

DOSAGE

Adult euthyroid hypercholesterolemic patient: Initial daily dose is 1 mg to 2 mg; increased in 1-mg to 2-mg increments at intervals of not less than 1 month to a maximum level of 4 mg/day to 8 mg/day. Recommended maintenance dosage is 4 mg/day to 8 mg/day.

Pediatric hypercholesterolemic patients: Initial daily dose is approximately 0.05 mg/kg; increased in up to 0.05-mg/kg increments at monthly intervals. Recommended maintenance dose is approximately 0.1 mg/kg. *Recommended maximum dosage*—4 mg/day.

NURSING IMPLICATIONS

HISTORY

See Appendix 4. Note allergy to iodides, seafoods. In diagnosis of hypercholesterolemia, note dietary history, family history of this disorder, heart disease, and vascular disease.

PHYSICAL ASSESSMENT

Based on symptoms (if any); monitor vital signs, weight. Pretreatment tests may include ECG, pregnancy test (when applicable), renal- or hepatic-function tests. Other tests may also be appropriate.

ONGOING ASSESSMENTS AND NURSING MANAGEMENT

Record vital signs daily; observe for adverse drug effects; inspect skin for evidence of rash (especially if patient has history of allergies), because rash or itching may be indicative of sensitivity to iodine (iodism).

Observe for cardiac symptoms (*e.g.,* chest pain or discomfort, palpitations, tachycardia, or other cardiac arrhythmia) and notify physician if these should occur.

Patient with history of cardiac disease is closely observed, especially during initial therapy. Observe for aggravation of angina or increased myocardial ischemia, cardiac failure, or development of an arrhythmia. If these should occur, notify physician because dosage may be reduced or drug discontinued.

Laboratory monitoring of drug effect is usually performed at monthly intervals.

Diabetic patient: Check urine for glucose, ketones qid. Adjustment (usually an increase) in insulin or oral hypoglycemic agent may be necessary.

PATIENT AND FAMILY INFORMATION

NOTE: Patient should be supplied with diet prescribed by physician. When necessary, review diet with patient. Physician may also recommend strict birth control procedures to women of childbearing age.

Notify physician or nurse if chest pain, palpitations, sweating, diarrhea, headache, or skin rash occurs.

If pregnancy is suspected, stop taking drug and notify physician immediately.

Adherence to prescribed dietary restrictions is important part of therapy. Intake of dietary cholesterol and saturated fats must be restricted.

Follow prescribed dosage schedule.

Inform other physicians and dentist of therapy with this drug.

Do not use any nonprescription drug without first checking with physician.

Diabetic patient: Check urine daily (or as recommended by physician). If test results (increase in or absence of glucose in urine) are different from what was normally acceptable before therapy with this drug, notify physician. A change in insulin/oral hypoglycemic dose may be necessary.

Diazepam

See Benzodiazepines; Anticonvulsants.

Diazoxide, Oral Rx

capsules: 50 mg	Proglycem
oral suspension: 50 mg/ml	Proglycem

INDICATIONS

Management of hypoglycemia due to hyperinsulinism in adults with inoperable islet cell adenoma or carcinoma or extrapancreatic malignancy. *In infants and children*—Leucine sensitivity, islet cell hyperplasia, nesidioblastosis, extrapancreatic malignancy, islet cell adenoma, or adenomatosis. May be used preoperatively as a temporary measure and postoperatively if hypoglycemia persists.

Use only after a diagnosis of hypoglycemia due to the above conditions has been definitely established; consider when other medical therapy or surgical management is unsuccessful or not feasible.

CONTRAINDICATIONS

Functional hypoglycemia. Not used in patients hypersensitive to drug or other thiazides unless potential benefits outweigh possible risks.

ACTIONS

Produces a prompt dose-related increase in blood glucose level, due primarily to an inhibitor of insulin release from the pancreas and also to an extrapancreatic effect. Hyperglycemic effect begins within an hour and generally lasts no more than 8 hours in the presence of normal renal function. Decreases excretion of sodium and water, resulting in fluid retention, which may be clinically significant. Effects on blood pressure are usually not marked with oral preparation. Other pharmacologic actions include increased pulse rate; increased serum uric acid levels due to decreased excretion; increased serum levels of free fatty acids; decreased chloride excretion; decreased para-aminohippuric acid (PAH) clearance with no appreciable effect on glomular filtration rate. Hyperglycemic effects also potentiated in presence of hypokalemia. Diazoxide-induced hyperglycemia is reversed by administration of insulin or tolbutamide.

Is extensively bound to serum proteins and excreted by the kidneys.

WARNINGS

Fluid retention: Antidiuretic property may lead to significant fluid retention in patients with compromised cardiac reserve. This may lead to congestive heart failure (CHF). Fluid retention will respond to conventional diuretic therapy.

Ketoacidosis and nonketotic hyperosmolar coma: Have been reported, usually during intercurrent illness. Prompt recognition and treatment essential (see *Overdosage*), and prolonged surveillance following acute episode necessary because of long half-life. Occurrence of these serious events may be reduced by careful patient education.

Use in pregnancy: Safety not established.

PRECAUTIONS

Serum uric acid levels may be elevated, particularly in those with hyperuricemia or history of gout.

In some patients higher blood levels have been observed with the liquid than with the capsule form. Dosage may need adjustment when patient is changed from one form to another.

Plasma half-life is prolonged in those with impaired renal function; a reduced dosage may be ordered and serum electrolyte levels evaluated.

DRUG INTERACTIONS

Inhibition of insulin release by diazoxide is antagonized by **alpha-adrenergic blocking agents.** Is highly bound to serum protein and may displace other protein-bound agents (*e.g.,* **bilirubin** or **coumarin** and its derivatives), resulting in higher blood levels of these substances. Administration of diazoxide and coumarin or its derivatives may require reduction in anticoagulant dosage. Diazoxide may displace bilirubin from albumin; this should be noted especially when treating newborns with increased bilirubinemia. Concomitant administration of **thiazides** or other potent **diuretics** may potentiate its hyperglycemic and hyperuricemic effects. The antihypertensive effect of other drugs may be enhanced; this should be considered when administering concomitantly with **antihypertensive agents.** Concomitant administration of **phenytoin** may result in loss of seizure control.

ADVERSE REACTIONS

Frequent and serious: Sodium and fluid retention are most common in young infants and adults and may precipitate CHF in those with compromised cardiac reserve.

Infrequent but serious: Hyperglycemia or glycosuria may require dosage reduction to avoid ketoacidosis or hyperosmolar coma. Diabetic ketoacidosis and hyperosmolar nonketotic coma may develop very rapidly. Conventional therapy with insulin and restoration of fluid and electrolyte balance are usually effective if instituted promptly. Prolonged surveillance is essential because of long half-life of diazoxide.

Other frequent adverse reactions: Hirsutism of the lanugo type, mainly on forehead, back, and limbs; occurs most commonly in children and women and may be cosmetically unacceptable. It subsides on discontinuation of drug.

GI intolerance may include anorexia, nausea and vomiting, abdominal pain, ileus, diarrhea, and transient loss of taste. Tachycardia, palpitations, and increased levels of serum uric acid are common. Thrombocytopenia with or without purpura may require discontinuation of drug. Neutropenia is transient, not associated with increased susceptibility to infection, and ordinarily does not require discontinuance. Skin rash, headache, weakness, and malaise may occur.

Other adverse reactions observed are the following.

Cardiovascular: Occasional hypotension, which may be augmented by thiazide diuretics given concurrently. Rarely, chest pain.

Hematologic: Eosinophilia, decreased hemoglobin/hematocrit, excessive bleeding, decreased IgG.

Hepatorenal: Increased SGOT, alkaline phosphatase; azotemia; decreased creatinine clearance; reversible nephrotic syndrome; decreased urinary output; hematuria; proteinuria.

Neurologic: Anxiety, dizziness, insomnia, polyneuritis, paresthesia, pruritus, extrapyramidal signs.

Ophthalmologic: Transient cataracts, subconjunctival hemorrhage, ring scotoma, blurred vision, diplopia, lacrimation.

Skeletal, integumentary: Monilial dermatitis, herpes, advance in bone age, loss of scalp hair.

Systemic: Fever, lymphadenopathy.

Other: Gout, acute pancreatitis/pancreatic necrosis, galactorrhea, enlargement of lump in breast.

OVERDOSAGE

Symptoms—marked hyperglycemia, which may be associated with ketoacidosis. *Treatment*—Prompt insulin administration and restoration of fluid and electrolyte balance. Because of drug's prolonged half-life (30 hours), symptoms of overdosage require prolonged surveillance for up to 7 days.

DOSAGE

Adults and children: Usual dose is 3 mg/kg/day to 8 mg/kg/day divided into two or three equal doses q8h to q12h. Some patients may require higher doses. Appropriate starting dose is 3 mg/kg/day divided into three equal doses q8h. An average adult would receive about 200 mg/day.

Infants and newborns: Usual dose is 8 mg/kg/day to 15 mg/kg/day divided into two or three equal doses q8h to q12h. Appropriate starting dose is 10 mg/kg/day divided into three equal doses q8h.

NURSING IMPLICATIONS

HISTORY (from patient's chart)
Diagnosis; health history; allergy history; current treatment modalities.

PHYSICAL ASSESSMENT
Review recent laboratory and diagnostic tests; evaluate general physical status; weight. Pretreatment laboratory tests may include serum electrolytes, blood glucose, CBC, urinalysis.

ADMINISTRATION
May be ordered in capsule or oral suspension form. Oral suspension available as 50 mg/ml and is flavored.

Administered two or three times daily q8h to q12h.

Special care is necessary to assure accuracy of dosage in infants and young children. Use calibrated dropper (provided with product) for measuring dose. Read physician's order carefully because dosage may be written in milligrams (mg) or milliliters (ml).

Shake suspension before pouring dose.

ONGOING ASSESSMENTS AND NURSING MANAGEMENT

Check urine for glucose, ketones qid; record vital signs q4h to q8h or as ordered; record weight; measure intake and output, especially during initial therapy. Observe for signs of fluid retention: weight gain, edema of extremities.

Blood glucose, serum electrolytes may be monitored daily during initial therapy and periodically thereafter. Dosage is based on severity of hypoglycemia and adjusted until desired clinical and laboratory effects are produced with the least amount of drug.

Patient's condition usually stabilizes within several days. If administration is not effective after 2 to 3 weeks, drug is usually discontinued.

Hyperglycemic effects are potentiated in presence of hypokalemia and may be reversed by administration of insulin or tolbutamide.

Notify physician before next dose is administered if recent laboratory test results indicate hypokalemia: if urine is positive for glucose or ketones, or percentage of glucose in urine is markedly increased over previous samples; or if fluid retention is apparent.

Patients with compromised cardiac reserve may develop CHF if significant fluid retention occurs. If history indicates cardiac disease, observe for signs of CHF (Appendix 6, section 6-9).

Ketoacidosis and nonketotic hyperosmolar coma have been reported in patients treated with recommended doses, usually during intercurrent illness.

In some patients, higher blood levels have been observed with the liquid than with the capsule formulation and dosage may need to be adjusted when patient is switched from one formulation to the other.

PATIENT AND FAMILY INFORMATION

Monitor urine for glucose and ketones as recommended by physician (patient or family member may require instruction in use of testing materials). Report any abnormalities of urine testing to physician.

Weigh self daily.

Contact physician or nurse immediately if any of the following occurs: increased thirst, lethargy, nausea, vomiting, abdominal pain or cramps, mental confusion, difficulty breathing (air hunger), marked weight gain, swelling of extremities.

Physician will order periodic blood tests to monitor therapy.

Diazoxide, Parenteral Rx

injection: 300 mg/20 ml   Hyperstat IV

INDICATIONS

Emergency reduction of blood pressure in malignant hypertension when urgent decrease of diastolic pressure is required. Treatment with oral agents is instituted as soon as hypertensive emergency is controlled. Is ineffective against hypertension due to pheochromocytoma. See also Antihypertensives.

CONTRAINDICATIONS

Treatment of compensatory hypertension, such as associated with aortic coarctation or arteriovenous shunt; coronary artery disease; dissecting aortic aneurysm; hypersensitivity to diazoxide, thiazides, or other sulfonamide derivatives.

ACTIONS

Related to thiazides but has no diuretic activity. Promptly reduces blood pressure by relaxing smooth muscle in peripheral arterioles, which neither impairs cardiac function nor seriously diminishes kidney perfusion. Reflex increases in heart rate, cardiac output, and stroke volume occur as blood pressure is reduced. A beta-adrenergic blocker may be used if these effects become clinically significant. Coronary and cerebral blood flow are maintained. Renal blood flow is increased after an initial decrease. Produces hyperglycemia, increased serum free fatty acids, and decreased plasma insulin levels by suppression of insulin release and enhanced catecholamine action. Patients refractory to other antihypertensives usually remain responsive to diazoxide.

Is bound to serum protein; plasma half-life is approximately 28 hours. Duration of antihypertensive effect is variable, generally less than 12 hours.

WARNINGS

Hypotensive effects: Use in severe hypertension has been associated with cerebral and myocardial infarction, angina, and permanent blindness secondary to optic nerve infarction. Observe caution when reducing severely elevated blood pressure. The desired blood pressure should be achieved over a period of days if compatible with patient's status. If hypotension severe enough to require therapy occurs, it will usually respond to administration of sympathomimetic agents.

Hyperglycemic effects: Special attention is required for those with diabetes mellitus. Nondiabetic patients may have transient, reversible, and clinically insignificant increase in blood glucose following injection. Hyperglycemia occurs in majority of patients, but usually requires treatment only in patients with diabetes.

Fluid and electrolyte balance: Drug causes sodium retention; repeat injections may precipitate edema and congestive heart failure (CHF). This retention responds to diuretic agents if adequate renal function exists. Increased extracellular fluid volume may be cause of treatment failure in nonresponsive patients; increased volume reduced by use of a diuretic.

Use in pregnancy and lactation: Safety not established. Does cross placental barrier and appears in cord blood. It may produce fetal or neonatal hyperbilirubinemia, thrombocytopenia, altered carbohydrate metabolism, and possibly other adverse reactions.

Use in children: Safety not established.

PRECAUTIONS

This is a potent antihypertensive agent; close monitoring of patient's blood pressure is required. Administration may occasionally cause hypotension, requiring treatment with sympathomimetic drugs.

Maximal antihypertensive effects occur with rapid administration; a slower injection may fail to reduce blood pressure or produce a very brief response. Use with care in those with impaired cerebral or cardiac circulation. Patients undergoing peritoneal dialysis or hemodialysis may require more than one injection because dialysis can reduce diazoxide blood levels.

DRUG INTERACTIONS

Bilirubin, coumarin anticoagulants, phenytoin interactions—see *Drug Interactions* under Diazoxide, Oral. Concomitant administration with **thiazides** or other potent diuretics may potentiate the hyperglycemic, hyperuricemic, and antihypertensive effects of diazoxide.

Administer with caution to patients treated concurrently with **methyldopa** or **reserpine** or other drugs that act by direct peripheral vasodilatation, especially **hydralazine,** the **nitrates,** and **papaverine-like compounds.**

ADVERSE EFFECTS

Frequent and serious: Sodium and water retention after repeated injections, especially in those with impaired cardiac reserve; hyperglycemia frequently requiring treatment in diabetic patients, especially after repeated injections.

Infrequent but serious: Hypotension to shock levels; myocardial or cerebral ischemia, usually transient but possibly leading to thrombosis; persistent

retention of nitrogenous wastes after repeated injections; hypersensitivity reactions such as rash, leukopenia, fever. Rarely, acute pancreatitis.

Other: Orthostatic hypotension, sweating, flushing, generalized or localized sensations of warmth; supraventricular tachycardia, palpitations; various neurologic findings secondary to alterations in regional blood flow to brain such as headache, dizziness, lightheadedness; ringing in the ears, momentary hearing loss; chest discomfort; transient hyperglycemia in nondiabetic patients; transient retention of nitrogenous wastes; various respiratory and GU findings secondary to relaxation of smooth muscle such as dyspnea, cough, nausea, vomiting. Also, warmth and pain along injected vein; cellulitis without sloughing and/or phlebitis at site of extravasation; back pain; increased nocturia.

OVERDOSAGE

May cause undesirable hypotension that can be controlled with sympathomimetic agents such as norepinephrine. Failure of blood pressure to rise may suggest that the hypotension is caused by something other than diazoxide. Excessive hyperglycemia will respond to conventional therapy. Diazoxide may be removed by peritoneal dialysis or hemodialysis.

DOSAGE

1 mg/kg to 3 mg/kg up to a maximum of 150 mg by IV push. May be repeated at intervals of 5 to 15 minutes until satisfactory response in blood pressure is achieved. Minibolus administration of doses of 1 mg/kg to 3 mg/kg repeated at intervals of 5 to 15 minutes is as effective as administration of 300 mg in a single dose.

Repeated administration every 4 to 24 hours will usually maintain blood pressure below pretreatment levels until oral antihypertensive agent becomes effective. Interval between injections may be adjusted by the duration of response to each injection. Treatment is usually unnecessary for more than 4 to 5 days. Because repeated administration can lead to sodium and water retention, administration of a diuretic may be necessary both for maximal blood pressure reduction and to avoid CHF.

NURSING IMPLICATIONS

HISTORY (from patient's chart)
When possible, review diagnosis, recent blood pressure determinations, weight, general history.

PHYSICAL ASSESSMENT
Obtain blood pressure, pulse, respirations, general physical status. Additional assessments are based on current symptoms.

ADMINISTRATION

Dose is based on weight; if weight is unknown, an estimate will have to be made.

Ampule contains 20 ml with total dose of 300 mg (15 mg/ml).

Place patient in a recumbent position.

Select site of IV injection.

Using opposite arm, obtain pretreatment blood pressure, pulse, and respirations. Leave deflated sphygmomanometer cuff in place.

Warn patient that a feeling of warmth or discomfort (and sometimes pain) may be felt as drug is injected.

Administer drug only into peripheral vein. *Do not* administer IM, subcutaneously, or into body cavities. Subcutaneous administration has produced inflammation and pain without subsequent necrosis; this is treated conservatively.

Dose is given by IV push in 15 to 30 seconds. Slow IV injection may fail to reduce blood pressure or may produce an exceedingly short response.

Drug may also be given by minibolus at repeated intervals of 5 to 15 minutes.

Storage: Protect from light and freezing. Store between 2°C and 30°C (36°F–86°F).

ONGOING ASSESSMENTS AND NURSING MANAGEMENT

Patient response varies. Blood pressure generally decreases within 5 minutes, and sometimes within 1 to 2 minutes, to lowest level achieved. The blood pressure then increases relatively rapidly in the next 10 to 30 minutes and then more slowly over the following 2 to 12 hours, nearly reaching but rarely exceeding pretreatment levels.

Begin to monitor blood pressure and pulse as soon as injection is completed. Obtain blood pressure and pulse every minute until response is noted; then monitor q5m to q10m for next hour (physician may also specify intervals for measuring blood pressure). Continue to monitor blood pressure and pulse at least every hour for 12 to 24 hours or as ordered. In ambulatory patients, measure the blood pressure with the patient standing before surveillance is ended.

CLINICAL ALERT: Severe hypotension may occur following administration. Notify physician immediately because treatment with sympathomimetic drugs may be necessary. Observe closely when reducing severely elevated blood pressure. Drug may be ordered to produce a desired response over a period of days if this is compatible with the patient's status. If successive injections are given, response frequently exceeds response to initial injection.

A further decrease in blood pressure 30 minutes or more after drug administration requires notifying the physician because investigation into possible other causes of the hypotensive response may be necessary.

Drug may be repeated at intervals of 4 to 24 hours. Close monitoring of blood pressure is necessary for each injection.

Measure intake and output. Report any decrease in output to physician.

When diazoxide and hydralazine are given concomitantly, observe patient closely. Profound hypotensive episodes may occur.

If patient is allowed to ambulate before treatment, check with physician about ambulation following drug administration. Patient should remain recumbent for at least 30 minutes after drug is administered. If ambulation is allowed, assistance should be given.

Concomitant administration of diazoxide with thiazides or other potent diuretics may potentiate the hyperglycemic, hyperuricemic, and antihypertensive effects of diazoxide. Patient should remain recumbent for a longer period of time. Check with physician about length of time patient should remain recumbent and when ambulation may be allowed. Patient should be assisted with ambulation, especially the first time out of bed after drug is administered.

Blood glucose levels may be monitored, especially in patients with diabetes or in those requiring multiple injections.

Myocardial ischemia, usually transient but possibly leading to thrombosis, may occur. Observe for atrial and ventricular arrhythmias, patient complaints of chest pain.

Cerebral ischemia, usually transient but possibly leading to thrombosis, may occur. Observe for change in level of consciousness, convulsions, paralysis, confusion, or focal neurologic deficit, such as numbness of the hands. Notify physician immediately if signs of myocardial or cerebral ischemia occur.

Weigh patient daily if possible.

Observe for signs of CHF (Appendix 6, section 6-9).

Diabetic patients: Test urine for glucose and ketones qid and observe for signs of hyperglycemia (Appendix 6, section 6-14). Dosage of insulin or oral hypoglycemic agent may require adjustment.

Dibasic Calcium Phosphate Dihydrate

See Calcium Preparations.

Dibucaine

See Anesthetics, Local, Injectable; Anesthetics, Local, Topical.

Dichlorphenamide

See Carbonic Anhydrase Inhibitors.

Dicloxacillin Sodium

See Penicillins.

Dicumarol

See Coumarin and Indandione Derivatives.

Dicyclomine Hydrochloride

See Gastrointestinal Anticholinergics/Antispasmodics.

Dienestrol

See Estrogens, Vaginal.

Diethylpropion Hydrochloride

See Anorexiants.

Diethylstilbestrol

See Estrogens; Estrogens, Vaginal.

Diethylstilbestrol Diphosphate

See Estrogens, Antineoplastic.

Diflorasone Diacetate

See Corticosteroids, Topical.

Diflunisal Rx

tablets, film coated: Dolobid
    250 mg, 500 mg

INDICATIONS
Acute or long-term symptomatic treatment of mild to moderate pain and osteoarthritis.

CONTRAINDICATIONS
Hypersensitivity; patients in whom acute asthmatic attacks, urticaria, or rhinitis is precipitated by aspirin or other nonsteroidal anti-inflammatory drugs.

ACTIONS
Is a nonsteroidal analgesic, anti-inflammatory, and antipyretic drug. Is a peripherally acting nonnarcotic analgesic. Diflunisal is a derivative of salicylic acid that chemically differs from aspirin and is not metabolized to salicylic acid. Mechanism of analgesic and anti-inflammatory actions not known. Diflunisal is a prostaglandin synthetase inhibitor. It is well absorbed following oral administration. Peak plasma concentrations occur between 2 and 3 hours, producing significant analgesia within 1 hour and maximum analgesia within 2 to 3 hours. Time required to achieve steady state increases with dosage, from 3 to 4 days with 125 mg bid to 7 to 9 days with 500 mg bid, because of its long half-life. An initial loading dose shortens the time to reach steady-state levels. The drug is excreted in the urine; little or no drug appears in the feces.

Doubling the dosage more than doubles drug accumulation. Plasma half-life is 8 to 12 hours; it increases in renal impairment.

Analgesic efficacy: 500 mg was comparable in analgesic efficacy to aspirin 650 mg, acetaminophen 600 mg or 650 mg, and acetaminophen 650 mg with propoxyphene napsylate 100 mg; 1000 mg is comparable to acetaminophen 600 mg with codeine 60 mg. Patients treated with diflunisal had more long-lasting responses than those who received acetaminophen with codeine. Patients treated with diflunisal generally continue to have good analgesic effect 8 to 12 hours after dosing.

Osteoarthritis: Diflunisal 500 mg/day or 750 mg/day was comparable in effectiveness to aspirin 2000 mg/day or 3000 mg/day. Patients treated with diflunisal had a lower overall incidence of digestive system adverse effects and of dizziness, edema, and tinnitus.

Uricosuric effect: Patients on long-term diflunisal therapy, 500 mg/day or 1000 mg/day, showed increased renal clearance of uric acid and a prompt and consistent reduction in mean serum uric acid levels. It is not known if diflunisal interferes with the activity of other uricosuric agents.

Effect on platelet function: As an inhibitor of prostaglandin synthetase, has a dose-related effect on platelet function and bleeding time. When recommended dose is exceeded, it inhibits platelet function. In contrast to those of aspirin, these effects were reversible. Bleeding time was not altered by 250 mg bid and was only slightly increased at 500 mg bid.

Effect on fecal blood loss: At 500 mg bid, fecal blood loss was not different than from a placebo. Diflunisal given at 1000 mg bid (which exceeds recommended dosage) caused a significant increase in fecal blood loss that was only one-half as large as that associated with aspirin 1300 mg bid.

WARNINGS

Peptic ulceration and GI bleeding have been reported. In those with active GI bleeding or an active peptic ulcer, weigh benefits of therapy against possible hazards; institute an appropriate ulcer regimen and monitor patient closely. When administering to those with a history of upper GI disease, monitor closely.

Use in pregnancy: Safe use during pregnancy has not been established. Use only when potential benefits justify the potential risk to the fetus; use during the third trimester is not recommended.

Use in lactation: Is excreted in breast milk. Because of potential for adverse effects in nursing infants, decision should be made whether to discontinue nursing or the drug.

Use in children: Safety and effectiveness in infants and children not established. Use in children under 12 not recommended.

PRECAUTIONS

Platelet function and bleeding time are inhibited by diflunisal at higher doses. Because of reports of adverse eye findings, ophthalmologic studies are recommended in those developing eye complaints during treatment. Use a lower daily dosage in patients with significantly impaired renal function. Peripheral edema has been observed; use drug with caution in those with compromised cardiac function, hypertension, or other conditions predisposing them to fluid retention.

Laboratory tests: Borderline elevations of **liver tests** may occur; these abnormalities may progress, remain essentially unchanged, or be transient with continued therapy. Severe hepatic reactions, including jaundice and cases of fatal hepatitis, have occurred rarely with other nonsteroidal anti-inflammatory drugs. If abnormal liver tests persist or worsen, if clinical signs and symptoms of liver disease develop, or if systemic manifestations occur (*e.g.,* eosinophilia, rash), drug is discontinued.

DRUG INTERACTIONS

Oral anticoagulants: Administration of **warfarin** or **phenprocoumon** may prolong the prothrombin time. When drug is administered with oral anticoagulants, prothrombin time is closely monitored during and for several days after concomitant drug administration. Dosage adjustment of oral anticoagulant may be required.

Hydrochlorothiazide and furosemide: Significantly increased levels of **hydrochlorothiazide** may occur. Diflunisal may decrease the hyperuricemic effects of **hydrochlorothiazide** and **furosemide.**

Antacids: Concomitant administration may reduce plasma levels of diflunisal. Effect is small with occasional doses of antacids, but may be clinically significant when antacids are used on a continuous schedule.

Acetaminophen: Diflunisal may increase plasma levels.

Nonsteroidal anti-inflammatory drugs: A small decrease in diflunisal levels was seen when multiple doses of **aspirin** and diflunisal were given. Administration of diflunisal with **indomethacin** decreased renal clearance and significantly increased plasma levels of indomethacin. Concomitant administration of diflunisal and **sulindac** resulted in substantial, but not significant, lowering of plasma levels of the active sulindac sulfide metabolite. Concomitant administration of diflunisal and **naproxen** had no effect on plasma levels of naproxen.

ADVERSE REACTIONS

Incidence greater than 1%

GI: Nausea, dyspepsia, GI pain, diarrhea (3%–9%); vomiting, constipation, flatulence (1%–3%).

CNS: Headache (3%–9%); dizziness, somnolence, insomnia (1%–3%).

Dermatologic: Rash (3%–9%).

Miscellaneous: Tinnitus, fatigue/tiredness (1%–3%).

Incidence less than 1% (causal relationship known)

GI: Peptic ulcer, GI bleeding, anorexia, eructation, cholestatic jaundice.

CNS: Vertigo, nervousness.

Dermatologic: Pruritus, sweating, dry mucous membranes, stomatitis, erythema multiforme, Stevens-Johnson syndrome.

Miscellaneous: Asthenia, edema.

Incidence less than 1% (causal relationship unknown)

CNS: Paresthesias, transient visual disturbances, depression.

Cardiovascular: Palpitations, syncope.

Miscellaneous: Chest pain, fever, malaise, hypersensitivity (including interstitial nephritis with renal failure), anaphylactic reaction with bronchospasm, dyspnea, dysuria, muscle cramps, thrombocytopenia.

OVERDOSAGE

Symptoms: Most common signs and symptoms were drowsiness, disorientation, and stupor.

Treatment: Empty stomach by inducing vomiting or by gastric lavage. Observe patient and give symptomatic and supportive treatment. Hemodialysis may not be effective because of high degree of protein binding.

DOSAGE

Mild to moderate pain: Initial dose of 1000 mg followed by 500 mg q12h; some patients may require 500 mg q8h. A lower dosage (*e.g.,* 500 mg initially followed by 250 mg q8h–q12h) may be appropriate.

Osteoarthritis: 500 mg/day to 1000 mg/day in two divided doses.

Maintenance doses higher than 1500 mg/day not recommended.

NURSING IMPLICATIONS

HISTORY
See Appendix 4.

PHYSICAL ASSESSMENT
Osteoarthritis: Examine involved joints of extremities and describe joint deformities; look for Heberden's nodes in distal joints, Bouchard's nodes in proximal joints; evaluate ability of patient to carry out activities of daily living (ADL); note if enlargement or malalignment interferes with joint range of motion. Physician may order x-rays of involved joints.

Acute or chronic pain: Determine location, intensity, type of pain (*e.g.,* sharp, dull, radiating, throbbing), what factors (if any) influence the pain (*e.g.,* movement, exposure to cold, damp weather, exercise).

ADMINISTRATION
If GI upset occurs, give drug with meals or food.
Do not break or crush tablets.

ONGOING ASSESSMENTS AND NURSING MANAGEMENT
When administering to patient with history of upper GI disease, observe for epigastric pain or distress, melena, hematemesis.

Drug is eliminated primarily by the kidneys. When administering to patients with significantly impaired renal function, observe for signs of overdosage. Usually, lower daily dosages are prescribed to avoid drug accumulation.

If dizziness occurs, patient may need assistance with ambulation.

Because of drug's long duration of action, 2 to 3 days of observation are necessary for evaluating changes in treatment regimens if a loading dose is not used.

Observe for adverse reactions; notify physician if they occur.

Osteoarthritis: Evaluate response to drug (relief of pain, increased joint movement, decrease in joint stiffness). Evaluate ability to carry out ADL and compare to baseline data.

Severely deformed or malaligned joints may be less painful, but patient's ability to participate in ADL may or may not significantly increase.

Encourage moderate exercise and movement. Physician may prescribe a physical or occupational therapy program.

If morning stiffness persists, patient should be allowed to bathe, ambulate, or perform other daily activities at time of day when stiffness is at a minimum.

Mild to moderate pain (acute, chronic): Drug has long duration of action and produces significant analgesia within 1 hour and maximum analgesia in 2 to 3 hours.

Evaluate analgesic effect of drug at time of expected effect. If pain remains the same or only slight relief is obtained, discuss with physician before next dose is due.

PATIENT AND FAMILY INFORMATION
May cause GI upset; may be taken with water, milk, or meals.

Do not take aspirin or acetaminophen with this medication, except on advice of physician. When purchasing nonprescription drugs, check with a pharmacist regarding aspirin or acetaminophen content of the drug.

Notify physician if GI upset persists despite taking drug with food or milk.

Notify physician or nurse if the following occur: nausea, vomiting, diarrhea, constipation, dizziness, rash. If pain is not controlled after several days of use of drug, contact physician.

Digestive Enzymes

Pancreatin *Rx, otc*

tablets, enteric coated: 1000 mg (2000 units lipase, 25,000 units protease, 25,000 units amylase) (*otc*)	Pancreatin Enseals
tablets: 325 mg (650 units lipase, 8125 units protease, 8125 units amylase) (*otc*)	*Generic*
tablets: 6500 units lipase, 32,000 units	Viokase

protease, 48,000 units amylase (*Rx*)

powder: 15,000 units lipase, 75,000 units protease, 112,500 units amylase per 0.75 g (*Rx*)   Viokase

Pancrelipase *Rx*

capsules: 8000 units lipase, 30,000 units protease, 30,000 units amylase, 25 mg calcium carbonate	Cotazym
capsules: 5000 units lipase, 20,000 units protease, 20,000 units amylase	Cotazym-S
capsules: 8000 units lipase, 30,000 units protease, 30,000 units amylase	Ku-Zyme HP
capsules: 4000 units lipase, 25,000 units protease, 20,000 units amylase	Pancrease
powder packets, regular: 16,000 units lipase, 60,000 units protease, 60,000 units amylase, 50 mg calcium carbonate	Cotazym
powder packets, flavored: 40,000 units lipase, 150,000 units protease, 150,000 units amylase, 50 mg calcium carbonate	Cotazym
tablets: 11,000 units lipase activity and not less than 30,000 units of protease and 30,000 units of amylase activity	Ilozyme

INDICATIONS

Used in patients with deficient exocrine pancreatic secretions. May be used as enzyme replacement therapy in cystic fibrosis, chronic pancreatitis, post-pancreatectomy, ductal obstructions caused by cancer of the pancreas, pancreatic insufficiency, steatorrhea of malabsorption syndrome, postgastrectomy (Billroth II and Total). Also used as a presumptive test for pancreatic function, especially in pancreatic insufficiency due to chronic pancreatitis.

CONTRAINDICATIONS

Hypersensitivity.

ACTIONS

Digestive enzymes exert their primary effects in the duodenum and upper jejunum. An enteric coating is often used to prevent destruction or inactivation by gastric pepsin and acid *p*H, but enteric coatings may partially or totally inhibit delivery of the enzymes to the duodenum. Pancrelipase is of porcine origin; pancreatin is of bovine or porcine origin.

WARNINGS

Pancreatic enzyme replacement therapy should not delay or supplant treatment of the primary disorder. Safety for use in pregnancy is not established.

PRECAUTIONS

A proper balance of fat, protein, and starch intake must be maintained to aovid temporary indigestion. A careful ratio of drug dosage to food intake is desirable.

Use pork products with caution in those sensitive to pork protein. Discontinue use if symptoms of sensitivity appear. Sensitivity may develop in those taking these drugs and others who come into contact with these products.

ADVERSE REACTIONS

High doses may cause nausea and diarrhea. Extremely high doses have been associated with hyperuricosuria and hyperuricemia.

DOSAGE

PANCREATIN
Tablets: One to three tablets with meals.
Powder: 0.75 g with meals.

PANCRELIPASE
Capsules and tablets, 1 to 3 before or with meals and snacks. In severe deficiencies, dose may be increased to 8 if no nausea, cramps, or diarrhea results. *Powder*—1 or 2 packets before meals or snacks.

NURSING IMPLICATIONS

HISTORY
See Appendix 4. Note allergy to pork.

PHYSICAL ASSESSMENT

Monitor general physical status, weight. Pretreatment examination of stool for fecal fat may be ordered.

ADMINISTRATION

Powder form may be sprinkled on food (especially for children). Do not sprinkle on large portions, especially if anorexia is a problem, because entire dose may not be consumed.

Instruct patient not to chew capsules or enteric-coated tablets.

Do not crush enteric-coated microspheres (Pancrease) or enteric-coated tablets.

An antacid or cimetidine may be prescribed to help increase the amount of available pancreatin in the duodenum. An antacid may also be used to control steatorrhea in those with deficient pancreatic bicarbonate secretion.

Avoid inhalation of powder dosage form when preparing it for administration.

ONGOING ASSESSMENTS AND NURSING MANAGEMENT

Observe for nausea and diarrhea and notify physician if these occur because dosage may need to be reduced.

Check patient's tray after each meal; if diet is taken poorly, or only certain types of foods are consumed, discuss with physician. (See _Precautions._)

Weigh weekly or as ordered. Report weight loss to physician.

Note appearance of each stool and record in chart. Physician may order periodic stool examinations.

Patients with chronic pancreatitis, pancreatectomy: Test urine for glucose, ketone bodies qid. Insulin or oral hypoglycemic agents may be necessary to control hyperglycemia.

PATIENT AND FAMILY INFORMATION

Take before or with meals.

Powder may be sprinkled over small portions of food. Avoid inhaling powder dosage form.

Do not exceed recommended dose.

PANCREASE

Do not crush or chew the microspheres.

PANCREATIN ENSEALS

Do not crush or chew tablets.

Digitalis

See Cardiac Glycosides.

Digitalis Glycoside Mixture

See Cardiac Glycosides.

Digitoxin

See Cardiac Glycosides.

Digoxin

See Cardiac Glycosides.

Dihydroergotamine Mesylate Rx

injection: 1 mg/ml   D.H.E. 45

INDICATIONS

To abort or prevent vascular headaches such as migraine, migraine variant, and cluster headaches (histamine cephalalgia) when rapid control is desired or when other routes of administration are not feasible.

CONTRAINDICATIONS

Peripheral vascular disease, coronary heart disease, hypertension, impaired hepatic or renal function, sepsis, hypersensitivity to ergot alkaloids. Contraindicated in pregnancy.

ACTIONS

An alpha-adrenergic blocking agent. Has direct stimulating effect on smooth muscle of peripheral and cranial blood vessels and produces depression of central vasomotor centers. Also has properties of serotonin antagonism. In comparison to ergotamine, adrenergic blocking actions are more pronounced, vasoconstrictive actions somewhat less pronounced, and incidence and degree of nausea and vomiting are reduced.

ADVERSE REACTIONS

Signs of ergotism (_e.g.,_ numbness, tingling of fingers and toes, muscle pains in extremities, weakness in legs, precordial distress and pain, transient tachycardia or bradycardia, nausea, vomiting, localized edema and itching).

OVERDOSAGE

Symptoms: Failure to observe upper limits of repeated parenteral dosage may result in eventual onset of peripheral toxic signs and symptoms of ergotism (see _Adverse Reactions_).

Treatment: Discontinue drug, apply warmth, administer vasodilators (such as nitroprusside) to prevent tissue damage.

DOSAGE

IM: 1 mg at first warning sign of headache, repeated at 1-hour intervals to a total of 3 mg.

IV: Where more rapid effect is desired, use IV route to a maximum of 2 mg. Do not exceed 6 mg/week.

NURSING IMPLICATIONS

HISTORY
See Appendix 4.

PHYSICAL ASSESSMENT
Monitor vital signs.

ADMINISTRATION
May be ordered IM or IV.

Rotate IM injection sites; record site used. Rotation is necessary to prevent localized vasoconstriction, which may occur from repeated use of one site.

ONGOING ASSESSMENTS AND NURSING MANAGEMENT
Onset of action occurs in 15 to 30 minutes following IM administration and persists for 3 to 4 hours. Repeated dosage at 1-hour intervals up to 3 hours may be required to obtain maximal effect.

Assess drug effect 30 to 45 minutes after IM administration or 5 to 10 minutes after IV injection; record response to drug.

Accurate recording of patient's response to drug (*i.e.,* relief of vascular headache) is essential. Physician obtains optimal results by adjusting the dose for several headaches to find the minimal effective dose for each patient. This dose is then used at onset of subsequent attacks.

Dihydrotachysterol

See Vitamin D.

Dihydroxyaluminum Sodium Carbonate

See Antacids.

Diltiazem Hydrochloride Rx

tablets: 30 mg,   Cardizem
   60 mg

INDICATIONS

Angina pectoris due to coronary artery spasm: Treatment of spontaneous coronary artery spasm presenting as Prinzmetal's variant (resting angina with ST segment elevation occurring during attack).

Chronic stable angina (classic effort-associated angina): For those who cannot tolerate therapy with beta-adrenergic blocking agents or nitrates or who remain symptomatic despite adequate doses of these agents.

CONTRAINDICATIONS

Sick sinus syndrome, except in presence of a functioning ventricular pacemaker; second- or third-degree atrioventricular (AV) block; hypotension (less than 90 mm Hg systolic blood pressure).

ACTIONS

Therapeutic benefits are related to drug's ability to inhibit the influx of calcium ions during membrane depolarization of cardiac and vascular smooth muscle. Prevents spontaneous and ergonovine-provoked coronary artery spasm. It causes a decrease in peripheral vascular resistance and a modest fall in blood pressure.

Like other calcium antagonists, diltiazem decreases sinoatrial (SA) and AV conduction and has a negative inotropic effect in isolated preparations. Chronic oral administration of doses up to 240 mg/day has resulted in small increases in the P–R interval but has not usually produced abnormal prolongation.

Diltiazem is about 80% absorbed and is subject to extensive first-pass effect, giving an absolute bioavailability of about 40%; it is 70% to 80% bound to plasma proteins. Binding is not altered by therapeutic concentrations of digoxin, hydrochlorothiazide, phenylbutazone, propranolol, salicylic acid, or warfarin. Single oral doses of 30 mg to 120 mg result in detectable plasma levels within 30 to 60 minutes and peak plasma levels in 2 to 3 hours. Diltiazem undergoes extensive hepatic metabolism; 2% to 4% of unchanged drug appears in urine. Plasma elimination half-life following single or multiple doses is approximately 3.5 hours.

WARNINGS

Cardiac conduction: Prolongs AV node refractory periods without significantly prolonging sinus node recovery time, except in those with sick sinus syndrome. This effect may rarely result in abnormally slow heart rate (particularly in patients with sick sinus syndrome) or second- or third-degree AV block. Concomitant use with beta-adrenergic blockers or digitalis may result in additive effects on cardiac conduction.

Hypotension: Therapy may occasionally result in symptomatic hypotension.

Use in pregnancy, lactation: Use only when

clearly needed and when potential benefits outweigh the potential hazards to the fetus. It is not known whether drug is excreted in human milk. Exercise caution when administering to nursing women.

Use in children: Safety and efficacy not established.

PRECAUTIONS

Drug is extensively metabolized by the liver and excreted by the kidneys. Use with caution in those with impaired renal or hepatic function.

DRUG INTERACTIONS

There may be additive effects in prolonging AV conduction with concomitant use of **beta-adrenergic blocking agents** or **digitalis. Sublingual nitroglycerin** may be taken as required to abort acute anginal attacks during diltiazem therapy. May be safely administered with **short-** and **long-acting nitrates.**

ADVERSE REACTIONS

Serious adverse reactions are rare. The following have been reported infrequently and represent adverse reactions that can be reasonably associated with the pharmacology of calcium influx inhibition, but their relationship to diltiazem is not established.

Cardiovascular: Swelling/edema (2.4%), arrhythmia (2%), flushing, congestive heart failure (CHF), bradycardia, hypotension, syncope, pounding heart (<1%).

CNS: Headache (2%), fatigue (1.1%), drowsiness, dizziness, lightheadedness, nervousness, depression, weakness, insomnia, confusion, hallucinations (<1%).

GI: Nausea (2.7%), vomiting, diarrhea, gastric upset, constipation, indigestion, pyrosis (<1%).

Dermatologic: Rash (1.8%), pruritus, petechiae, urticaria (<1%).

Other: Photosensitivity, nocturia, thirst, paresthesia, polyuria, osteoarticular pain.

Altered laboratory findings: Rarely, mild to moderate transient elevations of alkaline phosphatase, SGOT, SGPT, LDH, and CPK reported during therapy.

OVERDOSAGE

Symptoms: None reported; toxic dose unknown.

Treatment: In event of overdosage or exaggerated response, employ appropriate supportive measures in addition to gastric lavage. The following may be considered: *Bradycardia*—Atropine (0.6 mg–1 mg). If no response to vagal blockade, administer isoproterenol cautiously. *High degree AV block*—Treat as for bradycardia. Fixed high-degree AV block should be treated with cardiac pacing. *Cardiac failure*—Administer inotropic agents (isoproterenol, dopamine, dobutamine) and diuretics. *Hypotension*—Vasopres-

sors (*e.g.,* dopamine, norepinephrine). Actual treatment and dosage should depend on severity of the clinical situation.

DOSAGE

Exertional angina pectoris due to atherosclerotic coronary artery disease or angina pectoris at rest due to coronary artery disease: Start with 30 mg qid A.C. and H.S.; increase to 240 mg (given in divided doses 3–4 times/day) at 1- to 2-day intervals until optimum response is obtained. Dosage is adjusted to suit patient's needs. If drug is used in those with impaired renal or hepatic function, titration is carried out with caution.

NURSING IMPLICATIONS

HISTORY

See Appendix 4. Note thorough history of angina, exercise tolerance, description of angina pain.

PHYSICAL ASSESSMENT

Record vital signs (take apical and radial pulse), general physical status. Pretreatment ECG is usually ordered. Laboratory studies may include renal- and hepatic-function tests; other tests may also be appropriate.

ADMINISTRATION

Administer before meals and at bedtime.

ONGOING ASSESSMENTS AND NURSING MANAGEMENT

Obtain vital signs q4h or as ordered. Record all episodes of angina including onset, duration, location, intensity and radiation of pain, and possible precipitating factors (*e.g.,* ambulation, emotional stress). Notify physician immediately if there is an increase in the frequency of angina or an increase in the degree of pain experienced during an attack.

Other antianginal agents such as nitroglycerin and long-acting nitrates may be used concomitantly. If sublingual nitroglycerin is used, see p 776.

Observe for adverse drug effects, especially changes in cardiac rate and rhythm, hypotension, signs of CHF (Appendix 6, section 6-9). Notify physician immediately if these should occur.

Dizziness may occur. Patient should be assisted with ambulatory activities, especially during initial therapy.

Physician may order limited ambulation, especially if patient has resting angina. Ambulatory activities may be gradually increased once optimal drug response is attained.

Measurement of intake and output may be ordered if patient concomitantly receiving a diuretic or has a history of CHF.

PATIENT AND FAMILY INFORMATION

Notify physician or nurse if any of the following occurs: Irregular heartbeat, shortness of breath, swelling of hands and feet, pronounced dizziness, constipation, nausea, hypotension.

If dizziness or lightheadedness occurs, sit or lie down immediately. Do not attempt to walk without assistance if these symptoms persist.

If angina pain becomes worse, notify physician immediately.

Follow physician's recommendation about exercise.

Keep a record of each angina attack (if they occur). Make note of the date, time of onset, duration and intensity of pain (as compared with attacks before therapy with this drug), possible precipitating factors (*e.g.,* exercise, emotional stress). Bring this record with you at time of each office/clinic visit.

Dimenhydrinate

See Antiemetic/Antivertigo Agents.

Dimercaprol Rx

injection: 100 mg/ml   Bal In Oil

INDICATIONS

Treatment of arsenic, gold, and mercury poisoning. Also indicated in acute lead poisoning when used concomitantly with edetate calcium disodium. Is effective for use in acute poisoning by mercury salts if therapy is begun within 1 to 2 hours following ingestion. It is not very effective for chronic mercury poisoning. Is of questionable value in poisoning caused by other heavy metals such as antimony and bismuth.

CONTRAINDICATIONS

Most instances of hepatic insufficiency, with exception of postarsenical jaundice. Discontinue or use only with extreme caution if acute renal insufficiency develops during therapy. Not used in iron, cadmium, or selenium poisoning; the resulting dimercaprol–metal complexes are more toxic than the metal alone, especially to the kidneys.

ACTIONS

Promotes excretion of arsenic, gold, and mercury by chelation. Because of affinity of arsenic to dimer-

caprol, sulfhydryl enzyme inhibition is prevented. To a lesser degree, dimercaprol may reactivate affected enzymes; it is most effective when administered before significant enzyme damage. Also used in combination with edetate calcium disodium to promote excretion of lead. Following IM administration of a 10% solution in oil, peak concentrations are attained in 30 to 60 minutes. Has a short half-life and excretion is complete within 4 hours.

WARNINGS

Use in pregnancy: Not used unless necessary in treatment of life-threatening acute poisoning.

Use in children: A reaction apparently peculiar to children is fever, which may persist during therapy; occurrence is approximately 30%. A transient reduction of the percentage of polymorphonuclear leukocytes may also be seen.

PRECAUTIONS

Urinary alkalinization: Because the dimercaprol–metal complex breaks down easily in an acid medium, production of alkaline urine affords protection to the kidney during therapy.

Use with caution in those with glucose-6-phosphate dehydrogenase deficiency, especially in presence of infection or other stressful situations; hemolysis may occur.

DRUG INTERACTIONS

Do not administer **iron** to patients under therapy with dimercaprol.

ADVERSE REACTIONS

One of the most consistent responses is a rise in blood pressure accompanied by tachycardia. Rise is roughly proportional to dose administered. Doses larger than those recommended may cause other transitory signs and symptoms as follows, in approximate order of frequency: nausea and vomiting; headache; burning sensation of lips, mouth, throat; a feeling of constriction, even pain, in the throat, chest, or hands; conjunctivitis; lacrimation; blepharal spasm; rhinorrhea and salivation; tingling of hands; burning sensation in the penis; sweating of the forehead, hands, and other areas; abdominal pain; occasional appearance of painful sterile abscesses. Many of these are accompanied by a feeling of anxiety, weakness, and unrest and are often relieved by administration of an antihistamine.

DOSAGE

Give deep IM only. Injections are begun as soon as possible. Other supportive measures may be used in conjunction with dimercaprol therapy.

Mild arsenic or gold poisoning: 2.5 mg/kg qid

for 2 days, then twice on the third day and once daily thereafter for 10 days.

Severe arsenic or gold poisoning: 3 mg/kg q4h for 2 days, then 4 times on the third day, then twice daily thereafter for 10 days.

Mercury poisoning: 5 mg/kg initially, followed by 2.5 mg/kg one or two times daily for 10 days.

Acute lead encephalopathy: 4 mg/kg given alone in the first dose and thereafter at 4-hour intervals in combination with edetate calcium disodium administered at a separate site. For less severe poisoning, dose may be reduced to 3 mg/kg after first dose. Treatment is maintained for 2 to 7 days, depending on clinical course.

NURSING IMPLICATIONS

HISTORY

History depends on type of poisoning (*e.g.,* from drugs [gold for treatment of arthritis], environmental [mercury may be present in fish caught in water contaminated by some industries], accidental or deliberate ingestion [arsenic is found in weed killers, insecticides, etc.]). In some instances, an extremely thorough history may be necessary.

PHYSICAL ASSESSMENT

Record vital signs, weight. Additional assessments depend on symptoms and possible body systems involved. Depending on heavy metal, baseline urinalysis, CBC, hemoglobin, heavy-metal blood level, and so on may be ordered.

ADMINISTRATION

Drug is in oil. Use 19-gauge needle to withdraw from vial and 20- to 21-gauge needle to administer drug.

Give deep IM. Rotate injection sites; record site used.

Warn patient that pain or discomfort may be noted at injection site.

If edetate calcium disodium is given with dimercaprol for lead poisoning, use a different injection site for each drug. Record site used for each.

ONGOING ASSESSMENTS AND NURSING MANAGEMENT

Record vital signs q4h or as ordered; measure intake and output; assess body systems affected by poisoning (*e.g.,* CNS, skin, GI tract, GU tract, cardiovascular system).

A rise in blood pressure and tachycardia are common responses to dimercaprol therapy; degree of elevation is roughly proportional to dose

administered. Notify physician if blood pressure or pulse rate rises significantly.

Check previous injection sites for induration and evidence of sterile abscess formation, and notify physician if these should occur.

Alkalinization of urine is recommended. Physician may order sodium bicarbonate, potassium citrate and sodium citrate, potassium citrate and citric acid, or sodium citrate and citric acid solution.

Notify physician if any change in the intake–output ratio occurs.

A reaction peculiar to children is fever. Keep physician informed of all temperature elevations and assess child for evidence of dehydration (Appendix 6, section 6-10).

Daily laboratory monitoring of therapy is usually necessary and may include urinalysis, CBC, hemoglobin, heavy-metal blood levels, and so on.

Other therapies appropriate to the type and severity of heavy metal poisoning are also instituted and may include IV therapy for fluid replacement, treatment of renal failure, and treatment of anemia or leukopenia.

Dimethyl Sulfoxide (DMSO) Rx

solution: 50% in   Rimso-50
  50 ml

INDICATIONS

For symptomatic relief of interstitial cystitis.

Investigational uses: Dimethyl sulfoxide (DMSO) has been used in topical treatment of a wide variety of musculoskeletal disorders and related collagen diseases and to enhance the percutaneous absorption of other drugs. Other uses investigated (for topical or systemic administration) include treatment of scleroderma, arthritis, tendinitis, breast and prostate malignancies, retinitis pigmentosa, herpesvirus infections, head and spinal cord injury, stroke.

DMSO is available in a variety of forms not intended for human use (*i.e.,* veterinary and industrial solvents). Human use of such products should be discouraged because of their unknown purity. Because of drug's cutaneous transport characteristics, impurities and contaminants may be systemically absorbed when it is used topically.

CONTRAINDICATIONS

None known.

WARNINGS

Hypersensitivity reaction: Can liberate histamine; there have been hypersensitivity reactions with topical administration, but this has not occurred in those receiving drug intravesically. If anaphylactoid symptoms develop, institute appropriate therapy. Some data indicate DMSO potentiates other concomitantly administered medications.

Use in pregnancy, lactation: Safety not established. Use only when clearly needed and when potential benefits outweigh the unknown potential hazards to the fetus. It is not known if drug is excreted in human milk. Exercise caution in administering to nursing women.

Use in children: Safety and efficacy not established.

PRECAUTIONS

Ophthalmic effects: Full eye examinations, including slit-lamp examinations, are recommended before and periodically during treatment.

Hepatic and renal effects: Hepatic- and renal-function tests and CBC are recommended at 6-month intervals.

Intravesical instillation: May be harmful to those with urinary-tract malignancy because of DMSO-induced vasodilatation.

ADVERSE REACTIONS

Patient may note garliclike taste within a few minutes after instillation. This taste may last for several hours and an odor on the breath and skin may remain for 72 hours. Transient chemical cystitis has been noted following instillation. When drug is applied topically, a garliclike breath, local dermatitis, sedation, nausea, vomiting, headache, and burning or aching eyes may occur.

OVERDOSAGE

In case of accidental ingestion, induce emesis. Additional measures that may be considered are gastric lavage, activated charcoal, and forced diuresis.

DOSAGE

Not for IM or IV injection. Standard dose for bladder instillation is 50 ml. After retention for 15 minutes the medication is expelled by spontaneous voiding. Discard any remaining solution. Repeat treatment every 2 weeks until maximum symptomatic relief is obtained. Thereafter, time intervals between treatments may be increased. In those with severe interstitial cystitis and very sensitive bladders, the initial treatment, and possibly the second and third (depending on patient response), should be done under anesthesia (saddle block is suggested).

NURSING IMPLICATIONS

HISTORY
See Appendix 4.

PHYSICAL ASSESSMENT
Physician performs diagnostic cystoscopy, other GU evaluations prior to treatment. Hepatic- and renal-function tests, CBC may also be ordered. A complete eye examination is recommended before treatment.

ADMINISTRATION
Drug is instilled by physician. Treatment is carried out in physician's office, outpatient clinic, or hospital urology department.

Place patient in lithotomy position on treatment table; cover with a drape. Prepare equipment necessary for instillation.

If 500 ml solution is used to distend bladder, mix in a *glass* container immediately before use.

For direct instillation by catheter, an analgesic lubricant gel such as lidocaine jelly is usually applied to the urethra before the catheter is inserted.

Warn patient that moderately severe discomfort may be experienced on administration. A garliclike taste experienced a few minutes after administration may last for several hours.

The physician may prescribe an oral analgesic or a rectal suppository containing belladonna and opium before instillation to reduce bladder spasm in sensitive patients.

Instruct patient to hold the solution (500 ml or 50 ml) in the bladder for 15 minutes, after which time it is expelled by spontaneous voiding.

ONGOING ASSESSMENTS AND NURSING MANAGEMENT
Patient remains in office or urology department until drug is voided.

If patient is unable to retain solution for 15 minutes, inform physician.

An analgesic may be prescribed for posttreatment discomfort.

PATIENT AND FAMILY INFORMATION
Do not use nonprescription products without prior approval of physician because some products are excreted in the urine and may increase bladder irritability. Topical nonprescription drugs are also avoided, unless use has been approved by the physician.

Dinoprost Tromethamine

(Prostaglandin F₂ Alpha) Rx

injection: 5 mg/ml   Prostin F2 alpha

INDICATIONS
For aborting pregnancy between 16th and 20th weeks of gestation as calculated from the first day of

the last normal menstrual period. Not indicated if fetus *in utero* has reached stage of viability. Should not be considered a feticidal agent. Does not appear to affect the fetoplacental unit directly. The possibility does exist that the previable fetus aborted by dinoprost could exhibit transient life signs.

CONTRAINDICATIONS

Hypersensitivity; acute pelvic inflammatory disease; patients with known active cardiac, pulmonary, renal, or hepatic disease.

ACTIONS

Administered intra-amniotically. Stimulates myometrium of the gravid uterus to contract in a manner similar to contractions seen in the term uterus during labor. Whether or not this action results from a direct effect of drug on the myometrium has not been determined. Contractions induced are sufficient to produce evacuation of the uterus in a majority of cases. The mean abortion time is 20 hours.

WARNINGS

For use only with strict adherence to recommended dosages by medically trained personnel in hospital surroundings that provide intensive care and acute surgical facilities.

Any failed pregnancy termination should be completed by some other means.

Drug is not injected if amniocentesis is bloody or blood-tinged. Severe reactions that may include bronchospasm, hypertension, vomiting, and anaphylaxis can occur if medication is injected intravascularly.

PRECAUTIONS

It is recommended that concomitant intra-amniotic administration of dinoprost and IV oxytocin be used with caution in absence of adequate cervical dilatation.

Use with caution in patients with history of asthma, glaucoma, hypertension, cardiovascular disease, history of epilepsy, or previously compromised (scarred) uteri.

ADVERSE REACTIONS

Most commonly seen include vomiting, nausea, diarrhea.

Rare but serious include hypersensitivity, uterine rupture, cardiac arrest.

Events occurring in approximately 1%–5%: Blood loss, fever, uterine infections.

Rare: Disseminated intravascular coagulation, hypovolemic shock, bronchospasm, hypertension or hypotension, perforation of cervix, headache, dyspnea, urinary-tract infections, syncope or dizziness, chills, uterine pain, unspecified pain, coughing,

tachycardia, drowsiness, pulmonary embolism, perforated uterus—post instrumentation, pelvic thrombophlebitis, hypokalemia, congestive heart failure, second-degree heart block, ventricular arrhythmia, aggravation of diabetes, chest pain, back pain, skin eruption, paralytic ileus, weakness, bradycardia, urinary incontinence, dysuria, hematuria, unspecified muscle spasm, uterine atony or hypertonicity, hiccups, malaise, diplopia, polydipsia, hyperventilation, burning sensation in eye or breast, pupil constriction, paresthesias, pruritus, petechiae, breast engorgement, sweating, nosebleed, dehydration, excitement, cyanosis.

DOSAGE

A transabdominal tap of the amniotic sac usually is accomplished and at least 1 ml of amniotic fluid withdrawn. Then 40 mg of dinoprost is slowly injected into amniotic sac. The first 5 mg is injected very slowly and only if amniotic tap fluid is clear (not blood-tinged). If this procedure is followed, chances of anaphylaxis are reduced as is chance of inadvertent intravascular injection of a bolus of drug that may cause hypertension, bronchospasm, or severe vomiting.

NURSING IMPLICATIONS

HISTORY

Take health history; allergy history; pregnancy history.

PHYSICAL ASSESSMENT

Record vital signs, general mental and physical status. Review physical examination performed by physician.

ADMINISTRATION

Drug is administered by physician.

Prepare materials for administration according to hospital procedure manual.

Have patient void immediately before administration.

Obtain vital signs immediately before administration.

Physician may prescribe antiemetic and antidiarrheal agents before administration.

Storage: Must be refrigerated.

ONGOING ASSESSMENTS AND NURSING MANAGEMENT

Monitor vital signs q2h or as ordered.

Observe for onset of labor. Monitor uterine response (contractions) q½h to q1h or as ordered. Note and record onset of labor as well as time between contractions and intensity and duration of contractions. Keep physician informed of patient's progress.

Following administration, the mean abortion time is 20 hours. If within 24 hours the abortion process has not been established or completed and membranes are intact, an additional 10 mg to 40 mg may be administered.

Save all tissue expelled for physician to inspect or for laboratory identification of the fetus and placenta.

Observe for rare but serious adverse reactions (*e.g.,* hypersensitivity to drug, uterine rupture, and cardiac arrest).

Notify physician if any of the following is noted: significant changes in blood pressure or pulse rate, hypertonic uterine contractions, fever, profuse vaginal bleeding.

A few primigravida patients have experienced cervical perforation during induced abortion. This was usually associated with concomitant use of IV oxytocin, resulting in uterine hypertonus in the presence of an undilated or minimally dilated cervix.

A complete vaginal and cervical examination is performed following passage of the fetus and placenta because cervical trauma can occur without remarkable symptoms. Depending on hospital or unit policy, examination may be performed by nurse in absence of bleeding or other complications such as intrauterine infection, vaginal bleeding.

Dinoprost-induced abortion may be sometimes incomplete. In such cases other measures are taken to assure complete abortion. When treatment is not successful, an attempt to use hypertonic saline should be delayed until uterus is no longer contracting.

PATIENT INFORMATION

Contact physician if any of the following occurs: fever, vaginal bleeding (other than normal lochia), abdominal cramps or pain, passage of additional clots or pieces of tissue, foul-smelling lochia.

Discuss with physician when sex and use of douches or tampons may be resumed.

Reexamination will be necessary (usually 2–4 weeks).

NOTE: Following an abortion, depression may occur. Advise patient to discuss problem with her physician.

Dinoprostone (Prostaglandin E₂) Rx

vaginal suppository: Prostin E2
   20 mg

INDICATIONS

For termination of pregnancy from 12th through 20th gestational week as calculated from the first day of the last menstrual period.

For evacuation of the uterine content in management of missed abortion or intrauterine fetal death up to 28 weeks of gestational age as calculated from the first day of the last normal menstrual period.

In management of nonmetastatic gestational trophoblastic disease (benign hydatidiform mole).

Not indicated if the fetus *in utero* has reached stage of viability. Drug should not be considered a feticidal agent. Does not appear to affect the fetoplacental unit directly. Therefore, the possibility does exist that a previable fetus aborted by dinoprostone could exhibit transient life signs.

CONTRAINDICATIONS

Hypersensitivity; acute pelvic inflammatory disease; patients with known cardiac, pulmonary, renal, or hepatic disease.

ACTIONS

Administered intravaginally, drug stimulates the myometrium of the gravid uterus to contract in a manner similar to contractions seen in the term uterus during labor. Whether or not action results from a direct effect of the drug on myometrium is not determined. Myometrial contractions induced by vaginal administration are sufficient to produce evacuation from the uterus in majority of cases.

Drug is also capable of stimulating smooth muscle of the GI tract; this activity may be responsible for vomiting or diarrhea during use. Large doses can lower blood pressure, probably as a consequence of the drug's effect on smooth muscle of the vascular system. With doses used for terminating pregnancy, this effect has not been clinically significant. Drug can elevate body temperature.

WARNINGS

Use only with strict adherence to recommended dosages and only by medically trained personnel in hospital surroundings that provide intensive care and acute surgical facilities. Any failed pregnancy termination should be completed by some other means.

PRECAUTIONS

Use with caution in those with history of asthma; hypotension; hypertension; cardiovascular, renal, or hepatic disease; anemia; jaundice; diabetes; history of epilepsy; previously compromised (scarred) uteri; presence of cervicitis; infected endocervical lesions; acute vaginitis.

When pregnancy diagnosed as missed abortion is

electively interrupted with intravaginal administration, obtain confirmation of intrauterine fetal death in respect to a negative pregnancy test for chorionic gonadotropin activity (U.C.G. test or equivalent). When pregnancy with late fetal intrauterine death is interrupted with intravaginal administration, obtain confirmation of intrauterine fetal death prior to treatment.

Vaginal therapy is associated with transient pyrexia that may be due to hypothalamic thermoregulation. Temperature returns to normal on discontinuation of therapy.

ADVERSE REACTIONS
Most frequent reactions are related to contractile effect on smooth muscle and include vomiting, temperature elevation, diarrhea, some nausea, headache, shivering, and chills. Transient diastolic blood pressure decreases of greater than 20 mm Hg may be seen. Other adverse effects, in decreasing order of frequency (not all are clearly drug related), include fever; backache; joint inflammation or pain, new or exacerbated; flushing or hot flashes; dizziness; arthralgia; vaginal pain; chest pain; dyspnea; endometritis; syncope or fainting sensation; vaginitis or vulvitis; weakness; muscular cramp or pain; tightness in chest; nocturnal leg cramps; uterine rupture; breast tenderness; blurred vision; coughing; rash; myalgia; stiff neck; dehydration; tremor; paresthesia; hearing impairment; urine retention; pharyngitis; laryngitis; diaphoresis; eye pain; wheezing; cardiac arrhythmia; skin discoloration; vaginismus; and tension.

DOSAGE
Insert one suppository (20 mg) high into vagina. Additional administration of each suppository should be at 3- to 5-hour intervals until abortion occurs. With these recommended intervals, administration time should be determined by abortifacient progress, uterine contractility response, and patient tolerance.

▌ NURSING IMPLICATIONS

HISTORY
See Appendix 4. Obtain complete pregnancy history, previous uterine surgery.

PHYSICAL ASSESSMENT
Obtain vital signs, general mental and physical status. Review physical examination performed by physician. Pregnancy test for chorionic gonadotropin activity may be ordered if pregnancy

is diagnosed as missed abortion to confirm intrauterine fetal death.

ADMINISTRATION
Remove suppository from freezer; allow to reach room temperature just prior to use.

Physician may order antiemetic and antidiarrheal agents prior to administration of dinoprostone.

Carefully remove foil wrapper from suppository; avoid contact with fingers.

Obtain vital signs immediately prior to administration.

Place patient in supine position. Wearing glove, insert suppository high into vagina.

Storage: Store in freezer not above −20°C (−4°F); bring to room temperature just before use.

ONGOING ASSESSMENTS AND NURSING MANAGEMENT
Patient should remain in supine position for 10 minutes following insertion. Physician may allow patient to ambulate after this time.

Monitor vital signs q2h to q4h or as ordered.

Observe for onset of labor. Monitor uterine response (contractions) q1/2h to q1h or as ordered. Note and record onset of labor as well as time between contractions, intensity and duration of contractions. Keep physician informed of patient's progress.

Save all tissue expelled for physician to inspect or for laboratory identification of the fetus and placenta.

An approximate 2°F temperature elevation occurs in approximately 50% of patients. Supportive therapy for drug-induced fevers includes forcing of fluids. If temperature exceeds 2°F elevation, additional antipyretic measures may be employed.

If patient is vomiting, fluids may not be retained. Observe for signs of dehydration (Appendix 6, section 6-10), further rise in temperature; notify physician if these should occur.

Notify physician if there are significant changes in blood pressure or pulse rate, if temperature exceeds anticipated 2°F elevation, or if vaginal bleeding is profuse.

A complete vaginal and cervical examination is performed following passage of the fetus and placenta because cervical trauma can occur without remarkable symptoms. Depending on hospital or unit policy, examination may be performed by nurse in absence of bleeding or other complications such as intrauterine infection, vaginal bleeding.

Dinoprostone-induced abortion may sometimes be incomplete. In such cases, other measures are taken to assure complete abortion.

PATIENT INFORMATION

Contact physician if any of the following occurs: fever, vaginal bleeding (other than normal lochia), abdominal cramps or pain, passage of additional clots or pieces of tissue, foul-smelling lochia.

Discuss with physician when sex and use of douches or tampons may be resumed.

Reexamination will be necessary (usually 2–4 weeks).

NOTE: Following an abortion, depression may occur. Advise patient to discuss problem with her physician.

Diphenhydramine Hydrochloride

See Anticholinergic Antiparkinsonism Agents; Antiemetic/Antivertigo Agents; Antihistamines.

Diphenidol

See Antiemetic/Antivertigo Agents.

Diphenoxylate Hydrochloride With Atropine Sulfate Rx C-V

tablets: 2.5 mg diphenoxylate HCl and 0.025 mg atropine sulfate
liquid: 2.5 mg diphenoxylate HCl and 0.025 mg atropine sulfate per 5 ml

Diphenatol, Enoxa, Lofene, Lomotil, Lonox, Lo-Trol, Low-Quel, Nor-Mil, SK-Diphenoxylate, *Generic* Enoxa, Lomotil, Lo-Trol

INDICATIONS

Adjunctive therapy in management of diarrhea.

CONTRAINDICATIONS

Children under 2 years because of decreased margin of safety; known hypersensitivity to diphenoxylate or atropine; obstructive jaundice; diarrhea associated with pseudomembranous enterocolitis following therapy with antibiotics.

ACTIONS

A constipating meperidine congener that lacks analgesic activity. High doses (40 mg–60 mg) cause typical opioid activity, including euphoria, suppression

of the morphine abstinence syndrome, and physical dependence after chronic administration. A subtherapeutic dose of atropine is present in products containing diphenoxylate to discourage abuse.

Diphenoylate is rapidly and extensively metabolized by ester hydrolysis to diphenoxylic acid, which is biologically active and the major circulating metabolite in the blood. An average of 14% of the drug and its metabolites are excreted over a 4-day period in the urine and 49% in the feces. Serum half-life of parent drug is about 2.5 hours; elimination half-life is approximately 12 to 14 hours.

Has been demonstrated to be comparable to codeine phosphate (45 mg/day), paregoric and loperamide (10 mg/day) in chronic diarrhea. Diphenoxylate has a shorter duration of action than loperamide.

WARNINGS

Antiperistaltic agents may prolong or aggravate diarrhea associated with organisms that penetrate the intestinal mucosa (*e.g.,* toxigenic *Escherichia coli, Salmonella* and *Shigella* species) or in pseudomembranous enterocolitis associated with broadspectrum antibiotics and should not be used in these conditions. In some patients with acute ulcerative colitis, agents that inhibit intestinal motility or delay intestinal transit time may induce toxic megacolon.

Use in hepatic impairment: Use with extreme caution in those with cirrhosis and advanced hepatorenal disease and in all patients with abnormal hepatic-function tests, because hepatic coma may be precipitated.

Fluid and electrolyte balance: Use does not obviate need for appropriate fluid and electrolyte therapy.

Use in pregnancy, lactation: Use in women of childbearing potential only when clearly needed and when potential benefits outweigh the unknown potential hazards to the fetus. Effects of diphenoxylate or atropine may be evident in infants of nursing mothers; these compounds are excreted in breast milk.

Use in children: Contraindicated in children under 2 years. Use with caution, because signs of atropinism may occur even with recommended doses, particularly in those with Down's syndrome. Dosage recommendations should be strictly adhered to in children.

PRECAUTIONS

In doses used for treatment of acute and chronic diarrhea, drug has not produced addiction. Is devoid of morphinelike subjective effects at therapeutic doses. At high doses it exhibits codeinelike subjective effects. Because addiction is possible at high doses, recommended doses should not be exceeded. Administer with caution to patients receiving addicting drugs, to individuals known to be addiction prone, and to those whose histories suggest they may increase dosage on their own.

DRUG INTERACTIONS
Chemical structure is similar to that of meperidine; therefore, concurrent use with **monoamine oxidase inhibitors** may precipitate hypertensive crises. Diphenoxylate may potentiate depressant action of **barbiturates, tranquilizers,** and **alcohol.** Patient should be closely observed when these medications are used concurrently.

ADVERSE REACTIONS
Atropine effects such as dryness of skin and mucous membranes, flushing, hyperthermia, tachycardia, and urinary retention may occur, especially in children. Other reported adverse reactions reported are the following.

GI: Anorexia, nausea, vomiting, abdominal discomfort, paralytic ileus, toxic megacolon.

Allergic: Pruritus, swelling of gums, angioneurotic edema, giant urticaria.

CNS: Dizziness, drowsiness, sedation, headache, malaise, lethargy, restlessness, euphoria, depression, respiratory depression, coma, numbness of extremities.

OVERDOSAGE
Symptoms: Accidental overdosage may result in severe, even fatal, respiratory depression. Initial signs of overdosage may include dryness of skin and mucous membranes, flushing, hyperthermia, and tachycardia followed by lethargy or coma, hypotonic reflexes, nystagmus, pinpoint pupils, and respiratory depression. Although signs of overdosage and respiratory depression may not be evident soon after ingestion, respiratory depression may occur from 12 to 30 hours later.

Treatment: Gastric lavage, induction of emesis, establishment of patent airway, and possibly mechanically assisted respiration are advised. Naloxone should be used in treatment of respiratory depression. *Adults*—Usual initial dose is 0.4 mg naloxone IV. If respiratory function is not adequately improved after initial dose, repeat same IV dose at 2- to 3-minute intervals. *Children*—Usual initial dose is 0.01 mg/kg naloxone IV, repeated in 2- to 3-minute intervals if necessary.

Following initial improvement of respiratory function, repeat dose may be required in response to recurrent respiratory depression. Supplemental IM doses may be used to produce a more long-last-

ing effect. Diphenoxylate's duration of action is longer than that of naloxone; therefore improvement of respiration following administration may be followed by recurrent respiratory depression. Continuous observation is necessary for at least 48 hours, until effect of diphenoxylate on respiration has passed.

DOSAGE
Recommended initial dosage is 5 mg qid. Most patients will require this dosage until initial control is achieved, after which dosage may be reduced to meet individual requirements. Control is often maintained with as little as 5 mg/day.

Children: Contraindicated in children under 2 years. Use with special caution in young children because of variable response. In children 2 to 12 years, use liquid form only. Recommended initial dosage is 0.3 mg/kg/day to 0.4 mg/kg/day, in divided doses. See Table 25 for children's dosages.

Reduction of dosage may be made as soon as initial control of symptoms achieved. Maintenance dose may be as low as one fourth of initial daily dosage; do not exceed recommended dosage. If there is no response in 48 hours, drug is unlikely to be effective.

NURSING IMPLICATIONS

HISTORY
See Appendix 4. A thorough history is necessary to identify probable cause of diarrhea (if cause unknown) and should include travel history; type of foods eaten recently (and where eaten); any changes in dietary pattern such as eating of raw or uncooked food, eating foods different from normal diet; changes in bowel habits before onset of diarrhea; history of constipation; occupational history.

PHYSICAL ASSESSMENT
Monitor vital signs; weight; look for evidence of dehydration. Examine or have patient describe, stools. Auscultate abdomen for bowel sounds (may be hyperactive); palpate abdomen, looking for tenderness or pain, distention, rigidity,

Table 25. Recommended Dosages of Diphenoxylate for Children

Age (yr)	Weight (kg)	Frequency	Dose (mg/ml)
2–5	13–20	3 times/day	2 mg/4 ml
5–8	20–27	4 times/day	2 mg/4 ml
8–12	27–36	5 times/day	2 mg/4 ml

masses. Stool examination (blood, mucus, color) and stool culture and sensitivity are usually ordered. Stool may also be examined for ova and parasites. Other laboratory tests may include serum electrolytes, CBC, hemoglobin, and hematocrit.

ADMINISTRATION

Liquid form is recommended for children 2 to 12.

Use dropper supplied with product to measure liquid preparation.

Each milliliter of liquid preparation contains 0.5 mg.

ONGOING ASSESSMENTS AND NURSING MANAGEMENT

Record vital signs q4h to q8h (depending on severity of illness); record weight; examine and record time each stool passed, as well as note general appearance, color, odor, consistency, estimated amount of stool, and presence of blood, mucus, pus, undigested food, or other matter.

CLINICAL ALERT: If diarrhea is severe, observe for signs of dehydration (Appendix 6, section 6-10), hypokalemia (Appendix 6, section 6-15), hyponatremia (Appendix 6, section 6-17). Dehydration, especially in younger children, may further influence variability of drug response and may predispose the patient to delayed diphenoxylate intoxication.

Drug-induced inhibition of peristalsis may result in fluid retention in the intestine, which may further aggravate dehydration and electrolyte imbalance. If severe dehydration or electrolyte imbalance occurs, withhold drug and notify the physician because appropriate corrective therapy (IV fluids, electrolyte replacement) may be necessary.

Notify physician if any of the following occurs: fever, severe drowsiness, decreased respiratory rate, vomiting, abdominal pain or distention, pruritus, urticaria, angioneurotic edema, or palpitation.

If drug is administered to young child, observe closely for signs of atropinism (flushed hot dry skin, dry mucous membranes, urinary retention, fever, tachycardia with weak pulse, restlessness, confusion, CNS stimulation, skin rash), even when recommended doses are used.

Drowsiness may occur; assist patient with ambulation as needed.

Dry mouth may be relieved by sips of water.

Wash anal area thoroughly after each stool is passed to prevent irritation, skin breakdown. If area becomes excoriated, notify physician.

Physician may order a clear liquid diet for 24 hours, then a soft bland diet until diarrhea is controlled. Other dietary measures may be instituted depending on type and severity of diarrhea.

If diarrhea is severe, offer fluids hourly to prevent dehydration. IV fluid replacement may be necessary in some cases.

Serum electrolytes and other laboratory tests such as repeat stool culture, hemoglobin, and hematocrit may be ordered if diarrhea persists.

Carefully observe patients with ulcerative colitis for signs of toxic megacolon. Notify physician if abdominal distention, pain, or tenderness or vomiting develops because drug may be discontinued.

If diarrhea is due to food poisoning or infection with organisms such as *Salmonella,* notify public health authorities.

PATIENT AND FAMILY INFORMATION

Do not exceed recommended dosage.

May cause drowsiness or dizziness; use caution while driving or performing tasks requiring alertness.

Avoid alcohol and other CNS depressants; do not use other nonprescription drugs unless use is approved by physician.

May cause dry mouth, which may be relieved by sips of water.

Notify physician if diarrhea persists or fever or palpitations develop.

Diphenylpyraline Hydrochloride

See Antihistamines.

Diphtheria Antitoxin

See Antitoxins and Antivenins.

Diphtheria Toxoid, Adsorbed

See Immunizations, Active.

Diphtheria and Tetanus Toxoids, Combined

See Immunizations, Active.

Diphtheria and Tetanus Toxoids and Pertussis Vaccine, Adsorbed

See Immunizations, Active.

Dipivefrin Hydrochloride Rx

solution: 0.1%   Propine

INDICATIONS
Initial therapy for control of intraocular pressure (IOP) in chronic open-angle glaucoma. Those responding inadequately to other antiglaucoma therapy may respond to addition of dipivefrin.

CONTRAINDICATIONS
Hypersensitivity; narrow-angle glaucoma, because any dilation of the pupil may predispose the patient to an attack of glaucoma.

ACTIONS
Is a prodrug of epinephrine formed by diesterification of epinephrine and pivalic acid. Is converted to epinephrine inside the human eye by enzyme hydrolysis. Penetration of the human cornea is approximately 17 times that of epinephrine. The liberated epinephrine, an adrenergic agonist, appears to exert its action by decreasing aqueous production and by enhancing outflow facility. The prodrug delivery system is a more efficient way of delivering the therapeutic effects of epinephrine with few side-effects that are associated with conventional epinephrine therapy. Onset of action with 1 drop occurs about 30 minutes after treatment, with maximal effect seen at about 1 hour.

WARNINGS
Safety for use in pregnancy not established. Use only when clearly needed and when potential benefits outweigh unknown hazards to the fetus. It is not known whether drug is excreted in human milk; exercise caution when administering to nursing mothers. Safety and efficacy for use in children not established.

ADVERSE REACTIONS
Cardiovascular: Tachycardia, arrhythmias, and hypertension have been reported with ocular administration of epinephrine.

Local: Burning and stinging most frequently reported (6%) with dipivefrin alone. Conjunctival irritation observed in 6.5%. Epinephrine therapy can lead to adrenochrome deposits in the conjunctiva and cornea.

Aphakic patients: Macular edema occurs in up to 30% of those treated with epinephrine. Discontinuation of epinephrine generally results in reversal of maculopathy.

DOSAGE
Initial glaucoma therapy: 1 drop in eye(s) q12h.
Replacement therapy: When patient is being transferred to dipivefrin from antiglaucoma agents other than epinephrine, on first day continue previous medication and add 1 drop of dipivefrin in each eye q12h. On following day, discontinue previously used antiglaucoma agent and continue with dipivefrin. In transferring patient from conventional epinephrine therapy, discontinue epinephrine and institute dipivefrin regimen.

Concomitant therapy: When patient on other antiglaucoma agent requires additional therapy, add 1 drop of dipivefrin q12h. For difficult-to-control cases, addition of dipivefrin to other agents such as pilocarpine, carbachol, echothiophate iodide, or acetazolamide has been shown to be effective.

NURSING IMPLICATIONS

HISTORY
See Appendix 4.

PHYSICAL ASSESSMENT
Monitor vital signs; evaluate older patient's ability to carry out activities of daily living. Physician performs complete ophthalmologic examination.

ADMINISTRATION
Advise patient that slight stinging or burning on initial instillation may occur.

Place in upright position. Tilt head back.

Instill in eye(s). Apply light finger pressure on lacrimal sac for 1 minute following instillation.

ONGOING ASSESSMENTS AND NURSING MANAGEMENT
If symptoms are not relieved, notify physician because additional therapy may be necessary.

Monitor vital signs daily. If tachycardia, arrhythmias, or hypertension occurs, notify physician immediately.

Periodic IOP determinations may be performed by the physician.

PATIENT AND FAMILY INFORMATION
NOTE: Instruct patient in technique of administration.

Slight stinging or burning in initial instillation may occur.

Apply light finger pressure on lacrimal sac for 1 minute following instillation.

To avoid contamination, do not touch eyelids or surrounding area with dropper tip. Replace dropper in bottle immediately after use. Do not wash tip of dropper.

Dipyridamole Rx

tablets: 25 mg   Persantine (contains tartrazine), Pyridamole, *Generic*

tablets: 50 mg	Persantine-50, Pyridamole, *Generic*
tablets: 75 mg	Persantine-75, Pyridamole, *Generic*

INDICATIONS

"Possibly effective" for long-term therapy of chronic angina pectoris. Prolonged therapy may reduce frequency or eliminate anginal episodes, improve exercise tolerance, and reduce nitroglycerin requirements. Not intended to abort an acute anginal attack.

Investigational uses: Antiplatelet effect of dipyridamole, alone or in combination with aspirin, is being evaluated in the prevention of reinfarction and reduction of mortality following myocardial infarction.

ACTIONS

Therapeutic doses usually produce no significant alteration of systemic blood pressure or of blood flow in peripheral arteries. Increases coronary blood flow primarily by a selective dilation of coronary arteries.

Acts predominantly on small-resistance vessels of the coronary bed. Increases coronary vascular resistance and increases coronary blood flow and coronary sinus oxygen saturation without significantly altering myocardial oxygen consumption. Produces an accumulation of the potent vasodilators adenosine and adenine nucleotides by inhibiting the activity of adenosine deaminase and by blocking its uptake by erythrocytes and other tissues. Also inhibits phosphodiesterase and thus possibly produces vasodilatation through an accumulation of cyclic adenosine monophosphate (cAMP). A mild positive inotropic effect has been demonstrated. Also inhibits platelet aggregation and may inhibit platelet function by increasing the effects of prostacycline or by inhibiting phosphodiesterase activity, thus increasing intracellular concentration of cAMP in platelets.

PRECAUTIONS

Excessive doses can produce peripheral vasodilatation; use cautiously in those with hypotension.

Tartrazine sensitivity: See Appendix 6, section 6-23.

ADVERSE REACTIONS

Are minimal and transient at recommended dosages. Instances of headache, dizziness, nausea, flushing, weakness or syncope, mild GI distress, and skin rash have been noted. Rare cases of what appeared to be aggravation of angina pectoris have been reported, usually at initiation of therapy.

DOSAGE

Recommended dosage is 50 mg tid, 1 hour A.C.; higher doses may be necessary, but increased incidence of side-effects is associated with increased dosage.

NURSING IMPLICATIONS

HISTORY
See Appendix 4.

PHYSICAL ASSESSMENT
Record vital signs. ECG, serum enzymes may be ordered before initial therapy.

ADMINISTRATION
Give 1 hour before meals with full glass of water.

ONGOING ASSESSMENTS AND NURSING MANAGEMENT
Obtain vital signs q4h to q8h; record all episodes of angina including onset, duration, location, intensity and radiation of pain, possible precipitating factors (*e.g.,* ambulation, emotional stress). Notify physician immediately if there is an increase in frequency of angina or increase in degree of pain experienced during an attack.

Clinical response may not be evident before second or third month of continuous therapy.

If gastric distress occurs, notify physician.

Assist with ambulatory activities if patient experiences dizziness, weakness, or syncope.

PATIENT AND FAMILY INFORMATION
Take 1 hour before meals with full glass of water.

May cause headache, dizziness, or nausea. If these persist, contact physician.

Follow recommendations of physician about exercise, diet.

If angina becomes worse or there is an increase in degree of pain, notify physician immediately.

Disopyramide Rx

capsules: 100 mg, 150 mg	Norpace
capsules, controlled release: 100 mg, 150 mg	Norpace CR

INDICATIONS

Suppression and prevention of unifocal or multifocal (ectopic) ventricular contractions; paired ventricular contractions (couplets); episodes of ventricular tachycardia (persistent ventricular tachycardia ordinarily treated with D.C. cardioversion).

Investigational uses: Drug is being evaluated for

treatment of ventricular arrhythmias in emergency situations and in paroxysmal supraventricular tachycardia.

CONTRAINDICATIONS

Cardiogenic shock; preexisting second- or third-degree atrioventricular (AV) block (if no pacemaker is present); sick sinus syndrome; hypersensitivity.

ACTIONS

Is a Type I antiarrhythmic, pharmacologically similar to but not chemically related to procainamide and quinidine. It decreases the rate of diastolic depolarization (phase 4) in cells with augmented automaticity, decreases the upstroke velocity (phase O) and increases the action potential duration of normal cardiac cells. Also decreases the disparity in refractoriness between infarcted and adjacent normally perfused myocardium and has no effect on alpha- or beta-adrenergic receptors. Disopyramide shortens sinus node recovery time, lengthens the refractory period of the atrium, and has minimal effect on the effective refractory period of the AV node. Little effect has been shown on AV nodal or His-Purkinje conduction time, or on QRS duration; prolongation of conduction in accessory pathways occurs. Rarely produces significant alterations in blood pressure except in those with congestive heart failure (CHF).

Following oral administration, it is rapidly and almost completely absorbed. Peak plasma levels are attained in 2 to 3 hours after a single oral dose. Steady-state concentrations are achieved in approximately 35 hours in healthy adults. About 50% is excreted in the urine as unchanged drug and 30% as metabolites. The mean plasma half-life is about 7 hours, with a range of 4 to 10 hours. Patients with a recent myocardial infarction (MI) or ventricular arrhythmias may have a longer elimination half-life. The dose must be decreased in renal failure to avoid drug accumulation and an increased intensity of effect.

Disopyramide is equally effective in digitalized and nondigitalized patients. Also equally effective in treatment of primary cardiac arrhythmias and those that occur in association with organic heart disease, including coronary artery disease.

WARNINGS

Negative inotropic properties

Heart failure/hypotension: May cause or aggravate CHF or produce severe hypotension, primarily in primary cardiomyopathy or inadequately compensated CHF. Not used in patients with uncompensated or marginally compensated CHF or hypotension unless secondary to cardiac arrhythmia. Patients with history of heart failure may be treated with careful attention to maintenance of cardiac function, including optimal digitalization.

QRS widening: Although unusual, significant widening (greater than 25%) of the QRS complex may occur; discontinue drug in such cases.

Q-T prolongation: Prolongation of the Q-T interval (corrected) and worsening of the arrhythmia, including ventricular tachycardia and fibrillation, may occur. Those with Q-T prolongation in response to quinidine may be at particular risk. If Q-T prolongation greater than 25% and ectopy continue, monitor patient closely and consider discontinuing drug.

Atrial tachyarrhythmias

Those with atrial flutter are digitalized prior to administration of drug to ensure that enhancement of AV conduction does not result in an increase of ventricular rate beyond acceptable limits.

Conduction abnormalities

Use caution in those with sick sinus syndrome, Wolff-Parkinson-White (WPW) syndrome, bundle branch block.

Cardiomyopathy

Patients with myocarditis or other cardiomyopathy may develop significant hypotension. Loading dose is not given and initial dosage and subsequent adjustments are closely monitored.

Heart block

If first-degree heart block develops, reduce dosage. If block persists, continuation of drug depends on weighing benefit against risk of higher degrees of heart block. Development of second- or third-degree AV block or unifascicular, bifascicular, or trifascicular block requires discontinuation of drug, unless ventricular rate is controlled by a ventricular pacemaker.

Hypoglycemia

Rarely, significant lowering of blood glucose values is reported. Blood glucose levels are monitored in those with CHF, chronic malnutrition, or hepatic or renal disease and in those taking drugs (*e.g.,* beta-adrenoceptor blockers, alcohol) that could compromise normal glucoregulatory mechanisms in the absence of food.

Concomitant antiarrhythmic therapy

Concomitant use of disopyramide with other Type I antiarrhythmic agents or propranolol is reserved for life-threatening arrhythmias unresponsive to a single agent. Use may produce serious negative inotropic effects or excessively prolong conduction, particularly in those with cardiac decompensation.

Anticholinergic activity

Not used in patients with glaucoma, myasthenia gravis, or urinary retention unless adequate overriding measures are taken. In those with family history of glaucoma, measure intraocular pressure before therapy. Dose-dependent anticholinergic effects on glaucoma and urinary retention may be transitory or disappear with dose reduction. Those with myasthenia gravis require special care because drug's anticholinergic properties could precipitate myasthenia crisis.

Use in pregnancy, lactation: Use only when clearly needed and when potential benefits outweigh the hazards to the fetus. Drug is reported to stimulate contractions of the pregnant uterus. Monitor patient closely to avoid fetal or maternal effects. Drug has been detected in human milk at a concentration not exceeding that in plasma. If use is essential, an alternate method of infant feeding should be instituted.

PRECAUTIONS

Renal impairment: Reduce dosage; monitor ECG for signs of overdosage.

Hepatic impairment: Causes increase in plasma half-life. Reduce dosage in such patients; monitor ECG for signs of overdosage.

Potassium imbalance: May be ineffective in hypokalemia and toxic effects may be enhanced by hyperkalemia.

DRUG INTERACTIONS

Other antiarrhythmics (*e.g.,* quinidine, procainamide, lidocaine, propranolol) have occasionally been used with disopyramide. Widening of the QRS complex or Q–T prolongation may occur. **Phenytoin** may stimulate metabolism of disopyramide, reducing disopyramide's plasma levels and antiarrhythmic effects. Other **enzyme inducers** (*e.g.,* barbiturates, glutethimide, primidone, rifampin) may also induce disopyramide metabolism.

ADVERSE REACTIONS

Most serious are hypotension and CHF. Most common that are dose dependent are anticholinergic. These may be transitory but may be persistent or severe. Urinary retention is the most serious anticholinergic effect.

The following have been seen in 10% to 40% of patients.

Anticholinergic: Dry mouth (32%), urinary hesitancy (14%), constipation (11%).

The following have been seen in 3% to 9% of patients.

Anticholinergic: Blurred vision; dry nose, eyes, throat.

GU: Urinary frequency and urgency.

GI: Nausea, pain, bloating and gas.

General: Dizziness, fatigue, muscle weakness, headache, malaise, aches, pain.

The following reported in 1% to 3% of patients.

Anticholinergic: Urinary retention.

GU: Impotence.

Cardiovascular: Hypotension with or without CHF, increased CHF, edema, weight gain, cardiac conduction disturbances, shortness of breath, syncope, chest pain.

GI: Anorexia, diarrhea, vomiting.

Dermatologic: Generalized rash, dermatoses, itching.

CNS: Nervousness.

Other: Hypokalemia, elevated cholesterol and triglycerides.

The following have been observed in less than 1%.

Depression; insomnia; dysuria; numbness; tingling; elevated liver enzymes; AV block; elevated BUN; elevated creatinine; decreased hemoglobin, hematocrit; hypoglycemia. Rarely, acute psychosis has been reported following therapy, with prompt return to normal mental status when drug is discontinued.

There have been reports of severe myocardial depression (with an increase in venous pressure and hypotension) and unexplained severe epigastric pain following normal doses. Infrequent reversible cholestatic jaundice, fever, and respiratory difficulty have been reported as have rare instances of reversible agranulocytosis. Discontinue drug promptly if these occur. Angle-closure glaucoma and anaphylactoid reactions also have been reported.

OVERDOSAGE

Symptoms: Deliberate overdosage has produced early loss of consciousness after an apneic period, followed by arrhythmias and loss of spontaneous respiration, leading to death. Toxic plasma levels might be expected to produce widening of the QRS complex and Q–T interval, worsening of CHF, hypotension, varying conduction disturbances, bradycardia, and finally asystole. Obvious anticholinergic effects may also be observed.

Treatment: May include administration of isoproterenol, dopamine, cardiac glycosides, diuretics, intra-aortic balloon counterpulsation, and mechanically assisted respiration. Hemodialysis or hemoperfusion with charcoal may be used. Monitor the ECG. If progressive AV block develops, implement endocardial pacing. In impaired renal function, measures to increase the glomerular filtration rate may reduce toxicity. Anticholinergic effects may be reversed with neostigmine.

DOSAGE

Adults: Usual dosage is 400 mg/day to 800 mg/day in 4 divided doses. Recommended schedule is 150 mg q6h or 300 mg controlled release q12h. For those weighing less than 110 pounds, recommended dosage is 100 mg q6h or 200 mg controlled release q12h.

Pediatric: Divide total daily dosage and adminis-

Table 26. Suggested Total Daily Dosage of Disopyramide in Children

Age (yr)	Dosage (mg/kg/day)
<1	10–30
1–4	10–20
4–12	10–15
12–18	6–15

ter equal doses q6h or at intervals according to patient's needs (Table 26). Hospitalize patients during initial treatment period; dose titration started at lower end of range.

Initial loading dose: When rapid control of ventricular arrhythmia is essential, an initial loading dose of 300 mg (200 mg for patients under 110 lb) is recommended. If there is no response or evidence of toxicity within 6 hours of loading dose, 200 mg q6h may be prescribed instead of usual 150 mg. If there is no response in 48 hours, discontinue drug or monitor patient for subsequent doses of 250 mg or 300 mg q6h.

Severe refractory tachycardia: A limited number of patients have tolerated up to 1600 mg/day (400 mg q6h), resulting in plasma levels up to 9 mcg/ml. Patient should be hospitalized for close evaluation and continuous monitoring.

Cardiomyopathy: Loading dose not used. Initial dosage limited to 100 mg q6h. Subsequent dosage adjustments made gradually, with close monitoring for hypotension and CHF.

Use in renal failure: Initial and maintenance dosages based on creatinine clearance.

Use in hepatic failure: 100 mg q6h is recommended, with or without an initial loading dose of 200 mg.

Transfer to disopyramide: Disopyramide may be started using regular maintenance schedule without a loading dose 6 to 12 hours after last dose of quinidine sulfate or 3 to 6 hours after last dose of procainamide. When withdrawal of these drugs is likely to produce life-threatening arrhythmias, patient is usually hospitalized. When transferring to the controlled-release form, start the maintenance schedule of the controlled-release form 6 hours after the last dose of the immediate-release form.

NURSING IMPLICATIONS

HISTORY
See Appendix 4. Note family history of glaucoma.

PHYSICAL ASSESSMENT
Record vital signs including apical rate, weight. Review chart for recent diagnostic studies (*e.g.,* ECG, chest x-ray), laboratory tests. Baseline studies such as serum electrolytes and ECG are usually ordered. Renal- and hepatic-function tests as well as other appropriate studies may also be ordered. Any potassium deficit is corrected before instituting therapy.

ADMINISTRATION
Check apical and radial pulse rate before administration. Withhold drug if pulse is below 60/minute in adults or 80/minute in children (unless physician orders otherwise) and notify physician. Drug should also be withheld and physician notified if pulse is above 120/minute, there is a change in pulse rhythm or quality, or the rate significantly varies from previous pulse rates.

Pediatric administration: Pharmacist can prepare a 1 mg/ml to 10 mg/ml liquid suspension by adding content of capsule to cherry syrup. The resulting suspension is stable for 1 month and should be thoroughly shaken before measurement of each dose.

ONGOING ASSESSMENTS AND NURSING MANAGEMENT
Record blood pressure, pulse, and respirations q2h to q4h during initial therapy; take temperature q4h; observe for adverse effects; record weight; monitor intake and output (especially in those with CHF, renal or hepatic impairment, history of prostatic hypertrophy or other problem with voiding, cardiomyopathy, or those receiving cardiotonics).

CLINICAL ALERT: The most serious adverse reactions are hypotension and CHF (Appendix 6, section 6-9). Urinary retention is the most serious anticholinergic effect.

If hypotension occurs or CHF worsens, notify physician immediately because drug may be discontinued and later restarted at a lower dosage after cardiac compensation is established.

Hypotension may occur in a small percentage. Advise patient to make position changes slowly during early therapy.

Hypokalemia may decrease disopyramide's effectiveness and hyperkalemia may enhance its toxic effects (see Appendix 6, section 6-15). Observe for these symptoms and notify the physician should they occur.

Urinary retention may occur in either sex, but males with benign prostatic hypertrophy are at particular risk. Any decrease in the intake and output ratio is reported to the physician and the patient's abdomen palpated for evidence of bladder distention. Those not on measured intake and output should be assessed daily during first few weeks of therapy for evidence of possible urinary retention.

D

Some patients receiving this drug may be placed on a cardiac monitor to evaluate drug response or detect widening of the QRS interval or Q–T prolongation (see *Warnings*). If either of these is noted, contact physician immediately because drug may be discontinued.

Serum levels of disopyramide may be obtained. Therapeutic plasma levels of disopyramide free base are 2 mcg/ml to 6 mcg/ml. Levels above 9 mcg/ml are usually toxic. Notify physician immediately if plasma level exceeds 6 mcg/ml because dosage may be reduced or one or more doses omitted.

Dry mouth may be relieved by sips of water, hard candy, or gum. The physician may allow use of a saliva substitute (p 957) if condition persists.

Rarely, significant lowering of blood glucose has been reported. Observe patient for signs of hypoglycemia (Appendix 6, section 6-14) and, if it is evident, report findings to physician before next dose is due.

Periodic laboratory tests may include serum electrolytes, renal- and hepatic-function tests, fasting blood glucose.

PATIENT AND FAMILY INFORMATION

Photosensitivity may occur. Avoid exposure to ultraviolet light and prolonged exposure to sunlight.

Follow the dosage schedule printed on the drug container. Do not omit or increase a dose or stop the medication except on advice of a physician.

Do not take any nonprescription drug (especially cold or cough preparations) without first checking with physician.

May cause dry mouth, difficult urination, constipation, or blurred vision. Notify physician or nurse if these persist.

If dizziness, fatigue, blurred vision, or muscle weakness occurs, do not attempt to drive or perform tasks requiring alertness.

Disulfiram Rx

tablets: 250 mg,   Antabuse, *Generic*
  500 mg

INDICATIONS

Aid in management of selected chronic alcoholic patients who want to remain in a state of enforced sobriety. Effectiveness in promoting abstinence is limited. The threat of illness as a result of alcohol ingestion is just as important as the action of the drug. Compliance with a disulfiram regimen and regular follow-up care has been shown to correlate with abstinence.

CONTRAINDICATIONS

Patients receiving or having recently received metronidazole, paraldehyde, alcohol, or alcohol-containing preparations should not receive disulfiram. Contraindicated in presence of severe myocardial disease or coronary occlusion, psychosis, or hypersensitivity.

ACTIONS

Provides a sensitivity to alcohol that results in a highly unpleasant reaction when patient under treatment ingests even small amounts of alcohol. It blocks oxidation of alcohol at the aldehyde stage. Concentration of acetaldehyde in blood may be 5 to 10 times higher than normal alcohol metabolism. Accumulation of acetaldehyde produces the complex of highly unpleasant symptoms referred to as the disulfiram-alcohol reaction, which will persist as long as alcohol is being metabolized. Disulfiram does not appear to influence the rate of alcohol elimination.

WARNINGS

Patient must be fully informed of the disulfiram-alcohol reaction and cautioned against the consequences of drinking while taking this drug.

Disulfiram-alcohol reaction: Disulfiram plus alcohol (even small amounts) produces flushing, throbbing in head and neck, respiratory difficulty, nausea, copious vomiting, sweating, thirst, chest pain, palpitation, dypsnea, hyperventilation, tachycardia, hypotension, syncope, marked uneasiness, weakness, vertigo, blurred vision, and confusion. In severe reactions there may be respiratory depression, cardiovascular collapse, arrhythmias, myocardial infarction, acute congestive heart failure, unconsciousness, convulsions, and death. Intensity of the reaction is proportional to the amounts of disulfiram and alcohol ingested. Mild reactions may occur in sensitive individuals when blood alcohol concentration is as little as 5 mg/dl to 10 mg/dl. Symptoms are fully developed at 50 mg/dl and unconsciousness usually results when level reaches 125 mg/dl to 150 mg/dl. Duration of reaction varies from 30 to 60 minutes to several hours in more severe cases.

Disulfiram inhibits the metabolism, and thus enhances the carcinogenicity, of ethylene dibromide. Patients having environmental or occupational exposure to ethylene dibromide (which is used in leaded fuels, as a fumigant-insecticide, and as a nematocide) should not receive disulfiram.

Because of possibility of an accidental reaction, use with caution in those with diabetes mellitus, hypothyroidism, epilepsy, cerebral damage, chronic or acute nephritis, and hepatic cirrhosis or insufficiency. Safety for use in pregnancy is not established.

DRUG INTERACTIONS

Disulfiram decreases the rate at which certain drugs are metabolized and may increase serum levels and possibility of toxicity. Decreases plasma clearance of **diazepam** and **chlordiazepoxide.** The possibility of exaggerated clinical effects should be considered. When benzodiazepine therapy is indicated, oxazepam, alprazolam, or lorazepam may be more appropriate because they have short half-lives and are not metabolized to active metabolites.

Use with caution in those receiving **phenytoin** and its congeners, since concomitant therapy can lead to phenytoin intoxication. Before administering disulfiram to a patient on phenytoin therapy, a baseline phenytoin serum level is recommended. After initiation of therapy, serum levels of phenytoin are obtained on different days for evidence of an increase in levels; dosage is adjusted accordingly.

It may be necessary to adjust dosage of **oral anticoagulants** on beginning or stopping disulfiram, because disulfiram may prolong prothrombin time. Patients taking **isoniazid** should be observed for appearance of unsteady gait or marked changes in behavior; discontinue disulfiram if such signs appear. Patients taking **metronidazole** may exhibit acute toxic psychosis in combination with disulfiram. See _Warnings_ for **alcohol**-disulfiram reaction.

PRECAUTIONS

Alcoholism may accompany or be followed by dependence on narcotics or sedatives. Barbiturates have been administered with disulfiram without untoward effects, but the possibility of initiating a new abuse should be considered.

ADVERSE REACTIONS

Optic neuritis, peripheral neuritis, and polyneuritis may occur. Peripheral neuropathies have been reported. Occasional skin eruptions are usually controlled with antihistamines. In a small number of patients transient mild drowsiness, fatigability, impotence, headache, acneiform eruptions, allergic dermatitis, or a metallic or garliclike aftertaste may be experienced during first 2 weeks of therapy. These usually disappear with continued therapy or reduced dosage.

DOSAGE

Initial dosage schedule: 500 mg/day in single dose for 1 to 2 weeks.

Maintenance regimen: Average dose is 250 mg/day (range 125 mg–500 mg), not to exceed 500 mg/day.

Duration of therapy: Use must be continued until patient is fully recovered socially and a basis for permanent self-control is established. Therapy may be required for months or even years.

Trial with alcohol: The test reaction has been largely abandoned. Do not administer test reaction to a patient over 50. A clear, detailed, and convincing description of the reaction is sufficient in most cases. When test reaction is necessary, suggested procedure is as follows: After 1 to 2 weeks' therapy with 500 mg/day, 15 ml of 100 proof whiskey or equivalent is taken slowly. Test dose may be repeated once only, when patient is hospitalized and facilities are available.

NURSING IMPLICATIONS

HISTORY

Obtain alcohol history, including time of last drink taken; health history; allergy history; prescription and nonprescription drug history.

NOTE: History may or may not be reliable. When possible, obtain some or all of information from family. Review chart for recent psychological evaluation, patient's condition when admitted to inpatient or outpatient unit; review previous treatment records (when appropriate).

PHYSICAL ASSESSMENT

Record vital signs, weight. Evaluate general physical and mental status. Evaluation of mental status may include general appearance, orientation, affectivity and mood, thought content, memory, judgment, socialization, motor behavior. Baseline transaminase tests are suggested to detect any hepatic dysfunction that may result with therapy. CBC, SMA-12, and other laboratory tests relevant to individual patient may be ordered. Physician performs thorough physical and psychological examination prior to therapy.

ADMINISTRATION

May be given as whole tablet or crushed and mixed with liquid beverages.

If patient is suspected of not taking medication, crush tablet and mix well with a liquid beverage.

Do _not_ administer until patient has abstained from alcohol for at least 12 hours. If consumption of alcohol is suspected, withhold drug and contact physician.

ONGOING ASSESSMENTS AND NURSING MANAGEMENT

Without proper motivation and supportive therapy, disulfiram is not a cure for alcoholism.

Evaluate mental status (see _Physical Assess-_

ment, above) and compare to data base; write daily summary on chart. Observe for adverse reactions.

If drowsiness occurs, discuss with physician. Administration may be ordered for H.S. or dosage adjusted downward.

Occasional patients, while seemingly on adequate maintenance doses, report that they are able to drink alcoholic beverages with impunity and without any symptomatology. Such patients must be presumed to be disposing of their tablets in some manner without actually taking them. Until such patients have been reliably observed taking their daily tablets (preferably crushed and well mixed with liquid), it cannot be concluded that disulfiram is ineffective.

Psychotic reactions have occurred, attributable in most cases to high dosage, combined toxicity (with metronidazole or isoniazid), or unmasking of underlying psychosis. Notify physician immediately of any behavior changes.

Follow-up transaminase tests (10–14 days) are recommended to detect any hepatic dysfunction that may result with therapy. CBC and SMA-12 are recommended every 6 months.

Management of disulfiram-alcohol reaction: In severe reactions, institute supportive measures to restore blood pressure and treat shock. Other recommendations include oxygen or carbogen (95% oxygen, 5% carbon dioxide), vitamin C IV in massive doses (1 g), and ephedrine sulfate. Antihistamines have also been used IV. Monitor potassium levels, particularly in patients on digitalis, because hypokalemia has been reported.

PATIENT AND FAMILY INFORMATION

NOTE: Patient should be informed of serious nature of a disulfiram-alcohol reaction (see *Warnings*) and consequences of alcohol use. Physician or nurse may recommend Alcoholics Anonymous for the patient, Al-Anon for the family, or Alateen for teenage children of alcoholic parents. The family should also be advised that abuse of other drugs (*e.g.,* marijuana, tranquilizers, cocaine) has been known to occur in some individuals participating in an alcohol abstinence program.

Tablets may be crushed and added to liquid beverages; stir thoroughly before drinking.

Drug may cause a metallic or garliclike aftertaste during first 2 weeks of therapy.

Disulfiram should not be taken for at least 12 hours after ingestion of alcohol. A reaction may occur up to 2 weeks after discontinuation of disulfiram.

Avoid ingestion of alcohol in all forms, including beer, wine, liquor, cough mixtures, sauces, aftershave lotions, liniments, colognes, and so on. Read labels of all nonprescription drug products before use or, preferably, check with a pharmacist regarding alcohol content of preparation before purchase.

If drowsiness occurs, use caution when driving or performing other tasks requiring alertness.

Carry identification (such as Medic-Alert) indicating use of disulfiram; include phone numbers of physician or medical facility to be contacted if a reaction should occur. If unable to contact physician or medical facility, patient should be taken to nearest hospital for treatment.

Dobutamine Rx

injection: 250 mg/   Dobutrex
vial

INDICATIONS

For inotropic support in short-term treatment of adults with cardiac decompensation due to decreased contractility, resulting either from organic heart disease or from cardiac surgical procedures. In those who have atrial fibrillation with rapid ventricular response, a digitalis preparation is used before therapy with dobutamine is instituted.

Investigational use: Doses of 2 mcg/kg/minute and 7.75 mcg/kg/minute infused for 10 minutes each have been used in children with congenital heart disease undergoing diagnostic cardiac catheterization. Appears effective in augmenting cardiovascular function in children and no adverse effects were noted.

CONTRAINDICATIONS

Idiopathic hypertrophic subaortic stenosis (IHSS).

ACTIONS

Is chemically related to dopamine. Primary activity results from stimulation of $beta_1$ receptors of the heart while producing comparatively mild chronotropic, hypertensive, arrhythmogenic, and vasodilative effects. Has minor alpha (vasoconstrictor) and $beta_2$ (vasodilator) effects; these opposing effects minimize any direct vascular activity. Does not cause release of endogenous norepinephrine, as does dopamine.

In those with depressed cardiac function, both dobutamine and isoproterenol increase cardiac output to a similar degree. With dobutamine, the increase is usually not accompanied by marked increases in heart rate (although tachycardia is occasionally observed), and cardiac stroke volume is usually increased. In contrast, isoproterenol increases the cardiac index primarily by increasing the heart rate while stroke volume changes little or declines. Dobutamine produces less increase in heart rate and less decrease in peripheral vascular resistance for a given inotropic effect than does isoproterenol.

Facilitation of atrioventricular conduction has been observed in patients with atrial fibrillation. Systemic vascular resistance is usually decreased; occasionally, minimal vasoconstriction has been observed.

Onset of action is 1 to 2 minutes, but as much as 10 minutes may be required to obtain peak effect of a particular infusion rate. Plasma half-life is 2 minutes. Drug is excreted in the urine.

Most clinical experience with drug is short term (up to several hours' duration). In a limited number of patients studied for 24 to 72 hours, a persistent increase in cardiac output occurred in some, whereas the output of others returned toward baseline values.

WARNINGS

Increase in heart rate or blood pressure: May cause marked increase in heart rate or blood pressure, especially systolic pressure. Because drug facilitates atrioventricular conduction, those with atrial fibrillation are at risk of developing rapid ventricular response. Patients with preexisting hypertension appear to face an increased risk of developing an exaggerated pressor response.

Ectopic activity: May precipitate or exacerbate ventricular ectopic activity, but rarely has caused ventricular tachycardia.

Use in pregnancy: Use only when clearly needed and potential benefits outweigh the unknown hazards to the fetus.

Use in children: Safety and efficacy not established.

PRECAUTIONS

Not a substitute for replacement of blood, plasma, fluids, and electrolytes, which should be restored promptly when loss has occurred. Hypovolemia should be corrected with volume expanders before treatment is started. No improvement may be seen in presence of marked mechanical obstruction such as valvular aortic stenosis. Clinical experience in use following myocardial infarction is insufficient to establish safety of drug.

DRUG INTERACTIONS

Studies indicate concomitant use of dobutamine and **nitroprusside** results in a higher cardiac output

and, usually, a lower pulmonary wedge pressure than when either drug is used alone. **Cyclopropane** or **halogenated hydrocarbon anesthetics** may sensitize the myocardium to the effects of catecholamines. Use of vasopressors may lead to serious arrhythmias; use with extreme caution.

In obstetrics, if vasopressors are either used to correct hypotension or added to local anesthetic solutions, some **oxytocic drugs** may cause persistent hypertension; even rupture of a cerebral blood vessel may occur during the postpartum period.

The pressor effect of pressor amines is markedly potentiated in those receiving a **monoamine oxidase inhibitor (MAOI).** Use dobutamine with extreme caution and reduce initial dose to at least one tenth of usual dose, beginning with fractional (1/10) doses. Pressor effects may also be enhanced in patients taking **tricyclic antidepressants.** Insulin requirements may be increased by dobutamine.

ADVERSE REACTIONS

Increased heart rate, blood pressure, ventricular ectopic activity: A 10 mm Hg to 20 mm Hg increase in systolic blood pressure and an increase in heart rate of 5 to 15 beats/minute have been noted in most patients. See *Warnings* regarding exaggerated chronotropic and pressor effects. Approximately 5% of patients have had increased premature ventricular beats during infusions. These effects are dose related.

Miscellaneous (uncommon, 1%–3%): Nausea, headache, anginal pain, nonspecific chest pain, palpitations, shortness of breath.

Long-term safety: Infusions up to 72 hours have revealed no adverse effects other than those seen with shorter infusions.

OVERDOSAGE

Symptoms: Excessive alteration of blood pressure or tachycardia.

Treatment: Reduce rate of administration or temporarily discontinue until condition stabilizes. Because duration of action is short, usually no additional measures are necessary.

DOSAGE

Rate of administration: Rate of infusion needed to increase cardiac output usually ranges from 2.5 mcg/kg/minute to 10 mcg/kg/minute. Rarely, infusion rates up to 40 mcg/kg/minute have been required.

Concentrations up to 5000 mcg/ml (250 mg/50 ml) have been administered. Final volume administered is determined by fluid requirements of patient. See *Administration.*

NURSING IMPLICATIONS

HISTORY
Review chart for diagnosis, health history, allergy history, recent treatment modalities, and diagnostic tests.

PHYSICAL ASSESSMENT
Record general status of patient, blood pressure, pulse, respirations, weight. Review chart for physician's assessments.

ADMINISTRATION
Cardiac monitor is attached.

A CVP line or Swan-Ganz catheter is recommended.

The Swan-Ganz (4-lumen) catheter is used to measure pulmonary artery wedge pressure and cardiac output (by thermodilution method). A CVP line is used to measure central venous pressure.

An indwelling catheter may be inserted to measure urine flow.

A blood pressure cuff is applied to arm. Obtain blood pressure and pulse rate immediately before administration of drug.

Obtain central venous and/or pulmonary wedge pressure prior to administration. Cardiac output may also be obtained at this time.

Patients with atrial fibrillation are usually given a digitalis preparation before administration of dobutamine.

Hypovolemia, if present, is corrected before treatment is instituted.

Preparation of solution: Reconstitute with Sterile Water for Injection or 5% Dextrose Injection by adding 10 ml of diluent to 250-mg vial. If material is not completely dissolved, add an additional 10 ml of diluent. Store reconstituted solution under refrigeration for 48 hours or at room temperature for 6 hours.

Reconstituted solution must be further diluted to at least 50 ml before administration in 5% Dextrose Injection, 0.9% Sodium Chloride Injection, or Sodium Lactate Injection.

Physician orders IV solution for administration and rate of infusion. Dosage is based on weight (kg).

Rate of infusion may be slowed or infusion temporarily discontinued if signs of overdosage occur. Usually a volume-control set used to administer drug. See Table 27 for recommended infusion rates.

Admixture incompatibility: Incompatible with alkaline solutions; do not mix with products such as 5% Sodium Bicarbonate Injection. Also physically incompatible with hydrocortisone sodium succinate, cefazolin, cefamandole, neutral cephalothin, penicillin, sodium ethacrynate, and sodium heparin.

Admixture compatibility: Compatible when administered through common tubing with dopamine, lidocaine, tobramycin, nitroprusside, potassium chloride, or protamine sulfate.

Stability: After dilution (in glass or Viaflex containers), solution is stable for 24 hours at room temperature. Use IV solutions within 24 hours. Solutions containing dobutamine may exhibit a color that, if present, will increase with time. Color change is due to slight oxidation of drug but there is no significant loss of potency. Freezing is not recommended because of possible crystallization.

ONGOING ASSESSMENTS AND NURSING MANAGEMENT
The rate of administration and duration of therapy are adjusted according to patient response.

Patient response is determined by heart rate,

Table 27. Recommended Infusion Rates for Desired Delivery Rates of Dobutamine

Desired Delivery Rate (mcg/kg/min)	Infusion Rate (ml/kg/min)		
	250 mcg/ml*	500 mcg/ml†	1000 mcg/ml‡
2.5	0.01	0.005	0.0025
5.0	0.02	0.01	0.005
7.5	0.03	0.015	0.0075
10.0	0.04	0.02	0.01
12.5	0.05	0.025	0.0125
15.0	0.06	0.03	0.015

* 250 mg/liter of diluent
† 500 mg/liter or 250 mg/500 ml of diluent
‡ 1000 mg/liter or 250 mg/250 ml of diluent

presence of ectopic activity, blood pressure, urine flow, and whenever possible measurement of central venous or pulmonary wedge pressure and cardiac output.

Obtain blood pressure every 1 to 2 minutes or as ordered.

ECG and heart rate are monitored continuously (cardiac monitor).

Urinary output is measured every 15 to 30 minutes or as ordered.

Central venous and/or pulmonary wedge pressure is obtained every 15 minutes or as ordered. If performed, physician orders specific intervals for measuring cardiac output.

Dobutamine may cause a marked increase in heart rate or blood pressure, especially systolic pressure (see *Warnings*). Physician will specify upper limits of these parameters, with infusion rate adjusted accordingly.

The pulmonary artery wedge pressure approximates the left ventricular end-diastolic pressure and is elevated in cardiogenic shock. Pulmonary artery wedge pressure is normally between 4.5 mm Hg and 13 mm Hg.

Insulin requirements in diabetics may be increased by dobutamine. Monitor urine glucose and ketones q4h or as ordered.

Dobutamine plasma levels may be obtained. Therapeutic levels are between 40 ng/ml and 190 ng/ml.

Treatment is terminated when patient is stabilized or drug administration is ineffective.

Docusate Calcium, Sodium, Potassium

See Laxatives.

Dopamine Hydrochloride Rx

injection: 80 mg/ 100 ml, 160 mg/ 100 ml, 320 mg/ 100 ml	Dopamine HCl in 5% Dextrose
injection: 40 mg/ml	Dopastat, Intropin, *Generic*
injection: 80 mg/ml	Intropin, *Generic*
injection: 160 mg/ml	Intropin

INDICATIONS

Correction of hemodynamic imbalances present in the shock syndrome due to myocardial infarction, trauma, endotoxic septicemia, open heart surgery, renal failure, and chronic cardiac decompensation as in congestive heart failure. Patients most likely to respond adequately are those in whom physiological parameters such as urine flow, myocardial function, and blood pressure have not profoundly deteriorated. The shorter the time between onset of signs and symptoms of shock and initiation of therapy with volume correction and dopamine, the better the prognosis.

CONTRAINDICATIONS

Pheochromocytoma, tachyarrhythmias, ventricular fibrillation.

ACTIONS

Is an endogenous catecholamine and a precursor of norepinephrine. Acts both directly and indirectly (releases norepinephrine stores) on alpha and beta$_1$ receptors and has dopaminergic effects. Beta$_1$ actions produce an inotropic effect on the myocardium, resulting in increased cardiac output. Causes less increase in myocardial oxygen consumption than isoproterenol and is usually not associated with a tachyarrhythmia. Systolic and pulse pressure usually increase with either no effect or slight increase in diastolic pressure. Total peripheral resistance at low and intermediate doses is usually unchanged. Blood flow to peripheral vascular beds may decrease while mesenteric flow increases. Dopamine dilates the renal and splanchnic vasculature presumptively by activation of a dopaminergic receptor. This is accompanied by increases in glomerular filtration rate, renal blood flow, and sodium excretion. An increase in urinary output is usually not associated with a decrease in urine osmolarity.

When administered before urine flow has diminished to levels approximately 0.3 ml/minute, prognosis is more favorable. In oliguric or anuric patients, administration has resulted in an increase in urine flow, which has reached normal levels. May also increase urine flow in those whose output is within normal limits, reducing preexisting fluid accumulation. Increased cardiac output is related to direct inotropic effect on the myocardium and, at low or moderate doses, appears to be related to a favorable prognosis.

Has an onset of action within 2 to 4 minutes and a duration of less than 10 minutes. Is metabolized to homovanillic acid and other metabolites; very little is excreted as unchanged dopamine.

WARNINGS

Drug may be used in pregnant women when expected benefits outweigh potential risk to the fetus. Safety and efficacy for use in children not established.

PRECAUTIONS

Hypovolemia: Not a substitute for replacement of blood, plasma, fluids, and electrolytes, which are restored promptly when loss occurs.

Decreased pulse pressure: If a disproportionate rise in the diastolic pressure (a marked decrease in pulse pressure) occurs, decrease infusion rate and observe for further evidence of predominant vasoconstriction, unless such effect is desired.

Occlusive vascular disease: Closely monitor those with history of occlusive vascular disease (*e.g.,* atherosclerosis, arterial embolism, Raynaud's disease, cold injury, frostbite, diabetic endarteritis, Buerger's disease) for any changes in color or temperature of the extremities. If change occurs and is thought to be the result of compromised circulation to the extremities, benefits of continued use are weighed against possible necrosis. This condition can be reversed by either decreasing the infusion rate or discontinuing the drug.

DRUG INTERACTIONS

Those treated with **monoamine oxidase (MAO) inhibitors** before administration of dopamine will require substantially reduced dosage. Dopamine is metabolized by MAO; inhibition of this enzyme prolongs and potentiates the effect of dopamine. Starting dose should be reduced to at least one tenth of the usual dose. Pressor response to adrenergic agents may be potentiated by **tricyclic antidepressants.**

Concurrent administration with **diuretic agents** may produce an additive or potentiating effect. **Cyclopropane** or **halogenated hydrocarbon anesthetics** may sensitize the myocardium to the action of IV catecholamines; this appears to be related both to pressor activity and to beta-adrenergic stimulating properties of catecholamines. In obstetrics, if vasopressor drugs are used to correct hypotension or added to the local anesthetic solution, some **oxytocic drugs** may cause severe persistent hypertension. Rupture of a cerebral blood vessel may occur during the postpartum period.

Concomitant infusion of dopamine and **phenytoin** has been reported to lead to seizures, hypotension, and bradycardia. An alternative to phenytoin is recommended if anticonvulsant therapy is needed.

The effects of **beta-adrenergic agents** can be reversed by dopamine.

ADVERSE REACTIONS

Most frequent: Ectopic beats, nausea, vomiting, tachycardia, anginal pain, palpitation, dyspnea, headache, hypotension, vasoconstriction.

Infrequent: Aberrant conduction, bradycardia, piloerection, widened QRS complex, azotemia, elevated blood pressure.

High doses reported to cause dilated pupils.

OVERDOSAGE

Symptoms: Manifested by excessive blood pressure elevation.

Treatment: Reduce rate of administration or temporarily discontinue until condition stabilized. Duration of action is short and no additional measures are usually necessary. If these measures fail to stabilize patient's condition, phentolamine may be given.

DOSAGE

Rate of administration: After dilution, administer IV. A metering device is essential for controlling rate of flow. Titrate drug to desired hemodynamic or renal response. In titrating to the desired increase in systolic blood pressure, optimum dosage rate for renal response may be exceeded, necessitating a reduction in rate after hemodynamic condition has stabilized. Administration at rates greater than 50 mcg/kg/minute have been used in advanced circulatory decompensation states.

Suggested regimen: Begin administration at 2 mcg/kg/minute to 5 mcg/kg/minute for those likely to respond to modest increments of cardiac contractility and renal perfusion. In more seriously ill patients, begin administration at 5 mcg/kg/minute and increase gradually using 5- to 10-mcg/kg/minute increments, up to rate of 20 mcg/kg/minute to 50 mcg/kg/minute as needed. In patients not responding to these doses, additional increments may be used.

See *Administration.*

NURSING IMPLICATIONS

HISTORY

Review chart for diagnosis, health history, allergy history, recent treatment modalities, and diagnostic tests.

PHYSICAL ASSESSMENT

Record general status of patient, blood pressure, pulse, respirations, weight. Review chart for physician's assessments.

ADMINISTRATION

CVP line and/or Swan-Ganz catheter may be inserted before administration of dopamine. When appropriate, blood volume may be increased with whole blood or plasma until CVP is 10 cm to 15 cm water or pulmonary wedge pressure 14 mm Hg to 18 mm Hg.

Urinary output is usually monitored closely; an indwelling catheter may be ordered.

Cardiac monitor may be used to detect tachycardia, development of dysrhythmias.

This is a potent drug; dilute before use if not prediluted. The prediluted forms are labeled 80 mg/100 ml and 160 mg/100 ml.

CAUTION: *Labeling similarities*—80 mg/ml and 80 mg/100 ml; 160 mg/ml and 160 mg/100 ml.

Keep covered in box until ready to use (*i.e.,* dilute or add to IV infusion).

Use a metering device such as a Microdrip. This is essential for controlling rate of flow. An IV line with a secondary port allowing the administration of primary and secondary solutions should be used. Dopamine should be administered as a secondary solution.

Use large vein for venipuncture to prevent extravasation. Large veins of the antecubital fossa are preferred to veins in the hand or ankle.

The physician orders dose of drug; infusion rate and/or guidelines for adjusting rate of infusion; and type and amount of IV fluids to be used in the primary and secondary lines. The primary line is used to administer IV solutions or other drugs before and after administration of dopamine.

Obtain blood pressure, pulse, and respirations before administration of infusion containing dopamine.

Preparation of solution: Add 200 mg to 400 mg dopamine to 250 ml to 500 ml of one of the following IV solutions: Sodium Chloride Injection, USP; 5% Dextrose Injection, USP; 5% Dextrose and 0.9% Sodium Chloride Injection, USP; 5% Dextrose in 0.45% Sodium Chloride, USP; 5% Dextrose in Lactated Ringer's Solution; Sodium Lactate (⅙ Molar) Injection, USP; Lactated Ringer's Injection, USP.

Commonly used concentrations are 800 mcg/ml (200 mg in 250 ml) and 1600 mcg/ml (400 mg in 250 ml).

The 160 mg/100 ml concentrate may be preferred in those with fluid retention or when a slower rate of infusion is desired.

Stability: Solution is stable for 24 hours after dilution but manufacturer recommends diluting just before administration.

Admixture incompatibilities: Do not mix dopamine infusions with other drugs. *Do not* add to 5% Sodium Bicarbonate or other alkaline IV solutions, oxidizing agents, or iron salts because

drug is inactivated in an alkaline solution (solutions become pink to violet).

Storage: Protect from light. Store at room temperature 15°C to 30°C (59°F–86°F).

ONGOING ASSESSMENTS AND NURSING MANAGEMENT

Monitor blood pressure and pulse q2m to q5m or as ordered; measure urine output q15m or as ordered; check sign color q15m; check temperature in toes q15m; observe for adequacy of nailbed capillary filling q15m; check peripheral pulse q15m. Record all observations and monitoring parameters on flow sheet.

CLINICAL ALERT: Continually observe for signs of extravasation of IV fluid. Monitor infusion site closely for free flow. If extravasation occurs, follow procedure outlined by physician or hospital policy (see also below).

Before administration of dobutamine, physician should establish guidelines for treatment of extravasation. Manufacturer recommends infiltration of area as soon as possible with 10 ml to 15 ml saline solution containing 5 mg to 10 mg phentolamine using a syringe with a fine hypodermic needle to infiltrate liberally throughout ischemic area.

If extravasation should occur, IV should be immediately discontinued and another IV line established as soon as possible. Follow hospital or unit policy or physician's orders about intervention if extravasation occurs.

Loss of pallor, increase in temperature of toes, and adequacy of nailbed capillary filling may be used as indices of adequate dosage.

Check level of consciousness and observe for signs of reversal of confusion or comatose condition; record findings.

Urine flow is reported to be one of the better monitoring parameters of vital organ perfusion.

If doses in excess of 16 mcg/kg/minute are used, check urine output frequently. If urine flow decreases in absence of hypotension, reduce infusion rate and contact physician.

If there is a rise in diastolic pressure, infusion rate should be slowed and patient observed closely. Notify physician immediately and monitor blood pressure q1m to q2m with particular attention to changes in the diastolic pressure.

Also notify the physician immediately if any of the following occurs: decrease in urinary output; rapid increase in urinary output; tachycardia or cardiac dysrhythmia; signs of peripheral vasoconstriction (pallor, cyanosis, mottling, cool or cold extremities, lack of peripheral pulses); development of adverse reactions (see *Adverse Reactions, Most frequent*).

If vomiting should occur, suctioning may be necessary to prevent aspiration.

Doxapram Hydrochloride Rx

injection: 20 mg/ml   Dopram

INDICATIONS

Postanesthesia: When possibilities of airway obstruction and hypoxia have been eliminated, may be used to stimulate respiration in those with drug-induced postanesthesia respiratory depression or apnea other than that due to muscle relaxant drugs. May also be used to stimulate deep breathing in the "stir-up" regimen in postoperative patient. Simultaneous administration of oxygen is desirable.

Drug-induced CNS depression: May be used to stimulate respiration, hasten arousal and encourage return of laryngopharyngeal reflexes in those with mild to moderate respiratory and CNS depression due to overdosage.

NOTE: Respiratory depression due to overdosage of CNS depressants is best managed by mechanical ventilatory support.

Chronic pulmonary disease associated with acute hypercapnia: Indicated as a temporary measure in hospitalized patients with acute respiratory insufficiency superimposed on chronic obstructive pulmonary disease. Used for short period of time (approximately 2 hours) as an aid in prevention of elevation of arterial CO_2 tension during administration of oxygen. Not used in conjunction with mechanical ventilation.

CONTRAINDICATIONS

Epilepsy or other convulsive states; incompetence of the ventilatory mechanism due to muscle paresis, flail chest, pneumothorax, airway obstruction, extreme dyspnea; severe hypertension or cerebrovascular accidents; hypersensitivity; head injury.

Pulmonary disease: Suspected or confirmed pulmonary embolism, pneumothorax, acute bronchial asthma, respiratory failure due to neuromuscular disorders, restrictive diseases such as pulmonary fibrosis.

Cardiovascular disease: Coronary artery disease; frank uncompensated heart failure.

ACTIONS

Produces respiratory stimulation mediated through the peripheral carotid chemoreceptors. As dosage level is increased, central respiratory centers in the medulla are stimulated with progressive stimulation of other parts of the brain and spinal cord. A pressor response, due to improved cardiac output, may occur. If there is no impairment of cardiac function, the pressor effect is greater in hypovolemic than in normovolemic states. Although opiate-induced respiratory depression is antagonized by doxapram, analgesia is not affected.

Onset of respiratory stimulation following recommended single IV dose usually occurs in 20 to 40 seconds, with peak effect at 1 to 2 minutes. The duration of effect may vary from 5 to 12 minutes.

WARNINGS

Postanesthetic use: Not an antagonist to muscle relaxants or a specific narcotic antagonist. Administer with care to those with cerebral edema, history of bronchial asthma, severe tachycardia, cardiac arrhythmia, cardiac disease, hyperthyroidism, pheochromocytoma.

Drug-induced CNS and respiratory depression: Doxapram alone may not stimulate adequate spontaneous breathing or provide sufficient arousal in those severely depressed due to either respiratory failure or CNS depressant drugs. Should be used as an adjunct to established supportive measures.

Chronic obstructive pulmonary disease: In an attempt to lower pCO_2, rate of infusion is not increased in severely ill patients because of associated increased work in breathing.

Use in pregnancy: Safety not established. Used only when clearly needed and potential benefits outweight the unknown potential hazards to the fetus.

Use in children: Not recommended for children 12 years and under.

PRECAUTIONS

Lowered pCO_2—induced hyperventilation produces cerebral vasoconstriction and slowing of cerebral circulation.

Blood pressure increases are generally modest, but significant increases have been noted in some patients.

Postanesthetic use: In some patients who have received muscle relaxants, doxapram may temporarily mask residual effects of muscle relaxant drugs.

Chronic obstructive pulmonary disease: Arrhythmias seen in some patients in acute respiratory failure secondary to chronic obstructive pulmonary disease are probably the result of hypoxia. Use drug with caution in these patients. Arterial blood gases should be drawn before initiation of doxapram infusion and oxygen administration and at least q½h thereafter. Use of doxapram does not lessen need for careful monitoring and supplemental oxygen in those with acute respiratory failure. Discontinue use if arterial blood gases deteriorate and mechanical ventilation is initiated.

DRUG INTERACTIONS

Administer cautiously to those receiving **sympathomimetic** or **monoamine oxidase inhibiting drugs,** because additive pressor effect may occur. Because an increase in epinephrine release has been noted, it is recommended that initiation of therapy be delayed for at least 10 minutes following discontinuance of **anesthetics** known to sensitize the myocardium to catecholamines.

ADVERSE REACTIONS

Central and autonomic nervous systems:
Headache, dizziness, apprehension, disorientation, pupillary dilatation, hyperactivity, involuntary movements, convulsions, muscle spasticity, increased tendon reflexes, clonus, bilateral Babinski; pyrexia, flushing, sweating; pruritus and paresthesia such as feeling of warmth, burning, or hot sensation, especially in area of the genitalia and perineum.

Respiratory: Cough, dyspnea, tachypnea, laryngospasm, bronchospasm, hiccups, rebound hypoventilation.

Hematologic: Decrease in hemoglobin, hematocrit, or RBC has occurred in postoperative patients. In presence of leukopenia, a further decrease in WBC has occurred following anesthesia and treatment with doxapram. Elevations of BUN and proteinuria have also occurred.

Cardiovascular: Phlebitis, variations in heart rate, lowered T-waves, arrhythmias, chest pain, tightness in chest. A mild to moderate increase in blood pressure is commonly noted but is of concern only in hypertensive patients.

GI: Nausea, vomiting, diarrhea, desire to defecate.

GU: Urinary retention, spontaneous voiding.

OVERDOSAGE

Excessive pressor effect, tachycardia, skeletal muscle hyperactivity, and enhanced deep tendon reflexes may be early signs of overdosage. Blood pressure, pulse rate, and deep tendon reflexes should be evaluated periodically and dosage or infusion rate adjusted accordingly. Convulsive seizures are unlikely at recommended dosages, but IV anticonvulsants, oxygen, and resuscitative equipment should be available.

DOSAGE

Postanesthetic use: May be administered as single IV injection of 0.5 mg/kg to 1 mg/kg, not to exceed 1.5 mg/kg or 2 mg/kg when given as multiple injections at 5-minute intervals.

May be administered by infusion of 250 mg doxapram in 250 ml of dextrose or saline solution (1 mg/ml). Infusion rate is initiated at approximately 5 mg/minute (5 ml/minute) until satisfactory response is seen. Maintain rate at 1 mg/minute to 3 mg/minute, (1 ml/minute to 3 ml/minute), and adjust to sustain desired level of respiratory stimulation with minimal side-effects. Recommended maximum dosage by infusion is 4 mg/kg, not to exceed 3 g.

Management of drug-induced CNS depression:
For intermittent injection use single or repeat single IV injections. Give priming dose of 1 mg/lb (2 mg/kg); repeat in 5 minutes. Repeat same dose q1h to q2h until patient awakens. Watch for relapse into unconsciousness or development of respiratory depression, because doxapram does not affect the metabolism of CNS depressant drugs. If relapse occurs, q1h to q2h injections are resumed until arousal is sustained or total maximum daily dose (3 g) is given. Allow patient to sleep for 24 hours after first injection, using assisted or automatic respiration if needed. Repeat procedure until patient breathes spontaneously and sustains desired level of consciousness or maximum daily dose is given. Repetitive doses are administered only when response is shown to initial dose.

For intermittent IV infusion, give priming dose as above. If patient awakens, watch for relapse; if there is no response, continue supportive treatment for 1 to 2 hours and repeat doxapram. If some respiratory stimulation occurs, give IV infusion of 250 mg (12.5 ml) in 250 ml of saline or dextrose. This dilution gives 1 mg/ml. Administer at 1 mg/minute to 3 mg/minute (60 ml/hour to 80 ml/hour) according to patient size and depth of coma. Discontinue use at end of 2 hours or if patient begins to awaken.

Continue supportive treatment for ½ to 2 hours and repeat steps; do not exceed 3 g.

Chronic obstructive pulmonary disease associated with acute hypercapnia: Mix 400 mg in 180 ml of IV solution (2 mg/ml) and start infusion at 1 mg/minute to 2 mg/minute (0.5 ml/minute to 1 ml/minute). If indicated, increase to 3 mg/minute. Additional infusions beyond the maximum 2-hour administration period are not recommended.

NURSING IMPLICATIONS

HISTORY

Review chart for probable cause of respiratory depression, previous treatment modalities (if any), health history.

PHYSICAL ASSESSMENT

Obtain blood pressure, pulse, and respirations. Obtain weight from chart. Arterial blood gases may be ordered before institution of therapy and recommended for those with chronic pulmonary obstructive disease.

ADMINISTRATION

An adequate airway and oxygenation must be assured before administration.

May be administered by intermittent IV injection or infusion.

For administration by IV infusion, physician orders IV solution and rate of infusion. See *Dosage* for details.

If administering by intermittent IV infusion, use an IV line with a piggyback port or a secondary port.

IV short-acting barbiturates, oxygen, and resuscitative equipment should be available to manage overdosage manifested by excessive CNS stimulation.

If arterial blood gases are to be drawn q½h, inform laboratory before IV administration of doxapram is initiated.

Compatibilities: Doxapram is compatible with 5% and 10% Dextrose in water or normal saline. Admixture with alkaline solutions such as 2.5% thiopental sodium or sodium bicarbonate will result in precipitation.

ONGOING ASSESSMENTS AND NURSING MANAGEMENT

Monitor level of consciousness and rate and depth of respirations continuously when administering for CNS depression (drug induced or postanesthesia).

Monitor blood pressure, pulse, respirations, and deep tendon reflexes q10m to q15m or as ordered.

Check IV rate of infusion q5m to q10m.

Arterial blood gases are recommended q½h for those with chronic obstructive pulmonary disease with acute hypercapnia.

Blood pressure, pulse, respiratory rate, deep tendon reflexes, and arterial blood gases are used to determine effective dosage and identify overdosage. Use flow sheet to record observations.

Keep physician informed of patient response because increase or decrease in infusion rate or repeat of single injections may be necessary.

CLINICAL ALERT: If sudden hypotension or dyspnea develops, discontinue infusion and notify physician. Run primary IV line to KVO until physician examines patient.

Avoid vascular extravasation or use of a single injection site over an extended period; either may lead to thrombophlebitis or local skin irritation. Rapid IV infusion may result in hemolysis.

Exercise care to prevent vomiting and aspira-

tion when administering for CNS depression. Have suction machine available should vomiting occur.

Because narcosis may recur after stimulation with doxapram, postanesthetic patients should be observed until fully alert for ½ to 1 hour.

Doxepin Hydrochloride

See Antidepressants, Tricyclic Compounds.

Doxorubicin Hydrochloride (ADR) Rx

injection: 10 mg/vial,   Adriamycin
    50 mg/vial

INDICATIONS

Has been used to produce regression in acute lymphoblastic leukemia, acute myeloblastic leukemia, Wilms' tumor, neuroblastoma, soft-tissue and bone sarcomas, breast carcinoma, ovarian carcinoma, transitional cell bladder carcinoma, lymphomas of both Hodgkin's and non-Hodgkin's types, and bronchiogenic carcinoma. A number of other solid tumors have also shown some responsiveness.

CONTRAINDICATIONS

Should not be started in those with marked myelosuppression induced by previous treatment with other antiblastic agents or radiotherapy. Conclusive data are not available on preexisting heart disease as a cofactor of increased risk of drug-induced toxicity. Data suggest that in such cases cardiac toxicity may occur in doses lower than the recommended cumulative limit and drug is not recommended in such cases. Treatment is also contraindicated in those who have received previous treatment with complete cumulative doses of doxorubicin or daunorubicin.

ACTIONS

Is a cytotoxic anthracycline antibiotic isolated from cultures of *Streptomyces peucetius.* Although not completely understood, mechanism of action is related to drug's ability to bind to DNA and inhibit nucleic acid synthesis. IV administration is followed by rapid plasma clearance and significant tissue binding. Urinary excretion accounts for approximately 4% to 5% of the administered dose in 5 days. Biliary excretion represents the major excretion route; 40% to 50% of administered dose is recovered in bile and feces in 7 days. Impairment of hepatic function slows excretion and consequently increases retention and accumulation in plasma and tissues. Drug does not cross the blood–brain barrier.

WARNINGS

Myelosuppression: There is high incidence of bone-marrow depression, primarily of leukocytes. With recommended dosage schedule, leukopenia is usually transient. WBC counts as low as $1000/mm^3$ are to be expected during treatment with appropriate doses. RBC and platelet levels may also be depressed. Hematologic toxicity may require dose reduction or suspension or delay of therapy. Persistent severe myelosuppression may result in superinfection or hemorrhage.

Cardiac toxicity: Although uncommon, acute left ventricular failure has occurred, particularly in those who have received total dosage exceeding the recommended limit of 550 mg/m². This limit appears to be lower in those who received radiotherapy to the mediastinal area. Total dose administered should also take into account any previous or concomitant therapy with other potentially cardiotoxic agents such as cyclophosphamide or related compounds such as daunorubicin. Congestive heart failure (CHF) or cardiomyopathy may occur several weeks after discontinuation of drug and is often not favorably affected by presently known medical or physical therapy for cardiac support.

Early diagnosis of drug-induced CHF appears to be essential for successful treatment with digitalis, diuretics, low-salt diet, and bedrest. Severe cardiac toxicity may occur precipitously without antecedent ECG changes. Transient ECG changes such as T-wave flattening, S–T depression, and arrhythmias are not presently considered indications for suspension of therapy. Cardiomyopathy has been reported to be associated with persistent reduction in voltage of the QRS wave, a prolongation of the systolic time interval, and reduction of the ejection fraction. Acute life-threatening arrhythmias have been reported to occur during or within a few hours of administration.

Use in impaired hepatic function: Toxicity to recommended doses is enhanced by hepatic impairment. Evaluation of hepatic function is recommended before individual dosing.

Use in pregnancy: Safety not established. Use only when clearly needed and when potential benefits outweigh potential hazards to the fetus.

PRECAUTIONS

Initial treatment requires close observation of patient and extensive laboratory monitoring. Drug may induce hyperuricemia secondary to rapid lysis of neoplastic cells.

DRUG INTERACTIONS

May potentiate toxicity of other anticancer therapies. Exacerbation of **cyclophosphamide**-induced hemorrhagic cystitis and enhancement of hepatotoxicity of **6-mercaptopurine** have been reported. **Radiation**-induced toxicity to the myocardium, mucosa, skin, and liver have reportedly been increased by administration of doxorubicin.

ADVERSE REACTIONS

Dose-limiting toxicities are myelosuppression and cardiotoxicity. Other reactions are the following.

Cutaneous: Reversible, complete alopecia occurs in most cases. Hyperpigmentation of nailbeds and dermal creases, primarily in children, has been reported. Recall of skin reaction due to prior radiotherapy has occurred.

GI: Acute nausea and vomiting occur frequently and may be severe. Mucositis may occur 5 to 10 days after administration and may be severe, leading to ulceration and a site of origin for severe infections. Incidence and severity of mucositis is greater with the regimen of three successive daily dosages. Anorexia and diarrhea have occasionally been reported.

Vascular: Phlebosclerosis has been reported, especially when small veins are used or a single vein is used for repeated administration. Facial flushing may occur if injection is given too rapidly.

Local: Severe cellulitis, vesication, and tissue necrosis will occur if drug extravasates during administration. Erythematous streaking along the vein proximal to the site of injection has been reported.

Hypersensitivity: Fever, chills, and urticaria have been reported. Anaphylaxis may occur.

Other: Conjunctivitis and lacrimation (rare).

DOSAGE

Recommended dosage schedule: 60 mg/m² to 75 mg/m² as single IV injection administered at 21-day intervals. Lower dose is recommended for those with inadequate marrow reserves due to old age, prior therapy, or neoplastic marrow infiltration.

Alternate dosage schedule: 30 mg/m² on each of 3 successive days repeated every 4 weeks.

Dosage in patients with elevated bilirubin: ½ to ¼ the normal dose.

Combination therapy: Drug has been used in combination therapy (see Appendix 10).

NURSING IMPLICATIONS

HISTORY

See Appendix 4.

PHYSICAL ASSESSMENT

Record physical, emotional status; vital signs; weight. Baseline studies may include hepatic-function studies, serum uric acid, CBC, and platelet count. An ECG may also be performed.

ADMINISTRATION

An antiemetic may be ordered before administration of drug.

A Kold Kap or scalp tourniquet may be used to prevent alopecia. An outpatient may have purchased his own cap, which is brought to the physician's office or clinic for each treatment in a cold state (placing the cap in a small foam cooler keeps it cold). The cap is put into place just before injection of the drug and may be left in place approximately 1 hour, or as directed by the physician, after the drug is injected. The outpatient may wear his cap while returning home.

Physician orders dose, IV solution. Other administration instructions may include running the IV solution after administration of drug to flush tubing and steps to be taken if extravasation occurs.

IV line should be attached to a Butterfly needle inserted into a large vein. If possible, veins in extremities with compromised venous or lymphatic drainage are avoided. If there is a question about which vein to use, discuss with physician.

It is recommended that drug be administered slowly into tubing of a freely running IV infusion of Sodium Chloride Injection, USP or 5% Dextrose Injection, USP.

CLINICAL ALERT: Determine patency of IV line and correct placement of needle in vein before attempting to administer doxorubicin. *Do not administer drug if there is any question regarding correct placement of the IV needle because tissue necrosis may occur.*

Rate of administration depends on size of vein and dosage, but dose should be administered in not less than 3 to 5 minutes.

Local erythematous streaking along the vein as well as facial flushing may be indicative of too-rapid administration.

Instruct patient to mention immediately if burning is felt at injection site.

A burning or stinging sensation may be indicative of perivenous infiltration and the infusion should be *immediately terminated* and restarted in another vein.

NOTE: Perivenous infiltration may occur painlessly. It also may occur even if blood returns well on aspiration of the infusion needle. Notify physician immediately if extravasation occurs or is suspected.

If it is known or suspected that subcutaneous extravasation has occurred, local infiltration with an injectable corticosteroid and flooding of the site with normal saline have been reported to lessen local reaction.

Preparation of solution: Reconstitute with Sodium Chloride, USP. Dilute the 10-mg vial with 5 ml and the 50-mg vial with 25 ml to give final concentration of 2 mg/ml.

Bacteriostatic diluents are not recommended for dilution.

Stability: Reconstituted solution is stable for 24 hours at room temperature and 48 hours under refrigeration ($4°C–10°C$). Protect from exposure to sunlight and discard unused portion.

Incompatibilities: Should not be mixed with heparin or 5-fluorouracil because it has been reported that these drugs are incompatible to the extent that a precipitate may form. It is recommended doxorubicin *not* be mixed with other drugs.

GENERIC NAME SIMILARITY

Daunorubicin and doxorubicin.

ONGOING ASSESSMENTS AND NURSING MANAGEMENT

Patient may be hospitalized during the first phase of treatment; drug may later be given on an outpatient basis.

Life-threatening arrhythmias have been reported to occur during or within a few hours of drug administration. Monitor pulse and general status q½h to q1h beginning immediately after administration and continue to monitor for 4 to 6 hours. Then monitor vital signs q4h or as ordered. Resuscitation equipment must be available for emergency treatment of life-threatening arrhythmias.

Acute nausea and vomiting occur frequently. An antiemetic is usually ordered q4h until GI distress subsides. If vomiting is severe, an antiemetic should be given by the parenteral route or as a suppository.

A liquid diet, sips of water, or carbonated beverages may be offered.

If vomitus exceeds approximately 700 ml to 800 ml in 8 hours, notify physician.

Measure intake and output. If vomiting is severe, observe for signs of dehydration (Appendix 6, section 6-10).

A red coloration in the urine occurs for 1 to 2 days after administration.

Careful hematologic monitoring is essential. Leukopenia reaches its nadir 10 to 14 days after treatment, with recovery usually occurring by the 21st day. WBC may be as low as 1000/mm^3; RBC and platelets may also be depressed.

Observe for signs of bone-marrow depression

(Appendix 6, section 6-8) and report findings to physician immediately. If bone-marrow depression is severe, observe for signs of superinfection (Appendix 6, section 6-22).

CLINICAL ALERT: Early recognition of cardiac toxicity is essential (see *Warnings*). Observe for development of dyspnea, tachycardia, ankle edema, decreased urinary output, paroxysmal nocturnal dyspnea, fatigue, distention of jugular veins, and dry cough. Notify physician immediately if one or more of these are present because early treatment is essential.

Mucositis may occur 5 to 10 days after administration and may be severe. Beginning 3 to 4 days after administration of drug inspect oral cavity daily for erythema, ulcerations. If stomatitis is apparent, begin stomatitis care (Appendix 6, section 6-21) and notify physician.

Xylocaine Viscous, 15 ml q3h to q4h prn, may be prescribed for pain due to stomatitis. Instruct patient to swish solution around in mouth. Drug may be swallowed if pharynx is also sore. A topical local anesthetic ointment or spray may also be prescribed.

Anorexia may occur. Food intake may improve if food is given in small amounts. A high-protein, high-calorie diet may be ordered.

Weigh every 2 to 3 days or as ordered.

Notify physician if diarrhea occurs. An antidiarrheal agent may be prescribed.

Hyperuricemia secondary to rapid lysis of neoplastic cells may occur. Blood uric-acid levels are obtained at periodic intervals. Physician may prescribe allopurinol and suggest an increase in fluid intake.

PATIENT AND FAMILY INFORMATION

NOTE: The patient should receive a full explanation of all possible adverse reactions and what specific reactions should be reported immediately to the physician. The possibility of alopecia and use of a wig, scarf, or cap should be discussed. This information may be given by the physician or by nurse with physician approval.

Keep all physician and clinic appointments for administration of drug as well as tests necessary to monitor therapy.

Inform physician or nurse in any of the following occurs: fever, chills, sore throat, abscess formation, easy bruising or bleeding, fatigue, shortness of breath, swelling of the ankles, severe nausea and vomiting, diarrhea, pronounced weight gain or loss, prolonged anorexia (beyond 2–3 days), anogenital or vaginal itching, black furry tongue.

Inform other physicians and dentist of therapy with this drug.

Avoid use of nonprescription drugs unless use is approved by physician.

Alopecia may occur (usually in 3–4 weeks). Hair loss may be partial or total and may include scalp hair, eyebrows, and underarm and pubic hair. Hair will grow back but may be a different color or texture.

Physician may prescribe drugs (*e.g.,* antiemetic, Xylocaine Viscous, allopurinol) to be taken or used between treatments. Take or use these drugs exactly as directed.

A liquid diet, dry toast, unsalted crackers, or carbonated beverages may be taken if nausea and vomiting occurs.

Good oral care is essential. Rinse mouth thoroughly after taking food or beverages. Avoid use of mouthwashes or other oral products unless use is approved by physician. Follow physician's recommendations about treatment of mucositis.

Urine may appear red for 1 to 2 days after drug is administered. This is not unusual.

Hyperpigmentation of nailbeds and dermal creases and red streaking along vein used for injection may occur.

NOTE: If patient has received previous radiotherapy, skin reaction seen at time of x-ray therapy may occur again during therapy with this drug. Tell patient to notify physician if redness occurs in area of previous x-ray treatment.

Doxycycline

See Tetracyclines.

Dromostanolone Propionate Rx

injection: 50 mg/ml   Drolban

INDICATIONS

Palliative treatment of advanced or metastatic carcinoma of the breast in inoperable cases in women who are 1 to 5 years postmenopausal at time of diagnosis or who have hormone-dependent cancer proven by previous beneficial response to castration.

CONTRAINDICATIONS

Carcinoma of the male breast; premenopausal women.

ACTIONS

Is a synthetic steroid, a variant of testosterone (p 49).

PRECAUTIONS

Usual precautions pertaining to testosterone propionate (p 49) should apply, although androgenic effects of dromostanolone appear to be significantly less marked. Increase in libido is unusual, but if it occurs sedation may be helpful.

Objective evidence of tumor progression is evaluated periodically by physical examination, x-ray examination of known or suspected metastases, and determination of serum calcium and alkaline phosphatase levels. The latter determination may reflect improvement in osseous lesions if there is a slight to moderate rise after initiation of therapy, or it may be indicative of extensive hepatic metastasis if level is markedly elevated.

Drug-induced jaundice and masculinization of the fetus reported with use of other anabolic agents have not been seen. Use with caution in presence of liver disease, cardiac decompensation, nephritis, nephrosis, and carcinoma of the prostate. Not indicated for use during pregnancy.

DRUG INTERACTIONS

May increase effects of **oral anticoagulants;** adjust dosage accordingly.

ADVERSE REACTIONS

Most likely are mild virilism such as deepening of voice, acne, facial hair growth, and enlargement of the clitoris. At times, marked virilism will occur after prolonged treatment. Edema occasionally occurs. Hypercalcemia has been noted but usually has accompanied progression of the disease. Local reaction at site of injection may occur rarely. Significantly fewer side-effects appear wtih this drug than with comparable doses of testosterone propionate.

DOSAGE

100 mg IM three times weekly. Treatment should probably be continued as long as satisfactory response is obtained. After treatment is begun, 8 to 12 weeks should elapse before any conclusions are drawn as to efficacy of drug. If significant progression of disease occurs during first 6 to 8 weeks of therapy, another form of treatment may be considered.

▌ NURSING IMPLICATIONS

HISTORY

See Appendix 4.

PHYSICAL ASSESSMENT

Record general physical and emotional status, weight; vital signs; check extremities for edema. Baseline laboratory and diagnostic studies include serum calcium, alkaline phosphatase, hepatic-function studies, and x-ray examination of known or suspected metastases.

ADMINISTRATION

Give deep IM; record site used. Rotate injection sites.

Storage: Do not refrigerate.

ONGOING ASSESSMENTS AND NURSING MANAGEMENT

Monitor vital signs, weight; check extremities for edema; observe for hypercalcemia (Appendix 6, section 6-13). Inform physician if weight gain or edema is noted.

Check previous injection sites for evidence of a local reaction (*e.g.,* inflammation, warmth, swelling). If reaction persists, notify physician.

Patients with edema may require diuretics before or during treatment.

Serum calcium levels are determined periodically during treatment. Hypercalcemia may require other management such as corticosteroid therapy.

If hypercalcemia develops and patient is confined to bed, daily range-of-motion exercises should be instituted to prevent mobilization of calcium from the bone.

Observe for signs of virilism (see *Adverse Reactions*).

Patient may be aware of diagnosis and prognosis. Provide emotional support, an understanding attitude, and willingness to listen. Referral to support groups (with physician approval) may be indicated.

PATIENT AND FAMILY INFORMATION

NOTE: Patient should have possibility of virilism explained before therapy.

Keep all appointments for therapy (injections) and laboratory studies.

Weigh self daily; report weight gain to physician.

Inform physician if swelling in extremities is noted.

Droperidol Rx

injection: 2.5 mg/ml   Inapsine

INDICATIONS

To produce tranquilization and reduce incidence of nausea and vomiting in surgical and diagnostic procedures; for premedication, for induction, and as an adjunct in maintenance of general and regional anesthesia; in neuroleptanalgesia, in which droperidol is given concurrently with a narcotic analgesic such as fentanyl, to aid in producing tranquility and decreasing anxiety and pain.

CONTRAINDICATIONS
Known intolerance to droperidol.

ACTIONS
Produces marked tranquilization, sedation, and an antiemetic effect. It potentiates other CNS depressants. Also produces mild alpha-adrenergic blockade, peripheral vascular dilatation, and reduction of the pressor effect of epinephrine. Can produce decreased peripheral vascular resistance and hypotension. May decrease pulmonary arterial pressure (particularly if it is abnormally high). May reduce incidence of epinephrine-induced arrhythmias but does not prevent other arrhythmias. Onset of action is from 3 to 10 minutes following IM or IV administration. The full effect may not be apparent for 30 minutes. Duration of sedative and tranquilizing effects is generally 2 to 4 hours. Alteration of consciousness may persist for as long as 12 hours.

WARNINGS
Fluids and other countermeasures to manage hypotension should be available.

Concomitant narcotic analgesic therapy: If administered with a narcotic analgesic such as fentanyl, user should be familiar with both drugs. When a combination is used, resuscitative equipment and a narcotic antagonist should be readily available.

Use in pregnancy: Safety not established. Use only when clearly needed and when potential benefits outweigh the unknown potential hazards to the fetus. Data are insufficient about placental transfer and fetal effects; safety for the infant in obstetrics not established.

Use in children: Safety and efficacy for use in children less than 2 years of age have not been established.

PRECAUTIONS
Initial dose is reduced in elderly, debilitated, and other poor-risk patients. Effect of initial dose is considered in determining incremental doses.

Hypotension: If hypotension occurs, possibility of hypovolemia is considered and managed with appropriate parenteral fluid therapy. Reposition patient to improve venous return to the heart when operative condition permits. In spinal and peridural anesthesia, tilting patient into a head-down position may result in a higher level of anesthesia as well as impair venous return to the heart. Exercise care in moving and positioning patients because of possibil-

ity of orthostatic hypotension. If volume expansion with fluids and other countermeasures do not correct hypotension, administration of pressor agents other than epinephrine is considered.

DRUG INTERACTIONS
The respiratory depressant effect of narcotics persists longer than the measured analgesic effect. When narcotics are used with droperidol the total dose of **narcotic analgesics** is considered. When narcotics are required, initial dose is reduced as low as ¼ to ⅓ of that usually recommended.

Certain forms of **conduction anesthesia** (spinal anesthesia, some peridural anesthetics) can cause peripheral vasodilatation and hypotension because of sympathetic blockade. Through other mechanisms, circulation may be altered by droperidol. Other **CNS depressants** (*e.g.,* barbiturates, tranquilizers, narcotics, general anesthetics) have additive or potentiating effects with droperidol. When patients have received such drugs, the dose of droperidol should be reduced. Following the administration of droperidol, the dose of a CNS depressant should be reduced.

ADVERSE REACTIONS
Most common: Mild to moderate hypotension; occasionally tachycardia. These usually subside without treatment.

Extrapyramidal symptoms (dystonia, akathisia, oculogyric crisis): Have been observed following administration. Restlessness, hyperactivity, and anxiety that can be result of inadequate dosage or part of the symptom complex of akathisia may occur. Extrapyramidal symptoms can usually be controlled with antiparkinsonian agents.

Respiratory depression: When used with a narcotic analgesic such as fentanyl, respiratory depression, apnea, and muscular rigidity can occur; if these remain untreated, respiratory arrest could occur.

Elevated blood pressure: Has been reported following administration of droperidol combined with fentanyl or other parenteral analgesics.

Other: Dizziness, chills and/or shivering, laryngospasm, bronchospasm, postoperative hallucinatory episodes (sometimes associated with transient periods of mental depression).

OVERDOSAGE
Symptoms: Manifestations are extension of drug's pharmacologic actions.

Treatment: In presence of hypoventilation or apnea, administer oxygen and assist or control respiration as indicated. A patent airway must be maintained; an oropharyngeal airway or endotracheal tube may be indicated. Observe patient for 24 hours; maintain body warmth and adequate fluid intake. If hypotension occurs and is severe or persists, possibility of hypovolemia is considered and managed with appropriate fluid therapy.

DOSAGE

Dosage is individualized. Factors considered are body weight, physical status, underlying pathologic condition, use of other drugs, type of anesthesia to be used, surgical procedure involved.

Premedication (modified in the elderly, debilitated, and those who have received other depressant drugs): 2.5 mg to 10 mg IM, 30 to 60 minutes preoperatively.

Adjunct to general anesthesia: Average dose is 2.5 mg per 9 kg to 11 kg (20 lb–25 lb) IV for induction and 1.25 mg to 2.5 mg (usually IV) for maintenance.

Diagnostic procedures: Usual premedication administered IM 30 to 60 minutes before procedure. An additional 1.25 mg to 2.5 mg may be administered (usually IV).

Adjunct to regional anesthesia: 2.5 mg to 5 mg IM or slowly IV when additional sedation is required.

Children (2–12 yr): A reduced dose as low as 1 mg to 1.5 mg per 9 kg to 11 kg (20 lb–25 lb) is recommended for premedication or induction of anesthesia.

NURSING IMPLICATIONS

HISTORY

Review chart for general history and surgery or diagnostic procedure to be performed.

PHYSICAL ASSESSMENT

Record blood pressure, pulse, and respirations.

ADMINISTRATION

Nurse is responsible for premedication administration only.

Blood pressure, pulse, and respirations are taken immediately before administration of drug. Withhold drug and contact anesthesiologist or surgeon if respiratory rate is 12 or below.

Administer drug at time ordered (usually 30–60 minutes before surgery or diagnostic procedure) because sufficient time must elapse for adequate drug effect. Chart exact time drug is administered.

ONGOING ASSESSMENTS AND NURSING MANAGEMENT

If drug is administered with a narcotic analgesic such as fentanyl, be familiar with special properties of both drugs. Resuscitative equipment and a narcotic antagonist should be readily available.

Premedication: Monitor blood pressure, pulse, and respirations q15m before transportation of patient to operating room.

CLINICAL ALERT: If signs of respiratory depression occur, maintain patent airway (use oropharyngeal airway if necessary), administer oxygen, and contact physician immediately.

Exercise care in moving and positioning patient when preparing for transportation to operating room because of possibility of orthostatic hypotension.

Postoperative (when used as adjunct to anesthesia or without anesthetic for diagnostic purposes): Postoperative hallucinatory episodes may be lessened by minimizing stimulation (light, touch, sound).

Monitor blood pressure, pulse, and respirations q15m or as ordered. Observe for respiratory depression (see *Clinical Alert,* above). Notify physician if hypotension or tachycardia occurs.

Do not place patient in a head-down (Trendelenburg) position if hypotension occurs, especially if patient has received spinal or peridural anesthesia. This position should be used only on specific recommendation of a physician.

Narcotic analgesics (when required) are initially given in reduced doses (usually ¼ to ⅓ of those usually recommended) during recovery from anesthesia.

When EEG is used for postoperative monitoring, EEG pattern may be slow to return to normal.

If extrapyramidal symptoms are noted, contact physician.

Dyclonine Hydrochloride

See Anesthetics, Local, Topical.

Dyphylline

See Bronchodilators and Decongestants, systemic.

E

Echothiophate Iodide
Econazole Nitrate
Edetate Calcium Disodium
Edetate Disodium
Edrophonium Chloride
Electrolyte Mixtures, Oral
Emetine Hydrochloride
Enflurane
Ephedrine
Epinephrine
Ergocalciferol
Ergoloid Mesylates
Ergonovine Maleate
Ergotamine Preparations
    Ergotamine Tartrate
    Ergotamine Combinations
Erythrityl Tetranitrate
Erythromycin Preparations
  Intravenous Preparations
    Erythromycin Gluceptate
    Erythromycin Lactobionate
  Oral Preparations
    Erythromycin Base
    Erythromycin Estolate
    Erythromycin Ethylsuccinate

Erythromycin Stearate
Erythromycin Ethylsuccinate
    and Sulfisoxazole
Estramustine Phosphate Sodium
Estrogens
    Chlorotrianisene
    Combined Estrogens
      Aqueous
    Conjugated Estrogens
      (Oral)
    Conjugated Estrogens (Parenteral)
    Diethylstilbestrol
    Esterified Estrogens
    Estradiol
    Estradiol Cypionate in Oil
    Estradiol Valerate in Oil
    Estrogenic Substance
      Aqueous
    Estrogenic Substance
      (Mainly Estrone) in Oil
    Estrone Aqueous Suspension
    Estropipate

Ethinyl Estradiol
    Quinestrol
Estrogens, Antineoplastic
    Diethylstilbestrol Diphosphate
    Polyestradiol Phosphate
Estrogens, Vaginal
Ethacrynic Acid
Ethambutol Hydrochloride
Ethaverine Hydrochloride
Ethchlorvynol
Ethinamate
Ethinyl Estradiol
Ethionamide
Ethopropazine Hydrochloride
Ethosuximide
Ethotoin
Ethylene
Ethylestrenol
Ethylnorepinephrine Hydrochloride
Etidronate Disodium
Etomidate
Etoposide

Echothiophate Iodide

See Miotics, Cholinesterase Inhibitors.

Econazole Nitrate Rx

cream: 1%   Spectazole

INDICATIONS

Treatment of tinea pedis, tinea cruris, and tinea corporis caused by *Trichophyton rubrum, T. mentagrophytes, T. tonsurans, Microsporum canis, M. audouini, M. gypseum,* and *Epidermophyton floccosum;* cutaneous candidiasis; tinea versicolor.

CONTRAINDICATIONS

Hypersensitivity.

ACTIONS

Exhibits broad-spectrum antifungal activity against dermatophytes (see *Indications*), *Candida albicans, Pityrosporum orbiculare,* and certain gram-positive bacteria. Systemic absorption is very low following topical application.

WARNINGS

Do not use in first trimester of pregnancy unless essential to patient's welfare. Use during second and third trimesters only if clearly needed. It is not known whether drug is excreted in human milk. Exercise caution when administering to nursing women.

PRECAUTIONS

If reaction suggesting sensitivity or chemical irritation occurs, discontinue use.

ADVERSE REACTIONS

Burning, itching, stinging, erythema.

DOSAGE

Tinea pedis, tinea cruris, tinea corporis, cutaneous candidiasis: Apply sufficient quantity to cover affected area bid (morning and evening).
Tinea versicolor: Apply once daily.

NURSING IMPLICATIONS

HISTORY
See Appendix 4.

PHYSICAL ASSESSMENT
Examine and describe lesions and their locations.

ADMINISTRATION
Prior to application cleanse area with soap and warm water, rinse thoroughly, and gently pat dry.

Apply as directed by physician; cover affected areas.

Do not use an occlusive dressing unless directed by physician.

ONGOING ASSESSMENTS AND NURSING MANAGEMENT
Inspect lesions at time of each application. If redness or irritation is noted or patient complains of itching or stinging, do not apply next dose and contact physician.

Record appearance of lesions daily. Compare with data base.

Early relief of symptoms is experienced by majority of patients. Clinical improvement may be seen fairly soon after treatment is begun.

Candidal infections and tinea cruris and corporis are treated for 2 weeks and tinea pedis for 1 month, to reduce possibility of recurrence. Patients with tinea versicolor exhibit clinical and mycologic clearing after 2 weeks.

If patient shows no clinical improvement after treatment period, physician reevaluates diagnosis.

PATIENT AND FAMILY INFORMATION
If condition persists or worsens, or if irritation (burning, stinging, redness) occurs, discontinue use and notify physician.

Use medication for full treatment time, even though symptoms may have improved. Notify physician if there is no improvement after 2 weeks (tinea cruris and corporis, tinea versicolor, candidal infections) or 4 weeks (tinea pedis).

Clean area with soap and warm water, rinse thoroughly, and gently pat dry, unless directed otherwise by physician.

Do not apply a dressing over area unless directed by physician.

Tinea infections
Keep towels, facecloths, and bedding separate from those of other family members. Launder clothing, linens daily; use hot water and detergent. Do not wash clothes or bedding used by other family members at same time.

Tinea corporis, cruris: Change clothing contacting infected area after each application.

Tinea pedis: Keep feet dry; change socks daily or whenever damp or wet. Expose feet to air as much as possible. Follow directions of physician regarding shoes and care of feet until infection has cleared.

Edetate Calcium Disodium

(Calcium EDTA), Parenteral Rx

injection: 200 mg/ml   Calcium Disodium Versenate

INDICATIONS
For reduction of blood levels and depot stores of lead in lead poisoning (acute and chronic) and lead encephalopathy.

CONTRAINDICATIONS
Not given during periods of anuria.

ACTIONS
The calcium in edetate calcium disodium is readily displaced by heavy metals such as lead to form stable complexes that are excreted in the urine. The elimination half-life from circulation is 20 to 60 minutes. Approximately 50% is excreted in urine within 1 hour, 95% within 24 hours.

WARNINGS
Is capable of producing toxic and potentially fatal effects. *Do not* exceed recommended dosage. In lead encephalopathy, IM route is preferred. Safe use during pregnancy is not established. Not used in women of childbearing potential and particularly during early pregnancy unless potential benefits outweigh the unknown potential hazards to the fetus.

PRECAUTIONS
Renal damage: Severe acute lead poisoning may cause proteinuria and microscopic hematuria. Calcium EDTA may produce the same degree of renal damage. Presence of large renal epithelial cells, increasing numbers of red cells in urinary sediment, or greater proteinuria in daily urinalysis samples requires immediate discontinuation of drug.

Hydration: Excess fluids are avoided in those with lead encephalopathy and increased intracranial pressure. In such cases, mix a 20% solution with procaine (0.5% final concentration) and give IM. Acutely ill patients may be dehydrated from vomiting. Because this drug is excreted almost exclusively in urine, it is important to establish urine flow by IV infusion before administering first dose of the chelating agent. Once urine flow is established, further IV fluid is restricted to basal water and electrolyte requirements. Administration should be stopped when urine flow ceases.

ADVERSE EFFECTS
Principal toxic effect is renal tubular necrosis.

DOSAGE
Effective IV, subcutaneously, or IM. Because of convenience and greater safety in treating symptomatic children, IM route may be preferred and is recommended in those with overt or incipient lead encephalopathy. Rapid IV infusion may be lethal by suddenly increasing intracranial pressure in this group of patients with cerebral edema.

IV: Administer diluted solution (see *Administration*) over period of at least 1 hour. Doses may be administered bid for up to 5 days. Therapy is interrupted for 2 days and followed with an additional 5 days of treatment, if needed. In mildly affected or asymptomatic patients, do not exceed 50 mg/kg/day. In symptomatic adults, keep fluids to basal levels and increase administration time to 2 hours. Give second daily infusion 6 or more hours after the first.

IM: This is the route of choice for children. Do not exceed 35 mg/kg (0.5 g/30 lb) bid; total, approximately 75 mg/kg/day (1 g/30 lb/day). *Mild cases*—50 mg/kg/day should not be exceeded. For young children, total daily dose may be given in divided doses q8h to q12h for 3 to 5 days. A second course may be given after a rest period of 4 or more days. Add procaine to produce a concentration of 0.5% to minimize pain at injection site.

NURSING IMPLICATIONS

HISTORY
See Appendix 4. Obtain occupational and residential history to identify environmental sources of lead.

PHYSICAL ASSESSMENT
Monitor vital signs, weight. Assess general areas identified in history of symptoms. Review recent laboratory studies—renal-function studies, CBC, urinalysis, 24-hour urine for lead, blood lead level.

Symptoms of acute lead poisoning: Abdominal pain, vomiting, diarrhea, tarry stools, oliguria, metallic taste, coma.

Symptoms of chronic lead poisoning

Early: Anorexia, weight loss, blue-black lead line along gingival margin, anemia, metallic taste.

More advanced: Intermittent vomiting; irritability; vague pains in legs, arms; sensory disturbances.

Severe: Vomiting, lethargy, stupor, ataxia, elevated blood pressure, delirium, convulsions, coma.

ADMINISTRATION

The acutely ill patient may be dehydrated from vomiting. Physician may order IV fluids to establish urine flow before administration of first dose. Once urine flow is established, restrict IV fluid administration to basal water and electrolyte requirements.

Begin measuring intake and output on acutely ill patient before administration of drug.

IM: Addition of procaine to IM dose is recommended to minimize pain at injection site. Physician must order amount and strength of procaine to be mixed with IM dose.

Give deep IM. Rotate injection sites and record site used.

When administered concurrently, dimercaprol and edetate calcium disodium should be injected at separate deep IM sites.

Subcutaneous: Select area with adequate subcutaneous tissue.

IV: Dilute 5-ml ampule (200 mg) with 250 ml to 500 ml of Normal Saline or 5% Dextrose solution. In asymptomatic adults, administer diluted solution over a period of 1 hour. In symptomatic adults, recommended infusion time is 2 hours. Physician orders IV infusion and infusion rate.

GENERIC NAME SIMILARITY

Edetate calcium disodium and edetate disodium. Both also known by initials EDTA.

TRADE NAME SIMILARITY

Calcium Disodium Versenate and Sodium Versenate.

ONGOING ASSESSMENTS AND NURSING MANAGEMENT

Monitor IV infusion rate q15m.

Obtain vital signs q4h; measure intake and output (in acutely ill patients, physician may order output measured hourly); assess systems (GI, CNS) affected by lead poisoning and compare to baseline data.

Contact physician immediately if any of the following occurs: irregularity in cardiac rhythm, a marked decrease in urinary output, increased severity of CNS symptoms (*e.g.,* stupor, coma, convulsions, hypertension, persistent vomiting).

Urinalysis is recommended daily during therapy to monitor for progression of renal tubular damage.

Periodic BUN determinations are recommended during each course of therapy.

PATIENT AND FAMILY INFORMATION

NOTE: Education regarding prevention is imperative and based on the probable or known cause of lead poisoning. The environmental sources of lead should be eliminated and require cooperation of one or more agencies or individuals such as the Public Health Department, landlords, and so on.

Keep all follow-up clinic appointments for administration of drug and monitoring of therapy. Therapy must be continued until lead levels are below acceptable limits.

Follow suggestions of physician about elimination of sources of lead. If difficulty is experienced in eliminating the source, discuss problem with physician.

Edetate Disodium (Disodium EDTA) Rx

injection: 150 mg/ml   Chealamide, Endrate
injection: 200 mg/ml   Sodium Versenate

INDICATIONS

Emergency treatment of hypercalcemia in selected patients and control of ventricular arrhythmias and heart block associated with digitalis toxicity.

CONTRAINDICATIONS

Anuric patients. Not indicated for treatment of generalized arteriosclerosis associated with advancing age.

ACTIONS

Chelates with cations of calcium and many divalent and trivalent metals. Because of its affinity for calcium, edetate disodium will produce a lowering of serum calcium level during IV infusion. Slow infusion over a protracted period may cause mobilization of extracirculatory calcium stores. The chelate thus formed is excreted in the urine. Drug exerts a negative inotropic effect on the heart. Additionally, drug forms chelates with other polyvalent metals and produces increases in urinary excretion of magnesium, zinc, and other trace elements. Does not form a chelate with potassium but may reduce the serum level and a twofold to sixfold increase of potassium excretion may occur.

WARNINGS

Rapid IV infusion or attainment of high serum concentration of drug may cause a precipitous drop in the serum calcium level and may result in fatality. Toxicity appears to depend on total dosage and speed of administration. Renal function should be assessed prior to treatment and there should be periodic BUN and creatinine determinations; daily urinalysis should be performed.

Electrolyte imbalance: Because of possibility of inducing an electrolyte imbalance during treatment, appropriate laboratory determinations and studies to evaluate status of cardiac function should be performed. Repetition of these tests is recommended as clinically indicated, particularly in those with ventricular arrhythmia and those with a history of seizure disorders or intracranial lesions. If clinical evidence suggests disturbance in hepatic function during treatment, appropriate laboratory determinations should be performed. Withdrawal of drug may be required.

Use in pregnancy: Safety is not established. Use only when clearly needed and when potential benefits outweigh unknown potential hazards to the fetus.

PRECAUTIONS

Cardiac effects: When administering drug to those with heart disease, consider the possibility of an adverse effect on myocardial contractility. Caution is dictated in use of drug in patients with limited cardiac reserve or incipient congestive failure.

Hypokalemia: Use with caution in those with clinical or subclinical potassium deficiency states; checking serum potassium blood levels for possible hypokalemia and monitoring ECG for changes are recommended.

The possibility of hypomagnesemia is kept in mind during prolonged therapy. Treatment may cause a lowering of blood glucose and insulin requirements in those with diabetes who are treated with insulin.

ADVERSE REACTIONS

Gastrointestinal symptoms such as nausea, vomiting, and diarrhea are fairly common. Transient symptoms such as circumoral paresthesia, numbness, and headache and a transient drop in systolic and diastolic blood pressure may occur. Thrombophlebitis, febrile reactions, hyperuricemia, anemia, exfoliative dermatitis, and other toxic skin and mucous-membrane reactions have been reported.

Nephrotoxicity and damage to the reticuloendothelial system with hemorrhagic tendencies have been reported with excessive dosages.

OVERDOSAGE

Because of possibility that drug may produce a precipitous drop in the serum calcium level, a source of calcium replacement for IV administration should be immediately available. Extreme caution is necessary in use of IV calcium in the treatment of tetany, especially in digitalized patients, because action of the drug and replacement of calcium ions may produce a reversal of the desired digitalis effect.

DOSAGE

Adults: Recommended daily dose is 50 mg/kg (IV infusion) to a maximum of 3 g in 24 hours. A suggested regimen includes five consecutive daily doses followed by 2 days without medication, with repeated courses as necessary to a total of 15 doses. See _Administration._

Children: Recommended daily dose is 40 mg/kg (1 g/55 lb) (IV infusion). Maximum dose is 70 mg/kg/24 hours. See _Administration._

NURSING IMPLICATIONS

HISTORY
See Appendix 4.

PHYSICAL ASSESSMENT
Obtain vital signs, including apical pulse rate (if not presently on cardiac monitor), weight (may be obtained from chart).

ADMINISTRATION
Drug _must_ be diluted before administration because of its irritant effect on tissues and because of serious side-effects if administered in the undiluted form.

Physician orders IV solution to be used. For children, physician must order volume of IV solution to be used for dilution.

Because drug may cause a precipitous drop in serum calcium, an intravenous source of calcium replacement (_e.g.,_ calcium gluconate) must be instantly available before drug is administered.

Adults: Dose should be dissolved in 500 ml of 5% Dextrose Injection or Sodium Chloride Injection. The IV infusion should be regulated so that 3 or more hours are required for completion and the patient's cardiac reserve is not exceeded.

Children: Dissolve in a sufficient volume of 5% Dextrose Injection or Sodium Chloride Injection to bring final concentration to not more than 3%. The IV infusion should be regulated so that 3 or more hours are required for completion and the patient's cardiac reserve is not exceeded.

Obtain blood pressure, pulse, and respirations prior to administration of drug.

Infusion time is usually 3 or more hours. Apply timing label.

Rotate IV infusion sites. Record site used.

GENERIC NAME SIMILARITY

Edetate disodium and edetate calcium disodium. Both also known by initials EDTA.

TRADE NAME SIMILARITY

Sodium Versenate and Calcium Disodium Versenate.

ONGOING ASSESSMENTS AND NURSING MANAGEMENT

CLINICAL ALERT: Monitor IV infusion rate q5m to q15m and adjust rate of flow as needed. Rapid infusion rate or attainment of high serum concentration of edetate disodium may cause a precipitous drop in serum calcium and may result in fatality.

Monitor blood pressure and pulse q15m to q30m during infusion. *In those with heart disease*—Observe for changes in pulse rate, rhythm, or amplitude or signs of congestive heart failure (Appendix 6, section 6-9). Contact physician immediately if these changes or signs occur.

Patients with ventricular arrhythmias and heart block associated with digitalis toxicity should be placed on a cardiac monitor and continuously surveyed for changes in heart rate and rhythm, development of a new arrhythmia, and abolishment of the arrhythmia for which this drug is used.

Monitor intake and output. Report any change in the intake–output ratio to the physician.

Following termination of infusion, obtain blood pressure, pulse, and respirations. Have patient remain in bed for 30 minutes and assist with ambulation (if allowed) because of possibility of postural hypotension.

Treatment may cause lowering of blood glucose and insulin requirements in patients with diabetes who are treated with insulin. Monitor urine glucose and ketones qid; notify physician if percentage of glucose in urine changes.

Observe for signs of hypomagnesemia (Appendix 6, section 6-16), if patient is receiving prolonged therapy, and hypocalcemia (Appendix 6, section 6-13).

Nausea, vomiting, and diarrhea are fairly common. Observe for signs of dehydration (Appendix 6, section 6-10) if vomiting or diarrhea is prolonged.

Urinalysis and serum calcium levels may be obtained daily. Other laboratory tests (*e.g.,* serum potassium, hepatic- and renal-function studies) and diagnostic studies may also be appropriate.

Enter note on laboratory request slip regarding therapy with edetate disodium because modification of the laboratory method used in determining serum calcium may be necessary.

Edrophonium Chloride

See Muscle Stimulants, Anticholinesterase.

Electrolyte Mixtures, Oral otc

Infalyte, Lytren Solution, Pedialyte Solution, Pedialyte RS Solution

INDICATIONS

To supply water and electrolytes for maintenance and to replace mild to moderate fluid losses when food and liquid intake are discontinued. Also used in fluid management of diarrhea in forestalling dehydration and in postoperative states.

CONTRAINDICATIONS

Severe, continuing diarrhea or other critical fluid losses requiring parenteral therapy; intractable vomiting, adynamic ileus, intestinal obstruction, or perforated bowel; depressed renal function (anuria, oliguria); impaired homeostatic mechanisms.

ACTIONS

Electrolyte mixtures containing electrolytes, water, and glucose are used to prevent dehydration or achieve rehydration. They aid in maintaining strength and feeling of well-being and prevent potentially serious consequences of severe dehydration. These products contain sodium, chloride, potassium, and bicarbonate to replace depleted electrolytes and restore acid–base balance. Glucose or sucrose is included to facilitate sodium transport, aiding in absorption of sodium and water. Lytren Solution also contains sulfate and phosphate.

PRECAUTIONS

Use only in recommended volume intakes to avoid excessive electrolyte ingestion. Urgent needs in severe electrolyte imbalances must be met parenterally. When oral as well as parenteral fluid is given, total water and electrolyte requirements should not be exceeded. Intake of these solutions should be reduced when other electrolyte-containing foods are reintroduced into the diet.

DOSAGE

Adjust according to clinical indications. Only enough solution should be given to supply calculated water requirement. Additional liquid needed to satisfy thirst should be given as water or as other non–electrolyte containing fluids.

Infants, young children: Intake should approximate water requirement, which is calculated on basis of body surface area. The following estimated daily requirements may be used as a guide:

Maintenance in illness—1500 ml/m^2
Maintenance plus replacement of moderate losses
   (e.g., diarrhea, vomiting)—2400 ml/m^2.

Older children, adults: For mild to moderate *fluid loss*—Children (5–10 years), 1 qt to 2 qt daily. Children and adults (10 years and older), 2 qt to 3 qt daily.

NURSING IMPLICATIONS

HISTORY
Note duration of symptoms; approximate number of bowel movements per day and/or number of times vomiting occurs daily; general health history; prescription, nonprescription drugs taken to control nausea or vomiting.

PHYSICAL ASSESSMENT
Monitor vital signs, weight; examine or have patient describe stools and/or emesis; look for signs of dehydration. Serum electrolytes, CBC, and other appropriate tests or studies may be ordered.

ADMINISTRATION
Give undiluted unless ordered otherwise.
   Refrigerated solution is usually more palatable.

ONGOING ASSESSMENTS AND NURSING MANAGEMENT
Obtain vital signs q4h or as ordered; measure intake and output; record number, type, approximate amount, and appearance of each bowel movement; measure (when possible) and describe emesis; observe for signs of dehydration (Appendix 6, section 6-10), hypokalemia (Appendix 6, section 6-15), hyponatremia (Appendix 6, section 6-17).
   Additional fluids to satisfy thirst should be given as water. If patient desires other types of fluid, consult physician. In some instances certain nonelectrolyte beverages (*e.g.,* cola drinks, ginger ale) may be appropriate for a specific patient.
   If patient is unable to retain oral electrolyte solution, notify physician; parenteral fluid therapy may be necessary.

PATIENT AND FAMILY INFORMATION
Take as directed; do not exceed recommended dose.
   Fluid should be taken (or offered) at frequent intervals (*e.g.,* every ½–1 hour).
   To satisfy thirst, drink water. Do not drink other beverages (juice, milk) unless use is approved by physician.
   Notify physician if vomiting or diarrhea persists or becomes worse.
   Refrigerated solution may be more palatable.

Emetine Hydrochloride Rx

injection: 65 mg/ml   *Generic*

INDICATIONS
Intestinal amebiasis: Symptomatic management of acute fulminating amebic dysentery or acute exacerbations of chronic amebic dysentery. Not indicated in treatment of mild symptoms or carriers. Effect is symptomatic; cure can be expected in only 10% to 15% of cases with use of emetine alone. Patient should be given another antiamebic preparation simultaneously.

Extraintestinal amebiasis: Highly effective against amebae in tissues; is of value in treatment of amebic abscess and "amebic hepatitis." Increased efficacy in amebic hepatitis has been attributed to high concentration of drug in liver. Other amebicidal treatment instituted simultaneously or as immediate follow-up to guarantee *Entamoeba histolytica* is eradicated from primary lesions in the intestine.

Other parasitic infections: Useful in certain cases of balantidiasis, fascioliasis, and paragonimiasis.

CONTRAINDICATIONS
Patients with organic disease of the heart or kidney, except those with amebic abscess or hepatitis not controlled by chloroquine; patients who have received a course of emetine less than 6 weeks to 2 months previously. Contraindicated in pregnancy. Contraindicated in children except those with severe dysentery not controlled by other amebicides.

ACTIONS
Has lethal action on *E. histolytica.* Is an alkaloid related to ipecac that acts primarily in the bowel wall and liver. Inhibits polypeptide chain elongation, thereby blocking protein synthesis in parasitic and mammalian cells, but not in bacteria.
   Emetine is a general protoplasmic poison that, because of its slow elimination following parenteral administration, tends to accumulate in the body.

Subcutaneous and IM doses are concentrated primarily in the liver; appreciable levels are also found in the kidney, spleen, and lungs. Drug tends to accumulate and persist in these tissues for several months. Very little of drug is excreted into the bowel; however, it may continue to be eliminated in the urine 40 to 60 days after administration because renal excretion is slow. Does not achieve significant levels in the GI tract and therefore is not effective in intestinal amebiasis. Combined therapy, with emetine given for 10 days and chloroquine given for 3 weeks, results in a satisfactory response with few relapses.

WARNINGS

Exercise caution in administering to elderly or debilitated patients. Is a potentially dangerous drug and requires strict supervision. No fatalities have been reported from a single dose but some have been reported following repeated doses. May cause fetal harm when administered to a pregnant woman. Contraindicated in women who are or may become pregnant. If used during pregnancy or if patient becomes pregnant during therapy, she should be apprised of the potential hazard to the fetus. Safety for use in the nursing mother is not established.

PRECAUTIONS

Discontinue therapy on appearance of tachycardia, precipitous fall in blood pressure, neuromuscular symptoms, marked GI effects, or considerable weakness. ECG changes (*e.g.,* widening of QRS complex and prolongation of P–R interval) may be considered an indication for immediate cessation of therapy.

ADVERSE REACTIONS

Toxic manifestations may occur at any dose level.

Local: Aching, tenderness, muscle weakness in area of injection site. Eczematous, urticarial, or purpuric lesions may also appear. Subcutaneous administration produces pain at injection site.

GI: Severe GI effects are unusual; nausea and vomiting, in association with dizziness and headache, are more common.

Neuromuscular: Weakness, aching, tenderness, skeletal muscle stiffness. Weakness and muscle pain tend to persist until therapy is discontinued; they usually appear before more serious symptoms develop and thus serve as a guide for avoiding overdosage.

Cardiovascular: The most severe toxic effects are related to this system. Hypotension, tachycardia, precordial pain, dyspnea, ECG abnormalities, gallop rhythm, cardiac dilatation, congestive failure, and death have been reported. ECG patterns observed under emetine therapy sometimes resemble those of myocardial infarction. Changes appear about 7 days after drug is administered and are reversible. Average time for complete return of the tracing to normal is over 6 weeks.

OVERDOSAGE

Symptoms: Lethal dose is 10 mg/kg to 25 mg/kg. Poisoning is characterized by muscular tremors, weakness, and pain, especially in the extremities. Purpura, dermatitis, or hemoptysis may occur in severe cases. Neuritis may be due to muscle damage; vertigo may occur. GI symptoms such as nausea, vomiting, and diarrhea are not infrequent. Bloody diarrhea occurs accompanied by prostration and may be mistaken for recurrence of the amebic dysentery. The myotoxic effect is especially detrimental to the heart and may result in arrhythmias, myocardial weakness with congestive failure, or at times sudden cardiac failure.

Treatment: Discontinue drug and begin supportive measures.

DOSAGE

Do *not* give IV. This route is dangerous and contraindicated. May be given IM or subcutaneously.

Maximum dosage: Do not exceed 65 mg per day or 10 days of therapy (650 mg total dosage). Do not repeat course of therapy in less than 6 weeks. Some recommend a dose of 1 mg/kg/day, not to exceed 65 mg. May be administered as a single 65-mg dose or as 32 mg in A.M. and P.M.

Children: Use *only* in severe dysentery not controlled by other amebicides. *Under 8 years*—Do not exceed 10 mg/day. *Over 8 years*—Do not exceed 20 mg/day.

Acute fulminating amebic dysentery: Administer only long enough to control diarrheal or dysenteric symptoms, usually 3 to 5 days.

Amebic hepatitis or abscess: Administer for 10 days.

NURSING IMPLICATIONS

HISTORY

See Appendix 4. Drug is contraindicated in pregnancy; when appropriate, inquire about possibility of pregnancy. Local health department regulations may require investigation into recent travel to foreign countries. If patient has not traveled, further investigation of local travel, use of restaurants, water source, and so on may be necessary.

PHYSICAL ASSESSMENT

Obtain vital signs, weight, general physical status. Look for signs of dehydration (Appendix 6, section 6-10). Record appearance and consistency of stools. ECG is recommended before initial dose is administered.

ADMINISTRATION

May be ordered subcutaneous or IM; deep subcutaneous injection is usually preferred. Aspirate needle before injection because IV administration is dangerous and contraindicated. If blood return is noted, select alternate site.

Drug is very irritating and should not be allowed to come into contact with the cornea or mucous membranes, especially the conjunctiva. Be sure the needle is firmly attached to the syringe to avoid accidental separation of the needle and syringe during administration. Wash hands thoroughly immediately after preparation and administration of drug.

Warn patient that pain (subcutaneous route) or discomfort (IM route) at injection site may occur.

Rotate injection sites; record site used.

ONGOING ASSESSMENTS AND NURSING MANAGEMENT

Record vital signs q4h or as ordered; record number and appearance of stools; measure intake and output; inspect previous injection sites for local reactions (see *Adverse Reactions*). Closely observe patient q1h to q2h for adverse reactions, especially those listed below.

CLINICAL ALERT: Contact physician immediately if tachycardia, precipitous fall in blood pressure, neuromuscular symptoms, marked GI effects, or considerable weakness occurs.

Contact physician if vomiting is severe or prolonged or signs of dehydration (Appendix 6, section 6-10) are noted.

Patient is kept on complete bedrest during and for several days after administration.

Isolation is usually not necessary. Stool precautions may or may not be necessary (discuss with physician advisability of instituting stool precautions if order is not written). Follow hospital procedure for disposal of feces. Wash hands thoroughly after attending to patient following bowel movement, linen changes, anal care, and obtainment of stool specimen.

Deliver all stool specimens to laboratory immediately because specimen must be kept warm until examined.

If patient is acutely ill, IV fluids or total parenteral nutrition may be necessary.

Physician may prescribe special diet (*e.g.,* low residue, high calorie).

ECG is recommended before initiation of therapy, after fifth dose, at completion of therapy, and 1 week later.

Examination of stool specimens from all household members may be necessary.

PATIENT AND FAMILY INFORMATION

Stool specimens and other diagnostic tests may be required at periodic intervals.

Enflurane

See Anesthetics, General, Volatile Liquids.

Ephedrine* Rx

injection: 25 mg/ml, 50 mg/ml	*Generic* (as ephedrine sulfate)
injection: 50 mg/ml	*Generic* (as ephedrine)

INDICATIONS

To combat acute hypotensive states, especially those associated with spinal anesthesia; Stokes-Adams syndrome with complete heart block; as a CNS stimulant in narcolepsy and depressive states; occasionally, acute bronchospasm. Also as a pressor agent in hypotensive states following sympathectomy or following overdosage of ganglionic-blocking agents, antiadrenergic agents, or other drugs used for lowering blood pressure in treatment of arterial hypertension.

CONTRAINDICATIONS

Hypersensitivity; angle-closure glaucoma; patients anesthetized with cyclopropane or halothane; cases in which vasopressor drugs are contraindicated (*e.g.,* thyrotoxicosis, diabetes, obstetrics when maternal blood pressure is in excess of 130/80, hypertension, other cardiovascular disorders).

ACTIONS

A potent sympathomimetic that stimulates both alpha and beta receptors and has clinical uses related to both actions. Peripheral actions, owed in part to the release of norepinephrine, stimulate responses that are obtained when adrenergic nerves are stimulated. These include an increase in blood pressure,

---

* Ephedrine is also used as a systemic bronchodilator and decongestant and as a topical nasal decongestant. For other indications and preparations, see Bronchodilators and Decongestants, Systemic; Decongestants, Nasal, Topical.

stimulation of heart muscle, constriction of arterioles, relaxation of smooth muscles of the bronchi and GI tract, and dilation of pupils. In the bladder, relaxation of the detrusor muscle is not prominent, but tone of the trigone and vesicle sphincter is instimulates the cerebral cortex and subcortical centers.

Cardiovascular responses include moderate tachycardia, unchanged or augmented stroke volume, enhanced cardiac output, variable alterations in peripheral resistance, and usually a rise in blood pressure. Action of ephedrine is more prominent on the heart than on blood vessels. It increases the flow of coronary, cerebral, and muscle blood.

Hepatic glycogenolysis is increased but not as much as by epinephrine; usual doses are unlikely to produce hyperglycemia. Ephedrine increases oxygen consumption and metabolic rate, probably by central stimulation.

In myasthenia gravis, ephedrine produces a real but modest increase in motor power; the exact mechanism by which it affects skeletal muscle contraction is unknown.

Ephedrine is rapidly and completely absorbed following parenteral administration. Onset of action by the IM route is more rapid (within 10–20 minutes) than by subcutaneous injection. Pressor and cardiac responses persist for 30 to 60 minutes following IM or subcutaneous administration of 25 mg to 50 mg. Small amounts are slowly metabolized in the liver. Drug and its metabolites are excreted in the urine. Rate and percentage of urinary excretion are dependent on urinary pH, which is increased by acidification of the urine. Elimination half-life is about 3 hours when urine is acidified to a pH of 5 and about 6 hours when urinary pH is 6.3.

WARNINGS

May cause hypertension resulting in intracranial hemorrhage, angina pain in those with coronary insufficiency or ischemic heart disease, potentially fatal arrhythmias in patients with organic heart disease or who are receiving drugs that sensitize the myocardium. Initially, parenteral ephedrine may produce constriction of renal blood vessels and decreased urine formation.

Use in pregnancy: Safety not established. Use only when clearly needed.

Use in labor and delivery: Parenteral administration to maintain blood pressure during low or other spinal anesthesia for delivery can cause acceleration of fetal heart rate and is not used when maternal blood pressure exceeds 130/80. It is not known what effect it may have on the newborn or on child's later growth and development when administered to the mother just before or during labor.

Use in lactation: It is not known if drug is excreted in human milk. Exercise caution when administering to a nursing mother.

PRECAUTIONS

Administer cautiously to patients with heart disease, coronary insufficiency, cardiac arrhythmias, angina pectoris, diabetes, hyperthyroidism, prostatic hypertrophy, hypertension, or unstable vasomotor system. Prolonged use may produce a syndrome resembling an anxiety state. Tolerance may develop, but temporary cessation of drug usually restores its original effectiveness.

Hypovolemia: Not a substitute for replacement of blood, plasma, fluids, and electrolytes, which should be restored promptly when loss has occurred.

Drug abuse and dependence: Prolonged abuse can lead to symptoms of paranoid schizophrenia (*e.g.,* tachycardia, poor nutrition and hygiene, fever, cold sweat, dilated pupils). Some measure of tolerance develops but addiction does not occur.

DRUG INTERACTIONS

Use cautiously in patients taking **monoamine oxidase (MAO) inhibitors.** The pressor response of adrenergic drugs may be potentiated by **tricyclic antidepressants.** Not administered concomitantly with other **sympathomimetic drugs** because of possible additive effects and increased toxicity. Use cautiously with other drugs (*e.g.,* **digitalis glycosides**) that sensitize the myocardium to actions of sympathomimetic agents.

Alpha-adrenergic blocking agents may reduce vasopressor response to ephedrine by causing vasodilation. **Beta-adrenergic blocking drugs** may block cardiac and bronchodilating effects of ephedrine. The effects of these drugs may be reversed by direct-acting sympathomimetic amines.

Administration to patients receiving anesthesia with **cyclopropane** or **halogenated hydrocarbons** such as halothane, which sensitize the myocardium, may induce cardiac arrhythmias.

Drugs such as **reserpine** and **methyldopa,** which reduce the amount of norepinephrine in sympathetic nerve endings, may reduce the pressor response to ephedrine. **Diuretic agents** may also decrease vascular responses to pressor drugs. Therapeutic doses of ephedrine can inhibit the hypotensive action of **guanethidine.** The effect is a relative or complete blockade of the antihypertensive drug by a sudden rise in blood pressure. In obstetrics some **oxytocic drugs** may cause severe persistent hypertension, and even rupture of a cerebral blood vessel may occur during the postpartum period.

ADVERSE REACTIONS

Cardiovascular: Palpitation, tachycardia, precordial pain, cardiac arrhythmias.

CNS: Headache, insomnia, sweating, nervousness, vertigo, confusion, delirium, restlessness, anxiety, tension, tremor, weakness, dizziness, hallucinations.

GI: Nausea, vomiting, anorexia.

GU: Vesical sphincter spasm resulting in difficult and painful urination; urinary retention may develop in males with prostatism.

Miscellaneous: Respiratory difficulty, pallor.

OVERDOSAGE

Symptoms: Principal manifestation of poisoning is convulsions. In acute poisoning, nausea, vomiting, chills, cyanosis, irritability, nervousness, fever, suicidal behavior, tachycardia, dilated pupils, blurred vision, opisthotonos, spasms, convulsions, pulmonary edema, gasping respirations, coma, and respiratory failure have occurred. Initially, patient may have marked hypertension, followed later by hypotension accompanied by anuria. Large doses may lead to personality changes, with a psychic craving for the drug. Chronic use can also cause symptoms of tension and anxiety progressing to psychosis.

Treatment: Discontinue drug. If respirations are shallow or cyanosis is present, administer artificial respiration. Vasopressors are contraindicated. In cardiovascular collapse, maintain blood pressure. For hypertension, 5 mg phentolamine mesylate diluted in saline may be administered slowly IV, or 100 mg may be given orally. Convulsions may be controlled by diazepam or paraldehyde. Cool applications and dexamethasone 1 mg/kg administered slowly IV will control pyrexia.

DOSAGE

May be administered subcutaneously, IM, or by slow IV.

Adults: Usual dose is 25 mg to 50 mg. Absorption by IM route is more rapid (10–20 minutes) than by subcutaneous injection. IV route may be used if immediate effect is desired.

Pediatric dose: 25 mg/m^2 to 100 mg/m^2 IM or subcutaneously, divided into 4 to 6 doses.

Labor: Administer only sufficient dosage to maintain blood pressure at or below 130/80 mm Hg.

Acute attacks of asthma: Administer smallest effective dose (0.25 ml to 0.5 ml).

NURSING IMPLICATIONS

HISTORY

When possible, review chart for vital signs, current treatment modalities.

PHYSICAL ASSESSMENT

Obtain blood pressure, pulse, and respirations; general assessment of patient's condition (_e.g.,_ color, responsiveness, patent airway).

ADMINISTRATION

Obtain blood pressure, pulse, and respirations prior to administration of drug.

If drug is given for complete heart block, cardiac monitor may be used to observe drug response.

Ephedrine and ephedrine sulfate are both available as 50 mg/ml. Check physician's order and label of drug carefully.

Do not administer unless solution is clear. Discard unused portion.

Stability and storage: Is subject to oxidation. Protect against exposure to light.

ONGOING ASSESSMENTS AND NURSING MANAGEMENT

When used for hypotension, other supportive measures such as oxygen, support of respiration, and IV fluids may be employed.

Monitor blood pressure, pulse, and respirations q5m until condition is stabilized.

Monitor urinary output q15m to q30m. If output decreases, inform physician.

Continuously assess response to drug. Look for improvement in color, increase in blood pressure. If drug is given for complete heart block, look for increase in pulse rate.

Notify physician immediately if patient complains of anginal pain, a cardiac arrhythmia develops, the heart rate drastically increases, or other adverse effects are noted.

Observe for signs of overdosage if administered IM or subcutaneously for hypotension. As circulation improves, drug may be absorbed at a faster rate from subcutaneous tissues or muscle.

Epinephrine* Rx

solution: 1:1000	Adrenalin Chloride, _Generic_
solution: 1:10,000	_Generic_
solution: 1:100,000	_Generic_

* Epinephrine is also used for the following: Treatment of nasal congestion of hay fever, rhinitis, acute sinusitis; syncope due to heart block or carotid sinus sensitivity; symptomatic relief of serum sickness, urticaria, and angioneurotic edema; as a hemostatic agent; for resuscitation in cardiac arrest following anesthetic accidents; in simple (open-angle) glaucoma; relaxation of uterine musculature and inhibition of uterine contractions; prolongation of action of intraspinal and local anesthetics. For other indications and preparations, see Bronchodilators and Decongestants, Systemic; Decongestants, Nasal, Topical; Ophthalmic Vasoconstrictors/Mydriatics.

E

INDICATIONS

Intravenous epinephrine: Treatment and prophylaxis of cardiac arrest and attacks of transitory atrioventricular (AV) heart block with syncopal seizures (Stokes-Adams syndrome); acute hypersensitivity (anaphylactoid reactions to drugs, animal serums, insect stings, other allergens); treatment of acute asthmatic attacks to relieve bronchospasms not controlled by inhalation or subcutaneous administration of other solutions of the drug. In acute attacks of ventricular standstill, apply physical measures first. When external cardiac compression and attempts to restore circulation by electrical defibrillation or use of a pacemaker fail, intracardiac puncture and intramyocardial injection may be effective.

CONTRAINDICATIONS

Hypersensitivity; narrow-angle glaucoma; shock (nonanaphylactic); during general anesthesia with halogenated hydrocarbons or cyclopropane; individuals with organic brain damage; with local anesthesia of certain areas (fingers, toes); in labor; in cardiac dilatation and coronary insufficiency. Not used when vasopressor drugs may be contraindicated (*e.g.,* thyrotoxicosis, diabetes); in obstetrics when maternal blood pressure is in excess of 130/80; or in hypertension or other cardiac disorders.

ACTIONS

Actions resemble the effects of stimulation of adrenergic nerves. To a variable degree epinephrine acts on both alpha- and beta-receptor sites of sympathetic effector cells. Most prominent actions are on beta receptors of the heart and on vascular and other smooth muscle. When given by rapid IV injection, it produces a rapid rise in blood pressure, mainly systolic, and direct stimulation of cardiac muscle, which increases the strength of ventricular contraction, increases the heart rate, and constricts arterioles in the skin, mucosa, and splanchnic areas of circulation. It also relaxes smooth muscle of the bronchi and iris, is a physiologic antagonist of histamine, and produces an increase in blood glucose and glycogenolysis in the liver.

Given by slow IV injection, it usually produces a moderate rise in systolic and a fall in diastolic pressure. IV injection produces an immediate and intensified response. Following injection, epinephrine disappears rapidly from the bloodstream and is inactivated chiefly by enzymic transformation to metanephrine and normetanephrine, either of which is subsequently conjugated and excreted in the urine.

WARNINGS

May initially produce constriction of renal blood vessels and decrease in urine formation. Use with caution in the elderly, in those with cardiovascular disease, in psychoneurotic individuals, and in bronchial asthma and emphysema patients with degenerative heart disease. May induce potentially serious cardiac arrhythmias. Fatalities may result from pulmonary edema because of the peripheral constriction and cardiac stimulation produced by the drug. Use during pregnancy only when potential benefit justifies the potential risk to the fetus. Administer with caution to infants and children. Syncope has occurred following administration to asthmatic children.

PRECAUTIONS

Can produce ventricular fibrillation, but its actions in restoring electrical activity in asystole are well documented. However, use with caution in patients with ventricular fibrillation. In those with prefibrillatory rhythm, drug must be used with extreme caution because of its excitatory action on the heart.

DRUG INTERACTIONS

Do not administer concomitantly with other **sympathomimetic drugs** because of possible additive effects and increased toxicity. Combined effects may induce serious cardiac arrhythmias. Effects of epinephrine may be potentiated by **tricyclic antidepressants,** certain **antihistamines** (*e.g.,* diphenhydramine, tripelennamine, chlorpheniramine), and **sodium l-thyroxine.** In obstetrics, if vasopressor drugs are used to correct hypotension or are added to the local anesthetic solution, some **oxytocic drugs** may cause severe persistent hypertension; even rupture of a cerebral blood vessel may occur during the postpartum period. Use cautiously in those taking **monoamine oxidase (MAO) inhibitors. Cyclopropane** or **halogenated hydrocarbon anesthetics** may induce cardiac arrhythmias. **Diuretic agents** may decrease vascular response. Epinephrine may antagonize neuron blockade produced by **guanethidine,** resulting in decreased antihypertensive effect and requiring increased dosage of the latter. Use of epinephrine with excessive doses of **digitalis, mercurial diuretics,** and other drugs that sensitize the heart to arrhythmias is not recommended. Rapidly acting vasodilators such as **nitrites** or **alpha-blocking agents** may counteract marked pressor effects of epinephrine. **Propranolol** administered concomitantly may block the beta-adrenergic effects of epinephrine, causing hypertension.

ADVERSE REACTIONS

Cardiac arrhythmias and excessive risk in blood pressure; cerebral hemorrhage; hemiplegia; subarachnoid hemorrhage; anginal pain in those with angina pectoris; respiratory difficulty; nausea, vomiting.

OVERDOSAGE

Symptoms: Precordial distress, vomiting, headache, dyspnea, elevated blood pressure.

Treatment: Injection of an alpha-adrenergic blocker and a beta-adrenergic blocker. In event of a sharp rise in blood pressure, rapid-acting vasodilators such as the nitrites or alpha-adrenergic blocking agents can counteract marked pressor effects. If prolonged hypotension follows, another pressor drug such as norepinephrine may be used. If pulmonary edema occurs, treatment consists of a rapidly acting alpha-adrenergic blocking drug such as phentolamine or intermittent positive pressure respiration. Treatment of cardiac arrhythmias consists of a beta-adrenergic blocking drug such as propranolol.

Overdosage can also cause transient bradycardia followed by tachycardia; these may be accompanied by potentially fatal arrhythmias. Ventricular premature contractions may appear within 1 minute after injection and may be followed by multifocal ventricular tachycardia (prefibrillation rhythm). Ventricular effects may be followed by atrial tachycardia and occasionally AV block. Overdosage may also result in extreme pallor and coldness of the skin, metabolic acidosis, and kidney failure. Suitable corrective measures are taken.

DOSAGE

Administer by IV injection or, in cardiac arrest, by intracardiac injection into left ventricular chamber.

Cardiac arrest: 0.5 mg to 1 mg (5 ml to 10 ml of 1:10,000 solution). During resuscitation effort, administer 0.5 mg (5 ml) IV every 5 minutes.

Intracardiac injection: Administered only by trained personnel, if there has not been time to establish an IV route. Dose usually ranges from 0.3 mg to 0.5 mg (3 ml to 5 ml of 1:10,000 solution).

Intraspinal use: Usual dose is 0.2 ml to 0.4 ml of 1:1000 solution added to anesthetic spinal fluid mixture (may prolong anesthetic action by limiting absorption).

Concomitant use with local anesthetics: 1:100,000 to 1:200,000 is usual concentration employed.

NURSING IMPLICATIONS

HISTORY

Review of events (when possible) leading to ventricular standstill, anaphylactoid reaction, asthma attack. Brief history of events may also be obtained from those present when problem occurred.

PHYSICAL ASSESSMENT

Because administration of drug is of an emergency nature, assessment consists of a rapid survey of patient's present clinical condition, as well as blood pressure, pulse, and respirations.

ADMINISTRATION

Check label carefully. Solution is available as 1:1000, 1:10,000, and 1:100,000.

Solution strength and mg/ml are as follows:

1:1000 is 1 mg/ml.
1:10,000 is 0.1 mg/ml.
1:100,000 is 0.01 mg/ml.

Some products are available in 5-ml or 10-ml disposable syringe with an intracardiac needle.

Use cardiac monitor if emergency is related to cardiovascular system.

Do not use drug if it is brown or contains a precipitate. Do not use unless solution is clear and seal is intact. Discard unused portion.

When possible obtain blood pressure, pulse, and respirations immediately prior to administration.

Storage: Protect from light, extreme heat, and freezing.

ONGOING ASSESSMENTS AND NURSING MANAGEMENT

Monitor blood pressure, pulse, and respirations q1m to q2m.

Observe patient's response to drug.

Other emergency measures such as oxygen, IV fluids, pulmonary resuscitation, suctioning, and drugs may be employed.

Continue to monitor patient closely until condition is corrected and all danger has passed.

Record all events (*e.g.,* drug administration, other emergency measures, vital signs, assessments) on flow sheet.

Ergocalciferol

See Vitamin D.

Ergoloid Mesylates

(Dehydrogenated Ergot Alkaloids) Rx

tablets, sublingual: 0.5 mg	Circanol, Gerimal, H.E.A., Hydergine, *Generic*
tablets, sublingual: 1 mg	Circanol, Deapril-ST (contains tartrazine), Gerimal, H.E.A., Hydergine, *Generic*
tablets, oral: 1 mg	Hydergine
liquid: 1 mg/ml	Hydergine
liquid capsules: 1 mg	Hydergine

INDICATIONS

Some individuals over 60 who manifest signs and symptoms of an idiopathic decline in mental capacity can experience some symptomatic relief with this drug. Individuals who do respond come from groups of patients who have some ill-defined process related to aging or who have some underlying dementing condition (*e.g.,* primary progressive dementia, Alzheimer's dementia, senile-onset, multi-infarct dementia).

CONTRAINDICATIONS

Hypersensitivity; acute or chronic psychosis, regardless of etiology.

ACTIONS

Contains equal portions of dihydroergocornine mesylate, dihydroergocristine mesylate, and dihydroergocryptine mesylate. There is no evidence establishing the mechanism by which ergoloid mesylates produce their mental effects, nor is there conclusive evidence that they directly affect cerebral arteriosclerosis or cerebrovascular insufficiency. Drug undergoes rapid first-pass biotransformation in the liver; less than 50% reaches systemic circulation. Oral tablets are rapidly but incompletely absorbed from the GI tract with peak plasma levels occurring 1 hour after a single dose; by 24 hours, plasma levels are not detectable.

PRECAUTIONS

Ergot preparations have been reported to precipitate attacks of acute intermittent porphyria and are used with caution in susceptible patients.

Tartrazine sensitivity: Some products contain tartrazine (see Appendix 6, section 6-23).

ADVERSE REACTIONS

Has not been found to produce serious side-effects. Some sublingual irritation, transient nausea, and gastric disturbances have been reported. Does not possess vasoconstrictor properties of natural ergot alkaloids.

DOSAGE

Usual starting dose is 1 mg tid.

NURSING IMPLICATIONS

HISTORY

See Appendix 4.

PHYSICAL ASSESSMENT

Obtain general physical status, vital signs, weight; evaluate mental status (*e.g.,* cognitive and interpersonal skills, mood, orientation, grooming, alertness, memory).

ADMINISTRATION

Instruct patient in placement of sublingual tablet; advise not to eat, drink, or smoke until tablet is dissolved.

Stay with patient first few times sublingual form is used to be sure tablet dissolves under tongue and is not swallowed.

If patient has difficulty using sublingual tablet or his mouth is exceptionally dry, discuss with physician; oral tablets and liquid preparations are available.

ONGOING ASSESSMENTS AND NURSING MANAGEMENT

Record vital signs bid or as ordered; inspect oral cavity for sublingual irritation (if sublingual form is used); assess mental status, compare to baseline data, and record observations.

Weigh weekly. Report steady weight loss to physician.

Alleviation of symptoms is usually gradual and results may not be observed for 3 to 4 weeks.

Contact physician if patient complains of nausea, heartburn.

Reevaluation of patient is usually conducted at end of 12 weeks of therapy. Changes may be noted in the following areas: mental alertness, confusion, recent memory, orientation, emotional lability, self-care, depression, anxiety/fears, cooperation, sociability, appetite, dizziness, fatigue, bothersomeness.

PATIENT AND FAMILY INFORMATION

May cause transient nausea and heartburn. If these become severe, discuss with physician.

Allow sublingual tablets to dissolve completely under tongue. Do not swallow.

Ergonovine Maleate Rx

tablets: 0.2 mg	Ergotrate Maleate, *Generic*
injection: 0.2 mg/ml	Ergotrate Maleate, *Generic*

INDICATIONS

An oxytocic agent used in prevention and treatment of postpartum and postabortal hemorrhage due to uterine atony. Parenteral ergonovine is generally not as effective as ergotamine in treatment of migraine headache; however, it may be found more useful than ergotamine when use of ergotamine has caused paresthesias.

Investigational uses: Diagnostically to identify Prinzmetal's angina. Doses of 0.05 mg to 0.2 mg IV during coronary arteriography provoke spontaneous coronary arterial spasms responsible for Prinzmetal's angina. Arrhythmias, ventricular tachycardia, and myocardial infarction have been precipitated.

CONTRAINDICATIONS
Induction of labor; cases of threatened spontaneous abortion; patients who have shown allergic or idiosyncratic reactions to the drug.

ACTIONS
When used after placental delivery it increases strength, duration, and frequency of uterine contractions and decreases uterine bleeding. Exerts pharmacologic effects by acting as a partial agonist or antagonist at adrenergic, dopaminergic, and tryptaminergic receptors. Has a rapid onset of action, which varies with the route of administration; _IV_—40 seconds; _IM_—7 to 8 minutes; _oral_—10 minutes. Contractions continue for 3 or more hours after injection.

WARNINGS
Parenteral oxytocics are potentially dangerous. Patients have been injured, and some have died, because of their injudicious use. Hyperstimulation of the uterus during labor may lead to uterine tetany with marked impairment of the uteroplacental blood flow, uterine rupture, cervical and perineal lacerations, amniotic fluid embolism, and trauma to the infant (_e.g.,_ hypoxia, intracranial hemorrhage). In some calcium-deficient patients, the uterus may not respond to ergonovine. In such cases, responsiveness can be immediately restored by cautious IV injection of calcium salts. Calcium should not be given IV to those under the influence of digitalis.

PRECAUTIONS
Not recommended for routine use prior to delivery of the placenta. Prolonged use is avoided; drug is discontinued if symptoms of ergotism appear. Use cautiously in patients with hypertension, heart disease, venoatrial shunts, mitral valve stenosis, obliterative vascular disease, sepsis, or hepatic or renal impairment.

ADVERSE REACTIONS
Nausea, vomiting, and diarrhea may occur but are uncommon. Allergic phenomena, including shock, have been reported. Ergotism also has been reported. Elevations of blood pressure (sometimes extreme) and headache appear in a small percentage of patients, most frequently associated with regional anesthesia, previous administration of a vasoconstrictor, and IV administration of an oxytocic; however, they may occur in the absence of any of these. Blood pressure elevations are no more frequent with ergonovine than with other oxytocics and usually

subside following IV administration of 15 mg chlorpromazine. Drug may lower prolactin, which may decrease lactation.

OVERDOSAGE
Symptoms: Principal manifestations are convulsions and gangrene. Symptoms include vomiting, diarrhea, dizziness, rise or fall in blood pressure, weak pulse, dyspnea, loss of consciousness, numbness and coldness of the extremities, tingling, chest pain, gangrene of fingers and toes, hypercoagulability.

Treatment: Treat convulsions. Control hypercoagulability with heparin and maintain blood-clotting time at approximately three times normal. Give a vasodilator such as tolazoline as an antidote; rate of administration may be controlled by monitoring pulse rate and blood pressure. For emergency measures, delay absorption of tablets by giving tap water, milk, or activated charcoal; then remove by gastric lavage or emesis followed by catharsis. Gangrene requires surgical amputation.

DOSAGE
Parenteral: Intended primarily for routine IM injection. Usually produces a firm contraction of the uterus within a few minutes. Usual IM (or emergency IV) dose is 0.2 mg. Severe uterine bleeding may require repeated doses but rarely more than one injection every 2 to 4 hours. IV administration leads to quicker response, but incidence of nausea and other side-effects is higher. IV route is recommended for emergencies such as excessive uterine bleeding.

Oral: To minimize later postpartum bleeding, give one or two tablets q6h to q12h until danger of uterine atony has passed (usually 48 hours).

NURSING IMPLICATIONS

HISTORY
Review patient's chart for admission history and physical examination, health and pregnancy history, labor record. If administered postpartum, review delivery record.

PHYSICAL ASSESSMENT
Record blood pressure, pulse, and respirations.

ADMINISTRATION
In delivery room, administer drug at direction of physician, usually during third stage of labor after placenta has separated. Drug may also be administered prior to delivery of the placenta.

Postpartum administration: Assess uterine

fundus for firmness and position immediately prior to administration.

ONGOING ASSESSMENTS AND NURSING MANAGEMENT
Administration during third stage of labor:
Monitor blood pressure, pulse, and respirations q15m to q30m, as well as uterine response, until patient is transferred to postpartum (postdelivery) unit.

Administration during postpartum: Monitor blood pressure, pulse, and respirations; check uterine fundus for firmness and position q1h to q2h or as ordered.

Severe cramping is evidence of effectiveness, but inform physician because dosage may be reduced.

Notify physician immediately if blood pressure increases or decreases, the pulse rate changes, or uterine atony or hemorrhage occurs.

Signs of ergotism, although rare, include pale, cold, or numb fingers and toes; nausea, vomiting; diarrhea; headache; and muscle pain or weakness.

Drug is usually administered for 48 hours, until danger of uterine atony has passed.

Ergotamine Preparations

Ergotamine Tartrate *Rx*

tablets: 1 mg	Gynergen
tablets, sublingual: 2 mg	Ergomar, Ergostat
aerosol: 9 mg/ml	Medihaler Ergotamine

Ergotamine Combinations *Rx*

tablets: 1 mg ergotamine tartrate, 100 mg caffeine	Cafergot Tablets, Cafertabs Tablets, Cafetrate Tablets, Ercaf Tablets, Ercatab Tablets, Ergo-Caff, Wigraine Tablets
tablets: 1 mg ergotamine tartrate, 100 mg caffeine, 0.125 mg l-alkaloids of belladonna, 30 mg sodium pentobarbital	Cafergot P-B Tablets
suppositories: 2 mg ergotamine tartrate, 100 mg caffeine	Cafergot Suppositories
suppositories: 2 mg ergotamine tar-	Cafergot P-B Suppositories
trate, 100 mg caffeine, 0.25 mg l-alkaloids of belladonna, 60 mg pentobarbital	
suppositories: 2 mg ergotamine tartrate, 100 mg caffeine, 21.5 mg tartaric acid	Wigraine Suppositories

INDICATIONS
Vascular headaches such as migraine, migraine variant, and cluster headache (histaminic cephalalgia).

In the combinations: Ergotamine tartrate is used for its specific action against migraine.

Caffeine, a cranial vasoconstrictor, is added to enhance vasoconstrictor effects. Caffeine is reported to enhance the absorption of ergotamine.

Belladonna alkaloids are used for their anticholinergic and antiemetic effects for those with excessive nausea and vomiting during attacks.

Barbiturates are used for sedation.

CONTRAINDICATIONS
Hypersensitivity; sepsis; peripheral vascular disease; hepatic or renal disease; severe pruritus; coronary artery disease; hypertension; infectious states; malnutrition. Contraindicated in pregnancy.

ACTIONS
Is an alpha-adrenergic blocking agent with direct stimulating effect on smooth muscle of peripheral and cranial blood vessels. Produces depression of central vasomotor centers. Also has serotonin antagonist properties. Causes vasoconstriction with concomitant decrease in pulsations that are probably responsible for migraine and other vascular headache symptoms. Is considered a specific agent for this condition. GI absorption is slow and incomplete following oral administration. Sublingual absorption is dependent on oral pH. Ergotamine is metabolized by the liver and excreted in bile. Trace amounts of unmetabolized drug are excreted in feces and urine.

WARNINGS
Not known if drug is excreted in breast milk. Nursing should not be undertaken while taking this drug. Safety and efficacy for use in children not established.

PRECAUTIONS
Avoid prolonged administration or dosage in excess of that recommended because of danger of ergotism and gangrene.

ADVERSE REACTIONS

Side-effects usually do not necessitate interruption of therapy; however, serious toxicity may occur, especially with large doses.

Numbness and tingling of fingers and toes, muscle pains in the extremities, pulselessness, weakness in legs, precordial distress and pain, transient tachycardia or bradycardia, diarrhea, nausea, vomiting, localized edema, and itching. In large doses, drug raises blood pressure, causes arterial insufficiency, produces vasoconstriction, and slows the heart both by direct action and by its effect on the vagus. Also has oxytocic and spasmolytic properties. The above conditions are seen as a consequence of overdosage and may occur at dosage recommended for control of headaches. The vasoconstriction caused by ergot may be overcome by a vasodilator, such as nitroprusside, which has been used in ergot poisoning.

DOSAGE

ERGOTAMINE TARTRATE

Oral tablets: Two to six tablets per attack. Do not exceed ten tablets weekly.

Sublingual tablets: Initiate therapy as soon as possible after first symptoms of an attack. Place tablet under tongue; subsequent doses may be taken at ½-hour intervals if necessary. Do not exceed three tablets each 24 hours. Limit dosage to not more than 10 mg/week.

Inhalation: Start with one inhalation; repeat if not relieved in 5 minutes. Space additional inhalations at least 5 minutes apart. Do not exceed six inhalations every 24 hours.

ERGOTAMINE COMBINATIONS

One or two tablets or suppositories at onset, then one or two every 15 minutes to 1 hour. Do not exceed six tablets or two suppositories per attack or ten tablets or five suppositories per week.

NURSING IMPLICATIONS

HISTORY

See Appendix 4. Note symptoms experienced during prodromal stage (*e.g.,* scintillating scotomas, visual disturbances, nausea, vomiting, fatigue).

PHYSICAL ASSESSMENT

Obtain vital signs.

ADMINISTRATION

When patient states that prodromal symptoms are occurring, drug therapy is usually instituted. Physician usually writes order to begin therapy once prodromal symptoms or headache occurs.

Patient will require instruction for first-time use of a sublingual tablet or Medihaler.

Medihaler is self-administered and delivers 0.36 mg/dose.

Instruct patient to remain quiet after drug is administered.

ONGOING ASSESSMENTS AND NURSING MANAGEMENT

Monitor vital signs daily; record drug effect and compare to baseline data describing symptoms, severity, and length of previous migraine headaches.

Keep room semidark and free from disturbance and noise (patient is sensitive to noise and light during a migraine attack).

Observe for adverse drug reactions; notify physician if they occur.

PATIENT AND FAMILY INFORMATION

A patient package insert is available with product.

Follow physician's directions regarding initiating therapy at first sign of attack. Do *not* exceed recommended dosage because this drug can cause serious problems if dosage is exceeded.

Notify physician or nurse if any of the following occurs: irregular heartbeat, nausea, vomiting, numbness or tingling of fingers or toes, or pain or weakness of the extremities (signs of ergotism).

If pregnant, or pregnancy is suspected, do *not* take this drug. Consult physician about therapy for migraine during pregnancy.

Erythrityl Tetranitrate

See Nitrates.

Erythromycin Preparations* Rx

Intravenous Preparations

Erythromycin Gluceptate

powder for injection: Ilotycin Gluceptate
250 mg, 500 mg,
1 g

* This monograph discusses parenteral and oral erythromycin preparations. For other indications and preparations, see Antibiotics, Ophthalmic; Antibiotics, Topical.

Erythromycin Lactobionate

powder for injection: 500 mg, 1 g	Erythrocin Lactobionate-IV
piggyback—powder for injection: 500 mg	Erythrocin Piggyback

Oral Preparations

Erythromycin Base

tablets, enteric coated: 250 mg	E-Mycin, Ery-Tab, Ilotycin, Robimycin, Robitabs, RP-Mycin, *Generic*
tablets, enteric coated: 333 mg, 500 mg	E-Mycin, Ery-Tab
tablets, film coated: 250 mg, 500 mg	Erythromycin Base Film-tabs
capsules, enteric-coated pellets: 250 mg	Eryc

Erythromycin Estolate

tablets, chewable: 125 mg, 250 mg	Ilosone
capsules, 125 mg, 250 mg	Ilosone Pulvules
tablets: 250 mg	*Generic*
tablets: 500 mg	Ilosone
drops: 100 mg/ml	Ilosone Ready-Mixed
powder for oral suspension: 125 mg/5 ml when reconstituted	Ilosone
suspension: 125 mg/5 ml, 250 mg/5 ml	Ilosone, *Generic*

Erythromycin Ethylsuccinate

tablets, chewable: 200 mg	E.E.S.
tablets, film coated: 400 mg	E.E.S. 400, *Generic*
suspension: 200 mg/5 ml	E.E.S. 200, E-Mycin E, Pediamycin, Wyamycin E, *Generic*
powder for oral suspension: 200 mg/5 ml when reconstituted	E.E.S. Granules, Pediamycin Granules
powder for oral suspension: 400 mg/5 ml when reconstituted	EryPed
suspension: 400 mg/5 ml	E.E.S. 400, E-Mycin E, Pediamycin 400, Wyamycin E 400, *Generic*
powder for drops: 100 mg/2.5 ml when reconstituted	E.E.S., Pediamycin

Erythromycin Stearate

tablets, film coated: 250 mg	Bristamycin, Eramycin, Erypar, Erythrocin Stearate, Ethril '250,' Pfizer-E, SK-Erythromycin, Wyamycin S, *Generic*
tablets, film coated: 500 mg	Erypar, Erythrocin Stearate, Ethril '500' (contains tartrazine), Pfizer-E, SK-Erythromycin, Wyamycin S, *Generic*

INDICATIONS

Streptococcus pyogenes *(group A β-hemolytic streptococci):* Upper and lower respiratory tract, skin and soft-tissue infections of mild to moderate severity.

α-hemolytic streptococci (*Viridans *group): Prophylaxis against bacterial endocarditis prior to dental or other operative procedures in those with history of rheumatic fever or congenital heart disease who are hypersensitive to penicillin. Not suitable prior to GU or GI surgery.

Staphylococcus aureus: Acute infections of skin and soft tissue of mild to moderate severity.

Streptococcus pneumoniae: Upper respiratory tract infections (*e.g.,* otitis media, pharyngitis) and lower respiratory tract infections (*e.g.,* pneumonia) of mild to moderate degree.

Mycoplasma pneumoniae *(Eaton agent, PPLO):* Respiratory infections.

Haemophilus influenzae: Upper respiratory tract infections of mild to moderate severity when used concomitantly with sulfonamides. Not all strains susceptible.

Corynebacterium diphtheriae *and* C. minutissimum: As adjunct to antitoxin and in treatment of erythrasma.

Listeria monocytogenes: Infections due to this organism.

Neisseria gonorrhoeae: Erythromycin lactobionate or gluceptate injection given with erythromycin stearate or base orally, as alternative in treatment of acute pelvic inflammatory disease in those hypersensitive to penicillin.

Legionella pneumophila: Effective in treating legionnaires' disease.

In addition, oral erythromycin is indicated in treatment of intestinal amebiasis, as an alternative drug for primary syphilis in those allergic to penicillin, and elimination of *Bordetella pertussis* from the nasopharynx of infected individuals.

CONTRAINDICATIONS
Hypersensitivity. Erythromycin estolate is contraindicated in patients with preexisting liver disease.

ACTIONS
May be bactericidal or bacteriostatic at normal therapeutic concentrations. Binds to 50 S ribosomal subunits of susceptible bacteria and suppresses protein synthesis.

Erythromycin base is acid labile and usually formulated in enteric-coated forms. Acid-stable salts and esters (estolate, ethylsuccinate, stearate) are well absorbed. Parenteral administration is restricted to those in whom oral administration is not possible or when severity of the infection requires immediate high serum levels.

Erythromycin is approximately 70% bound in plasma. It diffuses into most body fluids, including prostatic fluid. Low concentrations are normally achieved in spinal fluid, but passage of drug across the blood–brain barrier increases in meningitis. It crosses the placental barrier, but fetal plasma levels are generally low. Drug is excreted in breast milk.

In normal hepatic function, drug is concentrated in the liver and excreted via bile. Plasma half-life is approximately 1.4 hours in those with normal renal function; it is prolonged (4.8–5.8 hours) in anuric patients. Erythromycin is not removed by peritoneal dialysis or hemodialysis.

WARNINGS
Use in impaired hepatic function: Exercise caution; there have been reports of hepatic dysfunction, with or without jaundice.

Hepatotoxicity: Administration has been associated with infrequent occurrence of cholestatic hepatitis. This effect is most common with use of erythromycin estolate but has been reported with other erythromycins. Laboratory findings are characterized by abnormal hepatic-function tests, peripheral eosinophilia, and leukocytosis. Symptoms may include malaise, nausea, vomiting, abdominal cramps, and fever; jaundice may or may not be present. In some instances, severe abdominal pain may simulate pain of biliary colic, pancreatitis, perforated ulcer, or an acute abdomen. In other instances, clinical symptoms and results of hepatic-function tests have resembled findings in extrahepatic jaundice.

Initial symptoms have developed in some cases after a few days of treatment but generally have followed 1 to 2 weeks of continuous therapy. The syndrome seems to result from a form of sensitization, occurs chiefly in adults, and has been reversible when drug is discontinued.

Use in pregnancy, lactation: Safety not established. Erythromycin crosses the placental barrier and is excreted in breast milk.

PRECAUTIONS
Superinfection: Use of antibiotics (especially prolonged or repeated therapy) may result in bacterial or fungal overgrowth of nonsusceptible organisms. Such overgrowth may lead to a secondary infection. Appropriate measures should be taken if superinfection occurs.

Tartrazine sensitivity: Some products contain tartrazine. See Appendix 6, section 6-23.

DRUG INTERACTIONS
Synergy between erythromycin and **sulfonamides** against *H. influenzae* has been demonstrated.
Use of erythromycin in those receiving high doses of **theophylline** may result in increased serum theophylline levels and potential theophylline toxicity; appropriate dosage adjustments are made. Erythromycin may elevate plasma **carbamazepine** levels.

Drug/lab tests: Erythromycin interferes with the fluorometric determination of **urinary catecholamines.**

ADVERSE REACTIONS
Allergic reactions: Serious allergic reactions, including anaphylaxis, have been reported. Mild allergic reactions such as rashes with or without pruritus, urticaria, bullous fixed eruptions, and eczema have occurred.

Parenteral

Side-effects following use of IV erythromycin are rare. Occasional venous irritation has been seen. If solution is given slowly, in dilute solution, preferably by continuous IV infusion or intermittent infusion in no less than 20 to 60 minutes, pain and vessel trauma are minimized.

Ototoxicity: Rarely, reversible hearing loss with use of IV infusion of 4 g or more per day of erythromycin lactobionate or gluceptate.

Hepatotoxicity: Erythromycin gluceptate IV has been associated with variations in hepatic function following daily doses at high levels or after prolonged therapy. Hepatic-function tests are recommended when such therapy is given.

Oral

Most frequent dose-related side-effects are gastrointestinal, such as abdominal cramping and discomfort. Nausea, vomiting, and diarrhea occur infrequently with usual oral doses. Psuedomembranous colitis associated with erythromycin therapy has been reported.

Ototoxicity: Reversible ototoxicity has been reported following administration of 4 g/day of erythromycin stearate.

Hepatotoxicity: Most commonly associated with erythromycin estolate (see *Warnings*).

Isolated instances of psychiatric complications (*e.g.,* uncontrollable crying, hysterical laughter, fear, confusion, abnormal thinking, and a feeling of impending loss of consciousness) have been reported during treatment with erythromycin.

OVERDOSAGE

Allergic reactions associated with acute overdosage should be handled in the usual manner (*i.e.,* administration of epinephrine, corticosteroids, antihistamines) as needed and the prompt elimination of the unabsorbed drug, in addition to supportive measures.

DOSAGE

Parenteral

Continuous infusion is preferable, but intermittent infusion at intervals not greater than q6h is also effective. Because of irritative properties, IV push is an unacceptable route of administration.

Severe infections (adults and children): 15 mg/kg/day to 20 mg/kg/day IV. Higher doses (up to 4 g/day) may be given in very severe infections.

Acute pelvic inflammatory disease caused by N. gonorrhoeae: 500 mg IV q6h for 3 days followed by 250 mg erythromycin stearate or base orally q6h for 7 days.

Legionnaires' disease: Optimal doses not established. Doses used have been 1 g/day to 4 g/day, in divided doses.

Oral

Dosages and product strengths are expressed as erythromycin base equivalents. Because of differences in absorption and biotransformation, 400 mg of the ethylsuccinate ester is required to achieve serum levels comparable to those with 250 mg of the base, stearate, or estolate forms.

Adults: Usual dose is 250 mg (400 mg of ethylsuccinate) q6h. This may be increased up to 4 g/day, according to severity of the infection. If twice-a-day dosage is desired, recommended dose is 500 mg q12h. Twice-a-day dosing is not recommended when doses larger than 1 g/day are administered.

Children: Age, weight, and severity of infection are important factors in determining proper dosage. Usual regimen is 30 mg/kg/day to 50 mg/kg/day in three or four divided doses. For more severe infections, dosage may be doubled.

Streptococcal infections: For treatment of group A β-hemolytic streptococcal infections in those allergic to penicillin, give 20 mg/kg/day to 50 mg/kg/day in divided doses for 10 days. In continuous prophylaxis for those with history of rheumatic heart disease who are allergic to penicillin and sulfonamides, dosage is 250 mg (400 mg of ethylsuccinate) twice daily. For prophylaxis of bacterial endocarditis in penicillin-allergic patients and patients with congenital heart disease or rheumatic or other acquired valvular heart disease, undergoing dental procedures or upper respiratory tract surgery or instrumentation, dosage is 1 g given 1½ to 2 hours prior to procedure, then 500 mg q6h for 8 doses. Children should receive 20 mg/kg prior to the procedure, then 10 mg/kg q6h for 8 doses. Alternatively, high-risk patients (those with prosthetic heart valves) should receive vancomycin 1 g IV over 30 to 60 minutes beginning ½ to 1 hour prior to the procedure, then erythromycin 500 mg q6h for 8 doses. Pediatric doses are vancomycin 20 mg/kg; erythromycin 10 mg/kg. Pediatric dose should not exceed recommended single dose or 24-hour dose for adult.

Primary syphilis: 30 g to 40 g (or 48 g to 64 g ethylsuccinate or 20 g estolate for 10 days) given in divided doses over period of 10 to 15 days.

Dysenteric amebiasis: Adult dosage is 250 mg (400 mg ethylsuccinate) 4 times/day for 10 to 14 days. *Children*—30 mg/kg/day to 50 mg/kg/day in divided doses for 10 to 14 days.

Acute pelvic inflammatory disease caused by N. gonorrhoeae: 500 mg erythromycin lactobionate or gluceptate IV q6h for 3 days, followed by 250 mg erythromycin stearate or base PO q6h for 7 days.

Legionnaires' disease: Although optimal doses are not established, doses used are 1 g to 4 g erythromycin stearate, estolate, or base daily in divided doses, or 1.6 g to 4 g erythromycin ethylsuccinate daily in divided doses.

Pertussis: Optimal dosage and duration are not established; doses of erythromycin (stearate, ethylsuccinate) used are 40 mg/kg/day to 50 mg/kg/day in divided doses for 5 to 14 days.

CDC-recommended treatment schedules for syphilis and gonorrhea

Early syphilis (primary, secondary, latent of less than 1 year's duration): In those allergic to penicillin, 500 mg erythromycin (stearate, ethylsuccinate or base) four times a day for 15 days.

Syphilis of more than 1 year's duration: In those allergic to penicillin, 500 mg erythromycin (stearate, ethylsuccinate or base) four times a day for 30 days.

Syphilis in pregnancy: Efficacy not established. Documentation of penicillin allergy important before treatment with erythromycin. Erythromycin estolate not recommended because of potential adverse effects on mother and fetus.

Disseminated gonococcal infection: 0.5 g four times a day for 7 days.

NURSING IMPLICATIONS

HISTORY
See Appendix 4.

PHYSICAL ASSESSMENT
Obtain vital signs. In skin and soft-tissue infections, observe area for appearance, drainage. In lower respiratory infections, auscultate lungs, note quantity and appearance of sputum. Additional assessments based on symptoms may also be appropriate. Hepatic-function tests may be ordered prior to therapy. Culture and sensitivity tests are recommended prior to institution of therapy unless drug is used for prophylaxis.

ADMINISTRATION
Parenteral
Generic name similarity: Erythromycin IV is available as lactobionate or glucleptate. Check physician's order carefully.

Reconstitute only with Sterile Water for Injection without preservatives to prevent precipitation.

Using Sterile Water for Injection, prepare initial solution by adding at least 10 ml to the 250-mg or 500-mg vials or at least 20 ml to the 1-g vials.

Piggyback solution: Prepare by adding 100 ml of 0.9% Sodium Chloride Injection, Lactated Ringer's Injection, or Normosol-R Solution to the dispensing vial. Shake well until all of drug is dissolved.

Intermittent infusion: One fourth of total daily dose given in 20 to 60 minutes by slow IV injection of 250 mg to 500 mg in 100 ml to 250 ml of 0.9% Sodium Chloride Injection or 5% Dextrose in Water. Administer slowly to avoid pain along the vein.

Continuous infusion: When all of drug is dissolved, solution may be added to 0.9% Sodium Chloride Injection, Lactated Ringer's Injection, or 5% Dextrose in Water to give 1 g/liter for slow, continuous infusion. If period of administration is prolonged, contact pharmacy for preparation of the IV solution because solution must be buffered to neutrality with a sterile agent such as 4% Sodium Bicarbonate Additive Solution. The buffered solution is administered within 24 hours after dilution. Apply timing label. If given in 100 ml or 250 ml of fluid by a volume control set, pharmacy buffers the IV fluid in its primary container before it is added to a volumetric administration set.

Administer intermittent infusion over period of 20 to 60 minutes. Check rate of infusion q5m to q10m and adjust rate of flow as necessary.

If pain or discomfort along the vein occurs, slow the infusion rate as well as check for signs of extravasation. If pain or discomfort is not relieved, contact physician.

Oral
Trade name similarity: Ilosone (erythromycin estolate) and Ilotycin (erythromycin base).

It is preferable to administer erythromycin base, stearate, and ethylsuccinate preparations in the fasting state or immediately before meals. Erythromycin estolate absorption is not appreciably altered by food.

Give with a full glass of water. Do not offer juice with medication. *Do not* crush enteric- or film-coated tablets. Instruct patient not to chew tablet. If patient is unable to swallow tablet whole, a liquid preparation (erythromycin estolate and ethylsuccinate) is available.

Chewable tablets must be chewed and not swallowed whole.

ONGOING ASSESSMENTS AND NURSING MANAGEMENT
Record vital signs q4h or as ordered; observe for adverse drug reactions. If more than 4 g/day of oral or parenteral form is administered, observe for signs of ototoxicity (*e.g.,* tinnitus, hearing loss). High dosage or prolonged therapy requires observation for hepatotoxicity (*e.g.,* jaundice, dark urine, pale stools, fatigue, abdominal pain, or discomfort). Observe for signs of superinfection (Appendix 6, section 6-22); notify physician at first sign of a superinfection because appropriate therapy is necessary.

If GI upset occurs, contact physician. Dose may be reduced or drug ordered to be given with food or meals.

Repeat culture and sensitivity studies may be ordered; periodic hepatic-function tests may be ordered during prolonged therapy.

In patients with *S. aureus* infections, observe for sudden onset of fever, increased drainage, or change in appearance of site of infection because resistant organisms may emerge.

When used for prophylaxis prior to surgery or

dental procedures, observe patient following the procedure for signs of bacterial endocarditis (*e.g.,* fatigue, anorexia, intermittent fever, arthralgia, night sweats); report symptoms promptly to physician.

Patients with syphilis usually have a microscopic examination for *Treponema pallidum* before therapy as well as monthly serologic tests for a minimum of 4 months.

PATIENT AND FAMILY INFORMATION

Preferably taken on empty stomach at least 1 hour before or 2 hours after meals with a full glass of water. Avoid taking medication with juice. Erythromycin estolate, ethylsuccinate, and certain brands of erythromycin base enteric-coated tablets may be taken without regard to food. Follow directions on prescription container, or ask pharmacist.

If GI upset occurs, contact physician. If unable to contact physician and next dose is due, take with food.

Complete full course of therapy. Do not stop taking drug even if symptoms improve or disappear.

Take at evenly spaced intervals, preferably around the clock (day and night), unless physician orders otherwise.

May cause nausea, vomiting, diarrhea, stomach cramps. Notify physician if these effects persist.

Notify physician if severe abdominal pain, yellow discoloration of the skin or eye, darkened urine, pale stools, or unusual tiredness occurs.

Erythromycin Ethylsuccinate and Sulfisoxazole Rx

powder for oral sus-	Pediazole
pension: 200 mg	
erythromycin ac-	
tivity and 600 mg	
sulfisoxazole/5 ml	

INDICATIONS

In children, acute otitis media caused by susceptible strains of *Haemophilus influenzae.*

CONTRAINDICATIONS

See Erythromycin; Sulfisoxazole.

ACTIONS

Erythromycin inhibits protein synthesis without affecting nucleic acid synthesis. Sulfonamides, including sulfisoxazole, exert bacteriostatic activity by

competitively inhibiting bacterial synthesis of folic acid from para-aminobenzoic acid. Resistance to erythromycin has been demonstrated by some strains of *H. influenzae.* Drug combination is usually active against *H. influenzae,* including ampicillin-resistant strains.

PRECAUTIONS, WARNINGS, DRUG INTERACTIONS, ADVERSE REACTIONS

See Erythromycin; Sulfisoxazole.

DOSAGE

Reconstituted powder results in an oral suspension containing erythromycin ethylsuccinate (equivalent to 200 mg erythromycin activity) and sulfisoxazole acetyl (equivalent to 600 mg sulfisoxazole) per 5 ml.

Not administered to infants under 2 months of age because systemic sulfonamides are contraindicated in this group.

Acute otitis media: Dosage may be based on erythromycin (50 mg/kg/day) or sulfisoxazole (150 mg/kg/day to a maximum of 6 g/day). Give in equally divided doses four times a day for 10 days. May be administered without regard to meals. See Table 28 for recommended dosage schedule.

NURSING IMPLICATIONS

HISTORY

See Appendix 4.

PHYSICAL ASSESSMENT

Examination of ear is performed by physician. Inspect outer ear canal for drainage.

ADMINISTRATION

Shake well before using.

Suspension is flavored and may be given without mixing with other vehicles.

ONGOING ASSESSMENTS AND NURSING MANAGEMENT

Obtain vital signs daily; observe for adverse drug reactions; note patient's response to medication (*e.g.,* relief of pain, decrease in temperature [fe-

Table 28. Recommended Dosage Schedules for Erythromycin Ethylsuccinate and Sulfisoxazole for Treatment of Acute Otitis Media in Children

Weight	Dose q6h
8 kg	2.5 ml
16 kg	5.0 ml
24 kg	7.5 ml
>45 kg	10.0 ml

ver usually accompanies otitis media], improvement in hearing [hearing loss may occur in acute secretory otitis media], relief of other symptoms such as dizziness, nausea, vomiting, drainage in the outer ear canal).

In infants, observe for prolonged or frequent crying, pulling at or holding ear, rolling of head side to side, failure to take formula or baby foods, drainage in the outer ear canal, restlessness, and irritability as signs of otitis media. As infection is controlled, symptoms should begin to lessen.

Additional treatment may include administration of an analgesic, antipyretic agent; use of a decongestant; myringotomy or insertion of myringotomy tubes.

FAMILY INFORMATION

Administer drug as prescribed by physician.

Complete full course of therapy. Do not discontinue medication even if child appears to improve.

Contact physician if symptoms become worse or condition does not improve. Follow physician's recommendations about administration of nonprescription preparations for pain or fever.

Esterified Estrogens

See Estrogens.

Estradiol

See Estrogens.

Estradiol Cypionate in Oil

See Estrogens.

Estradiol Valerate in Oil

See Estrogens.

Estramustine Phosphate Sodium Rx

capsules: equivalent   EMCYT
   to 140 mg estra-
   mustine phosphate

INDICATIONS

Palliative treatment of patients with metastatic and/or progressive carcinoma of the prostate.

CONTRAINDICATIONS

Known hypersensitivity to either estradiol or nitrogen mustard. Active thrombophlebitis or thromboembolic disorders, except in those cases in which the actual tumor mass is the cause of the thrombembolic phenomenon and benefits of therapy outweigh the risks.

ACTIONS

Is an antineoplastic agent combining estradiol (p 453) and nornitrogen mustard. Major metabolites in plasma are estramustine, the estrone analogue, estradiol, and estrone. Prolonged treatment produces elevated total estradiol plasma concentrations that fall within ranges similar to elevated estradiol levels found in prostatic cancer patients given conventional estradiol therapy. Estrogenic effects are similar in patients treated with either estramustine phosphate or conventional estradiol.

WARNINGS

There is an increased risk of thrombosis, including nonfatal myocardial infarction (MI), in men receiving estrogens for prostatic cancer. Use with caution in those with a history of thrombophlebitis, thrombosis, or thromboembolic disorders, especially if they were associated with estrogen therapy. Use caution in patients with cerebral vascular or coronary artery disease.

Glucose tolerance: Because glucose tolerance may be decreased, diabetic patients should be carefully observed while receiving this drug.

Elevated blood pressure: Because hypertension may occur, monitor blood pressure periodically during therapy.

PRECAUTIONS

Fluid retention: Exacerbation of preexisting or incipient peripheral edema or congestive heart disease has been seen. Other conditions that may be influenced by fluid retention, such as epilepsy, migraine, or renal dysfunction, require careful observation.

Use in impaired renal function: Drug may be poorly metabolized and should be administered with caution.

Calcium/phosphorus metabolism: Drug may influence metabolism of calcium and phosphorus and is used with caution in those with metabolic bone diseases that are associated with hypercalcemia or in patients with renal insufficiency.

Laboratory tests: Certain endocrine and hepatic-function tests may be affected by estrogen-containing drugs. Abnormalities of hepatic enzymes and of bilirubin have occurred but seldom have been severe enough to require cessation of therapy. Such tests should be done at appropriate intervals during therapy and repeated after drug is withdrawn for 2 months.

Carcinogenesis, mutagenesis, impairment of fertility: Estradiol and nitrogen mustard are mutagenic. For this reason and because some patients who have been impotent while on estrogen therapy have regained potency while taking the drug, patient is advised to use contraceptive measures.

ADVERSE REACTIONS

Cardiovascular-respiratory: Cerebrovascular accident, MI, thrombophlebitis, pulmonary emboli, congestive heart failure, edema, dyspnea, leg cramps, upper respiratory discharge, hoarseness.

GI: Nausea, diarrhea, minor GI upset, anorexia, flatulence, vomiting, GI bleeding, burning throat, thirst.

Hematologic: Leukopenia, thrombopenia.

Hepatic laboratory abnormalities: Bilirubin alone; bilirubin and SGOT; bilirubin, LDH, and SGOT; LDH and/or SGOT.

Integumentary: Rash, pruritus, dry skin, easy bruising, peeling skin or fingertips, thinning hair.

Miscellaneous: Lethargy, emotional lability, insomnia, headache, anxiety, chest pain, tearing of eyes, breast tenderness, mild to moderate breast enlargement.

OVERDOSAGE

May produce pronounced manifestations of the known adverse reactions. In event of overdosage, evacuate stomach contents by gastric lavage and initiate symptomatic therapy. Monitor hematologic and hepatic parameters for at least 6 weeks.

DOSAGE

Recommended daily dose is 14 mg/kg (*i.e.,* one 140-mg capsule for each 10 kg or 22 lb of body weight) given in three or four divided doses. Average dosage range is 10 mg/kg/day to 16 mg/kg/day. Patient is treated for 30 to 90 days before possible benefits of continued therapy are determined. Therapy is continued for as long as favorable response lasts. Some patients have been maintained on therapy for more than 3 years at doses ranging from 10 mg/kg/day to 16 mg/kg/day.

NURSING IMPLICATIONS

HISTORY
See Appendix 4.

PHYSICAL ASSESSMENT
Obtain vital signs; weight; general physical and emotional status. Baseline studies include hepatic- and renal-function tests, CBC, platelet count, serum calcium. Other laboratory tests may also be appropriate.

ADMINISTRATION
If nausea or GI upset occurs, check with physician whether drug can be given with food.

Storage: Refrigerate at 2°C to 8°C (36°F to 46°F).

ONGOING ASSESSMENTS AND NURSING MANAGEMENT
Monitor vital signs daily. If rise in blood pressure is noted, notify physician.

Weigh weekly. Inform physician if weight significantly increases or decreases.

Check extremities daily for evidence of edema. If fluid retention occurs, physician may prescribe a diuretic and recommend a salt-restricted diet. Patient may require list of foods high in sodium.

CLINICAL ALERT: Observe for signs and symptoms of thromboembolic episodes: pain or tenderness in calf of leg or groin; chest pain; sudden dyspnea; sudden severe headache, dizziness, or fainting; visual or speech disturbances; weakness or numbness in arm or leg; personality changes.

If bone metastasis is present, encourage ambulation to decrease mobilization of calcium from the bone. If patient is unable to ambulate, institute range-of-motion exercises.

Periodic hepatic-function and hematologic tests are performed.

Diabetic patients: Test urine for glucose qid; inform physician if glucose is present in urine. Adjustment in insulin or oral hypoglycemic dosage may be necessary.

PATIENT AND FAMILY INFORMATION
Take drug exactly as directed. If nausea or GI upset occurs, contact physician.

Inform physician or nurse if any of the following occurs: pain or tenderness in calf of leg or groin; chest pain; sudden shortness of breath; sudden severe headache, dizziness, or fainting; visual or speech disturbances; weakness or numbness in arm or leg; easy bruising or bleeding; swelling of feet or ankles.

Weigh self weekly. Inform physician if significant weight gain or loss occurs.

Contraceptive measures are recommended. Discuss methods with physician.

Keep drug in refrigerator at 36°F to 46°F; remove only to take medication.

Periodic laboratory or other diagnostic tests or studies will be necessary.

Estrogenic Substances

See Estrogens.

Estrogens*

Chlorotrianisene *Rx*

capsules: 12 mg, 25   Tace
mg, 72 mg

Combined Estrogens Aqueous *Rx*

injection: 2 mg   Gynogen R.P.
estrone, 0.1 mg
estradiol/ml

Conjugated Estrogens *(Oral) Rx*

tablets: 0.3 mg, 0.625   Premarin, *Generic*
mg, 1.25 mg,
2.5 mg

Conjugated Estrogens *(Parenteral) Rx*

injection: 25 mg/vial   Premarin Intravenous

Diethylstilbestrol *(DES) Rx*

tablets (regular or en-   *Generic*
teric coated): 0.1
mg, 0.25 mg, 0.5
mg, 1 mg, 5 mg

Esterified Estrogens *Rx*

tablets: 0.3 mg	Estratab, Menest
tablets: 0.625 mg, 1.25 mg	Estratab, Evex, Menest
tablets: 2.5 mg	Estratab, Menest

Estradiol *Rx*

tablets: 1 mg, 2 mg   Estrace
(contains tartra-
zine)

Estradiol Cypionate in Oil *Rx*

injection: 1 mg/ml   Depo-Estradiol Cypionate
injection: 5 mg/ml   Depanate, Depestro, dep-

Gynogen, Depo-Estradiol
Cypionate, Depogen, Dura-
Estrin, E-Ionate P.A., Es-
tra-D, Estro-Cyp, Estroject-
L.A., Hormogen Depot,
Generic

Estradiol Valerate in Oil *Rx*

injection: 10 mg/ml	Delestrogen, Dioval, Dura-gen-10, Estradiol L.A., Es-trate, Estraval P.A., Femi-nate-10, Gynogen L.A. 10, Valergen-10, *Generic*
injection: 20 mg/ml	Delestrogen, Dioval XX, Duragen-20, Estradiol L.A. 20, Estra-L 20, Estraval 2X, Feminate-20, Gynogen L.A. 20, L.A.E. 20, Valer-gen-20, *Generic*
injection: 40 mg/ml	Delestrogen, Dioval 40, Duragen-40, Estradiol L.A. 40, Estra-L 40, Estraval 4X, Feminate-40, Valer-gen-40, *Generic*

Estrogenic Substance Aqueous
(Mainly Estrone) Rx

| injection: 2 mg/ml | Estaqua, Estrofol, Estroject-2, Foygen Aqueous, Gravi-gen Aqueous, Gynogen, Hormogen-A, Kestrin Aqueous, Theogen, Unigen Aqueous, Wehgen, *Generic* |
| injection: 5 mg/ml | *Generic* |

Estrogenic Substance (Mainly Estrone) in Oil *Rx*

| injection: 2 mg/ml | Gravigen in Oil, *Generic* |

Estrone Aqueous Suspension *Rx*

| injection: 2 mg/ml | Bestrone, Estronol (Im-proved), Theelin Aqueous, *Generic* |
| injection: 5 mg/ml | Bestrone, Estrone "5," Kes-trone-5, *Generic* |

Estropipate *(Piperazine Estrone Sulfate) Rx*

tablets: 0.625 mg,   Ogen
1.25 mg, 2.5 mg,
5 mg

---

* For diethylstilbestrol diphosphate and polyestradiol phosphate, estrogens specifically indicated in the palliative therapy of advanced
prostatic carcinoma, see Estrogens, Antineoplastic. For vaginal
products, see Estrogens, Vaginal.

Ethinyl Estradiol Rx

| tablets: 0.02 mg, 0.5 mg | Estinyl |
| tablets: 0.05 mg | Estinyl, Feminone |

Quinestrol Rx

| tablets: 100 mcg | Estrovis |

INDICATIONS

CHLOROTHIANISENE

Postpartum breast engorgement, prostatic carcinoma, moderate to severe vasomotor symptoms associated with menopause, atrophic vaginitis and kraurosis vulvae, female hypogonadism.

COMBINED ESTROGENS AQUEOUS

Replacement therapy for estrogen deficiency, abnormal uterine bleeding due to hormone imbalance, inoperable progressing prostatic carcinoma, inoperable progressing breast carcinoma.

CONJUGATED ESTROGENS (ORAL)

Moderate to severe vasomotor symptoms associated with menopause, atrophic vaginitis and kraurosis vulvae, female hypogonadism, female castration, primary ovarian failure, osteoporosis, mammary carcinoma (for palliation), prostatic carcinoma (for palliation), prevention of postpartum breast engorgement.

CONJUGATED ESTROGENS (PARENTERAL)

Abnormal uterine bleeding due to hormonal imbalance in absence of organic pathology.

DIETHYLSTILBESTROL (DES)

Moderate to severe vasomotor symptoms, atrophic vaginitis, kraurosis vulvae associated with menopause; female hypogonadism, female castration or primary ovarian failure; inoperable progressing prostatic carcinoma; inoperable progressing breast carcinoma.

Investigational use: FDA has concluded that use as a postcoital contraceptive measure is safe for emergency treatment only. Not used as a routine method of birth control. Repeated courses of therapy are avoided. Effectiveness depends on time lapse between coitus and drug administration.

ESTERIFIED ESTROGENS

Moderate to severe vasomotor symptoms associated with menopause, atrophic vaginitis and kraurosis vulvae, female hypogonadism, female castration, primary ovarian failure, inoperable progressing prostatic carcinoma, inoperable progressing breast carcinoma.

ESTRADIOL

Moderate to severe vasomotor symptoms, atrophic vaginitis, kraurosis vulvae, female hypogonadism, female castration, primary ovarian failure, inoperable progressing prostatic carcinoma, inoperable progressing breast carcinoma.

ESTRADIOL CYPIONATE IN OIL

Moderate to severe vasomotor symptoms associated with menopause, female hypogonadism.

ESTRADIOL VALERATE IN OIL

Moderate to severe vasomotor symptoms, atrophic vaginitis or kraurosis vulvae associated with menopause, female hypogonadism, female castration, primary ovarian failure, prevention of postpartum breast engorgement, prostatic carcinoma.

ESTROGENIC SUBSTANCE AQUEOUS

Moderate to severe vasomotor symptoms, atrophic vaginitis or kraurosis vulvae associated with menopause; female hypogonadism; female castration; primary ovarian failure; inoperable progressing prostatic carcinoma.

ESTROGENIC SUBSTANCE IN OIL

Same as Estrogenic Substance Aqueous.

ESTRONE AQUEOUS SUSPENSION

Same as Estrogenic Substance Aqueous.

ESTROPIPATE (PIPERAZINE ESTRONE SULFATE)

Moderate to severe vasomotor symptoms, atrophic vaginitis or kraurosis vulvae associated with menopause; female hypogonadism; female castration; primary ovarian failure.

ETHINYL ESTRADIOL

Moderate to severe vasomotor symptoms associated with menopause, female hypogonadism, inoperable progressing breast carcinoma, inoperable progressing prostatic carcinoma.

QUINESTROL

Moderate to severe vasomotor symptoms associated with menopause, atrophic vaginitis, kraurosis vulvae, female hypogonadism, female castration, primary ovarian failure.

CONTRAINDICATIONS

Estrogens are contraindicated in known or suspected breast carcinoma, except in appropriately selected patients being treated for metastatic disease; known or suspected estrogen-dependent neoplasia; undiagnosed abnormal genital bleeding; active thrombophlebitis or thromboembolic disorders; history of thrombophlebitis, thrombosis, or thromboembolic disorders associated with previous estrogen use (except when used in treatment of breast or prostatic malignancy); hypersensitivity.

ACTIONS

The naturally occurring estrogenic hormone (follicular hormone) is composed of several closely related chemical substances: estradiol, estrone, and estriol. The most potent is estradiol; it undergoes rapid oxidation to estrone, which is approximately one-half as potent. Hydration of estrone produces estriol, which is much weaker.

Estrogens are important in development and maintenance of the female reproductive system and primary and secondary sex characteristics. They promote growth and development of the vagina, uterus, and fallopian tubes and enlargement of the breasts. They also affect release of pituitary gonadotropins; cause capillary dilatation, fluid retention, and protein anabolism; thin cervical mucus; inhibit ovulation; and prevent postpartum breast discomfort. Indirectly, estrogens contribute to shaping of the skeleton (conserve calcium and phosphorus and encourage bone formation), maintenance of tone and elasticity of urogenital structures, changes in the epiphysis of long bones that allow for the pubertal growth spurt and its termination, growth of axillary and pubic hair, and pigmentation of the nipples and genitals.

Estrogens induce proliferation in the epithelium of the fallopian tubes, endometrium, cervix, and vagina and increase vascularity. They are responsible for deposition of glycogen in vaginal epithelium and therefore for vaginal acidity. They encourage cornification of superficial vaginal cells to give a characteristic vaginal smear.

Estrogens do not induce ovulation. In the preovulatory phase they produce changes in tubular mucosa and stimulate contraction and motility of the fallopian tubes, which promote transport of the ovum. Estrogens restore the endometrium, including its coiled arteries, after menstruation, but do not induce the glands to secrete. An endometrium suddenly deprived of estrogen breaks down and bleeds. Growth and secretory activity of cervical epithelium are determined in part by estrogens; they also modify the physical and chemical properties of cervical mucus.

Decline of estrogenic activity at ends of the menstrual cycle can bring on menstruation, although cessation of progesterone secretion is the most important factor in the mature ovulatory cycle. In the preovulatory or nonovulatory cycle, estrogen is the primary determinant of the onset of menstruation.

Cessation of cyclic function is the basic ovarian event in menopause. Functional changes can be attributed to depletion of follicles, although a few follicles have been shown to persist for as long as 5 years after the last menses. The beginning is marked by decreasing frequency of ovulation, associated with irregular menses or variable periods of amenorrhea; later it is marked by decreasing estrogen secretion. Estrogen production, first to appear at the menarche, is last to decline at menopause. The declining estrogen secretion is accompanied by signs and symptoms of hormone deficits in estrogen-dependent organs, including the pituitary, uterus, cervix, vagina, and breasts. Pituitary gonadotropin secretion rises, reflected by increased quantities of gonadotropin in blood and urine. The endometrium becomes atrophic, myometrial mass decreases, and vaginal epithelium becomes thin; deficient in glycogens, it fails to become keratinized.

Naturally occurring estrogens are poorly absorbed orally and are therefore used parenterally. Conjugated and esterified derivatives and synthetic estrogens are active orally. In responsive tissues (female genital organs, breasts, hypothalamus, pituitary), estrogens enter the cell and are transported into the nucleus. As a result of estrogen activity, specific RNA and protein synthesis occurs. Metabolism and inactivation occur primarily in the liver. Some estrogens are secreted in the bile but are reabsorbed from the intestine and returned to the liver through the portal venous system.

Estrogens circulate in the blood in free and conjugated forms, which are 50% to 80% bound to plasma proteins. Estrogens are excreted in the urine; tubular absorption is minimal.

Equipotent doses of various estrogens produce similar pharmacologic effects and side-effects. Approximate equivalent doses of some of the estrogens are conjugated estrogens 5 mg, diethylstilbestrol (DES) 1 mg, mestranol 80 mcg, and estradiol 50 mcg.

WARNINGS

Estrogens have been reported to increase the risk of endometrial carcinoma in postmenopausal women exposed to exogenous estrogens for prolonged periods. When estrogens are used for treatment of postmenopausal symptoms, the lowest dose that will control symptoms should be used and medication should be discontinued as soon as possible. When prolonged treatment is indicated, patient is reassessed at least twice a year to determine need for continued therapy. Cyclic administration of low doses of estrogen may carry less risk than continuous administration. There is no evidence that "natural" estrogens are more or less hazardous than "synthetic" estrogens at equiestrogenic doses. Close surveillance of all women taking estrogens is important. In all cases of undiagnosed persistent or recurring abnormal vaginal bleeding, malignancy is ruled out.

There is no evidence that estrogens given to post-menopausal women increase the risk of breast cancer. Because research has raised this possibility, estrogens are used with caution in those with a strong family history of breast cancer and in those who have breast nodules, fibrocystic disease, or abnormal mammograms.

There is a twofold to threefold increase in the risk of gallbladder disease in women receiving post-menopausal estrogens.

Estrogens should *not* be used during pregnancy because use during early pregnancy may seriously damage the offspring. Females exposed *in utero* to DES have increased risk of developing vaginal or cervical cancer. A high percentage of such exposed women have epithelial changes of the vagina and cervix. Although these changes are histologically benign, it is not known if they are precursors of malignancy. Data are not available for other estrogens, but it cannot be presumed that they would not induce similar changes.

In addition to the effects of DES in females, there have also been congenital anomalies reported in male offspring whose mothers ingested the drug. Primary abnormalities noted have related to structural problems of the genitourinary tract and abnormal semen quality. How these lesions will affect future carcinoma development and fertility has yet to be determined.

Several studies suggest association between intra-uterine exposure to female sex hormones and congenital anomalies, including congenital heart defects and limb reduction defects.

Female sex hormones have been used in an attempt to treat threatened or habitual abortion. There is evidence that estrogens are ineffective for these indications and no evidence that progestins are effective. If estrogens are used during pregnancy or if the patient becomes pregnant while taking estrogens, she should be apprised of the potential risk to the fetus.

Effects similar to those caused by estrogen-progestin oral contraceptives

There are several serious adverse effects of oral contraceptives (OCs), most of which have *not* been documented as consequences of postmenopausal estrogen therapy. This may reflect the comparatively low doses of estrogen used in postmenopausal women. There is an increased risk of thrombosis in men receiving estrogens for prostatic cancer and in women receiving estrogens for postpartum breast engorgement, presumably because large doses are used in these instances. The following effects noted in OC users (see also p 457) are considered as potential risks of estrogen use.

Hepatic adenoma: Is considered in estrogen users having abdominal pain and tenderness, abdominal mass, or hypovolemic shock.

Elevated blood pressure: Although the average increase in blood pressure in women taking OCs is small, an occasional patient may have a significant increase. This may also occur with use of estrogens in menopause.

Thromboembolic disease: Users of OCs have an increased risk of thrombophlebitis, pulmonary embolism, stroke, and myocardial infarction. Retinal thrombosis, mesenteric thrombosis, and optic neuritis have also been reported with OC use. An increased risk of postsurgical thromboembolic complications has also been reported. If feasible, estrogens are discontinued at least 4 weeks before surgical procedures associated with an increased risk of thromboembolism or during periods of prolonged immobilization. Although an increased rate of thromboembolitic and thrombotic disease in postmenopausal users of estrogen has not been found, it is possible that such an increase may be present in some women or in those receiving large doses of estrogens. Therefore, estrogens are not recommended for those with a history of such disorders associated with estrogen use (except in treatment of malignancy). Also used with caution in those with cerebral vascular or coronary artery disease and only used when clearly needed. Cigarette smoking increases risk of serious cardiovascular side-effects from OCs and is marked in women over 35 years. Smoking should be considered an additional risk factor for such complications in estrogen users.

Large doses of estrogen comparable to those used in treatment of malignancy have been shown in men to increase the risk of nonfatal myocardial infarction, pulmonary embolism, and thrombophlebitis.

Glucose tolerance: A decrease in glucose tolerance has been observed in OC users; diabetic patients are observed closely while receiving estrogens.

Hypercalcemia: Estrogens may lead to severe hypercalcemia in those with breast cancer and bone metastases. If this occurs, drug is discontinued and appropriate measures taken to reduce serum calcium level.

Photosensitivity: Caution patient against exposure to ultraviolet light and prolonged exposure to sunlight.

Use in lactation: Estrogens are secreted in breast milk. Administer to nursing mother only when clearly needed.

PRECAUTIONS

Certain patients may develop undesirable manifestations of excessive estrogenic stimulation (*e.g.,* abnormal or excessive uterine bleeding, mastodynia).

Preexisting uterine leiomyoma may increase in size during estrogen use.

Fluid retention: Some degree may occur. Conditions that might be influenced by this factor (*e.g.,* asthma, epilepsy, migraine, cardiac or renal dysfunction) may require close observation.

Mental depression: OCs appear to be associated with an increased incidence of mental depression. Although not clear whether due to the contraceptive's estrogenic or progestogenic component, observe those with a history of mental depression.

Impaired hepatic function: Those with a history of jaundice during pregnancy have an increased risk of recurrence of jaundice while receiving estrogen-containing OCs. If jaundice develops in any patient receiving estrogen, drug is discontinued and cause is investigated. Estrogens may be poorly metabolized in those with impaired hepatic function and should be administered with caution.

Others: Estrogens influence metabolism of calcium and phosphorus and are used with caution in those with metabolic bone diseases associated with hypercalcemia or in those with renal insufficiency.

Because of the effects of estrogen on epiphyseal closure, estrogens are used judiciously in young patients in whom bone growth is not complete.

Estrogens are reported to precipitate attacks of acute intermittent porphyria.

Tartrazine sensitivity: Some products contain tartrazine. See Appendix 6, section 6-23.

DRUG INTERACTIONS

Drug/lab tests: Certain endocrine and hepatic-function tests may be affected by estrogen-containing OCs; the following similar changes may be expected with larger doses of estrogens:

Increased **prothrombin** and **factors VII, VIII, IX, X;** decreased **antithrombin 3;** increased norepinephrine-induced **platelet aggregability.**

Increased **thyroid-binding globulin (TBG)** leading to increased circulating total thyroid hormone, as measured by **PBI, T$_4$** by column, or T$_4$ by radioimmunoassay. **Free T$_3$ resin uptake** is decreased, reflecting the elevated TBG; **free T$_4$** concentration is unaltered.

Impaired **glucose tolerance;** decreased **pregnanediol** excretion; reduced response to **metyrapone test;** reduced **serum folate** concentration; increased **serum triglyceride** and **phospholipid** concentration.

ADVERSE REACTIONS

See *Warnings* regarding induction of neoplasia; adverse effects on fetus; increased incidence of gallbladder disease; adverse effects similar to those of OCs including thromboembolism, hepatic adenoma, elevated blood pressure, decreased glucose tolerance, hypercalcemia.

GU: Breakthrough bleeding, change in menstrual flow, dysmenorrhea, premenstrual-like syndrome, amenorrhea during and after treatment, increase in size of uterine fibromyomata, vaginal candidiasis, change in cervical eversion and in degree of cervical secretion, cystitislike syndrome, hemolytic uremic syndrome, endometrial cystic hyperplasia.

Breast: Tenderness, enlargement, secretion.

GI: Nausea, vomiting, abdominal cramps, bloating, cholestatic jaundice, colitis.

Dermatologic: Chloasma, which may persist when drug is discontinued; erythema multiforme or nodosum; hemorrhagic eruption; loss of scalp hair; hirsutism; urticaria; localized dermatitis.

Ophthalmologic: Steepening of corneal curvature, intolerance to contact lenses.

CNS: Headache, migraine, dizziness, mental depression, chorea, convulsions.

Localized reactions: Pain at injection site, sterile abscess, postinjection flare.

Miscellaneous: Increase or decrease in weight, reduced carbohydrate tolerance, aggravation of porphyria, edema, changes in libido.

OVERDOSAGE

Serious effects have not been reported following ingestion of large doses of estrogen-containing OCs by young children. Overdosage of estrogen may cause nausea; withdrawal bleeding may occur in females.

DOSAGE

CHLOROTRIANISENE
Give orally.

Postpartum breast engorgement: Usual dose is 12 mg qid for 7 days, or 50 mg q6h for 6 doses. The 72-mg capsule is administered bid for 2 days. First dose is given within 8 hours of delivery.

Prostatic carcinoma: 12 mg/day to 25 mg/day.

Moderate to severe vasomotor symptoms associated with menopause: Usual dose is 12 mg/day to 25 mg/day given cyclically for 30 days; one or more courses may be prescribed.

Atrophic vaginitis and kraurosis vulvae: Usual dosage is 12 mg/day to 25 mg/day given cyclically for 30 to 60 days.

Female hypogonadism: Usual dosage is 12 mg/day to 25 mg/day given cyclically for 21 days. May be followed immediately by IM injection of 100 mg progesterone or by an oral progestin during last 5 days of therapy. Next course may begin on the fifth day of induced uterine bleeding.

COMBINED ESTROGENS AQUEOUS
Give IM only.

Replacement therapy of estrogen deficiency–associated conditions: Initially 0.1 mg to 1 mg in single or divided doses. Some patients require 0.5 mg to 2 mg weekly. *For senile vaginitis and kraurosis vulvae*—0.1 mg to 0.5 mg 2 to 3 times/week. Continuous therapy with estrogen alone may induce functional bleeding.

Abnormal uterine bleeding due to hormonal imbalance: May respond to brief courses of intensive therapy. *Dosage*—2 mg to 5 mg for several days.

Prostatic cancer (inoperable, progressing): 2 mg to 4 mg 2 to 3 times/week.

Breast cancer (inoperable, progressing): 5 mg three or more times a week according to severity of pain.

CONJUGATED ESTROGENS, ORAL

Administer cyclically (3 weeks of daily estrogen and 1 week off) for all indications except selected cases of carcinoma and prevention of postpartum breast engorgement.

Moderate to severe vasomotor symptoms associated with menopause: 1.25 mg/day. If patient has not menstruated in 2 months or more, administration is started arbitrarily. If patient is menstruating, drug is given on day 5 of bleeding.

Atrophic vaginitis and kraurosis vulvae: 0.3 mg to 1.25 mg or more daily.

Female hypogonadism: 2.5 mg/day to 7.5 mg/day, in divided doses for 20 days, followed by a rest period of 10 days. If bleeding does not occur by end of this period, dosage schedule is repeated. Number of courses necessary to produce bleeding may vary. If bleeding occurs before end of 10-day rest period, a 20-day estrogen–progestin cyclic regimen is begun with estrogen 2.5 mg/day to 7.5 mg/day in divided doses. During the last 5 days of estrogen therapy, an oral progestin is given. If bleeding occurs before this regimen is concluded, therapy is discontinued and may be resumed on the fifth day of bleeding.

Female castration and primary ovarian failure: 1.25 mg/day. Dosage is adjusted according to severity of symptoms and patient's response. Maintenance dosage is adjusted to lowest level that produces effective control.

Osteoporosis: To retard progression, 1.25 mg/day cyclically.

Breast carcinoma (palliation): 10 mg tid for at least 3 months.

Prostatic carcinoma (palliation): 1.25 mg to 2.5 mg tid.

Prevention of postpartum breast engorgement: 3.75 mg q4h for five doses or 1.25 mg q4h for 5 days.

CONJUGATED ESTROGENS, PARENTERAL

Give for treatment of abnormal uterine bleeding due to hormonal imbalance in absence of organic pathology. IV administration produces more rapid response. Usual dose is one 25-mg injection IV or IM; repeat in 6 to 12 hours if necessary.

DIETHYLSTILBESTROL (DES)

Give orally.

Moderate to severe vasomotor symptoms, atrophic vaginitis or kraurosis vulvae associated with menopause: Give cyclically for short-term use. Usual dosage is 0.2 mg/day to 0.5 mg/day. Atrophic vaginitis may require up to 2 mg/day; cyclic administration may be necessary for several years. Those with atrophic vaginitis may notice relief if up to 1 mg/day of the suppository form is administered 10 to 14 days concomitantly with oral DES.

Female hypogonadism, female castration, primary ovarian failure: Usual dosage is 0.2 mg/day to 0.5 mg/day given cyclically.

Prostatic carcinoma (inoperable, progressing): Usual dosage is 1 mg/day to 3 mg/day initially, increased in advanced cases; dosage may later be reduced to an average of 1 mg/day.

Breast cancer (inoperable, progressing): In appropriately selected men and postmenopausal women, usual dosage is 15 mg/day.

Postcoital contraception: Emergency use only. Effectiveness depends on time lapse between coitus and drug administration. Recommended dosage is 25 mg bid for 5 consecutive days, beginning preferably within 24 hours and not later than 72 hours after exposure. Pregnancy test is performed prior to use.

ESTERIFIED ESTROGENS

Give orally.

Moderate to severe vasomotor symptoms associated with menopause: Cyclic therapy for short-term use recommended. Average dose is 0.3 mg/day to 1.25 mg/day. May be increased to 2.5 mg/day to 3.75 mg/day if needed.

Kraurosis vulvae: 0.3 mg/day to 3.75 mg/day.

Atrophic vaginitis and kraurosis vulvae: Cyclic therapy for short-term use recommended. Usual dosage range is 0.3 mg/day to 1.25 mg/day.

Female hypogonadism: 2.5 mg/day to 7.5 mg/day cyclically in divided doses for 20 to 21 days, followed by a 7- to 10-day rest period. If patient has not menstruated in the past 2 months or more, cyclic administration is started arbitrarily. If patient is menstruating, drug is started on day 5 of bleeding. In the following cycle, employ dosage level used to stop breakthrough bleeding in the previous cycle. In subsequent cycles, dosage is gradually reduced to the lowest level that will maintain patient without symptoms. If bleeding does not occur by end of this period, same dosage schedule is repeated. Number of courses of estrogen therapy to produce bleeding will vary. If bleeding occurs before end of 10-day rest period, a 20-day estrogen–progestin cyclic regimen as in primary ovarian failure is begun.

Female castration and primary ovarian failure: 20-day estrogen–progestin cycle begins with 2.5 mg/day to 7.5 mg/day of estrogen in divided doses. During last 5 days of estrogen therapy, oral progestin is given. If bleeding occurs before regimen is concluded, therapy is discontinued and resumed on fifth day of bleeding.

Prostatic carcinoma (inoperable, progressing): 1.25 mg to 2.5 mg tid for several weeks.

Breast cancer (inoperable, progressing): In appropriately selected men and postmenopausal women, 10 mg tid for 3 months.

ESTRADIOL
Administer orally.

Moderate to severe vasomotor symptoms, atrophic vaginitis, kraurosis vulvae, female hypogonadism, female castration, primary ovarian failure: Initially 1 mg/day or 2 mg/day, adjusted to control symptoms. Cyclic therapy is recommended. Usual regimen consists of 3 weeks of drug followed by 1 week without drug. Only short-term therapy is used for vasomotor symptoms, atrophic vaginitis, and kraurosis vulvae.

Prostatic cancer (inoperable, progressing): 1 mg to 2 mg tid.

Breast cancer (inoperable, progressing): In appropriately selected men and women, usual dose is 10 mg tid for at least 3 months.

ESTRADIOL CYPIONATE IN OIL
Give IM only.

Moderate to severe vasomotor symptoms associated with menopause: 1 mg to 5 mg every 3 to 4 weeks.

Female hypogonadism: 1.5 mg to 2 mg at monthly intervals.

ESTRADIOL VALERATE IN OIL
Provides 2 to 3 weeks of estrogenic effect from single IM injection.

Moderate to severe vasomotor symptoms, atrophic vaginitis, or kraurosis vulvae associated with menopause: 10 mg to 20 mg every 4 weeks.

Female hypogonadism, female castration, or primary ovarian failure: 10 mg to 20 mg every 4 weeks.

Prevention of postpartum breast engorgement: 10 mg to 25 mg as single injection at end of first stage of labor.

Prostatic carcinoma: 30 mg or more every 1 to 2 weeks.

ESTROGENIC SUBSTANCE (ESTROGENS AQUEOUS SUSPENSION)
Give IM only.

Moderate to severe vasomotor symptoms, atrophic vaginitis or kraurosis vulvae associated with menopause: Usual dosage range is 0.1 mg to 0.5 mg 2 to 3 times/week.

Female hypogonadism, female castration, primary ovarian failure: Initially 0.1 mg to 1 mg weekly in single or divided doses. Some patients may require 0.5 mg/week to 2 mg/week.

Prostatic cancer (inoperable, progressing): 2 mg to 4 mg two or three times a week.

ESTROGENIC SUBSTANCE IN OIL
Same as Estrogenic Substance.

ESTRONE AQUEOUS SUSPENSION
Same as Estrogenic Substance.

ESTROPIPATE (PIPERAZINE ESTRONE SULFATE)
Give orally.

Moderate to severe vasomotor symptoms, atrophic vaginitis or kraurosis vulvae associated with menopause: Give cyclically for short-term use. Usual dosage is 0.625 mg/day to 5 mg/day.

Female hypogonadism, female castration, or primary ovarian failure: Administer cyclically, 1.25 mg to 7.5 mg for first 3 weeks followed by a rest period of 8 to 10 days. Repeat if bleeding does not occur by end of rest period. Duration of therapy to produce withdrawal bleeding will vary. If satisfactory withdrawal bleeding does not occur, an oral progestin may be given in addition to estrogen during third week of cycle.

ETHINYL ESTRADIOL
Give orally.

Moderate to severe vasomotor symptoms associated with menopause: Give cyclically for short-term use. Usual dosage is 0.02 mg/day or 0.05 mg/day. In some instances, 0.02 mg every other day may be given. A dosage schedule for early menopause, while spontaneous menstruation continues, is 0.05 mg/day for 21 days followed by a 7-day rest period. This can be continued cyclically, adding a progestational agent during the latter part of the cycle. For late menopause, the same regimen is indicated with 0.02 mg for first few cycles, after which 0.05 mg may be substituted. In more severe cases, such as surgical or roentgenologic castration, 0.05 mg tid is given at the start of treatment. With adequate improvement, usually in a few weeks, dosage may be reduced to 0.05 mg/day. A progestational agent may be added during the latter part of a planned cycle.

Female hypogonadism: 0.05 mg one to three times a day during first 2 weeks of theoretical men-

E

strual cycle and followed with progesterone during last half of arbitrary cycle. Continue for 3 to 6 months; then patient is allowed to go untreated for 2 months. Additional courses of therapy may be prescribed if cycle is not maintained without hormonal therapy.

Female breast cancer (inoperable, progressing): 1 mg tid.

Prostatic cancer (inoperable, progressing): 0.15 mg/day to 2 mg/day.

QUINESTROL

Give orally.

Moderate to severe vasomotor symptoms associated with menopause, atrophic vaginitis, female hypogonadism, female castration, primary ovarian failure: 100 mcg daily for 7 days, followed with 100 mcg once weekly for maintenance starting 2 weeks after treatment begins. Dosage may be increased to 200 mcg/week if therapeutic response is not desirable or is not considered optimal.

NURSING IMPLICATIONS

HISTORY

See Appendix 4. When drug is used for symptoms of menopause, female hypogonadism, primary ovarian failure, or female castration, obtain menstrual history (menarche, menstrual pattern, onset of change in menstrual pattern); health history including history of thromboembolic disease, liver disease; smoking history.

PHYSICAL ASSESSMENT

Obtain vital signs, weight. *Females*—Physician performs pretreatment examination, which may include examination of breasts, abdomen, and pelvic organs and Pap smear. Hepatic-function tests may also be ordered. Other tests (*e.g.,* serum calcium) may be ordered for patient with a malignancy.

ADMINISTRATION

Read label carefully because some of these products have similar names but are different estrogens (*e.g.,* Gynogen and Gynogen R.P.; Estro-ject-L.A. and Estroject-2).

Parenteral

Estrogens are administered IM except for conjugated estrogens, which may be administered IV or IM.

Estrogenic substance in oil, estradiol cypionate or valerate in oil: Use 20-gauge or 21-gauge needle to withdraw drug from vial and administer drug.

Aqueous suspension: Rotate vial between palms to be sure drug is uniformly dispersed immediately before withdrawing solution.

Give deep IM (preferably in gluteus muscle); inject slowly. Advise patient that pain or discomfort may be noted at injection site.

Conjugated estrogens (parenteral) (Premarin Intravenous): Infusion with other agents is not recommended. In emergencies, when an infusion is already started, make injection into tubing just distal to infusion needle. Solution is compatible with normal saline, dextrose, and invert sugar. It is not compatible with protein hydrolysate, ascorbic acid, or any solution with an acid *p*H. Before reconstitution, store in refrigerator at 2°C to 8°C. Use reconstituted solution within a few hours. When stored under refrigeration, solution is stable for 60 days. Label vial with date of reconstitution. Do not use if darkening or precipitation occurs.

Oral

If GI upset occurs, may be taken with food.

TRADE NAME SIMILARITIES

Gynogen and Gynergen; Kestrin and Kestrone, Theelin and Theogen.

ONGOING ASSESSMENTS AND NURSING MANAGEMENT

If patient has diabetes mellitus, notify physician if glucose is present in urine. Adjustment in insulin or oral hypoglycemic dosage may be necessary.

Observe for mental changes (especially severe depression), jaundice, and elevation of blood pressure and report promptly to physician.

CLINICAL ALERT: Observe for signs of thromboembolic episodes. Notify physician immediately if any of the following occurs: pain or tenderness in calf of leg or groin; chest pain; sudden dyspnea; sudden severe headache, dizziness, or fainting; visual or speech disturbance; weakness or numbness in arm or leg; personality changes.

Symptoms of menopause, female hypogonadism, primary ovarian failure, female castration: Drug is usually prescribed for outpatient use. See also *Patient and Family Information,* below.

At time of each office or clinic visit, obtain blood pressure; weigh patient; inquire about relief of symptoms, occurrence of adverse reactions.

Periodic (at least yearly) history and physical examination are performed by physician and include special reference to blood pressure, breasts, abdomen, and pelvic organs. A Pap smear is also recommended. Include name of estrogen on

E

specimen request slip because pathologist should be advised of estrogen therapy.

If fluid retention occurs, physician may prescribe diuretic and recommend a salt-restricted diet. Patient may require list of foods high in sodium.

Prostatic carcinoma, breast carcinoma: Drug may be administered in hospital or prescribed for outpatient use. See also *Patient and Family Information,* below.

Obtain vital signs daily; observe for adverse drug reactions.

Weigh weekly or as ordered. Bring significant weight gain or loss to attention of physician.

Observe patient for response to drug (*e.g.,* relief of pain, increase in appetite, weight gain, feeling of well-being). In prostatic carcinoma, response to therapy is usually rapid. In breast carcinoma, response to therapy is slow and may not be seen for several months.

Patient may have many questions about therapy and prognosis of the disease. Although these questions should be directed to the physician, the nurse should allow the patient time to express thoughts about the present and future.

Physician periodically evaluates drug response by physical examination, laboratory tests.

Gynecomastia is frequent and may be disturbing. Loose shirts, open jackets, or sweaters may be used to disguise breast enlargement. Encourage patient to discuss this or other sexual problems (*e.g.,* loss of libido) with physician if concern is expressed.

Estrogens may lead to severe hypercalcemia in those with bone metastasis. If this occurs, drug is discontinued and appropriate measures taken to reduce serum calcium levels. Observe for symptoms of hypercalcemia (Appendix 6, section 6-13). If patient is immobilized for prolonged periods, institute range-of-motion exercises to decrease mobilization of calcium from the bone.

Postpartum breast engorgement: Physician may order a compression breast binder applied for 3 days in addition to estrogen administration. This may be followed by wearing of a firm brassiere.

Remove and reapply a fresh breast binder q4h or as needed.

Ice packs and analgesics may also be necessary until lactation is suppressed, usually in 2 to 3 days.

PATIENT AND FAMILY INFORMATION
Patient package insert is available with product. Read insert carefully. If there are any questions about this material, discuss with physician.

If GI upset occurs, drug may be taken with food. If condition persists, contact physician.

Notify physician or nurse if any of the following occurs: pain in calves of legs or groin; sharp chest pain or sudden shortness of breath; abnormal vaginal bleeding; missed menstrual period or suspected pregnancy; lumps in the breast; sudden severe headache, dizziness, or fainting; vision or speech disturbance; weakness or numbness in an arm or leg; severe abdominal pain or yellowing of the skin or eyes; severe depression.

If pregnancy is suspected, do not take drug; contact physician.

Follow-up visits will be necessary to monitor therapy.

Weigh self weekly. Contact physician if weight gain is significant or if swelling of ankles is noted.

Avoid prolonged exposure to sunlight or ultraviolet light because photosensitivity may occur. If exposure to sunlight is unavoidable, discuss with physician possibility of using a sunscreen.

Diabetic patient: Glucose tolerance may be decreased; monitor urine glucose and report abnormalities to physician. More frequent blood glucose tests may be necessary.

Estrogens, Antineoplastic

Diethylstilbestrol Diphosphate Rx

tablets: 50 mg	Stilphostrol
injection: 0.25 g/5 ml	Stilphostrol

Polyestradiol Phosphate Rx

injection: 40 mg/secule	Estradurin

INDICATIONS
Inoperable, progressing prostatic carcinoma (for palliation only when castration is not feasible or when castration failures or delayed escape following a response to castration have occurred).

CONTRAINDICATIONS
Not used in men with any of the following conditions: known or suspected cancer of the breast except appropriately selected patients being treated for metastatic disease; known or suspected estrogen-dependent neoplasia; active thrombophlebitis or thromboembolic disorders; markedly impaired hepatic function.

ACTIONS

These agents are synthetic estrogens. In male patients with androgenic hormone–dependent conditions such as metastatic carcinoma of the prostate, estrogens counter the androgenic influence by competing for receptor sites. As a result of treatment, metastatic bone lesions may show improvement. See also Estrogens.

WARNINGS

Thromboembolic disorders: Large doses of estrogen, comparable to those used to treat prostate cancer, have been shown to increase risk of nonfatal myocardial infarction, pulmonary embolism, and thrombophlebitis in men.

Ophthalmologic effects: Discontinue drug if there is sudden onset of proptosis, diplopia, or migraine. If examination reveals papilledema or retinal vascular lesions, medication should be withdrawn.

PRECAUTIONS

Hypercalcemia: Because estrogens influence metabolism of calcium and phosphorus, they should be used with caution in those with metabolic bone diseases associated with hypercalcemia and in patients with renal insufficiency.

Because of estrogen-induced salt and water retention, these drugs are used with caution in those with epilepsy, migraine, asthma, and cardiac or renal disease. Because of possibility of decrease in glucose tolerance, diabetic patients should be followed closely.

ADVERSE REACTIONS

A statistically significant association between use of estrogen-containing drugs and thrombophlebitis, pulmonary embolism, and cerebral thrombosis has been demonstrated. Although evidence suggests an association between estrogen use and coronary thrombosis and neuro-ocular lesions (retinal thrombosis, optic neuritis), none has been confirmed.

CNS: Aggravation of migraine headaches, nervousness, fatigue, irritability, malaise.

Dermatologic: Allergic rash, itching.

GI: Anorexia, changes in appetite, nausea and vomiting.

GU: Gynecomastia, changes in libido.

Hepatic: Hepatic cutaneous porphyria.

Other: Backache, sterile abscesses, pain at injection site, postinjection flare.

For additional adverse reactions, see Estrogens.

DOSAGE

DIETHYLSTILBESTROL DIPHOSPHATE

Oral: 50 mg tid initially; increased to 200 mg or more tid, depending on tolerance of patient. If relief is not obtained with higher doses, drug may be administered IV.

Parenteral: On first day, 0.5 g IV dissolved in 300 ml of saline or 5% dextrose. On subsequent days, 1 g dissolved in 300 ml of saline or dextrose. Infusion administered slowly (20–30 drops/minute) during first 10 to 15 minutes and then rate adjusted so entire amount is given in 1 hour. This procedure should be followed for 5 days or more depending on response of patient. Following this intensive course of therapy, 0.25 g to 0.5 g may be administered in a similar manner once or twice weekly.

POLYESTRADIOL PHOSPHATE

40 mg IM every 2 to 4 weeks or less frequently, depending on clinical response. If response is not satisfactory, doses up to 80 mg may be used. Increasing the dose may prolong the action but does not significantly increase the amount of estrogen available at any one time.

NURSING IMPLICATIONS

HISTORY

See Appendix 4.

PHYSICAL ASSESSMENT

Obtain vital signs, weight, general physical and emotional status. Hepatic-function tests, CBC, serum calcium may be ordered. Other laboratory tests may also be appropriate.

ADMINISTRATION

DIETHYLSTILBESTROL DIPHOSPHATE

Parenteral form given IV by intermittent infusion.

Dose dissolved in 300 ml of saline or 5% dextrose.

If patient has IV line, solution may be piggybacked into primary line.

If patient does not have IV line, a daily IV line is established and discontinued after drug is infused. Rotate sites; record site used.

Infusion rate determined by physician. Recommended rate is 20 to 30 drops per minute during first 10 to 15 minutes; then rate of flow is adjusted so that entire amount is given in 1 hour.

POLYESTRADIOL PHOSPHATE

Use diluent supplied with drug. Introduce diluent into sterile ampule using a 20-gauge needle affixed to a 5-ml syringe. Swirl gently until a solution is effected. *Do not* agitate violently.

After reconstitution, if storage is desired, solution should be kept at room temperature and away from direct light. Under these conditions solution is stable for about 10 days as long as cloudiness or evidence of a precipitate has not occurred.

Warn patient that a burning sensation may be experienced at site of injection. This is transitory and may not recur with subsequent injections.

Give deep IM in gluteus muscle. Rotate injection sites; record site used.

ONGOING ASSESSMENTS AND NURSING MANAGEMENT

Monitor vital signs daily; observe for adverse reactions; note patient's response to therapy (*i.e.,* relief of pain).

CLINICAL ALERT: Notify physician immediately if any of the following occurs: pain or tenderness in calf of leg or groin; chest pain; sudden dyspnea; sudden severe headache, dizziness, or fainting; visual or speech disturbance; weakness or numbness in arm or leg; personality changes.

Clinical response should be apparent within 3 months of beginning of therapy.

If pain persists after repeated injections of polyestradiol, inform physician. A local anesthetic may be ordered for concomitant administration.

Inspect previous injection sites for sterile abscess formation; notify physician if abscess is noted.

Weigh weekly or as ordered. Inform physician of significant weight increase or decrease or swelling of the ankles or feet.

If edema occurs, physician may prescribe a diuretic. A salt-restricted diet may also be recommended.

PATIENT AND FAMILY INFORMATION

May cause nausea, vomiting, headache, abdominal pain, or painful swelling of breasts. Notify physician or nurse if these become pronounced.

Weigh self weekly. Contact physician if a significant weight increase or decrease occurs or if swelling of the feet or ankles is noted.

Contact physician immediately if any of the following occurs: pain or tenderness in calf of leg or groin; chest pain; sudden shortness of breath; sudden severe headache, dizziness, or fainting; visual or speech disturbance; weakness or numbness in arm or leg.

Contraceptive measures are recommended during therapy. Discuss with physician method to be used.

Periodic laboratory or diagnostic tests will be necessary to monitor therapy.

Estrogens, Combined

See Estrogens.

Estrogens, Conjugated

See Estrogens; Estrogens, Vaginal.

Estrogens, Esterified

See Estrogens.

Estrogens, Vaginal Rx

	suppositories
dienestrol 0.7 mg w/lactose	DV
diethylstilbestrol 0.1 mg, 0.2 mg	*Generic*
	creams
conjugated estrogens 0.625 mg/g	Premarin
dienestrol 0.01%	Ortho Dienestrol
dienestrol 0.01% w/lactose	DV, Estraguard
estropipate 1.5 mg/g	Ogen

INDICATIONS

Treatment of atrophic vaginitis and kraurosis vulvae associated with menopause.

ACTIONS

Depletion of endogenous estrogens occurs postmenopausally as a result of a decline in ovarian function and may cause symptomatic vulvovaginal epithelial atrophy. Signs and symptoms of these atrophic changes may be alleviated by topical application of an estrogenic hormone.

WARNINGS

Systemic absorption: Degree of systemic absorption from use of vaginal preparations may be less than that following oral or parenteral administration but information given for estrogens (p 455) should be considered when using these products.

Vaginal bleeding: Because there is a possibility of absorption through vaginal mucosa, uterine bleeding may be provoked by excessive administration in menopausal women. Cytologic study or D and C may be required to differentiate this uterine bleeding from carcinoma. Tenderness of the breasts and vaginal discharge due to hypersecretion of mucus may result from excessive estrogenic stimulation;

endometrial withdrawal bleeding may occur if use is suddenly discontinued. Such reactions indicate overdosage. May cause serious bleeding in sterilized women because of endometriosis and because remaining foci of endometrium could be activated.

Use in pregnancy: Safety and efficacy are not established. Not recommended for any condition during pregnancy.

DOSAGE

Suppositories: One or two daily; those with atrophic vaginitis may require up to 2 mg daily and cyclic administration may be necessary for several years. Patients with atrophic vaginitis may notice relief of symptoms sooner if up to 1 mg of suppository form is administered daily for 10 to 14 days concomitantly with oral diethylstilbestrol (DES). Also, patients with atrophic vaginitis and kraurosis vulvae may receive the suppository form as the only means of estrogenic therapy, in which case dosage may be increased up to 5 mg/week to 7 mg/week.

Creams: One or two applicatorsful intravaginally daily; dosage is reduced gradually.

Dienestrol maintenance dose: One applicatorful or 1 suppository, 1 to 3 times/week after vaginal mucosa restored.

NURSING IMPLICATIONS

HISTORY

See Appendix 4. A history of patient's menopause should also be obtained and should include age at onset, present menstrual pattern, symptoms experienced, age at menarche, mother's menstrual history (if known), and family history of carcinoma.

PHYSICAL ASSESSMENT

Physician performs vaginal examination. A Pap smear may also be obtained at this time.

ADMINISTRATION

Patient may insert suppository or cream. If she is unable to do so, drug is administered by nurse.

Calibrated applicator available with cream (Premarin and Ortho Dienestrol also available without applicator). Insert supplied with DV suppositories.

ONGOING ASSESSMENTS AND NURSING MANAGEMENT

Inquire about relief of symptoms.

If uterine bleeding occurs, withhold next administration and notify physician.

PATIENT INFORMATION

Lying on back, insert high into vagina with applicator provided.

It may be necessary to wear a small sanitary pad to prevent drug from getting on clothing.

Do not exceed recommended dosage.

Discontinue use of drug and notify physician if vaginal bleeding occurs.

Estrone Aqueous Suspension

See Estrogens.

Estropipate

See Estrogens; Estrogens, Vaginal.

Ethacrynic Acid

See Loop Diuretics.

Ethambutol Hydrochloride Rx

tablets: 100 mg,   Myambutol
    400 mg

INDICATIONS

Treatment of pulmonary tuberculosis. Used in conjunction with at least one other antituberculous drug. In those who have received previous therapy, mycobacterial resistance to other drugs used in initial therapy is frequent.

CONTRAINDICATIONS

Hypersensitivity; known optic neuritis unless clinical judgment determines that it may be used.

ACTIONS

Diffuses into actively growing mycobacterium cells such as tubercle bacilli. It inhibits synthesis of one or more metabolites, causing impairment of cell metabolism, arrest of multiplication, and cell death. No cross-resistance with other agents has been demonstrated. Absorption is not influenced by food. Following a single oral dose of 15 mg/kg to 25 mg/kg, ethambutol attains a peak of 2 mcg/ml to 5 mcg/ml in serum 2 to 4 hours after administration. Serum levels are similar after prolonged dosing. The serum level falls to undetectable levels by 24 hours after last dose. Approximately 50% of dose is excreted unchanged in urine, 8% to 15% as metabolites, and 20% to 25% unchanged in the feces. Accumulation may occur in renal insufficiency.

WARNINGS

Use in pregnancy only when clearly needed and when potential benefits outweigh unknown potential hazards to the fetus. Not recommended for use in children under 13.

PRECAUTIONS
Patients with decreased renal function need reduced dosage (as determined by serum levels) because drug is excreted by kidney.

Because drug may have adverse effect on vision, physical examination should include ophthalmoscopy, finger perimetry, and testing of color discrimination. In those with visual defects such as cataracts, recurrent inflammatory conditions of the eye, optic neuritis, and diabetic retinopathy, evaluation of changes in visual acuity may be more difficult because variations in vision may be due to the underlying disease condition.

Periodic assessment of organ system functions, including renal, hepatic, and hematopoietic, is recommended during long-term therapy.

DRUG INTERACTIONS
The effectiveness of ethambutol may be decreased when taken concomitantly with **aluminum salts** because of decreased GI absorption.

ADVERSE REACTIONS
May produce decreases in visual acuity, which appear to be due to optic neuritis and related to dose and duration of treatment. Effects are generally reversible when drug is discontinued promptly. Rarely, recovery may be delayed for up to 1 year or more and effect may possibly be irreversible.

Acuity changes may be unilateral or bilateral. Testing should be performed before beginning therapy and periodically during administration. Snellen eye charts are recommended for testing visual acuity.

If evaluation confirms visual change and fails to reveal other causes, drug is discontinued and patient reevaluated at frequent intervals.

Patients developing visual abnormality during treatment may show subjective visual symptoms before, or simultaneously with, the demonstration of decreases in visual acuity. Recovery of visual acuity generally occurs over a period of weeks to months after drug is discontinued. Patients have then received the drug again without recurrence of loss of visual acuity.

Other adverse reactions reported include anaphylactoid reactions, dermatitis, pruritus, joint pain, anorexia, nausea, vomiting, gastrointestinal upset, abdominal pain, fever, malaise, headache and dizziness, mental confusion, disorientation, and possible hallucinations. Numbness and tingling of the extremities due to peripheral neuritis also have been reported.

Elevated serum uric acid levels occur and precipitation of acute gout has been reported. Transient impairment of hepatic function as indicated by abnormal hepatic-function tests is not unusual. Because drug is recommended for therapy in conjunction with one or more agents, these changes may be related to concurrent therapy.

DOSAGE
Not used alone in initial treatment or in retreatment. Drug is administered once every 24 hours only. Absorption is not significantly altered by administration with food.

Initial treatment: In patients who have not received previous antituberculous therapy, 15 mg/kg (7 mg/lb) once every 24 hours. Isoniazid may be administered concurrently as a single oral dose once every 24 hours.

Retreatment: In those who have received previous therapy, 25 mg/kg (11 mg/lb) as a single oral dose once every 24 hours. Concurrent administration of at least one other antituberculous drug, to which the organisms have been demonstrated to be susceptible, is recommended. After 60 days of administration, dose is decreased to 15 mg/kg once every 24 hours.

NURSING IMPLICATIONS

HISTORY
See Appendix 4.

PHYSICAL ASSESSMENT
Obtain vital signs, weight. Pretreatment diagnostic tests may include ophthalmologic examination, CBC, renal- and hepatic-function tests, culture and sensitivity tests.

ADMINISTRATION
Administer once every 24 hours. Give drug at same time each day.

Administer with food.

ONGOING ASSESSMENTS AND NURSING MANAGEMENT
Patient may or may not be hospitalized during time of initial diagnostic testing and initiation of treatment. Outpatients may require hospitalization for additional diagnostic tests or other treatment (*e.g.,* surgery).

Obtain vital signs daily or at time of each office or clinic visit.

Weigh weekly or at time of each office or clinic visit.

Observe for patient complaints of visual changes. Thoroughly question patient weekly or at time of each office or clinic visit about any type of visual change such as blurred vision or changes in color perception.

Changes in color perception are probably the first sign of toxicity. Color perception changes may be detected with use of hue charts. Testing of color perception should be conducted at time of each office or clinic visit. Testing of visual acuity with a Snellen eye chart is also recommended.

Monthly eye examinations are recommended when patient is on a daily dose of 25 mg/kg.

Know adverse effects, warnings, precautions, administration, and dosage of other antituberculous drugs included in the therapeutic regimen.

Monitor intake and output if patient has renal impairment; report any decrease in the intake–output ratio to the physician.

Periodic CBC, renal- and hepatic-function tests are recommended during therapy.

Therapy is usually continued until bacteriologic conversion has become permanent and maximal clinical improvement has occurred.

PATIENT AND FAMILY INFORMATION
May cause GI upset; take with food.

Take drug at same time each day. Avoid missing doses. Do not double the dose on the following day if a dose is missed.

Do not discontinue therapy except on advice of a physician.

Notify physician or nurse if changes in vision (*e.g.,* blurring, red-green color blindness) or skin rash occurs.

Periodic testing or examinations will be necessary to monitor therapy.

Ethaverine Hydrochloride Rx

tablets: 100 mg	Ethaquin, Ethatab
capsules: 100 mg	Isovex-100
capsules, timed release: 150 mg	Circubid

INDICATIONS
Peripheral and cerebral vascular insufficiency associated with arterial spasm; as a smooth muscle spasmolytic in spastic conditions of the GI and GU tracts. Studies do not show these drugs to be effective in the conditions for which they are labeled.

CONTRAINDICATIONS
Complete atrioventricular dissociation.

ACTIONS
Ethaverine is closely related to papaverine and has similar actions and uses.

WARNINGS
Safety for use in pregnancy or in nursing mother is not established. Do not use in pregnant women or in women of childbearing age unless essential to welfare of patient.

PRECAUTIONS
Administer with caution to patients with glaucoma or hypotension. Hepatic hypersensitivity has been reported with GI symptoms, jaundice, eosinophilia, and altered hepatic-function tests. Discontinue drug if these occur.

ADVERSE REACTIONS
Nausea, anorexia, abdominal distress, dryness of throat, hypotension, malaise, lassitude, drowsiness, flushing, sweating, constipation or diarrhea, skin rash, vertigo, respiratory depression, cardiac depression, cardiac arrhythmia, headache.

DOSAGE
Most effective if given early in course of vascular disorder. Because of chronic nature of disease, long-term therapy is required.

Capsules, timed release: 150 mg q12h. In more difficult cases, increase to 300 mg q12h.

Capsules and tablets: 100 mg tid. In more difficult cases, increase to 200 mg tid.

NURSING IMPLICATIONS

HISTORY
See Appendix 4.

PHYSICAL ASSESSMENT
Obtain vital signs; when applicable, assess problem areas (*e.g.,* legs [color, peripheral pulses]).

ADMINISTRATION
Instruct patient not to chew capsule (timed release or regular).

ONGOING ASSESSMENTS AND NURSING MANAGEMENT
Obtain vital signs daily; observe for adverse reactions.

If dizziness or drowsiness occurs, patient may require assistance with ambulation.

Summarize patient's symptoms and drug response (if any) once or twice a week.

PATIENT AND FAMILY INFORMATION
May cause dizziness or drowsiness; use caution when driving or performing other tasks requiring alertness. Alcohol may intensify these effects.

May also cause flushing, sweating, headache,

tiredness, jaundice, skin rash, or GI effects (nausea, anorexia, abdominal distress, constipation, diarrhea). Notify physician if these become pronounced.

Ethchlorvynol Rx C-IV

capsules: 100 mg, 200 mg, 500 mg, 750 mg (contains tartrazine)   Placidyl

INDICATIONS

Short-term hypnotic therapy for periods up to 1 week in the management of insomnia. If retreatment becomes necessary after drug-free intervals of 1 or more weeks, it should be undertaken only upon further patient evaluation.

CONTRAINDICATIONS

Hypersensitivity; porphyria.

ACTIONS

Has sedative-hypnotic, anticonvulsant, and muscle relaxant properties. It produces EEG patterns similar to those produced by barbiturates. Is rapidly absorbed from the GI tract, with peak plasma concentrations usually occurring within 2 hours after a single dose. Maximum blood concentrations occur in 1 to 1½ hours; approximately 90% of drug is destroyed in the liver. There is extensive tissue concentration, particularly in adipose tissue. Within 24 hours, 33% of a single 500-mg dose is excreted in the urine, mostly as metabolites. The free and unconjugated forms of the metabolites in the urine account for about 40% of the dose. Plasma half-life of the parent compound is approximately 10 to 20 hours.

The usual hypnotic dose induces sleep within 15 to 60 minutes. Duration of effect is about 5 hours.

WARNINGS

Psychological and physical dependence: Administer with caution to mentally depressed patients, with or without suicidal tendencies, and to those who have a psychological potential for drug dependence. The least amount of drug practical is prescribed. Prolonged use may result in tolerance and psychological and physical dependence.

Intoxication symptoms: Intoxication has been reported with prolonged use of doses as low as 1 g/day. Signs and symptoms may include incoordination, tremors, ataxia, confusion, slurred speech, hyperreflexia, diplopia, and generalized muscle weakness. Toxic amblyopia, scotoma, nystagmus,

and peripheral neuropathy have also been reported with prolonged use; these symptoms are usually reversible.

Withdrawal symptoms: Severe withdrawal symptoms, similar to those seen during barbiturate and alcohol withdrawal, have followed abrupt discontinuance after prolonged use. Symptoms may appear as late as 9 days after sudden withdrawal and may include convulsions, delirium, schizoid reaction, perceptual distortion, memory loss, ataxia, insomnia, slurring speech, unusual anxiety, irritability, agitation, tremors, anorexia, nausea, vomiting, weakness, dizziness, sweating, muscle twitching, and weight loss.

Withdrawal management: Involves readministration of drug to approximately the same level of chronic intoxication that existed before the abrupt discontinuance. (Phenobarbital may be substituted for ethchlorvynol.) A gradual, stepwise reduction of dosage may then be made over a period of days or weeks. A phenothiazine compound may be used in addition to this regimen for those who exhibit psychotic symptoms during the withdrawal period. Patient must be hospitalized or closely observed and given general supportive care as indicated.

Use in pregnancy: Not recommended during the first and second trimesters. Ethchlorvynol crosses the placental barrier and clinical experience has indicated that use during the third trimester may produce CNS depression and transient withdrawal symptoms in the newborn.

Use in lactation: Safety not established.

Use in children: Not recommended.

PRECAUTIONS

Use in elderly or debilitated patients: These patients should receive the smallest effective dose.

Use in impaired hepatic or renal function: Exercise caution.

CNS effects: Patients who exhibit unpredictable behavior or paradoxical restlessness or excitement in response to barbiturates or alcohol may react in this manner to ethchlorvynol. Drug is not used in management of insomnia in the presence of pain, unless insomnia persists after pain is controlled with analgesics. Do not heavily sedate patients with unrelieved pain.

Tartrazine sensitivity: Some of these products contain tartrazine (see Appendix 6, section 6-23).

DRUG INTERACTIONS

Exaggerated depressant effects will occur when used concomitantly with **alcohol, barbiturates, MAO inhibitors,** or other **CNS depressants.** May cause a decreased prothrombin time response to **coumarin anticoagulants;** dosage of these drugs may require adjustment at initiation and discontinuation of therapy. Transient delirium has been reported with use of ethchlorvynol and **amitriptyline;** administer with caution to patients receiving **tricyclic antidepressants.**

ADVERSE REACTIONS

GI: Nausea, vomiting, gastric upset.

CNS: Dizziness; facial numbness; mild stimulation; marked excitement; hysteria; prolonged hypnosis; profound muscular weakness. Transient giddiness and ataxia have occurred when absorption of drug is rapid; these effects can sometimes be controlled by administering the drug with food.

Cardiovascular: Hypotension; syncope without marked hypotension.

Hypersensitivity: Skin rash; urticaria; thrombocytopenia; cholestatic jaundice.

Miscellaneous: Mild "hangover"; aftertaste; blurred vision. Pulmonary edema has resulted from IV abuse.

OVERDOSAGE

Symptoms: Acute intoxication characterized by prolonged deep coma, severe respiratory depression, hypothermia, relative bradycardia. Nystagmus and pancytopenia have been reported. Death has occurred following ingestion of 6 g, but patients have survived overdoses of 50 g and more with intensive care.

Treatment: Immediate gastric evacuation. In the unconscious patient, precede gastric lavage by tracheal intubation with a cuffed tube. Supportive care (assisted ventilation, frequent monitoring of vital signs, control of blood pressure) is essential. Place emphasis on pulmonary care and monitoring of blood gases. Hemodialysis and peritoneal dialysis are reported to be of some value (aqueous and oil dialysate have been used); hemoperfusion with charcoal or XAD-4 resin has also been effective. Forced diuresis with maintenance of a high urinary output is of value.

DOSAGE

Hypnotic: Usual adult dose is 500 mg H.S. A dose of 750 mg may be required for those whose sleep response to 500 mg is inadequate or for patients being changed from barbiturates or other nonbarbiturate hypnotics.

Severe insomnia: Up to 1000 mg may be given as a single H.S. dose.

Supplemental dose: 100 mg to 200 mg may be given to reinstitute sleep in those who awaken after the original H.S. dose of 500 mg or 750 mg.

Insomnia: A single dose of 100 mg to 200 mg taken upon awakening may be adequate. Give small

effective dose to elderly or debilitated patients. It is recommended that drug not be prescribed for more than 1 week.

NURSING IMPLICATIONS

HISTORY
See Appendix 4.

PHYSICAL ASSESSMENT
Determine if specific factors that may be controlled or eliminated are interfering with sleep. Factors may include noise, bright lights, pain, or discomfort.

ADMINISTRATION
Obtain blood pressure prior to administration, especially if patient is elderly or baseline blood pressure is low normal.

Patient's immediate area should be free from disturbance (*e.g.,* noise, lights) before a hypnotic is given.

Do not administer drug if patient has pain, which should be controlled by administration of an analgesic.

Do not administer a hypnotic shortly before or after administration of a narcotic analgesic (both are CNS depressants; see *Drug Interactions*) or any other CNS depressant. If patient has an order for a narcotic analgesic (or other CNS depressant) and a hypnotic, check with physician regarding time interval between administration of these agents. Usually 2 or more hours should elapse between administration of a hypnotic and a CNS depressant, but interval may vary with a specific CNS depressant and the dose administered.

May be given with food if giddiness or GI upset occurs.

Raise the siderails. Advise patient to remain in bed and to call for assistance if it is necessary to get out of bed during nighttime hours.

ONGOING ASSESSMENTS AND NURSING MANAGEMENT
Observe patient in 60 to 90 minutes to evaluate effect of drug.

If no order for a supplemental dose is written and patient wakes during the night, record length of sleep from H.S. dose and discuss with physician.

Observe for adverse reactions.

If paradoxical restlessness or excitement occurs, patient should be closely observed until effect of drug has worn off. Do not administer another dose of drug until problem is discussed with the physician.

Observe elderly patient frequently during sleep. If the duration of the drug appears prolonged (*e.g.,* patient remains sleepy during morning hours) or if paradoxical effects occur, discuss problem with physician.

PATIENT AND FAMILY INFORMATION

Do not exceed the prescribed dose. *Do not* repeat the dose upon awakening during the night, unless a repeat dose is approved by the physician.

May cause drowsiness, dizziness, or blurred vision. It is advisable to remain in bed once drug has been taken for sleep. *Do not* attempt to drive or perform other tasks requiring alertness after taking this drug.

Do not drink alcoholic beverages before or after taking this drug because the combination of alcohol and this drug can be dangerous.

Avoid use of other CNS depressants while taking this drug.

Inform other physicians of use of this drug.

Symptoms of giddiness, ataxia, or GI upset may be reduced if medication is taken with food.

Ethinamate Rx C-IV

capsules: 500 mg	Valmid Pulvules

INDICATIONS

Short-acting hypnotic in management of insomnia. Prolonged administration is generally not recommended, because it is not effective for more than 7 days. Should insomnia persist, drug-free intervals of 1 week or more should elapse before retreatment is considered.

CONTRAINDICATIONS

Hypersensitivity.

ACTIONS

Is a hypnotic agent and nonselective CNS depressant. Site and mechanism of action and effect on REM sleep are unknown. A hypnotic dose of 500 mg is about as effective as 100 mg of secobarbital. Is rapidly absorbed from the GI tract and primarily inactivated in the liver and excreted in urine. Following a single dose of 1 g, peak plasma levels are reached in approximately 36 minutes and decline to negligible values over 8 hours. Approximately 36% of the dose appears in the urine within 24 hours. Onset of action is 20 to 30 minutes; it is more effective in inducing sleep than in maintaining sleep. Duration of action is approximately 4 hours.

WARNINGS

Physical and psychological dependence: Drug dependence has occurred when drug was taken at higher than recommended doses for prolonged intervals. Exercise caution in individuals who are addiction prone and in those whose history suggests that they may increase the dosage on their own. If drug dependence occurs, withdrawal must be accomplished with extreme care. Abrupt withdrawal may cause an abstinence syndrome accompanied by convulsions. Withdrawal may be accomplished by hospitalization and reduction of the addictive dose at a rate of 500 mg to 1000 mg every 2 to 3 days.

Use in pregnancy: Safety not established. Use only when clearly needed and when potential benefits outweigh unknown risks.

Use in lactation: Safety not established.

Use in children: Safety and efficacy for use in children below age 15 not established.

PRECAUTIONS

Use in elderly or debilitated: Risks of oversedation, dizziness, confusion, and ataxia substantially increase with administration of large doses. A single 500-mg dose should be given to elderly or debilitated individuals.

The usual precautions are indicated for severely depressed patients or those in whom there is any evidence of latent depression, particularly when it is recognized that suicidal tendencies may be present and that protective measures may be necessary.

Patients with unrelieved pain should not be heavily sedated.

Use drug with caution in those with acute intermittent porphyria.

DRUG INTERACTIONS

Additive depressant effects will occur when used concurrently with **alcohol, CNS depressants,** or other agents with CNS depressant or hypnotic effects.

ADVERSE REACTIONS

Rare: Thrombocytopenic purpura, drug idiosyncrasy with fever.

Miscellaneous: Paradoxical excitement in children, mild GI symptoms, skin rashes.

OVERDOSAGE

In suicidal overdosage, death has been reported after ingestion of 15 g, but recovery was noted after 28 g. Treat CNS and respiratory depression in same manner as barbiturate intoxication (p 169). Hemodialysis is effective.

DOSAGE
500 mg or 1000 mg taken 20 minutes before retiring.

NURSING IMPLICATIONS

HISTORY
See Appendix 4.

PHYSICAL ASSESSMENT
Determine whether specific factors that may be controlled or eliminated are interfering with sleep. Factors may include noise, bright lights, pain, or discomfort.

ADMINISTRATION
Patient's immediate area should be free from disturbance (*e.g.,* noise, lights) before hypnotic is given.

Do not administer drug if patient has pain, which should be controlled by administration of an analgesic.

Do not administer a hypnotic shortly before or after administration of a narcotic analgesic (both are CNS depressants; see *Drug Interactions*) or any other CNS depressant. If patient has an order for a narcotic analgesic (or other CNS depressant) and a hypnotic, check with physician about time interval between administration of these agents. Usually 2 or more hours should elapse between administration of a hypnotic and another CNS depressant, but interval may vary with a specific CNS depressant and the dose administered.

Advise patient to swallow capsule whole.

Raise the siderails and advise patient to remain in bed and call for assistance if it is necessary to get out of bed during nighttime hours.

ONGOING ASSESSMENTS AND NURSING MANAGEMENT
Observe patient in 45 to 60 minutes to evaluate effect of drug.

Observe for adverse reactions.

If paradoxical restlessness or excitement occurs, patient should be closely observed until effect of drug has worn off. Do not administer another dose of drug until problem is discussed with physician.

Observe elderly patient for oversedation, dizziness, and confusion. If these occur or if duration of the drug appears prolonged (*i.e.,* patient remains sleepy during morning hours), discuss problem with physician.

PATIENT AND FAMILY INFORMATION
Do not exceed the prescribed dose. *Do not* repeat the dose upon awakening during the night.

May cause drowsiness or dizziness. It is advisable to remain in bed once the drug has been taken for sleep. *Do not* attempt to drive or perform other tasks requiring alertness after taking this drug.

Do not drink alcoholic beverages before or after taking this drug because the combination of alcohol and this drug can be dangerous.

Avoid use of other CNS depressants while taking this drug.

Inform other physicians of use of this drug.

Ethinyl Estradiol

See Estrogens.

Ethionamide Rx

tablets: 250 mg   Trecator-SC

INDICATIONS
Recommended for any form of active tuberculosis when treatment with first-line drugs (isoniazid, rifampin) has failed. Should be given only with other effective antituberculous agents.

CONTRAINDICATIONS
Severe hypersensitivity; severe hepatic damage.

ACTIONS
Bacteriostatic against *Mycobacterium tuberculosis.*

WARNINGS
Use in pregnancy: Use only when clearly needed and when potential benefits outweigh the unknown potential hazards to the fetus.

Use in children: Optimal dosage not established. This does not preclude use when crucial to therapy.

PRECAUTIONS
Pretreatment examinations should include susceptibility tests of recent cultures of *M. tuberculosis* from the patient as measured against ethionamide and the usual primary antituberculous drugs.

Determination of serum transaminase (SGOT, SGPT) should be made prior to and every 2 to 4 weeks during therapy.

In those with diabetes mellitus, management of diabetes may be more difficult and hepatitis occurs more frequently.

DRUG INTERACTIONS
May intensify adverse effects of **other antituberculous agents** administered concomitantly. Convulsions have been reported and special care should be

taken, particularly when ethionamide is administered with **cycloserine.**

ADVERSE REACTIONS
Gastrointestinal intolerance, peripheral neuritis, optic neuritis, psychic disturbances (including mental depression), postural hypotension, skin rashes, thrombocytopenia, pellagralike syndrome, jaundice or hepatitis, increased difficulty in management of diabetes mellitus, gynecomastia, impotence.

DOSAGE
Should be administered with at least 1 other antituberculous drug. *Average adult dose*—0.5 g/day to 1 g/day in divided doses. Concomitant administration of pyridoxine is recommended.

NURSING IMPLICATIONS

HISTORY
See Appendix 4.

PHYSICAL ASSESSMENT
Obtain vital signs, weight. Pretreatment diagnostic tests include susceptibility tests of recent cultures from the patient, serum transaminase. Other laboratory tests may also be appropriate.

ADMINISTRATION
Give with food to reduce GI upset.

Concurrent administration of pyridoxine (vitamin B_6) is recommended to prevent peripheral neuritis.

ONGOING ASSESSMENTS AND NURSING MANAGEMENT
Patient may or may not be hospitalized during time of initial therapy with this drug.

Obtain vital signs daily or at time of each office or clinic visit.

Weigh weekly or at time of each office or clinic visit.

If GI disturbance persists even when drug is given with food, notify physician.

Determination of serum transaminase is recommended every 2 to 4 weeks during therapy.

If postural hypotension occurs, advise patient to make position changes slowly.

Psychic disturbances, including mental depression, may occur. If patient appears withdrawn, is noncommunicative, or has other personality changes, notify physician before next dose is due. Depression may require more frequent observation of the patient.

Know adverse effects, warnings, precautions, administration, and dosage of other antituberculous drugs included in the therapeutic regimen.

Inform patient that drug may cause a metallic taste, which may be alleviated by hard candy, chewing gum, and warm- or cool-water mouth rinses.

Diabetic patients: Check urine for glucose, ketone bodies qid. Notify physician if percentage of glucose in urine increases or urine is positive for ketones. Dosage of insulin or oral hypoglycemic agent may require adjustment. Frequent monitoring of fasting blood glucose may also be required. Observe signs of hyperglycemia and hypoglycemia (Appendix 6, section 6-14).

PATIENT AND FAMILY INFORMATION
May cause GI upset (nausea, vomiting, diarrhea), loss of appetite, metallic taste, or salivation. Notify physician if these effects become bothersome or increase in severity.

Take medication with food to reduce GI upset.

Take drug exactly as prescribed. Do not discontinue therapy except on advice of physician.

Periodic testing or examinations will be necessary to monitor therapy.

Ethopropazine Hydrochloride

See Anticholinergic Antiparkinsonism Agents.

Ethosuximide

See Anticonvulsants, Succinimides.

Ethotoin

See Anticonvulsants, Hydantoins.

Ethylene

See Anesthetics, General, Gases.

Ethylestrenol

See Anabolic Hormones.

Ethylnorepinephrine Hydrochloride

See Bronchodilators and Decongestants, Systemic.

Etidronate Disodium Rx

tablets: 200 mg   Didronel

INDICATIONS

Symptomatic Paget's disease of bone (osteitis deformans): Effectiveness has been demonstrated primarily in those with polyostotic Paget's disease with symptoms of pain and significant elevations of urinary hydroxyproline and serum alkaline phosphatase.

Heterotopic ossification due to spinal cord injury: Has been shown to significantly reduce severity of clinically important heterotopic ossification masses (*i.e.,* masses of sufficient size to restrict range of motion, require surgical removal, or be of other clinical significance).

Heterotopic ossification complicating total hip replacement: Drug reduces incidence of clinically significant heterotopic lesions, which are of sufficient size to restrict range of motion or require reoperation.

CONTRAINDICATIONS

None known.

ACTIONS

Acts primarily on bone to modify crystal growth of calcium hydroxyapatite by chemisorption onto the crystal surface. Depending on concentration, drug may inhibit either crystal resorption or crystal growth. Absorption of drug is dose dependent. Most of drug is cleared from the blood in 6 hours. The remainder is chemically adsorbed on the bone and slowly eliminated. Unabsorbed drug is excreted in the feces.

Serum phosphate elevations occur at doses of 10 mg/kg/day or above and occasionally at 5 mg/kg/day. This is not an indication for discontinuing therapy because elevation appears to be the result of increased tubular reabsorption of phosphate.

Paget's disease: Slows rate of bone turnover (bone resorption and new bone accretion) in pagetic bone lesions and in the normal remodeling process. Bone from patients on therapy shows a reduction in excessive cellular activity accompanied by a suppression of bone resorption and accretion and a return toward normal.

Heterotopic ossification: Drug chemisorbs to calcium hydroxyapatite crystals, blocking further crystal growth and mineralization; this is thought to be the mechanism of action that prevents or retards heterotopic bone formation during the active stage.

WARNINGS

Paget's disease: Response to therapy may be slow and may continue for months after treatment is discontinued. Dosage should not be increased prematurely, nor should treatment be resumed before there is evidence of reactivation of the disease process. Retreatment is not initiated until patient has had at least a 3-month drug-free interval. The incidence of osteogenic sarcoma is increased in Paget's disease. Pagetic lesions, with or without therapy, may appear by x-ray examination to progress markedly, possibly with some loss of definition of periosteal margins. Such lesions should be evaluated to differentiate them from osteogenic sarcoma.

PRECAUTIONS

Patient should maintain an adequate nutritional status, particularly an adequate intake of calcium and vitamin D. Those with restricted vitamin D and calcium intake may be particularly sensitive to drugs affecting calcium homeostasis and are followed closely.

Caution is advised in treating patients with renal impairment.

Therapy has been withheld from patients with enterocolitis because increased frequency of bowel movements and diarrhea are seen in some patients when this drug is administered at 20 mg/kg/day, and these may be seen occasionally at lower doses.

Paget's disease: Drug retards mineralization of osteoid laid down during accretion. This effect is dose and time dependent. There may be an overlap of beneficial and mineralization inhibition effects in some patients at higher doses. Extended periods of medication are approached cautiously. When administered at doses of 20 mg/kg/day, drug suppresses bone turnover and essentially stops mineralization of new bone in pagetic lesions, and, to a lesser extent, in uninvolved skeleton. Mineralization of pagetic lesions has been demonstrated to occur normally after drug is discontinued.

Heterotopic ossification due to spinal cord injury: Concomitant fractures are common in those with spinal cord injury. In controlled studies, no problems of fracture healing or stabilization of the spine were encountered. In cases with multiple long-bone fractures, therapy may be delayed for a short time until formation of callus is evident.

Use in pregnancy, lactation: Use only when clearly needed and when potential benefits outweigh unknown potential hazards to the fetus. It is not known if drug is excreted in human milk. Exercise caution when drug is administered to a nursing woman.

Use in children: Safety and effectiveness not established.

ADVERSE REACTIONS

GI complaints (loose bowel movements, nausea) are increased in some patients when doses greater than

5 mg/kg/day are given. In those with Paget's disease, increased or recurrent bone pain at existing pagetic sites and the appearance of pain at a site that was previously asymptomatic have been reported. Fractures are recognized as a common feature in those with Paget's disease. The risk of fracture may be increased when drug is taken at a dose level of 20 mg/kg/day in excess of 3 months. Risk may be greater in those with extensive and severe disease, a history of multiple fractures, or rapidly advancing osteolytic lesions. Discontinue drug when fractures occur; do not reinstate therapy until fracture healing is complete.

OVERDOSAGE
There is no experience with acute overdosage. Theoretically, hypocalcemia could occur.

DOSAGE
Administer as a single oral dose 2 hours before meals.

Paget's disease: Initially, recommended dose is 5 mg/kg/day. Treatment should not exceed 6 months. Doses above 10 mg/kg should be reserved for use when there is an overriding requirement for suppression of increased bone turnover or when prompt reduction of elevated cardiac output is required. Retreatment is undertaken only after a drug-free period of at least 3 months and after it is evident that reactivation of the disease has occurred.

Heterotopic ossification due to spinal cord injury: Recommended dose is 20 mg/kg/day for 2 weeks, followed by 10 mg/kg/day for 10 weeks. Total treatment period is 12 weeks. This recommended dosing regimen should be instituted as soon as feasible following injury, preferably before any radiographic evidence of heterotopic ossification.

Heterotopic ossification complicating total hip replacement: Recommended dose is 20 mg/kg/day for 1 month preoperatively, followed by 20 mg/kg/day for 3 months postoperatively. Total treatment period is 4 months.

NURSING IMPLICATIONS

HISTORY
See Appendix 4.

PHYSICAL ASSESSMENT
When applicable, evaluate general status.

ADMINISTRATION
Administer as a single oral dose 2 hours before meals.

May be given with fruit juice or water. Food, particularly materials high in calcium content such as milk, in the stomach or upper portion of the small intestine may reduce absorption.

Food should not be taken within 2 hours before or after drug administration.

ONGOING ASSESSMENTS AND NURSING MANAGEMENT
Monitor food intake. If anorexia occurs, a dietary consultation may be necessary.

Observe for GI complaints (_e.g.,_ nausea, diarrhea, loose bowel movements). If these occur, notify physician before next dose is due because drug may be discontinued.

Paget's disease: Increased or recurrent bone pain at existing pagetic sites and the appearance of pain at previously asymptomatic sites have occurred. Periodically inquire about pain and discomfort and record findings.

Monitor intake and output of those with known renal impairment. Notify physician of any change in the intake–output ratio.

Periodic urinary hydroxyproline and serum alkaline phosphatase levels are recommended during the course of therapy.

PATIENT AND FAMILY INFORMATION
Take on an empty stomach 2 hours before meals; may be taken with fruit juice or water. Do not take tablet with milk.

Do not eat food or drink milk for 2 hours after taking drug.

A balanced diet, particularly with an adequate intake of calcium and vitamin D, is important. Milk and dairy products provide calcium and vitamin D. If anorexia occurs, or if these foods are disliked, discuss problem with physician.

May cause GI upset (nausea, diarrhea, abdominal cramps). Notify physician if these persist for more than 1 to 2 days.

Periodic evaluation of drug response will be necessary. Keep all clinic or office appointments.

Etomidate

See Anesthetics, General, Nonbarbiturates.

Etoposide _(VP-16-213)_ Rx

injection: 20 mg/ml   VePesid

INDICATIONS
In combination chemotherapy with other chemotherapeutic agents in those with refractory testicular tumors who have already received appropriate surgical, chemotherapeutic, and radiotherapeutic therapy.

CONTRAINDICATIONS
Hypersensitivity.

ACTIONS
Is a semisynthetic derivative of podophyllotoxin. Its main effect appears to be at the G_2 portion of the cell cycle. The predominant macromolecular effect appears to be DNA synthesis inhibition. The adult terminal half-life is 7 hours with a range of 3 to 12 hours; pediatric terminal half-life is 5.7 hours plus or minus 1.3 hours. Drug is excreted primarily in the urine; a small amount is excreted in feces.

WARNINGS
Myelosuppression: Patient is observed for myelosuppression during and after therapy. Dose-limiting bone-marrow suppression is the most significant toxicity.

Anaphylaxis: An anaphylactic reaction may occur; treatment is symptomatic.

Administer by slow IV infusion because hypotension may occur.

Use in pregnancy: Can cause fetal harm.

Use during lactation and in children: Safety not established.

PRECAUTIONS
Most adverse reactions are reversible if detected early. If severe reactions occur, reduce dosage or discontinue drug and institute appropriate corrective measures. Therapy is reinstituted with caution.

Carcinogenesis: Because of its mechanism of action, etoposide is a possible carcinogen.

ADVERSE REACTIONS
Hematologic: Myelotoxicity is most often dose limiting, with granulocyte nadirs occurring in 7 to 14 days and platelet nadirs occurring in 9 to 16 days after drug administration. Bone-marrow recovery is usually complete by day 20; no cumulative toxicity has been reported. Leukopenia (60%–91%); severe leukopenia of less than 1000 WBC (7%–17%); thrombocytopenia (28%–41%); and severe thrombocytopenia, less than 50,000 platelets/mm^3 (4%–20%) have been reported.

GI: Nausea and vomiting (32%) are the major GI toxicities and can usually be controlled with antiemetics. Also reported are anorexia (10%–13%); diarrhea (1%–13%); stomatitis (1%); and liver toxicity (3%).

Alopecia: Reversible alopecia, sometimes progressing to total baldness (8%–20%).

Hypotension: Temporary hypotension following rapid IV administration (1%–2%). To prevent this occurrence, drug is given by slow IV infusion.

Allergic reactions: Anaphylacticlike reactions characterized by chills, fever, tachycardia, bronchospasm, dyspnea, and hypotension (0.7%–2%). These reactions usually respond promptly to cessation of therapy and administration of pressor agents, corticosteroids, antihistamines, or volume expanders.

Neurotoxicity: Peripheral neuropathy (0.7%); CNS toxicity, including somnolence and fatigue (3%).

Other toxicities: Rare—Aftertaste, hypertension, rash.

DOSAGE
Dosage is modified to account for the myelosuppressive effects of other drugs in the combination, the effects of prior x-ray therapy or chemotherapy that may have compromised bone-marrow reserve.

Usual dose: 50 mg/m^2/day to 100 mg/m^2/day, days 1 to 5, or 100 mg/m^2/day, days 1, 3, and 5, every 3 to 4 weeks in combination with other appropriate agents.

NURSING IMPLICATIONS

HISTORY
See Appendix 4.

PHYSICAL ASSESSMENT
Obtain vital signs, weight. Baseline laboratory tests may include CBC, differential, platelet count, hemoglobin.

ADMINISTRATION
The use of gloves in preparing the solution is recommended because skin reactions associated with accidental exposure may occur.

If solution contacts the skin or mucosa, immediately wash the skin or mucosa thoroughly with soap and water.

Final concentration and diluent ordered by the physician. Drug may be diluted with either 5% Dextrose Injection or 0.9% Sodium Chloride Injection to give a final concentration of 0.2 mg/ml or 0.4 mg/ml.

Drug is available as 20 mg/ml. To make a 0.2-mg/ml solution, add 99 ml to the drug to give a final volume of 100 ml. To make a 0.4-mg/ml solution, add 199 ml to drug to give a final volume of 200 ml.

Check with physician and have drugs available that may be used to treat hypotensive episodes or anaphylaxis (*e.g.,* a corticosteroid, antihistamine, pressor agent, volume expander).

An antiemetic may be ordered before the infusion.

Obtain vital signs immediately before administration.

Administer the diluted solution by IV infusion (IV piggyback) over a 30- to 60-minute period, or as ordered by the physician.

CLINICAL ALERT: Closely supervise patient during time of infusion. Check rate of infusion and obtain blood pressure and pulse every 5 to 10 minutes. Observe continuously (especially first 2–3 times drug is given) for hypotensive episodes and anaphylaxis (manifested by fever, chills, tachycardia, bronchospasm, dyspnea, and hypotension).

If hypotension or anaphylaxis occurs, terminate the infusion, run the primary line to KVO, and contact the physician immediately. Treatment of hypotension includes administration of IV fluids and other appropriate therapy prescribed by the physician. Once this is controlled, the infusion may be restarted at a slower rate. Treatment of anaphylaxis may include administration of corticosteroids, antihistamines, pressor agents, and volume expanders.

Stability: Unopened ampules are stable for 3 years at room temperature. Diluted solutions (concentration of 0.2 mg/ml or 0.4 mg/ml) are stable for 96 and 48 hours, respectively, at room temperature under normal room fluorescent light in both glass and plastic containers.

ONGOING ASSESSMENTS AND NURSING MANAGEMENT

Record vital signs q4h or as ordered. Notify physician immediately of any change in vital signs.

Nausea and vomiting may occur and can usually be controlled by administration of an antiemetic. A liquid diet, unsalted crackers, or carbonated beverages may be offered until GI symptoms are controlled. If vomiting persists or nausea remains severe despite antiemetic therapy, notify the physician as well as observe for signs of hypokalemia, hyponatremia, and dehydration. Administration of IV fluids and electrolytes may be necessary.

Measure intake and output. Notify the physician of any change in the intake–output ratio.

CBC, differential, platelet count, and hemoglobin are usually ordered daily. Notify the physician immediately when a decrease in these values begins to occur because the dosage schedule may be changed or the drug discontinued.

Weigh weekly or as ordered. Notify the physician of any significant weight loss.

CLINICAL ALERT: Myelotoxicity is most often dose limiting. The granulocyte nadir occurs in 7 to 14 days and the platelet nadirs occur in 9 to 16 days after drug administration. Observe for signs of bone-marrow suppression daily.

Protective (reverse) isolation may be necessary if severe leukopenia develops.

Inspect oral cavity daily for evidence of stomatitis. Institute stomatitis care at the first sign of changes in the oral mucosa or patient complaint of burning of the oral mucosa.

If thrombocytopenia occurs, protect the patient from injury by padding siderails, taking temperatures orally (to prevent injury to the rectal mucosa), and using prolonged pressure on venipuncture or IM or subcutaneous administration sites.

If anorexia is severe or persists for more than 2 days, consult the physician. A high-protein, high-calorie diet in small frequent feedings may be ordered.

Reversible alopecia, often progressing to total baldness, may occur. Hair loss is often distressing and patient will require understanding from both the family and the medical team. A cap may be worn to disguise hair loss and patient is told that the hair may grow back but may be a different color or texture.

PATIENT AND FAMILY INFORMATION

NOTE: When drug is given on an outpatient basis or patient is discharged shortly after a course of therapy is completed, patient and family should receive a full explanation of all possible adverse reactions, what can be done to control or alleviate these reactions, and what specific reactions should be reported immediately to the physician.

Contact the physician immediately if any of the following occurs: easy bruising, petechiae, blood in the urine or stool, bleeding (*e.g.*, cuts, gums), fever, sore throat, sores or ulcerations on any part of the body, sores in the mouth or on the lips, burning of the mouth, anorexia, weight loss.

Inform other physicians and dentist of therapy with this drug.

Do not take nonprescription drugs unless use is approved by the physician.

Frequent laboratory tests will be necessary to monitor results of therapy.

F

Factor IX Complex (Human) Rx

Dried plasma fraction of coagulation Factors II, VII, IX, and X with minimal amount of total protein. Heparin free. In 500-unit bottles w/ diluent.	Konȳne
Dried plasma fraction of coagulation Factors II, VII, IX, and X. Heparin free. In single-dose bottles.	Profilnine
Dried plasma fraction of coagulation Factors II, VII, IX, and X with small amount of heparin as stabilizing agent. In 30-ml vials with diluent and needles.	Proplex
Dried plasma fraction of coagulation Factors II, VII, IX, and X (lower VII content). In single-dose bottle w/diluent, needles.	Proplex SX

INDICATIONS

For Factor IX deficiency (hemophilia B, Christmas disease). IV administration intended to prevent or control bleeding episodes in patients with this deficiency. Not used in those with mild Factor IX deficiency for whom fresh plasma is effective. Proplex is also indicated for bleeding episodes in patients with inhibitors to Factor VIII.

CONTRAINDICATIONS

Cases of liver disease in which there are signs of intravascular coagulation or fibrinolysis.

ACTIONS

Human Factor IX complex consists of stable dried purified plasma fractions. Factor IX complex (plasma thromboplastin component) is involved in the intrinsic pathway of blood coagulation. It contains coagulation Factors II, VII, IX, and X and small amounts of other plasma proteins. These vitamin-K-dependent factors are synthesized in the liver. When the four factors are considered together, Factor X plays a key role in the clotting mechanism. In the intrinsic clotting system, Factor IX is essential for activating factor VIII, which in turn activates factor X. In the extrinsic clotting system, Factor X is activated directly by Factor VII and tissue thromboplastin. Activated Factor X causes conversion of Factor II (prothrombin) to its activated form (thrombin).

Deficiency of Factor IX complex results in a hemorrhagic condition known as hemophilia B or Christmas disease. Congenital deficiencies of each of the four factors occur in the absence of liver disease, and each results in a hemorrhagic condition. Acquired deficiencies of Factor II are common and are almost always associated with deficiencies of Factors VII, IX and X.

Severe congenital deficiency of Factor VII is rare; partial deficiency is more common. Severe deficiency causes a prolonged one-stage prothrombin time.

Factor X resembles factor VII. Both show a similar incidence of congenital deficiency, both are essential to a normal one-stage prothrombin time, and both are low in liver disease and vitamin-K-deficient states. The clotting time of blood that is deficient in Factor X is very prolonged in contrast to the clotting time of blood deficient in Factor VII.

The human Factor IX complex has a biphasic half-life; it takes 4 to 6 hours to equilibrate within the extravascular space and 22.5 hours for biodegradation.

WARNINGS

Hepatitis: Use in liver disease must be considered only in cases in which the expected benefits far outweigh the potential hazard of superimposing viral hepatitis on an already damaged liver. Because of the risks of hepatitis, Factor IX complex should not be used when fresh frozen plasma would be satisfactory.

Thrombosis: Thrombosis is a well-known risk of the postoperative period. Until more data are available, do not use in patients undergoing elective surgery unless expected beneficial effects outweigh increased risk of thrombosis, especially in those predisposed to thrombosis. In emergency cases and when large quantities of factor IX concentrate are needed, a prophylactic anticoagulant regimen may be used.

In any instance in which intravascular coagulation is suspected, stop infusion promptly. The risk of enhancing intravascular coagulation may be reduced by not attempting to raise the patient's Factor IX level to more than about 50% of normal.

PRECAUTIONS

Do not administer at a rate exceeding 10 ml/minute. Rapid administration may result in vasomotor reactions.

ADVERSE REACTIONS

Adverse reactions characterized by either thrombosis or disseminated intravascular coagulation have been reported.

Pyrogenic reactions: Chills, fever (particularly when large doses are used).

Rapid infusion rate: If drug is infused too rapidly, flushing, increased pulse rate, and decreased blood pressure may occur, caused by the presence of vasoactive substances, which varies from lot to lot. In some patients, rapid administration can cause, on rare occasions, transient fever, chills, headache, flushing, tingling, urticaria, nausea, vomiting, somnolence, or lethargy. Stopping the infusion allows symptoms to disappear promptly. Except for in the most reactive individuals, the infusion may be resumed at a slower rate. A different lot may prove satisfactory.

OVERDOSAGE

Factor X has a long postinfusion half-life. Repeated administrations generally result in successively larger increases in blood levels, particularly of Factors IX and X. Unnecessarily high levels of Factors II, IX and X can occur, which may increase the risk of intravascular coagulation.

DOSAGE

One unit is defined as the activity present in 1 ml of average normal plasma (less than 1 hour old). The actual number of units is shown on each bottle. Potency is adjusted in terms of Factor IX because Factors II, VII, and X are present in approximately the same amount.

Factor-IX-deficient patients (bleeding or nonbleeding): 2 units/kg will produce an average increase of 4% measured 15 minutes after administration.

Factor-VII-deficient patients (bleeding or nonbleeding): 2 units/kg will result in an average increase of 4% measured 15 minutes after administration.

Factor-VII-deficient and factor-IX-deficient patients: When patient is undergoing extensive surgical or dental procedures, levels of these factors are maintained above 20% of normal. An initial large dose makes it easier to maintain hemostatic levels later, using smaller and fewer doses. A critical period is about 5 days postsurgery, and full protection should be provided for about 8 days. Each patient

presents a specific problem, and no specific directions can be given.

Hemarthroses: In using Proplex in treatment of hemarthroses occuring in hemophiliacs with inhibitors to Factor VIII, dosage levels of approximately 75 units/kg may be used.

Prophylaxis: 500 units may be administered every week to prevent spontaneous bleeding episodes. A schedule of 500 units to 1000 units every 2·weeks may lessen the severity of spontaneous bleeding episodes.

NURSING IMPLICATIONS

HISTORY

Review chart for type of coagulation deficiency, physician's history, recent laboratory tests; obtain general health history.

PHYSICAL ASSESSMENT

Obtain vital signs (exercise care in applying and removing blood-pressure cuff, taking temperature); weight. Assess areas of bleeding (if present), noting location, size, and appearance. Appropriate coagulation studies are ordered prior to treatment with Factor IX.

ADMINISTRATION

Warm to room temperature before reconstituting.

Diluent is supplied with product. Needles for adding diluent and administration are supplied with Proplex and Proplex SX.

Actual number of units is shown on each bottle.

Administer within 3 hours of reconstitution.

Follow directions on package for IV administration. IV piggyback may be used to administer drug.

Record drug lot number on patient's chart.

CLINICAL ALERT: Do not administer at a rate exceeding 10 ml/minute. Rapid administration may result in vasomotor reactions.

Storage: Store under refrigeration between 2°C and 8°C (between 35°F and 46°F) until reconstituted. *Do not freeze.*

ONGOING ASSESSMENTS AND NURSING MANAGEMENT

Monitor infusion continuously.

Flushing, increased pulse rate, and decreased blood pressure are signs of too-rapid infusion. If these occur, stop the infusion, allow primary IV line to infuse at KVO, monitor patient closely, and notify the physician. Usually, stopping the infusion allows symptoms to disappear promptly. Physician may then order infusion resumed at a slower rate. In highly reactive individuals, a different lot number may be used to relieve symptoms.

Pyrogenic reactions may occur. Observe for chills, headache, flushing, tingling, and transient fever. If these occur, notify physician promptly.

In any instance in which intravascular coagulation is suspected, the physician may constantly monitor the infusion to detect any related signs and symptoms. Changes in blood pressure and pulse, respiratory distress, chest pain, or cough requires stopping the infusion immediately.

Physician will order coagulation assays during treatment.

Inform laboratory personnel of the importance of applying prolonged pressure at site following venipuncture. A pressure dressing may be required if oozing persists.

Other treatment, such as application of ice packs to areas of bleeding, may be ordered.

Continue to monitor patient for signs of bleeding in GI tract, CNS, skin, oral cavity, surgical incision, and so on.

Fenfluramine Hydrochloride

See Anorexiants.

Fenoprofen Calcium

See Nonsteroidal Anti-inflammatory Agents.

Fentanyl

See Narcotic Analgesics.

Fentanyl Citrate and Droperidol

See Anesthetics, General, Nonbarbiturate.

Ferrous Fumarate

See Iron Products.

Ferrous Gluconate

See Iron Products.

Ferrous Sulfate

See Iron Products.

Ferrous Sulfate Exsiccated

See Iron Products.

Fibrinolysin and Desoxyribonuclease Rx

dry powder: 25 units fibrinolysin, 15,000 units desoxyribonuclease	Elase
ointment: 1 unit fibrinolysin, 666.6 units desoxyribonuclease/g	Elase
ointment: 10 mg chloramphenicol, 1 unit fibrinolysin, 666.6 units desoxyribonuclease/g	Elase-Chloromycetin

INDICATIONS

Topical: As a debriding agent in a variety of inflammatory and infected lesions, including general surgical wounds; ulcerative lesions (trophic, decubitus, stasis, arteriosclerotic); second- and third-degree burns; circumcision; episiotomy. In infected lesions for which a topical antibiotic is desired, a product containing the enzymes plus chloramphenicol is indicated. Except in very superficial infections, systemic antibiotics are also indicated.

Intravaginal: Cervicitis (benign, postpartum, postconization) and vaginitis.

Irrigating agent: In infected wounds (abscesses, fistulae, sinus tracts); otorhinolaryngologic wounds; superficial hematomas (except when hematoma is adjacent to or within adipose tissue).

CONTRAINDICATIONS

History of hypersensitivity to any component. Not recommended for parenteral use because bovine fibrinolysin may be antigenic.

ACTIONS

Purulent exudates consist largely of fibrinous material and nucleoprotein. Desoxyribonuclease attacks the desoxyribonucleic acid (DNA) and fibrinolysin principally attacks fibrin of blood clots and fibrous exudates.

PRECAUTIONS

Observe usual precautions against allergic reactions, particularly in those with a history of sensitivity to materials of bovine origin or mercury compounds. To be maximally effective, solutions must be freshly prepared before use. Loss in activity is reduced by refrigeration; however, solution should not be used 24 hours or more after reconstitution even when stored under refrigeration.

ADVERSE REACTIONS

Side-effects attributable to the enzymes have not been a problem at the recommended dose for the recommended indications. With higher concentrations, side-effects have been minimal, consisting primarily of local hyperemia.

DOSAGE

General topical uses: Local application should be repeated for as long as enzyme action is desired. See *Administration* below for recommended application.

Recommended application of ointment—2 to 3 times a day.

Recommended application of gauze impregnated with solution (wet-to-dry procedure)—3 or 4 times a day.

Intravaginal use: In mild to moderate vaginitis and cervicitis, aply 5 g of ointment deep in the vagina H.S. for approximately five applications. In more severe cases, instill 10 ml of solution intravaginally, wait 1 to 2 minutes for enzyme to disperse, then insert cotton tampon into the vaginal canal. Remove tampon the next day. Continuing therapy should then be initiated with the ointment.

Abscesses, empyema cavities, fistulae, sinus tracts, and subcutaneous hematomas: Drain and replace solution at intervals of 6 to 10 hours to reduce amount of by-product accumulation and minimize loss of enzymatic activity. Traces of blood in discharge usually indicate active filling in of the cavity.

NURSING IMPLICATIONS

HISTORY (from chart or patient)
Duration of symptoms; health history; allergy history; prescription, nonprescription drug history; previous treatment modalities (if any).

PHYSICAL ASSESSMENT
Inspect involved area and describe location, size, appearance, and drainage (if any) of external lesion. Review physician's findings for cervicitis, vaginitis.

ADMINISTRATION

After application, these products become rapidly and progressively less active and insignificant activity remains after 24 hours.

For successful use of enzymatic debridement, (1) dense dry eschar, if present, should be removed surgically before enzymatic debridement is attempted; (2) the enzyme must be in constant contact with the substrate; (3) accumulated necrotic debris must be periodically removed; (4) the enzyme must be replenished at least once daily; and (5) secondary closure or skin grafting must be employed as soon as possible after optimal debridement is attained.

Topical: Application of ointment or solution and wound dressing must be carried out with aseptic technique.

Ointment: Clean wound with water, peroxide, or normal saline (physician orders agent to be used); dry area gently with sterile compress.

Apply a thin layer of ointment; cover with petrolatum or other type of nonadhering dressing (physician orders type of dressing to be used).

Reapplication—Flush away necrotic debris and fibrinous exudates with saline, peroxide, or warm water (physician orders agent to be used) so that newly applied ointment is in direct contact with the substrate.

Solution: The solution form may be applied as a liquid, spray, or wet dressing. Application of a spray can be accomplished by using a conventional atomizer.

Recommended procedure is to mix one vial of powder with 10 ml to 50 ml of saline and saturate strips of fine-mesh gauze or unfolded sterile gauze sponge with solution. Pack the ulcerated area with gauze, making sure the gauze remains in contact with the necrotic substrate. As gauze dries, necrotic tissues slough and become enmeshed in gauze. This mechanically debrides the area.

Reapplication—Gently remove dried gauze.

Intravaginal use: Disposable vaginal applicators are available in separate package with 30 g size used for gynecologic use.

Patient may self-administer drug; provide instructions for administration and fill applicator with ointment.

If patient is unable to self-administer, place in dorsal recumbent position with knees flexed.

See *Dosage.*

Abscesses, empyema cavities, fistulae, sinus tracts, subcutaneous hematomas: Prepared solution is used to irrigate these conditions. Pharmacist usually prepares solution.

Provide equipment for instillation. Solution is

drained and replaced q6h to q8h. Procedure may be performed by physician or nurse.

ONGOING ASSESSMENTS AND NURSING MANAGEMENT
Observe and record appearance of topical lesion each time ointment or solution is applied.

When solution is instilled in cavity, fistula, sinus tract, or abscess, record appearance of drainage when drained and replaced with fresh solution. Traces of blood in discharge usually indicate active filling of the cavity.

Inform physician if lesion does not appear to improve or if a different odor or appearance is noted in drainage.

PATIENT AND FAMILY INFORMATION
NOTE: If prescribed for outpatient application, patient or family member will require explanation of application.

Notify physician if area does not improve or drainage increases.

Flavoxate Hydrochloride Rx

tablets: 100 mg   Urispas

INDICATIONS
Symptomatic relief of dysuria, nocturia, suprapubic pain, urinary frequency, and incontinence as may occur in cystitis, prostatitis, urethritis, or urethrocystitis/urethrotrigonitis. *Not* indicated for definitive treatment, but is compatible with drugs used for treatment of urinary-tract infections.

CONTRAINDICATIONS
Pyloric or duodenal obstruction, obstructive intestinal lesions or ileus, achalasia, GI hemorrhage, obstructive uropathies of the lower urinary tract.

ACTIONS
Counteracts smooth muscle spasm of urinary tract. Exerts its effect directly on the muscle. Also has anticholinergic, local anesthetic, and analgesic properties.

WARNINGS
Give cautiously to those with suspected glaucoma.

Use in pregnancy: Safety is not established. Use only when clearly needed and when potential benefits outweigh the unknown potential hazards to the fetus.

Use in children: Safety and efficacy for use in children under 12 are not established.

ADVERSE REACTIONS
Nausea, vomiting; dry mouth; nervousness; vertigo; headache; drowsiness; blurred vision; increased ocular tension; disturbance in accommodation; urticaria, other dermatoses; mental confusion, especially in elderly; dysuria; tachycardia, palpitation; hyperpyrexia; eosinophilia; leukopenia.

DOSAGE
Adults, children over 12: 100 mg or 200 mg tid or qid.

NURSING IMPLICATIONS

HISTORY
See Appendix 4.

PHYSICAL ASSESSMENT
Urinalysis is usually ordered. GU evaluation may include cystoscopy, prostatic smear, and culture and sensitivity studies.

ONGOING ASSESSMENTS AND NURSING MANAGEMENT
Observe for adverse drug reactions and therapeutic drug effect, (*e.g.,* alleviation of symptoms of dysuria, nocturia, suprapubic pain, frequency, or incontinence).

May cause dry mouth, which may be alleviated by frequent sips of water, hard candy, or chewing gum.

May cause drowsiness, dizziness, or blurred vision. Patient (especially elderly) may require assistance in ambulation.

Inform physician if symptoms persist or become worse.

PATIENT AND FAMILY INFORMATION
May cause drowsiness, dizziness, or blurred vision; observe caution while driving or performing other tasks requiring alertness.

May cause dry mouth; sips of water, hard candy, or chewing gum may relieve problem.

Notify physician if symptoms persist or become worse.

Floxuridine Rx

injection: 500 mg   FUDR
  powder

INDICATIONS
Palliative management of GI adenocarcinoma metastatic to the liver, when given by continuous regional intra-arterial infusion in carefully selected pa-

tients considered incurable by surgery or other means. Patients with known disease extending beyond an area capable of infusion via a single artery should, except in unusual circumstances, be considered for systemic therapy with other agents.

CONTRAINDICATIONS
See Fluorouracil (parenteral).

ACTIONS
When administered by intra-arterial injection, it is apparently rapidly catabolized to 5-fluorouracil. Thus, rapid injection produces the same toxic and antimetabolic effects as fluorouracil (parenteral).

WARNINGS, PRECAUTIONS, DRUG INTERACTIONS, ADVERSE REACTIONS
See Fluorouracil (parenteral).

DOSAGE
For intra-arterial infusion only. Recommended therapeutic dose schedule by continuous arterial infusion is 0.1 mg/kg/day to 0.6 mg/kg/day. Higher dose ranges (0.4 mg to 0.6 mg) are usually employed for hepatic artery infusion because liver metabolizes the drug, reducing the potential for systemic toxicity. Therapy can be given until adverse reactions appear. When side-effects subside, therapy may be resumed. Therapy is maintained as long as response to drug continues.

NURSING IMPLICATIONS

HISTORY
See Appendix 4.

PHYSICAL ASSESSMENT
General physical and emotional status; vital signs; weight. Baseline laboratory studies usually include CBC, differential, platelet count, liver- and renal-function tests. Other tests may also be appropriate.

ADMINISTRATION
An intra-arterial catheter is inserted by the physician and placement verified by x-ray.

Powder is reconstituted with 5 ml sterile water; label vial with date of reconstitution.

Dose is removed from vial and added to IV infusion (usually 5% Dextrose or 0.95% Sodium Chloride).

Physician orders IV fluid, rate of infusion. Additional orders may be written regarding care of intra-arterial catheter, additional IV fluids, antiemetics, and so on.

Administration is best achieved with use of an infusion pump to overcome pressure in large arteries and ensure uniform rate of infusion.

Storage: Reconstituted vials stored under refrigeration for not more than 2 weeks.

ONGOING ASSESSMENTS AND NURSING MANAGEMENT
Patient must be hospitalized for initiation of treatment.

Drug given by intra-arterial infusion daily until toxicity occurs.

Discuss with physician specific toxic effects to be reported immediately because treatment is usually terminated when toxic effects appear. Toxic effects usually requiring discontinuance of therapy include stomatitis or esophagitis; rapidly falling WBC; leukopenia (WBC under 3500); intractable vomiting; diarrhea (frequent bowel movements or watery stools); GI ulceration and bleeding; thrombocytopenia (platelets under 100,000); hemorrhage from any site.

Procedural complications of regional arterial infusion include arterial aneurysm; arterial ischemia, arterial thrombosis; bleeding at catheter site; blocked, displaced, or leaking catheter; embolism; fibromyositis; abscesses; infection at catheter site; thrombophlebitis.

Assess vital signs q4h or as ordered; monitor infusion-pump performance; change dressing around arterial catheter site (if ordered); check catheter site for signs of infection, leakage; check mouth for early evidence of stomatitis (erythema, patient reports of dry mouth, burning, difficulty in swallowing); inspect skin for purpura; look for bleeding in mouth, GI tract (emesis, stools).

If stomatitis develops, begin q4h stomatitis care (Appendix 6, section 6-21).

CBC, platelet count usually obtained daily.

Depending on patient's condition and extent of metastasis, additional assessments and nursing management may be required.

Flucytosine (5-FC, 5-Fluorocytosine) Rx

capsules: 250 mg,   Ancobon
500 mg

INDICATIONS
Treatment of serious infections caused by susceptible strains of _Candida_ or _Cryptococcus._

Candida _species:_ Septicemia, endocarditis, and urinary-tract infections have been effectively treated. Trials in pulmonary infections have been limited.

Cryptococcus *species:* Meningitis and pulmonary infections have been treated effectively. Studies in septicemias and urinary-tract infections are limited, but good responses have been reported.

CONTRAINDICATIONS
Known hypersensitivity.

ACTIONS
Has activity against *Candida* and *Cryptococcus* species. Exact mode of action is unknown. It may enter the fungus cell and is converted by cytosine deaminase to 5-fluorouracil, which acts as a competitive inhibitor of nucleic acid synthesis. Because man lacks cytosine deaminase, host cells are not exposed to 5-fluorouracil.

Is well absorbed after oral administration. Drug concentrations in the cerebrospinal fluid reach 50% to 100% of serum levels. Drug also penetrates the aqueous humor, joints, bronchial secretions, peritoneal fluid, brain, bone, and bile. Minimum therapeutic serum concentrations are 20 mcg/ml to 25 mcg/ml; toxicity occurs at levels above 100 mcg/ml. Flucytosine is not significantly metabolized when given orally; 90% is excreted in the urine unchanged. Serum half-life is 2.5 to 6 hours. Drug is minimally bound to plasma proteins and easily removed by hemodialysis or peritoneal dialysis.

WARNINGS
Give with extreme caution to patients with impaired renal function. Because drug is excreted primarily by the kidneys, renal impairment may lead to accumulation of the drug. Assays for blood levels should be done to determine adequacy of renal excretion in such patients.

Give with extreme caution to those with bone-marrow depression. Patients may be more prone to depression of bone-marrow function if they have hemorrhagic disease, are being treated with radiation or drugs that depress the bone marrow, or have a history of treatment with such drugs or radiation. Frequent monitoring of hepatic function and the hematopoietic system is indicated during therapy.

Use in pregnancy: Safety not established. Use in pregnancy, lactation, and women of childbearing age only when clearly needed and when potential benefits outweigh the unknown potential hazards to the fetus or infant.

PRECAUTIONS
Before therapy is initiated, hematologic and renal status should be determined; close monitoring of patient is essential. Liver enzyme levels (alkaline phosphatase, SGOT, SGPT) should be determined at frequent intervals during therapy.

ADVERSE REACTIONS
Nausea, vomiting, diarrhea, rash, anemia, leukopenia, thrombocytopenia, and elevation of hepatic enzymes, BUN, and creatinine have been reported. Less frequently reported are confusion, hallucinations, headache, sedation, and vertigo.

DOSAGE
Usual dosage is 50 mg/kg/day to 150 mg/kg/day in divided doses q6h. If the BUN or serum creatinine level is elevated, or if there are other signs of renal impairment, initial dose should be at the lower level.

NURSING IMPLICATIONS

HISTORY
See Appendix 4.

PHYSICAL ASSESSMENT
Obtain vital signs, weight, general physical status. Culture and sensitivity studies are obtained prior to therapy. CBC and hepatic- and renal-function tests are recommended prior to therapy.

ADMINISTRATION
Average number of capsules administered to a patient may range from two to five q6h.

Nausea and vomiting may be reduced or avoided if capsules are given a few at a time over a 15-minute period.

If patient is unable to swallow capsules, check with pharmacist about administration of capsule contents in a fluid or on food.

GENERIC NAME SIMILARITY
5-FC (flucytosine) and 5-FU (5-fluorouracil).

ONGOING ASSESSMENTS AND NURSING MANAGEMENT
Record vital signs q2h to q4h; observe for adverse drug reactions; note patient's response to therapy by comparing daily observations to baseline data; monitor intake and output.

Weigh weekly or as ordered. Inform physician of any significant increase or decrease in weight.

If GI upset occurs despite giving drug over a 15-minute period, notify physician before next dose is due.

Notify physician if nausea, vomiting, diarrhea, or skin rash occurs or if urinary output decreases despite adequate intake.

Close monitoring of renal, hepatic, and hematopoietic systems is recommended. Periodic renal- and hepatic-function tests, CBC, and platelet count are usually ordered.

In those with renal impairment, assays for blood levels of flucytosine should be done to determine adequacy of renal excretion.

PATIENT AND FAMILY INFORMATION

May cause GI upset (nausea, vomiting, diarrhea). Notify physician if these effects persist or become intolerable or if skin rash occurs.

Nausea and vomiting may be reduced or avoided by taking capsules a few at a time over a 15-minute period.

Physician will monitor results of drug therapy. Keep all office or clinic appointments.

Fludrocortisone Acetate _Rx_

tablets: 0.1 mg   Florinef Acetate

INDICATIONS

Partial replacement therapy for primary and secondary adrenocortical insufficiency in Addison's disease and for treatment of salt-losing adrenogenital syndrome. Because of its marked effect on sodium retention, use in treatment of conditions other than those indicated is not advised. This compound may cause sodium and water retention, edema, and hypokalemia.

ACTIONS

A potent mineralocorticoid with high glucocorticoid activity used only for Addison's disease and in adrenogenital syndrome. The physiological action of fludrocortisone acetate is similar to those of hydrocortisone (p 515). However, the effects of fludrocortisone acetate, particularly on electrolyte balance, but also on carbohydrate metabolism, are considerably heightened and prolonged. In small oral doses, it produces marked sodium retention and increased urinary potassium excretion. It also causes a rise in blood pressure, apparently because of these effects on electrolyte levels. In larger doses, it inhibits endogenous adrenal cortical secretion, thymic activity, and pituitary corticotropin excretion; promotes the deposition of liver glycogen; and, unless protein intake is adequate, induces negative nitrogen balance.

CONTRAINDICATIONS, WARNINGS, DRUG INTERACTIONS, ADVERSE REACTIONS

See Glucocorticoids.

DOSAGE

Addison's disease: The combination of fludrocortisone acetate with a glucocorticoid such as hydrocortisone or cortisone provides substitution therapy approximating normal adrenal activity with minimal risk of unwanted effects. Usual dose is 0.1 mg/day, although doses ranging from 0.1 mg three times a week to 0.2 mg/day have been employed. If transient hypertension develops as a consequence of therapy, dose should be reduced to 0.05 mg/day. Administration in conjunction with cortisone (10 mg/day to 37.5 mg/day in divided doses) or hydrocortisone (10 mg/day to 30 mg/day) is preferable.

Salt-losing adrenogenital syndrome: 0.1 mg/day to 0.2 mg/day.

NURSING IMPLICATIONS

HISTORY

See Appendix 4.

PHYSICAL ASSESSMENT

Obtain vital signs, weight; note and record overt physical symptoms of disorder. Review recent laboratory and diagnostic tests, physician's physical examination.

ONGOING ASSESSMENTS AND NURSING MANAGEMENT

See Desoxycorticosterone; Glucocorticoids.

Flumethasone Pivalate

See Corticosteroids, Topical.

Flunisolide

See Corticosteroids, Intranasal.

Fluocinolone Acetonide

See Corticosteroids, Topical.

Fluocinonide

See Corticosterooids, Topical.

Fluorescein Sodium

Topical Preparations _Rx_

solution: 2%   _Generic_
strips: 0.6 mg   Ful-Glo
strips: 1 mg   Fluor-I-Strip-A.T.

Parenteral Preparations Rx

injection: 5%	Fluorescite
injection: 10%	Fluorescite, Funduscein-10
injection: 25%	Ak-Fluor, Fluorescite, Funduscein-25

INDICATIONS

Topical: Used in fitting hard contact lenses, performing applanation tonometry, and disclosing corneal injury.

Parenteral: Diagnostic aid in ophthalmic angiography, including examination of the fundus, evaluation of the iris vasculature, distinction between viable and nonviable tissue, observation of aqueous flow, differential diagnosis of malignant and nonmalignant tumors, and determination of circulation time and adequacy.

CONTRAINDICATIONS

Hypersensitivity. Topical form not used with hydrogel (soft) contact lenses.

ACTIONS

Instilled into the eye, it stains abraded or ulcerated areas of the cornea. Such defects appear green under normal light and bright yellow if viewed under cobalt blue illumination. Foreign bodies (if not epithelialized) are surrounded by a green ring. Similar lesions of the conjunctiva are delineated in orange-yellow.

WARNINGS

Exercise caution in those with a history of hypersensitivity, allergies, or asthma. If signs of sensitivity develop, discontinue use. Avoid parenteral use in pregnancy, especially in the first trimester. There have been no reports of fetal complications during pregnancy.

ADVERSE REACTIONS

Injectable form may produce nausea and headache, GI distress, vomiting, hypotension, and other symptoms and signs of hypersensitivity; cardiac arrest, basilar artery ischemia, thrombophlebitis at injection site, severe shock, convulsions, and temporary yellowish skin discoloration. Syncope, bronchospasm, anaphylaxis, pyrexia, transient dyspnea, urticaria, pruritus, angioneurotic edema, and slight dizziness may occur occasionally. A strong taste may develop following high dosage. Urine stains a bright yellow color. Discoloration of skin fades in 6 to 12 hours, urine fluorescence in 24 to 36 hours.

DOSAGE

Topical

Solution: 1 drop of 2% solution, followed by a 60-second interval with the lids closed before irrigation, produces the desired effect. Irrigate. The irrigation of excess stain is easily accomplished, and undesirable discoloration does not occur. Increased penetration of the dye may be produced by additional instillations and delayed irrigations.

Strips: Moisten strip with sterile water or irrigating solution. Touch conjunctiva or fornix as required with moistened tip. Patient should blink several times after application to distribute stain.

Injection

To avoid possible allergic reaction, a small test dose is injected before diagnostic injection. In 9 to 30 seconds, luminescence, which can be observed by standard viewing equipment, appears in the retinal and choroidal vessels. *Adults*—500 mg to 700 mg injected rapidly into the anticubital vein. *Children*—3.5 mg/lb injected into the anticubital vein.

NURSING IMPLICATIONS

HISTORY

Inquire about allergies, asthma, and history of hypersensitivity (see *Warnings*); inform physician immediately if patient has allergy history. In eye injury, obtain information about time of injury, type of injury (*e.g.,* foreign body, abrasion), where injury occurred (*e.g.,* home, place of employment).

PHYSICAL ASSESSMENT

Eye exam is performed by physician. In eye injury, inspect area around eye for signs of trauma.

ADMINISTRATION

Topical: See *Dosage* above.

Obtain materials (drug, irrigating equipment, and solution) per physician's order.

Depending on hospital or emergency department policy, physician or nurse may instill solution or apply moistened strip.

Patient with eye injury experiences severe pain and requires emotional support during diagnosis and treatment of injury.

Pediatric patient usually requires restraining measures during examination and treatment period. Some adult patients may also require restraining measures.

Injection: Epinephrine 1:1000 for IV or IM use, an antihistamine, and oxygen should be immediately available for treatment of a hypersensitivity reaction.

Physician administers test dose before diagnostic injection.

PATIENT AND FAMILY INFORMATION
Injection will cause discoloration of skin; this will fade in 6 to 12 hours. Urine attains a bright yellow color for 24 to 36 hours.

Fluorouracil

(5-Fluorouracil, 5-FU) (Parenteral)   Rx

injection: 500 mg/   Adrucil, *Generic*
    10 ml

INDICATIONS
Palliative management of carcinoma of the colon, breast, stomach, and pancreas in carefully selected patients considered incurable by surgery or other means.

CONTRAINDICATIONS
Patients in a poor nutritional state, those with depressed bone-marrow function, or those with potentially serious infections.

ACTIONS
Mechanism of action is competitive inhibition of thymidylate synthetase. Consequent thymidine deficiency results in inhibition of deoxyribonucleic acid (DNA) synthesis, inducing cell death. The effects of DNA and ribonucleic acid (RNA) deprivation are most marked on those cells that grow rapidly and take up fluorouracil at a more rapid pace. Inactive degradation products result from the extensive catabolic metabolism of fluorouracil. Following IV administration, no intact drug was detected in plasma after 3 hours. Approximately 15% is excreted intact in the urine in 6 hours, over 90% in the first hour; 60% to 80% is excreted as respiratory CO_2 in 8 to 12 hours. See also Antineoplastic Agents.

WARNINGS
Use with extreme caution in poor-risk patients who have history of high-dose pelvic irradiation or previous use of alkalyting agents or who have widespread involvement of bone marrow by metastatic tumors or impaired hepatic or renal function. Drug is not intended as adjuvant to surgery.

Combination therapy: Any form of therapy that adds to the stress of the patient, interferes with nutrition, or depresses bone-marrow function will increase toxicity.

Use in pregnancy: Do not use during pregnancy (particularly first trimester) unless potential benefits outweigh hazards.

PRECAUTIONS
Discontinue promptly if any of the following signs of toxicity appears: stomatitis or esophagopharyngitis (at first visible sign); rapidly falling WBC count; leukopenia (WBC under 3500); intractable vomiting; diarrhea (frequent bowel movements or watery stools); GI ulceration and bleeding; thrombocytopenia (platelets under 100,000); hemorrhage from any site.

These are highly toxic drugs with a narrow margin of safety. Therapeutic response is unlikely to occur without some evidence of toxicity. Inform patients of expected toxic effects, particularly oral manifestations. WBC count with differential is recommended before each dose. Severe hematologic toxicity, GI hemorrhage, and even death may result. Although severe toxicity is more likely in poor-risk patients, fatalities may be encountered in patients in good condition.

DRUG INTERACTIONS
Drug/lab tests: **5-Hydroxyindoleacetic acid (5-HIAA)** urinary excretion may be increased by fluorouracil. **Plasma albumin** may be decreased because of fluorouracil-induced protein malabsorption. Elevations in **alkaline phosphatase, serum transaminase, serum bilirubin,** and **lactic dehydrogenase** may occur.

ADVERSE REACTIONS
Cardiovascular: Myocardial ischemia, angina.

GI: Diarrhea, anorexia, nausea and vomiting, cramps, pain, enteritis, duodenal ulcer, duodenitis, gastritis, gastroenteritis.

Hematologic: Leukopenia, thrombocytopenia. Myelosuppression almost uniformly accompanies a course of adequate therapy. Low WBC counts are usually first observed between the ninth and fourteenth days after the first course of treatment, with nadir occurring in the third week but at times delayed for as long as 25 days. The count is usually within the normal range by the thirtieth day.

Dermatologic: Alopecia; dermatitis, often as a maculopapular rash usually appearing on the extremities and less frequently on the trunk (usually reversible and responsive to symptomatic treatment); erythema; nonspecific skin toxicity and rash; photosensitivity; nail changes including loss of nails; dry skin and fissuring; increased skin pigmentation.

CNS: Lethargy, malaise, weakness, euphoria, acute cerebellar syndrome (which may persist following discontinuation of treatment).

Ocular: Photophobia, lacrimation.

Other: Fever, epistaxis, glossitis, stomatitis, pharyngitis, esophagopharyngitis (which may lead to sloughing and ulceration).

DOSAGE

Administer IV only. All dosages based on patient's actual weight. Estimated lean body weight (dry weight) is used if patient is obese or if there is a spurious weight gain due to edema, ascites, or other abnormal fluid retention.

Initial dosage: 12 mg/kg IV once daily for 4 successive days. Daily dose should not be more than 800 mg. If no toxicity is observed, 6 mg/kg is given on the 6th, 8th, 10th, and 12th days. No therapy given on the 5th, 7th, 9th, or 11th day. Therapy is discontinued at end of the 12th day, even if no toxicity apparent. Poor-risk patients or those not in an adequate nutritional state should receive 6 mg/kg/day for 3 days. If no toxicity is observed, 3 mg/kg on the 5th, 7th, and 9th days is given. No therapy given on the 4th, 6th, or 8th day. Daily dose should not exceed 400 mg.

A sequence of injections on either schedule constitutes a "course of therapy."

Discontinue therapy promptly when any signs of toxicity listed under *Precautions* appear.

Maintenance therapy: In instances in which toxicity has not been a problem, it is recommended that therapy be continued using either of the following schedules: (1) Repeat dosage of first course every 30 days after last day of previous course of treatment; (2) When toxic signs resulting from the initial course have subsided, administer a maintenance dosage of 10 mg/kg/week to 15 mg/kg/week as a single dose. Do not exceed 1 g/week. Reduced dosages used for poor-risk patients.

NURSING IMPLICATIONS

HISTORY

See Appendix 4.

PHYSICAL ASSESSMENT

Physical, emotional status; vital signs; weight. Laboratory studies include CBC, differential, platelet count, renal- and hepatic-function tests.

ADMINISTRATION

Physician may order antiemetic to be administered prior to injection of drug.

No dilution required. Should not be mixed with IV additives or other chemotherapeutic agents.

Avoid contact with skin when preparing for administration.

Drug administered by slow IV push. Care must be taken to avoid extravasation.

If extravasation occurs, discontinue injection immediately and use another vein to administer the remaining dose. Physician may order ice packs applied to area to relieve pain/discomfort.

Storage: Solution may discolor during storage; potency and safety are not adversely affected. Store at room temperature, 59°F to 86°F (15°C to 30°C) and protect from light. If precipitate forms because of exposure to low temperatures, heat to 140°F with vigorous shaking; cool to body temperature before use.

ONGOING ASSESSMENTS AND NURSING MANAGEMENT

Hospitalization is recommended during initial course of therapy because of possible severe toxic reactions. Maintenance therapy may be given on an outpatient basis.

Assess vital signs q4h or as ordered; weight; administer antiemetic as ordered; measure intake and output; observe for toxic reactions (see below) as well as other adverse drug reactions.

Daily CBC and differential and platelet counts are obtained to monitor drug's effect on the bone marrow.

CLINICAL ALERT: Discontinue drug promptly if any signs of toxicity appear. First visible sign is usually stomatitis, which may initially cause a dry mouth or burning sensation. Examine oral cavity daily; inform patient to report dryness or burning sensation in the mouth.

Additional toxic symptoms include a rapidly falling WBC, leukopenia, intractable vomiting, diarrhea, GI ulceration, and bleeding.

Notify physician promptly if signs of toxicity are apparent.

Inspect each bowel movement for evidence of GI bleeding (*e.g.,* bright red blood in stool, black tarry stools). Report these findings immediately.

Physician may order stool tested daily for occult blood.

If nausea occurs, a liquid diet, unsalted crackers, dry toast, or cola syrup may relieve nausea.

If anorexia persists more than 2 days, inform physician. A high-calorie, high-protein diet may be ordered.

If diarrhea develops, notify physician. An antidiarrheal agent may be ordered.

Check patient for signs of dehydration (Appendix 6, section 6-10), especially when vomiting and diarrhea occur and/or patient is taking fluids poorly. Notify physician if dehydration is apparent.

If stomatitis develops, give stomatitis care (Appendix 6, section 6-21) q4h.

Low WBC counts usually seen between 9th and 14th day (after first course of treatment), with nadir occurring in the 3rd week. Reverse (protective) isolation may be necessary if WBC falls below 3500.

If thrombocytopenia occurs, protect patient from injury. Pad siderails, take oral or axillary temperatures, apply prolonged pressure over site of IM or IV injections or venipuncture site.

Acute cerebellar syndrome results in dizziness, ataxia, weakness, vertigo. Patient will require assistance with ambulation, activities of daily living.

Photophobia may be relieved by keeping the room semidark or by wearing sunglasses.

Good skin care is essential, especially if leukopenia and thrombocytopenia occur. If patient is unable to ambulate, change position q2h and inspect pressure points (over bony prominences) for early signs of skin breakdown.

PATIENT AND FAMILY INFORMATION

NOTE: The patient should receive a full explanation of all possible adverse reactions and what specific reactions should be reported immediately to the physician, the probable number of treatments, and the results expected.

Notify physician or nurse immediately if any of the following occurs: burning sensation of the mouth, throat; sores (ulcerations) in the mouth; fever; cough; sore throat; pain or burning on urination; abscess formation; extreme fatigue, weakness; easy bruising; petechiae; bleeding from nose, gums; rectal bleeding; blood in urine; prolonged vomiting, diarrhea (more than 2 days); severe loss of appetite (more than 3 days).

Good oral care is essential. Use a soft toothbrush, rinse mouth thoroughly after taking food or beverages. Avoid use of mouthwashes or other oral products unless use approved by physician.

Do not use any nonprescription drug, including aspirin, without obtaining prior approval of the physician.

Inform other physicians and dentists seen concurrently of therapy with 5-FU.

Physician may prescribe drugs (*e.g.,* antiemetic, Xylocaine Viscous) to be taken before or after each treatment. Take these drugs exactly as directed.

Avoid prolonged exposure to sunlight; photosensitivity may occur.

Physician may advise contraceptive measures during therapy (female patient).

Nail changes (including loss of nails), loss of hair, dry skin and fissuring, and increased skin pigmentation may occur. (*Note:* These changes should be discussed individually, including the methods that may be used to disguise them.)

Fluorouracil (Topical) Rx

solution: 1%	Fluoroplex
solution: 2%, 5%	Efudex
cream: 1%	Fluoroplex
cream: 5%	Efudex

INDICATIONS

Topical treatment of multiple actinic or solar keratoses. The 5% strength is also useful in treating superficial basal cell carcinoma when conventional methods are impractical, as with multiple lesions or difficult treatment sites. Diagnosis should be established before treatment because this new method has not been proven effective in other types of basal cell carcinomas. With isolated, easily accessible lesions, conventional techniques are preferred.

CONTRAINDICATIONS

Known hypersensitivity.

ACTIONS

There is evidence that the metabolism of fluorouracil in the anabolic pathway blocks the methylation reaction of deoxyuridylic acid to thymidylic acid. In this way it interferes with the synthesis of DNA and, to a lesser extent, inhibits formation of RNA. Because DNA and RNA are essential for cell division and growth, the effect of fluorouracil may create a thymine deficiency, which provokes unbalanced growth and cell death. The effects of DNA and RNA deprivation are most marked on those cells that grow rapidly and take up fluorouracil at a rapid pace. The catabolic metabolism of fluorouracil results in degradative products that are inactive.

WARNINGS

If an occlusive dressing is used, there may be an increase in the incidence of inflammation reactions in adjacent normal skin. A porous gauze dressing may be applied for cosmetic reasons without increase in reaction. Safety for use in pregnancy has not been established.

PRECAUTIONS

Follow-up biopsies are recommended in management of superficial basal cell carcinoma.

ADVERSE REACTIONS

Most frequent local reactions are pain, pruritus, hyperpigmentation, and burning at site of application. Other local reactions include dermatitis, scarring,

F

soreness, tenderness, suppuration, scaling, and swelling. Also reported are insomnia, stomatitis, irritability, medicinal taste, photosensitivity, lacrimation, and telangiectasia (causal relationship is remote).

Laboratory abnormalities: Leukocytosis, thrombocytopenia, toxic granulation, and eosinophilia.

DOSAGE
Actinic or solar keratoses: Apply twice daily in sufficient amount to cover lesions. Continue until inflammatory response reaches erosion and ulceration stage; then discontinue use. Usual duration of therapy is 2 to 6 weeks. Complete healing may not be evident for 1 to 2 months following cessation of application.

Superficial basal cell carcinoma: Only 5% strength is recommended. Apply twice daily in sufficient amount to cover lesions. Continue treatment for at least 3 to 6 weeks. Therapy may be required for as long as 10 to 12 weeks before lesions are obliterated.

NURSING IMPLICATIONS

HISTORY
See Appendix 4. Note duration of lesions.

PHYSICAL ASSESSMENT
Describe and record appearance and location of lesions. Review patient's chart for biopsy report, physician's examination.

ADMINISTRATION
If order is not written, clarify with physician whether skin preparation before application of drug is necessary.

Wear plastic disposable gloves to apply solution or cream.

Advise patient at time of first treatment that there may be burning at the site of application.

Apply in sufficient amount to cover lesions; avoid application to surrounding skin.

Solution (2%) supplied with dropper for application; rinse dropper after use.

Exercise care in applying near eyes, nose, or mouth. Use a gauze pad to remove cream or soak up solution that may have touched skin around lesion.

If physician orders an occlusive dressing, a porous gauze dressing is recommended. Other types of dressing may increase the incidence of inflammatory reactions in the adjacent normal skin.

ONGOING ASSESSMENTS AND NURSING MANAGEMENT
Inspect lesion and surrounding skin at time of application; record appearance.

Drug response occurs as follows: erythema, followed by vesiculation, erosion, ulceration, necrosis, and epithelization.

Observe for adverse drug reactions, both localized and systemic.

Notify physician if patient complains of severe pain at lesion site or if stomatitis develops.

Physician may order periodic CBC and platelet count during time of therapy.

Medicinal taste may be alleviated by hard candy, chewing gum, or frequent warm-water mouth rinses. Avoid use of mouthwash.

PATIENT AND FAMILY INFORMATION
NOTE: If treatment is initiated on an outpatient basis, patient should receive thorough instructions and a demonstration of application.

Pretreat the lesion as directed by the physician.

Apply exactly as directed by physician.

If applied with fingers, wash hands immediately afterward. Plastic disposable gloves or fingercots may be purchased at a pharmacy and used to protect hands or finger.

Apply with care near the eyes, nose, and mouth. If medication is difficult to self-apply, have a family member assist.

Do not cover lesions with a dressing unless instructed to do so by physician. Use only the type of dressing recommended by the physician. Avoid use of Band-Aids.

Contact physician if pain at site of application is severe, if sores or ulcerations in the mouth develop, or if easy bruising is noted.

Avoid prolonged exposure to sunlight and ultraviolet rays while under treatment; intensity of reaction may be increased.

Treated area may be unsightly during therapy and, occasionally, for several weeks following therapy.

Physician will inspect treated area at periodic intervals during therapy as well as after therapy is discontinued.

Fluoxymesterone

See Androgens.

Fluphenazine Decanoate

See Antipsychotic Agents.

Fluphenazine Enanthate

See Antipsychotic Agents.

Fluphenazine Hydrochloride

See Antipsychotic Agents.

Flurandrenolide

See Corticosteroids, Topical.

Flurazepam Hydrochloride Rx C-IV

capsules: 15 mg,   Dalmane
    30 mg

INDICATIONS

Insomnia characterized by difficulty in falling asleep, frequent nocturnal awakenings, or early-morning awakening. Can be used for recurring insomnia or poor sleeping habits and in acute or chronic medical situations requiring restful sleep. Insomnia is often transient or intermittent; prolonged administration not recommended.

CONTRAINDICATIONS

Hypersensitivity, pregnancy. Benzodiazepines may cause fetal damage when administered during pregnancy. An increased risk of congenital malformations associated with use during first trimester has been suggested.

ACTIONS

A benzodiazepine derivative, useful as a hypnotic. It decreases sleep latency and awake time and increases total sleep time. Compared to other hypnotics it does not significantly suppress REM sleep, and REM rebound does not occur with chronic administration. Effectiveness is maintained up to 4 weeks of continuous therapy. Does not induce hepatic microsomal enzymes, and may be safely administered to patients receiving oral anticoagulants. The exact site and mode of action are unknown.

Is rapidly absorbed from the GI tract and rapidly metabolized by the liver. Following a single oral dose, peak plasma concentrations ranging from 0.5 ng/ml to 4 ng/ml occur in 30 to 60 minutes. Onset of sleep ranges from 15 to 45 minutes. Maximum effectiveness may not be achieved for two to three nights because of slow accumulation of the active metabolite; residual effects may persist after discontinuation.

WARNINGS

Dependence: Physical and psychological dependence not reported in those taking recommended doses. Withdrawal symptoms have been reported following abrupt discontinuance of benzodiazepines taken continuously, generally at higher therapeutic levels, for at least several months. These have not been specifically reported for flurazepam. However, if it is determined that a patient has been taking flurazepam for a prolonged period, particularly at excessive doses, abrupt discontinuation is avoided and dosage gradually tapered. Caution is exercised in administering to any individual known to be addiction prone or those whose history suggests that they may increase dosage on their own initiative.

Use in renal/hepatic impairment and pulmonary insufficiency: Observe usual precautions.

Use in elderly, debilitated patients: Limit dosage to 15 mg to preclude oversedation, dizziness, confusion, and ataxia.

Use in children: Not recommended for children under 15 years.

PRECAUTIONS

Caution observed in administration to those severely depressed or with latent depression or suicidal tendencies. Patients with unrelieved pain should not be heavily sedated.

DRUG INTERACTIONS

Additive effects will occur when used concomitantly with **alcohol, CNS depressants,** or other agents with CNS depressant or hypnotic effects (*e.g.,* antianxiety agents, antihistamines). An additive effect may occur if alcoholic beverages are consumed during the day following use of flurazepam for nighttime sedation. The potential for this reaction continues for several days following discontinuance of flurazepam, until serum levels of psychoactive metabolites have declined. Patients receiving **cimetidine** concurrently may require lower dose of flurazepam, because excessive sedation may occur.

ADVERSE REACTIONS

CNS: Dizziness; drowsiness; lightheadedness; staggering; ataxia; falling, particularly in elderly or debilitated patients; severe sedation; headache; nervousness; talkativeness; apprehension; irritability; lethargy; disorientation; coma, probably indicative of drug intolerance or overdosage.

GI: Heartburn, upset stomach, nausea, vomiting, diarrhea, constipation, GI pain.

Miscellaneous: Weakness, palpitations, chest pains, body and joint pain, GU complaints.

Rare: Leukopenia, granulocytopenia, sweating, flushes, difficulty in focusing, blurred vision, burning eyes, faintness, hypotension, shortness of breath, sleep apnea syndrome, pruritus, skin rash, dry mouth, bitter taste, excessive salivation, cholestatic jaundice, anorexia, euphoria, depression, slurred speech, confusion, restlessness, hallucinations, paradoxical reactions (excitement, stimulation, hyperactivity).

Clinical laboratory test findings: Elevated SGOT, SGPT, total and direct bilirubin, and alkaline phosphatase.

OVERDOSAGE

Symptoms: Somnolence, confusion, coma.

Treatment: Monitor respiration, pulse, blood pressure. Employ general supportive measures along with immediate gastric lavage. Administer IV fluids and maintain an adequate airway. Hypotension and CNS depression may be combated by judicious use of appropriate therapeutic agents. Value of dialysis not determined. If excitation occurs, barbiturates should not be used.

DOSAGE

Dosage individualized for maximal beneficial effects.

Adults: 15 mg to 30 mg H.S. In elderly and/or debilitated patients, therapy is initiated with 15 mg until individual responses are determined.

NURSING IMPLICATIONS

HISTORY
See Appendix 4.

PHYSICAL ASSESSMENT
Determine if specific factors that may be controlled or eliminated are interfering with sleep. Factors may include noise, bright lights, pain, and discomfort.

ADMINISTRATION
Patient's immediate area should be free from disturbance (*e.g.,* noise, lights) before a hypnotic is given.

Do not administer drug if patient has pain, which should be controlled by administration of an analgesic.

Do not administer a hypnotic shortly before or after administration of a narcotic analgesic (both are CNS depressants; see *Drug Interactions*) *or any other CNS depressant.* If patient has an order for a narcotic analgesic (or other CNS depressant) and a hypnotic, check with physician regarding time interval between administration of these agents. Usually 2 or more hours should elapse between administration of a hypnotic and a CNS depressant, but interval may vary with a specific CNS depressant and the dose administered.

Raise siderails and advise patient to remain in bed and call for assistance if it is necessary to get out of bed during nighttime hours.

ONGOING ASSESSMENTS AND NURSING MANAGEMENT
Observe patient in 60 to 90 minutes to evaluate effect of drug.

Closely observe elderly and/or debilitated patient for oversedation, dizziness, confusion.

If oversedation, confusion, or paradoxical reactions (excitement, stimulation, hyperactivity) occur, observe patient at frequent intervals until effect of drug has worn off. In some instances, restraining measures may be necessary. Inform physician of drug response as dosage may need to be reduced or a different hypnotic selected.

PATIENT AND FAMILY INFORMATION
Avoid alcohol while taking this drug as well as for several days after drug is discontinued. Discuss with physician when alcohol may be safely taken.

Avoid taking CNS depressants.

Do not exceed prescribed dosage.

Inform other physicians and dentist of use of this drug.

Do not attempt to drive or perform other tasks requiring alertness after taking this drug. It is advisable to remain in bed once drug has been taken for sleep. In addition, there may be impairment of the performance of activities such as driving or other tasks requiring alertness on the day following use of this drug.

If dizziness, staggering, oversedation (on the following day), or falling occurs, contact physician.

If drug is prescribed for several months, do not abruptly discontinue its use.

Folic Acid

(Folacin, Pteroylglutamic Acid, Folate) Rx, otc

tablets: 0.1 mg, 0.4 mg, 0.8 mg	*Generic*
tablets: 1 mg	Folvite, *Generic*
injection: 5 mg/ml	Folvite
injection: 10 mg/ml	*Generic*

INDICATIONS
Treatment of megaloblastic anemias due to deficiency of folic acid as seen in sprue and anemias of nutritional origin, pregnancy, infancy, or childhood.

Although most folic acid products carry the *Rx*

legend, products that provide 0.4 mg or less (0.8 mg for pregnant or lactating women) may be *otc* items.

CONTRAINDICATIONS

Not effective in treatment of pernicious, aplastic, or normocytic anemias.

ACTIONS

Exogenous folate is required for nucleoprotein synthesis and maintenance of normal erythropoiesis. Folic acid stimulates production of red and white blood cells and platelets in certain megaloblastic anemias.

Dietary folic acid is present in foods primarily as reduced folate polyglutamate. It must undergo hydrolysis, reduction, and methylation in the GI tract before it is absorbed. Conversion to tetrahydrofolate, the metabolically active form, may be vitamin-B_{12} dependent; supplies are maintained by food and enterohepatic recirculation of the vitamin. Oral synthetic folic acid is completely absorbed following administration, even in the presence of malabsorption syndrome.

DRUG INTERACTIONS

An increase in seizure frequency and a decrease in serum **phenytoin** concentration to subtherapeutic levels have been reported in patients receiving folic acid (particularly 15 mg/day to 20 mg/day) with phenytoin. Conversely, **phenytoin** and **primidone** are reported to cause a decrease in serum folate levels and may produce symptoms of folic acid deficiency on long-term therapy. **P-aminosalicylic acid** and **sulfasalazine** may cause a similar deficiency.

Oral contraceptives may impair folate metabolism and produce folate depletion, but the effect is mild and unlikely to cause anemia or megaloblastic changes.

Folic acid may interfere with the antimicrobial actions of **pyrimethamine** against toxoplasmosis.

Administration of **folic acid antagonists, pyrimethamine, trimethoprim,** or **triamterene** may interfere with folic acid utilization.

ADVERSE REACTIONS

Allergic sensitization has been reported.

DOSAGE

Given orally except in severe intestinal malabsorption. Given IM, IV, or subcutaneously if disease is very severe or GI absorption is impaired.

Usual therapeutic dosage: Up to 1 mg/day. Resistant cases may require large doses.

Maintenance dosage level
When clinical symptoms have subsided and

blood picture is normal, the following dosage may be used:

Infants: 0.1 mg/day.
Children under 4: Up to 0.3 mg/day.
Adults, children over 4: 0.4 mg/day.
Pregnant and lactating women: 0.8 mg/day.

NURSING IMPLICATIONS

HISTORY

See Appendix 4. Note dietary history, including usual foods eaten (dietary pattern), foods avoided or disliked, and average daily food intake.

PHYSICAL ASSESSMENT

Obtain vital signs, weight. Perform general assessment based on symptoms. Symptoms may include fatigue, shortness of breath, glossitis, headache, fainting, slight jaundice, and pallor. Laboratory studies include serum folate, Schilling test, and CBC. Other tests may also be appropriate.

ADMINISTRATION

Usually given orally. May also be given IM, subcutaneously, or IV.

ONGOING ASSESSMENTS AND NURSING MANAGEMENT

Monitor vital signs daily or as ordered.
Weigh weekly or as ordered.
Physician may order diet high in folic acid content.

PATIENT AND FAMILY INFORMATION

Take as directed. Folic acid should be taken only under medical supervision.

Avoid use of multivitamin preparations unless use is approved by physician.

Adhere to prescribed dietary intake recommended by physician.

Furazolidone Rx

tablets: 100 mg	Furoxone
liquid: 50 mg/15 ml	Furoxone

INDICATIONS

Specific and symptomatic treatment of bacterial or protozoal diarrhea and enteritis caused by susceptible organisms.

CONTRAINDICATIONS

Infants under 1 month; prior sensitivity. See *Drug Interactions* for other contraindications.

F

ACTIONS

Has a broad antibacterial spectrum covering the majority of GI pathogens including *Escherichia coli,* staphylococci, *Salmonella, Shigella,* and *Proteus* species, *Enterobacter aerogenes, Vibrio cholerae,* and *Giardia lamblia.* Bactericidal activity is via interference with several bacterial enzyme systems; this antimicrobial action minimizes development of resistant organisms. It neither significantly alters normal bowel flora nor results in fungal overgrowth.

WARNINGS

Safety for use in pregnancy and lactation not established.

PRECAUTIONS

Orthostatic hypotension and hypoglycemia may occur. Hemolysis may occur in those deficient in glucose-6-phosphate dehydrogenase (G6PD).

DRUG INTERACTIONS

Ingestion of **alcohol** should be avoided during and after therapy (see *Adverse Reactions*). Furazolidone inhibits the enzyme monoamine oxidase; use with caution if given concurrently with monoamine oxidase inhibitors (**MAOIs**).

Concomitant administration with indirect-acting **sympathomimetic amines** (*e.g.,* ephedrine, phenylpropanolamine, phenylephrine), **tyramine-containing foods** (see Antidepressants), and **levodopa** may result in hypertension, flushing, tachycardia, headache, and hyperpyrexia. Effects of these interactions may occur for several weeks after furazolidone is discontinued.

The antihypertensive effect of **guanethidine** may be reduced. Therapeutic and toxic effects of furazolidone and **tricyclic antidepressants** may be increased if given together. Nausea, dizziness, excitability, cardiovascular instability, and seizures may develop. Concurrent administration of **meperidine** and **furazolidone** may result in serious and unpredictable effects. Hypotension, hypertension, restlessness, agitation, seizures, and coma may develop rapidly.

Use **sedatives, antihistamines, tranquilizers,** and **narcotics** in reduced dosages and with caution. Orthostatic hypotension and hypoglycemia may occur.

The hypoglycemic effects of **insulin** and **sulfonylureas** may be increased by furazolidone.

ADVERSE REACTIONS

Allergic: A few hypersensitivity reactions have been reported, including falling blood pressure, urticaria, fever, arthralgia, and vesicular morbilliform rash. These reactions subside following withdrawal of the drug.

GI: Nausea, emesis, headache, or malaise occurs

occasionally and may be minimized by dosage reduction or withdrawal of the drug.

Disulfiramlike reaction: Rarely, patients have exhibited a disulfiramlike reaction to alcohol characterized by flushing, slight temperature elevation, dyspnea, and in some instances a sense of constriction in the chest. All symptoms disappeared within 24 hours with no lasting ill effects.

Hematologic: May cause mild reversible intravascular hemolysis in patients with G6PD deficiency. Observe such patients closely. Not administered to infants under 1 month because of possibility of producing hemolytic anemia due to immature enzyme systems in the early neonatal period.

DOSAGE

Adults: Usual dose is 100 mg qid.

Children: 5 years and older, 25 mg to 50 mg qid; 1 to 4 years, 17 mg to 25 mg qid; 1 month to 1 year, 8 mg to 17 mg qid.

Dosage based on average dose of 5 mg/kg/day given in four equally divided doses. Do not exceed maximal dose of 8.8 mg/kg/day because of possibility of producing nausea and emesis. If these are severe, reduce dosage.

If satisfactory response not obtained within 7 days, the pathogen is refractory to furazolidone and drug should be discontinued.

NURSING IMPLICATIONS

HISTORY

See Appendix 4. Note alcohol intake (see *Drug Interactions*).

PHYSICAL ASSESSMENT

Vital signs; weight; look for evidence of dehydration (Appendix 6, section 6-10); note type of stool passed (watery, semisolid, small or copious amount, color). Laboratory tests may include stool culture, CBC, serum electrolytes. Certain infections (*e.g., Salmonella, Shigella, Giardia lamblia*) may need to be reported to the local health department and may require an extensive history to identify possible or probable source of infection.

ADMINISTRATION

Children 5 or older may receive the drug in tablet or liquid form; children under 5 are given the liquid.

A minim glass may be necessary to measure smaller doses (8 mg is 2.4 ml or 36 minims).

ONGOING ASSESSMENTS AND NURSING MANAGEMENT

Record vital signs q4h or as ordered; record number of stools passed, approximate amount, color, type of each stool; look for evidence of dehydration (Appendix 6, section 6-10), signs of electrolyte imbalance (Appendix 6, sections 6-13 to 6-18); measure intake and output; observe for adverse reactions.

Infants, small children, and elderly and/or debilitated patients should be observed closely for signs of dehydration and electrolyte imbalance; notify physician immediately if these should occur.

If nausea and/or vomiting occurs, notify physician before next dose is due. Drug dosage may need to be reduced. If GI upset continues, the drug may be discontinued.

Fluid and electrolyte replacement may be necessary. Oral fluids should be encouraged to maintain hydration.

Orthostatic hypotension may occur. If patient is allowed out of bed, assist with all ambulatory activities.

The pharmacologic effects of insulin may be increased and hypoglycemia may occur. Diabetic patient may require a lower dose of insulin during concomitant administration of furazolidone. Test urine qid and observe patient for signs of hypoglycemia (Appendix 6, section 6-14).

PATIENT AND FAMILY INFORMATION

Avoid ingestion of alcohol during and within 4 days after therapy with this drug.

Medication may discolor urine brown; this is not abnormal.

Do not use nonprescription drugs, especially nasal decongestants, cold and hay fever remedies, and weight-reducing drugs, without prior approval of physician.

Inform other physicians and dentists of therapy with this drug.

May cause nausea, vomiting or headache. Notify physician or nurse if these symptoms become severe.

Record number of stools passed, color, and type (_e.g.,_ watery, semi-formed). Notify physician if diarrhea becomes worse or persists beyond 1 week.

If therapy extends beyond 5 days, avoid tyramine-containing foods. (_Note:_ supply list of foods for patient or family.)

Furosemide

See Loop Diuretics.

F

G

Dexamethasone Sodium
  Phosphate With Lido-
  caine Hydrochloride
Hydrocortisone
Hydrocortisone Acetate
Hydrocortisone Cypionate
Hydrocortisone Sodium
  Phosphate
Hydrocortisone Sodium
  Succinate
Methylprednisolone
Methylprednisolone Ace-
  tate
Methylprednisolone So-
  dium Succinate
Paramethasone Acetate
Prednisolone
Prednisolone Acetate
Prednisolone Acetate and
  Prednisolone Sodium
  Phosphate
Prednisolone Sodium
  Phosphate
Prednisolone Tebutate
Prednisone
Triamcinolone

Triamcinolone Acetonide
Triamcinolone Diacetate
Triamcinolone Hexaceto-
  nide
Glucose
Glutamic Acid Hydrochloride
  Combination Products
Glutethimide
Glyburide
Glycerin
Glycopyrrolate
Gold Compounds
  Aurothioglucose
  Gold Sodium Thiomalate
Griseofulvin
  Microsize
  Ultramicrosize
Guaifenesin
Guanabenz Acetate
Guanadrel Sulfate
Guanethidine Sulfate

Gallamine Triethiodide Rx

injection: 20 mg/ml   Flaxedil

INDICATIONS
A muscle relaxant used as an adjunct to anesthesia to induce skeletal muscle relaxation. May also be employed to facilitate management of patients undergoing mechanical ventilation.

CONTRAINDICATIONS
Absolutely contraindicated in patients with myasthenia gravis. Also contraindicated in those with previously demonstrated hypersensitivity to drug, those sensitive to iodine, and those in whom acceleration of the cardiac rate may be hazardous. Drug is eliminated by the kidneys and is not used in cases of impaired renal function or shock.

ACTIONS
Produces a nondepolarizing blockade of neuromuscular transmission in skeletal muscles and competes with acetylcholine at cholinergic receptors of the motor endplate. It prevents acetylcholine-induced changes in permeability and electric potential and therefore neuromuscular transmission is inhibited.

Drug does not cause bronchospasm and possesses no histaminelike action. It exhibits no known action on autonomic ganglia, nor does it alter tone and motility of the GI tract. It exhibits no known effect on pain threshold, consciousness, or cerebration.

WARNINGS
Administer in carefully adjusted dosage. Facilities for intubation, artificial respiration, oxygen therapy, and antidotes (neostigmine and edrophonium), should be immediately available.

Elimination half-life is prolonged and plasma clearance is decreased in those with renal failure.

PRECAUTIONS
A slight rise in blood pressure may be encountered but is not clinically significant. Tachycardia occurs regularly after doses of 0.5 mg/kg and reaches a maximum within 3 minutes; from this, it gradually declines towards control level. Use with caution in those with impaired pulmonary function. Sensitivity reactions are rare; administer with care to avoid allergic or other untoward reactions. Drug action may be altered by changes in body temperature, dehydration, electrolyte imbalance, or presence of bronchiogenic carcinoma.

DRUG INTERACTIONS
Gallamine may be potentiated by several anesthetic agents, particularly **ether, methoxyflurane,** and **fluoroxene.** Action may be potentiated by use of certain antibiotics (**aminoglycosides, polymyxins**).

ADVERSE REACTIONS
Consist primarily of an extension of drug's pharmacologic actions. Profound and prolonged muscle relaxation may occur, resulting in profound respiratory depression or apnea. Hypersensitivity to drug may exist. Severe anaphylactoid reactions have been reported and are more likely to appear in those with history of allergy, asthma, atopy, or previous drug reactions.

MANAGEMENT OF PROLONGED NEUROMUSCULAR BLOCKADE
Same antagonists as for curare preparations are used.

DOSAGE
Initial dose is about 1 mg/kg but may vary. Repeat doses are usually 0.5 mg/kg to 1 mg/kg.

NURSING IMPLICATIONS

HISTORY
Alert anesthesiologist to current drug therapy and history of allergies, especially to iodine, iodides, and seafoods. Notification may be made by attaching note on cover of chart prior to transporting patient to surgery.

ADMINISTRATION
Drug is administered by anesthesia department.

ONGOING ASSESSMENTS AND NURSING MANAGEMENT

CLINICAL ALERT: Patient must not be left unattended until responding fully from anesthesia. This includes a partially awake patient with adequate respiratory exchange, movement in the extremities, return of swallowing and gag reflexes, and adequate circulation (arterial blood pressure returns to preanesthetic level).

Postanesthesia: Monitor blood pressure, pulse, and respirations q15m (or as ordered) until full recovery from anesthesia.

Maintain patent airway until patient is able to swallow or speak or until gag reflex returns.

Complete recovery from muscle relaxant effect may require several hours. Check for movement in the extremities, chest muscles (on inspiration and expiration), jaw and neck muscles, swallowing and gag reflexes.

G

Notify anesthesia department immediately if any of the following occurs: prolonged muscle relaxation; choking, noisy respirations; cyanosis; or prolonged apnea.

Additional nursing management is based on individual factors, such as type of surgery, condition of patient, complications during surgery (*e.g.,* prolonged procedure, hemorrhage, episodes of hypotension, development of a cardiac arrhythmia), additional medical problems present before surgery (*e.g.,* diabetes mellitus, chronic obstructive pulmonary disease), and patient's age.

Gastrointestinal Anticholinergics/ Antispasmodics

Anisotropine Methylbromide *Rx*

tablets: 50 mg	Valpin 50, *Generic*

Atropine Sulfate *Rx*

injection: 0.05 mg/ ml, 0.1 mg/ml, 0.3 mg/ml, 0.4 mg/ml, 0.5 mg/ml, 0.6 mg/ml, 1 mg/ml, 1.2 mg/ml	*Generic*
tablets: 0.4 mg	*Generic*
tablets, soluble: 0.3 mg, 0.4 mg, 0.6 mg	*Generic*

Belladonna* *Rx*

tablets: 15 mg	*Generic* (Belladonna Extract)
liquid: 30 mg alkaloids/100 ml	*Generic* (Belladonna Tincture)

Clidinium Bromide *Rx*

capsules: 2.5 mg, 5 mg	Quarzan

Dicyclomine Hydrochloride *Rx*

capsules: 10 mg	Bentyl, Di-Spaz, *Generic*
capsules: 20 mg	*Generic*

* Belladonna is a crude botanical preparation containing anticholinergic alkaloids. The active principles include hyoscyamine, hyoscine (scopolamine), and several minor alkaloids. Belladonna extract contains 1.25 g alkaloids/100 g; belladonna tincture contains 30 mg alkaloids/100 ml.

tablets: 20 mg	Bentyl, Dibent, *Generic*
syrup: 10 mg/5 ml	Bentyl, *Generic*
injection: 10 mg/ml	Antispas, Bentyl, Dibent, Dicen, Dilomine, Di-Spaz, Neoquess, Nospaz, Or-Tyl, Spasmoject, *Generic*

Glycopyrrolate *Rx*

tablet: 1 mg	Robinul, *Generic*
tablets: 2 mg	Robinul Forte, *Generic*
injection: 0.2 mg/ml	Robinul

Hexocyclium Methylsulfate *Rx*

tablets: 25 mg	Tral Filmtabs (contains tartrazine)
tablets, timed release: 50 mg	Tral Gradumets (contains tartrazine)

L-Hyoscyamine Sulfate *Rx*

elixir: 0.125 mg/5 ml	Levsin
solution: 0.125 mg/ml	Levsin Drops
injection: 0.5 mg/ml	Levsin
tablets: 0.125 mg	Anaspaz, Levsin
tablets: 0.15 mg	Cystospaz
capsules, timed release: 0.375 mg	Cystospaz-M, Levsinex Timecaps

Isopropamide Iodide *Rx*

tablets: 5 mg	Darbid

Levorotatory Alkaloids of Belladonna *Rx*

tablets: 0.25 mg	Bellafoline
injection: 0.5 mg/ml	Bellafoline

Mepenzolate Bromide *Rx*

tablets: 25 mg	Cantil

Methantheline Bromide *Rx*

tablets: 50 mg	Banthine

Methscopolamine Bromide *Rx*

tablets: 2.5 mg	Pamine

Oxyphencyclimine Hydrochloride *Rx*

tablets: 10 mg	Daricon

Oxyphenonium Bromide *Rx*

tablets: 5 mg	Antrenyl Bromide

Propantheline Bromide Rx

tablets: 7.5 mg	Pro-Banthine
tablets: 15 mg	Norpanth, Pro-Banthine, SK-Propantheline Bromide, *Generic*

Scopolamine Hydrobromide

(Hyoscine Hydrobromide) Rx

injection: 0.3 mg/ml, 0.4 mg/ml, 1 mg/ml	*Generic*
tablets, soluble: 0.4 mg, 0.6 mg	*Generic*

Thiphenamil Hydrochloride Rx

tablets: 100 mg, 400 mg	Trocinate

INDICATIONS

General uses are as follows. See listings below for specific indications of individual drugs.

Peptic ulcer: Adjunctive therapy in conjunction with antacids, diet, and possibly a histamine H_2 antagonist. These agents suppress gastric acid secretion and delay gastric emptying.

Other GI conditions: May be beneficial in functional GI disorders (functional diarrhea, spastic constipation, cardiospasm, pylorospasm, general hypermotility, neurogenic colon), irritable bowel syndrome (spastic colon, mucous colitis), acute enterocolitis, mild ulcerative colitis, diverticulitis, mild dysenteries, acute pancreatitis, duodenitis, gastritis, splenic flexure syndrome, infant colic.

Biliary tract: For spastic disorders (biliary colic, biliary dyskinesia); given in conjunction with a narcotic analgesic.

GU tract: Relief of urinary frequency and urgency, nocturnal enuresis, ureteral colic in conjunction with a narcotic analgesic.

Parkinsonism: See Anticholinergic Antiparkinsonism Agents.

Preoperative medication: Some of these agents, particularly atropine, scopolamine, and glycopyrrolate, are used to control bronchial, nasal, pharyngeal, and salivary secretions, to prevent bronchospasm and laryngospasm, and to block cardiac vagal inhibitory reflexes during induction of anesthesia and intubation. Scopolamine is used for preanesthetic sedation and obstetric amnesia in conjunction with morphine ("twilight sleep") or meperidine.

Upper respiratory conditions: Used as drying agents to reduce nasal secretions in acute rhinitis, coryza, hay fever. Nonprescription cold medicines often contain belladonna alkaloids for this purpose.

Antidotes for poisoning by cholinergic drugs: Atropine sulfate is most commonly used to combat CNS and peripheral toxic effects.

Bronchial asthma: Some of these agents relax smooth muscle of bronchi and bronchioles and decrease airway resistance. Atropine is effective in treating parasympathomimetic-mediated bronchospasm. Use in those with chronic lung disease not recommended because of possibility of inspissation and formation of mucous plugs due to reduced bronchial secretions.

Miscellaneous: Motion sickness (belladonna alkaloids); suppression of vagally mediated bradyarrhythmias (atropine); management of cerebral excitation such as delirium tremens, hysteria, other maniacal states (scopolamine).

ANISOTROPINE METHYLBROMIDE

Adjunctive therapy in treatment of peptic ulcer.

ATROPINE SULFATE

To reduce salivation, bronchial secretions. Useful in pylorospasm and other spastic conditions of GI tract. For ureteral and biliary colic, atropine concomitantly with morphine may be indicated. Also used in treatment of excessive vagus-induced bradycardia.

BELLADONNA

Adjunctive therapy in peptic ulcer, functional digestive disorders, diarrhea, diverticulitis, pancreatitis. Also used for dysmenorrhea, nocturnal enuresis, parkinsonism (idiopathic, postencephalitic), nausea and vomiting of pregnancy, motion sickness.

CLIDINIUM BROMIDE

Adjunctive therapy in treatment of peptic ulcer.

DICYCLOMINE HYDROCHLORIDE

"Probably effective" for treatment of functional bowel/irritable bowel syndrome. Syrup also "probably effective" for treatment of infant colic.

GLYCOPYRROLATE

Oral: As adjunctive therapy in treatment of peptic ulcer.

Parenteral: IM or IV use in conjunction with anesthesia. To reduce salivary, tracheobronchial, pharyngeal secretions; to block cardiac vagal inhibitory reflexes during induction of anesthesia, intubation.

HEXOCYCLIUM METHYLSULFATE

Adjunctive therapy in treatment of peptic ulcer.

L-HYOSCYAMINE SULFATE

Adjunctive therapy in treatment of peptic ulcer; to aid in control of gastric hypersecretion, intestinal hypermotility and associated abdominal cramps. May be used to relieve symptoms in functional intestinal disorders, infant colic, and biliary colic. Adjunctive therapy in peptic ulcer, irritable bowel syndrome, neurogenic bowel disturbances. As a "drying agent" in relief of symptoms of acute rhinitis. In preanesthesia to control salivation, respiratory tract secretions. In therapy for parkinsonism to reduce muscular rigidity, tremors and control associated sialorrhea, hyperhidrosis. May be used to reduce pain and hypersecretion in pancreatitis and for poisoning by anticholinesterase agents. Also used for cystitis and renal colic.

ISOPROPAMIDE IODIDE

Adjunctive therapy in treatment of peptic ulcer. "Probably effective" in irritable bowel syndrome.

LEVOROTATORY ALKALOIDS OF BELLADONNA

Whenever belladonna is indicated.

MEPENZOLATE BROMIDE

Adjunctive therapy in treatment of peptic ulcer.

METHANTHELINE BROMIDE

Adjunctive therapy in treatment of peptic ulcer.

METHSCOPOLAMINE BROMIDE

Adjunctive therapy in treatment of peptic ulcer.

OXYPHENCYCLIMINE HYDROCHLORIDE

Adjunctive therapy in treatment of peptic ulcer.

OXYPHENONIUM BROMIDE

Adjunctive therapy in treatment of peptic ulcer.

PROPANTHELINE BROMIDE

Adjunctive therapy in treatment of peptic ulcer.
   Unlabeled uses: Has been used for its antisecretory and antispasmodic effects.

SCOPOLAMINE HYDROBROMIDE (HYOSCINE HYDROBROMIDE)

   Oral: Inhibits excessive GI motility, hypertonicity in irritable colon syndrome, mild dysentery, diverticulitis, pylorospasm, cardiospasm. It may also prevent motion sickness (see Antiemetic/Antivertigo Agents). Symptomatic treatment of postencephalitic parkinsonism and paralysis agitans; also used for calming delirium.
   Parenteral: Preanesthetic sedation, obstetric amnesia in conjunction with analgesics, calming delirium.

THIPHENAMIL HYDROCHLORIDE

Relief of smooth muscle spasm associated with spastic colitis, irritable colon, mucous colitis, acute enterocolitis, functional GI disorders. "Possibly effective" in treatment of irritable bowel syndrome, neurogenic bowel disturbances.

CONTRAINDICATIONS

Hypersensitivity to anticholinergic drugs; narrow-angle glaucoma; adhesions between iris and lens of eye; tachycardia; some cases of cardiac disease; unstable cardiac status in acute hemorrhage; obstructive disease of GI tract; paralytic ileus; intestinal atony of the elderly or debilitated patient; toxic megacolon complicating ulcerative colitis; severe ulcerative colitis; hiatal hernia associated with reflux esophagitis; hepatitis; bladder neck obstruction due to prostatic hypertrophy; myasthenia gravis; toxemia of pregnancy.

ACTIONS

Anticholinergic drugs, previously known as parasympatholytic drugs, exert their pharmacologic effects by competitive antagonism of acetylcholine at the postganglionic receptors of the parasympathetic branch of the autonomic nervous system. These receptors are also designated as muscarinic receptors; therefore, these agents are also known as antimuscarinic drugs.

   These agents inhibit muscarinic actions of acetylcholine at postganglionic parasympathetic neuroeffector sites including smooth muscle, secretory glands, and sites within the CNS. Large doses may block nicotinic receptors at the autonomic ganglia and at the neuromuscular junction.

   Specific anticholinergic responses are dose related. The following effects may occur: Small doses inhibit salivary and bronchial secretions and sweating; moderate doses will dilate the pupil, inhibit accommodation and increase the heart rate (vagal effect); larger doses will decrease motility of the GI and urinary tracts; and very large doses will inhibit gastric secretion.

   Belladonna alkaloids*: Naturally ocurring alkaloids of belladonna are rapidly absorbed following oral administration. These agents readily cross the blood–brain barrier and therefore exert both therapeutic and toxic effects in the CNS. The major pharmacologic difference among these agents is that at usual therapeutic doses atropine is a stimulant, whereas scopolamine is a CNS depressant. Significant undesirable peripheral and central effects are

---

* Atropine sulfate, belladonna, L-hyoscyamine sulfate, levorotatory alkaloids of belladonna, scopolamine hydrobromide.

produced when given in doses sufficient to control GI motility and gastric acid secretion.

Quarternary anticholinergics*: Synthetic or semi-synthetic derivatives are structurally related to the belladonna alkaloids. They are poorly and unreliably absorbed following oral administration. Because they do *not* cross the blood–brain barrier, CNS effects are negligible. They are also less likely to affect the pupil or ciliary muscle of the eye. Duration of action is more prolonged than the alkaloids. In addition to antimuscarinic effects, these agents may cause some degree of ganglionic blockade; neuromuscular blockade may occur at toxic doses.

Antispasmodics†: Tertiary ammonia compounds have little or no antimuscarinic activity and therefore no significant effect on gastric secretion. They exhibit a nonspecific direct relaxant effect on smooth muscle.

WARNINGS

In the presence of high environmental temperature, heat prostration (fever, heat stroke due to decreased sweating) can occur. Diarrhea may be an early symptom of incomplete intestinal obstruction, especially in those with an ileostomy or colostomy. Elderly patients may react with excitement, agitation, drowsiness, other untoward manifestations to even small doses. Theoretically, with overdosage a cura-relike action may occur (*i.e.,* neuromuscular blockade leading to muscular weakness and possible paralysis). Use of these drugs in treatment of gastric ulcer may produce a delay in gastric emptying time and complicate therapy.

These drugs are administered with caution if an increase in heart rate is undesirable. Safety for use in pregnancy, in the nursing mother, or in women of childbearing potential is not established. Use only when clearly needed and potential benefits outweigh the unknown potential hazards to the fetus. An inhibiting effect on lactation may occur.

PRECAUTIONS

Used with caution in the following.

CNS: Autonomic neuropathy.

Ocular: Glaucoma.

GI: Hepatic disease; early evidence of ileus, as in peritonitis; ulcerative colitis; hiatal hernia with reflux esophagitis.

---

* Anisotropine methylbromide, clidinium bromide, glycopyrrolate, hexocyclium methylsulfate, isopropamide iodide, mepenzolate bromide, methantheline bromide, methscopolamine bromide, oxyphenonium bromide, propantheline bromide.
† Dicyclomine hydrochloride, oxyphencyclimine hydrochloride, thiphenamil hydrochloride.

GU: Renal disease, nonobstructing prostatic hypertrophy. Urinary hesitancy may be evidenced by patients with prostatic hypertrophy.

Endocrine: Hyperthyroidism.

Cardiovascular: Coronary heart disease, congestive heart failure, cardiac arrhythmias, hypertension.

Other: Use cautiously in infants, small children, debilitated patients with chronic lung disease, patients over 40 (because of increased incidence of glaucoma).

Tartrazine sensitivity: Some of these products contain tartrazine (see Appendix 6, section 6-23).

DRUG INTERACTIONS

Antihistamines, antipsychotics, antiparkinsonism drugs, alphaprodine, buclizine, meperidine, orphenadrine, benzodiazepines, and **tricyclic antidepressants** may enhance the side-effects of atropine and its derivatives due to their secondary anticholinergic activities. **Nitrates, nitrites, alkalinizing agents, primidone, thioxanthenes, methylphenidate, procainamide,** and **quinidine** may also potentiate side-effects. **Monoamine oxidase inhibitors** block detoxification of anticholinergics and thus potentiate their actions. Concurrent long-term therapy with **corticosteroids** or **haloperidol** may increase intraocular pressure. Anticholinergics antagonize the miotic actions of **cholinesterase inhibitors.**

Bronchial relaxation produced by **sympathomimetics** is enhanced by anticholinergics. Inhibition of gastric acid secretion by anticholinergics is antagonized by **guanethidine, histamine, reserpine.** Because of the potential for adverse effects, anticholinergics should be used cautiously with **digitalis, digoxin, cholinergics, diphenhydramine, levodopa** (in parkinsonism), **neostigmine. Antacids** may interfere with absorption.

IV administration of any anticholinergic in the presence of **cyclopropane anesthesia** can result in ventricular arrhythmias.

Lab test interferences: Iodine content of isopropamide iodide may alter thyroid function tests and will suppress ^{131}I uptake. It is suggested therapy be discontinued 1 week prior to these tests.

ADVERSE REACTIONS

These effects may be physiologic or toxic depending on individual response.

GI: Xerostomia, loss of taste, nausea, vomiting, dysphagia, heartburn, constipation, bloated feeling, paralytic ileus, gastroesophageal reflux.

GU: Urinary hesitancy and retention, dysuria, impotence.

Ocular: Blurred vision, mydriasis, photophobia, cycloplegia, increased ocular tension.

G

Cardiovascular: Palpitation, bradycardia (following low doses of atropine), tachycardia (after higher doses) that may increase frequency and severity of anginal attacks in those with coronary artery disease.

CNS: Headache, flushing, nervousness, drowsiness, weakness, dizziness, insomnia, nasal congestion, fever. The elderly may exhibit some degree of mental confusion and/or excitement to even smaller doses. Large doses may produce CNS stimulation (restlessness, tremor, irritability, delirium, hallucinations), which may be followed by depression and death from medullary paralysis. In presence of pain, scopolamine often produces delirium if used without morphine or meperidine.

Other: Suppression of lactation. Decreased sweating may occur.

Dermatologic–hypersensitivity: Severe allergic reaction or drug idiosyncrasies including anaphylaxis, urticaria, other dermal manifestations. With use of **isopropamide iodide,** iodine skin rash may occur rarely. With the parenteral form of **dicyclomine HCl** there may be a temporary sensation of lightheadedness and occasionally local irritation.

OVERDOSAGE

Symptoms: Acute overdosage can produce dry mouth accompanied by a burning sensation, respiratory failure, difficult swallowing; headache; nausea, vomiting; dizziness; marked thirst; blurred vision, photophobia; flushed, hot, dry skin; rash, hyperthermia; palpitations, tachycardia with weak pulse, elevated blood pressure; hypotension; leukocytosis; urinary urgency with difficulty in micturition; abdominal distention; muscular incoordination; restlessness, CNS stimulation, confusion, delirium, paralysis; stupor; coma; other signs suggestive of acute organic psychosis.

Treatment: Remove remaining drug from stomach by inducing emesis or by gastric lavage, then administer activated charcoal slurry and supportive therapy as indicated. Physostigmine 0.5 mg to 2 mg IV (repeated as needed up to total of 5 mg), neostigmine methylsulfate (0.5 mg to 1 mg IM q2h to q3h or 0.5 mg to 2 mg IV repeated as needed) or pilocarpine (5 mg subcutaneously) may relieve peripheral symptoms. Benzodiazepines or short-acting barbiturates may control excitement. Levarterenol or metaraminol infusions control hypotension and circulatory collapse. Artificial respiration and oxygen therapy should be used for respiratory depression. Administer fluids to increase excretion and catheterize to prevent urinary retention if necessary. Treat hyperpyrexia with physical cooling measures. If photophobia occurs, keep patient in darkened room.

DOSAGE

ANISOTROPINE METHYLBROMIDE
50 mg tid.

ATROPINE SULFATE
May be given PO, subcutaneously, IM, or IV.
Adults: 0.4 mg to 0.6 mg.
Children: 7–16 lb—0.1 mg
     17–24 lb—0.15 mg
     24–40 lb—0.2 mg
     40–65 lb—0.3 mg
     65–90 lb—0.4 mg
     >90 lb—0.4 mg to 0.6 mg

BELLADONNA
Extract: 15 mg tid or qid.
Tincture: Adults, 0.6 ml to 1 ml tid or qid; children, 0.03 ml/kg (0.8 ml/m^2) tid.

CLIDINIUM BROMIDE
Adults: 2.5 mg to 5 mg tid or qid, A.C. and H.S.
Geriatric and/or debilitated patients: 2.5 mg tid A.C.

DICYCLOMINE HYDROCHLORIDE
Oral: *Adults*—10 mg to 20 mg tid or qid. *Children*—10 mg tid or qid. *Infants*—5 mg (syrup) tid or qid. Syrup may be diluted with equal volume of water.
Parenteral: IM only; not for IV use. *Adults*—20 mg q4h to q6h.

GLYCOPYRROLATE
Oral: 1 mg tid or 2 mg bid or tid. *Maintenance dose*—1 mg bid. This is not recommended for children.
Parenteral
Peptic ulcer: 0.1 mg to 0.2 mg administered IM or IV tid or qid. This is not recommended for children.
Preanesthetic medication: *Adults*—0.002 mg/lb IM given 30 minutes to 1 hour prior to anesthesia. *Children under 12*—0.002 mg/lb to 0.004 mg/lb IM.
Intraoperative medication: *Adults*—0.1 mg IV. Repeat as needed at 2- to 3-minute intervals. *Children*—0.002 mg/lb.
Reversal of neuromuscular blockade: *Adults and children*—0.2 mg for each 1 mg neostigmine or equivalent dose of pyridostigmine. Administer IV simultaneously.

HEXOCYCLIUM METHYLSULFATE
25 mg qid. Timed release, 50 mg bid. Not for use in children.

L-HYOSCYAMINE SULFATE

Oral: *Adults*—0.125 mg to 0.25 mg q4h PO or sublingually; 0.375 mg sustained release q12h. *Children*—Individualize according to weight.

Parenteral: 0.25 mg to 0.5 mg subcutaneously, IM, or IV three or four times a day as needed.

ISOPROPAMIDE IODIDE

5 mg q12h; 10 mg bid or more may be required. Not for use in children under 12.

LEVOROTATORY ALKALOIDS OF BELLADONNA

Oral: *Adults*—0.25 mg to 0.5 mg tid; *children (over 6 yr)*—0.125 mg to 0.25 mg tid.

Parenteral: *Adults*—0.5 ml to 1 ml subcutaneously once or twice daily.

MEPENZOLATE BROMIDE

25 mg to 50 mg qid with meals and H.S. Safety and efficacy in children not established.

METHANTHELINE BROMIDE

Adults: 50 mg to 100 mg q6h.

Pediatric: *Newborn*—12.5 mg bid, then tid; *infants 1 to 12 months*—12.5 mg qid, increased to 25 mg qid, *children over 1 year*—12.5 mg to 50 mg qid.

METHSCOPOLAMINE BROMIDE

2.5 mg ½ hr A.C. and 2.5 mg to 5 mg H.S.

OXYPHENCYCLIMINE HYDROCHLORIDE

10 mg bid in A.M. and H.S. Some patients respond to 5 mg bid while others require higher dosage on tid regimen. Not for use in children under 12.

OXYPHENONIUM BROMIDE

10 mg qid for several days; reduce dosage according to response. Not for use in children.

PROPANTHELINE BROMIDE

Adults: 15 mg 30 minutes A.C. and 30 mg H.S. For patients with mild manifestations, geriatric patients or those of small stature, 7.5 mg tid.

Children: Safety and efficacy for use in peptic ulcer not established.

Antisecretory: 1.5 mg/kg/day in divided doses 3 to 4 times/day.

Antispasmodic: 2 mg/kg/day to 3 mg/kg/day in divided doses every 4 to 6 hours and H.S.

SCOPOLAMINE HYDROBROMIDE (HYOSCINE HYDROBROMIDE)

Parenteral: Give subcutaneously or IM; may be given IV after suitable dilution with Sterile Water for Injection.

Adults: 0.32 mg to 0.65 mg.
Children: 0.006 mg/kg. Maximum dosage, 0.3 mg.

Oral: 0.4 mg to 0.8 mg; increase cautiously in spastic states, parkinsonism.

THIPHENAMIL HYDROCHLORIDE

400 mg initially; may be repeated in 4 hours. Safety, efficacy in children not established.

NURSING IMPLICATIONS

HISTORY

See Appendix 4. Note family history of GI disorders; allergy history (if isopropamide iodide prescribed, inquire about iodine allergy, allergy to seafood).

PHYSICAL ASSESSMENT

Will depend on symptoms, diagnosis, rationale for drug use. Vital signs; palpation, auscultation of abdomen if lower GI tract disease suspected; examination of stool for melena, appearance; look for evidence of dehydration if diarrhea prominent symptom (especially in children, elderly); weight. Additional laboratory, diagnostic tests, such as GI series, CBC, and stool for occult blood, may be ordered.

ADMINISTRATION

If dry mouth persists, have patient take a few sips of water prior to swallowing tablet form.

These drugs may be ordered taken before or with meals.

Preoperative: Have patient void before drug is administered; give at exact time ordered because drug must be allowed to exert maximal effects prior to anesthesia; advise patient to remain in bed; raise siderails.

Emergency treatment of vagus-induced bradycardia: Atropine sulfate 0.5 mg is given by IV push; dose may be repeated every 5 minutes or as ordered until arrhythmia abolished. Patient should be on a cardiac monitor during and after administration. If arrhythmia persists, emergency insertion of a cardiac pacemaker may be necessary because results of atropine administration are variable.

Dicyclomine HCl: Given as syrup to infants; may be diluted with equal amounts of water.

ONGOING ASSESSMENTS AND NURSING MANAGEMENT

Vital signs daily; record therapeutic drug effects (or lack of anticipated drug response) by evaluation of symptoms/complaints related to diagnosis of peptic ulcer or other GI, GU, biliary tract disease or disorder; observe for adverse drug effects.

Urinary retention may be avoided if patient is advised to void before taking drug. If patient has history of urinary problems (*e.g.,* nocturia, dysuria) or is elderly, measure intake and output during first few days of therapy. If urinary retention is suspected, palpate abdomen (above symphysis pubis) for enlarged bladder.

Report any changes in pulse rate to physician. If severe tachycardia or bradycardia occurs, withhold next dose of drug and contact physician immediately.

Antacids may interfere with absorption. Do not give simultaneously; doses should be staggered.

If patient is scheduled for thyroid function tests, isopropamide iodide should be discontinued 1 week prior to tests.

Caution should be exercised when giving these drugs, for any reason, to the elderly (see *Warnings*). Observe these patients frequently following administration. If excitement, agitation, or other untoward effects occur, withhold next dose and contact physician. If administered as a preoperative medication, contact anesthesiologist or surgeon immediately.

These drugs may cause drowsiness, dizziness, blurred vision. Patient (especially elderly) should be assisted with ambulatory activities. For elderly patients or those experiencing visual difficulty, furniture (*e.g.,* footstools, chairs) obstructing ambulatory areas in room should be placed against a wall to prevent accidents, falls.

If photophobia occurs, patient may be more comfortable in a semidarkened room.

Cycloplegia and mydriasis may interfere with reading and similar activities; if upsetting, advise patient to discuss problem with physician.

In hot weather, decreased sweating followed by heat prostration may occur. Observe patient frequently, especially if elderly or debilitated, and contact physician immediately if fever, hot dry skin, mental confusion occurs.

Report any eye complaints, especially pain or unexpected visual changes, to the physician immediately.

PATIENT AND FAMILY INFORMATION
Take at times ordered by physician (*e.g.,* before or with meals).

May cause drowsiness, dizziness, blurring of vision; observe caution while driving or performing tasks requiring alertness.

Notify physician or nurse if skin rash, flushing, eye pain occurs.

May cause dryness of mouth, difficulty in urination, constipation, increased sensitivity to light; notify physician or nurse if these effects persist or become severe.

Dry mouth may be relieved by frequent sips of water, gum, hard candy; sensitivity to light can be avoided by wearing sunglasses, keeping room semidark.

Family of elderly patient: Remove objects that may cause falls (*e.g.,* throw rugs, footstools) because vision may be impaired during early therapy.

Do not use nonprescription drugs, especially cold, hay-fever, and cough remedies, without prior approval of physician.

Gelatin Hemostatics

Gelatin Film, Absorbable, Sterile otc

film	Gelfilm, Gelfilm Ophthalmic

Gelatin Powder, Absorbable, Sterile otc

powder	Gelfoam

Gelatin Sponge, Absorbable otc

sponges, packs, dental packs, prostatectomy cones	Gelfoam

INDICATIONS
GELATIN FILM, ABSORBABLE, STERILE
Used in neurosurgery, as a dural substitute, in thoracic surgery to repair pleural defects in connection with thoracotomies, thoracoplasties, and extrapleural procedures and in ocular surgery.

GELATIN POWDER, ABSORBABLE, STERILE
For hemostasis in control of bleeding from cancellous bone when ligatures or other conventional procedures are ineffective or impractical; chronic leg ulcers, decubitus ulcers.

GELATIN SPONGE, ABSORBABLE
In surgical procedures as adjunct to hemostasis when control of bleeding by ligature or conventional procedures is ineffective or impractical. Also used in oral and dental surgery as an aid in providing hemostasis. In open prostatic surgery, insertion into prostatic cavity provides hemostasis.

CONTRAINDICATIONS

Gelatin film is contraindicated in presence of purulent exudate and is not recommended for use in grossly contaminated or infected surgical wounds. Gelatin powder and sponge are not used in closure of skin incisions; may interfere with healing of skin edges.

ACTIONS

Gelatin film is a sterile absorbable product. In the dry state it has the appearance and texture of cellophane of equivalent thickness; when moistened, it assumes a rubbery consistency and can be cut to desired size. Rate of absorption ranges from 1 to 6 months, depending on size and site of implantation. Pleural and muscle implants are completely absorbed in 8 to 14 days, whereas dural and ocular implants usually require 2 to 3 months.

Gelatin powder possesses hemostatic and tissue-stimulating properties. When implanted, it is absorbed completely in 4 to 6 weeks without excessive scar formation. When applied to bleeding areas of skin or nasal, rectal, or vaginal mucosa, it completely liquefies within 2 to 5 days. Locally applied, it promotes growth of granulation tissue and healing of indolent, radiation, and decubitus ulcers and slowly healing wounds. It is nonirritating and has no deleterious effect on the activity of penicillin, streptomycin, or neomycin.

Gelatin sponge is a sterile, pliable surgical sponge prepared from purified gelatin solution and capable of absorbing and holding many times its weight in blood. When implanted into tissues, it is absorbed completely within 4 to 6 weeks. When applied to bleeding areas of skin or nasal, rectal, or vaginal mucosa it completely liquefies within 2 to 5 days.

WARNINGS

Do not resterilize by heat because heating may change absorption time. Ethylene oxide is not recommended for resterilization; it may be trapped in the interstices of the foam and may cause burns or irritation to tissue in trace amounts.

PRECAUTIONS

Gelatin powder and sponge are not recommended in presence of infection. If signs of infection or abscess develop in area where sponge has been placed, reoperation may be necessary to remove infected material and allow drainage. Not used for controlling postpartum bleeding or menorrhagia. Absorbable gelatin powder is also not recommended as the sole hemostatic agent in those with blood dyscrasias characterized by abnormal bleeding; concurrent therapeutic measures are also employed.

DOSAGE
See *Administration.*

NURSING IMPLICATIONS

PHYSICAL ASSESSMENT
Record size and appearance of decubitus or leg ulcer.

ADMINISTRATION
Storage: Once package or jar is opened, contents are subject to contamination. Unused portions are discarded.

GELATIN FILM
Immerse in sterile saline; soak until quite pliable. Surgeon cuts to desired size and shape and applies.

GELATIN POWDER
Hemostasis: To make paste, open jar and pour contents into sterile beaker. A puttylike paste is made by adding a total of approximately 3 ml to 4 ml of sterile saline to the powder. Avoid dispersion of powder by compressing with gloved fingers into bottom of beaker and then kneading to desired consistency. Paste is then applied by surgeon to cancellous bone.

Chronic leg ulcers: Pack ulcer with powder; cover with dry gauze and apply an elastic bandage. Repeat weekly until healing ensues. Severe secondary infection should be treated before application of powder. When secondary infection is moderate, a suitable topical antibiotic may be applied directly to the ulcer base prior to packing with powder. In the absence of obvious secondary infection, powder may be used alone. Excoriated areas around the ulcer zone may be covered with a mild paste, such as zinc oxide, before application of dressing.

Decubitus ulcers: Area is filled with powder and a dressing is applied. Dressings may be changed daily or left intact for maximum of 7 days. Leave powder in contact with the ulcer surface undisturbed, without cleansing, and add new powder as required. If infection develops, treatment is discontinued and appropriate therapy instituted. Check with physician about preferred type of dressing and frequency of dressing changes.

GELATIN SPONGE
Product is available in assorted sizes and is cut to desired size as needed. Applied dry or satu-

rated with sodium chloride injection. When bleeding is controlled, pieces are left in place.

ONGOING ASSESSMENTS AND NURSING MANAGEMENT

Sponge may expand and impinge on neighboring structures. Note patient complaints of pain or discomfort. In some postoperative patients it may be difficult to distinguish between the pain of surgery and pain due to sponge expansion.

Observe for signs of infection when applied to skin, oral or nasal cavity, or rectal or vaginal mucosa. Notify physician if signs of infection are apparent.

When an elastic bandage is applied, check bandage q8h (or more frequently if patient is active) and reapply as needed. Bandage should not interfere with circulation of the extremity.

Chronic leg ulcers, decubitus ulcers: Note size and appearance of ulcer at time of dressing change or when powder is added to area; compare with data base.

Gemfibrozil Rx

capsules: 300 mg   Lopid

INDICATIONS

Treatment of adult patients with very high serum triglyceride levels (type IV hyperlipidemia) who present a risk of abdominal pain and pancreatitis and who do not respond adequately to a determined dietary effort to control them. Patients with triglyceride levels in excess of 750 mg/dl are likely to present such risks. Not useful for hypertriglyceridemia of type I hyperlipidemia. Has little effect on elevated cholesterol levels in most subjects. A minority of subjects show a more pronounced response. There is no evidence that use of any lipid-altering drug will be beneficial in preventing death from coronary heart disease. Treatment with gemfibrozil confined to those with clearly defined risk due to severe hypercholesterolemia (*e.g.,* individuals with familial hypercholesterolemia starting in childhood) who respond inadequately to appropriate diet and more effective cholesterol-lowering drugs.

The biochemical response is variable and it is not always possible to predict which patient will obtain favorable results. Lipid levels are assessed and drug discontinued in 3 months in those who do not show significant improvement.

CONTRAINDICATIONS

Hepatic or severe renal dysfunction, including primary biliary cirrhosis; preexisting gallbladder disease; hypersensitivity.

ACTIONS

Lowers elevated serum lipid levels primarily by decreasing serum triglycerides with a variable reduction in total serum cholesterol. These decreases occur primarily in the very low-density lipoprotein (VLDL) fraction and less frequently in the low-density lipoprotein (LDL) fraction. May increase the high-density lipoprotein (HDL) cholesterol fraction, an action considered of possible benefit in inhibition of the atherosclerotic process. Mechanism of action not definitely established. It inhibits peripheral lipolysis and decreases hepatic extraction of free fatty acids, thus reducing hepatic triglyceride production. Also inhibits synthesis of VLDL carrier apoprotein, leading to decreased VLDL production.

Is well absorbed from the GI tract after oral administration. Peak plasma levels occur in 1 to 2 hours with plasma half-life of 1.5 hours following single doses and 1.3 hours following multiple doses. Plasma levels appear proportional to the dose and do not accumulate following multiple doses.

WARNINGS

May increase cholesterol excretion into bile, leading to cholelithiasis. Therapy should be discontinued if gallstones occur. Use during pregnancy is reserved for those in whom benefit outweighs the possible risk to the fetus; in lactation, decision should be made to discontinue nursing or discontinue drug.

Use in children: Safety and efficacy not established.

PRECAUTIONS

Before therapy is instituted, effort should be made to control serum lipids with appropriate diet, exercise, weight loss in obese patients, and other medical problems such as diabetes mellitus and hypothyroidism.

Pretreatment laboratory studies are recommended to ensure patients have abnormal serum levels.

Mild hemoglobin, hematocrit, and WBC decreases have been occasionally observed following initiation of therapy; these levels stabilize during long-term administration. Periodic blood counts are recommended during first 12 months of therapy.

Gemfibrozil is not expected to alter seasonal variations of high serum lipid values in midwinter and late summer or lower values in fall and spring.

Hepatic function: Abnormal hepatic-function tests have been observed occasionally during therapy, including elevations in SGOT, SGPT, LDH, and alkaline phosphatase. These are usually reversible when drug is discontinued. Periodic hepatic-function studies are recommended and therapy is terminated if abnormalities persist.

DRUG INTERACTIONS

Exercise caution when **anticoagulants** are given in conjunction with gemfibrozil. Dosage of anticoagulant is reduced to maintain prothrombin time at desired level to prevent bleeding complications. Frequent prothrombin time determinations are recommended until prothrombin level has stabilized.

ADVERSE REACTIONS

Most frequently reported involve GI system.

GI: Abdominal pain, epigastric pain, diarrhea, nausea, vomiting, flatulence.

Integumentary: Rash, dermatitis, pruritus, urticaria.

CNS: Headache, dizziness, blurred vision.

Musculoskeletal: Painful extremities.

Hematopoietic: Anemia, eosinophilia, leukopenia.

Other

Other reactions have been reported in which causal relationship is difficult to establish; these include reports of viral and bacterial infection (common cold, urinary-tract infections). Other reactions reported were the following.

GI: Dry mouth, constipation, anorexia, gas pain, dyspepsia.

Musculoskeletal: Back pain, arthralgia, muscle cramps, myalgia, swollen joints.

CNS: Vertigo, insomnia, paresthesia, tinnitus.

Clinical laboratory: Hypokalemia, hepatic-function abnormalities (increased SGOT, SGPT, LDH, CPK, alkaline phosphatase).

Miscellaneous: Fatigue, malaise, syncope.

OVERDOSAGE

None reported. Symptomatic supportive measures should be taken if overdosage occurs.

DOSAGE

Recommended adult dose is 1200 mg/day in two divided doses 30 minutes before morning and evening meal. Some patients will experience therapeutic effects on 900 mg/day; a few may require 1500 mg/day.

NURSING IMPLICATIONS

HISTORY

See Appendix 4. Note family history of hypertriglyceridemia, heart disease; dietary pattern; previous treatment modalities (*e.g.,* diet, weight loss).

PHYSICAL ASSESSMENT

Vital signs; weight. Pretreatment serum lipid levels will be ordered. CBC, hepatic-function tests may also be obtained.

ADMINISTRATION

Give 30 minutes before morning and evening meal.

ONGOING ASSESSMENTS AND NURSING MANAGEMENT

Vital signs daily; observe for adverse reactions.

Diet low in cholesterol as well as low in calories (if weight loss necessary) is usually prescribed.

Periodic laboratory monitoring is recommended and includes serum lipid level, CBC, hepatic-function tests.

If nausea and/or vomiting occurs, notify physician.

May cause dizziness, blurred vision. Patient may require assistance with ambulation.

Visitors may need to be reminded that patient is receiving a special diet that is an important part of treatment. Food should not be brought to the hospital.

PATIENT AND FAMILY INFORMATION

Adherence to prescribed diet is important. (Patient may be required to restrict dietary intake of saturated fats, sugar, and/or cholesterol.)

Alcohol intake should be limited. Discuss with physician amount that may be consumed daily.

May cause dizziness or blurred vision. Observe caution while driving or performing other tasks requiring alertness.

May cause abdominal or epigastric pain, diarrhea, nausea, vomiting, or flatulence. Notify physician or nurse if these become pronounced.

Periodic examination and laboratory studies will be necessary during therapy.

Gentamicin

See Aminoglycosides, Parenteral; Antibiotics, Ophthalmic; Antibiotics, Topical.

Gentian Violet Rx

tampons: 5 mg   Genapax

INDICATIONS

Treatment of vulvovaginal candidiasis.

G

CONTRAINDICATIONS

Hypersensitivity; other vaginal infections.

ACTIONS

A rosaniline dye static and cidal against some gram-positive bacteria and many fungi (yeasts and dermatophytes). Mechanism of antifungal action is unknown. Is effective for many strains of *Candida.*

WARNINGS

Can provoke acute chemical vulvovaginitis. Not used in presence of extensive excoriation or ulceration.

PRECAUTIONS

Intractable candidiasis may be the presenting symptom of unrecognized diabetes mellitus. Urine and blood glucose studies should be carried out on those who do not respond to treatment. A persistently resistant infection may be evidence of reinfection rather than strain resistance. If infection persists following treatment, discontinue use and use another agent.

ADVERSE REACTIONS

Acute chemical vulvovaginitis; staining of skin.

DOSAGE

Insert one or two times nightly or until signs and symptoms of vulvitis have disappeared. Treatment should continue until cultures become negative.

NURSING IMPLICATIONS

HISTORY

See Appendix 4. Note family history of diabetes (see *Precautions*).

PHYSICAL ASSESSMENT

Take vaginal smear to confirm diagnosis. Laboratory tests to rule out diabetes may also be appropriate in some patients.

ADMINISTRATION

Instruct patient to insert tampon; provide instructions, if necessary. Provide supply of sanitary napkins to prevent staining of gown and bed linen.

ONGOING ASSESSMENTS AND NURSING MANAGEMENT

Question patient about relief of symptoms. Notify physician if patient complains of burning or irritation.

PATIENT INFORMATION

Read directions supplied with the product.

Complete full course of therapy.

Notify physician or nurse if burning or irritation occurs.

During treatment it is usually necessary to refrain from sexual intercourse or to have partner wear a condom to avoid reinfection.

Drug will stain clothing. Use a sanitary napkin to prevent staining of clothing or bedding.

If infection persists after treatment or recurs, notify physician.

Gitalin

See Cardiac Glycosides.

Glipizide

See Sulfonylureas.

Glucagon Rx

powder for injection: *Generic*
1 mg/vial, 10 mg/
vial

INDICATIONS

Useful in counteracting severe hypoglycemic reactions in diabetic patients or during insulin shock therapy in psychiatric patients. Is helpful in hypoglycemia only if liver glycogen is available. Is of little or no help in states of starvation, adrenal insufficiency, or chronic hypoglycemia. Also indicated as a diagnostic aid in radiologic examination of the stomach, duodenum, small bowel, and colon when a hypotonic state would be advantageous.

ACTIONS

A polypeptide hormone produced by the alpha cells of the pancreatic islets. It accelerates glycogenolysis in the liver by stimulating synthesis of cyclic AMP and increasing phosphorylase kinase activity. Increased breakdown of glycogen to glucose and inhibition of glycogen synthetase result in blood glucose elevation. Also stimulates hepatic gluconeogenesis by promoting uptake of amino acids and converting them to glucose precursors. Lipolysis in the liver and adipose tissue is also enhanced, providing free fatty acids and glycerol to further stimulate ketogenesis and gluconeogenesis.

WARNINGS

Because glucagon is a protein, hypersensitivity may occur. Administer with caution to patients with a history of insulinoma and/or pheochromocytoma. In those with insulinoma, IV administration will produce an initial increase in blood glucose, but because of its insulin-releasing effect, may subsequently cause hypoglycemia. Exogenous glucagon also stimulates the release of catecholamines, which can cause a marked increase in blood pressure in patients with pheochromocytoma.

PRECAUTIONS

In treatment of hypoglycemic shock with glucagon, liver glycogen must be available. Glucose by the IV route or by gavage should be considered in the hypoglycemic patient.

ADVERSE REACTIONS

Is relatively free of adverse reactions except for occasional nausea and vomiting, which may also occur with hypoglycemia.

DOSAGE

Hypoglycemia: 0.5 mg to 1 mg subcutaneously, IM, or IV usually produces a response in 5 to 20 minutes. If response is delayed, there is no contraindication to the administration of one or two additional doses. In view of the deleterious effects of cerebral hypoglycemia and depending on the duration and depth of coma, use of parenteral glucose must be considered. IV glucose must be given if patient fails to respond to glucagon.

Insulin shock therapy: After 1 hour of coma, inject 0.5 mg to 1 mg subcutaneously, IM, or IV. Larger doses may be employed if desired. The patient will usually awaken in 10 to 25 minutes. If no response occurs, dose may be repeated. In a very deep state of coma, give IV glucose in addition to glucagon for a more immediate response. Glucagon and glucose may be used together without decreasing the efficacy of glucose administration.

Diagnostic aid: ¼ to 2 units (0.25 mg to 2 mg) IV; 1 to 2 units (1 mg to 2 mg) IM. Administration of 2-unit doses produces a higher incidence of nausea and vomiting.

▌ NURSING IMPLICATIONS

PHYSICAL ASSESSMENT

Recognition of signs of hypoglycemia (Appendix 6, section 6-14) is followed by immediate intervention (*exception*—insulin shock therapy). Depending on hospital or unit policy, a blood glucose sample may be drawn immediately prior to administration of an agent to correct hypoglycemia.

ADMINISTRATION

Powder is reconstituted with diluent supplied with the product.

May be given subcutaneously, IM, IV according to physician's order.

Glucagon may be injected into the tubing of a running IV infusion of dextrose in water solutions. A precipitate will form when mixed with solutions containing sodium chloride, potassium chloride, or calcium chloride.

ONGOING ASSESSMENTS AND NURSING MANAGEMENT

Administration usually produces a response in 5 to 20 minutes. Note and record time first response is noted. Continue to record patient responses until hypoglycemia is corrected.

Stay with patient until response occurs. If response is delayed, physician may order an additional dose.

If the patient fails to respond, IV glucose must be given.

Nausea and vomiting may occur. Have suction machine, emesis basin readily available.

CLINICAL ALERT: It is important that hypoglycemia be recognized and corrected as soon as possible. Prolonged hypoglycemia reactions may result in cortical damage.

When patient responds, oral carbohydrates are given to restore liver glycogen and prevent secondary hypoglycemia. Record the type and amount of carbohydrate administered.

Obtain urine sample; test for glucose and ketones. Continue to test urine at 1- to 2-hour intervals or as ordered, until patient stabilizes. Blood glucose samples may also be ordered.

The physician must be notified when hypoglycemic reactions occur so that the dose of insulin may be adjusted more accurately.

Review events preceding hypoglycemic reaction, including dietary intake, time insulin was administered, dose of insulin, urine test results.

Continue to monitor patient at q1h to q2h intervals for next 6 to 8 or more hours (depending on type of insulin administered).

Insulin shock therapy: Patient should awaken in 10 to 25 minutes. Upon his awakening, feed patient orally as soon as possible, and follow usual dietary regimen. Monitor patient closely during coma as well as 1 to 2 hours after he awakens.

Glucocorticoids*

Betamethasone *Rx*

tablets: 0.6 mg	Celestone
syrup: 0.6 mg/5 ml	Celestone

Betamethasone Sodium Phosphate *Rx*

injection: 4 mg/ml	Celestone Phosphate, Cel-U-Jec, Selestoject, *Generic*

Betamethasone Sodium Phosphate and Betamethasone Acetate *Rx*

injection: 3 mg of each/ml	Celestone Soluspan

Cortisone Acetate *Rx*

tablets: 5 mg, 10 mg	*Generic*
tablets: 25 mg	Cortone Acetate, *Generic*
injection: 25 mg/ml, 50 mg/ml	Cortone Acetate, *Generic*

Dexamethasone *Rx*

tablets: 0.25 mg	Decadron, *Generic*
tablets: 0.5 mg, 0.75 mg, 1.5 mg	Decadron, Dexone, Hexadrol, SK-Dexamethasone, *Generic*
tablets: 2 mg	*Generic*
tablets: 4 mg	Decadron, Dexone, Hexadrol, *Generic*
tablets: 6 mg	Decadron
tablets (therapeutic pack): six 1.5-mg and eight 0.75-mg tablets	Hexadrol
elixir: 0.5 mg/5 ml	Decadron, Hexadrol, *Generic*
oral solution: 0.5 mg/0.5 ml	Dexamethasone Intensol

* This monograph covers systemic preparations. For other dosage forms, see Corticosteroids, Intranasal; Corticosteroids, Ophthalmic; Corticosteroids, Topical; Corticosteroid Respiratory Inhalants.

Dexamethasone Acetate *Rx*

injection: 2 mg/ml	Dalalone I.L.
injection: 8 mg/ml	Dalalone L.A., Decadron-LA, Decaject-L.A., Decameth L.A., Demasone-LA, Dexacen LA-8, Dexasone-LA, Dexon LA, Dexone LA, L.A. Dezone, Solurex-LA, *Generic*
injection: 16 mg/ml	Dalalone D.P.

Dexamethasone Sodium Phosphate *Rx*

injection: 4 mg/ml	Ak-Dex, Dalalone, Decadrol, Decadron Phosphate, Decaject, Decameth, Delladec, Demasone, Dexacen-4, Dexasone, Dexon, Dexone, Dezone, Hexadrol Phosphate, Savacort-D, Solurex, Wexaphos "4," *Generic*
injection: 10 mg/ml, 20 mg/ml	Hexadrol Phosphate
injection: 24 mg/ml	Decadron Phosphate, *Generic*

Dexamethasone Sodium Phosphate With Lidocaine Hydrochloride *Rx*

injection: 4 mg dexamethasone, 10 mg lidocaine/ml	Decadron w/Xylocaine

Hydrocortisone (Cortisol) *Rx*

tablets: 5 mg	Cortef
tablets: 10 mg, 20 mg	Cortef, Hydrocortone, *Generic*
injection: 25 mg/ml	*Generic*
injection: 50 mg/ml	Cortef, *Generic*
retention enema: 100 mg/60 ml unit	Cortenema

Hydrocortisone Acetate *Rx*

injection: 25 mg/ml	Hydrocortone Acetate, *Generic*
injection: 50 mg/ml	Biosone, Cortef Acetate, Hydrocortone Acetate, *Generic*
intrarectal aerosol foam: 90 mg/applicatorful	Cortifoam

Hydrocortisone Cypionate Rx

oral suspension: 10 mg/5 ml	Cortef Fluid

Hydrocortisone Sodium Phosphate Rx

injection: 50 mg/ml	Hydrocortone Phosphate

Hydrocortisone Sodium Succinate Rx

injection: 100 mg/ vial	A-hydroCort, Lifocort-100, Solu-Cortef, _Generic_
injection: 250 mg/ vial	A-hydroCort, Solu-Cortef, _Generic_
injection: 500 mg, 1000 mg/vial	A-hydroCort, Solu-Cortef

Methylprednisolone Rx

tablets: 2 mg, 8 mg, 16 mg, 24 mg (contain tartrazine), 32 mg	Medrol
tablets: 4 mg	Medrol, _Generic_

Methylprednisolone Acetate Rx

injection: 20 mg/ml	Depo-Medrol, _Generic_
injection: 40 mg/ml	depMedalone, Depo-Medrol, Depopred-40, Duralone-40, Dura-Meth, Med-Depo, Medralone-40, Medrone-40, Mepred-40, Methylone, M-Prednisol-40, Pre-Dep-40, Rep-Pred 40, _Generic_
injection: 80 mg/ml	depMedalone, Depo-Medrol, Depo-Pred-80, D-Med-80, Duralone-80, Medralone-80, Medrone-80, Mepred-80, M-Prednisol-80, Pre-Dep-80, Rep-Pred 80, _Generic_
retention enema: 40 mg/bottle	Medrol Enpak

Methylprednisolone Sodium Succinate Rx

injection: 40 mg, 125 mg, 500 mg, 1000 mg/vial	A-methaPred, Solu-Medrol, _Generic_

Paramethasone Acetate Rx

tablets: 1 mg, 2 mg	Haldrone

Prednisolone Rx

tablets: 1 mg	Panisolone, _Generic_
tablets: 5 mg	Cortalone (contains tartrazine), Delta-Cortef, Fernisolone-P, Predoxine-5, Sterane, _Generic_

Prednisolone Acetate Rx

injection: 25 mg/ml	Fernisolone, Key-Pred-25, Predcor-25, _Generic_
injection: 50 mg/ml	Articulose 50, Key-Pred-50, Predaject-50, Predcor-50, Savacort-50, _Generic_
injection: 100 mg/ml	Key-Pred-100, Savacort-100, _Generic_

Prednisolone Acetate and Prednisolone Sodium Phosphate Rx

injection: 80 mg prednisolone acetate, 20 mg prednisolone sodium phosphate/ml	Di-Pred, Duapred, Predalone R.P., Soluject, _Generic_

Prednisolone Sodium Phosphate Rx

injection: 20 mg/ml	Hydeltrasol, Key-Pred-SP, PSP-IV, SoluPredalone, _Generic_

Prednisolone Tebutate Rx

injection: 20 mg/ml	Hydeltra-T.B.A., Metalone T.B.A., Predcor-TBA, _Generic_

Prednisone Rx

tablets: 1 mg	Meticorten, Orasone, _Generic_
tablets: 2.5 mg	Deltasone, _Generic_
tablets: 5 mg	Cortan, Deltasone, Meticorten, Orasone, Panasol, Prednicen-M, SK-Prednisone, _Generic_
tablets: 10 mg, 20 mg, 50 mg	Deltasone, Orasone, _Generic_
tablets: 25 mg	_Generic_
syrup: 5 mg/5 ml	Liquid Pred

Triamcinolone Rx

tablets: 1 mg, 2 mg, 16 mg	Aristocort

tablets: 4 mg	Aristocort, *Generic*
tablets: 8 mg	Aristocort, Kenacort (contains tartrazine)
syrup: 2 mg/5 ml	Aristocort
syrup: 4 mg/5 ml	Kenacort

Triamcinolone Acetonide Rx

injection: 10 mg/ml	Kenalog-10
injection: 40 mg/ml	Acetospan, Cenocort A-40, Kenalog-40, Tramacort-40, Triamonide 40, Tri-Kort, Trilog, *Generic*

Triamcinolone Diacetate Rx

injection: 25 mg/ml	Aristocort Intralesional
injection: 40 mg/ml	Amcort, Aristocort Forte, Articulose L.A., Cenocort Forte, Cino-40, Tracilon, Triacin 40, Triacort, Triam-Forte, Triamolone 40, Trilone, Tristoject, Trylone D, *Generic*

Triamcinolone Hexacetonide Rx

injection: 5 mg/ml	Aristospan Intralesional
injection: 20 mg/ml	Aristospan Intra-articular

INDICATIONS

Endocrine disorders: Primary or secondary adrenal cortical insufficiency; congenital adrenal hyperplasia, nonsuppurative thyroiditis; hypercalcemia associated with cancer. Parenteral use is necessary for acute adrenal cortical insufficiency; preoperatively or in the event of serious trauma or illness in those with known adrenal insufficiency or when adrenal cortical reserve is doubtful; and shock that is unresponsive to conventional therapy if adrenal cortical insufficiency exists or is suspected.

Rheumatic disorders: As adjunctive therapy for short-term administration (acute episode or exacerbation) in ankylosing spondylitis; acute and subacute bursitis; acute nonspecific tenosynovitis; acute gouty arthritis; psoriatic arthritis; rheumatoid arthritis, including juvenile rheumatoid arthritis (some may require low-dose maintenance therapy); posttraumatic osteoarthritis; osteoarthritis; synovitis of osteoarthritis; and epicondylitis.

Collagen diseases: During exacerbation or as maintenance therapy in selected cases of lupus erythematosus; acute rheumatic carditis; and systemic dermatomyositis.

Dermatologic diseases: Pemphigus; bullous dermatitis herpetiformis; severe erythema multiforme (Stevens-Johnson syndrome); exfoliative dermatitis; mycosis fungoides; severe psoriasis; severe seborrheic dermatitis; and angioedema or urticaria.

Allergic states: Control of severe or incapacitating allergic conditions intractable to adequate trials of conventional treatment in seasonal or perennial allergic rhinitis; bronchial asthma (including status asthmaticus); contact dermatitis; atopic dermatitis; serum sickness; and drug hypersensitivity reactions.

Ophthalmic diseases: Severe acute and chronic allergic and inflammatory processes involving the eye and its adnexa such as allergic conjunctivitis; keratitis; allergic corneal marginal ulcers; herpes zoster ophthalmicus; iritis and iridocyclitis; chorioretinitis; diffuse posterior uveitis and choroiditis; optic neuritis; sympathetic ophthalmia; and anterior segment inflammation.

Respiratory diseases: Symptomatic sarcoidosis; Löffler's syndrome not manageable by other means; berylliosis; fulminating or disseminated pulmonary tuberculosis when concurrently accompanied by appropriate and adequate antituberculous therapy; and aspiration pneumonia.

Hematologic disorders: Idiopathic thrombocytopenic purpura in adults (IV only; IM use contraindicated); secondary thrombocytopenia in adults; acquired (autoimmune) hemolytic anemia; erythroblastopenia (RBC anemia); and congenital (erythroid) hypoplastic anemia.

Neoplastic diseases: Palliative management of leukemias and lymphomas in adults and acute leukemia of childhood.

Edematous states: To induce diuresis or remission of proteinuria in the nephrotic syndrome (without uremia) of the idiopathic type or that due to lupus erythematosus.

GI diseases: During critical period of disease in ulcerative colitis, regional enteritis, and intractable sprue.

Nervous system: Acute exacerbations of multiple sclerosis.

Miscellaneous: Tuberculous meningitis with subarachnoid block or impending block when concurrently accompanied by appropriate antituberculous therapy; in trichinosis with neurologic or myocardial involvement.

Intra-articular or soft-tissue administration: As short-term adjunct in synovitis of osteoarthritis; rheumatoid arthritis; acute gouty arthritis; epicondylitis; acute nonspecific tenosynovitis; and posttraumatic osteoarthritis.

Intralesional administration: Keloids; localized hypertrophic, infiltrated, inflammatory lesions of lichen planus, psoriatic plaques, granuloma annulare, lichen simplex chronicus; discoid lupus erythematosus; necrobiosis lipoidica diabeticorum; and alopecia areata. May also be helpful in cystic tumors of an aponeurosis or tendon (ganglia).

Others: Dexamathasone is also indicated for diagnostic testing of adrenal cortical hyperfunction and to treat patients with cerebral edema associated with primary or metastatic brain tumor, craniotomy, or head injury.

Triamcinolone is also indicated for treatment of pulmonary emphysema when bronchospasm or bronchial edema plays a significant role and diffuse interstitial pulmonary fibrosis; in conjunction with diuretic agents to induce a diuresis in refractory congestive heart failure (CHF) and in cirrhosis of the liver with refractory ascites; and for dental postoperative inflammatory response.

Unlabeled uses: Septic shock (very controversial; drug most commonly used is methylprednisolone, IV); antiemetic (dexamethasone for cisplatin-induced vomiting); prevention of respiratory distress syndrome in premature neonates (betamethasone most common); diagnosis of depression (dexamethasone).

Retention enema: Adjunctive therapy in treatment of ulcerative colitis.

Intrarectal foam: Adjunctive therapy in the treatment of ulcerative proctitis of the distal portion of the rectum in patients who cannot retain corticosteroid enemas.

CONTRAINDICATIONS

Systemic fungal infections (except as maintenance therapy in concomitant adrenal insufficiency); hypersensitivity. IM preparations are contraindicated in idiopathic thrombocytopenic purpura. Retention enema is contraindicated in ileocolostomy during the immediate or early postoperative period. Intrarectal foam is contraindicated in obstruction; abscess; perforation, peritonitis; fresh intestinal anastomoses; extensive fistulas; and sinus tracts.

ACTIONS

Naturally occurring adrenal cortical steroids have both anti-inflammatory (glucocorticoid) and salt-retaining (mineralocorticoid) properties. Glucocorticoids cause profound and varied metabolic effects. In addition, they modify the body's immune responses to diverse stimuli. These compounds, including hydrocortisone and cortisone, are used as replacement therapy in adrenocortical deficiency states. Naturally occurring compounds may be used for their anti-inflammatory effects in addition to use in adrenal hypofunction. The synthetic steroid compounds prednisone, prednisolone, and fludrocortisone also have both glucocorticoid and mineralocor-

ticoid activity. Prednisone and prednisolone are used primarily for their glucocorticoid effects.

In addition to compounds having both mineralocorticoid and glucocorticoid activity, a group of synthetic compounds with marked glucocorticoid activity is distinguished by the absence of any salt-retaining activity. These compounds include triamcinolone, dexamethasone, methylprednisolone, paramethasone, and betamethasone. These agents are used for their potent anti-inflammatory effects.

The glucocorticoids may be distinguished by their duration of action. Cortisone and hydrocortisone are short-acting; prednisone, prednisolone, methylprednisolone, and triamcinolone are intermediate-acting. Long-acting agents include paramethasone, betamethasone, and dexamethasone.

WARNINGS

Infections: Corticosteroids may mask signs of infection; new infections may appear during their use. There may be decreased resistance and inability of the host defense mechanisms to prevent dissemination of the infection. If infection occurs during therapy, it should be controlled with antimicrobial therapy. Use of systemic glucocorticoids in active tuberculosis is restricted to cases of fulminating or disseminated disease in which the corticosteroid is used for management of the disease in conjunction with appropriate chemotherapy. If corticosteroids are indicated in those with latent tuberculosis or tuberculin reactivity, close observation is necessary because reactivation of the disease may occur. Corticosteroids may exacerbate systemic fungal infections and should not be used in the presence of such infections unless needed to control drug reactions due to amphotericin B. Corticosteroids may also activate latent amebiasis.

Ocular effects: Prolonged use may produce posterior subcapsular cataracts, may cause glaucoma with possible damage to optic nerves, and may enhance establishment of secondary ocular infections due to fungi or viruses. Use cautiously in ocular herpes simplex because of possible corneal perforation.

Fluid and electrolyte balance: Average and large doses of hydrocortisone and cortisone can cause elevation of blood pressure, salt and water retention, and increased excretion of potassium. These effects are less likely to occur with synthetic derivatives except when used in large doses. All corticosteroids increase calcium excretion.

Hypersensitivity: Rare instances of anaphylactoid reactions have occurred with parenteral corticosteroid therapy; precautionary measures are taken before administration, especially in those with history of allergies.

G

Immunosuppression: While on corticosteroid therapy, patient should not be vaccinated against smallpox. Other immunization procedures should not be undertaken, especially when patient is receiving high doses of steroid, because of possible hazards of neurologic complications and a lack of antibody response. This does not apply to those receiving corticosteroids as replacement therapy (*e.g.,* for Addison's disease). Corticosteroids may suppress reactions to skin tests.

Adrenal suppression: Prolonged therapy (over 5 days) of pharmacologic doses of corticosteroids may lead to hypothalamic–pituitary–adrenal (HPA) suppression. The degree of suppression varies with dosage and duration of therapy. Adrenal suppression may be minimized by use of short-acting agents on an alternate-day schedule (see *Administration*). Doses of 15 mg of prednisone, given once per day, have caused minimal adrenal suppression.

Following prolonged therapy: Abrupt discontinuation may result in a withdrawal syndrome with fever, myalgia, arthralgia, and malaise and may occur without evidence of adrenal insufficiency. Discontinuance of exogenous corticosteroid therapy must be gradual.

Stress: In patients on corticosteroid therapy or recently withdrawn from therapy, increased dosage of rapidly acting corticosteroids is indicated before, during, and after stressful situations, except in patients on high-dosage therapy. Relative adrenocortical insufficiency may persist for months after therapy ends; stress occurring during that period may require reinstitution of hormone therapy. If the patient is receiving steroids already, the dosage may need to be increased. Because mineralocorticoid secretion may be impaired, salt and a mineralocorticoid should be administered concurrently.

Use in pregnancy: Possible benefits must be weighed against potential hazards to the fetus. Corticosteroids appear in breast milk and could suppress growth, interfere with endogenous corticosteroid production, or cause other unwanted effects in the nursing infant. Mothers taking these drugs should be advised not to nurse.

Retention enema: In severe ulcerative colitis, it is hazardous to delay needed surgery while awaiting response to medical treatment. Damage to the rectal wall can result from careless or improper insertion of the enema tip. If clinical or proctologic improvement fails to occur in 2 to 3 weeks, therapy should be discontinued. Syptomatic improvement may be misleading and is not used as the sole criterion in judging efficacy. Sigmoidoscopic examination and x-ray visualization are essential for adequate monitoring.

Intrarectal foam: Because the foam is not ex-pelled, absorption of systemic hydrocortisone may be greater than that of corticosteroid enema formulations. If there is no evidence of clinical or proctologic improvement within 2 or 3 weeks, or if the patient's condition worsens, discontinue use. Administer with caution to patients with severe ulcerative disease because these patients are predisposed to perforation of the bowel wall.

PRECAUTIONS

Lowest possible dose should be used because complications of treatment are dependent on the size of dose and duration of treatment. A benefit/risk decision must be made in each individual case.

Monitor therapy: Observe patient for weight increase, edema, hypertension, and excessive potassium excretion, as well as less obvious signs of untoward effects of adrenocortical steroid.

Caution in use: There is an enhanced effect in patients with hypothyroidism and those with cirrhosis. Use steroids with caution in nonspecific ulcerative colitis if there is a probability of impending perforation, abscess, or other pyogenic infection; diverticulitis; fresh intestinal anastomoses; active or latent peptic ulcer; renal insufficiency; hypertension; osteoporosis; acute glomerulonephritis; exanthema; Cushing's syndrome; antibiotic-resistant infections; CHF; chronic nephritis; thromboembolitic tendencies; thrombophlebitis; convulsive disorders; metastatic carcinoma; and myasthenia gravis. May precipitate manifestations of latent diabetes mellitus and may aggravate diabetes, requiring adjustment in diet, insulin, or hypoglycemic agents. Because of risk of disseminating viral infection, corticosteroids should be used only in life-threatening vaccinia or varicella.

Psychic effects: Psychic derangements may appear, ranging from euphoria, insomnia, mood swings, personality changes, and severe depression to frank psychotic manifestations. Existing emotional instability or psychotic tendencies may be aggravated.

Menstrual irregularities: May occur and should be mentioned to females past menarche.

Tartrazine sensitivity: Some products contain tartrazine (see Appendix 6, section 6-23).

Parenteral therapy: Rare instances of anaphylactoid reactions have occurred. Take precautionary measures in those with history of drug allergy.

Repository injections: Atrophy may occur at site of injection. To minimize occurrence and/or severity of atrophy, do not inject subcutaneously, avoid injection into the deltoid, and avoid repeated IM injections into the same site when possible.

Local injections: Intra-articular injection may produce systemic as well as local effects. Joint fluid should be examined for a septic process. A marked increase in pain accompanied by local swelling, further restriction of joint motion, fever, and malaise is suggestive of septic arthritis. If this occurs and diagnosis of sepsis is confirmed, appropriate antimicrobial therapy is instituted.

Retention enema: Use with caution when there is a probability of impending perforation, abscess, or intestinal anastomoses; obstruction or extensive fistulas; and sinus tracts.

DRUG INTERACTIONS

Increased requirements for **insulin** or **oral hypoglycemic agents** in diabetics have occurred. **Phenytoin, phenobarbital, rifampin,** and possibly **ephedrine** may enhance the metabolic clearance of corticosteroids, resulting in decreased blood levels and lessened physiologic activity, requiring adjustment in corticosteroid dosage. **Oral contraceptives** and **troleandomycin** may increase the physiologic activity of corticosteroids by inhibiting the hepatic metabolism of corticosteroids.

The prothrombin time should be checked frequently in those receiving corticosteroids and **oral anticoagulants** concomitantly; corticosteroids have altered response to these anticoagulants. When corticosteroids are administered concomitantly with **potassium-depleting diuretics,** the patient should be observed closely for development of hypokalemia. **Aspirin** should be used cautiously in conjunction with corticosteroids, especially in hypoprothrombinemia. Steroids may increase renal clearance of aspirin. Steroid-induced hypokalemia may enhance the possibility of **digitalis** toxicity.

The pharmacologic effects of corticosteroids may be decreased because of interference of their GI absorption induced by **anion-exchange resins** (cholestyramine, colestipol). The antitubercular effectiveness of **isoniazid** may be decreased.

Drug/lab tests: **Urine glucose** and **serum cholesterol levels** may be increased. Decreased serum levels may be seen for **potassium** and **triiodothyronine;** a minimal decrease in **thyroxine** may occur. **Thyroid** ^{131}**I** uptake may be decreased.

ADVERSE REACTIONS

Fluid and electrolyte disturbances: Sodium and fluid retention, CHF in susceptible patients, potassium loss and hypokalemic alkalosis, hypertension, hypocalcemia, hypotension or shocklike reactions.

Musculoskeletal: Muscle weakness; steroid myopathy; loss of muscle mass; tendon rupture; osteoporosis; aseptic necrosis of femoral and humeral heads; spontaneous fractures, including vertebral compression fractures and pathologic fractures of long bones.

Cardiovascular: Thromboembolism or fat embolism, thrombophlebitis, necrotizing angiitis, syncopal episodes, arteriosclerosis in the ankles (in rheumatoid arthritis). There are reports of cardiac arrhythmias and circulatory collapse following rapid administration of large IV doses of methylprednisolone.

_GI:_ Pancreatitis, abdominal distention, ulcerative esophagitis, nausea, increased appetite and weight gain. Peptic ulcer with perforation and hemorrhage has been associated with steroid therapy; this has been disputed in the literature.

Dermatologic: Impaired wound healing; thin, fragile skin; petechiae and ecchymoses; erythema; increased sweating; suppression of skin-test reactions; subcutaneous fat atrophy; purpura; striae; hyperpigmentation; hirsutism; acneiform eruptions; other cutaneous reactions such as allergic dermatitis, urticaria, angioneurotic edema.

Neurologic: Convulsions; steroid-induced catatonia; increased intracranial pressure with papilledema, usually after treatment is discontinued; vertigo; headache; neuritis or paresthesias; steroid psychosis; steroid-induced catatonia; insomnia; hiccups (dexamethasone).

Endocrine: Amenorrhea, other menstrual irregularities; development of cushingoid state; suppression of growth in children; secondary adrenocortical and pituitary unresponsiveness, particularly in times of stress (trauma, surgery, illness); decreased carbohydrate tolerance; manifestations of latent diabetes mellitus; increased requirements for insulin or oral hypoglycemic agents in diabetes.

Ophthalmic: Posterior subcapsular cataracts; increased intraocular pressure; glaucoma; exophthalmos.

Metabolic: Negative nitrogen balance due to protein catabolism.

Other: Anaphylactoid or hypersensitivity reactions, aggravation or masking of infections, malaise. Epidural lipomatosis (fat accumulation) has been reported. Steroids may increase or decrease motility and number of spermatozoa.

Parenteral therapy: Rare instances of blindness associated with intralesional therapy around face and head; hyperpigmentation or hypopigmentation; subcutaneous and cutaneous atrophy; sterile abscess; postinjection flare following intra-articular use; Charcotlike arthropathy; burning or tingling, especially in the perineal area (after IV injection); scarring, induration, inflammation, paresthesia, and delayed pain or soreness. Muscle twitching, ataxia, hiccups, and nystagmus have also been reported.

Retention enema: Local pain or burning, rectal bleeding, and apparent exacerbations or sensitivity reactions have been reported rarely.

G

OVERDOSAGE

Symptoms: May produce CNS changes (anxiety, other signs of stimulation or depression); elevated blood glucose; elevated blood pressure; edema. Symptoms include mental confusion, anxiety, depression, GI cramping or bleeding, ecchymosis, "moon" facies, and hypertension.

Treatment: No specific therapy. General management consists of symptomatic and supportive therapy, including gastric lavage, oxygen, IV fluids, and maintenance of body temperature. If GI bleeding is present, treatment is the same as for peptic ulcer. Adrenal insufficiency may occur and become manifest as effects wear off or when patient is subjected to stress.

DOSAGE

For specific dosages of each agent, see separate discussions below.

Maximal activity of the adrenal cortex is between 2:00 A.M. and 8:00 A.M.; it is minimal between 4:00 P.M. and midnight. Exogenous corticosteroids suppress adrenocortical activity the least when given at the time of maximal activity (in the A.M.). In order to minimize adrenocortical suppression, these drugs should be administered before 9:00 A.M. When large doses are given, an antacid may be administered between meals to help prevent peptic ulcers.

Initiation of therapy: Initial dosage depends on the specific disease entity. In situations of less severity, lower doses generally suffice; for others, higher doses may be necessary. Initial dose is maintained or adjusted until satisfactory response is noted. Dosage requirements are variable and must be individualized.

Maintenance therapy: After favorable response is noted, maintenance dosage is determined by decreasing the initial dosage in small amounts at appropriate time intervals until the lowest dosage that will maintain an adequate response is reached. Situations that may make dosage adjustments necessary are changes in clinical status secondary to remissions and exacerbations in the disease process, the patient's individual drug responsiveness, and the effect of patient exposure to stressful situations not directly related to the disease under treatment.

Withdrawal therapy: If the drug is to be stopped after long-term therapy, it must be withdrawn gradually to avoid the consequence of adrenal suppression. Continued supervision of the patient after cessation of therapy is essential, because there may be a sudden reappearance of severe manifestations of the disease for which patient was treated.

Alternate-day therapy: A dosing regimen in which twice the usual daily dose is administered every other morning. The purpose of this mode of therapy is to provide the patient requiring long-term treatment with the beneficial effects of corticosteroids while minimizing certain undesirable effects, including pituitary–adrenal suppression, the cushingoid state, corticoid withdrawal symptoms, and growth suppression in children. The benefits of alternate-day therapy are achieved only by use of short-acting agents. Rationale for this treatment schedule is based on two premises: (1) The anti-inflammatory or therapeutic effect of short-acting corticoids persists longer than their physical presence and metabolic effects, and (2) administration every other morning allows for reestablishment of more nearly normal HPA activity on the off-steroid day.

Intra-articular injections: Dose depends on size of joint and varies with severity of the condition. In chronic cases, injections may be repeated at intervals of 1 to 5 or more weeks. Injection must be made into the synovial space. Unstable joints should not be injected. Repeated injections may result in instability of the joint. Suitable sites for injection include the knee, wrist, elbow, shoulder, phalangeal, and hip joints. Following therapy, care should be taken to avoid overuse of joints in which symptomatic benefit has been obtained. Negligence at this time may permit an increase in joint deterioration.

Miscellaneous (ganglion, tendinitis, epicondylitis): Drug is injected into tendon sheath for tendonitis and tenosynovitis. When treating epicondylitis, the drug is infiltrated into the area of greatest tenderness. For ganglia, drug is injected directly into the cyst.

Injections for local dermatologic conditions: Care is taken to avoid injection of sufficient material to cause blanching, because this may be followed by a small slough. The intervals between injections vary with the type of lesion and duration of improvement produced by the initial injection.

BETAMETHASONE

Initial dosage may range from 0.6 mg/day to 7.2 mg/day PO.

BETAMETHASONE SODIUM PHOSPHATE

Is highly soluble, has prompt onset of action, and may be given IV.

Systemic and local: Initial dose may vary up to 9 mg/day depending on the specific disease entity being treated.

BETAMETHASONE SODIUM PHOSPHATE AND BETAMETHASONE ACETATE

Betamethasone sodium phosphate provides prompt activity; betamethasone acetate affords sustained activity.

Systemic

Not for IV use. Initial dose may vary from 0.5 mg/day to 9 mg/day IM, depending on specific disease entity being treated. Usual dosage ranges are ⅓ to ½ the oral dose given q12h. In certain situations, dosages exceeding the usual dosages may be justified.

Intrabursal, intra-articular, periarticular, intradermal, intralesional

Bursitis, tenosynovitis, peritendinitis: 1 ml

Rheumatoid arthritis, osteoarthritis: Very large joints—1 ml to 2 ml; *large joints*— 1 ml; *medium joints*—0.5 ml to 1 ml; *small joints*—0.25 ml to 0.5 ml.

Dermatologic conditions: 0.2 ml/cm² intradermally. Do not exceed more than 1 ml/week.

Disorders of the foot: Bursitis—dose range is 0.25 ml to 0.5 ml; *tenosynovitis, periostitis of cuboid*—0.5 ml; *acute gouty arthritis*—0.5 ml to 1 ml.

CORTISONE

Cortisone acetate saline suspension has a slow onset but long duration of action. It is insoluble in water. Parenteral form is not for IV use.

Initial dosage: Varies from 20 mg/day to 300 mg/day IM or PO. In less severe diseases, oral doses lower than 25 mg or 20 mg IM may suffice.

Physiologic replacement: 0.25 mg/kg/day to 0.35 mg/kg/day or 12 mg/m²/day to 15 mg/m²/day IM or 0.5 mg/kg/day to 0.75 mg/kg/day or 25 mg/m²/day, divided q8h, PO.

DEXAMETHASONE

Initial dosage: May vary from 0.75 mg/day to 9 mg/day PO depending on disease entity.

Suppression tests: For Cushing's syndrome, give 1 mg at 11:00 P.M. Draw blood for plasma cortisol at 8:00 A.M. the following morning. For greater accuracy, give 0.5 mg q6h for 48 hours. Twenty-four-hour urine collections are made for determination of 17-hydroxycorticosteroid excretion. Test to distinguish Cushing's syndrome due to pituitary ACTH excess from Cushing's due to other causes: Give 2 mg q6h for 48 hours. Twenty-four-hour urine collections are made for determination of 17-hydroxycorticosteroid excretion.

DEXAMETHASONE ACETATE

A long-lasting repository preparation.

Systemic: 8 mg to 16 mg IM; repeated in 1 to 3 weeks if necessary.

Intralesional: 0.8 mg to 1.6 mg.

Intra-articular and soft tissue: 4 mg to 16 mg; may be repeated at 1- to 3-week intervals.

DEXAMETHASONE SODIUM PHOSPHATE

Has rapid onset and short duration of action as compared with the acetate salt.

Systemic: Initial dosage may vary from 0.5 mg/day to 9 mg/day. Usual dose ranges are from ⅓ to ½ the oral dose given q12h. Dosages exceeding the usual may be justified in certain situations.

Cerebral edema: In adults, an initial IV dose of 10 mg is recommended, followed by 4 mg IM q6h until maximal response is noted. This regimen may be continued for several days postoperatively in those requiring brain surgery. Oral form, 1 mg to 3 mg three times a day should be given as soon as possible and dosage tapered over a period of 5 to 7 days. Nonoperative patients may require continuous therapy to remain free of symptoms of increased intracranial pressure. The smallest effective dose should be used in children, preferably orally. This may approximate 0.2 mg/kg/24 hours in divided doses.

Unresponsive shock: High doses are currently recommended. Reported regimens range from 1 mg/kg to 6 mg/kg as a single IV injection, to 40 mg initially followed by repeated IV injections q2h to q6h while shock persists.

Intra-articular, intralesional, soft tissue: Large joints—2 mg to 4 mg; *small joints*—0.8 mg to 1 mg; *bursae*—2 mg to 3 mg; *tendon sheaths*—0.4 mg to 1 mg; *soft-tissue infiltration*—2 mg to 6 mg; *ganglia*—1 mg to 2 mg.

DEXAMETHASONE SODIUM PHOSPHATE WITH LIDOCAINE HYDROCHLORIDE

Dexamethasone sodium phosphate provides prompt activity. Lidocaine HCl is a local anesthetic with a rapid onset and duration of 45 to 60 minutes. Steroid activity usually begins by the time the anesthesia wears off.

Acute, subacute bursitis: 0.5 ml to 0.75 ml.

Acute, subacute nonspecific tenosynovitis: 0.1 ml to 0.25 ml.

HYDROCORTISONE

Oral: Initial dosage varies from 20 mg/day to 240 mg/day depending on disease entity treated.

Parenteral: Not for IV use. Usually ⅓ to ½ the oral dose is administered IM q12h. In certain situations, doses exceeding the usual dosages may be justified.

Retention enema: Usual course of therapy is 100 mg nightly for 21 days, or until remission occurs both clinically and proctologically. Clinical symptoms usually subside promptly within 3 to 5 days. Improvement in the appearance of the mucosa may lag behind clinical improvement. Difficult cases may require 2 or 3 months of treatment. When course of therapy extends beyond 21 days, discontinue gradually.

HYDROCORTISONE ACETATE

Parenteral

Provides a prolonged effect. For intralesional, intra-articular, or soft-tissue injection. Not for IV use.

Large joints: 25 mg, occasionally 37.5 mg.

Small joints: 10 mg to 25 mg.

Bursae: 25 mg to 37.5 mg.

Tendon sheaths: 5 mg to 12.5 mg.

Soft-tissue infiltration: 25 mg to 50 mg; occasionally 75 mg.

Ganglia: 12.5 mg to 25 mg.

Intrarectal foam

Usual dose is 1 applicatorful once or twice daily for 2 or 3 weeks, and every second day thereafter. Do not insert any part of the aerosol container into the anus. Satisfactory response usually occurs within 5 to 7 days. Sigmoidoscopy is recommended to judge dosage adjustment, duration of therapy, and rate of improvement.

HYDROCORTISONE CYPIONATE

Initial dosage varies from 20 mg/day to 240 mg/day.

HYDROCORTISONE SODIUM PHOSPHATE

A water-soluble salt that has a rapid onset but short duration of action. May be given IV, IM, or subcutaneously. Initial dosage varies from 15 mg/day to 240 mg/day. Usually ⅓ to ½ the oral dose is administered q12h.

Acute adrenal insufficiency: *Adults*—100 mg IV injection followed by 100 mg q8h in IV fluids. *Older children*—1 mg/kg to 2 mg/kg IV bolus, then 150 mg/kg/day to 250 mg/kg/day IV in divided doses. *Infants*—1 mg/kg to 2 mg/kg IV bolus, then 25 mg/kg/day to 150 mg/kg/day in divided doses.

HYDROCORTISONE SODIUM SUCCINATE

A water-soluble salt that is rapidly active. May be given IM or IV. Initial dose is 100 mg to 500 mg.

METHYLPREDNISOLONE

Initial dose varies from 4 mg/day to 48 mg/day.

METHYLPREDNISOLONE ACETATE

Because of low solubility, has a sustained effect.

Systemic: Not for IV use. When used as temporary substitute for oral therapy, total daily dose is administered as a single IM injection. For prolonged effect, a single weekly dose may be given.

Adrenogenital syndrome: 40 mg (as single injection) every 2 weeks.

Rheumatoid arthritis: Weekly IM maintenance dose will vary from 40 mg to 120 mg.

Dermatologic lesions: 40 mg/week to 120 mg/week for 1 to 4 weeks. In severe dermatitis (due to poison ivy), relief may result within 8 to 12 hours following single dose of 80 mg to 120 mg. In chronic dermatitis, repeated injection at 5- to 10-day intervals may be necessary. *Seborrheic dermatitis*—Weekly dose of 80 mg may be adequate.

Asthma, allergic rhinitis: 80 mg to 120 mg.

Intra-articular, soft tissue: *Large joints*—20 mg to 80 mg; *medium joints*—10 mg to 40 mg; *small joints*—4 mg to 10 mg; *ganglia, tendinitis, epicondylitis, bursitis*—4 mg to 30 mg.

Intralesional: 20 mg to 60 mg.

Retention enema: Usual dose is 40 mg given as a retention enema or by continuous drip, three to seven times weekly, for 2 or more weeks.

METHYLPREDNISOLONE SODIUM SUCCINATE

Highly soluble; has rapid effect by IV or IM route.

Initial dose: May vary from 10 mg/day to 40 mg/day IV over 1 to several minutes. Subsequent doses are given IV or IM. Dosages for infants and children should not be less than 0.5 mg/kg q24h. *For high-dose therapy*—30 mg/kg IV, infused over 10 to 20 minutes. May be repeated q4h to q6h for 48 hours.

PARAMETHASONE ACETATE

Initial dosage may vary from 2 mg/day to 24 mg/day.

PREDNISOLONE

Initial dosage may vary from 5 mg/day to 60 mg/day.

Multiple sclerosis: In treatment of acute exacerbations, daily doses of 200 mg for a week are followed by 80 mg every other day for 1 month.

PREDNISOLONE ACETATE

Relatively insoluble and slowly absorbed.

Systemic: Not for IV use. Initial dosage may vary from 4 mg/day to 60 mg/day IM.

Intralesional, intra-articular, soft-tissue injection: Dosage varies depending on size and site of lesion and severity of condition. May range from 5 mg up to 100 mg for large joints.

PREDNISOLONE ACETATE AND PREDNISOLONE SODIUM PHOSPHATE

Combined acetate and phosphate salts provide both rapid onset and prolonged activity.

Systemic: Not for IV use. Treatment is initiated with 0.25 ml to 1 ml IM; this is repeated within several days, up to 3 to 4 weeks, or more often as necessary. In dermatologic conditions, results are often achieved with 1 ml IM at intervals of several days, up to 3 to 4 weeks, or more often as necessary. In respiratory tract disorders, onset of relief of symptoms and effective control have occurred with injections of 0.5 ml to 1 ml, at intervals of several days, up to 3 to 4 weeks or more often as necessary.

Intra-articular or intrasynovial injection: 0.25 ml to 1 ml.

PREDNISOLONE SODIUM PHOSPHATE

Highly soluble and rapid acting; has short duration of action.

Systemic: For IV or IM use. Initial dose may vary from 4 mg/day to 60 mg/day.

Intra-articular, intralesional, soft tissue: Large joints—10 mg to 20 mg; *small joints*—4 mg to 5 mg; *bursae*—10 mg to 15 mg; *tendon sheaths*—2 mg to 5 mg; *soft-tissue infiltration*—10 mg to 30 mg; *ganglia*—5 mg to 10 mg.

PREDNISOLONE TEBUTATE

An insoluble salt of prednisolone having a slow onset and prolonged duration of action.

Intra-articular, intralesional, soft tissue: Large joints—20 mg to 30 mg; *small joints*—8 mg to 10 mg; *bursae*—20 mg to 30 mg; *tendon sheaths*—4 mg to 10 mg; *ganglia*—10 mg to 20 mg.

PREDNISONE

Initial dosage may vary from 5 mg/day to 60 mg/day. Prednisone is inactive and must be converted to prednisolone. This conversion may be impaired in those with liver disease.

Physiologic replacement, children: 0.1 mg/kg/day to 0.15 mg/kg/day or 4 mg/m^2/day to 5 mg/m^2/day, divided q12h.

TRIAMCINOLONE

Initial daily dosage in specific disorders is as follows.

Adrenocortical insufficiency—4 mg to 12 mg in addition to mineralocorticoid therapy. *Rheumatic and dermatologic disorders, bronchial asthma*—8 mg to 16 mg. *Systemic lupus erythematosus*—20 mg to 32 mg. *Acute rheumatic carditis*—20 mg to 60 mg. *Allergic states*—8 mg to 12 mg. *Ophthalmologic diseases*—12 mg to 40 mg. *Respiratory diseases*—16 mg to 48 mg. *Hematologic disorders*—16 mg to 60 mg. *Acute leukemia in children*—1 mg/kg to 2 mg/kg. *Acute leukemia and lymphoma in adults*—16 mg to 40 mg, although it may be necessary to give as much as 100 mg/day in leukemia. *Edematous states*—16 mg to 20 mg (up to 48 mg)

until diuresis occurs. *Tuberculous meningitis*—32 mg to 48 mg.

TRIAMCINOLONE ACETONIDE

Relatively insoluble; is slowly absorbed and has prolonged action.

Systemic: Not for IV use. Initial IM dose may vary from 2.5 mg/day to 60 mg/day depending on disease entity treated.

Intra-articular or intrabursal and injection into tendon sheaths: Initial dose may vary from 2.5 mg to 5 mg for smaller joints and from 5 mg to 15 mg for larger joints. For adults, doses up to 10 mg for smaller areas and up to 40 mg for larger areas have usually been sufficient.

Intradermal: Only 10 mg/ml solution is used. Initial dose will vary but is limited to 1 mg/injection site.

TRIAMCINOLONE DIACETATE

Slightly soluble, providing an intermediate onset and duration of effect.

Systemic: Not for IV use. May be given IM for initial therapy, which provides a sustained or depot action that can be used to supplement or replace initial oral therapy. Average dose is 40 mg IM once a week. A single parenteral dose four to seven times the oral daily dose may be expected to control patient from 4 to 7 days up to 3 to 4 weeks.

Intra-articular, intrasynovial: 5 mg to 40 mg.

Intralesional, sublesional: 5 mg to 48 mg. No more than 12.5 mg per injection site should be used. An average of 25 mg per lesion is the usual limit.

TRIAMCINOLONE HEXACETONIDE

Relatively insoluble; is slowly absorbed and has prolonged action. Not for IV use.

Intra-articular: 2 mg to 20 mg average. *Large joints*—10 mg to 20 mg; *small joints*—2 mg to 6 mg.

Intralesional, sublesional: Up to 0.5 mg/sq in of affected area.

NURSING IMPLICATIONS

HISTORY

See Appendix 4. Note history of psychiatric disorders, travel history.

PHYSICAL ASSESSMENT

Base on diagnosis and symptoms; assess systems involved. Obtain vital signs, weight. Baseline laboratory studies may include CBC, serum electrolytes, and urinalysis. Other laboratory tests and diagnostic studies may also be appropriate.

ADMINISTRATION

Parenteral administration: Take proper precautions (availability of oxygen, vasopressors, antihistamines) in administration by this route to those with history of allergies.

Generally, glucocorticoids are not administered subcutaneously (*exception*—hydrocortisone sodium phosphate).

Hydrocortisone sodium succinate and some brands of methylprednisolone sodium succinate are supplied with a separate diluent or as a single vial with a diluent (Univial, monovial, Mix-O-Vial). Reconstitute powder according to manufacturer's directions supplied with the drug.

Suspension solutions must be agitated immediately before withdrawing from the vial.

IV administration: Read label carefully because some parenteral forms may *not* be administered intravenously.

IM injections: Avoid use of the deltoid muscle; rotate sites of injection and chart site used.

Intralesional, intra-articular, soft-tissue administration: Performed by physician. Large needle (20 gauge to 22 gauge) may be used to withdraw drug from vial. Inquire of physician needle size required for administration.

Retention enema: Physician may order sedation or antidiarrheal agent (especially early in therapy) before administration to facilitate retention of the enema.

Administer retention enema H.S. Place patient on left side during administration. Exercise care in inserting enema tip to avoid trauma to rectal mucosa.

Instruct patient to remain lying on left side for at least 30 minutes and to retain liquid for at least 1 hour and preferably all night.

Alternate-day therapy: Drug must be given before 9:00 A.M. Be sure medication card is clearly labeled, showing that drug is given every other day. To avoid errors, write "every other day" instead of "qod." Select odd or even dates for administration. At end of months with 31 days, change from even to odd or from odd to even dates.

GENERIC NAME SIMILARITY

Prednisone and prednisolone.

TRADE NAME SIMILARITY

There are many similar trade names. Some examples are Dexone and Dezone, Decadrol and Decadron (dexamethasone sodium phosphate), Dexone (dexamethasone sodium phosphate) and Dexone LA (dexamethasone acetate). PSP-IV (brand of prednisolone sodium phosphate) should not be confused with initials for phenolsulfonphthalein (PSP) test for renal function, which is also given IV.

The physician's order and drug labels should be checked carefully when administering glucocorticoids because of the many trade name similarities.

ONGOING ASSESSMENTS AND NURSING MANAGEMENT

Daily assessments and the frequency of some assessments depend on disease entity being treated.

CLINICAL ALERT: Glucocorticoids must *never* be abruptly discontinued following prolonged therapy (more than 5 days). When therapy is to be terminated, the dose *must be tapered* (decreased) *gradually* and in *small increments.* Tapered dose schedules are variable and dependent on dose administered and length of therapy. If there is any question or doubt about the physician's order for discontinuing the drug or tapering the dose, the nurse has an obligation to pursue proper channels in clarifying these orders.

Doses of glucocorticoid preparations are *not* to be omitted. Ensure continuity of prescribed therapy by notation on the Kardex, informing health-team members responsible for drug administration.

During withdrawal therapy following long-term or high-dose administration, observe patient for signs of adrenal insufficiency (Appendix 6, section 6-3), even when dosage is being tapered gradually.

Following prolonged therapy, abrupt discontinuation may result in withdrawal syndrome with fever, myalgia, athralgia, and malaise, which may occur without evidence of adrenal insufficiency (Appendix 6, section 6-3).

During withdrawal therapy, increased supplementation of glucocorticoids may be necessary during periods of stress (*e.g.*, surgery, physical or emotional trauma).

Patients scheduled for surgery or in a prolonged fasting state for laboratory or diagnostic studies must *not* have glucocorticoid therapy interrupted. If parenteral administration has not been ordered, contact physician immediately.

Record vital signs daily to q4h or more often if condition warrants. Notify physician if blood pressure increases.

Evaluate drug response daily (more frequently if glucocorticoid is used for emergency situations). Base evaluation on patient's original symptoms, disease entity being treated. Record observations.

Weigh daily to weekly. Notify physician if significant weight gain occurs or edema of extremities is noted.

Observe for signs of electrolyte imbalance, especially hypocalcemia, hypokalemia, and hypernatremia (Appendix 6, sections 6-13, 6-15, and 6-17). Notify physician if signs of these occur because drug dosage may need to be decreased or other treatment instituted.

When glucocorticoids are administered for shock, monitor blood pressure, pulse, and respiratory rate q3m to q10m. Keep physician continually informed of patient's response to drug.

Observe for adverse effects, many of which occur during long-term therapy or when high doses are administered. Development of some adverse effects (*e.g.,* cushingoid appearance) may be gradual.

Observe for signs of mental changes (especially in those with history of psychiatric disorders); document accurately. Keep physician informed of behavioral changes. Depression requires close patient observation.

Observe for signs of infection, which may be masked by glucocorticoid therapy. Report any slight rise in temperature, sore throat, other signs of infection.

Because of possible decreased resistance to infection, nursing personnel and visitors with an infection (*e.g.,* sore throat, upper respiratory infection) or recent exposure to a communicable disease (*e.g.,* chickenpox) should avoid patient contact.

Diabetics may require adjustments of diet or dose of insulin or oral hypogycemic agent. Check urine for glucose and ketone bodies qid. Notify physician of any increase in urine glucose or if urine is positive for ketones.

Check urine of nondiabetic patient for glucose weekly because glucocorticoids may aggravate latent diabetes.

Encourage a liberal protein intake. Contact dietitian if diet is taken poorly because protein supplements may be necessary.

Dietary adjustment to compensate for sodium retention or increased potassium excretion may be prescribed.

Children on prolonged glucocorticoid therapy during growth years may experience growth retardation. Measure and record height and weight at time of clinic or office visit.

Infants born of mothers receiving these drugs should be frequently assessed for signs of hypoadrenalism (Appendix 6, section 6-3). Any change in the neonate's condition must be reported to the physician immediately.

Patients on long-term therapy, especially if immobilized or allowed only limited activity, are observed for signs of compression fractures of the vertebrae (back, chest, neck pain) and pathologic fractures of long bones, especially if patient falls or is injured. Extra supervision may be necessary if the patient is confused or prone to accidents.

Periodic laboratory tests and diagnostic studies may be performed during prolonged therapy and may include CBC, serum electrolytes, 2-hour postprandial blood glucose, fasting blood sugar, and chest x-ray examination.

Monitor laboratory studies, especially serum electrolytes and CBC; bring increases or decreases to the attention of the physician.

Peptic ulcer has been associated with glucocorticoid therapy. Observe for epigastric burning, discomfort, or pain; tarry stools. If tarry stools are noted, save specimen for physician's inspection and laboratory confirmation of melena.

Oral administration: If patient experiences nausea, vomiting, or diarrhea, contact physician immediately because drug may need to be given by the parenteral route.

Parenteral administration: Observe for anaphylactoid reactions, especially in those with history of allergies.

When administered IV for acute respiratory disorder (*e.g.,* bronchial asthma, drug hypersensitivity reactions) monitor drug response q5m to q15m. Additional treatment (*e.g.,* antihistamines, oxygen) may also be instituted.

Intra-articular administration: May require limitation of motion of involved joints. Clarify with physician limitations to be imposed and the correct alignment of the resting joint. Depending on joint involved, patient may require assistance with ambulation and activities of daily living. Observe for marked increase in joint pain with local swelling; further restriction of motion; fever; malaise. If these occur, notify physician because additional treatment may be necessary.

Retention enema: Record number and appearance of bowel movements daily.

Glucocorticoid can be absorbed systemically. Observe for adverse effects of glucocorticoid administration (p 517).

Record length of time enema is retained.

Notify physician if patient complains of local pain or burning or rectal bleeding is apparent.

Patient may, through trial and error, develop methods to prolong retention of the enema solution (*e.g.,* elevating hips on pillows, refraining from any food or drink for 2 or more hours before administration, lying quietly for 30 to 60 minutes before administration. The nurse should encourage the patient to discover those methods that may encourage retention.

Short-term therapy: Take exactly as directed on prescription container. Taper the dose as directed.

Do not omit, increase, or decrease dose during treatment or withdrawal period.

If problem does not improve, contact physician.

Intra-articular injection: Follow physician's recommendations about exercise and activity. Do not overuse or subject the treated area to stress until problem is corrected.

If problem does not improve or there is a marked increase in pain or local swelling, contact physician.

Intralesional injection: Do not use other medications on the treated area unless use has been approved or prescribed by the physician.

Retention enema: Use as directed by physician.

Directions are included with product.

If symptoms (diarrhea and bleeding) do not improve in approximately 5 days, notify physician.

Notify physician or nurse if local pain or burning occurs.

Alternate-day therapy: Take before 9:00 A.M. every other day.

Use a calendar to identify days, or take the drug on odd- or even-numbered days. When month has 31 days, change from even- to odd- or from odd- to even-numbered days at the end of the month.

Do not stop taking drug unless advised to do so by physician.

If problem is not relieved or becomes worse (especially on "off" days), contact physician.

NOTE: Some teaching points given under long-term or high-dose therapy may apply to those on alternate-day therapy.

Long-term and/or high-dose therapy: Drug must not be omitted or dosage increased or decreased except on advice of a physician.

Inform other physicians, dentist, and other health-care personnel of therapy with this drug *before* any examination, treatment (including administration or prescribing of other drugs), or therapy is instituted.

Do not take any nonprescription drug unless use has been approved by physician.

Whenever possible, avoid exposure to infections. Contact physician if minor cuts or abrasions fail to heal, persistent joint swelling or tenderness is noted, or fever, sore throat, upper respiratory infection, or other signs of illness or infections occur.

If drug cannot be taken orally (due to nausea, vomiting) or if diarrhea occurs, contact physician immediately. If unable to contact physician before next dose is due, go to the emergency department of a hospital (preferably the hospital where treatment originated) because parenteral administration of drug and other treatment may be required.

Weigh self weekly. If weight gain or swelling of the extremities is noted, contact physician.

Dietary modification may be recommended by the physician and is an important part of therapy. (Patient may need to be given printed dietary instructions, diet plan, or list of foods to be avoided.)

Wear a medical identification tag or bracelet, such as Medic-Alert, to provide medical personnel with full information if an emergency occurs.

Adhere to physician's recommendations about periodic eye examinations and laboratory tests. Keep all clinic or office visits.

Children on long-term or lifetime replacement therapy: Physician may recommend periodic height and weight measurements. Measure height in bare feet standing against a wall (printed charts are available in stores). Weigh with approximately same type and amount of clothing (*e.g.,* underwear, pajamas) each time. Keep a record of all measurements.

Diabetic patients: Follow physician's recommendations about frequency of urine testing, dietary adjustments, and insulin or oral hypoglycemic dose changes.

Female patient: Menstrual irregularities may occur. Consult physician if there is a significant change in menstrual pattern or flow.

Glucose otc

| gel: liquid glucose (40% dextrose) | Glutose, Insta-Glucose, Monojel |
| tablets, chewable: 5 g | B-D Glucose |

INDICATIONS
Management of hypoglycemia.

ACTIONS
Is a monosaccharide that is absorbed from the intestine after administration and then utilized, distributed, and stored by the tissues. Direct absorption takes place, giving an increased blood glucose

concentration quickly. Is effective in small doses; no evidence of toxicity reported.

ADVERSE REACTIONS
Isolated reports of nausea, which may also occur with hypoglycemia.

DOSAGE
Give 10 g to 15 g PO; repeat in 10 minutes if necessary. Response should be noted in 10 minutes. Must be swallowed to be effective because glucose is not absorbed from the buccal cavity. Not given to children under 2 years.

NURSING IMPLICATIONS

PHYSICAL ASSESSMENT
Recognition of signs of hypoglycemia (Appendix 6, section 6-14) is followed by immediate intervention. Depending on hospital or unit policy, a blood glucose sample may be drawn immediately prior to administration of an agent to correct hypoglycemia.

ADMINISTRATION

CLINICAL ALERT: Do not give to an unconscious or semiconscious patient. Swallowing and gag reflexes must be present. Lack of the gag reflex may result in aspiration.

A suction machine should be immediately available when oral carbohydrate is administered. Suction patient if gagging or apparent aspiration of solution occurs.

Products are flavored. Insta-Glucose is packaged in unit-dose tube; Glutose is packaged in a bottle.

ONGOING ASSESSMENTS AND NURSING MANAGEMENT
Administration usually produces a response in 10 minutes. Dosage may be repeated, if necessary.

Stay with patient until response occurs.

Have emesis basin also available because nausea and vomiting may occur.

CLINICAL ALERT: It is important that hypoglycemia be recognized and corrected as soon as possible. Prolonged hypoglycemia can result in cortical damage.

Obtain urine sample; test for glucose and ketones. Continue to test urine at 1- to 2-hour intervals or as ordered, until patient stabilizes. Blood glucose sample may also be ordered.

The physician must be notified when hypoglycemic reactions occur so that the dose of insulin may be adjusted more accurately.

Review events preceding the hypoglycemic reaction, including dietary intake, time insulin was administered, dose of insulin, and urine test results.

Continue to monitor patient at q1h to q2h intervals for next 6 to 8 or more hours (depending on type of insulin administered).

PATIENT AND FAMILY INFORMATION
Use according to instructions of physician.

Physician may advise product be carried at all times.

Notify physician when a hypoglycemic reaction has occurred; an adjustment in insulin dose or dietary allowances may be necessary.

Glutamic Acid Hydrochloride *otc*

tablets: 325 mg	*Generic*
capsules: 340 mg	Acidulin Pulvules

Combination Products

tablets: 500 mg glutamic acid hydrochloride and 35 mg pepsin	Muripsin
tablets: 325 mg glutamic acid, 195 mg betaine hydrochloride, 65 mg pepsin, and 167 mg pancreatic enzyme concentrate in an enteric-coated core	Milco-Zyme

INDICATIONS
These products are gastric acidifiers administered to counterbalance a deficiency of hydrochloric acid in the gastric juice and to destroy or inhibit growth of putrefactive microorganisms in ingested food. A deficiency of hydrochloric acid is often associated with pernicious anemia, certain allergies, chronic gastritis, gastric carcinoma, and congenital achlorhydria.

CONTRAINDICATIONS
Should not be used in patients with gastric hyperacidity or peptic ulcer.

OVERDOSAGE
Massive overdosage may produce systemic acidosis. Treatment includes alkalies, such as sodium bicarbonate or sodium r-lactate solution, one molar (to be diluted).

G

DOSAGE

Glutamic acid HCl: One to three capsules or tablets tid before meals.

Muripsin: One to two tablets with each meal. Swallow whole with water.

Milco-Zyme: One after each meal.

NURSING IMPLICATIONS

HISTORY

Obtain description and duration of symptoms; review chart for history (*e.g.,* gastric carcinoma, pernicious anemia).

ADMINISTRATION

See *Dosage* above.

ONGOING ASSESSMENTS AND NURSING MANAGEMENT

Deficiency of hydrochloric acid may result in vague GI symptoms, which may or may not be relieved by these drugs.

PATIENT INFORMATION

If gastrointestinal symptoms persist, consult a physician.

Glutethimide Rx C–III

tablets: 250 mg, 500 mg	Doriden, *Generic*
capsules: 500 mg	*Generic*

INDICATIONS

Short-term relief (3–7 days) of insomnia. Not indicated for chronic administration. Should insomnia persist, a drug-free interval of 1 or more weeks should elapse before retreatment is considered. Attempts should be made to find alternative nondrug therapy in chronic insomnia.

CONTRAINDICATIONS

Hypersensitivity.

ACTIONS

Produces CNS depression similar to that produced by barbiturates; precise mechanism of action not known. Exhibits profound anticholinergic activity, which is manifested by mydriasis, inhibition of salivary secretions, and intestinal motility. Suppresses REM sleep and its associated with REM rebound. It is erratically absorbed from the GI tract; following single dose of 500 mg, erratic and wide variations in absorption observed. Peak plasma concentrations occur from 1 to 6 hours after administration. Average plasma half-life is 10 to 12 hours. About 50% of drug is bound to plasma proteins. Glutethimide stimulates hepatic microsomal enzymes. Drug is excreted in the urine.

WARNINGS

Physical and psychological dependence: Both occur; therefore, patient is carefully evaluated before drug is prescribed. Usually, an amount for 1 week is sufficient. Patient is reevaluated before represcribing, after an interval of 1 or more weeks. Withdrawal symptoms include nausea, abdominal discomfort, tremors, convulsions, and delirium. Newborn infants of mothers dependent on glutethimide may also exhibit withdrawal symptoms. In the presence of dependence, dosage reduced gradually.

Use in pregnancy: Not recommended.

Use in children: Safety, efficacy not established.

PRECAUTIONS

May impair ability to perform hazardous tasks requiring alertness or physical coordination.

DRUG INTERACTIONS

Additive depressant effects may occur when used concomitantly with **CNS depressants** (including **alcohol**). Glutethimide induces hepatic microsomal enzymes, resulting in increased metabolism of **coumarin anticoagulants** and decreased anticoagulant response. Additive effects may occur when used with other **anticholinergic agents.**

ADVERSE REACTIONS

Most common: Osteomalacia after long-term use; generalized skin rash, occasionally purpuric or urticarial. Rash usually clears within a few days after withdrawal.

Rare: Nausea; hangover; paradoxical excitation; blurred vision; acute hypersensitivity reactions; porphyria; blood dyscrasias (*i.e.,* thrombocytopenic purpura, aplastic anemia, leukopenia); exfoliative dermatitis.

OVERDOSAGE

Acute overdosage: Lethal dose ranges from 10 g to 20 g; patients have died from 5 g and others survived doses as high as 35 g. A single dose of 5 g usually produces severe intoxication. A plasma level of 3 mg/dl is indicative of severe poisoning but level may be lower because of sequestration of drug in body fat depots and in the GI tract. A lower level does not preclude the possibility of severe poisoning. Serial plasma levels are mandatory for proper patient evaluation.

Symptoms: Are dose dependent and indistinguishable from those of barbiturate intoxication. The degree of CNS depression often fluctuates.

Symptoms include CNS depression, including coma (profound and prolonged in severe intoxication); hypothermia, which may be followed by fever; depressed or lost deep-tendon reflexes; depression or absence of corneal and pupillary reflexes; dilatation of pupils; depressed or absent response to painful stimuli; inadequate ventilation (even with relatively normal respiratory rate), sometimes with cyanosis; sudden apnea, especially with manipulation such as gastric lavage or endotracheal intubation; diminished or absent peristalsis. Severe hypotension unresponsive to volume expansion, tonic muscular spasms, twitching, and convulsions may occur.

Treatment: Cardiopulmonary supportive measures should include maintenance of a patent airway with assisted ventilation, if needed; monitoring of vital signs and level of consciousness; continuous ECG monitoring to detect arrhythmias; maintenance of blood pressure with plasma volume expanders; and, if absolutely essential, pressor drugs.

Vomiting is induced only if patient conscious. Institute gastric lavage in all cases, regardless of elapsed time since ingestion; use caution to prevent aspiration or respiratory arrest. Lavage with a 1:1 mixture of castor oil and water is more effective than an aqueous lavage. Leave 50 ml of castor oil in the stomach as a cathartic. Delay absorption by giving activated charcoal and water. Follow up as soon as possible with production of emesis or lavage. Intestinal lavage may be used to remove unabsorbed drug. Use 100 ml to 250 ml of 20% to 40% sorbitol or mannitol.

If coma is prolonged, monitor and maintain urinary output while preventing overhydration, which might contribute to pulmonary or cerebral edema. Hemodialysis or hemoperfusion may be considered in Grade III or Grade IV coma, when renal shutdown or impaired renal function is manifest, and in life-threatening situations complicated by pulmonary edema, heart failure, circulatory collapse, significant liver disease, major metabolic disturbances, or uremia. While aqueous hemodialysis is less effective, blood levels may decline more rapidly with hemodialysis and the duration of coma may be shortened. Use of pure food grade soybean oil as dialysate enhances removal by hemodialysis. Peritoneal dialysis is of minimal value. Charcoal hemoperfusion has been reported to be simpler and more effective than hemodialysis.

Continue drug extraction techniques for at least 2 hours after patient regains consciousness. As the drug is removed from the bloodstream by any technique, it is gradually released from fat storage back into the bloodstream. Even after substantial quantities have been extracted, this blood-level rebound can cause coma to persist or recur.

Chronic overdosage: Symptoms include impairment of memory and ability to concentrate; impaired gait; ataxia; tremors; hyporeflexia; slurred speech. Abrupt discontinuation frequently causes withdrawal reactions including nervousness; grand mal seizures; abdominal cramping; chills; numbness of extremities; and dysphagia. Treatment includes gradual, stepwise reduction of dosage over a period of days or weeks; if withdrawal symptoms occur, drug is readministered or pentobarbital is substituted and subsequently withdrawn gradually.

DOSAGE

Dosage is individualized. Usual adult dose is 250 mg to 500 mg H.S. For elderly or debilitated patients, the initial daily dosage should not exceed 500 mg H.S. Patients with unrelieved pain should not be heavily sedated.

NURSING IMPLICATIONS

HISTORY
See Appendix 4.

PHYSICAL ASSESSMENT
Determine if specific factors that may be controlled or eliminated are interfering with sleep. Factors may include noise, bright lights, pain, and discomfort.

ADMINISTRATION
Patient's immediate area should be free from disturbance (*e.g.,* noise, lights) before a hypnotic is given.

Do not administer if patient has pain, which should be controlled by administration of an analgesic.

Do not administer a hypnotic shortly before or after administration of a narcotic analgesic (both are CNS depressants). If patient has an order for a narcotic analgesic (or any other CNS depressant) and a hypnotic, check with physician regarding time interval between administration of these agents. Usually 2 or more hours should elapse between administration of a hypnotic and administration of an other CNS depressant, but interval may vary with a specific CNS depressant and the dose administered.

Raise siderails and advise patient to remain in bed and call for assistance if it is necessary to get out of bed during the night.

ONGOING ASSESSMENTS AND NURSING MANAGEMENT
Observe patient in 1 hour to evaluate effect of drug.

G

If skin rash occurs, notify physician before next dose is due. Purpuric or urticarial skin manifestations require discontinuing drug.

If paradoxical excitation occurs, patient should be closely observed until effect of drug has worn off. In some instances, restraints may be required to protect patient from injury. Inform physician if paradoxical response occurs, because different drug or lower dose may be required.

PATIENT AND FAMILY INFORMATION

Medication will cause drowsiness, dizziness, or blurred vision. It is advisable to remain in bed once drug is taken for sleep. *Do not* attempt to drive or perform tasks requiring alertness after taking this drug.

Do not drink alcohol before or after taking this drug because the combination can be dangerous.

Avoid use of CNS depressants while taking this drug.

Do not exceed the prescribed dosage. If drug is ineffective, discuss problem with physician.

Notify physician if skin rash occurs.

Glyburide

See Sulfonylureas.

Glycerin (Glycerol) Rx

| solution: 50% | Osmoglyn |
| solution: 75% | Glyrol |

INDICATIONS

For use before surgery done under local anesthesia, such as glaucoma surgery, cataract surgery, and other ocular surgery, when a preoperative reduction of intraocular pressure is indicated. See also Laxatives.

CONTRAINDICATIONS

Hypersensitivity.

ACTIONS

An oral osmotic agent for reducing intraocular pressure. The 50% solution contains 0.6 g glycerin/ml; 75% solution contains 0.94 g glycerin/ml.

WARNINGS

For oral use only; not for injection.

PRECAUTIONS

Use cautiously in hypervolemia, confused mental states, and congestive heart disease; also, in the elderly, senile, and diabetic patient and severely dehydrated individuals. Take measures to avoid acute urinary retention in the preoperative period.

ADVERSE REACTIONS

Occasionally, nausea, vomiting, diarrhea, headache, confusion, disorientation. Severe dehydration, cardiac arrhythmia, and hyperosmolar nonketotic coma, which may result in death, have been reported.

DOSAGE

1 g to 1.5 g of glycerin/kg, 1 to 1½ hours before surgery.

NURSING IMPLICATIONS

HISTORY

See Appendix 4.

PHYSICAL ASSESSMENT

Review chart for physician's examination. Obtain routine preoperative vital signs.

ADMINISTRATION

Administer orally as preoperative medication. Give only when a local anesthetic is being administered.

ONGOING ASSESSMENTS AND NURSING MANAGEMENT

If nausea, vomiting, diarrhea, confusion, or disorientation occurs before transportation to surgery, notify surgeon immediately.

Glycopyrrolate

See Gastrointestinal Anticholinergics/Antispasmodics.

Gold Compounds

Aurothioglucose Rx

| injection: 50 mg/ml | Solganal |

Gold Sodium Thiomalate Rx

| injection: 10 mg/ml, 25 mg/ml, 50 mg/ml | Myochrysine |

INDICATIONS

Adjunctive treatment of selected cases of active rheumatoid arthritis, both adult and juvenile types.

Greatest benefit occurs in the early active stages of the illness. In late stages, when cartilage and bone damage have occurred, gold can only check the progression of rheumatoid arthritis and prevent further structural damage to joints. It cannot repair damage caused by previously active disease.

CONTRAINDICATIONS
Uncontrolled diabetes; severe debilitation; renal disease; hepatic dysfunction or history of infectious hepatitis; marked hypertension; heart failure; systemic lupus erythematosus; agranulocytosis or hemorrhagic diathesis; blood dyscrasias; those who have recently had radiation; those who have developed severe toxicity from previous exposure to gold or other heavy metals; urticaria; eczema; colitis. Gold therapy usually contraindicated in pregnancy.

ACTIONS
Gold suppresses or prevents, but does not cure, arthritis and synovitis. Localized high concentrations of gold are found in Kupffer cell and synoviocyte lysosomes, which suggests that gold may inhibit lysosomal activity in macrophages and decrease macrophage phagocytic activity. Accumulation occurs and levels persist for many years in subsynovial tissues and in the macrophages of many tissues. Macrophages are involved in the antigen process and in the interaction of helper T-lymphocytes with antibody forming B-lymphocytes. However, the exact mode of action in rheumatoid arthritis is unknown.

Gold is rapidly absorbed; after IM administration peak levels are produced in 4 to 6 hours. Gold compounds are 95% bound to serum albumin. Storage in human tissues is dependent on organ mass as well as the concentration of gold. Major depots, in decreasing order of total gold content, are bone marrow, liver, skin, and bone. Highest concentrations are found in lymph nodes, adrenal glands, liver, kidneys, bone marrow, and spleen. Relatively small concentrations are found in articular structures. Concentrations in synovial fluid are about one-half that of serum. Arthritic joints contain more than twice as much gold as uninvolved joints. An initial 10 mg IM dose has a half-life of 1 day; this extends to 3 to 7 days after a 50-mg dose. Half-life increases with successive weekly injections. After the initial injection, serum level of gold rises sharply and declines over the next week. Weekly administration produces a continuous rise in basal value for several months, after which the serum level becomes relatively stable. A steady decline in gold levels occurs when the interval between injections is lengthened; small amounts may be found in the serum for months after discontinuance of therapy. Incidence of toxic reactions is apparently unrelated to the plasma level of gold but may be related to the cumulative body content.

WARNINGS
Rapid reduction of hemoglobin, leukopenia below 4000 WBC/mm^3, eosinophilia above 5%, platelet decrease below 100,000/mm^3, proteinuria, hematuria, pruritus, skin eruption, stomatitis, jaundice, and petechiae are considered signs of possible gold toxicity. Additional injections are not given until further studies show these abnormalities are caused by conditions other than gold toxicity.

Diabetes mellitus or congestive heart failure should be under control before therapy is instituted. Extreme caution is indicated in those with history of blood dyscrasias such as granulocytopenia or anemia caused by drug sensitivity; allergy or hypersensitivity to drugs; previous kidney or liver disease; marked hypertension, compromised cerebral or cardiovascular circulation.

Effects that may occur immediately after an injection or at any time during therapy include anaphylactic shock; syncope; bradycardia; thickening of the tongue, difficulty in swallowing and breathing; angioneurotic edema. If such effects are observed, treatment is discontinued.

Concomitant therapy: Use of salicylates, nonsteroidal anti-inflammatory agents, and systemic corticosteroids may be continued when gold therapy is instituted. After improvement begins, these agents may be slowly discontinued as symptoms permit.

Use in elderly: Tolerance to gold usually decreases with age.

Use in pregnancy: Use only when clearly needed and when potential benefits outweigh the unknown potential hazards to the fetus.

Use in lactation: Gold has been demonstrated in the milk of lactating mothers. Because of the potential for serious adverse reactions in nursing infants, a decision should be made whether to discontinue nursing or discontinue gold therapy.

Use in children: Safety and efficacy for use of aurothioglucose in children under 6 are not established.

DRUG INTERACTIONS
Do not use **penicillamine** or **antimalarials** with gold salts. Safety of coadministration with immunosuppressive agents other than corticosteroids not established. Safety of coadministration with **cytotoxic drugs** not established.

ADVERSE REACTIONS
May occur at any time during treatment or many months after therapy is discontinued. Adverse reactions are most frequently observed when the cumu-

lative dose of gold thiomalate is between 400 mg and 800 mg. Severe effects from aurothioglucose therapy are most common after 300 mg to 500 mg has been used.

Cutaneous: Dermatitis is most common reaction. Any eruption, especially if pruritic, should be considered a reaction to gold until proven otherwise. Pruritus often exists before dermatitis becomes apparent and is considered a warning sign of impending cutaneous reaction. Erythema and occasionally more severe reactions, such as papular, vesicular, and exfoliative dermatitis leading to alopecia and shedding nails, may occur. Chrysiasis (gray to blue pigmentation caused by deposition of gold in tissues) has been reported, especially on photoexposed areas. Gold dermatitis may be aggravated by exposure to sunlight or an actinic rash may develop.

Mucous membranes: Stomatitis is the second most common adverse reaction. Shallow ulcers on the buccal membranes, on borders of the tongue, and on the palate or in the pharynx may occur. Diffuse glossitus or gingivitis may develop. A metallic taste may precede these reactions and should be considered a warning signal. Inflammation of the upper respiratory tract, pharyngitis, gastritis, colitis, tracheitis, vaginitis, and rarely conjunctivitis have been reported.

Pulmonary: Interstitial pneumonitis and fibrosis have been reported. Fever, rash, cough, shortness of breath, and mouth ulcers that develop during therapy may be indicative of widespread interstitial and alveolar infiltrates. Pulmonary symptoms may or may not resolve after therapy is discontinued.

Renal: May produce a nephrotic syndrome or glomerulitis with hematuria. These reactions are usually mild and subside completely if recognized early and treatment is discontinued. They may become severe and chronic if treatment is continued after onset of the reaction. Gold is sometimes implicated in acute renal failure secondary to acute tubular necrosis, acute nephritis, or degeneration of the proximal tubular epithelium. It is important to perform a urinalysis before each injection; therapy is discontinued if proteinuria or hematuria develops.

Hematologic: Blood dyscrasia due to toxicity is rare but because of the potentially serious consequences, it must be watched for and recognized early by frequent blood examinations throughout treatment. Granulocytopenia; thrombocytopenia with or without purpura; leukopenia; eosinophilia; panmyelopathy; hemorrhagic diathesis; hypoplastic and aplastic anemia have been reported and may occur separately or in combinations.

Nitritoid and allergic: Reactions of the "nitritoid" type, which may resemble anaphylactic effects, have been reported. Flushing, fainting, dizziness, and sweating are most frequently reported. Other symptoms may include nausea, vomiting, malaise, weakness. More severe, but less common, effects include anaphylactic shock; syncope; bradycardia; thickening of the tongue; difficulty in swallowing and breathing; angioneurotic edema. These occur almost immediately after injection or as late as 10 minutes following injection. They may also occur any time during the course of therapy. If observed, treatment is discontinued.

Miscellaneous: GI reactions have been reported and include nausea, vomiting, colic, anorexia, abdominal cramps, diarrhea, and ulcerative enterocolitis. Some of these can be severe or even fatal. There have been reports of reactions involving the eye such as iritis, corneal ulcers, and gold deposits in ocular tissues. Hepatitis with jaundice, toxic hepatitis, cholestatic hepatitis, acute yellow atrophy, encephalitis, immunologic destruction of the synovia, EEG abnormalities, peripheral neuritis, gold bronchitis, partial or complete hair loss, fever, and headache also have been reported. Sometimes arthralgia occurs for a day or two after injection; this reaction usually subsides after the first few injections.

MANAGEMENT OF ADVERSE REACTIONS

Treatment should be discontinued immediately if toxic reactions occur. Minor complications such as localized dermatitis, mild stomatitis, or slight proteinuria generally require no other therapy and resolve spontaneously with suspension of therapy. Moderately severe skin and mucous membrane reactions often benefit from topical corticosteroids, oral antihistamines, and soothing or anesthetic lotions. If stomatitis or dermatitis becomes severe or more generalized, systemic corticosteroids may provide relief.

For serious renal, hematologic, pulmonary, and enterocolitic complications, high doses of systemic corticosteroids are recommended. Duration of corticosteroid treatment varies with response of individual patient but therapy may be required for many months when adverse effects are severe or progressive. In those whose complications do not improve with corticosteroid treatment or who develop significant steroid-related adverse reactions, a chelating agent may be given to enhance gold excretion. Dimercaprol has been used. Corticosteroids and a chelating agent may be used concomitantly. Adjunctive use of an anabolic steroid with other drugs (*e.g.,* dimercaprol, penicillamine, corticosteroids) may contribute to recovery of bone-marrow deficiency.

Therapy is not reinstituted after severe or idiosyncratic reactions, but may be readministered following resolution of mild reactions, using a reduced dosage schedule.

OVERDOSAGE

Symptoms: Overdosage resulting from too-rapid increases in dosing is manifested by rapid appearance of toxic reactions, particularly those relating to renal damage, such as hematuria and proteinuria, and to hematologic effects, such as thrombocytopenia and granulocytopenia. Other toxic effects, including fever, nausea, vomiting, diarrhea, and various skin disorders such as papulovesicular lesions, urticaria, and exfoliative dermatitis, all with severe pruritus, may develop.

Treatment: Promptly discontinue drug and administer dimercaprol. Specific supportive therapy should be given for renal and hematologic complications.

DOSAGE

Both drugs contain approximately 50% gold.

AUROTHIOGLUCOSE

Adults: Usual dosage schedule for IM administration is as follows: 1st dose, 10 mg; 2nd and 3rd doses, 25 mg; 4th and subsequent doses, 50 mg. Interval between doses is 1 week. The 50 mg dose is continued at weekly intervals until 0.8 g to 1 g has been given. If patient improved and exhibited no signs of toxicity, 50 mg dose may be continued many months longer, at 3- to 4-week intervals. A weekly dose above 50 mg is contraindicated. If no improvement is demonstrated after total administration of 1 g, therapy is reevaluated.

Children (6–12 years): One-fourth the adult dose, governed by body weight, not to exceed 25 mg/dose.

GOLD SODIUM THIOMALATE

Adults: Weekly injections as follows: 1st injection, 10 mg; 2nd injection, 25 mg; 3rd and subsequent injections 25 mg to 50 mg until major clinical improvement or toxicity occurs, or until cumulative dose reaches 1 g. If significant clinical improvement occurs before a cumulative dose of 1 g is administered, dose may be decreased or interval between injections increased as with maintenance therapy. Maintenance doses of 25 mg to 50 mg every other week for 2 to 20 weeks is recommended. If clinical course remains stable, injections of 25 mg to 50 mg may be given every third and subsequently every fourth week indefinitely. Should the arthritis exacerbate during maintenance therapy, weekly injections may be resumed temporarily until disease activity is suppressed. If patient fails to improve after 1 g, several options are available: (1) Patient may be considered unresponsive and drug discontinued; (2) the same dose (25 mg to 50 mg) may be continued for approximately 10 additional weeks; or (3) the dose may be increased in increments of 10 mg every 1 to 4 weeks, not to exceed 100 mg/injection. If significant clinical improvement occurs using the second or third option, the maintenance schedule (see above) is initiated.

Children: Pediatric dose is proportional to adult dose on a weight basis. After an initial test dose of 10 mg, recommended dose for children is 1 mg/kg, not to exceed 50 mg/injection. Guidelines given above for adults apply to children.

NURSING IMPLICATIONS

HISTORY

See Appendix 4. Note current treatment modalities (*e.g.,* drugs, diet, physical therapy, exercise allowed).

PHYSICAL ASSESSMENT

Examine and record description of involved joints noting appearance of joint, limitation of motion, appearance of skin over joint; evaluate ability to carry out activities of daily living. Pretreatment hemoglobin, RBC, WBC and differential, platelet count, and urinalysis are recommended. In women of childbearing age, pregnancy test is recommended.

ADMINISTRATION

Inspect vial of gold sodium thiomalate prior to use. Drug should not exceed pale yellow in color. Do not use if material has darkened.

Aurothioglucose must be thoroughly shaken in a horizontal position in order to suspend all active material. Heating vial to body temperature by immersing in warm water facilitates withdrawal from the vial. Use an 18-gauge 1½-inch needle for withdrawal and administration of the drug. A 2-inch needle should be used on obese patients. The syringe and needle must be dry.

Drug is administered deep IM, preferably in the upper outer quadrant of the gluteus muscle. These drugs are *never* given IV.

Rotate injection sites; record site used.

Patient should be lying down when injection given and remain recumbent for approximately 10 to 15 minutes after the injection.

Patient may require assistance in lying down, especially if arthritis involves the hip or back.

Storage: Both drugs should be stored in original containers and protected from light. Do not remove until ready for use.

ONGOING ASSESSMENTS AND NURSING MANAGEMENT

Obtain vital signs daily; observe for adverse reactions (see below); evaluate drug response (de-

G

crease in pain and stiffness, increase in joint mobility, decrease in joint swelling).

CLINICAL ALERT: Adverse reactions may occur any time during treatment or many months after therapy is discontinued. Review *Warnings* and *Adverse Reactions* carefully. Observe for the following: pruritus, which is a warning signal of impending cutaneous reaction; a metallic taste, which is a warning signal of mucous membrane reactions; fever, cough, and shortness of breath, which may indicate pulmonary toxicity; GI reactions (nausea, vomiting, diarrhea, colic, anorexia, abdominal cramps), which can be severe and sometimes fatal; and hematologic reactions including purpura, ecchymosis, and signs of bone-marrow depression (Appendix 6, section 6-8). Other severe (but less common) reactions include anaphylactic shock, syncope, bradycardia, thickening of the tongue, and difficulty in swallowing and breathing. Always notify the physician immediately if *any* adverse reaction is noted or suspected.

Good oral care is important. Patient may need assistance in brushing teeth, using a mouth rinse after each meal.

Short- and long-term goals should be established with primary consideration given to prevention of deformities and improvement in joint function.

If physical and occupational therapy are ordered, consult with therapists about methods that may be used to prevent joint deformity and increase range of joint motion.

Prior to each weekly injection, physician usually orders a urinalysis. Patient is also questioned thoroughly regarding development of adverse effects and the results of therapy (*e.g.,* relief of stiffness, pain, and improvement in joint function).

A CBC and platelet count is recommended prior to every second injection.

Periodic chest x-rays and pulmonary-function studies may be ordered.

PATIENT AND FAMILY INFORMATION

NOTE: The possibility of toxic reactions should be explained to patient before starting therapy. Patient should be warned to promptly report any symptoms suggesting toxicity.

Notify the physician or nurse promptly if any of the following occurs: itching, skin rash, hives, a metallic taste, sores in the mouth, redness of the mouth or tongue, fever, cough, shortness of breath, blood in the urine, sore throat, easy bruising or bleeding (gums, skin, cuts), malaise, weakness, nausea, vomiting, diarrhea, anorexia, abdominal cramping, yellowing of the skin, dark urine, fainting, or dizziness.

Arthralgia may occur for 1 to 2 days after an injection and this usually subsides after the first few injections.

Avoid exposure to sunlight.

If pregnancy is suspected, notify physician immediately. Brush teeth and rinse mouth well each time food is eaten. Physician will order frequent laboratory tests to monitor therapy. Before each injection, physician will evaluate response to drug.

Gold Sodium Thiomalate

See Gold Compounds.

Griseofulvin

Microsize Rx

capsules: 125 mg	Grisactin
capsules: 250 mg	Grisactin, *Generic*
tablets: 250 mg	Fulvicin-U/F, Grifulvin V
tablets: 500 mg	Fulvicin-U/F, Grifulvin V, Grisactin
oral suspension: 125 mg/5 ml	Grifulvin V

Ultramicrosize Rx

tablets: 125 mg, 250 mg	Fulvicin P/G, Grisactin Ultra, Gris-PEG
tablets: 165 mg, 330 mg	Fulvicin P/G

INDICATIONS

Management of ringworm infections of skin, hair, and nails, namely tinea corporis, tinea pedis, tinea cruris, tinea barbae, tinea capitis, and tinea unguium (onychomycosis) when caused by one or more of the following: *Trichophyton rubrum, T. tonsurans, T. mentagrophytes, T. interdigitale, T. verrucosum, T. megninii, T. gallinae, T. crateriforme, T. sulphureum, T. schoenleinii, Microsporum audouinii, M. canis, M. gypseum, and Epidermophyton floccosum.* Before therapy, the type of fungi responsible for the infection should be identified. Use of drug is not justified in minor or trivial infections that will respond to topical agents alone. Drug is not effective in bacterial infections, candidiasis (moniliasis), histoplasmosis, actinomycosis, sporotrichosis, chromoblastomycosis, coccidioidomycosis, North American blastomycosis, cryptococcosis, tinea versicolor, or nocardiosis.

CONTRAINDICATIONS

Hypersensitivity; porphyria; hepatocellular failure.

ACTIONS

Griseofulvin is deposited in keratin precursor cells, which are gradually exfoliated and replaced by non-infected tissue; it has greater affinity for diseased tissue. Drug is tightly bound to the new keratin, which becomes highly resistant to fungal invasions. Peak serum level in fasting adults given 0.5 g of the microsize occurs in about 4 hours. Some individuals are "poor absorbers" and tend to attain lower blood levels at all times. Serum level may be increased by giving drug with a meal high in fat content. GI absorption varies considerably among individuals due to insolubility of the drug in aqueous media of the upper GI tract. The efficiency of the absorption of the ultramicrosize is approximately 1.5 times that of the microsize formulation. This permits intake of two-thirds as much ultramicrosize form as the microsize form.

WARNINGS

Safety and efficacy for prophylaxis of fungal infections are not established. Safety during pregnancy is not established.

PRECAUTIONS

Patients on prolonged therapy should be under close observation. Renal, hepatic, and hematopoietic systems are periodically monitored.

Griseofulvin is derived from a species of *Penicillium;* the possibility of cross-sensitivity with penicillin exists.

Lupus erythematosus and lupuslike syndromes have been reported in patients receiving this drug.

DRUG INTERACTIONS

Griseofulvin decreases the activity of **warfarin-type anticoagulants;** patients receiving these drugs concomitantly may require anticoagulant dosage adjustment. **Barbiturates** usually depress griseofulvin activity; concomitant administration may require dosage adjustment of the antifungal agent. The effects of **alcohol** may be potentiated by griseofulvin, producing tachycardia and flush.

ADVERSE REACTIONS

Most common: Hypersensitivity-type reactions such as skin rashes, urticaria, and rarely, angioneurotic edema. Occurrence may necessitate withdrawal of drug and appropriate countermeasures.

Occasional: Oral thrush, nausea, vomiting, epigastric distress, diarrhea, headache, fatigue, dizziness, insomnia, mental confusion, impairment of performance of routine activities.

Rare: May precipitate acute intermittent porphyria. Proteinuria, leukopenia, and paresthesias of the hands and feet have been seen after extended therapy. Discontinue drug if granulocytopenia oc-

curs. When rare, serious reactions occur, they are usually associated with high dosages, long periods of therapy, or both.

DOSAGE

Adults: For tinea corporis, tinea cruris, and tinea capitis, a single or divided daily dose of 500 mg griseofulvin microsize or 250 mg of griseofulvin ultramicrosize. For tinea pedis and tinea unguium, daily dosage of 0.75 g to 1 g griseofulvin microsize or 500 mg griseofulvin ultramicrosize. The microsize dosage may be gradually reduced to 0.5 g after a response is noted.

Children: Approximately 5 mg griseofulvin microsize/lb/day (11 mg/kg/day) or approximately 2.5 mg griseofulvin ultramicrosize/lb/day. The following dosage schedule is suggested: *Children 30–50 lb (13.5–23 kg)*—125 mg to 250 mg griseofulvin microsize/day or 62.5 mg to 125 mg griseofulvin ultramicrosize/day. *Children weighing over 50 lb (over 23 kg)*—250 mg to 500 mg griseofulvin microsize/day or 125 mg to 250 mg griseofulvin ultramicrosize/day. *Children under 2 years*—Dosage not established.

NURSING IMPLICATIONS

HISTORY

See Appendix 4. Note allergy to penicillin (see *Precautions*).

PHYSICAL ASSESSMENT

Examine and describe infected area. Infecting organism is determined by examination of area under a Wood's light (hairs infected by certain fungi fluoresce) or by scrapings of infected area or the vinyl tape method (to strip layers from the epidermis) for microscopic examination.

ADMINISTRATION

Note difference in dosages of microsize and ultramicrosize preparations.

If serum levels are inadequate, physician may order drug taken with or immediately after a meal high in fat content.

ONGOING ASSESSMENTS AND NURSING MANAGEMENT

Inspect area daily or at time of each clinic or office visit. Record findings.

Notify physician if adverse reactions occur.

Periodic studies of renal, hepatic, and hematopoietic function are recommended.

PATIENT AND FAMILY INFORMATION

Beneficial effects may not be noticeable for some time; continue taking medication for entire course of therapy.

Photosensitivity reactions may occur; avoid prolonged exposure to sunlight or sunlamps.

Notify physician or nurse if fever, sore throat, or skin rash occurs.

Guaifenesin *(Glyceryl Guaiacolate)* otc

tablets: 100 mg	Glycotuss, Hytuss
tablets: 200 mg	Gee-Gee, Glytuss
capsules: 200 mg	Breonesin, Hytuss-2X
syrup: 100 mg/5 ml	Anti-Tuss, Baytussin, Colrex Expectorant, 2/G, GG-CEN, GG-Tussin, Glyate, Glycotuss, Liquitussin, Malotuss, Nortussin, Robitussin, S-T Expectorant, *Generic*

INDICATIONS
Symptomatic relief of respiratory conditions characterized by dry, nonproductive cough and in the presence of mucus in the respiratory tract.

CONTRAINDICATIONS
Hypersensitivity.

ACTIONS
Is claimed to have an expectorant action that enhances output of respiratory tract fluid by reducing adhesiveness and surface tension and facilitates removal of inspissated mucus. As a result, dry, nonproductive coughs become more productive and less frequent. There is a lack of convincing studies to document clinical efficacy.

WARNINGS
Not for persistent or chronic cough such as occurs with smoking, asthma, or emphysema, or when cough is accompanied by excessive secretions.

PRECAUTIONS
Persistent cough may indicate a serious condition. If cough persists for more than 1 week, tends to recur, or is accompanied by high fever, rash, or persistent headache, consult physician. Extremely large amounts may cause nausea and vomiting.

Laboratory test interferences: May cause a color interference with certain laboratory determinations of 5-hydroxyindoleacetic acid and vanillylmandelic acid.

ADVERSE REACTIONS
Vomiting, occasional nausea, gastric disturbance, and drowsiness have occurred.

DOSAGE
Adults, children 12 and over: 100 mg to 400 mg q4h to q6h. Do not exceed 2.4 g/day.

Children 6–12: 50 mg to 100 mg q4h to q6h. Do not exceed 600 mg/day.

Children 2–6: 50 mg q4h. Do not exceed 300 mg/day.

NURSING IMPLICATIONS

PATIENT AND FAMILY INFORMATION
Follow manufacturer's directions on package or physician's instructions regarding use.

Swallow capsules whole; do not chew.

See a physician if any of the following occurs: cough persisting for more than 1 week; fever; rash; persistent headache; bloody sputum; chest pain (on inspiration or expiration).

Guanabenz Acetate Rx

tablets: 4 mg, 8 mg	Wytensin

INDICATIONS
Treatment of hypertension, alone or in combination with a thiazide diuretic.

CONTRAINDICATIONS
Sensitivity to guanabenz.

ACTIONS
An orally active alpha$_2$ adrenergic agonist. Antihypertensive action appears to be mediated via stimulation of central alpha-adrenergic receptors, resulting in a decrease of sympathetic outflow from the brain at the bulbar level to the peripheral circulatory system. The acute antihypertensive effect occurs without major changes in peripheral resistance, but its chronic effect appears to be a decrease in peripheral resistance. A decrease in blood pressure is seen in both supine and standing positions without alterations of normal postural mechanisms, so that postural hypotension has not been observed. Decreases the pulse rate by about 5 beats/minute. Cardiac output and left ventricular ejection fraction are unchanged during long-term therapy.

About 75% of drug is absorbed; the effect of meals on absorption has not been studied. Peak plasma concentrations of unchanged drug occur between 2 hours and 5 hours after a single oral dose; average half-life is about 6 hours. The sites of metabolism and the consequences of renal or hepatic insufficiency on excretion have not been determined, but less than 1% of unchanged drug is recovered from the urine.

After a single oral dose, the onset of the antihypertensive action begins within 60 minutes, reaches a peak effect within 2 to 4 hours, and is reduced appreciably 6 to 8 hours after administration, and blood pressure approaches baseline values within 12 hours after administration.

No changes in serum electrolytes, uric acid, BUN, calcium, or glucose have been observed. Guanabenz and hydrochlorothiazide have been shown to have at least partially additive effects in patients not responding adequately to either drug alone.

WARNINGS
Use in pregnancy: May have adverse effects on the fetus when administered to pregnant women. Use during pregnancy only if potential benefit outweighs the potential hazards to the fetus.

Use in lactation: No information is available on excretion in human milk; not administered to nursing mothers.

Use in children: Safety and efficacy for use in children less than 12 have not been demonstrated; use is not recommended.

PRECAUTIONS
Causes sedation or drowsiness in large fraction of patients. Use with caution in those with severe coronary insufficiency, recent myocardial infarction, cerebrovascular disease, or severe hepatic or renal failure. Sudden cessation of therapy may rarely result in "overshoot" hypertension and more commonly produces an increase in serum catecholamines and subjective symptomatology.

Laboratory tests: No clinically significant test abnormalities have been identified. During long-term administration, there may be a small decrease in serum cholesterol and total triglycerides without any change in the high-density lipoprotein fraction. Rarely, an occasional nonprogressive increase in liver enzymes has been observed.

DRUG INTERACTIONS
Concomitant administration with **CNS depressants** may cause increased sedation.

ADVERSE REACTIONS
Most common
Drowsiness/sedation (20%–39%); dry mouth (28%–38%); dizziness (12%–17%); weakness (10%); headache (5%). Although these side-effects are not serious, they may lead to discontinuation of therapy.

Other
Other adverse effects reported, with a frequency of 3% or less, include the following.
Cardiovascular: Chest pain, edema, arrhythmias, palpitations.
GI: Nausea, epigastric pain, diarrhea, vomiting, constipation, abdominal discomfort.
CNS: Anxiety, ataxia, depression, sleep disturbances.
EENT: Nasal congestion, blurred vision.
Musculoskeletal: Aches in extremities, muscle aches.
Respiratory: Dyspnea.
Dermatologic: Rash, pruritus.
GU: Urinary frequency, disturbances in sexual function.
Other: Gynecomastia, taste disorders.

OVERDOSAGE
Symptoms: Accidental ingestion has caused hypotension, somnolence, lethargy, irritability, miosis, and bradycardia in two subjects (children). Gastric lavage and administration of pressor substances, fluids, and oral activated charcoal resulted in complete recovery in 12 hours.

Treatment: Experience is limited; suggested treatment is mainly supportive while drug is being eliminated from body and until patient is no longer symptomatic. Vital signs and fluid balance should be carefully monitored. Maintain an adequate airway; if indicated, institute assisted respiration.

DOSAGE
Dosage is individualized. Starting dose of 4 mg bid is recommended whether used alone or with a thiazide diuretic. Dosage may be increased in increments of 4 mg/day to 8 mg/day every 1 to 2 weeks, depending on patient response. Maximum dose to date has been 32 mg bid; doses as high as this are rarely needed.

NURSING IMPLICATIONS

HISTORY
See Appendix 4.
Female patient (childbearing age): Question whether known to be pregnant or if pregnancy is a possibility.

PHYSICAL ASSESSMENT
Take blood pressure with patient standing, sitting, and lying down (have patient rest 20–30 minutes before taking blood pressure); record pulse, respirations, weight. Baseline renal and hepatic studies and other laboratory tests may be ordered.

G

ADMINISTRATION

If GI distress (nausea, vomiting, epigastric distress) occurs, check with physician whether drug may be given with food (effect of meals on absorption is unknown).

ONGOING ASSESSMENTS AND NURSING MANAGEMENT

Take temperature daily; record blood pressure q4h to q8h or as ordered (especially early in therapy). Use same arm and place patient in same position (sitting, standing, lying down) for each measurement. Record arm used and position of patient.

Antihypertensive action begins in about 60 minutes, reaches a peak in 2 to 4 hours, is reduced in 6 to 8 hours, and approaches baseline values in 12 hours. Early in therapy, physician may order blood pressure taken at specific times after drug is administered to evaluate effectiveness of drug therapy.

Drowsiness/sedation is a common adverse reaction; dizziness and weakness may also occur. Advise patient to seek assistance with ambulatory activities, especially early in therapy.

Observe for adverse effects and report occurrence to physician.

Weigh weekly or as ordered.

Physician may prescribe dietary restrictions (*e.g.,* sodium, calories if patient is overweight).

Drug may be given alone or with a thiazide diuretic. Know adverse effects of both agents if combination therapy is prescribed.

Therapy should *not* be discontinued abruptly. If patient is unable to take medication, notify physician because other antihypertensive measures may be necessary.

PATIENT AND FAMILY INFORMATION

NOTE: Physician may wish patient to monitor own blood pressure between office visits. Patient or family member will require instruction.

Take as directed. Do not abruptly discontinue drug except on advice of physician.

May produce drowsiness or dizziness; observe caution while driving or performing other tasks requiring alertness.

Tolerance to alcohol and CNS depressants may be diminished and use should be avoided. If this presents a problem, discuss with physician.

Inform other physicians and dentists of therapy with this drug.

Notify physician or nurse if drowsiness, dizziness, or weakness becomes severe and interferes with daily activities.

Dry mouth may be relieved by frequent sips of water, hard candy, or chewing gum.

Guanadrel Sulfate Rx

tablets: 10 mg,   Hylorel
25 mg

INDICATIONS

Treatment of hypertension in those not responding adequately to a thiazide-type diuretic. Add to a diuretic regimen for optimum blood pressure control.

CONTRAINDICATIONS

Known or suspected pheochromocytoma; concurrently with, or within 1 week of, monoamine oxidase (MAO) inhibitors; sensitivity to guanadrel; frank congestive heart failure (CHF).

ACTIONS

Guanadrel, an adrenergic neuron-blocking agent, inhibits sympathetic vasoconstriction by inhibiting norepinephrine release from neuronal storage sites in response to nerve stimulation and causes depletion of norepinephrine from the nerve ending. This causes a relaxation of vascular smooth muscle, which decreases total peripheral resistance and decreases venous return. A hypotensive effect results that is greater in the standing than in the supine position by about an average of 10 mm Hg systolic and 3.5 mm Hg diastolic. Heart rate is decreased by about 5 beats/minute. Fluid retention occurs, particularly when not accompanied by a diuretic. The drug does not inhibit parasympathetic nerve function nor does it enter the CNS. No significant change in cardiac output accompanies the blood pressure decline in normal individuals.

Guanadrel is rapidly absorbed after oral administration. Plasma concentrations peak 1.5 to 2 hours after ingestion. Half-life is about 10 hours, but individual variability is great. Approximately 85% of the drug is excreted in the urine.

WARNINGS

Orthostatic hypotension: Is frequent in occurrence. Rarely, fainting upon standing or exercise occurs. Patients with known regional vascular disease (cerebral, coronary) are at particular risk from marked orthostatic hypotension; avoid hypotensive episodes even if this requires accepting a poorer degree of blood pressure control.

Surgery: To reduce the possibility of vascular collapse during anesthesia, discontinue guanadrel 48 to 72 hours before elective surgery. If emergency surgery is required, advise the anesthesiologist the patient has been taking guanadrel and administer preanesthetic and anesthetic agents cautiously in reduced dosage. Use vasopressors cautiously, because guanadrel can enhance the pressor response to such agents and increase their arrhythmogenicity.

Asthma: Special care is needed in those with bronchial asthma, because their condition may be aggravated by catecholamine depletion, and sympathomimetic amines may interfere with the hypotensive effect of guanadrel.

Use in pregnancy, lactation: Safety not established. Used only when clearly needed and when potential benefits outweigh the unknown potential hazards to the fetus.

Use in children: Safety and efficacy not established.

PRECAUTIONS

Salt and water retention may occur. Patients with heart failure have not been studied, but guanadrel could interfere with the adrenergic mechanisms that maintain compensation. Use cautiously in those with a history of peptic ulcer, which could be aggravated by a relative increase in parasympathetic tone.

DRUG INTERACTIONS

Tricyclic antidepressants and **indirect-acting sympathomimetics,** such as ephedrine or phenylpropanolamine and possibly phenothiazines, can reverse the effects of neuronal blocking agents. Guanadrel enhances the activity of **direct-acting sympathomimetics** such as norepinephrine by blocking neuronal uptake. Drugs that affect the adrenergic response by the same or other mechanisms may potentiate the effects of guanadrel, causing excessive postural hypotension and bradycardia. These include **alpha-** or **beta-adrenergic blocking agents** and **reserpine.**

ADVERSE REACTIONS

Cardiovascular/respiratory: Shortness of breath on exertion, palpitations, chest pain, coughing, shortness of breath at rest.

CNS/special senses: Fatigue, headache, faintness, drowsiness, visual disturbances, paresthesias, confusion, psychological problems, depression, sleep disorders, syncope.

GI: Increased bowel movements; gas pain/indigestion; constipation; anorexia; glossitis; nausea and/or vomiting; abdominal distress or pain; dry mouth, dry throat.

GU: Nocturia, urinary frequency or urgency, peripheral edema, ejaculation disturbances, impotence, hematuria.

Musculoskeletal: Aching limbs; leg cramps during the night or day; backache, neckache; joint pain or inflammation.

Miscellaneous: Excessive weight gain or loss.

OVERDOSAGE

Usually produces marked dizziness and blurred vision related to postural hypotension, which may progress to syncope on standing. The patient should lie down until symptoms subside. If excessive hypotension occurs and persists despite conservative treatment, intensive therapy may be needed to support vital functions. A vasoconstrictor such as phenylephrine will ameliorate the effect of guanadrel, but is used carefully because patients may be hypersensitive to such agents.

DOSAGE

Usual starting dosage is 10 mg/day in divided doses. Most patients will require a daily dosage in the range of 20 mg to 75 mg, usually in twice-daily doses. For larger doses, dosing three or four times a day may be needed. Because the half-life is approximately 10 hours, dosage is adjusted weekly or monthly until blood pressure is controlled.

NURSING IMPLICATIONS

HISTORY
See Appendix 4.

PHYSICAL ASSESSMENT
Obtain blood pressure with patient standing, sitting, lying down (have patient rest 20–30 minutes before taking blood pressure); obtain pulse, respirations, weight. Baseline laboratory tests and diagnostic studies may include serum electrolytes, ECG.

ADMINISTRATION
If GI distress (nausea, vomiting, indigestion) occurs, check with physician whether drug may be given with food.

ONGOING ASSESSMENTS AND NURSING MANAGEMENT
Obtain temperature, blood pressure, pulse q4h to q8h or as ordered (especially early in therapy). Use same arm and take blood pressure in a standing and supine position for each measurement, especially early in therapy or during period of dosage adjustment.

The drug's hypotensive effect is greater in the standing than in the supine position; a decrease in the pulse rate may also be noted.

Antihypertensive action begins in about 2 hours and produces maximal decreases in 4 to 6 hours. Early in therapy physician may order blood pressure taken at specific times after drug is administered to evaluate effectiveness of therapy.

G

Faintness due to orthostatic hypotension or other causes (fever, hot weather) is a common adverse reaction occurring in about half the patients. Rarely, fainting upon standing or exercise may occur. Assist patient with all ambulatory activities, especially early in therapy or during period of dosage adjustment.

If faintness or dizziness occurs, have patient sit or lie down immediately. Report the occurrence of these adverse effects to the physician, because dosage adjustment may be necessary.

The frequencies of adverse drug reactions may be higher during the first 8 weeks of therapy. Report all adverse effects to the physician. If adverse effects are severe or cause unusual patient discomfort, dosage adjustment or discontinuation of the drug may be necessary.

Weigh weekly or as ordered. Report any weight gain or loss to physician.

Dietary restriction of sodium or calories (if patient is overweight) may be necessary.

Guanadrel may be given with a thiazide diuretic. Know adverse effects of both agents if combination therapy is prescribed.

Therapy should not be discontinued abruptly. If patient is unable to take medication, notify physician because other antihypertensive measures may be necessary.

Drug is discontinued 48 to 72 hours before elective surgery. If emergency surgery is required, notify the anesthesiologist of the patient's therapy with guanadrel because preanesthetic and anesthetic agents are given in reduced dosages.

PATIENT AND FAMILY INFORMATION

NOTE: Physician may wish patient to monitor own blood pressure between office visits. Patient or family member will require instruction. The patient must be advised of the risk of orthostatic hypotension.

Episodes of hypotension may be exaggerated by alcohol, fever, hot weather, prolonged standing, or exercise.

Sit or lie down immediately at the onset of weakness or dizziness to prevent a loss of consciousness.

Take as directed. Do not abruptly discontinue drug except on advice of physician.

Do not take any nonprescription drug unless use of a specific product is approved by the physician. Some nonprescription preparations contain ingredients (sympathomimetic amines) that may interfere with the action of this drug.

Avoid use of alcohol, unless use has been approved by the physician.

May produce drowsiness, dizziness, or faint-

ness; observe caution while driving or performing other tasks requiring alertness.

Inform other physicians and dentists of therapy with this drug.

Notify physician if drowsiness, dizziness, or weakness becomes severe and interferes with daily activities.

Guanethidine Sulfate Rx

tablets: 10 mg (contains tartrazine), 25 mg   Ismelin Sulfate

INDICATIONS

Moderate to severe hypertension, either alone or as an adjunct. Renal hypertension, including that secondary to pyelonephritis, renal amyloidosis, or renal artery stenosis.

CONTRAINDICATIONS

Known or suspected pheochromocytoma; hypersensitivity; frank congestive heart failure (CHF) not due to hypertension; use of monoamine oxidase (MAO) inhibitors.

ACTIONS

Exerts its potent antihypertensive effects at postganglionic adrenergic nerve endings. It inhibits norepinephrine release and depletes norepinephrine stores in adrenergic nerve endings. Effector cells are sensitized to the effects of exogenous catecholamines. Peak antihypertensive effects occur within 8 hours of a single dose. Because of long half-life (approximately 5 days), drug accumulates slowly. Up to 2 weeks may be required to evaluate response to daily administration adequately. Guanethidine is partially metabolized and excreted primarily in the urine. Reduced dosages may be adequate in patients with impaired renal function.

WARNINGS

This is a potent drug that can lead to disturbing and serious clinical problems.

Orthostatic hypotension can occur frequently and is most marked in the morning and accentuated by hot weather, alcohol, or exercise. Dizziness or weakness may be particularly bothersome during initial period of dosage adjustment and with postural changes.

Therapy is withdrawn 2 weeks before surgery to reduce possibility of vascular collapse and cardiac arrest during anesthesia. If emergency surgery is indicated, preanesthetic and anesthetic agents are administered cautiously in reduced dosage. Oxygen, atropine, vasopressors, and adequate solutions for volume replacement should be ready to counteract vascular collapse. Vasopressors are used with extreme caution.

Dosage requirements may be reduced in the presence of fever. Special care is exercised in administration to patients with a history of bronchial asthma; asthmatics are more likely to be hypersensitive to catecholamine depletion and their condition may be aggravated. In those with impaired renal function, reduced dosages are required. Drug is used cautiously in those with renal disease and nitrogen retention or rising BUN levels, because decreased blood pressure may further compromise renal function.

Use in pregnancy: Safety is not established. Use only when clearly needed and when potential benefits outweigh the unknown potential hazards to the fetus.

PRECAUTIONS

The effects of guanethidine are cumulative; initial doses should be small and increased gradually in small increments. To minimize sodium retention and compensatory fluid retention, drug is usually used in combination with a thiazide diuretic.

Use cautiously in hypertensive patients with coronary disease with insufficiency or recent myocardial infarction (MI) or cerebral vascular disease, especially with encephalopathy. Do not give to those with severe cardiac failure except with great caution, because drug may interfere with the compensatory role of the adrenergic system in producing circulatory adjustment in those with CHF. Both digitalis and guanethidine slow the heart rate. Patients with incipient cardiac decompensation are watched for weight gain or edema, which may be averted by concomitant administration of a thiazide.

Use cautiously in those with history of peptic ulcer or other disorders that may be aggravated by a relative increase in parasympathetic tone.

Tartrazine sensitivity: Some of these products contain tartrazine (see Appendix 6, section 6-23).

DRUG INTERACTIONS

Concurrent use with **rauwolfia derivatives** may cause excessive postural hypotension, bradycardia, and mental depression. Both **digitalis** and guanethidine slow the heart rate. **Amphetaminelike compounds, stimulants,** (*e.g.,* ephedrine, methylphenidate), **tricyclic antidepressants** (*e.g.,* amitriptyline, imipramine, desipramine) and other **psychopharmacologic agents** (*e.g.,* phenothiazines and related compounds), and **oral contraceptives** may reduce the hypotensive effect of guanethidine. **MAO inhibitors** are discontinued at least 1 week before starting guanethidine therapy. Guanethidine augments responsiveness to exogenously administered **norepinephrine** and **vasopressors** with respect to blood pressure and their propensity for production of cardiac arrhythmias.

ADVERSE REACTIONS

Frequent reactions due to sympathetic blockade: Dizziness, weakness, lassitude, syncope resulting from either postural or exertional hypotension.

Frequent reactions due to unopposed parasympathetic activity: Bradycardia, increase in bowel movements, and diarrhea that may be severe at times and necessitate discontinuance of drug.

Other common reactions: Inhibition of ejaculation, a tendency toward fluid retention, edema with occasional development of CHF.

Less common reactions: Dyspnea, fatigue, nausea, vomiting, nocturia, urinary incontinence, dermatitis, scalp hair loss, dry mouth, rise in BUN, ptosis of the eyelids, blurred vision, parotid tenderness, myalgia, muscle tremor, mental depression, angina, chest paresthesias, nasal congestion, weight gain (secondary to fluid accumulation), asthma in susceptible individuals.

Causal relationship not established: A few instances of anemia, thrombocytopenia and leukopenia, and priapism have been reported.

OVERDOSAGE

Signs and symptoms: Postural hypotension (with dizziness, blurred vision, and so on, possibly progressing to syncope when standing) and bradycardia are most likely to occur; diarrhea, possibly severe, may also occur. Unconsciousness is unlikely if adequate blood pressure and cerebral perfusion can be maintained by appropriate positioning (supine) and by other treatment as required.

Treatment: In previously normotensive patients, restore normal blood pressure and heart rate by keeping patient in supine position. Normal homeostatic control usually returns gradually over a 72-hour period.

In previously hypertensive patients, particularly those with impaired cardiac reserve or other cardiovascular–renal disease, intensive treatment may be required to support vital functions and to control cardiac irregularities that might be present. Supine position must be maintained; if vasopressors are required, guanethidine may increase responsiveness to blood pressure rise and occurrence of cardiac arrhythmias. Severe or persistent diarrhea is treated symptomatically to reduce intestinal hypomotility and maintain hydration and electrolyte balance.

G

DOSAGE

Ambulatory patients: Begin with 10 mg/day; increase gradually, depending on patient response. Dosage increases are not made more often than every 5 to 7 days unless patient is hospitalized. Blood pressure is taken in the supine position, after standing for 10 minutes, and immediately after exercise, if feasible. Increase dosage only if there has been no decrease in standing blood pressure from previous levels. Average dosage is 25 mg/day to 50 mg/day; only 1 dose/day is required. Reduce dosage in any of the following situations: normal supine pressure, excessive orthostatic fall in pressure, or severe diarrhea.

Hospitalized patients: Initial oral dose is 25 mg to 50 mg; this is increased 25 mg/day to 50 mg every day or every other day as indicated. Because peak effects occur in 8 hours, additional doses may be given q8h until desired effect is obtained in hypertensive emergencies. Once blood pressure is normalized with this loading dose, proper daily maintenance dose must be determined.

Daily maintenance dosage may be estimated at one-seventh of the loading dose required. Dosage must be adjusted by monitoring response over several days. Unless absolutely impossible, take standing blood pressure regularly. Patient should not be discharged until the effect of the drug on standing blood pressure is known.

Combination therapy: Guanethidine may be added gradually to thiazides or hydralazine. Thiazide diuretics enhance the effectiveness of guanethidine. After control is established, dosage of all drugs is reduced to the lowest effective level. When replacing MAO inhibitors, at least 1 week should elapse before commencing treatment with guanethidine.

In many cases, ganglionic blockers will have been stopped before guanethidine is started. It may be advisable to withdraw the blocker gradually to prevent spiking blood pressure response during the transfer period.

NURSING IMPLICATIONS

HISTORY

See Appendix 4. Note history of bronchial asthma (see *Warnings*).

PHYSICAL ASSESSMENT

Blood pressure and pulse are taken with patient in the supine position and then again after patient is standing for 10 minutes. If patient is not allowed out of bed, take readings in supine position only. Take blood pressure on both arms. In addition, obtain weight. CBC, serum electrolytes, ECG, and renal-function tests may be ordered.

ADMINISTRATION

Drug is administered once daily.

Obtain blood pressure and pulse with patient in supine position and then again after patient is standing for 10 minutes. If patient is not allowed out of bed, take blood pressure in supine position only.

When ordered by physician, a third blood-pressure reading may be taken immediately after exercise.

Early in therapy, obtain blood pressure on both arms. When patient is on maintenance therapy, obtain blood pressure on one arm, using same arm each time. Record arm used.

Withhold drug and contact physician if a normal supine pressure is obtained, there is an excessive orthostatic (standing) fall in pressure, or severe diarrhea occurs.

ONGOING ASSESSMENTS AND NURSING MANAGEMENT

Obtain blood pressure and pulse with patient in standing and supine positions (see above) q4h or as ordered; take temperature daily; observe for adverse reactions q4h to q6h (early in therapy).

During initial therapy, dosage is adjusted to patient's individual response and based on standing and supine blood pressures.

Dizziness, weakness, lassitude, and syncope frequently result from either postural or exertional hypotension. Postural hypotension is most marked in the morning and is accentuated by hot weather, warm tub baths or showers, exercise, or alcohol. Early in therapy, have patient dangle legs 5 to 10 minutes before getting out of bed. Provide ambulatory assistance as necessary.

Bradycardia may occur. If pulse falls to 60 or below or decreases significantly from baseline levels, notify physician.

Early in therapy, monitor intake and output, especially if patient has impaired renal function, is elderly, is critically ill, or has incipient cardiac decompensation.

Weigh daily or as ordered at same time each day and with approximately same amount of clothing. Notify physician if weight gain or edema is noted.

If fever is present, notify physician; dosage may need to be reduced.

Observe for diarrhea, which may be severe and may necessitate discontinuance of the medication.

Physician may order salt-restricted or low-sodium diet.

To minimize sodium retention and compensatory fluid retention, a thiazide diuretic may be ordered. Be familiar with administration of both drugs when a thiazide is used concurrently.

In hypertensive emergencies, drug may be given q8h until blood pressure is controlled. Monitor patient closely; take blood pressure and pulse q1h to q2h.

Physician may order periodic serum electrolytes, CBC, and renal- and hepatic-function tests.

PATIENT AND FAMILY INFORMATION

NOTE: Physician may have patient or family member monitor blood pressure between office or clinic visits. Patient or family member will require full instruction in use of blood-pressure apparatus as well as positions assumed for blood-pressure readings. Advise patient to keep record of readings and bring to each office or clinic visit.

Do not discontinue medication unless directed by physician.

Avoid cough, cold, and allergy medications (containing sympathomimetics) except on professional recommendation.

Inform other physicians and dentist of therapy with this drug.

Notify physician or nurse immediately of severe diarrhea, frequent dizziness, or fainting. Do not attempt to drive or perform tasks requiring alertness until problem is corrected.

If dizziness (orthostatic hypotension) occurs, avoid sudden changes in posture. Rise slowly from a sitting position. Dangle legs 5 to 10 minutes before getting out of bed in the morning. Postural hypotension experienced during unassisted ambulation can usually be relieved by sitting or lying down. Assistance should then be sought for future ambulatory activities.

Alcohol, exercise, hot weather, and hot baths or showers may increase the incidence of dizziness and fainting.

Weigh self weekly, at same time of day and with approximately the same amount of clothing. Report significant weight gain to physician.

Periodic laboratory tests may be ordered.

Physician may prescribe dietary restrictions; adherence to diet is an important part of therapy.

Follow physician's recommendations about exercise, alcohol intake, use of caffeine-containing beverages (coffee, tea, colas), weight reduction, and clinic or office visits to monitor therapy.

G

H

Halazepam

See Benzodiazepines.

Halcinonide

See Corticosteroids, Topical.

Haloperidol

See Antipsychotic Agents.

Haloprogin Rx

cream, solution: 1%   Halotex

INDICATIONS
Topical treatment of tinea pedis, tinea cruris, tinea corporis, and tinea manuum due to infection with *Trichophyton rubrum, T. tonsurans, T. mentagrophytes, Microsporum canis, Epidermophyton floccosum.* Also useful in topical treatment of tinea versicolor due to *Malassezia furfur.*

CONTRAINDICATIONS
Hypersensitivity.

ACTIONS
A synthetic agent for treatment of superficial fungal infections of the skin.

WARNINGS
Safety for use in pregnancy not established.

PRECAUTIONS
In case of sensitization or irritation, treatment is discontinued and appropriate therapy instituted. If no improvement is shown after 4 weeks, diagnosis is reevaluated. In mixed infections when bacteria or nonsusceptible fungi are present, supplementary systemic anti-infective therapy may be indicated. Drug is for external use only. Keep out of eyes.

ADVERSE REACTIONS
Local irritation, burning sensation, vesicle formation, increased maceration, pruritus, exacerbation of preexisting lesions.

DOSAGE
Apply liberally to affected area bid for 2 to 3 weeks. Interdigital lesions may require up to 4 weeks of therapy.

NURSING IMPLICATIONS

HISTORY
See Appendix 4.

PHYSICAL ASSESSMENT
Inspect lesions; record size, color, location.

ADMINISTRATION
Exercise care in application if lesions are near eyes.

ONGOING ASSESSMENTS AND NURSING MANAGEMENT
Inspect affected areas every 2 to 3 days; note any change in size and appearance of lesions and record findings.

If patient complains of burning or irritation is apparent, notify physician before next application is due.

If condition does not improve, notify physician.

PATIENT AND FAMILY INFORMATION
Apply as directed by physician. Avoid contact with eyes.

If condition worsens, or if irritation or burning occurs, discontinue use and notify physician.

Tinea pedis (athlete's foot): Wash feet several times a day; dry thoroughly. Change socks as needed if feet perspire. Avoid footwear made of or coated with plastic or rubber; wear shoes that allow air to circulate. Expose shoes to air when not wearing them; do not wear shoes that are wet or damp.

Keep towels and facecloths separate from those of other family members to avoid spread of infection.

Tinea corporis, tinea cruris: Wear fresh clothes daily. Dry skin thoroughly after bath or shower.

Halothane

See Anesthetics, General, Volatile Liquids.

Heparin Preparations

Heparin Calcium Injection Rx

injection: 5000 units,   Calciparine
  12,500 units,
  20,000 units/dose

Heparin Sodium Injection, USP _Rx_

Multiple-Dose Vials

injection: 1000 units/ ml, 5000 units/ml, 10,000 units/ml, 20,000 units/ml, 40,000 units/ml	Lipo-Hepin, Liquaemin Sodium, _Generic_

Single-Dose Ampules and Vials

injection: 1000 units/ml	_Generic_
injection: 5000 units/ ml, 10,000 units/ ml, 20,000 units/ ml	Liquaemin Sodium, _Generic_
injection: 40,000 units/ml	Liquaemin Sodium

Unit-Dose

injection: 1000 units, 2500 units, 5000 units, 7500 units, 10,000 units, 15,000 units, 20,000 units/dose	_Generic_

Heparin Sodium Lock Flush Solution _Rx_

These dilute heparin sodium solutions are used as an IV flush to maintain patency of indwelling IV catheters used in intermittent IV therapy or blood sampling and are not intended for therapeutic use.

injection: 10 units/ ml, 100 units/ml	Heparin Lock Flush, Hep-Lock

INDICATIONS

Anticoagulant therapy in prophylaxis and treatment of venous thrombosis and its extension and pulmonary embolism.

In atrial fibrillation with embolization.

Diagnosis and treatment of acute and chronic consumptive coagulopathies (disseminated intravascular coagulation [DIC]).

Low-dose regimen for prevention of postoperative deep venous thrombosis and pulmonary embolism in patients undergoing major abdominothoracic surgery who are at risk of developing thromboembolic disease.

Prevention of clotting in arterial and heart surgery. In blood transfusions, extracorporeal circulation, dialysis procedures, and blood samples for laboratory purposes.

Prevention of cerebral thrombosis in the evolving stroke.

Adjunct in treatment of coronary occlusion with acute myocardial infarction and as an adjunct in prophylaxis and treatment of peripheral arterial embolism.

CONTRAINDICATIONS

Hypersensitivity; uncontrolled bleeding (except when used as indicated in therapy of consumptive coagulopathies); severe thrombocytopenia; any patient for whom suitable blood coagulation tests, such as whole blood clotting time (WBCT) or partial thromboplastin time (PTT), cannot be performed at required intervals.

ACTIONS

Commercial preparations are derived from bovine lung or porcine intestinal mucosa. The anticoagulant potency of Heparin Injection, USP is standardized and expressed in "units" of heparin activity. Because the number of USP units/mg may vary, dosage should always be expressed in units.

Heparin acts at multiple sites in the normal coagulation system. It inhibits formation of fibrin clots and therefore the clotting of blood, both _in vitro_ and _in vivo_. In combination with antithrombin III, heparin inactivates Factors IX, X, XI, and XII and thrombin, inhibiting conversion of fibrinogen to fibrin. Heparin also prevents formation of a stable fibrin clot by inhibiting the activation of Factor XIII (fibrin-stabilizing factor).

Heparin inhibits reactions that lead to clotting but does not significantly alter the concentration of normal clotting factors. Although clotting time is prolonged by therapeutic doses, bleeding time is usually unaffected. It does not have fibrinolytic activity and will not lyse existing clots but can prevent extension of existing clots.

Heparin is not active orally because it is inactivated by gastric acid; it must be given by IV or subcutaneous injection. IV bolus administration results in immediate anticoagulant effects. When it is administered by continuous IV infusion or by subcutaneous injection, an initial loading dose must be given by direct IV injection. Duration of action is dose dependent. Because of gradual absorption from site of subcutaneous administration, therapeutic effects may be maintained for 8 to 12 hours. Patients vary widely in response to various doses and plasma concentrations of heparin. Coagulation tests, WBCT, and activated partial thromboplastin time (APTT) are the best indicators of response.

Heparin is believed to be partially metabolized by the liver and by the reticuloendothelial system. It is excreted in the urine unchanged. Heparin clearance is decreased in those with renal disease.

H

WARNINGS

When heparin is administered in therapeutic amounts, dosage is regulated by frequent blood coagulation tests. If coagulation is unduly prolonged or if hemorrhage occurs, discontinue promptly (see *Overdosage*).

Do *not* administer IM because of the danger of hematoma formation. Larger doses may be necessary in febrile states. Increased resistance to drug is frequently encountered in thrombosis, thrombophlebitis, infections with thrombosing tendencies, myocardial infarction, cancer, and postoperative states. Use with caution during pregnancy, especially in the last trimester and immediate postpartum period, because of the risk of maternal hemorrhage.

Use heparin with extreme caution in disease states in which there is increased danger of hemorrhage. These include the following.

Cardiovascular: Subacute bacterial endocarditis; arterial sclerosis; dissecting aneurysm; increased capillary permeability; during and immediately after spinal tap, spinal anesthesia, or major surgery, especially of the brain, spinal cord, or eye; suspected intracranial hemorrhage; shock; severe hypertension.

Hematologic: Conditions in which there are increased bleeding tendencies such as hemophilia, some purpuras, jaundice, thrombocytopenia (exception is bleeding states associated with DIC), and postoperative oozing of blood. Before therapy, determine whether platelet count is adequate.

GI: Inaccessible ulcerative lesions (especially of GI tract), diverticulitis or ulcerative colitis, continuous tube drainage of stomach or small intestine.

Obstetric: Threatened abortion (unless complicated by DIC).

Other: Severe hepatic, renal, or biliary disease.

PRECAUTIONS

Heparin is derived from animal tissue; use with caution in those with history of allergy. Before therapeutic dose is given, a trial dose of 1000 units may be advisable. Use cautiously in presence of mild hepatic or renal disease, hypertension, during menstruation, or in patient with indwelling catheter. A higher incidence of bleeding may be seen in women over 60. Caution should be used when administering ACD (acid-citrate-dextrose)-converted blood because heparin anticoagulant activity persists without loss for as long as 22 days following conversion in blood stored at refrigeration temperatures. Heparin in the administered blood may produce alterations in the coagulation mechanism of the recipient, particularly when multiple transfusions of ACD-converted blood are given.

Heparin has been reported to produce thrombocytopenia due to platelet aggregation. In rare instances, this has been associated with clinically significant thromboembolism (white clot syndrome) presumed to be a result of platelet aggregates. If untreated, this may lead to complete arterial obstruction and organ infarction.

DRUG INTERACTIONS

May prolong one-stage **prothrombin time.** When given with **dicumarol** or **sodium warfarin,** a period of 4 to 5 hours after last IV dose or 12 to 24 hours after last subcutaneous dose should elapse if valid prothrombin time is to be obtained. Any drug that may induce prolongation of prothrombin time or delay coagulation by any means (*e.g.,* interfere with platelet aggregation) should be used with caution. These agents include **aspirin, dextran, phenylbutazone, ibuprofen, indomethacin, dipyridamole,** and **hydroxychloroquine.**

Heparin may antagonize the action of **ACTH, insulin,** and **corticosteroids,** but this effect has not been clearly defined. Heparin may increase plasma levels of **diazepam.** Use of **digitalis, tetracycline, nicotine,** and **antihistamines** may partially counteract the anticoagulant action of heparin.

ADVERSE REACTIONS

Hemorrhage: Is chief complication; an overly prolonged clotting time or minor bleeding during therapy can usually be controlled by withdrawing drug. Occurrence of significant GI or urinary-tract bleeding during anticoagulant therapy may indicate presence of underlying occult lesion. Adrenal hemorrhage resulting in acute adrenal insufficiency has occurred. Discontinue therapy in those developing signs and symptoms of acute adrenal hemorrhage or insufficiency. Plasma cortisol levels should be measured and vigorous IV corticosteroid therapy instituted.

Local: When heparin is administered IM, local irritation, mild pain, or hematoma may occur at injection site; avoid IM use. These effects are less frequent after deep subcutaneous (intrafat) administration. Histaminelike reactions have been observed at the injection site. Cutaneous necrosis has been reported.

Hypersensitivity: Reactions (chills, fever, urticaria) have been reported. Asthma, rhinitis, lacrimation, and anaphylactoid reactions also have been seen. Vasospastic reactions, independent of heparin origin, may develop 6 to 10 days after initiation of therapy and may last 4 to 6 hours. The affected limb is painful, ischemic, and cyanosed. After repeated injections, reaction may gradually increase to include generalized vasospasm with cyanosis, tachypnea, feeling of oppression, and headache. Chest pain, elevated blood pressure, arthralgias, and headache have been reported in the absence of definite peripheral vasospasm.

Other: Acute reversible thrombocytopenia has occurred following IV administration. Localized and disseminated venous and arterial thrombosis have been reported. Osteoporosis and suppression of renal function have occurred following long-term, high-dose administration. Suppression of aldosterone synthesis, delayed transient alopecia, and rebound hyperlipemia have been reported following discontinuation of heparin. Priapism has been reported.

OVERDOSAGE

Protamine sulfate (1% solution) by slow infusion will neutralize heparin. No more than 50 mg should be administered very slowly in any 10-minute period. Each milligram neutralizes approximately 100 USP heparin units. Decreasing amounts of protamine are required as the time from last heparin injection increases. Thirty minutes after a dose of heparin, approximately 0.5 mg of protamine is sufficient to neutralize each 100 units of heparin administered. Protamine has anticoagulant activity and a longer half-life than heparin. As heparin is eliminated, excess protamine may cause bleeding. In some cases, blood transfusions may be necessary; these dilute heparin and provide uninhibited clotting factors but do not neutralize heparin.

DOSAGE

Continuous IV infusion is generally preferable to intermittent IV therapy because of the higher incidence of bleeding complications associated with intermittent therapy. In addition, higher daily doses are usually required to achieve adequate anticoagulation with intermittent therapy. Intermittent injections produce periods of overcoagulation or undercoagulation; continuous infusion provides constant therapeutic effect.

Adjust dosage to coagulation test results, which are determined just before each injection. There usually is no need to monitor effect of low-dose heparin in those with normal coagulation parameters. Dosage is adequate when WBCT is approximately 2.5 to 3 times the control value or when PTT is 1.5 to 2.5 times the control value. When heparin is given by continuous IV infusion, perform coagulation tests q4h in early stages. When administered by intermittent IV or subcutaneous injection, perform coagulation tests before each dose during early stages and daily thereafter.

Concomitant oral anticoagulation therapy: When an oral anticoagulant is administered with heparin, perform coagulation tests and determine prothrombin activity at start of therapy. For immediate anticoagulation effect, give heparin in usual therapeutic doses. When result of initial prothrombin determination is known, administer oral anticoagulant in the usual initial amount. Thereafter, perform coagulation tests and prothrombin activity at appropriate intervals. To obtain valid prothrombin time, draw blood at least 5 hours after last IV dose or 24 hours after last subcutaneous dose of heparin. When prothrombin activity reaches the desired therapeutic range, heparin may be discontinued and therapy continued with the oral anticoagulant.

General anticoagulant therapy: Dosage is adjusted to individual patient; Table 29 may be used as a guide.

Low-dose prophylaxis of postoperative thromboembolism: Give just prior to and after surgery to reduce incidence of postoperative deep-vein thrombosis in legs and clinical pulmonary embolism. Usual dose is 5000 units subcutaneously 2 hours before surgery and 5000 units q8h to q12h thereafter for 7 days or until patient is fully ambulated. Appropriate coagulation tests are performed before therapy.

Surgery of heart and blood vessels: Patients un-

Table 29. Recommended Heparin Dosage Schedules for Different Routes of Administration for Anticoagulant Therapy

Route of Administration	Frequency	Recommended Dosage (based on 150-lb patient)
Subcutaneous	Initial dose	10,000–20,000 units (immediately preceded by IV loading dose of 5000 units)
	q8h or	8000–10,000 units
	q12h	15,000–20,000 units
Intermittent IV	Initial dose	10,000 units
	q4h to q6h	5000–10,000 units
IV infusion	Continuous	20,000–40,000 units/day in 1000-ml isotonic sodium chloride solution

dergoing total body perfusion for open heart surgery should receive an initial dose of not less than 150 units/kg. Frequently 300 units/kg is used for procedures lasting less than 60 minutes, and 400 mg/kg is used for procedures lasting longer than 60 minutes. Heparin should be added to fluids in the pump oxygenator to prevent blood from clotting in the tube system.

Extracorporeal dialysis: Follow manufacturers' operating directions.

Blood transfusion: Add 400 units/dl to 600 units/dl whole blood. Usually 7500 units are added to 1000 ml Sodium Chloride Injection; from this sterile solution, 6 ml to 8 ml is added per 1 dl of whole blood.

Laboratory samples: 70 units to 150 units added to a 10-ml to 20-ml sample of whole blood to prevent coagulation of sample.

NURSING IMPLICATIONS

HISTORY
See Appendix 4.

PHYSICAL ASSESSMENT
Obtain vital signs. In venous thrombosis of extremity, examine involved area above and below site of suspected thrombus for color and temperature, examine superficial veins and describe appearance, check peripheral pulses, and note if edema is present. Laboratory studies pertinent to heparin therapy include PTT and WBCT. If an oral anticoagulant will be administered concomitantly, a prothrombin time may be ordered. Additional laboratory tests and diagnostic studies pertinent to the diagnosis or clinical findings may also be ordered.

ADMINISTRATION
Heparin may be given subcutaneously or IV (continuous or intermittent). IM administration is avoided.

Dosage is measured in *units;* read label carefully because various strengths are available.

Baseline coagulation tests (PTT, WBCT) must be drawn and results obtained before administration of initial dose. In an emergency, physician may order drug given before test results are obtained.

Intermittent IV administration (heparin lock, heparin trap): An intermittent infusion set is used for administration. Following insertion of an intermittent infusion set, write date, time inserted, and needle size on a small piece of tape and gently apply on top of tape used to anchor loop of tubing and injection port. At the time of each heparin administration, wipe injection port

with antiseptic before inserting the needle. Check for patency by drawing back on the syringe. If no blood backflow is present, do *not* inject the heparin; a new intermittent infusion set will need to be inserted. If the needle and tubing are patent, inject the drug slowly. Heparin administered in this manner is given undiluted.

Use of a heparin lock flush solution before and after administration of heparin by intermittent IV administration may be ordered by the physician or may be a written hospital policy. Usually 1 ml or 2 ml of the solution is used. Hospital policy or the physician's order may prescribe the use of 1 ml to 2 ml of normal saline before and after heparin administration instead of a heparin lock flush solution.

Continuous IV infusion: An infusion pump is recommended to control rate and volume of administration; add prescribed amount of heparin to 1 liter of isotonic sodium chloride. If infusion pump is not used, flow rate must be monitored at frequent intervals (q15m–q30m) because position changes may vary flow rate.

Subcutaneous administration: Withdraw drug from vial with 20-gauge to 22-gauge needle. Dispose of needle and replace with a ½-inch 25-gauge or 26-gauge needle for administration. Select injection site. Preferred site is fatty layer of abdomen, above the level of anterior iliac spine. Pinch a fold of tissue approximately ½ inch between thumb and forefinger; insert needle at 90-degree angle. Do *not* draw back (aspirate) the syringe to check for possible entry into a blood vessel. Inject drug slowly. Shallow subcutaneous injection is avoided because of pain resulting from injection and greater incidence of hematoma formation. Apply gentle pressure to injection site for approximately 1 minute. If continuous oozing of blood or hematoma formation occurs, contact physician.

Ice may be applied to subcutaneous injection site for 10 to 15 minutes before injection; this requires a physician's order or a written hospital policy.

Subcutaneous administration sites are rotated. Record site of injection on patient's chart.

NOTE: A flow sheet is used to record IV and subcutaneous heparin administration as well as blood coagulation test results. *Always* check this flow sheet before drug is administered, and enter the required data immediately after heparin is administered.

ONGOING ASSESSMENTS AND NURSING MANAGEMENT
Monitor vital signs q2h to q4h or as ordered. If a drop in blood pressure or rise in pulse is

noted, look for signs of hemorrhage (see below) and notify physician of findings.

CLINICAL ALERT: Monitor patient for signs of hemorrhage, which may begin as a slight bleeding or bruising tendency. Look for bleeding gums, unexplained nosebleeds, bruises, petechiae, and hematemesis. Visually inspect urine for hematuria and stool for melena or bright red blood; observe for complaints of abdominal or lumbar pain (ovarian hemorrhage, adrenal hemorrhage), severe headache (epidural hematoma), and signs of adrenal insufficiency (Appendix 6, section 6-3). If any of these occurs, it is reported to the physician immediately. Protamine sulfate (see *Overdosage*) must be available in case administration is necessary.

Observe for evidence of new thrombosis. Because symptoms will vary and depend on the area or organ involved, consider each patient complaint or change in condition carefully and report findings to physician.

Each time drug is administered, inspect previous subcutaneous injection sites for signs of inflammation (redness, swelling, pain along pathway of vein) and hematoma formation; inspect needle site of continuous IV infusion q2h to q4h for signs of hematoma formation and inflammation; inspect intermittent infusion needle site for hematoma formation and inflammation each time drug is administered.

Continued blood coagulation tests are usually ordered. Blood is drawn ½ hour before administration of subcutaneous or intermittent IV dose, with the frequency of tests dependent on the dose administered and condition treated, as well as other factors. Early in therapy, blood coagulation tests may be performed before each heparin administration by the intermittent IV or subcutaneous route and q4h when heparin is administered by continuous IV infusion; once dosage is stabilized, coagulation tests are usually performed on a daily basis.

If each heparin dose is to be adjusted according to coagulation test results, inform laboratory personnel that test must be performed immediately. Once results are obtained, contact physician because intermittent IV or subcutaneous heparin administration must be given on time to maintain therapeutic anticoagulant effect.

Apply prolonged pressure to the needle or catheter site following venipuncture, removal of central or peripheral IV lines, and IM or subcutaneous injections. In some instances, a pressure dressing may be required. Laboratory personnel should be made aware of anticoagulant therapy.

When applicable, advise patient to stop smoking because nicotine may alter the anticoagulant action of heparin.

The physician may order periodic platelet counts because heparin administration may result in thrombocytopenia due to platelet aggregation. Contact physician immediately if recent platelet count is below normal value.

Do not piggyback other drugs into continuous heparin IV infusion line or mix heparin for subcutaneous or intermittent IV administration with any other drug unless specifically directed to do so by the physician.

Patient may be receiving concomitant oral anticoagulant therapy. Prothrombin time will be ordered before initial dose as well as daily during early therapy. See also Coumarin and Indandione Derivatives.

Hepatitis B Immune Globulin

See Immunizations, Passive.

Hepatitis B Vaccine

See Immunizations, Active.

Hetacillin

See Penicillins.

Hetastarch (Hydroxyethyl Starch) Rx

injection: 6% in 0.9%   Hespan
    sodium chloride

INDICATIONS
When plasma volume expansion is desired as an adjunct in shock due to hemorrhage, burns, surgery, sepsis, or other trauma. It is not a substitute for blood or plasma. Adjunctive use in leukapheresis has also been shown to improve harvesting and increase the yield of granulocytes by centrifugation.

CONTRAINDICATIONS
Patients with severe bleeding disorders or with severe congestive cardiac and renal failure with oliguria or anuria.

ACTIONS
Colloidal properties approximate those of human albumin. IV infusion results in expansion of plasma volume slightly in excess of the volume infused.

WARNINGS
Large volumes may alter coagulation. Administration may result in transient prolongation of pro-

thrombin, partial thromboplastin, and clotting times. With large doses, observe for the possibility of transient prolongation of bleeding time. Hematocrit may be decreased and plasma protein diluted excessively by administration of large volumes of hetastarch.

Use in leukapheresis: Significant declines in platelet count and hemoglobin levels have been observed in donors undergoing repeated leukapheresis procedures because of volume-expanding effects of hetastarch. Hemoglobin levels usually return to normal within 24 hours. Hemodilution by hetastarch and saline may also result in 24-hour declines of hemoglobin, total protein, albumin, calcium, and fibrinogen values.

Use in pregnancy: Not used in pregnant women unless potential benefits outweigh the unknown potential hazards to the fetus.

Use in children: No data available.

PRECAUTIONS

The possibility of circulatory overload should be kept in mind. Take special care in those with impaired renal clearance, because this is the principal way in which hetastarch is eliminated. Use caution when risk of pulmonary edema or congestive heart failure is increased.

Indirect bilirubin levels of 0.83 mg/dl have been reported; total bilirubin was within normal limits. Indirect bilirubin returned to normal by 96 hours after infusion. The significance of these elevations is not known, but caution should be observed in administration of hetastarch to those with liver disease.

Laboratory determinations are necessary to monitor use during leukapheresis. Studies should include CBC, total leukocyte and platelet counts, leukocyte differential count, hemoglobin, hematocrit, prothrombin time, and partial thromboplastin time.

Allergic or sensitivity reactions have been reported. If such reactions occur, discontinue use; if necessary, administer an antihistamine.

ADVERSE REACTIONS

Vomiting, mild temperature elevation, chills, itching, submaxillary and parotid gland enlargement, mild influenzalike symptoms, headache, muscle pains, peripheral edema (lower extremities), anaphylactoid reactions consisting of periorbital edema, urticaria, and wheezing.

DOSAGE

Plasma volume expansion: Total dosage and rate of infusion depend on amount of blood lost and resultant hemoconcentration. Amount usually administered is 500 ml to 1000 ml. Total dosage does not usually exceed 1500 ml/day (20 ml/kg). In acute hemorrhagic shock, administration rates approaching 20 ml/kg/hour may be used. In burn or septic shock, give at slower rates.

Leukapheresis: In continuous-flow centrifugation (CFC) procedures, 250 ml to 700 ml is typically infused at a constant fixed ratio, usually 1:8, to venous whole blood. Multiple CFC procedures using hetastarch of up to 2 per week and a total of 7 to 10 have been reported to be safe and effective.

NURSING IMPLICATIONS

HISTORY
Etiology of shock.

PHYSICAL ASSESSMENT
Monitor blood pressure, pulse, and respirations; review most recent vital signs. Note general condition of patient (skin color, level of consciousness, site of blood loss, extent of burns or other trauma). Laboratory tests may be ordered to determine extent of blood loss; other tests may also be appropriate.

ADMINISTRATION
Administer IV only.

Safety and compatibility of other additives are not established; do not add drugs or mix with other IV fluids.

Physician orders total dose and rate of infusion.

Product is available in 500-ml IV infusion bottles.

Usually administered by use of a secondary IV line.

Discard partially used bottles.

ONGOING ASSESSMENTS AND NURSING MANAGEMENT
Monitor blood pressure, pulse, and respirations q5m to q15m or as ordered. Keep physician informed of patient response.

If periorbital edema, urticaria, wheezing, or itching occurs (signs of sensitivity or allergic reaction), discontinue use immediately and run primary line IV fluid at KVO. Notify physician immediately.

Measure intake and output. Report oliguria, anuria, or significant change in intake–output ratio to physician immediately.

Large volumes may alter coagulation. Observe for increase in bleeding and unusual bleeding or bruising.

Observe for signs of fluid (circulatory) overload (Appendix 6, section 6-12). If symptoms are apparent, slow IV infusion rate to KVO and notify physician immediately.

Physician may order laboratory tests such as coagulation tests, hemoglobin, and hematocrit.

Leukapheresis: CBC, WBC and differential, platelet count, hemoglobin, hematocrit, prothrombin time, and partial thromboplastin time are recommended to monitor use of hetastarch during this procedure.

Hexachlorophene

See Antiseptics and Germicides.

Hexafluorenium Bromide Rx

20 mg/ml   Mylaxen

INDICATIONS
A muscle relaxant that is an adjunct for use with succinylcholine to prolong neuromuscular blockade and obviate muscular fasciculations sometimes induced by succinylcholine.

CONTRAINDICATIONS
Hypersensitivity to hexafluorenium or bromides.

ACTIONS
Prolongs neuromuscular blockade of succinylcholine and obviates muscular fasciculations sometimes seen when succinylcholine is used alone. Is a plasma cholinesterase inhibitor; its anticholinesterase activity is limited to plasma esterases. Its chemical structure is such that it apparently does not have access to intracellular cholinesterase. Has no known effect on consciousness, pain threshold, or cerebration. Duration of effect ranges from 20 to 30 minutes.

WARNINGS
Do not administer unless facilities for intubation, artificial respiration, and administration of oxygen therapy are instantaneously available.

Safety for use in pregnancy is not established. Use in women of childbearing potential, particularly in early pregnancy, only when clearly needed and when potential benefits outweigh unknown potential hazards.

PRECAUTIONS
Use with caution in those with cardiovascular, renal, hepatic, pulmonary (*e.g.,* asthma), or metabolic disorders, patients with glaucoma or during ocular surgery, those with fractures, muscle spasm,

or any type of neuromyopathy (*e.g.,* amyotrophic lateral sclerosis, muscular dystrophy, myasthenia gravis). Give with great caution to those with severe burns and to those who recently have been digitalized or who may have digitalis toxicity, because serious cardiac arrhythmias or arrest may result.

DRUG INTERACTIONS
If **other relaxants** are to be used during the same procedure, the possibility of synergistic or antagonistic effects should be considered.

ADVERSE REACTIONS
Profound and prolonged muscle paralysis, resulting in respiratory depression, apnea, bronchospasm; bradycardia; tachycardia; hypertension; hypotension; cardiac arrest; arrhythmias; hypersensitivity; hyperthermia; increased intraocular pressure; salivation.

DOSAGE
Give in ratio of 2 mg of hexafluorenium for each milligram of succinylcholine. Administer only after patient is unconscious.

Intermittent administration: 0.4 mg/kg IV, followed in 3 minutes by 0.2 mg/kg succinylcholine IV. In long surgical procedures, may repeat at doses of 0.1 mg/kg to 0.2 mg/kg at necessary intervals.

NURSING IMPLICATIONS
See Succinylcholine Chloride.

Hexocyclium Methylsulfate

See Gastrointestinal Anticholinergics/Antispasmodics.

Hexylcaine Hydrochloride

See Anesthetics, Local, Topical.

Histamine Phosphate Rx

injection: 0.55 mg   *Generic*
(gastric test), 0.275
mg (pheochromo-
cytoma test)

INDICATIONS
For subcutaneous administration to test ability of gastric mucosa to produce hydrochloric acid and IV administration for presumptive diagnosis of pheochromocytoma.

CONTRAINDICATIONS

Hypersensitivity to histamine products; severe hypertension; vasomotor instability; bronchial asthma (past or present); urticaria (past or present); severe cardiac, pulmonary, or renal disease.

ACTIONS

Acts on the vascular system, smooth muscle, and exocrine glands. Increases volume and acidity of gastric juice.

WARNINGS

Attacks of severe asthma or other serious allergic conditions may be precipitated by administration; extreme caution is advised in using histamine in susceptible patients.

Gastric test: Avoid accidental injection into vein or artery. Benefit-to-risk ratio is considered in performing the gastric test on patients with pheochromocytoma.

Safety for use in pregnancy not established; benefits must be weighed against the possible hazards to mother and child.

PRECAUTIONS

Average or large doses may cause flushing, dizziness, headache, nervousness, local or generalized allergic manifestations, marked hypertension, tachycardia, abdominal cramps. These reactions may be alarming and are potentially dangerous. Histamine increases the acid of the gastric juice and may cause symptoms of peptic ulcer. A large dose may cause severe occipital headache, blurred vision, anginal pain, a rapid drop in blood pressure, cyanosis of the face. Local reactions at site of injection for the gastric test may include erythema and edema. Histamine is used with caution in patients with any cardiac abnormalities.

ADVERSE REACTIONS

Average or large doses may produce flushing, dizziness, headache, bronchial constriction, dyspnea, visual disturbances, faintness, syncope, urticaria, asthma, marked hypertension or hypotension, palpitation, tachycardia, nervousness, abdominal cramps, diarrhea, vomiting, metallic taste, localized or general allergic manifestations, or collapse with convulsions.

Gastric test: Erythema, edema, weakness, nausea.

OVERDOSAGE

Symptoms: May cause severe symptoms, including circulatory or vasomotor collapse, shock, and even death.

Treatment: If accidental overdosage is discovered early, temporary application of a tourniquet proximally to the injection site may be tried to slow down drug absorption. Antidotes to histamine are epinephrine HCl 0.1 ml to 0.5 ml of 1:1000 aqueous solution subcutaneously in case of emergency due to severe reactions. An antihistamine preparation may be given PO in case of mild allergic reactions caused by usual dose of the drug.

DOSAGE

Histamine test: After basal gastric secretion is collected, give 0.0275 mg (or 0.01 mg of histamine base)/kg subcutaneously. Gastric contents are then collected in four 15-minute specimens for 1 hour and analyzed for volume, acidity, pH, and acid output.

Augmented histamine test: Initially, a suitable dose of antihistamine is administered IM (*e.g.,* 10 mg chlorpheniramine maleate, 50 mg pyrilamine maleate, or 50 mg diphenhydramine HCl). After conclusion of the basal study, 0.04 mg/kg is given subcutaneously.

Pheochromocytoma histamine test: Withhold antihypertensive drugs, sympathomimetic agents, sedatives, and narcotics for at least 24 hours, preferably 72 hours, before test is performed. Food is not withheld. This test is used only in patients whose resting blood pressure does not exceed 150/110.

Patient rests in bed while a slow IV infusion of either 5% dextrose or isotonic saline solution is established. The blood pressure is recorded until it is stable. At that time, a 2-hour period of urine collection for catecholamine assay is started. At the end of the period, histamine is rapidly administered through the infusion and another 2-hour collection started.

The first IV dose should be 0.01 mg (10 mcg). If no response is observed in 5 minutes, administer 0.05 mg (50 mcg). Record blood pressure and pulse every 30 seconds for 15 minutes. The expected responses in both positive and negative tests are headache, flushing, and a decrease in blood pressure, followed within 2 minutes by an increase.

NURSING IMPLICATIONS

HISTORY

See Appendix 4. Question patient about allergies, bronchial asthma (see *Contraindications*).

PHYSICAL ASSESSMENT

Obtain vital signs, weight.

ADMINISTRATION

Review hospital procedure manual.

Physician will calculate dose.

The ampules are labeled "gastric test" and "pheochromocytoma test." The gastric test ampule contains 0.55 mg (equivalent to 0.2 mg histamine base)/ml. The pheochromocytoma test ampule contains 0.275 mg (equivalent to 0.1 mg histamine)/ml.

Clarify if dosage is written in milligrams of histamine or histamine base.

Gastric test is administered subcutaneously; pheochromocytoma test is administered IV through running IV infusion.

See *Dosage* above.

Obtain required baseline blood pressure and pulse.

Have epinephrine HCl 1:1000 aqueous solution and needle and syringe for administration readily available before test is started. In addition, have phentolamine readily available for the pheochromocytoma histamine test to reverse any alarming increase in blood pressure.

Physician usually administers IV histamine for pheochromocytoma test; nurse monitors blood pressure before and after administration of drug.

ONGOING ASSESSMENTS AND NURSING MANAGEMENT

CLINICAL ALERT: Be aware of adverse reactions for average or large doses and symptoms of overdosage. Because some may be serious and potentially dangerous, notify physician immediately if one or more should occur.

Marked hypotension or hypertension during these tests requires immediate notification of the physician.

Gastric histamine test: Follow procedure (see *Dosage* or hospital procedure manual) for obtaining specimens. Label and number specimens.

Pheochromocytoma test: Follow procedure (see *Dosage* or hospital procedure manual) for obtaining blood pressure and pulse. Take and record measurements at required time interval (usually every 30 seconds for 15 minutes following administration of histamine). Physician will require this record to interpret test results.

Homatropine Hydrobromide

See Mydriatics, Cycloplegic.

Hyaluronidase Rx

powder for injection: Wydase
150 units/1-ml
vial, 1500 units/
10-ml vial
injection: 150
units/ml

INDICATIONS

As adjuvant to increase absorption and dispersion of injected drugs; for hypodermoclysis; as an adjunct in subcutaneous urography for improving resorption of radiopaque agents.

CONTRAINDICATIONS

Do not inject into acutely inflamed or cancerous areas.

ACTIONS

Hydrolyzes hyaluronic acid, which obstructs diffusion of invasive substances, promoting diffusion and absorption of fluids in tissues.

PRECAUTIONS

Discontinue if sensitization occurs. Sensitivity occurs infrequently. A preliminary skin test for sensitivity should be conducted. When epinephrine is injected along with hyaluronidase, observe usual precautions for use of epinephrine in cardiovascular disease, thyroid disease, diabetes, digital nerve block, ischemia of the fingers and toes, and so on.

ADVERSE REACTIONS

When solutions devoid of inorganic electrolytes are administered by hypodermoclysis, hypovolemia may occur. This can be avoided by using solutions containing adequate amounts of inorganic electrolytes or by controlling the volume and rate of fluid administered.

DOSAGE

Absorption and dispersion of injected drugs: May be enhanced by adding 150 units hyaluronidase.

Hypodermoclysis: Inject solution into rubber tubing close to the needle or injection port (close to needle) of plastic tubing. An alternate method is to inject subcutaneously prior to clysis into the same area that will be used for clysis. One-hundred-fifty units will facilitate absorption of 1000 ml or more of solution. May also be added to small volumes of IV solution (up to 200 ml) such as a small clysis for infants or solutions of drugs for subcutaneous injection. For children under 3 years, the volume of a single clysis should be limited to 200 ml; in premature infants or during the neonatal period, daily dosage should not exceed 25 ml/kg; rate should not be greater than 2 ml/minute. For older patients, rate and volume of administration should not exceed those employed by IV infusion.

Subcutaneous urography: Subcutaneous route of administration of urographic contrast media is indicated when IV administration cannot be accomplished, particularly in infants and small children. With patient prone, inject 75 units of hyaluronidase subcutaneously over each scapula; then inject the contrast medium at the same sites.

NURSING IMPLICATIONS

HISTORY
See Appendix 4.

PHYSICAL ASSESSMENT
Obtain vital signs; examine for signs of dehydration (Appendix 6, section 6-10). Review recent laboratory tests, diagnostic studies.

ADMINISTRATION
Preliminary skin test for sensitivity may be ordered. Administer an interdermal injection of 0.02 ml of 150 units/ml (3 units). A positive reaction consists of a wheal with pseudopods appearing in 5 minutes and persisting for 15 to 20 minutes, accompanied by localized itching. Transient vasodilatation (erythema) at test site is not a positive reaction.

Absorption and dispersion of injected drugs: The lyophilized powder is reconstituted with Sodium Chloride Injection, USP, immediately before use.

Check with physician about exact administration.

May be added to drug in syringe before administration or injected at site of drug injection. Usually, hyaluronidase is injected subcutaneously before injection of drug.

Hypodermoclysis (H clysis): Needle tip is inserted between skin and muscle, usually the dorsal surface of the thigh. Fluid should start in readily without pain or lump.

Physician orders method of administration (see *Dosage*) and infusion rate.

Subcutaneous urography: See *Dosage.*

ONGOING ASSESSMENTS AND NURSING MANAGEMENT
Observe site of hypodermoclysis q15m to q30m. Observe for signs of fluid and electrolyte imbalance (Appendix 6, sections 6-13 to 6-18), and of hypovolemia if nonelectrolyte solutions are administered.

If patient reports moderate to severe pain or discomfort or if solution fails to run at prescribed rate, notify physician.

Hydralazine Hydrochloride Rx

tablets: 10 mg, 50 mg	Apresoline (10 mg contains tartrazine), *Generic*
tablets: 25 mg	Apresoline, *Generic*
tablets: 100 mg	Apresoline (contains tartrazine)
injection: 20 mg	Apresoline

INDICATIONS
Orally for essential hypertension, usually in combination with other drugs. Parenterally for severe essential hypertension when drug cannot be given orally or when there is an urgent need to lower blood pressure.

CONTRAINDICATIONS
Hypersensitivity; coronary artery disease; mitral valvular rheumatic heart disease.

ACTIONS
Lowers blood pressure by exerting a peripheral vasodilating effect through direct relaxation of vascular smooth muscle, primarily arteriolar, with little effect on the venous capacitance vessels. This results in a decrease in arterial blood pressure (diastolic more than systolic); decreased peripheral vascular resistance; a reflex increased heart rate, stroke volume, and cardiac output. Drug also maintains or increases renal and cerebral blood flow. Because of reflex increases in cardiac function, hydralazine is commonly used in combination with a drug that inhibits sympathetic activity (*e.g.,* beta blockers, clonidine, or methyldopa).

Concomitant administration of food can increase bioavailability. Oral tablets produce peak concentrations in the blood within 1 hour. A very small portion is excreted as unchanged drug. Elimination half-life averages 3 hours (range 2–8 hours). Following oral administration, onset of action is within 45 minutes and effect lasts for a minimum of 6 hours.

WARNINGS
Lupus erythematosus: In a few patients, hydralazine may produce a clinical picture simulating acute systemic lupus erythematosus (LE) (*e.g.,* arthralgia, myalgia, dermatoses, fever, anemia, splenomegaly, and rarely cutaneous necrotizing vasculitis). If this occurs, discontinue drug and employ alternate antihypertensive therapy. Symptoms usually regress when drug is discontinued, but residual effects have been detected many years later. Long-term treatment with steroids may be necessary.

Use in pregnancy: Safety not established. Use only when clearly needed and when potential benefits outweigh the unknown potential hazards to the fetus.

Thrombocytopenia, leukopenia, petechial bleeding, and hematomas have been reported in newborns of women taking hydralazine. In all cases symptoms resolved spontaneously within 1 to 3 weeks.

PRECAUTIONS

Coronary artery disease: Myocardial stimulation produced by hydralazine can cause anginal attacks and ECG changes of myocardial ischemia. Drug has been implicated in production of myocardial infarction. Is used with caution in patients with suspected coronary artery disease.

Cardiovascular: The "hyperdynamic" circulation caused by hydralazine may accentuate specific cardiovascular inadequacies (*e.g.,* increased pulmonary artery pressure in those with mitral valve disease). May reduce the pressor responses to epinephrine. Postural hypotension may result from hydralazine but is less common with ganglionic blocking agents. Use with caution in those with cerebral vascular accidents.

Withdrawal: In those with marked reduction in blood pressure, withdraw drug gradually to avoid sudden rise in pressure.

Dosage increase: In those with severe forms of hypertension and with uremia, too rapid an increase in dosage may produce a marked fall in blood pressure. In these cases, certain cerebral symptoms, from mild anxiety to depression to acute anxiety or severe depression and coma, may appear.

Renal effects: In those with normal kidneys, there is evidence of increased renal flow and a maintenance of glomerular filtration. In some instances, improved renal function has been noted when control values were below normal prior to administration. Use with caution in those with advanced renal damage.

Neuritis: Peripheral neuritis, evidenced by paresthesias, numbness, and tingling, has been seen. The addition of pyridoxine to the regimen, if symptoms develop, has been recommended.

Hematologic effects: Blood dyscrasias, consisting of reduction in hemoglobin and red cell count, leukopenia, agranulocytosis, and purpura have been reported. If such abnormalities develop, discontinue therapy. Periodic blood counts are recommended.

Tartrazine sensitivity: Some products contain tartrazine (see Appendix 6, section 6-23).

DRUG INTERACTIONS

MAO inhibitors are used with caution in those receiving hydralazine. Because hydralazine alone may induce tachycardia and angina, **sympathomimetics** are used with caution. When other potent **parenteral antihypertensive drugs** (*e.g.,* diazoxide) are used in combination with hydralazine, observe patient continuously for several hours for any excessive fall in blood pressure. Profound hypotensive

episodes may occur when diazoxide injection and hydralazine are used concomitantly.

ADVERSE REACTIONS

Are usually reversible when dosage is reduced; in some cases it may be necessary to discontinue drug.

Most common: Headache, palpitations, anorexia, nausea, vomiting, diarrhea, tachycardia, angina pectoris.

Ophthalmic: Lacrimation, conjunctivitis.

Neurologic: Peripheral neuritis, evidenced by paresthesias, numbness, tingling; dizziness; tremors; psychotic reactions characterized by depression, disorientation, or anxiety.

Hypersensitivity: Rash, urticaria, pruritus, fever, chills, arthralgia, eosinophilia; rarely, hepatitis and obstructive jaundice.

GI and GU: Constipation, paralytic ileus, difficulty in micturition.

Hematologic: Blood dyscrasias, consisting of reduction in hemoglobin and RBC, leukopenia, agranulocytosis, purpura.

Miscellaneous: Nasal congestion, flushing, edema, muscle cramps, lymphadenopathy, splenomegaly, hypotension, paradoxical pressor response, dyspnea.

OVERDOSAGE

Symptoms: Hypotension, tachycardia, and general skin flushing are to be expected. Myocardial ischemia and cardiac arrhythmia can develop; profound shock can occur in severe overdosage.

Treatment: Evacuate gastric contents, taking adequate precautions against aspiration and for protection of the airway; instill activated charcoal slurry, if conditions permit. These manipulations may have to be omitted or carried out after cardiovascular status has been stabilized, because they might precipitate cardiac arrhythmias or increase depth of shock. Support of the cardiovascular system is of primary importance. Treat shock with volume expanders without resorting to vasopressors, if possible. If a vasopressor is required, use one that is least likely to precipitate or aggravate tachycardia and cardiac arrhythmias. Digitalization may be necessary. Renal function must be monitored and supported as required.

DOSAGE

Initial therapy: Initiate therapy in gradually increasing dosages and adjust according to individual response. Start with 10 mg qid for the first 2 to 4 days, and increase to 25 mg qid for balance of the first week.

Second and subsequent weeks: Increase dosage to 50 mg qid.

Maintenance: Adjust dosage to lowest effective level. During chronic administration, tolerance may develop and higher dosages may be necessary. Twice daily dosage may be adequate. In a few resistant patients, up to 400 mg/day may be required for significant antihypertensive effect. Incidence of toxic reactions, particularly the LE cell syndrome, is high in those receiving large doses of hydralazine. A lower dosage combined with other agents should be used. When combining therapy, individual titration is essential.

Parenteral: When there is an urgent need, therapy in the hospitalized patient may be initiated IV or IM. Use parenterally only when drug cannot be given orally. Usual dose is 20 mg to 40 mg, repeated as necessary. Certain patients (especially those with marked renal damage) may require lower dose.

NURSING IMPLICATIONS

HISTORY
See Appendix 4.

PHYSICAL ASSESSMENT
Obtain blood pressure on both arms with patient in standing and sitting positions; obtain temperature, pulse, respiratory rate, weight. Laboratory studies include serum electrolytes and CBC. An LE cell preparation and antinuclear antibody titer are also recommended prior to therapy. Other laboratory tests and diagnostic studies may also be appropriate.

ADMINISTRATION
Obtain blood pressure and pulse immediately prior to administration.

Do not administer and notify physician if there has been a significant decrease in the systolic and/or diastolic pressure.

Administer oral form with food or meals.

Parenteral form may be administered IM or IV.

Following parenteral administration, monitor blood pressure and pulse q5m until stabilized, or as ordered. There may be a decrease in blood pressure within a few minutes after injection, with an average maximal decrease in 10 to 80 minutes. In cases when there is a previously existing increased intracranial pressure, lowering the blood pressure may increase cerebral ischemia. Notify physician if there is a significant decrease in the systolic or diastolic pressure.

ONGOING ASSESSMENTS AND NURSING MANAGEMENT
Record vital signs (see above) daily; observe for adverse reactions. Measure intake and output if patient has history of renal impairment or drug is administered parenterally.

Postural hypotension may occur. Have patient dangle legs 5 to 10 minutes before getting out of bed. Assist with ambulation as needed.

A few patients may produce a clinical picture resembling acute systemic LE. Notify physician if patient develops arthralgia, fever, chest pain, continued malaise, or other unexplained signs or symptoms.

Periodic CBC, LE cell preparations, and antinuclear antibody titer determinations are recommended during therapy. A positive antinuclear antibody titer or positive LE cell reaction requires implications of test results be weighed against benefits to be derived from therapy with this drug.

Patients receiving parenteral therapy are observed closely until condition stabilizes. Most patients can be transferred to oral form in 24 to 48 hours.

If peripheral neuritis occurs (numbness, tingling, paresthesias of extremities) physician may prescribe pyridoxine (vitamin B_6). Pyridoxine may also be prescribed prophylactically.

Urinary output may be increased in some patients because of improved renal flow.

Psychotic reactions (depression, disorientation, anxiety) may occur. Observe mental status; notify physician if changes are noted. Depression may require more frequent observation of patient.

Physician may order salt-restricted diet as part of management of hypertension. In some patients, a weight-reduction diet may also be ordered.

PATIENT AND FAMILY INFORMATION
Take with meals or food.

Do not discontinue medication unless directed by physician.

Avoid cough, cold, or allergy medications (some contain sympathomimetics) except on professional recommendation.

A slight increase in urine output may be noted, especially early in therapy.

Notify physician of any unexplained prolonged general tiredness or fever, muscle or joint aching, or if chest pain (angina) occurs.

If dizziness (orthostatic hypotension) occurs, avoid sudden changes in posture. Arise from a sitting or lying position slowly and avoid standing in one place for prolonged periods. Do not attempt to drive or perform other potentially hazardous tasks if dizziness occurs.

May cause headache or palpitations, especially

during first few days of therapy. If these persist, notify physician.

Follow physician's recommendations regarding diet, exercise, weight reduction (if necessary).

Weigh self weekly. If significant weight gain or edema is noted, contact physician.

Hydrochlorothiazide

See Thiazides and Related Diuretics.

Hydrocortisone

See Corticosteroids, Topical; Glucocorticoids.

Hydrocortisone Acetate

See Corticosteroids, Ophthalmic; Corticosteroids, Topical; Glucocorticoids.

Hydrocortisone Cypionate

See Glucocorticoids.

Hydrocortisone Sodium Phosphate

See Glucocorticoids.

Hydrocortisone Sodium Succinate

See Glucocorticoids.

Hydrocortisone Valerate

See Corticosteroids, Topical.

Hydroflumethiazide

See Thiazides and Related Diuretics.

Hydrogen Iodide

See Iodine Expectorants.

Hydromorphone Hydrochloride

See Narcotic Analgesics.

Hydroxocobalamin, Crystalline

See Vitamin B_{12}.

Hydroxyamphetamine Hydrobromide

See Mydriatics/Ophthalmic Vasoconstrictors.

Hydroxychloroquine Sulfate

See 4-Aminoquinoline Compounds.

Hydroxyprogesterone Caproate

See Progestins.

Hydroxyurea Rx

capsules: 500 mg   Hydrea

INDICATIONS

An antineoplastic indicated in melanoma, resistant chronic myelocytic leukemia, and recurrent, metastatic, or inoperable carcinoma of the ovary. Concomitant administration with irradiation therapy in local control of primary squamous cell (epidermoid) carcinomas of the head and neck, excluding the lip.

CONTRAINDICATIONS

Patients with marked bone-marrow depression (_i.e._, leukopenia [less than 2500 WBC] or thrombocytopenia [less than 100,000 WBC]) or severe anemia.

ACTIONS

Precise mechanism is unknown. Studies support the hypothesis that hydroxyurea causes immediate inhibition of DNA synthesis without interfering with the synthesis of RNA or of protein. Is readily absorbed from the GI tract. Drug reaches peak serum concentration within 2 hours; by 24 hours, concentration in the serum is essentially zero.

WARNINGS

Patients who have received irradiation therapy in the past may have an exacerbation of postirradiation erythema.

Bone marrow: Bone-marrow suppression may occur, and leukopenia is generally the first and most common manifestation. Thrombocytopenia and anemia occur less often and seldom are seen without a preceding leukopenia. Recovery from myelosuppression is rapid when therapy is interrupted. Bone-marrow depression is more likely in those who have previously received radiotherapy or cyto-toxic cancer chemotherapeutic agents; use cautiously in such patients. Severe anemia must be corrected with whole blood replacement before initiating therapy.

Erythrocytic abnormalities: Megaloblastic eryth-ropoiesis, which is self-limiting, is often seen early in the course of therapy. Morphologic changes resemble those of pernicious anemia but are not related to vitamin B_{12} or folic acid deficiency. Drug may also delay plasma iron clearance and reduce rate of iron utilization by erythrocytes but does not appear to alter RBC survival time.

Use in impaired renal function: Hydroxyurea is excreted by the kidneys; use with caution in those with marked renal dysfunction. Elderly patients may be more sensitive to the effects of hydroxyurea and may require lower dosage regimen.

Abnormal changes in clinical laboratory data are often difficult to explain in cancer patients during drug therapy. Changes toward normal are often due to improvement in the function of an organ; changes to abnormal levels are more likely due to progressive disease.

Use in pregnancy: Drugs that affect DNA synthesis may be mutagenic. Drug is not recommended for use in women who are or who may become pregnant, unless potential benefits outweigh the possible hazards.

PRECAUTIONS

Determination of hemoglobin, total leukocyte counts, and platelet counts should be performed at least once a week throughout the course of therapy. If WBC decreases to less than 2500/mm³ or platelet count to less than 100,000/mm³, therapy should be interrupted until values rise significantly toward normal levels. Anemia, if it occurs, is managed with whole blood replacement without interruption of therapy.

DRUG INTERACTIONS

Drug/lab tests: **Serum uric acid, BUN,** and **creatinine levels** may be increased.

ADVERSE REACTIONS

Most frequent: Bone-marrow depression (leuko-penia, anemia, and occasionally thrombocytopenia).

Less frequent: GI symptoms (stomatitis, anorexia, nausea, vomiting, diarrhea, constipation) and dermatologic reactions (maculopapular rash, facial edema). Dysuria and alopecia occur very rarely. Large doses may produce moderate drowsiness.

Neurologic: Disturbances are extremely rare and are limited to headache, dizziness, disorientation, hallucinations, and convulsions.

Renal impairment: May cause temporary impairment of renal tubular function accompanied by elevations in serum uric acid, BUN, and creatinine levels.

Combination therapy: Adverse reactions observed with combined hydroxyurea and irradiation therapy are similar to those reported using hydroxyurea alone, primarily bone-marrow depression (anemia, leukopenia) and gastric irritation. Almost all patients receiving an adequate course of combined therapy will demonstrate concurrent leukopenia. Platelet depression has occurred rarely and only in the presence of marked leukopenia. Gastric distress has also been reported with irradiation alone and in combination with hydroxyurea therapy. Therapeutic doses of irradiation therapy alone produce the same adverse reactions as hydroxyurea; combined therapy may cause an increase in incidence and severity of these side-effects. Although inflammation of the mucous membranes at the irradiated site (mucositis) is attributed to irradiation, some believe that the more severe cases are due to combination therapy. If mucositis is severe, hydroxyurea therapy may be temporarily interrupted; if it is extremely severe, the irradiation dosage may be temporarily postponed.

Severe gastric distress, such as nausea, vomiting, and anorexia, may be controlled by temporary interruption of hydroxyurea administration; rarely has the additional interruption of irradiation been necessary.

DOSAGE

Dosage is based on patient's actual or ideal weight, whichever is less. An adequate trial period for determining effectiveness is 6 weeks. When there is regression of tumor size or arrest in tumor growth, therapy should be continued indefinitely. See *Warnings* and *Adverse Reactions* (combination therapy) for interruption of therapy in the event of hematologic changes.

Solid tumors: Patients on intermittent therapy have rarely required complete discontinuation of therapy because of toxicity.

Intermittent therapy: 80 mg/kg PO as single dose every third day.

Continuous therapy: 20 mg/kg to 30 mg/kg PO as a single daily dose.

Concomitant therapy with irradiation (carcinoma of the head and neck): 80 mg/kg/day PO as single dose every third day. Administration of hydroxyurea should begin at least 7 days before initiation of irradiation and continue during radiotherapy as well as indefinitely afterward, provided patient is kept under adequate observation and exhibits no unusual or severe reactions.

Resistant chronic myelocytic leukemia:
Continuous therapy (20 mg/kg to 30 mg/kg PO as single daily dose) is recommended.

Use in children: Dosage regimens are not established.

NURSING IMPLICATIONS

HISTORY
See Appendix 4.

PHYSICAL ASSESSMENT
Record physical, emotional status; vital signs; weight. Laboratory studies include CBC, differential, platelet count, and renal- and hepatic-function studies. Bone-marrow examination may be performed.

ADMINISTRATION
If patient prefers, or if he is unable to swallow capsules, the contents of the capsule may be emptied into a glass of water and taken immediately. Some inert material may not dissolve and may float on the surface.

ONGOING ASSESSMENTS AND NURSING MANAGEMENT
Monitor vital signs daily; observe for adverse reactions. Force fluids; patient should drink 10 to 12 glasses (8 oz each) per day. If fluid intake is below this amount, discuss with physician.

Measure intake and output if patient is taking fluids poorly, is elderly, is debilitated, or has renal impairment.

CLINICAL ALERT: Observe for signs of bone-marrow depression (Appendix 6, section 6-8).

An exacerbation of postirradiation erythema may occur in those who have received previous radiotherapy. Report this occurrence to the physician. Inspect sites daily; bring any changes to the attention of the physician. Keep areas clean and dry.

Drowsiness may occur with large doses. Patient may require assistance with ambulation.

Nausea and vomiting are reported to the physician. An antiemetic may be necessary.

Weigh weekly or as ordered. Report any significant weight loss to the physician.

Anorexia may occur. Monitor dietary intake. If anorexia persists for more than 2 days, notify physician. A diet high in calories, vitamins, and protein may be ordered.

Pain or discomfort from inflammation of the mucous membrane at the irradiated area (head and neck cancers) is usually controlled by measures such as topical anesthetics and orally administered analgesics. See also stomatitis care (Appendix 6, section 6-21).

The complete status of the blood, including bone-marrow examination (if indicated), as well as serum uric acid and renal- and hepatic-function tests, is recommended during treatment.

Serum uric acid levels may increase. Physician may order allopurinol.

PATIENT AND FAMILY INFORMATION
Notify physician or nurse if fever, chills, sore throat, nausea, vomiting, loss of appetite, diarrhea, sores in the mouth or on the lips, or unusual bleeding or bruising occurs.

Inform other physicians and dentist of therapy with this drug.

Medication may cause drowsiness, constipation, redness of the face, skin rash, itching, loss of hair; notify physician or nurse if these become pronounced.

If drowsiness does occur, do not attempt to drive or perform other tasks that are potentially hazardous.

Frequent laboratory tests will be necessary to monitor therapy.

It will be important to drink 8 to 10 glasses (8 oz each) of fluid daily. If unable to drink this amount, discuss with physician. Foods that are liquid at room temperature (Jell-O, ice cream) may be included as part of fluid intake.

Keep all clinic, office, or laboratory appointments because therapy must be monitored closely.

Female patient of childbearing age: Contraceptive measures may be recommended by the physician.

Hydroxyzine Rx

tablets (as HCl): 10 mg	Atarax, Atozine, Durrax, *Generic*
tablets (as HCl): 25 mg	Anxanil, Atarax, Atozine, Durrax, *Generic*
tablets (as HCl): 50 mg	Atarax, Atozine, *Generic*
tablets (as HCl): 100 mg	Atarax, *Generic*
syrup (as HCl): 10 mg/5 ml	Atarax, *Generic*
capsules (as pa-	Hy-Pam, Vamate, Vistaril,

moate): 25 mg,   *Generic*
50 mg

capsules (as pa-   Vamate, Vistaril, *Generic*
moate): 100 mg

oral suspension (as   Vistaril
pamoate): 25 mg/
5 ml

injection (as HCl):   Vistacon, Vistaject-25, Vis-
25 mg/ml   taril, *Generic*

injection (as HCl):   BayRox, E-Vista, Hydroxa-
50 mg/ml   cen, Hyzine-50, Orgatrax,
Quiess, Vistacon, Vistaject-
50, Vistaquel 50, Vistaril,
Vistazine 50, *Generic*

INDICATIONS

Symptomatic relief of anxiety and tension associated with psychoneurosis and as an adjunct in organic disease states in which anxiety is manifested;
in alcoholism and asthma. Useful in management
of pruritus due to allergic conditions such as
chronic urticaria and atopic and contact dermatoses, and in histamine-related pruritus.

As a sedative when used as premedication and
following general anesthesia.

IM administration is indicated for the acutely disturbed or hysterical patient; the acute or chronic
alcoholic with anxiety withdrawal symptoms or delirium tremens; as pre- and postoperative and pre-
and postpartum adjunctive medication to permit reduction in narcotic dosage, allay anxiety, and control emesis.

CONTRAINDICATIONS

Hypersensitivity. Contraindicated in early pregnancy because safety is not established.

WARNINGS

It is not known whether drug is excreted in human
milk; it should not be given to nursing mothers.

PRECAUTIONS

Inject IM form into relatively large muscle; inadvertent subcutaneous injection may result in significant
tissue damage.

DRUG INTERACTIONS

Potentiating action is considered when drug is used
in conjunction with **CNS depressants** such as narcotics, barbiturates, alcohol, antidepressants, and
antipsychotics. When CNS depressants are administered concomitantly with hydroxyzine, their dosage
should be reduced up to 50%.

ADVERSE REACTIONS

Dry mouth may occur. Drowsiness is usually transitory and may disappear in a few days of continued

therapy or with dosage reduction. Involuntary motor activity, including instances of tremor and convulsions, has been reported, usually with higher
than recommended dosage. Hypersensitivity reaction (wheezing, dyspnea, chest tightness) has been
reported.

OVERDOSAGE

Symptoms: Most common manifestation is oversedation. As in the management of any overdosage,
consider that multiple agents may have been taken.

Treatment: If vomiting has not occurred spontaneously, it should be induced. Immediate gastric lavage has also been recommended. General supportive care, including frequent monitoring of vital
signs and close observation of the patient, is indicated. Hypotension may be controlled with IV
fluids and norepinephrine or metaraminol. Do not
use epinephrine as hydroxyzine counteracts its pressor action. There is no specific antidote. It is doubtful that hemodialysis would be of value.

DOSAGE

Start patient on IM therapy when indicated and
maintain on oral therapy whenever practical. Dosage is adjusted to patient response.

Oral

Symptomatic relief of anxiety: *Adults*—Ranges
from 50 mg to 100 mg qid. *Children over 6*—50
mg/day to 100 mg/day in divided doses. *Children
under 6*—50 mg/day in divided doses.

**Management of pruritus due to allergic condi-
tions:** *Adults*—25 mg tid or qid. *Children over 6*—
50 mg/day to 100 mg/day in divided doses. *Children under 6*—50 mg/day in divided doses.

**Sedative as premedication and following general
anesthesia:** *Adults*—50 mg to 100 mg. *Children*—
0.6 mg/kg.

Intramuscular

**Adult psychiatric and emotional emergencies, in-
cluding acute alcoholism:** 50 mg to 100 mg immediately and q4h to q6h as needed.

Nausea and vomiting: 25 mg to 100 mg for
adults and 1.1 mg/kg (0.5 mg/lb) for children.

**Preoperative and postoperative adjunctive medica-
tion:** 25 mg to 100 mg for adults and 1.1 mg/kg
(0.5 mg/lb) for children.

**Prepartum and postpartum adjunctive ther-
apy:** 25 mg to 100 mg.

NURSING IMPLICATIONS

HISTORY
See Appendix 4.

PHYSICAL ASSESSMENT

Depends on reason for use.

Relief of anxiety, tension: Evaluate emotional status; note and record overt symptoms.

Allergic conditions (urticaria, dermatoses, pruritus): Examine skin; describe lesions.

Psychiatric and emotional emergencies: Observe and record patient behavior.

ADMINISTRATION

Parenteral form is for IM use only. Do not inject subcutaneously, IV, or intra-arterially. Inadvertent subcutaneous injection may result in significant tissue damage.

In adults, preferred site is the upper outer quadrant of the buttock or the midlateral thigh.

In children, recommended site is the midlateral muscles of the thigh. In infants and small children, the periphery of the upper outer quadrant of the gluteal region should be used only when necessary, such as in burn patients, in order to minimize possibility of damage to the sciatic nerve.

The deltoid area is used only if well developed, such as in certain adults and older children, and then only with caution to avoid radial-nerve injury. IM injections should *not* be made into the lower and mid-third of the upper arm.

Aspiration is necessary to help avoid inadvertent injection into a blood vessel.

Rotate injection sites; record site used.

When CNS depressants are administered concomitantly (*e.g.,* a narcotic as part of the preoperative medication), dosage of the depressants should be reduced up to 50%.

Preoperative administration: Advise patient to remain in bed following administration; raise siderails.

Psychiatric and emotional emergencies: Assistance may be required to restrain patient while injection is being given.

ONGOING ASSESSMENTS AND NURSING MANAGEMENT

Record vital signs daily; observe for therapeutic results (*e.g.,* relief of pruritus, relief of anxiety and tension, calming effect in psychiatric and emotional emergencies).

In psychiatric and emotional emergencies, observe patient q1h (in some instances more frequent observation may be warranted) until drug has produced a calming effect and patient is manageable.

If drug does not produce desired response, inform physician.

Dry mouth may be relieved by frequent sips of water, hard candy, or chewing gum. If dry mouth is severe and patient complains of discomfort, notify physician.

Severe dryness of the mouth requires good oral care. Inspect oral mucous membranes and tongue daily for abrasions, redness, ulcerations, and signs of irritation. Inform physician of changes in oral mucosa because dose reduction or treatment of mucous membranes may be required. This is especially important in the psychiatric patient.

Drowsiness may occur. If it is severe and persists after several days of therapy, inform physician. Patient may require assistance with ambulation and activities of daily living.

PATIENT AND FAMILY INFORMATION

May cause drowsiness; observe caution while driving or performing other tasks requiring alertness.

Do not drink alcoholic beverages while taking this drug; alcohol may intensify this drug's effect and the combination could be dangerous.

Inform other physicians and dentist of therapy with this drug because CNS depressants must be avoided.

Do not discontinue this drug or increase or decrease the dosage, except on advice of a physician.

Dry mouth may be relieved by frequent sips of cool water, hard candy, or chewing gum. Avoid use of commercial mouth rinses. If dry mouth is severe or if mouth becomes irritated, contact physician.

Female patient of childbearing age: This drug is contraindicated in early pregnancy. If pregnancy is suspected or known, contact physician immediately.

L-Hyoscyamine Sulfate

See Gastrointestinal Anticholinergics/Antispasmodics.

IJK

Ibuprofen

See Nonsteroidal Anti-inflammatory Agents.

Idoxuridine (IDU) Rx

ophthalmic solution: Herplex Liquifilm, Stoxil
  0.1%
ophthalmic oint-   Stoxil
   ment: 0.5%

INDICATIONS
Treatment of herpes simplex keratitis. Epithelial infections (especially initial attacks), characterized by presence of a dendritic figure, respond better than stromal infections. Recurrences are common. Drug will control infection, but will have no effect on accumulated scarring, vascularization, or resultant progressive loss of vision.

CONTRAINDICATIONS
Hypersensitivity.

ACTIONS
Blocks production of herpes simplex by alteration of normal DNA synthesis.

WARNINGS
May be sensitizing; sensitization is more common with dermal use than with use in the eye. Drug should be regarded as being potentially carcinogenic. Administer with caution in pregnancy or in women of childbearing potential. Safety for use in the nursing mother not established.

PRECAUTIONS
Some strains of herpes simplex appear to be resistant. If there is no response in epithelial infections after 7 to 8 days of treatment, other forms of therapy are considered. Not effective in corneal inflammations following herpes simplex keratitis, in which the virus is not present. Corticosteroids can accelerate the spread of viral infection and are usually contraindicated in herpes simplex keratitis. There may be a recurrence if medication is not continued 5 to 7 days after lesion is apparently healed.

DRUG INTERACTIONS
Boric acid should not be administered during course of therapy because it may cause irritation in the presence of idoxuridine.

ADVERSE REACTIONS
Occasionally, some irritation, pain, pruritus, inflammation, or edema will be experienced in the eyes or lids. Allergic reactions, although rare, have been reported. Photophobia has occurred. The occasional appearance of corneal clouding, stippling, and small punctate defects in the corneal epithelium have been seen. The punctate effects may be a manifestation of the infection, because healing usually takes place without interruption of therapy. These defects have also been observed in untreated herpes siplex keratitis. Squamous cell carcinoma has been reported at the site of topical treatment.

DOSAGE
Ophthalmic solution: Initially instill 1 drop in each infected eye q1h during the day and q2h at night. Initial dosage is continued until definite improvement has taken place as evidenced by loss of staining with fluorescein. Dosage may then be reduced to 1 drop q2h during the day and q4h during the night. In order to minimize recurrences, therapy is continued at this reduced dosage for 3 to 5 days after healing appears to be complete.

Ophthalmic ointment: Recommended dosage is 5 instillations daily, given approximately q4h, with last dose H.S. Therapy is usually continued for 3 to 5 days after healing appears to be complete.

▌ NURSING IMPLICATIONS

HISTORY
Description and duration of symptoms; allergy history.

PHYSICAL ASSESSMENT
Examine adjacent structures of the eye for signs of inflammation and infection.

ADMINISTRATION
Solution: Instill prescribed amount of solution in the lower conjunctival sac. Apply light finger pressure on lacrimal sac for 1 minute.

Ointment: Place prescribed amount in lower conjunctival sac. Instruct patient to close eye gently for 1 to 2 minutes. Warn patient that a temporary visual haze will be noted.

Inform patient that pain, irritation, itching, and swelling in the eye or eyelids may be noted.

Storage: Solutions stored under refrigeration; refrigeration not required for Herplex Liquifilm ophthalmic solution.

ONGOING ASSESSMENTS AND NURSING MANAGEMENT
Antibiotics may be ordered with idoxuridine to control secondary infections; atropine or topical corticosteroids may be also prescribed. Idoxuridine is not mixed with other medications. If

other drugs are ordered, physician will select a dosage schedule for ophthalmic instillations.

Inspect eye daily for evidence of secondary infection; notify physician if redness, exudate, or other abnormalities are noted.

If photosensitivity occurs, darken room or advise patient to wear sunglasses.

PATIENT AND FAMILY INFORMATION

NOTE: If first dose is to be instilled by the patient, administration technique should be explained. If possible, nurse or physician should instill first dose, explaining the technique of administration during instillation.

Follow instillation schedule exactly. Drug must be used as directed by physician. This includes instillation during nighttime hours. The medication will not be effective if this schedule is not followed.

Take care not to contaminate tip of ointment tube or dropper. Replace dropper in bottle immediately after instilling medication.

Store medication as directed on bottle (drug is refrigerated with exception of Herplex Liquifilm). Keep bottle tightly closed.

Do not discontinue use without consulting physician.

May cause sensitivity to bright light; this may be minimized by wearing sunglasses.

Ointment may produce a temporary visual haze. Observe caution when driving or performing other potentially hazardous tasks until vision clears.

Notify physician if improvement is not seen after 7 to 8 days, if condition worsens, if pain, itching, or swelling persists, or if pus is noted.

Imipramine

See Antidepressants, Tricyclic Compounds.

Immune Globulin

See Immunizations, Passive.

Immunizations, Active

Agents for active immunization include specific antigens that induce the endogenous production of antibodies. Agents that induce active immunity include vaccines and toxoids. Vaccines contain whole, either killed or attenuated live, microorganisms that are capable of inducing antibody formation but that are not pathogenic. Toxoids contain detoxified byproducts derived from organisms that induce disease primarily through the elaboration of exotoxins. Although toxoids are not toxic, they are antigenic and therefore stimulate specific antibody production. Active immunization induced through inoculation with vaccines and toxoids provides prolonged immunity, whereas passive immunization with immune sera or antitoxins is of short duration. See Table 30 for the recommended immunization schedules for infants and children. For use of vaccine for active immunization against rabies, see Rabies Prophylaxis Products.

BCG Vaccine Rx

injection: 1 ml amps   *Generic*

INDICATIONS
Persons with negative tuberculin skin tests who are repeatedly exposed to sputum-positive cases of pulmonary tuberculosis.

CONTRAINDICATIONS
Tuberculin-positive individuals; those with fresh smallpox vaccinations; burn patients; those on prolonged treatment with corticosteroids; those with hypogammaglobulinemia or other disorders in

Table 30. Recommended Immunization Schedules

Immunization	Age					
	2 mo	4 mo	6 mo	15 mo	18 mo	4–6 yr
Diphtheria toxoid	*	*	*		*	*
Tetanus toxoid	*	*	*		*	*
Pertussis vaccine	*	*	*		*	*
Trivalent oral polio vaccine	*	*			*	*
Measles vaccine				*		
Rubella vaccine				*		
Mumps vaccine				*		

which the natural immunologic capacity is altered. Those with chronic skin disease are vaccinated in a healthy area of skin. Not effective during isoniazid administration. Not used during pregnancy unless there is excessive risk of infectious tuberculosis.

ADVERSE REACTIONS

Incidence low. Severe or prolonged ulceration at vaccination site, lymphadenitis, osteomyelitis, disseminated BCG infection, and death have been seen. Granulomas appearing 4 to 6 weeks following vaccination have been reported.

ADMINISTRATION AND DOSAGE

0.1 ml intradermally; 0.05 ml for infants under 28 days old.

Normal local reaction: Initial lesion appears in 7 to 10 days and consists of a small red papule at injection site that reaches maximum diameter in 5 weeks. Lesion shrinks to smooth or scaly pink or bluish scar in 3 months and becomes a pitted white scar in 6 months.

Preparation: Add 1 ml Sterile Water to ampule; allow to stand 1 minute; avoid shaking. Withdrawing solution will yield a homogeneous suspension.

Storage: 2°C to 8°C. Do not expose to light. Use immediately after reconstitution. Sterilize unused portion before disposal.

NURSING IMPLICATIONS
See p 576.

Cholera Vaccine Rx

injection   *Generic*

INDICATIONS

Travel to countries requiring evidence of cholera vaccination.

CONTRAINDICATIONS

Acute respiratory or other active infection; immune deficiency conditions; patients who have experienced serious reaction to previous vaccination with cholera.

WARNINGS/PRECAUTIONS

Take precautions to control allergic and other reactions. Safety for use in pregnancy is not established. Not recommended for infants under 6 months. Not used to treat actual cholera infection.

ADVERSE REACTIONS

No evidence of serious major reactions, but post-vaccinal neurologic disorders have been reported.

Local: Transitory soreness; erythema, swelling, pain, tenderness, induration; rarely necrosis and ulceration.

Systemic: Malaise, low-grade fever, headache, generalized aches and pains, flushing, generalized urticaria, tachycardia, and hypotension may occur.

ADMINISTRATION AND DOSAGE

Given subcutaneously or IM in 2 doses, 1 week to 1 month apart. *First dose*—0.5 ml; second dose 0.5 ml. *Children 6 months to 4 years*—0.2 ml both doses; *children 5–10 years*—0.3 ml both doses; *children over 10 years*—adult dose.

NURSING IMPLICATIONS
See p 576.

Diphtheria Toxoid, Adsorbed (Pediatric) Rx

injection: 5-ml vials   *Generic*

INDICATIONS

Active immunization against diphtheria in infants and children under 6.

CONTRAINDICATIONS

Any acute or active infection; those receiving corticosteroids or other immunosuppressive agents.

WARNINGS

Not used for treatment of actual diphtheria infections. Take precautions for prevention of allergic or other reactions. Infants and children with cerebral damage, neurologic disorders, or history of febrile convulsions are injected cautiously.

ADVERSE REACTIONS

Mild to moderate local redness, tenderness, and induration surrounding injection site.

Systemic: Transient fever, malaise, generalized aches and pains, flushing, generalized urticaria or pruritus, tachycardia, hypotension.

Uncommon: Postvaccinal neurologic disorders.

ADMINISTRATION AND DOSAGE

Primary immunization: 2 injections of 0.5 ml 6 to 8 weeks apart with third dose of 0.5 ml 1 year later. Injections given IM.

Booster: 0.5 ml at 5- to 10-year intervals. Shake well before withdrawing each dose.

Storage: 2°C to 8°C.

NURSING IMPLICATIONS
See p 576.

Diphtheria and Tetanus Toxoids, Combined *Rx*

for adult use: 2 Lf units diphtheria toxoid
for pediatric use: 15 Lf units diphtheria toxoid

INDICATIONS
Pediatric form for active immunization through 6 years of age. Adult form for active immunization of adults and children 7 years of age and older.

CONTRAINDICATIONS
Adults and children receiving immunosuppressive agents (corticosteroids, antimetabolites, alkylating compounds, or irradiation) may not respond optimally to active immunization procedures. When possible, interrupt this treatment when immunization is contemplated with an injury.

Any acute respiratory infection or other active infection is reason to defer administration of routine immunizing or booster doses but not emergency booster doses.

Elective immunization should be deferred during an outbreak of poliomyelitis.

WARNINGS/PRECAUTIONS
Should not be used for actual treatment of tetanus or diphtheria. Safety for use in pregnancy is not established. Take precautions for prevention of allergic and other reactions. A history of CNS damage or convulsions is an indication to postpone primary immunization until the second year of life.

Adult type is used only as a prophylactic agent in those over 6 years. Only healthy individuals are injected. Local and systemic reactions may be seen somewhat more frequently and may be more severe in those who have had numerous previous injections of tetanus toxoid.

ADVERSE REACTIONS
Stinging sensation after injection; mild to moderate local reactions (redness, edema, erythema, tenderness, induration) persisting for a few days.

Systemic: Fretfulness, drowsiness, anorexia, vomiting, persistent crying, fever, malaise, generalized aches and pains, flushing, generalized urticaria or pruritus, rash, tachycardia, hypotension. Frequently there is itching of the edematous area and it may resemble a giant hive. Edema is occasionally extensive; axillary lymphadenopathy has also been reported. Persistent nodules and sterile abscesses may occur.

Uncommon: Postvaccinal neurologic disorders.

ADMINISTRATION AND DOSAGE
Give IM.

Pediatric, adsorbed toxoids: For primary immu-

nization give two 0.5-ml doses at interval of 4 to 8 weeks. *Reinforcing dose*—0.5 ml 6 to 12 months later. *Booster dose*—0.5 ml at time of entry into school. If initial dose gives severe local or systemic reactions, subsequent doses are divided into smaller fractions.

Adult, adsorbed toxoids: For immunizing dose, give 2 doses of 0.5 ml 4 to 8 weeks apart. *Reinforcing dose*—0.5 ml 6 to 12 months later. *Booster dose*—0.5 ml every 10 years.

Tetanus prophylaxis in wound management: See Tetanus Toxoid.

NURSING IMPLICATIONS
See p 576.

Diphtheria and Tetanus Toxoids and Pertussis Vaccine, Adsorbed *(DTP)* *Rx*

injection   Tri-Immunol, Ultrafined
                             Triple Antigen, *Generic*

INDICATIONS
Active immunization of infants and children through age 6. Recommended for primary immunization and routine recall.

CONTRAINDICATIONS
Not for use in adults or children over 7. Defer administration during any acute illness. Routine immunization is not attempted if child has personal or family history of CNS disease or convulsions. Not indicated during immunosuppressive therapy; outbreak of poliomyelitis; fever over 39°C (103°F); convulsions; alterations of consciousness; focal neurologic signs; screaming episodes; shock; collapse; thrombocytopenic purpura; somnolence; encephalopathy.

WARNINGS/PRECAUTIONS
When infant or child returns for next dose, question parent about occurrence of any symptoms or signs of a severe adverse reaction after last dose. If such are reported, further doses are contraindicated and active immunization is completed with Diphtheria and Tetanus Toxoids. Take precautions to prevent allergic and other reactions.

ADVERSE REACTIONS
Local: Erythema, induration with or without tenderness; palpable nodule at injection site for a few weeks; abscess at injection site.

Systemic: Mild to moderate temperature elevation with malaise occurring several hours after administration and persisting for 1 to 2 days; chills; irritability. Severe systemic reactions require reduction of volume of next injection or use of single antigens. Sudden infant death syndrome (SIDS) has been reported but significance is unclear.

Severe and occasionally fatal reactions have been reported following administration of pertussis vaccine; such reactions almost always appear in 24 to 48 hours. Reactions include severe temperature elevation; collapse with recovery; collapse followed by prolonged prostration and a shocklike state; screaming episodes of a prolonged period of peculiar crying during which infant cannot be comforted; isolated convulsions with or without fever; encephalopathy with changes in the level of consciousness, focal neurologic signs, and convulsions, which may be fatal or with or without permanent neurologic or mental deficit; thrombocytopenic purpura.

ADMINISTRATION AND DOSAGE

Give IM into midlateral muscles of thigh or deltoid.

Primary immunization: In infants and children 2 months to 6 years old, give three 0.5-ml doses at 4- to 8-week intervals. Give a reinforcing dose approximately 1 year after third injection. A fourth reinforcing dose is necessary to complete basic immunizing course.

Booster or recall doses: Given when child is 4 to 6 years old, preferably before starting kindergarten or elementary school. For booster doses thereafter use Diphtheria and Tetanus Toxoids, Adsorbed (adult) every 10 years. A booster dose (0.5 ml) can be administered to children under 6 exposed to diphtheria. Children over 6 should receive Diphtheria and Tetanus Toxoids, Adsorbed (adult). If it is necessary to reinforce pertussis immunity in children 6 or under, a recall dose of 0.5 ml is given. Children over 7 should not be immunized with pertussis.

NURSING IMPLICATIONS
See p 576.

Hepatitis B Vaccine Rx

injection: 20 mcg/ml   Heptavax-B

INDICATIONS

Immunization against infection caused by all known subtypes of hepatitis B virus. Will not prevent hepatitis caused by other agents. Recommended for those 3 months or older, especially those at increased risk of infection. Recommended for healthcare personnel (*e.g.,* physicians, dentists, nurses, laboratory personnel, patients, and staff in hemodialysis, hematology, and oncology units, residents and staff of institutions for mentally retarded); morticians; military personnel identified as being at increased risk; prisoners; persons at increased risk of

the disease because of sexual practices (*e.g.,* prostitutes, homosexually active males); users of illicit injectable drugs; populations with high incidence of the disease (*e.g.,* Alaskan Eskimos, Haitian and Indochinese refugees).

CONTRAINDICATIONS
Hypersensitivity.

WARNINGS/PRECAUTIONS

Not recommended for use in pregnant women; use caution when administering to nursing women. Safety and efficacy for children under 3 months are not established. Take precautions to prevent allergic and other reactions. Do not give if serious active infection is present. Exercise caution when giving to those with severely compromised cardiopulmonary status or to those in whom a febrile or systemic reaction could pose a risk.

ADVERSE REACTIONS

Generally well tolerated.

Local: Soreness, erythema, swelling, warmth, induration.

Systemic: Malaise, fatigue, headache, nausea, dizziness, myalgia, and arthralgia are infrequent and limited to the first few days following vaccination. Rarely, rash occurs. Low-grade fever occurs occasionally and is confined to the 48 hours following vaccination.

ADMINISTRATION AND DOSAGE

IM use only. Immunization regimen is three doses. Administered as initial dose, second dose in 1 month, and third 6 months after first dose.

Volume: Age 3 months to 10 years—0.5 ml each dose. *Adults, older children*—1 ml each dose. Dialysis or immunocompromised patients receive 2 ml (two 1-ml doses at different sites) each dose.

REVACCINATION

Duration is unknown at present; it is probably 5 years in those receiving all three doses.

Preparation: Shake well before use; thorough agitation is necessary. Inspect visually for particulate matter, discoloration. After agitation, vaccine is a slightly opaque, white suspension. Store at 2°C to 8°C.

NURSING IMPLICATIONS
See p 576.

Influenza Virus Vaccine Rx

injection (split virus)   Influenza Virus Trivalent, Types A & B; Fluogen; Fluzone

injection (whole   Fluzone
    virus)

INDICATIONS

Annual vaccination of individuals at increased risk of adverse consequences from infections of lower respiratory tract, older persons, and persons providing essential community services.

CONTRAINDICATIONS

In those with allergy to eggs, chicken, chicken feathers, chicken dander, those with an allergic condition (scratch test recommended first), and those with acute respiratory disease or other active infection.

WARNINGS/PRECAUTIONS

Take precautions to prevent allergic and other reactions. Avoid use during first trimester of pregnancy. Not effective against all strains of influenza virus; protection is afforded to most persons only against those strains from which vaccine is prepared. Exercise caution in immunizing those with history of febrile disorders.

ADVERSE REACTIONS

Local: Tenderness, redness, induration lasting 1 to 2 days.

Systemic: Fever, malaise, myalgia, and other systemic symptoms of toxicity (infrequent) beginning 6 to 12 hours after vaccination and persisting 1 to 2 days; immediate (presumably allergic) responses such as flare, wheal, various respiratory expressions of hypersensitivity; Guillain-Barré syndrome (uncommon); other neurologic disorders, including encephalopathies.

ADMINISTRATION AND DOSAGE

IM, preferably in deltoid or midlateral thigh. Split virus appears to be associated with fewer side-effects in children. Because vaccine is prepared for use during a specific year, see package insert for recommended dosage schedule.

▌ NURSING IMPLICATIONS
See p 576.

Measles (Rubeola) Virus Vaccine, Live, Attenuated Rx

injection   Attenuvax

INDICATIONS

Vaccine given immediately after exposure to natural measles may provide protection. If given a few days before exposure, substantial protection may be provided. Recommended for active immunization against measles for children 15 months or older. Booster is not needed. Infants less than 15 months may not respond. Children vaccinated before 12 months should be revaccinated at about 15 months. Vaccination may be advisable for high-school or college students in epidemic situations and for adults in isolated communities where measles are not endemic.

CONTRAINDICATIONS

Hypersensitivity to egg, chicken, chicken feathers, neomycin; acute respiratory or other active infections; immunodeficiency conditions.

WARNINGS/PRECAUTIONS

Not given to pregnant women. Pregnancy should be avoided for 3 months following vaccination because of fetal risk. Vaccination of postpubertal females entails potential for inadvertent immunization during pregnancy. Exercise caution in giving to children with history of febrile convulsions, cerebral injury, or other conditions in which stress due to fever should be avoided. Take precautions to prevent allergic and other reactions. Do not give within 1 month of immunization with other live virus vaccines, (exception monovalent or trivalent polio, rubella, or mumps vaccine, which may be given simultaneously). Defer use for at least 3 months after blood or plasma transfusions or administration of more than 0.02 ml/lb of human immune serum globulin.

ADVERSE REACTIONS

Occasional: Moderate fever during month of vaccination; generally fever and rash appear between fifth and twelfth days. Rash, when it occurs, is usually minimal. Children with fever may (rarely) exhibit febrile convulsions. Very rarely, CNS reactions (encephalitis, encephalopathy) may occur within 30 days postvaccination but risk is far less than with natural measles.

Local: Marked swelling, redness, and vesiculation in children previously vaccinated with killed measles.

ADMINISTRATION AND DOSAGE

Use only diluent supplied with product. After reconstitution give total volume of ampule subcutaneously. Before reconstitution, store at 2°C to 8°C. After reconstitution, discard if not used in 8 hours.

▌ NURSING IMPLICATIONS
See p 576.

Measles (Rubeola) and Rubella Virus Vaccine, Live Rx

injection   M-R-Vax II

INDICATIONS

Children 15 months to puberty for simultaneous immunization against measles and rubella. Infants less than 15 months may fail to respond. No revaccination is necessary when child is originally vaccinated at 12 months or older.

WARNINGS/PRECAUTIONS, ADVERSE EFFECTS

See Measles (Rubeola) Virus Vaccine, Live, Attenuated.

ADMINISTRATION AND DOSAGE

Use only diluent supplied with product. After reconstitution, inject total volume of vial subcutaneously into outer aspect of upper arm. Before reconstitution, store at 2°C to 8°C. Protect from light. Use as soon as possible after reconstitution. Discard if not used in 8 hours.

NURSING IMPLICATIONS

See p 576.

Measles, Mumps, and Rubella Virus Vaccine, Live Rx

injection (mixture of   M-M-R II
  3 viruses)

INDICATIONS

Simultaneous immunization against measles, mumps, and rubella for children 15 months to puberty. Infants less than 15 months may not respond. There is no reason to revaccinate children originally vaccinated when 12 months or older.

WARNINGS/PRECAUTIONS, ADVERSE REACTIONS

See Measles (Rubeola) Virus Vaccine, Live, Attenuated; Rubella Virus Vaccine, Live; Mumps Virus Vaccine, Live.

ADMINISTRATION AND DOSAGE

Inject total volume of reconstituted vaccine subcutaneously into outer aspect of upper arm. Before reconstitution, store at 2°C to 8°C. Protect from light. To reconstitute, use only diluent supplied with product. Agitate vial thoroughly after adding diluent. Use as soon as possible. Discard if not used in 8 hours.

NURSING IMPLICATIONS

See p 576.

Meningitis Vaccines Rx

Meningococcal Polysaccharide Vaccine, Group A	Menomune-A
Meningococcal Polysaccharide Vaccine, Group C	Menomune-C
Meningococcal Polysaccharide Vaccine, Groups A & C	Menomune-A/C, Meningovax-AC
Meningococcal Polysaccharide Vaccine, Groups A, C, Y & W-135	Menomune-A/C/Y/W-135

INDICATIONS

General use is not recommended. Vaccination of household contacts of meningococcal disease as adjunct to appropriate antibiotic therapy is considered. Use in children under 2 years is not recommended except with Group A vaccine. Use of Groups Y and W-135 in individuals under 18 years is not recommended.

Group A: Children over 3 months; adults at risk in epidemic or highly endemic areas.

Group C & Groups A & C: Children over 2 years; adults at risk in epidemic or highly endemic areas.

Groups A, C, Y & W-135: Adults 18 and older at risk in epidemic or highly endemic areas; medical and laboratory personnel at risk of exposure.

CONTRAINDICATIONS

Acute respiratory or other active infections; immunodeficiency conditions; pregnancy.

PRECAUTIONS

Take precautions to prevent allergic and other reactions.

ADVERSE REACTIONS

Systemic: Headache, malaise, chills, cramps, febrile reactions (may appear within hours and persist for 24–48 hours).

Local: Soreness, tenderness, pain, erythema, induration, local axillary lymphadenopathy; transient local immediate wheal-and-flare reaction and hypersensitivity reactions occur rarely.

ADMINISTRATION AND DOSAGE

Reconstitute using diluent supplied with product. Shake until dissolved. Store freeze-dried and reconstituted vaccine between 2°C to 8°C. Discard unused vaccine within 5 days after reconstitution.

Adults 18 years or older (Groups A, C, Y, & W-135): One 0.5-ml subcutaneous injection.

Age 2 years or older (Group A, Groups A & C only): One 0.5-ml subcutaneous injection.

Age 3–24 months (Group A only): Two 0.5-ml subcutaneous injections at least 1 month apart.

NURSING IMPLICATIONS

See p 576.

Mumps Virus Vaccine, Live Rx

injection   Mumpsvax

INDICATIONS

Immunization against mumps in children 15 months or older and adults. May be given as early as 12 months. Not recommended for infants under 1 year. There is no reason to revaccinate those originally vaccinated when 12 months or older.

CONTRAINDICATIONS

Hypersensitivity to neomycin, eggs, chicken, chicken feathers; immunodeficiency conditions; infections; pregnancy.

PRECAUTIONS

Take precautions to prevent allergic and other reactions. Do not give less than 1 month before or after immunization of other live virus vaccines, with exception of live attenuated measles, live rubella virus, or live oral monovalent or trivalent polio vaccines. Defer use at least 3 months following blood or plasma transfusions or administration of more than 0.02 ml/lb of human immune serum globulin.

ADVERSE REACTIONS

Occasionally mild fever; fever above 39.4°C (103°F) is uncommon. Parotitis has occurred in very low incidence, and rarely orchitis has occurred in persons who were vaccinated. In most instances, prior exposure to natural mumps was established. Rarely, purpura and allergic reactions such as urticaria occur. CNS reactions such as febrile seizures, unilateral nerve deafness, and encephalitis have occurred rarely, within 30 days of vaccination.

ADMINISTRATION AND DOSAGE

Reconstitute using diluent supplied with product; agitate thoroughly. Protect from light at all times. Store reconstituted vaccine in dark place at 2°C to 8°C; discard if not used in 8 hours. Inject total volume of reconstituted vaccine subcutaneously into outer aspect of upper arm.

NURSING IMPLICATIONS

See p 576.

Plague Vaccine Rx

injection   Generic

INDICATIONS

Immunization for those who must be in known plague areas. Known plague areas in the United States are California, New Mexico, Arizona, Utah, Colorado, Idaho, Oregon, and Nevada. Countries include Mongolia, southwestern Russia, central China, southern India, Pakistan, Nepal, Java, Vietnam, South Africa, Saudi Arabia, Brazil, Bolivia, and Peru. Use of plague vaccine greatly increases chances of recovery in those who may develop insect-borne (bubonic) form; the degree of protection afforded against pneumonic form is unknown, and vaccinated persons exposed to the pneumonic form should be given adequate daily doses of a suitable sulfonamide over a 6-day period.

CONTRAINDICATIONS

Administration is deferred in presence of acute respiratory or other active infection. If possible, avoid administration to immunodeficient individuals.

WARNINGS

Take precautions to prevent allergic and other reactions. Safety for use in pregnancy is not established.

ADVERSE REACTIONS

Primary immunization: General malaise, headache, local erythema and induration, mild lymphadenopathy, hyperpyrexia.

Booster injections: Depend on number received, how administered, and individual reactivity of patient; booster-injections will generally result in increased frequency of reactions.

Sensitivity reactions: Urticarial and asthmatic phenomena have been reported.

ADMINISTRATION AND DOSAGE (CDC-RECOMMENDED SCHEDULES)

Primary immunization: Give IM. For adults and children 11 years and over, primary series consists of three doses. First dose is 1 ml, followed by second dose of 0.2 ml 4 weeks later. Third dose of 0.2 ml is administered 6 months after first dose. If an accelerated schedule is necessary, three doses of 0.5 ml each are administered 1 week apart (efficacy of this schedule is not determined). For children 10 years and under, primary series is also three doses; intervals are the same as for adults. Dosage is as follows: Under 1 year, give first dose of 0.2 ml; second and third doses are 0.04 ml. For ages 1 to 4, give 0.4 ml in the first dose; the second and third doses are 0.08 ml. For ages 5 to 10, give first dose of 0.6 ml; second and third doses are 0.12 ml.

Booster doses: When needed, give three booster

doses at 6-month intervals. Thereafter, antibody levels decline slowly and booster doses are given at 1- to 2-year intervals, depending on degree of continuing exposure. Recommended booster doses for children and adults are the same as the second and third doses in the primary series. If severe side-effects are noted, smaller dose volume may be used.

| NURSING IMPLICATIONS
See p 576.

Pneumococcal Vaccine, Polyvalent Rx

injection   Pneumovax 23, Pnu-Immune 23

INDICATIONS
Immunization against pneumococcal pneumonia and pneumococcal bacteremia caused by type of pneumococci included in the vaccine. Used in selected individuals over 2 years of age. These include those with anatomic asplenia or those who have splenic dysfunction due to sickle-cell disease or other causes; those with chronic illnesses in which there is increased risk of pneumococcal disease (diabetes, functional impairment of cardiorespiratory, hepatic, or renal systems); those over 50; those in communities of closed groups (_e.g.,_ nursing homes, institutions); groups epidemiologically at risk in a community where there is a generalized outbreak; and those at high risk of influenza complications, particularly pneumonia.

CONTRAINDICATIONS
Acute respiratory or other active infections; immunodeficiency conditions; patients with Hodgkin's disease who have received extensive chemotherapy or nodal radiation.

WARNINGS/PRECAUTIONS
Take precautions to prevent allergic and other reactions. Intradermal reactions may cause severe local reactions. Safety for use in pregnancy is not established. Exercise caution in administration to nursing women. Not recommended for children under 2. Exercise caution in giving to those with cardiac/pulmonary disease and to patients who have had previous pneumococcal infections in the preceding 3 years.

ADVERSE REACTIONS
Local: Erythema, soreness usually of less than 48 hours duration; local induration.
Systemic reactions: Low-grade fever (usually confined to 24 hours after administration); acute febrile reactions, anaphylactoid reactions seen rarely.
Revaccination: Do not give a repeat (booster) injection of pneumococcal vaccine to previously vaccinated subjects, regardless of the time interval from the previous injection. Revaccination may result in more frequent and severe local reactions at the site of injection.

ADMINISTRATION AND DOSAGE
Administer subcutaneously or IM (preferably in deltoid muscle or lateral midthigh). Give one 0.5 ml dose. Store at 2°C to 8°C. Use as supplied; no dilution is necessary.

| NURSING IMPLICATIONS
See p 576.

Poliomyelitis Vaccine, Inactivated
(IPV, Salk) Rx

injection   Poliomyelitis Vaccine (Purified)

INDICATIONS
Immunizing agent for prevention of poliomyelitis. Is vaccine of choice for those with compromised immune systems. Trivalent Oral Poliovirus Vaccine (Sabin) is the vaccine of choice for primary vaccination of children in the United States.

CONTRAINDICATIONS
Acute respiratory or other active infection; immunodeficiency conditions.

WARNINGS/PRECAUTIONS
Vaccine should be clear and cherry red in color; discard vaccine showing turbidity, particulate matter, or change in color. Take precautions to prevent allergic and other reactions. Safety for use in pregnancy is not established. Does not protect all persons against paralytic manifestations of the disease; paralytic poliomyelitis may occur in rare instances in vaccinated individuals, particularly those with certain immunodeficiencies. Vaccine contains streptomycin, neomycin, and traces of animal protein; allergic reactions may occur in individuals sensitive to these substances.

ADMINISTRATION AND DOSAGE
Give by subcutaneous injection near insertion of deltoid muscle. Store at 2°C to 8°C.
Primary immunization: Three doses, 1 ml each, at 4- to 6-week intervals, followed by a fourth 1-ml dose 6 to 12 months after the third dose. For preschoolers, this schedule may be integrated with DTP immunization (p 568) beginning at 6 to 12 weeks of age. Administer subsequent booster doses of 1 ml every 2 to 3 years.
Supplementary immunization: Before entering

school, children previously immunized with four doses of IPV should be given one dose of OPV or one additional dose of IPV. Children immunized with IPV vaccine should obtain a booster dose every 5 years until age 18.

Unvaccinated adults: Primary immunization with IPV is recommended for those at increased risk of poliomyelitis. IPV is preferred because the risk of vaccine-associated paralysis following OPV is slightly higher in adults than in children. Give three doses at intervals of 1 to 2 months; fourth dose should follow 6 to 12 months after third dose.

Incompletely immunized adults at increased risk of exposure to poliomyelitis and who have received less than a full primary course should be given remaining required doses, regardless of the interval since the last dose. Adults previously given a complete primary course of IPV may be given IPV or OPV. If IPV is used exclusively, additional doses may be given every 5 years but their need has not been established.

▎ NURSING IMPLICATIONS
See p 576.

Poliovirus Vaccine, Live, Oral, Trivalent
(TOPV, Sabin) Rx

---

oral vacine   Orimune

INDICATIONS
Prevention of poliomyelitis caused by poliovirus Types 1, 2, and 3. Infants starting at 6 to 12 weeks of age; all unimmunized children and adolescents through age 18. Routine immunization of adults residing in the United States is not necessary because of unlikelihood of exposure, but primary immunization with IPV is recommended whenever feasible for unimmunized adults subject to increased risk of exposure.

CONTRAINDICATIONS
Presence of persistent vomiting or diarrhea; advanced debilitated patients; acute respiratory or other active infections; immunodeficiency conditions.

WARNINGS/PRECAUTIONS
Take precautions to prevent allergic and other conditions. Safety for use in pregnancy is not established. Other viruses (including poliovirus and other enterovirus) may interfere with this vaccine. Not administered shortly after immune serum globulin (ISG) unless such procedure is unavoidable. If given with or shortly after ISG, the dose should be repeated after 3 months if immunization is still indi-

cated. Vaccine is not effective in modifying or preventing cases of existing or incubating poliomyelitis.

ADVERSE REACTIONS
Paralytic disease has been reported in those receiving the vaccine and, in some instances, in persons in close contact with subjects given the vaccine. The risk of vaccine-associated paralysis is very small, but the parent should be advised of this possibility before administration. If adults in household were never vaccinated, physician may administer two doses of IVP a month apart.

ADMINISTRATION AND DOSAGE
Each single oral dose contains 0.5 ml.

Initial (primary) series: Three doses are recommended to be started at 6 to 12 weeks of age, commonly with DTP inoculation. Second dose is given not less than 6, and preferably 8, weeks later. Third dose is administered 8 to 12 months after second dose. The American Academy of Pediatrics recommends that the vaccine be administered at 2, 4, and 18 months of age. *Older children (up to age 18)—* Administer 2 doses not less than 6, and preferably 8, weeks apart; third dose 6 to 12 months after second dose.

Booster doses: On entering elementary school, all children who have completed primary series are given a single follow-up dose. All others should complete the primary series. Routine booster doses after the dose given upon entering school are not recommended. If an individual who has completed a primary series is subjected to a substantially increased risk, a single dose may be given.

Store at a temperature that will maintain ice continuously in a solid state. If it is frozen, thaw vaccine before use. An unopened container that has been frozen and then is thawed may be carried through a maximum of 10 freeze–thaw cycles, provided temperature does not exceed 8°C (46°F) during periods of thaw and provided total cumulative duration of thaw does not exceed 24 hours. If 24-hour period is exceeded, vaccine must be used within 30 days, during which time it must be stored at 2°C to 8°C.

▎ NURSING IMPLICATIONS
See p 576.

Rubella Virus Vaccine, Live Rx

---

injection   Meruvax II

INDICATIONS
Immunization against rubella in children 15 months to puberty (may be given as early as 12

months); adolescent and adult males; nonpregnant adolescent and adult females. Revaccination is not necessary.

CONTRAINDICATIONS

Hypersensitivity to neomycin; immunodeficiency conditions; pregnancy; acute respiratory or other active infections.

PRECAUTIONS

Take precautions to control allergic and other reactions. Not given within 1 month before or after immunization with other live virus vaccines, with the exceptions of live attenuated measles virus and live mumps virus vaccines. There is no evidence that this vaccine given after exposure will prevent illness; there is no contraindication to vaccinating children already exposed to natural rubella. Vaccination is deferred at least 3 months after blood or plasma transfusion or administration of more than 0.02 ml/lb of human immune serum globulin. This vaccine may result in a temporary depression of tuberculin skin sensitivity.

ADVERSE REACTIONS

Usually are mild and transient. Lymphadenopathy, urticaria, rash, malaise, sore throat, fever, headache, polyneuritis, and occasionally temporary arthralgia may be seen. Local pain, induration, and erythema may occur. Moderate fever occurs occasionally; high fever is less common. Very rarely, encephalitis and other CNS effects have occurred; cause-and-effect relationship is not established. Thrombocytopenic purpura is a theoretical hazard because of decreases in platelet counts that have been reported.

ADMINISTRATION AND DOSAGE

Inject supplied diluent into vial; agitate. Inject total volume of reconstituted vaccine subcutaneously, preferably into outer aspect of upper arm. Before reconstitution, store at 2°C to 8°C. Protect vaccine from light at all times. Store reconstituted vaccine in a dark place at 2°C to 8°C. Discard if not used in 8 hours.

NURSING IMPLICATIONS
See p 576.

Rubella and Mumps Virus Vaccine, Live Rx

injection   Biavax II

INDICATIONS

Simultaneous immunization against rubella and mumps in children 15 months to puberty; may be given as early as 12 months. Not recommended for infants under 12 months. Routine revaccination is not needed.

CONTRAINDICATIONS, WARNINGS/PRECAUTIONS, ADVERSE REACTIONS

See Rubella Virus Vaccine, Live; Mumps Virus Vaccine, Live.

ADMINISTRATION AND DOSAGE

Reconstitute with supplied diluent. Inject total volume of reconstituted vaccine subcutaneously. Store unreconstituted vaccine at 2°C to 8°C; protect from light. After recontitution, use as soon as possible. Store reconstituted vaccine in a dark place at 2°C to 8°C. Discard if not used in 8 hours.

NURSING IMPLICATIONS
See p 576.

Tetanus Toxoid, Fluid and Tetanus Toxoid, Adsorbed Rx

injection   *Generic*

INDICATIONS

Active immunization against tetanus in adults and children. Tetanus toxoid, adsorbed is the preferred agent. Those with known sensitivity to horse serum or with asthma or other allergies should be urged to maintain immunity with tetanus toxoid and avoid potential complications of antitoxin treatment. Usually administered at the time of injury, for recall, and can be used at all ages for establishing primary immunization and for booster injections. Routine prophylaxis is now usually accomplished between 2 months and 6 years of age by use of DTP vaccine, (p 568).

CONTRAINDICATIONS

Prior systemic reaction to tetanus toxoid; acute respiratory or other active infection unless emergency administration is necessary; outbreak of poliomyelitis (elective immunization). Occurrence of any type of neurologic signs or symptoms following administration is an absolute contraindication to further use.

WARNINGS/PRECAUTIONS

Not to be used in treatment of tetanus or for immediate prophylaxis of unimmunized individuals. Use is generally avoided in the first trimester of pregnancy. Use is also avoided in those receiving concomitant immunosuppressive therapy. Take precautions to prevent allergic and other reactions. Infants and children with cerebral damage, neurologic disorders, or history of febrile convulsions are given vaccine with caution.

DRUG INTERACTIONS

Chloramphenicol may interfere with response; concomitant administration of this antibiotic should be avoided.

ADVERSE REACTIONS

There is an increased incidence of local and systemic reactions to booster doses given to those over 25.

Local: Erythema, redness, and induration surrounding injection site, persisting for a few days. A nodule may be palpable at injection site for a few weeks. Increased local reactions seen in those over 25 or in children who have received several doses of toxoid in the past are Arthus-type hypersensitivity reactions characterized by severe local reactions (starting 2–8 hours after injection).

Systemic: Fever, chills, malaise, generalized aches and pains, flushing, generalized urticaria or pruritus, tachycardia, hypotension.

Neurologic: Paralysis of the radial or recurrent nerve, cochlear lesions, brachial plexus neuropathies, difficulty in swallowing, accommodation paresis, EEG disturbances.

ADMINISTRATION AND DOSAGE

Tetanus toxoid, adsorbed is given IM, preferably into deltoid or midlateral muscles of thigh. For infants, the vastus lateralis is the preferred site. Tetanus toxoid fluid is given IM or subcutaneously in the vastus lateralis or deltoid muscle.

Primary immunization for adults, children

Tetanus toxoid, adsorbed: Two doses of 0.5 ml 4 to 6 weeks apart; third dose of 0.5 ml given approximately 1 year after second injection. Booster doses of 0.5 ml every 10 years.

Tetanus toxoid, fluid: Three doses of 0.5 ml at 4- to 8-week intervals; fourth dose of 0.5 ml given approximately 6 to 12 months after third injection. Booster doses of 0.5 ml every 10 years.

Tetanus prophylaxis wound management: Dose is 0.5 ml. See package insert about information on wound status, immunization history, and other decisions entering into administration.

NURSING IMPLICATIONS
See this page.

Typhoid Vaccine Rx

injection   *Generic*

INDICATIONS

Active immunization against typhoid under the following conditions: intimate exposure to known typhoid carrier, foreign travel to areas where typhoid is endemic.

CONTRAINDICATIONS

Acute respiratory or other active infections.

WARNINGS/PRECAUTIONS

A severe systemic or allergic reaction following a prior dose is a contraindication to further use. Take precautions to prevent allergic and other reactions. Safety for use in pregnancy is not established. Review patient's history for possible sensitivity.

DRUG INTERACTIONS

Corticosteroids or **immunosuppressive agents** may alter immune response.

ADVERSE REACTIONS

Some degree of local or systemic response begins within 24 hours.

Local: Erythema, induration, tenderness.

Systemic: Malaise, headache, myalgia, elevated temperature.

ADMINISTRATION AND DOSAGE

Primary immunization for adults, children over 10: Two doses of 0.5 ml each, subcutaneously, at an interval of 4 or more weeks.

Children less than 10: Two doses of 0.25 ml each, subcutaneously, at interval of 4 or more weeks. When there is insufficient time for two doses at 4-week intervals, three doses of the same volume 1 week apart may be given.

Booster doses (every 3 years): *Adults and children over 10*—0.5 ml subcutaneously or 0.1 ml intradermally. *Children 6 months to 10 years*—0.25 ml subcutaneously or 0.1 ml intradermally.

NURSING IMPLICATIONS
See below.

NURSING IMPLICATIONS: IMMUNIZATIONS, ACTIVE

HISTORY

Question patient or parent about any previous serious reactions to other vaccines or a serious reaction to the first dose of present vaccine being administered. Do not administer if there is a history of serious reactions; inform physician. Obtain a thorough allergy history or review patient's record for known allergies.

Some patients with severe allergies or asthma may be at risk for some immunizations. In some instances, the physician may perform tests to determine possible sensitivity to a vaccine or its additional contents (e.g., neomycin).

Other disease states and drugs require that caution be exercised in administering the vaccine. A thorough history or review of the patient's clinical records is required. Immunodeficiency conditions due to corticosteroid therapy (_exception_—those receiving corticosteroids as replacement therapy in Addison's disease, etc.), irradiation therapy, and treatment with alkylating agents or antimetabolites may alter vaccine response or require postponement of immunization.

Persons with blood dyscrasias, leukemias, lymphomas, malignant neoplasms affecting bone marrow, or primary immunodeficiency states, including cellular immune deficiencies and hypogammaglobulinemic and dysgammaglobulinemic states, may be given vaccines with caution or not at all.

Alert physician to any segment of the patient history that may require specific precautions or be a contraindication to vaccine administration.

ADMINISTRATION

Have epinephrine 1:1000 available for treatment of possible allergic or other reactions. Physician may also request other drugs (_e.g.,_ antihistamine) available.

Follow manufacturer's directions about reconstitution, administration, and storage. (See also _Administration and Dosage_ sections for specific vaccines, above.)

When diluent is supplied with product, use _only_ this diluent. Use of other diluents may affect the product. Diluent may be supplied in a vial or in a disposable syringe. Do not mistake diluent supplied in a syringe with the vaccine.

Injections are usually given in sites not previously used for immunization. In some instances there may be no record of sites used for other immunizations.

When reconstituted, vaccine must be discarded after 8 hours; apply label with time of reconstitution.

Emergency department and clinic or physician's office personnel may wish to keep package inserts collated and posted for easy reference.

Refer to package inserts for more detailed information.

Immunizations, Passive

(Immune Serums)

Hepatitis B Immune Globulin Rx

injection	H-BIG, Hep-B-Gammagee, HyperHep

Immune Globulin Intramuscular
(Gamma Globulin, ISG) Rx

injection	Gamastan, Gammar, Immuglobin

Immune Globulin Intravenous Rx

injection	Gamimune

Lymphocyte Immune Globulin, Antithymocyte Globulin (Equine) Rx

injection	Atgam

Pertussis Immune Globulin Rx

injection	Hypertussis

RH₀ (D) Immune Globulin Rx

injection	Gamulin Rh, HypRho-D, RhoGAM

RH₀ (D) Immune Globulin Micro-dose Rx

injection	MICRhoGAM

Tetanus Immune Globulin Rx

injection	Homo-Tet, Hu-Tet, Hyper-Tet

Varicella-Zoster Immune Globulin
(Human) (VZIG) Rx

injection	_Generic_

INDICATIONS
HEPATITIS B IMMUNE GLOBULIN

Postexposure prophylaxis following either parenteral exposure (_e.g.,_ accidental "needle-stick"), direct mucous membrane contact (_e.g.,_ accidental splash), or oral ingestion (_e.g.,_ pipetting accident) involving HB$_s$Ag-positive materials such as blood, plasma, or serum. Use in other conditions continues to be evaluated.

IMMUNE GLOBULIN INTRAMUSCULAR (GAMMA GLOBULIN, ISG)

Hepatitis A (prophylactic value greatest when given before or soon after exposure); hepatitis B (hepatitis B immune globulin is preferred); measles (rubeola) for prevention and modification in susceptible contacts exposed less than 6 days previously; immunoglobulin deficiency; passive immunization for varicella in immunosuppressed patients (varicella-zoster immune globulin is preferred); prophylaxis of rubella in early pregnancy (use is of dubious value and cannot be justified).

IMMUNE GLOBULIN INTRAVENOUS

Immunodeficiency syndrome.

LYMPHOCYTE IMMUNE GLOBULIN, ANTITHYMOCYTE GLOBULIN (EQUINE)

Management of allograft rejection in renal transplant patients. Has also been administered as adjunct to other immunosuppressive therapy to delay onset of first rejection episode.

PERTUSSIS IMMUNE GLOBULIN

Prophylaxis and treatment of pertussis.

RH_O (D) IMMUNE GLOBULIN

To prevent sensitization to the Rh_O (D) factor and prevent hemolytic disease of the newborn (erythroblastosis fetalis) in a subsequent pregnancy. Also administered to all nonsensitized Rh-negative women after spontaneous or induced abortions, after ruptured tubal pregnancies, or after any occurrence of transplacental hemorrhage unless blood type of fetus is determined to be Rh_O (D) negative and D^U negative. In cases when Rh typing of fetus is not possible, fetus must be assumed to be Rh_O positive or D^U positive. Then patient is considered a candidate for administration of Rh_O (D) immune globulin. If father can be determined to be Rh_O (D) negative and D^U negative, immune globulin is not needed. Can be used to prevent Rh_O (D) sensitization in Rh_O (D)-negative patients accidentally transfused with Rh_O (D)-positive blood; is administered within 72 hours following incompatible transfusion.

RH_O (D) IMMUNE GLOBULIN MICRO-DOSE

Prevention of maternal Rh immunization following abortion or miscarriage after up to 12 weeks of gestation.

TETANUS IMMUNE GLOBULIN

Injured persons not actively immunized or in whom immunization status is undetermined and who would be candidates for tetanus antitoxin. Will not interfere with the primary immune response to tetanus toxoid given at same time at different site.

VARICELLA-ZOSTER IMMUNE GLOBULIN (HUMAN) (VSIG)

Passive immunization of susceptible immunodeficient children after exposure to varicella. Supply of vaccine is limited therefore use is restricted to individuals meeting criteria (see package insert).

CONTRAINDICATIONS

Individuals known to have an allergic response to gamma globulin or known to have anti-immunoglobulin A (anti-IgA) antibodies.

WARNINGS

Those with isolated IgA deficiency have potential for developing antibodies to IgA and could have anaphylactic reactions to subsequent administration of blood products that contain IgA; therefore, immune globulin is given only when expected benefits outweigh risks. In those with severe thrombocytopenia or any coagulation disorder contraindicating IM injections, immune globulin is given only if expected benefits outweigh potential risks. These products are not given IV (except immune globulin IV). Pregnancy is not a contraindication to administration.

PRECAUTIONS

Give with caution to those with history of prior systemic allergic reactions following administration of human immunoglobulin preparations. Incidence may be increased in those receiving large IM doses or repeated injections. Skin tests not done with these products.

DRUG INTERACTIONS

Defer **live virus vaccines** until 3 months after administration because antibodies in globulin preparation may interfere with immune response to the vaccination.

ADVERSE REACTIONS

Local: Occasionally tenderness and stiffness of muscles at injection site, which may persist for several hours.

Systemic: Urticaria, angioedema. Occasionally patient may react with erythema, low-grade fever. Anaphylactic reactions are rare. In highly allergic individuals, repeated injections may lead to anaphylactic shock.

DOSAGE

HEPATITIS B IMMUNE GLOBULIN

0.06 ml/kg IM; usual adult dose is 3 ml to 5 ml. Appropriate dose is administered as soon as possible after exposure (preferably within 7 days) and repeated 28 to 30 days after exposure.

IMMUNE GLOBULIN INTRAMUSCULAR (GAMMA GLOBULIN, ISG)

Give IM. Store at 2°C to 8°C. Do not freeze.

Hepatitis A: 0.01 ml/lb (0.02 ml/kg) as soon as possible after exposure (within 14 days).

Persons who plan to travel where hepatitis A is common: *Length of stay under 3 months*—0.02 ml/kg; *length of stay over 3 months*—0.05 ml/kg, repeated every 4 to 6 months.

Hepatitis B: 0.06 ml/kg as soon as possible after exposure (preferably within 7 days) and repeated 25 to 30 days after exposure.

Measles (rubeola): To prevent or modify measles in a susceptible person exposed less than 6 days previously, give 0.11 ml/lb (0.25 ml/kg). If a susceptible child exposed to measles has leukemia, lymphoma, or loss of cell-mediated immunity, or is undergoing chronic immunosuppression, give 0.5 ml/kg (15 ml maximum) immediately.

Immunoglobulin deficiency: 1.2 ml/kg followed in 3 to 4 weeks by 0.66 ml/kg to be given every 3 to 4 weeks. Some may require more frequent injections.

Varicella: 0.6 ml/kg to 1.2 ml/kg promptly (when varicella-zoster immune globulin is unavailable).

Rubella: Routine use for prophylaxis of rubella in early pregnancy is of dubious value; 20 ml has been suggested.

IMMUNE GLOBULIN INTRAVENOUS

Usual dose for prophylaxis in immunodeficiency syndromes is 100 mg/kg (*i.e.,* 2 ml/kg) administered once a month by IV infusion. May be diluted in 5% dextrose. Dosage may be increased to 200 mg/kg or infusion repeated more frequently than monthly if response is inadequate.

Recommended infusion rate: 0.01 ml/kg/minute to 0.02 ml/kg/minute for 30 minutes by itself. If no discomfort is experienced, rate may be increased to 0.02 ml/kg/minute to 0.04 ml/kg/minute. If side-effects occur, reduce rate of infusion until symptoms subside. Store at 2°C to 8°C. Do not use solution that has been frozen. Discard partially used vials. Do not use if turbid.

LYMPHOCYTE IMMUNE GLOBULIN, ANTITHYMOCYTE GLOBULIN

Warning: Only physicians experienced in immunosuppressive therapy and management of renal transplant patients should use this product.

Patients receiving this drug should be managed in facilities equipped and staffed with adequate laboratory and supportive medical resources.

Adults: 10 mg/kg/day to 30 mg/kg/day.

Children: 5 mg/kg/day to 25 mg/kg/day.

Delaying onset of renal allograft rejection: 15 mg/kg/day for 14 days, then every other day for 14 days for total of 21 doses in 28 days. Administer first dose within 24 hours before or after transplant.

Treatment of allograft rejection: 10 mg/kg/day to 15 mg/kg/day for 14 days. Additional alternate-day therapy up to total of 21 doses can be given.

Infusion instructions: Give IV. Dilute in saline solution before IV infusion. Invert IV bottle of saline so undiluted drug does not contact air inside. Add total daily dose to sterile 0.45% or 0.9% saline. Adding to dextrose solutions is not recommended. Do not infuse in less than 4 hours. An in-line filter with pore size of 0.2 to 1 micron is recommended.

PERTUSSIS IMMUNE GLOBULIN

Give IM.

Therapy: 1.25 ml, repeated at 24 to 48 hours, depending on response. In critically ill infants, child's dose should be doubled.

Prophylaxis: 1.25 ml as soon after exposure as possible.

Larger children: 2.5 ml. A second dose may be given 1 to 2 weeks later.

RH$_O$ (D) IMMUNE GLOBULIN

Obstetric usage: One vial is sufficient to prevent maternal sensitization to the Rh factor if fetal packed red blood cell volume that entered mother's blood due to fetomaternal hemorrhage is less than 15 ml (30 ml whole blood); if it is more than 15 ml, more than one vial may be given.

Transfusion accidents: Number of vials depends on volume of packed cells or whole blood transfused.

One-vial dose: Give entire contents IM.

Two or more vials: Use 5-ml to 10-ml syringes, withdraw contents from vials at one time, and administer IM. May be injected as a divided dose at different injection sites at same time or total dosage may be divided and injected at intervals within 72 hours postpartum or after a transfusion accident.

RH$_O$ (D) IMMUNE GLOBULIN MICRO-DOSE

One vial will suppress the immunogenic challenge of 2.5 ml of Rh$_O$ (D)-positive or D^U-positive packed red cells.

TETANUS IMMUNE GLOBULIN

Give IM.

Prophylaxis (adults, children): 250 units. More may be indicated if risk is great.

Therapy: No specific dosage recommended; use of 3000 units to 6000 units reported.

VARICELLA-ZOSTER IMMUNE GLOBULIN

Give deep IM.

Dosage according to weight: To 10 kg, give 125

units; 10.1 to 20 kg, give 250 units; 20.1 to 30 kg, give 375 units; 30.1 to 40 kg, give 500 units; over 40 kg, give 625 units. Administer entire contents of each vial (*e.g.,* 5 vials are required for those over 40 kg). Each vial contains 125 units in 2.5 ml or less.

NURSING IMPLICATIONS

HISTORY

When possible, obtain careful allergy history because these products are given with caution to those with a history of prior systemic allergic reactions following administration of human immunoglobulin preparations.

If outpatient is returning for a second dose, question patient regarding any reaction. Do not administer and inform physician if there is a history of severe reaction after first dose.

ADMINISTRATION

Have epinephrine 1:1000 available for possible allergic or other reactions.

Read package inserts carefully. See also *Dosage* sections, above.

Do not mix these products with other medications.

Follow manufacturer's directions regarding storage.

Advise outpatient receiving immune serums to notify physician if any systemic or local reactions become severe.

LYMPHOCYTE IMMUNE GLOBULIN

Anaphylaxis is uncommon but serious and may occur at any time during therapy. Keep tray with epinephrine, antihistamines, corticosteroids, syringes, needles, and airway at patient's bedside while drug is being administered. If anaphylaxis occurs, stop infusion immediately. Manufacturer recommends 0.3 ml aqueous epinephrine 1:1000 IM immediately, followed by steroids, assisted respiration, and other resuscitative measures. Therapy is not resumed.

Chills and fever occur frequently with administration of lymphocyte immune globulin. Monitor vital signs q4h; notify physician of temperature elevation.

Indapamide

See Thiazides and Related Diuretics.

Indomethacin

See Nonsteroidal Anti-inflammatory Agents.

Influenza Virus Vaccine

See Immunizations, Active.

Insulin Injection Concentrated Rx

injection: 500 units/ml   Regular (Concentrated) Iletin II (purified pork)

INDICATIONS

Treatment of diabetic patients with marked insulin resistance (requirement of more than 200 units/day), because a large dose may be administered in a small volume.

ACTIONS

Under usual circumstances, diabetes can be controlled with doses of 40 units/day to 60 units/day of insulin. An occasional patient will develop insulin resistance or become so unresponsive to the effect of insulin that daily doses of several hundred or even several thousand units are required. There seems to be no condition of absolute resistance; all patients respond to some dose if it is large enough. Occasionally, the cause of insulin resistance can be found (hemochromatosis, cirrhosis, a complicating disease of the endocrine glands other than the pancreas, allergy, or infection); in other cases no cause of high insulin requirement can be found.

Concentrated insulin injection is not modified by any agent that might prolong its action; experience shows that it frequently has a time action similar to that of repository insulin; a single dose may show activity over a 24-hour period. This effect has been credited to the high concentration of the preparation.

WARNINGS

Any change of insulin is made cautiously under medical supervision; patient is monitored closely. Changes in purity, brand, strength, or source species may result in need for change in dosage. Some patients may require one daily dose; others may require two or three injections. Most patients will show a "tolerance" to insulin. In some patients, minor variations in dosage can occur without development of untoward symptoms of hypoglycemia; a small number of patients may require dosage adjustment. Adjustment may be needed with the first dose or may occur over a period of several weeks. Be aware of symptoms of hypoglycemia or hyperglycemia.

Observe extreme caution in the measurement of dosage because inadvertent overdose may result in irreversible hypoglycemia.

PRECAUTIONS

Dose of pork insulin for those with insulin resistance due to antibodies to beef insulin may be only a fraction of that of beef insulin. Insulin resistance is frequently self-limited; after several weeks or months of high dosage, responsiveness to the pharmacologic effect of insulin may be regained and dosage can be reduced.

ADVERSE REACTIONS

Hypoglycemic reactions may occur. Deep secondary hypoglycemic reactions may develop 18 to 24 hours after injection. Patients should be carefully observed and prompt treatment initiated with glucagon injections and/or glucose by IV or gavage.

DOSAGE

Dosage variations are frequent in the insulin-resistant patient, because the individual is unresponsive to pharmacologic effect of insulin. Accuracy of measurement is encouraged because of potential danger of the preparation.

NURSING IMPLICATIONS

HISTORY

Obtain complete diabetic history, including insulin and dose used in past. See also Insulin Preparations.

PHYSICAL ASSESSMENT

See Insulin Preparations.

ADMINISTRATION

Give as per physician's order; can be administered by subcutaneous or IM route. IV route not advised because of possible development of allergic or anaphylactoid reactions.

A tuberculin (minim) syringe is used for administration. *Do not* use an insulin syringe because these are used only with U40 or U100 insulins.

Use the following to determine number of minims to be given:

$$\frac{D}{H} \times Q \text{ (15 or 16 minims)}$$

Dosage must be accurate because of potential danger of the preparation.

Storage: Cool place, preferably a refrigerator. Do not inject if not water clear. Discoloration, turbidity, or unusual viscosity indicates deterioration or contamination.

See also Insulin Preparations.

ONGOING ASSESSMENT AND NURSING MANAGEMENT

Patient is almost always hospitalized until dosage is established and control achieved.

Initially, patient may require repeated doses until blood glucose level decreases. Once patient is stabilized, dosage may be daily or several times per day.

CLINICAL ALERT: Even though patient is insulin resistant, inadvertent overdosage can result in irreversible hypoglycemia.

Blood glucose is monitored at frequent intervals. Initially, urine may be tested q1h to q2h for glucose and ketones. An indwelling catheter may be necessary.

Blood pressure, pulse, and respirations are monitored q1h to q2h or as ordered until patient's condition has stabilized, then q2h to q4h or as ordered.

Observe patient for signs of hypoglycemia (Appendix 6, section 6-14). Check with physician before insulin therapy is initiated regarding procedure to terminate hypoglycemia (physician may or may not order variation of standard procedure to terminate hypoglycemia). Contrary to U40 or U100 regular insulin, duration of activity may be prolonged. Deep secondary hypoglycemic reactions can occur 18 to 24 hours after injection; patient should be closely observed during this time period.

See also Insulin Preparations.

PATIENT AND FAMILY INFORMATION

NOTE: Patient and/or family member will require practice with tuberculin syringe in measuring dosage.

Following physician's recommendations regarding treatment of hypoglycemic reactions, frequency of urine testing, dietary changes (if any).

If a hypoglycemic reaction does occur, treat immediately and then notify physician. A second hypoglycemic reaction may occur 18 to 24 hours after injection of insulin. (Family member may need to observe patient at this time.)

See also Insulin Preparations.

Insulin Preparations*

Insulin Injection (Regular Insulin) otc

injection: 40 units/ml	Insulin (pork), Regular Iletin I (beef and pork)
injection: 100 units/ml	Actrapid (pork), Actrapid Human, Beef Regular Iletin II (purified beef), Hu-

---

* Insulin Injection Concentrated is discussed in the preceding monograph.

mulin R (recombinant DNA origin), Insulin (purified pork), Pork Regular Iletin II (purified pork), Regular Iletin I (beef and pork), Velosulin (purified pork)

Insulin Zinc Suspension

(Lente) (70% extended and 30% prompt insulin suspension) otc

injection: 40 units/ml	Lente Iletin I (beef and pork), Lente Insulin (beef)
injection: 100 units/ml	Beef Lente Iletin (beef), Lentard (purified pork and beef), Lente Iletin I (beef and pork), Lente Iletin II (purified beef or purified pork), Lente Insulin (beef), Monotard (purified pork), Monotard Human, Purified Beef Insulin Zinc (purified beef)

Insulin Zinc Suspension, Extended

(Ultralente) otc

injection: 40 units/ml	Ultralente Iletin I (beef and pork)
injection: 100 units/ml	Ultralente Iletin I (beef and pork), Ultralente Insulin (beef), Ultratard (purified beef)

Insulin Zinc Suspension, Prompt

(Semilente) otc

injection: 40 units/ml	Semilente Iletin I (beef and pork)
injection: 100 units/ml	Semilente Iletin I (beef and pork), Semilente Insulin (beef), Semitard (purified pork)

Isophane Insulin Suspension *(NPH) otc*

injection: 40 units/ml	Isophane Insulin NPH (beef), NPH Iletin I (beef and pork)
injection: 100 units/ml	Beef NPH Iletin II (purified beef), Humulin N (recombinant DNA origin), Insulatard NPH (purified pork), Isophane NPH (beef or purified beef), NPH Iletin I

(beef and pork), Pork NPH Iletin II (purified pork), Protaphane NPH (purified pork)

Isophane Insulin Suspension and Insulin Injection

(70% isophane insulin and 30% insulin) otc

injection: 100 units/ml	Mixtard (purified pork)

Protamine Zinc Insulin Suspension

(PZI) otc

injection: 40 units/ml	Protamine, Zinc & Iletin I (beef and pork)
injection: 100 units/ml	Beef Protamine, Zinc & Iletin II (purified beef); Pork Protamine, Zinc & Iletin II (purified pork); Protamine, Zinc & Iletin I (beef and pork); Protamine Zinc Insulin (beef)

INDICATIONS

Diabetes mellitus that cannot be properly controlled by diet alone; insulin injection (regular injection) may be given IV or IM for rapid effect in severe ketoacidosis or diabetic coma. In hyperkalemia, infusion of glucose and insulin produces a shift of potassium into cells and lowers serum potassium levels.

ACTIONS

Insulin, which is derived from beta cells of the pancreas, is the principal hormone required for proper glucose utilization in normal metabolic processes. Insulin preparations used to replace endogenous insulin deficiency are extracted from either beef or pork pancreas. The amino acid sequence of porcine insulin more closely resembles that of human insulin; pork insulins are generally less immunogenic than are bovine or mixed insulins.

Human insulin is now available. It is derived from synthetic processes (recombinant DNA technology using strains of *Escherichia coli*). Data are sparse, but human insulin has been shown to have characteristics very similar to those of the highly purified animal (particularly pork) insulins. Absolute indications for human insulin may be rare.

Modified insulins: Have been developed to delay the onset and prolong the duration of action and are classified as being rapid-acting, intermediate-acting, or long-acting (Table 31). Combining insulin with a large insoluble protein molecule (protamine)

Table 31. Onset, Peak, and Duration of Action of Various Insulin Preparations

Preparation	Onset (hr)	Peak (hr)	Duration (hr)
Rapid-Acting			
Insulin injection (regular)	½–1	2–5	6–8
Prompt insulin zinc suspension	½–1½	5–10	12–16
Intermediate-acting			
Isophane insulin suspension (NPH)	1–1½	8–12	24
Insulin zinc suspension (lente)	1–2½	7–15	24
Long-Acting			
Protamine zinc insulin suspension (PZI)	4–8	14–20	36
Extended insulin zinc suspension (Ultralente)	4–8	10–30	>36

slows absorption and prolongs duration of action. Insulin zinc suspensions have modified absorption characteristics because of the presence of zinc and control of particle size and physical state (amorphous or crystalline form) of the insulin. Insulin zinc suspension (lente) contains no protein modifiers and may be useful in those allergic to zinc, isophane, or protamine zinc insulins.

Individual response to insulin may vary and may be affected by diet, exercise, concomitant drug therapy, and other factors.

Purified insulins: Macromolecular protein contaminants in insulin preparations contribute to adverse immunogenic responses, including local or systemic allergic reactions and antibody-mediated insulin resistance. Purification techniques have been used to reduce the amount of proinsulin and noninsulin protein contaminants significantly. As a result, all commercially available insulin products now marketed in the United States are "single-peak" insulins, which are less likely to produce lipoatrophy. Further refinement may be applied to produce "purified" insulin. Purified pork insulins are the least immunogenic of currently available preparations.

PRECAUTIONS

Diet: Patients must follow diet prescribed by physician. Insulin is best administered 15 to 30 minutes before a meal.

Hypoglycemia: Excessive doses of insulin cause hypoglycemia. This condition may also occur following increased work or exercise; when food is not being absorbed in the usual manner (because of postponement or omission of a meal or in illness with vomiting, diarrhea, or delayed digestion); when insulin is administered too long before a meal; when insulin requirements decline; and when large doses are given at insufficient or irregular intervals.

An early symptom of hypoglycemia may be mere fatigue. Other vague symptoms include headache, drowsiness, lassitude, tremulousness, and nausea and demand immediate attention (see Appendix 6, section 6-14 for additional symptoms of hypoglycemia). Symptoms of hypoglycemia call for prompt and, if necessary, repeated administration of some form of carbohydrate. If the patient becomes delirious or mentally confused, corn syrup or orange juice with sugar may be given orally. In severe hypoglycemia, it may be desirable to administer 10 g to 20 g of dextrose in sterile solution IV.

Regular insulin (insulin injection) is required in dealing with acidosis and emergencies.

DRUG INTERACTIONS

Insulin may affect serum potassium levels; therefore, exercise caution when **cardiotonic glycosides** are administered concurrently. **Oral contraceptives, corticosteroids, epinephrine,** initiation of **thyroid hormone** replacement therapy, **dobutamine,** and **smoking** may increase insulin requirements. **Thiazide diuretics** elevate blood glucose levels and may antagonize the hypoglycemic effects of insulin. The hypoglycemic effects of insulin may be potentiated by **monoamine oxidase inhibitors, phenylbutazone, sulfinpyrazone, tetracycline, alcohol,** and **anabolic steroids.** Guanethidine may alter the hypoglycemic effects produced by insulin. **Beta-adrenergic blockers** (atenolol, metoprolol, nadolol, pindolol, propranolol, timolol) may increase the pharmacologic effects of insulin, resulting in possible hypoglycemia.

DOSAGE

The number and size of daily doses, time of administration, and diet and exercise all require continuous medical supervision.

Administer maintenance doses subcutaneously. Regular insulin injection may be given IV or IM in severe ketoacidosis or diabetic coma.

I
J
K

NURSING IMPLICATIONS

HISTORY

See Appendix 4. Note description and duration of symptoms (new diabetic), dietary history, and family history of diabetes mellitus.

PHYSICAL ASSESSMENT

Record vital signs, weight. Review chart for physician's physical examination, recent laboratory and diagnostic tests. Perform general assessment of skin, mucous membranes, extremities. If patient is using insulin, look for lipodystrophy at injection sites. If diagnosis is diabetic ketoacidosis (DKA), review chart for history (from family or previous hospital records) and physical assessment performed by physician.

ADMINISTRATION

The insulin order: The physician may order insulin by trade name rather than generic name (*e.g.,* Ultralente Iletin instead of insulin zinc suspension, extended). Do not substitute one brand for another (*e.g.,* Ultralente Iletin for Ultralente Insulin) unless substitution is approved by physician; some patients may be sensitive to changes in brands.

Read insulin label *carefully* for name, type (*e.g.,* beef, pork, beef and pork, purified beef, purified pork) and number of units/ml. U40 insulin has 40 units/ml; U100 insulin has 100 units/ml.

Note similarity in generic and trade names of some insulins. If physician's written order is unclear, obtain clarification.

Lente Iletin II is available as purified beef or purified pork. If this insulin is ordered and beef or pork is not specified, contact physician. Isophane insulin suspension (NPH) is available as beef or purified beef. If this insulin is ordered and beef or purified beef is not specified, contact physician.

If a new diabetic is to receive regular and NPH or regular and lente insulins, clarify with physician whether two separate injections are to be given or whether the insulins may be mixed in the same syringe.

If patient has been using the above insulins before admission, inquire whether insulins were administered separately or mixed in the same syringe.

Preparation for administration: Standardized color codes for insulin bottles are a red cap, red label, and red letters for U40; an orange cap and black letters are on the label for U100.

Check expiration date on label. Do not use outdated insulin.

When opening a new vial of insulin, write date on label.

Discard partially empty vials if not used for several weeks time. To prevent having vials unused for an undetermined length of time, avoid keeping several vials of the same type and strength on hand at any one time. Do not open new vials without checking all the insulin available for administration.

For insulins that are suspensions, ensure a uniform suspension by rotating the vial and inverting it from end to end several times immediately before withdrawing each dose. Avoid vigorous shaking, which may result in frothing of material and inaccurate dose.

Regular insulin may be mixed with crystalline PZI insulins in any proportion. Semilente, ultralente, and lente insulins may also be combined.

Recent evidence indicates that mixtures of regular and NPH insulins or regular and lente insulins may not be stable beyond 5 or 15 minutes, respectively. To achieve the same effect that would be expected from separate administration of the two insulins (for patients who previously administered these insulins separately and for whom it is now desirable to mix the insulins), use such mixtures within 5 minutes of mixing.

Once the interaction of regular insulin with NPH (5–15 minutes) or lente insulins (30 minutes to 24 hours) occurs, these insulin mixtures remain stable for 1 month at room temperature or 3 months under refrigeration. Patients stabilized on such mixtures should be expected to have a consistent response if the method of mixing is standardized. The potential for an unexpected response is most likely to occur when switching from separate injections to use of a mixture or vice versa.

Each different type of insulin used to prepare insulin mixtures must be of the same concentration (units/ml) and the insulins mixed in the same order (*e.g.,* regular insulin followed by NPH or a lente insulin) each time.

Always use a syringe that matches the concentration of the insulin (*i.e.,* a U100 syringe with U100 insulin, a U40 syringe with U40 insulin).

Insulin syringes have a 25-gauge or 26-gauge ½-inch or ¾-inch needle.

All air bubbles must be eliminated from the syringe barrel and hub of needle ("dead space") before the syringe is withdrawn from the vial.

Administration: Insulin is given subcutaneously; *only* insulin injection (regular) may be given IV or IM.

Regular insulin is given 15 to 30 minutes before a meal; longer-acting preparations are usually given before breakfast.

Select injection site. Insulin may be injected into the arms, thighs, abdomen, or buttocks. Clean skin with alcohol; allow to dry.

Pinch skin and insert needle at 45-degree angle. In areas containing more fatty tissue or in the obese individual, the skin may be spread tautly between the thumb and forefinger and the needle injected at a 90-degree angle. Aspirate syringe; if blood appears, discard needle, syringe, and insulin and prepare again for administration. If blood does not appear, inject insulin slowly.

Superficial injection of insulin may result in irritation or local allergic reactions.

Develop a plan for rotation of injection sites to prevent lipodystrophy, which may interfere with insulin absorption. The same injection site should not be used more than approximately once every 2 months. Charts may be used to develop a plan of rotation.

Storage: Although insulin preparations are generally stable when stored at room temperature (and not exposed to extreme temperatures or direct sunlight) for up to 2 years, it is recommended that insulin be stored in a cool place, preferably a refrigerator. Avoid exposure to either freezing or high temperatures. Vials in use should be kept cold; protect from strong light and use contents as continuously as possible. Discard partially empty vials if not used for several weeks. Insulin prefilled in plastic or glass syringes is stable for 1 week under refrigeration.

ONGOING ASSESSMENTS AND NURSING MANAGEMENT

Close observation of the diabetic patient is important, especially with juveniles; those who have been recently diagnosed and are being regulated with insulin; those with a medical illness or surgery; the pregnant diabetic; those who fail to adhere to physician's instructions (_e.g.,_ diet, weight loss, exercise); and those who have been difficult to regulate. Observe for possible hypoglycemic reactions at onset and at peak of insulin activity (see Table 31).

Hypoglycemia may occur when insulin is administered too long before a meal, when insulin requirements decline, when large insulin doses are given at insufficient or irregular intervals, or when a meal is omitted because of nausea, vomiting, or another cause.

Patients in the fasting state (for laboratory tests or diagnostic studies) must have their insulin withheld until the test is completed. Notify the dietary department when the meal may be served. If the patient is receiving regular insulin and there is the possibility that the meal will not be available in 30 minutes, it may be necessary to withhold the insulin until the meal arrives.

If the patient is receiving an intermediate- or long-acting insulin and the diagnostic test requires several hours, the physician may order regular insulin given for the remainder of the day. The dosage of insulin will depend on urine test results (glucose, ketones).

Patients going to surgery do not receive their daily insulin the morning of surgery (unless a specific dose is ordered for the day of surgery). The physician usually orders regular insulin to be added to each IV infusion.

Insulin absorption onto plastic IV sets has been reported to remove up to 80% of a dose; however, 20% to 30% is more common. The percentage absorbed is inversely proportional to the concentration of insulin, and the absorption takes place within 30 to 60 minutes. This phenomenon cannot be accurately predicted.

When a patient is receiving an IV infusion with insulin added, observe for signs of hyperglycemia (Appendix 6, section 6-14) and check urine for glucose q3h to q4h (in critical situations, the urine may be checked hourly). Notify the physician if the urine is positive for glucose because addition of more insulin to the IV infusion may be necessary. If additional insulin is added to the IV infusion, observe for signs of hypoglycemia (Appendix 6, section 6-14).

If patient received an intermediate- or long-acting insulin in the morning and one or more meals are not eaten (for any reason), the patient will need to be observed for hypoglycemia throughout the duration of insulin activity (see Table 31), including nighttime hours. Restlessness and diaphoresis during sleep may indicate a hypoglycemic reaction; wake patient and assess for signs of hypoglycemia.

Early signs of hypoglycemia may be vague and may vary from patient to patient. Early signs may include fatigue, headache, drowsiness, and lassitude. See also Appendix 6, section 6-14 for other signs of hypoglycemia.

CLINICAL ALERT: It is important that hypoglycemia be recognized and corrected as soon as possible. Prolonged hypoglycemia can result in cortical damage.

Methods of terminating a hypoglycemic reaction include administration of dilute corn syrup, orange juice with sugar, a lump of sugar dissolved in the mouth, commercial glucose products, glucagon subcutaneously, IM, or IV (p 510), or glucose 10% to 50% IV (50% more commonly used). Epinephrine 1:1000 may also be administered because it stimulates glycogenolysis but also has additional cardiac effects.

CLINICAL ALERT: _Never_ give a patient an oral fluid or substance to terminate a hypoglycemic reaction unless swallowing and gag reflexes are present. Lack of these reflexes may result in aspiration.

Hospital or clinical unit policies or a physician's written order may dictate the procedure to be followed (*e.g.,* types of fluids to be administered, obtaining blood samples) when hypoglycemia occurs.

If hypoglycemia occurs, notify the physician because insulin dosage and dietary intake may need to be changed.

Observe for the Somogyi effect, which may occur when insulin dosage is increased to control rising blood glucose levels. The glucose level drops but the body attempts to oppose the excessive insulin by releasing epinephrine (glycogenolysis), adrenal corticosteroids (glyconeogenesis), and growth hormone, all of which produce rebound hyperglycemia. Suspect the Somogyi effect if blood glucose levels are above normal but the patient exhibits signs of hypoglycemia or the patient exhibits marked swings of hyperglycemia and hypoglycemia.

Inspect most recent and previous injection sites daily for evidence of localized allergic reactions. Inform physician if local reaction is noted because insulin brand or type may be changed or an antihistamine ordered.

Weigh daily or as ordered.

Observe for signs of diabetic ketoacidosis (DKA) (Appendix 6, section 6-11), a state of acute insulin deficiency. Precipitating causes include fever, infection, pregnancy, severe emotional stress, surgery, undiagnosed diabetes mellitus, rapid growth in juveniles, steroid therapy, and certain disease states such as pancreatitis.

Treatment of DKA: Regular insulin IV and correction of fluid and electrolyte imbalance. Blood glucose is monitored frequently. Nursing management includes checking urine for glucose and ketone bodies hourly; taking blood pressure, pulse, and respirations q15m to q30m or as ordered; measuring intake and output; assessing patient's response to therapy including level of consciousness; observing for signs of fluid and electrolyte imbalance (Appendix 6, sections 6-10, 6-12, and 6-15); and looking for evidence of hypoglycemia (Appendix 6, section 6-14), because patient can pass from hyperglycemia to hypoglycemia as insulin is being administered. Other treatment may include use of an indwelling catheter, cardiac monitor, and oxygen.

Hyperosmolar hyperglycemic nonketotic coma (HHNK) may occur in non–insulin dependent diabetes mellitus (NIDDM), the undiagnosed diabetic, and disease states such as myocardial infarction, acute pancreatitis, and use of total parenteral nutrition (TPN) solutions.

Symptoms of HHNK are often insidious and include dehydration, polyuria, thirst, elevated blood glucose, increased serum osmolarity, and neurologic signs such as lethargy to coma, convulsions, positive Babinski, paresis, and hyperthermia.

Treatment of HHNK includes reduction of blood glucose (with regular insulin), correction of fluid and electrolyte imbalances, and close patient observation.

Urine is tested for glucose and ketone bodies qid (A.C. and H.S.). Because of variables in brands of urine glucose test materials (*e.g.,* 0.1% is reported as trace with Diastix and + (plus 1) with Tes-Tape), test results are recorded in percent. Most test materials range from 0% to 2% glucose concentration. Tests for ketones (acetone) are recorded as negative, small, moderate, and large. Consult package inserts for proper use and interpretation of test results. Record test results on a flow sheet.

Urine testing: Obtain urine for testing as second voided sample. When patient has an indwelling catheter, collect fresh urine from the catheter (and not from the collection bag).

If patient has difficulty in producing a second voided sample, encourage a liberal fluid intake for 30 or more minutes.

To prevent the Somogyi effect, physician may prefer to have urine show 0.1% (a trace) of glucose rather than have every sample negative.

Notify the physician if urine test is positive for ketones or glucose is more than 0.25%.

Patient may receive regular insulin based on each urine test's results for glucose. Often, 5 units of regular insulin is administered for each percentage increment (0.1%, 0.25%, 0.5%, 1% or 2%), that is, a patient with urine showing 0.25% would receive 10 units of regular insulin. The physician may also prefer the urine to show more than 0.1% before insulin is administered.

PATIENT AND FAMILY INFORMATION

A well-formulated teaching plan is necessary for all new diabetics as well as for those who have had any change in the management of their diabetes (*e.g.,* diet, insulin type or dosage) and those whose management is changed because of illness or disability (*e.g.,* loss of sight, disabling arthritis). The teaching plan must be individualized.

Inquire about physician preference for urine testing materials, frequency of urine testing, brand of needle and syringe, and materials or foods to be used to terminate hypoglycemic episodes. A diabetic teaching plan should include the following.

Urine testing: Materials to use and where purchased, a review of instructions included with urine test materials, patient's ability to read and interpret the color charts, techniques of urine testing, testing of the second voided specimen, when to notify the physician of test results, bringing a record of test results to the clinic or physician's office.

Insulin: Types, how dosage is expressed, where to purchase, prescription not required, color coding of caps and labels, location of expiration date, using only the brand recommended, advisability of not changing brands without physician approval, keeping a spare vial on hand, finishing one vial before opening the next.

Storage of insulin: Recommended temperatures, avoiding direct sunlight and warm temperatures.

Needle and syringe: Purchase of same brand and needle size each time, parts of the syringe, reading the scale of the syringe, prescription required for purchase of needle and syringe.

Preparation for administration: Principles of aseptic technique; how to withdraw insulin from vial; measurement of dosage in the syringe; when appropriate, mixing insulin in one syringe and using same order of mixing insulins each time; elimination of dead space and air bubbles; what to do if needle or syringe is contaminated.

Administration: Sites to be used, rotation of sites, angle of injection, technique of injection, administration at time of day prescribed by physician, proper disposal of needle and syringe.

Diet: Importance in management of diabetes, calories allowed, food exchanges, measuring (and, when applicable, weighing) foods, planning daily menus, selecting from a restaurant menu, reading food labels, establishing a meal schedule, dietary adjustments made only by physician, use of artificial sweeteners.

Traveling: Importance of carrying extra supply of insulin and prescription for needles and syringes, storage of insulin, protecting needles and syringes from theft, importance of discussing travel plans (especially foreign travel or travel to different time zones) with physician.

Hypoglycemia: Signs and symptoms, materials to take to terminate hypoglycemia, materials or foods to carry on person to terminate hypoglycemia, testing of urine, importance of relating hypoglycemic episodes to physician.

Hyperglycemia: Signs and symptoms, importance of notifying physician immediately.

Personal hygiene: Importance of good skin and foot care and frequent dental checkups, routine ophthalmologic examinations.

Exercise: Physician outlines amount of exercise allowed and activities that should be avoided (if any).

When to notify physician: Increase in glucose in urine; urine positive for ketones; if pregnancy occurs; hypoglycemic or hyperglycemic episodes; occurrence of illness, infection, or diarrhea (insulin dosage may require adjustment); appearance of new medical problems (*e.g.,* paresthesia of extremities, development of leg ulcers).

Visually impaired patient: Aids available for preparation of insulin for administration.

Other points: Importance of avoiding nonprescription drugs unless use is approved by physician.

Importance of routine medical supervision, laboratory tests.

Wearing of Medic-Alert or other identification.

Address of local chapter of American Diabetes Foundation.

Intrauterine Progesterone Contraceptive System Rx

intrauterine system: Progestasert
  38 mg proges-
  terone

INDICATIONS
Contraception in parous and nulliparous women.

CONTRAINDICATIONS
Pregnancy or suspected pregnancy; presence or history of pelvic inflammatory disease; presence or history of venereal disease; previous pelvic surgery; presence or history of postpartum endometritis or infected abortion; abnormalities of the uterus that result in uterine cavity distortion; known or suspected uterine or cervical malignancy including, but not limited to, an unresolved Pap smear; genital bleeding of unknown etiology; acute cervicitis unless infection is completely controlled and shown to be nongonococcal.

ACTIONS
Mechanism of action has not been conclusively demonstrated. It is possibly progesterone-induced inhibition of sperm capacitation or survival and alteration of the uterine milieu so as to prevent nidation. During use of system, endometrium shows progestational influence. Progesterone from the system suppresses proliferation of endometrial tissue (antiestrogenic effect). Following system's removal,

I
J
K

the endometrium rapidly returns to its normal cyclic pattern and can support pregnancy. Contraceptive effectiveness is enhanced by continuous release of progesterone into the uterine cavity at an average of 65 mcg/day for 1 year. The mechanism is local, not systemic. The concentrations of luteinizing hormone, estradiol, and progesterone in systemic venous plasma follow regular cyclic patterns indicative of ovulation during use of the system.

WARNINGS

Pregnancy: Long-term effects on the fetus are unknown. Reports indicate an increased incidence of septic abortion, associated in some instances with septicemia, septic shock, and death, in patients becoming pregnant with an intrauterine device (IUD) in place. Most of these reports were associated with the second trimester. In some cases initial symptoms were insidious and not easily recognized. If pregnancy occurs with a system *in situ,* the system is removed if the thread is visible; if removal is difficult, termination of pregnancy is considered. If pregnancy is maintained and the system remains *in situ,* the patient is warned of the increased risk of spontaneous abortion and sepsis. Patient is observed closely and instructed to report all abnormal symptoms immediately (*e.g.,* flulike syndrome, fever, abdominal cramping and pain, bleeding, or vaginal discharge) because generalized symptoms of septicemia may be insidious.

Ectopic pregnancy: Pregnancy that occurs while the woman is wearing an IUD is much more likely to be ectopic. Patients with delayed menses, slight menorrhagia, or unilateral pelvic pain and patients wishing to terminate an unplanned pregnancy are checked for ectopic pregnancy.

Pelvic infection: Increased risk reported with use of IUDs; patients should be taught to recognize symptoms.

Embedment: Partial embedment or lodging in the endometrium can result in difficult removal.

Perforation: Partial or total perforation of the uterine wall or cervix may occur; system must be removed because adhesions, foreign body reactions, and intestinal obstruction may result.

Congenital anomalies: It is not known if there is an increased or decreased risk when pregnancy is continued with the system in place.

PRECAUTIONS

The possibility of insertion in the presence of existing undetermined pregnancy is reduced if insertion is performed during or shortly after menstruation. System should not be inserted postpartum or postabortion until involution of uterus is complete because incidence of perforation and expulsion is greater. Use cautiously in those with anemia or history of menorrhagia or hypermenorrhea.

Syncope, bradycardia, or other neurovascular episodes may occur during insertion or removal, especially in those with a previous disposition to these conditions. Use in those with valvular or congenital heart disease may represent a potential for septic emboli. Insertion should be postponed in those with acute cervicitis until infection has cleared.

Because IUD may be expelled or displaced, patient is reexamined shortly after first postinsertion menses or at least 3 months after insertion.

DRUG INTERACTIONS

Use with caution in patients receiving **anticoagulants** or having coagulopathy.

ADVERSE REACTIONS

Endometritis, spontaneous abortion, septic abortion, perforation of uterus and cervix, pelvic infection, cervical erosion, vaginitis, leukorrhea, pregnancy, ectopic pregnancy, uterine embedment, difficult removal, complete or partial expulsion, intermenstrual spotting, prolongation of menstrual flow, anemia, amenorrhea or delayed menses, pain and cramping, dysmenorrhea, backache, dyspareunia, neurovascular episodes.

DOSAGE

Single system is inserted into uterine cavity and replaced 1 year after insertion.

NURSING IMPLICATIONS

HISTORY

Obtain complete menstrual history including date of last menstrual period, average length and type of flow (heavy, moderate, light), history of metrorrhagia; health history including venereal diseases (including herpes simplex II); pregnancy, spontaneous or therapeutic abortion history; prescription, nonprescription drug history. Alert physician to any abnormals in history. Obtain vital signs.

PHYSICAL ASSESSMENT

Physician performs pelvic examination, Pap smear, gonorrhea culture (and when appropriate other tests for venereal disease), sounding of the uterus to determine patency of endocervical canal, internal os, and the direction and depth of the uterine cavity. CBC and urinalysis may also be ordered. Other tests or diagnostic studies may also be appropriate.

ADMINISTRATION

System is inserted by physician with provided inserter.

Place patient on examining table with stirrups; drape. Obtain materials necessary for examination and insertion of IUD.

ONGOING ASSESSMENTS AND NURSING MANAGEMENT

Stay with patient while device is inserted. Observe for neurovascular episode (bradycardia, syncope).

Obtain blood pressure and pulse following insertion.

PATIENT INFORMATION

Patient package insert and patient instructions are available with product.

Notify physician or nurse immediately if any of the following occurs: fever, flulike syndrome, acute abdominal cramping and pain, bleeding, vaginal discharge, suspected pregnancy.

Some bleeding and cramps may occur during the first few weeks after insertion; if symptoms continue or become severe, contact physician immediately.

After menstrual period, make certain that the threads still protrude from the cervix. *Do not* pull on the threads. If threads cannot be felt, contact physician for examination.

If the IUD is partially expelled, *do not* remove. Contact physician for removal and insertion of a new system.

Physician may recommend other birth control measures for approximately 2 months after insertion of the IUD.

Physician will check placement of IUD after next menstrual period or within next 3 months. This examination is necessary to assure that the system is in place.

Iodinated Glycerol

See Iodine Expectorants.

Iodine Antiseptics

See Antiseptics and Germicides.

Iodine Expectorants

Hydrogen Iodide *otc*

syrup: 70 mg/5 ml   Hydriodic Acid

Iodinated Glycerol *Rx*

tablets: 30 mg	Organidin
elixir: 60 mg/5 ml	Organidin
solution: 50 mg/ml	Organidin

Potassium Iodide *Rx*

liquid: 500 mg/15 ml	*Generic*
solution: 1 g/ml	SSKI, *Generic*
syrup: 325 mg/5 ml	Pima
tablets, enteric coated: 300 mg	*Generic*
tablets: 135 mg potassium iodide, 25 mg niacinamide hydroiodide	Iodo-Niacin

INDICATIONS

As expectorants in symptomatic treatment of chronic pulmonary diseases in which tenacious mucus complicates the problem, including bronchial asthma, chronic bronchitis, bronchiectasis, and pulmonary emphysema. Also used as adjunctive treatment in respiratory tract conditions such as cystic fibrosis and chronic sinusitis and after surgery to help prevent atelectasis.

CONTRAINDICATIONS

Hyperthyroidism; hypersensitivity to iodides; hyperkalemia; acute bronchitis.

ACTIONS

Enhance secretion of respiratory fluids, decreasing viscosity of mucus. Objective evidence of clinical efficacy is lacking. Because of potential for adverse effects, other agents are preferred.

WARNINGS

Not administered continually or in the presence of certain types of goiter. If skin rash appears, discontinue use. Those with high fever or persistent cough should not use iodides unless directed by physician.

There have been reports of small-bowel lesions associated with administration of enteric-coated potassium salts. These lesions have caused obstruction, hemorrhage, perforation, and death.

Use in pregnancy, lactation: Potassium iodide can cause fetal harm, abnormal thyroid function, and goiter when administered to pregnant women. Because of possible fetal goiter, if drug is used during pregnancy or patient becomes pregnant while taking drug, patient is apprised of the potential hazard. Potassium iodide is excreted in breast milk; use by nursing mothers may cause skin rash and thyroid suppression in the infant.

Safety and effectiveness in children are not established.

PRECAUTIONS

Occasionally some patients are markedly sensitive to iodides; exercise care during initial administration. In some patients, prolonged use can lead to hypothyroidism. In those sensitive to iodides and in hyperthyroidism, iodine-induced goiter may occur. Some authorities consider tuberculosis a contraindication; use with caution in such cases and in those with Addison's disease, cardiac disease, hyperthyroidism, myotonia congenita, and renal impairment. Iodides have been reported to cause a flare-up of adolescent acne. Children with cystic fibrosis appear to have an exaggerated susceptibility to the goitrogenic effects of iodides. Dermatitis and other reversible manifestations of iodism have been reported with chronic use.

DRUG INTERACTIONS

Concurrent use with **lithium** and **antithyroid drugs** may potentiate the hypothyroid and goitrogenic effects of iodides. **Potassium-containing medications** may increase potential for hyperkalemia, and **potassium-sparing diuretics** may increase the effects of potassium, possibly resulting in hyperkalemia and cardiac arrhythmias or cardiac arrest.

Drug/lab tests: Thyroid-function tests may be altered. High intake of inorganic iodides has been shown to interfere with laboratory determination of protein-bound iodine (PBI). Although these have not been reported to be a problem clinically with use of iodinated glycerol in recommended doses, they should be kept in mind when a patient is receiving these preparations for prolonged periods.

ADVERSE REACTIONS

Thyroid adenoma and myxedema are possible side-effects. See also Iodine Thyroid Products.

OVERDOSAGE

Acute toxicity is rare. An occasional individual may show marked sensitivity, and the onset of acute poisoning may occur immediately or hours after administration. Angioedema, laryngeal edema, and cutaneous hemorrhages may occur. Symptoms of iodism disappear soon after drug is discontinued. Abundant fluid and salt intake aids in elimination of iodide.

DOSAGE

IODINATED GLYCEROL
5 ml tid or qid.

IODINATED GLYCEROL
Adults: 60 mg qid with liquid.
Children: Up to one-half adult dosage, based on weight.

POTASSIUM IODIDE
Liquid: 500 mg q4h to q6h.
Solution: 0.3 ml (300 mg) to 0.6 ml (600 mg) tid or qid diluted in water.
Tablets, enteric coated: 300 mg or 600 mg tid.
Syrup: *Adults*—5 ml to 10 ml q4h to q6h; *children*—2.5 ml to 5 ml q4h to q6h.

POTASSIUM IODIDE AND NIACINAMIDE HYDROIODIDE
Adults: Two tablets tid, P.C. with water.
Children (over 8): One tablet P.C. with water.

NURSING IMPLICATIONS

HISTORY

See Appendix 4. Note duration of cough, amount and appearance of mucus raised; allergy to iodine, seafoods.

PHYSICAL ASSESSMENT

If possible, visually examine sputum specimen; auscultate lungs. Chest x-ray and appropriate laboratory tests may be ordered.

ADMINISTRATION

If patient complains of taste when drug is diluted in water, check with physician whether drug can be administered with fruit juice, because manufacturers recommend administration with water.

Discard solutions that are discolored.

POTASSIUM IODIDE

Give solution diluted in full glass of water. Give tablets after meals, with water. Syrup is flavored and does not require dilution.

IODINATED GLYCEROL

Give with liquid.

ONGOING ASSESSMENTS AND NURSING MANAGEMENT

Observe patient for therapeutic drug effects, adverse reactions. Withhold dose and notify physician if adverse reactions are noted. Unless contraindicated, encourage increased fluid intake to help liquefy secretions.

Periodic serum potassium levels may be ordered.

Take only as prescribed. Do not increase dose.

Discontinue use and notify physician or nurse if epigastric pain, rash, fever, metallic taste, nausea, or vomiting occurs.

Do not use nonprescription drugs unless use is approved by physician (some drugs may contain iodides).

If problem continues, contact physician.

Iodine Thyroid Products

Potassium Iodide

tablets: 130 mg	IOSAT, Thyro-Block
solution: 21 mg potassium iodide/drop	Thyro-Block Solution

Sodium Iodide _Rx_

injection: 10%, 20%	_Generic_

Strong Iodine Solution _(Lugol's Solution)_ _Rx_

solution: 5% iodine, 10% potassium iodide	_Generic_

INDICATIONS

Used adjunctively with an antithyroid drug in hyperthyroid patients in preparation for thyroidectomy and to treat thyrotoxic crisis or neonatal thyrotoxicosis. IOSAT and Thyro-Block are available only to state and federal agencies; they are for thyroid blocking in a radiation emergency only.

CONTRAINDICATIONS

Hypersensitivity to iodides. Sodium iodide is contraindicated in pulmonary edema, pulmonary tuberculosis.

ACTIONS

Adequate intake of iodine is necessary for normal thyroid function and synthesis of thyroid hormone. Elemental iodine (from diet or medication) is reduced in the GI tract and enters the circulation in the form of iodide, which is actively transported and concentrated by the thyroid gland. Hormone synthesis requires oxidation of iodide and iodination of tyrosyl residues in thyroglobulin to form iodotyrosine precursors. These precursors undergo a "coupling reaction" to yield the active thyroid hormones triiodothyronine (T_3) and thyroxine (T_4). High concentrations of iodide greatly influence iodine metabolism by the thyroid gland. Large doses of iodides are capable of inhibiting thyroid hormone synthesis and release. This effect forms the basis for use of large doses of IV iodides in treating thyrotoxicosis. Iodides have a short half-life; an escape effect may occur with poor compliance. Effects of iodides are evident within 24 to 48 hours in the thyroid; maximum effects are attained after 10 to 15 days of therapy. Therapeutic effects may persist up to 6 weeks with chronic administration after the crisis has abated.

WARNINGS

It is not known if iodine can cause fetal harm or affect reproductive capacity. Administer to pregnant women only if clearly needed. It is not known if drug is excreted in human milk. Exercise caution in administering to nursing women. Safety and efficacy for use of parenteral form in children are not established.

PRECAUTIONS

Testing for idiosyncrasy to iodides is strongly recommended for all patients who are to receive parenteral iodide.

DRUG INTERACTIONS

Iodide preparations and **lithium carbonate** may have synergistic hypothyroid activity; concomitant use may result in hypothyroidism.

ADVERSE REACTIONS

Reactions are seldom seen after IV injection of sodium iodide. Occasionally, an individual will show marked sensitivity to iodide. Onset of acute iodide poisoning may occur immediately or several hours after administration. Angioneurotic phenomena are outstanding symptoms; edema of the larynx may lead to suffocation. Multiple hemorrhages of skin and mucous membranes, serum sickness, and fatalities have been reported. Possible side-effects of oral potassium iodide include skin rashes; swelling of the salivary glands; "iodism" (metallic taste, burning mouth and throat, sore teeth and gums, symptoms of head cold, sometimes stomach upset and diarrhea); allergic reactions (_i.e.,_ fever and joint pains, swelling of parts of the face and body, and at times severe shortness of breath requiring immediate medical attention). Overactivity, underactivity, or enlargement of the thyroid gland may occur rarely.

I
J
K

OVERDOSAGE

Acute poisoning

Symptoms: Iodine is corrosive; toxic symptoms are mainly a result of local irritation in GI tract. Vomiting, abdominal pain, and diarrhea (sometimes bloody) may be seen. Fatalities may occur from circulatory collapse due to shock, corrosive gastritis, or asphyxiation from swelling of glottis or larynx.

Treatment: Gastric lavage with soluble starch solution (15 g cornstarch or flour in 500 ml water) is recommended for removing iodine from the stomach. A 5% oral solution of sodium thiosulfate is a specific antidote because it reduces iodine to iodide. Milk may relieve gastric irritation. Correction of fluid and electrolyte imbalance and treatment of shock may be necessary.

Chronic toxicity

Chronic iodide toxicity, iodism, is a poorly understood phenomenon that is possibly related to the quantity of iodide administered. Manifestations include acneiform, maculopapular, vegetative (including frambesiform, fungating, and granulomatous), vesicular, or bullous eruptions; coryza; conjunctivitis; bronchial irritation; general swelling; inflammation; edema (including angioneurotic edema); erythema; purpura, or erythema multiforme (which may affect skin, mucous membranes); fever; nervous irritability. Discontinue use.

DOSAGE

Recommended daily allowance (RDA) for iodine is 150 mcg (adults).

Oral

Preparation for thyroidectomy: 2 to 6 drops strong iodine solution tid for 10 days prior to surgery.

Parenteral

Adjunct in management of thyroid crisis: 2 g IV/day.

Radiation emergency (Thyro-Block, IOSAT)

Adults, children over 1 year: 1 tablet/day (crush tablets for small children) or 6 drops added to ½ glass of liquid/day.

Infants under 1 year: ½ crushed tablet or 3 drops solution in small amount of liquid/day. Give for 10 days unless directed otherwise by state or local public health authorities.

NURSING IMPLICATIONS

HISTORY

If patient is scheduled for thyroidectomy, inquire number of days drug is taken prior to admission and whether any adverse reactions are noted.

Thyrotoxic crisis: Note allergy to iodine, seafoods.

PHYSICAL ASSESSMENT

Obtain vital signs; perform general assessment of body systems according to patient's symptoms; evaluate hydration. Laboratory and diagnostic studies include ECG, serum electrolytes, thyroid-function tests.

ADMINISTRATION

Oral solution (prescribed in drops): Add to fruit juice or water to improve taste. Patient may find that certain fruit juices disguise taste better than others; allow patient to experiment with various fruit juices.

Parenteral: Administered IV (usually used if patient vomiting).

ONGOING ASSESSMENTS AND NURSING MANAGEMENT

Preoperative preparation for thyroidectomy: Observe patient for signs of iodism (see *Overdosage*) and for adverse reactions, even if patient experienced no problem taking drug prior to admission. If adverse reactions occur, withhold drug and notify physician.

Thyrotoxic crisis: Other treatment modalities are usually used and may include other drugs, sedation, IV fluids, close observation of patient, vital signs.

Observe patient for signs of iodism, adverse reactions. Notify physician immediately if these occur.

PATIENT AND FAMILY INFORMATION

Dilute with water or fruit juice to improve taste.

Discontinue use and notify physician or nurse if fever, skin rash, metallic taste, swelling of throat, burning of mouth and throat, sore gums and teeth, head-cold symptoms, severe GI distress, or enlargement of the thyroid gland, swelling, or soreness of the salivary glands occurs.

Iodochlorhydroxyquin (Clioquinol) otc

cream: 3%	Torofor, Vioform, *Generic*
ointment: 3%	Vioform, *Generic*

INDICATIONS

Inflamed conditions of skin such as eczema, athlete's foot, and other fungal infections.

ACTIONS

Has antibacterial and antifungal properties.

PRECAUTIONS

Rarely, may prove irritating to skin. If itching, redness, irritation, swelling, or pain persists or increases or if infection occurs, discontinue use.

DRUG/LAB TESTS

May be absorbed through skin and interfere with **thyroid-function tests.**

DOSAGE

Apply to affected areas bid or tid. Not for use over 1 week.

NURSING IMPLICATIONS

HISTORY

Obtain description and duration of symptoms; allergy history; concurrent use of other skin preparations.

PHYSICAL ASSESSMENT

Examine and describe affected areas.

ADMINISTRATION

Wash affected area gently with soap and water; rinse and pat dry. Previous application must be removed before new application.

Physician may also order a different preapplication skin preparation.

Apply as directed by physician.

Do not apply occlusive dressing unless ordered by physician.

ONGOING ASSESSMENTS AND NURSING MANAGEMENT

Observe affected areas at time of each application.

If irritation or rash is apparent, discontinue use and notify physician.

Notify physician if infection is apparent or if pain persists or increases.

PATIENT AND FAMILY INFORMATION

Wash area with soap and warm water (or as directed by physician). Rinse and pat dry. Avoid rubbing area.

Apply as directed by physician or manufacturer's directions on container. Do not use for more than 1 week.

Exercise care when applying to face; avoid application near eyes.

Do not apply dressing unless directed to do so by physician.

May stain fabric, skin, or hair.

If itching, redness, irritation, swelling, or pain persists or increases or if infection occurs, discontinue use. Do not apply to deep or puncture wounds or burns; consult physician.

Iodoquinol (Diiodohydroxyquin) Rx

tablets: 210 mg	Yodoxin
tablets: 650 mg	Moebiquin, Yodoxin, *Generic*
powder	Yodoxin

INDICATIONS

Treatment of acute and chronic intestinal amebiasis. Not indicated for treatment of nonspecific diarrhea, particularly in children, because of potential toxicity.

CONTRAINDICATIONS

Hypersensitivity; hepatic damage.

ACTIONS

Is effective against the trophozoites and cysts of *Entamoeba histolytica* located in the large intestine. Because it is poorly absorbed from the GI tract, it can reach high concentrations in the intestinal lumen and produce its potent amebicidal effect precisely at the site of infection, without significant systemic absorption. Drug is not effective in amebic hepatitis and amebic abscess of the liver.

WARNINGS

Optic neuritis, optic atrophy, and peripheral neuropathy have been reported following prolonged high-dosage therapy; long-term therapy is avoided.

PRECAUTIONS

Use with caution in those with thyroid disease.

DRUG INTERACTIONS

Protein-bound iodine levels may be increased during treatment and interfere with results of certain thyroid-function tests. These effects may persist for as long as 6 months after discontinuance of therapy.

ADVERSE REACTIONS

Dermatologic: Various forms of skin eruptions (acneiform, papular, pustular, bullae, vegetating or tuberous iododerma), urticaria, pruritus.

GI: Nausea, vomiting, abdominal cramps, diarrhea, pruritus ani.

Other: Fever, chills, headache, vertigo, thyroid enlargement. Optic neurtis, optic atrophy, and peripheral neuropathy reported in association with prolonged high-dosage 8-hydroxyquinoline therapy.

ADMINISTRATION AND DOSAGE

Adults—650 mg two or three times a day, after meals for 20 days. *Children*—40 mg/kg/day in three divided doses for 20 days.

NURSING IMPLICATIONS

HISTORY

See Appendix 4. Local health department regulations may require investigation into recent travel to foreign countries. If patient has not traveled, further investigation of local travel, use of restaurants, water source, and so on may be necessary.

PHYSICAL ASSESSMENT

Obtain vital signs, weight, general physical status. Look for signs of dehydration (Appendix 6, section 6-10). Record appearance, consistency of stools.

ADMINISTRATION

Give after meals.

If patient has difficulty swallowing tablet it may be crushed; check with pharmacist regarding addition to foods or liquid.

ONGOING ASSESSMENTS AND NURSING MANAGEMENT

Obtain vital signs daily; observe for adverse reactions.

Measure intake and output. Record color, consistency of stools; note appearance of blood and mucus.

If nausea or vomiting occurs, notify physician.

If vomiting or diarrhea is severe, observe for signs of dehydration (Appendix 6, section 6-10) and notify physician if they are apparent. Fluid and electrolyte replacement may be necessary.

Isolation is usually not necessary. Follow hospital procedure for disposal of feces (stool precautions). Wash hands thoroughly after attending to patient following bowel movement, linen changes, anal care, obtainment of stool specimen.

Deliver all stool specimens to the laboratory immediately because specimens must be kept warm until examined.

Examination of stool specimens from all household members may be necessary.

PATIENT AND FAMILY INFORMATION

Take drug exactly as prescribed; take full course of therapy.

May cause nausea, vomiting, GI upset. If these symptoms become severe, contact physician.

Stool specimens will be required at periodic intervals, usually three times after therapy is completed and monthly for 3 months.

It is important to wash hands thoroughly after each bowel movement and when preparing and eating food. Raw foods should be thoroughly washed before eating.

NOTE: Food handlers may not return to employment until course of treatment is completed and all stool specimens are negative.

Ipecac Syrup *otc*

syrup: in 15 ml and   *Generic*
30 ml

INDICATIONS

Emetic for emergency treatment of drug overdose and in certain cases of poisoning.

CONTRAINDICATIONS

Do not use in semiconscious, unconscious, or convulsing persons.

WARNINGS

May not be effective in those cases in which ingested substance is an antiemetic. Drug can exert a cardiotoxic effect if it is not vomited but is absorbed. Emesis is not the proper treatment in all cases of potential poisoning; it should not be induced when such substances as petroleum distillates, strong alkali, acids, and strychnine are ingested.

DRUG INTERACTIONS

Activated charcoal will absorb ipecac syrup. If both are to be used, give activated charcoal only after successful vomiting has been produced by the ipecac. Do not administer **milk** or **carbonated beverages** with this product.

DOSAGE

Children less than 1 year: 5 ml to 10 ml followed by ½ to 1 glass of tepid water.

Children over 1 year and adults: 15 ml followed by 1 to 2 glasses of water. Dosage may be repeated once if vomiting does not occur within 20 minutes.

NURSING IMPLICATIONS

Ipecac syrup is recommended for home use. Teaching family in proper use of drug in cases of poisoning is essential.

PATIENT AND FAMILY INFORMATION

Read directions on label after drug is purchased; be familiar with the directions before an emergency occurs. Write date of purchase on container label; replace yearly.

Keep telephone number of the nearest poison control center and hospital posted over or near the telephone.

In cases of accidental or intentional poisoning, contact nearest poison control center or hospital emergency department for instructions *before* giving drug. Not all poisonings can be treated with this drug.

If calling a hospital, ask for the emergency department or emergency room. Inform the telephone operator that the call is about a poison ingestion and is an emergency.

When calling a poison control center or hospital, the name of the ingested substance must be known. If it is unsure which substance might have been ingested, give the names of the possible substances.

Administer ipecac syrup only if recommended.

Do not give drug to semisconscious, unconscious, or convulsing person. If person has history of convulsions, relate this information to personnel answering call.

Vomiting should occur in 20 to 30 minutes. If vomiting does not occur, contact the agency originally called. Dose can be repeated, but if possible request advice before repeating dose.

Follow recommendations given by agency. Even if the ingested substance has been vomited, it is usually recommended that the individual be examined by a physician. In some instances, it may be recommended that ipecac be given and patient immediately taken to a hospital. It is very important that the ingested substance's container be taken to the hospital.

If individual is transported by car, keep in upright position because vomiting may occur in transit.

Iron Dextran Rx

| injection: 50 mg iron/ml | Feostat, Hematran, Hydextran, I.D. 50, Imferon, Irodex, K-Feron, Nor-Feran, Proferdex |

INDICATIONS
Treatment of iron-deficiency anemia. IM or IV administration is advisable only in those in whom iron-deficiency anemia is present and its cause has been demonstrated and, if possible, corrected, and in whom oral administration is unsatisfactory or impossible (*e.g.,* intolerance to oral preparations, resistance to oral iron therapy, rapid replenishment of iron stores when oral therapy is ineffective, selected hemorrhagic cases, to replace postoperative transfusion to some degree, those patients who cannot be relied on to take oral medication).

CONTRAINDICATIONS
Hypersensitivity; all anemias other than iron-deficiency anemia.

WARNINGS
Parenteral use of complexes of iron and carbohydrates has resulted in fatal anaphylactic-type reactions. Deaths associated with such administration have been reported. Iron dextran should be used only in those in whom clearly established indications exist and have been confirmed by appropriate laboratory investigations corroborating iron-deficiency anemia not amenable to oral therapy.

Large IV doses may be associated with an increased incidence of adverse effects, particularly delayed reactions typified by arthralgia, myalgia, and fever.

Use with extreme care in presence of serious impairment of liver function. Use during pregnancy or in women of childbearing potential only when clearly needed and when potential benefits outweigh the unknown potential hazards to the fetus.

PRECAUTIONS
Parenteral product should not be administered concomitantly with oral iron preparations. Unwarranted parenteral therapy will cause excess storage of iron with possibility of exogenous hemosiderosis. Such iron overload is likely to occur in those with hemoglobinopathies and other refractory anemias that might be erroneously diagnosed as iron-deficiency anemia.

Patients with iron-deficiency anemia and rheumatoid arthritis may have an acute exacerbation of joint pain and swelling following IV administration of iron dextran. Use with caution in those with histories of significant allergies or asthma.

DRUG INTERACTIONS
Patients with iron-deficiency anemia showed delayed retriculocyte responses while receiving **chloramphenicol** concurrently.

Drug/lab tests: Exercise caution in interpreting results of **serum iron** values when blood samples are obtained within 1 to 2 weeks following large doses (exceeding 2 ml) of iron dextran. Bone scans involving Tc 99m diphosphonate showed dense, crescentic areas of activity following contours of the iliac crest, visualized 1 to 6 days after IM injections.

ADVERSE REACTIONS

Hypersensitivity: Anaphylactic reactions including fatal anaphylaxis; other hypersensitivity reactions include dyspnea, urticaria, other rashes and itching, arthralgia and mylagia, febrile episodes, and allergic purpura.

IM administration: Variable degrees of soreness and inflammation at or near injection site, including sterile abscesses; brown skin discoloration at injection site.

IV administration: Lymphadenopathy, local phlebitis at injection site, peripheral vascular "flushing" with rapid IV administration.

Miscellaneous: Hypotensive reaction; convulsions; possible arthritic reactivation in those with quiescent rheumatoid arthritis; leukocytosis, frequently with fever. Minor reactions include headache, transitory paresthesias, nausea, vomiting, shivering, itching, and rash.

DOSAGE

Discontinue oral iron before administration of iron dextran. Serum ferritin is periodically obtained during prolonged therapy.

Test dose: 0.5 ml IV or IM given before initial therapeutic dose. Although anaphylactic reactions known to occur following administration are usually evident within a few minutes, an hour or longer should elapse before the remainder of the initial therapeutic dose is given. If no adverse reactions are noted, administer drug.

Iron-deficiency anemia: The following formula provides a convenient method of determining the approximate dose needed for restoration of hemoglobin and body stores of iron:

$$0.3 \times \text{weight in lb}$$
$$\times \left(100 - \frac{\text{hemoglobin in g\% } \times 100}{14.8} \right) = \text{mg iron}$$

(To calculate dose in ml, divide this result by 50)

The requirements for patients weighing 30 lb or less is reduced to 80% of the above formula.

IM: Each day's dose should not exceed 25 mg (0.5 ml) for infants under 10 lb (4.5 kg); 50 mg (1 ml) for children under 20 lb (9 kg); 100 mg (2 ml) for patients under 110 lb (50 kg); and 250 mg (5 ml) for others.

Intermittent IV: Use only single-dose ampules without preservatives. Individual doses of 2 ml or less may be given daily. Give undiluted and slowly (1 ml or less/minute).

Iron replacement for blood loss: The formula below is based on the approximation that 1 ml of nor-mocytic, normochromic red cells contains 1 mg of elemental iron.

Replacement iron (in mg)

= Blood loss (in ml) × hematocrit

NURSING IMPLICATIONS

HISTORY

See Appendix 4. Note allergy history (drug is used with caution in those with significant allergies or asthma). Inform physician if patient has history of allergies or asthma.

PHYSICAL ASSESSMENT

Obtain vital signs, weight (may be required for calculation of dosage). Laboratory tests may include CBC, hemoglobin, hematocrit, serum ferritin, reticulocyte count.

ADMINISTRATION

Physician determines dose by using formula (see *Dosage*).

A test dose of 0.5-ml IM or IV is recommended before initiation of therapy. The test dose is given by the same route by which drug will be administered.

Epinephrine 1:1000 should be immediately available for test dose as well as each administration of drug. Usual adult dose of epinephrine is 0.5 ml subcutaneously or IM.

Observe patient closely immediately after test dose is administered; continue to observe q5m to q10m for adverse reactions for next hour or until the remainder of the initial dose is given.

The 0.5 ml used for the test dose is part of the initial dose. If there is any question about the physician's order, request clarification.

The 2-ml and 5-ml ampules are used for IV and IM administration. Multidose vials (10 ml) are for IM use only. Read drug label carefully.

IM: Advise patient that soreness at or near injection site may be noted.

Inject only into upper outer quadrant of buttock; never use arm or other exposed area.

Use 19-gauge to 20-gauge, 2-inch or 3-inch needle for injection.

If patient is standing, weight bearing should be on the leg opposite the injection site. If patient is in bed, place in the lateral position with the injection site uppermost.

Use the Z-track technique to avoid injection or leakage into subcutaneous tissue.

Do not mix with other drugs in same syringe.

IV: Rotate injection sites; record site used.

Depending on hospital policy, drug may be administered by physician or nurse.

Administer undiluted; inject slowly (1 ml or less/minute).

Have patient remain in bed 30 to 45 minutes following injection. Observe for hypotensive reaction; monitor blood pressure and pulse q15m.

ONGOING ASSESSMENTS AND NURSING MANAGEMENT

Monitor vital signs daily; observe for adverse reactions. If drug is administered by intermittent IV, check previous injection sites for signs of phlebitis; if administered IM, check previous injection sites for inflammation, sterile abscess.

Notify physician of adverse reactions. Physician must be notified immediately if signs of hypersensitivity (see *Adverse Reactions*) occur.

Periodic laboratory tests will be ordered to determine patient response to therapy.

Patients with rheumatoid arthritis: Observe for possible reactivation of arthritis. Acute exacerbation of joint pain and swelling may occur following IV administration of iron dextran.

Iron Products, Oral

Ferrous Fumarate *(33% elemental iron) otc*

tablets: 195 mg (64 mg iron)	Fumerin
tablets: 200 mg (66 mg iron)	Fumasorb, Ircon, Palmiron
tablets: 300 mg (99 mg iron)	*Generic*
tablets: 324 mg (106 mg iron)	Hemocyte
tablets: 325 mg (107 mg iron)	*Generic*
tablets, chewable: 100 mg (33 mg iron)	Feostat
tablets, timed release: 324 mg (106 mg iron)	Feco-T
suspension: 100 mg/ 5 ml (33 mg iron)	Feostat
drops: 45 mg/0.6 ml (15 mg iron)	Feostat

Ferrous Gluconate *(11.6% elemental iron) otc*

tablets: 320 mg (37 mg iron)	Fergon, Ferralet
tablets: 325 mg (38 mg iron)	*Generic*
capsules: 325 mg (38 mg iron)	*Generic*
capsules: 435 mg (50 mg iron)	Fergon
elixir: 300 mg/5 ml (35 mg iron)	Fergon

Ferrous Sulfate *(20% elemental iron) otc*

tablets: 195 mg (39 mg iron)	Mol-Iron, *Generic*
tablets: 300 mg (60 mg iron)	*Generic*
tablets: 325 mg (65 mg iron)	*Generic*
capsules, timed release: 150 mg (30 mg iron)	*Generic*
capsules, timed release: 225 mg (45 mg iron)	*Generic*
capsules, timed release: 250 mg (50 mg iron)	Ferospace, *Generic*
capsules, timed release: 390 mg (78 mg iron)	Mol-Iron Chronosules
tablets: timed release: 525 mg (105 mg iron)	Fero-Gradumet Filmtabs
syrup: 90 mg (18 mg iron)	Fer-In-Sol
elixir: 220 mg/5 ml (44 mg iron)	Feosol, *Generic*
drops: 75 mg/0.6 ml (15 mg iron)	Fer-In-Sol
drops: 125 mg/ml (25 mg iron)	Fer-Iron

Ferrous Sulfate Exsiccated *otc*

capsules: 190 mg (60 mg iron)	Fer-In-Sol
tablets: 200 mg (65 mg iron)	Feosol, Hematinic
capsules, timed release: 167 mg (50 mg iron)	Feosol Spansules

Polysaccharide-Iron Complex *otc*

tablets: 50 mg iron	Niferex
capsules: 150 mg iron	Hytinic-UD, Niferex-150, Nu-Iron 150

I
J
K

elixir: 100 mg iron/   Hytinic, Niferex, Nu-Iron
    5 ml

Soy Protein Complex *otc*

tablets: 50 mg iron   Fe-Plus

INDICATIONS
Prevention and treatment of iron-deficiency anemia.

CONTRAINDICATIONS
Hemochromatosis, hemosiderosis, chronic hemo-lytic anemias, known hypersensitivity to any ingre-dient, pyridoxine responsive anemia, cirrhosis of the liver. Usually contraindicated in peptic ulcer, re-gional enteritis, and ulcerative colitis.

ACTIONS
Iron, an essential mineral, is a component of hemo-globin, myoglobin, and a number of enzymes. Total body content is approximately 50 mg/kg in men and 35 mg/kg in women. About 30% is stored as hemosiderin or ferritin, found primarily in reticulo-endothelial cells of the liver, spleen, and bone mar-row. Approximately two-thirds of total body iron is in the circulating red blood cell mass in hemoglo-bin, the major factor of oxygen transport.

Average daily intake of iron is 18 mg/day to 20 mg/day; only 5% to 10% is absorbed (1 mg/day–2 mg/day). Anemic patients may absorb up to 30% of dietary iron. Iron is absorbed from the small intes-tine (primarily the duodenum). Sustained-release or enteric-coated preparations reduce the amount of available iron. They interfere with absorption by transporting iron beyond the duodenum where ab-sorption is most efficient. Iron is transported via the blood and bound to transferrin. Daily iron excre-tion is approximately 0.5 mg to 1 mg. An addi-tional 0.5 mg to 1 mg may be lost daily in the men-struating female.

In the products listed above the amount of ele-mental iron is given in parentheses.

WARNINGS
Individuals with normal iron balance should not chronically take iron. Prolonged therapeutic use of iron salts may produce iron storage disease.

PRECAUTIONS
Discontinue if symptoms of intolerance occur. Oc-casional GI discomfort, such as nausea, may be minimized by taking with meals and building up to recommended dosage.

DRUG INTERACTIONS
Vitamin C, 200 mg/30 mg iron, enhances the ab-sorption of iron from the GI tract. Oral iron inter-feres with absorption of oral **tetracyclines;** these products should not be taken within 2 hours of each other. **Chlormaphenicol** has been shown to de-lay iron clearance from plasma, delay iron incorpo-ration into red blood cells, and interfere with eryth-ropoiesis. Those with iron-deficiency anemia showed delayed reticulocyte responses to iron dex-tran injections while receiving chloramphenicol. **Magnesium trisilicate** containing antacids given concomitantly with iron compounds will decrease absorption of iron. Iron absorption is inhibited by ingestion of **eggs** and **milk.**

ADVERSE REACTIONS
May occasionally cause GI irritation, nausea, vomit-ing, constipation, diarrhea, allergic reactions. Stools may appear darker in color. When liquid iron is given to young babies, some darkening of mem-brane covering the teeth may occur.

OVERDOSAGE
Symptoms: May occur one-half to several hours after ingestion. Symptoms of massive overdose in-clude lethargy; melena; vomiting; diarrhea; GI dis-tress; dyspnea; weak, rapid pulse; and low blood pressure. Coma and metabolic acidosis may occur. Local erosion of the stomach and small intestine may result; sufficient iron may then be absorbed through the injured mucosa to produce systemic damage. Shock is commonly present. Stools are black and tarry. Bronchial pneumonia may be a complication. Increased capillary permeability, re-duced plasma volume, increased cardiac output, and sudden cardiovascular collapse may occur in acute iron intoxication. Chronic administration of large doses may lead to hemosiderosis.

Treatment: Quickly induce vomiting, then feed eggs and milk (to form iron complexes) until gastric lavage can be done. Lavage with 1% sodium bicar-bonate and administer iron-chelating agent (*e.g.,* de-feroxamine mesylate). Dimercaprol should not be used. Gastric lavage should not be performed after first hour because of danger of perforation due to gastric necrosis. Following emesis, administer a sa-line cathartic to speed passage through GI tract. It may be necessary to take measures to combat shock, acidosis, dehydration, blood loss, respiratory failure.

DOSAGE
Recommended dietary allowance (RDA) for adult males is 10 mg; adult females, 18 mg; during preg-nancy and lactation, 30 mg to 60 mg.

Iron-replacement therapy in deficiency states re-quires 90 mg to 300 mg of elemental iron daily (6 mg/kg/day).

NURSING IMPLICATIONS

HISTORY
See Appendix 4.

PHYSICAL ASSESSMENT
Obtain vital signs. Base additional assessment on patient's symptoms. Laboratory studies include CBC, hemoglobin. Other diagnostic tests may be performed to determine etiology of anemia.

ADMINISTRATION
Preferably administered between meals (on empty stomach) with water. May be given after meals or with food (exception milk, eggs) if GI upset occurs.

Avoid administration with tetracyclines. If patient is concurrently receiving tetracyclines, schedule administration of iron 2 hours before or 2 hours after.

Avoid administration with antacids containing magnesium trisilicate.

If patient has difficulty swallowing tablets or capsules, inform physician. A liquid preparation may be ordered.

Liquid preparations may be added to 2 oz to 4 oz of water or juice to prevent staining of teeth and mask taste.

ONGOING ASSESSMENTS AND NURSING MANAGEMENT
Patient with anemia may be asymptomatic or present various symptoms such as fatigue, listlessness, irritability, pallor, dyspnea, and headache. Chronic iron deficiency may result in spoon-shaped brittle nails, dysphagia, numbness and tingling of extremities, neuralgia.

Observe for relief of symptoms, which in some instances may be noted several days after therapy is initiated.

Check daily for constipation or diarrhea; withhold next dose and inform physician if either problem occurs.

Periodic CBC, hemoglobin, and reticulocyte counts are usually ordered to evaluate response to therapy. If improvement is not noted, further diagnostic studies may be performed.

Physician may prescribe vitamin C or an iron preparation containing vitamin C to enhance absorption of iron from the GI tract.

PATIENT AND FAMILY INFORMATION
Take drug exactly as recommended. Do not discontinue therapy even if symptoms are relieved.

Preferably take on empty stomach with water; may be taken after meals or with food (exception milk, eggs) if GI upset occurs.

Do not take tetracycline 2 hours before or after taking iron.

Do not take antacids while taking iron. If an antacid is recommended by physician, follow specific directions regarding time interval between these drugs.

Liquid preparation may be taken with small amount (especially for children, elderly) of water or juice to prevent staining of teeth and to mask taste.

May cause black stools, constipation, or diarrhea. If constipation or diarrhea is severe, contact physician.

Physician will perform periodic laboratory tests to monitor results of therapy.

Avoid indiscriminate use of advertised iron products. If true iron-deficiency anemia occurs, the cause of the anemia must be determined and therapy should be under the direction of a physician.

Isocarboxazid

See Antidepressants, Monoamine Oxidase Inhibitors.

Isoflurane

See Anesthetics, General, Volatile Liquids.

Isoflurophate

See Miotics, Cholinesterase Inhibitors.

Isoniazid _(Isonicotinic Acid Hydrazine) (INH)_ Rx

tablets: 50 mg	Laniazid, Teebaconin, _Generic_
tablets: 100 mg	Laniazid, Nydrazid, Teebaconin, _Generic_
tablets: 300 mg	Teebaconin, _Generic_
injection: 100 mg/ml	Nydrazid
powder	_Generic_

INDICATIONS
Recommended for all forms of tuberculosis in which organisms are susceptible. Also recommended as preventive therapy (chemoprophylaxis) for specific situations. The following priorities have been recommended for chemoprophylaxis:

1. Household members, other close associates of persons with recently diagnosed tuberculosis
2. Positive tuberculin skin test reactors whose chest x-ray findings are consistent with nonprogressive, healed, or quiescent lesions and in whom there are neither positive bacteriologic findings nor history of adequate chemotherapy
3. Persons whose tuberculin reaction has become positive within the last 2 years
4. Tuberculin reactors at risk of developing tuberculous disease (*i.e.,* prolonged glucocorticoid therapy, immunosuppressive therapy, diabetes mellitus, silicosis, leukemia, Hodgkin's disease, postgastrectomy)
5. Any positive tuberculin reactor under age 35 and particularly children up to age 7

Widespread prophylactic treatment is still questioned because of the inherent risk of hepatitis caused by isoniazid. Isoniazid prophylaxis is indicated during pregnancy by some for recent tuberculin converters and in any tuberculin reactor with inactive disease. Therapy for nearly all other pregnant candidates should probably be withheld during pregnancy until the postpartum period.

CONTRAINDICATIONS

Those with previous isoniazid-associated hepatic injury; severe adverse reactions to drug, such as drug fever, chills, arthritis; acute liver disease of any etiology.

ACTIONS

Acts against actively growing tubercle bacilli. Is bactericidal and interferes with lipid and nucleic acid biosynthesis in the growing organism. After oral administration, produces peak blood levels in 1 to 2 hours; these decline to 50% or less within 6 hours. It diffuses readily into all body fluids, tissues, organs, and excreta and also crosses the placental barrier and into milk. Drug is excreted by the kidneys. Pyridoxine (vitamin B_6) deficiency is sometimes seen in adults taking high doses of isoniazid.

WARNINGS

Severe and sometimes fatal hepatitis associated with therapy has been reported and may occur or develop even after many months of treatment. Risk is age related and highest in the 50 to 64 age group. Risk is increased with daily consumption of alcohol. Patient should be carefully monitored and interviewed at monthly intervals. If symptoms of hepatic damage are detected, drug is discontinued promptly because continued use has been reported to cause a more severe form of liver damage. Patient with tuberculosis should be given appropriate treatment with alternative drugs. If isoniazid must be reinstituted, it should be done only after symptoms and laboratory abnormalities have cleared. Drug is then restarted in very small and gradually increasing doses and withdrawn immediately if there is indication of recurrent liver involvement. Preventive treatment is deferred in those with acute hepatic diseases.

Use in pregnancy, lactation: Use only when necessary. The benefit of preventive therapy should be weighed against possible risks to the fetus. Preventive treatment should be started after delivery because risk of tuberculosis for new mothers is increased during the postpartum period. Neonates and breast-fed infants of isoniazid-treated mothers should be observed for any evidence of adverse effects.

DRUG INTERACTIONS

Isoniazid may decrease metabolism of **phenytoin;** dosage adjustment may be necessary to avoid phenytoin intoxication. Daily ingestion of **alcohol** may be associated with higher incidence of isoniazid-related hepatitis. The pharmacologic effects and toxicity of **carbamazepine** may be increased; dose of carbamazepine may need to be decreased. Effectiveness of isoniazid may be decreased when administered concurrently with **corticosteroids,** perhaps due to increased metabolism or clearance of isoniazid; the dose of isoniazid may have to be increased. The pharmacologic effects of **benzodiazepines** may be increased; their dose may need to be lowered. There is a possibility that the combination of isoniazid and **cycloserine** may result in an increased cycloserine-induced CNS toxicity. The hepatic toxicity of isoniazid and/or **rifampin** may be increased and may be reason for one or both to be discontinued when administered concomitantly. Isoniazid may act as an MAO inhibitor, raising the possibility of all of those attendant interactions, including with tyramine-containing foods (pp 99–100).

PRECAUTIONS

All drugs should be stopped and evaluation made at first sign of hypersensitivity. If isoniazid must be reinstituted, drug is given after symptoms have cleared and restarted in very small and gradually increasing doses. Discontinue drug if there is any indication of recurrent hypersensitivity reaction. Patients with active chronic liver disease or renal dysfunction are monitored closely. Periodic ophthalmologic examinations are recommended when visual symptoms occur.

Pyridoxine is recommended in those likely to develop peripheral neuropathies secondary to isoniazid administration.

ADVERSE REACTIONS

Toxic effects are usually encountered with higher doses; the most frequent affect the nervous system and liver.

Nervous system: Peripheral neuropathy is the most common toxic effect. It is dose related, occurs most often in malnourished and in those predisposed to neuritis (*e.g.,* alcoholics, diabetics), and is usually preceded by paresthesias of feet and hands. Other neurotoxic effects uncommon with conventional doses are convulsions, toxic encephalopathy, optic neuritis and atrophy, memory impairment, toxic psychosis.

GI: Nausea, vomiting, epigastric distress.

Hepatic: Elevated serum transaminase levels (SGOT, SGPT), bilirubinemia, bilirubinuria, jaundice, occasionally severe and sometimes fatal hepatitis. Mild hepatic dysfunction, evidenced by mild and transient elevation of serum transaminase levels occurs in 10% to 20% of patients. This abnormality usually appears in the first 4 to 6 months of treatment but can develop any time during therapy. Enzyme levels return to normal in most instances and medication need not be discontinued. Occasionally, progressive liver damage with accompanying symptoms may occur. In such cases, drug is discontinued immediately.

Hematologic: Agranulocytosis; hemolytic, sideroblastic, or aplastic anemia; thrombocytopenia; eosinophilia.

Hypersensitivity: Fever, skin eruptions (morbilliform, maculopapular, purpuric, or exfoliative), lymphadenopathy, vasculitis.

Metabolic and endocrine: Pyridoxine deficiency, pellagra, hyperglycemia, metabolic acidosis, gynecomastia.

Miscellaneous: Rheumatic syndrome, syndrome resembling systemic lupus erythematosus. Local irritation seen at site of IM injection.

Overdosage

Signs and symptoms: Overdosage signs and symptoms are seen within 30 minutes to 3 hours. Nausea, vomiting, dizziness, slurring of speech, blurred vision, and visual hallucinations (including bright colors and strange designs) are early manifestations. With marked overdosage, respiratory distress and CNS depression, progressing rapidly from stupor to profound coma, are to be expected, along with severe intractable seizures. Severe metabolic acidosis, acetonuria, and hyperglycemia are seen.

Treatment: Untreated or inadequately treated cases of gross overdosage can terminate fatally; good response is reported in most patients with adequate therapy within first few hours after ingestion.

Secure airway and establish adequate respiratory exchange. Gastric lavage is advised within the first 2 to 3 hours but is not attempted until convulsions are under control. Convulsions may be controlled with a short-acting barbiturate IV, followed by pyridoxine IV (usually 1 mg per each milligram of isoniazid ingested). Obtain blood samples for immediate determination of gases, electrolytes, BUN, glucose, and soon; type and cross-match blood in preparation for possible hemodialysis. Rapid control of metabolic acidosis is necessary. Give sodium bicarbonate IV immediately and repeat as needed. Forced osmotic diuresis must be started early and continued for some hours after clinical improvement is noted to hasten renal clearance of drug and prevent relapse. Monitor intake and output.

Hemodialysis is advised for severe cases; if not available, peritoneal dialysis can be used with forced diuresis.

DOSAGE

Treatment of tuberculosis: Used in conjunction with other effective antituberculosis agents. *Adults*— 5 mg/kg/day (up to 300 mg total) in a single dose. *Infants, children*—10 mg/kg/day to 20 mg/kg/day (up to 300 mg to 500 mg total) in a single dose, depending on severity of infection.

Preventive treatment: Adults—300 mg/day in a single dose. *Infants and children*—10 mg/kg/day (up to 300 mg total) in a single dose.

Concomitant administration of 6 mg/day to 50 mg/day of pyridoxine is recommended in the malnourished and in those predisposed to peripheral neuropathy (*i.e.,* alcoholics, diabetics).

NURSING IMPLICATIONS

HISTORY

See Appendix 4. Note history of hepatic disease. When prescribed for preventive treatment, question patient thoroughly regarding known or possible contacts.

PHYSICAL ASSESSMENT

Obtain vital signs, weight. Diagnostic studies include sputum culture and sensitivity, chest x-ray, CBC.

ADMINISTRATION

Oral preparation is best administered on an empty stomach at least 1 hour before or 2 hours after meals as a single daily dose. If patient develops GI upset, give with food.

Injection form is administered IM. Advise patient that discomfort or pain may be noted at injection site.

ONGOING ASSESSMENTS AND NURSING MANAGEMENT
Obtain vital signs daily; observe for adverse reactions and inform physician of occurrence.

CLINICAL ALERT: Observe patient for prodromal symptoms of hepatitis (*e.g.,* anorexia, nausea, vomiting, fatigue, malaise, weakness). If one or more of these occur, inform physician.

Signs of hypersensitivity include fever, skin eruptions, lymphadenopathy, vasculitis. If hypersensitivity is apparent, withhold all drugs and notify physician immediately.

Peripheral neuropathy may occur and is usually preceded by paresthesias of feet and hands. Physician may order 5 mg pyridoxine/day.

Weigh weekly or as ordered.

Periodic CBC may be ordered. Periodic ophthalmologic examinations are recommended during therapy if visual symptoms occur.

PATIENT AND FAMILY INFORMATION
Continuous therapy for the prescribed period is an essential part of treatment. Take medication regularly; avoid missing doses. Do not discontinue drug except on advice of physician.

Take on an empty stomach, at least 1 hour before or 2 hours after meals; may be taken with food to decrease GI upset.

Notify physician if weakness, fatigue, loss of appetite, nausea and vomiting, yellowing of the skin or eyes, darkening of the urine, or numbness or tingling of the hands and feet occurs.

Avoid foods containing tyramine (pp 99–100).

Reduce daily alcohol consumption (or preferably avoid alcohol entirely) while taking this drug.

Weigh self weekly; if weight loss is significant, inform physician.

Keep all appointments for physician or clinic visits or laboratory or diagnostic tests.

Isophane Insulin Suspension (NPH)

See Insulin Preparations.

Isophane Insulin Suspension and Insulin Injection

See Insulin Preparations.

Isopropamide Iodide

See Gastrointestinal Anticholinergics/Antispasmodics.

Isoproterenol Hydrochloride Rx

injection: 1:5000 (0.2   Isuprel, *Generic*
   mg/ml)
glossets (for sublin-   Isuprel
   gual or rectal use):
   10 mg, 15 mg

INDICATIONS
Parenteral form used as adjunct in management of shock (hypoperfusion syndrome) and in treatment of cardiac standstill or arrest; carotid sinus hypersensitivity; Adams-Stokes syndrome; ventricular tachycardia and ventricular arrhythmias that require increased inotropic cardiac activity for therapy. Sublingual or rectal use for Adams-Stokes syndrome and atrioventricular (AV) heart block. For other preparations and uses, see Bronchodilators and Decongestants, Systemic.

CONTRAINDICATIONS
Tachycardia caused by digitalis intoxication. Use in those with cardiac arrhythmias associated with tachycardia is generally contraindicated because the chronotropic effect may aggravate such disorders. Exceptions consist only of those ventricular tachycardias and ventricular arrhythmias that require increased inotropic cardiac activity for therapy.

ACTIONS
Has $beta_1$- and $beta_2$-adrenergic receptor activity. Primary actions are on beta receptors of heart and smooth muscle of the bronchi, skeletal muscle and splanchnic bed vasculature, and alimentary tract. The increased perfusion of skeletal muscle in the shock syndrome may be at the expense of more vital organs. Relaxes most smooth muscles, with the most pronounced effect on bronchial and GI smooth muscles. Produces marked relaxation in smaller bronchi and may dilate the trachea and main bronchi past the resting diameter.

Is not reliably absorbed following sublingual or oral administration. Onset of activity is approximately 30 minutes after sublingual administration and immediate after IV administration; duration is brief, 1 to 2 hours and less than 1 hour, respectively. Oral form is quickly inactivated in GI tract and rapidly and extensively metabolized in the liver; 50% of IV dose is excreted unchanged in urine.

WARNINGS

Infusions may produce increase in myocardial work and oxygen consumption. These effects may be detrimental to myocardial metabolism and functioning in those in cardiogenic shock secondary to coronary artery occlusion and myocardial infarction. Use in pregnancy only when clearly needed and when benefits outweigh unknown potential hazards to the fetus.

PRECAUTIONS

Hypovolemia: Use is not a substitute for replacement of blood, plasma, fluids, and electrolytes, which should be restored promptly when loss has occurred. Hypovolemia should be corrected by suitable volume expanders before treatment with isoproterenol.

Use with caution in those with cardiovascular disorders (*e.g.,* coronary insufficiency, diabetes, hyperthyroidism) and in patients sensitive to sympathomimetics.

Cardiac effects: Dose sufficient to increase heart rate to more than 130 beats/minute may induce ventricular arrhythmia. If cardiac rate increases sharply, those with angina pectoris may experience anginal pain.

DRUG INTERACTIONS

Do not administer isoproterenol and **epinephrine** simultaneously, because combined effects may induce serious arrhythmia. Drugs may be administered alternatively, provided proper interval has elapsed between doses. **Cyclopropane** or **halogenated hydrocarbon anesthetics** may sensitize myocardium to the effects of catecholamines. Use of vasopressors may cause severe persistent hypertension; rupture of a cerebral blood vessel may occur during postpartum period. The pressor effect of sympathomimetic amines is markedly potentiated in patients receiving of **monoamine oxidase (MAO) inhibitor.** When initiating pressor therapy, initial dosage should be small. Pressor response of adrenergic agents may also be potentiated by **tricyclic antidepressants,** although isoproterenol may be less likely to do so than some others. Use with caution and monitor ECG in patients receiving **digitalis,** especially in large doses, because arrhythmias may occur. The effects of **beta-adrenergic blocking agents** can be reversed by administration of isoproterenol.

ADVERSE REACTIONS

Serious reactions are infrequent, disappear quickly, and usually do not require discontinuation of treatment. No cumulative effects have been reported. The following have been reported.

Cardiac: Tachycardia with palpitation manifested by sensation of pounding in chest; precordial distress or anginal-type pain occurs rarely. In a few patients, presumably with organic disease of the A-V node and its branches, drug has been reported, paradoxically, to precipitate Adams-Stokes seizures during normal sinus rhythm or transient heart block.

CNS: Flushing of face, sweating, mild tremors, nervousness, headache, dizziness, weakness.

GI: Nausea, vomiting.

DOSAGE

Parenteral

Shock: Dilute 1:5000 solution in 5% Dextrose Injection, USP. A convenient dilution is 1 mg isoproterenol (5 ml) in 500 ml diluent (final concentration, 1:500,000 or 2 mcg/ml). Concentrations up to 10 times greater have been used. Infusion rates of 0.5 mcg/minute to 5 mcg/minute (0.25 ml to 2.5 ml diluted solution 1:500,000) are recommended. Rates greater than 30 mcg/minute have been used in advanced cases of shock.

Rate of infusion is adjusted on basis of heart rate, central venous pressure (CVP), systemic blood pressure, and urine flow. If heart rate exceeds 110 beats/minute, it may be advisable to decrease infusion rate or temporarily discontinue the infusion.

Cardiac standstill, arrhythmias: Adults—See Table 32. *Children*—Half initial adult dose of 0.1 mcg/kg/minute to 1.5 mcg/kg/minute. In all patients, subsequent dosage and method of administration depend on response of the ventricular rate and rapidity with which the cardiac pacemaker can take over when drug is gradually withdrawn. Usual route of administration is by IV injection or infusion. If time is not of utmost importance, initial therapy by IM or subcutaneous injection is preferred.

Sublingual or rectal

Suggested dosage for heart block in adults: Initial dose of 10 mg sublingually or 5 mg rectally; subsequent dose range is 5 mg to 50 mg sublingually or 5 mg to 15 mg rectally.

Children: Half the initial adult dose.

Usual route of administration in emergency treatment of those with severe heart block is IV injection or infusion. If time is not of the utmost importance, initial therapy by IM or subcutaneous injec-

Table 32. Dosage of Isoproterenol for Cardiac Standstill and Arrhythmias in Adults

Route	Dilution	Initial Dose	Subsequent Dose Range
IV injection	Dilute 1 ml of 1:5000 solution (0.2 mg) to 10 ml with Sodium Chloride or 5% Dextrose	0.02 mg–0.06 mg (1 ml–3 ml of diluted solution 1:50,000)	0.01 mg–0.2 mg (0.5 ml–10 ml of diluted solution)
IV infusion	Dilute 10 ml of 1:5000 solution (2 mg) in 500 ml of 5% Dextrose	5 mcg/min (1.25 ml/min of diluted solution (1:250,000)	
IM	Undiluted 1:5000 solution	0.2 mg (1 ml)	0.02 mg–1 mg (0.1 ml– 5 ml)
Subcutaneous	Undiluted 1:5000 solution	0.2 mg (1 ml)	0.15 mg–0.2 mg (0.75 ml–1 ml)
Intracardiac	Undiluted 1:5000 solution	0.02 mg (0.1 ml)	

tion preferred. If further maintenance therapy is necessary, glossets may be administered sublingually. Monitor ECG.

Sublingual or rectal administration is effective in control of mild stabilized symptomatic heart block and ventricular arrhythmias. In acute symptomatic heartblock, particularly in those with postcardiac surgery block, electrical pacing is the preferred method of treatment for maintenance of adequate ventricular rate. In ventricular arrhythmias, electroshock may be used and usually is the treatment of choice.

If given in acute symptomatic heart block, IV administration with constant ECG monitoring is preferred. This avoids irregular absorption, which is possible with sublingual and rectal administration. Rectal administration is more satisfactory for long-term therapy because effect is produced within 30 minutes and lasts 2 to 4 hours. Sinus rhythm sometimes occurs and persists for a variable period but often relapses again into complete block. In other cases, isoproterenol merely maintains an acceptable heart rate between 90 and 100 beats/minute.

Carotid sinus sensitivity with reflex cardiac standstill can be abolished by the cardiac stimulative action of isoproterenol until normal automaticity returns. From 10 mg to 30 mg, sublingually, 4 to 6 times a day may prevent heart block in these patients.

NURSING IMPLICATIONS

HISTORY
When possible, review events leading up to shock, cardiac standstill or arrest, or other cardiac arrhythmia.

PHYSICAL ASSESSMENT
Obtain blood pressure, pulse rate and rhythm, and respiratory rate; record general status (*e.g.,* color, level of consciousness).

ADMINISTRATION
Attach cardiac monitor to continuously monitor ECG during parenteral administration.

ECG monitoring may also be necessary when drug is given by sublingual or rectal route.

CVP monitoring is recommended. If line not presently in place, physician may insert CVP line. When applicable, keep tray and materials available for insertion.

Parenteral solution is available as 1:5000 solution (0.2 mg/ml) in 1-, 5-, or 10-ml vials.

IV infusion: Use large vein. Secure needle or catheter with tape.

Physician must order dose and rate of infusion and supply guidelines for adjusting rate of infusion (see *Dosage*). Recommended infusion dose is 10 ml added to 500 ml of 5% Dextrose and infused at 5 mcg/min (1.25 ml/minute).

Guidelines for regulating infusion rate may include blood pressure, CVP, and pulse rate range and urine flow.

Physician adjusts dosage according to ECG response.

Infuse IV solution containing drug by means of IV piggyback or a secondary IV line. The primary line can be used to administer an IV solution to keep vein open (KVO) if secondary or piggyback line containing isoproterenol is temporarily discontinued.

In some instances it may be advisable to use a

controlled infusion pump to administer by IV infusion.

IV injection: Initial dose is prepared by diluting 1 ml to 10 ml with Sodium Chloride or 5% Dextrose. From this solution, 1 ml to 3 ml (0.02 mg–0.06 mg) is administered by direct IV.

Subsequent doses are prepared by diluting 0.5 ml to 10 ml. From this solution, 0.5 ml to 10 ml (0.01 mg–0.2 mg) is administered by direct IV.

Drug is injected slowly. Patient must be on continuous cardiac monitor.

Intracardiac: Draw up 0.1 ml of undiluted solution using 20-gauge to 21-gauge needle; attach an intracardiac needle to syringe.

Sublingual: Instruct patient to place glosset under tongue and allow to dissolve. Drug should not be chewed or swallowed.

Rectal: Using a lubricated glove or fingercot, place tablet on finger and gently insert past rectal sphincter. If rectum contains feces (which may delay absorption), notify physician because other route may be necessary.

ONGOING ASSESSMENTS AND NURSING MANAGEMENT

Dosage and route of administration of subsequent doses depend on response of ventricular rate and the rapidity with which cardiac pacemaker can take over when drug is gradually withdrawn.

Hypoperfusion syndrome

(shock): Administration of volume expanders precedes administration of isoproterenol. Physician orders blood pH, and CO_2 to monitor patient response to treatment.

Monitor urinary output qh or as ordered until condition is stabilized. An indwelling catheter will be necessary to monitor urine output. Notify physician immediately if urinary output decreases.

Observe for adverse reactions; notify physician if any should occur.

IV administration

CLINICAL ALERT: Patient is monitored continuously. IV infusion should be temporarily stopped or slowed (depending on physician's guidelines) if any of the following occurs: anginal pain or other precordial distress; a pulse rate exceeding 110 beats/minute; development of a new arrhythmia. Other guidelines (*e.g.,* CVP, blood pressure) established by physician may also require adjustment in infusion rate.

Monitor blood pressure, pulse (from cardiac monitor), and respirations q5m or as ordered. Record on flow sheet.

IM, subcutaneous administration

Monitor blood pressure, pulse, and respirations q5m to q15m or as ordered until condition is stabilized. Patient should be on cardiac monitor until condition is stabilized.

Sublingual or rectal administration

Monitor blood pressure, pulse, and respirations during initial therapy q½h to q1h or as ordered.

Cardiac monitor may be indicated until condition is stabilized.

When isoproterenol is administered rectally, check patient ½ hour after administration to be sure drug has not been expelled from rectum. Check bed linen thoroughly (tablet is white and small).

Isosorbide Rx

solution: 100 g/ 220 ml	Ismotic

INDICATIONS

Short-term reduction of intraocular pressure prior to and after completion of intraocular surgery for glaucoma and cataract, chronic simple glaucoma, primary angle-closure glaucoma, certain types of secondary glaucoma.

CONTRAINDICATIONS

Well-established anuria due to severe renal disease, severe dehydration, frank or impending acute pulmonary edema, hemorrhagic glaucoma.

ACTIONS

An oral osmotic agent for reducing intraocular pressure with physical action similar to other osmotic agents. Is rapidly absorbed after oral administration. Is essentially nonmetabolized, and in the circulation contributes to the tonicity of the blood until it is eliminated unchanged by the kidney. While in the blood, it acts as an osmotic agent to promote redistribution of water toward the circulation with ultimate elimination in the urine.

WARNINGS

With repeated doses, consideration is given to maintaining adequate fluid and electrolyte balance. If urinary output continues to decrease, patient's clinical status is reviewed. Accumulation may result in overexpansion of extracellular fluid. There is no adequate information on whether drug has adverse effects on fetus.

PRECAUTIONS

Repetitive doses are used with caution, particularly in those with diseases associated with salt retention.

ADVERSE REACTIONS

Nausea, vomiting, diarrhea, headache, anorexia; rare occurrences of syncope, gastric discomfort, lethargy, vertigo, thirst, dizziness, hiccups, hypernatremia, hyperosmolality, irritability, rash, and lightheadedness have been reported.

DOSAGE

For oral use only.

Recommended initial dose: 1.5 g/kg (equivalent to 1.5 ml/lb). Onset of action is usually in 30 minutes; maximum effect expected at 1 to 1½ hours. Useful dose range is 1 g/kg to 3 g/kg. Drug's effect will persist up to 5 or 6 hours. Use 2 to 4 times a day as indicated.

NURSING IMPLICATIONS

HISTORY

See Appendix 4.

PHYSICAL ASSESSMENT

Review chart for ophthalmologic examination, surgical report (when applicable).

ADMINISTRATION

Drug administered orally.

Palatability may be improved if drug is poured over cracked ice and sipped. If patient refuses to take drug (because of taste), discuss with physician.

Patient with impaired vision may need assistance in taking drug. Do not fill glass to top because spillage may result. In some instances it may be necessary to dispense drug (over cracked ice) in two glasses.

GENERIC NAME SIMILARITY

Isosorbide and isosorbide dinitrate (an antianginal agent).

ONGOING ASSESSMENTS AND NURSING MANAGEMENT

With repeated doses, monitor intake and output. Notify physician of change in intake–output ratio; observe for symptoms of electrolyte imbalance.

Notify physician if patient experiences any adverse reactions, especially nausea and vomiting.

Isosorbide Dinitrate

See Nitrates.

Isotretinoin (13-cis-Retinoic Acid) Rx

capsules: 10 mg,   Accutane
    20 mg, 40 mg

INDICATIONS

Treatment of severe recalcitrant cystic acne; a single course of therapy results in complete and prolonged remission in many patients. If a second course is needed, 8 weeks should elapse after completion of the first course. Patients may continue to improve while off the drug. Because of significant adverse effects, treatment is reserved for those with severe cystic acne that is unresponsive to conventional drugs, including systemic antibiotics.

Unlabeled uses: Isotretinoin has been used in the treatment of numerous cutaneous disorders of keratinization, such as keratosis follicularis (Darier-White disease), pityriasis rubra pilaris, lamellar ichthyosis, congenital ichthyosiform erythroderma, hyperkeratosis palmaris et plantaris, and other ichthyotic conditions. Although improvement is observed in most patients, response is variable and higher than usual doses are required. Success has also been recorded for treating cutaneous T-cell lymphoma (mycosis fungoides).

CONTRAINDICATIONS

Not given to women of childbearing potential unless an effective form of contraception is used. Patients who are pregnant or who intend to become pregnant must not receive isotretinoin because major fetal abnormalities including hydrocephalus, microcephaly, abnormalities of the external ear, and cardiac abnormalities have occurred. In addition, several spontaneous abortions have been reported.

Do not give to those sensitive to parabens (perservatives in the formulation).

ACTIONS

Isotretinoin is related to retinoic acid and retinol (vitamin A). Exact mechanism of action is unknown. Clinical improvement in cystic acne patients occurs in association with reduction of sebum secretion. The decrease in sebum secretion is temporary and related to dose and duration of treatment; the decrease reflects a reduction in sebaceous gland size and an inhibition of sebaceous gland differentiation. Isotretinoin also inhibits keratinization.

WARNINGS

Hypertriglyceridemia: Approximately 25% of patients experience elevation in plasma triglycerides, 15% a decrease in high-density lipoproteins, and 7%

an increase in cholesterol. These effects are reversible on cessation of therapy. Patients with increased tendency to develop hypertriglyceridemia include those with diabetes mellitus, obesity, increased alcohol intake, and familial history. Some patients are able to reverse triglyceride elevation by weight reduction, restriction of dietary fat and alcohol, and reduction in dose while continuing therapy.

Musculoskeletal: Approximately 16% of patients develop musculoskeletal symptoms. In general, these are mild to moderate and have occasionally required discontinuation of drug. These symptoms generally clear rapidly after discontinuation of isotretinoin.

Ophthalmic: In 72 patients with keratinization disorders who have normal pretreatment ophthalmologic examinations, 5 developed corneal opacities. Corneal opacities have also been reported in cystic acne patients.

Use in pregnancy, lactation: See _Contraindications_ for use in pregnancy. Because abnormalities of the human fetus have been reported, continue contraception for one month or until a normal menstrual period has occurred following discontinuation of therapy. It is not known if drug is excreted in human milk. Because of the potential for adverse affects, do not give to nursing mothers.

PRECAUTIONS

An occasional exaggerated healing response, manifested by exuberant granulation with crusting, has been reported.

A transient exacerbation of acne has occurred generally during the initial period of therapy.

DRUG INTERACTIONS

To avoid additive toxic effects, do not take **vitamin A supplements** concomitantly.

Pseudotumor cerebri and papilledema have been reported in patients receiving isotretinoin; some patients were receiving concomitant **minocycline** or **tetracycline.**

Concomitant ingestion of **alcohol** may potentiate serum triglyceride elevations.

ADVERSE REACTIONS

Dose relationship and duration: Most adverse reactions appear to be dose related, with the more pronounced effects occurring at doses above 1 mg/kg/day. Adverse reactions seen in cystic acne patients were reversible when therapy was discontinued.

Most frequent: Cheilitis (90%); eye irritation (50%); conjunctivitis (40%); skin fragility (31%). Dry skin, pruritus, epistaxis, dry nose, and dry mouth may occur in up to 80% of cystic acne patients.

Dermatologic: Cheilitis (90%); dry skin, pruritus (80%); skin fragility (31%); xerosis, facial skin desquamation, drying of mucous membranes (30%); nail brittleness (10%); rash, temporary thinning of hair (<10%); peeling palms and soles, skin infections, photosensitivity, palmoplantar desquamation (5%); erythema nodosum, paronychia, hypo- or hyperpigmentation, urticaria (<1%); exaggerated healing response manifested by exuberant granulation tissue with crusting.

GI: Dry mouth (80%); nausea, vomiting, abdominal pain (20%); nonspecific GI symptoms (5%); anorexia (4%); inflammatory bowel disease including regional ileitis, mild GI bleeding, weight loss (<1%).

Ophthalmic: Eye irritation (50%); conjunctivitis (38%); corneal opacities (see _Warnings_).

CNS: Lethargy (10%); insomnia, fatigue, headache (5%); paresthesias, dizziness (<1%); pseudotumor cerebri including headache, visual disturbances, and papilledema (usually associated with concomitant tetracycline therapy; see _Drug Interactions_).

GU: White cells in urine (10% to 20%); proteinuria, hematuria, nonspecific urogenital findings (5%).

Musculoskeletal: Skeletal hyperostosis; arthralgia; bone, joint, muscle pain and stiffness (16% to 17%). Two children showed x-ray findings suggesting premature closing of the epiphysis. (See _Warnings_).

Miscellaneous: Epistaxis, dry nose (80%); mild bleeding (4%); bruising, disseminated herpes simplex, edema, respiratory infections, abnormal menses (<1%).

Laboratory abnormalities: Elevated sedimentation rate (40%); triglyceride elevation (25%); mild to moderate decrease in high-density lipoproteins (16%); decreased red blood cell parameters, white blood cell counts; elevated platelet counts, increased alkaline phosphatase, SGOT, SGPT, LDH (10% to 20%); increased fasting serum glucose, hyperuricemia (<10%); minimal elevation of cholesterol (7%). Approximately 4% to 11% showed triglyceride elevation above 500 mg/dl. Abnormalities of serum lipids are reversible on cessation of therapy.

DOSAGE

Initial dose is individualized according to patient's weight and severity of disease. After 2 weeks, dosage is adjusted according to clinical side-effects and disease response.

Recommended course of therapy is 1 mg/kg/day to 2 mg/kg/day, divided into two doses, for 15 to 20 weeks. If the total cyst count has been reduced by more than 70% before this time period, drug may be discontinued. After a period of 2 months off therapy, and if warranted by persistent severe cystic acne, a second course may be initiated. Patients whose disease is primarily manifested on the chest and back, as well as those who weigh more than 70 kg, may require doses at the higher end of the range.

NURSING IMPLICATIONS

HISTORY
See Appendix 4.

PHYSICAL ASSESSMENT
Obtain weight; inspect involved areas and describe appearance, number, and location of cysts. Baseline laboratory studies may include serum cholesterol, serum triglycerides, and lipoprotein-cholesterol fractionation. After consumption of alcohol, at least 36 hours should elapse before these determinations are made.

ADMINISTRATION
Advise patient not to chew capsules.

Storage and stability: Isotretinoin is photosensitive. Store in tight, light-resistant containers at 15°C to 30°C (59°F to 86°F).

ONGOING ASSESSMENTS AND NURSING MANAGEMENT
At time of each office or clinic visit, inspect involved areas and determine number and location of cysts; compare with data base.

Inquire of patient whether any new cysts have formed and record appearance and location.

When total cystic count is reduced by more than 70% during treatment period, physician may discontinue the drug.

Question patient about adverse drug reactions. Inspect lips for cheilitis (inflammation) and eyes for conjunctivitis, which are the two most common adverse reactions.

Periodic follow-up blood lipid studies are recommended.

PATIENT AND FAMILY INFORMATION
Do not take vitamin supplements containing vitamin A. Check with physician before using any vitamins.

Avoid use of alcohol, unless use is approved by the physician.

Avoid excessive exposure to sunlight; increased susceptibility to sunburn may occur.

Notify physician if any of the following occurs: extreme soreness or inflammation of the lips, infections or redness of the eyes, skin rash.

Women of childbearing potential: Effective contraceptive measures must be used and continued for 1 month after drug is discontinued or until a normal menstrual period has occurred.

If believed to be pregnant, stop the drug *immediately* and notify the physician.

Isoxsuprine Hydrochloride Rx

| tablets: 10 mg, 20 mg | Vasodilan, *Generic* |
| injection: 5 mg/ml | Vasodilan |

INDICATIONS
"Possibly effective" for relief of symptoms associated with cerebral vascular insufficiency; in peripheral vascular disease of arteriosclerosis obliterans, thromboangiitis obliterans (Buerger's disease), and Raynaud's disease.

CONTRAINDICATIONS
None known when used PO in recommended doses. Do not give immediately postpartum or in presence of arterial bleeding. IV administration should not be given because of increase likelihood of side effects.

ACTIONS
A vasodilator acting primarily on blood vessels within skeletal muscle. The drug also causes cardiac stimulation (increased contractility, heart rate, and cardiac output) and uterine relaxation. Isoxsuprine has been advocated for use in the treatment of dysmenorrhea and threatened premature labor, but efficacy in these conditions has not been established.

WARNINGS
Crosses placental barrier and may cause hypotension in newborn. Safety for use in pregnancy not established.

PRECAUTIONS
Parenteral administration not recommended in presence of hypotension or tachycardia.

ADVERSE REACTIONS
On rare occasions, oral administration has been associated with hypotension, tachycardia, nausea, vomiting, dizziness, abdominal distress, and severe rash. If rash appears, discontinue use. Incidence of nervousness and weakness tends to increase as dose increases. Administration of single doses of 10 mg IM may result in hypotension and tachycardia. These symptoms are more pronounced in higher doses.

DOSAGE

Oral: 10 mg to 20 mg tid or qid.

IM: 5 mg to 10 mg bid or tid. IM administration may be used initially in severe or acute conditions.

NURSING IMPLICATIONS

HISTORY

See Appendix 4.

PHYSICAL ASSESSMENT

Cerebral vascular insufficiency: Evaluate patient's mental status (memory, orientation, contact with reality); vital signs.

Peripheral vascular disease: Examine involved extremities for color, warmth, skin changes; palpate peripheral pulses; vital signs.

ADMINISTRATION

Obtain blood pressure, pulse prior to IM or oral administration. Withhold drug and notify physician if hypotension and/or tachycardia is noted.

ONGOING ASSESSMENTS AND NURSING MANAGEMENT

Vital signs daily; observe for adverse effects.

Withhold next dose and notify physician if adverse effects are noted because drug may be discontinued or dosage reduced.

If dizziness occurs, patients may require assistance with ambulation. This is especially important in elderly patients.

Cerebral vascular insufficiency: Observe patient and compare behavior to data base.

Peripheral vascular disease: Question patient about relief of symptoms; examine extremities and compare with data base.

PATIENT AND FAMILY INFORMATION

May cause flushing, palpitations, or skin rash. Notify physician if these symptoms become bothersome.

If dizziness occurs, avoid sudden changes in posture. Arise from sitting or lying positions slowly.

K

Kanamycin Sulfate

See Aminoglycosides, Oral; Aminoglycosides, Parenteral.

Ketamine Hydrochloride

See Anesthetics, General, Nonbarbiturate.

Ketoconazole Rx

tablets: 200 mg   Nizoral

INDICATIONS

Management of the following systemic fungal infections: candidiasis, mucocutaneous candidiasis, oral thrush, candiduria, blastomycosis, coccidioidomycosis, histoplasmosis, chromomycosis, paracoccidioidomycosis.

CONTRAINDICATIONS

Hypersensitivity. Not used for fungal meningitis because it penetrates poorly into cerebral spinal fluid.

ACTIONS

A synthetic broad-spectrum antifungal. Is active against infection with *Candida* species, *Coccidioides immitis, Histoplasma capsulatum, Paracoccidioides brasiliensis,* and *Phialophora* species. Development of resistance to ketoconazole has not been reported. Following absorption from the GI tract, drug is converted into several inactive metabolites. About 13% of dose is excreted in urine, but major route of excretion is through the bile into the intestinal tract.

WARNINGS

This drug has been associated with hepatic toxicity, including some fatalities. Hepatic injury has usually been reversible on discontinuation of treatment. Prompt recognition of hepatic injury is essential; hepatic-function tests recommended before treatment and monthly or more frequently during therapy.

Use in pregnancy only if potential benefit justifies the potential risk to the fetus. Mothers who are on treatment should not breast-feed.

DRUG INTERACTIONS

Antacids, anticholinergics, or **H$_2$-blockers** will increase GI *p*H and thus inhibit absorption of ketoconazole (which requires acidity for dissolution). Administer ketoconazole at least 2 hours before use of other agents that will affect gastric *p*H.

ADVERSE REACTIONS

Drug is usually well tolerated. Most reported adverse reactions have been mild and transient and rarely required withdrawal of therapy.

Most frequent: Nausea, vomiting; abdominal pain; pruritus.

Less frequent: Headache, dizziness, somnolence, fever and chills, photophobia, diarrhea, jaundice, gynecomastia.

Infrequent: Transient increases in serum liver enzymes observed in majority of cases (see *Warnings*).

OVERDOSAGE
In event of accidental overdosage, employ supportive measures, including gastric lavage with sodium bicarbonate.

DOSAGE
Adults: Recommended starting dosage is single daily administration of 200 mg. In very serious infections or if clinical responsiveness is insufficient within expected time, dosage may be increased to 400 mg once daily.

Children: Over 2 years, 3.3 mg/kg to 6.6 mg/kg; dosage for children under 2 years is not established.

Treatment is generally continued until all clinical and laboratory tests indicate that active fungal infection has subsided. Inadequate treatment may yield poor response and lead to early recurrence of clinical symptoms. Minimum duration of treatment of candidiasis is 1 or 2 weeks. Patients with chronic mucocutaneous candidiasis usually require maintenance therapy. Minimum treatment duration for other indicated systemic mycoses is 6 months.

NURSING IMPLICATIONS

HISTORY
See Appendix 4.

PHYSICAL ASSESSMENT
When applicable, examine and describe affected areas; obtain weight (children); review chart for laboratory identification of infecting organism (infecting organism must be identified, but treatment may be initiated before obtaining laboratory results). Baseline laboratory tests may include hepatic-function tests.

ADMINISTRATION
For those with achlorhydria, tablet should be dissolved in 4 ml of aqueous solution of 0.2 N HCl (physician must write order for use of HCl to dissolve tablet). For ingestion of resulting mixture, use a glass or plastic straw to avoid contact of liquid with the teeth. Administration is followed with a cup of tap water.

If antacids, anticholinergics, or H_2-blockers are prescribed, ketoconazide should be given at least 2 hours before these drugs are administered. Because dosage is once daily, drug can be given in early morning.

ONGOING ASSESSMENTS AND NURSING MANAGEMENT
Observe affected areas; record findings in patient's record.

If adverse effects are noted, contact physician before next dose is due.

CLINICAL ALERT: Observe for signs of liver dysfunction: unusual fatigue, fever, nausea, vomiting, jaundice, dark urine, pale stools. Notify physician immediately if one or more of these should occur.

Hepatic-function tests (SGOT, SGPT, SGGT, alkaline phosphatase. bilirubin) are recommended at monthly intervals.

PATIENT AND FAMILY INFORMATION
Take as prescribed for full course of therapy, even though infection may appear to be controlled. Failure to complete the prescribed course of therapy may result in poor control of infection and early recurrence of symptoms.

Do not take with antacids. If antacid therapy is required, take this drug early in the morning and at least 2 hours before first dose of antacid. (*Note:* This instruction also applies if patient is taking an anticholinergic agent or H_2-blocker).

Avoid use of nonprescription drugs unless use is approved by physician. Some nonprescription drugs may contain antacids or anticholinergic agents.

May produce headache, dizziness, and drowsiness; observe caution while driving or performing other tasks requiring alertness.

Notify physician or nurse if abdominal pain, fever, or diarrhea becomes pronounced or if any of the following occurs: unusual fatigue, nausea, vomiting, jaundice, dark urine, or pale stools.

L

Laxatives

Laxatives are agents that act to promote evacuation of the bowel. Because of lack of proper understanding of normal bowel function, nonprescription laxative products are frequently misused for a variety of nonspecific problems. Self-medication with laxatives should be restricted to short-term therapy of constipation. It should be emphasized that chronic use of laxatives (particularly stimulants) may lead to dependence. Before institution of laxative use, consideration should be given to living habits that affect bowel function. Rational therapy and prevention of constipation should include adequate fluid intake (6–8 full glasses of water daily), proper dietary habits including sufficient bulk or roughage, and daily exercise to promote normal bowel function.

Bulk-Producing Laxatives

Barley Malt Extract   otc

tablets: 750 mg	Maltsupex
powder	Maltsupex
liquid	Maltsupex

DOSAGE

Tablets (adults only): 4 tablets with meals and H.S.

Powder and liquid: Adults—2 tbsp bid for 3 or 4 days, then 1 to 2 tbsp H.S.; *children*—1 or 2 tbsp in milk or cereal once or twice a day; *infants (over 1 month)*—½ to 2 tbsp in day's total formula or 1 to 2 tsp in a single feeding.

Methylcellulose   otc

liquid: 450 mg/5 ml	Cologel

DOSAGE

5 ml to 20 ml tid with a glass of water.

Psyllium   otc

flakes	Mucilose
granules	Mucilose, Perdiem Plain
powder	Hydrocil Instant, Konsyl, Metamucil, Modane Bulk, Mucillium, Orange Flavor Metamucil, Regacilium, Reguloid, Saraka, Syllact, V-Lax
powder, effervescent	Effersyllium Instant Mix, Metamucil Instant Mix, Metamucil – Orange Flavor Instant Mix

DOSAGE

Flakes or granules—1 or 2 tsp in full glass of water bid. *Powder*—1 rounded tsp stirred into glass of liquid 1 to 3 times a day. *Effervescent powder*—1 packet in water 1 to 3 times a day.

Emollient Laxatives

Mineral Oil   otc

liquid	Nujol, *Generic*
jelly	Neo-Cultol
emulsion	Agoral Plain, Kondremul Plain, Zymenol
suspension	Petrogalar Plain

DOSAGE

Adults—5 ml to 30 ml H.S.; *children*—5 ml to 10 ml H.S.

Enemas

disposable enema: sodium phosphate, sodium biphosphate	Fleet
disposable enema: mineral oil	Fleet Mineral Oil
disposable enema: bisacodyl	Fleet Bisacodyl
disposable enema: docusate potassium, benzocaine	Therevac
enema: bisacodyl, aqueous hydroxypropyl methylcellulose	Fleet Bisacodyl Prep

DOSAGE

Disposable enemas are available in plastic squeeze bottles. Administer 1 unit. Pediatric size is available in Fleet and Fleet Mineral Oil.

Fleet Bisacodyl Prep: Add 1 packet to 1500 ml water.

Fecal Softeners

Docusate Calcium
(Dioctyl Calcium Sulfosuccinate)   otc

capsules: 50 mg	Surfak
capsules: 240 mg	Pro-Cal-Sof, Surfak, *Generic*

DOSAGE

Adults—240 mg/day until bowel movements are normal. *Children and adults with minimal needs*—50 mg/day to 150 mg/day.

Docusate Potassium

(Dioctyl Potassium Sulfosuccinate) otc

capsules: 100 mg	Dialose
capsules: 240 mg	Kasof

DOSAGE

100 mg/day to 300 mg/day until bowel movements are normal. It is helpful to increase the daily fluid intake by drinking a glass of water with each dose.

Docusate Sodium

(Dioctyl Sodium Sulfosuccinate, DSS) otc

capsules: 50 mg	Colace, *Generic*
capsules: 60 mg	Disonate, Doxinate
capsules: 100 mg	Afko-Lube, Bu-Lax 100, Colace, Coloctyl, Diosuccin, Dio-Sul, Disonate, D-S-S, Duosol, Laxinate 100, *Generic*
capsules: 120 mg	Modane Soft
capsules: 240 mg	Disonate, Doxinate
capsules: 250 mg	Afko-Lube, Bu-Lax 250, Dilax-250, Dioeze, Diosuccin, Duosol, *Generic*
capsules: 300 mg	Doss 300
tablets: 50 mg	Di-Sosul
tablets: 100 mg	Molatoc, Regutol, Stulex, *Generic*
drops: 10 mg/ml	Colace, Diocto, Disonate
syrup: 20 mg/5 ml	Afko-Lube Dioctyl, Colace, Disonate, Doss, *Generic*
syrup: 50 mg/15 ml	*Generic*
solution: 50 mg/ml	Doxinate

DOSAGE

Take with full glass of water. *Adults, older children*—50 mg to 240 mg. *Children 6–12 years*—40 mg to 120 mg; *children 3–6 years*—20 mg to 60 mg; *children under 3 years*—10 mg to 40 mg.

Higher doses are recommended for initial therapy; dosage is adjusted to individual response. Give liquid in milk, fruit juice, or infant formula to mask taste. In enemas, add 50 mg to 100 mg in water to a retention or flushing enema.

Poloxamer 188 otc

capsules: 240 mg	Alaxin

DOSAGE

Adults—480 mg H.S.; *children*—240 mg to 480 mg H.S.

Hyperosmolar Agents

Glycerin otc

suppositories	*Generic*
liquid: 4 ml/applicator	Fleet Babylax

DOSAGE

One suppository inserted high into rectum and retained for 15 minutes.

Rectal liquid: 1 applicator.

Irritant or Stimulant Laxatives

Bisacodyl otc

tablets, enteric coated: 5 mg	Cenalax, Deficol, Dulcolax, Fleet Bisacodyl, *Generic*
suppositories: 10 mg	Bisco-Lax, Cenalax, Deficol, Dulcolax, Fleet Bisacodyl, Theralax, *Generic*

DOSAGE

Tablets: Adults—10 mg to 15 mg; *children over 6 years*—5 mg to 10 mg.

Suppositories: Adults and children over 2 years—10 mg; *children under 2 years*—5 mg.

Cascara Sagrada otc

tablets: 325 mg	*Generic*
liquid (fluid extract)	*Generic*
liquid (aromatic fluid extract)	*Generic*

DOSAGE

325 mg to 650 mg in tablets; 1 ml of fluid extract; 5 ml of aromatic fluid extract.

Castor Oil otc

liquid	Kellogg's Castor Oil, *Generic*
emulsion	Alphamul, Emulsoil, Neoloid

DOSAGE

Liquid: Adults—15 ml to 30 ml; *children over 2 years*—5 ml to 15 ml; *children under 2 years*—1 ml to 5 ml.

Emulsion: Dose of emulsion depends on brand

used because percentage of castor oil may vary. *Alphamul*—15 ml to 45 ml for adults; 1.25 ml to 15 ml for children. *Emulsoil*—15 ml to 60 ml for adults; 5 ml to 10 ml for children. *Neoloid*—30 ml to 60 ml for adults; 2.5 ml to 30 ml for children.

Danthron *otc*

tablets: 37.5 mg	Modane Mild
tablets: 75 mg	Dorbane, Modane, *Generic*
liquid: 37.5 mg/5 ml	Modane

DOSAGE
37.5 mg to 150 mg with or 1 hour after evening meal.

Phenolphthalein *otc*

tablets, chewable: 30 mg	Prulet Liquitab
tablets, chewable: 60 mg	Prulet
tablets, chewable: 90 mg	Ex-Lax
tablets, chewable: 97.2 mg	Evac-U-Gen, Feen-a-Mint Gum
tablets: 60 mg	Alophen Pills
tablets: 90 mg	Ex-Lax Pills
tablets: 97.5 mg	Espotabs
wafers: 64.8 mg	Phenolax
wafers: 80 mg	Evac-U-Lax
liquid: 65 mg/15 ml	Correctol

DOSAGE
30 mg to 195 mg, preferably H.S.

Senna *otc*

tablets	Black-Draught, Senexon, Senokot, Senolax
granules	Black-Draught, Senokot
syrup	Senokot
liquid, powder	X-Prep
suppositories	Senokot

DOSAGE
Varies according to product used. Consult package labeling.

Saline Laxatives

Citrate of Magnesia *(Magnesium Citrate)* *otc*

solution	Citroma, Citro-Nesia, *Generic*

DOSAGE
Adults—1 glassful (approximately 240 ml); *children*—0.5 ml/kg/dose.

Magnesium Sulfate *(Epsom Salt)* *otc*

powder	*Generic*

DOSAGE
Adults—15 g in glass of water; *children*—0.25 g/kg/dose.

Magnesium Hydroxide *(Milk of Magnesia)* *otc*

liquid	*Generic*

DOSAGE
Adults—15 ml to 30 ml taken with liquid; *children*—0.5 ml/kg/dose.
   Concentrate: *Adults*—10 ml to 20 ml.

Sodium Phosphate *otc*

powder	*Generic*

DOSAGE
4 g to 8 g dissolved in water.

Sodium Phosphate and Sodium Biphosphate *otc*

solution	Phospho-Soda, *Generic*

DOSAGE
   Adults: 20 ml to 40 ml mixed with ½ glass cold water.
   Children: 5 ml to 15 ml.

CO$_2$-Releasing Suppositories

Sodium Bicarbonate and Potassium Bitartrate *otc*

suppositories (water-soluble polyethylene glycol base)	Ceo-Two

DOSAGE
One suppository. Moisten with warm water before inserting.

Laxative Combinations

Capsules and Tablets

50 mg docusate sodium, 187 mg senna	Gentlax S, Senokot S

100 mg docusate sodium, 30 mg casanthranol	Di-Sosul Forte, Molatoc-CST
100 mg docusate sodium, 37.5 mg danthron	Valax
100 mg docusate sodium, 50 mg danthron	Modane Plus
100 mg docusate sodium, 65 mg phenolphthalein	Correctol
150 mg docusate sodium, 75 mg danthron	Unilax

Capsules

50 mg docusate calcium, 50 mg danthron	Doxidan
50 mg docusate sodium, 25 mg danthron	Dorbantyl
50 mg docusate sodium, 163 mg senna	Senokap DSS
100 mg docusate potassium, 30 mg casanthranol	Dialose Plus
100 mg docusate sodium, 30 mg casanthranol	Afko-Lube Lax, Bu-Lax Plus, Diothron, Disanthrol, D-S-S plus, Peri-Colace, *Generic*
100 mg docusate sodium, 50 mg casanthranol	Diolax, *Generic*
100 mg docusate sodium, 50 mg danthron	Dorbantyl Forte

Emulsions

4.2 g mineral oil, 0.2 g phenolphthalein/15 ml	Agoral
3.3 mg docusate sodium, 4.75 ml mineral oil/5 ml	Milkinol
55% mineral oil, 147 mg phenolphthalein/15 ml	Kondremul w/Phenolphthalein
55% mineral oil, 660 mg cascara extract/15 ml	Kondremul w/Cascara
25% mineral oil, magnesium hydroxide	Haley's M-O

Syrup

60 mg docusate sodium, 30 mg casanthranol/15 ml	Peri-Colace, *Generic*

Powders, Granules

powder: 4 g malt soup extract, 3 g psyllium seed/tsp	Syllamalt
granules: psyllium, senna	Perdiem

DOSAGE

Tablets, capsules: 1 or 2 H.S. with full glass of water.

Emulsions, syrup: Usual adult dose is 7.5 ml to 30 ml H.S. with full glass of water.

Powder, granules: Usual adult dose is 1 or 2 tsp 1 to 3 times a day with full glass of water.

INDICATIONS

Short-term treatment of constipation. Certain stimulant and saline laxatives may be used to evacuate the colon in preparation for rectal or bowel examinations. Emollients or fecal softeners are useful prophylactically in patients who should not strain during defecation (*e.g.,* following anorectal surgery or myocardial infarction). The bulk-producing laxative psyllium is also used in the management of irritable bowel syndrome.

CONTRAINDICATIONS

Hypersensitivity to any ingredient, abdominal pain, vomiting or other signs or symptoms of appendicitis, acute surgical abdomen, fecal impaction, intestinal or biliary tract obstruction, acute hepatitis.

Castor oil is not used as a cathartic in treatment of infestation with fat-soluble vermifuge because it may increase toxicity by increasing absorption of the vermifuge.

ACTIONS

These agents act by a variety of mechanisms and are classified as follows.

Saline laxatives: Are hyperosmolar compounds that attract or retain water in the lumen of the intestine. Fluid accumulation alters stool consistency, distends the bowel, and induces peristaltic movement. These agents may significantly alter fluid and electrolyte balance with repeated use and should therefore be limited to short-term or occasional use.

Irritant or stimulant laxatives: Increase motor activity by direct action on the intestine and should be used only occasionally because prolonged use can lead to laxative dependence and loss of normal bowel function. Castor oil acts in the small intestine, whereas other stimulant laxatives act primarily on the colon. Castor oil may be preferred when more complete evacuation is required.

Bulk-producing laxatives: Are natural or synthetic polysaccharides and cellulose derivatives that increase the frequency of bowel movements and soften stools by holding water in the stool. Are considered the safest and most physiologic type of laxative. Dietary sources of bulk include bran and other cereals, fresh fruits, and fresh vegetables.

Emollient laxatives (mineral oil): Lubricate the intestinal mucosa and soften the stool, facilitating passage of fecal material.

Fecal softeners: Are anionic surfactants that promote water retention in the fecal mass, softening the stool. These agents are most beneficial when feces are hard and dry or in anorectal conditions in which passage of a firm stool is painful.

Hyperosmolar agents (glycerin): Cause dehydration of exposed tissues to produce irritation, which results in a laxative effect. Useful for lower bowel evacuation.

WARNINGS

Fluid and electrolyte balance: Excessive use of laxatives may lead to significant fluid and electrolyte imbalances. Do not use products containing phosphate, magnesium, or potassium salts in the presence of renal dysfunction. Preparations containing sodium salts should not be used by individuals on a sodium-restricted diet or in the presence of edema, congestive heart failure (CHF), megacolon, impaired renal function, or hypertension.

Dependency: Chronic use of stimulant laxatives may lead to laxative dependency.

Use in pregnancy, lactation: Castor oil and mineral oil should not be used during pregnancy. Danthron and cascara sagrada are excreted in breast milk.

Use in children: In general, stimulant cathartics such as danthron should seldom be used in children. Enemas should not be administered to children under 2 years.

PRECAUTIONS

Rectal bleeding or failure to respond to therapy may indicate a serious condition that may have to be treated surgically. If skin rash appears, do not use any preparation containing phenolphthalein. Prolonged use of danthron or cascara may cause discoloration of the rectal mucosa. Impaction or obstruction may occur if a bulk-forming agent is temporarily arrested in its passage through parts of the alimentary canal. In this case, water is absorbed and the bolus may become inspissated. Use of bulk-forming laxatives in those with narrowing of the intestinal lumen may be hazardous.

The following products are listed as containing tartrazine (see Appendix 6, section 6-23):

Tablets—Dulcolax, Modane, Modane Mild, Modane Plus, Phenolax
Capsules—Dorbantyl Forte, Modane Soft
Solutions—Phospho-Soda

DRUG INTERACTIONS

The absorption of **danthron** from the GI tract or its uptake by hepatic cells may be increased by the coadministration of **docusate.** Concomitant administration of **milk, antacids,** or **cimetidine** with **bisacodyl** tablets may cause the enteric coating to dissolve prematurely, resulting in gastric or duodenal stimulation. Concomitant administration of psyllium with **salicylates, nitrofurantoin,** and **digitalis** or **other cardiac glycosides** is not recommended. **Surfactant fecal softeners** may enhance absorption of **mineral oil;** this combination is not recommended. Absorption of **lipid-soluble vitamins** (A, D, E, and K) may decrease during prolonged concomitant administration with **mineral oil. Anionic surfactants** may increase GI absorption, hepatic uptake, and possibly the toxicity of concomitantly administered drugs.

ADVERSE REACTIONS

In order of frequency, excessive bowel activity (griping, diarrhea, nausea, vomiting), perianal irritation, weakness, dizziness, fainting, palpitations, and sweating. There has also been a suspected allergic reaction with facial swelling, redness, and discomfort.

Abdominal cramps may be noted, especially in severely constipated individuals.

Esophageal, gastric, small intestinal, and rectal obstruction due to accumulation of mucilaginous components of bulk laxatives have been reported. Frequently this is due to inadequate water intake or underlying organic disease.

Mineral oil may cause lipid pneumonitis if aspirated into the lungs. The elderly, debilitated, and dysphagic are at greatest risk. Mineral oil may also interfere with postoperative healing following anorectal surgery by causing pruritus ani.

DOSAGE

See individual product listings, above.

NURSING IMPLICATIONS

HISTORY

If laxative is given for chronic constipation, obtain history of recent bowel changes; health history; dietary history (including types of food usually eaten, amount of liquids consumed/day); allergy history; prescription and nonprescription drug history.

PHYSICAL ASSESSMENT
In some instances, a digital examination of the rectum (for fecal impaction) or auscultation of bowel sounds (presence or absence of peristalsis) may be indicated.

ADMINISTRATION
Bulk-producing laxatives or fecal softeners: Give with full glass of water or juice. Bulk-producing laxatives should be followed by an additional glass of liquid.

Barley malt extract may be mixed with liquid, added to milk, or sprinkled over cereal. When given to infants, it may be added to the total day's formula or given in a single feeding, as directed by physician.

Mineral oil: Preferably administered on an empty stomach H.S.

Bisacodyl tablets: Instruct patient to swallow whole and not to chew. Do not administer with milk or give within 1 hour of antacids or milk.

Granules, powders, or flakes: Add to liquid, stir, and have patient drink immediately.

Castor oil: Mix with ½ to 1 glass of liquid. Juice may be used to mask taste. Some products are flavored and patient may prefer drug mixed with water.

Suppositories: Lubricate with water-soluble lubricant and insert high into rectum.

Enemas: Remove cap covering tip; tip is usually prelubricated (check package instructions). Use additional water-soluble lubricant if needed, especially if patient has hemorrhoids. Place patient in a left lateral recumbent position, insert tip, and squeeze bottle gently (a small amount of fluid may remain in bottle after liquid is dispensed). Instruct patient to remain on side and retain fluid as long as possible.

General considerations: Patient should be informed if product has an unpleasant taste, even when mixed with a fluid such as juice. Chilling of some preparations or (when applicable) adding to cold water or juices or pouring over cracked ice may help to disguise taste.

Inform patient when laxative may be expected to produce results (see below). If a saline or irritant laxative is administered, warn patient that abdominal discomfort and diarrhea may occur.

ONGOING ASSESSMENTS AND NURSING MANAGEMENT
Expected onset of laxative action
Saline laxatives: ½ to 3 hours.

Irritant or stimulant laxatives: 6 to 10 hours. Given rectally, bisacodyl has an onset of 15 to 60 minutes.

Bulk-producing laxatives: 12 to 24 hours; may be delayed up to 72 hours.

Lubricant laxatives: 6 to 8 hours.

Fecal softeners: May require up to 72 hours before effects are seen.

Glycerin suppositories: 15 to 30 minutes.

Observe for therapeutic effects; record laxative results, describing type of stool (*e.g.,* loose, watery, solid, semisolid, soft) and time of evacuation.

Observe for adverse reactions, including excessive laxative effects (severe, prolonged diarrhea).

When laxative is administered daily or at frequent intervals, observe patient for fluid and electrolyte imbalance, especially dehydration, hypokalemia, and hyponatremia (Appendix 6, sections 6-10, 6-15, and 6-17).

Encourage liberal fluid intake when a laxative is administered (unless patient is in a fasting state).

When applicable, patient should be encouraged to ambulate frequently.

If constipation is chronic, physician may prescribe a diet containing additional bulk or roughage foods such as bran, vegetables, and fruits.

Bowel-training program: Follow procedure outlined by physician or hospital policy. *Bed patient*—Keep on side; place waterproof pad under buttocks. Check for evacuation q30m and record results.

PATIENT AND FAMILY INFORMATION
Do not use in presence of abdominal pain, nausea, or vomiting.

Prolonged, frequent, or excessive use may result in laxative dependence or electrolyte imbalance.

Notify physician or nurse if unrelieved constipation, rectal bleeding, or symptoms of electrolyte imbalance (*i.e.,* muscle cramps or pain, weakness, dizziness) occur.

Pink-red, red-violet, or red-brown discoloration of alkaline urine may occur with cascara sagrada, phenolphthalein, danthron, or senna.

Yellow-brown discoloration of acid urine may occur with cascara sagrada, phenolphthalein, or senna.

Bulk-producing or fecal-softening laxatives: Take with a full glass of water or juice. Drink several more glasses of water or juice in the next few hours.

Mineral oil: Best taken on an empty stomach at bedtime.

Bisacodyl tablets: Swallow whole; do not take within 1 hour of antacids or milk.

Prevention of future constipation: Increase fluid intake, exercise regularly, eat foods high in bulk or roughage (*e.g.,* whole grain cereals and bread, fresh or cooked fruits and vegetables; stewed fruit or fruit juices may also be helpful).

Elderly patient: Avoid foods with high bran content (may cause impaction).

Leucovorin Calcium

(Folinic Acid, Citrovorum Factor) Rx

tablets: 5 mg, 25 mg   Wellcovorin
injection: 3 mg/ml   *Generic*
injection: 5 mg/ml   Wellcovorin
powder for injection: *Generic*
   50 mg/vial

INDICATIONS

To diminish toxicity and counteract effect of overdosage of folic acid antagonists. Parenteral form also used in treatment of megaloblastic anemias due to sprue, nutritional deficiency, pregnancy, and infancy, when oral therapy is not feasible.

CONTRAINDICATIONS

Pernicious anemia or other megaloblastic anemias in which vitamin B_{12} is deficient.

ACTIONS

Is the formyl derivative and active reduced form of folic acid. Useful clinically in circumventing the action of folate reductase.

"Folinic acid rescue" is used to prevent or decrease the toxicity of massive doses of methotrexate used in some resistant neoplasms. Large doses of methotrexate can cause severe life-threatening toxicity. Maximum tolerated doses of methotrexate have ranged from 80 mg/m^2 to 900 mg/m^2 when given alone and from 900 mg/m^2 to 18,000 mg/m^2 when folinic acid rescue is employed. Folinic acid prevents severe toxicity by preferentially "rescuing" normal cells without reversing the oncolytic effect of methotrexate. See Methotrexate *Overdosage,* p 688, for general guidelines for use of leucovorin.

WARNINGS

Drug is improper therapy for pernicious anemia and other megaloblastic anemias secondary to lack of vitamin B_{12}. A hematologic remission may occur while neurologic manifestations remain progressive. In treatment of overdosage of folic acid antagonists, administer leucovorin within 1 hour, if possible; drug is usually ineffective after a delay of 4 hours.

Safety for use during pregnancy and lactation has not been established.

ADVERSE REACTIONS

Allergic sensitization has been reported.

DOSAGE

Megaloblastic anemia: Up to 1 mg daily. There is no evidence that IM doses greater than 1 mg/day have greater efficacy than those of 1 mg.

Overdosage of folic acid antagonists: A conventional dosage schedule is 10 mg/m^2 PO or parenterally, followed by 10 mg/m^2 PO q6h for 72 hours. If, at 24 hours following methotrexate administration, the serum creatinine is 50% or greater than the premethotrexate serum creatinine, dose of leucovorin is increased to 100 mg/m^2 q3h until the serum methotrexate level is below 5×10^{-8} M. The dose of leucovorin to counteract hematologic toxicity from folic acid antagonists with less affinity for mammalian dihydrofolate reductase than methotrexate (*i.e.,* trimethoprim, pyrimethamine) is less; 5 mg/day to 15 mg/day has been recommended.

NURSING IMPLICATIONS

HISTORY

See Appendix 4. Note etiology, concomitant treatment modalities.

PHYSICAL ASSESSMENT

Obtain vital signs; weight. Base additional assessments on etiology of anemia (*e.g.,* pregnancy, nutritional deficiency, sprue) or reason for use of drug (*e.g.,* methotrexate therapy). Baseline laboratory studies for overdosage of folic acid antagonists include serum creatinine levels.

ADMINISTRATION

Drug is available as 3 mg/ml in 1-ml ampules and 50 mg per vial for reconstitution.

Reconstitute powder in 50-mg vial with 5 ml Bacteriostatic Water for Injection, USP, which contains benzyl alcohol. This yields 10 mg/ml. Use within 7 days. If powder is reconstituted with Water for Injection, USP it must be used immediately. Any remaining drug is discarded.

Drug is administered IM for megaloblastic anemia. Administration for folinic acid rescue may be IM, IV infusion, or PO.

ONGOING ASSESSMENTS AND NURSING MANAGEMENT

Megaloblastic anemia: Diet high in folic acid (folacin) usually prescribed and includes protein (liver, meat, fish, nuts, whole grains, legumes) and green leafy vegetables. Notify physician if diet is taken poorly.

In those with severe anemia, observe for bleeding episodes, congestive heart failure, signs of infection (malaise, fever, chills).

Duration of therapy will depend on etiology and severity of anemia and response to therapy.

Folinic acid rescue following methotrexate therapy: Following administration of an (intentional) overdose of methotrexate, leucovorin is administered. The time interval between administration of methotrextae and leucovorin is established by the physician, but it is usually administered within 1 hour.

Routes of administration may vary according to the protocol established by the physician and may include IV infusion and/or IM or oral administration.

The physician must write specific orders regarding the dosage, route of administration, and time of each dose.

Administration of leucovorin is usually accompanied by fluid loading and urine alkalinization to reduce the nephrotoxicity of methotrexate.

CLINICAL ALERT: Drug must be administered at prescribed intervals to avoid possible fatal methotrexate toxicity. If patient is receiving leucovorin orally and is unable to retain the drug, contact the physician immediately because parenteral administration will be necessary.

PATIENT AND FAMILY INFORMATION

Megaloblastic anemia: Adhere to the diet prescribed by the physician. If unable to purchase recommended foods (some protein foods can be expensive), discuss with physician.

Laboratory tests and examination by physician will be necessary to monitor therapy.

Folinic acid rescue therapy: Occasionally, high-dose methotrexate therapy is administered in select individuals on an outpatient basis. Patient will be instructed to take leucovorin (PO) at home (_i.e.,_ told times drug is taken and what to do if nausea and/or vomiting occurs). Physician may prescribe an antiemetic to be taken as needed.

Levallorphan Tartrate

See Narcotic Antagonists.

Levodopa _Rx_

| capsules: 100 mg, 250 mg | Dopar (contains tartrazine), Larodopa |

| capsules: 500 mg | Dopar (contains tartrazine), Larodopa, _Generic_ |
| tablets: 100 mg, 250 mg, 500 mg | Larodopa |

INDICATIONS

Treatment of idiopathic Parkinson's disease (paralysis agitans), postencephalitic parkinsonism, and symptomatic parkinsonism that may follow injury to the nervous system by carbon monoxide intoxication and manganese intoxication. Indicated in those elderly patients believed to develop parkinsonism in association with cerebral arteriosclerosis. Also available in combination with carbidopa (p 240).

CONTRAINDICATIONS

Known hypersensitivity; narrow-angle glaucoma; patients on monoamine oxidase inhibitor (MAOI) therapy. Because levodopa may activate a malignant melanoma, it is not used in those with undiagnosed skin lesions or history of melanoma.

ACTIONS

Symptoms of Parkinson's disease are related to depletion of striatal dopamine. Dopamine does not cross the blood–brain barrier. Levodopa, the metabolic precursor of dopamine, does cross the blood–brain barrier and is converted into dopamine in the basal ganglia. It is well absorbed from the GI tract; peak plasma levels occur in 1 to 2 hours and may be delayed in the presence of food. Drug is extensively metabolized in the GI tract and by the liver and excreted primarily in the urine. The major urinary metabolites of levodopa appear to be dihydroxyphenylacetic acid (DOPAC) and homovanillic acid (HVA).

WARNINGS

Administer cautiously to those with severe cardiovascular or pulmonary disease, bronchial asthma, or renal, hepatic, or endocrine disease. Also administer with caution to those with a history of myocardial infarction who have residual atrial, nodal, or ventricular arrhythmias. In such patients, cardiac function is monitored during the period of dosage adjustment.

There is the possibility of upper GI hemorrhage in those with a history of peptic ulcer. All patients should be observed for development of depression with suicidal tendencies. Treat psychotic patients with caution.

Use in pregnancy, lactation: Safety is not established. Use only when clearly needed and potential benefits outweigh unknown potential hazards to the fetus. Do not use in nursing mothers.

Use in children: Safety for use in children under 12 not established.

DRUG INTERACTIONS

In some, concomitant administration of levodopa and **anticholinergic drugs** results in a mild degree of synergy and increased efficacy. Levodopa is often used concomitantly with anticholinergic drugs. If it is decided to withdraw or reduce dosage of these drugs, it is done gradually. Gradual reduction in anticholinergic dosage is necessary both during initiation of levodopa therapy and after optimum dosage is attained.

Postural hypotensive episodes have been reported as adverse reactions. Levodopa is given cautiously to those on antihypertensive drugs; dosage adjustment of antihypertensive drug may be necessary. Dosage requirements of **guanethidine** or of a **diuretic** may be reduced in hypertensive patients receiving concomitant levodopa therapy. **Methyldopa** has a mild inhibitory effect on dopa decarboxylase, and as it enters the brain it may potentiate the effects of levodopa. It is possible that the efficacy of levodopa may be reduced by concurrent administration of **benzodiazepines.**

Control of diabetes with **hypoglycemic agents** may be adversely affected by treatment with levodopa; blood glucose should be monitored frequently and the treatment regimen adjusted if necessary.

Concomitant administration of levodopa and an **MAOI** may cause considerable increase in blood pressure. MAOIs should be withdrawn at least 14 days before the institution of levodopa therapy.

The efficacy of levodopa may be reduced by concurrent administration of low dosages of **phenothiazines, butyrophenones,** or **thioxanthenes.** Beneficial effects of levodopa in Parkinson's disease have been reported to be reversed by **phenytoin** and **papaverine.**

Pyrodoxine HCl (vitamin B$_6$) in oral doses of 10 mg or 25 mg rapidly reverses the toxic and therapeutic effects of levodopa.

Levodopa may potentiate effects of the indirect-acting **sympathomimetic drugs** such as **ephedrine** and the **amphetamines** and the direct-acting sympathomimetic drugs such as **epinephrine** and **isoproterenol.** If levodopa is given concurrently with these drugs, the heart and circulation may be adversely affected; a reduction in sympathomimetic amine dosage may be necessary. Combine use of a **tricyclic antidepressant** and levodopa with caution.

Lab test interferences: Coombs' test has occasionally become positive during extended levodopa therapy. Elevations of serum uric acid have been noted with the colorimetric method. False-positive test results for urine glucose using the copper reduction method and false-negative results using the glucose oxidase method may occur. May also interfere with tests for urine ketones.

PRECAUTIONS

Patients with chronic wide-angle glaucoma are treated cautiously with levodopa, provided intraocular pressure is well controlled and patient is monitored carefully for changes in intraocular pressure.

Some products contain tartrazine. See Appendix 6, section 6-23.

ADVERSE REACTIONS

Most serious: Frequent—Adventitious movements, such as choreiform and dystonic movements. *Less frequent*—Cardiac irregularities or palpitations; orthostatic hypotensive episodes, bradykinetic episodes (the "on–off" phenomena); mental changes including paranoid ideation and psychotic episodes, depression with or without development of suicidal tendencies, dementia; urinary retention. *Rare*—GI bleeding, development of duodenal ulcer, hypertension, phlebitis, hemolytic anemia, agranulocytosis, convulsions.

Less serious: Frequent—Anorexia, nausea and vomiting with or without abdominal pain and distress, dry mouth, dysphagia, sialorrhea, ataxia, increased hand tremor, headache, dizziness, numbness, weakness and faintness, bruxism, confusion, insomia, nightmares, hallucinations and delusions, agitation and anxiety, malaise, fatigue, euphoria. *Less frequent*—Muscle twitching and blepharospasm (which may be taken as an early sign of overdosage), trismus, burning sensation of tongue, bitter taste, diarrhea, constipation, flatulence, flushing, skin rash, increased sweating, bizarre breathing patterns, urinary incontinence, diplopia, blurred vision, dilated pupils, hot flashes, weight gain or loss, dark sweat or urine. *Rare*—Oculogyric crisis, sense of stimulation, hiccups, development of edema, loss of hair, hoarseness, priapism, activation of Horner's syndrome.

Elevations of BUN, SGOT, SGPT, LDH, bilirubin, alkaline phosphatase, and protein-bound iodine have been reported; the significance is unclear. Occasional reduction in WBC, hemoglobin, and hematocrit has been noted.

OVERDOSAGE

For acute overdosage, general supportive measures should be employed, along with immediate gastric lavage. IV fluids should be administered judiciously and adequate airway maintained. ECG monitoring should be instituted and patient observed for possible development of arrhythmias. If required, appropriate antiarrhythmic therapy should be given. Consideration should be given to possibility of multiple drug ingestion.

DOSAGE

The optimal daily dose is carefully titrated for each patient. Usual initial dosage is 0.5 g to 1 g daily, divided into two or more doses with food. Total daily dosage is then increased gradually in increments of not more than 0.75 g/day every 3 to 7 days, as tolerated. The usual optimal therapeutic dosage should not exceed 8 g/day. The exceptional patient may be carefully given more than 8 g as required.

In the event of general anesthesia, levodopa therapy may be continued as long as the patient is able to take oral fluids and medication. If therapy is temporarily interrupted, usual daily dosage may be given as soon as the patient is able to take oral medication. Whenever therapy is interrupted for long periods, dosage should be adjusted gradually. In many cases the patient can be rapidly titrated to previous therapeutic dosage.

NURSING IMPLICATIONS

HISTORY

See Appendix 4. Note current treatment for parkinsonism (if any).

PHYSICAL ASSESSMENT

Look for neurologic alterations (_e.g.,_ tremor with head, hands at rest; masklike facial expression; muscular rigidity with resistance to passive movement; shuffling gait; monotone speech; postural deformities; drooling). Evaluate mental status, thought process, ability to participate in activities of daily living (ADL). If patient is presently receiving an antiparkinsonism agent, symptoms may be diminished.

ADMINISTRATION

Administer with food or meals.

Patient may require assistance in removing medicine from dispensing container and holding water glass.

If patient has difficulty swallowing tablet or capsule, encourage patient to take several sips of water before swallowing drug. If difficulty persists, discuss with physician or contact hospital pharmacist about the advisability of crushing tablet or opening capsule.

ONGOING ASSESSMENTS AND NURSING MANAGEMENT

Record vital signs q4h to q8h; observe for adverse drug effects, perform neurologic assessment, monitor intake and output daily during initial therapy.

Dosage adjustments, when necessary, are based on patient response and may be made every 3 to 7 days. Daily assessment of neurologic deficits identified during initial physical assessment aids physician in titrating dosage to patient's individual need.

In some patients, a significant response may not be obtained until after 6 months of treatment.

If cardiac irregularities or palpitations are noted, notify physician immediately.

Muscle twitching and blepharospasm may be signs of overdosage. If these are noted, withhold next dose of drug and notify physician. Dosage reduction may be necessary.

Check for urinary retention during initial therapy, especially in those with history of urinary tract obstruction (_e.g.,_ enlarged prostate).

Orthostatic hypotension may occur. Advise self-care patient to make position changes slowly. When assisting with ambulatory activities, allow patient to dangle legs 5 to 10 minutes before getting out of bed.

Adverse effects labeled as "less serious" (_e.g.,_ ataxia, anorexia, dizziness, confusion, insomnia) can present a problem for the elderly patient and may require reevaluation of nursing management if they occur.

CLINICAL ALERT: Observe closely for behavioral changes (paranoid ideation, psychotic episodes, depression with or without suicidal tendencies, dementia) and report occurrence to physician immediately. Patient must be observed at frequent intervals (q½h–q1h) when behavioral changes occur and an effort made to prevent patient from harming himself or others.

Adventitious movements, such as choreiform and dystonic movements (_e.g.,_ facial grimacing, protruding tongue, exaggerated chewing motion and head movement, jerking movements of arms and legs) may occur. Withhold next dose and notify physician because dosage may need to be reduced.

Weigh weekly or as ordered. Report weight loss to physician.

Adjust ADL to meet individual needs and capabilities. Patient may require longer time to eat, bathe, dress, and so on.

Develop short- and long-term goals for rehabilitation. Use occupational and physical therapists (with physician approval) in planning and implementing measures to prevent contractures, improve movement and self-care abilities, and promote independence.

Dry mouth may be relieved by offering frequent sips of water throughout day. Sialorrhea (excessive salivation) may also occur. Provide patient with ample supply of tissues.

Periodic tests of hepatic, hematopoietic, cardiovascular, and renal function are recommended during extended therapy.

Diabetic patient: May require adjustment of dosage of hypoglycemic agent. Observe patient for signs of hypoglycemia and hyperglycemia (Appendix 6, section 6-14). Monitor urine glucose and ketones closely and report all changes to physician. False positives and negatives may occur when testing for glucose and ketones (see *Drug Interactions, Lab Test Interferences*). Frequent blood glucose determinations are recommended.

PATIENT AND FAMILY INFORMATION

NOTE: In some instances it may be necessary to have a responsible family member administer medication until dosage is stabilized.

May cause GI upset; take with food or meals.

Do not take any vitamin preparation unless a specific brand is recommended or prescribed by the physician. Preparations containing vitamin B_6 may reverse the therapeutic effects of levodopa.

Observe caution while driving or performing other tasks requiring alertness.

If fainting, lightheadedness, or dizziness occurs, avoid sudden changes in posture; rise from sitting or lying positions slowly. Notify physician of this effect.

Medication may cause darkening of urine (on standing) or sweat. This is not harmful.

Notify physician or nurse if any of the following should occur: uncontrollable movements of face, eyelids, mouth, tongue, neck, arms, hands, or legs; mood or mental changes; irregular heartbeats or palpitations; difficult urination; severe or persistent nausea and vomiting.

Diabetic patient: Drug may interfere with urine tests for glucose or ketones. Report any abnormal tests to physician before adjusting dosage of antidiabetic medication.

Levorotatory Alkaloids of Belladonna

See Gastrointestinal Anticholinergics/Antispasmodics.

Levorphanol Tartrate

See Narcotic Analgesics.

Levothyroxine Sodium

See Thyroid Hormones.

Lidocaine Hydrochloride Rx

For IM Administration

injection: 300 mg/3 ml (automatic injection device)	LidoPen Auto-Injector
injection: 10% (100 mg/ml)	Xylocaine HCl IM for Cardiac Arrythmias

For Direct IV Administration

injection: 1% (10 mg/ml)	Generic
injection: 2% (20 mg/ml)	Xylocaine HCl IV for Cardiac Arrhythmias, *Generic*

For IV Admixtures

injection: 4% (40 mg/ml)	Xylocaine HCl IV for Cardiac Arrhythmias, *Generic*
injection: 10% (100 mg/ml)	Generic
injection: 20% (200 mg/ml)	Xylocaine HCl IV for Cardiac Arrhythmias, *Generic*

For IV Infusion

injection: 0.2% (2 mg/ml), 0.4% (4 mg/ml) 0.8% (8 mg/ml) in 5% Dextrose	Generic

INDICATIONS

IV: Used in management of acute ventricular arrhythmias occurring during cardiac manipulation, such as cardiac surgery; life-threatening arrhythmias, particularly those that are ventricular in origin, such as occur during acute myocardial infarction (MI).

IM: Single dose IM justified in the following exceptional circumstances: When ECG equipment not available to verify diagnosis but in physician's opinion the potential benefits outweigh the potential risks; when facilities for IV administration are not readily available; by paramedical personnel in a mobile coronary care unit under direction of a physician viewing the transmitted ECG.

See also Anesthetics, Local, Injectable; and Anesthetics, Local, Topical.

CONTRAINDICATIONS

Known hypersensitivity to local anesthetics of the amide type; Adams-Stokes syndrome; Wolff-Parkinson-White syndrome; severe degree of sinoatrial (SA), atrioventricular (AV), or intraventricular block.

ACTIONS

Exerts an antiarrhythmic effect by increasing electrical stimulation threshold of the ventricle during diastole. Not effective in atrial arrhythmias. In usual therapeutic doses, produces no change in myocardial contractility, systemic arterial blood pressure, or absolute refractory period.

Is ineffective orally. Is most commonly administered IV with an immediate onset (30–90 seconds) and brief duration (10–20 minutes) of action following a bolus dose. Continuous IV infusion (1–4 mg/min) is necessary to maintain antiarrhythmic effects. Following IM administration, therapeutic serum levels are achieved in 5 to 15 minutes and may persist for up to 2 hours. Higher and more rapid serum levels are achieved by injection into the deltoid muscle.

Lidocaine exhibits a biphasic half-life. The distribution phase (t½ is 7–8 minutes) accounts for short duration of action following IV bolus injection. The terminal elimination half-life is 1 to 2 hours. Therapeutic serum levels are 1.5 mcg/ml to 5 mcg/ml. Serum levels above 7 mcg/ml are usually toxic.

Extensive biotransformation in the liver (90%) results in two active metabolites. Hepatic insufficiency or reduction of hepatic blood flow may result in increased serum levels and may necessitate dosage adjustments. Only about 10% of the parent drug is excreted unchanged by the kidneys.

WARNINGS

Constant ECG monitoring is essential for proper administration. It is mandatory to have emergency resuscitative equipment and drugs immediately available to manage possible adverse reactions involving the cardiovascular, respiratory, or central nervous systems. Used with caution and in lower doses in those with congestive heart failure (CHF), those with reduced cardiac output, and the elderly.

Occasional acceleration of ventricular rate may occur when administered to those with atrial fibrillation.

IV use: Signs of excessive depression of cardiac conductivity, such as prolongation of P–R interval and QRS complex and appearance of arrhythmias, should be followed by prompt cessation of IV infusion.

IM use: Frequent aspirations are necessary to avoid possible inadvertent intravascular administration. In emergency situations when a ventricular rhythm disorder is suspected and ECG equipment is not available, a single dose is administered after determination of benefits and risks. IM use may result in an increase in CPK levels; use of this enzyme determination, without isoenzyme separation, as a diagnostic test for the presence of acute MI may be compromised by use of IM lidocaine.

Usage in impaired renal or hepatic function: Lidocaine is metabolized mainly in the liver and excreted by the kidney. Caution is used with repeated or prolonged use in those with severe liver or renal disease due to possible accumulation of lidocaine or its metabolites, which may lead to toxicity.

Electrolyte imbalance: Clinical evaluation and periodic laboratory determinations are necessary to monitor changes in fluid, electrolytes, and acid–base balance during prolonged therapy or whenever patient's condition warrants. Administration of IV solutions can cause fluid and/or solute overloading resulting in dilution of serum electrolytes, overhydration, congested states, or pulmonary edema. Excess administration of potassium-free solutions may result in significant hypokalemia.

Use in pregnancy: Safety not established. Use only when clearly needed and potential benefits outweigh the unknown potential hazards to the fetus.

Use in children: Not recommended for pediatric use.

PRECAUTIONS

Use with caution in hypovolemia and shock and all forms of heart block.

Cardiac effects: In those with sinus bradycardia or incomplete heart block, administration for elimination of ventricular ectopic beats without prior acceleration in heart rate (*e.g.,* by isoproterenol or electric pacing) may promote more frequent and serious ventricular arrhythmias or complete heart block.

Dextrose-containing solutions: Use with caution in those with known subclinical or overt diabetes mellitus. Do not give dextrose solutions without electrolytes simultaneously with blood through the same infusion set because of possibility that pseudoagglutination of red cells may occur. Additive medications should not be delivered via these solutions.

DRUG INTERACTIONS

During continuous lidocaine infusion, coadministration of **propranolol** impairs the clearance of lidocaine. Concomitant IV administration of **phenytoin** and lidocaine may produce excessive cardiac depression. Additive neurologic effects may be produced during concurrent administration of **procainamide** and lidocaine.

ADVERSE REACTIONS

CNS: Lightheadedness; drowsiness; dizziness; apprehension; euphoria; tinnitus; blurred or double vision; vomiting; sensations of heat, cold or numbness; twitching; tremors; convulsions; unconsciousness; respiratory depression and arrest.

Cardiovascular: Hypotension; cardiovascular collapse; bradycardia, which may lead to cardiac arrest.

Hypersensitivity: Are infrequent and characterized by cutaneous lesions, urticaria, edema, or anaphylactoid reactions and are managed by conventional means.

Other: Soreness at IM injection site reported. Other reactions occurring because of the solutions or technique of administration include febrile response, infection at site of injection, venous thrombosis or phlebitis extending from the site of injection, extravasation, hypovolemia.

MANAGEMENT OF TOXICITY

In case of severe reaction, discontinue drug. Institute emergency resuscitative procedures and administer emergency drugs necessary to manage the severe reaction. For severe convulsions, small increments of diazepam or an ultra-short-acting barbiturate (thiopental, thiamylal); if these not available, a short-acting barbiturate (pentobarbital, secobarbital); or if patient is under anesthesia, a short-acting muscle relaxant (succinylcholine) may be given IV. Should circulatory depression occur, vasopressors (*e.g.,* ephedrine, metaraminol) may be used.

DOSAGE

IM: Recommended dose in averge 150-lb man is 300 mg (approximately 4.3 mg/kg or 2 mg/lb). The deltoid muscle is preferred injection site. The LidoPen Auto-Injector unit for patient self administration is administered into the thigh. As soon as possible patient changed to an IV infusion of lidocaine or an oral antiarrhythmic preparation for maintenance therapy. If necessary, an additional IM injection may be made after an interval of 60 to 90 minutes.

IV bolus: Used to establish rapid therapeutic blood levels. Continuous IV infusion necessary to maintain steady state blood levels. Usual dose is 50 mg to 100 mg (1 mg/kg) given at rate of 20 mg to 50 mg/minute. Single IV bolus injections produce a brief therapeutic effect (10–20 minutes). If the initial injection does not produce the desired response, a second bolus (⅓–½ the initial dose) may be given after 5 minutes. No more than 200 mg to 300 mg of lidocaine should be administered during a 1-hour period. Loading dose reduced in those with CHF or reduced cardiac output from any cause and in those over 60.

IV continuous infusion: Used to maintain therapeutic plasma levels; is given following loading doses to those in whom arrhythmias tend to recur and who are incapable of receiving oral antiarrhythmic drugs. Continuous infusion may be administered at rate of 1 mg to 4 mg/minute (20–50 mcg/kg/minute). Maintenance doses should be reduced in those with heart failure or liver disease and in those over age 60. Infusion is terminated as soon as basic cardiac rhythm stabilizes or at earliest sign of toxicity. Patient is changed to oral antiarrhythmic agent for maintenance therapy as soon as possible.

NURSING IMPLICATIONS

PHYSICAL ASSESSMENT

Treatment of life-threatening arrhythmia is begun as soon as arrhythmia is identified. Obtain blood pressure and respiratory rate when possible. Weight, if obtained on admission, may be used to calculate dose.

ADMINISTRATION

Patient must be on a cardiac monitor to evaluate results of therapy.

Lidocaine is available for IM and IV use. Check label carefully; label identifies route of administration.

Lidocaine labeled for IM use must *not* be used IV.

Lidocaine without preservatives is used for IV administration. The 1% and 2% strengths are used for direct IV (bolus) injection. The 4% and 20% strengths are used for IV admixture. Drug is also available (premixed) in 500 ml of 5% Dextrose.

Patients with CHF, those with reduced cardiac output from any cause, or those over 60 years of age are given reduced dosages.

IM administration: The 10% injection (100 mg/ml) is available in 5-ml ampules.

Preferred site of injection is deltoid muscle because therapeutic blood levels occur faster and peak blood level is significantly higher as compared with injection into gluteus muscle or lateral thigh.

Injection is made with frequent aspiration to avoid possible inadvertent intravascular injection. If blood return is noted in syringe upon aspiration, withdraw, change needle, and inject into new site.

IV bolus: Usual dose is 50 mg to 100 mg.

Use 1% or 2% injection labeled for IV use. The 1% injection is 10 mg/ml and available in 5-ml (50 mg) and 10-ml (100 mg) disposable syringes. The 2% injection is 20 mg/ml and available in 5-ml (100 mg) disposable syringe and 5-ml ampules.

Inject drug by venipuncture or into injection port of IV line. Close IV line while drug is injected; open IV line as soon as all of drug is injected.

IV continuous infusion: Add 1 g or 2 g of lidocaine to 1000 ml of 5% Dextrose in Water.

Adding 1 g results in a 1% solution which is 1 mg of lidocaine/ml.

Adding 2 g results in a 2% solution which is 2 mg of lidocaine/ml.

Usual dose is 1 mg to 4 mg (1–4 ml) of lidocaine/minute.

If fluid restriction is necessary, a more concentrated solution may be prepared or the 0.2% (2 mg/ml) or 0.4% (4 mg/ml) premixed lidocaine in 5% Dextrose may be used.

Use a primary and secondary IV line or piggyback the lidocaine into a primary line.

Lidocaine is chemically stable for a minimum of 24 hours after dilution in 5% Dextrose in Water but it is advisable to dilute immediately prior to administration.

ONGOING ASSESSMENTS AND NURSING MANAGEMENT
Physician must prescribe dose administered and rate of infusion (expressed as mg or ml/minute). In some instances the hospital or unit may have a written policy regarding emergency administration of lidocaine until physician examines patient. Physician or hospital policy must also state specific guidelines for management of toxicity (see _Clinical Alert_).

Therapeutic effects: Seen in 30 to 90 seconds following IV bolus injection and 5 to 15 minutes following IM administration.

Duration of action: 10 to 20 minutes following IV bolus injection and up to 2 hours following IM administration.

Observe patient closely and monitor ECG continuously.

CLINICAL ALERT: Signs of excessive depression of cardiac conductivity, such as prolongation of the P–R interval and QRS complex and the appearance or aggravation of arrhythmias should be followed by prompt cessation of the IV infusion. Open primary line (_i.e.,_ the IV fluid without lidocaine) and run to KVO until physician examines patient.

Observe for convulsions. Keep an oropharyngeal airway at the bedside and insert (when possible) if convulsions occur; discontinue lidocaine infusion and run primary line; maintain a patent airway and ventilate as needed; notify physician immediately.

Observe for respiratory depression and respiratory arrest. Discontinue lidocaine infusion and run primary line; maintain a patent airway and ventilate as needed; notify physician immediately.

Observe for circulatory depression (decrease in blood pressure). If hypotension is pronounced, discontinue lidocaine infusion and run primary line; notify physician immediately.

Even though dosage is reduced, patients with CHF, patients with liver impairment, and patients over 60 should be carefully observed for toxicity.

It is important to follow the specific guidelines established by the physician and/or hospital (or unit) policy for nursing management of toxicity.

Clinical evaluation and periodic laboratory determinations may be necessary to monitor changes in fluid and electrolyte concentration and acid–base balance. Venipuncture should be performed on the arm opposite the infusion.

Therapeutic serum lidocaine levels are 1.5 mcg/ml to 5 mcg/ml.

Administration of IV solutions may result in fluid overload (Appendix 6, section 6-12), resulting in dilution of serum electrolytes, overhydration, congested states, or pulmonary edema. Auscultate lungs if fluid overload is suspected and notify physician immediately.

Patient is changed to oral antiarrhythmic therapy as soon as possible. It is rarely necessary to continue IV maintenance infusions beyond 24 hours.

PATIENT AND FAMILY INFORMATION
NOTE: Lidocaine 300 mg in 3-ml automatic injection device may be prescribed for self-administration by select patients. The drug is administered into the thigh (unless physician prescribes otherwise). There is a patient instruction sheet provided with the product. The physician must give a detailed explanation of when the drug should be used. The patient or a family member will require instruction and practice in administration of the drug under the guidance of the physician, or the nurse with physician approval.

Lincomycin Rx

capsules: 250 mg (pediatric), 500 mg	Lincocin
injection: 300 mg/ml	Lincocin

INDICATIONS
Treatment of serious infections due to susceptible strains of streptococci, pneumococci, and staphylococci. Use is reserved for penicillin-allergic patients or those for whom penicillin is inappropriate. Because of the risk of colitis, the nature of the infection and suitability of a less toxic alternative (_e.g.,_ erythromycin) are considered. Lincomycin is effec-

tive in the treatment of some staphylococcal infections resistant to other antibiotics. May be administered concomitantly with other antimicrobial agents, when indicated.

CONTRAINDICATIONS

Hypersensitivity to lincomycin or clindamycin. Not indicated for treatment of minor bacterial or viral infections.

ACTIONS

Derived from *Streptomyces lincolnensis.* Lincomycin binds exclusively to the 50S subunit of bacterial ribosomes and suppresses protein synthesis. Is bactericidal or bacteriostatic against most of the common gram-positive pathogens. Studies indicate spectrum of activity includes *Staphylococcus aureus, S. albus,* β-*hemolytic* streptococci, *S. viridans, S. pneumoniae, Clostridium tetani, C. perfringens, Corynebacterium diphtheriae,* and *C. acnes.*

Depending on the sensitivity of the organism and concentration of the antibiotic, lincomycin may be either bactericidal or bacteriostatic. Cross-resistance has not been demonstrated with penicillin, chloramphenicol, ampicillin, cephalosporins, or tetracyclines. Despite chemical differences, lincomycin exhibits antibacterial activity similar, but not identical, to that of the macrolide antibiotics (*e.g.,* erythromycin). Some cross-resistance with erythromycin and the phenomenon of dissociated cross-resistance have been reported. Microorganisms do not appear to develop resistance to lincomycin rapidly.

Lincomycin is absorbed rapidly after oral, IM, and IV administration; biological half-life is approximately 5.4 hours. Bile appears to be an important route of excretion. Significant levels have been demonstrated in the majority of body tissues. Oral administration produces peak levels in 2 to 4 hours. Levels above minimum inhibitory concentration (MIC) for most gram-positive organisms are maintained with 500 mg for 6 to 8 hours. IM administration of a single 600-mg dose produces peak serum level at 30 minutes with detectable levels persisting for 24 hours. IV infusion of 600 mg in 500 ml of 5% Dextrose in Water over a 2-hour period yields therapeutic levels for 14 hours. Hemodialysis and peritoneal dialysis do not effectively remove lincomycin.

WARNINGS

Studies indicate a toxin caused by *Clostridium* species is one primary cause of antibiotic-associated colitis. Mild cases of colitis and diarrhea may respond to drug discontinuation. Moderate to severe cases are managed promptly with fluid, electrolyte, and protein supplements as indicated. Systemic corticoids and corticoid retention enemas may help to relieve colitis. Other causes of colitis, such as previous sensitivities to drugs or other allergens, are also considered.

Use in pregnancy, lactation: Safety not established. Drug appears in breast milk in ranges of 0.5 mcg/ml to 2.4 mcg/ml.

Use in infancy: Not indicated for use in the newborn.

PRECAUTIONS

Older patients with associated severe illness may not tolerate diarrhea and are monitored carefully for change in bowel frequency. Is prescribed with caution in those with history of GI disease, particularly colitis, and in those with asthma or significant allergies.

Superinfection: Use of antibiotics (especially prolonged or repeated therapy) may result in bacterial or fungal overgrowth of nonsusceptible organisms. Such overgrowth may lead to secondary infection, and appropriate measures are taken if such superinfection occurs. When those with preexisting monilial infections require lincomycin therapy, concomitant antimonilial treatment is given.

During prolonged therapy, periodic hepatic-function studies and blood counts are recommended. Administration to those with impaired hepatic function is not recommended unless indicated by special clinical circumstances.

DRUG INTERACTIONS

Lincomycin has been shown to have neuromuscular blocking properties that may enhance the action of other **neuromuscular blocking agents.** Simultaneous administration of **kaolin** with lincomycin reduces GI absorption by as much as 90%. Concomitant administration with **chloramphenicol** or **erythromycin** may produce cross-interference because these drugs have a greater affinity for the 50S ribosomal unit of the bacterial cell. Administration of **antiperistaltic antidiarrheals** is not recommended because they may delay removal of toxins from the colon, prolonging or aggravating diarrhea.

ADVERSE REACTIONS

GI: Glossitis, stomatitis, nausea, vomiting, persistent diarrhea, enterocolitis, and pruritus ani.

Hematopoietic: Neutropenia, leukopenia, agranulocytosis, and thrombocytopenic purpura have been reported. There have been rare reports of aplastic anemia and pancytopenia.

Hypersensitivity: Angioneurotic edema, serum sickness, and anaphylaxis have been reported, some of these in known penicillin-sensitive patients. Drug is discontinued if an allergic reaction occurs. The usual agents (epinephrine, corticosteroids, antihistamines) should be available for emergency treatment. Rare instances of erythema multiforme, some resembling Stevens-Johnson syndrome, have been associated with lincomycin.

Skin, mucous membranes: Skin rashes, urticaria, vaginitis, and rarely exfoliative and vesiculobulbous dermatitis.

Hepatic: Rarely, jaundice and abnormal hepatic-function tests (particularly elevations of serum transaminases).

Cardiovascular: Hypotension has been reported, particularly after too-rapid IV administration. Rarely, cardiopulmonary arrest.

Special senses: Occasionally, tinnitus and vertigo.

Local reactions: IM administration is well tolerated. Reports of pain following injection are infrequent. IV administration in 250 ml to 500 ml 5% Dextrose in Water or normal saline produced no local irritation or phlebitis.

DOSAGE

Impaired renal function: When required, an appropriate dose is 25% to 30% of that recommended for those with normal renal function.

Oral

Adults: Serious infections—500 mg q8h. *More severe infections*—500 mg or more q6h. With β-hemolytic streptococcal infections, treatment is continued for at least 10 days to diminish likelihood of subsequent rheumatic fever or glomerulonephritis.

Children over 1 month: Serious infections—30 mg/kg/day (15 mg/lb) divided into three or four equal doses. *More severe infections*—60 mg/kg/day (30 mg/lb) divided into three or four equal doses.

Intramuscular

Adults: Serious infections—600 mg q24h. *More severe infections*—600 mg q12h or more often.

Children over 1 month: Serious infections—One injection of 10 mg/kg (5 mg/lb) q24h. *More severe infections*—One injection of 10 mg/kg (5 mg/lb) q12h or more often.

Intravenous

Dilute 1 g in a minimum of 100 ml and infuse over not less than 1 hour.

Adults: Dosage is determined by severity of infection. *Serious infections*—600 mg to 1 g q8h to q12h. *More severe infections*—Dose may be increased. *Life-threatening situations*—Doses as high as 8 g/day have been given.

Children over 1 month: 10 mg/kg/day to 20 mg/kg/day (5–10 mg/lb) depending on severity of infection. May be infused in divided doses as described above for adults.

Subconjunctival injection: 75 mg/0.25 ml in-

jected subconjunctivally results in ocular fluid levels of antibiotic (lasting for 5 hours).

NURSING IMPLICATIONS

HISTORY

See Appendix 4. Note drug allergies, asthma, significant other allergies. Inform physician if history reveals asthma or allergies to any drug or substance.

PHYSICAL ASSESSMENT

Base on symptoms, location of infection. Obtain vital signs, weight. Physician orders culture and sensitivity studies. Additional laboratory or diagnostic studies may include renal- and hepatic-function studies, CBC, platelet count, x-ray examinations.

ADMINISTRATION

Administer oral preparation at least 1 hour before or 2 hours after meals. Encourage patient to drink a full glass of water.

If administered orally to infants or small children, check with pharmacist about opening of capsule and vehicle (fluid, food) for administration of capsule contents.

If any patient is unable to swallow oral form (capsule), notify physician; parenteral administration may be necessary.

IV administration: Dilute dose in a minimum of 100 ml of solution. Physician must specify infusion solution to be used. Infuse over not less than 1 hour. A volume-control set or infusion pump is used to administer the drug.

CLINICAL ALERT: Severe cardiopulmonary reactions have occurred when drug is given at a concentration and rate greater than recommended. Monitor infusion rate q10m to q15m, even when a volume-control set or infusion pump is used. If a cardiopulmonary reaction (hypotension, tachycardia, altered respiratory pattern, difficulty in breathing, dyspnea, cardiopulmonary arrest) occurs, discontinue infusion immediately, open primary line, and notify physician immediately. If cardiopulmonary arrest occurs, begin resuscitative measures.

IM administration: Administer into large muscle mass, preferably the gluteus muscle. Rotate injection sites; record site used. Pain at injection site is infrequent, but advise patient that some soreness may be noted.

Physical compatibilities

Lincomycin is compatible in the following for 24 hours at room temperature unless otherwise indicated.

Infusion solutions: 5% and 10% Dextrose in

Water or Saline; Ringer's Solution; Sodium Lactate ⅙ Molar; Dextran in 6% saline.

Vitamins in infusion solutions: B-Complex; B-Complex with Ascorbic Acid.

Antibiotics in infusion solutions: Penicillin G sodium (satisfactory for 4 hours); cephalothin; tetracycline HCl; colistimethate; ampicillin; methicillin; chloramphenicol; polymyxin B sulfate.

Incompatibilities

Is incompatible with novobiocin, kanamycin, phenytoin sodium, and protein hydrolysates.

ONGOING ASSESSMENTS AND NURSING MANAGEMENT

Obtain temperature q4h; blood pressure, pulse, and respirations q2h to q4h or as ordered; observe for adverse reactions.

CLINICAL ALERT: Drug can cause severe and possibly fatal colitis, characterized by severe, persistent diarrhea and severe abdominal cramps, which may be associated with passage of blood and mucus. At first sign of diarrhea, notify physician immediately. Drug may be discontinued or drug continued and patient observed closely for continued diarrhea and severe abdominal cramps. If therapy is continued, do not hesitate to contact physician again if diarrhea persists or worsens.

Diarrhea, colitis, and pseudomembraneous colitis can begin up to several weeks following cessation of therapy; diarrhea must always be reported to the physician, even after lincomycin therapy has been terminated.

Physician may perform endoscopic examination for persistent diarrhea and passage of blood and mucus in the stool. Pseudomembraneous colitis has been reported.

Observe for signs of superinfection (Appendix 6, section 6-22); report occurrence to physician.

Periodic hepatic-function studies and CBC are recommended during prolonged therapy. A repeat culture and sensitivity study may also be ordered.

Observe for signs that may indicate infection is not controlled with therapy (*e.g.,* rise in temperature, increase in wound drainage when applicable, change in patient's general condition), and discuss observations with physician.

PATIENT AND FAMILY INFORMATION

Take on empty stomach at least 1 hour before or 2 hours after meals.

May cause diarrhea; notify physician immediately if this occurs. Do not use antidiarrheal medications to control diarrhea.

Do not take next dose, and notify physician immediately, if rash or other skin manifestations; swelling of face, tongue, or lips; vaginal or rectal itching; fever; black furry tongue; or ulcerations or soreness of the mouth occurs.

If problem is not improved or becomes worse, notify physician.

Lindane (Gamma Benzene Hexachloride) Rx

cream: 1%	Kwell
lotion: 1%	Kwell, Scabene, *Generic*
shampoo: 1%	Kwell, Scabene, *Generic*

INDICATIONS

Treatment of pediculosis capitis (head lice) and phthirus pubis (crab lice) and their ova. Cream and lotion forms also indicated for *Sarcoptes scabiei* (scabies).

CONTRAINDICATIONS

Hypersensitivity.

ACTIONS

An ectoparasiticide and ovicide.

WARNINGS

Use with caution in infants, children, and pregnant women. Lindane penetrates human skin and has potential for CNS toxicity. Seizures have been reported after use, but cause-and-effect relationship not established.

PRECAUTIONS

If irritation or sensitization occurs, discontinue use.

ADVERSE REACTIONS

Eczematous eruptions due to irritation from drug have been reported. Adverse systemic effects may occur with topical use (see *Warnings*).

OVERDOSAGE

If accidental ingestion occurs, prompt gastric lavage will rid body of large amounts of the toxicant. Because oils favor absorption, saline cathartics for intestinal evacuation should be given rather than oil laxatives. If CNS manifestations occur, they can be antagonized by administration of pentobarbital or phenobarbital.

DOSAGE

See *Administration.* In cases of pediculosis pubis, sexual contacts are treated concurrently.

NURSING IMPLICATIONS

HISTORY

Source of infestation should be determined, if possible. Investigate possibility of school, family members, sexual contact, and so on because concurrent treatment of others may be necessary. School may notify parents if pediculosis capitis is found in one or more pupils.

PHYSICAL ASSESSMENT

Examine affected area; note extent of infestation. Physician may employ skin scrapings to confirm scabies (see Crotamiton). Physician may examine patient for venereal disease, when applicable.

ADMINISTRATION

Apply early in the morning.

Clothing of patient should be removed prior to treatment and placed in a sealed plastic bag. If family member takes clothing, see *Patient and Family Information,* below.

A complete tub bath may be necessary prior to application of drug.

Gloves should be worn during application of drug.

Cream and lotion

Scabies: Apply thin layer to dry skin; rub in thoroughly. If crusted lesions are present, a warm bath preceding the medication is helpful; allow skin to dry and cool before application. Usually 1 oz is sufficient for an adult. Make total body application from the neck down. Scabies rarely affects the head of children or adults but may occur in infants. Leave on 8 to 12 hours; remove by thorough washing. One application is usually curative. Many patients exhibit persistent pruritus after treatment; this is not an indication for retreatment, unless living mites can be demonstrated.

Pediculosis pubis: Apply sufficient quantity only to cover hair and skin of pubic areas thinly and, if infested, the thighs, trunk, and axillary regions. Rub into skin and hair; leave in place 8 to 12 hours, then wash thoroughly. Retreatment usually unnecessary. Demonstrable living lice after 7 days is indication for retreatment.

Pediculosis capitis: Apply sufficient quantity to cover only the affected and adjacent hairy areas. Rub into scalp and hair; leave in place 8 to 12 hours followed by thorough washing. Retreatment usually unnecessary. Demonstrable living lice after 7 days indicates retreatment is necessary.

Shampoo

Pediculosis pubis and capitis: Apply sufficient quantity to wet hair and skin of infested and adjacent hairy areas thoroughly. Wet hair and skin thoroughly, add small quantities of water, and work shampoo into hair and skin until a good lather forms. Continue shampooing for 4 minutes. Rinse hair thoroughly and towel briskly.

Comb with a fine-toothed comb or use tweezers to remove any remaining nit shells. Retreatment usually not necessary. Demonstrable living lice after 7 days indicates retreatment is necessary. Do not use as a routine shampoo.

ONGOING ASSESSMENTS AND NURSING MANAGEMENT

Hospitalized patient should be isolated from others (when possible) to prevent transmission. Wash hands thoroughly after patient contact. Bed linens, hospital gown are placed in isolation linen bag and laundered separately.

Inspect skin for irritation once or twice during 8 to 12 hours drug remains on skin. If irritation noted, contact physician as drug may have to be removed.

Drug can be absorbed through the skin. Observe for CNS toxicity (seizures), especially when applied to young children. Notify physician immediately if a seizure occurs.

Drug must be left on skin/hair for prescribed number of hours to be effective.

Drug is removed by thorough washing.

Bedding, hospital gown should be changed before application of drug and when drug is removed.

PATIENT AND FAMILY INFORMATION

NOTE: Patient and/or family member may be embarrassed and refrain from asking questions. The nurse should have an understanding manner and make an effort to present information so that the patient or family member feels as comfortable as possible.

Do not apply to face. Avoid getting in eyes; if there is contact flush well with water.

Notify physician if condition worsens. If itching, burning, or skin rash occurs, remove drug (by washing area thoroughly) and contact physician.

Do not exceed prescribed dosage.

Clothing, bed linens should be washed in very hot water (boiling water is best), separately from clothes of other family members. Special attention should be given to clothing seams, which should be pressed with a hot iron.

Other family members or close contacts should be examined by a physician.

Patient instructions are supplied with the product. Follow these instructions carefully.

Liothyronine Sodium

See Thyroid Hormones.

Liotrix

See Thyroid Hormones.

Lithium Rx

capsules: 300 mg (as carbonate)	Eskalith, Lithonate, *Generic*
tablets: 300 mg (as carbonate)	Eskalith, Lithane, Lithotabs, *Generic*
tablets, slow release: 300 mg (as carbonate)	Lithobid
tablets, controlled release: 450 mg (as carbonate)	Eskalith CR
syrup: 8 mEq/5 ml (as citrate equivalent to 300 mg lithium carbonate)	Cibalith-S, *Generic*

INDICATIONS

Treatment of manic episodes of manic-depressive illness. Maintenance therapy prevents or diminishes the intensity of subsequent manic episodes in manic-depressive patients with history of mania.

Investigational uses: To improve the neutrophil count in those with chemotherapy-induced neutropenia and in children with chronic neutropenia. Lithium carbonate 300 mg/day to 1000 mg/day (effective serum levels appear to be between 0.5 and 1 mEq/liter) induces neutrophilic leukocytosis 7 to 10 days after initiation of therapy. Baseline values return 7 to 10 days after discontinuation. Also has been used in prophylaxis of cluster headache in doses of 600 mg/day to 900 mg/day.

ACTIONS

Lithium alters sodium transport in nerve and muscle cells and effects a shift toward intraneuronal metabolism of catecholamines. The specific mechanism of action in mania is unknown.

Is completely absorbed after oral administration. Peak serum levels usually occur at 1 to 4 hours. Therapeutic serum concentrations are usually in the range of 0.6 mEq/liter to 1.4 mEq/liter; toxicity may occur at these levels. Serum concentrations above 2 mEq/liter are associated with a significant increase in adverse reactions. Greater than 95% of the ion is excreted by the kidney; a negligible amount is recovered from feces and sweat. Renal excretion is proportionate to its plasma concentration. Renal clearance is 20% to 30% of creatinine clearance (15–30 ml/min under normal conditions).

The average plasma half-life is about 24 hours and prolonged in the elderly and renal impaired persons. Half-life may be as long as 36 hours in the elderly. Steady-state plasma concentrations are achieved in about 5 days.

WARNINGS

Lithium offers advantages in management of bipolar affective disorders because of its specificity, few adverse effects at stable therapeutic serum levels, prophylactic value, low sedation, high patient acceptability, and the availability of an objective blood level measurement for monitoring therapy. Use is associated with numerous side-effects; physician uses clinical judgement as to whether the patient's abnormal mood swings are significant enough to warrant continued long-term treatment. Suicidal or impulsive patients are poor candidates for therapy because of danger of overdosage.

Usually not given to those with significant renal or cardiovascular disease, severe debilitation, dehydration, or sodium depletion or to those receiving diuretics, because risk of toxicity is high. If psychiatric indication is life threatening and if patient fails to respond to other measures, treatment may be undertaken with extreme caution. Daily lithium determinations are recommended and hospitalization necessary.

Renal effects: Morphologic changes with glomerular and interstitial fibrosis have been reported in patients on chronic lithium therapy. Morphologic changes have also been seen in manic-depressive patients never exposed to lithium. The relationship between such changes and lithium has not been established.

Chronic lithium therapy may be associated with diminution of renal concentrating ability, occasionally presenting as nephrogenic diabetes insipidus, with polyuria and polydipsia. Such patients should be carefully managed to avoid dehydration with resultant lithium retention and toxicity. This condition is usually reversible. Progressive or sudden changes in renal function, even within the normal range, require reevaluation of treatment.

Use in pregnancy, lactation: Lithium crosses the placenta. An increased incidence of cardiovascular abnormalities has been reported in infants born of mothers who took lithium during pregnancy. Not used in pregnancy, especially during the first trimester, unless potential benefits outweigh possible hazards. Is found in breast milk. Nursing should not be undertaken during therapy except in rare and unusual circumstances when potential benefits to the mother outweigh possible hazards to the child.

Use in children: Safety and efficacy for children under 12 not established.

PRECAUTIONS

The ability to tolerate lithium is greater during the manic phase and decreases when manic symptoms subside. Concomitant infection with elevated temperature may necessitate a temporary reduction or cessation of medication.

Sodium depletion: Lithium decreases sodium reabsorption by the renal tubules, which could lead to sodium depletion. It is essential for the patient to maintain a normal diet (including salt) and adequate fluid intake (2500–3000 ml), at least during initial stabilization period. Low sodium intake causes a relative increase in lithium retention, and may predispose the patient to toxicity. Decreased tolerance to lithium has been reported to ensue from protracted sweating or diarrhea; if this occurs, supplemental fluid and salt are administered.

DRUG INTERACTIONS

Sodium bicarbonate, acetazolamide, urea, mannitol, and **aminophylline** all substantially increase renal clearance of lithium. Lithium excretion decreases with sodium depletion and increases when large doses of **sodium chloride** are given.

Long-term therapy with **thiazide diuretics, furosemide,** or **ethacrynic acid** has been shown to decrease renal clearance of lithium. Reduced urine output, paradoxical fluid retention, and a rise in serum lithium levels to toxic concentrations may occur during concomitant therapy. Dosage modification may be necessary. Undertake concomitant use of **amiloride, spironolactone,** and **triamterene** with great caution.

Indomethacin has been reported to increase steady-state plasma lithium levels. There is also evidence that other nonsteroidal anti-inflammatory agents may have a similar effect. When such combinations are used, increased plasma lithium level monitoring is recommended.

Isolated reports of drugs that appear to increase CNS toxicity of lithium include **mazindol, phenytoin, methyldopa, thioridazine, tetracycline,** and **carbamazepine.** An encephalopathic syndrome (characterized by weakness; lethargy; fever; tremulousness; confusion; extrapyramidal symptoms; leukocytosis; elevated serum enzymes, BUN, FBS) followed by irreversible brain damage has occurred rarely in those treated with lithium and **haloperidol.** A causal relationship has not been established. Patients receiving such combined therapy should be monitored closely for early evidence of neurologic toxicity and treatment discontinued promptly if such signs appear. The possibility of similar adverse interactions with other antipsychotic agents exists.

There is some evidence that lithium may produce a lowering of **chlorpromazine** levels in the blood and brain. Lithium may prolong the effects of **neuromuscular blocking agents;** these latter agents are given with caution to patients receiving lithium. Concomitant lithium carbonate and **potassium iodide** administration may act synergistically to produce hypothyroidism.

ADVERSE REACTIONS

Are seldom encountered at serum lithium levels below 1.5 mEq/liter. Mild to moderate toxic reactions may occur at levels from 1.5 mEq/liter to 2 mEq/liter; moderate to severe reactions may be seen from 2 mEq/liter to 2.5 mEq/liter. Serum levels of 2 mEq/liter are not exceeded during acute treatment phase. Lithium levels greater than 3 mEq/liter should be considered life threatening. There is considerable individual variability in response to the drug.

Fine hand tremor, polyuria, and mild thirst may occur during initial therapy for the acute manic phase and may persist throughout treatment. Transient and mild nausea and general discomfort may also appear during the first few days of administration. These usually subside with continued treatment or temporary dosage reduction.

Signs of lithium toxicity and the specific serum level at which they occur include the following.

Less than 1.5 mEq/liter: Nausea, vomiting, diarrhea, thirst, polyuria, lethargy, slurred speech, muscle weakness, fine hand tremor.

1.5 mEq/liter to 2 mEq/liter: Persistent GI upset, coarse hand tremor, mental confusion, muscle hyperirritability, ECG changes, drowsiness, incoordination.

2 mEq/liter to 2.5 mEq/liter: Ataxia, giddiness, large output of dilute urine, serious ECG changes, fasciculations, tinnitus, blurred vision, clonic movements, seizures, stupor, severe hypotension, coma. Fatalities are usually secondary to pulmonary complications.

Greater than 2.5 mEq/liter: A complex clinical picture may be produced, involving multiple organ systems.

The following toxic reactions have been reported and appear to be related to serum lithium levels, including levels in the therapeutic range.

Neuromuscular: Tremor, muscle hyperirritability (fasciculations, twitching, clonic movements of whole limbs), ataxia, choreoathetotic movements, hyperactive deep tendon reflexes, extrapyramidal symptoms.

CNS: Blackout spells, epileptiform seizures, slurred speech, dizziness, vertigo, incontinence of urine or feces, somnolence, psychomotor retardation, restlessness, confusion, stupor, coma, tongue movements, tics, tinnitus, hallucinations, poor memory, slowed intellectual functioning, startled response, fatigue, lethargy, tendency to sleep.

Cardiovascular: Cardiac arrhythmia, hypotension, peripheral circulatory collapse, bradycardia.

GI: Anorexia, nausea, vomiting, diarrhea, gastritis, salivary gland swelling, abdominal pain, excessive salivation, flatulence, indigestion.

GU: Proteinuria, oliguria, polyuria, glucosuria, decreased creatinine clearance.

Dermatologic: Drying and thinning of hair, anesthesia of skin, chronic folliculitis, dry skin, alopecia, exacerbation of psoriasis leading to generalized pustular psoriasis, itching, angioedema, exfoliative dermatitis.

Autonomic nervous system: Blurred vision, dry mouth.

Thyroid abnormalities: Euthyroid goiter or hypothyroidism (including myxedema) accompanied by decreasing serum T_3 and T_4 levels; elevation in ^{131}I uptake may occur. Underlying thyroid disorders are not a contraindication to lithium treatment. Careful monitoring of thyroid function during lithium stabilization and maintenance allows for correction of changing thyroid parameters and can be treated by thyroid agents. Rare cases of hyperthyroidism have been reported.

EEG changes: Diffuse slowing, widening of frequency spectrum, potentiation and disorganization of background rhythm.

ECG changes: Reversible flattening, isoelectricity, or inversion of T-waves.

Miscellaneous: Transient scotomata, dehydration, weight loss.

Reactions unrelated to dosage include transient EEG and ECG changes, hyperkalemia associated with ECG changes, syncope, tachy-bradycardia syndrome, megaloblastic anemia, leukocytosis, acute monocytic leukemia, headache, diffuse nontoxic goiter with or without hypothyroidism, hypercalcemia-associated hyperparathyroidism, transient hyperglycemia, generalized pruritus with or without rash, cutaneous ulcers, proteinuria, worsening of organic brain syndrome, excessive weight gain, edema of ankles or wrists, thirst or polyuria sometimes resembling those of diabetes insipidus, irreversible nephrogenic diabetes insipidus that improved with diuretic therapy, metallic taste, dysgeusia/taste distortion, salty taste, swollen lips, tightness in chest, impotence/sexual dysfunction, swollen and/or painful joints, fever, polyarthralgia, hypertoxicity, dental caries, reversible impairment of short-term memory.

OVERDOSAGE

Symptoms: Toxic levels are close to therapeutic levels.

Treatment: No specific antidote known. Early symptoms of toxicity can usually be treated with dosage reduction or cessation of therapy and resumption at a lower dose after 24 to 48 hours. In severe cases, the first goal is to eliminate drug from the patient. Treatment is essentially same as for barbiturate toxicity: gastric lavage; correction of fluid and electrolyte imbalance; regulation of kidney function. Urea, mannitol, and aminophylline all produce significant increases in lithium excretion. Infection prophylaxis, regular chest x-ray examination, and preservation of adequate respiration are essential. Hemodialysis is effective in lowering serum levels in severely toxic patients. Serum levels may continue to rise for several days in spite of treatment.

DOSAGE

Dosage is individualized according to serum levels and clinical response.

Acute mania: Optimal response is usually established and maintained with 600 mg tid or 900 mg bid for slow-release form. Such doses normally produce an effective serum level between 1 mEq/liter and 1.5 mEq/liter.

Long-term control: Desirable serum levels are 0.6 mEq/liter to 1.4 mEq/liter. Dosage will vary from one individual to another, but usually 300 mg tid or qid will maintain this level.

Slow-release form: Patients maintained on conventional dosage forms may be converted to slow-release form at the same total daily dosage is divided into twice daily.

NURSING IMPLICATIONS

HISTORY
See Appendix 4. Note mental health care history, previous drug therapies for psychiatric illness (if any).

MENTAL AND PHYSICAL ASSESSMENT
Obtain vital signs, weight. Observe overt symptoms: (1) general appearance and behavior, (2) response to immediate environment, (3) emotional status, (4) intellectual responses to verbal questions, and (5) thought content. Look for or inquire about typical symptoms of mania (*e.g.,* pressure of speech, motor hyperactivity, reduced need for sleep, flight of ideas, grandiosity, poor judgment, aggressiveness, and possibly hostility). Renal-function tests, pregnancy test (when applicable), CBC, urinalysis, and thyroid-function tests are usually ordered, along with a physical examination to detect cardiovascular, renal, or organic brain disease.

ADMINISTRATION

Check oral cavity after administration, especially if patient is elderly or resistant (physically or mentally) to treatment.

If patient has difficulty swallowing tablet or capsule, discuss with physician. A syrup form is available.

If nausea or vomiting occurs, discuss with physician about giving drug with meals.

ONGOING ASSESSMENTS AND NURSING MANAGEMENT

Obtain vital signs daily (monitor blood pressure, pulse, and respirations more frequently during initial therapy); observe behavior, compare to data base, and record observations; observe for adverse and toxic effects (review *Adverse Reactions,* signs of lithium toxicity). Report any marked changes in behavior to physician immediately.

Physician orders periodic lithium serum levels. During the acute phase, twice-weekly determinations are recommended until serum level and clinical condition of patient are stabilized. Blood samples are drawn immediately before next dose (8–12 hours after previous dose), when lithium concentrations are relatively stable.

Effective serum levels usually range between 1 mEq/liter and 1.5 mEq/liter. (See also *Adverse Reactions*).

CLINICAL ALERT: The toxic levels for lithium are close to the therapeutic levels. During initial therapy, observe patient closely for signs of lithium toxicity, even when serum levels appear to be in the normal range. Withhold next dose and notify physician immediately if lithium toxicity is suspected.

Elderly patients require close observation. They often respond to reduced dosage and may exhibit signs of toxicity at serum levels tolerated by other patients.

Encourage patient to maintain adequate fluid intake of 10 to 12 glasses of water a day. In some instances, fluid intake will have to be supervised.

An adequate salt intake is recommended. Check patient's food intake; inform physician if anorexia is noted. A low sodium intake causes a relative increase in lithium retention and may predispose the patient to toxicity. In some instances, a dietary consultation may be necessary to ensure adequate sodium intake.

Weigh weekly or as ordered. Report significant weight gain or loss to physician.

Observe for an increased urine output and persistent thirst (may indicate nephrogenic diabetes insipidus). If these symptoms are noted, inform physician and measure intake and output.

Dosage is individualized and based on serum levels and clinical response. Daily observation and recording of behavior assist physician in adjusting dosage.

Report temperature elevation to physician because infection with elevated temperature may necessitate temporary dosage reduction or cessation of medication.

Drowsiness may occur, especially early in therapy. Patient may require assistance with ambulation, activities of daily living.

Decreased tolerance to lithium may result from protracted sweating or diarrhea. If these occur, discuss with physician as well as increase patient's fluid and salt intake.

Lithium may induce thyroid enlargement or contribute to hypothyroidism. Observe for symptoms of hypothyroidism: fatigue, lethargy, weight gain, puffiness of face and eyes, intolerance to cold. Inform physician if these should occur.

Serum lithium levels are recommended every 2 months in uncomplicated cases receiving maintenance therapy during remission.

PATIENT AND FAMILY INFORMATION

NOTE: Some patients may fail to comply with their therapeutic regimen. Whenever possible, one or more family members should receive full instruction and information about treatment modalities and should be encouraged to discuss noncompliance with the physician. If the patient neglects to take drug or shows rapid deterioration in his mental or physical status, the physician should be contacted or the patient taken to a designated psychiatric center.

Take exactly as directed. Do not increase or decrease the dose or the interval between doses unless told to do so by physician.

Do not take next dose and notify physician immediately if any of the following occurs: diarrhea, vomiting, tremor, drowsiness, lack of coordination, or muscular weakness.

May cause drowsiness; observe caution while driving or performing other tasks requiring alertness.

Maintain adequate fluid and salt intake. Drink 10 to 12 large glasses of water a day. Eat a normal diet. Do not participate in weight loss programs (of any kind) or self-impose a restricted diet unless approved by physician.

Do not use nonprescription drugs unless use is approved by physician because some may contain excess sodium (large doses of sodium chloride may increase lithium excretion).

Inform other physicians and dentist of therapy with this drug.

L

Periodic laboratory tests will be required to monitor therapy. (*Note:* Some physicians only prescribe a sufficient number of tablets/capsules for the interval between laboratory tests. A new prescription is then written when the patient keeps the laboratory appointment.)

Female patient (when applicable): Physician may recommend contraceptive measures while taking this drug. If pregnancy is suspected, contact physician immediately.

Lomustine (CCNU) Rx

capsules: 10 mg, 40 mg, 100 mg	CeeNu
capsules, dose pack: two 100 mg, two 40 mg, two 10 mg	CeeNu

INDICATIONS

Palliative therapy employed in addition to other modalities, or in established combination therapy with other agents for the following.

Brain tumors: Both primary and metastatic; in patients who have already received appropriate surgical and/or radiotherapeutic procedures.

Hodgkin's disease: As secondary therapy.

CONTRAINDICATIONS

Hypersensitivity.

ACTIONS

Acts as an alkylating agent, but like other nitrosureas, it may also inhibit several key enzymatic processes. Serum half-life of lomustine and/or its metabolites range from 16 to 48 hours. It crosses the blood–brain barrier quite effectively because of high lipid solubility.

WARNINGS

Safe use in pregnancy not established.

DRUG INTERACTIONS

Drug/lab tests: Reversible elevation of **hepatic-function tests** may occur.

ADVERSE REACTIONS

GI: Nausea and vomiting may occur 3 to 6 hours after administration and usually last 24 hours. The frequency and duration may be reduced by use of antiemetics prior to dosing and by administration to fasting patient.

Hematologic: Thrombocytopenia occurs about 4 weeks after a dose and persists for 1 to 2 weeks. Leukopenia occurs about 6 weeks after a dose and

persists for 1 to 2 weeks. Approximately 65% of patients develop WBCs below 5000/mm^3 and 36% develop WBCs below 3000/mm^3. May produce cumulative myelosuppression manifested by more depressed indices or longer duration of suppression after repeated doses.

Other toxicities: Stomatitis, alopecia, anemia, and hepatic toxicity (manifested by transient reversible elevation of hepatic-function tests) are infrequent. Neurologic reactions such as disorientation, lethargy, ataxia, and dysarthria have been noted but relationship to medication is unclear.

Renal abnormalities consisting of decrease in kidney size, progressive azotemia, and renal failure have been reported in those who received large cumulative doses after prolonged therapy with lomustine and related nitrosureas. Kidney damage has also been occasionally reported in those receiving lower total doses.

DOSAGE

Recommended dose in adults and children is 130 mg/m^2 as a single oral dose every 6 weeks. In those with compromised bone-marrow function, dose should be reduced to 100 mg/m^2 every 6 weeks. A repeat course should not be given until circulating blood elements have returned to acceptable levels (platelets above 100,000/mm^3; leukocytes above 4000/mm^3). Blood counts recommended weekly and repeat courses not given before 6 weeks because hematologic toxicity is delayed and cumulative.

Doses subsequent to the initial dose should be adjusted according to hematologic response to the preceding dose (Table 33).

Concomitant therapy: When used with other myelosuppressive agents, dosage is adjusted accordingly.

NURSING IMPLICATIONS

HISTORY

See Appendix 4. Note previous therapy (radiation, chemotherapy, surgery).

Table 33. Recommended Doses Following Initial Dose of Lomustine, Based on Leukocyte and Platelet Counts

Nadir After Prior Dose		Percentage of Prior Dose to Be Given
Leukocytes	Platelets	
>4000	>100,000	100
3000–3999	75,000–99,999	100
2000–2999	25,000–74,999	70
<2000	<25,000	50

PHYSICAL ASSESSMENT
Physical, emotional status; vital signs; weight. Baseline studies include CBC, platelet count, renal- and liver-function tests.

ADMINISTRATION
Lomustine given as single oral dose every 6 weeks.

Administer on empty stomach.

Physician may prescribe an antiemetic administered prior to administration of lomustine.

ONGOING ASSESSMENTS AND NURSING MANAGEMENT
Vital signs q4h or as ordered. Observe for adverse drug reactions and report occurrence to physician.

Administer antiemetic as ordered for nausea and vomiting. Usually GI symptoms last 24 hours. Keep physician informed if vomiting is severe or persists beyond 24 hours and observe patient for signs of dehydration and electrolyte imbalance (Appendix 6, sections 6-10 and 6-13 to 6-18).

If nausea or vomiting occurs, patient may tolerate a liquid diet, dry toast or unsalted crackers or carbonated beverage.

CLINICAL ALERT: The major toxicity is delayed bone-marrow suppression. Thrombocytopenia occurs at about 4 weeks and leukopenia at about 6 weeks after administration of lomustine. Approximately 3 weeks after drug is administered, begin to observe patient closely for signs of bone-marrow suppression (Appendix 6, section 6-8). Keep physician informed of observations.

Stomatitis may occur, usually at the time bone-marrow suppression is noted. Examine oral cavity daily; observe for erythema, small ulcerations, patient complaints of tingling or soreness of oral mucous membranes. If stomatitis is noted, begin stomatitis care (Appendix 6, section 6-21).

Blood counts recommended weekly; periodic liver- and renal-function tests also recommended.

PATIENT AND FAMILY INFORMATION
NOTE: Patient should receive a full explanation of all possible adverse reactions, what can be done to control or alleviate these reactions, and what specific reactions should be reported immediately to the physician. This information may be given by the physician, or nurse with physician approval. The possible occurrence of alopecia should be explained; use of a wig or scarf for alopecia can be suggested.

Take on an empty stomach to reduce nausea.

Take drug prescribed for nausea as directed by physician.

Notify physician or nurse if fever, chills, sore throat, unusual bleeding or bruising, disorientation, sores on the mouth or lips, or unusual tiredness occurs.

Medication may cause loss of appetite, nausea, vomiting, skin rash, hair loss, or itching. Notify physician or nurse if these become pronounced.

A liquid diet, dry toast, unsalted crackers, carbonated beverages may be taken if nausea occurs.

Good oral care is essential. Use a soft toothbrush, rinse mouth thoroughly after taking food or beverages. Avoid use of mouthwashes or other oral products unless use is approved by physician.

Inform other physicians and dentist of therapy with this drug.

Periodic laboratory tests will be scheduled by the physician. Be sure to keep these appointments as they are necessary to monitor drug therapy.

Avoid use of nonprescription drugs unless use is approved by physician.

Loop Diuretics

Bumetanide _Rx_

| tablets: 0.5 mg, 1 mg | Bumex |
| injection: 0.25 mg/ml | Bumex |

Ethacrynic Acid _Rx_

| tablets: 25 mg, 50 mg | Edecrin |
| injection: 50 mg/vial | Sodium Edecrin |

Furosemide _Rx_

tablets: 20 mg, 40 mg	Lasix, SK-Furosemide, _Generic_
tablets: 80 mg	Lasix
oral solution: 10 mg/ml	Lasix (contains tartrazine)
injection: 10 mg/ml	Lasix, _Generic_

INDICATIONS
Treatment of edema associated with congestive heart failure (CHF), cirrhosis of the liver, and renal disease, including the nephrotic syndrome. Particu-

larly useful when greater diuretic potential is desired.

IV administration is indicated when rapid onset of diuresis is desired (*e.g.,* in acute pulmonary edema or when GI absorption is impaired) or when oral medication is not practical.

Ethacrynic acid is also indicated for short-term management of ascites due to malignancy, idiopathic edema, and lymphedema and for short-term management of hospitalized pediatric patients with congenital heart disease.

Furosemide is also used orally for treatment of hypertension alone or in combination with other antihypertensive agents. Hypertensive patients not adequately controlled with thiazides may not be adequately controlled with furosemide alone. See also Antihypertensive Agents.

CONTRAINDICATIONS

Anuria; hypersensitivity to these compounds. Infants and pregnant women should not be treated with ethacrynic acid until further studies are conducted.

Contraindicated in those with hepatic coma or in states of severe electrolyte depletion until condition is improved or corrected.

ACTIONS

These agents inhibit absorption of sodium and chloride, not only in the proximal and distal tubules, but also in the loop of Henle. Their high degree of efficacy is largely due to this unique site of action. Action on the distal tubule is independent of any inhibitory effect on carbonic anhydrase and aldosterone. Because these drugs inhibit reabsorption of a very high percentage of filtered sodium, they are often effective in those with markedly reduced glomerular filtration rates in whom other diuretics usually fail.

Bumetanide is more chloruretic than natriuretic and may have additional action in the proximal tubule. It does not appear to have noticeable action on the distal tubule.

All three drugs are metabolized and excreted primarily through the urine. Pharmacokinetics are summarized in Table 34.

WARNINGS

These are potent diuretics; if given in excess, they can lead to profound diuresis with water and electrolyte depletion.

Dehydration: Excessive diuresis may result in dehydration and reduction in blood volume, with circulatory collapse and the possibility of vascular thrombosis and embolism, particularly in elderly patients.

Table 34. Pharmacokinetic Variables of Loop Diuretics

Drug	Onset of Action (min)	Peak (min)	Duration of Action (hr)
Bumetanide PO	30–60	60–120	4
Bumetanide IV	Within minutes	15–30	3–6
Ethacrynic acid PO	Within 30	120	6–8
Ethacrynic acid IV	Within 5	15–30	2
Furosemide PO	Within 60	60–120	6–8
Furosemide IV	Within 5	30	2

Hepatic coma and states of electrolyte depletion: Therapy should not be instituted until the basic condition is improved. Sudden alterations of fluid and electrolyte balance in those with cirrhosis may precipitate hepatic encephalopathy, coma, and death. Strict observation is necessary during diuresis. Supplemental potassium chloride and, if needed, an aldosterone antagonist are helpful in preventing hypokalemia and metabolic alkalosis.

Use in impaired renal function: If increasing azotemia and oliguria occur during treatment of severe progressive renal disease, therapy is discontinued. If parenteral furosemide is administered to a patient with impaired renal function, controlled IV infusion is advised. For adults, an infusion rate not exceeding 4 mg/minute has been used.

Otoxicity: Tinnitus, reversible hearing impairment, deafness, and vertigo with a sense of fullness in the ears have been reported. Deafness is usually of a short duration (1–24 hours), but irreversible hearing impairment has occurred. Usually ototoxicity is reported when drug is injected rapidly into those with severe impairment of renal function at several times the usual dose and when other known ototoxic drugs have also been given.

Others: Observe for blood dyscrasias, liver damage, and idiosyncratic reactions. Systemic lupus erythematosus may be exacerbated or activated. Patients with known sulfonamide sensitivity may show allergic reactions to furosemide. In a few patients, ethacrynic acid has produced severe, watery diarrhea. If this occurs, drug should be discontinued and not readministered. Because of the amount of sorbitol present in the vehicle for furosemide solution, the possibility of diarrhea, especially in children, exists when higher dosages are given.

Use in pregnancy: Use only when clearly needed and when potential benefits outweigh the potential hazards to the fetus.

Use in lactation: Furosemide appears in breast milk; such transfer of ethacrynic acid and bumetanide is unknown. If use of loop diuretics is deemed essential, the patient should stop nursing.

Use in children, infants: Safety and efficacy of bumetanide in children under 18 are not established. Furosemide stimulates renal synthesis of prostaglandin E_2. When given to premature infants, furosemide may increase the incidence of patent ductus arteriosis and complicate neonatal respiratory distress syndrome.

PRECAUTIONS

Cardiovascular effects: Too vigorous diuresis, as evidenced by rapid and excessive weight loss, may induce an acute hypotensive episode. In elderly patients, to prevent thromboembolitic episodes such as cerebral vascular thrombosis and pulmonary emboli, avoid rapid contraction of plasma volume and resultant hemoconcentration.

Electrolyte imbalance: Effects of these agents on electrolytes are related to their renal pharmacologic activity and are dose dependent. The possibility of profound electrolyte and water loss may be avoided by weighing patient periodically, adjusting dosage, initiating treatment with small doses, and using drug on an intermittent schedule when possible. When excessive diuresis occurs, drug is withdrawn until homeostasis is restored. If excessive electrolyte loss occurs, dosage is reduced or drug is temporarily withdrawn.

Electrolyte depletion may occur, especially in those receiving higher doses and with restricted electrolyte intake. Serum electrolyte determinations are performed to detect possible imbalance. Observe patient for signs of fluid or electrolyte imbalance. Digitalis therapy may exaggerate metabolic effects of hypokalemia, especially with reference to myocardial activity. Serum and urine electrolyte determinations are important in those who are vomiting excessively, in those receiving parenteral fluids, during brisk diuresis, or when cirrhosis is present. Warning signs, irrespective of cause, are dry mouth, thirst, anorexia, weakness, lethargy, drowsiness, restlessness, paresthesias, muscle pain or cramps, muscle fatigue, tetany (rarely), hypotension, oliguria, tachycardia, arrhythmia, and GI disturbances such as nausea and vomiting.

Hypokalemia: Prevention requires particular attention to those receiving digitalis and diuretics for CHF, in states of aldosterone excess with normal renal function, potassium-losing nephropathy, certain diarrheal states, and other states in which hypokalemia represents added risk (_e.g.,_ ventricular arrhythmias).

A number of possible drug-related deaths have occurred with use of ethacrynic acid in critically ill patients refractory to other diuretics. They fall into 2 categories: (1) Patients with severe myocardial disease who have been receiving digitalis and presumably developed acute hypokalemia with fatal arrhythmia; and (2) patients with severely decompensated hepatic cirrhosis with ascites, with or without encephalopathy, who were in electrolyte imbalance and expired because of intensification of the electrolyte deficit.

Laboratory tests: Frequent serum electrolyte, calcium, glucose, uric acid, CO_2 and BUN determinations are recommended during the first few months of therapy and periodically thereafter. Asymptomatic hyperuricemia can occur, and rarely gout may be precipitated. Reversible elevations of BUN may be seen and observed in association with dehydration, which should be avoided, particularly in those with renal insufficiency.

These drugs may lower serum calcium levels and rare cases of tetany have been reported. Hypoproteinemia may reduce response to ethacrynic acid; use of albumin may be considered. When furosemide is administered to diabetics and those suspected of latent diabetes, periodic checks of urine and blood glucose are recommended. Increases in blood glucose and alterations in glucose tolerance tests with abnormalities of the fasting and 2-hour postprandial sugar have been seen. Rare cases of precipitation of diabetes mellitus have been reported.

Tartrazine sensitivity: Furosemide oral solution contains tartrazine. See Appendix 6, section 6-23.

DRUG INTERACTIONS

Effects of **antihypertensive drugs** may be potentiated; potentiation occurs with **ganglionic** or **peripheral adrenergic blocking drugs.** Excessive loss of potassium in patients receiving **digitalis glycosides** may precipitate digitalis toxicity.

The pharmacologic effects of **theophylline** may be increased during concomitant administration with **furosemide.**

Lithium generally should not be given with diuretics because the diuretics reduce its renal clearance and add a high risk of lithium toxicity. Concomitant administration of loop diuretics and **aminoglycoside antibiotics** increases potential for ototoxicity; in presence of impaired renal function, excessive use should be avoided.

Orthostatic hypotension may occur or be aggravated by **alcohol, barbiturates,** or **narcotics.** Hypokalemia may develop, especially during concomitant use of **corticosteroids** or **ACTH. Ethacrynic acid** may increase risk of corticosteroid-associated gastric hemorrhage.

Patients receiving high doses of **salicylates** in conjunction with **furosemide** may experience salicylate toxicity because of competitive renal excretory sites.

Pretreatment with **probenecid** reduces both the natriuresis and hyperreninemia produced by **bumetanide.** This antagonistic effect of probenecid on natriuresis is probably secondary to its inhibitory effect on renal tubular secretion of bumetanide.

Concomitant administration of **indomethacin** may reduce the natriuretic and antihypertensive effects of **furosemide** in some patients. This effect has been attributed to inhibition of prostaglandin synthesis by indomethacin. Indomethacin may also affect plasma renin levels and aldosterone excretion; this should be noted when a renin profile is evaluated in hypertensive patients. This effect may also occur with other **nonsteroidal anti-inflammatory agents** such as ibuprofen and naproxen. Indomethacin blunts the increases in urine volume and sodium excretion seen during **bumetanide** therapy and inhibits bumetanide-induced increase in plasma renin activity.

Metolazine appears to act synergistically with **furosemide** to stimulate profound diuresis in furosemide-resistant patients.

Furosemide may decrease arterial responsiveness to **norepinephrine,** but this is not sufficient to preclude effectiveness of the pressor agent for therapeutic use.

Furosemide has a tendency to antagonize the skeletal muscle relaxing effect of **tubocurarine** and may potentiate the action of **succinylcholine. Phenytoin** may reduce absorption of **furosemide. Ethacrynic acid** displaces **warfarin** from plasma protein binding sites; a reduction in the usual anticoagulant dosage may be required.

ADVERSE REACTIONS

GI: Anorexia, nausea, vomiting, diarrhea, acute pancreatitis, jaundice.

CNS: Vertigo, headache, blurred vision, tinnitus, irreversible hearing loss.

Hematologic: Thrombocytopenia, agranulocytosis.

Other: Occasionally, local irritation and pain have occurred with parenteral use.

Laboratory abnormalities: Hyperuricemia, hypochloremia, hypokalemia, azotemia, hyponatremia, increased serum creatinine, hyperglycemia, variations in phosphorus, CO_2 content, bicarbonate, calcium.

BUMETANIDE

CNS: Asterixis.

GI/GU: Abdominal pain, upset stomach, dry mouth, premature ejaculation, difficulty in maintaining erection, renal failure.

Musculoskeletal: Weakness, arthritic pain, musculoskeletal pain, muscle cramps, fatigue.

Cardiovascular: Hypotension, ECG changes, chest pain.

Other: Hives, pruritus, dehydration and sweating, hyperventilation, encephalopathy in those with preexisting liver disease, nipple tenderness.

Laboratory abnormalities: Diuresis may be accompanied by changes in LDH, total serum bilirubin, serum proteins, SGOT, SGPT, alkaline phosphatase, cholesterol, and creatinine clearance. Also reported are deviations in hemoglobin, prothrombin time, hematocrit, WBC, platelet counts, differential counts. Increase in urinary protein has also been seen.

ETHACRYNIC ACID

GI: Sudden watery profuse diarrhea; discontinue if diarrhea is severe and do not readminister. GI bleeding and dysphagia have occurred.

Hematologic: Severe neutropenia has been reported in a few critically ill patients also receiving agents known to produce this effect. Rare instances of Henoch-Schönlein purpura have been reported in patients with rheumatic heart disease receiving many drugs, including ethacrynic acid.

Other: Abnormal hepatic-function tests have been reported rarely in seriously ill patients on multiple drug therapy that included ethacrynic acid. Fever, chills, hematuria, apprehension, confusion, fatigue, and nystagmus have been reported.

FUROSEMIDE

GI: Oral and gastric irritation, constipation.

CNS: Paresthesia, xanthopsia.

Hematologic: Anemia, leukopenia. Rarely, aplastic anemia.

Dermatologic/hypersensitivity: Purpura, photosensitivity, urticaria, necrotizing angiitis (vasculitis, cutaneous vasculitis), exfoliative dermatitis, erythema multiforme, pruritus.

Cardiovascular: Orthostatic hypotension may occur and may be aggravated by alcohol, barbiturates, or narcotics.

Other: Glycosuria, muscle spasm, weakness, restlessness, urinary bladder spasm, thrombophlebitis.

OVERDOSAGE

Symptoms: Acute profound water loss, volume and electrolyte depletion, dehydration, reduction of blood volume, and circulatory collapse with the possibility of vascular thrombosis and embolism. Electrolyte depletion may be manifested by weakness, dizziness, mental confusion, anorexia, lethargy, vomiting, and cramps.

Treatment: Replacement of fluid and electrolyte losses by careful monitoring of the urine and electrolyte output and serum electrolyte levels.

DOSAGE

Therapy is individualized. Parenteral use is reserved for those in whom the oral route is not practical or in emergency situations. Replace with oral therapy as soon as practical for continued mobilization of edema.

BUMETANIDE

Because cross-sensitivity with furosemide is rare, bumetanide can be substituted at about a 1:40 ratio of bumetanide to furosemide in those allergic to furosemide.

Oral: Usual total daily dose is 0.5 mg to 2 mg given as a single dose. If diuretic response is not adequate, a second or third dose may be given at 4- to 5-hour intervals, up to a maximum daily dose of 10 mg. An intermittent dosage schedule, given on alternate days or for 3 or 4 days with rest periods of 1 to 2 days in between, is the safest and most effective method for continued control of edema. In those with hepatic failure, dosage is increased carefully.

Parenteral: Usual initial dose is 0.5 mg to 1 mg IV or IM. Administer IV over period of 1 to 2 minutes. If response to initial dose is insufficient, a second or third dose at intervals of 2 to 3 hours may be given. Do not exceed a daily dosage of 10 mg.

ETHACRYNIC ACID

Oral initial therapy: Onset of diuresis usually occurs at 50 mg to 100 mg for adults. Minimal effective dose (usually 50 mg–200 mg/day) is given on a continuous or intermittent dosage schedule to produce weight loss (1–2 lb/day). Dosage adjustments are usually in 25-mg to 50-mg increments. Higher doses, up to 200 mg bid, achieved gradually, are most often required in those with severe, refractory edema.

Children: Initial dose is 25 mg. Careful stepwise increments of 25 mg are made to achieve maintenance. Dosage for infants not established.

Oral maintenance therapy: Administer intermittently after effective diuresis is obtained using an alternate daily schedule or more prolonged periods of therapy interspersed with rest periods. This allows time to correct any electrolyte imbalance and may provide a more efficient diuretic response. The chloruretic effect may give rise to retention of bicarbonate and metabolic alkalosis, which may be corrected by giving ammonium chloride or arginine chloride. Ammonium chloride is not given to cirrhotic patients.

Concomitant diuretic therapy: Has additive effects when used with other diuretics. May potentiate action of carbonic anhydrase inhibitors; therefore, initial dose and changes in dose should be in 25-mg increments.

Parenteral: Do *not* give subcutaneously or IM because of local pain and irritation. Usual IV dose is 50 mg or 0.5 mg/kg to 1 mg/kg given slowly through tubing of a running IV infusion or by direct IV injection over several minutes. Usually only one dose is necessary; occasionally a second dose may be required. Use a new injection site to avoid thrombophlebitis. A single IV dose not exceeding 100 mg has been used. Insufficient pediatric experience precludes recommendation for this group.

FUROSEMIDE
Oral

Edema: Usual initial dose is 20 mg/day to 80 mg/day as a single dose. Depending on response, a second dose may be administered 6 to 8 hours later. If response is not satisfactory, increase by increments of 20 mg to 40 mg no sooner than 6 to 8 hours after the previous dose, until desired effect is obtained. Dose should then be given once or twice daily (*e.g.,* 8 A.M. and 2 P.M.). Dosage may be titrated up to 600 mg/day in those with severe edema. Intermittent dosage schedule may also be used, with drug given 2 to 4 consecutive days each week.

Hypertension: Usual initial dose is 40 mg bid, which is then adjusted according to patient response. If patient does not respond, other antihypertensive agents are added to regimen. Make careful observation for changes in blood pressure when furosemide is used with other antihypertensive agents, especially during initial therapy. To prevent excessive drop in blood pressure, dosages of other agents are reduced by at least 50% as soon as furosemide is added to regimen. As blood pressure falls, dosage is reduced or other antihypertensives are discontinued.

Infants and children: Usual initial dose is 2 mg/kg. If diuretic response is not satisfactory, dosage is increased by 1 mg/kg to 2 mg/kg not sooner than 6 to 8 hours. Doses greater than 6 mg/kg are not recommended. *Maintenance*—Dose is adjusted to minimum effective level.

Parenteral

Edema: Usual initial dose is 20 mg to 40 mg IM or IV. IV injection is given slowly (1–2 minutes). If response to single dose is not satisfactory, dose is increased in increments of 20 mg, no sooner than 2 hours after previous dose, until desired effect is obtained. This dose may then be given once or twice daily. High-dose parenteral therapy should be administered as a controlled infusion at a rate not exceeding 4 mg/minute.

Acute pulmonary edema: Usual initial dose is 40 mg injected slowly IV (1–2 minutes). If dose does not produce a satisfactory response within 1 hour, dose may be increased to 80 mg IV (given over 1–2 minutes). Additional therapy (*e.g.*, digitalis, oxygen) may be administered concomitantly.

Infants and children: Usual initial dose (IV or IM) is 1 mg/kg given slowly under close supervision. If response after initial dose is not satisfactory, dosage may be increased by 1 mg/kg no sooner than 2 hours after previous dose, until desired effect is obtained. Doses greater than 6 mg/kg not recommended.

NURSING IMPLICATIONS

HISTORY
See Appendix 4. Note allergy to sulfonamides if furosemide is prescribed (see *Warnings*).

PHYSICAL ASSESSMENT
Obtain weight, blood pressure (on both arms in sitting and lying position if patient is not acutely ill), pulse, respirations. Check extremities for edema; describe degree of edema. Baseline laboratory tests include CBC, serum electrolytes, renal- and hepatic-function studies.

ADMINISTRATION
Inform patient that drug will cause an increased volume and frequency of urination and the effect may last for 6 to 8 hours following oral administration and approximately 2 hours following parenteral administration.

Obtain blood pressure before administration. Withhold drug and contact physician if there has been a significant decrease in the systolic or diastolic pressure.

For once-daily oral administration, give early in A.M. to avoid nighttime diuresis and interruption of sleep. For twice-daily administration, recommended times are 8 A.M. and 2 P.M.

BUMETANIDE, PARENTERAL
May be given IM or IV. Administer IV over a period of 1 to 2 minutes.

ETHACRYNIC ACID, PARENTERAL
Give IV only. Subcutaneous or IM administration causes pain and local irritation.

To reconstitute, add 50 ml of 5% Dextrose Injection or Sodium Chloride Injection to vial. Occasionally, 5% Dextrose Injection solutions may have a low *p*H and the resulting solution may be hazy or opalescent; use is not recommended.

Do not mix reconstituted drug with whole blood or its derivatives.

Discard unused reconstituted soluton after 24 hours.

Administer slowly through injection port of IV tubing of a running infusion or by direct IV injection over period of several minutes.

FUROSEMIDE
Oral administration: Exposure to light may cause slight discoloration of tablets; do not use. Store oral solution in refrigerator (36°F–46°F).

Parenteral administration: Do not use solution that is discolored.

May be administered IM or IV. Give IV injection slowly over period of 1 to 2 minutes.

Do not mix with highly acid solutions of *p*H below 5.5. Isotonic saline, Lactated Ringer's Injection, and 5% Dextrose Injection have been used after *p*H is adjusted as necessary. If physician's order states drug is to be added to an IV solution, contact pharmacy about addition to a specific type and brand of parenteral fluid and whether *p*H adjustment is necessary.

If high-dose parenteral therapy is ordered for a patient with severely impaired renal function, controlled IV infusion at a rate not exceeding 4 mg/minute is recommended.

Store solution for injection at room temperature (59°F–86°F).

ONGOING ASSESSMENTS AND NURSING MANAGEMENT
Therapy is individualized according to patient response. Drug is titrated to gain maximal therapeutic response with minimal dose. Once dry weight is achieved (body weight without excess fluid accumulation), dosage may be reduced.

When an intermittent or alternate dosage schedule is employed, medicine cards must be clearly labeled to identify days drug is administered.

Monitor blood pressure, pulse, and respirations q4h to q8h; weigh (same time each day with approximately same amount of clothing); observe for adverse drug reactions including signs of dehydration, hypokalemia, hyponatremia (Appendix 6, sections 6-10, 6-15, 6-17); measure intake and output.

Close observation for changes in blood pressure must be made when furosemide is administered with other antihypertensive agents, especially during initial therapy. Monitor blood pressure and pulse q2h to q4h or as ordered. Notify physician of any significant decrease or increase in blood pressure.

If patient is acutely ill, blood pressure, pulse, and respirations may be taken at more frequent intervals, such as q1h to q2h.

In pulmonary edema, observe q½h to q1h for drug response (*e.g.,* decrease in respiratory rate, pulse; rise in blood pressure; general improvement in clinical status).

Onset of diuresis following oral administration is within 30 to 60 minutes for bumetanide, 30 minutes for ethacrynic acid, and 1 hour for furosemide. Duration of effect is 4 hours for bumetanide and 6 to 8 hours for ethacrynic acid and furosemide.

Onset of diuresis following IV administration of ethacrynic acid and furosemide is within 5 minutes.

If output decreases despite adequate intake, notify physician.

Ethacrynic acid has produced severe, watery diarrhea in a few patients. Notify physician immediately if this should occur because drug may be discontinued. Observe patient for signs of dehydration and electrolyte imbalance.

If excessive diuresis or electrolyte imbalance occurs, drug may be discontinued or dosage reduced.

Physician usually orders periodic determinations of serum electrolytes, including serum calcium. These are especially important in patients who are vomiting excessively, in those receiving parenteral fluids, during brisk diuresis, or in patients with cirrhosis.

Monitor current serum electrolyte determinations; report abnormals to physician as soon as possible.

CLINICAL ALERT: Observe for the following and contact physician immediately if one or more occurs: dry mouth, thirst, weakness, lethargy, drowsiness, restlessness, muscle pains or cramps, muscle fatigue, hypotension, oliguria, tachycardia, arrhythmia, and GI disturbances such as nausea and vomiting.

Excessive diuresis may result in dehydration and reduction in blood volume, with circulatory collapse and possibility of thrombosis and embolism, particularly in elderly patients. Observe for a sudden decrease in blood pressure, change in level of consciousness, confusion, or sudden onset of pain (chest, extremity) or headache.

Orthostatic hypotension may occur. Ambulatory patient should be instructed to dangle legs 5 to 10 minutes before getting out of bed as well as to make position changes slowly. If necessary, assist with ambulatory activities, especially early in therapy.

Ototoxicity has been reported. If patient complains of tinnitus, or if hearing appears to be impaired, notify physician.

Asymptomatic hyperuricemia can occur; rarely gout may be precipitated. If patient complains of sudden pain or tenderness in joints, contact physician.

Diabetic patient: Test urine qid. Report any increase in urinary glucose to physician. Periodic blood glucose and glucose tolerance tests may be ordered. Although increases in blood glucose and alterations in glucose tolerance tests have not been reported with bumetanide, the possibility of an effect on glucose metabolism exists.

PATIENT AND FAMILY INFORMATION

NOTE: Physician may wish hypertensive patient receiving furosemide to monitor own blood pressure between office/clinic visits. Patient and/or family member will require instruction.

May cause GI upset; take with food or milk.

Drug will increase urination; take early in day unless directed otherwise by physician. Frequent urination tends to lessen with therapy.

Notify physician or nurse if muscle weakness, cramps, nausea, or dizziness occurs.

Follow physician's recommendations about diet, exercise.

Weigh self weekly at same time of day and with approximately same amount of clothes. Keep record of weight and bring to next office or clinic visit.

Do not omit or increase the dose without physician approval.

Furosemide oral solution: Keep refrigerated.

Loperamide Hydrochloride Rx

capsules: 2 mg   Imodium

INDICATIONS

Control and symptomatic relief of acute nonspecific diarrhea and of chronic diarrhea associated with inflammatory bowel disease. Also indicated for reducing volume of discharge from ileostomies.

CONTRAINDICATIONS

Hypersensitivity; those in whom constipation must be avoided.

ACTIONS

Acts by slowing intestinal motility and by effecting water and electrolyte movement through the bowel. Inhibits peristaltic activity by direct effect on the circular and longitudinal muscles of the intestinal wall. Loperamide prolongs transit time of intestinal contents, reduces daily fecal volume, increases the viscosity and bulk density, and diminishes loss of fluid and electrolytes. Tolerance to its antidiarrheal effect not seen. Apparent elimination half-life ranges from 9.1 to 14.4 hours. Plasma levels are highest approximately 5 hours after administration. Drug is excreted mainly in the feces, with a small amount in urine.

WARNINGS

Do not use antiperistaltic agents in acute diarrhea associated with organisms that penetrate the intestinal mucosa (enteroinvasive *Escherichia coli, Salmonella, Shigella*) or in pseudomembranous colitis associated with broad-spectrum antibiotics.

Acute ulcerative colitis: In some patients, agents that inhibit intestinal motility or delay intestinal transit time have been reported to induce toxic megacolon. Therapy should be discontinued promptly if abdominal distention or other untoward symptoms develop.

Fluid/electrolyte balance: Fluid and electrolyte depletion may occur in those with diarrhea. Use of loperamide does not obviate need for appropriate fluid and electrolyte therapy.

Use in pregnancy, lactation: Safety not established. It is not known if drug is excreted in human milk.

Use in children: Safety and efficacy for use in children under 12 not established.

PRECAUTIONS

In acute diarrhea, if clinical improvement is not seen in 48 hours, discontinue use.

Abuse and dependence: Physical dependence not observed in humans.

ADVERSE REACTIONS

Adverse effects reported are difficult to distinguish from symptoms associated with diarrhea. Adverse experiences are generally minor and self-limiting and are more commonly observed during treatment of chronic diarrhea.

The following have been reported: abdominal pain, distention, or discomfort; constipation; drowsiness or dizziness; dry mouth; nausea and vomiting; tiredness; hypersensitivity reactions (including skin rash).

OVERDOSAGE

Symptoms: Overdosage may result in constipation, CNS depression, and GI irritation.

Treatment: If vomiting occurs spontaneously, a slurry of 100 g of activated charcoal should be administered PO as soon as fluids can be retained. If vomiting has not occurred, gastric lavage should be performed, followed by administration of 100 g of activated charcoal slurry through the gastric tube. Patient should be monitored for signs of CNS depression for at least 24 hours; if CNS depression is observed, naloxone may be administered. If responsive to naloxone, vital signs must be monitored carefully for recurrence of symptoms of drug over-

dose for at least 24 hours after last dose of naloxone. In view of the prolonged action of loperamide and short duration (1–3 hours) of naloxone, patient must be monitored closely and treated repeatedly with naloxone as indicated. Since relatively little drug is excreted in the urine, forced diuresis is not expected to be effective.

DOSAGE

Acute diarrhea: Recommended initial dosage is 4 mg followed by 2 mg after each unformed stool. Daily dosage should not exceed 16 mg. Clinical improvement usually observed within 48 hours.

Chronic diarrhea: Recommended initial dosage is 4 mg followed by 2 mg after each unformed stool until diarrhea is controlled, after which dosage should be reduced to meet individual requirements. When optimal daily dosage is established, this amount may be administered as a single dose or in divided doses. Average daily maintenance dosage is approximately 4 mg to 8 mg. If clinical improvement is not observed after treatment with 16 mg/day for at least 10 days, symptoms are unlikely to be controlled by further administration. Administration may be continued if diarrhea cannot be adequately controlled with diet or specific treatment.

NURSING IMPLICATIONS

HISTORY

Duration of diarrhea; number of stools/day; character of stools (color, consistency, amount); other related symptoms (*e.g.,* abdominal cramping, fever).

PHYSICAL ASSESSMENT

Vital signs; weight; look for evidence of dehydration (Appendix 6, section 6-10); auscultate abdomen for bowel sounds (which may be hyperactive). Serum electrolytes, stool culture, other diagnostic tests may be ordered.

ADMINISTRATION

Inspect each bowel movement (rather than rely on patient's description) before decision is made to administer or not to administer the drug.

Maximum daily recommended dosage is 16 mg (8 capsules). If physician orders drug to be given prn for each unformed stool, an accurate record must be kept and easily retreived to ensure maximum dosage not exceeded.

ONGOING ASSESSMENTS AND NURSING MANAGEMENT

Obtain vital signs q4h or as ordered if diarrhea acute. Notify physician if elevation in temperature occurs.

In acute ulcerative colitis, observe for abdominal distention, discomfort, pain, or fever. If one or more occur, withhold drug and notify physician.

Clinical improvement in acute diarrhea is usually seen in 48 hours. If diarrhea persists, notify physician.

CLINICAL ALERT: Severe diarrhea, especially in children or the elderly or debilitated patient, may result in dehydration and loss of electrolytes, especially sodium, potassium, and chloride (see Appendix 6, sections 6-10, 6-15, and 6-17). Notify physician immediately if symptoms of dehydration and electrolyte loss are apparent.

If diarrhea severe, additional treatment modalities (*e.g.,* IV fluids, electrolyte replacement) may be required.

If diarrhea is chronic, encourage a liberal oral fluid intake. In some instances the physician may prescribe oral electrolyte replacement.

If drowsiness or dizziness occurs, assist with ambulation. Tell patient not to get out of bed without assistance if these effects occur.

In chronic diarrhea associated with inflammatory bowel disease, periodic serum electrolyte studies may be ordered.

PATIENT AND FAMILY INFORMATION

Do not exceed prescribed dosage. When physician recommends a maximum number of capsules per day, make a note (use a small pad and keep next to prescription container) each time capsule is taken.

May cause drowsiness or dizziness. Observe caution while driving or performing other tasks requiring alertness.

May cause dry mouth, which may be relieved by frequent sips of water.

Notify physician if abdominal pain or fever occurs.

Do not drink alcoholic beverages or take nonprescription drugs unless use is approved by physician. Alcohol and the contents of some nonprescription drugs may enhance drowsiness.

Nonspecific diarrhea: If symptoms are not relieved in 48 hours, contact physician.

Chronic diarrhea associated with inflammatory bowel disease: Record number, consistency of stools.

Reducing volume of discharge from ileostomies: Keep daily record of volume of discharge (approximate estimation) and/or number of times ileostomy bag is emptied.

Lorazepam

See Benzodiazepines.

Loxapine

See Antipsychotic Agents.

Lymphocyte Immune Globulin

See Immunizations, Passive.

Lypressin Rx

nasal spray: 0.185 mg lypressin per ml (equivalent to 50 USP Posterior Pituitary [Pressor] Units per ml)   Diapid

INDICATIONS

Control or prevention of symptoms and complications of diabetes insipidus (including polydipsia, polyuria, dehydration) due to deficiency of endogenous posterior pituitary antidiuretic hormone (ADH). Particularly useful in those who have become unresponsive to other forms of therapy or who experience various types of local or systemic reactions, allergic reactions, or other undesirable effects (*e.g.,* excessive fluid retention) from preparations of posterior pituitary ADH of animal origin.

CONTRAINDICATIONS

None known.

ACTIONS

A synthetic lysine vasopressin analogue. Possesses antidiuretic activity with little vasopressor or oxytocic effect. Duration of action is 3 to 8 hours.

WARNINGS

Safety for use in pregnancy is not established. Use only when clearly needed and when potential benefits outweigh the unknown potential hazards to the fetus.

PRECAUTIONS

Cardiovascular pressor effects are minimal or absent when drug is administered as a nasal spray in therapeutic doses; nevertheless, use with caution in those for whom such effects would not be desirable. Large doses intranasally may cause coronary artery constriction; use caution in treating patients with coronary artery disease.

Effectiveness may be lessened in nasal congestion, allergic rhinitis, and upper respiratory infections, because of interference with absorption by the nasal mucosa; larger doses or adjunctive therapy may be needed.

Patients with known hypersensitivity to ADH should be tested.

DRUG INTERACTIONS

Other drugs known to potentiate ADH, such as **chlorpropamide, clofibrate,** or **carbamazepine,** may potentiate antidiuretic effects of lypressin.

ADVERSE REACTIONS

Have been infrequent and mild, including rhinorrhea, nasal congestion, irritation and pruritus of the nasal passages, nasal ulceration, headache, conjunctivitis, heartburn secondary to excessive nasal administration with drippage into the pharynx, abdominal cramps, and increased bowel movements. Inadvertent inhalation has resulted in substernal tightness, coughing, and transient dyspnea. Overdosage has caused marked, but transient, fluid retention. Tolerance or tachyphylaxis has not been reported to date. Hypersensitivity manifested by a positive skin test has occurred.

DOSAGE

One spray provides approximately 2 USP Posterior Pituitary (Pressor) Units. Usual dosage for adults and children is one or two sprays in each nostril qid. An additional H.S. dose is often helpful to eliminate nocturia, if it is not controlled with regular daily dosage. For those requiring more than two sprays per nostril q4h to q6h, it is recommended that time interval between doses be reduced rather than that the number of sprays per dose be increased. More than two or three sprays in each nostril usually result in wastage; the unabsorbed excess will drain posteriorly (by way of the nasopharynx) into the digestive tract, where it will be inactivated.

Although most patients require one or two sprays qid, dosage has ranged from one spray a day, H.S., to 10 sprays in each nostril q3h to q4h. Requirements of the larger doses may represent a greater severity of disease or other phenomena, such as poor nasal absorption. Requirement for large doses may be due to presence of mixed hypothalamic, hypophyseal, and nephrogenic diabetes insipidus, the latter being unresponsive to administration of ADH.

NURSING IMPLICATIONS

HISTORY

Record previous treatment modalities, etiology of diabetes insipidus (from chart).

PHYSICAL ASSESSMENT

Obtain vital signs; review recent intake and output and ratio of intake to output; check for signs of dehydration (Appendix 6, section 6-10); weight.

ADMINISTRATION

Medication is self-administered when patient is alert, cooperative, and old enough to understand administration. Patient will need instructions for first-time administration and should be supervised until able to self-administer drug correctly.

Effectiveness may be lessened in nasal congestion, allergic rhinitis, and upper respiratory infections. If nasal congestion is suspected, inspect both nares with a nasal speculum or have patient close one nostril with finger while inhaling and repeat maneuver on the opposite nostril.

If nasal congestion is apparent, notify physician because dosage adjustment or adjunctive therapy may be required.

Instruct patient to sit in an upright position and clear nasal passages (if necessary) by blowing nose with mouth open (to prevent nasal secretions from entering the middle ear).

Instruct patient not to inhale the spray.

Holding the spray bottle upright, insert nozzle into nares. Squeeze bottle to deliver prescribed number of sprays to each nostril.

Patient should remain upright for 1 to 2 minutes after administration.

ONGOING ASSESSMENTS AND NURSING MANAGEMENT

Obtain vital signs q4h or as ordered; record weight; measure intake and output; observe for adverse effects, signs of water retention (weight gain, edema) and notify physician if water retention is apparent.

Record total intake every 8 hours. Physician may also order measurement of each voided sample as well as time of voiding during the adjustment period. Use separate flow sheet to record time and amount of each voiding. Determination of specific gravity of each sample may also be ordered.

Dosage is adjusted to individual requirements. Accurate measurement of intake and output is important in determining individualized dosage.

If a marked increase in urinary output is noted, notify physician because dosage may need to be increased or it may be that drug is not being absorbed.

Periodic determinations of serum electrolytes may be ordered.

PATIENT AND FAMILY INFORMATION

NOTE: Administration technique must be explained to patient (see _Administration,_ above) when drug is prescribed for the first time on an outpatient basis. Physician may instruct patient to administer one or two sprays to one or both nostrils whenever frequency of urination becomes increased or significant thirst develops, as well as prescribe a specific daily dosage.

Follow physician's instructions about number of sprays per day. If there is any question about the dosage or if it appears that the dosage may need to be increased because of increased urinary output or marked thirst, contact physician immediately.

Notify physician or nurse if drowsiness, listlessness, headache, shortness of breath, heartburn, nausea, abdominal cramps, vulval pain, severe nasal congestion, upper respiratory infection, or persistent nasal congestion occurs.

L

M

Mafenide
Magaldrate
Magnesium
Magnesium Carbonate
Magnesium Hydroxide
Magnesium Oxide
Magnesium Salicylate
Magnesium Sulfate
Magnesium Trisilicate
Malathion
Mannitol
Maprotiline Hydrochloride
Mazindol
Measles Vaccine
Measles, Mumps, and Rubella
     Vaccine
Measles and Rubella Vaccine
Mebendazole
Mecamylamine Hydrochloride
Mechlorethamine Hydrochlo-
     ride (Nitrogen Mustard)
Meclizine Hydrochloride
Meclofenamate Sodium
Medroxyprogesterone Acetate
Medrysone
Mefenamic Acid
Megestrol Acetate

Melphalan
Menadiol Sodium Diphosphate
Menadione
Meningitis Vaccines
Menotropins
Mepenzolate Bromide
Meperidine Hydrochloride
Mephentermine Sulfate
Mephenytoin
Mephobarbital
Mepivacaine Hydrochloride
Meprobamate
Merbromin
Mercaptopurine
Mersalyl With Theophylline
Mesoridazine
Metaproterenol Sulfate
Metaraminol Bitartrate
Methacycline Hydrochloride
Methadone Hydrochloride
Methamphetamine Hydrochlo-
     ride
Methandriol
Methantheline Bromide
Metharbital
Methazolamide
Methdilazine Hydrochloride

Methenamine and Methena-
     mine Salts
   Methenamine
   Methenamine Hippurate
   Methenamine Mandelate
Methicillin Sodium
Methimazole
Methocarbamol
Methohexital Sodium
Methotrexate
Methotrimeprazine
Methoxamine Hydrochloride
Methoxyflurane
Methscopolamine Bromide
Methsuximide
Methyclothiazide
Methylcellulose
Methyldopa and Methyldopate
     Hydrochloride
Methylene Blue
Methylergonovine Maleate
Methylphenidate Hydrochlo-
     ride
Methylprednisolone
Methylprednisolone Acetate
Methylprednisolone Sodium
     Succinate

Methyltestosterone
Methyprylon
Methysergide Maleate
Metoclopramide
Metocurine Iodide
Metolazone
Metoprolol Tartrate
Metronidazole
Metyrapone
Metyrosine
Mezlocillin Sodium
Miconazole
Miconazole Nitrate
Microfibrillar Collagen Hemo-
stat
Mineral Oil
Minocycline Hydrochloride
Minoxidil
Miotics, Cholinesterase Inhib-
itors
Demecarium Bromide
Echothiophate Iodide

Isoflurophate
Physostigmine
Miotics, Direct Acting
Acetylcholine Chloride,
Intraocular
Carbachol, Intraocular
Carbachol, Topical
Pilocarpine Hydrochloride
Pilocarpine Nitrate
Pilocarpine Ocular Thera-
peutic System
Mitomycin
Mitotane
Molindone Hydrochloride
Morphine Sulfate
Moxalactam Disodium
Mumps Vaccine
Muscle Stimulants, Anticho-
linesterase
Ambenonium Chloride
Edrophonium Chloride

Neostigmine
Pyridostigmine Bromide
Mydriatics, Cycloplegic
Atropine Sulfate
Cyclopentolate Hydrochlo-
ride
Homatropine Hydrobro-
mide
Scopolamine Hydrobro-
mide
Tropicamide
Mydriatics/Ophthalmic Vaso-
constrictors
Epinephrine Hydrochloride
Hydroxyamphetamine Hy-
drobromide
Naphazoline Hydrochloride
Phenylephrine Hydrochlo-
ride
Tetrahydrozoline Hydro-
chloride

Mafenide Rx

cream: 85 mg/g   Sulfamylon

INDICATIONS
Adjunctive therapy of patients with second- and third-degree burns.

ACTIONS
Is structurally related to the sulfonamides. Applied topically, it produces a marked reduction in the bacterial population present in avascular tissues of second- and third-degree burns. Reduction in bacterial growth after application permits spontaneous healing of deep partial-thickness burns and thus prevents conversion of burn wounds from partial thickness to full thickness. It should be noted that delayed eschar separation has occurred in some cases.

Mafenide exerts bacteriostatic action against many gram-negative and gram-positive organisms, including _Pseudomonas aeruginosa_ and certain strains of anaerobes. Applied topically, it diffuses through devascularized areas and is absorbed and rapidly converted to a metabolite, which is cleared through the kidneys. It is active in the presence of pus and serum, and its activity is not altered by changes in the acidity of its environment.

WARNINGS
Hypersensitivity: Administer cautiously to those with history of hypersensitivity to mafenide. It is not known whether there is cross-sensitivity to other sulfonamides.

Fungal colonization in and below the eschar may occur concomitantly with reduction of bacterial growth in the burn wound. Fungal dissemination through the infected burn wound is rare.

Use in pregnancy: Safe use has not been established. Not recommended for treatment of women of childbearing potential unless the burned area covers more than 20% of total body surface or need for therapeutic benefit is greater than the potential hazard to the fetus.

PRECAUTIONS
Mafenide and its metabolite inhibit carbonic anhydrase, which may result in metabolic acidosis, usually comepensated by hyperventilation. In the presence of impaired renal function, high blood levels of mafenide and its metabolite may exaggerate the carbonic anhydrase inhibition. Close monitoring of the acid–base balance is necessary, particularly in those with extensive second-degree or partial-thickness burns and in those with pulmonary or renal dysfunction. Some burn patients treated with mafenide have been reported to manifest an unexplained syndrome of marked hyperventilation with resulting respiratory alkalosis (slightly alkaline blood pH, low arterial pCO_2 and decreased total CO_2); change in arterial pO_2 is variable. The etiology and significance of these findings are unknown.

If acidosis occurs and becomes difficult to control, particularly in those with pulmonary dysfunction, discontinuing therapy for 24 to 48 hours while continuing fluid therapy may aid in restoring acid–base balance.

Use drug with caution in those with acute renal failure.

ADVERSE REACTIONS
It is difficult to distinguish between an adverse reaction to mafenide and the effect of the severe burn.

Most frequent: Pain or a burning sensation.

Allergic manifestations: Rash, itching, facial edema, swelling, hives, blisters, erythema, and eosinophilia.

Miscellaneous (rare): Tachypnea or hyperventilation, acidosis, increase in serum chloride, decrease in arterial pCO_2, excoriation of new skin, bleeding of skin. Fatal hemolytic anemia with disseminated intravascular coagulation, presumably related to G6PD deficiency, has been reported following therapy. Accidental ingestion has been reported to cause diarrhea.

DOSAGE
See _Administration._

Duration of therapy: Depends on each patient's requirements. Treatment is usually continued until healing is progressing well or until burn site is ready for grafting. Mafenide is not withdrawn from the therapeutic regimen while there is a possibility of infection. If allergic manifestations occur during treatment, use is discontinued.

NURSING IMPLICATIONS

HISTORY AND PHYSICAL ASSESSMENT
Prompt institution of appropriate measures for controlling shock and pain is of prime importance. If initial treatment has been given, review patient's chart for type and extent of burns, recent laboratory determinations, health history, allergy history, and current treatment modalities.

ADMINISTRATION
Wound cleaning and removal of debris is usually ordered before each application; however, physicians' orders may vary on type of cleansing procedure.

M

Warn patient that a stinging or burning sensation may be noted. In some instances, the physician may order a narcotic analgesic or tranquilizer 30 to 60 minutes before cleaning of the burned area and application of mafenide.

Application: Apply with a sterile gloved hand. Satisfactory results can be achieved with application once or twice daily, to a thickness of approximately $\frac{1}{16}$ inch; thicker application is not recommended. Cover burned areas with mafenide at all times. Whenever necessary, reapply the cream to any areas from which it has been removed (*e.g.,* by patient activity).

Do not cover with occlusive dressing unless so ordered by physician. If occlusive dressing is ordered, a thin layer is recommended.

ONGOING ASSESSMENTS AND NURSING MANAGEMENT
Treatment is outlined by the physician and will vary according to extent of burned area, degree of burns, physical condition and age of the patient, and other medical problems such as pulmonary involvement (*e.g.,* smoke inhalation) and physical injuries (*e.g.,* fractures, lacerations).

A whirlpool bath, such as use of a Hubbard tank, may be employed once or twice daily to aid in removal of debris and cleansing of the burned area. The area may also be cleaned by bathing or showering.

Record appearance of area in patient's chart after each application.

Check burned areas q2h to q4h. If cream is removed because of patient's activity, reapply.

Monitor vital signs q1h to q4h, depending on patient's condition. Notify physician immediately of any changes in vital signs.

Monitor intake and output (in some instances hourly measurement may be necessary). Notify physician immediately of any change in the intake–output ratio.

CLINICAL ALERT: Observe patient for signs of metabolic acidosis (Appendix 6, section 6-1) or marked hyperventilation with resulting respiratory alkalosis (Appendix 6, section 6-5) and for signs of local or systemic infection (bacterial, fungal). Report findings to physician immediately.

A flow chart may be used to record treatments, burn care and appearance, vital signs, drug administration, intake and output, laboratory data, assessments of body systems (*e.g.,* neurologic, cardiopulmonary, renal), weight, and so on.

Magaldrate

See Antacids.

Magnesium Rx

| tablets: 500 mg magnesium gluconate (27 mg magnesium) | Almora, Magonate |
| tablets: 133 mg (as magnesium–protein complex) | Mg-PLUS |

INDICATIONS
Dietary supplement.

ACTIONS
Magnesium is an electrolyte necessary in a number of enzyme systems, muscular contraction, and nerve conduction. Deficiency is rare in well-nourished individuals, except in malabsorption syndromes. Although there are large stores of magnesium present intracellularly and in bone in adults, these stores are not mobilized sufficiently to maintain plasma levels.

PRECAUTIONS
Excessive dosage may cause a laxative effect.

DOSAGE
Recommended dietary allowances (RDAs): *Adult males*—350 mg; *adult females*—330 mg.

Dietary supplement: 27 mg to 133 mg one to three times a day.

NURSING IMPLICATIONS

HISTORY
Review chart for probable cause of hypomagnesemia. Possible causes include alcoholism, malnutrition, malabsorption syndrome, diabetic ketoacidosis, diuretic therapy, and magnesium-wasting renal disease.

PHYSICAL ASSESSMENT
Obtain vital signs. Assess for signs of hypomagnesemia (Appendix 6, section 6-16). Serum electrolytes will be ordered. Other laboratory tests and diagnostic studies may also be appropriate, depending on etiology of the deficiency.

ADMINISTRATION
Hypomagnesemia may cause tetany or athetoid or choreiform movements, which may interfere with swallowing. If difficulty in swallowing is suspected, have patient take a few sips of water before offering tablet. Withhold drug and notify physician if swallowing difficulty is encountered.

ONGOING ASSESSMENTS AND NURSING MANAGEMENT
Obtain vital signs daily; monitor dietary intake.

Look for improvement in symptoms (compare with data base).

If diarrhea occurs, withhold drug and notify physician.

PATIENT AND FAMILY INFORMATION

Take only as directed by physician.

If diarrhea occurs, stop taking drug and contact physician.

Magnesium Carbonate

See Antacids.

Magnesium Hydroxide

See Antacids; Laxatives.

Magnesium Oxide

See Antacids.

Magnesium Salicylate

See Salicylates.

Magnesium Sulfate (MgSO₄) Rx

injection: 10%,   *Generic*
   12.5%, 25%, 50%

INDICATIONS

Anticonvulsant: For prevention and control of seizures in severe preeclampsia or eclampsia and of convulsions associated with epilepsy, glomerulonephritis, and hypothyroidism (low plasma levels of magnesium may be contributing cause of convulsions in these conditions).

Hypomagnesemia: As replacement therapy. Total parenteral nutrition (TPN) patients may develop hypomagnesemia (magnesium levels less than 1.5 mEq/liter) within 3 to 4 days without supplementation. Magnesium sulfate is added to correct or prevent hypomagnesemia.

Unlabeled uses: Has demonstrated some effectiveness as an agent to inhibit premature labor; however, it is not a first-line agent.

See also Laxatives.

CONTRAINDICATIONS

Not administered to patients with heart block or myocardial damage. Because it is excreted by the kidneys, it should be given cautiously in the presence of serious renal impairment.

ACTIONS

Magnesium is an electrolyte necessary in a number of enzyme systems, muscular contraction, and nerve conduction. Magnesium prevents or controls convulsions by blocking neuromuscular transmission. It has a depressant effect on the CNS. Normal plasma levels range from 1.5 mEq/liter to 3 mEq/liter. As levels rise above 4 mEq/liter, deep tendon reflexes are first decreased, and they then disappear as plasma levels approach 10 mEq/liter. At this level, respiratory paralysis may occur. Heart block may also occur.

With IV use, onset of anticonvulsant action is immediate and lasts about 30 minutes. With IM use, onset occurs in 1 hour and persists for 3 to 4 hours. Effective serum levels range from 2.5 mEq/liter to 7.5 mEq/liter. Magnesium is excreted by the kidney.

Magnesium deficiency is rare in well-nourished individuals, except in malabsorption syndromes. Magnesium deficiency may occur in chronic alcoholism, malnutrition, intestinal bypass surgery, diuretic therapy, severe diarrhea, or prolonged nasogastric suction. Although large stores are found intracellularly and in bone in adults, they are often not mobilized sufficiently to maintain plasma levels. The normal adult body contains 20 g to 30 g (2000 mEq) of magnesium.

Predominant deficiency symptoms are neurologic: muscle irritability, clonic twitching, and tremors. Hypocalcemia and hypokalemia often accompany low serum magnesium levels.

Magnesium acts peripherally to produce vasodilation. With low doses, only flushing and sweating occur. Larger doses cause a lowering of blood pressure and CNS depression.

See also Magnesium.

WARNINGS

IV use in eclampsia is reserved for immediate control of life-threatening convulsions. Should not be given in toxemia of pregnancy during the 2 hours preceding delivery. When drug is used just before delivery, the newborn may manifest magnesium toxicity and require assisted ventilation and calcium administration.

Because magnesium is removed from the body solely by the kidneys, it is used with caution in those with renal impairment.

Magnesium sulfate has not been shown to increase the risk of fetal abnormalities if given during all trimesters. The possibility of fetal harm appears remote; however, use only if clearly needed.

M

PRECAUTIONS

Anticonvulsant therapy: Monitor patient's clinical status to avoid toxicity. Use with caution in impaired renal function; serum magnesium levels should be monitored. In severe renal insufficiency, do not administer more than 20 g in 48 hours. Studies have not shown that magnesium increases the risk of fetal abnormalities. If it is used, the possibility of fetal harm appears remote. However, studies cannot rule out the possibility of harm; use only if clearly needed.

Replacement therapy: Urine output should be maintained at a level of 100 ml q4h. Serum magnesium levels and the patient's clinical status are monitored to avoid overdosage.

DRUG INTERACTIONS

When used as an anticonvulsant, dosages of **barbiturates, narcotics, hypnotics,** and **systemic anesthetics** are adjusted because of additive depressant effects. Excessive neuromuscular blockade may occur if magnesium sulfate is used with **tubocurarine** or **succinylcholine.** Use with extreme caution in patients on **digitalis.** Treating toxicity with calcium in the digitalized patient may cause serious alterations in conduction and heart block.

ADVERSE REACTIONS

When used as an anticonvulsant, principal hazard is abnormally high magnesium levels. This may cause flushing, sweating, depressed reflexes, flaccid paralysis, hypotension, circulatory collapse, and cardiac and CNS depression. Hypocalcemia with tetany secondary to magnesium sulfate therapy has been reported. The most critical danger is respiratory depression.

Adverse effects seen with use as replacement therapy are usually the result of magnesium intoxication.

OVERDOSAGE

Symptoms: Sharp drop in blood pressure and respiratory paralysis. ECG changes reported include increased P–R interval, increased QRS complex, and prolonged Q–T interval. Heart block and asystole may occur.

Treatment: Artificial ventilation must be provided until a calcium salt can be injected IV to antagonize the effects of magnesium. A dose of 5 mEq to 10 mEq calcium will usually reverse the heart block and respiratory depression. Peritoneal dialysis and hemodialysis are also effective.

DOSAGE

Anticonvulsant therapy

Dosage is adjusted to patient requirements. Use is discontinued as soon as desired effect is obtained.

When repeated doses are given, test knee-jerk reflexes before each dose; if they are absent, do not give magnesium. Administration beyond the point of suppression of knee jerks may cause failure of the respiratory center and thus necessitate artificial respiration or the administration of IV calcium.

IM: 1 g to 5 g of a 25% to 50% solution 6 times a day as necessary.

IV: 1 g to 4 g of a 10% to 20% solution; not exceeding 1.5 ml/minute of 10% solution.

IV infusion: 4 g in 250 ml of 5% Dextrose, not exceeding 3 ml/minute.

Pediatric: IM—20 mg/kg to 40 mg/kg in a 20% solution; repeat as necessary.

Hyperalimentation: Magnesium maintenance requirements are not precisely known. *Maintenance dose range*—Adult, 8 mEq/day to 24 mEq/day; infant, 2 mEq/day to 10 mEq/day.

Mild magnesium deficiency: Adults—1 g (8.12 mEq or 2 ml of 50% solution) IM q6h for 4 doses (total of 32.5 mEq/24 hours).

Severe hypomagnesemia: IM—As much as 2 mEq/kg (0.5 ml of 50% solution) within 4 hours if necessary. *IV*—5 g (40 mEq)/1000 ml of 5% Dextrose in Water or Sodium Chloride for slow infusion over 3 hours.

NURSING IMPLICATIONS

HISTORY

Record etiology of hypomagnesemia or convulsant disorder; present symptomatology (when applicable); health history (especially history of cardiac or renal disease).

PHYSICAL ASSESSMENT

If used as an anticonvulsant, record neurologic symptoms and description of seizures. If used as replacement therapy in magnesium deficiency, record symptoms. Obtain vital signs. Depending on reason for use, serum electrolytes may be ordered before administration of magnesium sulfate.

ADMINISTRATION

Physician may order dosage in percentage and milliliters, in grams or in milliequivalents.

10% solution is 100 mg/ml or 0.8 mEq/ml.
12.5% solution is 125 mg/ml or 1 mEq/ml.
25% solution is 250 mg/ml or 2 mEq/ml.
50% solution is 500 mg/ml or 4 mEq/ml.

Check label and physician's order carefully when computing dose. If there is any question about clarity of the order or amount to be administered, check with the physician or hospital pharmacist.

For treatment of overdosage, have IV calcium preparation available before drug is administered IV or IM. Equipment for artifical ventilation is also recommended.

When repeated parenteral doses are given, test knee-jerk reflexes before each dose. If these reflexes are absent, do not give drug; notify physician.

IM: Usually 50% solution is used. If total volume of adult dose exceeds 5 ml, give in two separate sites. Give deep IM in gluteus muscle. *Pediatric administration*—Dilution of 50% solution to 20% concentration is recommended. Amount per injection site will depend on size of infant or child.

IV: Administer at a rate not exceeding 1.5 ml/minute of a 10% solution.

IV infusion: Prepare and administer according to physician's order (*e.g.,* volume and type of IV fluid, rate of administration). In severe hypomagnesemia, 5 g in 1000 ml of 5% Dextrose in Water or Sodium Chloride for infusion over 3 hours is recommended. *As anticonvulsant*—4 g in 250 ml of 5% Dextrose, not exceeding 3 ml/minute.

ONGOING ASSESSMENTS AND NURSING MANAGEMENT

When magnesium sulfate is given IV or by IV infusion as an anticonvulsant or for severe hypomagnesemia, patient requires constant observation. Obtain blood pressure, pulse, and respirations every 5 to 10 minutes.

CLINICAL ALERT: Observe patient for a sharp drop in blood pressure and respiratory paralysis (signs of overdosage). If these are observed, stop IV administration of drug immediately, run an IV solution (primary line) to KVO, and notify physician. Be prepared to provide artificial ventilation until calcium can be administered IV.

Early signs of hypermagnesemia are flushing, sweating, and drowsiness. Hypotension may also be seen at 3 mEq/liter to 5 mEq/liter. As magnesium level increases, weak to absent deep tendon reflexes and lethargy may be noted. Respiratory impairment may be noted when level reaches 10 mEq/liter.

When used before delivery, observe newborn for signs of magnesium toxicity (see above). If toxicity is noted, notify physician immediately. Be prepared to administer assisted ventilation until physician examines infant. IV calcium may be ordered.

When administered as replacement therapy or in TPN, urine output should be maintained at a level of 100 ml every 4 hours. Monitor intake and output; measure output hourly or as ordered. If urinary output drops below 25 ml/hour, notify physician. Do not administer repeat IM dose (replacement therapy) if urinary output is less than 100 ml/4 hours; contact physician.

Observe patient with hypomagnesemia and patient receiving replacement therapy for relief of symptoms (see Appendix 6, section 6-16 for symptoms of hypomagnesemia).

Frequent plasma magnesium levels are usually ordered. Laboratory requests are marked "emergency" because results should be obtained as soon as possible. Notify physician if magnesium level is higher or lower than normal range (1.5 mEq/liter–3 mEq/liter).

Magnesium Trisilicate

See Antacids.

Malathion Rx

lotion: 0.5%   Prioderm

INDICATIONS
Treatment of head lice and their ova.

CONTRAINDICATIONS
Hypersensitivity.

ACTIONS
Is lousicidal and ovicidal. Human safety studies have shown no evidence of sensitization and a very low level of irritation.

WARNINGS
Avoid open flames or hair dryers because this product is flammable. Allow hair to dry naturally and uncovered.

Use in pregnancy only if clearly needed. It is not known whether malathion is excreted in human milk; exercise caution when administering to a nursing mother.

PRECAUTIONS
If accidentally placed in eye, flush immediately with water.

ADVERSE REACTIONS
Scalp irritation.

OVERDOSAGE
Symptoms: Although a weaker cholinesterase inhibitor and therefore safer than other organophosphates, malathion may be expected to exhibit the

same symptoms of cholinesterase depletion after accidental oral ingestion.

Treatment: Induce vomiting promptly or lavage stomach with 5% sodium bicarbonate solution. Severe respiratory distress is the major and most serious symptom of organophosphate poisoning, requiring artificial respiration and large doses of IM or IV atropine. Usual starting dose of atropine is 1 mg to 4 mg with supplementation hourly, as needed, to counteract symptoms of cholinesterase depletion. Repeat analysis of serum and RBC cholinesterase assist in establishing the diagnosis and formulating a long-range prognosis.

DOSAGE

See *Administration*. If required, repeat with second application in 7 to 9 days. Further treatment is generally not necessary.

NURSING IMPLICATIONS

HISTORY

Source of infestation should be determined, if possible. Investigate possibility of school, family members, and so on because concurrent treatment may be necessary. School may notify parents if pediculosis is found in one or more pupils.

PHYSICAL ASSESSMENT

Examine affected area; note extent of infestation.

ADMINISTRATION

Apply early in morning. Sprinkle on hair and gently rub until soapy and thoroughly moistened. Allow to dry naturally; use no heat, and leave uncovered. After 8 to 12 hours, shampoo the hair. Rinse and use fine-tooth comb to remove dead lice and eggs.

ONGOING ASSESSMENTS AND NURSING MANAGEMENT

Hospitalized patient should be isolated from others (when possible) to prevent transmission. Wash hands thoroughly after patient contact. Bed linens and hospital gown are placed in isolation linen bag and laundered separately.

Shampoo hair at time ordered (see *Administration*).

If patient complains of itching or burning, inspect scalp for signs of irritation. If irritation is apparent, contact physician because lotion may have to be removed.

Bedding and hospital gown should be changed before application of drug and when drug is removed.

PATIENT AND FAMILY INFORMATION

NOTE: Patient and family members may be embarrassed and may refrain from asking questions. The nurse should have an understanding manner and make an effort to present information so that the patient or family member feels as comfortable as possible.

Avoid getting in or near eyes. If accidentally placed in eye, flush immediately with water.

Allow hair to dry naturally. Product is flammable; do *not* use hair dryers, and avoid open flames.

Clothing and bed linens should be washed in very hot water (boiling water is best), separately from clothes of other family members.

Other family members or close contacts should be examined by a physician.

Follow physician's instructions and instructions supplied with product for application and removal.

Mannitol Rx

| injection: 5%, 10%, 15%, 20% | Osmitrol, *Generic* |
| injection: 25% | *Generic* |

INDICATIONS

Therapeutic: Promotion of diuresis in the prevention and treatment of the oliguric phase of acute renal failure before irreversible renal failure becomes established. Also used for reduction of intracranial pressure and treatment of cerebral edema by reducing brain mass and promoting urinary excretion of toxic substances, and for reduction of elevated intraocular pressure when the pressure cannot be lowered by other means.

Diagnostic: Measurement of glomerular filtration rate.

CONTRAINDICATIONS

Well-established anuria due to severe renal disease; severe pulmonary congestion or frank pulmonary edema; active intracranial bleeding except during craniotomy; severe dehydration; progressive renal damage or dysfunction, including increasing oliguria and azotemia, after institution of mannitol therapy; progressive heart failure or pulmonary congestion after mannitol therapy.

ACTIONS

Mannitol is an obligatory osmotic diuretic. When administered parenterally, it is confined to the extracellular space. It is only slightly metabolized and is rapidly excreted by the kidneys. Approximately 80% of a 100-g dose appears in the urine in 3 hours. Mannitol is freely filtered by the glomeruli with less than 10% tubular reabsorption; it is not secreted by tubular cells. It induces diuresis by elevating the osmolarity of the glomerular filtrate, thereby hindering tubular reabsorption of water. Excretion of sodium and chloride is increased.

WARNINGS

Use in impaired renal function: Use with caution in those with significant renal dysfunction. In those with severe renal impairment, a test dose (see *Administration* and *Dosage*) is recommended. A second test dose may be tried if there is inadequate response. No more than two test doses are recommended. Urine output is monitored closely; infusion is discontinued promptly if output is low. If output continues to decline during infusion, the patient's clinical status is reviewed and the infusion is discontinued if necessary. Inadequate urinary output results in accumulation of mannitol and expansion of extracellular fluid volume, and it could result in water intoxication or CHF. Monitor renal function closely during mannitol infusion. Osmotic nephrosis, a reversible vacuolization of the tubules of no known clinical significance, may proceed to severe irreversible nephrosis.

The obligatory diuretic response following rapid infusion of 15%, 20%, or 25% mannitol may further aggravate preexisting hemoconcentration.

Use mannitol with caution in those with significant cardiopulmonary dysfunction.

Electrolyte imbalance: Excessive loss of water and electrolytes may lead to serious imbalances. With continued administration of mannitol, loss of water in excess of electrolytes can cause hypernatremia. Electrolyte measurements, including sodium and potassium, are important in monitoring the infusion of mannitol.

Use during pregnancy: Safety is not established. Not used in women of childbearing potential or, particularly, in early pregnancy unless potential benefits outweigh the possible hazards.

Use in children: Dosage requirements for children under 12 are not established.

PRECAUTIONS

Cardiovascular status is carefully evaluated before rapid administration of mannitol because sudden expansion of the extracellular fluid may lead to fulminating CHF.

Shift of sodium-free intracellular fluid into the extracellular compartment following mannitol infusion may lower sodium concentration and aggravate preexisting hyponatremia. By sustaining diuresis, mannitol administration may obscure and intensify inadequate hydration or hypovolemia.

ADVERSE REACTIONS

Isolated cases of adverse reactions, such as pulmonary congestion, fluid and electrolyte imbalance, acidosis, electrolyte loss, dry mouth, thirst, osmotic nephrosis, marked diuresis, urinary retention, edema, headache, blurred vision, convulsions, nausea, vomiting, rhinitis, diarrhea, arm pain, skin necrosis, thrombophlebitis, chills, dizziness, urticaria, dehydration, hypotension, hypertension, tachycardia, fever, and anginalike chest pains have been reported during and following mannitol infusion.

DOSAGE

Administer by IV infusion only. Total dosage, concentration, and rate of administration should be governed by the nature and severity of the condition treated, fluid requirement, and urinary output. Usual adult dose ranges from 50 g/24 hours to 200 g/24 hours; in most instances adequate response will be achieved with 100 g/24 hours. Rate of administration is usually adjusted to maintain a urine flow of at least 30 ml/hour to 50 ml/hour. Lower mannitol concentration and solutions containing sodium chloride are useful in preventing dehydration and electrolyte depletion. This dosage outline is only a general guide.

Test dose: Administered before therapy for those with marked oliguria or those believed to have inadequate renal function. Infuse 0.2 g/kg (about 50 ml of a 25% solution, 75 ml of a 20% solution, or 100 ml of a 15% solution) in 3 to 5 minutes to produce a urine flow of at least 30 ml/hour to 50 ml/hour. If urine flow does not increase, a second test dose may be given. If there is inadequate response, patient is reevaluated.

Prevention of acute renal failure (oliguria):
When used during cardiovascular and other types of surgery—50 g to 100 g as a 5% to 25% solution. Concentration depends on fluid requirements.

Treatment of oliguria: 300–400 mg/kg of 20% or 25% solution; up to 100 g of 15% or 20% solution.

Reduction of intracranial pressure and brain mass: A total dose of 1.5 g/kg to 2 g/kg is administered as a 15% to 25% solution, infused over 30 to 60 minutes, to reduce brain mass before or after neurosurgery. Circulatory and renal reserve are evaluated before and during administration at this relatively high dose and rapid infusion rate. Evaluate fluid and electrolyte balance, body weight, and total output before and after infusion. Evidence of reduced cerebral spinal fluid pressure must be observed within 15 minutes after starting infusion.

Reduction of intraocular pressure: 1.5 g/kg to 2 g/kg as a 25% solution (6 ml/kg to 8 ml/kg), as a 20% solution (7.5 ml/kg to 10 ml/kg), or as a 15% solution (10 ml/kg to 13 ml/kg) may be given over

M

30 minutes in order to obtain prompt and maximal effect. When using preoperatively, administer 1 to 1½ hours before surgery to achieve maximal effect.

Adjunctive therapy for intoxications: As an agent to promote diuresis. Concentration depends on fluid requirement and urinary output. IV water and electrolytes must be given to replace loss of these substances in the urine, sweat, and expired air. If benefits are not observed after administration of 200 g, infusion is discontinued.

Measurement of glomerular filtration rate (GFR): 100 ml of 20% solution (20 g) should be diluted with 180 ml of Sodium Chloride Injection (normal saline). The resulting 280 ml of 7.2% solution is infused at a rate of 20 ml/minute. Urine is collected by catheter for a specific period of time and analyzed for mannitol excreted in milligrams per minute. A blood sample is drawn at the start and end of the time period and the concentration of mannitol is determined in milligrams per milliliter of plasma. The GFR is the number of milliliters of plasma that must have been filtered to account for the amount excreted per minute in the urine. Normal clearance rates are approximately 125 ml/minute for men and 116 ml/minute for women.

NURSING IMPLICATIONS

HISTORY
See Appendix 4.

PHYSICAL ASSESSMENT
Obtain vital signs, weight. Review chart for recent urinary output. Laboratory tests include serum electrolytes and renal-function studies. Cardiac status is evaluated prior to administration. Other laboratory tests may also be appropriate.

ADMINISTRATION
Indwelling catheter is usually inserted before administration (reduction of intraocular pressure may not require indwelling catheter).

Physician must order percentage of solution (available as 5%, 10%, 15%, 20%, and 25%), amount of drug (in ml or g), and rate of infusion (as ml/minute or mg/minute) or the time period for administration (*e.g.,* 30 minutes, 3–5 minutes). The rate of infusion may also be adjusted according to the urinary output (as in treatment of oliguria). The physician must establish guidelines for minimal and maximal rate of infusion and the desired urinary output (see *Dosage*).

A test dose is given prior to therapy to those with marked oliguria (see *Dosage*). Amount of test (ordered by physician) is infused in 3 to 5 minutes. Expected response is 30 ml/hour to 50 ml/hour. Urinary output may be measured every 15, 30, or 60 minutes. Check with physician about desired interval for urine measurements.

Preparation of solution: When exposed to low temperatures, solution may crystallize. Concentrations greater than 15% have a greater tendency to crystallize. If crystals are observed, warm bottle in a hot water bath, and then cool to body temperature before administering. When infusing 10% and 20% mannitol, the administration set should include a filter.

When mannitol is infused over a short period of time (*e.g.,* 5–60 minutes), a primary and secondary infusion set may be advisable.

When mannitol is administered to measure GFR, see *Dosage,* above. Physician may also order slight variation of this procedure.

Electrolyte-free mannitol solutions should not be given conjointly with blood. If it is essential that blood be given simultaneously, at least 20 mEq of sodium chloride is added to each liter of mannitol to avoid agglutination.

ONGOING ASSESSMENTS AND NURSING MANAGEMENT
Intake and output are monitored closely during administration of mannitol.

Physician may order urine output measured at specific intervals (*e.g.,* q15m, q30m). Specific gravity of urine may also be ordered. Record intake and output on flow sheet. Keep physician informed of urinary output.

Rate of infusion is usually adjusted to maintain urine flow of at least 30 ml/hour to 50 ml/hour. If there is a question about increasing or decreasing the rate of infusion (based on hourly urine output), discuss with physician.

Monitor blood pressure, pulse, and respirations q30m or as ordered. Notify physician of any significant change in vital signs.

Check IV infusion site q15m to q30m. If extravasation is apparent, IV must be discontinued and a new site selected.

CLINICAL ALERT: Infusion of mannitol is discontinued if urinary output is low. If urinary output decreases below guidelines established by the physician, discontinue mannitol and run an IV infusion to KVO until physician examines patient. Failure to discontinue mannitol when urinary output is decreased may result in fluid overload and fulminating CHF.

Observe for signs of fluid and electrolyte imbalance, especially dehydration, fluid overload, hypokalemia, hyperkalemia, hyponatremia, and hypernatremia (see Appendix 6, sections 6-10, 6-12, 6-15, and 6-17).

Measurement of electrolytes, including sodium and potassium, is of vital importance in monitoring mannitol therapy. Keep physician informed of all abnormal laboratory results.

Oral fluids may or may not be allowed. If oral fluids are ordered, give in small amounts. If oral fluids are not allowed, check with physician whether ice chips may be given if patient complains of thirst or dry mouth.

Daily weight may be ordered to determine fluid retention or loss; a bed scale may be used if patient is on complete bedrest.

Dosage section is only a general guideline to administration. Infusion rates, time of infusion, and hourly urine output guidelines may vary in certain situations.

Maprotiline Hydrochloride

See Antidepressants, Tricyclic Compounds.

Mazindol

See Anorexiants.

Measles Vaccine

See Immunizations, Active.

Measles, Mumps, and Rubella Vaccine

See Immunizations, Active.

Measles and Rubella Vaccine

See Immunizations, Active.

Mebendazole Rx

tablets, chewable: Vermox
  100 mg

INDICATIONS
Treatment of *Trichuris trichiura* (whipworm), *Enterobius vermicularis* (pinworm), *Ascaris lumbricoides* (roundworm), *Ancylostoma duodenale* (common hookworm), or *Necator americanus* (American hookworm) in single or mixed infections. Efficacy varies as a function of such factors as preexisting

diarrhea and GI transit time, degree of infection, and helminth strains.

CONTRAINDICATIONS
Hypersensitivity. Also contraindicated in pregnancy because it may have a risk of producing fetal damage.

ACTIONS
Exerts its anthelmintic effect by blocking glucose uptake by the susceptible helminths, thereby depleting endogenous glycogen stored within the parasite. Glycogen depletion results in decreased formation of adenosine triphosphate (ATP), required for survival and reproduction of the helminth.

PRECAUTIONS
Safety and efficacy for use in children under 2 not established; the relative benefits and risks should be considered.

ADVERSE REACTIONS
Transient symptoms of abdominal pain and diarrhea have occurred in cases of massive infection and expulsion of worms. Fever, which may be a possible response to drug-induced tissue necrosis, has occurred.

DOSAGE (CHILDREN AND ADULTS)
Trichuriasis, ascariasis, hookworm infection: 1 tablet administered morning and evening on three consecutive days.
Enterobiasis: Single tablet given once.

NURSING IMPLICATIONS

HISTORY
See Appendix 4. A careful history of travel, eating habits, and sanitary facilities may be necessary to determine the source of infection. Because pinworm is easily transmitted from person to person, it is recommended that all family members be treated for complete parasite eradication. Family members should also have stool samples examined if the patient has whipworm, roundworm, or hookworm. Infection is usually reported to the public health department.

PHYSICAL ASSESSMENT
If patient is hospitalized or the outpatient appears ill or malnourished, obtain vital signs and weight. Examination of stools for ova and parasites will be ordered for confirmation of diagnosis. Pinworm specimen may be collected (in early A.M. before patient gets out of bed) by means of cellophane tape, wrapped with the

M

sticky side out around tongue blade or fingers; press against anal area (female pinworms deposit ova at night in perianal area). Transfer tape (sticky side down) to glass slide for microscopic examination. Other laboratory tests may include CBC and serum electrolytes, especially if patient shows evidence of weight loss or appears ill, or if massive infection is suspected.

ADMINISTRATION

Tablets may be chewed, swallowed, or crushed and mixed with food. If mixing with food, use only a small amount so that patient takes entire dose.

No special procedures, such as fasting or purging, are required.

ONGOING ASSESSMENTS AND NURSING MANAGEMENT

Isolation is rarely necessary; linen and stool precautions may be necessary in some instances. Wash hands thoroughly before and after each patient contact, especially when disposing of urine or feces or changing bed linens.

If patient is hospitalized, monitor vital signs daily (q4h if patient acutely ill or has a massive infection).

Diarrhea may occur with massive infection and expulsion of worms. Observe for signs of dehydration, hypokalemia, and hyponatremia (see Appendix 6, sections 6-10, 6-15, and 6-17). Notify physician if diarrhea is severe or signs of fluid or electrolyte imbalance occur.

Physician may order saving of all stool specimens for laboratory examination. Collect specimen in bedpan, transfer to stool-specimen container, and take to laboratory immediately. Advise patient to avoid urinating in bedpan, if possible.

If patient is anemic (anemia may be seen with hookworm, whipworm) blood transfusions or iron therapy may be necessary.

PATIENT AND FAMILY INFORMATION

NOTE: Patients with hookworm, roundworm, or whipworm should have a thorough investigation of sanitary facilities if family resides in an endemic area. A public health department referral may be necessary to help family establish proper disposal of urine and feces.

The tablet may be chewed, swallowed, or crushed and mixed with a small amount of food.

Wash hands thoroughly after defecation and urination and before handling food or eating.

Repeated stool examinations will be necessary until physician is sure that helminth is eradicated.

Change and launder undergarments, bed linen, towels, and nightclothes daily (to prevent reinfection). Bathe daily (showering is best). Disinfect toilet facilities daily.

Clean under fingernails daily. Avoid putting fingers in mouth; nail biting must be avoided (liquid preparations that have a bitter taste and are painted on the nails and fingertips to discourage nail biting are available if patient persists in biting nails).

Whipworm: Avoid contaminating soil with feces. Children should be discouraged from playing in areas where soil may be contaminated.

Hookworm: In endemic areas, shoes should be worn at all times because worm enters through skin, usually the sole of the foot.

Roundworm: Thoroughly wash all vegetables grown in contaminated soil.

Mecamylamine Hydrochloride Rx

tablets: 2.5 mg   Inversine

INDICATIONS

Management of moderately severe to severe essential hypertension and in uncomplicated cases of malignant hypertension. See also Antihypertensive Agents.

CONTRAINDICATIONS

Coronary insufficiency or recent myocardial infarction. Should not be used in mild, labile hypertension; may prove unsuitable in uncooperative patients. Give with discretion, if at all, when renal insufficiency is manifested by a rising or elevated BUN. Contraindicated in uremia. Those with chronic pyelonephritis receiving antibiotics and sulfonamides should not be treated with this or other ganglionic blockers. Additional contraindications are glaucoma, organic pyloric stenosis, or hypersensitivity to mecamylamine.

ACTIONS

A potent oral ganglionic blocker with antihypertensive effects. Although this antihypertensive effect is predominantly orthostatic, supine blood pressure is also significantly reduced. Reduces blood pressure in both normotensive and hypertensive individuals. Because of the many side-effects, ganglionic blockers are infrequently used.

Is almost completely absorbed from the GI tract. Has a gradual onset of action (30 minutes–2 hours) and a long-lasting effect (usually 6–12 hours or more).

WARNINGS

CNS effects: Mecamylamine, a secondary amine, readily penetrates into the brain and thus may produce CNS effects. Tremor, choreiform movements, mental abberations, and convulsions occur rarely. These have occurred most often when large doses are used, especially in patients with cerebral or renal insufficiency.

Discontinuation of therapy: When ganglionic blockers are discontinued suddenly, hypertensive levels return. In those with malignant hypertension and others, this may occur abruptly and may cause fatal cerebral vascular accidents or acute congestive heart failure (CHF). When drug is withdrawn, it is done so gradually and other antihypertensive therapy is substituted. The effects of mecamylamine can last from hours to days after therapy is discontinued.

PRECAUTIONS

Patient's condition, particularly renal and cardiovascular function, is evaluated carefully. When renal, cerebral, or coronary blood flow is deficient, any additional impairment, which might result from added hypotension, must be avoided. Use with caution in patients with marked cerebral and coronary arteriosclerosis or after a recent cerebrovascular accident (CVA).

The action of mecamylamine may be potentiated by excessive heat, fever, infection, hemorrhage, pregnancy, surgery, vigorous exercise, and salt depletion resulting from diminished intake or increased excretion due to diarrhea, vomiting, excessive sweating, or diuretics. During therapy, sodium intake is not restricted; if necessary, dosage of ganglionic blocker is adjusted.

Urinary retention may occur; therefore, caution is required in those with prostatic hypertrophy, bladder neck obstruction, and urethral stricture.

DRUG INTERACTIONS

Action of mecamylamine may be potentiated by **anesthesia, diuretics, other antihypertensive drugs,** or **alcohol.**

ADVERSE REACTIONS

GI: Anorexia, dry mouth and glossitis, nausea, vomiting, constipation (sometimes preceded by small, frequent, liquid stools), ileus. Constipation may be prevented by giving pilocarpine or neostigmine with each dose. Constipation is treated with milk of magnesia or similar laxative; bulk laxatives should not be used. Frequent loose bowel movements with abdominal distention and decreased borborygmi may be the first signs of paralytic ileus.

If these are present, drug is discontinued immediately and remedial steps taken.

Cardiovascular: Orthostatic dizziness, syncope, and paresthesia may occur. Interstitial pulmonary edema and fibrosis have been described after blood pressure reduction with potent antihypertensive agents. Postural hypotension due to excessive response may be corrected by adjustment of dosage.

CNS: Weakness, fatigue, sedation, dilated pupils, and blurred vision may occur. Rare instances of tremor, choreiform movements, mental aberrations, and convulsions have been reported.

Miscellaneous: Decreased libido, impotence, urinary retention.

OVERDOSAGE

Pressor amines may be used to counteract excessive hypotension. Because patients being treated with ganglionic blockers are more normally reactive to pressor amines, small doses are recommended to avoid excessive response.

DOSAGE

Therapy is usually started with 2.5 mg bid. Initial dose is modified in increments of 2.5 mg at intervals of not less than 2 days until desired blood-pressure response occurs (the criterion being a dosage just under that which causes signs of mild postural hypotension). Average total daily dosage is 25 mg, usually in three divided doses; as little as 2.5 mg/day may be sufficient for some patients. A range of two to four or even more doses may be required in severe cases when smooth control is difficult to obtain. In severe or urgent cases, larger increments at smaller intevals may be needed. Partial tolerance may develop, requiring an increase in the daily dosage.

Administration after meals may cause a more gradual absorption and smoother control of excessively high blood pressure. Timing of doses in relation to meals should be consistent. Because the blood-pressure response to antihypertensive drugs is increased in the early morning, larger doses are given at noontime and in the evening. The morning dose should be relatively small and in some instances may even be omitted.

Blood-pressure monitoring: Initial dosage is determined by blood-pressure readings in the erect position at time of maximal effect of the drug as well as by other signs and symptoms of orthostatic hypotension. Effective maintenance dosage is regulated by blood-pressure readings in the erect position and by limitation of dosage to that which causes slight faintness or dizziness in this position.

Concomitant antihypertensive therapy: When given with other antihypertensive drugs, dosage of

M

these other agents as well as that of mecamylamine should be reduced to avoid excessive hypotension. However, thiazides should be continued in their usual dosage while the dosage of mecamylamine is reduced by at least 50%.

NURSING IMPLICATIONS

HISTORY
See Appendix 4.

PHYSICAL ASSESSMENT
Obtain blood pressure on both arms with patient in the standing position after patient has rested for 5 to 10 minutes; obtain pulse, respiratory rate, weight; assess for evidence of peripheral edema. Renal-function studies and ECG are usually ordered. Other laboratory studies may also be appropriate.

ADMINISTRATION
Administer after meals; timing of administration after meals must be consistent (see *Dosage*).

Physician may order larger doses given at noontime and in the evening and smaller dose in the morning. Medicine card must clearly indicate dose for each time of day.

ONGOING ASSESSMENTS AND NURSING MANAGEMENT
Blood pressure and pulse are monitored frequently during initial dosage period. Obtain blood pressure on both arms with patient in standing position (after patient has rested 5–10 minutes if he has been active prior to obtaining blood pressure).

Discuss with physician time blood pressure is to be monitored. Readings may be ordered immediately prior to administration as well as 2 to 4 or more hours after administration.

During initial adjustment period, it is important that blood pressure is obtained at specific intervals. Use of a flow sheet aids in identifying changes.

CLINICAL ALERT: Withhold drug and contact physician if there is a significant change in the systolic or diastolic pressure or the pulse rate, or if patient experiences orthostatic hypotension. An immediate dosage adjustment may be necessary.

Drug is withdrawn gradually and other antihypertensive therapy substituted. Sudden discontinuation of therapy may result in abrupt return of hypertensive levels, resulting in fatal CVAs or acute CHF, especially in those with malignant hypertension. Ensure continuity of prescribed therapy by notation on the Kardex, informing health-team members responsible for drug administration.

Frequent loose bowel movements with abdominal distention and decreased bowel sounds may be early signs of paralytic ileus. Withhold next dose and notify physician immediately if these should occur.

When patient is arising from a lying position, have him sit on edge of bed and dangle legs for approximately 5 minutes. Once maintenance dosage is achieved, patient may be able to shorten time between position changes.

Observe for adverse reactions. Notify physician if lightheadedness or dizziness (especially on standing or making position changes), or constipation or diarrhea occurs.

A special diet (*e.g.,* weight reduction, low cholesterol) may be ordered. Sodium intake is not restricted.

Excessive heat, fever, infection, hemorrhage, surgery, diarrhea, vomiting, excessive sweating, diminished salt intake (*e.g.,* decreased dietary intake), diuretics, and pregnancy may necessitate dosage adjustment. Patients with these conditions should be closely observed for signs of excessive hypotension, orthostatic hypotension.

Observe for urinary retention in those with a history of prostatic hypertrophy, bladder neck obstruction, and urethral stricture. Elderly men without a history of a GU disorder should be observed for urinary retention.

Physician may prescribe pilocarpine or neostigmine with each dose to prevent constipation. Constipation may also be treated with milk of magnesia or a similar laxative. Bulk laxatives are not recommended.

Monitor dietary intake. If anorexia occurs, discuss with physician because salt depletion may require dosage adjustment.

Dry mouth may be relieved by frequent sips of water, hard candy, or chewing gum.

PATIENT AND FAMILY INFORMATION
NOTE: Complete patient compliance is necessary. Patient and family members must be given thorough instructions about dosage schedule, adverse reactions, and symptoms or problems requiring notification of the physician. The physician may recommend self-monitoring of blood pressure and may give specific instructions about omission or reduction of a dose if readings fall below a designated level or faintness or lightheadedness occurs. The patient or family member will require instructions in use of a sphygmomanometer and obtaining correct readings.

Take after meals.

Do not discontinue taking this medication or omit or change dosage unless directed by physician.

Avoid cough, cold, or allergy medications (some contain sympathomimetics), except on professional recommendation. Avoid use of laxatives or antidiarrheal medications should constipation or diarrhea occur, unless use is recommended by physician.

Notify physician of any side-effects.

If dizziness or lightheadedness occurs, avoid sudden changes in posture; rise slowly from a lying or sitting position.

Avoid alcohol because it potentiates the action of mecamylamine.

Notify the physician or nurse immediately if any of the following should occur, because dosage adjustment may be necessary: exposure to excessive heat, fever, infection, hemorrhage, pregnancy, vigorous exercise and salt depletion resulting from loss of appetite or increased excretion due to diarrhea, vomiting, excessive sweating.

Mechlorethamine Hydrochloride

(Nitrogen Mustard) Rx

injection: 10 mg/vial   Mustargen

INDICATIONS

When administered IV, used for palliative treatment of Hodgkin's disease (Stages III, IV), lymphosarcoma, chronic myelocytic or chronic lymphocytic leukemia, polycythemia vera, mycosis fungoides, and bronchogenic carcinoma. When given intrapleurally, intraperitoneally, or intrapericardially, indicated for palliative treatment of effusion secondary to metastatic carcinoma.

CONTRAINDICATIONS

Because of toxicity and unpleasant side-effects, potential risk and discomfort from use in those with inoperable neoplasms or in terminal stage of the disease must be balanced against the limited gains available. These gains will vary with the nature and status of the disease. Routine use in widely disseminated neoplasms is not recommended.

Use in those with leukopenia, thrombocytopenia, and anemia due to invasion of the bone marrow carries a greater risk. In these, a good response with disappearance of the tumor from the bone marrow may be associated with improvement of bone-marrow function. In the absence of a positive response or in patients who have previously been treated with chemotherapeutic agents, hematopoiesis may be further compromised; leukopenia, thrombocytopenia, and anemia may become more severe, leading to death of the patient.

Tumors of the bone and nervous system respond poorly. Also contraindicated in presence of known infectious diseases. Results are unpredictable in disseminated and malignant tumors of different types.

ACTIONS

An alkylating agent with cytotoxic, mutagenic, and radiomimetic actions that inhibit rapidly proliferating cells. Is rapidly transformed and excreted largely in the urine as inactive metabolites.

WARNINGS

Extravasation into subcutaneous tissue may result in painful inflammation. The area usually becomes indurated and sloughing may occur.

Use may contribute to extensive and rapid development of amyloidosis; use drug only if foci of acute and chronic suppurative inflammation are absent.

Use in pregnancy, lactation: There is evidence that nitrogen mustards have induced fetal abnormalities, particularly when used in early pregnancy. Possible benefits of administration to women of childbearing potential must be weighed against the risks. In pregnant patients requiring treatment for a life-threatening progressive tumor, use should be avoided at least until the third trimester. Breast-feeding should be stopped before beginning treatment.

PRECAUTIONS

Drug is highly toxic; both powder and solution must be handled and administered with care. It is a powerful vesicant and intended primarily for IV use. Inhalation of dust and vapors and contact with the skin or mucous membranes, especially the eyes, must be avoided.

Because drug toxicity, especially sensitivity to bone-marrow failure, seems to be more common in chronic lymphatic leukemia than in other conditions, drug is administered with great caution, if at all, for this disorder.

Concomitant therapy: Exercise caution in use of mechlorethamine and x-ray therapy or other chemotherapy in alternating courses. Hematopoietic function is characteristically depressed by either form of therapy; neither should be given until bone-marrow function has recovered. Irradiation of areas such as the sternum, ribs, and vertebrae shortly after a course of nitrogen mustard may lead to hematologic complications. Therapy with nitrogen mustard may be associated with an increased incidence of a second malignant tumor, especially when such therapy is combined with other antineoplastic agents or radiation therapy.

Urate precipitation may develop during therapy and should be anticipated (particularly in the treat-

M

ment of lymphomas); adequate methods for control of hyperuricemia should be instituted and careful attention directed toward adequate fluid intake before treatment.

ADVERSE REACTIONS

Use is usually accompanied by toxic manifestations.

Local toxicity: Thrombosis and thrombophlebitis may result from direct contact of drug with intima of the injected vein. High concentration and prolonged contact with the drug is avoided, especially in cases of elevated pressure in the antebrachial vein (*e.g.,* in mediastinal tumor compression from severe vena cava syndrome). Extravasation may cause inflammation and induration and may progress to tissue necrosis.

Systemic toxicity: Nausea, vomiting, and depression of formed elements in the circulating blood are dose-limiting side-effects that usually occur with full doses. Jaundice, alopecia, vertigo, tinnitus, and diminished hearing occur infrequently. Rarely, hemolytic anemia associated with such diseases as the lymphomas and chronic lymphocytic leukemia may be precipitated by treatment with alkylating agents. Various chromosomal abnormalities have been reported.

Given preferably at night in case sedation for side-effects is required. Nausea and vomiting usually occur 1 to 3 hours after administration. Anorexia, weakness, and diarrhea may also occur.

Hematologic: Usual course of treatment (total dose of 0.4 mg/kg) generally produces lymphocytopenia within 24 hours after first injection; significant granulocytopenia occurs within 6 to 8 days and lasts for 10 days to 3 weeks. Agranulocytosis appears to be relatively infrequent; recovery from leukopenia in most cases is complete within 2 weeks. Thrombocytopenia is variable, but the time course of the appearance and recovery from reduced platelet counts generally parallels the sequence of granulocyte levels. In some, severe thrombocytopenia may lead to bleeding from the gums and GI tract, petechiae, and small cutaneous hemorrhages. These symptoms appear to be transient and in most cases disappear with return to a normal platelet count. A severe and even uncontrollable depression of the hematopoietic system occasionally may follow the usual dose, particularly in those with widespread disease and debility and in patients previously treated with antineoplastic agents or x-ray therapy. Persistent pancytopenia has been reported in rare instances; hemorrhagic complications may be due to hyperheparinemia. Erythrocyte and hemoglobin levels may decline during the first 2 weeks after therapy but rarely significantly. Depression of the hematopoietic system may occur up to 50 days or more after starting therapy.

With total doses exceeding 0.4 mg/kg for a single course, severe leukopenia, anemia, thrombocytopenia, and hemorrhagic diathesis with subsequent delayed bleeding may develop. Death may follow. The only treatment in instances of excessive dosage appears to be repeated blood product transfusions, antibiotic treatment of complicating infections, and general supportive measures. Use extreme caution when exceeding the average recommended dose.

Immunosuppression: Nitrogen mustard is reported to have immunosuppressive activity. Use of the drug may predispose patient to bacterial, viral, or fungal infection. This is more likely to occur when concomitant stereoid therapy is employed.

Dermatologic: Occasionally, a maculopapular skin eruption occurs; this will not necessarily occur with subsequent courses. Herpes zoster, a common complicating infection in those with lymphomas, may first appear after therapy is reinstituted and on occasion may be precipitated by treatment. Further treatment is discontinued during the acute phase of this illness to avoid progression to generalized herpes zoster.

Reproductive: Because gonads are susceptible to mechlorethamine, treatment may be followed by delayed menses, oligomenorrhea, or temporary or permanent amenorrhea. Impaired spermatogenesis, azoospermia, and local germinal aplasia have been reported in males treated with alkylating agents, especially in combination with other drugs. In some instances, spermatogenesis may return in patients in remission, but this may occur several years after intensive chemotherapy is discontinued.

DOSAGE

IV: Dosage varies with clinical situation, therapeutic response, and magnitude of hematologic depression. A total dose of 0.4 mg/kg for each course is usually given as a single dose or in two or four divided doses of 0.1 mg/kg/day to 0.2 mg/kg/day. Dosage should be based on ideal body weight. Presence of edema or ascites may be considered so that dosage will be based on dry body weight.

Within a few minutes after IV injection, mechlorethamine undergoes chemical transformation, combined with reactive compounds, and is no longer present in its active form in the bloodstream. Subsequent courses are not given until patient has recovered hematologically from the previous course. It is often possible to give repeated courses as early as 3 weeks after treatment. Margin of safety is narrow and considerable care is exercised in the matter of dosage.

Intracavity: Used with varying success in certain malignant conditions for control of pleural, peritoneal, and pericardial effusions caused by malignant cells. Consult product labeling for details of administration; the technique and dose used by any of these routes varies.

NURSING IMPLICATIONS

HISTORY
See Appendix 4. Note previous therapy (radiation, chemotherapy).

PHYSICAL ASSESSMENT
Obtain physical, emotional status; vital signs; weight. Look for evidence of edema or ascites. CBC, differential, platelet count, and serum uric acid are usually ordered. Other laboratory tests may also be appropriate.

ADMINISTRATION
Usually given in evening.

Physician may order an antiemetic to be given immediately before administration of mechlorethamine. An analgesic may be ordered if drug is given intraperitoneally.

Adequate fluid intake prior to administration (usually for 24 hours) is recommended to prevent urate precipitation, particularly in those with lymphomas.

Solution should be prepared immediately before each injection because it decomposes on standing.

Physician orders IV infusion and diluent for reconstitution (water, sodium chloride).

Solution is best prepared under a laminar air flow hood. In some hospitals the solution may be prepared by a pharmacist. Notify pharmacy the day before or the morning of the day administration is scheduled.

Prior to preparation of the solution, have available isotonic ophthalmologic irrigating solution (should accidental eye contact occur), 2% thiosulfate solution (should accidental skin contact occur), and solution for decontamination of materials (equal volumes of 5% sodium thiosulfate and 5% sodium bicarbonate). These solutions are obtained from pharmacy.

CLINICAL ALERT: Drug is a powerful vesicant. Wear gloves when reconstituting drug. Both powder and reconstituted solution must be handled and administered with care.

Avoid inhalation of dust or vapors while preparing drug.

If accidental eye contact should occur, immediately irrigate with copious amounts of isotonic ophthalmic irrigation solution, followed by prompt ophthalmologic examination.

Should accidental skin contact occur, the affected part must be irrigated immediately with copious amounts of water for at least 15 minutes, followed by 2% sodium thiosulfate solution.

Preparation of solution: Each vial contains 10 mg. Using a sterile needle and syringe, reconstitute with 10 ml of Sterile Water for Injection or Sodium Chloride Injection. With the needle still in the rubber stopper (and the syringe attached), shake vial several times to completely dissolve the drug. The resultant solution contains 1 mg/ml.

Do not use if resulting solution is discolored or if droplets of water are visible within the vial.

When selecting site for IV infusion the forearm is preferred. The veins on the dorsum of the hand are avoided, when possible. If patient has had a mastectomy, use arm on the opposite side.

Drug may be injected into any suitable vein; preferably, drug is injected into the injection port of rubber or plastic tubing of a flowing IV infusion set. Check for blood return before and during injection of drug. Injection should be completed in a few minutes. The physician may order the IV infusion to run for several minutes following injection to flush the tubing.

CLINICAL ALERT: Extravasation of the drug into subcutaneous tissue results in painful inflammation. The area usually becomes indurated and sloughing may occur. Advise patient to mention immediately if pain or burning is noted during injection. If leakage of the drug is obvious, discontinue administration and promptly infiltrate area with sterile isotonic sodium thiosulfate ($\frac{1}{6}$ molar). Application of ice compresses for 6 to 12 hours may minimize local reaction. Have solution for treatment of extravasation available before drug is administered.

Intracavity administration: Paracentesis is performed and most of fluid removed from the pleural or peritoneal cavity prior to injection of mechlorethamine. For intrapleural or intrapericardial administration, drug is introduced through the thoracentesis needle. For intraperitoneal administration, drug is introduced through a rubber catheter inserted into the trocar used for paracentesis or through an 18-gauge needle inserted at another site. Check with physician regarding specific equipment required for intracavity administration.

Following administration, decontamination of the following is necessary: gloves, tubing, needle syringe, drug vial (whether empty or containing unused drug).

Soak used materials in solution of 5% sodium thiosulfate and 5% sodium bicarbonate for 45

M

minutes. Excess reagents and reaction products are washed away easily with water.

Any unused injection solution is neutralized by mixing with an equal volume of sodium thiosulfate/sodium bicarbonate solution; allow to stand 45 minutes. Empty vials are treated in the same manner before disposal.

ONGOING ASSESSMENTS AND NURSING MANAGEMENT

Following intracavity administration, the position of the patient is changed q5m to q10m for 1 hour. A side-to-back-to-side position change may be used; other position changes may be ordered.

Measure intake and output for 48 hours after drug is administered. In some instances, physician may order measurement 24 hours prior to, as well as 48 hours following, administration of mechlorethamine.

Monitor vital signs q4h; report any changes from baseline values to physician.

Observe for immediate adverse effects (*e.g.,* nausea and vomiting, anorexia, weakness, diarrhea).

Nausea and vomiting usually occur 1 to 3 hours after administration; vomiting may persist for 8 hours and nausea for 24 hours.

Physician usually prescribes an antiemetic and/or sedative for nausea and vomiting. If vomiting occurs, antiemetic should be given IM or as a suppository. Notify physician if vomiting is severe and/or not relieved by medication.

When vomiting or diarrhea is severe, observe for signs of dehydration, hypokalemia, and hyponatremia (Appendix 6, sections 6-10, 6-15, and 6-17). Notify physician immediately if these should occur.

Physician usually orders an analgesic q3h to q4h prn following intraperitoneal administration. If pain is not relieved, notify physician.

Hematologic toxicity is monitored by CBC daily or every other day.

Lymphocytopenia seen within 24 hours after first injection; granulocytopenia occurs within 6 to 8 days and lasts 10 days to 3 weeks. Thrombocytopenia is variable; appearance and recovery usually parallel the sequence of granulocyte levels.

Observe for signs of bone-marrow depression (Appendix 6, section 6-8); report findings immediately.

Thrombocytopenia: Assess for evidence of bleeding q4h. Look for bleeding gums; hematemesis; black, tarry stools; rectal bleeding; ecchymosis; epistaxis and hematuria, and report occurrence immediately. Use prolonged pressure on IM and venipuncture sites. Exercise care in applying blood pressure cuff to avoid bruising of area. Rectal temperatures usually avoided.

Give oral care q4h and as needed. Use a soft toothbrush and frequent mouth rinses with warm water. If stomatitis develops, see Appendix 6, section 6-21.

To prevent hyperuricemia, physician may order increased fluid intake, alkalinization of the urine, and allopurinol. Offer fluids at frequent intervals throughout day to keep intake 2000 ml or more per day. Observe for signs of urinary tract obstruction due calculus formation (*e.g.,* flank or abdominal pain, hematuria, difficulty in voiding).

Immunosuppression may occur and may predispose patient to bacterial, viral or fungal infections. If this occurs, visitors and hospital personnel with infections or exposure to infections should limit patient contact. Protective (reverse) isolation may be necessary.

A maculopapular rash may occur. Notify physician as symptomatic treatment may be necessary.

Observe for occurrence of herpes zoster, especially in those with lymphomas. Notify physician if lesions are noted or patient complains of pain or burning of any area. Symptomatic treatment is instituted and mechlorethamine therapy discontinued during acute phase of this illness.

If anorexia occurs, small, nutritious feedings 4 to 6 times a day may be given. A dietary consult may be necessary. A soft diet can be given if bleeding gums, stomatitis occurs. Dry toast, unsalted crackers may be offered during periods of nausea.

Report persistent anorexia or decreased fluid intake to physician; IV supplements may be necessary.

Thrombosis and thrombophlebitis may occur at the injection site. If patient complains of pain or burning in the area or if redness is noted, notify physician.

PATIENT AND FAMILY INFORMATION

NOTE: Prior to therapy, the physician should discuss the objectives of therapy and the possible adverse reactions that may be experienced. The patient should be made aware of the potential risk to reproductive capacity. Female patients should be told of the effect on the menstrual cycle and advised not to become pregnant during therapy.

Meclizine Hydrochloride

See Antiemetic/Antivertigo Agents.

Meclofenamate Sodium

See Nonsteroidal Anti-inflammatory Agents.

Medroxyprogesterone Acetate Rx

injection: 100 mg/   Depo-Provera
ml, 400 mg/ml

INDICATIONS
Adjunctive therapy and palliative treatment of inoperable, recurrent, and metastatic endometrial carcinoma or renal carcinoma. See Progestins for oral indications.

CONTRAINDICATIONS
Thrombophlebitis, thromboembolic disorders, cerebral apoplexy, or past history of any of these conditions; carcinoma of the breast; undiagnosed vaginal bleeding; missed abortion; known sensitivity to medroxyprogesterone acetate.

ACTIONS
Is a derivative of progesterone.

WARNINGS
Thrombotic manifestations: Early symptoms of thrombotic disorders (thrombophlebitis, cerebrovascular disorders, pulmonary embolism, retinal thrombosis) require discontinuation of drug.

Drug is discontinued pending examination if there is a sudden partial or complete loss of vision or sudden onset of proptosis, diplopia, or migraine. If papilledema or retinal vascular lesions are found, drug is withdrawn.

Following repeated injections, amenorrhea and infertility may persist for up to 18 months and occasionally longer. Not recommended during pregnancy; data indicate a possible association between administration of progestins during the first 4 months of pregnancy and congenital heart defects in the offspring. See also Progestins.

PRECAUTIONS
See Progestins.

ADVERSE REACTIONS
Injection site: Residual lump, change in color of skin, sterile abscess.

Breast: Breast tenderness, galactorrhea (rare).

CNS: Nervousness, insomnia, somnolence, fatigue, dizziness.

Thromboembolic phenomena: Thrombophlebitis, pulmonary embolism.

Skin and mucous membranes: Sensitivity reactions ranging from pruritus, urticaria, and angioneurotic edema to generalized rash and anaphylaxis. Acne, alopecia, and hirsutism have been reported in a few cases.

GI: Rarely, nausea. Jaundice has been noted in a few instances.

Miscellaneous: Rarely, headache, hyperpyrexia.

In addition to the above the following have been observed in women taking progestins: Breakthrough bleeding, spotting, change in menstrual flow; amenorrhea; edema; change in weight (increase or decrease); changes in cervical erosion and secretions; cholestatic jaundice; rash (allergic), with or without pruritus; melasma or chloasma; mental depression.

DOSAGE
Intended for IM administration only.

Endometrial or renal carcinoma: 400 mg/week to 1000 mg/week is recommended initially. If improvement is noted within weeks or months and disease appears stabilized, it may be possible to maintain improvement with as little as 400 mg/month. Not recommended as primary therapy, but as adjunctive and palliative treatment.

NURSING IMPLICATIONS

HISTORY
See Appendix 4. Note previous treatment modalities.

PHYSICAL ASSESSMENT
Obtain vital signs, weight; evaluate general emotional and physical status. Baseline laboratory and diagnostic studies include CBC, coagulation studies, Pap smear, renal-function tests, x-ray examinations (*e.g.,* renal, pelvic, bone).

ADMINISTRATION
Give deep IM. Rotate injection sites and record site used.

Advise patient that discomfort may be noted following injection.

ONGOING ASSESSMENTS AND NURSING MANAGEMENT
Obtain vital signs q4h or as ordered; record weight; observe for adverse drug reactions; monitor intake and output (especially if patient has renal carcinoma or takes food and fluids poorly).

M

Observe for signs and symptoms of thrombotic episodes: chest pain; sudden shortness of breath; sudden partial or complete loss of vision; migraine headache; diplopia; downward displacement of the eyeball (proptosis); local pain, swelling, tenderness, and redness. If any should occur, notify physician immediately.

Notify physician if sudden weight gain or oliguria is noted.

PATIENT AND FAMILY INFORMATION

NOTE: When applicable, describe the menstrual changes (breakthrough bleeding, spotting, change in menstrual flow, amenorrhea) that may occur.

Notify physician or nurse if any of the following occurs: shortness of breath; chest pain; sudden partial or complete loss of vision; double vision; migraine headache; localized pain, redness, or tenderness; sudden weight gain; swelling of the ankles, legs, or fingers; decrease in urinary output; nervousness; insomnia; somnolence, fatigue, dizziness; jaundice; rash.

Keep physician appointments for injections and monitoring of therapy.

Medrysone

See Corticosteroids, Ophthalmic.

Mefenamic Acid

See Nonsteroidal Anti-inflammatory Agents.

Megestrol Acetate Rx

tablets: 20 mg,   Megace, Pallace
  40 mg

INDICATIONS

Palliative treatment of advanced carcinoma of the breast or endometrium (*i.e.,* recurrent or metastatic disease). Not used in lieu of currently accepted procedures such as surgery, radiation, or chemotherapy.

CONTRAINDICATIONS

Not indicated as diagnostic test for pregnancy.

ACTIONS

Is a progestational agent. Exact mechanism by which megestrol produces antineoplastic effects against endometrial carcinoma is unknown; an antiluteinizing effect mediated via the pituitary has been postulated. Antineoplastic action on carcinoma of the breast is also unclear. See also Progestins; Appendix 10.

WARNINGS

Use in other types of neoplastic disease not recommended. Use of progestational agents during first 4 months of pregnancy is contraindicated.

PRECAUTIONS

Close surveillance indicated for any patient being treated for recurrent or metastatic cancer. Use with caution in patients with a history of thrombophlebitis.

ADVERSE REACTIONS

No untoward effects have been attributed to megestrol acetate therapy. There have been reports of some patients developing carpal tunnel syndrome, deep vein thrombophlebitis, and alopecia.

OVERDOSAGE

No serious side-effects resulted from studies involving administration as high as 800 mg/day.

DOSAGE

Breast cancer: 160 mg/day (40 mg qid).
Endometrial cancer: 40 mg/day to 320 mg/day in divided doses.

At least 2 months of continuous treatment is considered an adequate period for determining efficacy.

| NURSING IMPLICATIONS

HISTORY
See Appendix 4. Note history of thrombophlebitis, previous treatment modalities.

PHYSICAL ASSESSMENT
Monitor vital signs, weight; evaluate emotional and physical status.

ADMINISTRATION
Given orally in divided doses.

ONGOING ASSESSMENTS AND NURSING MANAGEMENT
Monitor vital signs daily; observe for back or abdominal pain, headache, nausea, vomiting, breast tenderness; inform physician if these become pronounced.

Weigh weekly or as ordered. Report significant weight gain or loss to physician.

PATIENT AND FAMILY INFORMATION
Take as directed. Do not omit dose.

May cause back or abdominal pain, headache, nausea, vomiting, or breast tenderness; notify physician or nurse if these become pronounced.

Periodic evaluation of therapy will be necessary.

When applicable, and with physician approval, contraceptive measures are recommended during therapy.

Melphalan _(PAM, L-PAM, Phenylalanine Mustard, L-Sarcolysin) Rx_

tablets: 2 mg	Alkeran

INDICATIONS

Palliative treatment of multiple myeloma and palliation of nonresectable epithelial carcinoma of the ovary.

CONTRAINDICATIONS

Hypersensitivity. There may be cross-sensitivity (skin rash) between melphalan and chlorambucil. Not used in those whose disease has demonstrated prior resistance to this drug.

ACTIONS

Is a phenylalanine derivative of nitrogen mustard. It is a highly reactive, bifunctional alkylating agent. Plasma levels are highly variable after oral dosing, with respect both to time of first appearance of melphalan and to the peak concentrations achieved. Whether this results from incomplete GI absorption or a variable "first-pass" hepatic metabolism is unknown.

WARNINGS

Bone-marrow depression: As with other nitrogen mustard drugs, excessive dosage will produce marked bone-marrow depression. Frequent blood counts are essential to determine optimal dosage and to avoid toxicity. Drug should be discontinued or dosage reduced on evidence of bone-marrow depression. If the leukocyte count falls below 3000/mm^3 or platelet count falls below 100,000/mm^3, discontinue drug until peripheral blood cell counts have recovered.

Safety for use in pregnancy has not been established. Use only when clearly needed, particularly during early pregnancy, and when potential benefits outweigh the unknown potential hazards to the fetus.

There are reports of patients with multiple myeloma who have developed acute, nonlymphatic leukemia following therapy with alkylating agents, including melphalan. Reports strongly suggest this drug is leukemogenic in those with multiple myeloma. There is increased evidence of acute, nonlymphatic leukemia in women with ovarian carcinoma treated with alkylating agents. Melphalan is a carcinogen in animals and must be presumed to be so in humans. Although the palliation anticipated is generally felt to outweigh greatly the possible induction of a second neoplasm, potential benefits and potential risk of carcinogenesis must be evaluated on an individual basis. Melphalan has been observed to produce chromosomal aberrations in human cells. It is potentially mutagenic and teratogenic in humans, although the extent of risk is unknown.

PRECAUTIONS

Use with extreme caution in those whose bone-marrow reserve may have been compromised by prior irradiation or chemotherapy or in those whose bone-marrow function is recovering from previous cytotoxic therapy. Whether dosage reduction should be made in those with impaired creatinine clearance cannot be determined because of individual variability in systemic availability of melphalan in those with normal renal function. Only a small amount of the administered dose appears as parent drug in the urine of patients with normal renal function. Patients with azotemia should be closely observed in order to make dosage reductions, if required, at the earliest possible time.

DRUG INTERACTIONS

Drug/lab tests: Uric acid levels may be increased. **Urinary 5-hydroxyindoleacetic acid (5-HIAA)** may be increased as a result of tumor cell destruction, with an accompanying release of metabolites.

ADVERSE REACTIONS

GI: Nausea and vomiting have followed high doses.

Hematologic: Dose-related bone-marrow depression produces anemia, neutropenia, and thrombocytopenia.

Dermatologic: Skin rashes, both maculopapular and urticarial, have been reported.

Pulmonary: Rare instances of bronchopulmonary dysplasia and pulmonary fibrosis have been reported.

DOSAGE

Multiple myeloma: Usual dosage is 6 mg/day. Entire daily dosage may be given at one time. It is adjusted, as required, on basis of weekly blood counts. After 2 to 3 weeks of treatment, drug should be discontinued for up to 4 weeks, during which time the blood count is followed carefully.

M

When WBC and platelet counts are rising, a maintenance dose of 2 mg/day may be given. Because of patient-to-patient variations in melphalan plasma levels, dosage is cautiously escalated until myelosuppression is observed, in order to assure therapeutic levels have been reached.

Alternative regimens: Initial course of 10 mg/day for 7 to 10 days. It has been reported that maximal suppression of leukocyte and platelet counts occurs within 3 to 5 weeks and recovery within 4 to 8 weeks. Continuous maintenance therapy with 2 mg/day is instituted when the WBC count is greater than 4000/mm^3 and platelet count is greater than 100,000/mm^3. Dosage is adjusted to between 1 mg/day and 3 mg/day depending on hematologic response. It is desirable to maintain a significant degree of bone-marrow depression in order to keep the leukocyte count in the range of 3000 to 3500 cells/mm^3.

Other investigators have started treatment with 0.15 mg/kg/day for 7 days, followed by a rest period of at least 2 weeks (but which may be as long as 5–6 weeks). Maintenance therapy is started when WBC and platelet counts are rising. Maintenance dose is 0.05 mg/kg/day or less and is adjusted according to the blood count.

Prednisone may be administered in combination with melphalan. One regimen has been to administer courses of melphalan at 0.25 mg/kg/day for 4 consecutive days (or 0.2 mg/kg/day for 5 consecutive days) for a total dose of 1 mg/kg/course. These 4- to 5-day courses are then repeated every 4 to 6 weeks if the granulocyte and platelet counts have returned to normal levels.

Melphalan has been used with other cytotoxic agents to increase the response rate. It is not known whether the addition of other agents to a combination of melphalan and prednisone significantly increases either response rate or duration of survival.

Response may be very gradual over many months. Repeated courses or continuous therapy is important because improvement may continue over many months and maximum benefit may be missed if treatment is abandoned too soon.

Epithelial ovarian cancer: One regimen consists of a dose of 0.2 mg/kg/day for 5 days as a single course. Courses are repeated every 4 to 5 weeks, depending on hematologic tolerance.

NURSING IMPLICATIONS

HISTORY
See Appendix 4. Note previous treatment modalities (if any).

PHYSICAL ASSESSMENT
Obtain physical, emotional status; vital signs; weight. Baseline laboratory tests include CBC, differential, platelet count, renal-function studies, and alkaline phosphatase.

ADMINISTRATION
Medicine card must clearly state dates therapy is to be initiated and discontinued (some regimens may be for 4–5 days only).

Physician may order drug given with meals.

ONGOING ASSESSMENTS AND NURSING MANAGEMENT
Obtain vital signs daily; observe for adverse effects.

Weight weekly. Report significant weight loss to physician.

Nausea and vomiting may occur with high doses. Notify the physician if these occur, because an antiemetic may be necessary.

Blood counts are ordered to follow hematologic response.

CLINICAL ALERT: Maximal suppression of leukocyte and platelet counts may occur at varying times, depending on treatment regimen used (see *Dosage*). Observe for signs of bone-marrow depression (Appendix 6, section 6-8) approximately 10 days after therapy is initiated; notify physician immediately if signs of bone-marrow depression are evident.

Encourage a high fluid intake of at least 10 to 12 glasses (8 oz each) daily. Some patients may require supervision of fluid intake. If patient does not appear to be taking sufficient oral fluids, measure intake and output and offer small amounts of liquid at frequent intervals.

Notify physician if patient takes fluids or food poorly or if patient complains of joint or flank pain (may be sign of hyperuricemia).

PATIENT AND FAMILY INFORMATION
NOTE: When drug is taken on an outpatient basis, patient or family requires a detailed explanation of signs of bone-marrow depression.

Notify physician or nurse immediately if unusual bleeding or bruising, chills, fever, sore throat, flank or stomach pain, joint pain, mouth sores, or black tarry stools occur.

May cause nausea, vomiting, or hair loss; notify physician or nurse if these become pronounced.

Drink at least 10 to 12 glasses (8 oz each) of water each day.

Contraceptive measures are recommended during therapy; discuss with physician methods to be used.

Periodic laboratory tests will be necessary to monitor therapy.

Menadiol Sodium Diphosphate

See Vitamin K Preparations.

Menadione

See Vitamin K Preparations.

Meningitis Vaccines

See Immunizations, Active.

Menotropins Rx

powder for injection:	Pergonal
75 IU follicle-stim-	
ulating hormone	
(FSH) and 75 IU	
luteinizing hor-	
mone (LH) activ-	
ity/ampule	

INDICATIONS

Women: Menotropins and human chorionic gonadotropin (HCG) (p 284) are given sequentially for induction of ovulation and pregnancy in the anovulatory infertile patient, in whom cause of anovulation is functional and not due to primary ovarian failure (*i.e.,* primary amenorrhea, secondary amenorrhea, secondary amenorrhea with galactorrhea, polycystic ovaries, and anovulatory cycles).

Men: Menotropins with concomitant HCG are indicated for stimulation of spermatogenesis in men who have primary or secondary hypogonadotropic hypogonadism. Effective with primary hypogonadotropic hypogonadism due to a congenital factor or prepubertal hypophysectomy and in secondary hypogonadotropic hypogonadism due to hypophysectomy, craniopharyngioma, cerebral aneurysm, or chromophobe adenoma.

CONTRAINDICATIONS

Women: High level of urinary gonadotropin indicating primary ovarian failure; overt thyroid or ad-

renal dysfunction; any cause of infertility other than anovulation; abnormal bleeding of undetermined origin; ovarian cysts or enlargement not due to polycystic ovary syndrome; organic intracranial lesion such as pituitary tumor; pregnancy.

Men: Normal gonadotropin levels indicating normal pituitary function; elevated gonadotropin levels indicating primary testicular failure; infertility disorders other than hypogonadotropic hypogonadism.

ACTIONS

A purified preparation of gonadotropins extracted from urine of postmenopausal women. It is biologically standardized for follicle-stimulating hormone (FSH) and luteinizing hormone (LH).

Women: Produces ovarian follicular growth in those who do not have primary ovarian failure. Treatment results only in follicular growth and maturation. In order to effect ovulation, HCG is given following menotropins, when sufficient follicular maturation has occurred.

Men: When administered concomitantly with HCG for at least 3 months, induces spermatogenesis in men with primary or secondary pituitary hypofunction who have achieved adequate masculinization with prior HCG therapy.

WARNINGS

Menotropins are capable of causing mild to severe adverse reactions.

PRECAUTIONS

Diagnosis prior to therapy

Women: A thorough gynecologic and endocrinologic evaluation is performed prior to therapy. Anovulation must be documented.

Men: Lack of pituitary function is documented.

Overstimulation of the ovary: To minimize hazard of abnormal ovarian enlargement, the lowest dose consistent with good results is used. Mild to moderate uncomplicated ovarian enlargement, with or without abdominal distention or abdominal pain, occurs in approximately 20% of those treated and generally regresses without treatment in 2 to 3 weeks. The hyperstimulation syndrome characterized by sudden ovarian enlargement and ascites, with or without pain or pleural effusion, occurs in approximately 0.4% of patients at recommended doses. If this syndrome occurs, treatment is discontinued and patient hospitalized.

Multiple pregnancy: Pregnancy following treatment may result in multiple births (incidence is 20%).

M

ADVERSE REACTIONS

Women: Ovarian enlargement; hyperstimulation syndrome; hemoperitoneum; arterial thromboembolism; sensitivity (febrile) reactions. Birth defects have been reported.

Men: Occasional gynecomastia.

DOSAGE

Women: To effect ovulation, HCG must be given following menotropins when clinical assessment indicates sufficient follicular maturation has occurred. This is indirectly estimated by changes in vaginal smear, appearance and volume of cervical mucus, and so on. Urinary excretion of estrogens is a more reliable index of follicular maturation.

Initial dosage: Dose is individualized. Initial dose should be 75 IU of FSH and 75 IU of LH (1 ampule) per day IM for 9 to 12 days, followed by HCG, 10,000 IU 1 day after last dose of menotropins. Hyperstimulation syndrome does not occur following this dosage schedule. Administration of menotropins should not exceed 12 days. Patient is treated until indices of estrogen activity are equivalent to, or greater than, those of the normal individual. If total estrogen excretion is less than 100 mcg/24 hours or estriol excretion less than 50 mcg/24 hours prior to HCG administration, hyperstimulation syndrome is less likely to occur. If estrogen values are greater than this, HCG is not advised because the hyperstimulation syndrome is more likely to occur. If ovaries are abnormally enlarged on last day of menotropin therapy, HCG is not administered in this course of therapy; this will reduce chances of development of the hyperstimulation syndrome. The couple should have intercourse daily beginning on the day prior to HCG administration, until ovulation occurs. Care should be taken to ensure insemination.

Repeat dosage: If there is evidence of ovulation but no pregnancy, regimen repeated for at least two courses before increasing dose to two ampules/day for 9 to 12 days. This is followed by 10,000 IU of HCG 1 day after last dose of menotropins. If ovulation is present but pregnancy does not ensue, same dose is repeated for two more courses. Larger doses not recommended.

Men: Prior to therapy, pretreatment with HCG alone (5000 IU three times/week) is required. HCG pretreatment should achieve serum testosterone levels within normal range and masculinization (appearance of secondary sex characteristics). Pretreatment may require 4 to 6 months. Recommended dose is one ampule menotropins IM three times/week and HCG 2000 IU twice/week. Therapy continued for minimum of 4 months to ensure detecting spermatozoa in the ejaculate. If patient has not responded with increased spermatogenesis at end of 4 months, pretreatment may continue or dose increased to two ampules three times/week, with the HCG dose unchanged.

NURSING IMPLICATIONS

HISTORY

Women: See Appendix 4. Obtain complete menstrual history, previous treatment modalities (if any) or methods used for induction of pregnancy.

Men: Review patient's chart for etiology of disorder.

PHYSICAL ASSESSMENT

Vital signs.

Women: Physician performs a thorough gynecologic and endocrinologic examination, which may include urinary estrogen, urinary pregnanediol, pregnancy test, pelvic examination, vaginal smear, hysterosalpingogram, cervical dilatation and curettage, and so on. Some drugs may interfere with test results. If patient is presently taking any drug, inform physician and write the name on all laboratory request slips. An evaluation of the husband's fertility potential is usually made.

Men: Physician performs thorough genitourinary and endocrinologic examination, which may include sperm count, serum testosterone, urinary gonadotropins, and so on.

ADMINISTRATION

Dissolve contents of one ampule in 1 ml to 2 ml of sterile saline. Discard any unused portion.

Give IM. See *Dosage* for various treatment regimens.

ONGOING ASSESSMENTS AND NURSING MANAGEMENT

Drug usually administered on outpatient basis.

Each time injection is given, question patient regarding adverse reactions.

Keep physician informed of laboratory test results as they become available.

Hyperstimulation syndrome (women): Develops rapidly over 3 to 4 days and generally occurs within 2 weeks following treatment.

Characterized by sudden ovarian enlargement and ascites, with or without pain or pleural effusion. Hospitalization is required.

Hemoconcentration associated with fluid loss in the abdominal cavity has occurred and should be thoroughly assessed by determination of intake and output and daily weight. Notify physician of any change in the intake and output ratio, decrease in urinary output, weight gain.

Daily hematocrit, serum and urinary electrolytes, and urine specific gravity are recommended.

Treatment is largely symptomatic and consists of bedrest, fluid and electrolyte replacement, and analgesics if needed.

In some instances, surgery may be required because of bleeding; usually a partial resection of the enlarged ovary is performed.

PATIENT AND FAMILY INFORMATION

NOTE: Patient must receive complete instructions regarding therapeutic regimen, number of injections, results expected. Female patient must have symptoms of hyperstimulation syndrome explained.

Keep all appointments for injections, examination, and laboratory tests. A full course of therapy is necessary to obtain desired results.

Women: Contact physician immediately if abdominal pain, abdominal distention, dyspnea (due to pleural effusion), sudden weight gain occurs.

Follow physician's recommendations regarding intercourse, taking daily basal temperature (temperature before arising in A.M.).

Mepenzolate Bromide

See Gastrointestinal Anticholinergics/Antispasmodics.

Meperidine Hydrochloride

See Narcotic Analgesics.

Mephentermine Sulfate Rx

injection: 15 mg/ml, Wyamine Sulfate
   30 mg/ml

INDICATIONS

Treatment of hypotension secondary to ganglionic blockade and occurring with spinal anesthesia. Although not recommended as corrective therapy for shock of hypotension secondary to hemorrhage, may be used as an emergency measure to maintain blood pressure until blood or blood substitutes are available.

CONTRAINDICATIONS

Hypersensitivity; in combination with any monoamine oxidase (MAO) inhibitor; in hypotension induced by chlorpromazine (see *Drug Interactions*).

ACTIONS

Is an indirect-acting sympathomimetic amine that releases norepinephrine and therefore affects both alpha and beta receptors. Increase in blood pressure is probably primarily due to an increase in cardiac output resulting from enhanced cardiac contraction; to a lesser degree, an increase in peripheral resistance due to peripheral vasoconstriction may also contribute to elevation in blood pressure.

Duration of action is prolonged; following subcutaneous administration, effects last 30 to 60 minutes. Pressor response is evident 5 to 15 minutes after IM injection and has a duration of up to 4 hours.

WARNINGS

Use with caution in those with known cardiovascular disease and in the chronically ill, because drug's action on the cardiovascular system may be profound. Safety for use in pregnancy, in the nursing mother, or in women of childbearing potential has not been established. Use only when clearly needed and when potential benefits outweigh the unknown potential hazards to the fetus.

PRECAUTIONS

Hypovolemia: Not a substitute for replacement of blood, plasma, fluids, and electrolytes, which should be restored promptly when loss has occurred (*i.e.,* during or after surgery).

Hemorrhagic shock: Use with caution in treatment of shock secondary to hemorrhage. For effective emergency treatment, infuse 300 mg to 600 mg in 5% Dextrose in Water. This will maintain blood pressure until volume replacement is effected.

Increased responsiveness to vasopressor agents may be seen in those with hyperthyroidism. Administer with care to known hypertensives.

DRUG INTERACTIONS

Cyclopropane and **halothane** are known to sensitize the heart to the arrhythmic action of catecholamines. Serious ventricular arrhythmias may occur in patients under general anesthesia with these agents if sympathomimetic drugs such as mephentermine are given to control hypotension. May be ineffective in those treated with **reserpine** or **guanethidine** because their mechanisms inhibit sympathetic nerve activity. In obstetrics, if vasopressor drugs are either used to correct hypotension or added to the local anesthetic solution, some **oxyto-**

M

cic drugs may cause severe persistent hypertension; even rupture of a cerebral blood vessel may occur during the postpartum period.

Sympathomimetic amines will act to potentiate, rather than correct, hypotension secondary to the adrenolytic effect of **chlorpromazine.** The effects of **beta-adrenergic blocking agents** may be reversed by sympathomimetic amines. Excessive pressor response may occur in those receiving **MAO inhibitors.** The pressor response of adrenergic agents may be potentiated or inhibited by **tricyclic antidepressants.**

ADVERSE REACTIONS

Side-effects following administration are minimal and result from central stimulatory effects. Following recommended doses, an occasional patient may display signs of anxiety. Cardiac arrhythmias may be produced and blood pressure raised excessively, particularly in those with heart disease.

DOSAGE

Can be administered IM without irritation or abnormal tissue reaction. Injection of an undiluted parenteral solution containing 30 mg/ml, or a continuous infusion of a 1 mg/ml solution in 5% Dextrose in Water, directly into the vein, is the preferable route for treatment of shock. IV administration of undiluted mephentermine does not produce vascular irritation, and no untoward tissue reaction will develop should extravasation occur.

Prevention of hypotension attendant to spinal anesthesia: 30 mg to 45 mg IM 10 to 20 minutes prior to anesthesia, operation, or termination of the operative procedure.

Hypotension following spinal anesthesia: 30 mg to 45 mg IV in a single injection. Repeat doses of 30 mg as necessary to maintain blood pressure. An immediate response and maintenance of blood pressure can be accomplished by continuous IV infusion of 0.1% solution of mephentermine in 5% Dextrose in Water (1 mg/ml). Regulate flow and duration of therapy according to patient response.

Hypotension secondary to spinal anesthesia in the obstetric patient undergoing cesarean section, who is known to be sensitive to drugs: Initial dose is 15 mg IV; may be repeated if response is not adequate.

Treatment of shock following hemorrhage: Although not recommended, continuous IV infusion of 0.1% solution in 5% Dextrose in Water may be useful in maintaining blood pressure until whole blood replacement can be accomplished.

NURSING IMPLICATIONS

HISTORY

If possible, review chart for diagnosis, health history, current treatment modalities (if any).

PHYSICAL ASSESSMENT

Obtain general status of patient; blood pressure, pulse, respirations.

ADMINISTRATION

Usual routes of administration are IM, IV, IV infusion.

Preparation of IV solution: Drug is available as 15 mg/ml or 30 mg/ml. To prepare a 0.1% solution, add 20 ml of mephentermine 30 mg/ml (*i.e.,* 600 mg) to 500 ml of 5% Dextrose and Water. Label infusion bottle with date and strength (approximately 1 mg/ml).

A microdrip may be used to facilitate the infusion rate.

A cardiac monitor may be used to detect arrhythmias, especially if patient is elderly or has a history of cardiovascular disease.

Depending on the reason for use, a primary and secondary line may be used with the primary line used to keep vein open when it is necessary to discontinue the mephentermine temporarily because of blood pressure response.

IV infusion rate is adjusted according to response of patient. Physician must order guidelines (*e.g.,* maximum systolic pressure) for regulating infusion rate.

ONGOING ASSESSMENTS AND NURSING MANAGEMENT

Monitor blood pressure, pulse, and respirations q2m to q5m until blood pressure is stabilized. Use flow sheet to record readings.

Adjust the rate of infusion based on blood pressure and guidelines established by the physician.

Notify physician immediately if blood pressure responds poorly (*i.e.,* the infusion rate is steadily increased and the blood pressure continues to decrease).

Notify physician immediately if a cardiac arrhythmia is noted.

Measure intake and output. Monitor urinary output qh until patient's condition stabilized. Notify physician immediately if urinary output is below 30 ml/hour.

After drug is discontinued and patient's condition is stabilized, monitor blood pressure, pulse, and respirations q10m to q15m for 1 to 2 hours if drug is given IV, or for 4 hours if drug given IM.

Mephenytoin

See Anticonvulsants, Hydantoins.

Mephobarbital

See Barbiturates.

Mepivacaine Hydrochloride

See Anesthetics, Local, Injectable.

Meprobamate Rx C–IV

tablets: 200 mg	Equanil, Miltown, Neuramate, SK-Bamate, *Generic*
tablets: 400 mg	Equanil, Miltown, Neuramate, Neurate-400, Sedabamate, SK-Bamate, Tranmep, *Generic*
tablets: 600 mg	Miltown 600, *Generic*
tablets, coated: 400 mg	Equanil Wyseals (contains tartrazine)
capsules: 400 mg	Equanil
capsules, sustained release: 200 mg, 400 mg	Meprospan

INDICATIONS

Management of anxiety disorders or short-term relief of symptoms of anxiety. Anxiety and tension associated with stress of everyday life usually do not require treatment.

CONTRAINDICATIONS

Acute intermittent porphyria, allergic or idiosyncratic drug reactions to these and related compounds such as carisoprodol or carbromal.

ACTIONS

Has effects on multiple sites in the CNS, including the thalamus and limbic system.

WARNINGS

Drug dependence: Physical and psychological dependence and abuse may occur. Chronic intoxication from prolonged use, usually of doses greater than recommended, is manifested by ataxia, slurred speech, and vertigo. Dose and amount prescribed should be carefully supervised and long use avoided, especially in alcoholics and addiction-prone persons.

Sudden withdrawal of meprobamate after prolonged and excessive use may precipitate recurrence of preexisting symptoms such as anxiety, anorexia, insomnia, or withdrawal reactions (*e.g.*, vomiting, ataxia, tremors, muscle twitching, confusional states, hallucinations, and, rarely, convulsive seizures). Seizures are more likely to occur in those with CNS damage or preexistent or latent convulsive disorders. Onset of withdrawal symptoms usually occurs within 12 to 48 hours after discontinuation. Symptoms usually cease in the next 12 to 48 hours.

When excessive dosage has continued for weeks or months, meprobamate should be withdrawn gradually over a period of 1 to 2 weeks. A short-acting barbiturate may be substituted and gradually withdrawn.

Use in pregnancy, lactation: An increased risk of congenital malformations during the first trimester has been suggested. The possibility that a woman of childbearing age may be pregnant at institution of therapy should be considered and patients should be advised that if they become pregnant during therapy, or intend to become pregnant, they should consult their physician. Meprobamate passes the placental barrier and is present in breast milk.

Use in children: Not recommended for children under 6.

PRECAUTIONS

This agent is metabolized in the liver and excreted by the kidney. To avoid excess accumulation, use with caution in those with compromised liver or kidney function. Avoid oversedation; use lowest effective dose in elderly or debilitated patients. May precipitate seizures in epileptics. May produce drowsiness, dizziness, blurred vision; patients should observe caution while driving or performing other tasks requiring alertness.

Tartrazine sensitivity: Some of these products contain tartrazine (Appendix 6, section 6-23).

DRUG INTERACTIONS

Additive effects with **alcohol** and other **CNS depressants** or **psychotropic drugs** should be anticipated.

ADVERSE REACTIONS

CNS: Drowsiness, ataxia, dizziness, slurred speech, headache, vertigo, weakness, paresthesias, impairment of visual accommodation, depressive reaction, confusion, panic reaction, insomnia, seizures, euphoria, overstimulation, paradoxical excitement, fast EEG activity.

GI: Nausea, vomiting, diarrhea, anorexia, dry mouth, glossitis.

Cardiovascular: Palpitations, tachycardia, various arrhythmias, transient ECG changes, syncope, hypotensive crisis, flushing.

Allergic or idiosyncratic: Usually seen between first and fourth dose in those having no previous contact with drug. *Milder reactions*—Itchy, urticarial, or erythematous maculopapular rash (generalized or confined to groin); leukopenia; acute non-thrombocytopenic purpura; petechiae; ecchymosis; eosinophilia; peripheral edema; adenopathy; fever; fixed drug eruption with cross-reaction to carisoprodol and cross-sensitivity between meprobamate and carbromal. *More severe*—Hyperpyrexia, chills, angioneurotic edema, bronchospasm, oliguria, anuria,

M

anaphylaxis, erythema multiforme, exfoliative dermatitis, stomatitis, proctitis. Stevens-Johnson syndrome and bullous dermatitis have also occurred.

Other: Exacerbation of symptoms of porphyria.

OVERDOSAGE

Symptoms: Suicide attempts with meprobamate have resulted in drowsiness, lethargy, stupor, ataxia, coma, shock, vasomotor, and respiratory collapse, and death.

Acute simple overdose: Death has been reported with ingestion of as little as 12 g and survival with as much as 40 g. Blood levels of 0.5 mg/dl to 3 mg represent usual range of therapeutic dosage. Blood levels of 3 mg/dl to 10 mg/dl usually correspond to findings of mild to moderate symptoms of overdosage such as stupor or light coma. Blood levels of 10 mg/dl to 20 mg/dl usually correspond to deeper coma, requiring more intensive treatment. Some fatalities occur. At levels greater than 20 mg/dl, more fatalities than survivals can be expected.

Acute combined overdose (meprobamate with other psychotropic drugs or alcohol): Effects are additive; a history of ingestion of a low dose of meprobamate plus any of these compounds (or a relatively low blood or tissue level of meprobamate) cannot be used as prognostic indicator.

Treatment: Excessive doses produce rapid sleep and reduce blood pressure, pulse, and respiratory rate to basal levels. Remove any drug remaining in stomach and give symptomatic treatment. Should respiration or blood pressure become compromised, respiratory assistance, CNS stimulants, and pressor agents may be ordered. Diuresis, osmotic (mannitol) diuresis, peritoneal dialysis, and hemodialysis have been used. Careful monitoring of urinary output is necessary; take caution to avoid overhydration. Relapse and death after initial recovery have been attributed to incomplete gastric emptying and delayed absorption.

DOSAGE

1200 mg/day to 1600 mg/day in three or four divided doses; doses above 2400 mg/day are not recommended.

Children (6 to 12 years): 100 mg to 200 mg bid or tid.

NURSING IMPLICATIONS

HISTORY

Record duration of symptoms; mental health history; drug history (because of drugs' potential for abuse, history of drug abuse may or may not be reliable). When applicable, inquire of female patient possibility of pregnancy or planned pregnancy in immediate future. See also Appendix 4.

PHYSICAL ASSESSMENT

Assess mental status: (1) motor responses (*e.g.,* trembling, tense, restless, unable to relax), (2) autonomic responses (*e.g.,* cold clammy hands, sweating, tachycardia). Inquire about symptoms such as diarrhea, insomnia, palpitations, frequent urination.

ADMINISTRATION

Withhold drug and contact physician if excessive sedation or drowsiness is apparent at time of next dose.

If gastric distress occurs, check with physician about administration with or immeditely after meals.

ONGOING ASSESSMENTS AND NURSING MANAGEMENT

Obtain vital signs daily; observe for adverse effects q2h to q4h early in therapy.

Report excessive drowsiness, sedation, or confusion to physician because dose or drug change may be necessary.

Have patient remain in bed with siderails raised if daytime sedation or drowsiness occurs.

The elderly may require assistance with ambulation.

Long-term therapy: Sudden withdrawal may precipitate recurrence of symptoms, withdrawal reactions (see *Warnings*). Ensure continuity of prescribed therapy by notation on Kardex, informing health-team members responsible for drug administration.

The physician usually prescribes a small number of tablets per prescription because of the possibility of suicide.

PATIENT AND FAMILY INFORMATION

May cause drowsiness, dizziness, blurred vision; use caution while driving or performing other tasks requiring alertness.

Avoid alcohol while taking drug.

Notify physician or nurse if skin rash, sore throat, or fever occurs.

Take drug as prescribed; do *not* increase dose or frequency.

Merbromin

See Antiseptics and Germicides.

Mercaptopurine

(6-Mercaptopurine, 6-MP) Rx

tablets: 50 mg   Purinethol

INDICATIONS

For remission induction, remission consolidation, and maintenance therapy of acute leukemia. Response depends on the particular subclassification (*e.g.,* lymphatic, myelogenous, undifferentiated) and age of patient (child or adult). Also indicated for palliative treatment of chronic myelogenous (granuylocytic) leukemia.

Acute lymphatic (lymphocytic, lymphoblastic) leukemia: Acute lymphatic leukemia responds, in general, more favorably to mercaptopurine in children than in adults. Given as a single agent for remission induction, it induces complete remission in approximately 25% of children and 10% of adults. These results can be improved by using multiple agents in combination. Duration of complete remission in children is brief without use of maintenance therapy; some form of drug therapy is essential following remission induction. As a single agent, drug is capable of significantly prolonging complete remission in children, but therapy with multiple agents produces results superior to mercaptopurine alone. Effectiveness in maintenance programs with adults not established.

Acute myelogenous (and acute myelomonocytic) leukemia: As a single agent, will induce complete remission in approximately 10% of children and adults. These results inferior to those achieved with combination chemotherapy.

Chronic myelogenous (granulocytic) leukemia: Is one of several agents with demonstrated efficacy. Approximately 30% to 50% of patients obtain an objective response. Busulfan usually preferred for initial therapy.

CNS leukemia: Not effective for prophylaxis or treatment.

Other neoplasms: Not effective in chronic lymphatic leukemia, the lymphomas, or solid tumors.

CONTRAINDICATIONS

Not used unless diagnosis is definitely established. Not used in patients whose disease has demonstrated prior resistance to drug. There is usually complete cross-resistance between mercaptopurine and thioguanine.

ACTIONS

Is an analogue of the purine bases adenine and hypoxanthine. It competes with hypoxanthine and guanine for the enzyme hypoxanthine-guanine phosphoribosyltransferase and is converted to thio-inosinic acid. This intracellular nucleotide inhibits several reactions involving inosinic acid, including conversion of inosinic acid to xanthylic acid and adenylic acid. In addition, 6-methylthioinosinate is formed by methylation of thio-inosinic acid. Both thio-iosinic acid and 6-methylthioinosinate have been reported to inhibit purine ribonucleotide synthesis. It is not known exactly which of the biochemical effects of mercaptopurine and its metabolites are directly or predominately responsible for cell death.

Oral absorption is incomplete and variable. Drug is excreted in the urine.

WARNINGS

Bone-marrow toxicity: Most consistent dose-related toxicity is bone-marrow suppression manifested by anemia, leukopenia, thrombocytopenia, or any combination of these. These findings may indicate progression of the underlying disease. Because drug may have a delayed effect, medication is withdrawn temporarily at first sign of an abnormally large fall in any of the formed elements of the blood. Toxic effects are often unavoidable during induction phase of adult acute leukemia if remission induction is to be successful. Life-threatening infections and bleeding have been seen as a consequence of mercaptopurine-induced granulocytopenia and thrombocytopenia. Severe hematologic toxicity may require supportive therapy with platelet transfusions for bleeding and antibiotics and granulocyte transfusions if sepsis is documented.

The decision to increase, decrease, continue, or discontinue a given dosage is based not only on absolute hematologic values but also on rate at which changes are occurring, particularly during the induction phase of acute leukemia. CBC is done frequently to evaluate effect of therapy. The dosage of mercaptopurine may need to be reduced when combined with other drugs whose primary toxicity is myelosuppression.

Hepatotoxicity: Deaths have been reported from hepatic necrosis. Hepatic injury may occur with any dosage, but occurs with greatest frequency when doses of 2.5 mg/kg/day are exceeded. The histologic pattern of hepatotoxicity includes features of both intrahepatic cholestasis and parenchymal cell necrosis, either of which may predominate. It is not clear how much may be due to direct drug toxicity and how much to hypersensitivity reaction. In some patients, jaundice has cleared following drug withdrawal and reappeared with introduction. Usually, detectable jaundice appears early in the course of treatment (1–2 months) but has been reported as early as 1 week and as late as 8 years after treatment.

Monitoring of serum transaminase, alkaline phosphatase, and bilirubin levels may allow early detection. Weekly monitoring of these tests is recommended when beginning therapy and monthly thereafter. More frequent liver-function tests are advisable in those receiving mercaptopurine with other hepatotoxic agents or those with preexisting liver disease.

M

Hepatotoxicity has been associated in some cases with anorexia, diarrhea, jaundice, and ascites. Hepatic encephalopathy has occurred. Onset of clinical jaundice, hepatomegaly, and anorexia with tenderness in the right hypochondrium are immediate indications for withholding drug until exact etiology is identified. Any evidence of deterioration in liver function, toxic hepatitis, or biliary stasis requires prompt discontinuation and a search for etiology of hepatotoxicity.

Immunosuppression: Patient may manifest decreased cellular hypersensitivities and impaired allograft rejection. Induction of immunity to infectious agents or vaccines will be subnormal. The degree of immunosuppression will depend on antigen dose and temporal relationship to the drug. This drug effect is similar to that of azathioprine and should be carefully considered with regard to intercurrent infections and risk of subsequent neoplasia.

Use in pregnancy: Women receiving this drug in the first trimester have an increased incidence of abortion; risk of malformation in offspring surviving the first trimester not known. Use during pregnancy only if the benefit justifies the risk to the fetus. Effect on fertility for both males and females unknown.

PRECAUTIONS

It is advisable to start with smaller doses in those with impaired renal function, owing to possibility of slower drug elimination and greater cumulative effect. Mercaptopurine causes chromosomal aberrations. Carcinogenic potential exists, but extent of risk unknown.

DRUG INTERACTIONS

When **allopurinol** is administered concomitantly, dosage of mercaptopurine is reduced to one-third to one-fourth of the usual dose. Failure to reduce dosage results in delayed catabolism of mercaptopurine and the likelihood of severe toxicity.

ADVERSE REACTIONS

Bone-marrow toxicity and hepatotoxicity: See *Warnings.*

Oral lesions: Rarely seen; when they occur, they resemble thrush rather than antifolic ulcerations.

GI: Intestinal ulcerations have been reported. Nausea, vomiting, and anorexia are uncommon during initial administration but may occur during toxicity. Mild diarrhea and spruelike symptoms have been noted occasionally.

Hyperuricemia: Occurs frequently as a consequence of rapid cell lysis. Adverse effects can be minimized by increased hydration, urine alkalinization, and prophylactic administration of a xanthine oxidase inhibitor such as allopurinol.

Drug fever: Has been reported rarely. Before attributing fever to mercaptopurine, attempt is made to exclude more common causes of pyrexia, such as sepsis, in those with acute leukemia.

OVERDOSAGE

There is no known pharmacologic antagonist; drug is discontinued when toxicity develops. If patient is seen immediately following overdosage, induced emesis may be useful. Hemodialysis is thought to be of marginal value due to the rapid cellular incorporation of mercaptopurine into active metabolites with long persistence.

DOSAGE

Induction and consolidation therapy: Dosage that will be tolerated or effective varies; careful titration is necessary to obtain optimum therapeutic effect without incurring toxicity.

Usual initial dose is approximately 2.5 mg/kg/day (100 mg to 200 mg in average adult and 50 mg in average 5-year-old child). Children with acute leukemia have tolerated this dose in most cases; it may be continued daily for several weeks or more in some patients. If after 4 weeks on this dosage there is no clinical improvement and no definite evidence of leukocyte or platelet depression, dosage may be increased up to 5 mg/kg/day.

A dosage of 2.5 mg/kg/day may result in a rapid fall in leukocyte count within 1 to 2 weeks in some adults with acute leukemia and high total leukocyte counts, as well as in certain adults with chronic myelocytic leukemia.

A total daily dosage may be given at one time and is calculated to closest multiple of 25 mg. The leukocyte count is carefully followed. Because drug may have a delayed action, it should be discontinued at first sign of an abnormally large fall in the leukocyte count. If leukocyte count remains constant for 2 to 3 days, or rises, treatment may be resumed.

Maintenance therapy: If complete hematologic remission is obtained with mercaptopurine alone or in combination with other agents, maintenance therapy should be considered. This is indicated in children with acute lymphatic leukemia. Use in maintenance schedules for adults with acute leukemia not established to be effective. If remission is achieved, maintenance doses vary from patient to patient. A usual daily dosage is 1.5 mg/kg to 2.5 mg/kg as a single dose. Mercaptopurine should rarely be relied on as a single agent for maintenance of remissions induced in acute leukemia.

NURSING IMPLICATIONS

HISTORY
See Appendix 4. Note previous treatment modalities, if any.

PHYSICAL ASSESSMENT
Evaluate physical and emotional status; vital signs; weight; look for evidence of dehydration (Appendix 6, section 6-10). Baseline studies usually include CBC, differential, platelet count, renal- and hepatic-function tests.

ADMINISTRATION
If patient is dehydrated, physician may order oral and/or IV fluids before therapy is initiated.

If ordered as 6-mercaptopurine, the "6" is part of the generic drug name and does _not_ designate the number of tablets to be administered. Dose is ordered in milligrams.

Given orally, usually as a single daily dose.

To prevent hyperuricemia, physician may order allopurinol as well as agent for alkalinization of urine (_e.g.,_ sodium bicarbonate, potassium citrate and sodium citrate, potassium citrate and citric acid). Dose of mercaptopurine is reduced by one-third to one-fourth when allopurinol is administered concurrently.

ONGOING ASSESSMENTS AND NURSING MANAGEMENT
Obtain vital signs q4h or as ordered; monitor intake and output (especially during initial therapy).

To prevent hyperuricemia, encourage daily oral intake of 10 to 12 glasses (8 oz each) or approximately 2400 ml to 2800 ml of fluid/day. If patient is receiving IV fluids, consult physician regarding oral fluid intake.

Oral fluid intake may need to be supervised (especially in children or acutely ill adults). Offer fluid at frequent intervals. If patient fails to take sufficient amount of oral fluids, notify physician.

CBC and platelet count may be monitored daily or every other day in hospitalized patient or weekly in outpatient.

CLINICAL ALERT: Onset of bone-marrow depression is variable. Plan to observe patient for signs of bone-marrow depression (Appendix 6, section 6-8) when therapy is initiated.

Withhold next dose and notify physician if most recent laboratory report shows evidence of any abnormally large fall in WBC count or if patient exhibits signs of bone-marrow depression or hepatotoxicity (jaundice, clay-colored stools, dark urine, pruritus).

Weigh weekly or as ordered. Notify physician of any significant weight change.

Nausea, vomiting, and anorexia are uncommon but may occur. Notify physician if these should occur because an antiemetic may be necessary.

If nausea and anorexia occur, a liquid diet or small frequent feedings may be offered. Carbonated beverages and unsalted crackers may also be offered.

When leukopenia occurs, patient must be protected from infection. Hospital personnel and visitors with upper respiratory or other infections or known exposure to a communicable disease should avoid contact with patient. Protective isolation may be necessary.

When thrombocytopenia occurs, protect patient from injury. Apply prolonged pressure on venipuncture sites, IM administration sites; wrap sphygmomanometer cuff gently on arm, avoid overinflation; avoid rectal temperatures when possible; pad siderails if patient is restless.

Observe for development of abdominal, flank, or joint pain or change in the intake and output ratio (may indicate urate deposits in joints or development of urate calculi); notify physician of findings.

Provide emotional support for patient and family.

PATIENT AND FAMILY INFORMATION
NOTE: Patient and family must have drug regimen and toxic effects explained in detail.

Take exactly as directed by physician. If unable to take medication for any reason, contact physician as soon as possible.

Notify physician or nurse if fever, sore throat, chills, unusual bleeding or bruising, yellow discoloration of the skin or eyes, abdominal pain, flank or joint pain, or swelling of the feet or legs occurs.

Medication may cause darkening of the skin, diarrhea, fever, headache, skin rash, itching, weakness, loss of hair. Notify physician or nurse if these become pronounced.

Drink at least 10 to 12 glasses of fluid (8 oz each) daily. This is an important part of therapy.

Weigh self weekly. If significant weight loss occurs or anorexia persists more than 2 to 3 days, contact physician. Small, frequent feedings may help overcome anorexia.

Adults: Discuss use of alcoholic beverages with physician because use should be limited.

Female patients: Contraceptive measures are recommended during therapy.

M

Mersalyl With Theophylline Rx

injection: 100 mg mersalyl, 50 mg theophylline/ml

Mercutheolin, Theo-Syl-R, *Generic*

INDICATIONS

Treatment of edema secondary to congestive heart failure (CHF); the nephrotic syndrome; the nephrotic state of glomerulonephritis; hepatic cirrhosis or portal obstruction.

CONTRAINDICATIONS

Acute nephritis, intractable oliguric states, ulcerative colitis, evidence of dehydration, hypersensitivity to mercury ion or theophylline, severe liver disease.

ACTIONS

Inhibits tubular reabsorption of sodium and chloride and, secondarily, water. Has dual action on potassium secretion. Urinary potassium is increased or decreased, depending on whether initial secretory rate is low or high. Diuretic action is related to liberation of mercuric ion, which combines with sulfhydryl groups on enzymes involved in ion transport. Release of the mercuric ion is *p*H dependent and occurs more readily in an acid medium. Acidifying salts, such as ammonium chloride, increase efficacy; alkalosis decreases efficacy. Patient may become refractory with continued administration. Responsiveness may be restored by lengthening interval between injections or by administration with ammonium chloride (avoid in those with liver disease). Theophylline potentiates diuretic effect of mercurials.

Is rapidly and completely absorbed from parenteral sites and mainly eliminated by the kidney. Diuresis begins within 1 to 2 hours, reaches its peak in 4 to 9 hours (depending on mode of injection), and is usually complete in 12 to 24 hours. Drug is used infrequently and has largely been replaced by thiazides and related diuretics and loop diuretics.

WARNINGS

A few instances of anaphylactic reactions have been reported. IV injection has caused rare, immediate cardiac reactions with sudden death. This route is reserved for severe edema and cardiac failure. Safety for use in pregnancy and lactation and in women of childbearing age has not been established. Use only when clearly needed and potential benefits outweigh the unknown potential hazards to the fetus or nursing infant.

PRECAUTIONS

Use may result in excessive loss of body water, sodium, potassium, and chloride. Excessive diuresis may result in dehydration and reduction in blood volume, with circulatory collapse and possibly vascular thrombosis and embolism, especially in elderly patients. Caution is advised in treating children. A small test dose may be given initially and increased gradually only if untoward effects such as chills, fever, malaise, morbilliform rash, vomiting, or convulsive episodes do not occur. Use with caution in elderly patients who are likely to have urologic disease. Acute urinary retention in men with large prostate glands may result from brisk diuresis. In rare cases of idiosyncrasy, may cause gastric disturbance, vertigo, febrile reactions, and cutaneous eruptions.

ADVERSE REACTIONS

Hypersensitivity: Flushing, pruritus, urticaria, cutaneous rash (which may become exfoliative), anaphylactic reactions.

GI: Nausea, vomiting, diarrhea (sometimes with bloody stools), abdominal pain.

Local: Ecchymoses, induration.

GU: Transient azotemia or increase in preexistent azotemia, acute urinary retention.

Hematologic: Bone-marrow depression manifested by neutropenia and agranulocytosis.

Miscellaneous: Mercurialism, from excessive therapy or in patients with advanced renal disease, as manifested by stomatitis, marginal gingivitis, metallic taste, diarrhea, proteinuria, renal tubular necrosis. Also, vertigo, headache, thromboembolism, febrile reactions. Rarely, hyperuricemia. Electrolyte disturbances include hypochloremic alkalosis, hyponatremia, and hypokalemia.

OVERDOSAGE

Discontinue at first signs of overdosage. Correct symptoms of digitalis intoxication, evidenced from diuretic overdose, by administration of potassium salts to normalize serum potassium levels. When hypochloremic alkalosis occurs and plasma sodium is normal, correct with ammonium chloride. Vasopressin and posterior pituitary injections exhibit antidiuretic actions that may assist in counteracting excessive diuresis.

DOSAGE

May be given IM or by slow IV injection. Also effective subcutaneously, but painful local reaction may result.

Adults: To test susceptibility of patient, first dose should be 0.5 ml or less. Usual dose for severe edema is 1 ml/day or 2 ml/day (or every other day) until "dry weight" is attained. Subsequent doses are individualized.

NURSING IMPLICATIONS

HISTORY
See Appendix 4. Note current treatment modalities.

PHYSICAL ASSESSMENT
Obtain vital signs, weight; examine extremities for edema, describe extent of edema; auscultate lungs. Laboratory tests include serum electrolytes, CBC. Renal- and hepatic-function tests may also be ordered.

ADMINISTRATION
May be given IM, subcutaneously, or IV. Administer early in morning (when possible) to avoid nighttime diuresis.

IM: Gluteus, deltoid, or thigh muscle may be used. Select nonedematous area for injection. Is preferred route of administration.

Subcutaneous: Inject over deltoid or thigh; painful local reaction may occur.

IV: Drug may be diluted with 5 ml or 10 ml of Sterile Water for Injection. Use median cephalic or other vein, at or below bend of elbow if possible. This is the route used in presence of marked general edema of tissues. Make injection slowly over a period of 3 to 5 minutes. ECG monitoring is advised to reduce risk of producing serious adverse effects.

To test susceptibility: Adults, 0.5 ml; children, 0.25 ml.

ONGOING ASSESSMENTS AND NURSING MANAGEMENT
Monitor vital signs q4h or as ordered; record weight; monitor intake and output; observe for adverse effects; check elderly patient or those with history of GU disorder for urinary retention.

Bedrest potentiates the diuretic effect. Physician may allow bathroom privileges.

A continued daily loss of 2 to 4 lb (1–2 kg) is preferable. If weight loss exceeds this amount, notify physician before next dose is given.

Ammonium chloride 6 g/day to 10 g/day may be prescribed concomitantly to prevent hypochloremic alkalosis. Ammonium chloride is contraindicated in severe hepatic or renal disease.

CLINICAL ALERT: Observe for signs of dehydration, hypokalemia (Appendix 6, sections 6-10 and 6-15), and hypochloremic alkalosis. Notify physician immediately if signs are apparent.

Patients receiving a digitalis preparation should be closely observed for hypokalemia, which can sensitize or exaggerate the response of the heart to the toxic effects of digitalis. Notify physician immediately if any cardiac arrhythmia is noted.

Excessive reduction of salt intake, especially in hot weather, is not necessary. Physician may order moderate sodium restriction for some patients.

Renal function is evaluated periodically during long-term therapy. An elevated BUN (>60 mg/100 ml) or definite proteinuria, hematuria, or oliguria may require discontinuation of therapy.

Mesoridazine

See Antipsychotic Agents.

Metaproterenol Sulfate

See Bronchodilators and Decongestants, Systemic.

Metaraminol Bitartrate Rx

injection: 10 mg/ml   Aramine, *Generic*

INDICATIONS
Prevention and treatment of acute hypotensive state occurring with spinal anesthesia; adjunctive treatment of hypotension due to hemorrhage; reactions to medications; surgical complications; shock associated with brain damage due to trauma or tumor. "Possibly effective" as adjunct in treatment of hypotension due to cardiogenic shock or septicemia.

CONTRAINDICATIONS
Use with cycloproane or halothane anesthesia is avoided, unless clinical circumstances demand such use; hypersensitivity.

ACTIONS
A potent sympathomimetic amine that increases both systolic and diastolic blood pressure, primarily by vasoconstriction; this effect is usually accompanied by reflex bradycardia. Has direct effect on alpha-adrenergic receptors. Does not depend on release of norepinephrine. It will deplete norepinephrine from sympathetic nerve endings and may function as a false transmitter. Repeated use may result in an overall diminution of sympathetic activity.

Renal, coronary, and cerebral blood flow are a function of perfusion pressure and regional resistance. In most instances of cardiogenic shock, beneficial effect of sympathomimetic amines is their positive inotropic effect. In those with insufficient or failing vasoconstriction, there is an additional advantage to the peripheral action of metaraminol, but in most patients with shock, vasoconstriction is adequate and any further increase unnecessary. Blood flow to vital organs may decrease if regional resistance increases excessively. It increases cardiac output in hypotensive patients. Also increases venous tone, causes pulmonary vasoconstriction and elevated pulmonary pressure even when cardiac output is reduced. Pressor effect is decreased, but not reversed, by alpha-adrenergic blocking agents. When pressor responses are due primarily to vasoconstriction, cardiac stimulation may play a small role. A fall in blood pressure and tachyphylaxis may occur with prolonged use. Use reserved for conditions in which hypotensive state likely to be of brief duration.

Pressor effect begins in 1 to 2 minutes after IV infusion, in about 10 minutes after IM injection, and in 5 to 20 minutes after subcutaneous injection. Effect lasts from 20 minutes to 1 hour.

WARNINGS

May cause cardiac arrhythmias. This may be particularly dangerous in those with myocardial infarction (MI) or in patients who have received anesthetics that sensitize the heart to catecholamines (*e.g.,* cyclopropane, halothane). Prolonged administration may reduce venous return and cardiac output and increase workload of the heart. Metabolic acidosis may ensue.

PRECAUTIONS

Use with caution in heart or thyroid disease, hypertension, or diabetes.

Hypovolemia: Not a substitute for replacement of blood, plasma, fluids, or electrolytes, which should be restored promptly when loss has occurred.

Vasoconstriction: When vasopressor amines are used for prolonged periods, resulting vasoconstriction may prevent adequate expansion of circulating volume and may perpetuate the shock state. Measurement of CVP and pulmonary wedge pressure useful in assessment of plasma volume. Blood or plasma volume expanders are employed when circulating volume is decreased.

Hypertension: Excessive blood pressure response is avoided. Rapidly induced hypertensive responses have been reported to cause acute pulmonary edema, arrhythmias, cardiac arrest.

Use in cirrhosis: Patients are treated cautiously and with adequate restoration of electrolytes if diuresis ensues. In several instances, ventricular extrasystoles that appeared during infusion subsided when rate of infusion reduced.

Cumulative effects: Because of prolonged action, cumulative effect is possible. With an excessive vasopressor response there may be prolonged elevation of blood pressure, even with discontinuation.

Malaria: Sympathomimetic amines may provoke a relapse in those with a history of malaria.

DRUG INTERACTIONS

If vasopressor drugs are used in obstetrics to correct hypotension or added to the local anesthetic solution, some **oxytocic drugs** may cause severe persistent hypertension; even rupture of a cerebral blood vessel may occur during the postpartum period. Use with caution in digitalized patients because combination of **digitalis** and sympathomimetic amines is capable of causing ectopic arrhythmic activity. Administration to patients receiving **MAO inhibitors, tricyclic antidepressants, reserpine,** or **guanethidine** may precipitate hypertensive crisis. Effects of beta-adrenergic blocking agents may be reversed by sympathomimetic amines. **Cyclopropane** or **halogenated hydrocarbon anesthetics** may sensitize the myocardium to the effects of catecholamines. Use of vasopressors may lead to serious arrhythmias.

ADVERSE REACTIONS

Cardiovascular: Sympathomimetic amines may cause sinus or ventricular tachycardia, or other arrhythmias, especially in those with MI. Hypertension and hypotension following cessation of the drug, cardiac arrhythmias, cardiac arrest, and palpitation have been reported.

Miscellaneous: Headache, flushing, sweating, tremors, dizziness, nausea, apprehension, abscess formation, tissue necrosis, sloughing at injection site.

OVERDOSAGE

May cause convulsions, cerebral hemorrhage, or cardiac arrhythmias. Patients with hyperthyroidism or hypertension are particularly sensitive to these effects.

DOSAGE

May be given IM, subcutaneously, or IV. Because maximum effect is not immediately apparent, allow at least 10 minutes to elapse before increasing dose. IV infusion is preferred in those in shock because IM and subcutaneous absorption may be impaired because of poor circulation. Response to vasopressors may be poor in those with coexistent shock and acidosis. Established methods of shock management and other measures directed to specific cause of shock also employed.

IM or subcutaneous injection (prevention of hypotension): Recommended dose is 2 mg to 10 mg. Wait at least 10 minutes before evaluating effects of initial dose prior to readministration.

IV infusion (adjunctive treatment of hypotension): Recommended dose is 15 mg to 100 mg in 500 ml of Sodium Chloride Injection or 5% Dextrose Injection; adjust rate of infusion to maintain blood pressure at desired level. Higher concentrations, 150 mg/500 ml to 500 mg/500 ml of infusion fluid, have been used. Concentration of drug in the infusion may be adjusted depending on patient's need for fluid replacement.

Direct IV injection: In severe shock, give by IV injection. Suggested dose is 0.5 mg to 5 mg, followed by infusion of 15 mg to 100 mg in 500 ml of infusion fluid, as described above.

Children: 0.01 mg/kg as a single dose or a solution of 1 mg/25 ml in dextrose or saline.

NURSING IMPLICATIONS

HISTORY

When possible, review chart for diagnosis, health history, allergy history, recent treatment modalities and diagnostic tests, recent vital signs.

PHYSICAL ASSESSMENT

General status of patient; blood pressure, pulse, respirations.

ADMINISTRATION

May be given IM, subcutaneously, or IV (infusion, direct injection). In severe shock drug given by direct IV injection. IM and subcutaneous routes are avoided (when possible) in shock because absorption may be impaired owing to poor circulation.

If circulating volume is decreased, blood or plasma volume expanders may also be administered. Measurement of CVP and pulmonary wedge pressure may also be used in assessment of plasma volume.

IV infusion: Establish IV line as soon as possible. When profound shock is present, a cutdown may be necessary.

Use larger vein if possible. Avoid those of the ankle or dorsum of the hand, especially in patients with peripheral vascular disease, diabetes mellitus, or hypercoagulability states.

Use primary and secondary or primary and piggyback IV set. Metaraminol is given through the secondary or piggyback set. Use a microdrip filter.

Support extremity used for IV infusion. Restraining measures may be necessary to avoid extravasation if patient is restless.

Physician orders dose, IV infusion fluid, and guidelines for maintenance of systolic blood pressure (usually 90 mm Hg to 110 mm Hg if patient was normotensive, higher if patient was hypertensive) (see *Dosage*).

Have phentolamine available as antidote for extravasation.

Compatibility: In addition to Sodium Chloride Injection, USP and 5% Dextrose Injection, USP, the following were found physically and chemically compatible with metaraminol when 5 ml (10 mg/ml) was added to 500 ml of infusion solution: Ringer's Injection, USP; Lactated Ringer's Injection, USP; 6% Dextran in Saline; Normosol-R *p*H 7.4; Normosol-M in D5-W.

Stability: Infusion solutions should be used in 24 hours.

ONGOING ASSESSMENTS AND NURSING MANAGEMENT

Pressor effect begins in 1 to 2 minutes after IV infusion, in about 10 minutes after IM injection, and in 5 to 20 minutes after subcutaneous injection. The effect lasts from 20 to 60 minutes.

Monitor blood pressure and pulse q3m to q5m if drug given IV, q5m to q10m if given IM or subcutaneously. Measure intake and output. Hourly output measurements may be ordered; keep physician informed of output.

Other assessments, such as CVP, pulmonary wedge pressure (with Swan-Ganz catheter), ECG monitoring may be ordered.

Drug has prolonged action; a cumulative effect is possible. It is recommended to allow at least 10 minutes to elapse before increasing dose. If blood pressure significantly decreases during this time, notify physician immediately. A change in dosage, administration interval, or other treatment modalities may be ordered.

CLINICAL ALERT: Avoid excessive blood pressure response. Rapidly induced hypertensive responses have been reported to cause acute pulmonary edema, arrhythmias, and cardiac arrest.

Observe for ectopic arrhythmic activity if patient has been digitalized prior to administration of metaraminol. Observe for cardiac arrhythmias, particularly in patients with MI and in those who have received cyclopropane or halogenated hydrocarbon anesthetics. ECG monitoring is usually necessary in these patients. Notify physician immediately if any arrhythmia is noted.

If shock is not due to hemorrhage, observe patient for signs of fluid overload (Appendix 6, section 6-12), especially if patient has cardiac disease, urinary output is decreased, or a large volume of IV fluid is administered.

M

When IM or subcutaneous administration is discontinued, monitor blood pressure and pulse q15m. Notify physician immediately if blood pressure falls rapidly.

IV infusion: Adjust rate of infusion to maintain blood pressure at prescribed level. Notify physician immediately if blood pressure fails to respond, pulse rate changes, or arrhythmia is noted.

Monitor infusion site closely for free flow. Extravasation may cause necrosis and sloughing of surrounding tissue.

If extravasation occurs, it is recommended that area be infiltrated as soon as possible with 10 ml to 15 ml of saline solution containing 5 mg to 10 mg of phentolamine. Use syringe with a fine needle (26- or 27-gauge) and infiltrate liberally throughout ischemic area. Treatment of extravasation must be ordered by the physician, preferably before metaraminol is administered.

When therapy is discontinued, run primary line as ordered or to KVO. Continue to monitor blood pressure and pulse q15m. If blood pressure falls rapidly, reinitiate therapy until physician examines patient.

Methacycline Hydrochloride

See Tetracyclines.

Methadone Hydrochloride

See Narcotic Analgesics.

Methamphetamine Hydrochloride

See Amphetamines.

Methandriol

See Anabolic Hormones.

Methantheline Bromide

See Gastrointestinal Anticholinergics/Antispasmodics.

Metharbital

See Barbiturates.

Methazolamide

See Carbonic Anhydrase Inhibitors.

Methdilazine Hydrochloride

See Antihistamines.

Methenamine and Methenamine Salts

Methenamine otc

tablets: 0.5 g	*Generic*

Methenamine Hippurate Rx

tablets: 1 g	Hiprex, Urex

Methenamine Mandelate Rx

tablets: 0.5 g, 1 g	Mandelamine, *Generic*
tablets, enteric coated: 0.25 g, 0.5 g, 1 g	*Generic*
oral suspension: 0.25 g/5 ml	Mandelamine
suspension forte: 0.5 g/5 ml	Mandelamine, *Generic*
granules: 0.5 g, 1 g packets	Mandelamine

INDICATIONS

Suppression or elimination of chronic bacteriuria associated with pyelonephritis, cystitis, and other chronic urinary-tract infections (UTI). Also indicated for infected residual urine sometimes accompanying neurologic diseases and in patients with anatomic abnormalities of the urinary tract requiring indwelling catheters.

CONTRAINDICATIONS

Renal insufficiency; severe dehydration; severe hepatic insufficiency because it facilitates ammonia production in the intestinal tract.

ACTIONS

In an acid urine is hydrolyzed to ammonia and formaldehyde, which is bactericidal. The nonspecific antibacterial action of formaldehyde is effective against both gram-positive and gram-negative organisms and fungi. *Escherichia coli,* enterococci, and staphylococci are usually susceptible. *Entero-*

bacter aerogenes and *Proteus vulgaris* are generally resistant. Urea-splitting organisms (*e.g., Proteus, Pseudomonas*) may be resistant because they raise the *p*H of urine. Is particularly suited for therapy of chronic infections, because bacteria and fungi do not develop resistance to formaldehyde.

Is readily absorbed and is excreted by glomerular filtration and tubular excretion. Antibacterial activity is confined to the urine and is dependent on urine *p*H. Maximum efficacy occurs when urine *p*H is 5.5 or lower. The proportion of formaldehyde liberated from methenamine decreases at higher *p*H levels. A urinary formaldehyde concentration of greater than 25 mcg/ml is necessary for antimicrobial activity. Increased urinary volume or flow rate decreases the concentration of free formaldehyde in the urine; high fluid intake may decrease therapeutic response. The acid salts (mandelate and hippurate) help maintain a low urine *p*H. Methenamine hippurate is effective in lower daily doses than methenamine mandelate. Supplementary acidification may be necessary, particularly if used against urea-splitting organisms. Urine *p*H should be monitored. If *p*H is above 4.5, acidification with ammonium chloride or ascorbic acid may be necessary. Ascorbic acid (not sodium ascorbate) 4 g/day to 12 g/day administered in divided doses q4h around the clock may be necessary.

WARNINGS
Should not be used alone for acute infections or infections with parenchymal involvement causing systemic symptoms. Safe use in early pregnancy not established. Safety in last trimester suggested but not definitely proven.

PRECAUTIONS
Large doses (8 g/day for 3–4 weeks) have caused bladder irritation, pain and frequent micturition, proteinuria, and gross hematuria. Dysuria can be controlled by reducing dosage and acidification.

Care should be taken to maintain acid *p*H of urine, especially when treating infections due to urea-splitting organisms. When acidification is contraindicated or unattainable (as with some urea-splitting bacteria), drug is not recommended. In a few instances, serum transaminase levels showed mild elevation during treatment but returned to normal while patients were still receiving methenamine hippurate. Periodic liver-function studies are recommended for patients receiving methenamine hippurate, especially those with liver dysfunction.

In those with gout, methenamine salts may cause precipitation of urate crystals in the urine.

DRUG INTERACTIONS
Concurrent use of **sulfonamides** is avoided because some sulfonamides may form insoluble precipitate with formaldehyde in the urine. **Sodium bicarbonate** and **acetazolamide** can decrease effectiveness of methenamine by alkalinizing the urine and inhibiting the conversion of methenamine to formaldehyde.

Drug/lab tests: May interfere with laboratory urine determinations of 17-hydroxycorticosteroids (false increase), catecholamines (false increase; VMA not affected) and 5-HIAA acid (false decrease). Urinary estriol concentration may be decreased owing to destruction of hormone by formaldehyde.

ADVERSE REACTIONS
GI disturbances, dysuria, bladder irritation, proteinuria, hematuria, generalized skin rash (pruritus).

DOSAGE
METHENAMINE
   Adults: 1 g qid.
   Children 6–12 years: 0.5 g qid.
   Children under 6: 50 mg/kg/day divided into 3 doses.

METHENAMINE HIPPURATE
   Adults, children over 12: 1 g bid.
   Children 6–12: 0.5 g to 1 g bid.

METHENAMINE MANDELATE
   Adults: 1 g qid.
   Children 6–12: 0.5 g qid.
   Children under 6: 0.25 g/30 lb qid.

NURSING IMPLICATIONS

HISTORY
See Appendix 4.

PHYSICAL ASSESSMENT
Obtain vital signs. Urine culture and sensitivity testing, hepatic-function tests may be ordered.

ADMINISTRATION
Give with meals or food to minimize GI upset.

If child is unable to swallow tablet, check with pharmacist regarding crushing of tablet. Methenamine mandelate is available as enteric-coated tablet (exception some 0.5-g tablets) and should not be crushed.

Observe caution in administering Mandelamine oral suspensions to children or to debilitated or otherwise susceptible patients because product has vegetable oil base. Aspiration may result in lipid pneumonia.

M

Evenly spaced intervals are recommended (*e.g.,* qid or q6h, tid or q8h, bid or q12h).

Physician may order ammonium chloride or ascorbic acid to acidify the urine.

ONGOING ASSESSMENTS AND NURSING MANAGEMENT
Daily, observe for adverse drug reactions; monitor intake and output.

Physician may order daily urinary *p*H. Maximum efficacy occurs when urinary *p*H is 5.5 or lower. Manufacturer recommends acidification of urine if urine *p*H is above 4.5. Keep physician informed of urine *p*H; if 4.5 or above, notify physician.

Dietary restriction of alkaline-producing foods (acid-ash diet) may be ordered.

Check with physician regarding fluid intake because an increased fluid intake is usually desirable in GU infections, but excessive hydration may also decrease therapeutic drug response.

PATIENT AND FAMILY INFORMATION
Take at intervals ordered by physician; drug is best taken at evenly spaced intervals around the clock.

Take with food to minimize gastric distress.

Avoid excessive intake of alkalinizing foods (citrus fruits and juices, milk and milk products, most vegetables).

Keeping urine acidic is important. Foods that acidify the urine include meats, fish, eggs, gelatin products, prunes, plums, cranberries, and cranberry juice.

Check with physician regarding use of nonprescription drugs (some may alkalinize the urine). Avoid use of sodium bicarbonate (baking soda).

Complete full course of therapy; take until gone.

Notify physician or nurse if skin rash, painful urination, or persistent GI upset occurs or if symptoms become worse.

Methicillin Sodium

See Penicillins.

Methimazole

See Antithyroid Agents.

Methocarbamol Rx

tablets: 500 mg   Delaxin, Robaxin, *Generic*

tablets: 750 mg   Marbaxin-750, Robaxin-750, *Generic*

injection: 100 mg/ml   Robaxin, *Generic*

INDICATIONS
As an adjunct to rest, physical therapy, and other measures for relief of discomfort associated with acute, painful musculoskeletal conditions.

CONTRAINDICATIONS
Hypersensitivity; administration of parenteral form to those with known renal pathology (because of presence of polyethylene glycol 300 in preparation, which is known to have increased preexisting acidosis and urea retention in those with renal impairment); when muscle spasticity is necessary to maintain an upright position and balance in locomotion or whenever spasticity is used to obtain or maintain locomotive function; comatose states or significant CNS depression from any cause.

ACTIONS
Mechanism of action is not established but may be due to general CNS depression. Has no direct effect on contractile mechanism of striated muscle, the motor endplate, or nerve fiber. Mode of action may be related to its sedative properties. Does not directly relax tense skeletal muscles. Any lessening of discomfort associated with muscle spasm following oral administration is most probably secondary to tranquilizing action with subsequent relief of anxiety and tension. No conclusive evidence is available to suggest drug is superior to sedatives, tranquilizers, or analgesics in relieving discomfort associated with skeletal muscle spasm.

Has an onset of action in 30 minutes. The half-life is from 1 to 2 hours; inactive metabolites are excreted in the urine and small amounts in the feces.

WARNINGS
Safety for use in pregnancy is not established. It is not known whether drug is excreted in human milk, but it should not be used in nursing mothers. Safety and efficacy for use in children under 12 are not established, except in tetanus.

PRECAUTIONS
Total parenteral dosage should not exceed 3 g/day for more than 3 days except in the treatment of tetanus. Rate of injection should not exceed 3 ml/minute. Exercise caution when using injectable form in suspected or known epileptics.

DRUG INTERACTIONS
Has a CNS depressant effect; ingestion of **alcohol** and **CNS depressants** should be avoided. Caution is

advised in myasthenia gravis patients receiving **pyridostigmine bromide.**

Drug/lab test: False increases in 5-hydroxyindoleacetic acid (5-HIAA) determinations, some urinary vanillylmandelic acid (VMA) determinations (depending on method used).

ADVERSE REACTIONS
Parenteral

Cardiovascular: Fainting, syncope, hypotension, and bradycardia. In most cases of syncope, there has been spontaneous recovery; in others, epinephrine, injectable steroids, and/or injectable antihistamines have been employed to hasten recovery.

CNS: Dizziness, lightheadedness, drowsiness, vertigo, headache, mild muscular incoordination. Onset of convulsive seizures has been reported, including instances in known epileptics. The psychic trauma of the procedure may have been a contributing factor. Administration to those with epilepsy is not recommended.

Ophthalmologic: Conjunctivitis, nystagmus, diplopia, blurred vision.

Dermatologic: Urticaria, pruritus, rash, flushing.

Special senses: Metallic taste, nasal congestion.

Miscellaneous: GI upset, thrombophlebitis, sloughing or pain at injection site, anaphylactic reaction, fever.

Oral

Lightheadedness; dizziness; drowsiness; vertigo; lassitude; nausea; allergic manifestations such as urticaria, pruritus, rash; conjunctivitis with nasal congestion, blurred vision, fever.

DOSAGE
Parenteral

For IV and IM use only; subcutaneous administration is not recommended. Total adult dosage should not exceed 3 g/day for more than 3 consecutive days, except in treatment of tetanus. This course may be repeated after a lapse of 48 hours if condition persists. Dosage and frequency of injection are based on severity of condition and therapeutic response.

For relief of symptoms of mild to moderate degree, 1 g may be adequate. Ordinarily, this need not be repeated, because oral administration will usually sustain the relief initiated by the injection. For severe cases or in postoperative conditions in which oral administration is not feasible, 2 g to 3 g may be required.

IV: May be administered undiluted directly into the vein at a maximum rate of 3 ml/minute. May also be added to an IV drip of Sodium Chloride Injection or 5% Dextrose Injection; one vial given as a single dose should not be diluted to more than 250 ml for IV infusion.

IM: Not more than 5 ml should be injected into each gluteal region. May be repeated at 8-hour intervals. As relief of symptoms is achieved, change to oral administration.

Tetanus: Drug may be beneficial in controlling neuromuscular manifestations but does not replace usual procedure of debridement, tetanus antitoxin, penicillin, tracheostomy, attention to fluid balance, and supportive care.

Adults: 1 g or 2 g directly into IV tubing. An additional 1 g or 2 g may be added to the infusion bottle so that a total of up to 3 g is given as initial dose. May be repeated q6h until conditions allow for insertion of nasogastric tube. Crushed tablets, suspended in water or saline, may be given through the tube. Total daily dose up to 24 g may be required.

Children: Minimum initial dose of 15 mg/kg is recommended. May be repeated q6h as needed. Maintenance dosage may be given by injection into IV tubing or IV infusion with appropriate quantity of fluid.

Oral (adults)

Initial dose: 1.5 g qid.

Maintenance: 1 g qid; 750 mg q4h; or 1.5 g 2 to 3 times daily. For the first 48 to 72 hours, 6 g/day is recommended. For severe conditions, 8 g/day may be administered. Thereafter, reduce to approximately 4 g/day.

NURSING IMPLICATIONS

HISTORY
See Appendix 4. Note etiology of musculoskeletal disorder (document accurately).

PHYSICAL ASSESSMENT
Obtain blood pressure, pulse, and respirations; evaluate limitations imposed by musculoskeletal disorder (*e.g.*, walking, sitting, movement or use of limbs).

ADMINISTRATION
Parenteral form for IV or IM use only; do not give subcutaneously.

Place patient in recumbent position during and for at least 10 to 15 minutes following IV injection to reduce possibility of fainting, syncope, hypotension.

May be administered undiluted directly into vein at maximum rate of 3 ml/minute.

May be added to IV infusion of Sodium Chloride Injection or 5% Dextrose injection. One vial (1 g) given as single dose should not be diluted to more than 250 ml for IV infusion. Physician orders dose, IV fluid, and IV infusion rate (see *Dosage*).

Exercise care to avoid vascular extravasation of this hypertonic solution, which may result in thrombophlebitis.

IM: Not more than 5 ml (500 mg) should be injected into each gluteal region. Advise patient that injection may be uncomfortable or painful. Rotate injection sites when administering more than one dose.

ONGOING ASSESSMENTS AND NURSING MANAGEMENT

IV: Monitor blood pressure, pulse, and respirations q1h to q2h; monitor IV infusion rate q15m.

IM: Monitor blood pressure, pulse and respirations q2h to q4h.

If extravasation occurs, discontinue IV infusion and notify physician; IM or oral administration or restarting of the IV infusion in another vein may be ordered.

Check IV infusion site for signs of thrombophlebitis daily if extravasation occurred. Notify physician if redness, soreness, or streaking along pathway of vein is noted. Check IM injection site daily for evidence of irritation.

Notify physician if adverse effects occur; in some instances, dosage change or discontinuation of drug may be necessary.

Assist patient with ambulatory activities (when allowed) for at least 2 hours after parenteral administration. If CNS effects are pronounced, patient should remain recumbent until symptoms abate.

Note response to therapy (*e.g.,* relief of pain or discomfort, muscle spasm).

If CNS symptoms occur during oral therapy, advise patient to make position changes slowly.

PATIENT AND FAMILY INFORMATION

May cause drowsiness, dizziness, or lightheadedness. Observe caution while driving or performing tasks requiring alertness.

Avoid alcohol or other CNS depressants.

Notify physician or nurse if skin rash, itching, fever, or nasal congestion occurs or symptoms are not improved or become worse.

Urine may darken to brown, black, or green on standing.

Methohexital Sodium

See Anesthetics, General, Barbiturates.

Methotrexate *(Amethopterin, MTX)* Rx

tablets: 2.5 mg	*Generic*
injection: 2.5 mg/ml, 25 mg/ml	*Generic*

powder for injection: 20 mg/vial for reconstitution	Mexate, *Generic*
powder for injection: 25 mg/vial for reconstitution	Folex
powder for injection: 50 mg/vial, 100 mg/vial for reconstitution	Folex, Mexate, *Generic*
powder for injection: 250 mg/vial for reconstitution	Mexate

INDICATIONS

Antineoplastic chemotherapy: For treatment of gestational choriocarcinoma, and in those with chorioadenoma destruens and hydatidiform mole; for palliation of acute lymphocytic leukemia. Also indicated in treatment and prophylaxis of meningeal leukemia. Greatest effect seen in palliation of acute lymphoblastic (stem cell) leukemias in children. In combination with other anticancer drugs or suitable agents, may be used for induction of remission, but is most commonly used in maintenance of induced remissions.

May be used alone or in combination with other anticancer agents in management of breast cancer, epidermoid cancers of head and neck, and lung cancer, particularly squamous cell and small cell types. Also effective in treatment of the advanced stages (III and IV, Peters's Staging System) of lymphosarcoma, particularly in children, and in advanced cases of mycosis fungoides.

Psoriasis chemotherapy: Symptomatic control of severe, recalcitrant, disabling psoriasis not adequately responsive to other forms of therapy. Used only when diagnosis is established by biopsy and/or after dermatologic consultation.

CONTRAINDICATIONS

When used in treatment of psoriasis, contraindicated in severe renal or hepatic disorders; preexisting blood dyscrasias, such as bone marrow hypoplasia, leukopenia, thrombocytopenia, or anemia and pregnancy.

ACTIONS

Principal mechanism of action is competitive inhibition of folic acid reductase. Folic acid must be reduced to tetrahydrofolic acid by this enzyme in the process of DNA synthesis and cellular replication. Methotrexate inhibits the reduction of folic acid and therefore interferes with tissue-cell reproduction. Actively proliferating tissues such as malignant cells, bone marrow, fetal cells, dermal epithelium, buccal and intestinal mucosa, and cells of the urinary bladder are generally more sensitive to this effect of methotrexate. Cellular proliferation in malignant tissue is greater than in most normal tissue; thus methotrexate may impair malignant growth without irreversible damage to normal tissues.

Orally administered, it is rapidly absorbed in most patients, and reaches peak serum levels in 1 to 2 hours. After injection, peak serum levels seen in about one-half this period. Approximately 50% of absorbed drug is reversibly bound to serum protein, but exchanges with body fluids easily and diffuses into body tissue cells. Excretion of single daily doses occurs through the kidneys in amounts from 55% to 88% or more within 24 hours. Repeated daily doses result in more sustained serum levels and some drug retention over each 24-hour period, which may result in the accumulation of drug in tissues. Liver cells appear to retain certain amounts of drug for prolonged periods even after a single therapeutic dose. Drug is retained in the presence of impaired renal function and may accumulate rapidly. Does not penetrate the blood–cerebrospinal fluid barrier in therapeutic amounts when given orally or parenterally; high concentrations, when needed, may be attained by direct intrathecal administration.

WARNINGS

Because of possibility of fatal or severe toxic reactions, patient is informed of risks involved and kept under constant supervision. Deaths have been reported with use of methotrexate in psoriasis.

May produce marked depression of bone marrow, anemia, leukopenia, thrombocytopenia, and bleeding. May be hepatotoxic, particularly at high dosage or with prolonged therapy. Liver atrophy, necrosis, cirrhosis, fatty changes, and periportal fibrosis have been reported. Because changes may occur without previous signs of GI or hematologic toxicity, hepatic function must be determined prior to initiation of therapy and monitored regularly throughout therapy. Special caution is indicated in presence of preexisting liver damage or impaired hepatic function. Concomitant use of other drugs with hepatotoxic potential (including alcohol) should be avoided.

Has caused fetal death and/or congenital anomalies; not used in women of childbearing potential unless benefits outweigh possible risks.

Impaired renal function usually a contraindication; dosage modifications required.

Diarrhea and ulcerative stomatitis are frequent toxic effects and require interruption of therapy; otherwise, hemorrhagic enteritis and death from intestinal perforation may occur.

Has been administered in very high dosage followed by leucovorin rescue in experimental treatment of certain neoplastic diseases. This procedure is investigational and hazardous.

PRECAUTIONS

Has high toxicity potential, usually dose related. Patients should be under supervision so that signs and symptoms of possible toxic effects or adverse reactions may be detected and evaluated with minimal delay. Pretreatment and periodic hematologic studies are essential due to possibility of hematopoietic suppression. This may occur abruptly and on apparent safe dosage; any profound drop in blood cell count indicates immediate withdrawal of drug and appropriate therapy. Used with caution, if at all, in patients with malignant disease who have preexisting bone marrow aplasia, leukopenia, thrombocytopenia or anemia.

**Use in impaired renal function:** May result in accumulation of toxic amounts or additional renal damage. Renal status should be determined prior to and during therapy. Caution is exercised should additional renal impairment occur. Drug dosage should be reduced or discontinued until renal function improved or restored.

Use with extreme caution in presence of infection, peptic ulcer, ulcerative colitis, debility, and in extreme youth or old age.

If profound leukopenia occurs during therapy, bacterial infection may occur or become a threat. Cessation of drug and appropriate antibiotic therapy usually indicated. In severe bone-marrow depression, blood or platelet transfusions may be necessary.

May have immunosuppressive action; this is taken into consideration in evaluating use of drug when immune responses may be important or essential. Smallpox vaccination may produce generalized vaccinia and should not be undertaken.

Most adverse reactions are reversible if detected early. When such effects occur, dosage should be reduced or discontinued and appropriate corrective measures taken. Reinstitution of therapy should be done with caution.

Intrathecal therapy with large doses may cause seizures. Untoward side-effects may occur and are commonly neurologic. Intrathecal methotrexate appears in the systemic circulation and may cause systemic toxicity; adjust systemic antileukemic therapy appropriately.

DRUG INTERACTIONS

Methotrexate is bound in part to serum albumin after absorption. Toxicity may be increased because of displacement by certain drugs such as **salicylates, sulfonamides, phenytoin, phenylbutazone,** and some antibacterials such as **tetracycline, chloramphenicol,** and **para-aminobenzoic acid. Probenecid** and **salicylates** may also increase toxicity by blocking renal tubular excretion of methotrexate. These drugs, especially salicylates, phenylbutazone and sulfonamides (whether antibacterial, hypoglycemic, or di-

M

uretic) should not be given concurrently. Vitamin preparations containing **folic acid** or its derivatives may decrease response to methotrexate. **Pyrimethamine,** because of similar folic acid antagonist actions, may increase methotrexate toxicity. **Alcohol** may increase risk of methotrexate-induced hepatotoxicity; consumption should be restricted. Methotrexate may enhance hypoprothrombinemic effect of oral anticoagulants.

ADVERSE REACTIONS

Most common include ulcerative stomatitis, leukopenia, nausea, and GI distress. Others reported are malaise, fatigue, chills and fever, dizziness, and decreased resistance to infection. Incidence and severity are dose related.

Dermatologic: Erythematous rashes, pruritus, urticaria, photosensitivity, depigmentation, alopecia, ecchymosis, telangiectasia, acne, furunculosis. Lesions of psoriasis may be aggravated by concomitant exposure to ultraviolet radiation.

Hematologic: Bone-marrow depression, leukopenia, thrombocytopenia, anemia, hypogammaglobulinemia, hemorrhage from various sites, septicemia.

Alimentary: Gingivitis, pharyngitis, stomatitis, anorexia, vomiting, diarrhea, hematemesis, melena, GI ulceration and bleeding, enteritis, hepatic toxicity resulting in acute liver atrophy, necrosis, fatty metamorphosis, periportal fibrosis, or hepatic cirrhosis.

GU: Renal failure, azotemia, cystitis, hematuria, defective oogenesis or spermatogenesis, transient oligospermia, menstrual dysfunction, infertility, abortion, fetal defects, severe nephropathy.

Pulmonary: Interstitial pneumonitis deaths have been reported; chronic obstructive pulmonary disease has occasionally occurred.

CNS: Headaches, drowsiness, blurred vision. Aphasia, hemiparesis, paresis, and convulsions have occurred. Leukoencephalopathy following IV administration to those who have had craniospinal irradiation. After intrathecal use, CNS toxicity which may occur can be classified as (1) chemical arachnoiditis (headache, back pain, nuchal rigidity, fever); (2) transient paresis (paraplegia associated with involvement with spinal nerve roots); or (3) leukoencephalopathy (confusion, irritability, somnolence, ataxia, dementia, occasionally major convulsions).

Other: Pneumonitis, metabolic changes, precipitating diabetes, osteoporotic effects, abnormal tissue cell changes, anaphylaxis, sudden death.

OVERDOSAGE

Leucovorin (citrovorum factor) is a potent agent for neutralizing immediate toxic effects on the hematopoietic system. When large doses or overdoses given, calcium leucovorin may be administered by IV infusion in doses up to 75 mg within 12 hours, followed by 12 mg IM q6h for four doses. Where average doses of methotrexate appear to have an adverse effect, 6 mg to 12 mg of calcium leucovorin may be given IM q6h for four doses. In general, when overdosage is suspected, dose of leucovorin should be equal to or higher than dose of methotrexate and is best administered within the first hour. Use of leucovorin after an hour delay is much less effective. Alternatively, leucovorin may be administered orally: 10 mg/m^2 initially, followed by 10 mg/m^2 every 6 hours for 72 hours. See also Leucovorin.

DOSAGE

Antineoplastic

Oral administration is often preferred because absorption is rapid and effective serum levels are obtained. Parenterally it may be given IM, IV, intraarterially, or intrathecally.

Choriocarcinoma and similar trophoblastic diseases: Given orally or IM in doses of 15 mg/day to 30 mg/day for a 5-day course. Course is usually repeated 3 to 5 times as required, with rest periods of 1 or more weeks interposed between courses until any toxic symptoms subside. Effectiveness of therapy usually evaluated by 24-hour analysis of urinary chorionic gonadotropin hormone (CGH), which should return to normal or less than 50 IU/24 hours, usually after third or fourth course and usually followed by complete resolution of lesions in 4 to 6 weeks. One or two courses after normalization of CGH are recommended. Prophylactic chemotherapy for hydatidiform mole is recommended because lesion may precede or be followed by choriocarcinoma; doses similar to those for choriocarcinoma.

Leukemia: Acute lymphatic (lymphoblastic) leukemia in children and young adolescents is most responsive. In young adults and older patients, remission is more difficult and early relapse is common. In chronic lymphatic leukemia, adequate response is less encouraging. Corticosteroid therapy in combination with other antileukemic drugs or in cyclic combinations with methotrexate appears to produce rapid and effective remissions.

When used for induction, methotrexate doses of 3.3 mg/m^2 in combination with prednisone 60 mg/m^2 given daily produced remission in 50% of patients, usually within 4 to 6 weeks. Methotrexate alone or in combination with other agents appears to be drug of choice for maintenance of remissions. When remission achieved, maintenance therapy is initiated as follows: methotrexate 2 times/week PO or IM in doses of 30 mg/m^2; also may be given in doses of 2.5 mg/kg IV every 14 days.

Meningeal leukemia: Because of increased frequency of meningeal leukemia, methotrexate may be administered prophylactically in lymphocytic leukemia, as well as for treatment of meningeal leukemia.

Intrathecal injection: Sodium salt of methotrexate is administered in a solution in doses of 12 mg/m^2 or in an empirical dose of 15 mg. Drug is given at intervals of 2 to 5 days and usually repeated until cell count in the CSF returns to normal. For prophylaxis against meningeal leukemia, dose is the same, except for the intervals of administration.

Lymphomas: In some cases of Burkitt's tumor (Stages I and II), methotrexate has produced prolonged remission. Recommended dosage is 10 mg/day to 25 mg/day PO for 4 to 8 days. In Stage III, methotrexate is usually given concomitantly with other antitumor agents. Treatment in all stages generally consists of several courses interposed with 7- to 10-day rest periods. Lymphosarcomas in Stage III may respond to combined drug therapy with methotrexate given in doses of 0.625 mg/kg/day to 2.5 mg/kg/day. Hodgkin's disease responds poorly.

Mycosis fungoides: Dosage usually is 2.5 mg/day to 10 mg/day PO for weeks or months. May also be given IM in doses of 50 mg/week or 25 mg twice a week. Dosage and dose regimen are adjusted according to patient response.

Severe, recalcitrant, disabling psoriasis

Dosage is individualized. Test dose (5 mg to 10 mg parenterally) is performed 1 week prior to therapy.

Weekly single oral, IM or IV dose schedule: 10 mg/week to 25 mg/week until adequate response achieved. Do not exceed 50 mg/week.

Divided dose schedule: 2.5 mg q12h for three doses or q8h for four doses each week. Do not exceed 30 mg/week.

Daily oral dose schedule: 2.5 mg/day for 5 days followed by at least a 2-day rest period. Do not exceed 6.25 mg/day. This schedule may carry increased risk of serious liver pathology.

NURSING IMPLICATIONS

HISTORY
See Appendix 4.

PHYSICAL ASSESSMENT
Record general physical and emotional status, vital signs, weight.

Psoriasis: Examine lesions; record location, appearance.

General: Extensive baseline studies are ordered, including complete hemogram, hematocrit, urinalysis, renal- and hepatic-function tests, chest x-ray. Liver biopsy or bone-marrow aspiration is recommended when high-dose or long-term therapy is administered. These studies are also recommended when drug is used in treatment of psoriasis.

ADMINISTRATION
When administered parenterally, check physician's order and label carefully. Parenteral isotonic liquid form (generic from Lederle) is available as preservative free or preserved and physician must specify which form is to be used.

Reconstitution of powder for injection: For IV or IM use, dilute with 2 ml to 10 ml of a preservative-free solution such as 5% Dextrose Solution, USP or Sodium Chloride Injection, USP. Physician must specify diluent and amount used. For intrathecal use, physician will order amount and type of diluent. Recommended strength is 1 mg/ml.

Dilute drug immediately before use.

IV administration is by slow IV push.

Intra-arterial administration: An infusion pump will be necessary. Physician must specify diluent, volume, and rate of infusion.

NOTE: A variety of dosage schedules have been developed for induction and maintenance of remission in leukemia. Dosage prescribed may differ from those listed under *Dosage.*

A test dose (5 mg to 10 mg parenterally) is recommended 1 week prior to therapy for psoriasis.

ONGOING ASSESSMENTS AND NURSING MANAGEMENT

CLINICAL ALERT: Methotrexate may produce marked bone-marrow depression, may be hepatotoxic, and may cause hemorrhagic enteritis. Death has occurred as a result of administration. Most adverse reactions are reversible if detected early; therefore, careful observations are essential.

Record temperature q4h; blood pressure, pulse, and respirations q2h to q4h or as ordered; observe for adverse reactions (review *Adverse Reactions* carefully); measure intake and output.

In order to identify adverse reactions, the nurse should assess body systems most likely affected—skin and mucous membranes, blood (signs of bone-marrow depression), GI, GU, pulmonary, and CNS—every day. Each person responsible for care of patients receiving this drug should perform the same systematic assessment and record findings daily. Notify physician immediately if any adverse reactions are noted.

Observe for signs of bone-marrow depression (Appendix 6, section 6-8). CBC, differential, and platelet count are performed periodically during therapy (usually every 3–7 days) as well as on completion of a course of therapy. Blood cell counts may be performed every 1 to 2 weeks if drug is used for psoriasis.

Begin good oral care at time of initiation of therapy. Inspect mouth daily for signs of ulcerative stomatitis (erythema of mucous membranes, small white blisters; patient may initially complain of burning sensation in mouth). Inform physician of development immediately because therapy may need to be discontinued. Begin stomatitis care (Appendix 6, section 6-21). Check patient's stools and vomitus for blood, which may indicate GI ulceration and bleeding, hemorrhagic enteritis.

Profound leukopenia may result in bacterial infection or a threat of infection. Drug is discontinued and antibiotic therapy usually instituted. Protective isolation may be necessary. Hospital personnel and visitors with upper respiratory infections or recent exposure to a communicable disease should avoid patient contact.

Severe bone-marrow depression may require blood or platelet transfusions. Physician may order type and cross-match as soon as bone-marrow depression is noted.

Notify physician of any change in intake–output ratio. Impaired renal function may result in accumulation of toxic amounts of drug or even additional renal damage.

If thrombocytopenia occurs, protect patient from injury. Apply prolonged pressure on venipuncture sites, IM administration sites; wrap sphygmomanometer cuff gently on arm, avoid overinflation; avoid rectal temperatures when possible; pad siderails if patient is restless.

If diarrhea occurs, notify physician because antidiarrheal therapy may be necessary. If diarrhea is severe, observe patient for signs of dehydration, electrolyte imbalance (Appendix 6, sections 6-10 and 6-13 to 6-18).

Convulsions may occur. Keep oral airway at bedside. Notify physician immediately if a convulsion does occur.

Anorexia may occur. If it persists more than 2 days, discuss with physician.

Weigh daily or as ordered. Notify physician of any significant weight loss.

Nausea and vomiting may occur. If vomiting is severe or persists more than 4 hours, notify physician because an antiemetic may be necessary. Patients who have experienced severe nausea and vomiting during previous courses of therapy may receive an antiemetic prior to first dose and q4h prn during therapy. A liquid diet, carbonated beverages, and unsalted crackers may be offered.

Drug may be hepatotoxic, particularly at high dosage or with prolonged therapy. Liver-function studies are usually performed during therapy. Observe patient daily for evidence of jaundice, darkened urine, pale stools. If these occur, notify physician immediately.

Pneumonitis may occur. Notify physician promptly if fever, cough, or dyspnea occurs.

Diabetes may be precipitated. Check urine daily for glucose. Notify physician if glycosuria present or patient complains of polydipsia or polyuria.

Effectiveness of therapy in choriocarcinoma may be evaluated by 24-hour urines for CGH, which should return to normal or less after third or fourth course.

Intrathecal administration: CNS reactions may occur several hours after administration. Observe patient q2h to q4h for headache, backpain, nuchal rigidity, fever, transient paresis, confusion, irritability, somnolence, ataxia, dementia, major convulsions. Notify physician immediately if CNS symptoms are apparent.

Leucovorin rescue: Physician will write specific orders regarding administration of leucovorin following large dose of methotrexate. This procedure is hazardous; it is essential that the protocol outlined by the physician is followed. See also *Overdosage,* above, and Leucovorin.

Patient with severe, debilitating psoriasis: Inspect lesions daily and compare with data base; question patient regarding present symptoms as compared to original symptoms.

PATIENT AND FAMILY INFORMATION

NOTE: Patient and/or family member must receive full instructions regarding dosage, potential dangers associated with this drug, and those adverse effects requiring omission of the next dose and immediate notification of the physician.

Take exactly as directed on prescription container (physician may prescribe only a 7-day supply of drug at one time because of drug's potential toxicity).

Avoid alcohol and prolonged exposure to sunlight or sunlamps.

Do not use any nonprescription drug unless use is approved by physician. Salicylates and some vitamin preparations (may contain folic acid) must be avoided.

Inform other physicians, dentists of therapy with this drug.

May cause nausea, vomiting, anorexia, hair loss, skin rash, boils, or acne. Notify physician or nurse if these effects persist.

Notify physician or nurse immediately if any of the following occurs: diarrhea, abdominal pain, black tarry stools, fever and chills, sore throat, unusual bleeding or bruising, sores in or around the mouth, cough or shortness of breath, yellow discoloration of skin or eyes, darkened urine, bloody urine, swelling of the feet or legs, flank pain, or joint pain.

Strict supervision is necessary while taking this drug; keep all physician and laboratory appointments.

Drink plenty of fluids. If anorexia is severe, or significant weight loss is noted, inform physician.

Contraceptive measures are recommended during and for at least 8 weeks following cessation of therapy.

Psoriasis (in addition to the above): Contact physician if condition worsens.

Methotrimeprazine _Rx_

injection: 20 mg/ml   Levoprome

INDICATIONS

Relief of moderate to marked pain in nonambulatory patients; for obstetric analgesia and sedation when respiratory depression is to be avoided; as a preanesthetic for producing sedation, somnolence, and relief of apprehension and anxiety.

CONTRAINDICATIONS

Do not use concurrently with antihypertensive agents including monoamine oxidase (MAO) inhibitors, in patients with history of phenothiazine sensitivity, in presence of overdosage of CNS depressants or comatose states, in presence of severe myocardial infarction (MI) or renal or hepatic disease, in presence of clinically significant hypotension, or in patients under 12 years.

ACTIONS

A phenothiazine derivative and potent CNS depressant that produces suppression of sensory impulses, reduction of motor activity, sedation, and tranquilization. Raises pain threshold and produces amnesia. Also has antihistamine, anticholinergic, and antiadrenergic effects.

Low concentrations of drug occur in the serum. Is actively metabolized into sulfoxides and glucuronic conjugates and is largely excreted in the urine as such. Small amounts of unchanged drug

are excreted in feces and urine. Elimination into urine usually continues for several days after administration.

WARNINGS

Following administration, orthostatic hypotension, sedation, fainting, or dizziness may occur. Use of vasopressors is required rarely; when needed, phenylephrine and methoxamine are suitable agents. Epinephrine should not be used because paradoxical decrease in blood pressure may occur. Norepinephrine is reserved for hypotension not reversed by other vasopressors.

Use with caution in women of childbearing potential and during early pregnancy. A possible antifertility effect has been suggested. There is no evidence of adverse developmental effect when used during late pregnancy and labor.

PRECAUTIONS

Elderly and debilitated patients with heart disease are more sensitive to phenothiazine effects; low initial doses are recommended, with adjustment of subsequent doses based on patient response and tolerance.

Continued administration beyond 30 days is usually unnecessary and is advised only when narcotics are contraindicated or in terminal illness. When long-term use is anticipated, periodic blood counts and liver-function studies are recommended.

DRUG INTERACTIONS

Extra additive effects with **CNS depressants** including **narcotics, barbiturates, general anesthetics,** and certain drugs such as **meprobamate** and **reserpine.** The dose of methotrimeprazine and each drug should be reduced and adjusted when used concomitantly or when sequence of use results in overlapping drug effects. Not used concurrently with **antihypertensive drugs,** including **MAO inhibitors.** Use with caution with **atropine, scopolamine,** and **succinylcholine;** tachycardia and fall in blood pressure may occur, and undesirable CNS effects such as stimulation, delirium, and extrapyramidal symptoms may be aggravated.

ADVERSE REACTIONS

There is considerable variation in type and frequency of these effects; some may be dose related and many involve patient sensitivity. Most of these effects have occurred only on long-term, high-dosage administration and have not necessarily been reported with recommended analgesic doses.

Cardiovascular: Most important side-effects are associated with orthostatic hypotension and include fainting or syncope and weakness. See _Ongoing Assessments and Nursing Management_ (p 692).

M

CNS: Disorientation, dizziness, excessive sedation, weakness, slurred speech.

GI: Abdominal discomfort, nausea, vomiting.

GU: Difficulty in urination; rarely, uterine inertia.

Allergic: Local inflammation and swelling.

Hematologic: Agranulocytosis with long-term, high-dosage use.

Hepatic: Jaundice with long-term, high-dosage use.

Miscellaneous: Chills, dry mouth, nasal congestion, pain at injection site. See also Antipsychotic Agents for other adverse effects that may occur with use of phenothiazines.

DOSAGE

Administer deep IM into large muscle mass. Do not administer subcutaneously because local irritation may occur. IV administration is not recommended.

Adults: Usual dosage for analgesia is 10 mg to 20 mg q4h to q6h as required for pain relief. Dose per injection has varied from 5 mg to 40 mg at intervals of 1 to 24 hours. Flexible dosage schedule and low initial dose of 10 mg are advised until patient response and tolerance are determined.

Elderly patients: Initial recommended dose is 5 mg to 10 mg. If patient tolerates drug and requires greater relief from pain, subsequent doses may be gradually increased.

Analgesia for acute or intractable pain: Initial dose is 10 mg to 20 mg; subsequent doses are given q4h to q6h and adjusted as required.

Obstetric analgesia: During labor, an initial dose of 15 mg to 20 mg is usually satisfactory. May be repeated in similar or adjusted amounts at intervals needed for analgesia and sedation.

Preanesthetic medication: Preoperative dose has varied from 2 mg to 20 mg administered 45 minutes to 3 hours before surgery. A dose of 10 mg often is satisfactory; 15 mg to 20 mg may be used when more sedation is desired. Atropine sulfate or scopolamine hydrobromide may be used concurrently, but in lower than usual dosage.

Postoperative analgesia: In immediate postoperative period, initial dose of 2.5 mg to 7.5 mg is suggested, because residual effects of anesthetic agents and other medications may be additive to actions of methotrimeprazine. Subsequent doses are adjusted and administered at intervals of 4 to 6 hours as needed. Ambulation must be avoided or carefully supervised.

NURSING IMPLICATIONS

HISTORY

Review patient's record for health history, allergy history, concomitant drug therapy. When applicable, review chart for etiology of pain, length of time drug given, time of last administration, therapeutic effect of analgesic, date of drug order.

PHYSICAL ASSESSMENT

At time patient requests analgesic, determine exact location of pain, type of pain (sharp, dull, stabbing), when pain began. In addition, look for controllable factors (*e.g.,* uncomfortable position, thirst, noise, bright lights, cold) that may decrease patient's tolerance to pain.

ADMINISTRATION

If patient is receiving other CNS depressants or certain other drugs (see *Drug Interactions*), dosages must be adjusted. If patient received any drug listed in this section within last 2 to 4 hours, contact physician before administering methotrimeprazine because sequence of use may result in overlapping of drug effects.

Obtain blood pressure, pulse, and respirations immediately before preparing drug for administration. If these vital signs are significantly increased or decreased from average baseline values, withhold drug and notify physician immediately.

May be given IM in same syringe with either atropine sulfate or scopolamine hydrobromide. Do *not* mix with other drugs.

Doses of atropine or scopolamine are lower than usual dosage when these drugs are given concurrently with methotrimeprazine.

When multiple injections are used, rotate injection sites; record site used.

Place patient in supine position. Inform patient that drug may cause pain at injection site.

Proper injection technique is important to prevent inadvertent injection into a blood vessel into or in the region of a peripheral nerve trunk, and to avoid leakage along the needle track. Use Z-track technique for injection; aspirate prior to injection of drug.

Following administration keep patient in supine position and raise siderails.

ONGOING ASSESSMENTS AND NURSING MANAGEMENT

Cardiovascular adverse effects can usually be avoided by keeping patient supine for about 6 hours (occasionally as long as 12 hours) after injection. Advise patient to remain in bed in this position to avoid dizziness, lightheadedness.

Obtain blood pressure and pulse 20 to 30 minutes after administration. A drop in blood pressure often occurs, usually beginning 10 to 20 minutes after administration, and may last 4 to 6 hours (and occasionally 12 hours). If decrease in blood pressure is significant, notify physician immediately. Occasionally, fall in blood pressure may be profound and requires immediate restorative measures.

Continue to monitor blood pressure and pulse q1h to q2h, especially if significant decrease occurred, patient is elderly or acutely ill, or a high dose was administered, as well as during initial use of drug.

At end of 6 hours (if patient is allowed out of bed) assist to a sitting position. If lightheadedness or dizziness persists more than 2 to 3 minutes, place patient again in a supine position for several more hours.

Cardiovascular effects usually diminish or disappear with continued or intermittent administration.

Observe for other adverse drug reactions. If any such reaction occurs, notify physician before next dose is due because dosage may need to be reduced or drug discontinued and another analgesic ordered.

Observe and record analgesic effects of drug. Maximum analgesic effect usually occurs within 20 to 40 minutes and is maintained for about 4 hours. If drug fails to produce sufficient analgesia, discuss problem with physician because a different analgesic may be necessary.

Assist patient with all ambulatory activities when he is receiving this drug.

Once tolerance to the cardiovascular effects of the drug is obtained, it will usually be maintained unless more than several days elapse between subsequent doses.

Methoxamine Hydrochloride Rx

injection: 20 mg/ml   Vasoxyl

INDICATIONS

For supporting, restoring, or maintaining blood pressure during anesthesia (including cyclopropane anesthesia); for terminating some episodes of paroxysmal supraventricular tachycardia.

CONTRAINDICATIONS

In combination with local anesthetics to prolong their action at local sites.

ACTIONS

A vasopressor that produces prompt and prolonged rise in blood pressure by increasing peripheral resistance. Is especially useful for maintaining blood pressure during operations under spinal anesthesia. May also be used during general anesthesia. Has no direct effect on the heart and therefore is not useful

when cardiac failure is the major cause of hypotension.

Provides potent, prolonged pressor action. There is no increase in cardiac rate; occasionally a decrease develops as blood pressure increases. This bradycardia is apparently caused by a carotid sinus reflex mediated over the vagus nerve; this is abolished by atropine. Cardiac output may be decreased or unchanged.

PRECAUTIONS

Not used as a substitute for replacement of blood, plasma, fluids, and electrolytes, which should be restored promptly when loss has occurred.

Extravasation may cause necrosis and sloughing of surrounding tissue.

Use with care in those with hyperthyroidism or severe hypertension. In heart failure, increase in peripheral resistance produced by drug may produce or exacerbate heart failure associated with a diseased myocardium.

DRUG INTERACTIONS

Vasopressors may cause serious cardiac arrhythmias during **halothane anesthesia.** If vasopressors are used in obstetrics to correct hypotension or are added to the local anesthetic solution, some **oxytocic drugs** may cause severe persistent hypertension; even rupture of a cerebral blood vessel may occur during the postpartum period.

The pressor effect of sympathomimetic pressor amines is markedly potentiated in those receiving **MAO inhibitors** or **tricyclic antidepressants.** To prevent excessive rise in blood pressure, observe caution when used following parenteral injection of **ergot alkaloids.** Concomitant administration with **beta-adrenergic blocking agents, guanethidine,** or **reserpine** may precipitate a severe hypertensive response.

ADVERSE REACTIONS

Sustained hypertension with severe headache, pilomotor response, a desire to void, and projectile vomiting, particularly with high dosage.

OVERDOSAGE

Exercise caution to avoid overdosage so that undesirably high blood pressure or excessive bradycardia will not occur. Bradycardia may be abolished with atropine.

DOSAGE

Emergencies: 3 mg to 5 mg IV, injected slowly. IV injection may be supplemented by IM injection to provide prolonged effect.

Spinal anesthesia: Usual IM dose is 10 mg to 15 mg, shortly before or with spinal anesthesia to pre-

M

vent hypotension. A 10-mg dose may be adequate at lower levels; 15 mg to 20 mg may be required at higher levels of spinal anesthesia. Repeat doses if necessary, but allow time for previous dose to act (about 15 minutes).

Correction of a fall in blood pressure: 10 mg to 15 mg IM, depending on degree of decrease. When systolic pressure falls below 60 mm Hg or when an emergency exists, 3 mg to 5 mg is given IV. This may be accompanied by 10 mg to 15 mg IM for prolonged effect.

Pre- and postoperative use (moderate hypotension): 5 mg to 10 mg IM may be adequate.

Paroxysmal supraventricular tachycardia: Average dose is 10 mg IV, injected slowly.

NURSING IMPLICATIONS

HISTORY

When possible, review chart for diagnosis, health history, allergy history, recent treatment modalities and diagnostic tests, recent vital signs.

PHYSICAL ASSESSMENT

Obtain general status of patient; blood pressure, pulse, respirations.

ADMINISTRATION

May be given IV or IM. IV injection may be supplemented by IM injection.

When giving IV, inject slowly over period of 2 to 3 minutes. Monitor blood pressure during administration.

When methoxamine is administered for paroxysmal supraventricular tachycardia, patient should be on a cardiac monitor.

Have atropine sulfate available for correction of excessive bradycardia.

ONGOING ASSESSMENTS AND NURSING MANAGEMENT

Monitor blood pressure and pulse q5m until condition is stabilized, then q1/2h to q1h until possibility of repeat hypotensive episode has passed. If patient has received a spinal anesthetic, monitor vital signs until feeling and movement return and vital signs have stabilized.

If blood pressure decreases after drug is discontinued, notify physician immediately.

CLINICAL ALERT: Overdosage is to be avoided so that undesirably high blood pressure or excessive bradycardia will not occur. Repeat doses, when necessary, will be based on blood pressure and pulse. Allow at least 15 minutes for IM dose to act.

Observe for development of bradycardia; notify physician immediately if significant decrease in pulse rate occurs. Atropine sulfate may be ordered to correct bradycardia.

Observe for adverse reactions, particularly with high dosage, and notify physician should they occur.

Measure intake and output. Notify physician of change in intake–output ratio or if urinary output is less than 30 ml/hour to 50 ml/hour.

Methoxyflurane

See Anesthetics, General, Volatile Liquids.

Methscopolamine Bromide

See Gastrointestinal Anticholinergics/Antispasmodics.

Methsuximide

See Anticonvulsants, Succinimides.

Methyclothiazide

See Thiazides and Related Diuretics.

Methylcellulose

See Laxatives; Ocular Lubricants and Artificial Tears.

Methyldopa and Methyldopate Hydrochloride Rx

tablets: 125 mg, 250 mg, 500 mg	Aldomet
oral suspension: 250 mg/5 ml	Aldomet
injection: 250 mg/5 ml (as methyldopate HCl)	Aldomet

INDICATIONS

Hypertension. Treatment of acute hypertensive crisis may be initiated with parenteral methyldopate HCl. However, drug has a slow onset of action and other agents are preferred when rapid reduction of blood pressure is necessary.

CONTRAINDICATIONS

Active hepatic disease, such as acute hepatitis or active cirrhosis; if previous methyldopa therapy has been associated with liver disorders (see *Warnings*); hypersensitivity.

ACTIONS

Mechanism of action not conclusively demonstrated. Antihypertensive effect is probably due to its metabolism to alpha-methyl-norepinephrine, which then lowers arterial pressure by stimulation of central inhibitory alpha-adrenergic receptors, false neurotransmission, and/or reduction of plasma renin activity. Has been shown to cause net reduction in tissue concentrations of serotonin, dopamine, norepinephrine, and epinephrine.

Has no direct effect on cardiac function and usually does not reduce the glomerular filtration rate (GFR), renal blood flow, or filtration fraction. Cardiac output is usually decreased without cardiac acceleration. In some, the heart rate is slowed. Normal or elevated plasma renin activity may decrease. Reduces standing blood pressure, and, to a lesser degree, supine blood pressure. Usually produces highly effective lowering of supine pressure with infrequent symptomatic postural hypotension. Exercise hypotension and diurnal blood pressure variations may occur. Methyldopate HCl (parenteral form) possesses the same pharmacologic attributes as methyldopa (oral forms).

Absorption of methyldopa variable; peak antihypertensive effect is 4 to 6 hours after administration. Elimination half-life is approximately 2 hours; however, antihypertensive activity persists up to 24 hours. Approximately 2 days are required to establish maximal antihypertensive effects and for hypertension to return after therapy is discontinued. Effective IV doses cause a decline in blood pressure, which may begin in 4 to 6 hours and last 10 to 16 hours. Drug is removed by dialysis.

WARNINGS

A positive Coombs' test, hemolytic anemia, and liver disorders may occur. Rare occurrences of hemolytic anemia or liver disorders could lead to potentially fatal complications unless properly recognized and managed. If Coombs-positive hemolytic anemia occurs, drug is discontinued; usually the anemia remits promptly. If not, corticosteroids may be given and other causes of anemia considered. The positive Coombs' test may not revert to normal until weeks to months after drug is stopped. In addition to a positive direct Coombs' test, there is less often a positive indirect Coombs' test, which may interfere with cross-matching of blood.

Liver disorders: Fever has occasionally occurred within first 3 weeks of therapy, associated in some cases with eosinophilia or abnormalities in one or more liver-function tests. Jaundice, with or without fever, may occur with onset usually within first 2 to

3 months of therapy. In some, the findings are consistent with cholestatic jaundice. Fatal hepatic necrosis has been reported rarely. These hepatic changes may represent hypersensitivity reactions. If fever, abnormalities in liver-function tests, or jaundice appears, therapy is discontinued. Temperature and liver function revert to normal when drug is discontinued and therapy is not reinstituted.

Hematologic disorders: Rarely, a reversible reduction in WBC count with a primary effect on granulocytes has been seen. The granulocyte count promptly returned to normal when drug was discontinued. Reversible thrombocytopenia has occurred rarely.

Use in pregnancy: Safety for use not established. Use only when clearly needed and potential benefits outweigh the unknown potential hazards to the fetus. Neonates born of mothers receiving drug have demonstrated decreased blood pressure for 2 days after delivery. Methyldopa crosses the placental barrier and appears in cord blood and breast milk. Possibility of injury to the nursing infant cannot be excluded.

PRECAUTIONS

A paradoxical pressor response has been reported with IV use. Involuntary choreoathetotic movements have been observed rarely during therapy in those with severe bilateral cerebrovascular disease. Should these occur, therapy is discontinued. Use with caution in those with previous liver disease or dysfunction. Hypertension has occurred occasionally after dialysis in patients given methyldopa because drug is removed by this procedure.

DRUG INTERACTIONS

Concomitant **antihypertensive** therapy may potentiate the antihypertensive effect. Patient may require reduced doses of **anesthetics;** hypotension occurring during anesthesia usually can be controlled with vasopressors. Adrenergic receptors remain responsive during treatment with methyldopa.

Tolbutamide metabolism may be impaired, resulting in enhanced hypoglycemic effects. Concomitant administration of **phenoxybenzamine** and methyldopa may produce reversible total urinary incontinence. Symptoms of **lithium** intoxication (without elevated lithium blood levels) have been reported during concurrent administration of therapeutic doses of lithium and methyldopa. Concurrent administration of **haloperidol** and methyldopa may produce adverse psychiatric symptoms manifested by irritability, aggressiveness, assaultiveness, and dementia.

Drug/lab tests: May interfere with **urinary uric acid, serum creatinine,** and **SGOT** (depending on methods used). Falsely high levels of **urinary cate-cholamines** may be reported. Does not interfere with measurement of **vanillylmandelic acid (VMA)** by method that converts VMA to vanillin. Rarely, when urine is exposed to air after voiding, it may darken. A positive **Coombs'** test may occur.

ADVERSE REACTIONS

Significant adverse effects are infrequent; drug is usually well tolerated.

CNS: Sedation, usually transient, may occur during initial therapy or whenever dose is increased. Headache, asthenia, or weakness may be noted as early and transient symptom. Dizziness; lightheadedness; symptoms of cerebrovascular insufficiency; paresthesias; parkinsonism; Bell's palsy; decreased mental acuity; involuntary choreoathetotic movements; psychic disturbances including nightmares and reversible mild psychosis or depression; memory impairment.

Cardiovascular: Bradycardia; prolonged carotid sinus hypersensitivity; aggravation of angina; paradoxical pressor response (with IV use); myocarditis (fatal); orthostatic hypotension (decrease daily dosage); edema and weight gain, usually relieved by a diuretic. Drug is discontinued if edema progresses or signs of heart failure appear.

GI: Nausea; vomiting; distention; constipation; flatus; diarrhea; colitis; mild dryness of mouth; sore or "black" tongue; pancreatitis; sialadenitis.

Hepatic: Abnormal hepatic-function tests; jaundice; liver disorders; hepatitis.

Hematologic: Positive Coombs' test; hemolytic anemia; bone-marrow depression; leukopenia; granulocytopenia; thrombocytopenia; positive tests for antinuclear antibody, LE cells, rheumatoid factor.

Dermatologic: Rash as in eczema or lichenoid eruption; toxic epidermal necrolysis.

Allergic: Drug-related fever; lupuslike syndrome.

Other: Nasal stuffiness; rise in BUN; breast enlargement; gynecomastia; lactation; hyperprolactinemia; amenorrhea; galactorrhea; impotence; failure to ejaculate; decreased libido; myalgia; septic shock-like syndrome.

DOSAGE

Those with impaired renal function may respond to smaller doses. Syncope in older patients may be related to an increased sensitivity and advanced arteriosclerotic vascular disease. This may be avoided by lower doses.

Oral

Adults: Initiation of therapy—Usual starting oral dose is 250 mg two to three times/day in first 48 hours. Daily dosage is then increased or decreased, preferably at intervals of not less than 2 days, until adequate response is achieved. To minimize seda-

tion, dosage increases are started in evening. By adjustment of dosage, morning hypotension may be prevented without sacrificing control of afternoon blood pressure.

Maintenance—Usual oral daily dosage is 500 mg to 2 g given in two to four doses. *Maximum recommended dosage*—3 g/day. Once effective dosage range is attained, smooth blood pressure response occurs in most patients in 12 to 24 hours. Drug is usually administered in two divided doses; some patients may maintain adequate blood pressure control with a single daily dose H.S.

Concomitant drug therapy—When given with antihypertensives other than thiazides, initial dose should be limited to 500 mg/day in divided doses. When added to a thiazide, dosage of thiazide need not be changed.

Children: Initial oral dosage based on 10 mg/kg/day in two to four doses. Daily dosage is then increased or decreased until adequate response achieved. *Maximum dosage*—65 mg/kg or 3 g daily, whichever is less.

Tolerance: Occasionally may occur, usually between second and third month of therapy. Adding a diuretic or increasing dosage of methyldopa will frequently restore effective control of blood pressure. A thiazide may be added at any time during therapy and is recommended if therapy is not started with a thiazide or effective control cannot be maintained on 2 g of methyldopa a day.

Discontinuation: Drug has relatively short duration of action; withdrawal is usually followed by return of hypertension within 48 hours. This is not complicated by an overshoot of blood pressure above pretreatment levels.

IV

Add desired dose to 100 ml of 5% Dextrose or give in 5% Dextrose in water in a concentration of 100 mg/10 ml. Administer by slow IV infusion over period of 30 to 60 minutes. When control is obtained, oral therapy may be substituted, starting with same dosage schedule being used parenterally.

Adults: Usual dosage is 250 mg to 500 mg q6h as required. Maximum recommended dose is 1 g q6h.

Children: Recommended daily dosage is 20 mg/kg to 40 mg/kg in divided doses q6h. Maximum dosage is 65 mg/kg or 3 g daily, whichever is less.

NURSING IMPLICATIONS

HISTORY
See Appendix 4.

PHYSICAL ASSESSMENT
Obtain blood pressure, pulse on both arms in standing, sitting, and supine position; weight;

look for evidence of edema in extremities. Laboratory studies include hepatic-function tests, CBC, Coombs' test. Other tests may also be appropriate.

ADMINISTRATION

Larger oral dose may be given in evening during adjustment period. Medicine cards should be clearly labeled when divided doses are different.

IV: Dose may be added to 100 ml of 5% Dextrose or dose given in 5% Dextrose in Water in a concentration of 100 mg/10 ml. Physician must specify method of dilution to be used (see *Dosage*).

If concentration of 100 mg/10 ml is desired, 250 mg methyldopa is added to 25 ml or 500 mg is added to 50 ml of Dextrose in Water.

Obtain blood pressure and pulse immediately before and q5m to q10m during infusion of methyldopate HCl.

IV infusion is run slowly over period of 30 to 60 minutes. Calculate infusion rate based on final amount of solution and prescribed time of infusion. When 250 mg is administered over a period of 30 minutes, it should infuse at rate of 1 ml/minute; 500 mg added to 50 ml administered over a period of 60 minutes should infuse at rate of 1 ml/minute. If dose is added to 100 ml, run at 3 ml/minute to infuse in approximately 30 minutes. Physician may also order different infusion rate.

ONGOING ASSESSMENTS AND NURSING MANAGEMENT

Monitor vital signs q4h during period of adjustment. Take blood pressure on both arms in standing, sitting, and supine positions. Once dosage is stabilized, obtain temperature daily and blood pressure and pulse q8h or as ordered.

Weigh daily during period of adjustment and 1 to 2 times a week thereafter. Inform physician of any significant weight gain.

Measure intake and output during period of adjustment. Notify physician of any change in the intake–output ratio.

Sedation may occur during initial period or whenever dosage is increased. Assist patient with ambulatory activities.

Orthostatic hypotension may occur. Advise patient to make position changes slowly; assist with ambulatory activities and notify physician because dosage change may be necessary.

Daily, observe for adverse reactions and report occurrence to physician because dosage adjustment may be necessary. If edema of extremities is noted, contact physician because a diuretic may be necessary.

CLINICAL ALERT: If fever or jaundice occurs, notify physician before next dose is due because drug may need to be discontinued (see *Warnings*).

For 2 to 3 days, monitor blood pressure and pulse of neonates born to mothers receiving methyldopa; notify physician if changes are noted.

In addition to a (possible) positive direct Coombs' test, there is less often a positive indirect Coombs' test, which may interfere with cross-matching of blood.

Observe elderly patients closely for blood-pressure changes and adverse drug reactions. Syncope may occur and may require dosage adjustment.

Periodic hepatic-function tests are recommended during first 6 to 12 weeks of therapy or whenever unexplained fever occurs; drug may be discontinued if hepatic-function tests are abnormal. Periodic CBC is recommended to detect hemolytic anemia. Direct Coombs' test is recommended at 6 and 12 months after start of therapy.

Report any rise in blood pressure to physician. Tolerance to drug may occur, usually between second and third months of therapy. Dosage adjustment may be necessary.

Diabetic receiving tolbutamide: Observe for enhanced hypoglycemic effects and notify physician if hypoglycemia occurs.

IV administration: Monitor patient closely until infusion is terminated. Monitor blood pressure q5m to q10m. Slow infusion to KVO and notify physician immediately if significant drop or a rise (paradoxical response) in blood pressure occurs.

Following termination of infusion, continue to monitor blood pressure and pulse q1h to q2h or as ordered.

When control of blood pressure is obtained, oral therapy may be instituted.

PATIENT AND FAMILY INFORMATION

NOTE: Patient compliance is especially necessary during adjustment period.

Do not discontinue drug unless directed by physician.

Avoid cough, cold, or allergy medications (may contain sympathomimetics) unless use is approved by physician.

May cause drowsiness, especially during first few days of therapy or whenever dose is increased. Avoid driving and those tasks requiring alertness if drowsiness occurs.

Notify physician of any unexplained prolonged general tiredness or if fever occurs.

If dizziness (orthostatic hypotension) occurs, avoid sudden changes in posture and prolonged standing. Notify physician of this problem.

M

Weigh self weekly; notify physician of significant weight gain.

Urine may darken on standing.

Periodic laboratory tests will be necessary to evaluate therapy. Frequent physician appointments may be necessary during adjustment period.

Methylene Blue Rx

| tablets: 65 mg | Urolene Blue |
| injection: 10 mg/ml | *Generic* |

INDICATIONS

Oral: Mild GU antiseptic for cystitis and urethritis; treatment of idiopathic and drug-induced methemoglobinemia; as an antidote for cyanide poisoning; management of oxalate urinary-tract calculi.

Parenteral: Treatment of cyanide poisoning and drug-induced methemoglobinemia.

Unlabeled uses: Delineation of body structures and fistulas through its dye effect; diagnosis/confirmation of rupture of amniotic membranes.

CONTRAINDICATIONS

Allergy to drug; renal insufficiency; intraspinal injection.

ACTIONS

A dye that is a weak germicide. Has an oxidation reduction action. It has opposite actions on hemoglobin related to concentration. In high concentrations it converts the ferrous iron of reduced hemoglobin to the ferric form; as a result, methemoglobin is produced. This action is the basis for use in cyanide poisoning. In contrast, low concentrations of this drug are capable of hastening conversion of methemoglobin to hemoglobin.

PRECAUTIONS

May induce hemolysis in G6PD-deficient patients. Continued administration may cause marked anemia due to accelerated destruction of erythrocytes. Frequent checks of hemoglobin should be made. Cyanosis and cardiovascular abnormalities have accompanied treatment.

ADVERSE REACTIONS

Turns urine and sometimes stool blue-green. May cause bladder irritation and, in some cases, nausea, vomiting, and diarrhea. Large doses may produce abdominal and precordial pain, dizziness, headache, profuse sweating, fever, mental confusion, and formation of methemoglobin.

DOSAGE

Oral: 65 mg to 130 mg tid P.C. with full glass of water.

Parenteral: 1 mg/kg to 2 mg/kg (0.1 mg/kg–0.2 ml/kg). Inject IV slowly over period of several minutes.

NURSING IMPLICATIONS

HISTORY

See Appendix 4. If used for cyanide poisoning, obtain information (when possible) about approximate amount ingested, time of ingestion, substance ingested or inhaled (cyanide may be found in some fertilizers, fumigants, metal-refining processes, and seeds of stone fruits such as apricots).

PHYSICAL ASSESSMENT

CBC is usually done; renal-function tests may also be ordered. If cyanide poisoning is suspected, assess vital signs, general patient status (treatment is an emergency).

NOTE: Amyl nitrate is also an antidote for cyanide poisoning.

ADMINISTRATION

Give P.C. with full glass of water.

Parenteral: Inject slowly over period of 5 or more minutes or as directed by physician.

ONGOING ASSESSMENTS AND NURSING MANAGEMENT

Daily, observe for adverse reactions; compare symptoms with baseline data; record temperature.

Notify physician if condition is not improved or if symptoms become worse.

Frequent checks of hemoglobin are recommended (except in once-only use as in urologic procedures, treatment of cyanide poisoning).

Cyanide poisoning: Treatment is an emergency; physician orders specific therapies based on severity of poisoning.

PATIENT AND FAMILY INFORMATION

Take after meals with full glass of water.

May discolor urine and sometimes stool blue-green.

If symptoms are not improved or become worse, contact physician.

Methylergonovine Maleate Rx

| tablets: 0.2 mg | Methergine |
| injection: 0.2 mg/ml | Methergine |

INDICATIONS

Routine management after delivery of placenta; postpartum atony and hemorrhage; subinvolution. Under full obstetric supervision, may be given in second stage of labor following delivery of the anterior shoulder.

CONTRAINDICATIONS

Hypertension; toxemia; pregnancy; hypersensitivity.

ACTIONS

Increases strength, duration, and frequency of uterine contractions and decreases uterine bleeding following placental delivery. Induces a rapid and sustained tetanic uterotonic effect, which shortens third stage of labor and reduces blood loss.

WARNINGS

Should not be administered routinely IV because it may induce sudden hypertensive or cardiovascular accidents. If IV administration is considered essential as lifesaving measure, give slowly over period of not less than 60 seconds, with careful monitoring of blood pressure.

PRECAUTIONS

Caution is exercised in presence of sepsis, obliterative vascular disease, hepatic or renal involvement.

ADVERSE REACTIONS

Nausea, vomiting, dizziness, increased blood pressure, headache, tinnitus, diaphoresis, palpitation, temporary chest pain, dyspnea.

DOSAGE

IM: 0.2 mg after delivery of the placenta, after delivery of the anterior shoulder, or during the puerperium. May be repeated as required, at intervals of 2 to 4 hours.

IV: Dosage same as IM. See *Warnings*.

Oral: 0.2 mg three or four times a day in the puerperium for maximum of 1 week.

NURSING IMPLICATIONS

HISTORY

Review patient's chart for pregnancy history, labor and delivery history (when applicable).

PHYSICAL ASSESSMENT

Obtain blood pressure and pulse rate.

ADMINISTRATION

Given IM, at direction of physician, at time of delivery of the anterior shoulder or after delivery of the placenta. Obtain blood pressure immediately before administration.

May also be given IM or PO during the puerperium.

IV route reserved for lifesaving measures; give slowly over period of at least 60 seconds.

ONGOING ASSESSMENTS AND NURSING MANAGEMENT

Onset of action after IV administration is immediate; after IM administration is in 2 to 5 minutes; after oral administration is in 5 to 10 minutes.

Monitor blood pressure q15m (or as ordered) following IM administration and q3m to q5m following IV administration until stable. Monitor uterine response q15m or as ordered.

During puerperium (postpartum) monitor blood pressure q4h and uterine response q2h to q4h or as ordered. Patient with uterine atony and hemorrhage will require more frequent monitoring of vital signs, uterine response.

Observe for adverse reactions. Notify physician before next dose is due if adverse reactions become severe or bothersome to patient.

Notify physician if blood pressure increases or decreases or uterine relaxation occurs at frequent intervals.

Physician, unit policy, or patient's condition may dictate nursing observations at intervals other than given above.

PATIENT INFORMATION

May cause nausea, vomiting, dizziness, increased blood pressure, headache, ringing in the ears, chest pain, shortness of breath. Notify physician or nurse if these become severe or bothersome.

Methylphenidate Hydrochloride

Rx C–II

tablets: 5 mg, 10 mg, 20 mg	Ritalin, *Generic*
tablets, sustained release: 20 mg	Ritalin-SR

INDICATIONS

Attention deficit disorders (previously known as minimum brain dysfunction, or MBD, in children): As integral part of total treatment program, which typically includes other remedial measures (psychological, educational, social) for a stabilizing effect in children with behavioral syndrome characterized by the following group of developmentally inappropriate symptoms: moderate to severe distractibility, short attention span, hyperactivity, emotional lability, and impulsivity. Diagnosis is not final when these symptoms are of recent origin. Nonlocalized neurologic signs, learning disability, and abnormal EEG may or may not be present, and diagnosis of CNS dysfunction may or may not be warranted. Drug treatment is not indicated for all children with this syndrome.

Also used for narcolepsy and is labeled "possibly effective" for mild depression; apathetic or withdrawn senile behavior.

CONTRAINDICATIONS
Marked anxiety, tension, and agitation, because drug may aggravate these symptoms; hypersensitivity; glaucoma.

ACTIONS
A mild cortical stimulant with CNS actions similar to those of amphetamines. The exact mechanism of action is not fully understood. It is rapidly absorbed from the GI tract. Peak blood levels are achieved in 1 to 3 hours. Pharmacologic effects persist up to 4 to 6 hours. Most of the drug appears in the urine as metabolites. Plasma half-life ranges from 1 to 2 hours.

WARNINGS
Not to be used for severe depression of either exogenous or endogenous origin. Not used for prevention or treatment of normal fatigue.

Use in children: Not used in children under 6, because safety and efficacy are not established. In psychotic children, drug may exacerbate symptoms of behavioral disturbance and thought disorder. Sufficient data on safety and efficacy of long-term use are not established. Suppression of growth has been reported with long-term use of stimulants in children.

Use in seizure disorders: May lower convulsive threshold in those with prior history of seizures, prior EEG abnormalities in absence of seizures, and, very rarely, in absence of history of seizures and no prior EEG evidence of seizures. Safe concomitant use with anticonvulsants is not established. In presence of seizures, drug is discontinued.

Hypertension: Use cautiously in those with hypertension.

Drug dependence: Use cautiously in emotionally unstable patients, such as those with history of drug dependence or alcoholism, because patient may increase dosage on own initiative. Chronic abuse can lead to marked tolerance and psychic dependence with varying degrees of abnormal behavior. Careful supervision is required during drug withdrawal, because severe depression as well as the effects of chronic overactivity can be unmasked. Long-term

follow-up may be required because of patient's basic personality disturbances.

Visual effects: Symptoms of visual disturbances are encountered rarely. Difficulty with accommodation and blurred vision have been reported.

Use in pregnancy: Use in women of childbearing age only when clearly needed and when potential benefits outweigh the unknown potential hazards to the fetus.

PRECAUTIONS
Long-term effects in children are not well established. Agitated patients may react adversely; drug is discontinued if necessary. Periodic CBC, differential, and platelet count are recommended during therapy.

DRUG INTERACTIONS
May decrease hypotensive effect of **guanethidine.** Use cautiously with **pressor agents, monoamine oxidase (MAO) inhibitors.** May inhibit metabolism of **coumarin anticoagulants, anticonvulsants** (phenobarbital, phenytoin, primidone), **phenylbutazone, tricyclic antidepressants** (imipramine, desipramine). Dosage adjustments of these drugs may be required.

Drug/lab test: May increase urinary excretion of epinephrine.

ADVERSE REACTIONS
Nervousness and insomnia are the most common adverse reactions but are usually controlled by reducing dosage and omitting drug in afternoon or evening.

Hypersensitivity: Skin rash, urticaria, fever, arthralgia, exfoliative dermatitis, erythema multiforme with histopathologic findings of necrotizing vasculitis, thrombocytopenia purpura.

CNS: Dizziness, headache, dyskinesia, chorea, drowsiness.

Cardiovascular: Blood pressure and pulse changes (increase or decrease), tachycardia, angina, cardiac arrhythmia, palpitations.

GI: Anorexia, nausea, abdominal pain, weight loss during prolonged therapy.

Other: Toxic psychosis has been reported. Although definite relationship is not established, leukopenia, anemia, and a few instances of scalp hair loss have been reported.

Children: Anorexia, abdominal pain, weight loss during prolonged therapy, insomnia, and tachycardia may occur more frequently. Any of the above adverse reactions may also occur.

OVERDOSAGE
Symptoms: Symptoms of acute overdosage, resulting principally from overstimulation of the CNS

and from excessive sympathomimetic effects, may include vomiting, agitation, tremors, hyperreflexia, muscle twitching, convulsions (may be followed by coma), euphoria, confusion, hallucinations, delirium, sweating, flushing, headache, hyperpyrexia, tachycardia, palpitations, cardiac arrhythmias, hypertension, mydriasis, dry mucous membranes.

Treatment: Appropriate supportive measures are instituted. Protect patient from self-injury and against external stimuli that would aggravate overstimulation. If signs and symptoms are not too severe and patient is conscious, evacuate gastric contents by induction of emesis or gastric lavage. In presence of severe intoxication, use carefully titrated dosage of short-acting barbiturate before gastric lavage. Intensive care must be provided to maintain adequate circulation and respiratory exchange; external cooling procedures may be required for hyperpyrexia. Efficacy of peritoneal or extracorporeal hemodialysis has not been established.

DOSAGE
Adults: Dosage is individualized. Administer in divided doses two to three times a day, preferably 30 to 45 minutes A.C. Average dose is 20 mg/day to 30 mg/day. Some patients may require 40 mg/day to 60 mg/day. In others, 10 mg/day to 15 mg/day is adequate.

Children with attention disorders (6 years and over): Start with small doses (*e.g.,* 5 mg A.C., breakfast and lunch) with gradual increments of 5 mg/week to 10 mg/week. Daily dosage above 60 mg is not recommended. If improvement is not observed after dosage adjustment over 1 month, discontinue use. If paradoxical aggravation of symptoms or other adverse effects occur, dosage is reduced or drug is discontinued. Discontinue drug periodically to assess condition. Improvement may be sustained when drug is either temporarily or permanently discontinued. Drug treatment should not be indefinite and usually may be discontinued after puberty.

NURSING IMPLICATIONS

HISTORY
See Appendix 4.

PHYSICAL ASSESSMENT
Obtain vital signs; weight (and height in children). *Attention deficit disorder*—Observe behavior (if possible) and record observations. Baseline studies include CBC, differential, platelet count.

ADMINISTRATION
Drug is given before meals. Last daily dose is given before 6 P.M. to prevent insomnia.

If child resists taking medication, inform physician.

ONGOING ASSESSMENTS AND NURSING MANAGEMENT
Obtain vital signs daily; record behavior (activity, attention span, emotional lability, impulsivity, distractibility) if prescribed for attention deficit disorder; record general behavior if prescribed for depression, apathy, or withdrawn senile behavior; observe for adverse reactions.

Inform physician of blood-pressure and pulse changes (increase or decrease) or other cardiovascular reactions. More frequent monitoring of blood pressure and pulse is necessary if cardiovascular changes occur.

Weigh weekly or as ordered. In children, measure and record height monthly and weight weekly; height and weight gains are usually evaluated at 6-month intervals.

Periodic CBC, differential, and platelet counts are obtained during long-term therapy.

PATIENT AND FAMILY INFORMATION
Take last daily dose early in evening (before 6 P.M.) to avoid insomnia.

May mask symptoms of fatigue, impair physical coordination, or produce dizziness or drowsiness. Use caution while driving or performing other tasks requiring alertness.

Notify physician or nurse if nervousness, insomnia, palpitations, vomiting, fever, or skin rash occurs.

Children with attention deficit disorders: During initial therapy, parent should write a daily summary of child's activities, general behavior. This will aid physician in determining adequate drug dosage.

Methylprednisolone

See Glucocorticoids.

Methylprednisolone Acetate

See Corticosteroids, Topical; Glucocorticoids.

Methylprednisolone Sodium Succinate

See Glucocorticoids.

Methyltestosterone

See Androgens.

M

Methyprylon Rx C–III

capsules: 300 mg	Noludar
tablets: 50 mg, 200 mg	Noludar

INDICATIONS
Hypnotic. Prolonged administration generally not recommended.

CONTRAINDICATIONS
Hypersensitivity.

ACTIONS
Increases threshold of the arousal centers in the brain stem and produces CNS depression similar to barbiturates. It suppresses REM sleep and is associated with REM rebound following discontinuation of drug. It stimulates the hepatic microsomal enzyme system.

Plasma half-life is 4 hours; it is prolonged in acute intoxication. Approximately 3% is excreted in urine as intact drug and another 3% as the dihydrometabolite within first 24 hours. When taken H.S., induces sleep within 45 minutes and provides sleep for 5 to 8 hours.

WARNINGS
Physical and psychological dependence: Has been reported infrequently. Withdrawal symptoms, when they occur, resemble those associated with barbiturate withdrawal (see p 170). Exercise caution in giving to those known to be addiction prone or with history suggesting they may increase dosage on their own initiative. It is recommended repeated prescriptions have adequate medical supervision.

Use in pregnancy, lactation: Use only when clearly needed and when potential benefits outweight the unknown potential hazards to mother and child.

Use in children: Not recommended for children under 12 years.

PRECAUTIONS
Total daily intake should not exceed 400 mg; greater amounts do not significantly increase hypnotic benefits. Patients with unrelieved pain should not be heavily sedated. Usual cautions observed in presence of hepatic or renal disorders. Has been reported to precipitate attacks of acute intermittent porphyria and is used with caution in susceptible patients.

DRUG INTERACTIONS
Additive depressant effects will occur when used concomitantly with **alcohol** or other **CNS depressants.**

ADVERSE REACTIONS
Rare: Morning drowsiness; dizziness; mild to moderate gastric upset (including diarrhea, esophagitis, nausea, and vomiting); headache; paradoxical excitation; skin rash. There have been a few isolated reports of neutropenia and thrombocytopenia, but relationship to methyprylon is unclear.

OVERDOSAGE
Symptoms: Somnolence, confusion, coma, constricted pupils, respiratory depression, hypotension.

Treatment: Monitor respiration, pulse, blood pressure. Employ supportive measures, along with immediate gastric lavage with precautions to prevent pulmonary aspiration. Administer appropriate IV fluids; maintain adequate airway. Combat hypotension with norepinephrine, metaraminol, or other accepted antihypotensive measures. Hemodialysis may be of value and use is considered in those in whom supportive measures are failing and adequate urinary output cannot be maintained. There have been occasional reports of excitation and convulsions following overdosage, almost invariably during the recovery phase. Barbiturates may be used with great caution.

DOSAGE
Dosage is individualized for maximum beneficial effects.

Adults: Usual dosage is 200 mg to 400 mg H.S.

Children (over 12): Treatment may be initiated with 50 mg and increased up to 200 mg, if required. Give H.S.

NURSING IMPLICATIONS

HISTORY
See Appendix 4. If prescribed for treatment of insomnia, attempt to discover pattern and possible causes of insomnia.

PHYSICAL ASSESSMENT
Determine if specific factors that may be controlled or eliminated are interfering with sleep. Factors may include noise, bright lights, pain, and discomfort.

ADMINISTRATION
Patient's immediate area should be free from disturbance (*e.g.,* noise, lights) before hypnotic is given.

Following administration, raise siderails and advise patient to remain in bed and call for assistance if it is necessary to get out of bed during nighttime hours.

Do not administer if patient has pain, which should be controlled by administration of an analgesic.

Do not administer a hypnotic shortly before or after administration of a narcotic analgesic (both are CNS depressants; see *Drug Interactions*) or any other CNS depressant. If patient has an order for a narcotic analgesic (or other CNS depressant), check with physician regarding time interval between administration of these agents. Usually 2 or more hours should elapse between administration of a hypnotic and CNS depressant, but interval will vary with a specific CNS depressant and the dose administered.

ONGOING ASSESSMENTS AND NURSING MANAGEMENT
Sleep is usually induced in 45 minutes. Observe patient in 45 to 60 minutes to evaluate effect of drug.

Observe for adverse reactions. If paradoxical excitation occurs, evaluate situation; patient may require close observation. Contact physician if excitation is severe; restraints or other measures may be necessary to prevent injury or falls.

Evaluate drug effect during nighttime hours and the following morning. Notify physician if drug appears ineffective.

If used repeatedly over prolonged periods, periodic blood counts are recommended.

PATIENT AND FAMILY INFORMATION
May cause drowsiness or dizziness. Do not attempt to drive or perform other tasks requiring alertness after taking this drug.

Do not drink alcoholic beverages before or after taking this drug because the combination of alcohol and this drug can be dangerous.

Avoid use of other CNS depressants while taking this drug.

Do not exceed prescribed dosage.

Methysergide Maleate Rx

tablets: 2 mg   Sansert

INDICATIONS
Prevention or reduction of intensity or frequency of vascular headaches in the following: patients suffering from one or more severe vascular headaches a week; patients with vascular headaches that are uncontrollable or so severe that preventive therapy is indicated regardless of the frequency of attack. Drug is for prophylaxis of vascular headache and has no place in management of the acute attack. May prove beneficial in migraine prophylaxis in up to 65% of patients treated; adverse reactions occur in up to 40% of patients treated. Treatment is limited to short-term use in those with severe headaches refractory to other therapy.

CONTRAINDICATIONS
Peripheral vascular disease; severe arteriosclerosis; severe hypertension; coronary artery disease; phlebitis or cellulitis of lower limbs; pulmonary disease; collagen diseases or fibrotic processes; impaired hepatic or renal function; valvular heart disease; debilitated states and severe infections.

Contraindicated in pregnancy.

ACTIONS
Inhibits or blocks the effects of serotonin, a substance that may be involved in the mechanism of vascular headaches. Serotonin has been described as central neurohormonal agent or chemical mediator, as a "headache substance" acting directly or indirectly to lower pain threshold (others in this category include tyramine, polypeptides such as bradykinin, histamine, acetylcholine), as an intrinsic "motor hormone" of the GI tract, and as a hormone involved in connective tissue reparative processes. Serotonin is also a potent vasoconstrictor. Plasma serotonin levels are elevated during the pre-headache phase of classical migraine and decreased during an attack. Methysergide may replace serotonin on receptor sites of the walls of the cranial arteries during a migraine attack and thereby preserve the vasoconstriction afforded by serotonin. Mechanism by which this drug produces clinical effects is not established. One or two days are required for protective effects to develop; following termination, 1 to 2 days are required before effects subside.

WARNINGS
With long-term uninterrupted administration, retroperitoneal fibrosis or related conditions (pleuropulmonary fibrosis and cardiovascular disorders with murmurs or vascular bruits) have been reported. Continuous administration should not exceed 6 months. There must be a drug-free interval of 3 to 4 weeks after each 6-month course of treatment. Not recommended for use in children.

PRECAUTIONS
All patients receiving drug should remain under constant supervision and be examined regularly for development of fibrotic or vascular complications. Manifestations of retroperitoneal fibrosis, pleuropulmonary fibrosis and vascular shutdown have shown a high incidence of regression once drug withdrawn. Cardiac murmurs (may indicate endocardial fibrosis) have shown varying degrees of regression, with complete disappearance in some and persistence in others.

M

Drug contains tartrazine. See Appendix 6, section 6-23.

ADVERSE REACTIONS

Fibrosis: Fibrotic changes have been observed in retroperitoneal, pleuropulmonary, cardiac, and other tissues, either singly or, very rarely, in combination. *Retroperitoneal fibrosis*—May present clinically with one or more symptoms such as general malaise, fatigue, weight loss, backache, low-grade fever, urinary obstruction (girdle or flank pain, dysuria, polyuria, oliguria, elevated BUN), vascular insufficiency of lower limbs (leg pain, Leriche syndrome, edema, thrombophlebitis). The single most useful device for diagnosis is intravenous pyelography (IVP). Typical deviation and obstruction of one or both ureters may be seen. *Pleuropulmonary fibrosis*—Presents clinically with dyspnea, tightness and pain in chest, pleural friction rubs, and pleural effusion and is confirmed by chest x-rays. *Cardiac fibrosis*—Presents clinically with cardiac murmurs, dyspnea. *Other fibrotic complications*—Fibrotic plaques simulating Peyronie's disease.

Cardiovascular: Encroachment of retroperitoneal fibrosis on the aorta, inferior vena cava, and their common iliac branches may result in vascular insufficiency of lower limbs. Intrinsic vasoconstriction of large and small arteries, involving one or more vessels or a segment of vessel, may occur at any stage of therapy. Depending on vessel involved, this complication may present with chest pain, abdominal pain, or cold, numb, painful extremities with or without paresthesias and diminished or absent pulses. Drug is withdrawn promptly at first signs of impaired circulation. Postural hypotension and tachycardia have also been seen.

GI: Nausea, vomiting, diarrhea, heartburn, abdominal pain. These effects tend to appear early and may be relieved by gradual introduction of medication and administration with meals. Constipation and elevation of gastric hydrochloric acid have also been reported.

CNS: Insomnia, drowsiness, mild euphoria, dizziness, ataxia, lightheadedness, hyperesthesia, unworldly feelings (described as "dissociation," "hallucinatory experiences," etc.). Some symptoms may be associated with vascular headaches and may be unrelated to drug.

Dermatologic: Facial flush, telangiectasia, nonspecific rashes have been rarely reported. Increased hair loss may occur, but in many instances tendency has abated despite continued therapy.

Edema: Peripheral edema and, more rarely, localized brawny edema. Dependent edema has responded to lower doses, salt restriction, or diuretics.

Weight gain: Caution patients regarding caloric intake.

Hematologic: Neutropenia, eosinophilia.
Miscellaneous: Weakness, arthralgia, myalgia.

DOSAGE

Adults: Usual dose is 4 mg/day to 8 mg/day, with meals or food. There must be a medication-free interval of 3 to 4 weeks after each 6-month course of treatment. If, after a 3-week trial period, efficacy has not been demonstrated, longer administration is unlikely to be of benefit.

Children: No pediatric dosage established.

NURSING IMPLICATIONS

HISTORY

See Appendix 4. Note description, frequency, duration of vascular headache; factors that may increase frequency or severity; prodromal symptoms.

PHYSICAL ASSESSMENT

Vital signs; weight. Pretreatment chest x-ray, pregnancy test (when applicable), ECG, CBC, other tests may be ordered.

ADMINISTRATION

Give with meals or food.

To prevent GI distress, physician may initiate therapy with low dose and increase gradually.

ONGOING ASSESSMENTS AND NURSING MANAGEMENT

Daily or at time of physician's office or clinic visit, obtain vital signs, weight (especially early in therapy); observe for adverse reactions (base assessments on patient complaints as well as checking for edema of extremities).

If vascular headache does occur during therapy, record patient's description of headache and comparison to previous vascular headaches.

May cause dizziness. In some instances, patient may require assistance with ambulation.

Dosage is reduced gradually during last 2 to 3 weeks of each treatment course to avoid "headache rebound."

PATIENT AND FAMILY INFORMATION

May cause GI upset; take with meals or food.

One or two days will be required for protective effects to develop.

May cause drowsiness; use caution when driving or performing other tasks requiring alertness.

If dizziness occurs, avoid sudden changes in posture; rise from a sitting or lying position slowly.

Notify physician or nurse immediately if any of the following occurs: cold, numb, and painful hands and feet; leg cramps on walking; girdle, flank, or chest pain; shortness of breath; painful or difficult urination.

If headache should occur, note date, time of onset, duration, severity of symptoms (as compared with previous episodes); bring this information to next office or clinic visit.

If headaches persist or become worse (after 2 days of drug therapy), contact physician.

Weigh self weekly; notify physician if significant weight gain or edema of extremities is noted. In addition, watch caloric intake.

There will be a 3- to 4-week drug-free interval every 6 months. The dosage will be reduced during the last 2 to 3 weeks of this period.

Physician will evaluate effectiveness of therapy at periodic intervals.

Metoclopramide Rx

tablets: 10 mg	Reglan
injection: 10 mg/ 2 ml	Reglan
syrup: 5 mg/5 ml	Reglan

INDICATIONS

Oral: Relief of symptoms associated with acute and recurrent diabetic gastroparesis. Usual manifestations of delayed gastric emptying (*i.e.,* nausea, vomiting, persistent fullness after meals, anorexia) appear to respond within different time intervals. Significant relief of nausea appears early and continues to improve over a 3-week period. Relief of vomiting and anorexia may precede relief of abdominal fullness by 1 week or more.

Parenteral: Prophylaxis of vomiting associated with cisplatin cancer chemotherapy. Single dose may be used to facilitate small bowel intubation in those in whom the tube does not pass the pylorus with conventional maneuvers. Also used to stimulate gastric emptying and intestinal transit of barium in cases in which delayed emptying interferes with radiologic examination of the stomach or small intestine.

Unlabeled uses: Has been used investigationally to improve lactation. Doses of 30 mg/day to 45 mg/day have been shown to increase milk secretion, possibly by elevating serum prolactin levels. In addition, studies have indicated some potential value of metoclopramide in the following conditions: gastroesophageal reflux; nausea and vomiting of a variety of etiologies, including emesis during pregnancy and labor; gastric ulcer and anorexia nervosa (due to GI stimulation). It may also be of value in protecting against chemotherapy-induced vomiting from agents other than cisplatin.

CONTRAINDICATIONS

Hypersensitivity. Not used when stimulation of GI motility might be dangerous (*e.g.,* in presence of GI hemorrhage, mechanical obstruction, or perforation). Contraindicated in pheochromocytoma because drug may cause hypertensive crisis, probably because of release of catecholamines from the tumor. Such crisis may be controlled by phentolamine. Not used in epileptics or those receiving other drugs likely to cause extrapyramidal reactions, because frequency and severity of seizures or extrapyramidal reactions may be increased.

ACTIONS

Stimulates motility of upper GI tract without stimulating gastric, biliary, or pancreatic secretions. Mode of action is unclear. It appears to sensitize tissues to the action of acetylcholine. The effect on motility is not dependent on intact vagal innervation, but can be abolished by anticholinergic drugs. Increases the tone and amplitude of gastric (especially antral) contractions, relaxes the pyloric sphincter and duodenal bulb, and increases peristalsis of the duodenum and jejunum, resulting in accelerated gastric emptying and intestinal transit. It increases tone of the lower esophageal sphincter; has little, if any effect on motility of the colon or gallbladder.

Like phenothiazines and related drugs, which are also dopamine antagonists, metoclopramide produces sedation and may produce extrapyramidal reactions, although these are rare. Drug inhibits central and peripheral effects of apomorphine, induces release of prolactin, and causes a transient increase in circulating aldosterone levels.

Is well absorbed after oral administration but is subject to significant first-pass metabolism, with total bioavailability in range of 50% to 70%. Half-life is approximately 4 hours, and drug is excreted in the urine.

WARNINGS

Extrapyramidal reactions: Are rare. Occur most frequently in children and young adults and are even more frequent at higher doses used in prophylaxis of vomiting due to cancer chemotherapy. If reaction should occur, it is treated with 50 mg of diphenhydramine IM.

Use in pregnancy, lactation: Use only when clearly needed and when potential benefits outweigh the unknown potential hazards to the fetus. Readily enters into breast milk; exercise caution when administering to a nursing mother.

PRECAUTIONS

Elevates prolactin levels, which may be of significance in those with previously detected breast cancer because some breast cancers are prolactin de-

M

pendent. Gastroparesis (gastric stasis) may be responsible for poor diabetic control in some patients. Exogenously administered insulins may begin to act before food has left stomach and may lead to hypoglycemia.

DRUG INTERACTIONS
Effects of drug on GI motility are antagonized by **anticholinergic drugs** and **narcotic analgesics.** Additive effects can occur when drug is given with **alcohol, sedatives, hypnotics, narcotics,** or **tranquilizers.** Absorption of drugs from stomach may be diminished (*e.g.,* **digoxin, cimetidine**), whereas absorption of drugs from the small bowel may be increased (*e.g.,* **acetaminophen, tetracycline, levodopa, ethanol**). It influences delivery of food to the intestines and thus the rate of absorption; **insulin** dosage or timing of dosage may require adjustment.

ADVERSE REACTIONS
Approximately 20% to 30% of patients experience side-effects. These usually are mild and transient and are reversible on drug withdrawal. High doses of 2 mg/kg for control of cisplatin-induced vomiting have produced CNS and GI side-effects with an incidence of 81% and 43% respectively.

CNS (12%–24%): Drowsiness; restlessness; fatigue; lassitude; extrapyramidal reactions and parkinsonismlike reactions; akathisia; dizziness; anxiety; dystonia; insomnia; headache; rarely, depression and persistent dyskinesia.

GI (12%–24%): Nausea, diarrhea.

Other: Transient hypertension.

OVERDOSAGE
Symptoms: May include drowsiness, disorientation, extrapyramidal reactions. These are self-limiting and usually disappear within 24 hours.

Treatment: Anticholinergic or antiparkinsonism drugs or antihistamines with anticholinergic properties may be helpful in controlling extrapyramidal symptoms.

DOSAGE
Oral: For relief of symptoms associated with diabetic gastroparesis, give 10 mg 30 minutes before each meal and H.S. for 2 to 8 weeks, depending on response and likelihood of continued well-being upon drug discontinuation. Because problem is frequently recurrent, therapy is reinstituted at earliest manifestation.

May be given IM or IV for severe symptoms of nausea and vomiting in those with diabetic gastroparesis. Dose is 10 mg IM or IV 30 minutes A.C. and H.S. until symptoms subside and oral administration is tolerated.

Diluted IV infusion: For prevention of cisplatin-induced emesis, dilute injectable in 50 ml of large volume of parenteral solution (Dextrose 5% in Water, Sodium Chloride Injection, Dextrose 5% in 0.45% Sodium Chloride, Ringer's Injection, or Lactated Ringer's Injection). Infuse slowly, over period of not less than 15 minutes, 30 minutes before beginning cisplatin; repeat q2h for two doses, then q3h for three doses. Initial two doses should be 2 mg/kg. If vomiting is suppressed, a 1 mg/kg dose can be tried. If extrapyramidal symptoms occur, 50 mg of diphenhydramine may be given IM.

Direct IV injection: Recommended single dose is 10 mg (2 ml) for adults; 2.5 mg to 5 mg (0.5 ml–1 ml) for children 6 to 14 years; 0.1 mg/kg for children under 6 years.

For facilitation of small bowel intubation: If tube has not passed the pylorus with conventional maneuvers in 10 minutes, a single undiluted dose may be given direct IV over a period of 1 to 2 minutes.

Radiologic examinations: When delayed gastric emptying interferes with examination of stomach or small intestine, a single dose may be given by direct IV over a 1- to 2-minute period.

NURSING IMPLICATIONS

HISTORY
Diabetic with gastroparesis: Description and duration of symptoms; diabetic history (insulin or oral hypoglycemic agent, dose, dietary management).

Other indications: Review chart for health history; allergy history; current treatment modalities.

PHYSICAL ASSESSMENT
Obtain vital signs, weight.

Patient receiving cisplatin therapy: Evaluate general physical status, hydration.

Diabetic patient: Baseline blood glucose, urinalysis may be ordered.

ADMINISTRATION
Parenteral

Visually inspect parenteral drug for particulate matter and discoloration; do not use if discolored or particulate matter is present.

When administering by IV infusion, protect from light by placing brown paper bag or aluminum foil over infusion container.

Prevention of cisplatin-induced emesis: Dilute ordered dose in volume of parenteral solution as ordered by physician (usually dose diluted in 50 ml). Use piggyback or secondary IV line and volume control set for administration unless physician (or unit policy) orders otherwise. Administer at rate ordered by physician (usually over a period of not less than 15 minutes). Drug is given 30 minutes before administration of cisplatin and may be repeated (see *Dosage*).

Direct IV injection: Inject slowly over 1- to 2-minute period, because transient but intense feeling of anxiety and restlessness, followed by drowsiness, may occur with rapid administration.

May be given IM or IV for severe symptoms of nausea and vomiting (see *Dosage*).

Storage: Dilutions may be stored up to 48 hours after preparation if protected from light. Protect from light during storage and infusion.

Oral

Give 30 minutes A.C. and H.S.

ONGOING ASSESSMENTS AND NURSING MANAGEMENT

Onset of action is 1 to 3 minutes following IV dose, 10 to 15 minutes following IM administration, and 30 to 60 minutes following oral dose. Effects persist for 1 to 2 hours.

Observe for adverse reactions, especially extrapyramidal symptoms, which may be evidenced by feelings of restlessness and may occasionally include involuntary movements of limbs and facial grimacing; rarely, torticollis, oculogyric crisis, rhythmic protrusion of tongue, bulbar type speech, and trismus.

Diphenhydramine 50 mg IM may be ordered to control extrapyramidal symptoms.

Drowsiness or dizziness may occur. Ambulatory patient may require assistance.

Relief of symptoms of diabetic gastroparesis: Evaluate and record drug response (*e.g.,* relief of nausea, vomiting, anorexia, feeling of epigastric fullness after meals).

If drug is given parenterally, use oral route as soon as patient is able to tolerate this route of administration.

Measure intake and output; notify physician if oral intake is poor or vomiting persists.

Insulin dosage may require adjustment. Check urine for glucose, ketone bodies qid; report glycosuria and/or ketonuria to physician. Observe for signs and symptoms of hyperglycemia and hypoglycemia (Appendix 6, section 6-14) and manage according to physician's instructions or hospital policy (see also Insulin).

Patient receiving cisplatin: Monitor infusion rate q5m.

Evaluate drug effect (*e.g.,* relief from or reduced incidence of cisplatin-induced emesis); record observations and inform physician.

Observe for adverse drug effects, especially extrapyramidal symptoms (see above); report oc-

currence promptly because physician may order diphenhydramine 50 mg IM.

PATIENT AND FAMILY INFORMATION

Take 30 minutes before each meal and at bedtime.

May produce drowsiness and dizziness; observe caution while driving or performing other tasks requiring alertness.

Notify physician or nurse immediately if involuntary movement of eyes, face, or limbs occurs.

Check urine for glucose, ketones at least daily or as recommended by physician. Insulin dosage may require adjustment during administration of this drug; therefore, keep physician informed of hypoglycemic episodes, glycosuria.

Metocurine Iodide

See Curare Preparations.

Metolazone

See Thiazides and Related Diuretics.

Metoprolol Tartrate

See Beta-Adrenergic Blocking Agents.

Metronidazole Rx

tablets: 250 mg, 500 mg	Flagyl, Metryl, Protostat, Satric, *Generic*
injection: 500 mg/ vial (as HCl)	Flagyl IV
injection, ready to use: 500 mg per 100 ml (as HCl)	Flagyl IV RTU, Metro I.V.

INDICATIONS

Oral

Amebiasis: Treatment of acute intestinal amebiasis (amebic dysentery) and amebic liver abscess.

Symptomatic trichomoniasis: In females and males when presence of trichomonad is confirmed.

Asymptomatic trichomoniasis: Treatment of asymptomatic females when organism is associated with endocervicitis, cervicitis, or cervical erosion.

Treatment of asymptomatic partner: *Trichomonas vaginalis* infection is a venereal disease. Asymptomatic partners of treated patients

M

should be treated simultaneously if organism is found to be present, in order to prevent reinfection. Because there may be considerable difficulty in isolating the organism from the asymptomatic male carrier, negative smears and cultures cannot be relied upon. Women may become reinfected if male partners are not treated; it may be advisable to treat the asymptomatic male partner with negative culture or when no culture has been attempted.

Anaerobic bacterial infections: Treatment of serious infections caused by susceptible organisms (see *Parenteral,* below). In most serious infections, the parenteral form is usually administered initially; this may be followed by oral therapy.

Parenteral

Anaerobic bacterial infections: Treatment of serious infections caused by susceptible anaerobic bacteria. In mixed aerobic and anaerobic infection, antibiotics appropriate for treatment of the aerobic infection are also used. Effective in *Bacteroides fragilis* infections resistant to clindamycin, chloramphenicol, and penicillin.

Intra-abdominal infections (peritonitis, intra-abdominal abscess, liver abscess): Infections caused by *Bacteroides* species, *Clostridium* species, *Eubacterium* species, *Peptostreptococcus* species, *Peptococcus* species.

Skin, skin structure infections: Infections caused by *Bacteroides* species, *Clostridium* species, *Peptococcus* species, *Peptostreptococcus* species, *Fusobacterium* species.

Gynecologic infections (endometritis, endomyometritis, tubo-ovarian abscess, postsurgical vaginal cuff infection): Infections caused by *Bacteroides* species, *Clostridium* species, *Peptococcus* species, *Peptostreptococcus* species.

Bacterial septicemia: Septicemia caused by *Bacteroides* species, *Clostridium* species.

Other: Bone and joint infections (as adjunctive therapy), CNS infections, lower respiratory tract infections (pneumonia, empyema, lung abscess), and endocarditis caused by *Bacteroides* species.

Unlabeled uses: Has shown efficacy, alone and in combination, as a prophylactic agent in reducing infection rates in gynecologic, abdominal, and colonic surgery. Also has compared favorably with neomycin in treatment of hepatic encephalopathy. Metronidazole and some of its relatives have been investigated for action as radiosensitizers, rendering resistant tumors more susceptible to radiation therapy; however, more data are needed.

CONTRAINDICATIONS

Hypersensitivity. Oral form contraindicated in *first* trimester of pregnancy.

ACTIONS

Is a synthetic antibacterial compound. Disposition of drug in the body is similar for both oral and IV dosage forms. It appears in CSF, saliva, and breast milk in concentrations similar to those found in plasma. Major route of elimination is the urine. Drug has an average elimination half-life of 8 hours in healthy individuals. Plasma clearance is decreased in those with decreased liver function.

Oral: Possesses direct trichomonacidal and amebicidal activity against *T. vaginalis* and *Entamoeba histolytica.* It enters the bacterial cell more readily under anaerobic conditions. Is active against *T. vaginalis, E. histolytica, Giardia lamblia,* and obligate anaerobic bacteria. Gram-negative anaerobic bacilli and clostridia are also susceptible. Against susceptible organisms, it is bactericidal at concentrations equal to or slightly higher than the minimum inhibitory concentration (MIC). It is usually well absorbed; bioavailability does not appear to be significantly decreased by food.

Parenteral: Has been shown to be active against anaerobic gram-negative bacilli including *Bacteroides* species (*e.g., B. fragilis, B. distasonis, B. ovatus, B. thetaiotaomicron, B. vulgatus*), *Fusobacterium* species; anaerobic gram-positive bacilli, including *Clostridium* species and susceptible strains of *Eubacterium;* anaerobic gram-positive cocci, including *Peptococcus* species, *Peptostreptococcus* species.

WARNINGS

Oral

Crosses the placental barrier and rapidly enters fetal circulation; when administered to nursing mothers, drug is secreted in breast milk. Although metronidazole is not shown to be teratogenic, data are not adequate to rule out a possible teratogenic effect. Drug should not be used in the first trimester of pregnancy. In addition, it has been shown to be tumorigenic in rodents; use in trichomoniasis in the second and third trimesters and during lactation should be restricted to those in whom local palliative treatment has been inadequate to control symptoms. If used during lactation, an alternate method of infant feeding may be elected. Neurologic effects (see *Parenteral,* below) may also be seen.

Parenteral

Neurologic effects: Convulsive seizures and peripheral neuropathy have been reported.

Sodium retention: Administration of solutions containing sodium ions may result in sodium retention (Flagyl IV RTU contains 14 mEq sodium/vial). Metronidazole should be administered carefully to those receiving corticosteroids or predisposed to edema.

Use in impaired hepatic function: Accumulation of drug and its metabolites may occur in the plasma of those with severe hepatic disease. Doses below those usually recommended are given cautiously.

Use in pregnancy, lactation: Crosses the placental barrier and enters fetal circulation rapidly. Use during pregnancy only if clearly needed. Safety for use in the nursing mother is not established. Drug is secreted in breast milk in concentrations similar to those found in plasma.

Use in children: Safety and effectiveness are not established.

PRECAUTIONS

Oral: Mild leukopenia has been reported; total and differential leukocyte counts are recommended before and during treatment, especially if a second course is necessary. Abnormal neurologic signs require prompt discontinuation of therapy. Known or previously unrecognized candidiasis may present more prominent symptoms during therapy and require treatment with a candicidal agent. Vaginitis due to organims other than *T. vaginalis* does not respond to this drug. When used for amebic liver abscess, metronidazole does not obviate the need for aspiration of pus.

Parenteral: Known or previously unrecognized candidiasis may present more prominent symptoms during therapy and require treatment with a candicidal agent. Use with care in those with evidence or history of blood dyscrasia. Mild leukopenia has been reported during administration; total and differential leukocyte counts are recommended before and after therapy.

DRUG INTERACTIONS

Ingestion of **alcohol** may result in the occurrence of abdominal cramps, nausea, vomiting, headache, and flushing. May potentiate the anticoagulant effect of **warfarin** and other **coumarin anticoagulants** resulting in a prolongation of prothrombin time. Concurrent use with **disulfiram** may result in an acute psychotic reaction or confusional state caused by the combined toxicity. Antimicrobial effectiveness may be decreased when administered concurrently with **phenobarbital** or **phenytoin,** probably because of increased metronidazole metabolism; a higher dose of metronidazole may be required.

Drug/lab tests: May interfere with certain chemical analysis for **SGOT,** resulting in decreased values. A value of zero may be seen.

ADVERSE REACTIONS

CNS: The two most serious reactions reported have been convulsive seizures and peripheral neu-

ropathy, the latter being characterized mainly by numbness or paresthesia of an extremity. Less serious effects are dizziness, vertigo, incoordination, ataxia, confusion, irritability, depression, weakness, insomnia, headache, and syncope. Toxic encephalopathy has been associated with high dose or prolonged dosing; controversy exists as to whether it is concentration related.

GI: *Most common*—Nausea, sometimes accompanied by headache, anorexia, and occasionally vomiting; diarrhea; epigastric distress; abdominal cramping; constipation; proctitis; sharp, unpleasant, metallic taste; modification of taste of alcoholic beverages; furry tongue; glossitis; stomatitis (these may be associated with a sudden overgrowth of *Candida*). This drug has been paradoxically implicated in causing, curing, and failing to cure pseudomembranous colitis.

Hematopoietic: Reversible neutropenia (leukopenia).

Renal/GU: Dysuria, cystitis, polyuria, incontinence, sense of pelvic pressure. Darkened urine has been reported but has no clinical significance. Proliferation of *Candida* in the vagina, dyspareunia; decreased libido.

Cardiac: Flattening of the T-wave.

Hypersensitivity: Urticaria, erythematous rash, flushing, nasal congestion, dryness of mouth (or vagina or vulva), fever.

Local reactions: Thrombophlebitis after IV infusion can be minimized or eliminated by avoiding prolonged use of indwelling IV catheters.

Other: Fleeting joint pains, sometimes resembling serum sickness.

OVERDOSAGE

Symptoms of oral overdosage include nausea, vomiting, and ataxia. The oral form has been studied as a radiation sensitizer in treatment of malignant tumors. Neurotoxic effects, including seizures and peripheral neuropathy, have been reported. There is no specific antidote; management consists of symptomatic and supportive therapy.

DOSAGE

Anaerobic bacterial infections

In treatment of most serious anaerobic infections, the IV form is usually administered initially.

Loading dose (adults): 15 mg/kg infused over 1 hour (approximately 1 g for 70-kg adult).

Maintenance dose: 7.5 mg/kg infused over 1 hour q6h (approx 500 mg for 70-kg adult). First maintenance dose should be instituted 6 hours following the initial loading dose. Do not exceed a maximum of 4 g/24 hours. Usual duration of treatment is 7 to 10 days; however, infections of the bone and joint, lower respiratory tract, and endocardium may require longer treatment.

Parenteral therapy may be changed to the oral dosage form when conditions warrant, based on severity of disease and response of the patient to IV treatment. Usual adult oral dose is 7.5 mg/kg q6h.

Amebiasis

Acute intestinal amebiasis (acute amebic dysentery): 750 mg tid for 5 to 10 days.

Amebic liver abscess: 500 mg or 750 mg tid for 5 to 10 days.

Children: 35 mg/kg/24 hours to 50 mg/kg/24 hours, in three divided doses for 10 days.

Trichomoniasis

1-day treatment: 2 g given either as a single dose or in two divided doses of 1 g each given in the same day.

7-day treatment: 250 mg tid for 7 consecutive days.

Cure rates, as determined by vaginal smears, signs, and symptoms, may be higher after a 7-day course than after a 1-day course of treatment. Single-dose treatment can assure compliance, especially if administered under supervision, in those who cannot be relied on to continue the 7-day regimen. A 7-day course may minimize reinfection of the woman long enough to treat sexual contacts. Some patients may also tolerate one course of therapy better than the other.

Patients are *not treated* in the *first* trimester of pregnancy. If treated during the second and third trimesters in those in whom palliative treatment has been inadequate to control symptoms, the 1-day course is not used because it results in higher serum levels, which reach fetal circulation.

When a repeat course is required, 4 to 6 weeks should elapse between courses and the presence of the trichomonad should be reconfirmed. Total and differential leukocyte counts are recommended before and after retreatment.

Hepatic disease: Patients with severe hepatic disease metabolize this drug slowly; accumulation occurs in the plasma. Dosages are reduced below those usually recommended.

Renal disease: Dose is not specifically reduced in anuric patients because accumulated metabolites may be removed by dialysis.

NURSING IMPLICATIONS

HISTORY
See Appendix 4.

Trichomoniasis: Inquire of woman patient whether she is pregnant or pregnancy is sus-

pected. Treatment of male partner is recommended.

Amebiasis: Local health department regulations may require investigation into recent travel to foreign countries. If patient has not traveled, further investigation of local travel, use of restaurants, water source, and so on may be necessary.

PHYSICAL ASSESSMENT

Anaerobic infection: Obtain vital signs, weight; evaluate general status of patient. Laboratory studies include culture and sensitivity, CBC, and differential. Serum electrolytes and renal- and hepatic-function tests may also be ordered. Treatment is usually instituted while awaiting results of culture and sensitivity studies.

Trichomoniasis: Diagnosis made by wet smears and/or cultures.

Amebiasis: Obtain vital signs, weight. Diagnosis is made by stool examination. CBC and differential may be ordered. Other laboratory tests may also be appropriate.

ADMINISTRATION

Oral
May cause GI upset; administer with food.

Pediatric patient: If unable to swallow tablets whole, tablets may be crushed.

Parenteral
Physician must order infusion rate (see *Dosage*).

Flagyl IV: Is reconstituted before use and is prepared as follows; *order of mixing is important.* In most instances, the following procedure for reconstituting, diluting, and neutralizing is performed by a pharmacist. The nurse should be familiar with the procedure in order to interpret the label placed on the solution container as well as to be aware of the absolute necessity of preparing this IV solution in a specific manner before use.

1. Reconstitute by adding 4.4 ml of one of the following diluents to the vial and mix thoroughly: Sterile Water for Injection, USP; Bacteriostatic Water for Injection, USP; 0.9% Sodium Chloride Injection, USP; or Bacteriostatic 0.9% Sodium Chloride Injection, USP. Resultant volume is 5 ml with approximate concentration of 100 mg/ml. The *p*H of the reconstituted product will be between 0.5 and 2.0. Reconstituted, the solution is clear and pale yellow to yellow-green. Inspect visually for particulate matter and discoloration. Do not use if cloudy or precipitated.
2. *Dilution in IV solution*—Reconstituted drug may be added to glass or plastic IV container.

Do not exceed concentration of 8 mg/ml. The following IV solutions may be used: 0.9% Sodium Chloride Injection, USP; 5% Dextrose Injection, USP; Lactated Ringer's Injection, USP.

3. *Neutralization for IV infusion*—Neutralization is required prior to administration. Add approximately 5 mEq of Sodium Bicarbonate Injection for each 500 mg of metronidazole used; mix thoroughly. The *p*H of the neutralized solution will be approximately 6.0 to 7.0. Carbon dioxide gas will be generated with neutralization; it may be necessary to relieve gas pressure within the container. A concentration of 8 mg/ml should not be exceeded in the neutralized solution.

Do *not* refrigerate neutralized solutions; precipitation may occur. Use diluted and neutralized solutions within 24 hours. Reconstituted vials are stable for 96 hours when stored below 30°C in room light.

Flagyl IV RTU: The prepared metronidazole solution is ready to use (RTU). No dilution or buffering is required.

Do *not* use plastic containers in series connections (*i.e.*, primary and secondary IV lines). If used with a primary IV fluid system, the primary solution must be discontinued during infusion because air embolism may result as residual air is drawn down from the primary line before administration of secondary container is complete.

STORAGE: At room temperature; protect from light.

ONGOING ASSESSMENTS AND NURSING MANAGEMENT
Obtain vital signs q4h or as ordered; observe for adverse drug reactions.

IV infusion: Check infusion rate and site q15m.

CLINICAL ALERT: Occurrence of convulsive seizures or peripheral neuropathy (characterized by numbness or paresthesia of an extremity) is reported to the physician immediately. Abnormal neurologic signs may require discontinuation of therapy.

Notify physician of temperature elevation; administration of an antipyretic agent may be necessary.

Check IV site for evidence of thrombophlebitis (*e.g.*, redness, tenderness, or pain along pathway of vein).

Total and differential counts are recommended before and after therapy.

Physician may order stool examination following course of therapy for amebiasis.

Patient receiving concomitant anticoagulant therapy may require adjustment of anticoagulant dose (see *Drug Interactions*). Observe these patients closely for bleeding episodes (see also Coumarin), prolongation of prothrombin time.

Ambulatory patient: If dizziness or syncope occurs, patient may require assistance with ambulatory activities.

PATIENT AND FAMILY INFORMATION
May cause GI upset; take with food or meals.

Complete full course of therapy; take exactly as directed.

Avoid alcoholic beverages. Ingestion of any alcoholic beverage may result in nausea, vomiting, abdominal cramps, headache, flushing, or sweating.

May cause darkening of the urine; this is of no significance and need not be a cause of concern.

An unpleasant metallic taste may be noted and may be relieved by hard candy, chewing gum.

Trichomoniasis: During treatment, refraining from sexual intercourse is recommended or the male partner should wear a condom to avoid reinfection. Follow-up examination after completion of therapy may be necessary.

Amebiasis: Repeated stool examinations (usually for 3 or more months) are necessary to assure that amebae have been eliminated.

Metyrapone Rx

tablets: 250 mg   Metopirone

INDICATIONS
Diagnostic test drug for hypothalamico-pituitary function.

CONTRAINDICATIONS
Adrenal cortical insufficiency; hypersensitivity.

ACTIONS
Has immediate effect of reducing cortisol production by inhibition of adrenal 11-β-hydroxylation. In normal person, a compensatory increase in ACTH release follows and the secretion of 11-desoxycortisol and 11-desoxycorticosterone (17-hydroxycorticoids) is markedly accelerated.

WARNINGS
Safety for use in pregnancy not established.

PRECAUTIONS

All corticosteroid therapy is discontinued prior to and during testing. Ability of adrenals to respond to exogenous ACTH should be demonstrated before metyrapone is employed as a test. May induce acute adrenal insufficiency in those with reduced adrenal secretory capacity.

DRUG INTERACTIONS

Erroneous results in pituitary function as determined by the metyrapone test may occur in those taking **cyproheptadine** or **phenytoin** for as long as 2 weeks following cessation of therapy. A subnormal response may also occur in **pregnant women** and in patients on **estrogen** therapy.

ADVERSE REACTIONS

Nausea, abdominal discomfort, dizziness, headache, sedation, allergic rash.

DOSAGE

Day 1: Control period. Collect 24-hour urine specimen with measurement of 17-hydroxycorticosteroids (17-OHCS) or 17-ketogenic steroids (17-KGS).

Day 2: ACTH test. Standard ACTH test such as administering 50 units of ACTH by infusion over 8 hours and measurement of 24-hour urinary steroids.

Days 3–4: Rest period.

Day 5: Metyrapone administration. *Adults*—750 mg q4h for 6 doses. A single dose is approximately equivalent to 15 mg/kg. *Children*—15 mg/kg q4h for 6 doses. A minimal dose of 250 mg is recommended.

Day 6: Post–oral metyrapone measurement—24-hour steroid determination for effect.

Interpretation

ACTH: Normal 24-hour urinary excretion of 17-OHCS ranges from 3 mg to 12 mg. Following ACTH, the 17-OHCS excretion is increased to 15 mg/24 hours to 45 mg/24 hours.

Metyrapone: In those with normally functioning pituitary, metyrapone induces a twofold to fourfold increase of 17-OHCS excretion or doubling of 17-KGS excretion.

Subnormal response: In those without adrenal insufficiency, subnormal response indicates impairment of pituitary function: either panhypopituitarism or partial hypopituitarism.

Excessive response: Excessive excretion of 17-OHCS or 17-KGS above the normal range after metyrapone administration is suggestive of Cushing's syndrome associated with adrenal hyperplasia.

NURSING IMPLICATIONS

HISTORY

See Appendix 4. Inquire of female patient if pregnant or if pregnancy is suspected.

PHYSICAL ASSESSMENT

Obtain vital signs, weight. Perform general physical assessment based on symptoms; record findings.

ADMINISTRATION

See *Dosage* above.

All corticosteroid therapy is discontinued.

Physician orders specific 24-hour urine tests prior to and during metyrapone test and day 3 ACTH test (dose, drug used, time of administration, etc.).

GENERIC NAME SIMILARITIES

Metyrapone and metyrosine (see below).

ONGOING ASSESSMENTS AND NURSING MANAGEMENT

Explain test and urine collection to ambulatory patient. Each time a 24-hour urine specimen is collected, be sure patient understands procedure.

Collect urine specimens as ordered and as outlined in hospital or laboratory procedure book. Start and end specimen collection as directed.

Use only the container supplied by the laboratory. Label collection bottle with patient's name, name of test, time collection started and ended, and date. Send to laboratory immediately after 24-hour collection is finished.

If adverse reactions to metyrapone occur, notify physician because decision to continue dosage (on day 5) may be necessary.

If dizziness or sedation occurs, patient may require assistance with ambulation.

Metyrosine Rx

capsules: 250 mg   Demser

INDICATIONS

Treatment of patients with pheochromocytoma: preoperative preparation of patients for surgery, management of patients when surgery is contraindicated, and chronic treatment of patients with malignant pheochromocytoma.

CONTRAINDICATIONS

Hypersensitivity.

ACTIONS

Inhibits tyrosine hydroxylase, which catalyzes the first transformation in catecholamine biosynthesis (*i.e.,* conversion of tyrosine to dihydroxyphenylalanine [DOPA]). Because this is the rate-limiting step, blockade of tyrosine hydroxylase activity results in decreased endogenous levels of catecholamines, usually measured as decreased urinary excretion of catecholamines and their metabolites. In patients with pheochromocytoma, who produce excessive amounts of norepinephrine and epinephrine, administration of 1 g/day to 4 g/day has reduced catecholamine biosynthesis by about 35% to 80%. Maximum biochemical effect usually occurs within 2 to 3 days, and the urinary concentration of catecholamines and their metabolites usually returns to pretreatment levels within 3 to 4 days after discontinuation. In some, the total excretion of catecholamines and catecholamine metabolites may be lowered to normal or near normal levels (less than 10 mg/24 hours). Metyrosine is well absorbed from the GI tract and excreted in the urine.

WARNINGS

Maintenance of fluid volume during and after surgery: When metyrosine is used preoperatively, alone or especially in combination with alpha-adrenergic blocking agents, adequate intravascular volume must be maintained intraoperatively (especially after tumor removal) and postoperatively to avoid hypotension and decreased perfusion of vital organs resulting from vasodilatation and expanded volume capacity. Following tumor removal, large volumes of plasma may be needed to maintain blood pressure and central venous pressure (CVP) within normal range. In addition, life-threatening arrhythmias may occur during anesthesia and surgery and may require treatment.

Intraoperative effects: Although preoperative use is thought to decrease intraoperative problems with blood-pressure control, it does not eliminate danger of hypertensive crisis or arrhythmias during manipulation of the tumor; the alpha-adrenergic blocking drug phentolamine may be needed.

Use in pregnancy, lactation: Use only when potential benefits outweigh the potential hazards to the fetus. It is not known whether drug is excreted in human milk. If use is necessary, discontinue breastfeeding.

PRECAUTIONS

Crystalluria has been observed in a few patients. To minimize risk, maintain sufficient water intake to achieve daily urine volume of 2000 ml or more, particularly with doses greater than 2 g/day. Perform routine examination of urine; metyrosine will crystallize as needles or rods. If crystalluria occurs, increase fluid intake. If it persists, reduce dosage or discontinue drug. No evidence of effects on hepatic, hematologic, or other functions has been noted. A few instances of increased SGOT levels were noted; periodic laboratory tests in patients with impaired hepatic or renal function are recommended.

DRUG INTERACTIONS

Observe caution when administering to those receiving **phenothiazines** or **haloperidol** because extrapyramidal effects of these drugs may be potentiated by inhibiting catecholamine synthesis. Metyrosine may have additive effects with **alcohol** and other **CNS depressants.** Spurious increases in urinary catecholamines may be observed because of presence of metabolites.

ADVERSE REACTIONS

Sedation: Moderate to severe sedation is the most common adverse reaction. It occurs at both high and low dosages. Sedative effects begin within the first 24 hours of therapy, are maximal after 2 or 3 days, and tend to wane during the next few days. Sedation is usually not obvious after 1 week unless dosage is increased; at dosages greater than 2000 mg/day, some degree of sedation or fatigue may persist. In most patients who experience sedation, temporary changes in sleep pattern (insomnia lasting 2–3 days, feelings of increased alertness and ambition) occur following withdrawal of drug. Even those not experiencing sedation may report symptoms of psychic stimulation when drug is discontinued.

Extrapyramidal signs: Drooling, speech difficulty, and tremor (10%). These occasionally have been accompanied by trismus and frank parkinsonism.

Anxiety and psychic disturbances: Depression, hallucinations, disorientation, and confusion may occur. These effects usually disappear with dosage reduction.

Diarrhea: Occurs in about 12% of patients and may be severe. Antidiarrheal agents may be required if continuation of metyrosine is necessary.

Miscellaneous: Infrequent—Slight swelling of the breast, galactorrhea, nasal congestion, decreased salivation, dry mouth, nausea, vomiting, abdominal pain, impotence or failure of ejaculation. Crystalluria and transient dysuria and hematuria have been observed. Eosinophilia, increased SGOT, peripheral edema, and hypersensitivity reactions such as urticaria and pharyngeal edema have been reported rarely.

DOSAGE

Adults, children over 12: Recommended initial dosage is 250 mg qid. May be increased by 250 mg to 500 mg every day to a maximum of 4 g/day in divided doses. When used for preoperative preparation, the optimally effective dosage is given for at least 5 to 7 days (between 2 and 3 g/day); the dosage is titrated by monitoring of clinical symptoms and catecholamine excretion. In those who are hypertensive, dosage is titrated to achieve normalization of blood pressure and control of clinical symptoms. In those usually normotensive, dosage is ti-

M

trated to an amount that will reduce urinary metanephrines and/or vanillylmandelic acid (VMA) by 50% or more. In cases not adequately controlled by metyrosine, an alpha-adrenergic blocking agent (phenoxybenzamine) should be added.

Children under 12 years: Not recommended.

NURSING IMPLICATIONS

HISTORY
See Appendix 4.

PHYSICAL ASSESSMENT
Obtain vital signs. Obtain blood pressure and pulse in both arms with patient in standing, sitting, and lying positions; obtain weight. Baseline laboratory tests may include urinary catecholamines and catecholamine metabolites (VMA, metanephrine, homovanillic acid, etc.). Other tests may also be appropriate.

ADMINISTRATION
Obtain blood pressure immediately before administration; use same arm and position as for premedication measurements. Withhold drug and notify physician immediately if there is a significant decrease in blood pressure.

If patient has difficulty swallowing capsule, consult hospital pharmacist about advisability of opening capsule and sprinkling over food or in liquids.

Dry mouth may occur during therapy and may make swallowing of capsule difficult. Have patient take several sips of water to moisten oral cavity before swallowing capsule.

Have patient drink a full glass of water with each dose.

GENERIC NAME SIMILARITY
Metyrosine and metyrapone (pituitary-function test).

ONGOING ASSESSMENTS AND NURSING MANAGEMENT
Obtain blood pressure and pulse q4h or as ordered; have patient compare any symptoms presently experienced with pretreatment symptoms and record response; encourage liberal fluid intake.

Obtain blood pressure in same position and on same arm each time. Early in therapy, physician may request blood pressure on both arms with patient in standing, sitting, and lying positions.

Most patients experience decreased frequency and severity of hypertensive attacks with associated headache, nausea, sweating, and tachycardia. In those who respond, blood pressure de-

creases progressively during the first 2 days of therapy.

Moderate to severe sedation may occur, beginning within the first 24 hours of therapy, becoming maximal after 2 to 3 days, and tending to wane during the next few days. Assist patient with all ambulatory activities during initial therapy and until sedative effects abate.

Encourage a liberal fluid intake to achieve a daily urine volume of 2000 ml or more to minimize risk of crystalluria. In some patients it may be necessary to measure intake and output to ensure adequate fluid intake.

Periodic urinalysis is usually ordered to detect crystalluria. If crystalluria occurs, fluid intake is increased. Persistent crystalluria, despite increased fluid intake, may require dosage reduction or discontinuation of drug.

CLINICAL ALERT: Observe for signs of drooling, speech difficulty, trismus (contraction of muscles used for chewing), and frank parkinsonism. If any of these should occur, notify physician before next dose is due because dosage may need to be reduced or drug may be discontinued.

When administered for preoperative preparation for removal of pheochromocytoma, drug is given for 5 to 7 days. Dosage is adjusted by physician according to clinical symptoms and catecholamine excretion. Record patient response (blood pressure, pulse) and comparison of symptoms to baseline data; when ordered, obtain 24-hour urine for catecholamines.

PATIENT AND FAMILY INFORMATION
NOTE: Physician may wish patient or responsible family member to monitor blood pressure, pulse; instruction will be necessary.

Take each dose with a full glass of water. Drink at least 10 to 12 glsases (8 oz each) of fluid each day.

Avoid alcohol and other CNS depressants. Notify other physicians and dentist of therapy with this drug.

Avoid use of nonprescription drugs unless use is approved by physician.

May cause drowsiness; observe caution while driving or performing other tasks requiring alertness.

Notify physician or nurse if any of the following occurs: jaw stiffness, drooling, speech difficulty, tremors, disorientation, diarrhea, painful urination.

Mezlocillin Sodium

See Penicillins.

Miconazole Rx

injection: 10 mg/ml   Monistat i.v.

INDICATIONS

Treatment of the following severe systemic fungal infections: coccidioidomycosis, candidiasis, cryptococcosis, petriellidiosis, paracoccidioidomycosis, chronic mucocutaneous candidiasis. Drug is not recommended to treat common trivial forms of fungus diseases.

In treatment of fungal meningitis or urinary bladder infections, IV infusion alone is inadequate; it must be supplemented with intrathecal administration or bladder irrigation. Appropriate diagnostic procedures should be followed.

For topical preparations, see Miconazole Nitrate.

CONTRAINDICATIONS

Hypersensitivity.

ACTIONS

Exerts fungicidal effect by alteration of the permeability of the fungal cell membrane. Clinical efficacy demonstrated against *Coccidioides immitis, Candida albicans, Cryptococcus neoformans, Petriellidium boydii, Paracocciodioides brasiliensis.* Is rapidly metabolized by the liver and about 14% to 22% of administered dose is excreted in the urine, mainly as inactive metabolites. Elimination half-life is 20 to 25 hours.

WARNINGS

Rapid injection of undiluted miconazole may produce transient tachycardia or arrhythmia. There are no data on use of drug in pregnant women. Safety and efficacy for use in children under 1 year not established.

PRECAUTIONS

Drug should be given by IV infusion. Treatment should be started under stringent conditions of hospitalization, but subsequently may be given to suitable patients under ambulatory conditions with close clinical monitoring. An initial dose of 200 mg should be given with the physician in attendance.

DRUG INTERACTIONS

Drugs containing **cremophor-type vehicles** are known to cause electrophoretic abnormalities of the lipoproteins. These effects are reversible on discontinuation of treatment, but are usually not an indication that treatment should be discontinued. Interaction with **coumarin drugs** resulting in enhancement of the anticoagulant effect has also been reported; reductions of anticoagulant doses may be indicated.

ADVERSE REACTIONS

No serious renal or hepatic toxicity reported.

Integumentary: Phlebitis (29%), pruritus (21%), rash (9%). If pruritus and skin rashes are severe, discontinuation of treatment may be necessary.

GI: Nausea (18%), vomiting (7%), diarrhea, anorexia.

Hematologic: Transient increases in hematocrit have been observed following infusion. Thrombocytopenia, aggregation of erythrocytes, and rouleau formation on blood smears have been reported.

Miscellaneous: Febrile reactions (10%), drowsiness, flushes; transient decreases in serum sodium values have been observed following infusion. Hyperlipemia (increased serum triglycerides and cholesterol) has occurred in patients and is reported to be due to the vehicle Cremophor EL (PEG 40, castor oil).

DOSAGE

Adults: Doses vary with diagnosis and with infective agent, from 200 mg to 1200 mg per infusion. Table 35 gives recommended daily doses, which may be divided over 3 infusions.

Children: A total dosage of about 20 mg/day to 40 mg/kg/day is generally adequate. A dose of 15 mg/kg per infusion should not be exceeded.

Intrathecal: Administration of the undiluted solution by the various intrathecal routes (20 mg/dose) is indicated as adjunct to intravenous treatment in fungal meningitis. Succeeding intrathecal injections may be alternated between lumbar, cervical, and cisternal punctures every 3 to 7 days.

Bladder instillation: 200 mg of diluted solution is indicated in treatment of mycoses of the urinary bladder.

NURSING IMPLICATIONS

HISTORY

See Appendix 4. Note current treatment modalities.

Table 35. Recommended Dosages of Miconazole for Fungal Infections

Infection	Total Daily Range (mg)	Duration of Therapy (weeks)
Coccidioidomycosis	1800–3600	3 to >20
Cryptococcosis	1200–2400	3 to >12
Petriellidiosis	600–3000	5 to >20
Candidiasis	600–1800	1 to >20
Paracoccidioidomycosis	200–1200	2 to >16

M

PHYSICAL ASSESSMENT

Obtain vital signs, weight. Evaluate general physical status. Laboratory studies include CBC, serum electrolytes, hemoglobin, hematocrit, serum cholesterol, triglycerides. Diagnosis is confirmed by appropriate cultures. Depending on severity of infection and patient's condition, other laboratory tests may also be appropriate.

ADMINISTRATION

May be given by IV infusion, bladder instillation, intrathecal injection.

Dosing intervals and sites and duration of treatment may vary from patient to patient.

IV infusion: Dilute dose in volume (usually 200 ml) and diluent (0.9% Sodium Chloride or 5% Dextrose Solution) ordered by physician. Label container.

Physician must specify time of infusion (usually 30–60 minutes).

Daily dosage may be divided over three infusions.

It is recommended that an initial dose of 200 mg be given with the physician in attendance.

Depending on condition of patient and current treatment modalities, drug may be administered as a single IV infusion with the IV discontinued following administration of the drug or added to a secondary line. The primary line may be ordered to KVO (because daily dosage may be divided into three infusions a day) or may be used to administer parenteral fluids when oral intake is inadequate.

Bladder instillation: Usual dose is 200 mg (20 ml or 1 ampule). Drug must be diluted, according to physician's instructions, prior to instillation. Pharmacy usually prepares drug for instillation.

Physician gives specific directions for administration (methods may vary). Drug may be instilled by physician.

Intrathecal administration: Injections given every 3 to 7 days.

Sites may be alternated between lumbar, cervical, and cisternal punctures. Obtain appropriate trays for physician.

ONGOING ASSESSMENTS AND NURSING MANAGEMENT

In selected patients, drug may be given under ambulatory conditions following hospitalization.

Obtain vital signs daily. Assess patient's general condition and compare with baseline data; inspect IV infusion site for evidence of phlebitis (pain, redness); measure intake and output (especially during early therapy); observe for adverse drug reactions, especially pruritus, rash, nausea, vomiting, elevated temperature.

Inform physician of any adverse drug reactions before next dose is due; in some instances, discontinuation of drug therapy may be necessary.

If nausea and vomiting occur, physician may treat with antihistamines or antiemetics given prior to infusion or with reduction of dose, slowing of the rate of infusion, or avoidance of administration at mealtime. If nausea and vomiting are not controlled by any one or more of these measures, notify physician.

Inform physician of any change in intake–output ratio or if patient fails or is unable to take oral fluids.

Weigh 2 to 3 times a week or as ordered.

Generally, treatment is continued until all clinical and laboratory tests no longer indicate that active fungal infection is present. Inadequate periods of treatment may yield poor response and early recurrence of symptoms.

PATIENT AND FAMILY INFORMATION

Outpatients: Maintenance of the treatment schedule is essential. Failure to adhere to the treatment schedule may result in recurrence of clinical symptoms.

Miconazole Nitrate Rx, otc

cream (vaginal): 2%	Monistat 7 (*Rx*)
cream: 2%	Micatin (*otc*), Monistat-Derm (*Rx*)
lotion: 2%	Monistat-Derm (*Rx*)
powder: 2%	Micatin (*otc*)
vaginal suppositories: 100 mg	Monistat 7 (*Rx*)

INDICATIONS

Vaginal cream, suppository: Local treatment of candidiasis (moniliasis); effective in both pregnant and nonpregnant women and in women taking oral contraceptives (see *Warnings*).

Cream, powder, and lotion: Tinea pedis (athlete's foot), tinea cruris, and tinea corporis; cutaneous candidiasis (moniliasis); tinea versicolor.

For systemic preparation, see Miconazole.

CONTRAINDICATIONS

Hypersensitivity.

ACTIONS

Exhibits fungicidal activity against species of genus *Candida*. Inhibits growth of the common dermatophytes, *Trichophyton rubrum, T. mentagrophytes, Epidermophyton floccosum,* and the active organism in tinea versicolor (*Malassezia furfur*).

M

WARNINGS

Use in pregnancy: Because vaginal cream is absorbed in small amounts from the vagina, it should be used in the first trimester only when considered essential to the welfare of the patient.

Use in children: Cream, lotion, and powder are not used on children under 2 years.

Sensitivity: If a reaction suggesting sensitivity or chemical irritation occurs, discontinue use.

ADVERSE REACTIONS

Vaginal cream, suppository: Most complaints were reported during the first week of therapy and included vulvovaginal burning, itching, and irritation (6.6%). Other complaints such as vaginal burning, pelvic cramps, hives, skin rash, and headache occurred rarely.

Topical cream, powder, lotion: There have been isolated reports of irritation, burning, and maceration.

DOSAGE

Vaginal cream, suppository: One applicatorful of cream or one suppository intravaginally, daily H.S. for 7 days. Course of therapy may be repeated if necessary after other pathogens have been ruled out by appropriate smears and cultures.

Cream and lotion: Cover affected areas bid, morning and evening (once daily in those with tinea versicolor). Lotion is preferred in intertriginous areas; if cream is used, apply sparingly to avoid maceration.

Powder: Spray or sprinkle liberally over affected area in morning and evening.

NURSING IMPLICATIONS

HISTORY
See Appendix 4.

PHYSICAL ASSESSMENT
Vulvovaginitis: Smears and cultures are obtained for diagnosis.

Other fungus infections: Scrapings of affected area and microscopic examination or use of a Wood's light may be employed for tinea versicolor; scrapings and microscopic examination may also be employed for other superficial fungus infections. Inspect affected area; describe in patient's chart.

ADMINISTRATION
Vaginal cream: Directions for use and applicator are supplied with drug.

Place patient in supine position with knees flexed. Insert one applicatorful high in the va-

gina. Patient may also self-administer the drug after being given instructions for insertion.

Apply sanitary napkin to prevent staining of bed linen, clothing.

Cream, lotion, powder: Inquire of physician whether cleansing of area is desired before each application.

Apply to affected area as directed by physician. See *Dosage,* above.

ONGOING ASSESSMENTS AND NURSING MANAGEMENT
Early relief (2–3 days) of symptoms of topical fungal infections is usually seen in the majority of patients, and clinical improvement is seen soon after treatment is begun. *Candida* infections, tinea cruris, and tinea corporis are treated for 2 weeks; tinea pedis infections are treated for 1 month; vulvovaginal candidiasis is treated for 7 days. Patients with tinea versicolor usually exhibit clinical and mycologic clearing after 2 weeks.

Inspect (topical) area daily for evidence of improvement; record findings.

Withhold next application if patient complains of irritation, burning, or skin maceration (topical application) and notify physician.

Supply patient with sanitary napkins to change as desired between applications of vaginal cream.

PATIENT AND FAMILY INFORMATION
Vaginal cream

Insert high into vagina with applicator provided.

Complete full course of therapy.

Do not insert next dose, and notify physician immediately, if burning or irritation occurs.

Use a sanitary napkin to prevent staining of clothing, bed linens.

During treatment refrain from sexual intercourse, or have partner wear a condom to prevent reinfection.

Topical cream, lotion, powder

If condition persists or worsens, or if irritation (burning, itching, stinging, redness) occurs, discontinue use and notify physician.

Use for the full treatment prescribed by physician, even if symptoms have improved. Notify physician if there is no improvement after 2 weeks (tinea cruris and corporis) or 4 weeks (tinea pedis).

Keep towels, facecloths separate from those of other family members to avoid spread of infection.

Tinea pedis (athlete's foot): Wash feet several times a day; dry thoroughly. Change socks as needed if feet perspire. Avoid footwear made of or coated with plastic or rubber; wear shoes that allow air to circulate. Expose shoes to air when not wearing them; do not wear shoes that are wet or damp.

Tinea corporis, tinea cruris: Wear fresh clothes daily. Dry skin thoroughly after bath or shower.

Microfibrillar Collagen Hemostat Rx

1-g and 5-g sterile jars, nonwoven web form	Avitene

INDICATIONS

Used in surgical procedures as adjunct to hemostasis when control of bleeding by ligation or conventional procedures is ineffective or impractical.

CONTRAINDICATIONS

Not used in closure of skin incisions because it may interfere with healing of skin edges; not used on bone surfaces to which prosthetic materials are attached with methylmethacrylate adhesives.

ACTIONS

An absorbable hemostatic agent prepared as a dry, sterile, fibrous, water insoluble, partial hydrochloric acid salt of purified bovine corium collagen. In contact with bleeding surface, it attracts platelets, which adhere to the fibrils and undergo the release phenomena to trigger aggregation of platelets into thrombi in the interstices of the fibrous mass.

WARNINGS

Use in pregnancy only when clearly needed and potential benefits outweigh the unknown potential hazards to the fetus.

PRECAUTIONS

Only amount necessary to produce hemostasis is used. After several minutes, excess material is removed. Failure to remove excess material may result in bowel adhesion or mechanical pressure sufficient to compromise the ureter. In otolaryngologic surgery, precautions against aspiration should include removal of all excess dry material and thorough irrigation of the pharynx.

ADVERSE REACTIONS

Most common, which may be related to use of drug, is potentiation of infection, including abscess formation, hematoma, wound dihiscence, and mediastinitis. Other reported reactions that are possibly related are adhesion formation, allergic reaction, foreign body reaction.

ADMINISTRATION AND DOSAGE

Applied directly to source of bleeding by physician.

NURSING IMPLICATIONS

To facilitate handling, dry smooth forceps should be used. Product will adhere to wet gloves, instruments, tissue surfaces.

Do not autoclave or resterilize product.

Mineral Oil

See Laxatives.

Minocycline Hydrochloride

See Tetracyclines.

Minoxidil Rx

tablets: 2.5 mg, 10 mg	Loniten

INDICATIONS

Treatment of severe hypertension that is symptomatic or associated with target-organ damage and is not manageable with maximum therapeutic doses of a diuretic plus two other antihypertensive drugs. Use in milder degrees of hypertension is not recommended.

CONTRAINDICATIONS

Pheochromocytoma, because drug may stimulate secretion of catecholamines from the tumor through its antihypertensive action.

ACTIONS

Exact mechanism of action is unknown. Does not interfere with vasomotor reflexes and therefore does not produce orthostatic hypotension. Does not affect CNS function. Is an orally effective direct-acting peripheral vasodilator that reduces elevated systolic and diastolic blood pressure by decreasing peripheral vascular resistance. Blood-pressure response is dose related and is proportional to the extent of hypertension.

Because it causes peripheral vasodilatation, minoxidil elicits a reduction of peripheral arteriolar resistance. This action, with associated fall in blood pressure, triggers sympathetic, vagal inhibitory, and renal homeostatic mechanisms, including an increase in renin secretion, that leads to increased cardiac rate and output, and salt and water retention.

Is at least 90% absorbed from the GI tract. Plasma levels of the parent drug reach their maximum within the first hour and decline rapidly thereafter. Drug is not bound to serum proteins; it accumulates in arterial smooth muscles. Minoxidil is excreted in the urine; the drug and its metabolites are hemodialyzable. Average plasma half-life is 4.2 hours.

After an effective oral dose, blood pressure usually starts to decline within ½ hour, reaches a minimum between 2 and 3 hours, and recovers at a linear rate of about 30% per day. Total duration of effect is approximately 75 hours.

WARNINGS

Fluid and electrolyte balance; congestive heart failure: Administered with a diuretic to prevent fluid retention and possible congestive heart failure (CHF); a loop diuretic (furosemide) is almost always required. If used without a diuretic, retention of salt and corresponding volumes of water can occur within a few days, leading to increased plasma and interstitial fluid volume and local or generalized edema. Diuretic treatment alone, or in combination with restricted salt intake, will usually minimize fluid retention. Ascites has been reported. Diuretic effectiveness is limited mostly by impaired renal function. The condition of those with preexisting CHF occasionally deteriorates in association with fluid retention; because of the fall in blood pressure (reduction of afterload), more than twice as many may improve as may worsen. Under close medical supervision, it may be possible to resolve refractory salt retention by discontinuing drug for 1 to 2 days and then resuming treatment in conjunction with vigorous diuretic therapy.

Tachycardia: Drug increases heart rate; this can be partly or entirely prevented by concomitant administration of a beta-adrenergic blocking drug or other sympathetic nervous system suppressant (*e.g.,* clonidine, methyldopa). In addition, angina may worsen or appear for the first time during treatment, probably because of increased oxygen demands associated with increased heart rate and cardiac output. This can usually be prevented by sympathetic blockade.

Pericardial effusion and tamponade: Pericardial effusion, occasionally with tamponade, has been seen in about 3% of patients not on dialysis, especially those with inadequate or compromised renal function. Although many cases were associated with a connective tissue disease, uremic syndrome, CHF, or fluid retention, there were instances in which potential causes of effusion were not present. Echocardiographic studies are recommended if suspicion arises. More vigorous diuretic therapy, dialysis, pericardiocentesis, or surgery may be required. If effusion persists, drug may be discontinued.

Hazard of rapid control of blood pressure: In those with severely elevated blood pressure, too rapid control (especially with IV agents) can precipitate syncope, cerebrovascular accident (CVA), myocardial infarction (MI), and ischemia of special sense organs (vision, hearing). Patients with cryoglobulinemia may also suffer ischemic episodes of affected organs. Such events have not been unequivocally associated with minoxidil, but experience is limited. Any patient with malignant hypertension should have initial treatment with minoxidil carried out in a hospital setting, to assure both that blood pressure is falling and that it is not falling more rapidly than intended.

Use in pregnancy, lactation: Use only when clearly needed and when potential benefits outweigh the unknown potential hazards to the fetus. Safety for use in the nursing mother is not established. In general, do not breast-feed when taking drug.

Use in children: Use is limited, particularly in infants. Recommendations under *Dosage* can be considered only a rough guide; careful titration is necessary.

PRECAUTIONS

Has not been used in those who have had an MI within the preceding month. It is possible that a reduction of arterial pressure with the drug might further limit blood flow to the myocardium, although this might be compensated by decreased oxygen demand because of lower blood pressure. Possible hypersensitivity, manifested by skin rash, has been seen. Renal failure or dialysis patients may require smaller doses and should be under close supervision to prevent exacerbation of renal failure or precipitation of cardiac failure.

DRUG INTERACTIONS

Administration to those receiving **guanethidine** can result in profound orthostatic effects. If possible, guanethidine is discontinued well before minoxidil therapy is begun. When this is not possible, minoxidil therapy is started in the hospital, where the patient should remain until severe orthostatic effects are no longer present or he has learned to avoid activities that provoke them.

ADVERSE REACTIONS

Fluid and electrolyte balance: Temporary edema developed in 7% of patients not edematous at start of therapy.

Pericardial effusion and tamponade: See *Warnings.*

M

Hypertrichosis: Elongation, thickening, and enhanced pigmentation of fine body hair develops 3 to 6 weeks after starting therapy (approximately 80% of patients). This is usually first noticed on the temples, between eyebrows, between hairline and eyebrows, or in sideburn area of the upper lateral cheek, later extending to the back, arms, legs, and scalp. Upon discontinuation of drug, new hair growth stops, but 1 to 6 months are required for restoration to pretreatment appearance.

Allergic: Rashes have been reported, including rare reports of bullous eruptions and Stevens-Johnson syndrome.

Cardiac effects: Changes in direction and magnitude of T-waves occur in approximately 60%. In rare instances, a large negative amplitude of the T-wave may encroach upon the S–T segment, but the S–T segment is not independently altered. These changes usually disappear with continuance of treatment and revert to the pretreatment state if drug is discontinued. No symptoms have been associated with these changes.

Hematologic: Initially, hematocrit, hemoglobin, and erythrocyte count usually fall about 7%, then recover to pretreatment levels. Thrombocytopenia and leukopenia have been reported rarely.

GI: Nausea, vomiting.

Miscellaneous: Breast tenderness (<1%), fatigue, headache, and darkening of the skin have been reported occasionally. Rebound hypertension has been reported following gradual withdrawal of drug in children.

Altered lab findings: Alkaline phosphatase increased varyingly without other evidence of liver or bone abnormality. Serum creatinine increased an average of 6% and BUN slightly more, but these later declined to pretreatment levels.

OVERDOSAGE

Symptoms: Few instances of deliberate or accidental overdosage have been reported. When exaggerated hypotension is encountered, it is most likely to occur in association with residual sympathetic nervous system blockade from previous therapy (guanethidinelike effects or alpha-adrenergic blockade), which prevents usual compensatory maintenance of blood pressure.

Treatment: IV administration of normal saline will help maintain blood pressure and facilitate urine formation. Sympathomimetic drugs (*e.g.,* norepinephrine, epinephrine) are avoided because of their excessive cardiac-stimulating action. Phenylephrine, angiotensin II, vasopressin, and dopamine all reverse hypotension due to minoxidil, but these are used only if underperfusion of a vital organ is evident.

DOSAGE

Adults, children over 12: Initial dosage is 5 mg/day given as a single dose. Daily dosage can be increased to 10 mg, 20 mg, and then 40 mg in single or divided doses if required. Effective dosage range is usually 10 mg/day to 40 mg/day. *Maximum recommended dose*—100 mg/day.

Children under 12: Initial dose is 0.2 mg/kg/day as single dose. Dosage may be increased in 50% to 100% increments until optimum control is achieved. Effective dosage range is usually 0.25 mg/kg/day to 1 mg/kg/day. *Maximum recommended dose*—50 mg/day. Experience in children is limited; dosage is closely monitored with careful titration for optimal effects.

Dose frequency: Magnitude of within-day fluctuation of arterial pressure during therapy is directly proportional to the extent of pressure reduction. If supine diastolic pressure is reduced less than 30 mm Hg, drug is administered only once a day. If supine blood pressure is reduced by more than 30 mm Hg, daily dosage is divided into two equal parts.

Frequency of dosage adjustment· Should normally be at least three days. When more rapid management is required, adjustments can be made q6h if patient is carefully monitored.

Concomitant drug therapy

Diuretics: Used in conjunction with a diuretic in patients relying on renal function for maintaining salt and water balance. Recommended dosages are hydrochlorothiazide 50 mg bid or other thiazide at equieffective dosage; chlorthalidone 50 mg to 100 mg once daily; and furosemide 40 mg bid. If excessive salt and water retention result in a weight gain of more than 5 lb, diuretic is changed to furosemide. If patient is already taking furosemide, dosage is increased.

Beta-adrenergic blockers or other sympathetic nervous system suppressants: When therapy is begun, dosage of beta blocker should be the equivalent of 80 mg to 160 mg of propranolol a day in divided doses. If beta blockers are contraindicated, methyldopa 250 mg to 750 mg bid may be used and should be started 24 hours before the start of minoxidil therapy. Clonidine 0.1 mg to 0.2 mg bid may also be used.

Sympathetic nervous system suppressants may not completely prevent an increase in heart rate but usually do prevent tachycardia. Typically, patients receiving a beta blocker prior to minoxidil therapy have bradycardia and can be expected to have an increase in heart rate toward normal when minoxidil is added. When treatments with minoxidil and a beta blocker or other sympathetic nervous system suppressant are begun simultaneously, their opposing cardiac effects usually nullify each other, leading to little change in heart rate.

NURSING IMPLICATIONS

HISTORY
See Appendix 4. Note current treatment modalities.

PHYSICAL ASSESSMENT
Obtain vital signs; obtain blood pressure on both arms with patient in standing, sitting, and lying positions; obtain weight; check extremities for edema; auscultate lungs. Serum electrolytes, CBC, hemoglobin, and hematocrit may be ordered prior to therapy. Other laboratory tests may be ordered, depending on health history.

ADMINISTRATION
May be ordered as single daily dose or in divided doses. Concomitant administration of at least two other antihypertensive drugs (diuretic, beta blocker) is usual treatment modality.

Following initial dosage, daily dosage may be increased.

Obtain blood pressure and pulse with patient in standing, sitting, and lying positions (unless physician states that only one position is necessary) on both arms immediately prior to administration of drug.

Withhold drug and contact physician if pulse rate increases 20 or more beats/minute over baseline data or systolic or diastolic pressure decreases more than 20 mm Hg, unless physician has established other parameters.

CLINICAL ALERT: In those with severe hypertension, too rapid control (decrease) in blood pressure can precipitate syncope, CVA, MI, and ischemia of special sense organs (see _Warnings_).

ONGOING ASSESSMENTS AND NURSING MANAGEMENT
Obtain vital signs q4h or as ordered (in addition to blood pressure and pulse prior to administration); monitor weight; check extremities for edema; auscultate lungs for rales; measure intake and output; observe for development of adverse reactions.

Take pulse for 1 full minute; obtain blood pressure on both arms with patient in standing, sitting, and lying positions.

Notify physician immediately if any of the following occurs: rise in pulse rate of more than 20 beats/minute; significant increase or decrease in systolic or diastolic blood pressure, (rapid) weight gain of more than 5 lb, nausea or vomiting, edema of extremities, signs of CHF (Appendix 6, section 6-9), anginal pain, skin rash, respiratory distress, dizziness, lightheadedness, syncope.

Pericardial effusion and tamponade may occur. Symptoms may include distant or muffled heart sounds, distention of neck veins, reduced arterial blood pressure, paradoxical pulse (a drop in systemic blood pressure greater than 15 mm Hg on inspiration), and dyspnea. If these signs are apparent, notify physician immediately.

Closely monitor fluid and electrolyte balance during therapy; physician may order periodic serum electrolytes.

If patient is receiving a diuretic, observe for signs of hyponatremia (Appendix 6, section 6-17) and hypokalemia (Appendix 6, section 6-15).

Dietary restriction of sodium may be ordered for some patients; other dietary restrictions may also be applicable.

Experience with minoxidil therapy in children under 12 years is limited; these patients should be observed at more frequent intervals than adults.

If nausea or vomiting occur and patient is unable to take or retain drugs, notify physician immediately.

When used according to its indications, minoxidil reduced supine diastolic blood pressure by 20 mm Hg, or to 90 mm Hg or less in approximately 75% of patients. Full response to a given dose is not obtained for at least 3 days.

PATIENT AND FAMILY INFORMATION
NOTE: Patient package insert is available with product. Review material with patient or family member. Physician may also direct patient or family member to monitor blood pressure and pulse one or more times a day; instruction in these measurements is usually necessary.

Drug is usually taken together with at least 2 other antihypertensive medications. Take all medications (including minoxidil) exactly as prescribed. Do not discontinue any of these, except on advice of physician.

May cause nausea and vomiting; notify physician if vomiting is severe, persists for more than 1 day, or hinders taking medication.

Enhanced hair growth and darkening of fine body hair may occur within 3 to 6 weeks after starting therapy. Although this may be bothersome, do not discontinue medication without consulting physician.

**Female patient:** Some of the hair growth between the forehead and scalp may be disguised with scarves or a change in hair style. Do not at-

M

tempt to shave or bleach these areas without discussing problem with physician.

Males, children: Change in hair style may disguise some hair growth. Excess hair growth in certain areas must be tolerated.

Notify physician or nurse if any of the following occurs: increased pulse rate of 20 or more beats/minute over normal; rapid weight gain of more than 5 lb; unusual swelling of extremities, face, or abdomen; difficulty in breathing, especially when lying down; new or aggravated symptoms of chest, arm, or shoulder pain (angina); signs of severe indigestion; dizziness, lightheadedness, or fainting.

Inform other physicians and dentist of therapy with minoxidil and other antihypertensive agents.

Follow any specific directions given by the physician about this and other drugs presently taken. These directions may involve dietary restriction of salt, daily weight measurement, what to do if blood pressure or pulse increases or decreases (if these are being monitored), changes in dosage or frequency, use of nonprescription drugs, and so on.

Miotics, Cholinesterase Inhibitors

Demecarium Bromide Rx

| solution: 0.125%, 0.25% | Humorsol |

Echothiophate Iodide Rx

| powder for reconstitution: 1.5 mg (0.03%), 3 mg (0.06%), 6.25 mg (0.125%), 12.5 mg (0.25%) w/5 ml diluent | Phospholine Iodide |

Isoflurophate Rx

| ointment: 0.025% | Floropryl |

Physostigmine Rx

| ointment: 0.25% | Eserine Sulfate |
| solution: 0.25% | Isopto Eserine |

INDICATIONS

Physostigmine: Indicated only for reduction of intraocular tension in glaucoma.

Others: Therapy of open-angle glaucoma; conditions obstructing aqueous outflow, such as synechia formation, that are amenable to miotic therapy; following iridectomy; in accommodative esotropia (accommodative convergent strabismus).

CONTRAINDICATIONS

Active uveal inflammation, most cases of angle-closure (narrow-angle) glaucoma (prior to iridectomy) or in those with narrow angles, due to possibility of producing pupillary block and increasing angle blockage; glaucoma associated with iridocyclitis; hypersensitivity.

ACTIONS

Inhibits enzyme cholinesterase and thus enhances effects of endogenous acetylcholine. In the eye, increase in cholinergic activity leads to intense miosis and contraction of the ciliary muscle (accommodation). Decrease in intraocular pressure results primarily from increased facility of outflow of aqueous humor. In addition to reduction of intraocular pressure, these effects lead to myopia. These agents are reserved for use in those who fail to respond adequately to direct-acting cholinergics alone or in combination with epinephrine and/or a carbonic anhydrase inhibitor. Because of prolonged duration of action, administration is required only twice daily; some patients may achieve adequate control with administration daily or every other day. Because of tendency to produce more severe adverse effects, including systemic reactions, lowest effective dose is used. A cholinesterase inhibitor with epinephrine and/or a carbonic anhydrase inhibitor has additive effects, providing greater control of glaucoma at reduced doses of each agent.

Physostigmine has a duration of action of 12 to 36 hours. Demecarium, echothiophate, and isoflurophate have prolonged effects (up to 1 week or longer).

WARNINGS

Overdosage may produce systemic cholinergic effects. Safety for use in pregnancy not established. Use only when clearly needed and when potential benefits outweigh the unknown potential hazards to the fetus.

PRECAUTIONS

Except in aphakic patients, used in glaucoma only when shorter acting miotics are inadequate. When inflammatory process is present, abstention from or cautious use of these drugs is recommended; use with caution, if at all, if there is history of retinal detachment. These drugs are discontinued 3 weeks before ophthalmic surgery; after long-term use, dilatation of blood vessels and resultant greater permeability increases the possibility of hyphema during surgery.

Systemic effects are infrequent when drugs are instilled carefully. Despite observance of all precautions and use of recommended doses, repeated administration may cause depression of concentration of cholinesterase in the serum and erythrocytes with resultant systemic effects.

Anticholinesterase drugs are used with caution, if at all, in those with marked vagotonia, bronchial asthma, spastic GI disturbances, peptic ulcer, pronounced bradycardia and hypotension, recent MI, epilepsy, parkinsonism, other disorders that may respond adversely to vagotonic effects.

DRUG INTERACTIONS

Succinylcholine is administered with extreme caution before or during general anesthesia to those receiving these drugs because of possibility of respiratory and cardiovascular collapse. Because of possible additive effects, administer with extreme caution to those with myasthenia gravis who are receiving **systemic anticholinesterase** therapy; conversely, extreme caution is exercised in use of an anticholinesterase drug for myasthenia gravis in those already undergoing topical therapy with cholinesterase inhibitors. Those receiving cholinesterase inhibitors who are exposed to **carbamate** or **organophosphate-type insecticides** and **pesticides** should be warned of added systemic effects from possible absorption through the respiratory tract or skin.

ADVERSE REACTIONS

Ocular: Stinging, burning, lacrimation, lid muscle twitching, conjunctival and ciliary redness, browache, headache, and induced myopia with visual blurring may occur. Activation of latent iritis or uveitis may occur. Iris cysts may form, enlarge, and obscure vision. Occurrence is more frequent in children. The iris cyst usually shrinks upon discontinuation of drug, or following reduction in strength of dosage or frequency of administration. Rarely, the cyst may rupture or break free into the aqueous humor. Retinal detachment and vitreous hemorrhage have been reported occasionally. Prolonged use may cause conjunctival thickening and obstruction of nasolacrimal canals. Posterior synechiae to the lens may occur; dilatation of the pupil once or twice yearly will prevent synechiae formation. Lens opacities have been reported; routine slit lamp examinations, including lens, should accompany prolonged use. Paradoxical increase in intraocular pressure by pupillary block may follow instillation. This may be alleviated with pupil-dilating medication.

Systemic: Should systemic effects occur (*e.g.,* nausea, vomiting, abdominal cramps, diarrhea, urinary incontinence, salivation, difficulty breathing, bradycardia, cardiac irregularity), parenteral administration of atropine sulfate is indicated (see *Overdosage*).

OVERDOSAGE

If taken systemically by accident, or if systemic effects occur after topical application in the eye or from accidental skin contact, administer parenteral atropine sulfate (IV if necessary) 0.4 mg to 0.6 mg or more for adults. For children, use 0.01 mg/kg to 0.02 mg/kg to a maximum of 0.4 mg to 0.6 mg. The use of much larger doses of atropine in treating anticholinesterase intoxication in adults has been reported. Initially, give 2 mg to 6 mg followed by 2 mg qh or more often, as long as muscarinic effects continue. The greater possibility of atropinization with large doses, particularly in sensitive individuals, is considered. Pralidoxime has been reported to be useful in treating systemic effects; however, use is recommended in addition to, and not as a substitute for, atropine. A short-acting barbiturate is indicated if convulsions occur that are not entirely relieved by atropine. Dosage is carefully adjusted to avoid central respiratory depression. Promptly treat marked weakness or paralysis of muscles of respiration by artificial respiration and maintenance of a clear airway.

DOSAGE

Careful dosage adjustments are necessary to achieve maximal therapeutic benefit with minimal side-effects. Essentially equal visual acuity of both eyes is a prerequisite to successful treatment of accommodative esotropia.

DEMECARIUM BROMIDE

Closely observe patient during initial period; if response is not adequate in the first 24 hours, other measures are considered. Frequency of use is kept to a minimum, especially in children, to reduce chance of cyst development.

Glaucoma: Initially, 1 drop (children) or 1 to 2 drops (adults) in eye. Decrease in intraocular pressure should occur within a few hours. During this period, patient is kept under constant supervision and tonometric examinations made at least qh for 3 to 4 hours to be sure no immediate rise in pressure occurs. Dosage may be increased, if necessary, from 1 drop twice a week to 1 or 2 drops bid. Duration of effect varies. The 0.125% strength used bid usually results in smooth control of the physiological diurnal variation in intraocular pressure.

Accommodation esotropia: May be used as a diagnostic aid to determine if accommodation factor exists. Instill 1 drop a day for 2 weeks, then 1 drop every 2 days for 2 to 3 weeks. If eyes become straighter, an accommodative factor is demonstrated. *Therapy*—If esotropia is uncomplicated by amblyopia or anisometropia, instill in both eyes, not more than 1 drop at a time, every day for 2 to 3 weeks. Dosage is then reduced to 1 drop every other day for 3 to 4 weeks and patient is reevaluated. Continue in a dosage of 1 drop every 2 days to 1 drop twice a week. Patient is evaluated every 4 to 12 weeks. If improvement continues, dosage is reduced to 1 drop once a week and eventually trial without medication.

ECHOTHIOPHATE IODIDE

Tolerance may develop after prolonged use; a rest period will restore original drug activity.

Glaucoma

Lowest possible dosage administered that will control intraocular pressure around the clock. When tonometry around the clock is not feasible, measurements are made at different times of day so that inadequate control detected.

Early chronic, simple glaucoma: 0.03% solution instilled just before retiring and in the morning in cases not controlled with pilocarpine. Therapy may be changed if tension fails to remain at acceptable level.

Advanced chronic simple glaucoma, glaucoma secondary to cataract surgery: Instill 0.03% solution bid as above.

Concomitant therapy: May be used with epinephrine, a carbonic anhydrase inhibitor, or both.

Accommodative esotropia

For diagnosis, 1 drop of 0.125% solution daily in both eyes on retiring, for 2 to 3 weeks. If esotropia is accommodative, favorable response may begin in a few hours. *Treatment*—After initial period for diagnostic purposes, dosage is reduced to 0.125% every other day or 0.06% every day. Dosages may be lowered as treatment progresses. There is no definite limit of therapy if drug is well tolerated. If eyedrops, with or without glasses, are gradually withdrawn after a year or two and deviation recurs, surgery is considered.

ISOFLUROPHATE

When possible, applied before retiring to prevent blurring of vision.

Glaucoma: Initial therapy, ¼-in strip of ointment in eye q8h to q72h. A decrease in intraocular pressure should occur in a few hours. During this period patient kept under supervision and tonometric measurements made qh for at least 3 to 4 hours to be sure no immediate rise in pressure occurs.

Accommodative esotropia: For initial evaluation, may be used as diagnostic aid to determine if accommodative factor exists. Not more than ¼-in strip of ointment is administered every night for 2 weeks. If eyes become straighter, an accommodative factor is demonstrated. In esotropia uncomplicated by amblyopia or anisometropia, not more than ¼-in strip used at a time in both eyes every night for 2 weeks, because too severe a degree of miosis may interfere with vision. Dosage is then reduced from ¼-in strip every other day to ¼-in strip once a week for 2 months. Patient is then reevaluated. If benefit is not maintained with a dosage interval of at least 48 hours, therapy should be discontinued. Intervals between administration gradually increased to greatest length compatible with good results. Therapy may need to be continued indefinitely. Occasionally, drug may be needed only when eyes begin to turn in. In a few instances, it has been possible to discontinue therapy after several months.

PHYSOSTIGMINE

Follicular conjunctivitis occurs more frequently with chronic use of this drug.

Solution: 2 drops in eyes up to tid.

Ointment: Apply small quantity to lower eyelid as per physician's directions, up to tid.

NURSING IMPLICATIONS

HISTORY
See Appendix 4.

PHYSICAL ASSESSMENT
Obtain vital signs; evaluate older patient's ability to carry out ADL. Physician performs complete ophthalmologic examination; type of tests/examination performed depend on visual problem being treated.

ADMINISTRATION
If patient has history of allergy to iodides or iodine, check with physician before instilling echothiophate iodide.

Check label for percentage of solution, ointment carefully; compare with physician's written order. This is especially important when multiple strengths are stored in one area or on an eye tray.

Check label for expiration date.

Wash hands immediately before and after administration.

If patient is wearing contact lens following cataract surgery, consult physician about need to remove (or not remove) lens before instillation of drug.

Small children may require restraining measures while drug is being instilled.

Exercise care in instillation; do not touch the cornea with tip of dropper or tube. If drug is spilled on skin, remove immediately.

Solution: Instill in lower conjunctival sac. Have patient close eye without squeezing and apply light finger pressure on lacrimal sac 1 to 2 minutes following instillation (patient may be able to do this after instruction by nurse).

Ointment: Manufacturer recommends placing patient in supine position. Apply quantity prescribed in lower conjunctival sac. Inform patient vision will usually be blurred following instillation.

Concomitant administration of other ophthalmic drugs may also be prescribed.

Manufacturer recommends keeping tube of isoflurophate tightly closed to prevent absorption of moisture and loss of potency. The tip of the tube should not be washed or allowed to touch the eyelid or moist surface.

ONGOING ASSESSMENTS AND NURSING MANAGEMENT

If used for glaucoma, physician may perform tonometric examinations during first several hours of treatment. Patient should be closely observed for relief of symptoms.

Observe for adverse effects; report occurrence to physician because dosage adjustment or other treatment modalities may be necessary.

CLINICAL ALERT: Notify physician immediately if pain or other symptoms of glaucoma become worse.

Notify physician immediately if any of the following occurs: salivation, urinary incontinence, diarrhea, profuse sweating, muscle weakness, respiratory difficulties, shock, or cardiac irregularities.

Vision may be impaired at night or in dimly lit areas. Have patient seek assistance if it is necessary to get out of bed at night. Keep room well lit during evening hours and dimly lit at night, and remove obstacles (*e.g.,* slippers, stools, chairs) that may hinder ambulation or result in falls.

PATIENT AND FAMILY INFORMATION

NOTE: Patient and/or family member will need instruction in instillation of solution or ointment. If family member is to instill drug, allow time for observation as well as practice (under supervision) of the technique.

Do not exceed prescribed dose or frequency.

Wash hands immediately before and immediately after administration.

Apply light finger pressure on lacrimal sac for 1 to 2 minutes following instillation of solution. This will decrease risk of systemic absorption and side-effects.

Local irritation and headache may occur at start of therapy; these effects subside with continued use.

Keep bottle or tube tightly closed. Do not wash tip of tube or dropper. Do not lay dropper on table (or other surface); replace immediately in bottle after use. Replace cap on tube immediately after use.

Notify physician or nurse if abdominal cramps, diarrhea, or excessive salivation occurs.

Do not discontinue medication except on advice of physician.

If exposed to insecticides or pesticides (gardeners, warehouse workers, farmers, residents of communities undergoing insecticide spraying or dusting), added systemic effects are possible from absorption through skin, respiratory tract. Contact physician and give name of product. Respiratory masks, frequent washing, and clothing changes may be advised.

Observe caution driving a car at dusk or nighttime hours.

Miotics, Direct Acting

Acetylcholine Chloride, Intraocular Rx

solution: 1:100 when reconstituted	Miochol Intraocular

Carbachol, Intraocular Rx

solution: 0.01%	Miostat Intraocular

Carbachol, Topical Rx

solution: 0.75%, 1.5%, 3%	Carbacel, Isopto Carbachol
solution: 2.25%	Isopto Carbachol

Pilocarpine Hydrochloride Rx

solution: 0.25%	Isopto Carpine, Pilocel
solution: 0.5%	Isopto Carpine, Pilocar, Pilocel, *Generic*
solution: 1%, 2%, 4%	Adsorbocarpine, Akarpine, Almocarpine, Isopto Carpine, Pilocar, Pilocel, Pilomiotin, *Generic*
solution: 3%	Isopto Carpine, Pilocar, Pilocel, *Generic*

solution: 5%	Isopto Carpine, *Generic*
solution: 6%	Isopto Carpine, Pilocar, Pilocel, *Generic*
solution: 8%, 10%	Isopto Carpine

Pilocarpine Nitrate Rx

solution: 0.5%, 1%, 2%, 3%, 4%, 6%	P.V. Carpine Liquifilm

Pilocarpine Ocular Therapeutic System

See individual monograph.

INDICATIONS

ACETYLCHOLINE CHLORIDE, INTRAOCULAR

To obtain complete miosis in seconds, by irrigating the iris after delivery of the lens in cataract surgery, and in penetrating keratoplasty, iridectomy, and other anterior segment therapy when rapid miosis is required.

CARBACHOL, INTRAOCULAR

Pupillary miosis during surgery.

CARBACHOL, TOPICAL

Lowering intraocular pressure in treatment of glaucoma. Particularly useful as an alternative in those who have become intolerant or resistant to pilocarpine.

PILOCARPINE HYDROCHLORIDE

Chronic simple glaucoma: Medical management of glaucoma, especially open-angle glaucoma. Patient may be maintained on drug as long as intraocular pressure is controlled and there is no deterioration of visual fields. Choice of concentration is determined by severity of condition and patient response.

Acute (closed-angle) glaucoma: May be used alone or in combination with carbonic anhydrase inhibitors or hyperosmotic agents to decrease intraocular pressure prior to surgery.

Miosis: Used to counter effect of cycloplegics and mydriatics following surgery or ophthalmoscopic examination.

PILOCARPINE NITRATE

See Pilocarpine Hydrochloride, above.

CONTRAINDICATIONS

Hypersensitivity; when miosis is undesirable (*e.g.,* in some forms of secondary glaucoma, acute inflammatory disease of anterior chamber). Carbachol is contraindicated in presence of corneal abrasions.

ACTIONS

Are cholinergic agents that have effects on the muscarinic receptors of the eye. Pharmacologic effects include constriction of the pupil (miosis) and contraction of the ciliary muscle (accommodation). In narrow-angle glaucoma, miosis opens the anterior chamber angle to improve outflow of aqueous humor. In chronic open-angle glaucoma, increase in outflow is independent of the miotic effect. Contraction of the ciliary muscle enhances outflow of aqueous humor via indirect effects on the trabecular system. The exact mechanism of this action is not known.

WARNINGS

Carbachol penetrates the intact cornea poorly; administer with caution if the epithelial barrier of the conjunctiva and cornea has been reduced by topical anesthetics, tonometry, or trauma.

PRECAUTIONS

Although systemic effects are uncommon at usual doses, use with caution in those with acute cardiac failure, bronchial asthma, peptic ulcer, hyperthyroidism, GI spasm, urinary-tract obstruction, or Parkinson's disease.

ADVERSE REACTIONS

May produce ciliary spasm with temporary reduction in visual acuity; temporal or supraorbital headache; conjunctival vascular congestion; induced myopia. This is especially true in younger patients who have recently started administration. Reduced visual acuity in poor illumination is frequently experienced by older individuals and by those with lens opacity. Sensitivity is infrequent. Contact allergy or follicles in conjunctiva may develop after prolonged use. Lens changes have been reported with chronic use; increased pupillary block may occur. Retinal detachments and vitreous hemorrhages have been reported. Transient lenticular opacities have been reported after use of acetylcholine intraocular preparations.

OVERDOSAGE

Systemic effects may include flushing, sweating, epigastric distress, abdominal cramps, diarrhea, tightness of the urinary bladder, and headache.

DOSAGE

ACETYLCHOLINE CHLORIDE

During surgery, 0.5 ml to 2 ml instilled into anterior chamber before or after securing sutures. Because duration of action is short, pilocarpine may be applied topically before dressing to maintain miosis.

CARBACHOL, INTRAOCULAR

During surgery, 0.5 ml is instilled into anterior chamber before or after securing sutures. Miosis is usually maximal 2 to 5 minutes after application.

CARBACHOL, TOPICAL

One to two drops into eyes two to four times a day.

PILOCARPINE HCl AND PILOCARPINE NITRATE

Initial dose is one drop repeated up to six times a day, depending on response. Frequency of instillation and concentration are determined by severity of glaucoma and patient response. Usual range is 0.5% to 4%; concentrations above 4% are used less frequently. Concentrations greater than 4% are occasionally more effective, especially in patients with darkly pigmented eyes, but incidence of adverse reactions is also increased. The most widely used concentrations are 1% and 2%. During acute phases in narrow-angle glaucoma, drug must also be instilled into the unaffected eye to prevent an attack of angle-closure glaucoma. Dosage and strength to reverse mydriasis depend on the cycloplegic used.

NURSING IMPLICATIONS

HISTORY
See Appendix 4.

PHYSICAL ASSESSMENTS
Obtain vital signs; evaluate older patient's ability to carry out activities of daily living. Physician performs complete ophthalmologic examination.

ADMINISTRATION
Check label of drug; it must be labeled for "ophthalmic use."

Check percentage of solution carefully; compare with physician's order. This is especially important when multiple strengths are stored in one area or on an eye tray.

Check label for expiration date.

Physician administers acetylcholine chloride, intraocular and carbachol, intraocular during surgery. Nurse must show label to surgeon while at the same time stating drug name.

Acetylcholine must be reconstituted before use and is available in a dual-chamber univial with the upper chamber containing diluent. Prepare solution immediately before use; discard unused solution.

Wash hands immediately before administration.

Exercise care in instillation; do not touch the cornea with tip of dropper.

Instill in lower conjunctival sac. Have patient close eye without squeezing and apply light finger pressure on lacrimal sac for 1 to 2 minutes following instillation (patient may be able to do this after instruction by nurse).

In some instances hospitalized patient may be allowed to instill own medication as well as keep drug at bedside; this usually requires a physician's order.

BRAND NAME SIMILARITY
Pilocel and Pilocar (both pilocarpine HCl); Miochol (acetylcholine chloride) and Miostat (carbachol).

ONGOING ASSESSMENTS AND NURSING MANAGEMENT
Evaluate drug response at frequent intervals (each time drug is instilled) during initial therapy and daily when on maintenance therapy; observe for adverse reactions.

Therapeutic drug response results in relief of symptoms of glaucoma (symptoms vary with type of glaucoma).

CLINICAL ALERT: Notify physician immediately if pain or other symptoms of glaucoma become worse.

Drug-induced myopia may occur, with alteration of distance vision and decreased night vision. Patient should be warned that distant objects may be blurred.

Vision may be impaired at night or in dimly lit areas. Have patient seek assistance if it is necessary to get out of bed at night. Keep room well lit during evening hours and dimly lit at night, and remove obstacles (_e.g.,_ slippers, stools, chairs) that may hinder ambulation or result in falls.

When drug is used to reverse effect of drugs used for ophthalmoscopic examination, inform patient that full drug effect (reversal of mydriasis, cycloplegia) will take a few minutes; patient should wait for full effect before driving.

PATIENT AND FAMILY INFORMATION
NOTE: Patient or family member will need instruction in instillation of drug. If family member is to instill drug, allow time for observation as well as practice (under supervision) of the technique.

Do not exceed prescribed dose or frequency.

May sting on instillation, especially first few doses.

May cause headache, browache, alteration of distance vision, and decreased night vision. Observe caution while driving or performing other tasks requiring visual acuity.

M

Apply light finger pressure on lacrimal sac for 1 to 2 minutes after instillation.

Keep bottle tightly closed. Do not wash tip of dropper; do not lay dropper on table (or other surface). Replace dropper in bottle immediately after use.

Do not discontinue except on advice of physician.

Mitomycin (Mitomycin-C, MTC) Rx

injection: 5 mg/vial,   Mutamycin
20 mg/vial

INDICATIONS

Therapy of disseminated adenocarcinoma of the stomach or pancreas in combination with other chemotherapeutic agents and as palliative treatment when other modalities have failed. Not recommended as single agent, primary therapy. Not recommended to replace surgery and/or radiotherapy.

Unlabeled use: Has been given by the intravesical route for the management of superficial bladder cancer.

CONTRAINDICATIONS

Hypersensitivity or idiosyncratic reaction; those with thrombocytopenia, coagulation disorder, or increase in bleeding tendency due to other causes.

ACTIONS

Is an antibiotic isolated from broth of *Streptomyces caespitosus,* which has been shown to have antitumor activity. It selectively inhibits synthesis of DNA. The guanine and cytosine content correlates with the degree of mitomycin-induced cross-linking. At high concentrations, cellular RNA and protein synthesis are suppressed. IV mitomycin is rapidly cleared from the serum. Time required to reduce serum concentration by 50% after a 30-mg bolus injection is 17 minutes. Clearance is effected primarily by metabolism in the liver but metabolism occurs in other tissues as well. Approximately 10% of dose is excreted unchanged in urine.

WARNINGS

Bone marrow: Use of drug results in high incidence of bone-marrow suppression, particularly thrombocytopenia and leukopenia, which may contribute to overwhelming infection in an already compromised patient and is *most common* and *severe* toxic effect. Platelet count, WBC, differential, hemoglobin should be done repeatedly during ther-

apy and for at least 7 weeks after therapy. Platelet count below 150,000, a WBC below 4000, or a progressive decline in either is indication to interrupt therapy.

Renal function: Observe for evidence of toxicity. Not given to patients with serum creatinine greater than 1.7 mg/dl.

Use in pregnancy: Safety for use in pregnancy not established. Teratologic changes noted in animal studies. Effect on fertility unknown.

ADVERSE REACTIONS

Bone-marrow toxicity: Most common and serious toxicity, occurring in 64% of patients. Thrombocytopenia and/or leukopenia may occur any time within 8 weeks of therapy; average time is 4 weeks. Recovery after therapy was within 10 weeks. About 25% of patients who experienced leukopenic or thrombocytopenic episodes did not recover. Myelosuppression is cumulative.

Integument, mucous membrane toxicity: Occurs in 4% of patients. Cellulitis at injection site is occasionally severe. Stomatitis and alopecia occur frequently.

Renal toxicity: 2% of patients demonstrate a statistically significant rise in creatinine. There appears to be no correlation between total dose administered or duration of therapy and degree of renal impairment.

Pulmonary toxicity: Occurs infrequently but can be severe. Dyspnea with nonproductive cough and radiographic evidence of pulmonary infiltrates may be indicative of pulmonary toxicity. If other etiologies are eliminated, therapy is discontinued. Steroids have been used as treatment of this toxicity, but therapeutic value not determined.

Microangiopathic hemolytic anemia: A syndrome consisting of microangiopathic hemolytic anemia, thrombocytopenia, renal failure, and hypertension; occurred with long-term therapy (6–12 months) and frequently in combination with fluorouracil but also other drugs.

Acute side-effects: Fever, anorexia, nausea, and vomiting (14% of patients).

Other undesirable side-effects: Headache, blurred vision, confusion, drowsiness, syncope, fatigue, edema, thrombophlebitis, hematemesis, diarrhea, pain. These do not appear to be dose related and were not unequivocally drug related and may have been due to the primary or metastatic disease process.

DOSAGE

Given IV only; avoid extravasation. After hematologic recovery from previous chemotherapy, either of the following schedules may be used at 6- to 8-week intervals:

20 mg/m^2 IV as single dose via IV catheter

_or_

2 mg/m^2/day IV for 5 days. After a drug-free interval of 2 days, 2 mg/m^2/day for 5 days (total initial dose 20 mg/m^2 over 10 days)

Because of cumulative myelosuppression, patient is reevaluated after each course of therapy, and dose is reduced if patient experiences toxicity. Doses greater than 20 mg/m^2 are not shown to be more effective and are more toxic than lower doses. Dosage adjustments made on basis of leukocyte and platelet counts. No repeat dosage should be given until leukocyte count is returned to 3000 and platelet count to 75,000. If disease continues to progress after two courses, drug is discontinued because chances of response are minimal. When used in combination with other myelosuppressive agents, dosage is adjusted accordingly.

NURSING IMPLICATIONS

HISTORY
See Appendix 4. Review chart for diagnosis, recent laboratory/diagnostic studies, previous treatment modalities.

PHYSICAL ASSESSMENT
Physical and emotional status; vital signs; weight. Baseline studies include CBC, differential, platelet count, hemoglobin, renal-function studies. Chest x-ray may also be ordered (because of potential pulmonary toxicity).

ADMINISTRATION
Reconstitute 5-ml or 20-ml vial with 10 ml or 40 ml of Sterile Water for Injection, respectively. If product does not dissolve immediately, allow to stand at room temperature until solution is obtained.

Label vial with date and time of reconstitution.

Physician orders IV fluid, method of administration.

An antiemetic may be ordered to be given prior to administration of drug.

Administration methods vary according to physician, hospital protocol; may be given by IV push or through injection port of a rapidly running IV.

Use large vein for administration; when possible, avoid veins on back of hand. Be sure needle is correctly placed before administration of drug.

Following administration of drug, intermittent IV set (for administration by IV push) should be cleared of drug by administration of 5 ml or 10 ml of Sodium Chloride; IV line should be cleared by running additional IV fluid. Physician orders method of clearing tubing following administration.

CLINICAL ALERT: Observe closely for extravasation. Tell patient to mention pain or burning at injection site. If extravasation occurs, discontinue administration immediately and contact physician because treatment may be necessary. (Extravasation treatment may also be ordered by physician before administration of first dose. Materials for treatment should be immediately available.) Select new site for administration of remainder of dose.

Stability: When reconstituted as recommended solution, stable for 14 days under refrigeration or 7 days at room temperature. Diluted in various IV fluids at room temperature to a concentration of 20 mcg/ml to 40 mcg/ml: 5% Dextrose Injection stable for 3 hours; 0.9% Sodium Chloride Injection stable for 12 hours; Sodium Lactate Injection stable for 24 hours. Combination of 5 mg to 15 mg of mitomycin and heparin (1000–10,000 units) in 30 ml of 0.9% Sodium Chloride Injection stable for 48 hours at room temperature.

ONGOING ASSESSMENTS AND NURSING MANAGEMENT
Average time of appearance of bone-marrow suppression is 4 weeks, but may occur at any time.

Monitor vital signs q4h to q8h; observe for adverse reactions, especially signs of bone-marrow toxicity (Appendix 6, section 6-8); measure intake and output; inspect IV administration site for evidence of thrombophlebitis (redness, pain, discomfort) and cellulitis (redness, streaking along pathway of vein) and report occurrence immediately.

CLINICAL ALERT: Bone-marrow suppression, notably thrombocytopenia and leukopenia, is the most common and severe toxic effect. Physician must be notified immediately if signs of bone-marrow toxicity are apparent. Deaths have been reported because of septicemia resulting from leukopenia.

CBC, differential, platelet count, hemoglobin monitored frequently (frequency may vary and depend on previous test results). Notify physician immediately of a significant decrease (compared to previous results), and/or a platelet count below 150,000, and/or a WBC below 4000/mm^3.

M

Renal-function tests may be performed at periodic intervals.

Stomatitis occurs frequently. Inspect oral cavity daily for signs of erythema, ulcerations (patient may first complain of burning in oral cavity). Begin stomatitis care (Appendix 6, section 6-21) at first sign of oral mucosal changes.

At beginning of therapy, begin oral care q4h as well as after each meal.

If fever occurs, physician may order an antipyretic. Monitor temperature closely following administration of an antipyretic; if temperature does not decrease, notify physician.

If nausea and vomiting occur, an antiemetic may be ordered. Notify physician if vomiting exceeds 700 ml to 800 ml per 8 hours because fluid replacement may be necessary. Observe patient for signs of dehydration (Appendix 6, section 6-10). A liquid diet, carbonated beverages, and unsalted crackers may be offered.

If anorexia severe or persists more than 2 days, consult physician. A high-protein, high-calorie diet in small frequent feedings may be ordered.

Weigh 2 to 3 times a week or as ordered. Report significant weight loss to physician.

Alopecia occurs frequently. Physician or nurse should discuss purchase and use of a wig or scarf. Patient may wish to purchase wig before treatment or wait to see degree of alopecia. Hair loss is often distressing; patient will require understanding from both family and medical team.

Pulmonary toxicity occurs infrequently but can be severe. Observe for dyspnea, nonproductive cough and report occurrence immediately. Physician may order chest-ray and/or pulmonary-function studies.

Diarrhea (rare) may occur. If severe or persistent for more than 8 hours, notify physician; an antidiarrheal agent may be ordered. Observe patient for signs of dehydration if diarrhea persists or patient taking oral fluids poorly.

Protective (reverse) isolation may be necessary if leukopenia is severe.

PATIENT AND FAMILY INFORMATION

NOTE: Outpatient or discharged patient and/or family should receive a full explanation of all possible adverse reactions, what can be done to control or alleviate these reactions, and what specific reactions should be reported immediately to the physician.

Notify the physician or nurse immediately if any of the following occurs: easy bruising, petechiae, blood in urine or stool, bleeding (*e.g.,* cuts, gums), fever, sore throat, sore or ulcerations anywhere on body, cough, dyspnea, extreme fatigue, sores in mouth or on lips, burning of mouth, anorexia, weight loss.

Inform other physicians and dentist of therapy with this drug.

Do not take nonprescription drugs unless use is approved by physician.

Laboratory tests will be necessary to monitor results of therapy.

Hair loss may be complete or partial; hair will grow back but may be a different texture or color.

Mitotane (o, p'-DDD) Rx

tablets: 500 mg   Lysodren

INDICATIONS
Inoperable adrenal cortical carcinoma (functional and nonfunctional).

CONTRAINDICATIONS
Hypersensitivity.

ACTIONS
Is an adrenal cytotoxic agent, although it can cause adrenal inhibition, apparently without cellular destruction. Primary action is on the adrenal cortex. Biochemical mechanism of action is unknown. Data suggest that drug modifies the peripheral metabolism of steroids and directly suppresses the adrenal cortex. Administration alters extra-adrenal metabolism of cortisol, leading to reduction in measurable 17-hydroxycorticosteroids, even though plasma levels of corticosteroids do not fall. There is no evidence of a cure as a consequence of administration. A number of patients have been treated intermittently, restarting treatment when severe symptoms reappeared. Patients do not often respond after the third or fourth such course. Experience to date suggests continuous treatment with maximum possible dosage would be the best approach. A substantial number of patients showed signs of adrenal insufficiency; steroid therapy may be necessary. It has been shown that metabolism of exogenous steroids is modified with mitotane; somewhat higher doses than just replacement therapy may be needed.

There was a significant decrease in tumor mass in about 50% of patients, and a significant reduction in elevated steroid excretion in about 80%.

WARNINGS
Use in impaired hepatic function: Administer with care to those with liver disease other than met-

astatic lesion of the adrenal cortex. Interference with mitotane metabolism may occur, causing drug to accumulate.

All possible tumor tissue should be surgically removed from large metastatic masses before administration to minimize the possibility of tumor infarction and hemorrhage due to a rapid, positive effect of the drug.

Long-term therapy: Continuous administration of high doses may lead to brain damage and impairment of function. Behavioral and neurologic assessments should be made at regular intervals when continuous treatment exceeds 2 years.

Use in pregnancy, lactation: Safety for use is not established. Use only when clearly needed and potential benefits outweigh unknown potential hazards to the fetus.

PRECAUTIONS

Adrenal insufficiency may develop, and adrenal steroid replacement is considered for these patients. May produce sedation, lethargy, vertigo, or other CNS side-effects.

DRUG INTERACTIONS

Corticosteroid metabolism may be altered; higher doses may be required.

Drug/lab tests: **Protein-bound iodine (PBI)** levels and **urinary 17-hydroxycorticosteroids** may be decreased.

ADVERSE REACTIONS

A very high percentage of patients have shown at least one type of side-effect.

_GI:_ Anorexia, nausea or vomiting, diarrhea (80%).

CNS: Occurring in about 40%, these reactions consist primarily of depression as manifested by lethargy and somnolence (25%) and dizziness or vertigo (15%).

Skin toxicity: Observed in about 15%. In some instances this subsided while patient was maintained on the drug.

Eyes (infrequent): Visual blurring, diplopia, lens opacity, toxic retinopathy.

_GU_ (infrequent): Hematuria, hemorrhagic cystitis, proteinuria.

Cardiovascular (infrequent): Hypertension, orthostatic hypotension, flushing.

Miscellaneous (infrequent): Generalized aching, hyperpyrexia, lowered PBI.

DOSAGE

Patient is started on 9 g/day to 10 g/day in divided doses, three or four times a day. If severe side-effects appear, dosage is reduced until maximum tol-

erated dose is achieved. If patient can tolerate higher doses and improved clinical response appears possible, dosage is increased until adverse reactions interfere. Experience has shown that the maximum tolerated dose will vary from 2 g/day to 16 g/day but has usually been 8 g to 10 g. Highest doses used to date are 18 g/day to 19 g/day.

Treatment should be continued as long as clinical benefits are observed. Maintenance of clinical status or slowing growth of metastatic lesions can be considered clinical benefits if they have been shown to occur. If no benefits are observed after 3 months at maximum tolerated doses, the case may be considered a clinical failure. However, 10% of patients who showed a measurable response required more than 3 months at the maximum tolerated dose. Early diagnosis and prompt institution of treatment improve probability of positive clinical response.

NURSING IMPLICATIONS

HISTORY

See Appendix 4. Note recent and current treatment.

PHYSICAL ASSESSMENT

Evaluate general physical and emotional status; obtain vital signs, weight. Perform general neurologic assessment: gait, reflexes, speech. Physician may also perform a detailed behavioral and neurologic assessment. Baseline laboratory tests may include urine for 17-hydroxycorticosteroids and renal- and hepatic-function tests.

ADMINISTRATION

Given in divided doses three to four times a day.

Physician may prescribe antiemetic for nausea and vomiting; antiemetic is usually given ½ hour before mitotane is administered.

Notify physician if antiemetic is not effective and patient is unable to take or retain medication because of GI symptoms.

ONGOING ASSESSMENTS AND NURSING MANAGEMENT

Obtain vital signs q4h; measure intake and output; observe for adverse reactions; enter a daily behavioral summary on patient's chart.

CLINICAL ALERT: Monitor patient closely for signs of adrenal insufficiency (Appendix 6, section 6-3). Contact physician immediately if adrenal insufficiency is suspected, because steroid replacement therapy (larger than normal doses) may be necessary.

Perform weekly (or as ordered) neurologic assessments and daily behavioral assessments. Notify physician immediately if signs of depression (manifested by lethargy, somnolence) or any neurologic change occurs.

M

Notify physician immediately if vomiting is persistent or severe; fluid and electrolyte replacement as well as a decrease in drug dosage or discontinuation of therapy may be necessary. Observe patient for signs of dehydration (Appendix 6, section 6-10), electrolyte imbalances.

A liquid diet, unsalted crackers, and carbonated beverages may be offered if patient is experiencing nausea and vomiting.

Drug may produce sedation, lethargy, vertigo, or other CNS side-effects. Patient may require assistance with ambulation and activities of daily living.

If diarrhea occurs, notify physician; an antidiarrheal agent may be necessary. If diarrhea is severe, observe patient for signs of dehydration, electrolyte imbalances.

Weigh weekly or as ordered. Report significant weight changes to physician.

Clinical effectiveness of therapy is shown by reduction in tumor mass; reduction in pain, weakness, or anorexia; reduction of steroid. Record patient response to therapy by means of weekly summaries.

Physician may order periodic renal- and hepatic-function tests, urinary 17-hydroxycorticosteroids, serum electrolytes (if vomiting or diarrhea is severe).

Anorexia may occur. If it persists for more than 2 days, notify physician. A high-calorie, high-protein diet may be ordered and given in small frequent feedings.

If patient is receiving a steroid preparation, review nursing management of the specific agent.

CLINICAL ALERT: Steroid preparations must not be omitted or suddenly discontinued.

If patient has metastatic disease of the liver, a lower dosage of mitotane may be ordered. Patient is also observed for increased incidence of adverse reactions because drug may accumulate.

PATIENT AND FAMILY INFORMATION

NOTE: Hospitalization is recommended until stable dosage regimen is achieved. Patient and family should receive full explanation of adverse reactions (both frequent and infrequent), length of therapy, and other treatment modalities (medical, pharmacologic). The symptoms of adrenal insufficiency should be thoroughly explained and preferably given as printed material.

Contraceptive measures are recommended during therapy.

Notify physician or nurse immediately if nausea, vomiting, loss of appetite, diarrhea, mental depression, skin rash, or darkening of skin occurs.

Medication may cause muscle ache, fever, flushing, or muscle twitching; notify physician or nurse if these become pronounced.

May produce drowsiness, dizziness, tiredness. Observe caution when driving or performing other tasks requiring alertness.

Take additional prescribed medication exactly as directed. If taking a steroid, do not omit or change dosage unless directed to do so by the physician. (See also *Patient and Family Information,* Glucocorticoids.)

Molindone Hydrochloride

See Antipsychotic Agents.

Morphine

See Narcotic Analgesics.

Moxalactam Disodium

See Cephalosporins and Related Antibiotics.

Mumps Vaccine

See Immunizations, Active.

Muscle Stimulants, Anticholinesterase

Ambenonium Chloride Rx

tablets: 10 mg	Mytelase Caplets

Edrophonium Chloride Rx

injection: 10 mg/ml	Tensilon

Neostigmine Rx

tablets: 15 mg (as bromide)	Prostigmin Bromide, *Generic*
injection: 1:1000, 1:2000, 1:4000 (as methylsulfate)	Prostigmin Methylsulfate, *Generic*

Pyridostigmine Bromide Rx

tabletes: 60 mg	Mestinon Bromide

syrup: 60 mg/5 ml
sustained-release tab-
  lets: 180 mg
injection: 5 mg/ml

Mestinon Bromide
Mestinon Bromide

Mestinon Bromide,
Regonol

INDICATIONS

AMBENONIUM CHLORIDE
Treatment of myasthenia gravis.

EDROPHONIUM CHLORIDE
Differential diagnosis of myasthenia gravis and as
adjunct in evaluating treatment requirements in this
disease. May also be used for evaluating emergency
treatment in myasthenic crisis. Because of brief duration of action, it is not useful in maintenance
therapy.

  Also used when a curare antagonist is needed to
reverse neuromuscular block produced by curare,
tubocurarine, or gallamine triethiodide. Is not effective against succinylcholine. May be used adjunctively in treating respiratory depression caused by
curare overdosage.

NEOSTIGMINE
Symptomatic control of myasthenia gravis. Greatest
use of oral form is in prolonged therapy when no
difficulty in swallowing is present. In acute myasthenic crisis when difficulty in breathing and swallowing present, parenteral form is used and patient
transferred to oral therapy as soon as tolerated. Parenteral form can also be used as a diagnostic test
for myasthenia gravis; however, edrophonium is
preferred because of its more rapid onset and brief
duration of action. Can also be used as an antidote
for tubocurarine.

PYRIDOSTIGMINE BROMIDE
Treatment of myasthenia gravis. Injectable form
also used to reverse or antagonize nondepolarizing
muscle relaxants such as curariform drugs and gallamine triethiodide.

CONTRAINDICATIONS
Hypersensitivity; mechanical intestinal and urinary
obstructions. **Neostigmine bromide** or **pyridostigmine bromide** should not be used in patient with
history of reaction to bromides or urinary-tract infections.

ACTIONS
These drugs facilitate transmission of impulses
across the myoneural junction by inhibiting destruction of acetylcholine by cholinesterase. They differ
in duration of action and adverse effects. Table 36
summarizes onset and duration of action.

Table 36. Equivalent Doses and Onset and Duration of Action of Anticholinesterase Muscle Stimulants

Agent	Equivalent Dose (mg)	Onset (min)	Duration (hr)
Pyridostigmine	PO—60	30–45	3–6
	IM—2	<15	2–4
	IV—2	2–5	2–4
Ambenonium	PO—5–10	20–30	3–8
Neostigmine	PO—15	45–75	2–4
	IM—1.5	<20	2–4
	IV—0.5	4–8	2–4
Edrophonium	IM—10	2–10	0.2–0.7
	IV—10	<1	0.1–0.4

WARNINGS
Use with caution in those with bronchial asthma or
cardiac dysrhythmias. Transient bradycardia may be
relieved by atropine. Isolated instances of cardiac
and respiratory arrest following administration have
been reported; these are believed to be vagotonic effects.

  Because of possibility of occasional hypersensitivity, atropine and epinephrine should always be
available when using parenteral therapy.

  Cholinergic/myasthenic crisis: Overdosage may
result in cholinergic crisis, characterized by increasing muscle weakness, which, through involvement
of muscles of respiration, may lead to death. Myasthenic crisis, due to increased severity of the disease,
is also accompanied by extreme muscle weakness
and may be difficult to distinguish on a symptomatic basis. Differentiation is extremely important,
since increases in doses of these drugs in presence
of cholinergic crisis or of a refractory or "insensi-
tive" state could have serious consequences. Differentiated by using edrophonium and clinical judgement. Treatment of these two conditions differs rad-
ically; myasthenic crisis requires more intensive
anticholinesterase therapy while cholinergic crisis
calls for prompt withdrawal of all drugs of this type.
Immediate use of atropine in cholinergic crisis is
also recommended. Atropine may also be used to
abolish or obtund GI side-effects or other muscarinic reactions but such use may lead to inadvertent
induction of cholinergic crisis by masking signs of
overdosage.

  When used as antagonists to nondepolarizing
muscle relaxants, adequate recovery of voluntary
respiration and neuromuscular transmission is obtained prior to discontinuing therapy. Observe patient continuously; if there is doubt concerning adequacy of recovery, artificial ventilation is continued.

M

Use in pregnancy, lactation: Safety not established. Use only when clearly needed and when potential benefits outweigh unknown potential hazards to the fetus.

PRECAUTIONS

Patient may develop "anticholinesterase insensitivity" for brief or prolonged periods. During these periods patient is carefully monitored and may need respiratory assistance. Dosage reduced or withheld until patient again becomes sensitive.

DRUG INTERACTIONS

Aminoglycosides (neomycin, streptomycin, tobramycin, amikacin, kanamycin) have a mild but definite nondepolarizing blocking action which may accentuate neuromuscular block. Use only in myasthenic patients when definitely indicated; dosage of anticholinesterase drug is adjusted. Caution exercised in those with myasthenic symptoms who are receiving other **anticholinesterase drugs.** Because symptoms of anticholinesterase overdosage (cholinergic crisis) may mimic those of underdosage (myasthenic weakness), the condition may be worsened. Routine administration of **atropine** with these agents is contraindicated, because belladonna derivatives may suppress parasympathomimetic (muscarinic) symptoms of excessive GI stimulation, leaving only more serious symptoms of fasciculation and paralysis of voluntary muscles as signs of overdosage. Do not administer to patients receiving **mecamylamine,** a ganglionic blocking agent.

ADVERSE REACTIONS

Observe for cholinergic reactions in the hyperreactive individual. The following reactions may occur, although not all have been reported with each product.

Ocular: Lacrimation, myosis, spasm of accommodation, diplopia, conjunctival hyperemia.

CNS: Convulsions, dysarthria, dysphonia, dysphagia.

Respiratory: Increased tracheobronchial secretions, laryngospasm, bronchiolar constriction, paralysis of muscles of respiration, central respiratory paralysis.

Cardiac: Arrhythmias (especially bradycardia), fall in cardiac output leading to hypotension.

GI: Increased salivary, gastric, and intestinal secretions; nausea; vomiting; increased peristalsis; diarrhea; abdominal cramps.

Skeletal muscle: Weakness, fasciculations, muscle cramps.

Miscellaneous: Increased urinary frequency and incontinence, diaphoresis.

Pyridostigmine bromide or **neostigmine bromide** may occasionally cause skin rash, which usually subsides promptly upon discontinuation of drug. Thrombophlebitis reported after IV use. Alopecia has been reported following **pyridostigmine** administration.

OVERDOSAGE

Symptoms: Muscarinic symptoms (nausea, vomiting, diarrhea, sweating, increased bronchial and salivary secretions, bradycardia) often appear with overdosage (cholinergic crisis). Obstruction of the airway by bronchial secretions may occur.

Management: Suction (especially if tracheostomy has been performed) and atropine. If there are copious secretions, up to 1.2 mg atropine IV may be given initially and repeated every 20 minutes until secretions controlled; a total dose of 5 mg to 10 mg or more may be required. Avoid signs of atropine overdosage (*e.g.,* dry mouth, flush, tachycardia); tenacious secretions and bronchial plugs may form with overdose. Maintain adequate respiratory exchange by assuring an open airway and using assisted respiration with oxygen. Monitor cardiac function until stable. Pralidoxime chloride (a cholinesterase reactivator) may be given, 1 g to 2 g IV, followed by 250 mg every 5 minutes. Institute appropriate measures when shock or convulsions present.

DOSAGE

AMBENONIUM CHLORIDE

Dosage is individualized according to response. The amount required may fluctuate in each patient, depending on activity, current disease status, including spontaneous remission. Because point of maximum therapeutic effectiveness with optimal muscle strength and no GI disturbance is a highly critical one, close supervision is necessary. Has longer duration of action than other agents, requiring administration q3h to q4h, depending on clinical response. Medication usually is not required throughout the night.

Moderately severe myasthenia: 5 mg to 25 mg tid or qid. Dosage may range from 5 mg to as much as 50 mg to 75 mg per dose. Initially, 5 mg is given, with careful observation of effect of drug. Dosage is increased gradually to determine effective and safe dose. Dosage adjusted at 1- to 2-day intervals to avoid drug accumulation and overdosage.

A few patients require greater doses for control, but increasing dose above 200 mg/day requires exacting supervision to avoid overdosage.

Edrophonium chloride may be used to evaluate adequacy of maintenance dose (see below).

EDROPHONIUM CHLORIDE

Differential diagnosis of myasthenia gravis

Adults: Prepare tuberculin syringe containing 10 mg edrophonium with IV needle. Inject 2 mg IV in 15 to 30 seconds; leave needle *in situ.* If no reaction occurs after 45 seconds, inject remaining 8 mg. If a cholinergic reaction occurs after injection of 2 mg, test discontinued and atropine sulfate 0.4 mg to 0.5 mg administered IV. After ½ hour, test may be repeated. In those with inaccessible veins, test may be performed IM; dosage is 10 mg. Those who demonstrate hyperreactivity (cholinergic reaction) should be retested after ½ hour with 2 mg IM to rule out false-negative reactions.

Children: IV testing dose in children weighing up to 75 lb is 1 mg; over 75 lb dose is 2 mg. If there is no response after 45 seconds, dose may be titrated up to 5 mg in children under 75 lb and up to 10 mg in heavier children, given in increments of 1 mg every 30 to 45 seconds. In infants, recommended dose is 0.5 mg. IM route may also be used. In children weighing up to 75 lb, dose is 2 mg IM; children weighing more than 75 lb, dose is 5 mg IM. There is a 2- to 10-minute delay in reaction; all signs appearing with the IV test also appear in IM testing.

Evaluation of treatment requirements in myasthenia gravis: Recommended dose is 1 mg to 2 mg IV 1 hour after oral intake of drug being used in treatment. Response will be myasthenic in undertreated patients, adequate in controlled patients, and cholinergic in overtreated patients. Responses are summarized in Table 37.

Edrophonium test in crisis: The term *crisis* is applied to the myasthenic whenever severe respiratory distress with objective ventilatory inadequacy occurs and response to medication is not predictable. This state may be secondary to a sudden increase in severity (myasthenic crisis) or to overtreatment with anticholinesterase drugs (cholinergic crisis). When patient is apneic, secure controlled ventilation immediately to avoid cardiac arrest and irreversible CNS damage. Test is not attempted until respiratory exchange is adequate. Dosage at this time is most important. If the crisis is cholinergic, edrophonium will cause increased oropharyngeal secretions and further weakness in respiratory muscles. If crisis is myasthenic, respiration improves and patient can be treated with longer-acting IV anticholinesterase drug. When test is performed, there should be no more than 2 mg in the syringe. Initially give 1 mg IV; carefully observe patient's heart action. If after 1 minute this dose does not further impair patient, inject remaining 1 mg. If no clear improvement of respiration occurs after a 2-mg dose, discontinue all anticholinesterase therapy and secure controlled ventilation by tracheostomy and assisted respiration.

Curare antagonist: 10 mg by slow IV; repeated when necessary. *Maximal dose—40 mg.*

NEOSTIGMINE

Symptomatic control of myasthenia

gravis: Orally, usually total requirement for optimum benefits varies from 15 mg/day to 375 mg/day. In some instances these dosages may be exceeded. Average dosage is 150 mg given over 24 hours. Interval between doses is important; best dosage schedule must be ascertained by trial and error. Frequently, therapy is required day and night. Larger portions of total daily dose may be given at times of greater fatigue (*e.g.,* afternoon, mealtimes). *Parenteral*—1 mg of 1:2000 solution (0.5 mg) subcutaneously or IM. Subsequent doses based on patient response.

Antidote for tubocurarine: When given IV it is recommended atropine (0.6 mg–1.2 mg) also be given IV. Usual dose is 0.5 mg to 2 mg by slow IV injection, repeated as required. However, only in exceptional cases should the total dose exceed 5 mg.

PYRIDOSTIGMINE BROMIDE

Myasthenia gravis: Average dose is 600 mg/day, spaced to provide relief when maximum strength

---

Table 37. Responses to Edrophonium in Myasthenic and Nonmyasthenic Patients

Response to Test	Myasthenic	Adequate	Cholinergic
Muscle strength	Increased	No change	Decreased
Fasciculations	Absent	Present or absent	Present or absent
Side-effects (lacrimation, diaphoresis, salivation, abdominal cramps, nausea, vomiting, diarrhea)	Absent	Minimal	Severe

M

needed. In severe cases, as much as 1500 mg/day may be required; in mild cases 60 mg/day to 360 mg/day may suffice. *Sustained release*—Average dose is 180 mg to 540 mg once or twice a day; needs of individuals may vary from this average. Interval between doses should be at least 6 hours. For optimum control it may be necessary to use the more rapidly acting regular tablets or syrup in conjunction with sustained release therapy. *Parenteral*—Used to supplement oral dosage when this route impractical (*e.g.,* preoperatively, postoperatively, during myasthenic crisis). Approximately $\frac{1}{30}$ of the oral dose may be given IM or by very slow IV injection. Patient is observed closely for cholinergic reactions, especially when IV route is used.

Neonates of myasthenic mothers may have transient difficulty in swallowing, sucking, and breathing. Injectable form may be indicated (by symptoms, use of edrophonium test) until syrup can be taken. Dosage requirements may range from 0.05 mg/kg to 0.15 mg/kg IM. Giving parenterally 1 hour before second-stage labor is complete enables patient to have adequate strength during labor and provides protection to infant in the immediate postnatal state.

Reversal of nondepolarizing muscle relaxants: Atropine sulfate (0.6 mg–1.2 mg IV) recommended immediately prior to pyridostigmine. Pyridostigmine 10 mg or 20 mg IV will usually be sufficient for antagonism of the effects of nondepolarizing muscle relaxants.

NURSING IMPLICATIONS

HISTORY
See Appendix 4.

PHYSICAL ASSESSMENT
Obtain vital signs, weight. Additional assessment should be based on condition of patient (controlled on maintenance therapy, in possible myasthenic crisis or possible cholinergic crisis, or presumptive diagnosis of myasthenia gravis and untreated). Edrophonium may be ordered as diagnostic test. Other laboratory tests may also be appropriate.

ADMINISTRATION
Drug is administered by anesthesiologist when used as antidote for nondepolarizing muscle relaxant.

When used parenterally, have atropine sulfate available. Dose of atropine may range from 0.4 mg to 1.2 mg IV. Observe patient closely for cholinergic reactions, particularly when IV route is used.

Patient with myasthenia may experience difficulty swallowing tablet or syrup. To be sure patient is able to swallow drug, offer a sip of water before drug is administered. If patient has any difficulty swallowing a small amount of water, withhold drug and notify physician immediately because parenteral administration may be necessary.

Physician may order drug given 30 to 60 minutes A.C. (exception, sustained-release tablets) to facilitate chewing, swallowing.

CLINICAL ALERT: Obtain blood pressure, pulse, and respirations before administration of drug. If there is a significant decrease in pulse rate over baseline values or if respiratory difficulty or symptoms of cholinergic crisis are observed, withhold drug and notify physician immediately.

ONGOING ASSESSMENTS AND NURSING MANAGEMENT
Have suction equipment, oxygen, and atropine sulfate available at all times. If patient is newly diagnosed, is suspected or known to be in cholinergic or myasthenic crisis, or has additional medical problems, have a tracheostomy tray and ventilation equipment additionally available.

Myasthenia gravis: Symptoms of cholinergic crisis (overdosage of anticholinesterase muscle stimulant) include nausea, vomiting, diarrhea, sweating, increased bronchial and salivary secretions, bradycardia, increasing muscle weakness. Treatment includes withholding drug administration of atropine sulfate and treatment of symptoms (*e.g.,* suctioning, oxygen, assisted ventilation, possible tracheostomy).

Symptoms of myasthenic crisis include extreme muscle weakness and severe respiratory distress. Treatment is additional anticholinesterase therapy.

CLINICAL ALERT: Any change in the patient's condition, especially respiratory difficulty, increased respiratory secretions, or bradycardia, must be reported to the physician immediately. Institute measures to maintain a patent airway by suctioning excessive secretions and administering oxygen until patient is examined by physician.

At times, myasthenic crisis may be difficult to distinguish from cholinergic crisis. Differentiation may be made by the edrophonium test.

Obtain vital signs q4h (more frequently if patient in myasthenic or cholinergic crisis); observe for adverse drug reactions.

Following administration, note and record drug response and duration of therapeutic effect (see Table 36 for onset and duration of drug). Expected drug effects include increased muscle strength, decreased fatigue, improved ability to perform repetitive motions (such as chewing food, swallowing) without early fatigue. Facial drooping and lid ptosis may also improve.

To assist physician in adjusting dosage, have patient keep a daily record of periods of fatigue and times when muscle strength is increased or decreased. If patient is unable to keep own record, nurse should record patient's status following each assisted activity.

Space activities (bathing, grooming, eating, ambulating) at intervals to avoid fatigue. Allow patient to participate in activities of daily living at own pace.

Deep breathing, coughing, and range-of-motion exercises should be encouraged; consult physician regarding frequency. Auscultate lungs daily or when patient experiences muscular weakness or has difficulty coughing and deep breathing. Inform physician if prominent rales are noted.

Patients who have been taking medication for myasthenia gravis may have been allowed to adjust drug dosage according to their needs. If the patient states that more or less medication is needed at a particular time, contact the physician because some patients are able to detect drug over- or underdosage before overt clinical symptoms are apparent.

Neonates of myasthenic mothers: May have transient difficulty in swallowing, sucking, and breathing.

Have available drug (such as pyridostigmine, injectable) recommended by physician.

Observe neonate closely; notify physician immediately if respiratory, swallowing, or sucking difficulty or any other symptoms are noted.

Antidote for nondepolarizing neuromuscular blocking agents: Observe patient continuously until recovery.

Obtain blood pressure and pulse q15m.

Assisted ventilation is continued until recovery from nondepolarizing muscle relaxant is complete.

Following discontinuation of assisted ventilation, monitor respirations q5m to q10m. Notify physician immediately if any signs of respiratory depression are apparent.

PATIENT AND FAMILY INFORMATION

NOTE: Many patients learn to adjust dosage according to their needs as dosage may vary slightly from day to day in some of these patients. The patient and family members must be taught symptoms of overdose (cholinergic crisis) and myasthenic crisis and what steps the physician wishes them to take should these occur.

Myasthenia gravis may be controlled but not cured. Lifetime medication and close medical supervision are essential.

Follow physician's instructions regarding dosage and what to do if drug overdose or underdose is apparent.

Notify physician or nurse if any of the following occurs: nausea, vomiting, diarrhea, sweating, increased salivary secretions, irregular or slow heartbeat, muscle weakness, severe abdominal pain, difficulty in breathing.

Keep a record of response to drug (*e.g.,* time of day increased or decreased muscle strength and/or fatigue noted); bring this record to each physician or clinic visit. (Record keeping may not be necessary when patient is well controlled on maintenance therapy.)

Wear or carry identification (such as Medic-Alert) indicating myasthenia gravis and current drug therapy.

Mydriatics, Cycloplegic

Atropine Sulfate Rx

ointment: 1%	*Generic*
solution: 0.5%	Atropisol Ophthalmic, Isopto Atropine Ophthalmic
solution: 1%	Atropine-Care Ophthalmic, Atropisol Ophthalmic, Isopto Atropine Ophthalmic, *Generic*
solution: 2%	Atropisol Ophthalmic, *Generic*
solution: 3%	Isopto Atropine Ophthalmic

Cyclopentolate Hydrochloride Rx

solution: 0.5%, 2%	Cyclogyl Ophthalmic
solution: 1%	Ak-Pentolate, Cyclogyl Ophthalmic, *Generic*

Homatropine Hydrobromide Rx

solution: 2%, 5%	Homatrocel Ophthalmic, Isopto Homatropine Ophthalmic, *Generic*

Scopolamine Hydrobromide
(Hyoscine Hydrobromide) Rx

solution: 0.25%	Isopto Hyoscine Ophthalmic

Tropicamide Rx

solution: 0.5%, 1%	Mydriacyl Ophthalmic

M

INDICATIONS

Cycloplegic refraction and dilation of the pupil in inflammatory conditions of the iris and uveal tract. **Tropicamide** and **cyclopentolate HCl** are used for diagnostic purposes only.

CONTRAINDICATIONS

Glaucoma or tendency toward glaucoma (*e.g.,* narrow anterior chamber angle); hypersensitivity to belladonna alkaloids or any component.

ACTIONS

These anticholinergic agents block the responses of the sphincter muscle of the iris and the muscle of the ciliary body to cholinergic stimulation, producing pupillary dilation (mydriasis) and paralysis of accommodation (cycloplegia).

WARNINGS

For topical ophthalmic use only. Intraocular tension and depth of the anterior chamber are determined before and during use to avoid glaucoma attacks. Not used in glaucoma, in the elderly (in whom undiagnosed glaucoma may be present), or in children under 6 except when used under close medical supervision. Do not exceed recommended doses. Excessive use in children and certain susceptible individuals may produce general toxic symptoms.

PRECAUTIONS

Use with care in those with narrow anterior chamber angle, in infants and children, in the elderly, and in hypertensive, hyperthyroid, and diabetic patients. Use is discontinued if signs of hypersensitivity develop. These drugs may cause an increase of pressure in the normal eye.

ADVERSE REACTIONS

Increased intraocular pressure.

Prolonged use may produce local irritation characterized by follicular conjunctivitis, vascular congestion, edema, exudate, and an eczematoid dermatitis. Systemic atropine toxicity is manifested by flushing and dryness of the skin (a rash may be present in children), blurred vision, rapid and irregular pulse, fever, abdominal distention in infants, mental aberration (hallucinosis), loss of muscular coordination. Severe reactions are manifested by hypotension with progressive respiratory depression.

Transient stinging, dryness of mouth, photophobia with or without corneal staining, tachycardia, headache, parasympathetic stimulation, allergic reactions, and somnolence may occur.

Use of **cyclopentolate** and **tropicamide** has been associated with psychotic reactions and behavioral disturbances in children. Cardiorespiratory collapse in children has occurred with **tropicamide**. Ataxia, incoherent speech, restlessness, hallucinations, disorientation as to time and place, and failure to recognize people have been reported with **cyclopentolate.**

DOSAGE

ATROPINE SULFATE

Adults: For uveitis, instill one or two drops in eye up to three times a day. For refraction, instill one or two drops in eye 1 hour before examination.

Children: For uveitis, instill one or two drops of 0.5% solution in eye up to three times a day. For refraction instill one or two drops of 0.5% solution in eye twice daily for 1 to 3 days before examination and 1 hour before examination.

CYCLOPENTOLATE HCl

Adults: One drop of 0.5% solution followed by a second drop in 5 minutes or one drop of either 1% or 2% solution. In those with darkly pigmented irises, a 2% solution is recommended; the 1% solution also has produced satisfactory results. Although complete recovery usually occurs in 24 hours, one or two drops of 1% or 2% pilocarpine reduces recovery time to 3 to 6 hours in most eyes.

Children: Pretreatment on day prior to examination usually is not necessary. One drop of 0.5%, 1%, or 2% solution is instilled in each eye, followed 5 minutes later by a second application of 0.5% or 1% solution if necessary. On rare occasions, atropine-like symptoms have been produced in children as a result of overdosage with 2% solution.

HOMATROPINE HBr

Refraction: One or two drops; repeat in 5 to 10 minutes if necessary.

Uveitis: One or two drops up to q3h to q4h.

SCOPOLAMINE HBr

Refraction: One or two drops in eye 1 hour before refracting.

Uveitis: One or two drops in eye up to three times a day.

TROPICAMIDE

Refraction: One or two drops of 1% solution in eye, repeated in 5 minutes. If patient is not seen within 20 to 30 minutes, instill an additional drop to prolong mydriatic effect. For examination of fundus, one or two drops of 0.5% solution 15 or 20 minutes prior to examination.

NURSING IMPLICATIONS

HISTORY
See Appendix 4. Prior to refraction, a complete health history, allergy history, and prescription and nonprescription drug history is taken.

ADMINISTRATION
Place patient in upright position (when possible). Tilt head back.

Solution or ointment is instilled in lower conjunctival sac.

Solution: Apply light finger pressure on lacrimal sac for 1 to 2 minutes during and following instillation. Sac compression blocks passage of the drops to the wide absorption area of the nasal and pharyngeal mucosa. This is recommended in use of stronger solutions and especially in children.

Ointment: Have patient close eyes (without squeezing shut) for 1 to 2 minutes following instillation.

Advise patient receiving drug for ophthalmic examination that a time interval must elapse before refraction can be performed. Atropine, homatropine, and scopolamine require up to 1 hour; tropicamide requires 15 to 20 minutes.

ONGOING ASSESSMENTS AND NURSING MANAGEMENT
Notify physician immediately if eye pain occurs. Do not administer next dose until patient is seen by a physician.

Withhold next dose and notify physician if local irritation, systemic atropine toxicity, or other adverse reactions are noted (see *Adverse Reactions*).

PATIENT AND FAMILY INFORMATION
Apply light finger pressure on lacrimal sac for 1 minute after instillation of solution.

May cause blurred vision and increased sensitivity to light.

If eye pain occurs, discontinue use and consult physician immediately.

Exercise caution in driving or performing potentially dangerous tasks if vision is blurred.

To avoid contamination, do not touch the eyelids or surrounding area with ointment tube or dropper tip. Replace dropper in bottle immediately after use. Do not lay dropper on table.

Ointment: Replace cap immediately after use. Do not wash tip of tube or dropper.

Mydriatics/Ophthalmic Vasoconstrictors

Epinephrine Hydrochloride Rx

solution: 0.1%	Adrenalin Chloride, *Generic*
solution: 0.25%	Epifrin
solution: 0.5%, 1%, 2%	Epifrin, Glaucon

Hydroxyamphetamine Hydrobromide Rx

| solution: 1% | Paredrine 1% Ophthalmic |

Naphazoline Hydrochloride Rx, otc

solution: 0.1% (*Rx*)	Ak-Con Ophthalmic, Albalon Liquifilm Ophthalmic, Naphcon Forte Ophthalmic, Vasocon Regular Ophthalmic
solution: 0.02% (*otc*)	VasoClear
solution: 0.012% (*otc*)	Allerest Eye Drops, Clear Eyes, Degest 2 Ophthalmic, Naphcon

Phenylephrine Hydrochloride Rx, otc

solution: 10% (*Rx*)	Efricel 10% Ophthalmic, Neo-Synephrine 10% Plain or Viscous Ophthalmic, *Generic*
solution: 2.5% (*Rx*)	Ak-Dilate Ophthalmic, Efricel 2.5% Ophthalmic, 2.5% Mydfrin Ophthalmic, Neo-Synephrine 2.5% Ophthalmic
solution: 0.12% (otc)	Ak-Nephrin, Isopto Frin Ophthalmic, Prefrin Liquifilm, Tear-Efrin Eye Drops

Tetrahydrozoline Hydrochloride otc

| solution: 0.05% | Murine Plus Eye Drops, Optigene 3 Eye Drops, Tetracon, Tetrasine, Visine |

INDICATIONS
EPINEPHRINE HYDROCHLORIDE

The 0.1% solution is used in conjunctivitis, in operations to control bleeding, and for rapid dilatation of the pupil. The 0.25%, 0.5%, 1%, and 2% solu-

M

tions are used in management of open-angle (chronic simple) glaucoma, alone, or in combination with other agents.

HYDROXYAMPHETAMINE HYDROBROMIDE

To dilate pupil; produces pupillary dilatation that lasts for a few hours.

NAPHAZOLINE HYDROCHLORIDE

Topical ocular vasoconstrictor.

PHENYLEPHRINE HYDROCHLORIDE

The 10% solution is used as a decongestant and vasoconstrictor and for pupil dilatation in uveitis (posterior synechiae), wide-angle glaucoma, and surgery. The 2.5% solution is used for refraction, ophthalmoscopic examination, diagnostic procedures, and before intraocular surgery. The 0.12% solution is used as a decongestant to provide temporary relief of minor eye irritations caused by hay fever, colds, dust, wind, swimming, sun, smog, hard contact lenses, eye strain, glare, or smoke.

TETRAHYDROZOLINE HYDROCHLORIDE

Topical ocular decongestant.

CONTRAINDICATIONS

Hypersensitivity; narrow-angle glaucoma. Also contraindicated before peripheral iridectomy, in eyes capable of angle closure because their mydriatic action may precipitate angle block. Phenylephrine HCl 10% is contraindicated in infants, insulin-dependent diabetics, hypertensive patients receiving guanethidine or reserpine, and in those with advanced arteriosclerotic changes, aneurysms, organic cardiac disease, or intraocular lens implants.

WARNINGS

Discontinue before use of anesthetics that sensitize the myocardium to sympathomimetics (*e.g.,* cyclopropane, halothane). Because pupil dilatation may precipitate an acute attack of narrow-angle glaucoma, the anterior chamber angle is evaluated by gonioscopy.

PRECAUTIONS

Use with caution in presence of hypertension, diabetes, hyperthyroidism, heart disease, cerebral arteriosclerosis, or long-standing bronchial asthma.

Use with caution in the elderly. Because of the strong action of drug on the dilator muscle, older individuals may also develop transient pigment floaters in the aqueous humor 35 to 45 minutes following administration. The appearance of these may be similar to those of anterior uveitis or microscopic hyphema.

Ordinarily, any mydriatic is contraindicated in those with narrow-angle glaucoma. When temporary dilatation of the pupil may free adhesions, or when vasoconstriction of the intrinsic vessels may lower intraocular tension, these advantages may temporarily outweigh the danger from coincident dilatation of the pupil.

Phenylephrine 10% may cause corneal clouding if the corneal epithelium has been denuded or damaged.

Epinephrine may cause discoloration of soft contact lenses.

DRUG INTERACTIONS

As with all other adrenergic drugs, when administered simultaneously with, or up to 21 days after, administration of **monoamine oxidase inhibitors**, careful supervision and adjustment of dosages are required, because exaggerated adrenergic effects may result. The pressor response of adrenergic agents may also be potentiated by **tricyclic antidepressants, beta-adrenergic blocking agents, reserpine, guanethidine, methyldopa,** and **anticholinergics.**

ADVERSE REACTIONS

Ocular: Transitory stinging on initial instillation may occur. Headache or browache may occur, but will usually diminish as treatment is continued. Conjunctival allergy occurs occasionally. Pigmentary deposits in the lids, conjunctiva, or cornea may occur after prolonged use. In rare cases, maculopathy with a central scotoma results from use in aphakic patients; prompt reversal generally follows discontinuance.

Systemic: Systemic effects have occasionally been reported, such as palpitation, tachycardia, extrasystoles, cardiac arrhythmia, hypertension, anxiety, fear, trembling, sweating, and pallor. Elevated blood pressure and untoward cardiovascular effects are rare but can occur with conjunctival instillation of **phenylephrine 10%** solution. Exercise caution when administering this solution to those with marked hypertension (especially those taking reserpine or guanethidine), those with advanced arteriosclerotic changes or with insulin-dependent diabetes, and children of low body weight. Rebound miosis and decreased mydriatic response to therapy have been reported in older persons 1 day after receiving **phenylephrine HCl.** This may be of importance when dilating pupils of older subjects before retinal detachment or cataract surgery.

DOSAGE

EPINEPHRINE HCI

One or two drops in eye with frequency individualized.

Management of open-angle glaucoma: One drop of 0.25%, 0.5%, 1%, or 2% solution in each eye once or twice daily. Frequency of instillation is determined by tonometry.

HYDROXYAMPHETAMINE HBr

One or two drops of 0.1% solution into conjunctival sac.

NAPHAZOLINE HCl

One or two drops into conjunctival sac of affected eye q3h to q4h.

PHENYLEPHRINE HCl

Vasoconstriction and pupil dilatation: A drop of a suitable topical anesthetic may be applied, followed in a few minutes by one drop of 2.5% or 10% solution on the upper limbus. Anesthetic prevents stinging and consequent dilution by lacrimation. It may be necessary to repeat the instillation after 1 hour, again preceded by use of a topical anesthetic.

Uveitis and posterior synechiae: Formation of synechiae may be prevented by using 2.5% or 10% solution and atropine to produce wide dilatation of the pupil. To free recently formed synechiae, one drop of 2.5% or 10% solution is applied to upper surface of cornea. Treatment may be continued the following day, if needed. In the interim, apply hot compresses for 5 to 10 minutes tid using 1% or 2% solution of atropine sulfate before and after each series of compresses.

Glaucoma: One drop of 10% solution on upper surface of cornea. May be repeated as often as necessary. May be used with miotics in those with wide-angle glaucoma.

Surgery: When a short-acting mydriatic is needed for wide dilatation of the pupil before intraocular surgery, the 2.5% or 10% solution may be applied topically 30 to 60 minutes before the operation.

Refraction: 2.5% solution with homatropine HBr, atropine sulfate, or a combination of homatropine and cocaine HCl. *Adults*—one drop of the preferred cycloplegic in each eye; follow in 5 minutes with one drop phenylephrine 2.5% solution, and in 10 minutes with another drop of the cycloplegic. In 50 to 60 minutes, eyes are ready for refraction. *Children*—one drop of atropine sulfate 1% in each eye; follow in 10 to 15 minutes with one drop phenylephrine 2.5% solution and in 5 to 10 minutes with second drop of atropine sulfate 1%. In 1 to 2 hours, eyes are ready for refraction. For a "one-application method," combine 2.5% phenylephrine with a cycloplegic to elicit synergistic action. The additive effect varies depending on the patient.

Ophthalmoscopic examination: One drop of 2.5% solution in each eye. Sufficient mydriasis to permit examination is produced in 15 to 30 minutes. Dilatation lasts from 1 to 3 hours.

Diagnostic procedures

Provocative test for angle block in patients with glaucoma: 2.5% solution may be used when latent increased intraocular pressure is suspected. Tension is measured before application and again after dilatation. A 3 mm Hg to 5 mm Hg rise suggests presence of angle block in those with glaucoma. Failure to obtain such a rise does not preclude the presence of glaucoma from other causes.

Shadow test (retinoscopy): When dilatation of pupil without cycloplegic action is desired, the 2.5% solution may be used alone.

Blanching test: Apply one or two drops of 2.5% solution to the injected eye. After 5 minutes, examine for perilimbal blanching. If blanching occurs, congestion is superficial and probably does not indicate iritis.

TETRAHYDROZOLINE HCl

One or two drops in each eye two or three times a day.

NURSING IMPLICATIONS

HISTORY
See Appendix 4.

PHYSICAL ASSESSMENT
Physician performs ophthalmologic examination.

ADMINISTRATION
Check solution visually; do not use if it is discolored or if precipitate is present.

Place patient in upright position. Tilt head back.

Instill in conjunctival sac unless physician orders otherwise. Have patient close eyes without squeezing shut and apply light pressure on the lacrimal sac for 1 to 2 minutes.

EPINEPHRINE HCl

When epinephrine is used with a miotic in treatment of glaucoma, the miotic is instilled first.

Storage: Epinephrine solutions are inherently unstable. Keep container tightly sealed; protect from light; store in cool place (possibly under refrigeration).

PHENYLEPHRINE HCl

When used for refraction, advise patient of a 1-hour wait before examination can be performed. When used for ophthalmoscopic examination, a wait of approximately 30 minutes will be necessary.

M

Stability: Is incompatible with butacaine.

Storage: Prolonged exposure to air or strong light may cause oxidation and discoloration.

ONGOING ASSESSMENTS AND NURSING MANAGEMENT

CLINICAL ALERT: Withhold next dose and notify physician immediately if sudden eye pain or other symptoms of glaucoma occur.

Conjunctival administration of phenylephrine 10% may cause elevated blood pressure and untoward cardiovascular effects. Blood pressure and pulse should be monitored daily for those receiving this strength.

If adverse reactions are noted or if patient complains of itching and burning, withhold next dose and notify physician.

Pupil dilatation may result in sensitivity to light.

PATIENT AND FAMILY INFORMATION

If eye pain occurs, discontinue use and notify physician immediately.

Nonprescription products: Follow manufacturer's directions on label or recommendation of physician. Avoid overuse.

If eye problem persists, see a physician.

Prescription products: NOTE: Patient or family member will need instruction in instillation of drug. If family member is to instill drug, allow time for observation as well as practice (under supervision) of the technique.

Use as prescribed by physician. Follow physician's directions for instilling drug.

Transitory stinging may be noted initially. If this persists or worsens, notify physician.

Keep container tightly closed and away from strong light. Do not use solution if it is discolored or contains a precipitate. Physician may recommend that medication be refrigerated.

Do not wash tip of dropper; do not lay dropper on table (or other surface). Replace dropper in bottle immediately after use.

If sensitivity to bright light is noted, wear sunglasses or tinted lenses.

If eyelids become red or swollen, or if palpitations, anxiety, trembling, or sweating is noted, contact physician immediately.

N

Nadolol
Nafcillin Sodium
Nalbuphine Hydrochloride
Nalidixic Acid
Naloxone Hydrochloride
Nandrolone Decanoate
Nandrolone Phenpropionate
Naphazoline Hydrochloride
Naproxen
Narcotic Analgesics
> Alphaprodine Hydrochloride
> Codeine
> Fentanyl
> Hydromorphone Hydrochloride
> Levorphanol Tartrate
> Meperidine Hydrochloride
> Methadone Hydrochloride
> Morphine
> Opium
> Oxycodone Hydrochloride
> Oxymorphone Hydrochloride
Narcotic Analgesic Combinations
Narcotic Antagonists
> Levallorphan Tartrate
> Naloxone Hydrochloride

Natamycin
Neomycin Sulfate
Neostigmine
Neostigmine Methylsulfate
Netilmicin Sulfate
Niclosamide
Nicotinamide
Nicotinic Acid
Nicotinyl Alcohol
Nifedipine
Nikethamide
Nitrates
> Amyl Nitrite
> Erythrityl Tetranitrate
> Isosorbide Dinitrate, Oral
> Isosorbide Dinitrate, Sublingual and Chewable
> Nitroglycerin, Intravenous
> Nitroglycerin, Sublingual
> Nitroglycerin, Sustained Release
> Nitroglycerin, Topical
> Nitroglycerin, Transdermal Systems
> Nitroglycerin, Transmucosal
> Pentaerythritol Tetranitrate
> Combination Products
Nitrofurantoin

Nitrofurazone
Nitroglycerin
Nitroprusside Sodium
Nitrous Oxide
Nonsteroidal Anti-inflammatory Agents
> Fenoprofen Calcium
> Ibuprofen
> Indomethacin
> Meclofenamate Sodium
> Mefenamic Acid
> Naproxen
> Piroxicam
> Sulindac
> Tolmetin Sodium
Norepinephrine
Norethindrone, Norethindrone Acetate
Norethynodrel
Norgestrel
Nortriptyline Hydrochloride
Novobiocin
Nylidrin Hydrochloride
Nystatin

N

Nadolol

See Beta-Adrenergic Blocking Agents.

Nafcillin Sodium

See Penicillins.

Nalbuphine Hydrochloride Rx

injection: 10 mg/ml   Nubain

INDICATIONS
Relief of moderate to severe pain. Also used for preoperative analgesia, as a supplement to surgical anesthesia, and for obstetric analgesia during labor.

CONTRAINDICATIONS
Hypersensitivity.

ACTIONS
Is a potent analgesic with narcotic agonist and antagonist actions. Has a chemical structure similar to that of the phenanthrene derivatives oxymorphone and naloxone. Analgesic potency is essentially equivalent to that of morphine and about three times that of pentazocine on a milligram basis. Unlike other agonists–antagonists, it does not significantly increase pulmonary artery pressure or systemic vascular resistance. Onset of action occurs within 2 to 3 minutes after IV administration and in less than 15 minutes following subcutaneous or IM administration. Plasma half-life is 5 hours. Duration of activity is reported to range from 3 to 6 hours. The narcotic antagonist activity is ten times that of pentazocine.

WARNINGS
Drug dependence: Has shown to have low abuse potential that is approximately that of pentazocine. When compared with drugs that are not mixed agonist–antagonists, abuse potential is less than that of codeine and prophoxyphene. Psychological and physical dependence and tolerance may follow abuse or misuse. Caution is observed in prescribing to emotionally unstable patients or those with history of narcotic abuse. Care is exercised in increasing dosage or frequency of administration, which might result in physical dependence in susceptible individuals. Abrupt discontinuation following prolonged use has been followed by symptoms of narcotic withdrawal (*i.e.,* abdominal cramps, nausea and vomiting, rhinorrhea, lacrimation, restlessness, anxiety, elevated temperature, piloerection).

Head injury and increased intracranial pressure: The possible respiratory depressant effects and potential of potent analgesics to elevate CSF pressure may be markedly exaggerated in the presence of head injury, intracranial lesions, or preexisting increase in intracranial pressure. Potent analgesics can produce effects that may obscure clinical course of patients with head injuries; therefore, drug is used with extreme caution and only if use is deemed essential.

Ambulatory patients: May impair mental or physical abilities.

Use during labor and delivery: May produce respiratory depression in the neonate. Use with caution in women delivering premature infants.

Use in pregnancy (other than labor): Safety not established. Administer only when potential benefits outweigh the possible hazards.

Use in children: Administration to those under 18 years not recommended.

PRECAUTIONS
Respiratory depression: At usual adult doses of 10 mg/70 kg, nalbuphine causes some respiratory depression, approximately equal to that produced by equal doses of morphine. In contrast with morphine use, respiratory depression is not appreciably increased with higher doses. Respiratory depression can be reversed by naloxone, when indicated. Administer with caution at low doses to those with impaired respiration (*e.g.,* from other drugs, uremia, bronchial asthma, severe infection, cyanosis, respiratory obstructions).

Use in impaired renal or hepatic function: Drug is metabolized in the liver and excreted by the kidneys; those with renal or liver dysfunction may overreact to customary doses. Therefore, use with caution and in reduced amounts.

Use in myocardial infarction: Use with caution in patients with MI who have nausea and vomiting.

Biliary tract surgery: Use with caution in patients about to undergo surgery of the biliary tract because it may cause spasm of the sphincter of Oddi.

DRUG INTERACTIONS
Although drug possesses narcotic antagonist activity, there is evidence that in nondependent patients it will not antagonize a narcotic analgesic administered just before, concurrently with, or just after an injection of the drug. Patients receiving **narcotic analgesics, general anesthetics, phenothiazines,** other **tranquilizers, sedatives, hypnotics,** or **CNS depressants** (including alcohol) concomitantly with nalbuphine may exhibit an additive effect. When such

combined therapy is contemplated, the dosage of one or both agents should be reduced.

ADVERSE REACTIONS

Most frequent: Sedation (36%).

Less frequent: Sweaty/clammy (9%); nausea and vomiting (6%); dizziness and vertigo (5%); dry mouth (4%); headache (3%).

Other adverse reactions that may occur (reported incidence 1% or less)

CNS: Nervousness, depression, restlessness, crying, euphoria, floating feeling, hostility, unusual dreams, confusion, faintness, hallucinations, dysphoria, feeling of heaviness, numbness, tingling, unreality.

Cardiovascular: Hypertension, hypotension, bradycardia, tachycardia.

GI: Cramps, dyspepsia, bitter taste.

Respiration: Depression, dyspnea, asthma.

Skin: Itching, burning, urticaria.

Miscellaneous: Speech difficulty, urinary urgency, blurred vision, flushing, warmth.

OVERDOSAGE

Symptoms: Sleepiness, mild dysphoria.

Treatment: Immediate IV administration of naloxone. Oxygen, IV fluids, vasopressors, and other supportive measures should be used as indicated.

DOSAGE

Adults: Usual recommended dose is 10 mg for 70 kg individual, administered subcutaneously, IM, or IV; may be repeated q3h to q6h as necessary. Dosage is adjusted according to severity of pain, physical status of patient, and other medications patient may be receiving. In intolerant individuals, recommended single maximum dose is 20 mg with a maximum total daily dose of 160 mg.

Patients dependent on narcotics: May experience some withdrawal symptoms upon administration of this drug. If unduly troublesome, narcotic withdrawal symptoms can be controlled by slow IV administration of small increments of morphine until relief occurs. If previous analgesic was morphine, meperidine, codeine, or another narcotic with similar duration of activity, ¼ the anticipated dose of nalbuphine can be administered initially. Observe for signs of withdrawal. If untoward symptoms do not occur, progressively larger doses may be tried at appropriate intervals until the desired level of analgesia is obtained.

NURSING IMPLICATIONS

HISTORY

See Appendix 4. When applicable, review chart for etiology of pain, length of time drug given, time of last administration, therapeutic effect of analgesic, date of drug order.

PHYSICAL ASSESSMENT

At time patient requests analgesic, determine exact location of pain, type of pain (*e.g.,* sharp, dull, stabbing), when pain began. In addition, look for controllable factors (*e.g.,* uncomfortable position, thirst, noise, bright lights, cold) that may decrease patient's tolerance to pain.

ADMINISTRATION

Give subcutaneously, IM, or IV.

Obtain blood pressure, pulse, and respirations immediately before preparing drug for administration. If these vital signs are significantly increased or decreased from average baseline values, withhold drug and notify physician.

ONGOING ASSESSMENTS AND NURSING MANAGEMENT

Onset of analgesia is less than 15 minutes following subcutaneous or IM administration and 2 to 3 minutes following IV administration.

Assess patient 20 to 30 minutes after administration for relief of pain. Check blood pressure, pulse, and respirations (especially during initial use of drug). Notify physician if there is significant increase or decrease in these vital signs following administration of drug.

If administered to patient with known or suspected physical dependence on narcotics, observe for symptoms of narcotic withdrawal (*e.g.,* abdominal cramps, nausea and vomiting, rhinorrhea, lacrimation, restlessness, anxiety, elevated temperature, piloerection). Report these symptoms to physician immediately (see *Dosage*).

If drug fails to produce sufficient analgesia, discuss problem with physician because a different analgesic may be necessary.

If sedation occurs, patient should remain in bed or ambulate with assistance.

If patient is to be assisted out of bed at scheduled times during the day, attempt to schedule ambulatory activity for 30 to 60 minutes after administration of drug.

May produce respiratory depression in the neonate when used during labor and delivery. Observe neonate at frequent intervals; notify physician if respiratory depression is apparent or neonate is difficult to arouse (fails to cry when stimulated).

When administered to those with impaired respiration (see *Precautions*), check respiratory rate q15m for at least first hour after drug administered. Report respiratory depression to physician immediately.

N

Nalidixic Acid Rx

caplets: 250 mg, 500   NegGram
  mg, 1 g
suspension: 250 mg/   NegGram
  5 ml

INDICATIONS

Urinary-tract infections (UTIs) caused by susceptible gram-negative microorganisms including majority of *Proteus* strains, *Klebsiella* and *Enterobacter*
species, and *Escherichia coli.*

CONTRAINDICATIONS

Hypersensitivity; history of convulsive disorders.

ACTIONS

Is bactericidal against most gram-negative bacteria
that cause UTIs. DNA polymerization appears to be
inhibited, the primary target being the single-
stranded DNA precursors in the late stages of chromosomal replication. RNA synthesis may be partially inhibited as well.

Following administration, nalidixic acid is rapidly
absorbed from the GI tract, partially metabolized by
the liver, and rapidly excreted through the kidneys.

WARNINGS

Brief convulsions, increased intracranial pressure,
and toxic psychosis have rarely been reported.
These occurred in infants and children or in geriatric patients, usually from overdosage or in those
with predisposing factors, and completely and rapidly disappeared on discontinuation of drug. If these
reactions occur, drug should be discontinued and
appropriate therapeutic measures instituted.

Drug has been reported to induce clinically significant hemolysis in G6PD-deficient red cells.

Safe use during the first trimester of pregnancy
has not been established. Drug has been used during the last two trimesters without producing ill effects in mother or child.

PRECAUTIONS

Blood counts and renal- and hepatic-function tests
should be performed periodically if treatment is
continued for more than 2 weeks. Use with caution
in patients with liver disease, epilepsy, or severe cerebral arteriosclerosis.

Although caution should be used in those with
severe renal failure, therapeutic concentrations of
drug in urine, without increased toxicity due to
drug accumulation in the blood, have been observed in patients on full dosage with creatinine
clearances as low as 2 ml/minute to 8 ml/minute.

If bacterial resistance emerges during treatment, it

usually does so within 48 hours, permitting rapid
change to another antimicrobial. If clinical response
is unsatisfactory or relapse occurs, culture and sensitivity tests are recommended. Underdosage during
initial treatment (<4 g/day for adults) may predispose the patient to emergence of bacterial resistance.

DRUG INTERACTIONS

May enhance effects of **oral anticoagulants** (warfarin, dicumarol) by displacing significant amounts
from serum albumin binding sites.

Drug/lab tests: A false-positive reaction for urine
glucose may be seen when urine tested with Benedict's or Fehling's solution or Clinitest Reagent tablets. Clinistix Reagent Strips and Tes-Tape do not
give a false-positive reaction. Incorrect elevated values may be obtained for urinary 17-keto and keto-
genic steroids.

ADVERSE REACTIONS

CNS: Drowsiness, weakness, headache, dizziness,
vertigo. Toxic psychosis or brief convulsions have
been reported rarely (see *Warnings*). In infants and
children receiving therapeutic doses, increased intracranial pressure with bulging anterior fontanel, papilledema, and headache have occasionally been observed. A few cases of sixth cranial nerve palsy have
been reported. Although mechanisms of these reactions are unknown, signs and symptoms usually disappeared rapidly with no sequelae when treatment
was discontinued.

Visual: Reversible subjective visual disturbances
without objective findings have occurred infrequently and include overbrightness of lights, change
in color perception, difficulty in focusing, decrease
in visual acuity, and double vision. They usually
disappeared promptly when dosage was reduced or
therapy discontinued.

GI: Abdominal pain, nausea, vomiting, diarrhea.

Allergic: Rash, pruritus, urticaria, angioedema,
eosinophilia, arthralgia with joint stiffness and swelling, and rarely anaphylactoid reaction. Photosensitivity reactions (erythema and bullae on exposed
skin surfaces) usually resolve completely 2 to 8
weeks after discontinuation, but bullae may continue to appear with successive exposure to sunlight
or with mild skin trauma for up to 3 months.

Other: Rarely, cholestasis, paresthesia, metabolic
acidosis, thrombocytopenia, leukopenia, or hemolytic anemia, sometimes associated with G6PD deficiency.

OVERDOSAGE

Symptoms: Toxic psychosis, convulsions, increased intracranial pressure, or metabolic acidosis

may occur in those taking more than recommended dosage. Vomiting, nausea, and lethargy may also occur following overdosage.

Treatment: Reactions are short lived (2–3 hours) because drug is rapidly excreted. If overdosage is noted early, gastric lavage is indicated. If absorption has occurred, increase fluid administration and have supportive measures such as oxygen and means of artificial respiration available. Anticonvulsant therapy may be indicated in severe cases.

DOSAGE

Adults: *Initial therapy*—1 g qid for 1 or 2 weeks (total dose 4 g/day). *Prolonged therapy*—Total dose may be reduced to 2 g/day after initial treatment period.

Children: Do not administer to infants younger than 3 months. *Children 12 and under*—Dosage is calculated on basis of body weight. *Recommended total daily dosage for initial therapy*—25 mg/lb/day (55 mg/kg/day) given in four equally divided doses. *Prolonged therapy*—Total daily dose may be reduced to 15 mg/lb/day (33 mg/kg/day).

NURSING IMPLICATIONS

HISTORY
See Appendix 4.

PHYSICAL ASSESSMENT
Obtain vital signs, weight. Urine tests for culture and sensitivity, CBC, and renal- and hepatic-function tests may also be ordered.

ADMINISTRATION
Give with meals or food.

ONGOING ASSESSMENTS AND NURSING MANAGEMENT
Monitor blood pressure, pulse, and respirations daily, temperature q4h (during initial therapy or if previously elevated); observe for adverse reactions.

May produce drowsiness, dizziness, blurred vision. Patient may require assistance with ambulation.

Subjective reversible visual disturbances may occur during first few days of treatment. If patient complains of visual disturbances, notify physician before next dose is due because dosage may need to be reduced or therapy discontinued.

If symptoms of UTI persist beyond 2 days or become worse, notify physician because repeat urine culture and sensitivity may be ordered or a different antimicrobial prescribed.

CNS reactions (see *Warnings, Adverse Reactions*) may occur in infants, children, the elderly, or those with a history of convulsive disorders. Notify physician immediately if these reactions occur because drug may need to be discontinued.

Blood counts and renal- and hepatic-function tests may be performed periodically if treatment is continued for more than 2 weeks.

Diabetic patient: Test urine for glucose using Tes-Tape or Clinistix (see *Drug Interactions*).

Patient receiving anticoagulants: Dosage of anticoagulant may need to be adjusted. Observe patient for sudden fluctuations in prothrombin time and bleeding episodes (see Coumarin and Indandione Derivatives).

PATIENT AND FAMILY INFORMATION
May produce GI upset; take with food or meals.

May produce drowsiness, dizziness, or blurred vision. Observe caution while driving or performing other tasks requiring alertness.

Take exactly as ordered and complete full course of therapy. Do not increase or decrease dose unless advised to do so by physician.

If symptoms do not improve or if they become worse (allow at least 2 days of therapy), notify physician promptly.

Avoid direct exposure to sunlight or ultraviolet light; photosensitivity may occur. If exposure to sun is unavoidable, check with physician about use of a sunscreen preparation.

Naloxone Hydrochloride

See Narcotic Antagonists.

Nandrolone Decanoate

See Anabolic Hormones.

Nandrolone Phenpropionate

See Anabolic Hormones.

Naphazoline Hydrochloride

See Decongestants, Nasal, Topical; Mydriatics/Ophthalmic Vasoconstrictors.

Naproxen

See Nonsteroidal Anti-inflammatory Agents.

Narcotic Analgesics

Alphaprodine Hydrochloride Rx C–II

injection: 40 mg/ml, 60 mg/ml	Nisentil

Codeine Rx C–II

Codeine Sulfate

tablets: 15 mg, 30 mg, 60 mg	Generic
tablets, soluble: 15 mg, 30 mg, 60 mg	Generic

Codeine Phosphate*

injection: 30 mg/ml, 60 mg/ml	Generic
tablets, soluble: 15 mg, 30 mg, 60 mg	Generic

Fentanyl Rx C–II

injection: 0.05 mg/ml	Sublimaze

Hydromorphone Hydrochloride Rx C–II

tablets: 1 mg, 2 mg, 3 mg, 4 mg	Dilaudid (1-, 2-, and 4-mg tablets contain tartrazine)
injection: 1 mg/ml, 2 mg/ml, 4 mg/ml	Dilaudid, Generic
injection: 3 mg/ml	Generic
suppositories: 3 mg	Dilaudid

Levorphanol Tartrate Rx C–II

tablets: 2 mg	Levo-Dromoran
injection: 2 mg/ml	Levo-Dromoran

Meperidine Hydrochloride* Rx C–II

tablets: 50 mg, 100 mg	Demerol HCl, Pethadol, Generic
syrup: 50 mg/5 ml	Demerol HCl
multi-dose vials, injection: 50 mg/ml, 100 mg/ml	Demerol HCl, Generic
single-dose vials, syringes, ampules: 25 mg, 50 mg, 75 mg, 100 mg/dose	Demerol HCl, Generic

* For combination products, see the following monograph: Narcotic Analgesic Combinations.

Methadone Hydrochloride Rx C–II

injection: 10 mg/ml	Dolophine HCl
tablets: 5 mg, 10 mg	Dolophine HCl, Generic
dispersible tablets: 40 mg	Methadone HCl Diskets
oral solution: 5 mg/5 ml, 10 mg/5 ml	Generic

Morphine Rx C–II

injection: 2 mg/ml, 4 mg/ml, 5 mg/ml, 8 mg/ml, 10 mg/ml, 15 mg/ml	Generic (as sulfate)
soluble tablets: 10 mg, 15 mg, 30 mg	Generic (as sulfate)
oral solution: 10 mg/5 ml, 20 mg/5 ml	Generic (as sulfate)
oral solution: 20 mg/ml	Roxanol
oral tablets: 15 mg, 30 mg	Generic (as sulfate)
rectal suppositories: 5 mg, 10 mg, 20 mg	RMS Uniserts

Opium* Rx

injection: hydrochlorides of opium alkaloids: 20 mg/ml	Pantopon (C–II)
liquid: 10% opium, 19% alcohol	Opium Tincture, Deodorized (C–II)
liquid: 2 mg morphine equivalent per 5 ml; with 45% alcohol	Paregoric Tincture (C–III)
liquid: 12% paregoric (equivalent to 1.44 mg anhydrous morphine); with glycyrrhiza fluidextract, antimony potassium tartrate, and alcohol	Brown Mixture (C–V)

Oxycodone Hydrochloride* Rx C–II

tablet: 5 mg	Generic
solution: 5 mg/5 ml	Generic

Oxymorphone Hydrochloride Rx C–II

injection: 1 mg/ml, 1.5 mg/ml	Numorphan
suppositories: 5 mg	Numorphan

* For combination products, see the following monograph: Narcotic Analgesic Combinations.

INDICATIONS

ALPHAPRODINE HYDROCHLORIDE

Obstetric analgesia; urologic examinations and procedures, particularly cystoscopy; preoperatively in major surgery; in minor surgery when rapid analgesia of brief duration is desirable, particularly in children requiring analgesia during dental procedures. Drug is indicated in children only for analgesia during dental procedures.

CODEINE

Relief of mild to moderate pain and as an antitussive.

FENTANYL

For analgesic action of short duration during anesthesia (premedication, induction, maintenance) and in the immediate postoperative period (recovery room) as needed. Used as a narcotic analgesic supplement in general or regional anesthesia. May be administered with a neuroleptic such as droperidol. Also used as an anesthetic agent with oxygen in selected high-risk patients (undergoing open heart surgery or certain complicated neurologic or orthopedic procedures).

HYDROMORPHONE HYDROCHLORIDE

Relief of moderate to severe pain.

LEVORPHANOL TARTRATE

Relief of moderate to severe pain. Used preoperatively, it allays apprehension, provides prolonged analgesia, reduces thiopental requirements, and shortens recovery time. Is compatible with a wide range of anesthetic agents. Is a useful supplement to nitrous oxide–oxygen anesthesia.

MEPERIDINE HYDROCHLORIDE

Orally for relief of moderate to severe pain. Preoperatively to allay apprehension, provide prolonged analgesia, reduce thiopental requirements, and shorten recovery time.

METHADONE HYDROCHLORIDE

Relief of severe pain; detoxification and temporary maintenance treatment of narcotic addiction. Methadone is ineffective for relief of general anxiety. Methadone HCl Diskets are for detoxification and maintenance treatment only.

MORPHINE

Relief of severe pain. Also used preoperatively to sedate patient and allay apprehension, facilitate induction of anesthesia, and reduce anesthetic dosage. Is widely used in treatment of severe pain associated with myocardial infarction (MI) and for dyspnea associated with acute left ventricular failure and pulmonary edema.

Unlabeled uses: Given intrathecally and epidurally or by continuous IV infusion in treatment of acute and chronic pain.

OPIUM

For all disorders in which the analgesic, sedative-hypnotic narcotic, or antidiarrheal effect of an opiate is needed; for relief of severe pain in place of morphine.

OXYCODONE HYDROCHLORIDE

Relief of moderate to moderately severe pain.

OXYMORPHONE HYDROCHLORIDE

Relief of moderate to severe pain. Parenterally for preoperative medication, support of anesthesia, obstetric analgesia, and relief of anxiety in those with dyspnea associated with acute left ventricular failure and pulmonary edema.

ACTIONS

Stimulation of the opiate receptors in the CNS results in effective analgesia. These receptors are present in the brain, brain stem, and spinal cord. Narcotic agonists apparently occupy the same stereospecific receptors as endogenous opioid peptides (enkephalins and endorphins). Binding of the agonist to the opiate receptor decreases sodium permeability and thus inhibits transmission of pain impulses.

Pure agonists lead to tolerance and physical dependence with chronic use; abrupt withdrawal may lead to acute abstinence syndrome. Narcotic antagonists (p 762) block the opiate receptor, inhibit the pharmacologic activity of the agonist, and can precipitate withdrawal in dependent patients.

Agents with both agonist and antagonist properties provide effective analgesic effects; however, tolerance does not readily develop. These agents (pentazocine p 859, butorphanol p 218, and nalbuphine p 744) have a lower potential for abuse and can precipitate withdrawal when given to dependent patients.

In addition to analgesia, narcotic analgesics have a variety of secondary pharmacologic effects including the following.

CNS: Euphoria, drowsiness, lethargy, apathy, and mental confusion. Nausea and vomiting are secondary to stimulation of the emetic chemoreceptors located in the medulla.

Respiratory: Depressant effects first diminish tidal volume, followed by reduction of respiratory rate. This is secondary to reduced sensitivity of the respiratory center to CO_2.

Cardiovascular: Narcotics are known to depress responsiveness of the alpha-adrenergic receptors, which may lead to visceral pooling of blood; this may result in hypotension (especially while standing or in those with hypovolemia).

GI: Narcotics inhibit peristalsis and may cause spasm of the sphincter of Oddi. Constipation may also be induced.

Urinary tract: Urinary retention may occur as a result of increased sphincter tone in the bladder.

Table 38 compares the narcotic analgesics. Data are based on IM administration unless otherwise noted.

CONTRAINDICATIONS

Hypersensitivity to narcotics; diarrhea caused by poisoning, until toxic material has been eliminated from the GI tract; premature infants or during labor when delivery of a premature infant is anticipated.

Meperidine is contraindicated in those who are taking monoamine oxidase inhibitors (MAOIs) or those who have recently received such agents.

WARNINGS

Drug dependence: Narcotic analgesics have potential for abuse. Psychological dependence and physical tolerance may develop upon repeated use. Opiates produce relaxation, indifference to pain and stress, lethargy, and euphoria. Patients receiving narcotics for more than a few days may exhibit mild symptoms upon discontinuation. Most patients receiving opiates for medical reasons do not develop dependence syndromes.

Head injury and increased intracranial pressure: Respiratory depressant effects and the capacity to elevate CSF pressure may be markedly exaggerated in the presence of head injury, brain tumor, other intracranial lesions, or a preexisting increase in intracranial pressure. Narcotics may obscure the clinical course of head injuries. In such cases, these drugs are used with caution and only if deemed essential.

Parenteral therapy: Give by very slow IV injection, preferably as a dilute solution. Rapid IV injection increases incidence of adverse reactions; severe respiratory depression, hypotension, apnea, peripheral circulatory collapse, cardiac arrest, and anaphylactoid reactions have occurred. Do not administer IV unless a narcotic antagonist and facilities for assisted or controlled respiration are immediately available. When drug is given parenterally, especially IV, patient should be lying down. Use caution when injecting subcutaneously or IM in chilled areas or into those with hypotension or shock because impaired perfusion may prevent complete absorption. If repeated injections are administered, an excessive amount may be suddenly absorbed if normal circulation is reestablished. **Alphaprodine** is never administered IM because absorption is too unpredictable.

Asthma and other respiratory conditions: Use with extreme caution in those with acute asthma, those with chronic obstructive pulmonary disease or cor pulmonale, those with substantially decreased respiratory reserve, and those with preexisting respiratory depression, hypoxia, or hypercapnia. Even usual therapeutic doses may decrease respiratory drive while simultaneously increasing airway resistance to the point of apnea.

Hypotensive effect: Administration may result in severe hypotension in the postoperative patient or in any patient whose ability to maintain his blood pressure has already been compromised by hypovolemia or concurrent administration of phenothiazines or general anesthetics. Narcotics may pro-

Table 38. Comparison of Pharmokinetics of the Narcotic Analgesics

Drug	Onset (minutes)	Peak (hours)	Duration (hours)	Half-life (hours)
Alphaprodine	1–2*	—	½–1½	2
	2–30†	—	1–2	
Codeine	15–30	1–1½	4–6	3–4
Fentanyl	5–15	within ½	1–2	1½–6
Hydromorphone	15–30	½–1½	4–5	2–4
Levorphanol	within 60	within ⅓*	4–8	—
Meperidine	10–15	½–1	2–4	3–8
Methadone	10–15	1–2	4–6	22–25
Morphine	within 20	½–1½	up to 7	2–3
Oxycodone	—	—	4–5	—
Oxymorphone	5–10	½–1½	3–6	—

* IV administration
† Subcutaneous administration

duce orthostatic hypotension in ambulatory patients.

Use in pregnancy: Safety has not been established. The placental transfer of opiates is very rapid. Maternal addiction with subsequent neonatal withdrawal is well known during illicit use.

Use in labor: When used as obstetric analgesics, narcotics cross the placental barrier and can produce depression of respiratory and psychophysiologic functions in the newborn. **Methadone** is not recommended for obstetric analgesia because its long duration of action increases the probability of respiratory depression in the newborn. It has also been associated with low infant birth weight and subsequent development of sudden infant death syndrome (SIDS).

Use in lactation: These agents appear in breast milk; however, effects on the infant may not be significant. Some recommend waiting 4 to 6 hours after administration before breast-feeding. **Methadone** enters breast milk in concentrations approaching plasma levels and may prevent withdrawal symptoms in addicted infants. **Meperidine** also achieves an average milk–plasma ratio of about 1.0. Other narcotics are excreted into breast milk in small amounts.

PRECAUTIONS

Acute abdominal conditions: Diagnosis or clinical course may be obscured by narcotics.

Special-risk patients: Caution is exercised in elderly and debilitated patients and in those known to be sensitive to CNS depressants, including those with cardiovascular or pulmonary disease, myxedema, acute alcoholism, delirium tremens, cerebral arteriosclerosis, emphysema, fever, bronchial asthma, kyphoscoliosis, Addison's disease, prostatic hypertrophy or urethral stricture, and severe CNS depression or coma. **Fentanyl** may produce bradycardia, which may be treated with atropine. Caution is used when administering fentanyl to patients with bradyarrhythmia.

Renal and hepatic dysfunction: May cause a prolonged duration and cumulative effect.

Supraventricular tachycardias: Use with caution in those with atrial flutter and other supraventricular tachycardias because of possible vagolytic action, which may produce a significant increase in the ventricular response rate.

Seizures: May be aggravated or may occur in individuals without a history of convulsive disorders if dosage is substantially increased because of tolerance.

Cough reflex: These agents suppress the cough reflex. Exercise caution when using postoperatively and in those with pulmonary disease.

Tartrazine sensitivity: Hydromorphone (Dilaudid) tablets of 1 mg, 2 mg, and 4 mg contain tartrazine. See Appendix 6, section 6-23.

DRUG INTERACTIONS

Use with caution and in reduced doses in patients concurrently receiving **other narcotic analgesics, general anesthetics, antihistamines, phenothiazines, barbiturates, other tranquilizers, sedative-hypnotics, tricyclic antidepressants,** and **other CNS depressants** (including alcohol). Respiratory depression, hypotension, profound sedation, or coma may result.

Nitrous oxide and **diazepam** may produce cardiovascular depression when given with high doses of **fentanyl.** Certain forms of **conduction anesthesia,** such as spinal anesthesia and some peridural anesthesia, can alter respiration by blocking intercostal nerves. Through other mechanisms, fentanyl can also alter respiration. When used with a tranquilizer (*e.g.,* **droperidol**) blood pressure may be altered, hypotension can occur, and pulmonary arterial pressure may be decreased.

The analgesic effect of morphine is potentiated by **chlorpromazine** and **methocarbamol.** The depressant effects of morphine may be enhanced by **chloral hydrate, glutethimide, beta-adrenergic blockers** (propranolol), and **furazolidone.**

Case reports have described CNS toxicity (confusion, disorientation, respiratory depression, apnea, seizures) following concurrent administration of **cimetidine** and narcotic analgesics.

Meperidine has precipitated unpredictable and occasionally fatal reactions in those concurrently receiving **MAOIs** or those who have received such agents within 14 days. The mechanism is unclear. Some reactions have been characterized by symptoms of acute narcotic overdose; in others, the predominant reactions have been hyperexcitability, convulsions, tachycardia, hyperpyrexia, and hypertension. Virtually all of the reported reactions occurred with meperidine; however, other narcotics should also be given with caution to those receiving MAOIs.

Concurrent administration of **rifampin** or **phenytoin** may reduce plasma levels of **methadone** to a degree sufficient to produce withdrawal symptoms. Patients addicted to **heroin** or who are on the **methadone** maintenance program may experience withdrawal symptoms when given **pentazocine, butorphanol,** or **nalbuphine.**

Drug/lab tests: Because narcotic analgesics may increase biliary tract pressure, with resultant increases in plasma **amylase** or **lipase,** levels may be unreliable for 24 hours after narcotic administration.

N

ADVERSE REACTIONS

Major hazards: Respiratory depression, apnea, and (to a lesser degree) circulatory depression; respiratory arrest, shock, and cardiac arrest have occurred.

Most frequent: Lightheadedness, dizziness, sedation, nausea, vomiting, sweating. These effects seem more prominent in ambulatory patients and in those not suffering severe pain. In such individuals, lower doses are advisable.

CNS: Euphoria, dysphoria, weakness, headache, somnolence, drowsiness, miosis, pinpoint pupils, coma, insomnia, agitation, tremor, uncoordinated muscle movements, impairment of mental and physical performance, mental clouding, lethargy, anxiety, fear, psychic dependence, mood changes, transient hallucinations, disorientation, confusion, and visual disturbances have been reported. Injection near a nerve trunk may result in sensory-motor paralysis, which is usually, although not always, transitory. Choreiform movements have been reported with **methadone.** Deaths and cerebral damage have been reported with **alphaprodine,** especially when given concomitantly with other CNS depressants. Seizures have been reported following **fentanyl** administration.

GI: Dry mouth, anorexia, constipation, biliary tract spasms. Patients with chronic ulcerative colitis may experience increased colonic motility; toxic dilatation has been reported in those with acute ulcerative colitis.

Cardiovascular: Flushing of face, peripheral circulatory collapse, tachycardia, bradycardia, palpitation, faintness, hypotension, syncope, and phlebitis following IV injection.

GU: Ureteral spasm and spasms of vesical sphincters, urinary retention or hesitancy, oliguria, antidiuretic effect, reduced libido or potency.

Allergic: Pruritus, urticaria, other skin rashes, edema, rarely hemorrhagic urticaria. Wheal and flare over vein with IV injection may occur. Anaphylactoid reactions have been reported following IV administration.

Other: Muscular rigidity, pain at injection site; local tissue irritation and induration following subcutaneous injection, particularly when repeated.

ACUTE OVERDOSAGE

In general, the shorter the onset and duration of action of the opiate, the greater the intensity and rapidity of symptom onset. Infants and children may be relatively more sensitive to opiates on a body-weight basis. Elderly patients are comparatively intolerant of opiates.

Symptoms: In severe overdosage, mainly by the IV route, apnea, circulatory collapse, convulsions, cardiopulmonary arrest, and death may occur. The less severely poisoned patient often presents with the triad of CNS depression, miosis, and respiratory depression. Severe overdosage is characterized by respiratory depression, extreme somnolence progressing to stupor or coma, constricted pupils, skeletal muscle flaccidity, and cold and clammy skin. Hypotension, bradycardia, hypothermia, pulmonary edema, pneumonia, or shock may occur in up to 40% of patients.

Treatment: Primary attention should be given to adequate respiratory exchange through provision of a patent airway and institution of assisted or controlled ventilation. If depressed respiration is associated with muscle rigidity, an IV neuromuscular blocking agent may be required.

After assessing the patient's pulmonary status, administer a narcotic antagonist. The narcotic antagonists are specific antidotes for overdosage. Because the duration of action of most narcotics exceeds that of the narcotic antagonists, repeat the antagonist to maintain adequate respiration; keep the patient under surveillance. Do not give an antagonist in the absence of clinically significant respiratory or cardiac depression. Naloxone is the antagonist of choice.

Oxygen, IV fluids, vasopressors, and other supportive measures should be employed as indicated. In cases of oral overdose, the stomach should be evacuated by emesis or gastric lavage if treatment can be instituted within 2 hours following ingestion. The patient should be closely observed for a rise in temperature or pulmonary complications that may signal the need for institution of antibiotic therapy.

PHYSICAL DEPENDENCE

Narcotic analgesics can lead to physical dependence when used for prolonged periods. Dependence is recognized by increased tolerance to the analgesic effect and appearance of purposive phenomena (complaints, pleas, demands, manipulative actions) shortly before the time of the next scheduled dose. Withdrawal should be treated in a hospital.

Acute abstinence syndrome (withdrawal): Severity of the abstinence syndrome is related to the degree of dependence, abruptness of withdrawal, and the drug used. Generally, withdrawal symptoms develop at the time the next dose would ordinarily be given. For heroin or morphine, they gradually increase in intensity, reach a maximum in 36 to 72 hours, and subside over 5 to 10 days. In contrast, methadone withdrawal is slower in onset and the patient may not recover for 6 to 7 weeks. Meperidine withdrawal has often run its course within 4 to 5 days. Withdrawal precipitated by narcotic antagonist administration is manifested by an onset of symptoms within minutes and maximum intensity within 30 minutes. If administration of a narcotic antagonist must be used to treat serious respiratory depression in a physically dependent patient, administer with extreme care, using one-tenth to one-fifth the usual dose.

Signs and symptoms of opiate withdrawal are as follows:

Early—Yawning, lacrimation, rhinorrhea, "yen sleep," perspiration
Intermediate—Mydriasis, piloerection, flushing, tachycardia, twitching, tremor, restlessness, irritability, anorexia
Late—Muscle spasm, fever, nausea, diarrhea, vomiting, spontaneous orgasm

Treatment: Primarily symptomatic and supportive, including maintenance of proper fluid and electrolyte balance and administration of a tranquilizer to suppress anxiety. Severe symptoms may require narcotic replacement. Gradual withdrawal, using incrementally smaller doses, will minimize symptoms.

Methadone maintenance therapy to permit psychosocial rehabilitation before narcotic withdrawal may be beneficial. Because methadone is not a tranquilizer, patients maintained on this drug will react to problems and stresses with the same symptoms of anxiety as do other individuals. Such symptoms should not be confused with those of narcotic abstinence; do not treat them by increasing the dosage of methadone. During the induction phase of methadone maintenance, patients withdrawn from heroin may show withdrawal symptoms, to be differentiated from methadone-induced side-effects. During prolonged administration of methadone there is gradual progressive disappearance of side-effects over several weeks. However, constipation and sweating often persist.

DOSAGE

ALPHAPRODINE HCl

Usual adult dosage is 0.4 mg/kg to 0.6 mg/kg IV or 0.4 mg/kg to 1.2 mg/kg subcutaneously. Initially, a lower dosage range is recommended in order to evaluate patient response. Initial IV dosage should not exceed 30 mg and initial subcutaneous dose should not exceed 60 mg. Total dose administered by any route should not exceed 240 mg/24 hours.

Subcutaneous administration usually provides analgesic effects within 10 minutes, lasting from 1 to over 2 hours. If required, an additional ¼ dose may be given 30 minutes after initial dose. IV route is recommended when more rapid onset and shorter duration of action are desired. An additional amount of the ¼ initial dose may be injected after 15 minutes, if required.

Obstetrics: Initially, 40 mg to 60 mg subcutaneously after cervical dilatation has begun, repeated as required at 2-hour intervals. May be combined with scopolamine or atropine and used in conjunction with nerve block or inhalation anesthesia.

Urologic procedures: Initially, 20 mg to 30 mg IV.

Preoperatively in major surgery: Initially, 20 mg to 40 mg subcutaneously or 10 mg to 20 mg IV.

Minor surgery: Initially, 40 mg subcutaneously or 20 mg IV.

Pediatric dentistry: Recommended dose is 0.3 mg/kg to 0.6 mg/kg by submucosal route only. Routine reversal with naloxone should be performed following each procedure.

CODEINE

Adults: *Analgesic*—15 mg to 60 mg q4h PO, IM, IV, or subcutaneously. *Antitussive*—10 mg to 20 mg q4h to q6h. Do not exceed 120 mg in 24 hours.

Children: *Analgesic (1 yr of age or older)*—0.5 mg/kg or 15 mg/m² q4h to q6h PO, IM, or subcutaneously. *Antitussive (6–12 yr)*—5 mg to 10 mg PO q4h to q6h, not to exceed 60 mg/24 hours; *antitussive (2–6 yr)*—2.5 mg to 5 mg q4h to q6h, not to exceed 30 mg/24 hours.

FENTANYL

Dosage is individualized according to age, body weight, physical status, underlying pathologic condition, use of other drugs, type of anesthesia used, and surgical procedure involved.

Concomitant narcotic administration: The respiratory depressant effect of fentanyl persists longer than the measured analgesic effect. Other narcotics, when required, are used initially in lower doses (as low as one-fourth to one-third of those usually recommended).

Premedication: 0.05 mg to 0.1 mg administered IM 30 to 60 minutes prior to surgery.

Adjunct to general anesthesia: *Total low dosage*—0.002 mg/kg in small doses for minor, painful surgical procedures and postoperative pain relief.

Total moderate dosage—0.002 mg/kg to 0.02 mg/kg. In addition to adequate analgesia, some abolition of stress response should occur. Respiratory depression necessitates artificial ventilation.

Total high dosage—0.02 mg/kg to 0.05 mg/kg to produce stress-free anesthesia.

Maintenance low dosage—Infrequently needed in minor surgical procedures.

Maintenance moderate dosage—0.025 mg to 0.1 mg IM or IV when movement or changes in vital signs indicate surgical stress or lightening of analgesia.

Maintenance high dosage—Ranging from 0.025 mg; additional dosage individualized.

Adjunct to regional anesthesia: 0.05 mg to 0.1 mg IM or slowly IV over 1 to 2 minutes.

Postoperative (recovery room): 0.05 mg to 0.1 mg IM for control of pain, tachypnea, and emergence delirium; repeat dose in 1 to 2 hours if needed.

Children (2–12 yr): For induction and maintenance, 0.02 mg to 0.03 mg/20 to 25 lb recommended. Safety in children younger than 2 not established.

General anesthetic: 0.05 mg/kg to 0.1 mg/kg; doses up to 0.15 mg/kg may be used.

Storage: Protect from light; store at room temperature.

HYDROMORPHONE HCl

Oral: 2 mg q4h to q6h; more severe pain may require 4 mg or more q4h to q6h.

Parenteral: 2 mg subcutaneously or IM q4h to q6h as needed. For severe pain, 3 mg to 4 mg q4h to q6h as needed. May be given by slow IV injection.

Rectal: 3 mg q6h to q8h.

Children: Safety and effectiveness for children not established.

Storage: Store suppositories in refrigerator.

LEVORPHANOL TARTRATE

Average adult dose is 2 mg PO or subcutaneously. Dosage may be increased to 3 mg, if necessary. Has been given by slow IV injection.

MEPERIDINE HCl

Although subcutaneous administration is suitable for occasional use, IM administration is preferred for repeated doses. If IV administration is required, dosage is decreased and drug injected very slowly, preferably using a diluted solution. Is less effective when administered orally than when given parenterally.

Adults: 50 mg to 150 mg IM, subcutaneously, or PO q3h to q4h as necessary.

Children: 0.5 mg/lb to 0.8 mg/lb (1 mg/kg–1.8 mg/kg) IM, subcutaneously, or PO up to adult dose, q3h to q4h as necessary.

Preoperative medication: Given 30 to 90 minutes before beginning anesthesia. *Adults*—50 mg to 100 mg IM or subcutaneously. *Children*—0.5 mg/lb to 1 mg/lb (1–2 mg/kg) IM or subcutaneously, up to adult dose.

Support of anesthesia: May be administered in repeated doses diluted to 10 mg/ml by slow IV injection or by continuous infusion diluted to 1 mg/ml.

Obstetric analgesia: When pains become regular, 50 mg to 100 mg IM or subcutaneously; repeat at 1- to 3-hour intervals.

METHADONE HCl

Relief of pain: Although subcutaneous administration is suitable for occasional use, IM injection is preferred when repeated doses are required. Usual adult dose is 2.5 mg to 10 mg IM, subcutaneously, or PO q3h to q4h as needed.

Detoxification treatment: Daily dose is administered under close supervision. Detoxification treatment should not exceed 21 days and may not be repeated earlier than 4 weeks after completion of the preceding course. Oral form of administration is preferred, but parenteral form may be used initially. In detoxification, patient may receive methadone when there are significant withdrawal symptoms. Initially, 15 mg to 20 mg will often suppress withdrawal symptoms with additional methadone provided if withdrawal symptoms are not suppressed or if symptoms reappear. When patients are physically dependent on high doses, 40 mg/day in single or divided doses usually constitutes an adequate stabilizing dose. Stabilization is continued for 2 to 3 days; then dosage is gradually decreased on a daily basis or at 2-day intervals. In hospitalized patients, a daily reduction of 20% of the total daily dose may be tolerated.

Maintenance treatment: The initial dose should control abstinence symptoms that follow withdrawal of narcotic drugs but should not cause sedation, respiratory depression, or other effects of acute intoxication. If patient has been a heavy heroin user up to the day of admission, 20 mg of methadone may be given 4 to 8 hours after heroin has been stopped, or 40 mg may be given in a single oral dose. If treatment is entered with little or no narcotic tolerance, the initial dose may be one-half these quantities. When there is any doubt, smaller doses are used. If symptoms of abstinence are distressing, additional 10-mg doses may be given as needed. Dosage level is adjusted as required, up to 120 mg/day.

MORPHINE

Parenteral administration is more reliable than oral administration. Oral bioavailability is estimated to be one-sixth of IV dose. When used chronically, oral–parenteral ratio may be as low as 1.5:1.

Oral: 10 mg to 30 mg q4h or as directed by physician.

Subcutaneous or IM: *Adults*—10 mg/70 kg (range, 5 mg–20 mg). *Children*—0.1 mg/kg/dose to 0.2 mg/kg/dose (maximum dose, 15 mg).

IV: Usual adult dose is 4 mg to 10 mg given very slowly. Rapid IV use increases the incidence of adverse reactions.

Rectal: 10 mg to 20 mg q4h as directed by the physician.

Unlabeled uses: Administration intrathecally and epidurally in doses of 0.5 mg to 4 mg and by continuous IV infusion (wide range of doses, 0.5 mg–275 mg/hour) in treatment of acute and chronic pain.

Bromptom's cocktail: Bromptom's cocktail or mixture is an oral narcotic mixture used for chronic severe pain. The original formulation contained heroin or morphine (15 mg), cocaine (10 mg), alcohol, chloroform, water, and syrup and was given on a regular schedule as prophylaxis for pain, rather than on an "as-needed" basis. The term *Bromptom's mixture* is commonly used to designate any alcoholic solution containing morphine and either cocaine or a phenothiazine. However, a single-entity narcotic solution (usually morphine) is often as effective as Bromptom's cocktail; cocaine apparently does not add to the mixture's effectiveness. Methadone has also been recommended. Various adjunctive drugs may be effective given concomitantly with a narcotic solution; these include aspirin, acetaminophen, tricyclic antidepressants, stimulants (*e.g.,* dextroamphetamine) and sedatives (*e.g.,* diazepam). Use of Bromptom's cocktail established the value of regular administration of narcotic analgesics for chronic severe pain. Current recommendations stress the use of a simple narcotic analgesic administered on a regular basis; adjunctive drugs may be of benefit in selected patients, but "standard" combinations are not advocated.

OPIUM

Activity is primarily due to morphine content. When taken orally, drug is rapidly absorbed from the GI tract.

Brown mixture: *Adults*—5 ml q3h to q4h. *Children*—1.7 ml to 2.5 ml q3h to q4h.

Opium tincture, deodorized: 0.6 ml four times daily.

Pantopon (hydrochlorides of opium alkaloids): 5 mg to 20 mg q4h to q5h IM or subcutaneously.

Paregoric (camphorated tincture of opium): *Adults*—5 ml to 10 ml one to four times daily. *Children*—0.25 ml/kg to 0.5 ml/kg one to four times daily.

OXYCODONE HCl

Adults: 5 mg q6h as needed PO.
Children: Not recommended.

OXYMORPHONE HCl

Safety for use in children under 12 not established.
IV: 0.5 mg initially.

Subcutaneous or IM: Initially, 1 mg to 1.5 mg q4h to q6h as needed. In nondebilitated patients, dose can be cautiously increased until satisfactory pain relief is obtained. For analgesia during labor, 0.5 mg to 1 mg IM is recommended.

Rectal: 5 mg q4h to q6h.
Storage: Store suppositories in refrigerator.

NURSING IMPLICATIONS

HISTORY
Review patient's record for health history, allergy history, concomitant drug therapy. When applicable, review chart for etiology of pain, length of time drug has been given, time of last administration, therapeutic effect of analgesic, date of drug order.

Methadone clinic (treatment of narcotic withdrawal, maintenance treatment): Follow protocol of clinic regarding history.

PHYSICAL ASSESSMENT
At time patient requests analgesic, determine exact location of pain, type of pain (*e.g.,* sharp, dull, stabbing), when pain began. In addition, look for controllable factors (*e.g.,* uncomfortable position, thirst, noise, bright lights, cold) that may decrease patient's tolerance to pain.

Methadone clinic: Follow protocol of clinic regarding physical assessment (*e.g.,* obtaining urine specimen, vital signs).

ADMINISTRATION
Check label of preparation carefully because some preparations are available in a variety of dosages.

Do not mix these drugs with other pharmacologic agents without consulting a pharmacist.

Do not give **alphaprodine** IM because absorption is unpredictable.

CLINICAL ALERT: Major hazards of these drugs are respiratory depression, apnea, and, to a lesser degree, circulatory depression, respiratory arrest, shock, and cardiac arrest. Obtain blood pressure, pulse, and respirations immediately before preparing drug for administration. Withhold drug and contact the physician immediately if any

N

one or more of the following are present: a significant decrease in the respiratory rate or a respiratory rate of 12/minute or below; a significant increase or decrease in pulse rate or a change in pulse quality; a significant decrease in blood pressure (systolic or diastolic) or a systolic pressure below 100 mm Hg. Depending on clinical circumstances and nursing judgment, additional signs, symptoms, or factors may require contacting the physician.

When administering parenterally, IM administration is preferred when repeated doses are required.

If given IV, drug is almost always given in dilute form. A narcotic antagonist and facilities for assisted or controlled respiration must be immediately available.

When drug is administered parenterally, especially IV, patient should be lying down.

Aspirate syringe before injection; inadvertent IV administration of undiluted drug may result in serious adverse effects.

Oral form may be administered with food if GI upset occurs.

Bromptom's cocktail or mixture is usually administered around the clock at prescribed intervals rather than on a prn basis.

Keep Bromptom's cocktail or mixture refrigerated unless the pharmacist directs otherwise.

ONGOING ASSESSMENTS AND NURSING MANAGEMENT

Check blood pressure, pulse, and respirations 15 to 30 minutes after administration if given IM or subcutaneously, after 30 or more minutes if given PO, and after 5 to 10 minutes if given IV.

CLINICAL ALERT: Notify physician immediately if respiratory depression, decreased blood pressure, significant changes in pulse rate or quality, or serious CNS changes (e.g., somnolence, coma, agitation, delirium) are noted. Administration of a narcotic antagonist may be necessary.

Continue to monitor blood pressure, pulse, and respirations q30m following administration, because respiratory depression or changes in blood pressure or pulse may occur at variable intervals.

Assess patient for relief of pain approximately 1 hour after administration (see also Table 38 for onset, peak, and duration of drug). Physician adjusts dosage according to severity of pain and patient response. Notify physician if analgesic is not effective.

Elderly or debilitated patients, those sensitive to CNS depressants, and children should be observed closely for adverse drug reactions.

Analgesic effect is best achieved when a narcotic is administered *before* patient experiences intense pain. If patient is not receiving repeated doses, observe for signs indicating that patient

may be in pain (*Note:* Some patients fear injections, prefer to accept pain stoically, fear addiction).

Pain can cause hypotension as well as intensify shock.

Observe for restlessness, which may indicate hypoxia due to respiratory depression or may be due to inadequate analgesia. Restlessness, as well as delirium, hallucinations, agitation, and so on, may also be due to adverse drug reactions.

Observe patient for adverse reactions. Report all adverse reactions to physician; in some instances drug may be discontinued or dosage may need to be reduced.

If patient is receiving Bromptom's cocktail or mixture, check with pharmacist regarding ingredients. Patient is then observed for adverse reactions of all drugs used in the formulation of the mixture.

Measure intake and output (when repeated doses are given) because these drugs may cause urinary retention, ureteral spasm, oliguria, and antidiuretic effect.

If patient does not have an indwelling catheter, encouraging voiding q4h. To detect possible bladder distention, palpate lower abdomen q4h to q6h.

Notify physician if there is any change in the intake–output ratio, if bladder distention is apparent, or if patient experiences difficulty in voiding.

Narcotics may produce orthostatic hypotension in ambulatory patients. If patient is allowed out of bed, assist with ambulation. Have patient rise from a lying or sitting position slowly.

Narcotics may depress the cough reflex and result in pooling of secretions, especially in those confined to bed. Encourage deep breathing and coughing (unless contraindicated) q2h to q3h; change patient's position q2h. Auscultate lungs q8h for rales. Notify physician if rales are noted or if patient fails to deep-breathe and cough adequately.

Miosis or pinpoint pupils may occur and decrease ability to see in dim light as well as at night. Keep room well lit during daytime hours; advise patient to seek assistance when getting out of bed during nighttime hours.

Anorexia may occur. Monitor patient's food intake. If patient is eating poorly, notify physician.

Monitor bowel pattern; constipation may occur with repeated doses. Notify physician if constipation is apparent because a stool softener, enema, or other means of relieving constipation may be necessary.

If drug is used as an obstetric analgesic, observe neonate closely for CNS and respiratory depression. Resuscitation may be required; naloxone (p 772) should be immediately available.

Dependence may occur in a newborn whose mother took opiates during pregnancy. Withdrawal symptoms usually appear during the first few days of life and include irritability, excessive crying, yawning, sneezing, increased respiratory rate, tremors, hyperreflexia, fever, vomiting, increased stools, and diarrhea. Notify physician immediately if these symptoms are apparent.

When drug is used as an antitussive, note patient response to drug. Observe for pooling of respiratory secretions due to drug's antitussive action.

When drugs are used as antidiarrheal agents, note patient response to drugs. Record each bowel movement, as well as appearance, color, consistency. If diarrhea is not relieved or becomes worse, or if severe abdominal pain or blood in the stool is noted, notify physician immediately.

Morphine may be given by IV drip for severe pain. Physician orders IV solution, rate of infusion, and amount of drug added to IV solution.

CLINICAL ALERT: Drug dependence can occur (review *Warnings* section on drug dependence and *Physical Dependence*). If dependence appears to be occurring, this problem is discussed with the physician. In those with a terminal illness, drug dependence may be allowed.

Observe for signs of the abstinence syndrome (withdrawal) when a narcotic analgesic is discontinued, especially in those receiving these drugs for an extended period of time. Review section on acute abstinence syndrome under *Physical Dependence*. If one or more symptoms are noted, contact physician immediately.

The nurse should not deny a patient a narcotic, or allow the patient to wait for a narcotic, except in those situations when clinical judgement mandates withholding the drug and notifying the physician.

Methadone programs (detoxification, maintenance): These programs are governed by strict federal regulations. The hospitalized patient currently enrolled in a methadone program continues to receive methadone. The duration and half-life of methadone increase with repeated use of drug, owing to cumulative effects.

PATIENT AND FAMILY INFORMATION

NOTE: Narcotics for outpatient use are almost always prescribed in the oral form. In certain instances, such as in terminally ill patients being cared for at home, the family may receive instruction in parenteral administration of these drugs. In these instances, the material listed under *Ongoing Assessments and Nursing Management* may apply and should be included in a patient/family teaching plan.

May cause drowsiness, dizziness, blurring of vision; use caution while driving or performing tasks requiring alertness.

Avoid use of alcohol, other CNS depressants.

May cause nausea, vomiting, constipation; notify physician if these become prominent or bothersome.

If GI upset occurs, drug may be taken with food.

Notify physician if shortness of breath or troubled breathing occurs.

Do not increase dose; if pain is not relieved or becomes worse, notify physician.

Narcotic Analgesic Combinations Rx

COMPONENTS

Components of these combinations include the following:

Narcotic analgesics: Codeine, hydrocodone bitartrate, dihydrocodeine bitartrate, opium, oxycodone HCl, oxycodone terephthalate, meperidine HCl, propoxyphene HCl, and propoxyphene napsylate*

Nonnarcotic analgesics: Acetaminophen, salicylates, salicylamide

Caffeine, a traditional component of many analgesic formulations with subtle analgesic value; may be beneficial in certain vascular headaches

Magnesium-aluminum hydroxides and **calcium carbonate,** used as buffers

Barbiturates, used for their sedative effects

Promethazine HCl (a phenothiazine derivative with antihistaminic properties), used for its sedative effect

Belladonna alkaloids, used as antispasmodics

DOSE

The average adult dose is one or two tablets, capsules, or suppositories, or 15 ml liquid, every 4 to 6 hours as needed for pain.

Content is given per tablet, 5 ml liquid, capsule, 1 ml injection, or suppository.

---

* See Propoxyphene monograph for propoxyphene combination products.

	Product	Narcotic	Acetaminophen	Aspirin	Caffeine	Other Content
C–III	Tylenol w/Codeine No. 1 Tablets	7.5 mg codeine phosphate	300 mg			
C–V	Acetaminophen w/Codeine Elixir	12 mg codeine phosphate	120 mg			
C–V	Bayapap w/Codeine Elixir					7% alcohol
C–V	Capital w/Codeine Suspension					
C–V	Tylenol w/Codeine Elixir					7% alcohol
C–III	Acetaminophen w/Codeine Tablets	15 mg codeine phosphate	300 mg			
C–III	SK-APAP w/Codeine Tablets					
C–III	Tylenol w/Codeine No. 2 Tablets					
C–III	Anacin-3 w/Codeine No. 2 Tablets	15 mg codeine phosphate	325 mg			
C–III	Phenaphen w/ Codeine No. 2 Capsules					
C–III	Acetaminophen w/Codeine Tablets	30 mg codeine phosphate	300 mg			
C–III	Aceta w/Codeine Tablets					
C–III	Anacin-3 w/Codeine No. 3 Tablets					
C–III	Empracet w/Codeine No. 3 Tablets					
C–III	Panadol w/Codeine No. 3 Tablets					
C–III	SK-APAP w/Codeine Tablets					
C–III	Tylenol w/Codeine No. 3 Capsules					
C–III	Tylenol w/Codeine No. 3 Tablets					
C–III	Ty-Tab #3 Tablets					
C–III	Capital w/Codeine Tablets	30 mg codeine phosphate	325 mg			
C–III	Phenaphen w/ Codeine No. 3 Capsules					
C–III	Proval No. 3 Capsules					
C–III	Phenaphen-650 w/Codeine Tablets	30 mg codeine phosphate	650 mg			
C–III	Codap Tablets	32 mg codeine phosphate	325 mg			
C–III	Acetaminophen w/Codeine Tablets	60 mg codeine phosphate	300 mg			
C–III	Anacin-3 w/Codeine No. 4 Tablets					
C–III	Empracet w/Codeine No. 4 Tablets					
C–III	Panadol w/Codeine No. 4 Tablets					

	Product	Narcotic	Acetaminophen	Aspirin	Caffeine	Other Content
C–III	SK-APAP w/Codeine Tablets					
C–III	Tylenol w/Codeine No. 4 Capsules					
C–III	Tylenol w/Codeine No. 4 Tablets					
C–III	Ty-Tab #4 Tablets					
C–III	Phenaphen w/ Codeine No. 4 Capsules	60 mg codeine phosphate	325 mg			
C–III	Empirin w/Codeine No. 2 Tablets	15 mg codeine phosphate		325 mg		
C–III	Emcodeine #3 Tablets	30 mg codeine phosphate		325 mg		
C–III	Empirin w/Codeine No. 3 Tablets					
C–III	Emcodeine #4 Tablets	60 mg codeine phosphate		325 mg		
C–III	Empirin w/Codeine No. 4 Tablets					
C–III	A.S.A. & Codeine Compound Pulvules (Capsules) No. 3	30 mg codeine phosphate		380 mg	30 mg	
C–III	A.S.A. & Codeine Compound Tablets No. 3					
C–III	Anexsia w/Codeine Tablets	30 mg codeine phosphate		325 mg	32 mg	
C–III	Tega-Code-M Tablets	32.4 mg codeine phosphate	300 mg			200 mg salicylamide
C–III	G-2 Capsules	15 mg codeine phosphate	500 mg			50 mg butalbital
C–III	Bancap w/Codeine Capsules	30 mg codeine phosphate	325 mg			50 mg butalbital
C–III	G-3 Capsules	30 mg codeine phosphate	500 mg			50 mg butalbital
C–III	Maxigesic Capsules	30 mg codeine phosphate	325 mg			6.25 mg promethazine
C–III	Ascriptin w/Codeine No. 2 Tablets	15 mg codeine phosphate		325 mg		150 mg magnesium-aluminum hydroxide
C–III	Bufferin w/Codeine No. 3 Tablets	30 mg codeine phosphate		325 mg		48.6 mg aluminum glycinate & 97.2 mg magnesium carbonate
C–III	Ascriptin w/Codeine No. 3 Tablets	30 mg codeine phosphate		325 mg		150 mg magnesium-aluminum hydroxide
C–III	Codalan No. 1 Tablets	8 mg codeine phosphate	162.5 mg		32.5 mg	227.5 mg salicylamide
C–III	Codalan No. 2 Tablets	16.3 mg codeine phosphate	162.5 mg		32.5 mg	227.5 mg salicylamide
C–III	Codalan No. 3 Tablets	32.5 mg codeine phosphate	162.5 mg		32.5 mg	227.5 mg salicylamide
C–III	Amaphen w/Codeine #3 Capsules	30 mg codeine phosphate	325 mg		40 mg	50 mg butalbital
C–III	Tabloid APC w/Codeine No. 2 Tablets	15 mg codeine phosphate		227 mg	32 mg	162 mg phenacetin

N

	Product	Narcotic	Acetaminophen	Aspirin	Caffeine	Other Content
C–III	Tabloid APC w/Codeine No. 3 Tablets	30 mg codeine phosphate		227 mg	32 mg	162 mg phenacetin
C–III	Tabloid APC w/Codeine No. 4 Tablets	60 mg codeine phosphate		227 mg	32 mg	162 mg phenacetin
C–III	Fiorinal w/Codeine No. 1 Capsules	7.5 mg codeine phosphate		325 mg	40 mg	50 mg butalbital
C–III	Fiorinal w/Codeine No. 2 Capsules	15 mg codeine phosphate		325 mg	40 mg	50 mg butalbital
C–III	Fiorinal w/Codeine No. 3 Capsules	30 mg codeine phosphate		325 mg	40 mg	50 mg butalbital
C–III	Buff-A-Comp #3 Tablets	30 mg codeine phosphate		325 mg	40 mg	50 mg butalbital
C–III	Isollyl w/Codeine Capsules					
C–V	Rid-A-Pain w/ Codeine Tablets	1 mg codeine phosphate	97.2 mg	226.8 mg	32 4 mg	32.4 mg salicylamide
C–III	Lortab Liquid	2.5 mg hydrocodone bitartrate	120 mg			
C–III	Amacodone Tablets	5 mg hydrocodone bitartrate	500 mg			
C–III	Bancap HC Capsules					
C–III	Co-Gesic Tablets					
C–III	Duradyne DHC					
C–III	Hycodaphen Tablets					
C–III	Lortab 5 Tablets					
C–III	Vicodin Tablets					
C–III	Lortab 7 Tablets	7 mg hydrocodone bitartrate	500 mg			
C–III	Dolo-Pap Tablets	7.5 mg hydrocodone bitartrate	650 mg			
C–III	Hydrogesic Tablets					
C–III	Norcet Tablets					
C–III	T-Gesic Forte Tablets	7.5 mg hydrocodone bitartrate	1000 mg			
C–III	Lortab Tablets	2.5 mg hydrocodone bitartrate	325 mg			3.125 mg promethazine HCl
C–III	T-Gesic Capsules	5 mg hydrocodone bitartrate	325 mg		40 mg	50 mg butalbital
C–III	Anexsia-D Tablets	7 mg hydrocodone bitartrate		325 mg		
C–III	Damason-P Tablets	5 mg hydrocodone bitartrate		224 mg	32 mg	
C–III	Anodynos-DHC Tablets	5 mg hydrocodone bitartrate	150 mg	230 mg	30 mg	
C–III	Christodyne-DHC Tablets					

	Product	Narcotic	Acetaminophen	Aspirin	Caffeine	Other Content
C–III	Di-Gesic Tablets					
C–III	Synalgos-DC Capsules	16 mg dihydro-codeine bitartrate		356.4 mg	30 mg	
C–III	Compal Capsules	16 mg dihydro-codeine bitartrate	356.4 mg		30 mg	6.25 mg promethazine HCl
C–III	Sinodeine Capsules	16 mg dihydro-codeine bitartrate		357 mg	30 mg	6.25 mg promethazine HCl
C–III	Sycodeine Compound Capsules					
C–II	B & O Supprettes No. 15A	30 mg powdered opium				16.2 mg powdered belladonna extract
C–II	Opium and Belladonna Suppositories	60 mg powdered opium				15 mg belladonna extract
C–II	B & O Supprettes No. 16A	60 mg powdered opium				16.2 mg powdered belladonna extract
C–II	Oxycodone HCl and Acetaminophen Tablets	5 mg oxycodone HCl	325 mg			
C–II	Percocet-5 Tablets					
C–II	SK-Oxycodone w/Acetaminophen Tablets					
C–II	Tylox Capsules	4.5 mg oxycodone HCl & 0.38 mg oxycodone terephthalate	500 mg			
C–II	Oxycodone HCl, Oxycodone Terephthalate and Aspirin Tablets	4.5 mg oxycodone HCl & 0.38 mg oxycodone terephthalate		325 mg		
C–II	Codoxy Tablets					
C–II	Percodan Tablets					
C–II	SK-Oxycodone w/Aspirin Tablets					
C–II	Oxycodone HCl, Oxycodone Terephthalate and Aspirin Tablets, Half Strength	2.25 mg oxycodone HCl & 0.19 mg oxycodone terephthalate		325 mg		
C–II	Percodan-Demi Tablets					
C–II	Demerol APAP Tablets	50 mg meperidine HCl	300 mg			
C–II	Mepergan Fortis Capsules	50 mg meperidine HCl				25 mg promethazine HCl
C–II	Mepergan Injection	25 mg meperidine HCl				25 mg promethazine HCl

N

▮ NURSING IMPLICATIONS
See monograph for each component.

Narcotic Antagonists

Levallorphan Tartrate Rx

injection: 1 mg/ml   Lorfan

Naloxone Hydrochloride Rx

injection: 0.4 mg/ml   Narcan
injection, neonatal: Narcan
   0.02 mg/ml

INDICATIONS

Complete or partial reversal of narcotic depression, including respiratory depression, induced by opioids including natural and synthetic narcotics, propoxyphene, methadone, nalbuphine, butorphanol, and pentazocine. Also indicated for diagnosis of suspected acute opioid overdosage.

Investigational uses: Naloxone has been used to improve circulation in refractory shock. It antagonizes the effect of beta-endorphin and allows prostaglandins and catecholamines to reestablish control of circulation. It also has been used for reversal of alcoholic coma.

CONTRAINDICATIONS

Hypersensitivity. Not used in narcotic addicts in whom it may produce withdrawal symptoms.

ACTIONS

Naloxone, a pure narcotic antagonist, and levallorphan, which also has narcotic agonist properties, will precipitate abstinence syndrome in the presence of narcotic addiction. Because it is devoid of undesirable agonist properties, naloxone is the preferred agent in reversal of narcotic-induced respiratory depression.

Naloxone prevents or reverses the effects of opioids, including respiratory depression, sedation, and hypotension, and can reverse the psychotomimetic and dysphoric effects of agonist–antagonist agents such as pentazocine. In the presence of strong narcotic effect, levallorphan acts as a narcotic antagonist; in the absence of narcotic effect, it may cause respiratory depression and other effects.

The mechanism of naloxone's action is not fully understood. Evidence suggests that it antagonizes opioid effects by competing for the same receptor sites. Naloxone is an essentially pure antagonist (*i.e.,* it does not possess "agonistic" or morphinelike properties characteristic of levallorphan). Naloxone antagonizes all actions of morphine.

Naloxone does not produce respiratory depression, psychotomimetic effects, or pupillary constriction. In the absence of narcotics or agonistic effects of other narcotic antagonists, naloxone exhibits essentially no pharmacologic activity; doses up to 24 mg cause only slight drowsiness. Naloxone has not produced tolerance or caused physical or psychological dependence. Following administration, it is rapidly distributed in the body; it is metabolized in the liver and excreted in the urine. Onset of action of IV naloxone is generally apparent within 2 minutes; onset is only slightly less rapid when given subcutaneously or IM. Naloxone has a serum half-life of about 1 hour and a duration of action of 1 to 4 hours, depending on dose and route of administration. IM administration produces a more prolonged effect than IV administration. Requirement for repeat doses is also dependent on amount, type, and route of administration of the narcotic being antagonized.

WARNINGS

Drug dependence: Administer cautiously to those known or suspected to be physically dependent on opioids, including newborns of mothers with narcotic dependence. Reversal of effects may precipitate an acute abstinence syndrome.

Repeat administration: Repeat doses are administered as necessary, because the duration of action of some narcotics may exceed that of the narcotic antagonist.

Respiratory depression: Not effective against respiratory depression due to nonopioid drugs. Levallorphan does not counteract mild respiratory depression, and it may, in fact, increase it. Repeated doses result in decreasing effectiveness and may eventually produce respiratory depression equal to, or greater than, that produced by narcotics.

Use in pregnancy, lactation: Safety for use not established. Use in pregnancy only when clearly needed and when potential benefits outweigh the unknown potential hazards to the fetus.

PRECAUTIONS

Maintain a free airway and provide artificial ventilation, cardiac massage, and vasopressor agents; employ when necessary to counteract acute narcotic overdosage. Several instances of hypotension, hypertension, ventricular tachycardia and fibrillation, and pulmonary edema have been reported. These have occurred in postoperative patients, most of whom had preexisting cardiovascular disorders or had received other drugs that may have similar adverse cardiovascular effects. A direct cause-and-effect relationship not established; use naloxone with caution in those with preexisting cardiac disease or patients who have received potentially cardiotoxic drugs.

ADVERSE REACTIONS

Abrupt reversal of narcotic depression may result in nausea, vomiting, sweating, tachycardia, increased blood pressure, and tremulousness. In the postoperative patient, excessive dosage may result in significant reversal of analgesia and in excitement. Hypotension, hypertension, ventricular tachycardia and fibrillation, and pulmonary edema have been associated with postoperative use of **naloxone.** Seizures have been reported infrequently after administration of **naloxone,** but a causal relationship has not been established.

In high doses, **levallorphan** may produce psychotomimetic manifestations (weird dreams, visual hallucinations, disorientation, feelings of unreality). Dysphoria, miosis, pseudoptosis, lethargy, drowsiness, dizziness, sweating, gastric upset, pallor, nausea, and a sense of heaviness in the limbs may occur. In asphyxia neonatorum, irritability and a tendency toward increased crying may occur.

DOSAGE

LEVALLORPHAN

Adults: For narcotic overdose, give 1 mg IV; this may be followed by one or two additional doses of 0.5 mg at 10- or 15-minute intervals. Initial dose should not exceed 1 mg if there is doubt as to whether a narcotic produced the respiratory depression. Total dose should not exceed 3 mg. This regimen may also be used in narcotic-induced respiratory depression in parturient women.

Neonates: For narcotic-induced depression secondary to narcotic administration to the mother, inject 0.05 mg to 0.1 mg (approximately $^1/_{10}$ adult dose) into the umbilical cord vein immediately after delivery. If vein cannot be used, injection may be made IM or subcutaneously.

NALOXONE HCl

Administer IV, IM, or subcutaneously. Most rapid onset of action is with IV administration, which is recommended in emergency situations.

Adults

Narcotic overdose (known or suspected): Initial dose of 0.4 mg to 2 mg given IV. Additional doses may be repeated IV at 2- to 3-minute intervals. If no response is observed after 10 mg has been administered, diagnosis of narcotic-induced or partial narcotic-induced toxicity is questioned. IM or subcutaneous administration may be necessary if IV route is not available.

Postoperative narcotic depression (partial reversal): Smaller doses are usually sufficient. Dosage is titrated according to patient response. Excessive dosage may result in significant reversal of analgesia and increase in blood pressure. Too-rapid reversal may induce nausea, vomiting, sweating, or circulatory stress. *Initial dose*—Inject in increments of 0.1 mg to 0.2 mg IV at 2- to 3-minute intervals to desired degree of reversal (*i.e.,* adequate ventilation and alertness without significant pain or discomfort). *Repeat doses*—May be required within 1- or 2-hour intervals depending on the amount, type (*e.g.,* short- or long-acting), and time intervals since last administration of narcotic. Supplemental IM doses have been shown to produce longer-lasting effects.

Children

Narcotic overdose (known or suspected): Usual initial dose is 0.01 mg/kg IV; a subsequent dose of 0.1 mg/kg may be administered if needed. If IV route is not available, may be administered IM or subcutaneously in divided doses. If necessary, dilute with Sterile Water for Injection.

Postoperative narcotic depression: Follow recommendations and cautions under adult administration guidelines. For initial reversal of respiratory depression, 0.005 mg to 0.01 mg IV at 2- to 3-minute intervals to desired degree of reversal.

Neonates

Narcotic-induced depression: Usual initial dose is 0.01 mg/kg IV, IM, or subcutaneously; may be repeated in accordance with adult administration guidelines.

IV infusions

Dilute in normal saline or 5% dextrose solutions. Addition of 2 mg in 500 ml of either solution provides a concentration of 0.004 mg/ml. Administration rate is titrated according to patient response. Do not mix naloxone with preparations containing bisulfite, metasulfite, or long-chain or high–molecular weight anions, or with any solution having an alkaline *p*H. Do not add any drug or chemical agent unless its effect on the chemical and physical stability of the solution has been established.

NURSING IMPLICATIONS

HISTORY

Review patient's record for drug administered, dose, and time of administration. If possible, review chart for health history, allergy history, current treatment modalities.

PHYSICAL ASSESSMENT

Obtain blood pressure, pulse, respirations. Obtain neonate's, child's weight for calculation of

N

drug dosage. Drawing of arterial blood gasses may be ordered.

ADMINISTRATION

CLINICAL ALERT: Maintain a free airway. Depending on patient's condition, artificial ventilation, cardiac massage, and vasopressors may also be necessary.

Obtain baseline blood pressure, pulse, and respiratory rate (if artificial ventilation is not being used).

Have suction equipment readily available because abrupt reversal of narcotic depression can result in vomiting.

In some instances (*e.g.,* postoperative patients, those with preexisting cardiac disorder, those receiving cardiotoxic drugs), a cardiac monitor may be used.

LEVALLORPHAN

Given IV to adults. *Neonates*—May be given through the umbilical vein immediately after delivery or IM or subcutaneously.

NALOXONE

May be given IV, IM, or subcutaneously. May be given to children in divided doses IM or subcutaneously and may be diluted, if necessary, with Sterile Water for Injection.

May be given by IV infusion. Physician must order IV fluid (normal saline or 5% dextrose recommended) and amount, drug dosage. See also *Dosage,* above. Recommended dosage is 2 mg added to 500 ml, giving a concentration of 0.004 mg/ml. Infusion rate is titrated according to patient response, with physician establishing guidelines for rate of infusion, desired response, and when infusion can be discontinued.

To give by IV infusion, use secondary line or IV piggyback because infusion may be intermittent (depending on patient's response).

Stability: Use mixtures within 24 hours. After 24 hours, discard remaining unused solution.

ONGOING ASSESSMENT AND NURSING MANAGEMENT

Monitor blood pressure, pulse, and respirations q5m until patient responds. Patient should not be left unattended until full response to narcotic antagonist is confirmed.

Continue to monitor vital signs q10m to q15m following adequate drug response.

The duration of action of some narcotics may exceed that of the narcotic antagonist. The duration of close patient observation will depend on duration of narcotic's action, dose, and patient's current physical status. Guidelines for duration of observation should be established by the physician.

Repeat doses may be necessary and are based on patient response.

Abrupt reversal of narcotic depression may result in nausea, vomiting, sweating, tachycardia, increased blood pressure, and tremulousness. Notify physician if these should occur because additional medical management may be necessary.

When administering to a postoperative patient, observe for significant reversal of analgesia (*e.g.,* pain) and excitement. Notify physician if patient begins to experience pain or becomes restless.

CLINICAL ALERT: Suction as needed to maintain clear airway.

Monitor intake and output; notify physician of any change in the intake–output ratio.

When giving naloxone, observe for hypotension, hypertension, ventricular tachycardia and fibrillation, and pulmonary edema, especially in the postoperative patient (see *Precautions*), and report findings immediately.

Always notify physician if there is any sudden change in the patient's status.

Natamycin Rx

ophthalmic suspen-   Natacyn
   sion: 5%

INDICATIONS

Treatment of fungal blepharitis, conjunctivitis, and keratitis caused by susceptible organisms. Initial drug of choice in *Fusarium solani* keratitis.

CONTRAINDICATIONS

Hypersensitivity.

ACTIONS

An antibiotic derived from *Streptomyces natalensis* possessing activity against a variety of yeasts and fungi, including *Candida, Aspergillus, Cephalosporium, Fusarium,* and *Penicillium.* Mechanism of action appears to be through binding of the molecule to the sterol moiety of the fungal cell membrane. The polyene-sterol complex alters permeability of the membrane to produce depletion of essential cellular constituents. Although activity against fungi is dose related, drug is predominantly fungicidal. Topical administration appears to produce effective concentrations within the corneal stroma, but not in intraocular fluid. Is not absorbed from the GI tract. Systemic absorption should not be expected following topical administration.

WARNINGS

Safety for use in pregnancy has not been established. Use in pregnancy only when clearly needed and when potential benefits outweigh the unknown potential hazards to the fetus.

PRECAUTIONS

Failure of keratitis to improve following 7 to 10 days of administration suggests that the infection may be caused by a microorganism not susceptible to natamycin. Adherence of the suspension to areas of epithelial ulceration or retention in the fornices occurs regularly. Tolerance to drug should be monitored at least twice weekly. Should suspicion of drug toxicity occur, drug is discontinued.

DOSAGE

Fungal keratitis: One drop instilled in the conjunctival sac at 1- or 2-hour intervals. Frequency of application can usually be reduced to one drop six to eight times a day after the first 3 to 4 days. Therapy is generally continued for 14 to 21 days, or until there is resolution of active fungal keratitis. In many cases, dosage may be gradually reduced at 4- to 7-day intervals to assure that the organism has been eliminated.

Fungal blepharitis and conjunctivitis: Four to six daily applications may be sufficient.

NURSING IMPLICATIONS

HISTORY
See Appendix 4.

PHYSICAL ASSESSMENT
Inspect eye; record findings. Physician performs examination, obtains corneal scraping for culture and sensitivity.

ADMINISTRATION
Drug is a suspension; gently agitate container immediately before administration.

Place patient in sitting position with head tilted back. Instill prescribed amount into lower conjunctival sac.

Instruct patient to gently close eye for 1 to 2 minutes. Do not apply eye dressing unless instructed to do so by physician.

Storage: May be stored at room temperature or in refrigerator.

ONGOING ASSESSMENTS AND NURSING MANAGEMENT
Inspect eye daily; describe findings on patient's chart.

If patient complains of irritation, notify physician before next dose is due.

If improvement is not noted in 7 to 10 days, physician reevaluates therapy.

PATIENT AND FAMILY INFORMATION
NOTE: Patient must be instructed in proper instillation technique and frequency of administration (as prescribed by physician).

May be stored at room temperature or in refrigerator. Shake gently but thoroughly before each use. Do not touch tip of dropper to skin or lay dropper on table; replace in container immediately after use.

Notify physician if improvement is not seen after 7 to 10 days, if condition worsens, or if irritation occurs.

Neomycin Sulfate

See Aminoglycosides, Oral; Aminoglycosides, Parenteral; Antibiotics, Topical.

Neostigmine

See Muscle Stimulants, Anticholinesterase.

Neostigmine Methylsulfate Rx

injection: 1:1000,   Prostigmin, *Generic*
   1:2000, 1:4000

INDICATIONS
Prevention and treatment of postoperative distention and urinary retention. See also Muscle Stimulants, Anticholinesterase.

CONTRAINDICATIONS
Hypersensitivity; peritonitis; mechanical, intestinal, or urinary-tract obstruction.

ACTIONS
Inhibits hydrolysis of acetylcholine by competing with acetylcholine for attachment to acetylcholinesterase at sites of cholinergic transmission. Enhances cholinergic action by facilitating transmission of impulses across neuromuscular junctions. Also has direct cholinomimetic effect on skeletal muscle and possibly on autonomic ganglion cells and neurons of the central nervous system.

N

Following IM administration, drug is rapidly absorbed and eliminated. It undergoes hydrolysis by cholinesterase and is also metabolized by microsomal enzymes in the liver. Approximately 80% is eliminated in the urine within 24 hours. Following IV administration, plasma half-life ranges from 47 to 60 minutes. Clinical effects usually begin within 20 to 30 minutes after IM injection and last 2.5 to 4 hours.

WARNINGS

Use with caution in those with epilepsy, bronchial asthma, bradycardia, recent coronary occlusion, vagotonia, hyperthyroidism, cardiac arrhythmias, or peptic ulcer. When large doses are given, prior or simultaneous administration of atropine may be advisable. Because of possibility of hypersensitivity in an occasional patient, atropine and antishock medication should always be available.

Safety for use in pregnancy is not established. Use only when clearly needed and when potential benefits outweigh unknown potential risks to the fetus. It is not known whether drug is excreted in breast milk. Safety for use in the nursing mother not established.

Safety for use in children not established.

ADVERSE REACTIONS

Side-effects are generally due to an exaggeration of pharmacologic effect; salivation and fasciculation are most common.

Allergic: Allergic reactions and anaphylaxis.

Neurologic: Dizziness, convulsions, loss of consciousness, drowsiness, headache, dysarthria, miosis, visual changes.

Cardiovascular: Cardiac arrhythmias (including bradycardia, tachycardia, AV block, nodal rhythm) and nonspecific ECG changes have been reported, as well as cardiac arrest, syncope, and hypotension. These have been predominantly noted following use of injectable form.

Respiratory: Increased oral, pharyngeal, and bronchial secretions, dyspnea, respiratory depression, respiratory arrest, bronchospasm.

Dermatologic: Rash, urticaria.

GI: Nausea, emesis, flatulence, increased peristalsis, bowel cramps, diarrhea.

GU: Urinary frequency.

Musculoskeletal: Muscle cramps and spasms, arthralgia.

Miscellaneous: Diaphoresis, flushing, weakness.

OVERDOSAGE

Symptoms: Overdosage may result in cholinergic crisis, characterized by increasing muscle weakness, which may lead to death through involvement of the muscles of respiration.

Treatment: Prompt withdrawal of all drugs of this type and immediate use of atropine. Atropine may also be used to abolish or diminish GI side-effects or other muscarinic reactions, but such use, by masking signs of overdosage, can lead to inadvertent induction of cholinergic crisis.

DOSAGE

Prevention of postoperative distention and urinary retention: 1 ml of 1:4000 solution (0.25 mg) subcutaneously or IM as soon as possible after surgery; repeat q4h to q6h for 2 to 3 days.

Treatment of postoperative distention: 1 ml of 1:2000 solution (0.5 mg) subcutaneously or IM. If urination does not occur within 1 hour, patient should be catheterized. After patient has voided or bladder has been emptied by catheterization, 0.5 mg injections are continued q3h for at least 5 injections.

NURSING IMPLICATIONS

HISTORY

See Appendix 4. Review chart for surgery performed and concomitant drug therapy, including IV fluids.

PHYSICAL ASSESSMENT

Obtain blood pressure, pulse, and respirations. If prescribed for abdominal distention, palpate abdomen, auscultate abdomen for bowel sounds, and measure abdomen with tape measure (at approximately level of umbilicus). If used for urinary retention, palpate lower abdomen for bladder distention. Record findings.

ADMINISTRATION

May be given subcutaneously or IM.

Physician may order drug in milligrams; 1:1000 = 1 mg/ml; 1:2000 = 0.5 mg/ml; 1:4000 = 0.25 mg/ml.

Atropine and antishock medication should be readily available when this drug is administered.

If atropine and neostigmine are ordered concomitantly, use separate syringes and injection sites for each drug.

ONGOING ASSESSMENTS AND NURSING MANAGEMENT

CLINICAL ALERT: Observe closely for signs of cholinergic crisis (*e.g.,* increased muscle weakness, nausea, vomiting, diarrhea, sweating, increased bronchial or salivary secretions, bradycardia). Notify physician immediately if one or more of these occur; withhold further doses until patient is examined by physician.

Postoperative abdominal distention: Insertion of rectal tube may be ordered to facilitate passage of gas. Lubricate rectal tube with water-soluble lubricant; insert past rectal sphincter. Rectal tube may be left in place for 1 or more hours, depending on patient response.

Palpate abdomen, auscultate abdomen for bowel sounds; measure abdomen q1h to q2h; compare with data base.

Observe for adverse effects; if noted, contact physician.

Withhold next dose of drug if abdomen becomes further distended or becomes rigid or boardlike, and notify physician immediately.

Urinary retention: Place call light, as well as bedpan or urinal, within reach.

If patient voids (usually within 30–60 minutes), measure output; record amount and time of voiding.

If patient does not void in 1 hour, catheterization may be ordered.

Netilmicin Sulfate

See Aminoglycosides, Parenteral.

Niclosamide Rx

tablets, chewable: Niclocide
  500 mg

INDICATIONS
Treatment of tapeworm infections by *Taenia saginata* (beef tapeworm), *Diphyllobothrium latum* (fish tapeworm), and *Hymenolepis nana* (dwarf tapeworm).

CONTRAINDICATIONS
Hypersensitivity.

ACTIONS
Inhibits oxidative phosphorylation in the mitochondria of cestodes. The scolex (head) and proximal segments are killed on contact with the drug. The scolex, loosened from the gut wall, may be digested in the intestine and may not be identified in the feces even after extensive purging.

WARNINGS
Safety for use during pregnancy and in the nursing mother has not been established. Safety and efficacy for use in children under 2 years have not been established.

PRECAUTIONS
Drug affects the cestodes in the intestines only. It is without effect in cysticercosis.

ADVERSE REACTIONS
GI: Nausea/vomiting (4.1%); abdominal discomfort, including loss of appetite (3.5%); diarrhea (1.6%); constipation, rectal bleeding.
CNS: Drowsiness, dizziness, and/or headache (1.4%).
Dermatologic: Skin rash, including pruritus ani (0.3%).
Miscellaneous (decreasing order of frequency): Oral irritation, fever, weakness, bad taste in mouth, sweating, palpitations, alopecia, edema of an arm, backache, irritability.

OVERDOSAGE
Insufficient data available. In event of overdose, give fast-acting laxative and enema. Vomiting should be induced.

DOSAGE
T. saginata *and* D. latum
Adults: 2 g in a single dose.
Children weighing more than 34 kg (75 lb): 1.5 g in a single dose.
Children weighing between 11 kg and 34 kg (25–75 lb): 1 g in a single dose.
H. nana:
Adults: 2 g as single daily dose for 7 days.
Children weighing more than 34 kg: 1.5 g on first day, then 1 g daily for next 6 days.
Children weighing between 11 kg and 34 kg: 1 g on first day, then 0.5 g daily for next 6 days.

NURSING IMPLICATIONS

HISTORY
See Appendix 4. Source of infection should be determined, if possible, by thorough questioning. Sources of infection are as follows: beef tapeworm from uncooked or undercooked infected beef; fish tapeworm from uncooked or undercooked infected fish; dwarf tapeworm passes from person to person by means of ova passed in stool and is chiefly due to inadequate handwashing.

PHYSICAL ASSESSMENT
Stool sample is obtained to identify parasite. CBC and hemoglobin may also be ordered because anemia may be present.

N

ADMINISTRATION

Instruct patient to chew thoroughly, then swallow tablet with a little water.

Young children and incompetent adults should have tablets crushed into a fine powder and mixed with a small amount of water to form a paste.

Best time to administer drug is after a light meal (*e.g.,* breakfast).

Because dwarf tapeworm is more common among institutionalized mentally retarded individuals, tablets (as a paste) may need to be spoonfed. If patient fails to swallow paste or is uncooperative in other ways, notify physician.

ONGOING ASSESSMENTS AND NURSING MANAGEMENT

May be administered on ambulatory or outpatient basis.

No special dietary restrictions are necessary before or after treatment.

Physician may prescribe a mild laxative for constipated patient to achieve normal bowel movement. A laxative or enema may also be ordered following 1-day treatment for beef or fish tapeworm.

Drug action renders the tapeworm, especially the scolex and proximal segments, vulnerable to destruction during their passage through the intestine; it is not always possible to identify the scolex in stools.

Save all stool specimens for examination; take to laboratory immediately. The sooner the tapeworm is passed and examined after treatment, the better the chance of identification of the scolex.

Wear gloves when handling stool specimens, giving personal care, and handling bedpans and bed linens. Wash hands thoroughly after removing gloves. In some hospitals, linen precautions may be required.

Instruct patient to wash hands thoroughly following personal care and use of bedpan.

Segments and ova of beef or fish tapeworm may be present in the stool for up to 3 days after therapy.

Persistent beef or dwarf tapeworm segments or ova on the seventh day following therapy indicate failure. A second clinical course may be given at this time.

Patient is not considered cured unless stool has been negative for a minimum of 3 months. Physician will order periodic stool specimens for examination.

If anemia is present prior to therapy, physician may prescribe iron supplements. Periodic CBC and hemoglobin may also be ordered.

PATIENT AND FAMILY INFORMATION

Chew tablets, then swallow with small amount of water. *Children*—Thoroughly crush tablet, being careful not to lose crushed particles; mix with small amount of water to make a paste; spoonfeed.

May cause GI upset. Take with food after a light meal (*e.g.,* breakfast).

Physician may suggest a mild laxative to relieve constipation, should it occur.

Repeat stool examinations will be necessary; physician will give list of times stool specimen is to be examined. (*Note:* Patient should be provided with stool specimen containers.)

Patient with **H. nana:** Observe strict personal hygiene; wash hands thoroughly after using lavatory and following personal care because autoinfection is possible. Clean lavatory facilities thoroughly each day until stool is negative. Keep towels and bed linens separate from those of other family members; launder separately.

Patient with **T. saginata, D. bothrium:** Cook meat or fish thoroughly. Do not eat raw or partially cooked fish or meat.

Nicotinamide (Niacinamide) Rx, otc

tablets: 50 mg, 100 mg, 500 mg	*Generic (otc)*
capsules: 500 mg	*Generic (Rx)*
injection: 100 mg/ml	*Generic (Rx)*

INDICATIONS

Prophylaxis and treatment of pellagra.

ACTIONS

Nicotinamide is utilized by the body as a source of the vitamin niacin (B_3). Lipid metabolism, tissue respiration, and glycogenolysis require nicotinamide. Does *not* have hypolipidemic or vasodilating effects. Is useful as source of the vitamin without the flushing that may be caused by niacin. See also Nicotinic Acid.

DOSAGE

Oral: 500 mg/day or as directed by physician.

Parenteral: 100 mg to 200 mg one to five times daily depending on severity of deficiency. Therapeutic dose is 50 mg two to ten times daily.

Other: May also be included in some multivitamin preparations.

NURSING IMPLICATIONS

HISTORY

See Appendix 4.

PHYSICAL ASSESSMENT

Niacin deficiency can occur in carcinoid syndrome, isoniazid therapy, or Hartnup disease and can also be due to a dietary deficiency. When applicable, base assessment on patient's symptoms.

ADMINISTRATION

Usually given orally. If oral route is not feasible may be given IM or IV. May also be added to 0.9% Sodium Chloride as directed by physician.

When given IM, rotate injection sites; record site used.

ONGOING ASSESSMENTS AND NURSING MANAGEMENT

If deficiency is severe, symptoms usually clear rapidly (24–72 hours). Assess patient daily for relief of symptoms; record findings.

PATIENT AND FAMILY INFORMATION

Take as recommended by physician. Do not exceed recommended dose.

Nicotinic Acid Rx, otc

tablets: 50 mg, 100 mg	*Generic (otc)*
tablets: 500 mg	Nicolar (contains tartrazine), *Generic (Rx)*
tablets, timed release: 150 mg	Span-Niacin-150 *(Rx)*
capsules, timed release: 125 mg, 250 mg	Nicobid, *Generic (otc)*
capsules, timed release: 300 mg	Niac *(Rx)*
capsules, timed release: 400 mg	Nico-400, Nico-Span, Tega-Span, *Generic (otc)*
capsules, timed release: 500 mg	Nicobid *(otc)*
elixir: 50 mg/ml	Nicotinex *(otc)*
injection: 50 mg/ml, 100 mg/ml	*Generic (Rx)*

INDICATIONS

Correction of nicotinic acid deficiency; prevention and treatment of pellagra; those conditions associated with deficient circulation. Also indicated as adjunctive therapy in those with significant hyperlipidemia who do not respond adequately to diet and weight loss. Although these agents have been in use many years, it is still not clear whether drug-induced lowering of serum cholesterol or lipid levels has a detrimental effect, a beneficial effect, or no effect on morbidity or mortality due to atherosclerosis or coronary heart disease. Therapeutic value of use as a vasodilating agent is not well established.

CONTRAINDICATIONS

Hypersensitivity; hepatic dysfunction; active peptic ulcer; severe hypotension; hemorrhaging or arterial bleeding.

ACTIONS

Niacin functions in the body as a component of two coenzymes: nicotinamide adenine dinucleotide (NAD, coenzyme I) and nicotinamide adenine dinucleotide phosphate (NADP, coenzyme II). The niacin-deficiency state pellagra is characterized by cutaneous, mucous membrane, gastrointestinal, and CNS manifestations. In addition to its function as a vitamin, niacin exerts several distinctive pharmacologic effects that vary according to the dosage level employed. In large doses it causes a reduction in serum lipids (both cholesterol and triglycerides). The mechanism of this action is unknown.

In large doses, peripheral vasodilatation is produced, predominantly in the cutaneous vessels of the face, neck, and chest. Niacin acts directly on blood vessels by relaxing the musculature of peripheral vessels, producing vasodilation and increased blood flow.

Is rapidly absorbed from the GI tract; peak serum concentrations usually occur in 45 minutes. Plasma elimination half-life is about 45 minutes. Approximately one-third of oral dose is excreted in the urine.

WARNINGS

There is no convincing evidence to support use of megadoses in treatment of schizophrenia. High doses are associated with considerable toxicity including liver damage, hypotension, peptic ulceration, hyperglycemia, hyperuricemia, dermatoses, cardiac arrhythmias, tachycardia, heartburn, nausea, vomiting, diarrhea, and other effects commonly seen with lower doses such as flushing and pruritus.

Doses in excess of nutritional requirement during pregnancy or lactation or in women of childbearing age are used only when clearly needed and when potential benefits outweigh unknown potential hazards to the fetus or nursing infant. Safety and efficacy in children are not established in doses that exceed nutritional requirements.

PRECAUTIONS

Patients with gallbladder disease or glaucoma or a past history of jaundice, liver disease, or peptic ulcer should be observed closely while taking this

N

drug. Hepatic-function tests and blood glucose levels should be monitored frequently during therapy.

Diabetics or potential diabetics should be observed closely in the event of decreased tolerance. Adjustment of diet and/or hypoglycemic therapy may be necessary. Elevated uric acid levels have occurred; drug is used with caution in those predisposed to gout.

Tartrazine sensitivity: Some of these products contain tartrazine. See Appendix 6, section 6-23.

DRUG INTERACTIONS

In those receiving **antihypertensive drugs of the sympathomimetic blocking type,** niacin may have an additive vasodilating effect and produce postural hypotension.

ADVERSE REACTIONS

GI: Activation of peptic ulcer, jaundice, nausea, vomiting, abdominal pain, diarrhea, GI disorders.

Dermatologic: Severe generalized flushing, sensation of warmth, keratosis nigricans, pruritus, skin rash, dry skin, itching, tingling.

Clinical laboratory findings: Decreased glucose tolerance; abnormalities of hepatic-function tests; hyperuricemia.

Miscellaneous: Toxic amblyopia, hypotension, headache, allergy, cystoidedema of the macula.

DOSAGE

Recommended dietary allowances (RDAs): Adult males, 18 mg; adult females, 13 mg.

Oral: Niacin deficiency— 50 mg/day to 100 mg/day. *Pellagra—*Up to 500 mg/day. *Hyperlipidemia—*1 g to 2 g tid. Do not exceed 6 g/day.

Parenteral: Used only for vitamin deficiencies (not for treatment of hyperlipoproteinemia) and when oral therapy is impossible. Length of parenteral treatment depends on patient response and how soon oral medication and a complete and well-balanced diet can be taken. The IV route is the preferred parenteral route whenever possible.

NURSING IMPLICATIONS

HISTORY
See Appendix 4.

PHYSICAL ASSESSMENT
Obtain vital signs.

Niacin deficiency: Examine areas of involvement (skin, mucous membrane, CNS, GI). Baseline laboratory tests (*e.g.,* hepatic-function tests, blood glucose) are usually ordered. In those with hyperlipidemia, serum cholesterol and triglycer-

ides are also obtained. Additional laboratory tests may also be appropriate.

ADMINISTRATION
May cause GI upset; give with food or meals.

Offer cold water (not hot beverages) if necessary to facilitate swallowing.

If patient is unable to take oral medication, parenteral therapy (preferably IV) may be ordered.

ONGOING ASSESSMENTS AND NURSING MANAGEMENT
Because flushing, pruritus, and GI distress appear frequently, therapy is usually begun with small doses and increased in gradual increments.

Observe for adverse effects within the first 2 hours of each dose. If they become severe, notify physician before next dose is due.

In some instances, adverse effects are so severe or cause such extreme discomfort that therapy must be discontinued. Physician may also lower dose and attempt more gradual dosage increments.

Hepatic function and blood glucose are monitored at periodic intervals.

Observe patient for signs of hepatic dysfunction (*e.g.,* jaundice, dark urine, light stools, and pruritus [which also may be a drug side-effect]). Notify physician if these occur.

Diabetic or potentially diabetic patient: Observe closely for signs of hyperglycemia (Appendix 6, section 6-14). Test urine qid for glucose, ketone bodies. Notify physician if signs of hyperglycemia are apparent or if urine is positive for glucose and/or ketones; dosage of hypoglycemic agent and/or diet may require adjustment.

Niacin deficiency: Many physicians prefer to use nicotinamide (p 768) for prevention or correction of niacin deficiency because it lacks the vasodilating effects of nicotinic acid.

Therapeutic response is usually noted in 24 to 72 hours.

Observe for relief of clinical manifestations of niacin deficiency (*e.g.,* fatigue; anorexia; weight loss; headache; dermatitis; redness and soreness of mouth, tongue, and lips; nausea, vomiting, diarrhea; CNS symptoms including confusion, neuritis, and disorientation). Symptoms will vary according to severity of the deficiency.

A well-balanced diet with emphasis on foods high in niacin is usually prescribed.

Hyperlipidemia: Periodic determinations of serum cholesterol and triglycerides are usually obtained. Dosage may then be adjusted according to patient response.

Dietary management may also be necessary. Physician prescribes diet according to type and severity of hyperlipidemia (_e.g.,_ a diet restricting cholesterol, fats, or sugars).

PATIENT AND FAMILY INFORMATION

NOTE: A special diet may be prescribed. In niacin deficiency, encourage consumption of foods high in niacin (_e.g.,_ meat, fish, poultry, eggs, breads, cereals, some vegetables). If deficiency is due to inability to purchase those foods necessary for a well-balanced diet, use agencies that may offer assistance. In hyperlipidemias, review diet prescribed by physician. Those with hypertriglyceridemia should also be advised to limit intake of alcohol.

May cause GI upset; take with food or meals.

Cutaneous flushing and a sensation of warmth, especially in area of face, neck, and ears, may occur within first 2 hours after taking drug. Itching or tingling and headache may also occur. These effects are transient and will usually subside with continued therapy.

If effects become distressing, notify physician or nurse.

If dizziness occurs, avoid sudden changes in posture. Rise from a sitting or lying position slowly. Do not attempt to drive or engage in other hazardous tasks if dizziness persists.

Adhere to prescribed diet, which is an important part of therapy.

Diabetic patient: Check urine daily. If urine is positive for glucose or ketones, notify physician.

Nicotinyl Alcohol Rx

tablets: 50 mg (as tartrate)	Roniacol, _Generic_
tablets, timed release: 150 mg (as tartrate)	Roniacol, _Generic_
elixir: 50 mg/5ml	Roniacol

INDICATIONS

"Possibly effective" in conditions associated with deficient circulation (_e.g.,_ peripheral vascular disease, vascular spasm, varicose ulcers, decubitus ulcers, chilblains, Meniere's syndrome, vertigo).

ACTIONS

Acts directly by relaxing musculature of peripheral blood vessels, particularly cutaneous vessels in the blush area (face, neck, ears). Little effect is produced in vessels of lower extremities. Is converted to nicotinic acid (p 769) from which drug derives its

pharmacologic effects. Action is gradual in onset. Sustained-release form increases blood flow for up to 12 hours with a single dose. Patient usually does not develop tolerance on prolonged medication. Sustained-release form releases some of drug immediately and remainder continuously over a period of approximately 12 hours, increasing blood flow in ischemic extremities for 10 to 12 hours by dilation of peripheral vessels.

WARNINGS

Safety for use in pregnancy is not established. Use only when clearly needed and potential benefits outweigh unknown hazards to the fetus.

ADVERSE REACTIONS

Transient flushing, gastric disturbances (nausea, vomiting, heartburn), minor skin rashes, pruritus, and allergies may occur in some patients, seldom requiring discontinuation of drug. Tingling of extremities, faintness, dizziness, and a marked fall in blood pressure have also been reported.

DOSAGE

Tablets, elixir: 50 mg to 100 mg tid.
Timed-release tablets: 150 mg to 300 mg in A.M. and P.M.

NURSING IMPLICATIONS

HISTORY
See Appendix 4.

PHYSICAL ASSESSMENT
Obtain vital signs; examine involved areas for color, warmth, skin changes. If extremities are involved, palpate peripheral pulses. When prescribed for Meniere's syndrome or vertigo, base assessment on patient's present symptoms.

ADMINISTRATION
Physician may order drug given before or with meals or food.

If patient has difficulty swallowing tablet, contact physician; a liquid preparation is available.

Instruct patient not to chew timed-release tablet.

ONGOING ASSESSMENTS AND NURSING MANAGEMENT
Monitor vital signs daily; observe for adverse reactions; evaluate drug response by questioning patient about relief of original symptoms. If peripheral vascular disease is present, check extremities for color, warmth, skin changes, improvement in peripheral pulses.

N

May cause dizziness (orthostatic hypotension). If dizziness is severe (especially in the elderly), assist patient with ambulatory activities.

PATIENT AND FAMILY INFORMATION
May cause flushing and sensation of warmth, skin rash, and GI disturbances. Notify physician or nurse if these become particularly bothersome.

If dizziness occurs, avoid sudden changes in posture. Rise slowly (and with help, if needed) from a sitting or lying position. Avoid potentially dangerous tasks when dizziness occurs.

Nifedipine Rx

capsules: 10 mg   Procardia

INDICATIONS
Vasospastic angina: Management of this disorder confirmed by any of the following criteria: classic pattern of angina at rest accompanied by S–T segment elevation, angina, or coronary artery spasm provoked by ergonovine or angiographically demonstrated coronary artery spasm. May also be used when clinical presentation suggests a vasospastic component but vasospasm has not been confirmed (*e.g.*, when pain has a variable threshold on exertion, in unstable angina when ECG findings are compatible with intermittent vasospasm, or when angina is refractory to nitrates and/or adequate doses of beta blockers).

Chronic stable angina (classical effort-associated angina): Management of this disorder without vasospasm in those who remain symptomatic despite adequate doses of beta blockers and/or nitrates or who cannot tolerate those agents. Drug has been effective in controlled trials of up to 8 weeks, but confirmation of effectiveness and long-term safety is incomplete. Limited data suggest concomitant use with beta blocking agents may be beneficial.

CONTRAINDICATIONS
Hypersensitivity.

ACTIONS
Contractile processes of cardiac and vascular smooth muscle are dependent on movement of extracellular calcium ions into these cells through specific channels. Nifedipine selectively inhibits calcium influx across the cell membrane of cardiac and vascular smooth muscle without changing serum calcium concentrations.

Drug causes decreased peripheral vascular resistance and a fall in systolic and diastolic blood pressure, usually modest (5–10 mm Hg systolic) but sometimes larger. There is usually a small increase in heart rate, a reflex response to vasodilation.

Precise means by which slow channel inhibition relieves angina is not fully determined but includes at least the following two mechanisms:

1. *Relaxation and prevention of coronary artery spasm*—Nifedipine dilates coronary arteries and arterioles, in both normal and ischemic regions, and is a potent inhibitor of coronary artery spasm. This increases myocardial oxygen delivery in vasospastic (Prinzmetal's or variant) angina. Whether this effect plays any role in classical angina is not clear.
2. *Reduction of oxygen utilization*—Nifedipine regularly reduces arterial pressure at rest and at a given level of exercise by dilating peripheral arterioles and reducing total peripheral resistance (afterload) against which the heart works. This unloading of the heart reduces myocardial energy consumption and oxygen requirements and probably accounts for effectiveness in chronic stable angina.

Drug is rapidly and fully absorbed after administration. It is detectable in the serum in 10 minutes and peak blood levels occur in approximately 30 minutes. It is highly bound by serum proteins and extensively converted to inactive metabolites; approximately 80% of metabolites are eliminated via the kidneys. Plasma half-life is approximately 2 hours.

WARNINGS
Hypotension: Although hypotensive effect is usually modest and well tolerated, occasional patients have excessive and poorly tolerated hypotension. These responses usually occur during initial therapy or at the time of dosage increases and may be more likely in those taking concomitant beta blockers.

Increased angina/beta blocker withdrawal: Occasional patients have increased frequency, duration or severity of angina on starting drug or at time of dosage increases. Those recently withdrawn from beta blockers may develop a withdrawal syndrome with increased angina, probably related to increased sensitivity to catecholamines. Initiation of treatment will not prevent this occurrence and might be expected to exacerbate it by provoking reflex catecholamine release. If possible, it is important to taper beta blockers rather than stop them abruptly before beginning therapy.

Congestive heart failure: Rarely, patients usually receiving a beta blocker have developed CHF after beginning therapy. Patients with tight aortic stenosis may be at greater risk for such event.

Use in pregnancy: There are no well-controlled studies in pregnant women. Drug is used during pregnancy only if potential benefit justifies the potential risk to the fetus.

PRECAUTIONS

Mild to moderate edema, typically associated with arterial vasodilation and not due to left ventricular dysfunction, occurs in 10%. Edema occurs primarily in the lower extremities and usually responds to diuretics. In those with CHF, care is taken to differentiate this peripheral edema from effects of increasing left ventricular dysfunction. Nifedipine may be safely coadministered with long-acting nitrates but there are no controlled studies evaluating the effectiveness of this combination.

DRUG INTERACTIONS

Concomitant use of nifedipine and **beta blocking agents** is usually well tolerated. Occasionally this combination may increase the likelihood of CHF, severe hypotension, or exacerbation of angina.

ADVERSE REACTIONS

Are frequent but generally not serious and rarely require discontinuation of therapy or dosage adjustment. Most are expected consequences of vasodilator effects: dizziness, lightheadedness, giddiness, flushing, heat sensation, headache, weakness, nausea, heartburn, muscle cramps, tremor, peripheral edema, nervousness, mood changes, palpitation, dyspnea, cough, wheezing, nasal congestion, sore throat.

Most common adverse reactions include dizziness or lightheadedness, peripheral edema, nausea, weakness, headache, and flushing, each occurring in about 10% of patients, transient hypotension in about 5%, palpitation in about 2%, and syncope in about 0.5%. Syncopal episodes did not recur with reduction in dose or concomitant antianginal medication. Very rarely, introduction of therapy was associated with an increase in anginal pain, possibly due to associated hypotension. Several of these side-effects (peripheral edema, transient hypotension) appear to be dose related.

In addition, 2% or fewer patients reported the following:

Respiratory: Nasal and chest congestion, shortness of breath.

GI: Diarrhea, constipation, cramps, flatulence.

Musculoskeletal: Inflammation, joint stiffness, muscle cramps.

CNS: Shakiness, nervousness, jitteriness, sleep disturbances, blurred vision, difficulties in balance.

Other: Dermatitis, pruritus, urticaria, fever, sweating, chills, sexual difficulties.

More serious effects: In addition, more serious adverse effects were observed, not readily distinguishable from the natural history of the disease in these patients. It is possible these events were drug related. MI occurred in about 4%, CHF or pulmonary edema in about 2%, and ventricular arrhythmias and conduction disturbances each occurred in fewer than 0.5%.

Laboratory tests: Rare, mild to moderate, transient elevations of enzymes such as alkaline phosphatase, CPK, LDH, SGOT, SGPT reported. The relationship is uncertain.

OVERDOSAGE

Symptoms: Gross overdosage could result in excessive peripheral vasodilation with subsequent marked and probably prolonged systemic hypotension.

Treatment: Clinically significant hypotension calls for active cardiovascular support including monitoring of cardiac and respiratory function, elevation of extremities, and attention to circulating fluid volume and urine output. A vasoconstrictor (such as norepinephrine) may be helpful in restoring vascular tone and blood pressure, provided there is no contraindication to its use. Clearance would be expected to be prolonged in those with impaired liver function. Drug is highly protein bound; dialysis is not likely to be of benefit.

DOSAGE

Dosage needed to suppress angina and that can be tolerated by patient must be established by titration. Excessive doses can result in hypotension.

Starting dose is 10 mg tid. Usual effective dose range is 10 mg to 20 mg tid. Some patients, especially those with evidence of coronary artery spasm, respond only to higher doses, more frequent administration, or both. In such patients, 20 mg to 30 mg tid or qid may be effective. Doses above 120 mg/day are rarely necessary. More than 180 mg/day is not recommended.

In most cases, titration should extend over a 7- to 10-day period so response to each dose level and blood pressure can be assessed. If symptoms warrant, titration may proceed more rapidly provided patient is assessed more frequently. Based on patient's physical activity level, attack frequency, and sublingual nitroglycerin consumption, dose may be increased from 10 mg tid to 20 mg tid and then 30 mg tid over a 3-day period.

In hospitalized patients, dose may be increased in 10-mg increments over 4 to 6 hours as required to control pain and arrhythmias due to ischemia. A single dose should rarely exceed 30 mg.

No "rebound effect" is observed upon discontinuation, but if discontinuation is necessary dosage should be decreased gradually with close supervision. Sublingual nitroglycerin may be taken as required for control of acute manifestations of angina, particularly during titration.

NURSING IMPLICATIONS

HISTORY
Complete description of angina, duration of attack, what factors precipitate attack (*e.g.,* activity, emotion, rest). See also Appendix 4.

PHYSICAL ASSESSMENT
Obtain vital signs. Obtain blood pressure on both arms with patient in sitting and lying position. Based on health history, additional assessments (*e.g.,* examining extremities for peripheral edema, auscultating lungs) may be performed. ECG, CBC, serum enzymes may be ordered. Other laboratory and/or diagnostic tests may be appropriate to confirm type of angina.

ADMINISTRATION
During titration period, dosage changes may be ordered every few days (in severe angina more frequently). Be sure medicine card and Kardex clearly show dosage increments and length of time each dosage is to be administered.

Sublingual nitroglycerin (p 776) may be taken during titration period.

Obtain blood pressure and pulse (use same arm with patient in same position each time) immediately before administration.

CLINICAL ALERT: If blood pressure decreases more than 10 mm Hg or pulse significantly increases, withhold drug and contact physician.

ONGOING ASSESSMENTS AND NURSING MANAGEMENT
Monitor blood pressure, pulse, and respirations frequently with interval dependent on severity of angina; note past changes in blood pressure, pulse; note frequency in dosage increments; note whether patient is receiving concomitant medication known to lower blood pressure.

Keep record (or have patient keep record) of all anginal attacks because dosage adjustments may be required.

Occasional patients have increased frequency, duration, or severity of angina on starting the drug or at the time of dosage increases. Although this is known to occur, physician must still be informed of increased frequency of angina. At time of increased frequency, reassure patient that this is a known drug effect and that the physician will be contacted.

Mild to moderate edema of lower extremities may occur. Check extremities daily. If edema occurs, notify physician.

Dizziness and lightheadedness may occur. Assist with ambulatory activities as needed.

Keep physician informed of any adverse reactions that occur. In some instances, dosage may need to be reduced; in others, the reactions may need to be tolerated.

If discontinuation of drug is necessary, it is recommended that dosage be decreased gradually. Observe patient at frequent intervals for increase in angina attacks; monitor blood pressure and pulse q4h or as ordered.

PATIENT AND FAMILY INFORMATION
NOTE: If physician prescribes periodic dosage increments, dosage schedule must be carefully explained to the patient. Physician should explain possible increase in angina on starting drug or during dosage increases.

Follow dosage as written on prescription container. Do not increase dosage if angina becomes worse; instead, contact physician. Do not decrease or omit a dose unless advised to do so by the physician. Concomitant medication (if any) is also taken as directed.

May cause dizziness, lightheadedness. Avoid sudden changes in position; rise from a sitting or lying position slowly. Avoid potentially hazardous tasks if these symptoms occur.

Notify the physician or nurse if any of the following should occur: severe dizziness, lightheadedness; swelling of ankles; nausea. If weakness, headache, flushing, or other noted drug effects persist or become intolerable, notify physician or nurse.

Nikethamide Rx

injection: 25%	Coramine
solution, oral: 25%	Coramine

INDICATIONS
To overcome CNS depression, respiratory depression, and circulatory failure, particularly when due to effects of depressant drugs. Helps restore respiration with electroshock therapy and may reduce number of treatments required.

NOTE: Respiratory depression due to overdosage of CNS depressants is best managed by mechanical ventilatory support.

CONTRAINDICATIONS

Hypersensitivity.

ACTIONS

A CNS stimulant with direct medullary effects. Secondary indirect stimulation of peripheral chemoreceptors may contribute to its stimulatory effects on respiration. Has no direct effect on the heart or blood vessels. Has a narrow therapeutic margin and is less effective an analeptic than is doxapram. Is well absorbed after administration. Is converted to nicotinamide and excreted in urine.

WARNINGS

Do not inject intra-arterially; arterial spasm and thrombosis may result. Safety for use in pregnancy has not been established. Use only when clearly needed and potential benefits outweigh unknown potential hazards to the fetus.

ADVERSE REACTIONS

The difference between therapeutic and toxic doses varies. The following side-effects may be a result of overdosage: burning or itching, especially at the back of the nose; flushing or a subjective feeling of warmth; sneezing; coughing; sweating; nausea; vomiting; generalized restlessness; fear; changing depth and frequency of respiration; tachycardia; elevated blood pressure; muscle twitching (especially facial); and convulsions.

OVERDOSAGE

Symptoms: Coughing, sneezing, hyperpnea, muscle tremors. Cardiac rate and blood pressure may increase. With severe overdosage, generalized muscle spasms and convulsive seizures occur.

Treatment: A short-acting barbiturate is effective in controlling generalized muscle spasms and convulsions. Attempts to induce emesis or perform gastric lavage are of little value, and in the presence of paroxysmal coughing and sneezing, they could result in complications from aspiration.

DOSAGE

Although readily absorbed after oral, subcutaneous, or IM administration, it is most effective by IV route.

Anesthetic overdosage: To shorten narcosis—4 ml (1000 mg) IV or IM. *To increase amplitude of respiration*—2 ml to 5 ml (500–1250 mg) IV. *To overcome respiratory depression*—5 ml to 10 ml (1250–2500 mg) IV; repeat as necessary. *To combat respiratory paralysis*—15 ml (3750 mg) IV as minimal

initial dose; repeat as needed. Other methods of resuscitation, including artificial respiration, are employed as indicated. If cardiac arrest is present, 0.5 ml to 1 ml (125–250 mg) intracardially may be of some benefit.

Narcotic, hypnotic, and carbon monoxide poisoning: Initial dose is 5 ml to 10 ml (1250–2500 mg) IV, then 5 ml (1250 mg) every 5 minutes for the first hour, depending on response. Thereafter, administer 5-ml (1250-mg) booster doses every ½ to 1 hour if needed. Artificial respiration, gastric lavage, oxygen, and other measures should also be employed.

Cardiac decompensation and coronary occlusion: Emergencies—5 ml to 10 ml (1250–2500 mg) IV or IM.

Shock: Primary treatment requires oxygen and adequate solutions, including blood or plasma, for volume replacement. Drug may be of value in compensating peripheral circulation until blood or plasma is available. Dose is 10 ml or 15 ml (2500–3750 mg) IV or IM initially, repeated as indicated.

Acute alcoholism: Initial dose is 5 ml to 20 ml (1250–5000 mg) IV to overcome central depression; repeat as necessary.

Electroshock therapy: Dilute 5 ml (1250 mg) with equal volume of sterile water. Inject rapidly into anticubital vein. Apply electrical stimulus when patient's face is flushed and respiratory rate increases noticeably, within 1 minute.

Maintenance: 3 ml to 5 ml (750–1250 mg) of oral solution q4h to q6h.

NURSING IMPLICATIONS

HISTORY

When applicable, review patient's chart for possible cause of respiratory depression or circulatory failure, health history.

PHYSICAL ASSESSMENT

Obtain blood pressure, pulse, and respirations. Laboratory tests may be ordered to determine cause and extent of respiratory depression.

ADMINISTRATION

An adequate airway and oxygenation must be assured before administration.

Have available a short-acting barbiturate (check with physician about drug desired) to control convulsive seizures, which may occur with overdosage.

May be administered IV, IM, subcutaneously, or PO (oral solution).

N

ONGOING ASSESSMENTS AND NURSING MANAGEMENT

CLINICAL ALERT: Drug has a narrow therapeutic margin; difference between therapeutic and toxic dose varies. Review *Overdosage*. Inform physician immediately if signs of overdosage are apparent.

Monitor level of consciousness and respiratory rate and depth continuously until patient responds.

Monitor blood pressure and pulse q10m to q15m or as ordered.

Keep physician informed of patient response.

Other treatment modalities (*e.g.,* oxygen, artificial ventilation, IV fluids) may also be employed.

Exercise care to prevent vomiting and aspiration; have suction machine immediately available.

Laboratory tests (*e.g.,* arterial blood gases, barbiturate levels) may be drawn periodically to evaluate results of therapy.

Oral solution may be ordered once patient is conscious and able to swallow.

Nitrates

Amyl Nitrite *Rx*

inhalant: 0.18 ml	*Generic*
inhalant: 0.3 ml	*Generic*

Erythrityl Tetranitrate *Rx*

tablets, chewable: 10 mg	Cardilate
tablets, oral: 5 mg, 10 mg, 15 mg	Cardilate
tablets, sublingual: 5 mg, 10 mg	Cardilate

Isosorbide Dinitrate, Oral *Rx*

tablets: 5 mg	Isogard, Isordil Titradose, Sorbitrate (contains tartrazine), *Generic*
tabletes: 10 mg	Isogard, Isordil Titradose, Sorbitrate (contains tartrazine), *Generic*
tablets: 20 mg	Isordil Titradose, Sorbitrate, *Generic*
tablets: 30 mg	Isordil Titradose, Sorbitrate
tablets: 40 mg	Sorbitrate
tablets, sustained release: 40 mg	Isogard, Isordil Tembids, Sorbitrate SA (contains tartrazine), *Generic*

capsules, sustained release: 40 mg	Dilatrate-SR, Iso-Bid, Isordil Tembids, Isotrate Time-celles, Sorate-40, Sorbide T.D., *Generic*

Isosorbide Dinitrate, Sublingual and Chewable *Rx*

tablets, sublingual: 2.5 mg	Isogard, Isordil, Sorate-2.5, Sorbitrate, *Generic*
tablets, sublingual: 5 mg	Isogard, Isordil, Sorate-5, Sorbitrate, *Generic*
tablets, sublingual: 10 mg	Isordil, Sorbitrate
tablets, chewable: 5 mg	Isotrate, Onset-5, Sorate-5, Sorbitrate
tablets, chewable: 10 mg	Isordil, Onset-10, Sorbitrate

Nitroglycerin, Intravenous *Rx*

injection: 0.8 mg/ml	Nitrostat IV, Nitrol IV
injection: 5 mg/ml	Nitro-Bid IV, Tridil, *Generic*

Nitroglycerin, Sublingual *Rx*

tablets: 0.15 mg, 0.3 mg, 0.4 mg, 0.6 mg	*Generic*
tablets (stabilized): 0.3 mg, 0.4 mg, 0.6 mg	Nitrostat

Nitroglycerin, Sustained Release *Rx*

tablets: 2.6 mg, 6.5 mg	Klavikordal, Niong, Nitroglyn, Nitronet, Nitrong
tablets: 9 mg	Nitrong
capsules: 2.5 mg	Ang-O-Span, N-G-C, Nitro-Bid Plateau Caps, Nitrocap T.D., Nitrolin, Nitrospan, Nitrostat SR, Trates Granucaps (contains tartrazine), *Generic*
capsules: 6.5 mg	N-G-C, Nitro-Bid Plateau Caps, Nitrocap T.D., Nitrolin, Nitrospan, Nitrostat SR, *Generic*
capsules: 9 mg	Nitro-Bid Plateau Caps, Nitrostat SR

Nitroglycerin, Topical *Rx*

ointment: 2%	Nitro-Bid, Nitrol, Nitrong, Nitrostat, *Generic*

Nitroglycerin, Transdermal Systems Rx

transdermal system: 2.5 mg, 5 mg, 10 mg, or 15 mg/24 hours	Transderm-Nitro
transdermal system: 2.5 mg, 5 mg, 7.5 mg, 10 mg, or 15 mg/24 hours	Nitro-Dur
transdermal system: 5 mg or 10 mg/24 hours	Nitrodisc

Nitroglycerin, Transmucosal Rx

tablets: 1 mg, 2 mg, 3 mg	Susadrin

Pentaerythritol Tetranitrate *(P.E.T.N.)* Rx

tablets: 10 mg	Pentylan, Peritrate, Rate-10, *Generic*
tablets: 20 mg	Naptrate, Pentylan, Peritrate, Rate-20, *Generic*
tablets: 40 mg	Peritrate
capsules, sustained release: 30 mg	Duotrate Plateau Caps, Pentritol Tempules, *Generic*
capsules, sustained release: 45 mg	Duotrate 45 Plateau Caps
capsules, sustained release: 60 mg	Pentritol Tempules
capsules, sustained release: 80 mg	Vaso-80 Unicelles, *Generic*
tablets, sustained release: 80 mg	Peritrate SA, *Generic*

Combination Products

The combination products listed below contain two or more of the following:

Nitrates—The primary antianginal component of these formulations
Ethaverine (p 466)—Used for spasmolytic action
Barbiturates (p 165), Meprobamate (p 673), Hydroxyzine HCl (p 559)—Included for their sedative and antianxiety effects in patients in whom emotional excitement may contribute to or accompany angina.

Tablets

pentaerythritol tetranitrate 10 mg, phenobarbital 15 mg	Peritrate w/Phenobarbital, *Generic*
pentaerythritol tetranitrate 10 mg, hydroxyzine HCl 10 mg	Cartrax-10
pentaerythritol tetranitrate 10 mg, meprobamate 200 mg	Miltrate-10
pentaerythritol tetranitrate 10 mg, ethaverine HCl 30 mg	Papavatral 10
pentaerythritol tetranitrate 20 mg, phenobarbital 15 mg	Peritrate w/Phenobarbital, *Generic*
pentaerythritol tetranitrate 20 mg, hydroxyzine HCl 10 mg	Cartrax-20
pentaerythritol tetranitrate 20 mg, meprobamate 200 mg	Miltrate-20 (contains tartrazine)
pentaerythritol tetranitrate 20 mg, ethaverine HCl 30 mg	Papavatral 20
sodium nitrite 65 mg, phenobarbital 16 mg	Soniphen

Capsules and Tablets, Sustained Release

pentaerythritol tetranitrate 30 mg, secobarbital 50 mg	Corovas Tymcaps
pentaerythritol tetranitrate 50 mg, ethaverine HCl 30 mg	Papavatral L.A. Capsules
pentaerythritol tetranitrate 80 mg, phenobarbital 45 mg	Peritrate w/Phenobarbital SA Tablets

INDICATIONS

These drugs are antianginal agents and include rapid-acting nitrates used to relieve pain of acute angina and long-acting preparations used for prophylaxis or to decrease the severity of angina pectoris. See below for specific indications of individual drugs.

Investigational uses: Sublingual and topical nitroglycerin and oral nitrates have been used to reduce cardiac workload in patients with acute myocardial infarction (MI) and congestive heart failure (CHF).

N

AMYL NITRITE

Relief of angina pectoris.

ERYTHRITYL TETRANITRATE

Prophylaxis and long-term treatment of frequent or recurrent anginal pain and reduced exercise tolerance associated with angina pectoris.

ISOSORBIDE DINITRATE, ORAL

Prophylactic management of anginal pectoris. Not intended to abort acute angina episode, but may be useful in prophylactic treatment.

ISOSORBIDE DINITRATE, SUBLINGUAL AND CHEWABLE

Treatment of acute anginal attacks and prophylaxis in situations likely to provoke such attacks.

NITROGLYCERIN, INTRAVENOUS

Control of hypertension associated with surgical procedures, especially cardiovascular procedures, such as hypertension seen during intratracheal intubation, anesthesia, skin incision, sternotomy, cardiac bypass, and in the immediate postoperative period. Also used in CHF associated with MI, treatment of angina pectoris in those not responding to recommended doses of organic nitrates or a beta blocker, and production of controlled hypotension during surgical procedures.

NITROGLYCERIN, SUBLINGUAL

Prophylaxis, treatment, and management of angina pectoris.

NITROGLYCERIN, SUSTAINED RELEASE

"Possibly effective" for management or prophylaxis of angina pectoris.

NITROGLYCERIN, TOPICAL

Prevention and treatment of angina pectoris due to coronary artery disease.

NITROGLYCERIN, TRANSDERMAL SYSTEMS

Prevention and treatment of angina pectoris due to coronary artery disease.

NITROGLYCERIN, TRANSMUCOSAL

Prophylaxis, treatment, and management of angina pectoris.

PENTAERYTHRITOL TETRANITRATE (P.E.T.N.)

Prophylactic management of angina pectoris. Not intended to abort acute anginal episode, but may be useful in prophylactic treatment.

CONTRAINDICATIONS

Hypersensitivity or idiosyncrasy to nitrates; severe anemia. Because these drugs increase intracranial pressure, they are contraindicated or used with great caution in those with head trauma, cerebral hemorrhage, or postural hypotension.

IV nitroglycerin: Hypotension or uncorrected hypovolemia in IV use could produce severe hypotension or shock, inadequate cerebral circulation, constrictive pericarditis, and pericardial tamponade.

ACTIONS

Relaxation of smooth muscle is the principal pharmacologic action. Although venous effects predominate, nitroglycerin produces, in a dose-related manner, dilation of both arterial and venous beds. Dilation of postcapillary vessels, including large veins, promotes peripheral pooling of blood and decreases venous return to the heart, reducing left ventricular end-diastolic pressure (preload). Arteriolar relaxation reduces systemic vascular resistance and arterial pressure (afterload). Myocardial oxygen consumption or demand is decreased by both the arterial and the venous effects of nitroglycerin, and a more favorable supply–demand ratio can be achieved. In coronary circulation, nitrates redistribute circulating blood flow along collateral channels so that the inner layers of the myocardium are better perfused.

IV nitroglycerin: Therapeutic doses reduce systolic, diastolic, and mean arterial blood pressure. Effective coronary perfusion pressure is usually maintained but can be compromised if blood pressure falls excessively or increased heart rate decreases diastolic filling time. Elevated central venous and pulmonary capillary wedge pressures, pulmonary vascular resistance, and systemic vascular resistance are also reduced. Heart rate is usually slightly increased, presumably as a reflex response to the fall in blood pressure. Patients with elevated left ventricular filling pressure and systemic vascular resistance values in conjunction with a depressed cardiac index are likely to experience an improvement in cardiac index. On the other hand, when filling pressures and cardiac index are normal, cardiac index may be slightly reduced.

Nitroglycerin and isosorbide dinitrate are well absorbed from the sublingual mucosa. Nitroglycerin is also absorbed through the skin; nitroglycerin ointments and transdermal systems provide gradual release of the drug, which reaches target organs before hepatic inactivation. Transmucosal nitroglycerin passes directly into the bloodstream through the oral mucosa. Nitrates are metabolized by the liver. Approximately one-third of an inhaled dose of amyl nitrite is excreted in the urine. Nitroglycerin is widely distributed in the body. It is rapidly metabolized to dinitrates and mononitrates with a short half-life, estimated at 1 to 4 minutes. This results in a low plasma concentration after IV infusion.

The onset and duration of activity are given in Table 39.

See Table 39.

WARNINGS

Postural hypotension: Transient episodes of dizziness, weakness, syncope, or other signs of cerebral ischemia due to postural hypotension may develop, especially following administration of rapidly acting agents and particularly if patient is standing or immobile, and may occasionally progress to unconsciousness.

Transdermal nitroglycerin is not for immediate relief of anginal attacks. Those with acute MI or CHF are closely monitored.

Safety for use in pregnancy has not been established. Use with caution when administering to a nursing mother.

Safety and efficacy in children have not been established.

PRECAUTIONS

IV nitroglycerin: Use with caution in those with severe hepatic or renal disease. Excessive hypotension, especially for prolonged periods, must be avoided because of possible effects on the brain, heart, liver, and kidney from poor perfusion and the risk of ischemia, thrombosis, and altered function of these organs. Paradoxical bradycardia and increased angina pectoris may accompany nitroglycerin-induced hypotension. Patients with normal or low pulmonary capillary wedge pressure are especially sensitive to the hypotensive effects of IV nitroglycerin. A fall in wedge pressure precedes the onset of arterial hypotension and thus is a useful guide to safe titration of the drug.

Tolerance: Tolerance and cross-tolerance with other nitrates may develop with repeated use and may be minimized by using smallest effective dose and alternating with other coronary vasodilators.

Sustained-release products: Patients with gastric hypermotility, in whom the duration of drug passage through the GI tract may be less than normal, should take sublingual or oral rather than sustained-release medication.

Withdrawal: When discontinuing prolonged therapy, withdrawal is gradual because of the possibility of precipitation of angina.

Use in elderly: Occasionally, an elderly patient who has no untoward symptoms while recumbent may develop postural hypotension with faintness on suddenly arising.

Drug abuse: Volatile nitrates are abused for sexual stimulation. The effect of inhalation is almost instantaneous and causes lightheadedness, dizziness, and a feeling interpreted by some as euphoria. Headache is common.

Tartrazine sensitivity: Some of these products contain tartrazine; see Appendix 6, section 6-23.

Other: Excessive dosage may produce violent headache. Lowering the dosage and using analgesics will help control headaches, which usually diminish or disappear as therapy is continued. Drug should be discontinued if blurring of vision or dry mouth occurs.

Observe caution in administering to those with a history of recent cerebral hemorrhage because vasodilatation occurs in this area.

DRUG INTERACTIONS

Do not use **alcohol** concomitantly with **amyl nitrite;** severe hypotension and cardiovascular collapse may result.

N

Table 39. Onset and Duration of Action of Various Nitrate Preparations

Agent	Dosage Form	Onset (minutes)	Duration
Amyl nitrite	Inhalant	½	3–5 min
Nitroglycerin	Intravenous	1–2	3–5 min
	Sublingual	1–3	10–30 min
	Transmucosal	3	6 hr
	Oral, sustained release	40	8–12 hr
	Topical ointment	20–60	2–12 hr
	Transdermal	30–60	24 hr
Isosorbide dinitrate	Sublingual & chewable	2–5	1–2 hr
	Oral	15–40	4–6 hr
	Oral, sustained release	Slow	12 hr
Erythrityl tetranitrate	Sublingual & chewable	5	2 hr
	Oral	30	Variable
Pentaerythritol tetranitrate	Oral	30	4–5 hr
	Oral, sustained release	Slow	12 hr

ADVERSE REACTIONS

Cutaneous vasodilation with flushing. Headache is common and may be severe and persistent during initial therapy, especially with nitroglycerin. Transient episodes of dizziness, palpitation, vertigo, and weakness, as well as other signs of cerebral ischemia associated with postural hypotension, may occasionally develop and may be minimized by taking medication in a sitting or recumbent position. Occasionally there may be marked sensitivity to the hypotensive effects of nitrates, and severe responses (nausea, vomiting, weakness, restlessness, involuntary passing of urine and feces, tachycardia, syncope, apprehension, muscle twitching, retrosternal discomfort, abdominal pain, hypotension, pallor, perspiration, collapse) can occur even with therapeutic doses. **Alcohol** may enhance this effect.

Drug rash and exfoliative dermatitis may occur occasionally.

Sublingual nitroglycerin may cause a local burning sensation in the oral cavity at the point of dissolution. **Nitroglycerin ointment** may cause topical allergic eruptions, including localized pruritic eczematous eruptions; erythematous, vesicular, and pruritic lesions; and anaphylactoid reaction characterized by oral mucosal and conjunctival edema.

Excessively high doses of **amyl nitrite** may cause methemoglobinemia, especially in those with methemoglobin reductase deficiency or another metabolic abnormality that interferes with the normal conversion of methemoglobin back to hemoglobin.

OVERDOSAGE

Symptoms: Nitroglycerin overdosage can produce paralysis, followed by clonic convulsions. In fatal cases, death occurs from respiratory failure after 4 to 7 hours. Toxic effects may result from inhalation of the drug as dust as well as by ingestion. Such effects follow excessive absorption through intact skin; prolonged contact will produce skin eruptions.

Treatment: Ergotamine tartrate may be beneficial; do not employ depressants. Accidental overdosage of IV nitroglycerin may result in severe hypotension and reflex tachycardia and is treated by elevating the legs and decreasing or temporarily terminating the infusion until condition is stabilized. Because the duration of these effects is short, additional corrective measures are usually not required. If further therapy is indicated, administration of an IV alpha-adrenergic agonist (*e.g.,* phenylephrine) may be used.

DOSAGE

AMYL NITRITE

Usual adult dose is 0.18 ml or 0.3 ml by inhalation as required.

ERYTHRITYL TETRANITRATE

Therapy may be initiated with 5 mg to 10 mg sublingually before each anticipated incidence of physical or emotional stress. If oral administration is preferred, therapy may be initiated with 10 mg tid. Additional doses may be administered H.S. for those subject to nocturnal attacks. Dose may be increased or decreased as needed. Up to 100 mg/day is well tolerated, but temporary headache is more apt to occur with large doses of nitroglycerin.

ISOSORBIDE DINITRATE

Tablets: 5 mg to 30 mg qid. Average dose is 10 mg to 20 mg qid. Give smallest effective dose necessary for prevention and treatment of pain of anginal attack.

Sustained release: 40 mg q6h to q12h.

Sublingual: 2.5 mg to 10 mg is usual dose; doses up to 30 mg have been given. May be taken as needed for prompt relief of q4h to q6h prophylactically.

Chewable: No more than 5 mg initially, because an occasional severe hypotensive response may occur. The low dose may be effective in relieving the acute attack; if no significant hypotension is seen, dosage may be increased as necessary. For relief of an acute attack, take as needed; for prophylaxis give q2h to q3h.

NITROGLYCERIN, INTRAVENOUS

Preparation of infusion: See *Administration,* under *Nursing Implications.* IV nitroglycerin infusions may be used in dilutions ranging from 25 mcg/ml to 400 mcg/ml.

Dosage requirements: Initial dosage should be 5 mcg/minute, delivered through an infusion pump capable of exact and constant delivery of drug. Subsequent titration is adjusted to the clinical situation. Initial titration should be in 5-mcg/minute increments with increases every 3 to 5 minutes until response is noted. If no response is seen at 20 mcg/minute, increments of 10 mcg/minute and later 20 mcg/minute can be used. Once partial blood pressure response is observed, dosage increases should be made in smaller increments and at longer time intervals. Some patients with normal or low left ventricular filling or pulmonary capillary wedge pressure (*e.g.,* angina patients without other complications) may be hypersensitive and may respond to doses as small as 5 mcg/minute. These patients require careful titration and monitoring.

There is no fixed optimum dose because of the variations in responsiveness of individual patients. Continuous monitoring of physiological parameters (blood pressure and heart rate in all patients and other measurements such as pulmonary capillary wedge pressure as appropriate) must be performed to achieve correct dose. Adequate systemic blood pressure and coronary perfusion must be maintained.

NITROGLYCERIN, SUBLINGUAL

Dissolve one tablet under tongue or in buccal pouch at first sign of an acute attack. Repeat approximately every 5 minutes until relief is obtained. May be used prophylactically 5 to 10 minutes before activities that might precipitate an acute attack.

NITROGLYCERIN, SUSTAINED RELEASE

One capsule or tablet q8h to q12h on an empty stomach.

NITROGLYCERIN, TOPICAL

One inch of ointment contains approximately 15 mg nitroglycerin. See *Administration*, under *Nursing Implications*.

Usual therapeutic dose: One to two inches (25–50 mm) q8h; some may require 4 to 5 inches (100–125 mm) or application q4h. Start with ½ inch (12.5 mm) q8h; increase dose by ½ inch with each successive application to achieve desired clinical effects. Optimal dosage is based on clinical response, side-effects, and effects on blood pressure. The greatest attainable decrease in resting blood pressure that is not associated with clinical symptoms of hypotension, especially during orthostasis, indicates optimal dosage. To decrease adverse reactions, dose and frequency are tailored to individual needs.

In terminating treatment, both dose and frequency of application are gradually reduced over a 4- to 6-week period to prevent sudden withdrawal reactions. A 60-g tube delivers approximately 60 1-inch doses.

NITROGLYCERIN, TRANSDERMAL SYSTEMS

When pad is applied to skin, nitroglycerin is continuously absorbed into the systemic circulation. Transdermal absorption occurs in a continuous and well-controlled manner for a minimum of 24 hours. Therapeutic plasma levels are attained within 1 hour after application and remain in the therapeutic range for 24 hours.

Apply pad once each day (see *Administration*). Optimal dosage regimen is based on clinical response, side-effects, and effects on blood pressure and heart rate. Dosage may be increased by applying more systems or by using a system with a higher release rate.

Because of technical differences in the various transdermal systems, neither the amount of drug in the system nor the drug release rates can be directly compared.

NITROGLYCERIN, TRANSMUCOSAL

Usual dose: One tablet tid (on rising, after lunch, and after evening meal). Starting dose is 1 mg tid. Dosage may be titrated upward if necessary and adjusted as follows: If angina occurs while tablet is in place, increase dose. If angina occurs between tablet administrations, when no tablet is in place, increase the frequency to qid. Tablet dissolution may be expected to vary from 3 to 5 hours. If continuous nitration is desirable, the next tablet should be taken within 1 hour after the previous one dissolves, unless clinical response suggests a different regimen.

Acute prophylaxis: To cover periods of peak activity, one tablet (but no more than one tablet q2h).

PENTAERYTHRITOL TETRANITRATE (P.E.T.N.)

May be initiated at 10 mg to 20 mg tid or qid and titrated upward to 40 mg qid, ½ hour before or 1 hour after meals and H.S.

Sustained release: One tablet or capsule q12h on an empty stomach.

NURSING IMPLICATIONS

HISTORY

Obtain complete description and duration of symptoms: location of pain, whether pain radiates (and to where), type of pain (*e.g.*, sharp, dull, squeezing), events that appear to precipitate anginal episodes (*e.g.*, exercise, emotion), steps taken to relieve angina (*e.g.*, resting). See also Appendix 4.

PHYSICAL ASSESSMENT

Obtain blood pressure, apical/radial pulse rate, and respiratory rate (after patient is at rest for approximately 10 minutes). Depending on condition and diagnosis, other assessments (*e.g.*, weight, inspection of extremities for edema, auscultation of lungs) may be appropriate. ECG, laboratory tests (*e.g.*, serum electrolytes, serum transaminase, CBC), and other diagnostic studies may be ordered to evaluate extent of coronary disease.

ADMINISTRATION

AMYL NITRITE

Ampule is crushed and vapor inhaled. The woven fabric cover protects fingers; however, further protection by wrapping ampule in cloth, gauze, or several layers of tissue is advisable. Ampule crushes easily.

ISOSORBIDE DINITRATE, ORAL

Patient should take on an empty stomach. If vascular headache cannot be controlled by ordinary measures, drug can be taken with meals.

N

NITROGLYCERIN, INTRAVENOUS

This is a concentrated, potent drug and *must be diluted* in 5% Dextrose Injection, USP or 0.9% Sodium Chloride Injection, USP before infusion. Several preparations are available and differ in concentration or volume per vial. When switching from one preparation to another, attention must be paid to dilution, dosage, and administration instructions.

Label container with number of micrograms per milliliter.

Note that dose is expressed in micrograms (mcg) per milliliter (ml). Dose range is 25 mcg (0.025 mg)/ml to 400 mcg (0.4 mg)/ml. Manufacturer's package insert gives dilution recommendations.

Dosage is affected by the type of container and administration set used. Use *only* with glass IV bottles and the administration set provided with the product. Do *not* use standard plastic IV tubing because tubing will absorb 40% to 80% of the total amount of nitroglycerin in the final diluted solution. Two manufacturers offer the option of purchasing disposable IV tubing with the drug. Non-PVC (polyvinyl chloride) IV tubing that can be used with this drug is also available from other sources.

Because some IV filters absorb nitroglycerin, they should be avoided.

NITROGLYCERIN, SUBLINGUAL

Patients new to sublingual drugs must receive instructions on tablet placement. Tablet is placed under tongue or between cheek and gum (buccal pouch) and allowed to dissolve. Advise patient to wet tablet with saliva before placing under tongue, especially if mouth is dry. Placement site can be rotated (left side, right side).

Have patient sit or lie down at first indication of pain and before tablet is placed under the tongue. Patient should remain in this position for 15 to 20 minutes after taking tablet to minimize dizziness and lightheadedness.

Tablets may be left at bedside (physician's order is usually required). Usually six to ten tablets are left in a container and patient is instructed to take one tablet at the first sign of an acute anginal attack.

Dose may be repeated every 5 minutes until relief is obtained. Instruct patient to use call light to notify nurse if pain is not relieved after three doses (15 minutes). Failure of drug to relieve pain is reported to physician immediately.

Storage: Should be dispensed in manufacturer's original glass container and stored at normal room temperature. Conventional tablets are stable under normal storage conditions for 2 years

following manufacture; it is usually recommended that unused tablets be discarded 6 months after the original bottle is opened. The stabilized formulation is less subject to loss of potency and carries a 5-year expiration date.

NITROGLYCERIN, ORAL TABLETS, SUSTAINED-RELEASE CAPSULES

Give on empty stomach (½ hour A.C. or 1–2 hours P.C.) unless physician orders otherwise.

Take blood pressure and pulse prior to administration. If there is a significant decrease in blood pressure or a rise in pulse rate, withhold drug and contact the physician.

NITROGLYCERIN, CHEWABLE TABLETS

May be taken for an acute attack. Tablet must be thoroughly chewed.

NITROGLYCERIN, TOPICAL

Dose is ordered in inches or millimeters (mm); approximately 25 mm = 1 inch. Unit doses with 1 inch of ointment are also available.

Before drug is measured and applied, take blood pressure and pulse (first have patient rest 10–15 minutes if ambulatory); compare with baseline data. If blood pressure is appreciably lower or pulse higher than resting baseline, contact physician before applying drug.

Applicator paper is supplied with drug; use one paper for each application. Holding applicator paper with printed side down, express the prescribed amount of ointment from the tube onto the paper.

Remove the plastic wrap and tape from the previous application and cleanse the area as needed. Using applicator paper, apply ointment to skin and spread over a 6 × 6 inch (150 × 150 mm) area in a thin uniform layer; *do not* rub or massage into skin. Cover area with plastic wrap and hold in place with tape.

Ointment is effective regardless of site of application. Rotate sites to prevent dermal inflammation and sensitization; record site used. Areas that may be used are chest (front, back), abdomen, and arms and legs (upper and lower). Avoid using hirsute areas unless area is shaved.

Do not allow ointment to come into contact with the fingers or hands while measuring or applying because drug may be absorbed through the skin, resulting in mild dizziness, lightheadedness, and headache.

NITROGLYCERIN, TRANSDERMAL SYSTEMS

Drug is supplied as an impregnated pad and is applied at the same time each day. Skin site should be free of hair and not subject to excessive movement. Do not use irritated or abraded areas. If necessary, a suitable area should be shaved free of hair. *Do not* apply to distal parts of the extremities.

When removing pad applied the previous day, the area is cleansed as needed.

To avoid using more than one pad per day, schedule application after morning care (bed bath, shower, tub bath). Wait approximately ½ hour to be sure skin is thoroughly dry before applying pad. Rotate application sites and record site used.

NITROGLYCERIN, TRANSMUCOSAL

Patients new to transmucosal therapy must receive instructions on tablet placement. Tablet is placed between the lip and gum above the upper incisors; some will prefer the buccal pouch. Sites may be alternated. Tablet should be allowed to dissolve undisturbed. Dissolution time is 3 to 5 hours.

Tablet is inserted upon arising, after lunch, and after the evening meal. Fluids are allowed while tablet is in place because tablet adheres to the mucosa; however, food and excessive chewing may dislodge the tablet, which should be immediately replaced. Tablet is not used H.S. because of danger of aspiration during sleep.

Storage: Dispensed only in original container. Store below 30°C (86°F).

ONGOING ASSESSMENTS AND NURSING MANAGEMENT

Table 39 gives the onset and duration of action of various nitrate preparations and may be used as a guideline in determining the effectiveness of the drug administered.

Obtain blood pressure, pulse, and respirations q3h to q4h or as ordered (if patient is ambulatory, have him rest for approximately 10 minutes before taking vital signs); evaluate drug response by means of questions about relief of pain or chest discomfort.

It may be advisable early in therapy to check patient each time drug is used for an acute attack (instruct patient to use call light). Note time required for drug to relieve pain, adverse effects; monitor blood pressure and pulse.

Contact physician immediately if pain is not relieved, if pain becomes worse, or if hypotension occurs.

Those with nitroglycerin kept at the bedside should have their supply checked q4h to q8h and replenished as needed. Record time and number of tablets given.

Observe for adverse drug effects, especially early in therapy. If headache is severe or postural hypotension interferes with activity, inform physician of problem.

Postural hypotension may be minimized by taking the drug in a sitting or recumbent position. Measures that facilitate venous return, such as head-low posture, deep breathing, movements of the extremities, and elevation of the legs may be used to relieve dizziness, weakness, syncope, or other signs of cerebral ischemia.

If patient is self-administering drug for an acute anginal attack, provide him with a pad and pen or pencil to record the time the attack occurs, when it is relieved, and how many tablets are taken. If the patient does not have a watch, the family can be asked to bring in a watch or a small clock.

Although therapy permits more normal activity, the patient should not be allowed to misinterpret freedom from anginal attacks as a signal to drop all restrictions.

PATIENT AND FAMILY INFORMATION

Avoid alcohol.

May cause headache, dizziness, flushing. Notify physician or nurse if blurring of vision, dry mouth, or persistent headache occurs or if medication fails to relieve pain.

Take on an empty stomach.

Inhalants (amyl nitrite): Use when seated or lying down. Highly inflammable; do not use where it might be ignited.

Sublingual tablets: Keep in original container (the cotton filler may be removed once container is opened). Keep tightly closed at all times; do not handle tablets any more than necessary. Check expiration date before leaving pharmacy. Allow tablet to dissolve under tongue; do not swallow.

It is recommended that unused nitroglycerin (sublingual) tablets be discarded 6 months after container is opened. Write date container is opened on label. Nitrostat is less subject to loss of potency; if prescribed, check with physician about advisability of keeping drug beyond 6 months once container is opened.

Topical ointment: Spread thin layer on skin, using applicator; do not rub or massage into skin; wash medication from hands after application. Keep tube tightly closed.

Transdermal nitroglycerin: Instructions are available with product.

Transmucosal nitroglycerin: Place tablet under upper lip or in buccal pouch and permit to dissolve. Do not chew or swallow.

Store drug at room temperature.

Keep all oral tablets and capsules in original containers. *Do not* mix with other drugs.

N

Keep record of use for acute anginal attacks (*i.e.,* date and time of attack, number of tablets used to relieve pain), and bring this record to each clinic or physician's office visit.

Carry tablets used for an acute anginal attack on person at all times; make family aware of where medication is kept in house.

When drug is taken for an acute anginal attack, it is advisable to assume a sitting or recumbent position. Severe lightheadedness or dizziness often is relieved by lying down, elevating the extremities, moving the extremities, and deep breathing.

Wear Medic-Alert tag/bracelet or carry other identification that alerts others to medical problem (angina) and drug therapy.

Follow physician's recommendations about exercise, diet, and avoidance of stress-producing situations.

Nitrofurantoin Rx

tablets: 50 mg	Furadantin, Furalan, Furan, Furatoin, *Generic*
tablets: 100 mg	Furadantin, Furalan, Furan, *Generic*
capsules: 50 mg, 100 mg	*Generic*
suspension: 25 mg/ 5 ml	Furadantin
powder for injection: 180 mg/vial	Ivadantin
macrocrystals (capsules): 25 mg, 50 mg, 100 mg	Macrodantin

INDICATIONS

Treatment of urinary-tract infections (UTIs) due to susceptible strains of *Escherichia coli,* enterococci, *Staphylococcus aureus,* and certain strains of *Klebsiella, Enterobacter,* and *Proteus* species. Injection is used only in patients with clinically significant UTIs when oral administration cannot be given.

CONTRAINDICATIONS

Hypersensitivity. Anuria, oliguria, or significant impairment of renal function (creatinine clearance under 40 ml/min). Treatment of this type patient is much less effective and carries an increased risk of toxicity because of impaired excretion of drug.

Contraindicated in pregnant patients at term and in infants under 1 month because of possibility of hemolytic anemia due to immature enzyme systems.

ACTIONS

An antibacterial agent for specific UTIs. Is bacteriostatic in low concentrations and considered bactericidal in higher concentrations. Presumed mode of action is interference with bacterial carbohydrate metabolism via inhibition of acetylcoenzyme A. May also disrupt bacterial cell wall formation.

Most gram-negative bacilli and gram-positive cocci associated with UTIs are susceptible, including *E. coli; Klebsiella, Enterobacter,* and *Citrobacter* species; group B streptococci; enterococci; *S. aureus,* and *S. epidermidis.* Some strains of *Enterobacter* and *Klebsiella* are resistant. Usually, sensitive organisms develop only a limited resistance to drug.

Is well absorbed from GI tract after oral administration. The macrocrystalline form is absorbed more slowly because of slower dissolution and causes less GI distress. Absorption is enhanced by concomitant administration of food. Therapeutic serum and tissue concentrations are not achieved after usual IV or oral doses, except in the urinary tract. Drug is rapidly inactivated by body tissues and excreted in urine and bile. Renal excretion is via glomerular filtration and tubular secretion. About 40% of dose is excreted unchanged in urine. Plasma half-life is about 20 minutes in normal individuals. In those with impaired renal function, drug accumulates in the serum and may produce toxic symptoms on repeated dosing. Acid urine enhances tubular reabsorption, thereby increasing renal tissue levels and enhancing antibacterial activity. Tubular reabsorption is decreased and renal clearance enhanced in alkaline urine.

WARNINGS

Pulmonary reactions: Acute, subacute, and chronic pulmonary reactions have been reported. If these reactions occur, drug is withdrawn and appropriate measures instituted. Insidious onset of pulmonary reactions (diffuse interstitial pneumonitis, pulmonary fibrosis, or both) during long-term therapy warrants close monitoring. There have been isolated reports of pulmonary reaction as a contributing cause of death.

Hemolysis: Cases of hemolytic anemia of the primaquine sensitivity type have been induced by nitrofurantoin. Hemolysis appears to be linked to a G6PD deficiency in red blood cells of affected patients. Any sign of hemolysis is an indication to discontinue drug. Hemolysis ceases when drug withdrawn.

Hepatitis: Chronic active hepatitis has been observed. Onset may be insidious; therefore, monitor patients receiving long-term therapy for changes in liver function.

Use in pregnancy, lactation: Safety not established. Use in women of childbearing potential only when clearly needed and when potential benefits outweigh unknown possible hazards to the fetus. Drug should be administered with caution to pregnant patients with G6PD deficiency because of risk of hemolysis in the mother and fetus. Minimal concentrations are found in breast milk following therapeutic doses.

Safety for parenteral use in children under 12 not established.

PRECAUTIONS

Peripheral neuropathy may occur; this may become severe or irreversible. Fatalities have been reported. Predisposing conditions such as renal impairment, anemia, diabetes, electrolyte imbalance, vitamin B deficiency, and debilitating disease may enhance such occurrence.

Superinfection: Pseudomonas is the organism most commonly implicated in superinfections.

DRUG INTERACTIONS

Anticholinergic drugs and **food** increase bioavailability by delaying gastric emptying and increasing absorption. Nitrofurantoin may antagonize the antibacterial effects of **nalidixic acid.** The clinical significance of this is not known. **Magnesium trisilicate** may delay or decrease absorption.

Drug/lab tests: May cause false-positive tests for serum glucose, bilirubin, alkaline phosphatase, blood urea nitrogen. Elevation of urinary creatinine and a false-positive urine glucose determination using Benedict's reagent may also occur.

ADVERSE REACTIONS

GI: Most frequent are anorexia, nausea, emesis (with parenteral use, these are related to the infusion rate). Less frequent are abdominal pain and diarrhea.

Hepatic: Rarely, hepatitis is a dose-related toxic reaction that can be minimized by decreased dosage, especially in females. Active chronic hepatitis, cholestatic jaundice, and cholestatic hepatitis have been reported.

Pulmonary sensitivity reactions (acute, subacute, chronic): Acute reaction is manifested by fever, chills, cough, chest pain, dyspnea, pulmonary infiltration with consolidation of pleural effusion on x-ray, and eosinophilia. Acute reactions usually occur within the first week of treatment and resolve with cessation of therapy. Subacute or chronic pulmonary reaction is associated with prolonged therapy. Insidious onset of malaise, dyspnea on exertion, cough, altered pulmonary function, and x-ray or histologic findings of diffuse interstitial pneumonitis, fibrosis, or both are common manifestations. Fever is rarely prominent. Severity of these chronic pulmonary reactions and degree of their resolution appear to be related to duration of therapy after first clinical signs appear. Pulmonary function may be permanently impaired, even after cessation of drug therapy. This risk is greater when pulmonary reactions are not recognized early.

Dermatologic: Maculopapular, erythematous, or eczematous eruption; pruritus; urticaria; angioedema; rarely, exfoliative dermatitis and erythema multiforme.

Other sensitivity reactions: Anaphylaxis; asthmatic attack in those with history of asthma; drug fever; arthralgia.

Hematologic: Rarely, hemolytic anemia due to G6PD deficiency has been reported. Granulocytopenia, leukopenia, eosinophilia, megaloblastic anemia. Return of blood picture to normal has followed cessation of therapy.

Neurologic: Peripheral neuropathy, headache, dizziness, nystagmus, drowsiness, vertigo.

Miscellaneous: Transient alopecia, superinfections in GI tract by resistant organisms, hypotension, muscular aches, pancreatitis.

DOSAGE

Oral: May be given with food or milk to minimize GI upset. In acute infections, full doses should be given for 10 to 14 days. Continue for at least 3 days after sterile urine is obtained.

Adults: 50 mg to 100 mg qid (5–7 mg/kg/24 hours, not to exceed 400 mg). For long-term suppressive therapy, reduced dosage (25–50 mg qid) is usually sufficient.

Children: 5 mg/kg to 7 mg/kg/24 hours given in divided doses qid. For long-term suppressive therapy, 1 mg/kg/24 hours given in single or two divided doses is usually adequate. Contraindicated in children under 1 month.

Parenteral (IV use only): Patients weighing over 120 lb—180 mg bid. *Patients weighing less than 120 lb*—3 mg/lb/day in two equal doses.

NURSING IMPLICATIONS

HISTORY
See Appendix 4.

PHYSICAL ASSESSMENT
Obtain vital signs; weight may be needed to calculate dosage. Culture and sensitivity are usually ordered. Other laboratory tests (*e.g.,* CBC, uri-

N

nalysis, renal- and hepatic-function studies) may also be appropriate.

ADMINISTRATION

Oral

Give with food, milk, or meals.

Drug is best taken at evenly spaced intervals around the clock (q6h).

If patient is unable to take tablet or capsule, notify physician before next dose is due. An oral suspension is available.

Parenteral

Given IV only, bid, usually at 12-hour intervals.

Preparation of injection: Dissolve just prior to use as follows: Add 20 ml of 5% Dextrose Injection, USP, or Sterile Water for Injection, USP, to vial of dry sterile powder.

To prepare final solution, each milliliter of the initial solution should be added to a minimum of 25 ml of parenteral fluid. If 180 mg is the prescribed dose, the minimal volume of the final solution is 500 ml. Physician must order IV solution and dilution directions.

Do not use solutions containing methyl and propyl parabens, phenol or cresol perservatives; these compounds cause powder to be precipitated out of solution.

Recommended administration of final solution: Give by IV drip at rate of 50 to 60 drops (2–3 ml)/minute, but physician may prescribe different rate of infusion.

The final solution should be used within 24 hours and should be protected from ultraviolet light and excessive heat. Mixing other antibacterials in the same solution is not recommended.

ONGOING ASSESSMENTS AND NURSING MANAGEMENT

Monitor vital signs q4h; observe for adverse reactions; measure intake and output; compare present symptoms with data base.

If nausea or vomiting occurs despite giving drug with food or milk, notify physician.

CLINICAL ALERT: Observe for signs of a pulmonary reaction. An acute pulmonary reaction is manifested by fever, chills, cough, chest pain, and dyspnea. During prolonged therapy, observe for a subacute or chronic pulmonary reaction, manifested by an insidious onset of malaise, dyspnea on exertion, and cough. Report occurrence to physician immediately.

Peripheral neuropathy may occur and may become severe and irreversible (fatalities have been reported). Withhold next dose of drug and contact physician if patient complains of numbness, tingling, weakness, or other sensations in the extremities.

Although an increase in fluid intake is often recommended in UTIs, check with physician before forcing fluids because drug's antibacterial activity is dependent on its concentration in the urine.

Drug action is enhanced in acid urine. Physician may order urinary acidifiers (*e.g.,* ammonium chloride, ascorbic acid).

Observe for signs of superinfection of GU tract (*e.g.,* sudden onset of original symptoms or development of fever, dysuria, suprapubic abdominal pain or tenderness, frequent urination).

Culture and sensitivity tests are recommended during drug administration. They may also be performed if superinfection occurs.

Measure intake and output, especially if patient is acutely ill.

Diabetic patient: If urine glucose is being tested with Benedict's reagent, a false-positive reaction may occur; a different method of testing must be used.

PATIENT AND FAMILY INFORMATION

Take at evenly spaced intervals around the clock (preferably q6h) unless physician orders otherwise.

Complete full course of therapy even if symptoms are relieved. Do not discontinue drug without notifying the physician.

May cause GI upset (*e.g.,* nausea, vomiting, anorexia, abdominal pain); take with food or milk, which increases absorption and decreases GI upset.

Do not take antacids while taking this drug unless a specific product is approved by the physician.

May cause brown or rust-yellow discoloration of the urine; this is not harmful.

Notify physician or nurse immediately if fever, chills, cough, chest pain, difficult breathing, skin rash, numbness or tingling of fingers or toes, or intolerable GI upset occurs.

Nitrofurazone Rx

soluble dressing: 0.2%	Furacin, *Generic*
cream, topical: 0.2%	Furacin

INDICATIONS

Adjunctive therapy of second- or third-degree burns when bacterial resistance to other agents is a real or potential problem; skin grafting when bacterial contamination may cause graft rejection and/or donor site infection, particularly in hospitals with historical resistant bacterial epidemics. There is no known evidence of effectiveness in treatment of minor burns or surface bacterial infections involving wounds, cutaneous ulcers, or various pyrodermas.

CONTRAINDICATIONS
Hypersensitivity.

ACTIONS
A synthetic nitrofuran with a broad antibacterial spectrum. Bactericidal against most bacteria commonly causing surface infections, including many that have become antibiotic resistant. Acts by inhibiting enzymes necessary for carbohydrate metabolism. Topically it is without appreciable toxicity to human cells.

WARNINGS
Use the soluble burn dressing with caution in those with known or suspected renal impairment. The polyethylene glycol present in the base can be absorbed through denuded skin and may not be excreted normally by a compromised kidney. This may lead to symptoms of progressive renal impairment, increased BUN, anion gap, and metabolic acidosis.

Safety for use during pregnancy not established. Not recommended for treatment of women of childbearing potential unless need for therapeutic benefit is greater than the unknown hazards to the fetus.

PRECAUTIONS
Use may result in bacterial or fungal overgrowth of nonsusceptible organisms. Such overgrowth may lead to secondary infection. Take appropriate measures if superinfection occurs. Use with caution in individuals with G6PD deficiency.

ADVERSE REACTIONS
Not significantly toxic by topical application. Contact dermatitis and sensitivity may occur. Treatment of sensitization is not distinctive; general measures commonly used for a variety of sensitization reactions are adequate except for rare instance of severe contact dermatitis, in which steroid administration may be indicated.

DOSAGE
Soluble dressing: *Burns*—Apply directly to lesion or place on gauze. Reapply once daily or weekly. Also prepares burns and other lesions for grafting.

Cream: Apply directly to lesion or place on gauze. Reapply once daily or every few days.

NURSING IMPLICATIONS

HISTORY
Cause of burn (thermal, chemical, electrical, friction); health history; emergency measures used to treat burn (when applicable).

PHYSICAL ASSESSMENT
Note and record location and appearance of involved area(s). Physician determines degree of burn, percentage of body involvement. Depending on extent and severity, a variety of laboratory tests may be ordered (*e.g.,* serum electrolytes, renal-function studies, total protein, alkaline phosphatase).

ADMINISTRATION
Apply as directed by physician. See also *Dosage, above.*

Physician will order method of cleaning affected area prior to application of nitrofurazone.

Use aseptic technique when applying drug.

A dressing may or may not be ordered.

Apply drug only to affected area.

When removing previous dressing, take care to remove dressing slowly and *gently.* If dressing is firmly affixed to affected area, soaking the gauze with normal saline (or solution ordered by physician) may facilitate removal.

ONGOING ASSESSMENTS AND NURSING MANAGEMENT
If dressing is changed and drug applied daily, inspect affected area. If redness, irritation, or infection is noted, inform physician.

Note patient reports of irritation or itching (may indicate sensitivity), a new odor present around burned area, and presence of purulent exudate (may indicate superinfection). Notify physician if these should occur.

Depending on severity and extent of burn, additional treatment modalities and nursing management may be necessary.

PATIENT AND FAMILY INFORMATION
NOTE: If physician orders a dressing placed over burned area, patient should receive instructions regarding aseptic technique, type of dressing to be purchased (usually sterile gauze), and method of drug application.

Apply as directed by physician.

Notify physician if condition worsens or if irritation occurs.

N

Nitroglycerin

See Nitrates.

Nitroprusside Sodium Rx

powder for injection: 50 mg/vial	Nipride, Nitropress, *Generic*

INDICATIONS

Immediate reduction of blood pressure in hypertensive crisis. Concomitant oral antihypertensive medication should be started while hypertensive emergency is being brought under control. There are no contraindications to using nitroprusside simultaneously with oral antihypertensive medications.

Also indicated for producing controlled hypotension during anesthesia to reduce bleeding in surgical procedures when surgeon and anesthesiologist deem it appropriate.

Investigational uses: Vasodilator effect of drug, either alone or in combination with dopamine, has been used in those with severe refractory CHF. Concomitant administration of these agents has also been used in those with acute MI. Also used to treat lactic acidosis due to impaired peripheral perfusion. May be used to attenuate vasoconstrictor (alpha-adrenergic) effects of dopamine and norepinephrine.

CONTRAINDICATIONS

Not used in treatment of compensatory hypertension (*e.g.,* arteriovenous shunt or coarctation of the aorta). Use to produce controlled hypotension in surgery contraindicated in those with known inadequate cerebral circulation. Not intended for use during emergency surgery on moribund patients.

ACTIONS

A potent, immediately acting, IV hypotensive agent. Hypotensive effects are caused by peripheral vasodilatation (arterial and venous) as a result of a direct action on blood vessels, independent of autonomic innervation.

Has an immediate onset of action; within 30 to 60 seconds of beginning of infusion, a reduction in blood pressure may be seen. Hypotensive effects may become maximum in 1 to 2 minutes. The infusion flow rate may be increased gradually until the desired reduction in blood pressure is achieved. Following discontinuation of nitroprusside infusion, blood pressure returns to pretreatment levels within 1 to 10 minutes.

Nitroprusside is converted to cyanmethemoglobin and free cyanide, which is converted to thiocyanate in the liver. Thiocyanate is eliminated by the kidneys and has a half-life of approximately 4 days in those with normal renal function. The rate of conversion from cyanide to thiocyanate is dependent on the availability of sulfur, usually as thiosulfate.

WARNINGS

Not for direct injection. Use only as an infusion with 5% Dextrose in Water. If adequate reduction in blood pressure is not obtained in 10 minutes with 10 mcg/kg/minute, drug should be discontinued. Hypertensive patients are more sensitive than normotensive subjects to the effect of the drug.

If excessive amount of drug used or sulfur (*i.e.,* thiosulfate) supplies are depleted, cyanide toxicity can occur (see *Overdosage*).

If nitroprusside infusion is to be extended, and renal impairment is present, do not exceed recommended maximum infusion rates of 10 mcg/kg/minute. If, in the course of therapy, increased tolerance to the drug (as shown by the need for higher infusion rate) develops, monitor blood acid–base balance, because metabolic acidosis is the earliest and most reliable evidence of cyanide toxicity. If signs of metabolic acidosis appear, drug is discontinued and an alternate drug administered.

Although serum thiocyanate levels do not reflect cyanide toxicity, levels should be monitored daily, especially in those with renal dysfunction.

Because cyanide is metabolized by hepatic enzymes, it may accumulate in those with severe liver impairment. Nitroprusside is used with caution in these patients. Because thiocyanate inhibits uptake and binding of iodine, drug is used with caution in patients with hypothyroidism. Use with caution in those with severe renal impairment.

Safety for women who are or who may become pregnant not established. Use only when potential benefits outweigh possible hazards to mother and child. It is not known whether drug is excreted in human milk. Caution is used when administering to a nursing woman.

Use for controlled hypotension during anesthesia: Tolerance to blood loss, anemia, and hypovolemia may be diminished. If possible, preexisting anemia and hypovolemia should be corrected prior to using controlled hypotension.

PRECAUTIONS

Adequate facilities, equipment, and personnel should be available for frequent monitoring of blood pressure. Use with caution and initially in low doses in elderly patients, because they may be more sensitive to hypotensive effects. Young, vigorous males may require larger than ordinary doses for hypotensive anesthesia, but infusion rate of 10 mcg/kg/minute should not be exceeded.

DRUG INTERACTIONS

Ganglionic blocking agents, volatile liquid anesthetics (*e.g.,* halothane and enflurane), and **circulatory depressants** augment drug's hypotensive effect. Patient receiving concomitant **antihypertensive medications** is more sensitive to the hypotensive effect; dosage is adjusted accordingly.

ADVERSE REACTIONS

Nausea, diaphoresis, apprehension, headache, restlessness, perspiration, muscle twitching, retrosternal discomfort, palpitations, dizziness, and abdominal pain have been noted with too-rapid reduction of blood pressure. These symptoms rapidly disappeared with slowing or temporary discontinuation of the infusion and did not reappear with continued slower rate of administration. Irritation at infusion site may occur. Methemoglobinemia has been reported to occur following administration. Antiplatelet effects, which may cause bleeding, have been noted.

OVERDOSAGE

Symptoms: First signs are those of profound hypotension. Overdosage may lead to cyanide toxicity. Metabolic acidosis and increasing tolerance to drug are early signs of overdosage. These may be associated with or followed by dyspnea, headache, vomiting, dizziness, ataxia, loss of consciousness. Infusion should be immediately discontinued. Other signs of cyanide poisoning are coma, imperceptible pulse, absent reflexes, widely dilated pupils, pink color, distant heart sounds, and shallow breathing. Oxygen alone will not provide relief.

Treatment: In cases of massive overdosage, when signs of cyanide toxicity are present, use the following regimen: Discontinue nitroprusside administration. Administer amyl nitrite inhalations for 15 to 30 seconds each minute until a 3% sodium nitrite solution can be prepared for IV administration. Inject sodium nitrite 3% solution IV at a rate not exceeding 2.5 ml/minute to 5 ml/minute, up to a total dose of 10 ml to 15 ml. Monitor blood pressure. Following the above, inject sodium thiosulfate IV, 12.5 g in 50 ml of 5% Dextrose in Water over a 10-minute period. Because signs of overdosage may reappear, observe for several hours. If signs of overdosage reappear, repeat sodium nitrite and thiosulfate injections in one-half the above doses. During administration of nitrites and later when thiocyanate formation is taking place, blood pressure may drop but can be corrected with vasopressor agents.

It has been reported that hydroxocobalamin can prevent cyanide toxicity. The thiocyanate ion is readily removed by hemodialysis.

DOSAGE

For use *only* by continuous IV infusion.

Adults and children: In those not receiving antihypertensive drugs, average dose is 3 mcg/kg/minute (range—0.5–10 mcg/kg/min). At this rate, blood pressure can usually be lowered by about 30% to 40% below pretreatment diastolic levels and stabilized. In those receiving concomitant antihypertensive medications, smaller doses are required. In order to avoid excessive thiocyanate levels and lessen possibility of a precipitous drop in blood pressure, infusion rates greater than 10 mcg/kg/minute should rarely be used. See *Administration.*

NURSING IMPLICATIONS

HISTORY

When possible, obtain (from patient and/or chart) history of hypertension (including etiology, if known), concomitant drug therapy, and current treatment modalities.

PHYSICAL ASSESSMENT

Obtain blood pressure, pulse, and respirations. Obtain most recent weight from chart for dosage calculation. Laboratory tests may be ordered, based on patient's physical status, diagnosis, contributing factors, and so on.

ADMINISTRATION

Preparation of solution: Dissolve contents of 50-mg vial in 2 ml or 3 ml of 5% Dextrose in Water.

Dilute the prepared stock solution in 250 ml to 1000 ml of 5% Dextrose in Water and promptly wrap in aluminum foil or other opaque material to protect from light. Administration set need not be covered; tubing should be observed for color changes in the infusion.

The freshly prepared solution for infusion has a very faint brownish tint. If it is highly colored (blue, green, dark red), it should be discarded.

Administer by an infusion pump, microdrip regulator or other similar device that will allow precise measurement of flow rate.

Because infusion may be temporarily discontinued because of blood pressure response, signs of overdosage, and so on, drug should be administered by either a primary or secondary line.

Physician must order the following: volume of IV fluid to which stock solution is added (250–1000 ml); infusion rate (either as ml/min or mcg/min); additional IV fluid to run KVO. Physician may also specify whether an infusion pump, microdrip, or other device should be used.

N

50 mg added to 250 ml = 0.2 mg/ml or 200 mcg/ml

50 mg added to 500 ml = 0.1 mg/ml or 100 mcg/ml

50 mg added to 1000 ml = 0.05 mg/ml or 50 mcg/ml

The infusion fluid used for administration of nitroprusside should not be used for administration of any other drug.

Storage: Protect from light. Store below 30°C (86°F). Avoid freezing.

Administration: Have airway, suction equipment immediately available.

Physician may order amyl nitrite and 3% sodium nitrite solution, 12.5 g sodium thiosulfate, and equipment for administration kept at bedside for immediate use if cyanide toxicity occurs.

Use large vein, when possible.

Take care to avoid extravasation.

Obtain blood pressure, pulse, and respirations immediately before administration. Record on flow sheet.

Concomitant administration of an oral antihypertensive agent may be ordered.

ONGOING ASSESSMENTS AND NURSING MANAGEMENT

Hypotensive effects may become maximal in 1 to 2 minutes.

Monitor blood pressure and pulse frequently (every 30–60 seconds) during time of infusion of nitroprusside; record on flow sheets.

Record infusion rate.

Follow physician's guidelines regarding increase or decrease in infusion rate based on blood pressure. Rate of administration should be adjusted to maintain desired effect, as determined by frequent blood pressure determinations. Blood pressure should not be allowed to drop at a too-rapid rate and systolic pressure should not be lowered below 60 mm Hg in hypertensive emergencies. Infusion may be continued until patient can be safely treated with oral antihypertensive medications alone.

CLINICAL ALERT: Metabolic acidosis (see *Overdosage*) and increasing tolerance to drug are early indications of overdosage.

Closely observe patient for development of thiocyanate accumulation: tinnitus, blurred vision (subjective complaints) and delirium (confusion, hyperreflexia, convulsions). Also observe patient for signs of cyanide toxicity: coma, imperceptible pulse, absent reflexes, widely dilated pupils, pink color, distant heart sounds, shallow breathing. Closely observe for other signs of overdosage that may be associated with or follow signs of metabolic acidosis and increasing tolerance to the drug. These other signs include dyspnea, headache, vomiting, dizziness, ataxia, and loss of consciousness.

Notify physician immediately of development of any of the above.

If adequate blood-pressure reduction is not obtained in 10 minutes, administration should be stopped.

When administration is stopped (for any reason), run IV fluid to KVO or as ordered by physician.

Observe for adverse reactions that have been noted to occur with too-rapid infusion rate (see *Adverse Reactions*). Slow infusion rate and notify physician immediately if adverse reactions are noted.

Inspect infusion site for signs of irritation; inform physician if apparent.

A bleeding tendency may occur because of antiplatelet effects; notify physician if any type of bleeding is noted.

Measure intake and output.

Following discontinuation of infusion, continue to monitor blood pressure and pulse at 3- to 10-minute intervals for next 1 to 2 hours, or as ordered. Blood pressure returns to pretreatment levels within 1 to 10 minutes.

Additional nursing assessments and management may be necessary and are dependent on patient's clinical status, other concomitant treatment modalities, response to drug, and so on.

Nitrous Oxide

See Anesthetics, General, Gases.

Nonsteroidal Anti-inflammatory Agents

Fenoprofen Calcium Rx

capsules: 200 mg, 300 mg	Nalfon
tablets: 600 mg	Nalfon

Ibuprofen Rx, otc

tablets: 200 mg (*otc*)	Advil, Nuprin
tablets: 300 mg, 600 mg (*Rx*)	Motrin
tablets: 400 mg (*Rx*)	Motrin, Rufen

Indomethacin Rx

capsules: 25 mg, 50 mg	Indocin
capsules, sustained release: 75 mg	Indocin SR

Meclofenamate Sodium Rx

capsules: 50 mg, 100 mg	Meclomen

Mefenamic Acid Rx

capsules: 250 mg	Ponstel

Naproxen Rx

tablets: 275 mg	Anaprox (as naproxen sodium)
tablets: 250 mg, 375 mg, 500 mg	Naprosyn

Piroxicam Rx

capsules: 10 mg, 20 mg	Feldene

Sulindac Rx

tablets: 150 mg, 200 mg	Clinoril

Tolmetin Sodium Rx

tablets: 200 mg	Tolectin
capsules: 400 mg	Tolectin DS

INDICATIONS

See below for specific indications for individual drugs.

Concomitant therapy: Use of these agents in combination with gold salts has demonstrated additional therapeutic benefit. However, it cannot be inferred that these agents potentiate the effect of gold on the underlying disease. Whether they can be used in conjunction with partially effective doses of corticosteroid for a "steroid-sparing" effect, and result in greater improvement, has not been studied. Use in conjunction with salicylates is not recommended; there does not appear to be any greater benefit over that achieved with aspirin alone and the potential for adverse effects is increased. Use of aspirin with other anti-inflammatory agents may result in a decrease in blood levels of the nonaspirin drug.

Because of analgesic and anti-inflammatory effects, these agents may be used for relief of mild to moderate pain such as primary dysmenorrhea, post-extraction dental pain, postsurgical episiotomy pain, and soft-tissue athletic injuries such as strains and sprains.

FENOPROFEN CALCIUM

Relief of signs and symptoms of rheumatoid arthritis and osteoarthritis (acute flares and long-term management); relief of mild to moderate pain.

IBUPROFEN

Relief of signs and symptoms of rheumatoid arthritis and osteoarthritis (acute flares and long-term management); relief of mild to moderate pain; treatment of primary dysmenorrhea.

INDOMETHACIN

Moderate to severe rheumatoid arthritis (including flares of chronic disease); moderate to severe ankylosing spondylitis; moderate to severe osteoarthritis; acute painful shoulder (bursitis or tendinitis); acute gouty arthritis. Sustained-release form is not indicated for acute gouty arthritis.

Because of potential for adverse reactions, particularly at high dosage levels, use in rheumatoid arthritis or osteoarthritis in adults should be carefully considered for active disease unresponsive to adequate trial with salicylates and other measures, such as appropriate rest.

Investigational uses: Has been used for pharmacologic closure of persistent patent ductus arteriosus in infants as alternative to surgical ligation. Clinical closure has occurred within 24 to 30 hours without untoward effects in majority of neonates given single doses of 0.3 mg/kg or one or more doses of 0.1 mg/kg via retention enema or nasogastric tube. Higher doses, while also producing more dramatic improvement, have produced transient impairment of renal function. Isolated incidences of gastric perforation and GI bleeding also reported.

Indomethacin also suppresses uterine activity by inhibiting prostaglandin synthesis and has been used to prevent premature labor. Prolonged maternal administration for this purpose could result in prenatal ductal closure and increased neonatal morbidity. Such use should be avoided.

MECLOFENAMIDE SODIUM

Acute and chronic rheumatoid arthritis and osteoarthritis. Not recommended as initial drug for treatment because of GI side-effects including diarrhea, which is sometimes severe. Selection requires careful assessment of benefit–risk ratio.

MEFENAMIC ACID

Relief of moderate pain when therapy will not exceed 1 week; treatment of primary dysmenorrhea.

NAPROXEN

Treatment of signs and symptoms of mild to moderately severe, acute or chronic, musculoskeletal and soft-tissue inflammation; relief of mild to moderate pain; treatment of primary dysmenorrhea.

PIROXICAM

Acute or long-term use in relief of signs and symptoms of osteoarthritis and rheumatoid arthritis.

N

SULINDAC

Acute or long-term use in relief of signs and symptoms of the following: osteoarthritis, rheumatoid arthritis, ankylosing spondylitis, acute painful shoulder (acute subacromial bursitis/supraspinatus tendinitis), acute gouty arthritis.

TOLMETIN SODIUM

Treatment of acute flares and in long-term management of rheumatoid arthritis and osteoarthritis; treatment of juvenile rheumatoid arthritis.

CONTRAINDICATIONS

Hypersensitivity. Because potential exists for cross-sensitivity to other nonsteroidal anti-inflammatory drugs, do not give to patients in whom aspirin or other nonsteroidal anti-inflammatory drugs have induced symptoms of asthma, urticaria, nasal polyps, angioedema, or bronchospastic reaction.

Do not use **fenoprofen** or **mefenamic acid** in those with history of significantly impaired renal function. **Mefenamic acid** is contraindicated in those with ulceration or chronic inflammation of either the upper or the lower GI tract.

ACTIONS

These nonsteroidal anti-inflammatory agents also have analgesic and antipyretic activities. Exact mode of action not known; however, therapeutic effects are not due to pituitary–adrenal stimulation. Inhibition of prostaglandin synthetase has been demonstrated, but exact significance of this effect not fully understood. Although most are used primarily for their anti-inflammatory effects, they are effective analgesics and are useful for relief of mild to moderate pain.

These agents are rapidly and almost completely absorbed. In general, food delays absorption but does not affect the total amount absorbed. Excretion is via the kidney, primarily as metabolites. All of these agents are highly protein bound.

Studies in rheumatoid and osteoarthritis show these agents were comparable to aspirin in controlling signs and symptoms of disease activity and, with the exception of indomethacin, were associated with a significant reduction in milder GI side-effects. These agents may be well tolerated in some patients who have had GI side-effects with aspirin, but such patients should be followed for signs and symptoms of ulceration and bleeding. Indomethacin appears to have greatest incidence of GI and CNS side-effects.

Rheumatoid arthritis: These agents do *not* alter the progressive course of the underlying disease. In general, they may be used in conjunction with corticosteroid or gold compounds.

Juvenile rheumatoid arthritis: Tolmetin is the only agent specifically approved for this indication. It has been shown to be comparable to aspirin in controlling disease activity, with a similar incidence of side-effects.

Dysmenorrhea: An excess of prostaglandins is thought to produce uterine hyperactivity. Although exact mechanism of action is unknown, these agents appear to inhibit prostaglandin synthesis. Lower prostaglandin levels in plasma and endometrium prevent symptoms of primary dysmenorrhea.

WARNINGS

Anaphylactic reactions have occurred in those with known aspirin hypersensitivity.

GI effects: Administer under close supervision to those prone to upper GI disease. Peptic ulcer and GI bleeding, sometimes severe and occasionally fatal, have been reported. In patients with active peptic ulcer and active rheumatoid arthritis, attempts should be made to treat arthritis with nonulcerogenic drugs such as gold. If these agents must be given, an appropriate ulcer regimen is instituted and patient observed closely for signs of ulcer perforation or GI bleeding. The risk of continuing therapy in face of GI symptoms must be weighed against possible benefits. GI bleeding without obvious ulcer formation and perforation of preexisting sigmoid lesions (*e.g.*, diverticulum, carcinoma) have occurred. Increased abdominal pain in ulcerative colitis patients and development of ulcerative colitis and regional ileitis have been reported rarely.

Do not give **indomethacin** to those with active GI lesions or history of recurrent GI lesions except under circumstances that warrant the very high risk and when patient can be monitored very closely. If diarrhea occurs with **mefenamic acid,** dosage is reduced or drug temporarily discontinued. Some patients may be unable to tolerate further therapy with this drug.

Use in elderly: Age appears to increase possibility of adverse reactions; these drugs used with greater care and initiated with reduced dosages.

Use in impaired renal function: Use with caution because these drugs are primarily eliminated by the kidney. Monitoring of serum creatinine and/or creatinine clearance is advised. Dosage is reduced to avoid excessive drug accumulation.

Renal effects: Untoward renal effects are more likely to occur in those with preexisting renal dysfunction. Adverse renal effects, including glomerular nephritis, interstitial nephritis, nephrotic syndrome, and renal papillary necrosis and elevations of serum creatinine and BUN have been reported to occur with these agents. There have been reports of GU tract problems in those taking **fenoprofen.** Most frequently reported problems have been episodes of dysuria, cystitis, hematuria, allergic nephritis, and nephrotic syndrome. This syndrome may be preceded by appearance of fever, rash, arthralgia, oliguria, azotemia and may progress to anuria. Rapid recovery followed early recognition and withdrawal of drug. Treatment also included use of steroids and dialysis. In those with possibly compromised renal function, periodic renal-function tests are recommended. In those with impaired renal function, there have been reports of worsening of renal impairment and some development of hyperkalemia associated with therapy with **indomethacin.** In those with sodium retention associated with hepatic disease or CHF, precipitation of acute renal failure has been reported.

CNS effects: **Indomethacin** may aggravate depression or other psychiatric disturbances, epilepsy, and parkinsonism; use with caution in patients with these conditions. If severe CNS adverse reactions develop, discontinue drug. Indomethacin may also cause headaches. If headache persists despite dosage reduction, use is discontinued.

Use in pregnancy, lactation: Safety not established. Most of these drugs are excreted in breast milk; nursing should not be undertaken while patient taking these agents. Use during pregnancy, especially the third trimester, should be avoided because nonsteroidal anti-inflammatory agents, which inhibit prostaglandin synthesis, may cause constriction of the ductus arteriosis and possibly other untoward effects on the fetus.

PRECAUTIONS

Safety and effectiveness of these agents not established in those rheumatoid arthritis patients who are designated as Functional Class IV (incapacitated, largely or wholly bedridden, or confined to wheelchair, little or no self-care). If steroid dosage is reduced or eliminated during therapy, dosage is reduced slowly and patient observed for evidence of adverse effects, including adrenal insufficiency and exacerbation of symptoms.

Effects on platelet aggregation: The agents can inhibit platelet aggregation, but effect is quantitively less and of shorter duration than that seen with aspirin. These agents shown to prolong bleeding time (but within the normal range) in normal subjects. This effect may be exaggerated in those with underlying hemostatic defects; therefore these drugs are used with caution in persons with intrinsic coagulation defects and those on anticoagulant therapy.

Hematologic effects: Decreases in hemoglobin and/or hematocrit levels have occurred, but they rarely require discontinuation of therapy. If anemia suspected in patients on long-term therapy, hemo-globin and hematocrit are values determined. Those with initial hemoglobin of 10 g/dl or less who are to receive long-term therapy should have hemoglobin values determined frequently. Low WBC rarely observed. These were transient and usually returned to normal while therapy continued. Persistent leukopenia, granulocytopenia or thrombocytopenia warrants further evaluation and may require discontinuing drug.

Cardiovascular effects: These agents have been shown to cause some water retention. Peripheral edema has been reported. Use with caution in those with compromised cardiac function, hypertension, or other conditions predisposing them to fluid retention.

Ophthalmologic effects: Because of reported adverse eye findings, patients who develop eye complaints during therapy should have ophthalmologic studies performed. Reported effects included blurred and/or diminished vision, scotomata and/or changes in color vision, corneal deposits, and retinal disturbances including those of the macula. Therapy is discontinued if ocular changes are noted. Blurred vision may be a significant symptom and warrants a thorough ophthalmologic examination. Because these changes may be symptomatic, periodic ophthalmologic examinations are recommended during prolonged therapy.

Infection: **Indomethacin** may mask usual signs of infection and is used with care in presence of existing controlled infection.

Hepatic effects: Liver-function abnormalities include elevations in serum transaminase, LDH, and alkaline phosphatase values. These effects are usually transient and reversible. Use with caution and monitor hepatic-function tests in those with impaired liver function.

Safety for use of **fenoprofen** in those with impaired hearing is not established. Periodic auditory function tests are recommended during chronic therapy.

If rash occurs with **mefenamic acid** therapy, drug is discontinued promptly.

DRUG INTERACTIONS

These drugs have an affinity for serum albumin and may displace other drugs which are also bound to albumin. Patients receiving these agents concomitantly with **hydantoins, sulfonamides,** or **sulfonylureas** should be observed for signs of toxicity to these drugs.

In those receiving **coumarin-type anticoagulants,** these agents could prolong the prothrombin time. Daily prothrombin times are required whenever any drugs are added to or taken away from the treatment regimen of patients taking oral anticoagulants.

Meclofenamate enhances the effect of warfarin. To prevent excessive prolongation of the prothrombin time, reduce dosage of warfin when meclofenamate is given.

Do not administer **sodium bicarbonate** with **tolmetin. Phenobarbital** may be associated with a decrease in plasma half-life of **fenoprofen;** when added or withdrawn, dosage adjustment may be required. **Probenecid** has been reported to increase plasma half-life of some of these agents; a lower total daily dosage may produce a satisfactory therapeutic effect.

Indomethacin may reduce natriuretic and antihypertensive effect of **furosemide** and **thiazide diuretics** in some patients; may blunt antihypertensive effect of **beta-adrenergic blocking agents;** blocks **furosemide**-induced increase in plasma renin activity; elevates plasma **lithium** and reduces renal lithium clearance in those with steady-state plasma lithium concentrations. Concomitant administration of indomethacin and **triamterene** may result in reversible acute renal failure. Patients receiving indomethacin and these other agents are closely monitored.

Drug/lab test interactions: Administration of **naproxen** may result in increased urinary values for 17-ketogenic steroids; therapy should be discontinued 72 hours before **adrenal-function tests** are performed. May also interfere with some urinary assays of 5-HIAA. Metabolites of **tolmetin** in urine have been found to give positive tests for **proteinuria** when certain tests are used; no interference is seen in tests using dye-impregnated commercially available reagent test strips. A false-positive for urinary bile using the **diazo tablet test** may result after administration of **mefenamic acid.**

ADVERSE REACTIONS

GI

Nausea, vomiting, diarrhea, constipation. Diarrhea reported in those taking **sulindac** (3%–9%), **meclofenamate** (10%–33%). Vomiting reported in those taking **fenoprofen** (3%–9%) and **meclofenamate** (11%).

GI pain: Epigastric pain, heartburn, abdominal distress/discomfort, indigestion, abdominal cramps or pain, dyspepsia, gastritis, gastroenteritis, proctitis.

Ulcer: Gastric or duodenal ulcer with bleeding and/or perforation, intestinal ulceration associated with stenosis and obstruction, ulcerative stomatitis, gingival ulcers.

Bleeding: Occult blood in stool; GI bleeding without peptic ulcer; melena; perforation and hemorrhage of esophagus, stomach, duodenum, or small intestine; hematemesis; rectal bleeding.

Hepatic: Cholestatic jaundice; toxic hepatitis, and jaundice with some fatalities; mild hepatic toxicity; abnormal liver-function tests.

Other: Fullness of GI tract (bloating/flatulence), stomatitis, anorexia, dry mouth, sore or dry mucous membranes, pancreatitis.

CNS

Dizziness and headache are most common CNS reactions. Dizziness occurs in about 3% to 9%; headache reported in 10% taking **indomethacin** and **tolmetin.** Headache and somnolence reported in 15% taking **fenoprofen.** Drowsiness reported in 3% to 9% taking **naproxen.**

Dizziness/anxiety: Lightheadedness; vertigo; nervousness; tension.

Neurologic: Paresthesias; peripheral neuropathy; tremor; convulsions; aggravation of epilepsy, parkinsonism; myalgia; muscle weakness; asthenia; malaise; fatigue.

Sleep disturbances: Insomnia, somnolence, drowsiness, dream abnormalities.

Psychiatric: Confusion; inability to concentrate; depression; emotional lability; psychic disturbances, including psychotic episodes; depersonalization.

Cardiovascular

CHF, angiitis, fall in blood pressure, elevated blood pressure, palpitations, arrhythmias, dyspnea, peripheral edema, fluid retention, chest pain.

Renal

Hematuria; cystitis; UTI; symptoms of cystitis without UTI; azotemia; elevated BUN; elevated or decreased creatinine; polyuria; dysuria; oliguria; anuria; acute renal failure in those with impaired renal function; renal papillary necrosis; nephrosis; nephrotic syndrome; glomerular, interstitial, and allergic nephritis.

Hematologic

Neutropenia, eosinophilia, leukopenia, pancytopenia, thrombocytopenia, agranulocytosis, granulocytopenia, aplastic anemia, hemolytic anemia, anemia secondary to obvious or occult bleeding, epistaxis, hemorrhage, petechiae, bruising, bone-marrow depression.

Special senses

Visual disturbances, amblyopia (blurred and/or diminished vision), scotomata, diplopia, swollen or irritated eyes, photophobia, toxic optic neuropathy, corneal deposits, retinal degeneration, periorbital edema, reversible loss of color vision, tinnitus, hearing loss, ear pain. Tinnitus reported in 3% to 9% taking **naproxen.** Rhinitis and taste change also occurred.

Hypersensitivity

Asthma, anaphylaxis, bronchospasms, acute respiratory distress, dyspnea.

Dermatologic

Rash, erythema, urticaria, skin irritation and eruptions, vesiculobullous eruptions, toxic epidermal necrolysis, exfoliative dermatitis, erythema mul-

tiforme, Stevens-Johnson syndrome, erythema nodosum, angioneurotic edema, ecchymosis, purpura,
phototoxicity, onycholysis, alopecia, pruritus. Rash
reported in 3% to 9% taking **ibuprofen, sulindac,
meclofenamate.** Pruritus reported in 3% to 9% taking **naproxen, fenoprofen.**

Metabolic/endocrine

Decreased appetite, weight decrease or increase,
glycosuria, hyperglycemia, hypoglycemia, increased
need for insulin in a diabetic, flushing or sweating,
menstrual disorders, vaginal bleeding.

Miscellaneous

Thirst; pyrexia (fever, chills); vaginitis; aseptic
meningitis with fever and coma, syncope and coma.

Causal relationship unknown

Apthous ulceration of buccal mucosa, metallic
taste, cholelithiasis/cholecystitis, pseudomotor cerebri, disorientation, trigeminal neuralgia, neuritis, akathisia, hallucinations, personality changes, pulmonary edema, ECG changes, periarteritis, nocturia,
leukemia, conjunctivitis, optic neuritis, burning
tongue, serum sickness, lupus erythematosus, Henoch-Schönlein syndrome, gynecomastia, mastodynia, breast changes including enlargement and
tenderness, menorrhagia, lymphadenopathy, hemoptysis.

OVERDOSAGE

Employ supportive measures. Empty stomach by
inducing vomiting or by gastric lavage, followed by
administration of activated charcoal. Because these
agents are acidic and excreted in urine, it is theoretically beneficial to administer alkali and induce diuresis. Because these agents are strongly bound to
plasma proteins, hemodialysis and peritoneal dialysis may be of little value.

DOSAGE

FENOPROFEN CALCIUM

Do not exceed 3200 mg/day.

Rheumatoid arthritis, osteoarthritis: 300 mg to
600 mg tid or qid. Dosage is adjusted depending on
severity of symptoms. Improvement may be seen in
a few days but an additional 2 to 3 weeks may be
required to gauge full benefits of therapy.

Mild to moderate pain: 200 mg q4h to q6h, as
needed.

Children: Safety, efficacy not established.

IBUPROFEN

Do not exceed 2400 mg/day.

Rheumatoid arthritis, osteoarthritis: 300 mg to
600 mg tid or qid. Dosage is individualized. Therapeutic response may be seen in a few days to a
week but is most often observed within 2 weeks.

Mild to moderate pain: 200 mg to 400 mg q4h
to q6h as necessary.

Primary dysmenorrhea: 400 mg q4h as necessary.

Children: Safety, efficacy not established.

INDOMETHACIN

Adverse reactions appear to correlate with dose in
most, but not all, patients. Every effort is made to
determine smallest effective dose.

**Moderate to severe rheumatoid arthritis (includ-
ing acute flares of chronic disease), moderate to severe ankylosing spondylitis, moderate to severe osteoarthritis:** 25 mg two or three times a day. If this
is well tolerated, daily dose is increased by 25 mg or
50 mg if required by continuing symptoms at
weekly intervals until satisfactory response obtained
or total daily dose of 150 mg to 200 mg is reached.
Doses above this amount generally do not increase
drug effectiveness. In those with persistent night
pain and/or morning stiffness, giving a large portion, up to maximum of 100 mg of total daily dose,
H.S. may be helpful. In acute flares of chronic rheumatoid arthritis, it may be necessary to increase
dosage by 25 mg or 50 mg daily. If minor adverse
effects develop, dosage is reduced rapidly to a tolerated dose and patient observed closely. If serious
adverse reactions occur, drug discontinued. After
acute phase is under control, attempt is made to reduce daily dose.

Acute painful shoulder (bursitis and/or tendinitis): 75 mg/day to 150 mg/day in three or four divided doses. Drug is discontinued after signs of inflammation are controlled for several days. Usual
course of therapy is 7 to 14 days.

Acute gouty arthritis: 50 mg tid until pain is tolerable. Dose should then be rapidly reduced to
complete cessation of drug. Definite relief of pain
usually occurs within 2 to 4 hours. Tenderness and
heat usually subside in 24 to 36 hours; swelling
gradually disappears in 3 to 5 days.

Children: Not recommended for children under 14.

Sustained-release form: 75 mg sustained-release
capsule once a day can be used as alternate dosage
form for 25 mg to 50 mg capsules tid. One 75-mg
sustained-release capsule bid can be substituted for
one 50-mg capsule tid.

MECLOFENAMATE SODIUM

Usual dosage: 200 mg/day to 400 mg/day in
three or four equal doses.

Initial dosage: Therapy is initiated at lower dosage, then increased as needed to improve clinical response. Dosage is individualized. Do not exceed 400
mg/day. Improvement may be seen in some patients in a few days, but 2 to 3 weeks of treatment

N

may be required to obtain optimum therapeutic benefit. If intolerance occurs, dosage may need to be reduced. Therapy should be terminated if any severe reactions occur.

Children: Not recommended.

MEFENAMIC ACID

Acute pain in adults and children over 14: Initially 500 mg, followed by 250 mg q6h as needed.

Primary dysmenorrhea: 500 mg as initial dose, followed by 250 mg q6h starting with onset of bleeding and associated symptoms. Studies indicate effective treatment can be initiated with start of menses and should not be necessary for more than 2 to 3 days.

NAPROXEN

Do not exceed 1250 mg (1375 mg naproxen Na) per day.

Rheumatoid arthritis, osteoarthritis, ankylosing spondylitis: 250 mg to 375 mg (275 mg naproxen Na) bid. Dosage is adjusted depending on clinical response. Daily doses higher than 1000 mg (1100 mg naproxen Na) not studied. Morning and evening doses do not have to be equal in size. Symptomatic improvement usually begins within 2 weeks. If no improvement is seen, a trial of 2 more weeks is considered.

Acute gout: 750 mg (825 mg naproxen Na), followed by 250 mg (275 naproxen Na) q8h until attack has subsided.

Mild to moderate pain, primary dysmenorrhea, acute tendinitis and bursitis: 500 mg, followed by 250 mg q6h to q8h (550 mg naproxen Na, followed by 275 mg q6h–q8h).

Children: Safety and efficacy not established.

PIROXICAM

Rheumatoid and osteoarthritis: Initiate and maintain therapy at single daily dose of 20 mg. If desired, dosage may be divided. Because of long half-life, steady-state blood levels are not reached for 7 to 12 days. Therapeutic effect may be evident early in treatment; there is a progressive increase in response over several weeks. Effect of therapy should not be assessed for 2 weeks.

Children: Safety, efficacy not established.

SULINDAC

Usual maximum dosage is 400 mg/day. Doses above this not recommended.

Osteoarthritis, rheumatoid arthritis, and ankylosing spondylitis: Recommended starting dose is 150 mg bid. Dosage may be lowered or raised depending on response. A prompt response (within 1 week) can be expected in about one-half of those with osteoarthritis, ankylosing spondylitis, and rheumatoid arthritis; others may require longer to respond.

Acute painful shoulder, acute gouty arthritis: 200 mg bid. After satisfactory response is achieved, dosage is reduced. In acute painful shoulder therapy for 7 to 14 days, and in gouty arthritis therapy for 7 days, is usually adequate.

Children: Safety, efficacy not established.

TOLMETIN

Therapeutic response can be expected in a few days to a week. Progressive improvement can be anticipated during succeeding weeks of therapy.

Adults: Recommended initial dose for rheumatoid arthritis and osteoarthritis is 400 mg tid, preferably including a dose on rising and a dose H.S. To achieve optimal therapeutic effect, dose should be adjusted according to response. *Rheumatoid arthritis*—Control usually achieved at doses of 600 mg/day to 1800 mg/day in 3 to 4 divided doses. *Osteoarthritis*—Control is usually achieved at doses of 600 mg/day to 1600 mg/day in three to four divided doses. Doses larger than 2000 mg/day for rheumatoid arthritis or 1600 mg/day for osteoarthritis are not recommended.

Children: Recommended starting dose for children 2 years and older is 20 mg/kg/day in three or four divided doses. Doses higher than 30 mg/kg/day not recommended.

NURSING IMPLICATIONS

HISTORY

See Appendix 4. Note allergy to aspirin, current treatment modalities (*e.g.*, diet, exercise program, physical therapy). Inform physician if patient has a history of aspirin allergy.

PHYSICAL ASSESSMENT

For arthritic disorders and musculoskeletal and soft-tissue inflammation, examine joints/areas involved. Examine and record description of involved joints/areas, noting appearance, limitation of motion, and appearance of skin over joint or affected area. Evaluate ability to carry out ADL. X-ray of involved area(s), renal function tests, CBC, hemoglobin, hematocrit may be ordered. Depending on health history, other laboratory tests may also be appropriate.

ADMINISTRATION

Indomethacin is to be given with food, immediately after meals, or with antacids to reduce gastric irritation.

Sulindac, mefenamic acid are administered with food.

If GI upset occurs, **ibuprofen, fenoprofen, meclofenamate sodium** may be administered with meals or milk.

Indomethacin, sulindac, and **mefenamic acid** can be administered with an aluminum and magnesium hydroxide antacid (physician must order antacid).

If GI upset occurs despite giving drugs with food, meals, or milk, notify physician.

Patients with arthritis involving the hands may have difficulty removing drug from container, holding glass, or putting tablet/capsule in mouth. Provide assistance as needed.

ONGOING ASSESSMENTS AND NURSING MANAGEMENT

Observe patient closely (q4h–q8h) for adverse effects, especially during initial therapy. Because these drugs have many adverse reactions, observe for *any* complaint the patient may offer.

CLINICAL ALERT: GI reactions can occur with use of these drugs. These can be severe and sometimes fatal, especially in those prone to upper GI disease. Withhold next dose and notify physician immediately if any GI symptom, especially diarrhea, nausea, vomiting, evidence of GI bleeding (blood in stool, tarry stools), or abdominal pain, occurs.

Advise patient with arthritis that immediate clinical improvement may not be noted because drug may take several days or more to produce effect. The following may be used as a guideline:

Fenoproen—Few days; an additional 2 to 3 weeks may be required to gauge full benefits.

Ibuprofen—Few days to a week; most often observed within 2 weeks.

Indomethacin—Patients with acute gouty arthritis usually experience definite relief of pain within 2 to 4 hours; tenderness and heat usually subside in 24 to 36 hours; swelling gradually disappears in 3 to 5 days.

Meclofenamate sodium—Few days (some patients); 2 to 3 weeks may be required to obtain optimum therapeutic benefit.

Naproxen—Usually begins within 2 weeks.

Piroxicam—Steady-state blood levels not reached for 7 to 12 days; therapeutic effects may be evident early in treatment but effect of therapy should not be assessed for 2 weeks.

Sulindac—Within 1 week in ½ of patients; others may require longer.

Tolmetin—Few days to a week; progressive improvement can be anticipated during succeeding weeks.

Osteoarthritis: Clinical improvement is shown by reduction of tenderness with pressure, reduc-

tion of pain in motion and at rest, reduction of night pain, stiffness, swelling, and reduction of overall disease activity and by increase in range of motion in involved joints.

Rheumatoid arthritis: Clinical improvement is shown by reduction in joint swelling, pain, duration of morning stiffness, and disease activity and by increased functional capacity demonstrated by increase in grip strength, delay time in onset of fatigue, and a decrease in time to walk 50 feet.

Acute gouty arthritis, ankylosing spondylitis: Clinical improvement is shown by relief of pain, reduction of fever, swelling, redness, and tenderness and increase in range of motion in acute gouty arthritis.

Patient with arthritis should be allowed to parcipitate in ADL at own pace or as recommended by physician.

If dizziness or other CNS reactions occur, patient may require assistance with ambulatory activities.

If drug is administered to patient with impaired renal function, measure intake and output; observe for decrease in urinary output. Physician usually orders periodic renal-function studies.

GU tract problems have been reported with use of **fenoprofen.** The appearance of fever, rash, arthralgia, oliguria, or other GU complaints such as symptoms of cystitis and hematuria are reported to the physician immediately.

If steroid dosage is reduced (or the steroid is eliminated during therapy), it must be done gradually and patient observed for adverse effects, including signs of adrenal insufficiency (Appendix 6, section 6-3).

These drugs can inhibit platelet aggregation; this effect may be exaggerated in persons with underlying hemostatic effects. Report any evidence of easy bleeding or ecchymosis to physician immediately.

Anemia may occur in those on long-term therapy. Physician may order periodic hemoglobin and hematocrit determinations, especially if anemia is suspected.

Note eye complaints such as blurred vision, changes in color vision, diminished vision, and report to physician because ophthalmologic examination may be ordered. Therapy may be discontinued if ocular changes are noted.

Periodic auditory function tests recommended during therapy with **fenoprofen.**

If skin rash develops, notify physician. If patient is receiving **mefenamic acid,** drug should be discontinued at first signs of skin rash.

N

Patient receiving coumarin-type anticoagulants: These agents could prolong the prothrombin time. Daily prothrombin times are recommended whenever nonsteroidal anti-inflammatory agents are added to or taken away from the treatment regimen of patients receiving oral anticoagulants.

Diabetic patient: Insulin dosage may require adjustment while receiving these agents. Report to physician may change in urine glucose test results; observe for signs of hypoglycemia and hyperglycemia (Appendix 6, section 6-14).

PATIENT AND FAMILY INFORMATION

NOTE: Patient with arthritis should receive explanation about time interval necessary for drug to produce effect (see above).

Avoid aspirin while taking medication. Check with physician about use of any nonprescription drug because some drugs may contain multiple ingredients, some of which should not be taken with these drugs.

If GI upset occurs, take with food, milk. Antacids may also be used but check with physician regarding preferred brands. Do not use sodium bicarbonate as an antacid, unless physician approves use.

May cause drowsiness, dizziness, blurred vision; observe caution while driving or performing other tasks requiring alertness.

Notify physician or nurse if skin rash, itching, visual disturbances, weight gain, edema, diarrhea, black stools, nausea, vomiting, or persistent headache occurs.

If drug fails to relieve some or all of symptoms within 2 weeks, continue taking medication but contact physician.

If drug is being taken for mild to moderate pain (*e.g.,* dysmenorrhea, dental procedures), notify physician or dentist if pain is not relieved.

Patient with diabetes mellitus: Test urine daily. Notify physician or nurse if positive for glucose or episodes of hypoglycemia (Appendix 6, section 6-14) occur.

Mefenamic acid: If rash or diarrhea or other digestive problems occur, discontinue use and notify physician or nurse immediately.

Norepinephrine (Levarterenol) Rx

injection: 1 mg/ml   Levophed

INDICATIONS

Restoration of blood pressure in controlling certain acute hypotensive states (*e.g.,* pheochromocytomec-tomy, sympathectomy, poliomyelitis, spinal anesthesia, MI, septicemia, blood transfusion and drug reactions) and as adjunct in treatment of cardiac arrest and profound hypotension.

CONTRAINDICATIONS

Do not give to those who are hypotensive from blood volume deficits, except as emergency measure to maintain coronary and cerebral artery perfusion until blood volume replacement therapy can be completed. If continuously administered to maintain blood pressure in absence of blood volume replacement, the following may occur: severe peripheral and visceral vasoconstriction, decreased renal perfusion and urine output, poor systemic blood flow despite "normal" blood pressure, tissue hypoxia, and lactic acidosis.

Do not give to patients with mesenteric or peripheral vascular thrombosis because of risk of increasing ischemia and extending area of infarction, unless administration is necessary as a lifesaving procedure.

Use during cyclopropane and halothane anesthesia generally is contraindicated because of risk of producing ventricular tachycardia or fibrillation. The same type of arrhythmia may result from use in profound hypoxia or hypercarbia.

ACTIONS

Functions as a powerful peripheral vasoconstrictor acting on both arterial and venous beds (alpha-adrenergic action) and as a potent inotropic stimulator of the heart (beta$_1$ action). Coronary vasodilatation occurs secondary to enhanced myocardial contractility. These actions result in an increase in systemic blood pressure and coronary artery blood flow. Cardiac output will vary in response to systemic hypertension but is usually increased in hypotension when blood pressure is raised to an optimal level. Venous return is increased and the heart tends to resume a more normal rate and rhythm than in the hypotensive state. In hypotension that persists after correction of blood volume deficits, it helps raise blood pressure to an optimal level and establish more adequate circulation.

Is ineffective orally; subcutaneous absorption is poor. It is rapidly inactivated; only 4% to 16% is excreted in urine. Effects are transient when given by IV infusion.

PRECAUTIONS

Hypovolemia: Not a substitute for replacement of blood, plasma, fluids, or electrolytes, which should be restored promptly when loss has occurred.

Avoid hypertension: Because of drug's potency and varying response to pressor substances, dangerously high blood pressure may be produced with overdoses. Headache may be symptom of hypertension due to overdosage.

Infusion site: Whenever possible, infuse into a large vein to minimize necrosis of overlying skin from prolonged vasoconstriction. Occlusive vascular disease (*i.e.,* atherosclerosis, arteriosclerosis, diabetic endarteritis, Buerger's disease) are more likely to occur in the lower extremity; avoid use of veins of the leg in elderly or those suffering from such disorders.

Extravasation: May cause necrosis and sloughing of surrounding tissue.

DRUG INTERACTIONS

Use with extreme caution in persons receiving **mono-amine oxidase (MAO) inhibitors** or **tricyclic antide-pressants** of the triptyline or imipramine types, because severe, prolonged hypertension may result. In obstetrics, if vasopressor drugs are either used to correct hypotension or added to the local anesthetic solution, some **oxytocic drugs** may cause severe persistent hypertension; even rupture of a cerebral vessel may occur during the postpartum period.

Cyclopropane or **halogenated hydrocarbon anesthetics** may sensitize the myocardium to the effects of catecholamines. Use of vasopressors may lead to serious arrhythmias. The effects of **beta-adrenergic blocking agents** can be reversed by norepinephrine. **Furosemide** and **thiazide diuretics** may decrease arterial responsiveness to norepinephrine. The diminution is not sufficient to preclude effectiveness of the pressor agent.

ADVERSE REACTIONS

Norepinephrine's therapeutic index is four times that of epinephrine. Bradycardia sometimes occurs, probably as a reflex result of a rise in blood pressure. Headache may indicate overdosage and extreme hypertension. Gangrene was reported in a lower extremity when drug was infused into an ankle vein.

OVERDOSAGE

Symptoms: Overdosage may result in severe hypertension, reflex bradycardia, marked increase in peripheral resistance, decreased cardiac output. Prolonged administration of any potent vasopressor may result in plasma volume depletion.

Treatment: Correct by appropriate fluid and electrolyte replacement. If plasma volumes are not corrected, hypotension may occur when norepinephrine is discontinued, or blood pressure may be maintained at the risk of severe peripheral vasoconstriction with diminution of blood flow and tissue perfusion.

DOSAGE

Restoration of blood pressure in acute hypotensive states: Always correct blood volume depletion as fully as possible before any vasopressor administered. When, as an emergency measure, intra-aortic pressures must be maintained to prevent cerebral or coronary artery ischemia, drug can be administered before and concurrently with blood volume replacement.

Average IV dose: Add 4 ml of drug to 1000 ml 5% dextrose solution (4 mcg base/ml). This concentration may be adjusted depending on fluid requirements. Avoid catheter tie-in technique because this promotes stasis. After observing response to an initial dose of 2 ml/minute to 3 ml/minute, adjust rate of flow to establish and maintain a low normal blood pressure (usually 80–100 mm Hg systolic) sufficient to maintain circulation to vital organs. In previously hypertensive patients, raise blood pressure to no higher than 40 mm Hg below the preexisting systolic pressure. Average maintenance dose ranges from 2 mcg/minute to 4 mcg/minute.

Dosage adjustments: Great individual variation in dose occurs. Occasionally, enormous daily doses may be necessary if patient remains hypotensive, but occult blood volume depletion should always be suspected and corrected when present.

Duration of therapy: Infusion is continued until adequate blood pressure and tissue perfusion are maintained without therapy. Infusion is reduced gradually, avoiding abrupt withdrawal. In some cases of vascular collapse due to acute MI, treatment was required for up to 6 days.

Adjunctive treatment in cardiac arrest: Usually administered IV during cardiac resuscitation to restore and maintain adequate blood pressure after an effective heartbeat and ventilation established. Its powerful beta-adrenergic stimulating action is also thought to increase strength and effectiveness of systolic contractions once they occur.

NURSING IMPLICATIONS

HISTORY

Obtain history from chart or other personnel (nurse, ambulance attendant, family). When possible, history should include events leading up to hypotensive episode, possible cause of hypotension (*e.g.,* blood loss, heart disease), previous blood pressure range, history of hypertension, other health problems.

PHYSICAL ASSESSMENT

Obtain blood pressure, pulse rate and quality, respiratory rate and pattern. Perform general survey (*e.g.,* color, level of consciousness) to determine general status. Other assessments may be warranted if hypotensive episode is due to trauma, blood loss. ECG, other diagnostic and

N

laboratory tests may be ordered, based on the clinical situation.

ADMINISTRATION

Preparation

IV line is established as soon as possible. Use large vein, preferably vein in forearm or antecubital fossa.

A plastic intravenous catheter inserted through a suitable bore needle well advanced into the vein and securely fixed with adhesive tape is recommended. Avoid, if possible, catheter tie-in technique because this promotes stasis.

In an emergency, IV can be run to KVO until norepinephrine solution is prepared.

Administer drug in 1000 ml of 5% Dextrose in Distilled Water or 5% Dextrose in Saline solution. Fluids containing dextrose are protection against significant loss of potency due to oxidation. Administration in saline solution alone not recommended.

Dosage added to IV solution may be prescribed in ampules, or in milligrams or milliliters. One ampule contains 4 ml or 4 mg (1 mg/ml).

Physician prescribes dose and volume and type of IV fluid.

Physician may order phentolamine (5–10 mg) added to the infusion of norepinephrine, which may be an effective antidote against sloughing should extravasation occur.

In patients with severe hypotension following MI, physician may order heparin 1000 units added to each 500 ml of IV infusion fluid to prevent thrombosis in the infused vein and perivenous reactions and necrosis.

Administer whole blood or plasma, if indicated, separately.

Use Y-tubing (primary and secondary lines). One line is used to run IV at KVO when IV fluid containing norepinephrine is discontinued temporarily because of overdosage or adequate blood pressure response, or when drug is being gradually withdrawn while patient is closely observed for a repeat hypotensive episode.

An infusion pump or microdrip may be used to regulate infusion with flow rate adjusted according to blood pressure response.

Administration

Immediately prior to administration, obtain blood pressure, pulse; record on flow sheet.

Physician may prescribe initial rate of infusion, but rate is adjusted according to patient response. Recommended initial rate is 2 ml/minute to 3 ml/minute, with further dosage adjusted according to patient response.

Physician establishes guidelines for maximum systolic response (usually 80–100 mm Hg). Guidelines may be higher if patient has a history of hypertension. In such cases, blood pressure is raised no higher than 40 mm Hg below the preexisting systolic pressure.

ONGOING ASSESSMENTS AND NURSING MANAGEMENT

Physician may order antidote for extravasation. Have materials (usually phentolamine, normal saline) immediately available.

CLINICAL ALERT: Patient must be attended constantly during time of infusion.

Monitor blood pressure and pulse every 2 minutes until stabilized, then every 3 to 5 minutes during administration.

Infusion rate must be adjusted according to blood pressure response (see *Dosage*).

Observe for blanching along the course of the infused vein, and notify physician immediately if this occurs because it is recommended that the infusion site, when possible, be changed. Blanching may result in venous constriction with increased permeability of the vein wall, resulting in some leakage without signs of extravasation. This may progress to superficial sloughing of tissue.

Check infusion site closely for free flow. Extravasation can result in local necrosis and sloughing of tissue. If extravasation occurs, notify physician immediately. Because blood pressure must be maintained, immediately attempt to start another infusion in the opposite extremity while waiting for arrival of physician. Follow recommendations of physician (clarify before drug is administered) about exact procedure to follow should extravasation occur (*e.g.,* if IV should be slowed or discontinued while attempting to restart in another vein), as well as administration of antidote.

Antidote for extravasation—Infiltrate area as soon as possible with 10 ml to 15 ml of saline solution containing 5 mg to 10 mg of phentolamine. Use a syringe with a fine hypodermic needle.

Note patient complaint of headache, which may indicate overdosage. Slow infusion rate and monitor blood pressure closely.

During administration, constantly monitor patient's general status. Note presence of cyanosis, level of consciousness, urinary output, and temperature and color of extremities.

Measure urinary output q15m to q30m or as ordered. Notify physician of any change in intake–output ratio or decrease in urinary output.

Observe for signs of fluid overload (Appendix 6, section 6-12). Physician may order more concentrated solution of norepinephrine if fluid overload is suspected. If large volumes of fluid replacement are necessary, physician may order a less concentrated solution.

Physician orders procedure to be followed when therapy is discontinued. Usually, infusion rate is gradually reduced. Abrupt withdrawal is not recommended. Continue to monitor blood pressure and pulse q5m to q10m or as ordered. Continue to monitor patient's general status.

Norethindrone, Norethindrone Acetate

See Contraceptives, Oral; Progestins.

Norethynodrel

See Contraceptives, Oral.

Norgestrel

See Contraceptives, Oral.

Nortriptyline Hydrochloride

See Antidepressants, Tricyclic Compounds.

Novobiocin _Rx_

capsules: 250 mg   Albamycin

INDICATIONS
Treatment of serious infections due to susceptible strains of _Staphylococcus aureus_ when patient is sensitive to other effective antibiotics, such as penicillins, cephalosporins, vancomycin, lincomycin, erythromycin, and the tetracyclines, or when there are other contraindications to these antibiotics. May be useful in the few urinary tract infections caused by _Proteus_ species sensitive to novobiocin but resistant to other therapy.

CONTRAINDICATIONS
Hypersensitivity.

ACTIONS
Is principally bacteriostatic. It inhibits protein and nucleic acid synthesis and interferes with bacterial cell wall synthesis. May also effect cell membrane stability by complexing with magnesium within the bacterial cell. Shows no cross-resistance with penicillin against strains of _S. aureus_ but studies indicate _S. aureus_ rapidly develops resistance to novobiocin.

Is well absorbed from the GI tract. Peak serum levels, which occur in about 2 hours, are higher when drug is taken in the fasting state. Drug is highly bound to serum proteins; diffusion into body fluids is poor. Concentrations in pleural, ascitic, and joint fluids are usually lower than serum levels. Small amounts may penetrate into cerebral spinal fluid if meninges are inflamed. Excretion is primarily via bile and feces; 3% is excreted in urine.

WARNINGS
Use only for those serious infections in which other less toxic drugs are ineffective or contraindicated because of high frequency of (1) adverse reactions, principally urticaria and maculopapular dermatitis, and hepatic dysfunction and blood dyscrasias (which occur less frequently) and (2) the rapid and frequent emergence of resistant strains, especially staphylococci.

PRECAUTIONS
Novobiocin possesses a high index of sensitization. If allergic reactions develop during treatment and are not readily controlled by usual measures, drug is discontinued.

Hepatic and hematologic studies are recommended during therapy. Drug is discontinued in case of development of liver dysfunction and if hematologic studies show evidence of development of leukopenia or other blood dyscrasias.

Use in infants: Affects bilirubin metabolism adversely; avoid use in newborn or premature infants.

Superinfection: Use of antibiotics (especially prolonged or repeated therapy) may result in bacterial or fungal overgrowth of nonsusceptible organisms. Such overgrowth may lead to secondary infection. Appropriate measures should be taken if superinfection occurs.

ADVERSE REACTIONS
Hypersensitivity: There is a high incidence of hypersensitivity reactions consisting of skin eruptions, including urticarial, erythematous, maculopapular, and scarlatiniform rash. Erythema multiforme has occurred but is rare.

Hematopoietic: Blood dyscrasias, including leukopenia, eosinophilia (with or without fever), anemia, pancytopenia, agranulocytosis, and thrombocytopenia have occurred.

Hepatic dysfunction: Liver dysfunction, including jaundice and elevation of serum bilirubin concentration. Yellow discoloration of plasma, skin, and sclera may also occur as a result of a lipochrome pigment metabolite; a normal serum bilirubin distinguishes this effect from jaundice.

Miscellaneous: Nausea, vomiting, loose stools and diarrhea, intestinal hemorrhage, alopecia.

N

DOSAGE

Adults: 250 mg q6h or 500 mg q12h. Continue for at least 48 hours after temperature has returned to normal and evidence of infection has disappeared. In severe or unusually resistant infections, give 0.5 g q6h or 1 g q12h.

Children: 15 mg/kg/day for moderate acute infections; up to 30 mg/kg/day to 45 mg/kg/day for severe infections. Dosage should be given in divided doses q6h to q12h.

NURSING IMPLICATIONS

HISTORY

See Appendix 4. Review chart for previous and current treatment modalities, culture and sensitivity tests.

PHYSICAL ASSESSMENT

Obtain vital signs. If infection is external, note type and color of exudate (if present), appearance of area; record observations. Baseline laboratory tests may include hepatic-function tests, serum bilirubin, CBC, hematocrit, and platelet count. A repeat culture and sensitivity test may also be ordered.

Children: Obtain weight (for dosage calculation).

ADMINISTRATION

Administer on empty stomach (1 hour before or 2 hours after meals) unless physician orders otherwise.

If child has difficulty swallowing capsule, check with physician or pharmacist about sprinkling capsule's contents over a small amount of food.

ONGOING ASSESSMENTS AND NURSING MANAGEMENT

Obtain vital signs q4h; observe for adverse reactions (see below).

CLINICAL ALERT: There is a high incidence of hypersensitivity reactions. Observe q4h to q6h for development of skin rash or urticaria. Withhold drug and notify physician immediately if skin manifestations are apparent or if patient complains of itching.

Observe for signs of hepatic dysfunction (*e.g.,* jaundice, dark urine, clay-colored stools). Notify physician if these occur.

Observe for hematopoietic changes, which may be manifested by fever, sore throat, and unusual bleeding or bruising.

S. aureus may rapidly develop resistance to novobiocin. Observe for recurrence of symptoms of infection (fever, increased drainage, development of a purulent exudate).

Repeat culture and sensitivity tests may be ordered, as well as hepatic-function studies, CBC, and platelet count.

Observe for signs of superinfection (Appendix 6, section 6-22).

If nausea and vomiting develop, notify physician because it may be necessary to administer drug with food. Drug may be discontinued if these symptoms become severe.

Always inform physician if there is any change in the infection pattern (*e.g.,* sudden rise in temperature, development of a different odor of drainage, increase in amount of drainage) or any change in the patient's general condition.

PATIENT AND FAMILY INFORMATION

Complete full course of therapy; take until gone.

Take at times prescribed. Physician may recommend taking drug on an empty stomach.

Notify physician or nurse immediately if skin rash or hives; yellowish discoloration of skin or eyes; light-colored, black, or bloody stools; diarrhea; vomiting; nausea; fever; sore throat; or unusual bleeding or bruising occurs.

Nylidrin Hydrochloride Rx

tablets: 6 mg, 12 mg   Arlidin, *Generic*

INDICATIONS

"Possibly effective" whenever an increase in blood supply is desirable in vasospastic disease such as the following:

Peripheral vascular disease: Arteriosclerosis obliterans; thromboangiitis obliterans (Buerger's disease); diabetic vascular disease; night leg cramps; Raynaud's phenomena and disease; ischemic ulcer; frostbite; acrocyanosis; acroparesthesia; thrombophlebitis; cold feet, legs, hands.

Circulatory disturbances of the inner ear: Primary cochlear cell ischemia; cochlear stria vascular ischemia; macular or ampular ischemia; other disturbances due to labyrinthine artery spasm or obstruction.

CONTRAINDICATIONS

Acute myocardial infarction, paroxysmal tachycardia, progressive angina pectoris, thyrotoxicosis.

ACTIONS

Acts by beta-adrenergic stimulation to dilate arterioles in skeletal muscles and increase cardiac output.

Increases cerebral blood flow and diminishes vascular resistance associated with cerebrovascular insufficiency. May also have direct action on vascular smooth muscle. Effects on cutaneous blood flow are negligible.

WARNINGS
In those with cardiac disease such as tachyarrhythmias and uncompensated congestive heart failure, the benefit–risk ratio should be weighed before therapy and reconsidered at intervals throughout therapy. A significant increase in blood glucose has been reported with use during the last trimester of pregnancy; increases are more marked in diabetic women. Safety for use in pregnancy has not been established.

ADVERSE REACTIONS
CNS: Trembling, nervousness, weakness, dizziness (not associated with labyrinthine artery insufficiency), palpitations.

GI: Nausea, vomiting.

Cardiovascular: Postural hypotension, although not reported, may occur.

DOSAGE
3 mg to 12 mg tid or qid.

NURSING IMPLICATIONS

HISTORY
See Appendix 4.

PHYSICAL ASSESSMENT
Peripheral vascular disease: Examine involved areas, noting skin color, temperature, and appearance; palpate peripheral pulses, noting quality and amplitude.

Circulatory disturbance of inner ear: If dizziness is a prominent symptom, determine patient's ability to carry out activities of daily living (*e.g.,* walking, bathing, shaving, eating).

ADMINISTRATION
If patient has balance difficulty or dizziness, assistance in taking medication may be needed.

Advise patient that improvement may require several weeks of therapy.

ONGOING ASSESSMENTS AND NURSING MANAGEMENT
Observe for adverse effects daily; also, look for improvement in original symptoms by examination of involved extremities (in those with peripheral vascular disease) or inquiring of patient if symptoms are improved (circulatory disturbance of inner ear); compare with data base.

If dizziness occurs, patient (especially the elderly) may require assistance with ambulatory activities.

In peripheral vascular disease, physician may prescribe additional treatment modalities such as special exercises.

PATIENT AND FAMILY INFORMATION
May cause dizziness (orthostatic hypotension); avoid sudden changes in posture, and rise from a sitting or lying position slowly.

Use caution when driving or performing other tasks requiring alertness.

May cause trembling, nervousness, weakness, nausea, or vomiting. Notify physician or nurse if these symptoms become severe or if palpitations occur.

Follow physician's recommendations about smoking, avoiding exposure to cold, and exercise. Wear properly fitting shoes. Avoid constrictive clothing.

Nystatin Rx

tablets: 100,000 units	*Generic*
tablets: 500,000 units	Mycostatin, Nilstat, *Generic*
oral suspension: 100,000 units/ml	Mycostatin, Nilstat, *Generic*
cream: 100,000 units/g	Mycostatin, Nilstat, *Generic*
ointment: 100,000 units/g	Mycostatin, Nilstat
powder: 100,000 units/g	Mycostatin
tablets, vaginal: 100,000 units	Korostatin, Mycostatin, Nilstat, *Generic*
oral/vaginal therapy pack	O-V Statin

INDICATIONS
Oral suspension: Treatment of candidiasis of the oral cavity.

Oral tablets: Treatment of intestinal candidiasis.

Cream, ointment, and powder: Treatment of cutaneous or mucocutaneous mycotic infections caused by *Candida albicans* and other *Candida* species.

Vaginal tablets and oral/vaginal therapy pack: Contain 21 oral tablets (500,000 units nystatin) and 14 vaginal tablets (100,000 units nystatin) and are used for treatment of vulvovaginal candidiasis.

CONTRAINDICATIONS
Hypersensitivity.

ACTIONS
Is an antifungal antibiotic that is both fungistatic and fungicidal against a wide variety of yeasts and yeastlike fungi. It probably acts by binding to sterols in the cell membrane of the fungus with a resultant change in membrane permeability, allowing leakage of intracellular components. Following oral administration it is sparingly absorbed with no detectable blood levels. Most of the orally administered drug is passed unchanged in the stool.

No adverse effects or complications have been attributed to the drug in infants born to women treated with nystatin.

PRECAUTIONS
Should hypersensitivity reaction occur, drug is discontinued and appropriate measures taken. The 500,000-unit oral tablets marketed as Mycostatin contain tartrazine. See Appendix 6, section 6-23.

ADVERSE REACTIONS
Orally, drug is virtually nontoxic and is well tolerated by all age groups including debilitated infants, even on prolonged administration. Large oral doses have occasionally produced diarrhea, GI distress, nausea, and vomiting. Nausea, vomiting, GI distress, and diarrhea occur occasionally with large doses of the oral suspension. Rarely, sensitization occurs with vaginal use. If irritation occurs when applied topically to cutaneous and mucocutaneous structures, use is discontinued.

DOSAGE
Oral tablets for intestinal candidiasis
Usual therapeutic dosage is 500,000 to 1,000,000 units tid. Treatment should generally be continued for at least 48 hours after clinical cure to prevent relapse.
Oral suspension for oral candidiasis
Local treatment continued at least 48 hours after perioral symptoms have disappeared and cultures return to normal.
Adults and children: 400,000 to 600,000 units qid (½ of dose on each side of mouth, retaining drug as long as possible before swallowing).
Infants: 200,000 units qid (100,000 units on each side of mouth).
Premature and low-birth weight infants: 100,000 units qid.
Cream, ointment, powder for cutaneous and mucocutaneous use
Apply to affected areas two or three times a day or as indicated until healing complete. Continue use for 1 week after clinical cure. For fungal infection of the feet caused by *Candida* species, powder should be dusted freely on feet as well as in shoes and socks. The cream is usually preferred in candidiasis involving intertriginous areas; very moist lesions are best treated with powder.
Vaginal tablets
Usual dosage is one tablet (100,000 units) intravaginally daily for 2 weeks. Even though symptomatic relief may occur within a few days, treatment should be continued for the full course. Adjunctive measures such as therapeutic douches are unnecessary and sometimes inadvisable. Cleansing douches may be used by nonpregnant women, if desired.

NURSING IMPLICATIONS

HISTORY
See Appendix 4.

PHYSICAL ASSESSMENT
Examine affected cutaneous, mucocutaneous, or oral area and record observations. Physician confirms diagnosis of vaginal candidiasis by KOH smears and/or cultures. Other pathogens commonly associated with vulvovaginitis do not respond to nystatin and are ruled out by appropriate laboratory methods. Predisposing factors of vulvovaginal candidiasis (*e.g.,* diabetes, pregnancy, infection by sexual partner) may be ruled out with further testing. Use of birth control pills, antibiotics, or corticosteroids may also be a contributing cause.

ADMINISTRATION
Oral suspension
Usual total volume of dose is 4 ml to 6 ml/dose (adults, children). To prepare, divide dose into two containers for ease of administration.

Have patient rinse out mouth with tap water to remove any accumulated debris.

One-half of dose (1 container) is retained on each side. Instruct patient to retain liquid in side of mouth for as long as possible before swallowing.

Infants, premature and low-birth weight infants: Physician should specify method of administration because infant cannot retain liquid in mouth. One method that may be used is to paint the inside of the mouth with the oral suspension. Place infant in an upright or near upright position as *care must be taken to prevent aspiration of the liquid by a crying infant.*
Cream, ointment, lotion, powder
Area should be cleansed to remove previous application unless physician directs otherwise.

Cleansing is usually not necessary when cream is applied because it is in an aqueous base.

Apply as directed (see *Dosage*). Do not apply a dressing unless ordered.

Vaginal tablets

Place patient in supine position with knees flexed.

Using applicator provided with product, insert tablet high into vagina.

Hospitalized patient may prefer to self-administer medication; adequate instruction for insertion must be given and patient assisted, if necessary.

ONGOING ASSESSMENTS AND NURSING MANAGEMENT

Inspect involved areas each time cream, ointment, lotion, or powder is applied. If infection appears worse, or redness or irritation is noted, contact physician before next application.

In candidiasis of oral cavity, inspect oral cavity daily; record appearance of lesions. Give oral care after each meal or feeding. Have patient thoroughly rinse mouth with tap water. Avoid use of commercial mouthwash preparation unless use is ordered by physician.

If patient complains of burning and/or irritation with use of vaginal tablet, contact physician before next dose is due.

In intestinal candidiasis, record each bowel movement. If diarrhea persists, inform physician. Cleanse and dry perianal area thoroughly after each loose stool. If diarrhea is severe, observe for signs of dehydration (Appendix 6, section 6-10).

PATIENT AND FAMILY INFORMATION

Complete full course of therapy; take until gone.

If irritation or redness occurs, do not take or use next dose; notify physician immediately.

Intestinal candidiasis: Notify physician if diarrhea or other symptoms persist.

Cleanse perianal area thoroughly after each loose stool.

Oral candidiasis: One-half of dose is retained in each side of the mouth.

Retain drug in mouth as long as possible; drug may then be swallowed.

If nausea, vomiting or GI distress occurs, notify physician or nurse.

Infants, newborns—Follow recommendation of physician in applying in mouth. (*Note*—Family member should receive instruction in positioning infant, applying medication.)

After eating, brush teeth, or remove dentures and clean, followed by thoroughly rinsing the mouth with tap water.

Avoid use of commercial mouthwashes unless recommended by physician or dentist.

If dentures fit poorly, consult a dentist.

Cutaneous, mucocutaneous mycotic infection: Cleanse affected area as recommended by physician; dry gently but thoroughly.

Apply in the amount prescribed, to the affected area(s).

Change underclothing or socks/stockings daily.

Launder clothing separately from that of other family members until infection has cleared.

Avoid wearing tight-fitting clothing. Women with vulval candidiasis should avoid use of pantyhose.

If feet are affected, wear shoes that allow air to circulate. Bathe feet thoroughly one or more times per day or as directed by physician.

Avoid use of dressings, unless ordered by physician.

Vulvovaginal candidiasis: Insert tablet high into vagina with applicator supplied with product.

Should be used continuously, even during menstrual period.

Partner should use a condom to avoid reinfection.

Ask physician about douching. Usually a cleansing douche is permitted, but medicated douches are contraindicated.

N

O

O

Ocular Lubricants and Artificial Tears

Artificial Tears Rx

insert: 5 mg hydroxy-propyl cellulose	Lacrisert
solutions	Adsorbotear, Akwa Tears, Hypotears, Isopto (Alkaline, Plain, Tears), Lacril, Liquifilm Tears, Liquifilm Forte, Lyteers, Methopto-Forte ½% and 1%, Murocel, Muro Tears, Neo-Tears, Nu-Tears, Tearisol, Tears Naturale, Tears Plus, Ultra Tears

Ocular Lubricants otc

ointment	Akwa Tears, Duolube, Duratears, Lacri-Lube S.O.P., Nu-Tears

INDICATIONS

OCULAR LUBRICANTS

These products are ointments used for protection and lubrication of the eye in exposure keratitis; decreased corneal sensitivity; recurrent corneal erosions; keratitis sicca, particularly for nighttime use; after removal of a foreign body; following surgery.

ARTIFICIAL TEAR INSERT

Moderate to severe dry eye syndromes including keratoconjunctivitis sicca. Also used in exposure to keratitis, decreased corneal sensitivity, and recurrent corneal erosions.

ARTIFICIAL TEAR SOLUTIONS

Offer tearlike lubrication for relief of dryness and eye irritation associated with deficient tear production. Also used as ocular lubricants for artificial eyes and contact lenses.

Contain balanced amounts of salts to maintain tonicity compatible with the eye; buffers to adjust pH of the formulation; viscosity agents to prolong contact time with the eye; preservatives to maintain sterility of the solutions.

CONTRAINDICATIONS

Development of hypersensitivity.

ADVERSE REACTIONS

The following were reported with use of **artificial tear insert** and in most instances were mild and transient: ocular discomfort or irritation; matting or stickiness of eyelashes; photophobia; hypersensitivity; edema of eyelids; hyperemia.

DOSAGE

OCULAR LUBRICANTS

Instill small amount in conjunctival cul-de-sac as needed.

ARTIFICIAL TEAR INSERT

One daily into inferior cul-de-sac. This is usually sufficient to relieve symptoms associated with moderate to severe dry eye syndrome. Individual patients may require twice daily use for optimal results.

ARTIFICIAL TEAR SOLUTIONS

Usually one to three drops in eye tid, qid, or as needed.

NURSING IMPLICATIONS

ADMINISTRATION

Instill as ordered by physician or recommended by manufacturer (see *Dosage*).

ONGOING ASSESSMENTS AND NURSING MANAGEMENT

If hyperemia, exudate, or edema of eyelids occurs, or if patient complains of ocular discomfort or irritation, notify physician.

PATIENT AND FAMILY INFORMATION

Use as directed by physician or label of container.

If eye drainage, swelling of the eyelids, or eye irritation or discomfort occurs, discontinue use and see physician.

Artificial tear insert: May produce transient blurring of vision. Exercise caution while operating hazardous machinery or driving a motor vehicle. (*Note*—Patient instructions are available with product but patient may need further instructions in its use.)

Opium

See Narcotic Analgesics.

Orphenadrine Citrate Rx

tablets: 100 mg	Marflex, *Generic*
tablets, sustained release: 100 mg	Norflex, *Generic*
injection: 30 mg/ml	Banflex, Flexoject, Flexon, K-Flex, Myolin, Norflex, O'Flex, X-Otag, *Generic*

INDICATIONS

Adjunct to rest, physical therapy, and other measures for relief of discomfort associated with acute, painful musculoskeletal conditions.

CONTRAINDICATIONS

Glaucoma; pyloric or duodenal obstruction; stenosing peptic ulcers; prostatic hypertrophy; bladder neck obstruction; cardiospasm (megaesophagus) and myasthenia gravis; hypersensitivity.

ACTIONS

Mode of action has not been identified. Does not directly relax tense skeletal muscles. Possesses anticholinergic actions. Peak plasma levels occur 2 hours after administration of 100 mg; duration of action is 4 to 6 hours. Half-life is approximately 14 hours for parent drug, 2 to 25 hours for metabolites. Excretion is via urine and feces.

WARNINGS

May cause transient episodes of lightheadedness, dizziness, or syncope. Safety for use in pregnancy has not been established. Use during pregnancy, particularly early pregnancy, only when clearly needed and when potential benefits outweigh the unknown potential hazards to the fetus. Safety and efficacy for use in children have not been established; not recommended for use in the pediatric age group.

PRECAUTIONS

Use with caution in those with cardiac decompensation, coronary insufficiency, cardiac arrhythmias, or tachycardia. Safety for continuous long-term therapy is not established; periodic monitoring of blood, urine, and liver function is recommended.

DRUG INTERACTIONS

Confusion, anxiety, and tremors have been reported in patients receiving **propoxyphene** concomitantly. Because these symptoms may be due to an additive effect, reduction of dosage or discontinuation of one or both agents is recommended.

ADVERSE REACTIONS

Are mainly due to the anticholinergic action of drug and are usually associated with higher dosage.

Dryness of the mouth is the first side-effect to appear. When daily dose is increased, possible side-effects include tachycardia, palpitation, urinary hesitancy or retention, blurred vision, dilatation of the pupils, increased ocular tension, weakness, nausea, vomiting, headache, dizziness, constipation, drowsiness, hypersensitivity reactions, pruritus, hallucinations, agitation, tremor, gastric irritation, and rarely urticaria and other dermatoses. Infrequently, elderly patients may experience some degree of mental confusion. These reactions can usually be eliminated by dosage reduction.

Very rare cases of aplastic anemia have been reported, but no causal relationship has been established. Rare instances of anaphylactic reaction have been reported with IM use.

DOSAGE

Oral: 100 mg morning and evening.

Parenteral: 60 mg IV or IM. May be repeated in 12 hours.

NURSING IMPLICATIONS

HISTORY

See Appendix 4. Note etiology of musculoskeletal disorder (document accurately).

PHYSICAL ASSESSMENT

Obtain blood pressure, pulse, and respirations; evaluate limitations imposed by musculoskeletal disorder (_e.g.,_ walking, sitting, movement or use of limbs). If long-term therapy is planned, CBC, urinalysis, and liver-function tests may be ordered.

ADMINISTRATION

Parenteral form is for IM or IV use only.

GENERIC NAME SIMILARITY

Orphenadrine hydrochloride (antiparkisonism agent) and orphenadrine citrate.

ONGOING ASSESSMENTS AND NURSING MANAGEMENT

Note response to therapy (_e.g.,_ relief of pain or discomfort, muscle spasm).

Physician may prescribe additional treatment modalities such as physical therapy, limitation of activity.

Drowsiness or dizziness may occur. Assist patient with ambulatory activities as needed, especially early in therapy or when drug is given parenterally.

Dry mouth may be relieved by sips of water, chewing gum, hard candy.

Observe for adverse reactions; notify physician of occurrence because dosage may be reduced or drug discontinued.

Observe elderly patient for urinary retention, constipation. If urinary retention is suspected or patient has a history of urinary hesitancy or other bladder dysfunction, measure intake and output and palpate lower abdomen for enlarged bladder q4h to q6h. Record bowel movements. Notify physician if urinary retention is suspected or constipation occurs.

O

Periodic monitoring of blood, urine, and liver function is recommended for those on long-term therapy.

PATIENT AND FAMILY INFORMATION

May cause drowsiness, dizziness, blurred vision, or fainting. Observe caution while driving or performing tasks requiring alertness.

Avoid alcohol and other CNS depressants while taking drug.

May cause dry mouth, difficult urination, constipation, headache, GI upset, nervousness, or trembling. Notify physician or nurse if these effects persist or become bothersome, or if skin rash or aching, rapid heart rate, palpitations, or mental confusion occurs.

If discomfort is not relieved, notify physician or nurse.

Orphenadrine Hydrochloride

See Anticholinergic Antiparkinsonism Agents.

Otic Preparations

Antibiotics Rx

solution: 0.5% chlor-   Chloromycetin Otic
amphenicol

INDICATIONS
Used for treatment of superficial infections of the external auditory canal.

CONTRAINDICATIONS
Hypersensitivity.

ACTIONS
See Chloramphenicol, p 278.

WARNINGS
Bone-marrow hypoplasia, including aplastic anemia and death, has been reported following local application.

PRECAUTIONS
Superinfection: Use of antibiotics (especially prolonged or repeated therapy) may result in bacterial or fungal overgrowth of nonsusceptible organisms. Such overgrowth may lead to secondary infection. Appropriate measures should be taken if superinfection occurs. Except in superficial infections, therapy should include systemic medication.

ADVERSE REACTIONS
Signs of local irritation (itching or burning, angioneurotic edema, urticaria, vesicular and maculopapular dermatitis) have been reported in those sensitive to **chloramphenicol.** Blood dyscrasias may be associated with systemic absorption of **topical chloramphenicol.** Similar sensitivity reactions to other materials in topical preparations may also occur.

DOSAGE
Two or three drops tid.

NURSING IMPLICATIONS
See p 811.

Antibiotic and Steroid Combinations Rx

suspension: 1% hydrocortisone, 3.3 mg neomycin sulfate, 3 mg colistin sulfate/ml	Coly-Mycin S Otic
suspension, solution: 1% hydrocortisone, 5 mg neomycin sulfate, 10,000 units polymyxin B sulfate/ml	Cortisporin Otic
solution: 0.1% hydrocortisone, 5 mg neomycin sulfate, 2000 units polymyxin B sulfate, 5% antipyrine, 0.25% dibucaine HCl/ml	My Cort Otic #1-20
solution: 1% hydrocortisone, 5 mg neomycin sulfate, 10,000 units polymyxin B sulfate/ml	AK-Sporin H.C. Otic, Ortega Otic M, Otocort Ear Drops, Otoreid-HC
suspension: 1% hydrocortisone, 5 mg neomycin sulfate, 10,000 units polymyxin B sulfate/ml	AK-Sporin H.C. Otic, BaySporin Otic
suspension: 1% hydrocortisone, 5 mg neomycin sulfate/ml	Otic Neo-Cort-Dome
solution: 0.5% hydrocortisone, 10,000 units polymyxin B sulfate/ml	Otobiotic Otic, Pyocidin-Otic

INDICATIONS

Solutions: Treatment of superficial bacterial infections of the external auditory canal caused by susceptible organisms.

Suspensions: Treatment of superficial bacterial infections of the external auditory canal and treatment of infections of mastoidectomy and fenestration cavities caused by susceptible organisms.

CONTRAINDICATIONS

Hypersensitivity to any component; perforated eardrum; tuberculous, fungal, and viral conditions of the skin or ear (_e.g.,_ herpes simplex, vaccinia, varicella).

ACTIONS

In these combinations, steroids are used for their antiallergic, antipruritic, and anti-inflammatory effects and antibiotics are used for their antibacterial actions. See individual steroid and antibacterial monographs for actions.

DOSAGE

Usual adult dose is three to five drops three or four times a day.

NURSING IMPLICATIONS

See this page.

Miscellaneous Preparations Rx

solution: 1.4% benzocaine, 5.4% antipyrine	Auralgan Otic, Auromid, Oto Ear Drops

DOSAGE

Fill ear canal; insert saturated cotton pledget. Repeat three to four times a day or up to once every 1 to 2 hours.

solution: 0.05% desonide, 2% acetic acid	Otic Tridesilon

DOSAGE

Three to four drops three or four times a day.

solution: 5% benzocaine, 0.25% phenylephrine HCl, 5% antipyrine	Tympagesic

DOSAGE

Fill ear canal; plug with cotton. Repeat q2h to q4h.

solution: 1% hydrocortisone, 2% acetic acid	VōSoL HC Otic

DOSAGE

Insert saturated wick; keep moist 24 hours. Remove wick and instill five drops three or four times a day.

INDICATIONS

Auralgan, Auromid, Oto Ear Drops: For prompt relief of pain and as adjuvant therapy during systemic antibiotic administration for resolution of infection in acute otitis media.

Otic Tridesilon, VōSoL-HC: Superficial infections of the external auditory canal caused by susceptible organisms.

Tympagesic: Topical anesthetic to relieve ear pain. May be used with systemic antibiotics in treatment of acute otitis media.

CONTRAINDICATIONS

Hypersensitivity; perforated tympanic membrane.

PRECAUTIONS

Safety for use in pregnancy has not been established. It is not known whether these drugs are excreted in human breast milk.

DOSAGE

See individual drugs, above.

NURSING IMPLICATIONS: OTIC PREPARATIONS

HISTORY

See Appendix 4. Note previous treatment modalities (if any).

PHYSICAL ASSESSMENT

Examine external auditory canal. Culture and sensitivity tests may be ordered, especially for repeat infections.

ADMINISTRATION

See dosage given for individual products.

Although manufacturers may recommend insertion of a saturated or a dry cotton pledget, check with physician about exact procedure to follow.

Warm solution in hand immediately before use.

Advise patient that momentary dizziness may be noted after drug is instilled. Hearing may also be impaired if cotton is inserted following instillation of drug.

Children may require mild restraining measures.

ONGOING ASSESSMENTS AND NURSING MANAGEMENT

If patient complains of itching, burning, or sudden ear pain, or if exudate is noted, withhold drug and contact physician.

O

PATIENT AND FAMILY INFORMATION

NOTE: Patient should receive full instructions in technique of instillation and, when ordered, insertion of cotton pledget.

Warm solution in hand for a few minutes before using.

Do not touch external parts of ear with dropper tip. Do not wash dropper after use. Replace dropper in bottle immediately after use and keep cap tightly closed.

When inserting cotton pledget, do so gently. Do not pack or push the pledget into the ear canal.

Hearing may be impaired when cotton pledget is in place.

A momentary sense of dizziness may be noted following instillation, especially if solution is cold.

If sudden pain, itching, burning, or drainage is noted, contact physician as soon as possible.

Child: May require mild restraining measures.

Oxacillin Sodium

See Penicillins.

Oxandrolone

See Anabolic Hormones.

Oxazepam

See Benzodiazepines.

Oxidized Cellulose Rx

pellets	Novocell
pads, pledgets	Oxycel
strips	Oxycel, Surgicel

INDICATIONS

Used adjunctively in surgical procedures to assist in control of capillary, venous, and small arterial hemorrhage when ligation or other conventional methods of control are impractical or ineffective. Also indicated in dental and oral surgery.

CONTRAINDICATIONS

As packing or wadding as a hemostatic agent, as packing or implantation in fractures or laminectomies, or to control hemorrhage from large arteries or nonhemorrhagic oozing surfaces.

ACTIONS

An absorbable hemostatic agent prepared from cellulose. Oxidation of cellulose by nitrogen dioxide is controlled to yield an absorbable product of known acidity, soluble in alkali. Provides hemostatic action when applied to sites of bleeding. Mechanism of action is not completely understood, but it appears to be a physical effect, rather than an alteration of the physiologic clotting mechanism. On contact with blood, it becomes a dark reddish brown or almost black, tenacious, adhesive mass. It conforms and adheres readily to the bleeding surface. After 24 to 48 hours, it becomes gelatinous and can be removed, usually without causing additional bleeding. If left *in situ,* absorption depends on several factors, including amount used, degree of saturation with blood, and the tissue bed. It swells on contact with blood and the resultant pressure adds to its hemostatic action. It does not alter the clotting mechanism, but in a few minutes of contact with blood, it forms an artifically produced clot in the bleeding area. It is bactericidal against a wide range of gram-positive and gram-negative organisms, including aerobes and anaerobes.

WARNINGS

Closing oxidized cellulose in a contaminated wound without drainage may lead to complications. May be left *in situ* when necessary, but it is advisable to remove it once hemostasis is achieved. Hemostasis is not enhanced by materials such as buffering or hemostatic substances or by addition of thrombin.

ADVERSE REACTIONS

Encapsulation of fluid and foreign body reactions, with or without infection, has occurred. Possible prolongation of drainage in cholecystectomies and difficulty passing urine by the urethra in prostatectomies have been reported. Occasional reports of burning and stinging sensations and sneezing when used as a packing in epistaxis are believed to be due to the low pH of the product. Burning has been reported when applied after nasal polyp removal and after hemorrhoidectomy. Headache, burning, and stinging in epistaxis and other rhinologic procedures and stinging when applied on surface wounds have also been reported. Intestinal obstruction has occurred because of transmigration of a bolus of oxidized cellulose from gallbladder bed to terminal ileum or because of adhesions in a loop of denuded intestine to which it had been applied.

Other reactions include necrosis of nasal membrane or perforation of nasal septum due to tight packing; urethral obstruction following retropubic prostatectomy and introduction of oxidized cellulose within enucleated prostatic capsule.

DOSAGE

Laid on bleeding site or pressed against tissues until hemostasis obtained. Pellets applied with pressure. Undissolved portions can be removed several days later.

NURSING IMPLICATIONS

ADMINISTRATION

Sterile technique is observed in removing from container.

Glass container should be wiped with an antiseptic. Cap is then removed and product withdrawn from container with dry sterile forceps.

The hemostatic effect is greater when applied dry. Do not moisten with water or saline.

Physician applies to bleeding area.

Opened, unused oxidized cellulose should be discarded because it _cannot_ be resterilized.

Warn patient who is not anesthetized (general anesthesia) of possible burning or stinging when product is applied.

ONGOING ASSESSMENTS AND NURSING MANAGEMENT

If applied for epistaxis or other rhinologic procedure and sneezing occurs, observe for bleeding; inform physician if patient sneezes excessively or if bleeding is apparent.

Patient with prostatectomy should be closely observed for difficulty in urination once urethral catheter is removed.

Oxtriphylline

See Bronchodilators and Decongestants, Systemic.

Oxybutynin Chloride Rx

tablets: 5 mg   Ditropan
syrup: 5 mg/5 ml   Ditropan

INDICATIONS

Relief of symptoms associated with voiding in those with uninhibited neurogenic and reflex neurogenic bladder.

CONTRAINDICATIONS

Glaucoma; partial or complete GI obstruction; paralytic ileus; intestinal atony of the elderly or debilitated; megacolon; toxic megacolon complicating ulcerative colitis; severe colitis; myasthenia gravis; obstructive uropathy; unstable cardiovascular status in acute hemorrhage.

ACTIONS

Exerts direct antispasmodic effect on smooth muscle and inhibits muscarinic action of acetylcholine on smooth muscle. Exhibits only one-fifth the anticholinergic activity of atropine, but four to ten times the antispasmodic activity. No blocking effects occur at skeletal neuromuscular junctions or autonomic ganglia. In uninhibited neurogenic and reflex neurogenic bladder, cystometric studies demonstrated increased vesical capacity, diminished frequency of uninhibited contractions of the detrusor muscle, and delay of initial desire to void. These effects are more consistently improved in those with uninhibited neurogenic bladder. Tolerance has been demonstrated.

WARNINGS

When administered in presence of high environmental temperature, oxybutynin can cause heat prostration (fever, heat stroke due to decreased sweating). Diarrhea may be early sign of incomplete intestinal obstruction, especially in those with ileostomy or colostomy; in such cases treatment is discontinued.

Safety for use in pregnancy not established. Use only when clearly needed and when potential benefits outweigh unknown potential hazards to the fetus. Safety and efficacy for use in children under 5 not established. Not recommended for this age group.

PRECAUTIONS

Use with caution in the elderly and in those with autonomic neuropathy or hepatic or renal disease. Large doses given to those with ulcerative colitis may suppress GI motility, produce paralytic ileus, and precipitate toxic megacolon. Symptoms of hyperthyroidism, coronary heart disease, CHF, cardiac arrhythmias, tachycardia, hypertension, and prostatic hypertrophy may be aggravated. Administer with caution to persons with hiatal hernia associated with reflux esophagitis, because anticholinergic drugs may aggravate this condition.

ADVERSE REACTIONS

Dry mouth, decreased sweating, urinary hesitance and retention, blurred vision, tachycardia, palpitations, dilatation of the pupil, cycloplegia, increased ocular tension, drowsiness, insomnia, weakness, dizziness, nausea, vomiting, constipation, bloated feeling, impotence, suppression of lactation, severe allergic reactions or drug idiosyncrasies including urticaria and other dermal manifestations.

OVERDOSAGE

Symptoms: Intensification of CNS disturbances (from restlessness and excitement to psychotic be-

0

havior), circulatory changes (flushing, fall in blood pressure, circulatory failure), respiratory failure, paralysis, and coma.

Treatment: Immediately lavage stomach and inject physostigmine 0.5 mg to 2 mg IV, repeated as necessary up to 5 mg. Treat fever symptomatically. For excitement of a degree that demands attention, give 2% sodium thiopental slowly IV or chloral hydrate (100 ml to 200 ml of a 2% solution) by rectal infusion. If curarelike effect progresses to paralysis of respiratory muscles, artificial respiration is required.

DOSAGE
Adults: 5 mg bid or tid. Maximum is 5 mg qid.
Children over 5: 5 mg bid. Maximum is 5 mg tid.

NURSING IMPLICATIONS

HISTORY
See Appendix 4. Note previous and current treatment modalities.

PHYSICAL ASSESSMENT
Obtain vital signs; physician usually performs cystometry and other appropriate diagnostic procedures.

ADMINISTRATION
If child has difficulty swallowing tablet, break scored tablet in half to facilitate administration.

ONGOING ASSESSMENTS AND NURSING MANAGEMENT
Monitor vital signs daily; measure intake and output, especially early in therapy; record time and amount of each voiding on flow sheet. Palpate lower abdomen after each voiding. Note if bladder is distended; record findings on flow sheet. Inquire about relief of symptoms.

May cause drowsiness, dizziness. Assist with ambulatory activities as needed.

Observe for adverse reactions and report occurrence to physician.

Observe for development of diarrhea in patient with ileostomy or colostomy. If diarrhea occurs, withhold next dose and notify physician because diarrhea may be early symptom of intestinal obstruction.

Repeat cystometry may be performed to evaluate response to therapy.

PATIENT AND FAMILY INFORMATION
May cause drowsiness, dizziness, or blurred vision. Observe caution while driving or performing other tasks requiring alertness.

Avoid high temperatures because drug can cause heat prostration. In hot weather, use room or ceiling fans or air conditioning to keep cool, wear loose-fitting and lightweight clothing, and take in adequate fluids and eletrolytes. Symptoms of heat prostration may include headache; muscle cramps; nausea, vomiting; cool, pale skin that can progress to hot, red, dry skin as the heat syndrome progresses; mental confusion. If any of these symptoms occurs, notify physician immediately.

May cause dry mouth. Frequent sips of water, chewing gum, hard candy may relieve problem.

Keep record of voiding pattern (*e.g.,* time and amount of each voiding), as well as comparison of current symptoms with those present before therapy with this drug.

Oxycodone Hydrochloride

See Narcotic Analgesics.

Oxymetazoline Hydrochloride

See Decongestants, Topical, Nasal.

Oxymetholone

See Anabolic Hormones.

Oxymorphone Hydrochloride

See Narcotic Analgesics.

Oxyphenbutazone

See Phenylbutazone and Oxyphenbutazone.

Oxyphencyclimine Hydrochloride

See Gastrointestinal Anticholinergics/Antispasmodics.

Oxyphenonium Bromide

See Gastrointestinal Anticholinergics/Antispasmodics.

Oxytetracycline

See Tetracyclines.

Oxytocin Rx

| injection: 10 units/ml | Pitocin, Syntocinon |
| nasal spray: 40 units/ml | Syntocinon |

INDICATIONS

Antepartum: Parenteral oxytocin is used for initiation or improvement of uterine contractions, in order to achieve early vaginal delivery, for fetal or maternal reasons such as Rh problems, maternal diabetes, preeclampsia at or near term, when delivery is in best interest of mother and fetus, or when membranes are prematurely ruptured and delivery is indicated; stimulation or reinforcement of labor, as in selected cases of uterine inertia; management of inevitable or incomplete abortion. In the first trimester, curettage is generally considered primary therapy. In second-trimester abortion, oxytocin infusion will often be successful in emptying the uterus. Other means of therapy may be required in such cases.

Postpartum: Parenteral oxytocin is indicated to produce uterine contractions during third stage of labor and to control postpartum bleeding or hemorrhage.

Nasal oxytocin is indicated for initial milk letdown.

Investigational uses: Antepartum fetal heart rate testing (oxytocin challenge test); breast engorgement.

CONTRAINDICATIONS

Significant cephalopelvic disproportion; unfavorable fetal positions or presentations that are undeliverable without conversion before delivery; in obstetric emergencies when benefit-to-risk ratio for either fetus or mother favors surgical intervention; in cases of fetal distress when delivery is not imminent; prolonged use in uterine inertia or severe toxemia; hypertonic uterine patterns; hypersensitivity to drug; induction or augmentation of labor in those for whom vaginal delivery is contraindicated, such as invasive cervical carcinoma, cord presentation or prolapse, total placenta previa, and vasa previa. Nasal oxytocin is contraindicated in pregnancy.

ACTIONS

Is an endogenous hormone produced by the posterior pituitary gland that has uterine stimulating properties, especially on the gravid uterus, as well as vasopressive and antidiuretic effects. Exact role in normal labor as well as medically induced labor is not fully understood. It may act primarily on uterine myofibril activity, thus augmenting the number of contracting myofibril. Sensitivity of the uterus to oxytocin increases gradually during gestation and increases sharply before parturition. Has weak antidiuretic effects but has led to fetal water intoxication. It also has a definite but transient relaxing effect on vascular smooth muscle.

May be given parenterally or intranasally; the latter may be erratically absorbed. Plasma half-life of synthetic oxytocin is 1 to 6 minutes, but this decreases in late pregnancy and lactation. Elimination is through the liver, kidney, and functional mammary gland and by the enzyme oxytocinase.

WARNINGS

When used for induction or stimulation of labor, drug must be administered only by the IV route.

PRECAUTIONS

Uterine contractions: When properly administered, drug stimulates uterine contractions similar to those seen in normal labor. Overstimulation can be hazardous to both mother and fetus. Even with proper administration and supervision, hypertonic contractions can occur in persons whose uteri are hypersensitive to oxytocin.

Except in unusual circumstances, oxytocin should not be administered in the following conditions: fetal distress, partial placenta previa, prematurity, borderline cephalopelvic disproportion, previous major surgery on the cervix or uterus including cesarean section, overdistention of the uterus, grand multiparity, history of uterine sepsis, traumatic delivery, or invasive cervical carcinoma.

Maternal deaths due to hypertensive episodes, subarachnoid hemorrhage, and rupture of the uterus and fetal deaths due to various causes have been reported associated with use of parenteral oxytocic drugs for induction of labor or for augmentation of the first and second stages of labor.

Water intoxication: Oxytocin has been shown to have an intrinsic antidiuretic effect, acting to increase water reabsorption from the glomerular filtrate. Water intoxication is considered, particularly when oxytocin is administered continuously by infusion and patient is receiving fluids by mouth.

DRUG INTERACTIONS

If used in conjunction with oxytocic drugs, the pressor effect of **sympathomimetic pressor amines** is potentiated; severe persistent hypertension and even rupture of a cerebral blood vessel may occur during the postpartum period.

ADVERSE REACTIONS

Fetal bradycardia, neonatal jaundice, anaphylactic reaction, postpartum hemorrhage, cardiac arrhythmia, fatal afibrinogenemia, nausea, vomiting, premature ventricular contractions, and pelvic hematoma have been reported. Excessive dosage or hypersensitivity to drug may result in uterine hypertonicity, spasm, tetanic contraction, or rupture of the uterus. The possibility of increased blood loss and afibrinogenemia should be kept in mind when administering drug. Severe water intoxication with convulsions and coma has occurred, associated with a slow oxytocin infusion over a 24-hour period. Maternal death due to oxytocin-induced water intoxication has been reported.

DOSAGE
Dosage is determined by uterine response.
Induction or stimulation of labor
IV infusion (drip method): This is the only acceptable method of administration for induction and stimulation of labor. Use physiologic electrolyte solution, except under unusual circumstances.

Initial dosage: Should be no more than 1 mU/minute to 2 mU/minute (0.001–0.002 units/minute). Gradually increase dose in increments of no more than 1 to 2 mU/minute at 15- to 30-minute intervals until a contraction pattern has been established that is similar to that of normal labor. Maximum doses should rarely exceed 20 mU/minute. Discontinue infusion immediately in the event of uterine hyperactivity or fetal distress, and administer oxygen to the mother.
Control of postpartum uterine bleeding
IV infusion (drip method): 10 units to 40 units may be added to 1000 ml of nonhydrating diluent and run at a rate necessary to control uterine atony.

IM: 10 units given after delivery of the placenta.
Treatment of incomplete or inevitable abortion
IV infusion with 500 ml of physiologic saline solution, or 5% dextrose in physiologic saline solution with 10 units of oxytocin infused at rate of 20 mU/minute to 40 mU/minute.
Initial milk let-down
Using nasal spray, one spray into one or both nostrils 2 to 3 minutes before breast-feeding or pumping breasts.

▌ NURSING IMPLICATIONS

HISTORY
Obtain obstetric history (parity, gravidity, previous obstetric problems, type of labor, stillbirths, abortions, live-birth infant abnormalities); EDC; health history; allergy history; drugs taken during pregnancy.

PHYSICAL ASSESSMENT
Obtain vital signs. Review laboratory tests, physician's physical examination; pelvic adequacy and maternal and fetal conditions are evaluated before oxytocin administration.

ADMINISTRATION
IV
Physician must order IV fluid (usually 5% dextrose in water), number of units to be added to IV and volume of IV fluid, and initial infusion rate. Five percent dextrose in saline may be ordered as the second IV to be run, when necessary, at KVO. Normal saline may be used if the patient is a diabetic.

Following addition of oxytocin to IV fluid, rotate bottle gently to ensure even distribution.

Use of an infusion pump (or other device such as a microdrip) for accurate control of infusion flow is essential.

A primary and secondary line or IV piggyback is used. If the IV infusion of oxytocin is discontinued temporarily, IV fluid (without oxytocin) is run at KVO or as ordered.

The initial infusion rate should be no more than 1 mU/minute to 2 mU/minute (0.001–0.002 units/minute). If 10 units are added to 1000 ml of IV fluid, each milliliter contains 0.01 units. If 5 units are added to 1000 ml of IV fluid, each milliliter contains 0.005 units. The rate of infusion (in drops/minute) must be calculated according to the delivery system used.

Have available magnesium sulfate, which may be administered for oxytocin-induced uterine tetany.

Explain procedure to patient and family.

Obtain maternal blood pressure and pulse and fetal heart rate (FHR), and determine uterine activity (strength, duration, frequency of contractions) before starting infusion of oxytocin. A fetal monitor may also be used to obtain the FHR. Record on flow chart.

Place patient on side; usually a left lateral position is used.

The physician establishes guidelines about increasing the infusion rate. Usually the dosage is increased every 15 minutes, but this may vary according to patient response.
Nasal spray
Place patient in upright position.

Have patient clear nasal passages.

Hold squeeze bottle upright; deliver prescribed number of sprays.

Wait 2 to 3 minutes before nursing or pumping breasts.

Solution may also be instilled in drop form by inverting the squeeze bottle and exerting gentle pressure.

ONGOING ASSESSMENTS AND NURSING MANAGEMENT
IV infusion

All patients receiving IV oxytocin must be under continuous observation to identify complications. A qualified physician should be immediately available.

Monitor maternal blood pressure, pulse, and respirations and FHR q15m or as ordered. Monitor each contraction as well as the status of the uterus between contractions. Record all data on flow sheet.

CLINICAL ALERT: Notify physician immediately of any change in FHR or any evidence of fetal distress; change in rate, rhythm, or frequency of uterine contractions; or significant increase or decrease in maternal vital signs.

If hypertonic contractions occur or fetal distress is noted, discontinue IV oxytocin and run IV fluid to KVO until physician examines patient.

The following usually require discontinuation of oxytocin and infusion of IV fluid to KVO: intrauterine pressure exceeding 65 mm Hg to 75 mm Hg (or the limit established by the physician); contractions lasting over 60 seconds (or the length established by the physician); contractions occurring more frequently than every 2 to 3 minutes; fetal bradycardia, tachycardia, or arrhythmia.

Physician must establish guidelines for increasing or decreasing the rate of infusion or for discontinuing the procedure.

Observe patient closely for signs of fluid overload (Appendix 6, section 6-12).

Measure intake and output. Notify physician of any change in intake–output ratio.

Keep patient and her family aware of progress.

If uterine inertia persists beyond 8 hours, the physician may order the procedure terminated.

Following delivery, patients receiving oxytocin are closely observed because maternal deaths due to hypertensive episodes or subarachnoid hemorrhage have been reported.

If IV infusion is used in treatment of incomplete or inevitable abortion, patient and family will require added emotional support.

IM

Given after delivery of placenta.

Monitor blood pressure, pulse, and respirations q5m to q10m or as ordered.

Check fundus for drug response. Prolonged uterine tetany may require administration of magnesium sulfate.

Nasal spray

Oxytocin stimulates the milk ejection (letdown) reflex.

Record amount of milk pumped from breasts or whether sufficient milk is produced at time of breast-feeding.

Notify physician if milk drips from breast before nursing, if milk drips from the breast not being nursed, or if uterine cramps occur during nursing, because drug may be discontinued.

O

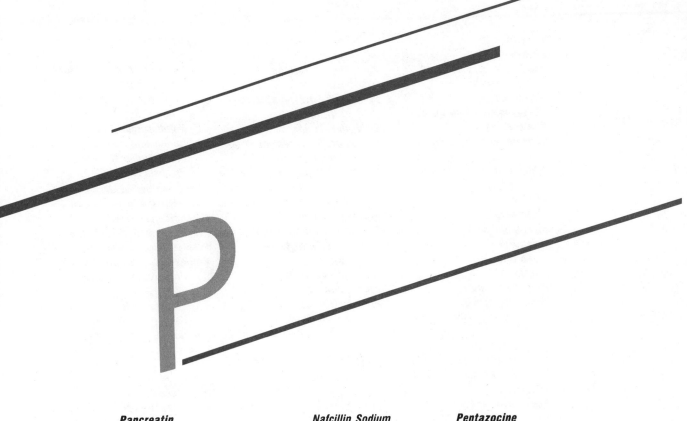

P

Pancreatin
Pancrelipase
Pancuronium Bromide
Papain
Papaverine Hydrochloride
Paraldehyde
Paramethadione
Paramethasone Acetate
Pargyline Hydrochloride
Paromomycin Sulfate
Pemoline
Penicillamine
Penicillins
    Amoxicillin
    Ampicillin, Oral
    Ampicillin Sodium, Parenteral
    Ampicillin With Probenecid
    Azlocillin Sodium
    Bacampicillin Hydrochloride
    Carbenicillin Disodium
    Carbenicillin Indanyl Sodium
    Cloxacillin Sodium
    Cyclacillin
    Dicloxacillin Sodium
    Hetacillin
    Methicillin Sodium
    Mezlocillin Sodium

    Nafcillin Sodium
    Oxacillin Sodium
    Penicillin G Benzathine, Oral
    Penicillin G Benzathine, Parenteral
    Penicillin G Benzathine and Procaine Combined
    Penicillin G (Aqueous), Parenteral
    Penicillin G Potassium, Oral
    Penicillin G Procaine, Aqueous (APPG)
    Penicillin V (Phenoxymethyl Penicillin)
    Penicillin V Potassium
    Piperacillin Sodium
    Ticarcillin Disodium
Penicillin G Benzathine
Penicillin G Benzathine and Procaine Combined
Penicillin G (Aqueous), Parenteral
Penicillin G Potassium
Penicillin G Procaine, Aqueous
Penicillin V
Penicillin V Potassium
Pentaerythritol Tetranitrate

Pentazocine
Pentobarbital and Pentobarbital Sodium
Perphenazine
Pertussis Immune Globulin
Phenacemide
Phenazopyridine Hydrochloride (Phenylazo Diamino Pyridine HCl)
Phendimetrazine Tartrate
Phenelzine Sulfate
Phenindamine Tartrate
Phenmetrazine Hydrochloride
Phenobarbital, Phenobarbital Sodium
Phenolphthalein
Phenoxybenzamine Hydrochloride
Phenprocoumon
Phensuximide
Phentermine Hydrochloride
Phentolamine
Phenylbutazone and Oxyphenbutazone
    Oxyphenbutazone
    Phenylbutazone
Phenylephrine Hydrochloride
Phenylpropanolamine Hydrochloride

Phenytoin
Phosphate
Phosphorus Replacement
    Products
Physostigmine
Physostigmine Salicylate
Phytonadione
Pilocarpine Hydrochloride, Ni-
    trate
Pilocarpine Ocular Therapeu-
    tic System
Pindolol
Piperacetazine
Piperacillin Sodium
Piperazine
Pipobroman
Piroxicam
Plague Vaccine
Plasma Protein Fractions
    Albumin Human (Normal
        Serum Albumin), 5%
    Albumin Human (Normal
        Serum Albumin), 25%
    Plasma Protein Fraction
Plicamycin
Pneumococcal Vaccine, Poly-
    valent
Poliomyelitis Vaccine
Poliovirus Vaccine
Poloxamer 188
Polyestradiol Phosphate
Polymyxin B Sulfate
Polysaccharide-Iron Complex
Polythiazide
Posterior Pituitary Injection
Potassium Acid Phosphate
    Preparations
    Potassium Acid Phosphate
    Potassium Acid Phosphate

and Sodium Acid Phos-
    phate
Potassium Citrate and Citric
    Acid
Potassium Citrate and Sodium
    Citrate
Potassium Iodide
Potassium Replacement Prod-
    ucts, Oral
Potassium Salts, Parenteral
    Potassium Acetate
    Potassium Chloride
Povidone-Iodine
Pralidoxime Chloride (PAM)
Pramoxine Hydrochloride
Prazepam
Prazosin Hydrochloride
Prednisolone
Prednisolone Acetate
Prednisolone Acetate and
    Prednisolone Sodium
    Phosphate
Prednisolone Sodium Phos-
    phate
Prednisolone Tebutate
Prednisone
Prilocaine Hydrochloride
Primaquine Phosphate
Primidone
Probenecid
Probenecid and Colchicine
    Combinations
Probucol
Procainamide Hydrochloride
Procaine Hydrochloride
Procarbazine Hydrochloride
Prochlorperazine
Procyclidine

Progesterone
Progestins
    Hydroxyprogesterone Cap-
        roate in Oil
    Medroxyprogesterone Ace-
        tate
    Norethindrone
    Norethindrone Acetate
    Progesterone Aqueous
    Progesterone in Oil
Promazine Hydrochloride
Promethazine Hydrochloride
Propantheline Bromide
Proparacaine Hydrochloride
Propiomazine Hydrochloride
Propoxyphene Preparations
    Propoxyphene Hydrochlo-
        ride
    Propoxyphene Napsylate
        Combination Products
Propranolol Hydrochloride
Propylthiouracil
Protamine Sulfate
Protamine Zinc Insulin Sus-
    pension
Protriptyline Hydrochloride
Pseudoephedrine Hydrochlo-
    ride, Pseudoephedrine
    Sulfate
Psyllium
Pyrantel Pamoate
Pyrazinamide
Pyridostigmine Bromide
Pyridoxine Hydrochloride
Pyrilamine Maleate
Pyrimethamine
Pyrvinium Pamoate

Pancreatin

See Digestive Enzymes.

Pancrelipase

See Digestive Enzymes.

Pancuronium Bromide Rx

injection: 1 mg/ml,   Pavulon
   2 mg/ml

INDICATIONS
Muscle relaxant used as an adjunct to anesthesia to induce skeletal muscle relaxation; to facilitate management of those undergoing mechanical ventilation.

CONTRAINDICATIONS
Known hypersensitivity to pancuronium or bromide ion.

ACTIONS
A nondepolarizing neuromuscular agent possessing all the characteristic actions of this class of drugs (curariform) on the myoneural junction (see also Curare Preparations). Is approximately five times as potent as tubocurarine.

Onset and duration of action are dose dependent. Administration of 0.04 mg/kg results in onset of action in 45 seconds and a peak effect within 4.5 minutes; recovery usually takes less than 1 hour.

WARNINGS
Administer in carefully adjusted dosage only by, or under the supervision of, those who are familiar with its actions and possible complications. Do not administer unless facilities for intubation, artificial respiration, oxygen therapy, and reversal agents are immediately available. Be prepared to assist or control respiration.

In those with myasthenia gravis, small doses may have profound effects. A peripheral nerve stimulator is especially valuable in such patients. Safety for use in pregnancy has not been established; use only when clearly needed and when potential benefits outweigh unknown potential hazards to the fetus. May be used in operative obstetrics (cesarean section), but reversal of drug may be unsatisfactory in those receiving magnesium sulfate for toxemia of pregnancy because magnesium salts enhance neuromuscular blockade.

PRECAUTIONS
Although it has been used successfully in many patients with preexisting pulmonary, hepatic, or renal disease, caution should be exercised in these situations. This is particularly true of renal disease because a major portion is excreted unchanged in the urine.

DRUG INTERACTIONS
Intensity and duration of action are increased in those receiving potent volatile **inhalation anesthetics** (halothane, diethyl ether, enflurane, methoxyflurane). Prior administration of **succinylcholine** enhances the relaxant effect and duration of action of pancuronium. Is antagonized by **acetylcholine, anticholinesterase,** and **potassium ion.** Action is increased by **quinine, magnesium salts,** and certain **antibiotics** such as neomycin, streptomycin, clindamycin, kanamycin, gentamicin, and bacitracin. Action may be altered by concomitant administration of other **neuromuscular agents.** Use in combination with **cardiac glycosides** may have additive cardiotoxic effects.

ADVERSE REACTIONS
Most frequent consist of an extension of pharmacologic actions beyond the time period needed for surgery and anesthesia. This may vary from skeletal muscle weakness to profound and prolonged skeletal muscle relaxation, resulting in respiratory insufficiency and apnea. Inadequate reversal of neuromuscular blockade by anticholinesterase agents has also been seen. These adverse reactions are managed by manual or mechanical ventilation until recovery is judged adequate. A slight increase in pulse rate is frequently noted. Salivation is sometimes noted during light anesthesia, especially if no anticholinergic premedication is used. An occasional transient rash may be seen.

MANAGEMENT OF PROLONGED NEUROMUSCULAR BLOCKADE
Pyridostigmine bromide or neostigmine, accompanied or preceded by atropine, may be used. See also Curare Preparations.

DOSAGE
Adults: Initial dose range is 0.04 mg/kg to 0.1 mg/kg. Incremental doses at 0.01 mg/kg may be used. If used to provide skeletal muscle relaxation for endotracheal intubation, 0.06 mg/kg to 0.1 mg/kg is recommended.

Children: Dosage requirement is the same as for adults. Neonates are especially sensitive to these drugs during the first month of life. A test dose of 0.02 mg/kg is recommended.

P

NURSING IMPLICATIONS

HISTORY
Alert the anesthesiologist to current drug therapy and history of allergies. Notification may be made by attaching note on cover of chart before transporting patient to surgery.

ADMINISTRATION
Drug is administered by anesthesia department.

ONGOING ASSESSMENTS AND NURSING MANAGEMENT

CLINICAL ALERT: Patient must not be left unattended until responding fully from anesthesia. This includes a partially awake patient with adequate respiratory exchange, movement in the extremities, return of swallowing and gag reflexes, and adequate circulation (arterial blood presure returns to preanesthetic level).

Postanesthesia: Monitor blood pressure, pulse, and respirations q15m (or as ordered) until full recovery from anesthesia.

Maintain patent airway until patient is able to swallow or speak, or until gag reflex returns.

Complete recovery from muscle relaxant effect may require several hours. Check for movement in the extremities, chest muscles (on inspiration and expiration), and jaw and neck muscles, and for swallowing and gag reflexes.

Notify anesthesia department immediately if any of the following occurs: erythema, edema, flushing, tachycardia, hypotension, bronchospasm (all are signs of histamine release); prolonged muscle relaxation; choking, noisy respirations; cyanosis; prolonged apnea.

Additional nursing management is based on individual factors, such as type of surgery, condition of patient, complications during surgery (*e.g.,* prolonged procedure, hemorrhage, episodes of hypotension, development of a cardiac arrhythmia), additional medical problems present prior to surgery (*e.g.,* diabetes mellitus, chronic obstructive pulmonary disease), patient's age.

Papain Rx

ointment: 10% papain, 10% urea	Panafil (also contains chlorophyll), Panafil White

INDICATIONS AND ACTIONS
For enzymatic debridement and promotion of normal healing in surface lesions, particularly when healing is retarded by local infection, necrotic tissue, fibrinous or purulent debris, or eschar.

PRECAUTIONS
Do not use in eyes.

ADVERSE REACTIONS
Itching or stinging sensation is sometimes associated with first application.

DOSAGE
Apply directly to lesion once or twice a day and cover with gauze. At each redressing, irrigate lesion with mild cleansing solution (not hydrogen peroxide, which may inactivate papain) to remove any accumulation of liquefied necrotic material.

NURSING IMPLICATIONS

HISTORY
See Appendix 4.

PHYSICAL ASSESSMENT
Note and record size and appearance of lesion, type and amount of drainage (if any).

ADMINISTRATION
Advise patient that itching or stinging may be noted, especially with the first application.

Irrigate area and apply to lesion as prescribed (see *Dosage*). Following application, apply gauze dressing unless physician orders otherwise.

ONGOING ASSESSMENTS AND NURSING MANAGEMENT
If itching or stinging persists on application, inform physician.

Note appearance of lesion each time drug is applied; compare with data base.

Notify physician if drainage increases, becomes more purulent, or develops a different odor or if lesion enlarges.

Papaverine Hydrochloride Rx

tablets: 30 mg, 60 mg, 100 mg, 200 mg	Generic
tablets: 300 mg	Pavabid HP Capsulets
tablets, timed release: 200 mg	P-200
capsules, timed release: 150 mg	Cerespan, Dilart, Pavabid Plateau, Pavatym, Generic
capsules, timed release: 300 mg	Dilart-300, PT-300
elixir: 100 mg/15 ml	Lapav
injection: 30 mg/ml	Generic

INDICATIONS

Oral: As a smooth muscle relaxant. For relief of cerebral and peripheral ischemia associated with arterial spasm and myocardial ischemia complicated by arrhythmias.

Parenteral: Has been used in various conditions accompanied by spasm of muscle, such as vascular spasm associated with acute myocardial infarction (MI); angina pectoris; peripheral and pulmonary embolism; peripheral vascular disease in which there is a vasospastic element; certain cerebral angiospastic states; visceral spasm as in ureteral, biliary, and GI colic.

Although papaverine has been used for many years for a number of conditions, there is insufficient evidence of any therapeutic value.

CONTRAINDICATIONS

Large doses can depress atrioventricular (AV) and intraventricular conduction and thereby produce serious arrhythmias. Contraindicated in presence of complete AV block. When conduction is depressed, may produce transient ectopic rhythms of ventricular origin, either premature beats or paroxysmal tachycardia.

ACTIONS

Most characteristic effect is relaxation of the tonus of all smooth muscle, especially when it has been spasmodically contracted. Action is apparently direct on the muscle itself. It has little effect on the CNS, although very large doses tend to produce some sedation and sleepiness in some patients. In some instances, mild respiratory stimulation can be seen. Possibly because of its direct vasodilating action on cerebral blood vessels, it may increase cerebral blood flow and at the same time decrease cerebral vascular resistance in normal subjects. These effects may explain the reported benefits in cerebral vascular encephalopathy.

Papaverine is effective by all routes of administration. It is metabolized by the liver. About 90% of the drug is bound to plasma protein. Reasonably constant plasma levels can be maintained with oral administration at 6-hour intervals. Drug is excreted in the urine in an inactive form.

WARNINGS

Safety for use in pregnancy has not been established. Use only when clearly needed and when potential benefits outweigh the unknown potential hazards to the fetus. It is not known whether drug is excreted in human milk. Safety for use in the nursing mother has not been established. Safety and effectiveness in children have not been established.

PRECAUTIONS

Use with caution in persons with glaucoma. Hepatic hypersensitivity has been reported with GI symptoms, jaundice, eosinophilia, and altered hepatic-function tests. Drug is discontinued if these symptoms appear.

Drug abuse and dependence: Drug dependence resulting from abuse of many of the selective depressants, including papaverine, has been reported.

ADVERSE REACTIONS

Nausea, abdominal distress, anorexia, sweating, flushing of face, vertigo, malaise, drowsiness, excessive sedation, headache, skin rash, constipation or diarrhea, increase in heart rate and depth of respiration. Hepatic hypersensitivity has been reported, resulting in jaundice, eosinophilia, and altered hepatic-function tests.

OVERDOSAGE

Toxicity of oral papaverine is very low; ingestion of more than ten times the usual therapeutic dose has not resulted in untoward effects. A single dose of 0.1 g/kg to 0.5 g/kg would be fatal to an adult.

Acute poisoning

Symptoms: Drowsiness, weakness, nystagmus, diplopia, incoordination, and lassitude, progressing to coma with cyanosis and respiratory depression.

Treatment: Give tap water, milk, or activated charcoal; then remove stomach contents by gastric lavage or emesis, followed by catharsis. If coma and respiratory depression occur, appropriate measures should be taken. Hemodialysis has been suggested. Blood pressure should be maintained. Concurrent administration of other depressant drugs should be avoided.

Chronic poisoning

Symptoms: Drowsiness, depression, weakness, anxiety, ataxia, headache, blurred vision, gastric upset, and pruritic skin rashes characterized by urticaria or erythematous macular eruptions. Laboratory findings show that any of the formed elements of the blood may be decreased in number.

Treatment: Discontinue medication. Severe hypotension may occur when any depressant, including papaverine, is used. Drug is discontinued at onset of any abnormal hematologic findings. Dosage is reduced if drowsiness occurs. Recovery should occur, except in patients with aplastic anemia.

DOSAGE

Oral: Usual dosage ranges from 100 mg to 300 mg, one to five times a day.

Oral, timed release: 150 mg q12h. In difficult cases, increase to 150 mg q8h or 300 mg q12h.

P

Parenteral: May be administered IV or IM. IV route is recommended when immediate effect is desired; inject slowly over 1 to 2 minutes. Parenteral administration in doses of 30 mg to 120 mg is repeated q3h as indicated. For cardiac extrasystoles, give two doses 10 minutes apart.

NURSING IMPLICATIONS

HISTORY
See Appendix 4.

PHYSICAL ASSESSMENT
Obtain blood pressure, pulse, and respirations. If drug is prescribed for peripheral ischemia, examine involved areas noting skin color, temperature, and appearance; palpate peripheral pulses. Depending on diagnosis and rationale for use, additional assessments may be warranted. Hepatic-function tests may be ordered.

ADMINISTRATION
Instruct patient not to chew timed-release capsules or tablets.

If patient has difficulty swallowing tablet or capsule, discuss with physician; an elixir is available.

If GI side-effects occur, discuss with physician about administration with food or meals.

When given IV, drug is injected slowly over 1 to 2 minutes. Parenteral form should not be added to Lactated Ringer's Injection because precipitation will result.

ONGOING ASSESSMENTS AND NURSING MANAGEMENT
Monitor blood pressure, pulse, and respirations daily; observe for drug effect as well as adverse reactions.

May cause dizziness (hypotension) or drowsiness. Assist patient with ambulatory activities as needed.

Withhold drug and notify physician if excessive drowsiness, skin rash, depression, weakness, anxiety, or ataxia is noted or if patient complains of headache or blurred vision. These may be signs of chronic poisoning (see *Overdosage*).

Jaundice may indicate hepatic hypersensitivity. Drug should be withheld until physician examines patient or hepatic-function tests are performed.

Hepatic-function tests, CBC may be performed at periodic intervals on those receiving long-term therapy.

When applicable, patient should be encouraged to stop smoking (nicotine constricts blood vessels).

PATIENT AND FAMILY INFORMATION
May cause dizziness or drowsiness. Observe caution when driving or performing other tasks requiring alertness. Alcohol may intensify these effects and use should be avoided.

May cause flushing, sweating, headache, tiredness, jaundice, skin rash, and GI effects (nausea, anorexia, abdominal distress, constipation, diarrhea). Notify physician or nurse if these become pronounced.

Do not increase dosage unless instructed to do so by physician.

Paraldehyde Rx C-IV

liquid (oral, rectal)	Paral, *Generic*
injection	Paral, *Generic*

INDICATIONS
Emergency treatment of tetanus, eclampsia, and status epilepticus, and of poisoning by convulsant drugs, particularly if a soluble barbiturate is not available. May be used as a sedative/hypnotic. Also used in treatment of delirium tremens and other psychiatric states characterized by excitement and is administered to quiet the patient and produce sleep. Large doses (15 ml–30 ml or more) may be needed for this purpose. It has been used IM to induce artificial sleep and facilitate EEG study, especially in children. Parenteral use as a sedative/hypnotic has largely been replaced by use of safer, more effective agents.

CONTRAINDICATIONS
May at times be contraindicated in bronchopulmonary disease because of excretion of drug by the lungs. Hepatic insufficiency constitutes a contraindication because approximately 80% of drug is metabolized by the liver. In persons with gastroenteritis, especially if ulceration is present, it may cause considerable irritation.

ACTIONS
Is a colorless, bitter-tasting liquid with a strong, unpleasant odor. Upon exposure to light and air it decomposes to acetaldehyde and oxidizes to acetic acid. Like other hypnotic drugs, it produces nonspecific, reversible depression of the CNS. With usual therapeutic doses, it has little effect on respiration and blood pressure; large doses may cause respiratory depression and hypotension.

It is rapidly absorbed after oral administration and produces sleep within 10 to 15 minutes after a 4-ml to 8-ml dose. It is detoxified in the liver; 11%

to 28% is excreted unchanged via the lungs. A negligible amount is excreted in urine.

WARNINGS

Drug abuse and dependence: Prolonged use of larger than therapeutic doses may result in tolerance and psychic or physical dependence. After prolonged administration, drug is gradually withdrawn to avoid possible precipitation of withdrawal symptoms.

Use in pregnancy and lactation: Safety has not been established. Crosses the placental barrier, producing appreciable fetal blood concentrations. Use during labor may cause respiratory depression of the neonate. Use only if clearly needed and if potential benefits outweigh the unknown potential hazards to the fetus.

PRECAUTIONS

So-called hypersensitivity may be due to presence of liver damage. IV use is dangerous and reserved for emergencies. See also _Overdosage_ for IV administration of toxic doses. The mechanism of the coughing that is frequently observed with IV use is unknown. When injecting IM, avoid vicinity of the nerve trunks. Like alcohol, the drug may cause nerve injury and paralysis.

DRUG INTERACTIONS

Concurrent use of **general anesthetics, monoamine oxidase (MAO) inhibitors,** or **tricyclic antidepressants** may increase the effects of either these agents or paraldehyde. Concurrent use of **disulfiram** may decrease metabolism of paraldehyde, resulting in increased blood levels and acetaldehyde; concomitant use should be avoided. Will have additive effects with other **CNS depressants.**

ADVERSE REACTIONS

Prolonged use: Continued use may result in addiction that resembles alcoholism. Withdrawal may produce delirium tremens and vivid hallucinations. Prolonged use may produce yellowing of eyes or skin (hepatitis).

Rarely, unusually slow heartbeat, shortness of breath, and troubled breathing occur. Local reactions include skin rash, redness, swelling, or pain at injection site (thrombophlebitis). Severe and permanent nerve damage including paralysis, particularly of the sciatic nerve, has occurred when drug was injected too close to nerve trunks.

Miscellaneous: Although medically insignificant, strong, unpleasant breath may occur. Coughing (IV use only).

OVERDOSAGE

Symptoms: Are similar to those of chloral hydrate overdosage and include coma, severe hypotension, respiratory depression, pulmonary edema, and cardiac failure. Coma may last for several hours because rate of drug metabolism is slow. Diagnosis of overdosage is facilitated by the characteristic odor of the drug on the breath. Although fatalities are rare, administration of 25 ml of paraldehyde PO or 12 ml rectally has caused death. Death is usually due to respiratory failure. A few fatalities have been attributed to pulmonary edema and right-sided heart failure or metabolic acidosis. Acute overdosage will produce rapid, labored respiration; rapid, feeble pulse; and hypotension. Toxic doses given by vein cause massive pulmonary hemorrhage, edema, and dilation of the right side of the heart. Chronic and acute overdosage may cause acidosis, bleeding gastritis, azotemia, oliguria, albuminuria, fatty infiltration of the liver and kidney, hepatitis and nephrosis, pulmonary hemorrhage with edema, and dilation of the right side of the heart. Metabolic acidosis has been associated with nausea, muscular tremor, severe epigastric cramps, mental confusion, agitation, pseudoketosis, and hyperacetaldehydemia.

Treatment: Give primary attention to reestablishment of adequate respiratory exchange by maintenance of an adequate airway, control of respiration, and oxygen administrtion. Other treatment measures consist of gastric lavage for oral overdosage (if an endotracheal tube with cuff inflated is in place to prevent aspiration of vomitus) or rectal lavage for rectal overdosage, followed by administration (oral or by nasogastric tube) of a demulcent (_e.g.,_ mineral oil) to relieve gastric irritation, maintaining body temperature and supporting circulation. Correct metabolic acidosis by IV administration of sodium bicarbonate or sodium lactate.

DOSAGE

Oral: Usual hypnotic dose is 4 ml to 8 ml given in milk or iced fruit juice to mask taste and odor. In delirium tremens, 10 ml to 35 ml may be necessary.

Rectal: Dissolve in oil as a retention enema. Mix 10 ml to 20 ml of paraldehyde with one or two parts olive oil or isotonic sodium chloride solution to avoid rectal irritation.

_IM:_ For hypnosis in adults, give 10 ml (maximum 5 ml per injection site). For hypnosis in children, give 0.3 ml/kg or 12 ml/m^2. For sedation in adults, give 2 ml to 5 ml. For sedation in children, give 0.15 ml/kg or 6 ml/m^2. As an anticonvulsant, usual dose is 5 ml.

_IV:_ For hypnosis in adults, give 10 ml diluted with at least 200 ml of 0.9% Sodium Chloride Injection, at a rate not exceeding 1 ml/minute. For sedation in adults, give 5 ml diluted with at least 100 ml of 0.9% Sodium Chloride Injection, at a rate not exceeding 1 ml/minute. As an anticonvulsant, give 3 ml to 5 ml. For IV infusion, dilute 5 ml with at least 100 ml Sodium Chloride Injection and infuse at a rate of not more than 1 ml/minute.

NURSING IMPLICATIONS

HISTORY
See Appendix 4.

PHYSICAL ASSESSMENT
Obtain blood pressure, pulse, and respirations. If patient has a convulsant disorder, record seizure pattern. If patient has delirium tremens or other psychiatric disorder, record behavior.

ADMINISTRATION
Do not use if solution has a brownish color or sharp, penetrating odor of acetic acid (vinegar). Because drug oxidizes more rapidly in opened, partially filled containers, do not use drug from a container that has been opened longer than 24 hours.

Paraldehyde is not compatible with most plastics. Use glass syringes, drinking glasses, measuring cups, and medicine cups. Paper drinking straws should be used when a straw is necessary. Use a rubber tube and metal or glass container for rectal administration. Do not use IV fluids available in plastic containers or plastic IV tubing without first checking with pharmacist.

Stability and storage: Store oral liquid at a temperature not exceeding 25°C (77°F). *Injection*—Keep away from heat, open flame, and sparks. Paraldehyde solidifies at approximately 12°C (54°F) and must be liquefied before use. Do not store in direct sunlight or expose to temperatures above 25°C (77°F). Protect from light by keeping covered in box until use. Discard unused portion.

Oral/rectal
When opening container for first time, write date and time on label.

Mix prescribed oral dose in iced fruit juice or milk to mask taste and odor.

For rectal administration, dissolve in oil as a retention enema. Mix prescribed dose with one or two parts of olive oil or isotonic sodium chloride to avoid rectal irritation.

Parenteral
Do *not* give subcutaneously.

In psychiatric states characterized by excitement, restraining measures may be necessary.

Patient should be restrained until injection is administered and needle is withdrawn.

IM: Administer deeply into the gluteus maximus, taking care to avoid nerve trunks (see *Adverse Reactions*). Do not give more than 5 ml at any one site. Because as much as 10 ml IM may be required and drug must be given into the gluteus muscle, it may be necessary in some instances to administer 5 ml per injection site.

IM injection is painful, but pain rapidly disappears with the onset of action of the drug. When applicable, warn patient that injection is painful.

IV: Drug must be diluted before administration. Physician orders IV fluid (usually 0.9% Sodium Chloride Injection) and volume and infusion rate. Infuse at a rate of not more than 1 ml/minute.

Have suction equipment available because bronchopulmonary secretions may be increased. When possible, keep patient on side to prevent aspiration of secretions.

When given IV, central depression may be preceded by a few seconds of excitement or coughing.

ONGOING ASSESSMENTS AND NURSING MANAGEMENT
Patient receiving IV infusion should be closely supervised until infusion is completed. Monitor blood pressure, pulse, and respirations q10m to q15m. Suction as necessary.

When given as a sedative/hypnotic, sleep is usually produced within 10 to 15 minutes.

When drug is given for delirium tremens and other psychiatric states, patient should be closely observed until drug produces calming effect. When possible, patient should remain in bed; siderails should be raised. Other protective restraining measures may also be necessary.

Patient should not be allowed to smoke.

Observe and record drug effects. If drug is ineffective in producing hypnosis or sedation or controlling convulsive disorder, notify physician.

When drug is used as an anticonvulsant, see also Anticonvulsants.

Patient's breath will have characteristic odor for several hours.

CLINICAL ALERT: When paraldehyde is given IV for emergency treatment of convulsive disorders, observe patient for severe dyspnea and signs of pulmonary edema. Notify physician immediately if patient experiences any respiratory difficulty.

Following prolonged administration, drug should be gradually withdrawn to avoid possible precipitation of withdrawal symptoms.

Paramethadione

See Anticonvulsants, Oxazolidinediones.

Paramethasone Acetate

See Glucocorticoids.

Pargyline Hydrochloride Rx

tablets: 10 mg,   Eutonyl Filmtabs
   25 mg

INDICATIONS

Treatment of moderate to severe hypertension. Not recommended for use in those with mild or labile hypertension. However, it does not interfere with or obviate use of diuretic therapy in hypertensive patients who may have associated edema. May be used alone or concurrently with most other antihypertensive agents. Is often effective at reduced dosage when administered with one of the thiazides and/or rauwolfia alkaloids. See also Antihypertensive Agents.

CONTRAINDICATIONS

Patients with pheochromocytoma, paranoid schizophrenia, hyperthyroidism, advanced renal failure. Not given to those with malignant hypertension or to children under 12.

The following drugs are contraindicated in those receiving pargyline: **centrally-acting sympathomimetic amines** (*e.g.,* amphetamine and its derivatives and anorectics) and **peripherally-acting sympathomimetic drugs** (*e.g.,* ephedrine and its derivatives), which are found in nasal decongestants, cold remedies, and hay fever preparations. Foods containing tyramine (p 99) are avoided. In some patients receiving pargyline, tyramine may precipitate an abrupt rise in blood pressure accompanied by all or some of the following: severe headache, chest pain, profuse sweating, palpitation, tachycardia or bradycardia, visual disturbances, stertorous breathing, coma, and intracranial bleeding (which could be fatal). Phentolamine may be administered parenterally for treatment of an acute hypertensive reaction.

Parenteral administration of **reserpine** or **guanethidine** may cause hypertensive reactions from the sudden release of catecholamines. Parenteral use of these drugs is contraindicated during and for at least 1 week following treatment with pargyline.

Tricyclic antidepressants should not be used with pargyline. Use of these drugs with an MAO inhibitor has been reported to cause vascular collapse and hyperthermia, which may be fatal. A drug-free interval (about 2 weeks) should separate therapy with pargyline and use of these agents. **Other MAO inhibitors** are contraindicated because they may augment the effects of pargyline.

Methyldopa or **dopamine** may cause hyperexcitability in patients receiving pargyline. There have been reports of potentiation of the pressor effects of **levodopa** by various MAO inhibitors; concomitant therapy is contraindicated and at least 1 month should elapse after discontinuation of a MAO inhibitor before levodopa is given.

ACTIONS

Pargyline is an MAO inhibitor. The mechanism of its antihypertensive activity is unknown. Like the antidepressant MAO inhibitors, the hypotensive effect is predominantly postural. Clinical response is slow and may take up to 2 to 3 weeks. After discontinuation of the drug, effects may persist for several weeks. The drug is excreted primarily in the urine.

WARNINGS

Concomitant administration of CNS depressants: When indicated, the following are prescribed in reduced dosages: antihistamines; hypnotics, sedatives, or tranquilizers; narcotics (meperidine should not be used). An increased response to central depressants may be manifested by acute hypotension and increased sedative effect.

Use in surgical patients: Drug is discontinued at least 2 weeks prior to elective surgery. In emergency surgery, dose of narcotics and other premedications should be reduced to one-fourth to one-fifth of usual amount. Response to all anesthetic agents can be exaggerated.

Use in diabetes: Drug may induce hypoglycemia. Administer with caution to diabetics because severe hypoglycemia may occur. If it is necessary to administer pargyline to patients receiving insulin or other hypoglycemic agents, dose of these agents is reduced and patient monitored closely.

Use in impaired renal function: Patient may experience cumulative effects as drug is excreted in the urine. Patient should be observed for elevated BUN, other evidence of progressive renal failure. If such alterations persist, drug is discontinued.

Use in pregnancy, lactation: Safety not established. Before prescribing in pregnancy, lactation, or women of childbearing age, potential benefit is weighed against the possible hazard to the mother and child.

PRECAUTIONS

All patients with impaired circulation to vital organs from any cause, including those with angina pectoris, coronary artery disease, and cerebral arteriosclerosis, should be closely observed for symptoms of orthostatic hypotension. If hypotension develops, dosage is reduced or drug discontinued because severe and/or prolonged hypotension may precipitate cerebral or coronary vessel thrombosis.

Hepatic effects: There have been no substantiated reports of hepatotoxicity, but because liver damage has resulted from use of other MAO inhibitors and because transient alterations in liver enzyme levels have occasionally occurred, it is recommended that patient have periodic liver-function tests.

Cardiovascular disease: The hypotensive effect of pargyline may be augmented by febrile illnesses; it may be advisable to withdraw drug during such diseases.

Psychic effects: Not used in those with hyperactive or hyperexcitable personalities; some of these patients show an undesirable increase in motor activity with restlessness, confusion, agitation, disorientation. Drug may unmask severe psychotic symptoms such as hallucinations or paranoid delusions in some patients with preexisting serious emotional problems. This can usually be controlled by administration of IM chlorpromazine or other phenothiazines.

Use in Parkinson's disease: Drug is used with caution, because it may increase symptoms. Great care is required if pargyline is administered in conjunction with antiparkinsonism agents.

Ophthalmologic effects: Nonspecific visual disturbances and aggravation of glaucoma have occurred; patients receiving drug should be examined for any change in color perception, visual fields, fundi, visual acuity.

Tartrazine sensitivity: 25 mg strength contains tartrazine. See Appendix 6, section 6-23.

DRUG INTERACTIONS

Caffeine, alcohol, antihistamines, barbiturates, chloral hydrate, other **hypnotics, sedatives,** and **tranquilizers,** and **narcotics** are used cautiously and at reduced dosages. **Meperidine** should not be used. Some individuals on prolonged therapy are refractory to the nerve blocking effects of **local anesthetics** (*e.g.,* lidocaine).

See also *Contraindications* and *Warnings.*

ADVERSE REACTIONS

Orthostatic hypotension (dizziness, weakness, palpitation, fainting); mild constipation; fluid retention (with or without edema); dry mouth; sweating; increased appetite; arthralgia; nausea, vomiting; headache; blurred vision; insomnia; difficulty in micturition; nightmares; impotence and delayed ejacula-

tion; rash and purpura; hyperexcitability; increased neuromuscular activity (muscle twitching); other extrapyramidal symptoms; weight gain. Drug fever, hypoglycemia, and CHF occur rarely.

OVERDOSAGE

Symptoms: Reported effects of MAO inhibitor overdosage includes agitation, hallucinations; hyperreflexia; hyperpyrexia; convulsions; and both hypotension and hypertension.

Treatment: Management must be attempted with great caution because of potential for interaction with antidotal drugs. Conservative treatment aimed at maintenance of normal temperature, respiration, blood pressure, and proper fluid and electrolyte balance is generally successful. If severe hypotension should occur, this can be controlled by small doses of a vasopressor such as epinephrine.

DOSAGE

Give PO as a single daily dose; there is no known advantage to taking more than once daily. Clinical response not immediate; 4 days to 3 weeks or more may be required to produce full effects of a given daily dosage. It is recommended that dosage not be increased more frequently than once a week. Drug effects may persist following dosage reduction or withdrawal. If therapy must be interrupted because of undesirable side-effects, drug should be withheld until all such effects have disappeared. Therapy is then reinstituted at a lower dosage. Because drug exerts an orthostatic effect on blood pressure, dosage adjustments are based on blood pressure response in the standing position. Not given to children under 12 years.

Initial dosage: Usual dosage in hypertensive patient not receiving other antihypertensive agents is 25 mg once daily. Dosage may be increased once a week by 10-mg increments until desired response obtained. Total daily dose should not exceed 200 mg.

Patients over 65 or those having undergone sympathectomy may be unusually sensitive to antihypertensive properties of drug. In such patients, initial dosage should be 10 mg to 25 mg. When added to established antihypertensive therapy, initial dose should not exceed 25 mg daily (less in sympathectomized and elderly patients).

Maintenance: Reduction of blood pressure is often maintained with daily dose of 25 mg to 50 mg. Larger doses may be tried in resistant cases. In general, dosage should be kept at the minimum level required to maintain a desirable reduction in blood pressure without encountering undue side-effects.

Concomitant antihypertensive therapy: A few patients may develop a relative tolerance to the antihypertensive effects; administration of additional antihypertensive agents may be considered in cases not controlled by pargyline alone.

NURSING IMPLICATIONS

HISTORY
See Appendix 4.

PHYSICAL ASSESSMENT
Obtain blood pressure on both arms with patient in standing position; obtain pulse and respiratory rates. Blood pressure may additionally be obtained with the patient in the sitting and lying position. Hepatic-, renal-function tests may be ordered.

ADMINISTRATION
Drug given once daily, at same time each day.

ONGOING ASSESSMENTS AND NURSING MANAGEMENT
Obtain blood pressure with patient in standing position on both arms; obtain pulse and respirations q4h to q8h or as ordered; take temperature; check ankles, tibia for edema; observe for adverse drug reactions.

Physician makes dosage adjustments based on blood pressure response in the standing position.

Weigh weekly or as ordered. Report significant weight gain or evidence of edema to physician.

Clinical response to drug is not immediate; 4 days to 3 weeks may be required.

CLINICAL ALERT: Withhold drug and notify physician if there is a significant change (increase or decrease) in the blood pressure or pulse rate.

Meperidine should not be administered to patients receiving this drug.

Patients over 65 or sympathectomized patients may be unusually sensitive to drug. Monitor blood pressure and pulse at more frequent intervals in these patients.

Have patient make position changes slowly to avoid symptoms of orthostatic hypotension. Patient should receive assistance in ambulatory activities, especially during dosage adjustment period.

Notify physician of temperature elevation; drug may need to be discontinued.

Notify physician of any behavior changes as drug may unmask severe psychotic symptoms (see _Precautions_).

Dietary restrictions include elimination of foods containing tyramine (pp 99–100).

Drug is discontinued at least 2 weeks prior to elective surgery. In emergency surgery, the dose of narcotics or other premedications should be reduced (see _Warnings_).

Dry mouth may be relieved by frequent sips of water, chewing gum, hard candy.

Periodic liver- and renal-function tests and ophthalmologic examination are recommended during therapy.

Notify physician if patient complains of any visual difficulties.

Diabetic patient should be monitored closely for signs of hypoglycemia (Appendix 6, section 6-14). Dosage of hypoglycemic agent is usually reduced but frequent adjustment may be necessary.

Patients with impaired renal function may experience cumulative drug effects. Frequent evaluation of renal function (BUN, serum creatinine) plus observation for evidence of renal failure recommended. Measure intake and output; notify physician of any decrease in urinary output.

PATIENT AND FAMILY INFORMATION
NOTE: Provide patient with list of foods containing tyramine (pp 99–100). Explain importance of checking labels of products containing multiple foods, including those foods to which a meat tenderizer has been added. In addition, patient should be warned not to eat foods brought or sent (_e.g.,_ gift baskets) to the hospital without checking with the nurse.

Drug does not take effect immediately; 4 days to 3 weeks may be required.

Do not discontinue drug or increase or decrease the dose unless directed by a physician. Inform other physicians, dentist of therapy with this drug.

Do not take cold, cough, or allergy medications, weight-control products, unless use of a specific product approved by the physician.

If dizziness occurs, avoid sudden changes in posture. Rise from a sitting or lying position slowly; avoid prolonged standing in one place. If dizziness does occur, sit or lie down until symptoms relieved.

Observe caution in driving or performing potentially dangerous tasks if dizziness occurs.

Notify physician or nurse immediately if fainting, severe headache, visual changes, or other unusual symptoms occur.

Avoid alcoholic beverages and coffee unless a specified amount is allowed by the physician.

Patient with angina, coronary artery disease: Do not increase physical activities in response to diminution of anginal symptoms or an increased sense of well-being occurring during therapy.

Patient with diabetes: Check urine daily or as recommended by physician. If hypoglycemia occurs, contact physician.

Paromomycin Sulfate

See Aminoglycosides, Oral.

Pemoline Rx C-IV

tablets: 18.75 mg, 37.5 mg, 75 mg	Cylert
chewable tablets: 37.5 mg	Cylert

INDICATIONS

Attention deficit disorder or hyperkinetic syndrome, as integral part of a total treatment program that includes other remedial measures (psychological, educational, social) for a stabilizing effect in children with a behavioral syndrome. See Methylphenidate *Indications* for behavioral syndrome characteristics and criteria for drug selection.

Investigational use: 50 mg to 200 mg in two divided doses daily has been used in treatment of narcolepsy and excessive daytime sleepiness.

CONTRAINDICATIONS

Hypersensitivity.

ACTIONS

Is a CNS stimulant structurally dissimilar to the amphetamines and methylphenidate. Pharmacologic activity is similar to that of other known stimulants but with minimal sympathomimetic effects. Although exact site and mechanism of action are unknown, studies indicate it may act through dopaminergic mechanisms. Peak serum levels occur within 2 to 4 hours after ingestion of a single dose. Serum half-life is approximately 12 hours. Steady state is reached in approximately 2 to 3 days. Pemoline and its metabolites are excreted primarily in urine. It has a gradual onset of action. Using the recommended dosage schedules, significant clinical benefit may not be seen until third or fourth week of administration.

WARNINGS

Administer with caution to those with impaired renal or hepatic function. Safety for use in pregnancy and lactation not established. Not recommended for use in children under 6 years. Clinical experience suggests that in psychotic children, administration may exacerbate symptoms of behavior disturbance and thought disorder. Data inadequate to determine whether chronic administration may be associated with growth inhibition. Long-term effects in children not well established.

PRECAUTIONS

Hepatic effects: Liver-function tests should be performed prior to and periodically during therapy. Use is discontinued if abnormalities are revealed and confirmed by follow-up tests (see *Adverse Reactions*).

Drug dependence: The pharmacologic similarity of pemoline to other psychostimulants with known dependence liability suggests psychological and/or physical dependence might also occur. There have been isolated reports of transient psychotic symptoms occurring in adults following long-term misuse of excessive doses. Give with caution to emotionally unstable patients who may increase dosage on their own initiative.

DRUG INTERACTIONS

Patients receiving pemoline concurrently with other agents, especially drugs with **CNS activity,** should be monitored carefully.

ADVERSE REACTIONS

Mild adverse reactions occurring early in treatment often remit with continuing therapy. If adverse reactions are of significant or protracted nature, dosage reduction or discontinuation of therapy is considered.

Most frequent: Insomnia usually occurs early in therapy prior to optimum therapeutic response, and in majority of cases is transient or responds to dosage reduction. Anorexia with weight loss may occur during first few weeks; in the majority of cases it is transient. Weight gain usually resumes within 3 to 6 months.

CNS: Dyskinetic movements of tongue, lips, face, and extremities; nystagmus and nystagmoid eye movements; and convulsive seizures. A definite causal relationship has not been established.

Other: Stomachache; skin rashes; irritability; mild depression; nausea; dizziness; headache; drowsiness; hallucinations.

Altered laboratory findings: Elevations of SGOT, SGPT, and serum LDH have occurred, usually several months after therapy. These effects appear to be reversible upon withdrawal of drug and are thought to be manifestations of a delayed hypersensitivity reaction. There have been a few reports of jaundice; a causal relationship has not been established.

OVERDOSAGE

Symptoms: Tachycardia, hallucinations, agitation, dyskinetic movements or restlessness; overactivity, irregular respiration, increased salivation, intermittent tongue protrusion, and generalized hyperreflexia have also been reported.

Treatment: Same as for overdosage of any CNS stimulant. Management is primarily symptomatic and may include induction of emesis, gastric lavage, sedation, or other supportive measures. Hemodialysis may be useful. Forced diuresis and peritoneal dialysis appear to be of little value.

DOSAGE

Give as a single oral dose each morning. Recommended starting dose is 37.5 mg/day. Gradually increase at 1 week intervals using increments of 18.75 mg until desired clinical response obtained. Mean effective doses range from 56.25 mg/day to 75 mg/day. Maximum recommended dose is 112.5 mg/day. When possible, drug administration should be interrupted occasionally to determine if there is a recurrence of behavioral symptoms sufficient to require continued therapy.

NURSING IMPLICATIONS

HISTORY
See Appendix 4.

PHYSICAL ASSESSMENT
Observe behavior (if possible) and record observations; height; weight. Hepatic-function tests may be ordered.

ADMINISTRATION
Given as single oral dose in morning to avoid insomnia.

If child resists taking medication, inform physician.

Chewable tablet: Instruct child to chew tablet thoroughly.

ONGOING ASSESSMENTS AND NURSING MANAGEMENT
Observe behavior and record daily or weekly summaries; observe for adverse effects.

Significant benefit may not be seen for 3 to 4 weeks.

Weigh weekly or as ordered. Inform physician if anorexia is apparent or significant weight loss is noted.

Insomnia usually occurs early in therapy. Hospitalized child may have difficulty adhering to usual hours of sleep and may disturb other pa-tients. Notify physician if insomnia persists because dosage may need to be reduced.

Liver-function tests are recommended at periodic intervals during therapy.

Measure height monthly.

PATIENT AND FAMILY INFORMATION
Take/give dose early in the morning.

Notify physician or nurse if insomnia occurs.

If dizziness or drowsiness occurs, it may be necessary to control child's activities that may be potentially hazardous (*e.g.*, climbing, playing on swings, swimming). Excessive drowsiness or sedation is reported to the physician.

Three or four weeks may elapse before clinical benefits are seen.

Early in therapy write a daily summary of child's activities, general behavior. This will assist physician in adjusting dosage.

Weigh weekly. If significant weight loss occurs, notify physician. Loss of appetite may also occur. Notify physician if this persists more than 1 to 2 weeks.

Penicillamine Rx

capsules: 125 mg, 250 mg	Cuprimine
tablets: 250 mg	Depen Titratabs

INDICATIONS
Treatment of rheumatoid arthritis. Use is restricted to those who have severe, active disease and who have failed to respond to an adequate trial of conventional therapy. Also used in treatment of Wilson's disease (hepatolenticular degeneration) to promote excretion of copper deposited in tissues. May be used in treatment of cystinuria when other measures inadequate to control recurrent stone formation.

Investigational uses: The benefits of drug's copper-chelating and immunologic effects have been investigated for use in treatment of primary biliary cirrhosis. Doses of 600 mg/day to 900 mg/day have been used. Some data suggest that penicillamine may be beneficial in scleroderma.

CONTRAINDICATIONS
History of penicillamine-related aplastic anemia or agranulocytosis. Because of potential for renal damage, not administered to rheumatoid arthritis patients with history or other evidence of renal insufficiency. *Contraindicated in rheumatoid arthritis patients who are pregnant.*

P

ACTIONS

Penicillamine is well absorbed from the GI tract and is rapidly excreted in the urine.

Cystinuria: Reduces excess cystine excretion.

Rheumatoid arthritis: Mechanism of action unknown. Unlike cytotoxic immunosuppressants, it markedly lowers IgM rheumatoid factor but produces no significant depression in absolute levels of serum immunoglobulins.

Wilson's disease: Is a chelating agent for removal of excess copper in those with Wilson's disease.

WARNINGS

Use has been associated with fatalities due to certain diseases such as aplastic anemia, agranulocytosis, thrombocytopenia, Goodpasture's syndrome, and myasthenic syndrome.

Because of potential for serious hematologic and renal adverse reactions, routine urinalysis, WBC and differential, hemoglobin, and platelet count are recommended every 2 weeks for first 6 months of therapy and monthly thereafter.

Proteinuria and/or hematuria may develop during therapy and may be warning signs of membranous glomerulopathy, which can progress to a nephrotic syndrome. In some patients, proteinuria disappears with continued therapy; in others, drug must be discontinued.

Rheumatoid arthritis patients who develop a moderate degree of proteinuria may be continued cautiously on therapy; quantitative 24-hour urinary protein determinations are recommended at 1- to 2-week intervals. Dosage of penicillamine is not increased under these circumstances. Proteinuria that exceeds 1 g/24 hours, or progressively increasing proteinuria, requires discontinuation of therapy. In some patients, proteinuria is reported to clear following dosage reduction. Drug is also discontinued if unexplained gross hematuria or persistent microscopic hematuria develops.

When used in cystinuria, an annual x-ray for renal stones advised; cystine stones form rapidly, sometimes in 6 months.

Up to 1 year or more may be required for any urine abnormalities to disappear after drug is discontinued. Because of rare reports of intrahepatic cholestasis and toxic hepatitis, liver-function tests are recommended every 6 months during year and a half of therapy.

Goodpasture's syndrome has occurred rarely. The development of abnormal urinary findings associated with hemoptysis and pulmonary infiltrates on x-ray requires immediate cessation of drug. Pemphigoid-type reactions characterized by bullous lesions clinically indistinguishable from pemphigus have occurred and require discontinuation of therapy and treatment with corticosteroids.

Once instituted for Wilson's disease or cystinuria, treatment with penicillamine should, as a rule, be continued on a daily basis. Interruptions for even a few days have been followed by sensitivity reactions after reinstitution of therapy.

Myasthenic syndrome sometimes progressing to myasthenia gravis has been reported. In most cases, symptoms have receded after withdrawal of drug.

Use in pregnancy: Do *not* administer to rheumatoid arthritis patients who are *pregnant;* therapy is discontinued *promptly* in those in whom pregnancy is suspected or diagnosed. Use only when clearly needed and potential benefits outweigh the unknown potential hazards to the fetus. There are no well-controlled studies in pregnant women with Wilson's disease, but experience does not include any positive evidence of adverse effects on the fetus. Experience shows that continued treatment with the drug protects the mother against relapse of Wilson's disease and that discontinuation of the drug has deleterious effects on the mother. It indicates that the drug does not increase the risk of fetal abnormalities, but it does not exclude the possibility of infrequent or subtle damage to the fetus. If administered during pregnancy it is recommended that daily dosage be limited to 1 g. If cesarean section is planned, daily dosage should be limited to 250 mg during the last 6 weeks of pregnancy and postoperatively until wound healing complete.

If possible, drug should not be given during pregnancy to women with cystinuria. If stones continue to form, benefits to mother must be weighed against risk to the fetus.

Use in children: Efficacy in juvenile rheumatoid arthritis not established.

DRUG INTERACTIONS

Drug should not be used in those receiving concurrent **gold therapy, antimalarial** or **cytotoxic drugs, oxyphenbutazone,** or **phenylbutazone** because these drugs are also associated with similar hematologic and renal adverse reactions. Absorption of penicillamine is significantly decreased by **iron salts, antacids,** and **food;** avoid concomitant administration. Serum levels of **digoxin** may be reduced; digoxin dose may need to be increased.

PRECAUTIONS

Some patients may experience drug fever, a marked febrile response to penicillamine, usually in the second or third week following initiation of therapy. Drug fever may sometimes be accompanied by a macular cutaneous eruption. In the case of drug fever with Wilson's disease or cystinuria, because no alternative treatment is available, drug should be temporarily discontinued until reaction subsides, and then reinstituted with a small dose and gradually increased until desired dosage is attained. Systemic steroid therapy may be necessary. In rheumatoid arthritis patients, because other treatment is available, drug should be discontinued and another therapeutic alternative tried.

The skin and mucous membranes should be observed for allergic reactions; early and late rashes have occurred. Early rash occurs during first few months and is more common. It is usually a generalized pruritic, erythematous, maculopapular or morbilliform rash and resembles the allergic rash seen with other drugs. Early rash usually disappears within days after stopping the drug and seldom recurs when drug is restarted at a lower dosage. The rash is often controlled with antihistamines. Less commonly, a late rash may be seen, usually 6 months after treatment, and requires discontinuation of the drug. It is usually on the trunk, accompanied by intense pruritus, and usually unresponsive to corticosteroid therapy. It may take weeks to disappear after drug is stopped and usually recurs after drug is restarted.

Certain patients develop a positive antinuclear antibody (ANA) test; some may show a lupus erythematosus–like syndrome. Some patients may develop oral ulcerations, which in some cases have the appearance of aphthous stomatitis that often clears on lower dosage. Rarely, cheilosis, glossitis, and gingivostomatitis have been reported. These lesions are frequently dose related.

Hypogeusia (blunting or diminution in taste perception) has occurred; this may last 2 to 3 months or more and may develop into a total loss of taste. It is usually self-limited despite continued treatment and is rare in those with Wilson's disease.

Patients allergic to penicillin may theoretically have cross-sensitivity to penicillamine.

Because of dietary restrictions, patients with cystinuria, Wilson's disease, or rheumatoid arthritis whose nutrition is impaired are given 25 mg/day of pyridoxine during therapy. Multivitamins may also be prescribed, but in Wilson's disease the preparation must be copper free. Mineral supplements should not be given, because they may block response to penicillamine.

Iron deficiency may develop, especially in children and menstruating women. In Wilson's disease, this may be the result of adding the effects of a low-copper diet, which is probably low in iron, and the penicillamine to the effects of blood loss or growth.

In cystinuria, a low-methionine diet may contribute to iron deficiency. Iron is given in short courses.

Penicillamine causes an increase in the amount of soluble collagen and may cause increased skin friability at sites especially subject to pressure or trauma. Extravasations of blood may occur and appear as purpuric areas, with external bleeding if the skin is broken, or as vesicles containing dark blood. Therapy may be continued and they may not recur if dosage is reduced.

The effects of penicillamine on collagen and elastin make it advisable to reduce dosage to 250 mg/day when surgery is contemplated. Reinstitution of full therapy should be delayed until wound healing is complete.

ADVERSE REACTIONS
Drug has high incidence of adverse reactions, some of which are potentially fatal.

Allergic: Generalized pruritus, early and late rashes; pemphigoid-type reactions, drug eruptions which may be accompanied by fever, arthralgia or lymphadenopathy, lupus erythematosus–like syndrome. Urticaria, exfoliative dermatitis have occurred. Thyroiditis reported but is very rare. Some patients may develop migratory polyarthralgia, often with subjective synovitis.

GI: Anorexia, epigastric pain, nausea, vomiting, occasional diarrhea. Isolated cases of peptic ulcer, hepatic dysfunction, cholestatic jaundice, pancreatitis have occurred. Increased serum alkaline phosphatase, LDH, positive cephalin flocculation, thymol turbidity tests reported. Hypogeusia, oral ulcerations, and rarely cheilosis, glossitis, gingivostomatitis reported.

Hematologic: May cause bone-marrow depression; leukopenia and thrombocytopenia have occurred. Fatalities reported as a result of thrombocytopenia, agranulocytosis, and aplastic anemia. Thrombotic thrombocytopenic purpura, hemolytic anemia, red cell aplasia, monocytosis, leukocytosis, eosinophilia, thrombocytosis reported.

Renal: Proteinuria and/or hematuria, which in some may progress to the nephrotic syndrome.

CNS: Tinnitus, reversible optic neuritis, which may be related to pyridoxine deficiency.

Other: Rarely, thrombophlebitis; hyperpyrexia; alopecia; myasthenic syndrome; polymyositis; mammary hyperplasia; toxic epidermal necrolysis; Goodpasture's syndrome; severe and ultimately fatal glomerulonephritis. Allergic alveolitis and obliterative bronchiolitis reported in patients with severe rheumatoid arthritis. Also increased skin friability, excessive wrinkling of skin, development of small white papules at venipuncture and surgical sites.

The chelating action of the drug may cause increased excretion of other heavy metals such as zinc, mercury, and lead.

DOSAGE

Cystinuria

Usual dosage is 2 g/day with range of 1 g/day to 4 g/day. For children, dosage based on 30 mg/kg/day. Divide total daily amount into four doses; if four doses not feasible, give larger portion H.S. If adverse reactions necessitate dosage reduction, it is important to retain the H.S. dose. Initiating dose at 250 mg/day and increasing gradually gives closer control of the effects of the drug and may help reduce incidence of adverse reactions. Dosage must be individualized.

Rheumatoid arthritis

Initial therapy: Single daily dose of 125 mg or 250 mg and increased at 1- to 3-month intervals by 125 mg/day or 250 mg/day according to patient response and tolerance. If remission is achieved, dose associated with remission is continued. If there is no improvement and no signs of potentially serious toxicity after 2 to 3 months with doses of 500 mg/day to 750 mg/day, increases of 250 mg/day at 2- to 3-month intervals may be continued until satisfactory remission occurs or signs of toxicity develop. If no improvement seen after 3 to 4 months with 1000 mg/day to 1500 mg/day, it may be assumed patient will not respond and drug is discontinued.

Maintenance therapy: Dosage individualized. Many patients respond to 500 mg/day to 750 mg/day or less. Some patients may subsequently require an increase in dosage to achieve maximal disease suppression. In those patients who do respond, but evidence incomplete suppression after the first 6 to 9 months of treatment, daily dosage may be increased by 125 mg/day to 250 mg/day at 3-month intervals. It is rarely necessary to use more than 1 g/day, but up to 1.5 g/day has sometimes been required.

Management of exacerbations: During course of treatment, some may experience exacerbation of disease activity following an initial good response. These may be self-limited and can subside within 12 weeks. They are usually controlled by addition of nonsteroidal anti-inflammatory drugs.

Duration of therapy: Not determined. If patient has been in remission for 6 months or more, a gradual dosage reduction in increments of 125 mg/day to 250 mg/day at approximately 3-month intervals may be tried.

Concomitant drug therapy: See *Drug Interactions.* Salicylates, other nonsteroidal anti-inflammatory drugs, or systemic corticosteroids may be continued when penicillamine is initiated. After improvement begins, analgesic and anti-inflammatory drugs may be discontinued slowly as symptoms permit. Corticosteroids are withdrawn gradually; many months of penicillamine treatment may be required before steroids can be completely eliminated.

Wilson's disease

Optimal dosage determined by measurement of urinary copper excretion. Given qid. Suggested initial dosage is 1 g/day for children and adults. This may be increased as indicated. It is seldom necessary to exceed 2 g/day. In those who cannot tolerate 1 g/day initially, initiating dosage with 250 mg/day and increasing gradually to the requisite amount gives closer control of the effects of the drug and may help reduce incidence of adverse reactions.

NURSING IMPLICATIONS

HISTORY

See Appendix 4. Note allergy to penicillin, dietary restrictions (if any).

PHYSICAL ASSESSMENT

Rheumatoid arthritis—examine involved joints; evaluate ability to carry out ADL and record findings. *Wilson's disease*—Because disease affects many organs and structures, base assessment on patient's symptoms. *Cystinuria*—Review x-ray, laboratory studies. In addition to laboratory tests to establish diagnosis, baseline laboratory studies may include WBC and differential, hemoglobin, platelet count, urinalysis, liver-function tests, pregnancy test (when appropriate). Those with Wilson's disease will have a measurement of urinary copper; those with cystinuria will have a determination of cystine excretion.

ADMINISTRATION

Given on an empty stomach ½–1 hour before meals.

Penicillamine is given at least 1 hour apart from any other drug, food, or milk.

If oral iron therapy is prescribed, a period of 2 hours should elapse between administration of penicillamine and iron.

Rheumatoid arthritis: Dosages up to 500 mg/day can be given as single daily dose; dosage over 500 mg/day given in divided doses.

Patient with rheumatoid arthritis may require assistance in holding water glass, removing tablet or capsule from dispensing cup.

GENERIC NAME SIMILARITY

Penicillin and penicillamine.

TRADE NAME SIMILARITY

Cylert and Cydel (cyclandelate).

ONGOING ASSESSMENTS AND NURSING MANAGEMENT

Monitor vital signs daily; observe for adverse drug reactions.

CLINICAL ALERT: Use of penicillamine has been associated with fatalities due to certain diseases such as aplastic anemia, agranulocytosis, thrombocytopenia, Goodpasture's syndrome, and myasthenic syndrome.

Patient should be observed closely for adverse reactions. Because there are many potentially serious adverse reactions, _any_ complaint offered by the patient is investigated.

Nursing management should include a daily surveillance of the areas or systems most commonly subject to adverse reactions (_e.g.,_ skin and mucous membranes, GI, hematologic, renal, CNS).

Observe for fever, a marked febrile response to penicillamine, usually in the second or third week following initiation of therapy. Notify physician of febrile response because drug may be discontinued.

The skin and mucous membranes should be checked daily for allergic reactions (_e.g.,_ rash of any type, oral lesions). Notify physician immediately if a rash or aphthous stomatitis is noted. See also _Precautions_ about early and late rashes.

The appearance of drug eruption accompanied by fever, arthralgia, lymphadenopathy, or other allergic manifestations usually requires discontinuation of therapy. Withhold next dose and notify the physician immediately if these reactions occur.

Increased skin friability at sites usually subject to pressure or trauma (shoulders, elbows, knees, buttocks) may occur. Patients with limited ambulatory activity must have a position change q2h; special care to the skin over bony prominences is necessary. Extravasation of blood may occur and appear as purpuric areas, with external bleeding if skin is broken, or as vesicles containing dark blood. Notify physician if these occur because dosage may need to be reduced.

Interruptions in therapy for cystinuria or Wilson's disease, even for a few days, have been followed by sensitivity reactions after reinstituting therapy. Ensure continuity of prescribed therapy by notation on Kardex, informing health-team members responsible for drug administration.

Cystinuria: Conventional treatment is directed at keeping urinary cystine diluted enough to prevent stone formation, keeping the urine alkaline enough (_p_H 7.5–8) to dissolve as much cystine as possible, and minimizing cystine formation by a diet low in methionine, the major dietary precursor of cystine.

Patient must drink enough fluid to keep urine specific gravity below 1.010. Determine urine specific gravity daily, in early A.M., midday, and H.S. unless physician directs otherwise.

Physician may prescribe sodium bicarbonate, potassium citrate and sodium citrate, sodium citrate and citric acid, or potassium citrate and citric acid to alkalinize the urine. Urine _p_H should be determined daily.

The greater the fluid intake, the lower the required dose of penicillamine.

Patient is encouraged to drink copious amounts of water during daytime hours. It is important to drink about a pint of fluid H.S. and another pint during the night when urine is more concentrated and more acid than during the day. If there is a question about patient compliance, measure intake and output. Daily urinary output should be approximately 3000 ml.

Cystine stones form rapidly, sometimes in 6 months. Observe for signs of stone formation: hematuria (gross or microscopic); flank, back, or abdominal pain (which can be severe); nausea; vomiting; fever; chills; pyuria; abdominal distention; symptoms of urinary-tract infection.

Rheumatoid arthritis: Therapeutic response may not be seen for 2 to 3 months. This must be explained to the patient to alleviate concern about therapeutic regimen.

Optimum duration of therapy has not been determined. If remissions occur, they may last from months to years, but usually require continued treatment.

In those who respond to the drug, first evidence of suppression of symptoms such as pain, tenderness, and swelling is generally apparent in 3 months.

Concomitant therapy with anti-inflammatory agents and/or corticosteroids may be employed. After improvement begins, analgesic and anti-inflammatory drugs may be discontinued slowly as symptoms permit.

Wilson's disease: Treatment has two objectives: (1) to minimize dietary intake and absorption of copper; and (2) to promote excretion of copper deposited in tissues.

Daily diet should contain no more than 1 mg to 2 mg of copper.

Distilled or demineralized water should be used if drinking water contains more than 0.1 mg copper. Provide patient with distilled or demineralized water unless physician approves of use of tap water (copper content will vary according to local water supply).

Noticeable improvement may not occur for 2 to 3 months. Occasionally neurologic symptoms become worse during initiation of therapy; this must be explained to the patient.

Urine for copper must be collected in copper-free glassware. Therapy is monitored by 24-hour urinary copper analysis approximately every 3 months for duration of therapy.

PATIENT AND FAMILY INFORMATION

NOTE: Patient must have therapeutic regimen thoroughly explained prior to institution of therapy in an outpatient setting as patient compliance is an important part of therapy. Patients with cystinuria or Wilson's disease will require a full explanation of necessary dietary restrictions. Parents of small children with Wilson's disease or cystinuria must closely supervise child's eating habits, especially outside the home. School-age children may be unable to participate in school lunch programs; lunches must usually be prepared by the parent. Compliance with dietary restrictions is often difficult because many foods liked by children (*e.g.,* chocolate, hamburger, pizza) may be restricted. Physician may wish patient to measure specific gravity of urine; patient will require instruction in using and reading a hydrometer.

Take on an empty stomach, 1 hour before or 2 hours after meals.

If iron therapy is prescribed, 2 hours must elapse between taking penicillamine and iron preparation.

If physician prescribes vitamins, do not use a different vitamin preparation unless use of a specific brand is approved by the physician.

Do not take any nonprescription preparation unless use is approved by physician.

Penicillamine should be taken 1 hour apart from any other drug, food or milk.

Notify physician or nurse if any of the following occurs: skin rash or other types of skin lesions; unusual bruising; sore throat; fever; sores in the mouth; persistent anorexia, nausea, vomiting, diarrhea; unusual fatigue; blood in the urine; any other unusual effects.

An impairment of taste perception may occur (in some instances a complete loss of taste may develop); this may last 2 to 3 months or more. (Taste impairment is rare in Wilson's disease.)

Observe skin over pressure areas such as knees, elbows, shoulders, toes, buttocks. If excessive bruising or bleeding or breaks in the skin occur, notify physician or nurse immediately.

Laboratory tests will be necessary to monitor therapy. Appointments should be kept.

Cystinuria: Drink copious amounts (4000 ml or more) of water every day. Drink 1 pint of water before retiring and 1 pint during the night, unless physician directs otherwise.

Adherence to the prescribed diet is an important part of therapy.

Yearly x-rays will be necessary. In some instances x-rays may be taken at more frequent intervals.

Notify physician or nurse immediately if any of the following occurs: blood in urine; fever; chills; nausea, vomiting; flank, back or abdominal pain or discomfort; abdominal distention; burning on urination, foul odor to urine, urinary frequency.

Rheumatoid arthritis: Drug is contraindicated in pregnancy. If pregnant or pregnancy is suspected, contact physician immediately.

Therapeutic effect may not be seen for 2 to 3 months.

Wilson's disease: Most important exclusions in low-copper diet are chocolate, nuts, shellfish, mushrooms, liver, molasses, broccoli, cereals enriched with copper, raisins, kidney, brains, dried legumes.

Adherence to diet low in copper is an important part of therapy.

Unless physician suggests otherwise, drink only distilled or demineralized water. (*Note—* The amount of copper in tap water will vary with geographic location.)

When collecting urine for analysis, use the container supplied by the laboratory. Do not void into household glassware or other containers before adding to the laboratory-provided container. Check with the laboratory about appropriate household collection containers for use in collection of voided specimen.

Penicillins

Amoxicillin Rx

tablets, chewable: 125 mg, 250 mg	Amoxil
capsules: 250 mg, 500 mg	Amoxil, Larotid, Polymox, Sumox, Trimox 250 or 500, Utimox, Wymox, *Generic*
powder for oral suspension: 50 mg/5 ml	Amoxil Pediatric Drops, Larotid Drops, Polymox Pediatric Drops
powder for oral suspension: 125 mg/5 ml, 250 mg/5 ml	Amoxil, Larotid, Polymox, Sumox, Trimox 125 or 250, Utimox, Wymox, *Generic*
powder for oral suspension: 125 mg/ unit dose, 250 mg/ unit dose	Amoxil, Larotid, Polymox, Trimox 125 or 250

Ampicillin, Oral Rx

capsules: 250 mg (as trihydrate)	Amcap, Amcill, Polycillin, Principen '250,' SK-Ampicillin, Supen, Totacillin, _Generic_
capsules: 250 mg, 500 mg (anhydrous)	Omnipen
capsules: 500 mg (as trihydrate)	Amcill, D-Amp, Pfizerpen-A, Polycillin, Principen '500,' SK-Ampicillin, Supen, Totacillin, _Generic_
powder for oral suspension: 100 mg/ml (as trihydrate)	Amcill Pediatric Drops, Omnipen Drops, Polycillin Pediatric Drops, SK-Ampicillin Drops
powder for oral suspension: 125 mg/5 ml, 250 mg/5 ml (as trihydrate)	Amcill, Omnipen, Pfizerpen-A, Polycillin, Principen '125,' SK-Ampicillin, Supen, Totacillin, _Generic_
powder for oral suspension: 125 mg/unit dose	Polycillin, Principen '125'
powder for oral suspension: 250 mg/unit dose	Omnipen, Polycillin, Principen '250'
powder for oral suspension: 500 mg/5 ml (as trihydrate)	Omnipen, Polycillin
powder for oral suspension: 500 mg/unit dose	Polycillin

Ampicillin Sodium, Parenteral Rx

powder for injection: 125-mg vials	Omnipen-N, Polycillin-N
powder for injection: 250-mg, 1-g, 2-g, 10-g vials; 500-mg, 1-g, 2-g piggyback vials	Omnipen-N, Polycillin-N, Totacillin-N
powder for injection: 500-mg vials	Omnipen-N, Polycillin-N, SK-Ampicillin-N, Totacillin-N

Ampicillin With Probenecid Rx

capsules: 3.5 g ampicillin, 1 g probenecid/9-capsule regimen	Principen w/Probenecid
oral suspension: 3.5 g ampicillin, 1 g probenecid/bottle	Polycillin-PRB, Probampacin

Azlocillin Sodium Rx

powder for injection: 2-g, 3-g, 4-g vials and infusion bottles	Azlin

Bacampicillin Hydrochloride Rx

tablets: 400 mg	Spectrobid
powder for oral suspension: 125 mg/5 ml	Spectrobid

Carbenicillin Disodium Rx

powder for injection: 1-g, 2-g, 5-g vials; 2-g, 5-g, 10-g piggyback units	Geopen, Pyopen

Carbenicillin Indanyl Sodium Rx

tablets, film coated: 382 mg	Geocillin

Cloxacillin Sodium Rx

capsules: 250 mg, 500 mg	Cloxapen, Tegopen, _Generic_
powder for oral solution: 125 mg/5 ml	Tegopen, _Generic_

Cyclacillin Rx

tablets: 250 mg, 500 mg	Cyclapen-W
powder for oral suspension: 125 mg/5 ml, 250 mg/5 ml	Cyclapen-W

Dicloxacillin Sodium Rx

capsules: 125 mg	Dynapen
capsules: 250 mg	Dycill, Dynapen, Pathocil, Veracillin, _Generic_
capsules: 500 mg	Dycill, Dynapen, Veracillin, _Generic_
powder for oral suspension: 62.5 mg/5 ml	Dynapen, Pathocil

Hetacillin Rx

powder for oral suspension: hetacillin equivalent to 112.5 mg or 225 mg ampicillin/5 ml	Versapen

P

capsules: hetacillin equivalent to 225 mg ampicillin	Versapen-K

Methicillin Sodium *Rx*

powder for injection: 1-g, 4-g, 6-g vials; 1-g, 4-g piggyback units	Staphcillin

Mezlocillin Sodium *Rx*

powder for injection: 1-g vial; 2-g, 3-g, 4-g vials and piggyback	Mezlin

Nafcillin Sodium *Rx*

capsules: 250 mg	Unipen
tablets: 500 mg	Unipen
powder for oral solution: 250 mg/5 ml	Unipen
powder for injection: 500-mg, 1-g, 2-g vials; 1-g, 2-g piggyback	Nafcil, Unipen
powder for injection: 1.5-g, 4-g piggyback	Unipen

Oxacillin Sodium *Rx*

capsules: 250 mg, 500 mg	Bactocill, Prostaphlin
powder for oral solution: 250 mg/5 ml	Prostaphlin
powder for injection: 250-mg vial	Prostaphlin
powder for injection: 500-mg, 1-g, 2-g, 4-g vials; 1-g, 2-g piggyback	Bactocill, Prostaphlin

Penicillin G Benzathine, Oral *Rx*

tablets: 200,000 units	Bicillin (contains tartrazine)

Penicillin G Benzathine, Parenteral *Rx*

injection: 300,000 units/ml; 600,000, 900,000, 2,400,000 units/dose	Bicillin L-A
injection: 1,200,000 units/dose	Bicillin L-A, Permapen

Penicillin G Benzathine and Procaine Combined *Rx*

injection: 300,000 units, 600,000 units/ml; 600,000 units, 1,200,000 units, 2,400,000 units/dose	Bicillin C-R
injection: 1,200,000 units/dose	Bicillin C-R 900/300

Penicillin G (Aqueous), Parenteral *Rx*

powder for injection: 200,000 units, 500,000 units, 10,000,000 units/ vial (as potassium)	*Generic*
powder for injection: 1,000,000 units, 5,000,000 units, 20,000,000 units/ vial (as potassium)	Pfizerpen, *Generic*
powder for injection: 5,000,000 units/ vial (as sodium)	*Generic*

Penicillin G Potassium, Oral *Rx*

tablets: 200,000 units	Pentids, Pfizerpen G, *Generic*
tablets: 250,000 units	Pfizerpen G, *Generic*
tablets: 400,000 units	Pentids '400,' Pfizerpen G, SK-Penicillin G, *Generic*
tablets: 500,000 units	*Generic*
tablets: 800,000 units	Pentids '800' (contains tartrazine), Pfizerpen G, SK-Penicillin G
powder for oral solution: 200,000 units/5 ml	Pentids (contains tartrazine)
powder for oral solution: 250,000 units/5 ml	*Generic*
powder for oral solution: 400,000 units/5 ml	M-Cillin B 400, Pentids '400' (contains tartrazine), *Generic*

Penicillin G Procaine, Aqueous *(APPG)* *Rx*

injection: 300,000 units/ml	Crysticillin 300 A.S., Duracillin A.S., Pfizerpen-AS, Wycillin
injection: 500,000 units/ml (600,000 units/1.2 ml)	Crysticillin 600 A.S., Wycillin

injection: 1,200,000 units/dose	Pfizerpen-AS, Wycillin
injection: 2,400,000 units/dose	Wycillin
combination package: two 4-ml doses of 2,400,000 units & two 500-mg probenecid tablets	Wycillin Injection & Probenecid Tablets

Penicillin V (Phenoxymethyl Penicillin) Rx

| tablets: 125 mg, 250 mg, 500 mg | _Generic_ |
| powder for oral solution: 125 mg, 250 mg/5 ml | _Generic_ |

Penicillin V Potassium Rx

tablets: 125 mg	Pen-Vee K, V-Cillin K
tablets: 250 mg	Beepen-VK, Betapen-VK, Deltapen-VK, Ledercillin VK, Penapar VK, Pen-Vee K, Pfizerpen VK, Repen-VK, Robicillin VK, SK-Penicillin VK, Uticillin VK, V-Cillin K, Veetids '250,' _Generic_
tablets: 500 mg	Beepen-VK, Betapen-VK, Ledercillin VK, Penapar VK, Pen-Vee K, Pfizerpen VK, Robicillin VK, SK-Penicillin VK, Uticillin VK, V-Cillin K, Veetids '500,' _Generic_
powder for oral suspension: 125 mg/ 5 ml	Beepen-VK, Betapen-VK, Ledercillin VK, Penapar VK, Pen-Vee K, Pfizerpen VK, Repen-VK, Robicillin VK, SK-Penicillin VK, V-Cillin K, Veetids '125' (contains tartrazine), _Generic_
powder for oral solution: 125 mg/unit dose	V-Cillin K
powder for oral solution: 250 mg/5 ml	Beepen-VK, Betapen-VK, Deltapen-VK, Ledercillin VK, Penapar VK, Pen-Vee K, Pfizerpen VK, Repen-VK, Robicillin VK, SK-Penicillin VK, Suspen, V-Cillin K, Veetids '250,' _Generic_
powder for oral solution: 250 mg/unit dose	Pen-Vee K, V-Cillin K

Piperacillin Sodium Rx

| powder for injection: 2-g, 3-g, 4-g vials; 3-g, 4-g infusion bottles | Pipracil |

Ticarcillin Disodium Rx

| powder for injection: 1-g, 3-g, 6-g vials; 3-g piggyback | Ticar |

INDICATIONS

See below for specific indications of individual drugs.

Parenteral: Patients with severe illness or when there is nausea, vomiting, gastric dilatation, or intestinal hypermotility. Parenteral aqueous penicillin is the dosage form of choice in severe infections caused by penicillin-sensitive microorganisms when rapid and high penicillin levels are required.

Oral: Penicillin G is indicated in treatment of mild to moderately severe infections due to penicillin-sensitive microorganisms that are sensitive to low serum levels achieved by this dosage form. Severe pneumonia, empyema, bacteremia, pericarditis, meningitis, and purulent or septic arthritis are not treated with oral penicillin during the acute stage. Penicillin V is preferred over penicillin G for oral administration because of better absorption.

Penicillinase-resistant penicillins (see _Actions_): Although principal indication for these agents is treatment of infections due to penicillinase-producing staphylococci, they may be used to initiate therapy in any patient with suspected staphylococcal infection. The percentage of staphylococcal isolates resistant to penicillin G outside the hospital is increasing, approximating the high percentage of resistant staphylococcal isolates found in the hospital. Use of a penicillinase-resistant penicillin as initial therapy for any suspected staphylococcal infection is recommended until culture and sensitivity results are known. The choice of a penicillinase-resistant penicillin before culture and sensitivity results are known takes into consideration that these penicillins have been shown to be effective only in treatment of infections caused by pneumococci, group A beta-hemolytic streptococci, and penicillin G–resistant and penicillin G–sensitive staphylococci.

AMOXICILLIN

Infections due to susceptible strains of the following organisms.

P

Gram negative: *Haemophilus influenzae, Escherichia coli, Proteus mirabilis, Neisseria gonorrhoeae.*
Gram positive: Streptococci (including *Streptococcus faecalis*), *S. pneumoniae,* and non–penicillinase-producing staphylococci.

AMPICILLIN, ORAL
See Ampicillin Sodium, Parenteral, below.

AMPICILLIN SODIUM, PARENTERAL
Infections caused by susceptible strains of the following: *Shigella, Salmonella, E. coli, H. influenzae, P. mirabilis, N. gonorrhoeae,* and enterococci. Also effective in treatment of meningitis due to *N. meningitidis.* May be used IV as initial therapy for meningitis before results of bacteriology are available. May also be indicated in infections caused by susceptible gram-positive organisms: penicillin G–sensitive staphylococci and pneumococci.

AMPICILLIN WITH PROBENECID
Treatment of uncomplicated infections (urethral, endocervical, or rectal) caused by *N. gonorrhoeae* in adults.

AZLOCILLIN SODIUM
Serious infections caused by susceptible strains of *Pseudomonas aeruginosa* in lower respiratory infections, urinary-tract infections, skin and skin-structure infections, bone and joint infections, and bacterial septicemia. Also effective for infections caused by *E. coli, H. influenzae, P. mirabilis,* and *S. faecalis.*

BACAMPICILLIN HYDROCHLORIDE
Upper and lower respiratory-tract infections due to streptococci, pneumococci, non–penicillinase-producing staphylococci, *H. influenzae.* Urinary-tract infections due to *E. coli, P. mirabilis, S. faecalis.* Skin and skin-structure infections due to streptococci and susceptible staphylococci. Gonorrhea (uncomplicated urogenital infections) due to *N. gonorrhoeae.*

CARBENICILLIN DISODIUM
Primarily indicated for infections due to *Pseudomonas aeruginosa, Proteus* species, and certain strains of *E. coli.* In treatment of infections due to *P. aeruginosa,* clinical efficacy may be enhanced by combined therapy of carbenicillin sodium with gentamicin or tobramycin in full therapeutic doses. Drug is particularly effective in urinary-tract infections because of very high urine levels achieved by IM use. Effectiveness demonstrated in severe systemic infections and septicemia including meningitis due to *H. influenzae* and *S. pneumoniae;* GU in-

fections including those due to *N. gonorrhoeae, Enterobacter,* and *S. faecalis;* acute and chronic respiratory infections, soft-tissue infections. Also indicated in the following infections due to susceptible anaerobic bacteria: septicemia; lower respiratory-tract infections; intra-abdominal infections; infections of the female pelvis and genital tract such as endometritis, pelvic inflammatory disease (PID), pelvic abscess, salpingitis; skin and soft-tissue infections.

CARBENICILLIN INDANYL SODIUM
Treatment of acute and chronic upper and lower urinary-tract infections and in asymptomatic bacteriuria due to susceptible strains of *E. coli, P. mirabilis, Morganella morganii, Providencia rettgeri, Proteus vulgaris, Pseudomonas, Enterobacter,* and enterococci. Also indicated in treatment of prostatitis due to susceptible strains of *E. coli,* enterococci, *P. mirabilis,* and *Enterobacter* species. When high rapid drug levels are indicated, therapy should be initiated with parenteral administration, followed by oral therapy.

CLOXACILLIN SODIUM
Although principal indication for penicillinase-resistant penicillins is treatment of infections due to penicillinase-producing staphylococci, they may be used to initiate therapy when staphylococci infection is suspected.

CYCLACILLIN
Respiratory-tract infections including tonsillitis and pharyngitis caused by group A beta-hemolytic streptococci; bronchitis and pneumonia caused by *S. pneumoniae;* otitis media caused by *S. pneumoniae,* group A beta-hemolytic streptococci and *H. influenzae;* acute exacerbations of chronic bronchitis caused by *H. influenzae.* Skin and skin-structure infections caused by group A beta-hemolytic streptococci and staphylococci, non–penicillinase-producing strains. Urinary-tract infections caused by *E. coli* and *P. mirabilis.*

DICLOXACILLIN SODIUM
See Cloxacillin Sodium.

HETACILLIN
Group A beta-hemolytic streptococcus: tonsillitis, otitis media, skin and soft-tissue infections. (Injectable benzathine penicillin is considered the drug of choice in treatment and prevention of streptococcal pharyngitis and in long-term prophylaxis of rheumatic fever. Hetacillin is effective in eradication of streptococci from the nasopharynx, but data establishing efficacy in subsequent prevention of rheu-

matic fever are not available.) _Streptococcus pneumoniae:_ bronchopneumonia, lobar pneumonia, otitis media. Non–penicillinase-producing _Staphylococcus aureus:_ skin and soft-tissue infections, otitis media. _H. influenzae:_ bronchitis, bronchopneumonia, otitis media. _E. coli:_ cystitis, pyelonephritis, prostatitis/urethritis, skin and soft-tissue infections. _P. mirabilis:_ cystitis, pyelonephritis, skin and soft-tissue infections. Enterococcus (_Streptococcus faecalis_): cystitis, pyelonephritis, prostatis/urethritis. _Shigella_ species: shigellosis.

METHICILLIN SODIUM
See Cloxacillin Sodium.

MEZLOCILLIN SODIUM
Lower respiratory-tract infections including pneumonia and lung abscesses caused by _H. influenzae; E. coli; P. mirabilis; Klebsiella, Pseudomonas,_ and _Bacteroides_ species. Intra-abdominal infections including acute cholecystitis, cholangitis, peritonitis, hepatic abscess and intra-abdominal abscess caused by susceptible _E. coli; P. mirabilis; S. faecalis; Klebsiella, Pseudomonas, Bacteroides, Peptococcus,_ and _Peptostreptococcus_ species. Urinary-tract infections caused by _E. coli; P. mirabilis;_ indole-positive _Proteus_ species; _M. morganii; S. faecalis; Klebsiella, Enterobacter, Serratia,_ and _Pseudomonas_ species; uncomplicated gonorrhea due to _N. gonorrhoeae._ Gynecologic infections including endometritis, pelvic cellulitis, and PID associated with susceptible _N. gonorrhoeae; E. coli; P. mirabilis; Peptococcus, Peptostreptococcus, Bacteroides, Klebsiella,_ and _Enterobacter_ species. Skin and soft-tissue infections caused by susceptible _S. faecalis; E. coli; P. mirabilis;_ indole-positive _Proteus_ species; _P. vulgaris; P. rettgeri; Klebsiella, Enterobacter, Pseudomonas, Peptococcus,_ and _Bacteroides_ species. Septicemia including bacteremia caused by susceptible _E. coli; Klebsiella, Enterobacter, Pseudomonas, Bacteroides,_ and _Peptococcus_ species. Streptococcal infections including group A beta-hemolytic streptococcus and _S. pneumoniae._ Severe infections when causative organism is unknown. Drug may be administered with an aminoglycoside or a cephalosporin as initial therapy until results of culture and sensitivity tests are known. _Pseudomonas_ infections in combination with an aminoglycoside for treatment of life-threatening infections caused by _P. aeruginosa._ For treatment of febrile episodes in immunosuppressed patients with granulocytopenia, mezlocillin is combined with an aminoglycoside or cephalosporin.

NAFCILLIN SODIUM
See Cloxacillin Sodium.

OXACILLIN SODIUM
See Cloxacillin Sodium.

PENICILLIN G BENZATHINE, ORAL
See general Indications, above.

PENICILLIN G BENZATHINE, PARENTERAL
See general Indications, above.

PENICILLIN G BENZATHINE AND PROCAINE COMBINED
Treatment of moderately severe infections due to microorganisms that are susceptible to serum levels of penicillin G achievable with this dosage form. Not used in treatment of venereal diseases, including syphilis and gonorrhea, or yaws, bejel, and pinta. The following usually respond to adequate doses of this drug:

  Streptococcal infections (group A without bacteremia): Moderately severe to severe infections of the upper respiratory tract, skin and soft-tissue infections, scarlet fever, erysipelas.

  Pneumococcal infections: Moderately severe to severe pneumonia and otitis media.

PENICILLIN G (AQUEOUS), PARENTERAL
See general Indications, above.

PENICILLIN G POTASSIUM, ORAL
See general Indications, above.

PENICILLIN G PROCAINE, AQUEOUS (APPG)
For IM use only. A long-acting penicillin indicated in treatment of moderately severe infections due to penicillin G–sensitive microorganisms sensitive to low and persistent serum levels achievable with this dosage form.

PENICILLIN V (PHENOXYMETHYL PENICILLIN)
See general Indications, above.

PENICILLIN V POTASSIUM
See general Indications, above.

PIPERACILLIN SODIUM
Useful in treatment of mixed infections and presumptive therapy prior to identification of the causative organisms. Also may be administered as single drug therapy in some situations in which two antibiotics might normally be employed. May be used in the following:

  Intra-abdominal infections (including hepatobiliary and surgical infections) caused by _E. coli; P. aeruginosa;_ enterococci; anaerobic cocci; _Clostridia, Bacteroides_ species.

  Urinary-tract infections caused by _E. coli; P. aeruginosa;_ enterococci; _Klebsiella, Proteus_ species.

P

Gynecologic infections caused by *Bacteroides* species; anaerobic cocci; *N. gonorrhoeae;* enterococci.

Septicemia caused by *E. coli; Klebsiella, Enterobacter, Serratia, Bacteroides* species; *P. mirabilis; S. pneumoniae;* enterococci; *P. aeruginosa;* anaerobic cocci.

Lower respiratory-tract infections caused by *E. coli; Klebsiella, Enterobacter, Serratia, Bacteroides* species; *P. aeruginosa; H. influenzae;* anaerobic cocci. Although improvement has been noted in those with cystic fibrosis, lasting bacterial eradication may not be achieved.

Skin and skin-structure infections caused by *E. coli; Klebsiella, Serratia, Bacteroides, Acinetobacter, Enterobacter,* indole-positive *Proteus* species; *P. aeruginosa; P. mirabilis;* anaerobic cocci; enterococci.

Bone and joint infections caused by *P. aeruginosa,* enterococci, *Bacteroides* species, anaerobic cocci.

Gonococcal infections—Treatment of uncomplicated gonococcal urethritis.

Streptococcal infections caused by streptococcus species including group A beta-hemolytic *Streptococcus* and *S. pneumoniae,* but these infections are normally treated with more narrow-spectrum penicillins.

Concomitant therapy: Has been successfully used with aminoglycosides, especially in patients with impaired host defenses. Both drugs should be used in full therapeutic doses.

TICARCILLIN DISODIUM

Treatment of bacterial septicemia, skin and soft-tissue infections, acute and chronic respiratory-tract infections caused by susceptible strains of *P. aeruginosa, Proteus* species, and *E. coli.* Although clinical improvement has been shown, bacteriologic cures cannot be expected in those with chronic respiratory disease or cystic fibrosis.

GU tract infections (complicated and uncomplicated) due to susceptible strains of *P. aeruginosa, Proteus* species, *E. coli, Enterobacter, Streptococcus faecalis.*

Infections due to susceptible anaerobic bacteria: bacterial septicemia; lower respiratory-tract infections; intra-abdominal infections; infections of the female pelvis and genital tract; skin and soft-tissue infections.

Based on synergism between ticarcillin and gentamicin or tobramycin against certain strains of *P. aeruginosa,* combined therapy has been successful using full therapeutic dosages.

CONTRAINDICATIONS

History of previous hypersensitivity to penicillins or cephalosporins. Do not inject parenteral solutions into or near an artery or nerve.

ACTIONS

Penicillins are bactericidal antibiotics that include natural and semisynthetic derivatives. All of these agents share cross-allergenicity and a similar mechanism of action. The significant differences among agents include resistance to gastric acid inactivation, resistance to inactivation by penicillinase, and spectrum of antimicrobial activity. In addition to the prototype penicillin G, this class includes the penicillins listed in Table 40.

Penicillins inhibit the biosynthesis of cell wall mucopeptide, rendering the cell wall osmotically unstable. They are bactericidal against sensitive organisms when adequate concentrations are reached and are most effective during the stage of active multiplication. Inadequate concentrations may produce only bacteriostatic effects.

Absorption: Oral preparations of penicillin G are only slightly affected by normal gastric acidity (*p*H 2.0–3.5); a *p*H below 2.0 may partially or totally inactivate it. Oral penicillin G is absorbed in the upper small intestine, chiefly the duodenum. Only 30% of dose is absorbed; therefore, 4 to 5 times the oral dose of penicillin G is needed to obtain a blood level comparable to that obtained with parenteral penicillin G. Because gastric acidity, stomach emptying time, and other factors affecting absorption may vary, serum levels may be reduced to nontherapeutic levels in some individuals. Penicillin V is preferred for oral therapy because it achieves blood levels 2 to 5 times higher than the same dose of penicillin G and shows less individual variation. Nafcillin's oral absorption is reported to be inferior

Table 40. Characteristics of Different Penicillins

Penicillin	Routes of Administration	Penicillinase Resistant	Acid Stable
Penicillin G	IM, IV, PO	no	no
Penicillin V	PO	no	yes
Cloxacillin	PO	yes	yes
Dicloxacillin	PO	yes	yes
Methicillin	IM, IV	yes	no
Nafcillin	IM, IV, PO	yes	yes
Oxacillin	IM, IV, PO	yes	yes
Ampicillins			
Amoxicillin	PO	no	yes
Ampicillin	IM, IV, PO	no	yes
Bacampicillin	PO	no	yes
Cyclacillin	PO	no	yes
Hetacillin	PO	no	yes
Extended spectrum			
Azlocillin	IV	no	—
Carbenicillin	IM, IV, PO	no	yes*
Mezlocillin	IM, IV	no	—
Piperacillin	IM, IV	no	—
Ticarcillin	IM, IV	no	—

* Indanyl derivative

to that of oxacillin, cloxacillin, or dicloxacillin. Ampicillin and carbenicillin indanyl have good GI absorption, although amoxicillin, bacampicillin, and cyclacillin are more completely absorbed. Cyclacillin and bacampicillin produce more rapid and higher serum concentrations than do equal doses of ampicillin or amoxicillin.

Absorption is affected by food; penicillin V is less affected than other penicillins. Peak serum levels occur 1 to 2 hours after oral administration. Parenteral penicillin G gives high but transient blood levels; derivatives provide prolonged penicillin blood levels with IM administration. Procaine penicillin G must be given IM; it dissolves slowly at the injection site and reaches a plateau in about 4 hours, with levels declining gradually over 15 to 20 hours. IM benzathine penicillin G is absorbed very slowly from the injection site; serum levels are lower but more prolonged, sustaining serum levels for up to 4 weeks. The sodium salts of penicillins produce rapid and high serum levels following parenteral administration.

Penicillins are bound to plasma proteins, primarily albumin, in varying degrees. They diffuse readily into most body tissues and fluids. Adequate penetration into CSF, brain, and eye occurs only with inflammation. Methicillin appears to achieve the highest CSF levels among the penicillinase-resistant penicillins and is found in pericardial and ascitic fluids. Bile levels of azlocillin are approximately 15 times greater than corresponding serum levels. Penicillins cross the placental barrier and are found in amniotic fluid, cord serum, and human milk.

Penicillins are excreted largely unchanged in the urine by glomerular filtration and active tubular secretion. Excretion by renal tubular secretion can be delayed by concurrent administration of probenecid. Excretion is delayed in neonates, infants, and those with impaired renal function. Elimination half-life for most penicillins is short; for ampicillin it is slightly longer. Impairment of renal function will prolong serum half-life of penicillins excreted primarily by renal excretion. Because piperacillin is excreted by the biliary route as well as by the renal route, it can be used in appropriate dosages in those with severely restricted kidney function and treatment of hepatobiliary infections.

WARNINGS

Hypersensitivity: Serious and occasionally fatal immediate hypersensitivity (anaphylactoid) reactions have been reported. Although more frequent following parenteral therapy, anaphylaxis may occur with oral use. Accelerated reactions (urticaria and occasionally laryngeal edema) and delayed reactions (most commonly involving skin and mucous membranes) may also occur. These reactions are more likely to occur in those with a history of sensitivity to multiple allergens. Individuals with a history of penicillin hypersensitivity have experienced severe reactions when treated with a cephalosporin.

Bleeding abnormalities: High doses of **ticarcillin, carbenicillin, mezlocillin, piperacillin, azlocillin,** or **nafcillin** may induce hemorrhagic manifestations associated with abnormalities of coagulation tests (_e.g.,_ bleeding time, prothrombin time, and platelet aggregation).

Use in pregnancy, lactation: Safety for use in pregnancy has not been established. These drugs are used only when clearly needed. Penicillins are excreted in breast milk; use may cause diarrhea or candidiasis in the nursing infant. Oral ampicillin-class antibiotics are generally poorly absorbed during labor. It is not known whether use has immediate or delayed adverse effects on the fetus or whether it alters normal labor.

Use in neonates: Because of incompletely developed renal function in infants, rate of elimination will be slow. Use caution in giving to newborns.

Streptococcal infections: Therapy must be sufficient to eliminate the organisms (a minimum of 10 days); otherwise, the sequelae of streptococcal disease (_e.g.,_ endocarditis, rheumatic fever) may occur. Cultures are taken following treatment to confirm that streptococci have been eradicated.

Venereal infections: When treating gonococcal infections in which primary and secondary syphilis are suspected, proper diagnostic procedures and monthly serologic tests for at least 4 months are recommended. All patients with penicillin-treated syphilis should receive clinical and serologic examinations every 6 months for 2 to 3 years.

Laboratory tests: Bacteriologic studies are performed to determine causative organisms and their susceptibility. Blood cultures, WBC, and differential are recommended prior to initiation of therapy and at least weekly during therapy with penicillinase-resistant penicillins. SGOT and SGPT are recommended periodically during therapy to monitor possible hepatic-function abnormalities. Periodic urinalysis, BUN, and creatinine determinations are recommended during therapy with penicillinase-resistant penicillins; dosage alterations are considered if these values become elevated. If impairment of renal function is suspected or known to exist, dosage is reduced and blood levels are monitored to avoid possible neurotoxic reactions. Monitoring is especially important in prematures, neonates, and other infants when high doses are used.

Superinfection: Use of antibiotics (especially prolonged or repeated therapy) may result in bacterial or fungal overgrowth of nonsusceptible organisms. Such overgrowth may lead to a secondary infection.

Resistance: Small ineffective doses of penicillin

P

are avoided, because resistant strains of organisms are more likely to emerge. Adequate dosage at proper time intervals in relation to meals is important. The number of strains of staphylococci resistant to penicillinase-resistant penicillins has been increasing. Widespread use of these penicillins may result in the appearance of an increasing number of resistant staphylococci strains.

Procaine sensitivity: If there is a history of sensitivity to procaine in **penicillin G procaine,** intradermal testing may be performed with 0.1 ml of a 1% or 2% procaine solution. Development of erythema, wheal, flare, or eruption indicates procaine sensitivity and procaine penicillin preparations are not used. Antihistamines may be used to treat procaine reactions.

Tartrazine sensitivity: Some of these products contain tartrazine. See Appendix 6, section 6-23.

Parenteral administration: Inadvertent intravascular administration, including inadvertent direct intra-arterial injection or injection immediately adjacent to arteries has resulted in *severe neurovascular damage,* including transverse myelitis with permanent paralysis, gangrene requiring amputation of digits and more proximal portions of extremities, and necrosis and sloughing at and surrounding the injection site. Such adverse effects have been reported following injections into the buttock, thigh, and deltoid areas. Other serious complications of suspected intravascular administration that have been reported include immediate pallor, mottling or cyanosis of the extremity both distal and proximal to the injection site, followed by bleb formation, and severe edema requiring anterior and posterior compartment fasciotomy in the lower extremity. These severe effects and complications have most often occurred in infants and small children. Quadraceps femoris fibrosis and atrophy have been reported following repeated IM injections of penicillin preparations into the anterolateral thigh. Injection into or near a nerve may result in permanent neurologic damage.

Particular care is taken with IV administration because of possibility of thrombophlebitis. Higher than recommended doses of most of the penicillins IV may cause neuromuscular excitability and convulsions.

DRUG INTERACTIONS

Concurrent administration of **bacteriostatic antibiotics** (*e.g.,* erythromycin, tetracycline) may diminish the bactericidal effects of penicillins by slowing rate of bacterial growth. Bactericidal agents work most effectively against the immature cell wall of rapidly proliferating microorganisms. Penicillin blood levels may be prolonged with administration of **probene-**

cid. Mixing penicillins with an **aminoglycoside** in solutions for parenteral administration can result in substantial inactivation of the aminoglycoside.

Carbenicillin and **ticarcillin** may be synergistic with **gentamicin** or **tobramycin** when used in combination for *Pseudomonas* infections. **Penicillin** acts synergistically with **gentamicin** or **tobramycin** against many strains of enterococci. **Tobramycin** and **carbenicillin** are synergistic against certain *Providencia* strains. These combinations should not be mixed in the same IV bottle because of physiochemical incompatibility. The expected half-life of **gentamicin** or **tobramycin** may be decreased in patients with impaired renal function because of inactivation by large doses of **carbenicillin** or **ticarcillin.** **Bacampicillin** should not be administered with **disulfiram.**

Concomitant use of **penicillin V potassium** and **oral neomycin** is avoided because malabsorption of penicillin V potassium has been reported. **Oral contraceptives** may be rendered less effective and an increased incidence of breakthrough bleeding may occur when administered with **ampicillin** or **penicillin V** (other studies indicate ampicillin may not be responsible for contraceptive failure).

The incidence of **ampicillin**-induced skin rash may increase when administered concomitantly with **allopurinol.**

Drug/lab tests: False-positive **urine glucose** reactions may occur with high urine levels of **ampicillin** if Clinitest, Benedict's solution, or Fehling's solution is used. It is recommended that enzymatic glucose oxidase tests (such as Clinistix or Tes-Tape) be used. Positive **Coombs' tests** have been reported after large IV doses of **penicillin, carbenicillin,** and **piperacillin.** High urine concentrations of **mezlocillin** or **azlocillin** may produce false-positive protein reactions with some testing methods. A transient decrease in plasma concentrations of **estrogens** has been reported in pregnant women following administration of **ampicillin.** The serum uric acid level was depressed in some patients receiving **azlocillin;** this appears to be transient.

ADVERSE REACTIONS

Hypersensitivity: Most likely to occur in individuals with previously demonstrated hypersensitivity and in those with history of allergy, asthma, hay fever, or urticaria. Anaphylaxis is the most serious reaction and is usually associated with parenteral dosage. Although incidence of reactions with oral use is lower, all degrees of hypersensitivity, including anaphylaxis, have been reported with oral penicillin.

Allergic symptoms, including wheezing and sneezing, urticaria, pruritus, angioneurotic edema, laryngospasm, bronchospasm, hypotension, vascular collapse, death, maculopapular to exfoliative dermatitis, vascular eruptions, erythema multiforme, reactions resembling serum sickness (chills, fever, edema, arthralgia, malaise, myalgia), laryngeal edema, various skin rashes, and prostration have been reported. A maculopapular rash, not representing true penicillin allergy, occasionally occurs with **ampicillin** and occurs more frequently in those taking allopurinol, patients with lymphatic leukemia, and those with infectious mononucleosis.

GI (usually associated with oral use): Glossitis, stomatitis, gastritis, sore mouth or tongue, dry mouth, furry tongue, black "hairy" tongue, abnormal taste sensation, nausea, vomiting, abdominal pain or cramp, epigastric distress, diarrhea or bloody diarrhea, flatulence, enterocolitis, pseudomembranous colitis. The incidence of GI symptoms, particularly diarrhea, is less with amoxicillin, bacampicillin, and cyclacillin than with ampicillin.

Hepatic: Transient symptomatic and asymptomatic elevations of SGOT, SGPT, and LDH have been noted in those receiving semisynthetic penicillins (particularly **oxacillin**); such reactions are more common in infants. Elevations of serum alkaline phosphatase, hypernatremia, and reduction in serum potassium and uric acid may occur. Evidence indicates glutamic oxaloacetic transaminase (GOT) is released at the site of IM injection of ampicillin; increased amounts of this enzyme in the blood does not necessarily indicate liver involvement. Changes in cephalin flocculation tests and hyperbilirubinemia have also been reported.

Hematopoietic and lymphatic systems: Anemia, hemolytic anemia, thrombocytopenia, thrombocytopenic purpura, eosinophilia, leukopenia, granulocytopenia, transient neutropenia with evidence of bone-marrow depression and agranulocytosis, reduction of hemoglobin and hematocrit, reduction in serum potassium, and prolongation of bleeding and prothrombin time have been reported during therapy with penicillins. These reactions are usually reversible on discontinuation of therapy and believed to be hypersensitivity phenomena. Hemorrhagic manifestations associated with abnormalities of coagulation tests have been reported.

Renal: Interstitial nephritis (oliguria, proteinuria, hematuria, casts, azotemia, pyuria, cylinduria) is infrequent and is associated with high doses of parenteral penicillin (most frequently **methicillin**); this has also been reported with oral ampicillin and has occurred with all penicillins. Such reactions are allergic and are usually associated with fever, skin rash, and eosinophilia. Acute glomerulonephritis, endarteritis, acute tubular necrosis, and elevations of creatinine or BUN have been rarely reported. Transient hematuria and azotemia have occurred in newborns and infants receiving high doses of **oxacillin.**

CNS: Neurotoxicity may occur with excessively high serum levels. **Penicillin, carbenicillin,** and **ticarcillin** have caused neurotoxicity (manifested as lethargy, neuromuscular irritability, hallucinations, convulsions, asterixis, seizures) when given in large doses and to patients in renal failure. Mental disturbances including anxiety, confusion, agitation, depression, hallucinations, weakness, seizures, combativeness, and expressed "fear of impending death" have been reported following single-dose therapy for gonorrhea with **penicillin G procaine.** Reactions have been transient, lasting 15 to 30 minutes. Headache, dizziness, giddiness, fatigue, and prolonged muscle relaxation have also been reported.

Electrolyte imbalance: Patients given continuous IV therapy with **potassium penicillin G** in high dosage (10–100 million units/day) may suffer severe and even fatal potassium poisoning, particularly if renal insufficiency is present. Hyperreflexia, convulsions, coma, cardiac arrhythmias, and cardiac arrest may be indicative of this syndrome. High dosage of **sodium salts of penicillins** may result in or aggravate congestive heart failure (CHF) because of high sodium intake. Patients with liver disease or those receiving cytotoxic drugs or diuretics have been reported rarely to demonstrate a decrease in serum potassium concentrations with high doses of **piperacillin.**

Local reactions: Pain (rarely accompanied by induration) at injection site, ecchymosis, deep-vein thrombosis, hematomas. Vein irritation and phlebitis can occur, particularly when undiluted solution is injected directly into a vein. Thrombophlebitis has been reported after IV therapy. Tissue necrosis due to extravasated **nafcillin** has been successfully modified with hyaluronidase.

Miscellaneous: Oral and rectal moniliasis, vaginitis, neuropathy, disturbed smell, sciatic neuritis caused by IM injection of penicillin, laryngeal stridor, high fever. Rapid IV administration of **azlocillin** is associated with transient chest discomfort; do not infuse drug in less than 5 minutes.

DOSAGE

AMOXICILLIN

Larger doses may be required for persistent or severe infections. Children's dose is intended for patients whose weight will not cause the calculated dosage to be greater than that recommended for adults.

Infections of ear, nose, throat, GU tract, skin and soft tissues: Adults and children over 20 kg—250 mg q8h. *Children*—20 mg/kg/day in divided doses q8h. *Severe infections or those caused by less sus-*

ceptible organisms—500 mg q8h for adults and 40 mg/kg/day in divided doses q8h for children.

Infections of lower respiratory tract: *Adults and children over 20 kg*—500 mg q8h. *Children*—40 mg/kg/day in divided doses q8h.

CDC-recommended treatment schedules for sexually transmitted diseases

Uncomplicated gonococcal infections in adults: 3 g with 1 g probenecid PO administered at same time.

Gonorrhea with coexisting chlamydial infection: 3 g with 1 g probenecid PO plus 500 mg tetracycline PO, qid for 7 days. Doxycycline hyclate, 100 mg PO bid for 7 days may be substituted for tetracycline.

Gonococcal urethritis and epididymitis: 500 mg tid for at least 10 days.

Disseminated gonococcal infection: 3 g plus 1 g probenecid PO, followed by 500 mg amoxicillin or ampicillin PO, qid for at least 7 days.

Uncomplicated vulvovaginitis and urethritis (children under 100 lbs): 50 mg/kg with 25 mg/kg probenecid PO.

Acute PID (ambulatory patients): 3 g with 1 g probenecid PO, followed by 100 mg doxycycline PO, bid for 10 to 14 days.

Rape victims (prophylaxis of infection): For pregnant women and patients allergic to tetracycline, give 3 g amoxicillin with 1 g probenecid as single oral dose.

AMPICILLIN, ORAL AND PARENTERAL

May be given IM or IV. Parenteral form is reserved for moderately severe to severe infections and for those unable to take oral medication. Patient is changed to oral therapy as soon as appropriate.

Respiratory-tract, soft-tissue infections

Parenteral: *Patients weighing 40 kg or more*—250 mg to 500 mg q6h. *Patients weighing less than 40 kg*—25 mg/kg/day to 50 mg/kg/day in equally divided doses q6h to q8h.

Oral: *Patients weighing 20 kg or more*—250 mg q6h. *Patients weighing less than 20 kg*—50 mg/kg/day in equally divided doses q6h to q8h.

GI and GU tract infections (including those caused by *N. gonorrhoeae* in females)

Higher doses may be used for persistent or severe infections. In persistent infections, therapy may be required for several weeks.

Parenteral: *Patients weighing 40 kg or more*—500 mg q6h. *Patients weighing less than 40 kg*—50 mg/kg/day in equally divided doses q6h to q8h.

Oral: *Patients weighing 20 kg or more*—500 mg q6h. *Patients weighing less than 20 kg*—100 mg/kg/day in equally divided doses q6h to q8h.

Urethritis due to N. gonorrhoeae

In treatment of complications of gonorrheal urethritis, such as prostatitis and epididymitis, prolonged and intensive therapy is recommended.

Parenteral (males): Two doses of 500 mg each at an interval of 8 to 12 hours. Treatment may be repeated if necessary or extended if required.

Oral (males or females): 3.5 g with 1 g probenecid, administered simultaneously as single dose.

Bacterial meningitis

Parenteral (adults, children): 150 mg/kg/day to 200 mg/kg/day in equally divided doses q3h to q4h. Treatment may be initiated with IV drip therapy and continued with IM injections.

Prevention of bacterial endocarditis

For GI and GU tract surgery or instrumentation: 1 g IM or IV, plus gentamicin 1.5 mg/kg IM or IV (not to exceed 80 mg) or streptomycin 1 g IM may be used. Give initial dose 30 to 60 minutes prior to procedure and give two additional doses q8h with gentamicin or q12h with streptomycin.

Pediatric doses: 50 mg/kg, plus gentamicin 2 mg/kg or streptomycin 20 mg/kg. Timing of doses for children is the same as for adults. Pediatric doses should not exceed recommended dose or 24-hour dose for adults.

Septicemia

Parenteral (adults, children): 150 mg/kg/day to 200 mg/kg/day. Administer IV for at least 3 days, then continue with IM route q3h to q4h.

CDC-recommended treatment schedules for sexually transmitted diseases

Uncomplicated gonococcal infections in adults: 3.5 g PO with probenecid 1 g PO administered at same time.

Gonorrhea with coexisting chlamydial infection: 3.5 mg with probenecid 1 g PO plus tetracycline 500 mg PO qid for 7 days. Doxycycline hyclate 100 mg PO bid for 7 days may be substituted for tetracycline.

Disseminated gonococcal infection: 3.5 g PO plus probenecid 1 g PO, followed by ampicillin or amoxicillin 500 mg PO qid for at least 7 days.

Gardnerella vaginalis: 500 mg PO qid for 7 days. This regimen is less effective than metronidazole but is suggested for pregnant patients or those for whom metronidazole is contraindicated. If indicated, male sexual partners are treated as above.

Acute PID (ambulatory patients): 3.5 g PO with probenecid 1 g PO, followed by doxycycline 100 mg PO bid for 10 to 14 days.

Rape victims (prophylaxis of infection): For pregnant patients and those allergic to tetracycline, 3.5 g with probenecid 1 g as single oral dose.

AMPICILLIN WITH PROBENECID

3.5 g ampicillin and 1 g probenecid as single oral dose.

AZLOCILLIN

Administer by slow IV injection (5 minutes or longer) or by IV infusion (30 minutes).

Adults

Serious infections: 200 mg/kg/day to 300 mg/kg/day given in 4 to 6 divided doses. Usual dose is 3 g q4h.

Life-threatening infections: Up to 350 mg/kg/day; total daily dose should not ordinarily exceed 24 g (4 g q4h).

Renal impairment: Dosage in renal impairment is adjusted to degree of impairment. Dosage in renal failure for patients undergoing hemodialysis is 3 g after each dialysis and then q12h. Measurement of serum levels is recommended for dosage adjustment.

Children

Not used in newborn. In children with acute pulmonary exacerbation of cystic fibrosis, 75 mg/kg q4h. Total daily dosage should not exceed 24 g. May be infused IV over a period of about 30 minutes.

BACAMPICILLIN

Because drug is hydrolyzed to ampicillin during absorption from GI tract and is more completely absorbed than ampicillin, it is given in lower total daily doses and sustains effective serum levels when given q12h. Tablets may be given without regard to meals; suspension is administered to fasting patients. Adult doses are for those persons weighing 25 kg or more.

Upper respiratory tract infections (including otitis media)

Adults: 400 mg q12h.

Children: 25 mg/kg/day in two equally divided doses q12h.

Severe infections or those caused by less susceptible organisms

Adults: 800 mg q12h.

Children: 50 mg/kg/day in two equally divided doses q12h.

Lower respiratory tract infections

Adults: 800 mg q12h.

Children: 50 mg/kg/day in two equally divided doses q12h.

Gonorrhea

Usual adult dose (male and female) is 1.6 g plus probenecid 1 g as single oral dose. No pediatric dosage is established. Larger doses may be needed for persistent or severe infections.

CARBENICILLIN DISODIUM

Higher IV doses are used in serious urinary-tract and systemic infections. Maximum recommended dose is 40 g/day. IM injections should not exceed 2 g/dose. Gentamicin or tobramycin may be used concurrently with carbenicillin for initial therapy until results of culture and sensitivity studies are known. Seriously ill patients should receive higher doses.

Adults

Urinary-tract infections: For serious infections, 200 mg/kg/day by IV drip. For uncomplicated infections, 1 g to 2 g IM or IV q6h.

Severe systemic infections, septicemia, respiratory infections, soft-tissue infections due to **Pseudomonas and anaerobes:** 400 mg/kg/day to 500 mg/kg/day (30–40 g) IV continuously or in divided doses.

Proteus *and* **E. coli:** 250 mg/kg/day to 400 mg/kg/day (15–30 g) IV continuously or in divided doses.

Infections complicated by renal insufficiency due to **Proteus** *and* **E. coli:** 2 g IV q8h.

Infections due to **Proteus** *and* **E. coli:** *During dialysis*—2 g IV q6h; *during hemodialysis*—2 g IV q4h.

Meningitis: 400 mg/kg/day to 500 mg/kg/day IV continuously or in divided doses.

Gonorrhea, acute uncomplicated anogenital and urethral infections: Single 4 g IM injection, divided between two sites. Give probenecid 1 g PO 30 minutes prior to injection.

Children

Urinary-tract infections: For *Pseudomonas, Enterobacter, S. faecalis,* 50 mg/kg/day to 200 mg/kg/day in divided doses q4h to q6h IM or IV. For infections due to *Proteus* and *E. coli,* 50 mg/kg/day to 100 mg/kg/day in divided doses q4h to q6h IM or IV.

Severe systemic infections, septicemia, respiratory infections, soft-tissue infections: For those due to *Pseudomonas* and anaerobes, 400 mg/kg/day to 500 mg/kg/day IV, continuously or in divided doses; due to *Proteus, E. coli,* 250 mg/kg/day to 400 mg/kg/day IV continuously or in divided doses.

Meningitis: 400 mg/kg/day to 500 mg/kg/day IV continuously or in divided doses.

Neonates

For severe systemic infections (sepsis) due to susceptible strains of **Pseudomonas, Proteus, H. influenzae, E. coli, S. pneumoniae:** The following dosages may be given IM or by 15-minute IV infusions: *Infants under 2 kg*—100 mg/kg initially; subsequent doses during first week 75 mg/kg/8 hours (225 mg/kg/day); after 7 days of age give 100 mg/kg/6 hours (400 mg/kg/day). *Infants over 2 kg*—100 mg/kg initially; subsequent doses during first 3 days 75 mg/kg/6 hours; after 3 days of age 100 mg/kg/6 hours (400 mg/kg/day).

CARBENICILLIN INDANYL SODIUM

Urinary tract infections

Due to **E. coli, Proteus** *species,* **Enterobacter:** 382 mg to 764 mg qid.

Due to **Pseudomonas**, *enterococci:* 764 mg qid.
Prostatitis
764 mg qid.

CLOXACILLIN SODIUM

Mild to moderate upper respiratory and localized skin and soft-tissue infections
Adults and children over 20 kg: 250 mg q6h.
Children less than 20 kg: 50 mg/kg/day in equally divided doses q6h.
Severe infections (lower respiratory-tract or disseminated infections)
Adults and children over 20 kg: 500 mg or more q6h.
Children less than 20 kg: 100 mg/kg/day or more in equal doses q6h.

CYCLACILLIN

Respiratory-tract infections
Tonsillitis and pharyngitis: In adults—250 mg q6h. *In children less than 20 kg*—125 mg q8h. *In children greater than 20 kg*—250 mg q8h.
Bronchitis and pneumonia: In adults—250 mg q6h for mild or moderate infections and 500 mg q6h for chronic infections. *Children*—50 mg/kg/day q6h for mild or moderate infections and 100 mg/kg/day q6h for chronic infections.
Otitis media and skin and skin structures
Adults: 250 mg to 500 mg q6h depending on severity.
Children: 50 mg/kg/day to 100 mg/kg/day depending on severity, given in equally spaced doses.
GU tract
Adults: 500 mg q6h.
Children: 100 mg/kg/day in equally spaced doses.
Renal failure
Dosage and dosage intervals are based on creatinine clearance.
Infants
Cyclacyllin is not indicated in children under 2 months.

DICLOXACILLIN

Mild to moderate upper respiratory and localized skin and soft-tissue infections
Adults, children over 40 kg: 125 mg q6h.
Children under 40 kg: 12.5 mg/kg/day in equal doses q6h.
More severe infections such as lower respiratory-tract or disseminated infections
Adults, children over 40 kg: 250 mg or more q6h.
Children under 40 kg: 25 mg/kg/day or more in equally divided doses q6h.
Newborns: Use in newborn not recommended.

HETACILLIN

Give on empty stomach to ensure maximum absorption.
Patients weighing 40 kg or more: 225 mg to 450 mg qid, depending on severity of infection.
Patients weighing less than 40 kg: 22.5 mg/kg/day to 45 mg/kg/day or 10 mg/lb/day to 20 mg/lb/day, depending on severity of infection.
Very severe infections: Treatment is initiated with parenteral ampicillin.

METHICILLIN SODIUM

IM administration
Adults: 1 g q4h to q6h.
Infants, children less than 20 kg: 25 mg/kg (12 mg/lb) q6h.
IV administration
Adults: Usual dose is 1 g q6h in 50 ml of Sodium Chloride Injection at rate of 10 ml/min.
Newborns: 50 mg/kg/day to 150 mg/kg/day.
Children: 200 mg/kg/day to 300 mg/kg/day.

MEZLOCILLIN

May be given IV or IM. For serious infections, IV route is used. IM doses should not exceed 2 g/injection.
Adults: Recommended dosage for serious infections is 200 mg/kg/day to 300 mg/kg/day given in four to six divided doses. Usual dose is 3 g q4h or 4 g q6h. For life-threatening infections, up to 350 mg/kg/day or 4 g q4h may be given, but total daily dosage should ordinarily not exceed 24 g. For acute, uncomplicated, gonococcal urethritis, usual dose is 1 g to 2 g given once by IV or IM injection. Probenecid 1 g PO may be given at time of dosing or up to ½ hour before.
Infants and children: Limited data are available on safety and effectiveness. If drug is judged appropriate, suggested dosage is 75 mg/kg q12h (150 mg/kg/day) in infants over or under 2000 g and less than 7 days of age. For infants over 7 days of age, give 75 mg/kg q8h for infants under 2000 g and 75 mg/kg q6h for infants over 2000 g. For infants over 1 month and children up to 12 years, 50 mg/kg may be given q4h; infuse IV over 30 minutes or administration by IM injection.
Patient with impaired renal function: Dosage is based on creatinine clearance. For life-threatening infections, 3 g may be given q6h to those with creatinine clearances between 10 ml/minute and 30 ml/minute and 2 g q6h to those with creatinine clearances less than 10 ml/minute. Patient with serious systemic infection undergoing hemodialysis for renal failure may receive 3 g to 4 g after each dialysis and then q12h. Patient undergoing peritoneal dialysis may receive 3 g q12h. For renal failure and

renal insufficiency, measurement of serum levels of mezlocillin with provide additional guidance for adjusting dosage.

NAFCILLIN

Parenteral route is used initially in severe infections and changed to oral therapy as condition warrants. Very severe infections may require very high doses.

Parenteral

_IV:_ 500 mg q4h; doubled if necessary in very severe infections. This route is used for short-term therapy (24–48 hours) because of occasional occurrence of thrombophlebitis, particularly in the elderly.

_IM:_ 500 mg q6h in adults, with dosage interval decreased to q4h in very severe infections. In infants and children, 25 mg/kg bid; neonates, 10 mg/kg bid.

Oral

Adults: 250 mg to 500 mg q4h to q6h for mild to moderate infections; in severe infections, 1 g q4h to q6h may be necessary.

Children: Staphylococcal infections—50 mg/kg/day in four divided doses; for neonates, 10 mg/kg three to four times a day is recommended and, if ineffective, change to parenteral form. _Scarlet fever and pneumonia_—25 mg/kg/day in four divided doses.

OXACILLIN SODIUM

Oral

Mild to moderate infections of skin, soft tissue or upper respiratory tract: _Adults_—500 mg q4h to q6h for minimum of 5 days. _Children weighing more than 40 kg_—Adult dosage. _Children weighing less than 40 kg_—50 mg/kg/day in equally divided doses q6h for at least 5 days.

Serious or life-threatening infections: Use of parenteral form or other penicillinase-resistant penicillin is advised for initial treatment. Following initial control, oral form may be given for follow-up therapy as follows: _Adults_—1 g q4h to q6h. _Children_—100 mg/kg/day or more in equally divided doses q4h to q6h. In serious systemic infections, therapy is continued for at least 1 to 2 weeks after patient is afebrile and cultures are sterile. Treatment of osteomyelitis may require several months of intensive therapy. Most appropriate use for oral medication is in prolonged follow-up therapy following successful initial parenteral treatment.

Parenteral

Use is considered for patient unable to take oral form. Change to oral therapy when parenteral therapy is no longer necessary.

Mild to moderate upper-respiratory and localized skin and soft-tissue infections: _Adults and children weighing 40 kg or more_—250 mg to 500 mg q4h to q6h. _Children weighing less than 40 kg_—50 mg/kg/day in equally divided doses q6h.

Severe infections (lower respiratory-tract or disseminated infections): _Adults and children weighing more than 40 kg_—1 g or more q4h to q6h. _Children weighing less than 40 kg_—100 mg/kg/day or more in equally divided doses q4h to q6h. Very severe infections may require very high doses and prolonged therapy.

PENICILLIN G BENZATHINE

Oral

Parenteral penicillin is recommended as initial therapy in moderately severe infections. Not used as adjunctive prophylaxis for GU instrumentation or surgery, lower intestinal-tract surgery, or childbirth.

Streptococcal infections: _Mild to moderately severe infections of upper respiratory tract including scarlet fever and erysipelas_—400,000 to 600,000 units q4h to q6h for 10 days.

Pneumococcal infections: _Mild to moderately severe infections of the respiratory tract, including otitis media_—400,000 to 600,000 units q4h to q6h until afebrile for at least 2 days.

Staphylococcal infections: _Mild skin and soft tissue_—400,000 to 600,000 units q4h to q6h.

Prevention of recurrence following rheumatic fever or chorea: 200,000 units bid on a continuing basis.

Children under 12: For infants and small children, suggested dose is 25,000 to 90,000 units/kg/day in three to six divided doses.

Parenteral

Children under 12: Adjust dosage in accordance with age and weight of child, severity of infection.

Streptococcal (group A) upper respiratory-tract infections: A single injection of 1.2 million units for adults; a single injection of 900,000 units for older children; a single injection of 300,000 to 600,000 units for infants and older children under 60 lb (27 kg).

Early syphilis (primary, secondary, latent syphilis of less than 1 year duration): 2,400,000 units IM at a single session.

Congenital syphilis (asymptomatic infants with normal CSF): 50,000 units/kg IM in a single dose.

Late syphilis (tertiary and neurosyphilis): 2.4 million to 3 million units at 7-day intervals for a total of 6 million to 9 million units.

Yaws, bejel, and pinta: 1.2 million units as single dose.

Prophylaxis (rheumatic fever, chorea, glomerulonephritis): Following an acute attack, 1.2 million units once a month or 600,000 units every 2 weeks.

PENICILLIN G BENZATHINE AND PROCAINE COMBINED

Streptococcal infections (group A): Treatment is usually given in a single session using multiple IM sites when indicated. An alternative dosage schedule may be used, giving one-half the total dose on day 1 and one-half on day 3. *Adults and children over 60 lb*—2.4 million units. *Children 30–60 lb*—900,000 to 1.2 million units. *Infants and children under 30 lb*—600,000 units.

Pneumococcal infections: 600,000 units in children and 1.2 million units in adults, repeated every 2 to 3 days until patient has been afebrile 48 hours.

PENICILLIN G (AQUEOUS), PARENTERAL

Severe infections due to susceptible strains of streptococci, pneumococci, staphylococci: Minimum of 5 million units/day.

Syphilis: Dosage and duration of therapy are determined by age of patient and stage of disease; hospitalization is recommended because of frequency of administration.

Gonorrheal endocarditis and arthritis: Minimum of 5 million units/day.

Meningococcal meningitis: 1 million to 2 million units IM q2h or by continuous IV drip of 20 million to 30 million units/day.

Actinomycosis: 1 million to 6 million units/day for cervicofacial cases; 10 million to 20 million units/day for thoracic and abdominal disease.

Clostridial infections: 20 million units/day, as adjunct to antitoxin.

Fusospirochetal infection: 5 million to 10 million units/day.

Rat-bite fever: 12 million to 15 million units/day for 3 to 4 weeks.

Listeria *infections:* 500,000 to 1 million units/day. *Adults with meningitis*—15 million to 20 million units/day for 2 weeks. *Adults with endocarditis*—15 million to 20 million units/day for 4 weeks.

Pasturella *infections:* 4 million to 6 million units/day for 2 weeks.

Erysipeloid: *Endocarditis*—2 million to 20 million units/day for 4 to 6 weeks.

Gram-negative bacillary bacteremia: 20 million to 30 million units/day.

Diphtheria: 300,000 to 400,000 units/day in divided doses for 10 to 12 days.

Anthrax: Minimum of 5 million units/day in divided doses.

Prophylaxis against bacterial endocarditis

For those with congenital heart disease or rheumatic or other acquired valvular heart disease when undergoing dental or surgical procedures.

Dental procedures: *Adults*—600,000 units aqueous procaine penicillin mixed with 1 million units of aqueous penicillin G ½ to 1 hour before procedure. *Children*—30,000 units/kg aqueous penicillin G IM combined with 600,000 units procaine pencillin G ½ to 1 hour before procedure; 500 mg of penicillin V PO or 250 mg for children under 60 lb is then given q6h for 8 doses. Alternatively, streptomycin 1 g IM for adults or 20 mg/kg IM for children may be added to regimen for high-risk patients (*e.g.,* those with prosthetic heart valves).

Patients undergoing GU tract surgery or instrumentation: *Adults*—2 million units aqueous penicillin G IM or IV plus 1.5 mg/kg gentamicin (not to exceed 80 mg) IM or IV or 1 g streptomycin IM. Give ½ to 1 hour prior to procedure and give two additional doses q8h with gentamicin or q12h with streptomycin. *Children*—30,000 units/kg aqueous penicillin G IM or IV, plus 2 mg/kg gentamicin IM or IV, or 20 mg/kg streptomycin IM ½ to 1 hour before procedure.

CDC-recommended treatment for syphilis

Neurosyphilis: 12 million to 24 million units IV/day (2–4 million units q4h) for 10 days, followed by benzathine penicillin G 2.4 million units IM weekly for three doses.

In symptomatic infants or asymptomatic infants with abnormal CSF: 50,000 units/kg IM or IV daily in two divided doses for minimum of 10 days.

CDC-recommended treatment for gonorrhea

Disseminated gonococcal infections in arthritis–dermatitis syndrome: 10 million units IV/day until improvement occurs, followed by 500 mg amoxicillin or ampicillin qid PO to complete 7 days of treatment.

Management of infants born to mothers with gonococcal infection: 50,000 units in a single IV or IM injection to full-term infants or 20,000 units to low–birth weight infants.

Adult gonococcal ophthalmia: 10 million units IV/day for 5 days. Irrigate eyes with saline or buffered solutions, as needed.

Neonatal gonococcal ophthalmia: 50,000 units/kg/day in two doses IV for 7 days. Irrigate eyes as for adults, as needed.

Neonatal arthritis and septicemia: 75,000 to 100,000 units/kg/day IV in four doses for 7 days.

Meningitis: 100,000 units/kg/day in three or four IV doses for at least 10 days.

PENICILLIN G POTASSIUM, ORAL

250 mg = 400,000 units. Give at least 1 hour before or 2 hours after meals.

Streptococcal infections: *Mild to moderately severe infections of upper respiratory tract, including otitis media, scarlet fever, and mild erysipelas*—200,000 to 250,000 units q6h to q8h for 10 days for mild infections; 400,000 to 500,000 units q8h for

10 days for moderately severe infections. Alternatively, 800,000 units q12h.

Pneumococcal infections: _Mild to moderately severe infections of respiratory tract, including otitis media_—400,000 to 500,000 units q6h until afebrile for at least 2 days.

Streptococcal infections: _Mild infections of skin and skin structures_—200,000 to 500,000 units q6h to q8h until infection is cured.

Vincent's gingivitis and pharyngitis of the oropharynx (fusospirochetosis): _Mild to moderately severe infections_—200,000 to 500,000 units q6h to q8h. Obtain necessary dental care in infections involving gum tissue.

Prevention of recurrence following rheumatic fever or chorea: 200,000 to 250,000 units bid on a continuing basis.

Children under 12: 25,000 to 90,000 units/kg/day in three to six divided doses.

PENICILLIN G PROCAINE, AQUEOUS (APPG)

600,000 to 1.2 million units/day given in the following: Pneumonia; streptococcal infections (group A): moderately severe to severe tonsillitis, erysipelas, scarlet fever, upper respiratory-tract infections including otitis media, and skin and skin-structure infections (for minimum of 10 days); staphylococcal infections: moderately severe to severe infections of skin and skin structure; bacterial endocarditis (only in extremely sensitive infections); anthrax (cutaneous); Vincent's gingivitis and pharyngitis; erysipeloid; _Streptobacillus moniliformis_ and _Spirillum minus_ (rat-bite fever).

Perioperative prophylaxis against bacterial endocarditis: _In those with rheumatic or congenital heart lesions undergoing dental or upper respiratory-tract surgery or instrumentation_—See Penicillin G (Aqueous), Parenteral, p 850.

Syphilis: _Primary, secondary, and latent with negative spinal fluid in adults, children over 12 yr_—600,000 units/day for 8 days. _Late (tertiary, neurosyphilis, latent syphilis with positive spinal fluid examination or no spinal fluid examination)_—600,000 units/day for 10 to 15 days. _In pregnancy_—treatment should correspond to stage of the disease. _For yaws, bejel, and pinta_—Treatment should correspond to stage of the disease.

CDC-recommended treatment schedules for sexually transmitted diseases

Acute PID (ambulatory patient): 4.8 million units IM at 2 sites, with probenecid 1 g PO, followed by doxycycline 100 mg PO bid for 10 to 14 days.

Neurosyphilis: 2.4 million units IM/day, with probenecid 500 mg PO qid for 10 days, followed by 2.4 million units benzathine penicillin G IM weekly for three doses.

Symptomatic infants or asymptomatic infants with abnormal CSF: 50,000 units/kg/day IM for minimum of 10 days.

Uncomplicated gonococcal infections in adults and pharyngeal, urethral, and anorectal gonococcal infections: 4.8 million units IM, divided at two different sites, together with probenecid 1 g PO.

Childhood proctitis or pharyngitis (uncomplicated): 100,000 units/kg IM and probenecid 25 mg/kg PO (maximum 1 g).

Retreatment: CDC recommends test of cure procedures at approximately 7 to 14 days after therapy. _Male_—A gram-stained smear is adequate if positive; otherwise a culture specimen should be obtained from the anterior urethra. _Female_—Culture specimens should be obtained from both the endocervical and anal canal sites. Retreatment in male is indicated if urethral discharge persists for 3 or more days following initial therapy and the smear or culture remains positive. Follow-up treatment consists of 4.8 million units IM, divided in two injection sites at a single visit. In uncomplicated gonorrhea of the female, retreatment is indicated if follow-up cervical or rectal cultures remain positive. Follow-up treatment consists of 4.8 million units daily on 2 successive days.

Syphilis: A serologic test for syphilis is performed at the time of diagnosis. Patients with gonorrhea who also have syphilis should be given additional treatment appropriate to the stage of syphilis.

PENICILLIN V

125 mg = 200,000 units.

Streptococcal infections: _Mild to moderately severe infections of upper respiratory tract, including scarlet fever and mild erysipelas_—125 mg to 250 mg q6h to q8h for 10 days.

Pneumococcal infections: _Mild to moderately severe infections of respiratory tract, including otitis media_—250 mg to 500 mg q6h until afebrile at least 2 days.

Staphylococcal infections: _Mild infections of skin and soft tissue_—250 mg to 500 mg q6h to q8h.

Vincent's infection of oropharynx: _Mild to moderately severe infections_—250 mg to 500 mg q6h to q8h. Obtain necessary dental care in infections involving gum tissue.

To prevent recurrence following rheumatic fever or chorea: 125 mg to 250 mg bid on a continuing basis.

To prevent bacterial endocarditis: _In patients with rheumatic, congenital, or other acquired valvular heart disease who are to undergo dental or upper_ *respiratory-tract surgery or instrumentation*—See Penicillin G (Aqueous), Parenteral, p 850.

Children under 12: Dosage is calculated on basis of body weight. Suggested dose is 25,000 to 90,000 units/kg/day in 3 to 6 divided doses.

PENICILLIN V POTASSIUM
Same as Penicillin V, above.

PIPERACILLIN SODIUM
May be given IM or IV; for serious infections, IV route is usually used. Usual dosage for serious infections is 3 g to 4 g q4h to q6h as a 20-minute infusion. Maximum daily dose for adults is usually 24 g/day; higher doses may be used. IM injections should be limited to 2 g/site. This route is used primarily in treatment of uncomplicated gonorrhea and urinary-tract infections.

The following dosages are recommended:

Severe infections: *Septicemia, nosocomial pneumonia, intra-abdominal infections, aerobic and anaerobic gynecologic infections, skin and soft-tissue infections*—12 g to 18 g IV (200–300 mg/kg) per day in divided doses q4h to q6h.

Complicated urinary-tract infections: 8 g to 16 g IV (125–200 mg/kg) per day in divided doses q6h to q8h.

Uncomplicated urinary-tract infections and most community-acquired pneumonia: 6 g to 8 g IM or IV (100–125 mg/kg) per day in divided doses q6h to q12h.

Uncomplicated gonorrhea: 2 g IM with probenecid 1 g PO ½ hour prior to injection as a single dose.

Renal impairment: Dosage in renal impairment adjusted according to creatinine clearance.

Patient on hemodialysis: Maximum dose is 6 g/day (2 g q8h). Hemodialysis removes 30% to 50% of piperacillin in 4 hours; a 1-g additional dose should be given following each dialysis period.

Renal failure and hepatic insufficiency: Measurement of serum levels provide guidance for adjusting dosage.

Infants, children under 12: Dosages not established.

Concomitant administration: When given concurrently with aminoglycosides, both drugs are used in full therapeutic dosages.

TICARCILLIN DISODIUM
IM injections should not exceed 2 g/injection. IV therapy in higher doses is used in serious urinary-tract and systemic infections. Seriously ill patients should receive higher doses. Drug is useful in infections in which protective mechanisms are impaired, such as acute leukemia, and during therapy with immunosuppressive or oncolytic drugs.

Bacterial septicemia, respiratory-tract infections, skin and soft-tissue infections, intra-abdominal infections, infections of the female pelvis and genital tract

Adults: 200 mg/kg/day to 300 mg/kg/day by IV infusion in divided doses every 3, 4, or 6 hours.

Children under 40 kg: 200 mg/kg/day to 300 mg/kg/day by IV infusion in divided doses q4h to q6h (not to exceed adult dosage).

Urinary-tract infections

Adults: In complicated infections, 150 mg/kg/day to 200 mg/kg/day by IV infusion in divided doses q4h to q6h. Usual recommended dose for average weight adult is 3 g qid. In uncomplicated infections, 1 g IM or direct IV q6h.

Children under 40 kg: In complicated infections, 150 mg/kg/day to 200 mg/kg/day by IV infusion; in uncomplicated infections, 50 mg/kg/day to 100 mg/kg/day IM or direct IV in divided doses q6h to q8h.

Dosage in neonates

For severe infections (sepsis), the following may be given IM or by 10- to 20-minute IV infusions:

Infants under 2 kg: Age 0–7 days, 75 mg/kg/12 hours; over 7 days of age, 75 mg/kg/8 hours.

Infants over 2 kg: Age 0–7 days, 75 mg/kg/8 hours; over 7 days of age, 100 mg/kg/8 hours.

Dosage in renal insufficiency

Half-life of ticarcillin in those with renal failure is approximately 13 hours. Initial loading dose should be 3 g IV, followed by IV doses based on creatinine clearance.

NURSING IMPLICATIONS

HISTORY
See Appendix 4.

PHYSICAL ASSESSMENT
Obtain vital signs; record overt signs of infection; assess patient's general status, especially if severely ill. Culture and sensitivity tests may be ordered before initiation of therapy (therapy may be instituted before results of testing known). Additional laboratory tests may include renal- and hepatic-function tests, blood culture, WBC and differential, urinalysis, and so on.

ADMINISTRATION
Obtain culture and sensitivity test *before* administration of first dose.

Check expiration date on label before preparing for administration; do not use outdated penicillin preparations.

Contact dermatitis may occur if the individual dispensing the drug is allergic to penicillin; wearing plastic disposable gloves may prevent contact dermatitis in these individuals.

Shake parenteral solutions thoroughly before withdrawing medication. Visually check vial or bottle to be sure medication is completely dissolved and has an even color and viscosity.

Following reconstitution, label the multidose vial or single-dose vial not used immediately with date and time of reconstitution and units per milliliter.

Once reconstituted, preparations should be stored under refrigeration until used. Return vial to refrigerator immediately after withdrawing dose.

Have materials ready for emergency treatment of anaphylaxis. Hospital protocol may vary; items that may be used include epinephrine, antihistamine (_e.g._, diphenhydramine), corticosteroids, suction equipment, and tracheostomy tray.

Always ask patient about allergy to penicillin and cephalosporins before administering first dose, even if a complete drug history has been obtained. Clearly tell patient that "penicillin" is being given (regardless of route of administration). This is especially important when administering drug for the first time to those who are under influence of CNS depressants such as narcotics, anesthetics, and so on.

Oral: Oral penicillins are best given on an empty stomach, 1 hour before or 2 hours after meals. **Bacampicillin** (tablets) and **amoxicillin** may be given without regard to meals or food. **Penicillin V** is less affected than other penicillins by food; check with physician before administering this penicillin with food.

Oral suspensions are kept refrigerated.

Shake oral suspensions well before pouring.

Give with full glass of water.

If a child is unable to take an oral tablet, discuss problem with physician because suspensions for oral products (_exception_—carbenicillin indanyl sodium) are available. Do not crush tablets and mix with food.

_IM:_ If there is a history of sensitivity to procaine in penicillin G procaine, an intradermal test may be performed with 0.1 ml of procaine 1% or 2%. Development of erythema, wheal, flare, or eruption indicates procaine sensitivity and procaine penicillin preparations are not administered.

Lidocaine HCl is available with and without epinephrine. When lidocaine is ordered as a diluent (to decrease pain/discomfort of IM injection), check drug name on label carefully. _Do not_ use lidocaine containing epinephrine; only lidocaine without epinephrine is used. Lidocaine is used as a diluent only for preparation of IM injections and is contraindicated in those sensitive to local anesthetics.

Adults—Inject deep IM into body of relatively large muscle. Preferred site is the upper outer quadrant of gluteus muscle or midlateral thigh. Use the deltoid only if well developed (adults, older children) and then only with caution, to avoid radial nerve injury. Do _not_ give injections into the lower or mid-third of the upper arm.

Children—Give in midlateral muscles of thigh. In infants and small children, use periphery of the upper outer quadrant of the gluteus muscle only when necessary, such as in burn patients, to minimize possibility of sciatic nerve damage.

When IM doses are repeated, rotate injection sites; record site used.

CLINICAL ALERT: Do _not_ inject parenteral solutions into or near an artery or nerve; severe neurovascular complications can occur. _Always_ aspirate before injection. Do not give drug if blood is returned in the syringe; withdraw needle, change needle, and give in different site.

During injection, observe for appearance of red wheal or flare around the injection site. If this occurs, patient is probably allergic to penicillin. Stop administration, withdraw needle, and contact physician immediately.

_IV:_ When giving direct IV, administer drug slowly over period of 3 to 5 minutes. Use injection port of IV tubing.

When giving by IV infusion (piggyback or secondary IV line), discontinue the IV fluid running in the primary line while drug is infusing. Check IV at frequent intervals so the primary line is opened immediately following infusion of the drug.

AMOXICILLIN

May be given without regard to meals.

AMPICILLIN, ORAL

Oral suspension: Powder for oral suspension is reconstituted by pharmacist.

Dosage similarity: Oral suspension—100 mg/ml and 125 mg/5 ml.

AMPICILLIN, PARENTERAL

Preparation of solutions: Use only freshly prepared solutions. Administer IM and IV injections within 1 hour after preparation, because potency may decrease significantly after this period.

Reconstitute with Sterile or Bacteriostatic Water for Injection. Piggyback vials may be reconstituted with Sodium Chloride Injection.

Direct IV administration: Give _slowly_ over 3 to 5 minutes. _Caution_—More rapid infusion may result in convulsive seizures.

IV drip (standard vials): Dilute as above for direct IV use prior to further dilution with compatible IV solutions (Table 41).

Table 41. Solutions Used to Dilute Ampicillin for IV Administration

IV solution	Concentrations up to (mg/ml)	Stability (hours)
0.9% Sodium Chloride	30	8
5% Dextrose in Water	2	4
5% Dextrose in Water	10–20	2
5% Dextrose in 0.45% Sodium Chloride	2	4
10% Invert Sugar in Water	2	4
M/6 Sodium Lactate	30	8
Lactated Ringer's	30	8
Sterile Water for Injection	30	8

IV drip (piggyback vials): After reconstitution, administer alone or further dilute with suitable IV solutions. To ensure compatibility and stability, use only the solutions listed in Table 41.

If reconstituted solution is to be further diluted, physician must specify IV solution, volume (or concentration in mg/ml), and rate of infusion.

IV drip is inserted piggyback into primary line and infused over period of 15 to 30 minutes unless physician orders otherwise. For infants and small children, physician should specify rate of infusion.

AMPICILLIN WITH PROBENECID

Single-dose bottle of nine capsules or bottle of oral suspension taken as single dose.

AZLOCILLIN SODIUM

Administer by slow IV injection (5 minutes or longer) or by IV infusion (30 minutes).

When given in combination with another antimicrobial, give each drug separately in accordance with the recommended dosage and routes of administration.

IV infusion: Reconstitute each gram by vigorous shaking with at least 10 ml of Sterile Water for Injection, 5% Dextrose Injection, or 0.9% Sodium Chloride Injection.

Dilute dissolved drug to volume ordered by physician (usually 50–100 ml) with appropriate IV solution (see Compatible IV Solutions, below).

Administer solution of reconstituted drug over a period of 30 minutes by direct infusion or through Y-tube infusion set. If Y-tube infusion set is used, temporarily discontinue administration of any other solutions during the infusion.

IV injection: Reconstituted solution may be injected directly into vein or into IV tubing; give slowly over period of 5 or more minutes. To minimize venous irritation, concentration of drug should not exceed 10%.

Compatible IV solutions: Sterile Water for Injection; 0.9% Sodium Chloride Injection; 5% Dextrose Injection; 5% Dextrose in 0.225% Sodium Chloride Injection; Lactated Ringer's Injection; 5% Dextrose in 0.45% Sodium Chloride Injection.

Stability: Concentrations of 10 mg/ml and 50 mg/ml are stable when stored at room temperature in compatible IV solutions for 24 hours. When stored under refrigeration, concentrations up to 100 mg/ml are stable for 24 hours. Discard unused portion after the time period stated.

Storage: Store at or below 30°C (86°F). Product may darken slightly depending on storage conditions, but potency is not affected.

BACAMPICILLIN

Tablets may be given without regard to meals; give oral suspension to fasting patient.

CARBENICILLIN DISODIUM

Preparation of solutions

IM: Reconstitute with Sterile Water for Injection. Solutions may be diluted with 0.5% lidocaine HCl (without epinephrine) or bacteriostatic water containing 0.9% benzyl alcohol (physician must specifically order lidocaine as diluent).

Dilution for IM Administration

1-g vial: Add 2 ml diluent, 2.5 ml = 1 g; add 2.5 ml diluent, 3 ml = 1 g; add 3.6 ml diluent, 4 ml = 1 g.

2-g vial: Add 4 ml diluent, 2.5 ml = 1 g; add 5 ml diluent, 3 ml = 1 g; add 7.2 ml diluent, 4 ml = 1 g.

5-g vial: Add 7 ml diluent, 2 ml = 1 g; add 9.5 ml diluent, 2.5 ml = 1 g; add 17 ml diluent, 4 ml = 1 g.

Administer deep IM into body of relatively large muscle.

Advise patient that pain at injection site may be noted.

Direct IV injection

Dilution for IV Administration

2-g vial: Add 100 ml diluent to = 1 g/50 ml; 50 ml diluent to = 1 g/25 ml; 20 ml diluent to = 1 g/10 ml.

5-g vial: Add 100 ml diluent to = 1 g/20 ml; 50 ml diluent to = 1 g/10 ml.
10-g vial: Add 95 ml diluent to = 1 g/10 ml.

Following reconstitution, further dilute each gram with at least 5 ml of Sterile Water for Injection.

Give as slowly as possible to avoid vein irritation.

IV infusion: When using 2-, 5-, and 10-g piggyback units, each unit should be reconstituted with a minimum of 10 ml of Sterile Water for Injection/gram of drug. A dilution of 1 g/20 ml or more will further reduce incidence of vein irritation.

Continuous IV infusion: After reconstitution, drug may be added to IV infusion solutions. Physician must order volume of IV solution to be used.

Compatibility: Carbenicillin should *not* be mixed together with gentamicin or tobramycin in the same IV solution.

Stability: Drug is stable for 24 hours at 21°C and 72 hours at 4°C when diluted to as low as 10 mg/ml with the following: Sterile Water for Injection; Sodium Chloride Injection; Dextrose 5% and Sodium Chloride (0.225%, 0.45% or 0.9%); Ringer's or Lactated Ringer's Injection; 5% Dextrose w/Electrolyte #48; 5% Fructose w/ Electrolyte #75; 10% Invert Sugar in Water; 5% Alcohol; 5% Dextrose in Water; 5% Dextrose in Alcohol; Maintenance Electrolyte Solution (Electrolyte #75); Pediatric Maintenance Electrolyte Solution (Electrolyte #48).

METHICILLIN SODIUM

Preparation of solutions: Reconstitute with Sterile Water for Injection or Sodium Chloride Injection.

Do *not* physically mix methicillin with other drugs.

IM: Diluted as follows, 1 ml = 500 mg. 1-g vial, add 1.5 ml diluent; 4-g vial, add 5.7 ml diluent; 6-g vial, add 5.6 ml diluent.

Direct IV administration: Dilute each milliliter of reconstituted solution with 20 ml to 25 ml Sodium Chloride Injection or Sterile Water for Injection. Administer at rate of 10 ml/minute through injection port of IV line.

Continuous IV infusion: Dilute reconstituted solution with IV solution, as ordered by physician (see Compatible IV Solutions, below). Administer at rate prescribed by physician. Drug is normally given q6h; therefore, infusion should be completed within this time period.

IV piggyback: Reconstitute according to directions on label of glass vial. Administer as directed by physician.

Compatible IV solutions: 0.9% Sodium Chloride Injection; 5% Dextrose in Water or Normal Saline; 10% D-Fructose in Water or Normal Saline; M/6 Sodium Lactate Solution; Lactated Ringer's Injection; Lactated Potassic Saline Injection; 5% Plasma Hydrolysate in Water; 10% Invert Sugar in Water or Normal Saline; 10% Invert Sugar plus 0.3% Potassium Chloride in Water; Travert 10% Electrolyte #1, #2, or #3.

MEZLOCILLIN SODIUM

May be administered IV or IM. IM dose should not exceed 2 g/injection.

IV administration

May be given by intermittent infusion or direct IV injection.

IV infusion: Reconstitute each gram with at least 10 ml Sterile Water for Injection, 5% Dextrose Injection, or 0.9% Sodium Chloride Injection. Shake vigorously.

Further dilute to desired volume (50–100 ml) with appropriate IV solution (see Compatible Diluents, below), as ordered by physician.

Solution may then be given over a period of 30 minutes by direct infusion or through a Y-type infusion set or by IV piggyback. Temporarily discontinue administration of any other IV solutions during the infusion.

IV injection: Reconstituted solution may be injected directly into a vein or into IV tubing. Inject slowly over period of 3 to 5 minutes.

IM administration

Each gram may be reconstituted with 3 ml to 4 ml of Sterile Water for Injection or 3 ml to 4 ml of 0.5% or 1% lidocaine HCl (without epinephrine). Lidocaine must be ordered by physician. Shake vigorously.

Inject well within body of a relatively large muscle. Slow injection (12–15 seconds) will minimize discomfort of administration.

Compatible diluents

Concentration of 10 mg/ml to 100 mg/ ml: Sterile Water for Injection; 0.9% Sodium Chloride Injection; 5% Dextrose Injection; 5% Dextrose in 0.225% Sodium Chloride Injection; Lactated Ringer's Injection; 5% Dextrose in Electrolyte #75 Injection; 5% Dextrose in 0.45% Sodium Chloride; Ringer's Injection; 5% Fructose Injection.

Concentration up to 250 mg/ml: Sterile Water for Injection; 0.9% Sodium Chloride Injection; 0.5% and 1% lidocaine HCl solution without epinephrine.

P

Storage

Reconstituted solutions may be kept at room temperature or under refrigeration. Stability is increased when refrigerated. If precipitation occurs under refrigeration, warm to 37°C for 20 minutes in a water bath and shake well. Consult package insert or pharmacist about time of stability for each diluent.

NAFCILLIN SODIUM

Preparation and administration of solutions

IV: Dilute in 15 ml to 30 ml Sterile Water for Injection or Sodium Chloride for Injection.

Inject over a period of 5 to 10 minutes by IV piggyback or by injection port of IV line.

Stability studies indicate drug at concentrations of 2 mg/ml to 40 mg/ml loses less than 10% activity at 21°C for 24 hours or 4°C for 96 hours in the following IV solutions: 0.9% Sodium Chloride; Sterile Water for Injection; 5% Dextrose in Water; 5% Dextrose in 0.4% Sodium Chloride Solution; Ringer's Solution; M/6 Sodium Lactate Solution. Discard unused portions of IV solution after time period stated. Use only solutions listed above for IV infusion. Concentration of antibiotic should be in the range of 2 mg/ml to 40 mg/ml.

IV piggyback: The diluent and volume are stated on the label of each package.

IM: Reconstitute with Sterile or Bacteriostatic Water for Injection or Sodium Chloride Injection.

Administer clear solution immediately by deep intragluteal injection.

After reconstitution, refrigerate (2°C–8°C) and use within 7 days or keep at room temperature (25°C) and use within 3 days or keep frozen (−20°C) for up to 3 months.

OXACILLIN SODIUM

Reconstitute vials only with Sterile Water for Injection or Sodium Chloride (normal saline) Injection.

IM: Reconstitute to a dilution of 250 mg/ml. Discard unused solution after 3 days at room temperature or 7 days under refrigeration.

Direct IV: Dilute reconstituted solution to maximum concentration of 1 g/10 ml; may be further diluted, if ordered. Administer slowly (3–5 minutes) to avoid vein irritation.

Continuous IV infusion: After reconstitution with water or saline, may be further diluted with suitable IV solution (see below).

Compatible IV solutions: Only the following solutions should be used for IV infusions. At concentrations from 0.5 mg/ml to 40 mg/ml,

these dilutions are stable for at least 6 hours at room temperature: Normal Saline Solution; 5% Dextrose in Water or Normal Saline; 10% D-Fructose in Water or Normal Saline; Lactated Ringer's Solution; Lactated Potassic Saline Injections; 10% Invert Sugar in Water or Normal Saline; 10% Invert Sugar plus 0.3% Potassium Chloride in Water; Travert 10% Electrolyte #1, #2, or #3.

PENICILLIN G BENZATHINE, PARENTERAL AND PENICILLIN G BENZATHINE AND PROCAINE COMBINED

Administer by deep IM injection.

PENICILLIN G (AQUEOUS), PARENTERAL

Given IM or by continuous IV infusion; 10 million or 20 million unit dosage given by IV infusion only.

Preparation of solutions: Depending on route of administration, use Sterile Water for Injection, Isotonic Sodium Chloride Injection, or Dextrose injection.

Directions for dilution to obtain desired concentration (in units)/ml are given on label. Following dilution, label vial with the number of units/ml.

Available in 5-million unit dose size as either penicillin G potassium or penicillin G sodium. Physician must specify which penicillin is to be administered.

Stability: Dry powder does not require refrigeration. Sterile solutions may be refrigerated for 1 week without loss of potency. Solutions prepared for IV infusion are stable at room temperature for at least 24 hours.

IM: Keep total volume of injection small. Solutions containing up to 100,000 units/ml may be used with minimum of discomfort.

Continuous IV infusion: Physician orders volume and rate of fluid administration and drug dosage for 24-hour period.

PENICILLIN G POTASSIUM, ORAL

250 mg = 400,000 units. Physician's order may be stated in milligrams or units.

PENICILLIN G PROCAINE, AQUEOUS (APPG)

Administer by deep IM injection.

PENICILLIN V (PHENOXYMETHYL PENICILLIN)

125 mg = 200,000 units. Physician may order dose in milligrams or units.

PIPERACILLIN SODIUM

IM: Reconstitute with Sterile or Bacteriostatic Water for Injection; Sodium Chloride Injection;

Sterile lidocaine HCl 0.5% to 1% (without epinephrine). *Amount of diluent added*—4 ml to 2-g vial, 6 ml to 3-g vial, and 7.8 ml to 4-g vial to equal 1 g/2.5 ml.

Give by deep IM injection.

Direct IV infusion: Reconstitute each gram with at least 5 ml of diluent such as Bacteriostatic Water for Injection; Sodium Chloride Injection; or Bacteriostatic Sodium Chloride Injection. Shake well until dissolved. May be further diluted, as specified by physician, to the desired volume.

Administer slowly over a period of 3 to 5 minutes into injection port of IV tubing.

Intermittent IV infusion: Reconstitute each gram with at least 5 ml, using suitable IV solution listed below; dilute the total content of the vial or infusion bottle. Then, further dilute to volume specified by physician (at least 50 ml). Administer by IV infusion (piggyback) over a period of about 30 minutes; discontinue primary infusion during infusion of drug.

Diluents for reconstitution—Sterile or Bacteriostatic Water for Injection; Sodium Chloride Injection; Bacteriostatic Sodium Chloride Injection.

IV solutions—Dextrose 5% in Water; 0.9% Sodium Chloride; Dextrose 5% and 0.9% Sodium Chloride; Lactated Ringer's Injection; Dextran 6% in 0.9% Sodium Chloride.

IV admixtures—Also compatible with Ringer's and the above IV solutions with 40 mEq potassium chloride added.

Incompatibilities: Should not be mixed with an aminoglycoside in a syringe or infusion bottle because this can result in inactivation of the aminoglycoside.

TICARCILLIN DISODIUM

IM: Reconstitute each gram with 2 ml Sterile Water for Injection, 1% lidocaine HCl solution (without epinephrine), or Bacteriostatic Water containing 0.9% benzyl alcohol. Each 2.5 ml of resulting solution will contain 1 g ticarcillin.

Inject well into a relatively large muscle. Discard IM solutions stored at room temperature after 24 hours, or after 60 hours if stored under refrigeration.

IV: Reconstitute each gram with at least 4 ml of Sterile Water for Injection. When dissolved, dilute further to volume specified by physician. When injecting solution directly, administer as slowly as possible to avoid vein irritation.

For IV infusions, dilute desired volume with suitable diluent, as ordered by physician (see compatibility, below), and administer by continuous or intermittent IV drip.

Intermittent infusion should be administered over a 30-minute to 2-hour period in six equally divided doses.

Piggyback vials should be reconstituted with a minimum of 10 ml of Sterile Water for Injection for each gram of ticarcillin. A dilution of approximately 1 g/20 ml will reduce incidence of vein irritation.

Compatibility: Ticarcillin solutions at concentrations between 10 mg/ml and 50 mg/ml lose less than 10% of their activity at room temperature over 72 hours in the following solutions: Sterile Water for Injection; Sodium Chloride Injection; 5% Dextrose in 0.225% or 0.45% Sodium Chloride Solution; 5% Dextrose Injection; 5% Alcohol; 5% Dextrose in 0.9% Sodium Chloride solution. Solutions are stable for 48 hours in the following: Ringer's Injection; Lactated Ringer's Injection; 10% Invert Sugar in Water; 5% Dextrose in Electrolyte #48 Solution; 5% Dextrose or 5% Fructose in Electrolyte #75 Solution.

Stability: Above solutions remain stable for 14 days if stored under refrigeration. Solutions stored longer than 72 hours should not be used for multidose purposes. Discard unused portions of solution after time periods mentioned above.

Incompatibilities: It is recommended that drug *not* be mixed together with gentamicin, amikacin, or tobramycin in the same IV solution. Therapeutic effects of these drugs remain unimpaired when administered separately.

GENERIC NAME SIMILARITY

Methicillin sodium and mezlocillin sodium; cloxacillin and cyclacillin; carbenicillin disodium and carbenicillin indanyl disodium; amoxicillin and ampicillin; penicillin V and penicillin V potassium; penicillin G benzathine and penicillin G benzathine and procaine combined; penicillin G (aqueous), parenteral, penicillin G potassium, oral, and penicillin G procaine, aqueous. Penicillin labels should be checked carefully with the physician's written order.

TRADE NAME SIMILARITY

Beepen-VK and Betapen-VK; Pfizerpen VK, Pfizerpen AS, Pfizerpen G, and Pfizerpen.

ONGOING ASSESSMENTS AND NURSING MANAGEMENT

CLINICAL ALERT: Hypersensitivity reactions are more likely to occur in those with previously demonstrated hypersensitivity to penicillin and in those with a history of asthma, hay fever, or urticaria.

Anaphylaxis is usually associated with parenteral dosage but may also occur with oral penicillin.

P

After administration of first and second doses of penicillin, closely observe patient for ½ to 1 hour for hypersensitivity reaction (*i.e.,* wheezing and sneezing, urticaria, pruritus, angioneurotic edema, laryngospasm, bronchospasm, hypotension, vascular collapse, maculopapular to exfoliative dermatitis, vesicular eruptions, erythema multiforme, reactions resembling serum sickness [chills, fever, edema, arthralgia, malaise, myalgia], laryngeal edema, skin rash, and prostration). The appearance of hypersensitivity reactions is unpredictable; some of these allergic reactions may occur immediately or hours after penicillin administration. Notify physician immediately if any one or more of these occur.

Continue to observe patient for hypersensitivity reactions after subsequent doses of penicillin. Hypersensitivity reactions may be rapid in onset or occur days (and sometimes weeks) after therapy.

If patient is found to be allergic to penicillin, a prominent notation is placed on the front of the patient's chart and on the Kardex. In some instances, hospitals may also require posting this information at the bedside.

Obtain vital signs q4h or as ordered; observe for adverse reactions. If adverse reactions are noted, withhold next dose and notify physician immediately.

In patients receiving oral penicillin, check oral cavity daily for signs of glossitis, sore mouth or tongue, furry tongue, and black "hairy" tongue.

Observe for development of superinfection (Appendix 6, section 6-22).

Always withhold next dose and notify physician if patient has any unusual complaints or any adverse reaction is noted.

Look for signs of drug effectiveness (*e.g.,* decrease in symptoms caused by infection such as fever, exudate, pain/discomfort, increase in appetite, patient looks and feels better).

In patients receiving penicillin by IV infusion, check needle site for signs of thrombophlebitis (*e.g.,* redness, warmth, patient complaints of pain or discomfort in area).

Measure intake and output on those with renal impairment, the elderly or pediatric patient, and the acutely ill patient; notify physician immediately of any change in the intake–output ratio.

High doses of **azlocillin, carbenicillin, mezlocillin, nafcillin, piperacillin,** or **ticarcillin** may induce hemorrhagic manifestations associated with abnormalities of coagulation tests. Upon withdrawal of drug, bleeding should cease and coagulation abnormalities should revert to normal. Observe those with renal impairment, in whom excretion of these drugs is delayed, for prolonged hemorrhagic manifestations.

Electrolyte imbalance may occur with **aqueous penicillin G IV** in high doses (above 10 million units). Drug is administered slowly and patient observed for signs of hyperkalemia, if potassium form is used (Appendix 6, section 6-15), or hypernatremia, if sodium form is used (Appendix 6, section 6-17).

Hypokalemia has been occasionally reported in those receiving **carbenicillin, mezlocillin, piperacillin,** and **ticarcillin** and may occur in patients who have potentially low potassium reserves and in those who are receiving cytotoxic therapy and diuretics. Serum potassium is monitored and supplemented when necessary.

When sodium restriction is necessary (as in cardiac patients), frequent electrolyte determinations are usually ordered and cardiac status is monitored. Observe for development of CHF and cardiac arrhythmias, and report occurrence immediately.

Neurotoxicity may occur with excessively high serum levels (see *Adverse Reactions*).

Culture and sensitivity tests may be performed during therapy.

Periodic evaluation of renal and hepatic function, urinalysis, and CBC may be performed during therapy. In some instances, blood cultures may also be ordered.

Diabetic patient: False-positive urine glucose may occur with high urine levels of ampicillin. It is recommended that glucose oxidase tests (such as Clinistix, Tes-Tape) be used for urine testing.

PATIENT AND FAMILY INFORMATION

Complete full course of therapy.

Take on an empty stomach 1 hour before or 2 hours after meals (*exceptions*—penicillin V, amoxicillin, and bacampicillin, which are not significantly affected by food).

Take each dose with a full glass of water.

Take at even intervals, preferably around the clock (unless physician orders otherwise). Do not skip doses.

Contact physician or nurse immediately if skin rash, itching, hives, severe diarrhea, sore mouth, black "furry" tongue, rectal or vaginal itching, or any other unusual symptom or problem occurs. If skin rash, itching, hives, or breathing difficulty occurs, do not take next dose. If breathing difficulty becomes severe, or swelling of the mouth or tongue is noted, seek medical attention immediately.

Discard any drug remaining after a full course of therapy (may occur with oral suspensions or if physician discontinues drug before course of therapy is completed). *Do not* save remaining drug for future use, use it for another illness, or give it to another person.

Notify physician if symptoms do not improve or condition becomes worse.

NOTE: If patient develops an allergy to penicillin, encourage wearing of Medic-Alert or other identification indicating allergy. Be sure patient fully understands allergy to penicillin and the importance of notifying all medical personnel of allergy before any treatment is given.

Penicillin G Benzathine

See Penicillins.

Penicillin G Benzathine and Procaine Combined

See Penicillins.

Penicillin G (Aqueous), Parenteral

See Penicillins.

Penicillin G Potassium

See Penicillins.

Penicillin G Procaine, Aqueous

See Penicillins.

Penicillin V

See Penicillins.

Penicillin V Potassium

See Penicillins.

Pentaerythritol Tetranitrate

See Nitrates.

Pentazocine *Rx C–IV*

injection: 30 mg/ml	Talwin
tablets: 50 mg pentazocine, 0.5 mg naloxone	Talwin NX
tablets: 12.5 mg pentazocine, 325 mg aspirin	Talwin Compound Caplets
tablets: 25 mg pentazocine, 650 mg acetaminophen	Talacen Caplets

INDICATIONS

Relief of moderate to severe pain. Parenteral form also may be used for preoperative and preanesthetic medication and as a supplement to surgical anesthesia.

CONTRAINDICATIONS

Hypersensitivity to pentazocine or naloxone.

ACTIONS

Is a potent analgesic. It weakly antagonizes the effects of morphine, meperidine, and other opiates. May precipitate withdrawal symptoms in patients taking narcotic analgesics regularly. In addition, it produces incomplete reversal of cardiovascular, respiratory, and behavioral depression induced by morphine and meperidine. Drug also has sedative activity. Parenterally, 30 mg to 60 mg is usually as effective an analgesic as 10 mg morphine or 75 mg to 100 mg meperidine. Orally, a 50-mg dose is equivalent to 60 mg of codeine.

Naloxone in Talwin NX prevents the effect of pentazocine if the product is misused by injection. Oral naloxone has no pharmacologic activity. Naloxone, given parenterally at the same dose, is an effective antagonist to pentazocine and a pure antagonist to narcotic analgesics.

Onset of action is 15 to 20 minutes after IM injection, 2 to 3 minutes after IV injection and 15 to 30 minutes after oral administration. Pentazocine is well absorbed from the GI tract and from subcutaneous and IM injection sites. It undergoes extensive first-pass hepatic metabolism and oral bioavailability is less than 20%. It is metabolized in the liver; excretion occurs via the kidney.

WARNINGS

Talwin NX is intended for oral use only. Severe, potentially lethal reactions (*e.g.,* pulmonary emboli, vascular occlusion, ulceration and abscesses, withdrawal symptoms in narcotic-dependent individuals) may result from misuse of the drug by injection or in combination with other substances.

Drug dependence: Care is exercised in prescribing to emotionally unstable patients and to those with history of drug abuse. These patients closely supervised when more than 4 to 5 days of therapy contemplated. There have been instances of psychological and physical dependence when using parenteral form in patients with such a history and, rarely, in those without such history. Abrupt discontinuance following extended use of parenteral form has resulted in withdrawal symptoms such as abdominal cramps, elevated temperature, rhinorrhea, restlessness, anxiety, lacrimation. Even when these occurred, discontinuance has been accomplished with minimal difficulty. In rare patient in whom minor difficulty has been encountered, reinstitution of parenteral pentazocine with gradual withdrawal has ameliorated symptoms. Substitution of methadone or other narcotics in treatment of withdrawal is avoided. There have been a few reports of dependence and withdrawal symptoms with the oral form.

"T's and blues": IV injection of oral preparations of pentazocine (Talwin, T's) and tripelennamine (PBZ, Blues), an antihistamine, has become a common form of drug abuse, used as a "substitute" for heroin. The tablets, usually in a 2 to 1 ratio, respectively, are dissolved in tap water, filtered, and injected IV. The most frequent and serious complication of addiction to this combination is pulmonary disease, due primarily to occlusion of pulmonary arteries and arterioles with unsterile particles of cellulose and talc used as tablet binders. The occlusion leads to granulomatous foreign body reactions, infections, increased pulmonary artery resistance, and pulmonary hypertension. Neurologic complications include seizures, strokes, and CNS infections. Replacement of oral pentazocine with the oral pentazocine/naloxone combination may decrease the popularity of this mixture.

Tissue damage: Severe sclerosis of the skin, subcutaneous tissues, and underlying muscle has occurred at injection sites of those who received multiple doses.

Head injury and increased intracranial pressure: The potential for elevating CSF pressure may be attributed to CO_2 retention due to the respiratory depressant effects of the drug. These effects may be markedly exaggerated in presence of head injury, other intracranial lesions, or preexisting increase in intracranial pressure. Drug can also produce effects that may obscure the clinical course of those with head injuries.

Myocardial infarction: Caution is exercised in IV use of drug for patients with acute MI accompanied by hypertension or left ventricular failure. IV administration increases systemic and pulmonary artery pressure and systemic vascular resistance in acute MI. Oral form is used with caution in MI patients who have nausea or vomiting.

Acute CNS manifestations: Patients receiving therapeutic doses have experienced hallucinations (usually visual), disorientation, and confusion,

which cleared spontaneously. Seizures have occurred with use of pentazocine.

Ambulatory patients: May produce sedation, dizziness, occasional euphoria.

Use in pregnancy: Safety during pregnancy (other than labor) not established and administered only when benefits outweigh the hazards. Mothers addicted to "T's and blues" have lower–birth weight infants who have problems similar to infants born of other narcotic-addicted mothers.

Use in labor: No adverse effects noted other than those that occur with commonly used analgesics. Rarely, abstinence syndromes in newborns reported after prolonged use during pregnancy. Drug is used with caution in women delivering premature infants.

Use in children: Safety and efficacy for use in children under 12 not established.

PRECAUTIONS

Use in respiratory conditions: Possibility of respiratory depression is considered in those with bronchial asthma; drug is administered with caution and in low dosage to those with respiratory depression (*e.g.,* from other medication, uremia, severe infection), severely limited respiratory reserve, obstructive respiratory conditions, or cyanosis. Although respiratory depression is reported rarely with oral use, it should still be used cautiously in the above conditions.

Use in impaired renal or hepatic function: Because drug is metabolized in the liver and excreted by the kidney, it is administered with caution to those with such impairment. Extensive liver disease appears to predispose to greater side-effects (*e.g.,* marked apprehension, anxiety, dizziness, drowsiness) from the usual clinical dose and may be result of decreased metabolism of drug by the liver.

Biliary surgery: Use with caution in those about to undergo surgery of the biliary tract because it may cause spasm of the sphincter of Oddi.

Patients receiving narcotics: Pentazocine is a mild narcotic antagonist. Some patients previously given narcotics, including methadone for daily treatment of narcotic dependence, have experienced withdrawal symptoms after receiving pentazocine.

DRUG INTERACTIONS

Due to the potential for increased CNS depressant effects, **alcohol** is used cautiously in those currently taking this drug. **Barbiturate anesthetics** may increase the respiratory and CNS depression of pentazocine because of additive pharmacologic activity.

ADVERSE REACTIONS

Most common: Nausea; dizziness; lightheadedness; vomiting; euphoria.

GI: Constipation; cramps; abdominal distress; anorexia; diarrhea; dry mouth; taste alteration.

CNS: Sedation; euphoria; headache; weakness; mood alteration (nervousness, apprehension, depression, floating feeling); disturbed dreams; insomnia; syncope; hallucinations; tremor; irritability; excitement; tinnitus; disorientation; faintness.

Ophthalmic: Blurred vision; focusing difficulty; nystagmus; diplopia; mioisis.

Allergic: Edema of the face.

Dermatologic: Soft-tissue induration; nodules; cutaneous depression; ulceration (sloughing); severe sclerosis of skin and subcutaneous tissue (and rarely underlying muscle) at injection site; diaphoresis; stinging on injection; flushed skin; dermatitis; pruritus; toxic epidermal necrolysis.

Cardiovascular: Hypotension; tachycardia; circulatory depression; shock; hypotension.

Respiratory: Respiratory depression, dyspnea; transient apnea in newborns whose mothers received parenteral form during labor.

Hematologic: Depression of WBC (especially granulocytes), usually reversible; moderate transient eosinophilia.

Other: Urinary retention; paresthesia; alterations in rate or strength of uterine contractions during labor (parenteral form).

OVERDOSAGE

Employ oxygen, IV fluids, vasopressors, and other supportive measures as indicated. Assisted or controlled ventilation should also be considered. For respiratory depression due to overdosage or unusual sensitivity to drug, parenteral naloxone is a specific and effective antagonist.

DOSAGE

Not recommended for children under 12 years.

PENTAZOCINE

Oral: Initially, 50 mg q3h to q4h; increased to 100 mg if needed. Do not exceed a total daily dosage of 600 mg. When anti-inflammatory or antipyretic effects are desired in addition to analgesia, aspirin can be given concomitantly.

Parenteral: 30 mg IM, subcutaneously, or IV; may be repeated q3h to q4h. Doses in excess of 30 mg IV or 60 mg IM or subcutaneously are not recommended. Do not exceed a total daily dosage of 360 mg. Use subcutaneously only when necessary because of possible severe tissue damage at injection sites. *Patients in labor*—A single 30-mg IM dose is most common. A 20-mg IV dose, given two or three times at 2- to 3-hour intervals, has resulted in adequate pain relief when contractions become regular.

PENTAZOCINE COMBINATIONS

Pentazocine and aspirin: Two tablets three or four times a day.

Pentazocine and acetaminophen: One tablet q4h, up to six tablets/day.

NURSING IMPLICATIONS

HISTORY
See Appendix 4.

PHYSICAL ASSESSMENT
At time patient requests analgesic, determine exact location of pain, type of pain (sharp, dull, stabbing), when pain began. Look for controllable factors (*e.g.,* uncomfortable position, thirst, noise, lights, cold) that may decrease patient's tolerance to pain.

ADMINISTRATION
Review chart for date of drug order, time of last administration, therapeutic effect of drug.

Obtain blood pressure, pulse, and respirations immediately prior to preparing for administration. Do not give drug if respiratory rate is below 12/minute; contact physician.

Do not mix pentazocine in the same syringe with soluble barbiturates; a precipitate may form.

May be given PO, IM, IV, or subcutaneously. Subcutaneous route used only when necessary because of possible severe tissue damage at injection sites.

When frequent injections are needed, IM route is recommended. Rotation of injection sites (*e.g.,* upper outer quadrants of buttocks, midlateral aspects of the thighs, deltoid areas) is essential. Record site used.

GENERIC NAME/TRADE NAME SIMILARITY
Pentazocine and Pentazine (trade name for promethazine HCl).

ONGOING ASSESSMENTS AND NURSING MANAGEMENT
Onset of action is 15 to 20 minutes after IM injection, 2 to 3 minutes after IV injection, 15 to 30 minutes after oral administration. Observe patient at time of or shortly after anticipated onset of action for analgesic effect.

If analgesia is not sufficient, contact physician because an increase in dosage or different analgesic may be required.

Ambulatory patient should be advised to remain in bed or seek assistance with ambulation if dizziness, lightheadedness, drowsiness occurs.

Observe patient for adverse reactions. If CNS

manifestations (visual hallucinations, disorientation, confusion) occur, observe patient at frequent intervals; monitor blood pressure, pulse, and respirations and inform physician of problem before next dose is administered. Discontinuation of drug may be necessary. Reinstitution of therapy requires caution because these CNS manifestations may recur.

When multiple injections are given, inspect skin over injection sites for changes.

Tolerance to drug may occur and is noted by decrease in analgesic effect and decrease in duration of drug action. Inform physician of apparent tolerance because an increase in dose or different analgesic may be required.

Seizures have occurred with administration of this drug. Patient is observed at frequent (30–45 minute) intervals, especially during initial use of the drug.

Newborns whose mothers received parenteral form during labor should be observed for transient periods of apnea for first 3 to 4 hours following delivery.

PATIENT AND FAMILY INFORMATION

NOTE: Physician may prescribe parenteral form for chronic use to be self-administered. Patient or family member must receive instruction in administration as well as warning not to increase dose or frequency or use drug in anticipation of pain rather than for pain relief.

May cause drowsiness; observe caution while driving or performing other tasks requiring alertness.

Avoid alcohol and other depressants.

Notify physician or nurse if skin rash, confusion, or disorientation occurs.

Do not increase dose or decrease intervals between doses. If pain is not relieved, contact physician.

Pentobarbital and Pentobarbital Sodium

See Barbiturates.

Perphenazine

See Antiemetic/Antivertigo Agents; Antipsychotic Agents.

Pertussis Immune Globulin

See Immunizations, Passive.

Phenacemide Rx

tablets: 500 mg   Phenurone

INDICATIONS

Control of severe epilepsy, particularly mixed forms of psychomotor seizures refractory to other drugs.

ACTIONS

Studies show that drug elevates threshold for minimal electroshock convulsions and abolishes the tonic phase of maximal electroshock seizures. It prevents or modifies seizures induced by convulsant agents. In animal tests, it was found to be equal to, or more effective than, other commonly used anticonvulsants against focal seizures of a psychomotor type.

Is well absorbed from the intestine; following a single dose, duration of action is about 5 hours. Is degraded by the liver with formation of inactive metabolites that are excreted by the kidney.

WARNINGS

Safe use in pregnancy and lactation is not established. Should not be given to women of childbearing age unless expected benefits outweigh the possible hazards.

PRECAUTIONS

Can produce serious side-effects as well as direct organ toxicity. Usually not administered unless other anticonvulsants are found ineffective in controlling seizures.

Behavioral effects: Extreme caution is essential if administered with any other anticonvulsant known to cause similar toxic effects. Extreme caution is also exercised in treating those who have previously shown personality disorders. Hospitalization of patient during first week of treatment is recommended. Personality changes, including suicide attempts and occurrence of psychoses requiring hospitalization, have been reported during therapy. Caution is exercised in administration with **ethotoin** because paranoid symptoms have been reported during therapy with this combination.

Hepatic function: Hepatic-function tests are recommended before and during therapy. Drug is used with caution in those with history of previous liver dysfunction. Death attributed to liver damage during therapy has been reported.

Hematologic effects: Complete blood counts should be made before instituting therapy and at monthly intervals thereafter. If no abnormality appears within 12 months, the interval between blood counts may be extended. Blood changes have been reported, with leukopenia (leukocyte count of ≤4000/mm³) the most commonly observed effect. Aplastic anemia has occurred and death from this condition has been reported.

Renal function: Nephritis occasionally has occurred; urine should be examined at regular intervals. Abnormal urinary findings are an indication to discontinue therapy.

Hypersensitivity: Give with caution to those with history of allergy, particularly in association with administration of other anticonvulsants. Discontinue use at first sign of skin rash or other allergic manifestation.

ADVERSE REACTIONS
GI disturbances, anorexia and weight loss, headache, drowsiness, dizziness, insomnia, paresthesias, psychic changes, hepatitis, blood dyscrasias, skin rash, nephritis.

OVERDOSAGE
Symptoms: Excitement or mania followed by drowsiness, ataxia, and coma.

Treatment: Induce emesis; gastric lavage may be considered as alternative or adjunct. General supportive measures will be necessary. A careful evaluation of liver and kidney function, mental state, and the blood-forming organs should be made following recovery.

DOSAGE
Adults: Usual starting dose is 1.5 g/day, in three divided doses of 500 mg each. After the first week, if seizures are not controlled and drug is well tolerated, an additional 500 mg may be taken upon arising. In the third week, if necessary, dosage may be further increased by another 500 mg H.S. Satisfactory results have been seen in some on an initial dose of 250 mg tid. Effective total daily dose for adults usually ranges from 2 g to 3 g; some patients may require as much as 5 g/day.

Children (5–10 yr): Approximately one-half adult dose, given at same intervals as for adults.

Concomitant anticonvulsant therapy: May be administered alone or in combination with other anticonvulsants.

Replacement therapy: When phenacemide is to replace other anticonvulsant medication, withdraw the latter gradually as dosage of phenacemide is increased to maintain seizure control.

NURSING IMPLICATIONS

HISTORY
See Appendix 4; obtain from family or review chart for history of seizure disorder, including average length of seizure, aura (if any), degree of impairment of consciousness, motor and psychic activity, previous drug therapy.

PHYSICAL ASSESSMENT
Obtain vital signs; if seizures are frequent, observe and record accurate description. CBC, urinalysis, and hepatic-function tests may be ordered.

ADMINISTRATION
If nausea occurs, consult physician about giving drug with food.

See also Appendix 1.

ONGOING ASSESSMENTS AND NURSING MANAGEMENT
Obtain vital signs daily; observe for adverse reactions; observe and record seizures (if any).

CLINICAL ALERT: Observe for changes in behavior or personality such as decreased interest in surroundings, depression, or aggressiveness, and notify physician immediately if these changes are noted because drug may need to be discontinued. If depression is noted, observe patient at frequent intervals (every 15–30 minutes). See _Precautions._

Notify physician immediately if skin rash or other allergic manifestation, malaise, sore throat, fever, stomatitis, jaundice, darkened urine, pale stools, abdominal pain, or unusual bleeding or bruising is noted.

Drowsiness and dizziness may occur. Assist patient as necessary with ambulatory activities.

See also Anticonvulsants.

PATIENT AND FAMILY INFORMATION
NOTE: Family should be made aware of possibility of personality or behavioral changes and that these changes must be reported to the physician immediately. If seizures become more frequent, physician should be notified as soon as possible.

Take drug exactly as directed. Do not stop drug or increase or decrease dosage except on advice of physician.

Inform dentist and other physicians of therapy with this drug.

Notify physician or nurse if jaundice, abdominal pain, pale stools, darkened urine, fever, sore throat, mouth sores, unusual bleeding or bruising, loss of appetite, or skin rash occurs.

May produce drowsiness or dizziness. Observe caution while driving or performing other tasks requiring alertness.

Close medical supervision is necessary. Periodic blood counts and other laboratory tests will be scheduled.

P

Phenazopyridine Hydrochloride

(Phenylazo Diamino Pyridine HCl) Rx

tablets: 100 mg	Azo-Standard, Baridium, Di-Azo, Phenazodine, Pyridiate, Pyridium, *Generic*
tablets: 200 mg	Phenazodine, Pyridiate, Pyridium, *Generic*

INDICATIONS
Symptomatic relief of pain, burning, urgency, frequency, and other discomforts arising from irritation of the lower urinary-tract mucosa. These symptoms may result from infection, trauma, surgery, endoscopic procedures, or passage of sounds or catheters. Drug's topical analgesic action may reduce or eliminate need for systemic analgesic or narcotics.

CONTRAINDICATIONS
Renal insufficiency; a yellowish tinge of the skin or sclerae may indicate accumulation due to impaired renal excretion and a need to discontinue therapy.

ACTIONS
Is excreted in the urine, where it exerts a topical analgesic effect on the urinary-tract mucosa; it should be used only for relief of symptoms. It is compatible with antibacterial therapy and can help relieve pain and discomfort during the interval before antibacterial therapy controls the infection.

Drug/lab test interferences: Is an azo dye that may interfere with colorimetric laboratory test procedures.

ADVERSE REACTIONS
Occasional GI disturbances. Methemoglobinemia, hemolytic anemia, and renal and hepatic toxicity have been reported, usually at overdose levels.

OVERDOSAGE
Exceeding recommended dose in those with good renal function or administering usual dose to those with impaired renal function (common in elderly patients) may lead to toxic reactions. Methemoglobinemia generally follows a massive acute overdose. Oxidative Heinz body hemolytic anemia may occur, and "bite cells" may be present in a chronic overdosage situation. Red blood cell G6PD deficiency may predispose the patient to hemolysis. Renal and hepatic impairment and failure, usually due to hypersensitivity, may also occur.

Treatment: Methylene blue, 1 mg/kg to 2 mg/kg IV, or 100 mg to 200 mg ascorbic acid PO should cause prompt reduction of methemoglobinemia and disappearance of the cyanosis that is an aid in diagnosis.

DOSAGE
Average adult dose is 200 mg tid P.C.

NURSING IMPLICATIONS

HISTORY
See Appendix 4.

PHYSICAL ASSESSMENT
Urinalysis and other diagnostic tests may be ordered, depending on reason for use.

ADMINISTRATION
Give after meals.

TRADE NAME SIMILARITY
Pyridium and Pyridiate.

ONGOING ASSESSMENTS AND NURSING MANAGEMENT
Inquire daily about relief of symptoms; drug is usually discontinued when pain and discomfort are relieved.

If yellow tinge to skin or sclera is noted, withhold next dose and notify physician.

If nausea or other GI symptoms occur despite giving drug after meals, or pain or discomfort increases, notify physician.

PATIENT AND FAMILY INFORMATION
May cause GI upset; take after meals.

May cause a reddish orange discoloration of the urine (this is not abnormal) and may stain underclothing.

If symptoms do not improve or become worse after several days or a yellowish tinge to skin or sclera is noted, notify physician or nurse.

Phendimetrazine Tartrate

See Anorexiants.

Phenelzine Sulfate

See Antidepressants, Monoamine Oxidase Inhibitors.

Phenindamine Tartrate

See Antihistamines.

Phenmetrazine Hydrochloride

See Anorexiants.

Phenobarbital, Phenobarbital Sodium

See Barbiturates.

Phenolphthalein

See Laxatives.

Phenoxybenzamine Hydrochloride Rx

capsules: 10 mg   Dibenzyline

INDICATIONS
Pheochromocytoma, to control episodes of hypertension and sweating. If tachycardia is excessive, it may be necessary also to use a beta-blocking agent. See also Antihypertensive Agents.

CONTRAINDICATIONS
Conditions in which a fall in blood pressure may be undesirable.

ACTIONS
An irreversible alpha-adrenergic receptor (both presynaptic and postsynaptic) blocking agent that can produce and maintain "chemical sympathectomy" by oral administration. It increases blood flow to the skin, mucosa, and abdominal viscera and lowers both supine and erect blood pressures. It has no effect on the parasympathetic system. Absorption from the GI tract is incomplete; between 20% and 30% is absorbed in the active form. Peak effects occur within 4 to 6 hours.

WARNINGS
Phenoxybenzamine-induced alpha-adrenergic blockade leaves beta-adrenergic receptors unopposed. Compounds that stimulate both types of receptors (*e.g.,* epinephrine) may produce an exaggerated hypotensive response and tachycardia.

PRECAUTIONS
Give with caution to those with marked cerebral or coronary arteriosclerosis or renal damage. Adrenergic blocking effects may aggravate symptoms of respiratory infections. Not used in diseases involving large blood vessels, in which direct-acting vasodilators are preferred.

ADVERSE REACTIONS
Nasal congestion, miosis, postural hypotension, tachycardia, and inhibition of ejaculation may occur. These are evidence of adrenergic blockade. They vary according to degree of blockade and tend to decrease as therapy is continued. GI irritation (nausea, vomiting) has also been reported.

OVERDOSAGE
Symptoms: These are largely the result of block of the sympathetic nervous system and of circulating epinephrine. They may include postural hypotension resulting in dizziness or fainting; tachycardia, particularly postural; lethargy; and shock.

Treatment: When symptoms and signs of overdosage exist, discontinue drug. Treatment of circulatory failure, if present, is prime consideration. In cases of mild overdosage, recumbent position with legs elevated usually restores cerebral circulation. In more severe cases, institute usual measures to combat shock, including normal saline infusion to expand plasma volume. Usual pressor agents are not effective. Epinephrine is contraindicated because it stimulates both alpha and beta receptors; because alpha receptors are blocked, the net effect of epinephrine administration is vasodilation and a further drop in blood pressure (epinephrine reversal). The patient may have to be kept flat for 24 hours or more. Leg bandages and an abdominal binder may shorten period of disability. IV infusion of norepinephrine may be used to combat severe hypotensive reactions.

DOSAGE
Dosage is adjusted to needs of the patient. Small initial doses should be slowly increased until desired effect is obtained or side-effects from blockade become troublesome. After each increase, patient is observed for at least 4 days before another increase is instituted. Dosage should be increased to a point at which symptomatic relief or objective improvement is obtained, but not so high that side-effects become troublesome.

Initial dose: 10 mg/day. After at least 4 days, may be increased by 10 mg, and similarly increased thereafter until optimum dosage is reached. Dosage range is usually 20 mg/day to 80 mg/day. At least 2 weeks are usually required to reach optimal dosage level. At this time improvement will usually be observed, but it may be several more weeks before full benefits are apparent.

NURSING IMPLICATIONS

HISTORY
See Appendix 4.

P

PHYSICAL ASSESSMENT

Obtain blood pressure in both arms with patient in standing and recumbent positions; obtain pulse and respiratory rates.

ADMINISTRATION

If nausea or vomiting occurs, check with physician about giving drug with food or meals.

ONGOING ASSESSMENTS AND NURSING MANAGEMENT

Take blood pressure (in both arms, standing and recumbent positions), pulse, and respirations q4h or as ordered; observe for adverse reactions; observe for relief of symptoms (hypertension, tachycardia, sweating).

Postural hypotension may occur. In some instances, assistance with ambulatory activities may be necessary.

Support stockings may be prescribed by physician if dizziness persists during ambulation.

PATIENT AND FAMILY INFORMATION

NOTE: Physician may advise patient to take own blood pressure daily. Patient or family member may require instruction.

Avoid alcoholic beverages, cough, cold, or allergy medications unless use of a specific product is approved by physician.

If dizziness occurs, avoid sudden changes in posture. Rise from a lying or sitting position slowly. Dangle legs for a few minutes when getting out of bed. If dizziness is severe, sit or lie down immediately. Contact physician if severe dizziness persists.

Medication may cause nasal congestion, inhibition of ejaculation, and small pupils, which may result in difficulty seeing in dim light or driving at night. Avoid driving after dusk if night vision is impaired.

Two weeks may be required before relief of symptoms is noted. Keep physician informed of relief or nonrelief of symptoms.

Phenprocoumon

See Coumarin and Indandione Derivatives.

Phensuximide

See Anticonvulsants, Succinimides.

Phentermine Hydrochloride

See Anorexiants.

Phentolamine Rx

| tablets: 50 mg | Regitine |
| injection: 5 mg/vial | Regitine |

INDICATIONS

Prevention or control of hypertensive episodes that may occur in patient with pheochromocytoma as a result of stress or manipulation during preoperative preparation and surgical excision.

Parenteral: Prevention and treatment of dermal necrosis and sloughing following IV administration or extravasation of norepinephrine or dopamine. Although phentolamine has been used as a pharmacologic test for pheochromocytoma, measurement of urinary or plasma catecholamines and urinary catecholamine metabolites is the preferred diagnostic method.

Investigational uses: Has been used to treat hypertensive crisis secondary to monoamine oxidase (MAO) inhibitor/sympathomimetic amine interactions and rebound hypertension on withdrawal of clonidine, propranolol, or other antihypertensive agents.

CONTRAINDICATIONS

Myocardial infarction, coronary insufficiency, angina, or other evidence suggestive of coronary artery disease; hypersensitivity.

ACTIONS

Is an alpha-adrenergic blocking agent; it blocks both presynaptic and postsynaptic alpha-adrenergic receptors. It also acts on both the arterial tree and the venous bed. Thus, total peripheral resistence is lowered and venous return to the heart diminished. Also causes cardiac stimulation and is a competitive antagonist of endogenous and exogenous alpha active agents. Has an immediate onset and short duration of action. It is not well absorbed after oral administration; oral dosage is considerably higher than parenteral dosage.

WARNINGS

MI, cerebrovascular spasm, and cerebrovascular occlusion have been reported following administration, usually in association with marked hypotensive episodes with shocklike states that occasionally follow parenteral administration. Safety for use in pregnancy or lactation not established. Use only when clearly needed and when potential benefits outweigh the unknown potential hazards to the fetus or nursing child.

PRECAUTIONS

Tachycardia and cardiac arrhythmias may occur with use of phentolamine or other alpha-adrenergic agents. Secondary cardiac stimulation may be controlled with a beta-adrenergic blocking agent. When possible, administration of cardiac glycosides is deferred until cardiac rhythm returns to normal.

ADVERSE REACTIONS

Acute and prolonged hypotensive episodes (secondary to vasodilatation), tachycardia, and cardiac arrhythmias have been reported, most frequently after parenteral administration. Weakness, dizziness, flushing, orthostatic hypotension, nasal congestion, nausea, vomiting, and diarrhea may also occur.

OVERDOSAGE

If blood pressure drops to a dangerous level or evidence of shock occurs, treat vigorously and promptly. Include IV infusion of norepinephrine, titrated to maintain blood pressure to normotensive level. Epinephrine is contraindicated because it stimulates both alpha and beta receptors; because alpha receptors are blocked, the net effect of epinephrine administration is vasodilation and a further drop in blood pressure (epinephrine reversal).

DOSAGE

Prevention or control of hypertensive episodes in pheochromocytoma: Prior to surgery, usual adult oral dosage is 50 mg four to six times a day. In certain severe cases, higher doses may be required. In children, smaller doses generally suffice: 25 mg PO four to six times a day.

Preoperative reduction of elevated blood pressure: 5 mg (1 mg for children) IV or IM 1 to 2 hours before surgery. Repeat, if necessary. _During surgery_—5 mg for adults (1 mg for children) IV as indicated to help prevent or control paroxysms of hypertension, tachycardia, respiratory depression, convulsions, or other effects of epinephrine intoxication. _Postoperatively_—norepinephrine may be given to control hypotension that commonly follows removal of pheochromocytoma.

Prevention and treatment of dermal necrosis and sloughing following administration or extravasation of norepinephrine: _Prevention_—Add 10 mg to each liter of solution containing norepinephrine. The pressor effect of norepinephrine is not affected. _Treatment_—Inject 5 mg to 10 mg in 10 ml saline into area of extravasation within 12 hours.

Diagnosis of pheochromocytoma: Sedatives, analgesics, and all other medications not considered essential are withheld for at least 24 hours (preferably 48–72 hours) prior to test. Withhold antihypertensive drugs until blood pressure returns to untreated, hypertensive level. Keep patient at rest in supine position throughout test, preferably in a darkened room. Injection is delayed until blood pressure has stabilized, as evidenced by readings taken every 10 minutes for at least 30 minutes.

IV test—Although 5 mg (1 mg for children) is recommended, use of 2.5-mg test dose will produce fewer false-positive tests and minimize dangerous drop in blood pressure in those with pheochromocytoma. If 2.5-mg dose is negative, a 5-mg test should be done. Positive response is indicated by drop in blood pressure of more than 35 mm Hg systolic and 25 mm Hg diastolic. Maximum decrease is usually evident within 2 minutes after injection. Return to preinjection pressure usually occurs within 15 to 30 minutes but may return more rapidly. A negative response is indicated when blood pressure is unchanged, elevated, or reduced by less than parameters given above.

IM test—Preparation same as for IV test. Adult dosage is 5 mg; for children, 3 mg. Positive response is indicated by drop in blood pressure as for IV test, within 20 minutes following injection.

NURSING IMPLICATIONS

HISTORY
See Appendix 4.

PHYSICAL ASSESSMENT
Pheochromocytoma: Obtain blood pressure in both arms with patient in standing and supine positions; obtain pulse, respirations.

Treatment of extravasation of norepinephrine or dopamine: Inspect and describe affected area.

ADMINISTRATION
Diluent is supplied with parenteral form; shake thoroughly until dissolved. Place patient in supine position when administering IV or IM.

Pheochromocytoma

Obtain blood pressure on both arms with patient in standing and supine positions; obtain pulse, respirations.

May be given PO, IM, or IV.

Preoperative preparation: Prescribed dose is given 1 to 2 hours before surgery or as ordered. Drug may also be administered during the operative procedure.

Dermal necrosis and sloughing following IV administration or extravasation of norepinephrine

Prevention: Add prescribed dose (usually 10 mg) to each liter; label infusion container.

Treatment: Prepare prescribed dose (usually 5 mg or 10 mg dissolved in 10 ml saline); use small needle (24 gauge–27 gauge) and inject around and into extravasated area.

Diagnosis of pheochromocytoma

See *Dosage* for patient preparation for test.

IV

Dissolve prescribed dose (2.5 mg or 5 mg for adults, 1 mg or less for children) in 1 ml Sterile Water for Injection.

Obtain blood pressure q5m; injection is delayed until pressor response to venipuncture has subsided.

Following injection, obtain and record blood pressure immediately and at 30-second intervals for first 3 minutes, then at 60-second intervals for next 7 minutes.

IM

Prepare prescribed dose as for IV administration, above.

Obtain baseline blood pressure, administer drug, and obtain and record blood pressure every 5 minutes following injection for 30 to 45 minutes.

ONGOING ASSESSMENTS AND NURSING MANAGEMENT

Prevention or control of hypotensive episodes in pheochromocytoma: Obtain blood pressure, pulse, and respirations q4h or as ordered; observe for adverse reactions, especially hypotensive episodes, tachycardia, and cardiac arrhythmias.

If dizziness or lightheadedness occurs, provide assistance in ambulation.

Withhold drug and notify physician is significant decrease in systolic or diastolic blood pressure occurs, cardiac arrhythmia is noted, dizziness or lightheadedness is severe, or nausea, vomiting, or diarrhea occurs.

Dermal necrosis and sloughing following administration of norepinephrine: *Prevention*—Use of phentolamine still requires close supervision of IV infusion and observing for signs of extravasation. *Treatment*—Physician may additionally order warm soaks to area or other treatment. Observe area daily for signs of tissue necrosis and sloughing.

Test for pheochromocytoma: Following completion of test, continue to monitor blood pressure, pulse, and respirations q½h for 3 to 4 hours or as ordered.

PATIENT AND FAMILY INFORMATION

Notify physician or nurse if any of the following occurs: weakness, nasal congestion, nausea, vomiting, diarrhea, palpitations.

May cause dizziness or fainting. Avoid sudden changes in posture; rise from a sitting or standing position slowly. If symptoms are severe, notify physician or nurse.

Avoid cough, cold, allergy, or weight-loss medications unless a specific product is approved by physician.

Phenylbutazone and Oxyphenbutazone

Oxyphenbutazone Rx

tablets: 100 mg	Oxalid, Tandearil

Phenylbutazone Rx

tablets: 100 mg	Azolid, Butazolidin (contains tartrazine), *Generic*
capsules: 100 mg	Azolid, Butazolidin

INDICATIONS

Acute gouty arthritis, active rheumatoid arthritis, and active ankylosing spondylitis; short-term treatment of acute attacks of degenerative joint disease of the hips and knees not responsive to other treatment; painful shoulder (peritendinitis, capsulitis, bursitis, acute arthritis of joint).

CONTRAINDICATIONS

Use in children under 14; use in senile patients; use in patients with history or suggestion of prior toxicity, sensitivity, or idiosyncrasy.

Other medical conditions: Patients with incipient cardiac failure, blood dyscrasias, pancreatitis, parotitis, stomatitis, polymyalgia rheumatica, temporal arteritis, drug allergy, hypertension, thyroid disease, systemic edema, severe renal, cardiac, or hepatic disease. Also, a history of peptic ulcer disease or symptoms of GI inflammation, including severe or recurrent or persistent dyspepsia, or active ulceration, because serious adverse reactions or aggravation of existing medical problems can occur.

Concomitant medications: Contraindicated in those receiving drugs that accentuate or share a potential for similar toxicity. These drugs are not recommended in combination with other potent drugs because of increased possibility of adverse reactions from these drugs and other agents (see *Drug Interactions*). **Phenylbutazone** is not given to patients on long-term anticoagulant therapy.

ACTIONS

Phenylbutazone and its analogue oxyphenbutazone have anti-inflammatory, antipyretic, analgesic, and mild uricosuric actions, resulting in symptomatic relief only. The disease is unaltered by these drugs. The exact mechanism of the anti-inflammatory effects has not been elucidated, but studies show that these drugs inhibit certain factors believed to be involved in the inflammatory process (*i.e.,* prostaglandin synthesis, leukocyte migration, and release or activity of lysosomal enzymes).

Both drugs are rapidly and completely absorbed after administration. Elimination of oxyphenbutazone is mainly by biotransformation in the liver. The plasma elimination half-life for phenylbutazone is approximately 84 hours; for oxyphenbutazone, approximately 72 hours. After therapeutic doses, approximately 98% is bound to serum albumin. The major metabolite of phenylbutazone is oxyphenbutazone; steady-state plasma levels are approximately 50% of those of phenylbutazone.

WARNINGS

GI effects: Upper GI tests are performed in those with persistent, severe dyspepsia. Peptic ulceration, reactivation of latent peptic ulcer, perforation, and GI bleeding, sometimes severe, have been reported.

Hematologic effects: Frequent and regular hematologic evaluations are performed on those receiving drug for periods over 1 week. Any significant change in total WBC, relative decrease in granulocytes, appearance of immature forms, or fall in hematocrit should be a signal for immediate cessation of therapy and a complete hematologic investigation. Serious, sometimes fatal, blood dyscrasias, including aplastic anemia, have been reported. Hematologic toxicity may occur suddenly or many days or weeks after cessation of treatment as manifested by appearance of anemia, leukopenia, thrombocytopenia, or clinically significant hemorrhagic diathesis.

Leukemia: Although a definite causal relationship to phenylbutazone has not been established, cases of leukemia have been seen in patients with history of short- and long-term therapy. The majority of patients were over 40. It should be noted that arthritic-type pains can be the presenting symptom of leukemia.

Blurred vision: Patients reporting visual disturbances during therapy should discontinue treatment and have an ophthalmologic examination.

Aging: In those over 40, there appears to be an increase in the possibility of adverse reactions. In elderly patients (over 60), treatment is restricted to 1 week. Treatment is discontinued in the event of clinical edema.

Asthma: These drugs may precipitate acute episodes of asthmatic attacks in patients with asthma.

Edema: These agents increase sodium retention. Evidence of fluid retention in those in whom there is danger of cardiac decompensation is an indication to discontinue use. In those under 60, swelling of the ankles and face alone may be prevented by reducing dosage.

Unexplained bleeding: Unexplained bleeding involving the CNS, adrenal glands, and GI tract has occurred because of therapy with phenylbutazone.

Use in pregnancy and lactation: Use during pregnancy, especially during the third trimester, should be avoided. Nonsteroidal anti-inflammatory agents that inhibit prostaglandin synthesis may cause constriction of the ductus arteriosus and possibly other untoward effects on the fetus. Phenylbutazone may result in prolonged labor when given to pregnant patients before delivery. These drugs may appear in cord blood and breast milk; use in nursing mothers is not recommended.

PRECAUTIONS

Some of these products contain tartrazine. See Appendix 6, section 6-23.

DRUG INTERACTIONS

These drugs are highly bound to serum proteins. If their affinity for protein binding is higher than other concurrently administered drugs, the actions and toxicity of the other drug may be increased. Both drugs accentuate the prothrombin depression produced by **coumarin-type anticoagulants.** Occasional instances of severe bleeding have been reported when these anticoagulants and phenylbutazone were given concurrently.

The pharmacologic action of **insulin, antidiabetics,** and **sulfonamide** drugs may be potentiated by the simultaneous administration of phenylbutazone or oxyphenbutazone. Administration of these drugs with **phenytoin** may increase serum levels and toxicity of phenytoin. Concomitant administration of **alcohol** may impair psychomotor skills. Microsomal enzymes that metabolize **digitoxin** in the liver are stimulated by a number of drugs including phenylbutazone. Introduction of this drug may lower digitoxin serum levels and discontinuation of phenylbutazone may lead to toxicity.

Drug/lab tests: These agents may reduce iodine uptake by the thyroid and may interfere with laboratory tests of thyroid function.

ADVERSE REACTIONS

Most frequent adverse reactions reported in those receiving phenylbutazone: Abdominal discomfort and edema, nausea, dyspepsia (including indigestion and heartburn), and rash.

The following have occurred in fewer than 1% of patients

GI: Vomiting; abdominal distention with flatulence; constipation; diarrhea; esophagitis; epigastric pain; gastritis; salivary gland enlargement; stomatitis, sometimes with ulceration; ulceration and perforation of large bowel; ulceration and perforation of the intestinal tract, including acute and reactivated peptic ulcer with perforation, hemorrhage, and hematemesis; anemia due to GI bleeding, which may be occult; hepatitis, (fatal and nonfatal), sometimes associated with evidence of cholestasis.

Hematologic: Anemia; leukopenia; thrombocytopenia with associated purpura, petechiae, and hemorrhage; pancytopenia; aplastic anemia; bone-marrow depression; agranulocytosis and agranulocytic anginal syndrome; hemolytic anemia.

Hypersensitivity: Urticaria, anaphylactic shock; arthralgia, drug fever, fever and rashes, hypersensitivity angiitis and vasculitis, Lyell's syndrome, serum sickness, Stevens-Johnson syndrome, toxic epidermal necrolysis, exfoliative dermatitis, activation of systemic lupus erythematosus, aggravation of temporal arteritis in those with polymyalgia rheumatica.

Dermatologic: Pruritus and toxic pruritus, drug rashes, erythema nodosum, erythema multiforme, nonthrombocytopenic purpura.

Cardiovascular, fluid and electrolyte: Sodium and chloride retention, fluid retention and plasma dilution, congestive heart failure (CHF) with edema and dyspnea, metabolic acidosis, respiratory alkalosis, hypertension, pericarditis, interstitial myocarditis with muscle necrosis and perivascular granulomata.

Renal: Hematuria, proteinuria, ureteral obstruction with uric acid crystals, anuria, oliguria, glomerulonephritis, acute tubular necrosis, cortical necrosis, renal stones, nephrotic syndrome, impaired renal function and renal failure associated with azotemia.

CNS: Headache, drowsiness, agitation, confusional states and lethargy, tremors, numbness, weakness.

Endocrine-metabolic: Hyperglycemia, thyroid hyperplasia, toxic or nontoxic goiter, myxedema.

Ophthalmic: Optic neuritis, superficial ulceration of the cornea, conjunctivitis, blurred vision, retinal hemorrhage, toxic amblyopia, retinal detachment.

Otic: Hearing loss, tinnitus.

Other: Generalized lymphadenopathy.

The following have been reported in fewer than 1% but occurred under circumstances in which causal relationship was not established: leukemia, goiters associated with hypo- or hyperthyroidism, pancreatitis, scotomata, oculomotor palsy.

OVERDOSAGE

Symptoms: Include any of the following: nausea and vomiting, epigastric pain, excessive perspiration, euphoria, psychosis, headaches, giddiness, vertigo, hyperventilation, insomnia, tinnitus, difficulty hearing, edema, hypertension, cyanosis, respiratory depression, agitation, hallucinations, stupor, convulsions, coma, hematuria, and oliguria. Hepatomegaly, jaundice, and ulceration of buccal or GI mucosa have been reported as late manifestations of massive overdosage. Reported laboratory abnormalities include respiratory or metabolic acidosis, impaired renal or hepatic function, and abnormalities of formed blood elements.

Treatment: In the alert patient, empty stomach promptly by induced emesis followed by lavage. In the obtunded patient, secure airway with a cuffed endotracheal tube before beginning lavage (do not induce emesis). Maintain adequate respiratory exchange; do not use respiratory stimulants. Treat shock with appropriate supportive measures. Control seizures with IV diazepam or short-acting barbiturates. Dialysis may be helpful if renal function is impaired. Hemoperfusion has also been used successfully.

DOSAGE

In elderly patients (60 and over), therapy is discontinued on, or as soon as possible after, the seventh day, because of exceedingly high risk of severe or fatal toxic reactions.

For the individual patient, efficacy and safety of therapy are unpredictable. Goal of therapy is short-term relief of severe symptoms to a level tolerable at the smallest possible dosage. When improvement occurs, dosage is reduced promptly until complete discontinuation of drug is achieved. Actions of these drugs usually manifest by third or fourth day of treatment.

Rheumatoid arthritis, ankylosing spondylitis, acute attacks of degenerative joint disease, painful shoulder: Initial daily dose in adults ranges from 300 mg to 600 mg divided into three or four doses. Maximum therapeutic response is usually obtained at a total daily dosage of 400 mg. When improvement is noted, dosage is promptly decreased. Maintenance dosage should not exceed 400 mg/day because of possible cumulative toxicity. Satisfactory clinical response is often achieved with 100 mg/day to 200 mg/day.

Acute gouty arthritis: Satisfactory results are obtained from initial dose of 400 mg followed by 100 mg q4h. Articular inflammation usually subsides within 4 days; treatment should be continued no longer than 1 week.

NURSING IMPLICATIONS

HISTORY
See Appendix 4.

PHYSICAL ASSESSMENT

Inspect and record appearance of affected joints, noting joint deformities (when applicable), appearance of skin over joints; evaluate ability to carry out activities of daily living; weight; vital signs. CBC (including WBC and differential) is usually ordered. Additional laboratory tests may be indicated.

ADMINISTRATION

Give with meals or full glass of milk. Physician may order drug given with an antacid.

ONGOING ASSESSMENTS AND NURSING MANAGEMENT

Obtain vital signs, weight daily; observe for adverse reactions, especially edema, abdominal discomfort, GI distress, and rash. Because there are potentially serious adverse reactions associated with these drugs, carefully evaluate *any* complaint the patient may have and report to physician before next dose is due.

CLINICAL ALERT: Withhold next dose and notify physician immediately if sore throat, sore mouth, stomatitis, unusual bleeding or bruising, blurred vision, fever, tarry stools, edema (legs, feet), or skin rash occurs.

Observe for relief of symptoms (*i.e.,* decrease in pain, increased joint mobility); record observations.

Hematologic evaluation is performed at frequent and regular intervals, especially if therapy extends beyond 1 week.

Therapeutic response may be seen in 3 to 4 days. If favorable response is not apparent after 1 week, drug is usually discontinued.

Once therapeutic response is obtained, dosage is reduced and drug discontinued as soon as possible.

If drowsiness occurs, assistance with ambulatory activities may be required.

A restricted sodium diet may be prescribed because these drugs increase sodium retention.

PATIENT AND FAMILY INFORMATION

Take drug exactly as directed. Do *not* increase dosage if pain becomes worse.

May cause GI upset. Take with food, meals, or full glass of milk. If physician recommends an antacid, use only the brand recommended.

May cause drowsiness. Observe caution while driving or performing other tasks requiring alertness.

Notify physician or nurse immediately if sore throat, mouth sores, unusual bleeding or bruising, blurred vision, fever, black stools, unusual

weight gain, swelling of the feet or legs, or skin rash occurs.

Phenylephrine Hydrochloride Rx

injection: 1%   Neo-Synephrine

INDICATIONS

Treatment of vascular failure in shock, shocklike states, drug-induced hypotension, or hypersensitivity; to overcome paroxysmal tachycardia; prolong spinal anesthesia; vasoconstrictor in regional anesthesia; maintain an adequate level of blood pressure during spinal and inhalation anesthesia. See also Decongestants, Nasal, Topical; Mydriatics/Ophthalmic Vasoconstrictors.

CONTRAINDICATIONS

Hypersensitivity; severe hypertension; ventricular tachycardia.

ACTIONS

Is a powerful postsynaptic alpha-receptor stimulator with little effect on beta receptors of the heart. Predominant actions are on the cardiovascular system. Parenteral administration causes a rise in systolic and diastolic pressures due to peripheral vasoconstriction. Accompanying the pressor response is a marked reflex bradycardia that can be blocked by atropine; after atropine, large doses of the drug increase the heart rate only slightly. Cardiac output is slightly decreased and peripheral resistance considerably increased. Circulation time is slightly prolonged and venous pressure slightly increased; venous constriction is not marked. Most vascular beds are constricted; renal splanchnic, cutaneous, and limb blood flows are reduced, but coronary blood flow is increased. Pulmonary vessels are constricted and pulmonary artery pressure is raised.

Phenylephrine is a powerful vasoconstrictor, with properties very similar to those of norepinephrine, but almost completely lacking the chronotropic and inotropic actions on the heart. Cardiac irregularities are seen only rarely, even with large doses. In contrast to epinephrine and ephedrine, it produces longer-lasting vasoconstriction and a reflex bradycardia and increases the stroke output, producing no disturbance in the rhythm of the pulse. In therapeutic doses, it produces little, if any, stimulation of either the spinal cord or the cerebrum. An advantage is that repeated injections produce comparable effects.

WARNINGS

Safety for use in pregnancy not established. Use only when clearly needed and when potential bene-

P

fits outweigh the unknown potential hazards to the fetus. If vasopressor drugs are either used to correct hypotension or added to the local anesthetic solution, some oxytocic drugs may cause severe persistent hypertension, and even rupture of a cerebral blood vessel may occur during the postpartum period. Safety for use in the nursing mother not established. Because many drugs are excreted in human milk, exercise caution when administering to a nursing woman.

PRECAUTIONS

Use with extreme caution in elderly patients and in patients with hyperthyroidism, bradycardia, partial heart block, myocardial disease, or severe arteriosclerosis. Extravasation may cause necrosis and sloughing of surrounding tissue.

DRUG INTERACTIONS

Vasopressors may cause serious cardiac arrhythmias during **halothane anesthesia.** If used in conjunction with **oxytocic drugs,** pressor effect of the sympathomimetic pressor amines is potentiated (see *Warnings*). The pressor effect of sympathomimetic amines is markedly potentiated in those receiving **monoamine oxidase inhibitors.** When initiating pressor therapy in these patients, initial dosage should be small and used with caution. The pressor response of adrenergic agents may also be potentiated by **tricyclic antidepressants.**

Use with caution and ECG monitored in patients receiving **digitalis,** especially large doses, because arrhythmias may occur. Other agents that may predispose to such a response are **beta-adrenergic blocking agents, guanethidine,** and **reserpine.**

ADVERSE REACTIONS

Headache, reflex bradycardia, excitability, restlessness; rarely, arrhythmias.

OVERDOSAGE

Symptoms: Ventricular extrasystoles, short paroxysms of ventricular tachycardia, sensation of fullness in the head, tingling of extremities.

Treatment: Relieve excessive elevation of blood pressure by an alpha-adrenergic blocking agent (*e.g.,* phentolamine).

DOSAGE

Inject subcutaneously, IM, or IV, or in dilute solution as continuous IV infusion. In those with paroxysmal supraventricular tachycardia and, if indicated, in case of emergency, administer directly IV. Dosage is adjusted according to pressor response.

Mild to moderate hypotension

Subcutaneous or IM: Usual dosage—2 mg to 5 mg. *Range*—1 mg to 10 mg. Initial dose should not exceed 5 mg. A 5-mg IM dose should raise blood pressure for 1 to 2 hours.

IV: Usual dose—0.2 mg. *Range*—0.1 mg to 0.5 mg. Initial dose should not exceed 0.5 mg. Do not repeat injections more often than every 10 to 15 minutes. A dose of 0.5 mg IV should elevate blood pressure for about 15 minutes.

Severe hypotension and shock, including drug-related hypotension

Blood volume depletion should always be corrected as fully as possible before any vasopressor is administered. When, as an emergency measure, intra-aortic pressures must be maintained to prevent cerebral or coronary artery ischemia, phenylephrine can be given before and concurrently with blood volume replacement. Hypotension and occasionally severe shock may result from overdosage or idiosyncrasy following administration of certain drugs; phenylephrine may be used as an adjunct in management of such episodes. Higher initial and maintenance doses are required in those with persistent or untreated severe hypotension or shock.

Continuous IV infusion: Add 10 mg to 500 ml of dextrose or sodium chloride solution (providing a 1:50,000 dilution). To raise blood pressure rapidly, start infusion at about 100 to 180 drops/minute. When blood pressure has stabilized (at low normal level for the individual), a maintenance rate of 40 to 60 drops/minute usually suffices. If prompt initial vasopressor response is not obtained, additional increments of the drug (10 mg or more) are added to the infusion bottle and rate of flow adjusted until desired response obtained.

Spinal anesthesia

Hypotension: Is best administered subcutaneously or IM 3 to 4 minutes before injection of the spinal anesthetic. Total requirement for high anesthetic levels is usually 3 mg; for lower levels, 2 mg. For hypotensive emergencies during spinal anesthesia: 0.2 mg IV, with any adjustment not exceeding the previous dose by more than 0.1 mg or 0.2 mg and not more than 0.5 mg administered as a single dose. *For hypotension during spinal anesthesia in children*—0.5 mg to 1 mg/25 lb subcutaneously or IM.

Prolongation of spinal anesthesia: Addition of 2 mg to 5 mg to the anesthetic solution increases the duration of motor block by as much as 50% without an increase in incidence of complications (*e.g.,* nausea, vomiting, blood-pressure disturbances).

Vasoconstrictor for regional anesthesia: Concentrations about 10 times those of epinephrine recommended. Optimal strength is 1:20,000 (made by adding 1 mg of drug to every 20 ml of local anesthetic solution). Some pressor responses may be expected when 2 mg or more are injected.

Paroxysmal supraventricular tachycardia

Rapid IV injection (within 20–30 seconds) is recommended; initial dose should not exceed 0.5 mg, and subsequent doses, which are determined by the initial blood pressure response, should not exceed the preceding dose by more than 0.1 mg to 0.2 mg and should never exceed 1 mg.

NURSING IMPLICATIONS

HISTORY
Review chart for most recent vital signs. When applicable, review health history.

PHYSICAL ASSESSMENT
Obtain blood pressure, pulse, and respirations. When administered to child to combat hypotension during spinal anesthesia, weight will be required.

ADMINISTRATION
Blood volume depletion is corrected before administration of drug, but drug can be administered before and concurrently with blood volume replacement as an emergency measure.

In emergency situations, physician may order CVP line, ECG monitoring and other measures for monitoring therapeutic response.

Do not use solutions that are cloudy or discolored.

Dosage calculations (using phenylephrine 1%): For doses of 10 mg, use 1 ml; for 5 mg, use 0.5 ml; for 1 mg, use 0.1 ml.

For convenience of intermittent IV administration, dilute 1 ml of phenylephrine with 9 ml Sterile Water for Injection, USP to make phenylephrine 0.1%. For doses of 0.1 mg, use 0.1 ml; for 0.2 mg, use 0.2 ml; for 0.5 mg, use 0.5 ml.

For continuous infusion, add 10 mg (1 ml) to 500 ml of dextrose or sodium chloride solution (providing a 1:50,000 dilution).

When given by continuous IV infusion, physician orders initial and maintenance infusion rates (either as drops/minute or mg/minute). Infusion rate also adjusted according to patient response. See *Dosage* for recommended guidelines.

Use Y-tubing or IV piggyback to administer by continuous IV infusion.

Have available phentolamine for treatment of overdosage.

Obtain blood pressure, pulse, and respirations immediately before administration.

ONGOING ASSESSMENTS AND NURSING MANAGEMENT
Monitor blood pressure and pulse every 3 to 5 minutes or as ordered following administration.

Rate of continuous IV infusion is adjusted according to blood-pressure response.

CLINICAL ALERT: Ventricular extrasystoles, short paroxysms of ventricular tachycardia, sensation of fullness in the head, and tingling of the extremities are signs of overdosage. Hypertension, headache, and bradycardia may also be seen. If any one or more of these occur, slow infusion rate, monitor patient closely, and notify physician.

IM administration may raise blood pressure for 1 to 2 hours; IV dose should raise blood pressure for about 15 minutes.

If restlessness is noted (adverse reaction), patient with continuous IV infusion may require restraining measures. Notify physician if this or other adverse reactions are noted.

Measure intake and output when patient is treated for severe hypotension and shock. Notify physician if oliguria or anuria is noted.

Phenylpropanolamine Hydrochloride *otc*

tablets: 25 mg	Diadax, Diet Gard
tablets: 37.5 mg	Westrim
capsules: 25 mg	Diet Gard
capsules: 37.5 mg	Resolution II Half-Strength
capsules, timed release: 75 mg	Control, Dex-A-Diet Caffeine Free, Dexatrim Caffeine Free, Dietac Maximum Strength, Resolution I Maximum Strength Caffeine Free, Unitrol, Westrim LA 75
tablets, precision release: 75 mg	Acutrim Maximum Strength

INDICATIONS
Management of exogenous obesity as short-term adjunct in a regimen of weight reduction based on caloric restriction. Nonprescription combination products promoted as diet aids, which contain phenylpropanolamine along with vitamins, caffeine, or other constituents, are also available. Phenylpropanolamine is also used as a nasal decongestant (see Bronchodilators and Decongestants, Systemic).

CONTRAINDICATIONS

Advanced arteriosclerosis; symptomatic cardiovascular disease; moderate to severe hypertension; hyperthyroidism; kidney disease; diabetes; known hypersensitivity or idiosyncrasy to sympathomimetic amines; glaucoma; during or within 14 days following administration of monoamine oxidase (MAO) inhibitors.

ACTIONS

Is an adrenergic agent similar to epinephrine and ephedrine but has longer duration of action than epinephrine and causes less CNS stimulation than ephedrine. It stimulates both alpha and beta receptors and part of its peripheral action is due to release of norepinephrine. Increase in blood pressure due primarily to vasoconstriction, but mostly to cardiac stimulation. Is readily absorbed from the GI tract with a half-life of 3 to 4 hours. While small amounts are metabolized in the liver, 80% to 90% is excreted as unchanged drug.

WARNINGS

Should not be used in pregnancy or lactation. Safety for use in children not established.

PRECAUTIONS

Avoid continuous use for longer than 3 months.

DRUG INTERACTIONS

Insulin requirements in diabetes mellitus may be altered and a decrease in the hypotensive effect of **guanethidine** may occur with use of phenylpropanoloamine. Do not use concomitantly with **antihypertensive** and **antidepressant** drugs containing **MAO inhibitors,** or with drugs containing **sympathomimetic amines** (*i.e.,* decongestants). Severe hypertensive episodes have occurred during concomitant administration with **propranolol** or **indomethacin.**

ADVERSE REACTIONS

Palpitation; tachycardia; elevation of blood pressure; overstimulation; restlessness; dizziness; insomnia; euphoria; dysphoria; headache; dry mouth; nausea; nasal dryness; diuresis. Has also been associated with severe hypertension and hypertensive crisis and possible renal failure in previously normotensive patients. Serious CNS effects (tremor, increased motor activity, agitation, hallucinations) have been reported.

OVERDOSAGE

Symptoms: Manifestations includes restlessness, tremor, hyperreflexia, rapid respiration, confusion, assaultive behavior, hallucinations, panic states. Fatigue and depression follow central stimulation.

Cardiovascular effects include arrhythmias, hypertension or hypotension, circulatory collapse. GI symptoms include nausea, vomiting, diarrhea, abdominal cramps. In fatal poisoning, death is usually preceded by convulsion and coma.

Treatment: Largely symptomatic and includes gastric lavage and sedation with a barbiturate. Acidification of the urine increases drug excretion.

DOSAGE

Immediate release: 25 mg tid. Do not exceed 75 mg/day.

Timed release: 75 mg once daily in the morning.

Precision release (16-hour duration): 75 mg after a light breakfast.

NURSING IMPLICATIONS

PATIENT AND FAMILY INFORMATION

Do not exceed recommended dosage or use continuously for longer than 3 months.

Must be used in conjunction with a restricted-calorie diet.

Discontinue use if rapid pulse, dizziness, or palpitations occur.

Do not use indiscriminately, especially if taking other prescription or nonprescription drugs on a regular basis or have health problems, without first consulting a physician.

Phenytoin

See Anticonvulsants, Hydantoins.

Phosphate Rx

potassium phosphate solution: Provides 3 mM phosphate, 4.4 mEq potassium/ml
sodium phosphate solution: Provides 3 mM phosphate, 4 mEq sodium/ml

INDICATIONS

A source of phosphate, for addition to large volume IV fluids, to prevent or correct hypophosphatemia in those with restricted or no oral intake.

CONTRAINDICATIONS

In diseases with high phosphate or low calcium levels. **Potassium phosphate** is contraindicated in diseases with high potassium levels. **Sodium phosphate** is contraindicated in those with hypernatremia.

ACTIONS

A prominent component of all tissues, phosphorus is necessary for a variety of essential biochemical factors, including deposition of bone, regulation of calcium metabolism, buffering effects on acid–base equilibrium, utilization of B-complex vitamins. It is also a component of various enzyme systems (*e.g.,* synthesis of carbohydrates, fats, proteins) and plays a primary role in renal excretion of the hydrogen ion. Normal serum inorganic phosphate levels are 3.0 mg/dl to 4.5 mg/dl for adults and 4.0 mg/dl to 7.5 mg/dl for children. Intravenously infused phosphate not taken up by tissues is excreted almost entirely in the urine.

WARNINGS

Dilute and mix thoroughly before use. To avoid phosphate or potassium intoxication, infuse solutions slowly. Infusion of high concentrations of phosphate reduce serum calcium levels and produce symptoms of hypocalcemic tetany. In those with severe renal or adrenal insufficiency, administration of **potassium phosphate** can cause potassium intoxication.

PRECAUTIONS

Replacement therapy should be guided by the serum inorganic phosphate level and the limits imposed by the accompanying sodium or potassium ion. High plasma potassium may cause death via cardiac depression, arrhythmia or arrest.

Sodium phosphate: Use with caution in those with renal impairment, cirrhosis, cardiac failure, and other edematous or sodium retaining states.

Potassim phosphate: Use with caution in presence of cardiac disease, particularly in digitalized patients, and in presence of renal disease.

ADVERSE REACTIONS

Phosphate intoxication results in a reduction of serum calcium, and the symptoms are those of hypocalcemic tetany.

OVERDOSAGE (POTASSIUM PHOSPHATE)

Symptoms: May involve combined potassium and phosphate intoxication and include paresthesias of the extremities, flaccid paralysis, listlessness, mental confusion, weakness and heaviness of the legs, hypotension, cardiac arrhythmias, heart block, ECG abnormalities.

Treatment: Immediately discontinue infusion; restore depressed serum calcium levels and reduce elevated potassium levels.

DOSAGE

For IV use only. Dilute and mix thoroughly in a larger volume of fluid. Dose and rate of administration depend on individual needs of patient. For total parenteral nutrition (TPN), approximately 10 mM to 15 mM of phosphorus per liter of TPN solution is usually adequate to maintain normal serum phosphate; larger amounts may be required in hypermetabolic states. Suggested dose for infants receiving TPN is 1.5 mM/kg/day to 2 mM/kg/day.

NURSING IMPLICATIONS

HISTORY

See Appendix 4.

ADMINISTRATION

Phosphate is usually added by pharmacist to TPN solution.

Infuse these solutions slowly. Physician orders infusion rate.

ONGOING ASSESSMENTS AND NURSING MANAGEMENT

Observe for signs of hyperphosphatemia and hypophosphatemia (Appendix 6, section 6-18) (which may be present when therapy is initiated), hypocalcemia (Appendix 6, section 6-13), hyperkalemia (Appendix 6, section 6-15) (when potassium phosphate is given), and hypernatremia (Appendix 6, section 6-17) (when sodium phosphate is given).

Serum inorganic phosphate and serum calcium levels are monitored at frequent intervals. Serum sodium and/or potassium may also be ordered.

Review *Overdosage,* above. If signs of overdosage are noted, slow infusion and notify physician.

Phosphorus Replacement Products otc

tablets: 173 mg phosphorus, 227 mg sodium, 50 mg potassium	Uro-KP-Neutral
tablets: 250 mg phosphorus, 298 mg sodium, 45 mg potassium	K-Phos Neutral
capsules, powder: 250 mg phosphorus, 164 mg sodium, 278 mg potassium	Neutra-Phos
capsules, powder: 250 mg phosphorus, 556 mg potassium	Neutra-Phos-K

P

INDICATIONS

Dietary supplements of phosphorus, particularly if diet is restricted or if needs are increased. Phosphate administration lowers urinary calcium levels and increases urinary stone inhibitors, phosphate, and pyrophosphate.

CONTRAINDICATIONS

Addison's disease, hyperkalemia.

PRECAUTIONS

Use with caution if on a sodium-restricted diet.

ADVERSE REACTIONS

Occasionally, a mild laxative effect may be noted for the first few days.

DOSAGE

Uro-KP-Neutral: Adults, 2 tablets, tid with full glass of water.

K-Phos Neutral: Adults, 1 or 2 tablets, qid with full glass of water.

Neutra-Phos, Neutra-Phos-K capsules: Contents of 1 capsule mixed with 75 ml water qid.

Neutra-Phos, Neutra-Phos-K powder: Mix content of 1 bottle with sufficient water to make 1 gallon of solution; take 75 ml qid.

NURSING IMPLICATIONS

HISTORY

See Appendix 4.

ADMINISTRATION

See *Dosage,* above.

Use of chilled or ice water for mixing capsule contents and refrigeration of solution made from powder may make solution more palatable.

ONGOING ASSESSMENTS AND NURSING MANAGEMENT

If diarrhea occurs and persists or becomes severe, notify physician because drug may need to be discontinued or dosage reduced.

PATIENT INFORMATION

Take as recommended by physician.

Powder, capsules: Directions for use are on label.

Tablets: Take with full glass of water.

Refrigeration of solution (from powder) or use of ice water may make solution more palatable.

If diarrhea occurs and persists or becomes severe, discontinue use and notify physician or nurse.

Physostigmine

See Miotics, Cholinesterase Inhibitors.

Physostigmine Salicylate Rx

injection: 1 mg/ml   Antilirium

INDICATIONS

Reversal of toxic effects on the CNS caused by drugs in clinical or toxic dosages capable of producing anticholinergic poisoning (including tricyclic antidepressants). It also has been reported that it may antagonize CNS depressant effects of diazepam.

CONTRAINDICATIONS

Do not use in presence of asthma, gangrene, diabetes, cardiovascular disease, mechanical obstruction of the intestine, urogenital tract, or any vagotonic state, or in those receiving choline esters or depolarizing neuromuscular blocking agents.

ACTIONS

Is a reversible anticholinesterase agent that effectively increases the concentration of acetylcholine at sites of cholinergic transmission. The action of acetylcholine is normally very transient because of its hydrolysis by the enzyme, acetylcholinesterase. Physostigmine salicylate inhibits the destructive action of acetylcholinesterase and prolongs and exaggerates the effects of acetylcholine. It reverses both central and peripheral anticholinergic effects.

Central toxic effects: Anxiety, delirium, disorientation, hallucinations, hyperactivity, seizures. Severe poisoning may produce coma, medullary paralysis, and death.

Peripheral toxic effects: Tachycardia, hyperpyrexia, mydriasis, vasodilatation, urinary retention, diminution of GI motility, decreased secretion in salivary and sweat glands, loss of secretions of the pharynx, bronchi, nasal passages.

Dramatic reversal of the effects of anticholinergic symptoms can be expected minutes after IV administration if diagnosis is correct and patient has not suffered anoxia or other trauma.

Numerous drugs and some plants produce the anticholinergic syndrome directly or as a side-effect. This potentially dangerous phenomenon may be brought about with either therapeutic doses or overdoses of drugs, including atropine, other derivatives of belladonna alkaloids, tricyclic antidepressants, phenothiazines, and antihistamines.

Short-acting physostigmine is readily absorbed and freely crosses the blood–brain barrier following administration. Peak effects are seen within 5 minutes and persist for approximately 1 to 2 hours following IV administration. It is rapidly hydrolyzed by cholinesterase, the enzyme which it inhibits. Renal impairment does not require dosage alteration.

WARNINGS

Discontinue if symptoms of excessive salivation or emesis, frequent urination, or diarrhea occurs. If excessive sweating or nausea occurs, dosage is reduced.

PRECAUTIONS

Because of possibility of hypersensitivity, atropine sulfate injection should be at hand because it is an antagonist and antidote for physostigmine.

DOSAGE

Adults: Usual dose is 0.5 mg to 2 mg IM or IV. It may be necessary to repeat dosages of 1 mg to 4 mg as life-threatening signs recur.

Pediatric: Should be reserved for life-threatening situations only. Initially, no more than 0.5 mg by very slow IV injection of at least 1 minute. If toxic effects persist and there is no sign of cholinergic effects, dose may be repeated at 5- to 10-minute intervals until therapeutic effect is obtained or a maximum dose of 2 mg is attained.

NURSING IMPLICATIONS

HISTORY

Obtain information about drug or substance producing symptoms of anticholinergic poisoning. If drug/substance was self-administered (intentionally or accidentally), attempt to obtain name of drug or substance and dosage or amount of substance ingested. If symptoms occur with clinical or toxic dosage of drug administered in a hospital, review pharmacology of involved agent.

PHYSICAL ASSESSMENT

Review *Actions* for central and peripheral toxic effects; obtain vital signs; check pupils for dilatation; evaluate mental state (look for delirium, confusion, anxiety, apparent hallucinations); check oral membranes and oral cavity for dryness, absence of saliva; auscultate bowel sounds; check for urinary retention.

ADMINISTRATION

Because of possibility of hypersensitivity, atropine sulfate should be on hand because it is an antagonist and antidote for physostigmine.

Each ampule contains 2 mg (1 mg/ml).

IV administration should be at a slow, controlled rate, no more than 1 mg/minute.

Rapid IV administration can cause bradycardia and hypersalivation leading to respiratory difficulties and, possibly, convulsions.

Use in pediatric patients is reserved for life-threatening situations only.

ONGOING ASSESSMENTS AND NURSING MANAGEMENT

Immediately after administration, monitor blood pressure, pulse, and respirations every 3 to 5 minutes or as ordered.

Observe for relief of central and peripheral anticholinergic effects present prior to administration of physostigmine.

Observe for symptoms of physostigmine overdosage: excessive salivation, emesis, frequent urination, diarrhea, abdominal cramps, muscle weakness.

Record response to drug on flow sheet, noting time each symptom is abolished.

Drug has brief duration of action; therefore, central and peripheral anticholinergic toxic effects may return. Continue to observe patient closely for next 2 to 3 or more hours (depending on severity of toxic effects being treated and substance involved). Monitor blood pressure, pulse, and respirations q15m or as ordered; observe for relief of central and peripheral symptoms.

Phytonadione

See Vitamin K.

Pilocarpine Hydrochloride, Nitrate

See Miotics, Direct Acting.

Pilocarpine Ocular Therapeutic System Rx

| ocular therapeutic system | Ocusert Pilo-20, Ocusert Pilo-40 |

INDICATIONS

Control of elevated intraocular pressure in pilocarpine-responsive patients.

Concurrent therapy: Ocusert has been used with various ophthalmic medications. Its release rate is not influenced by carbonic anhydrase inhibitors, epinephrine ophthalmic solutions, fluorescein, or anesthetic, antibiotic, or anti-inflammatory steroid ophthalmic solutions.

CONTRAINDICATIONS

When pupillary constriction is undesirable, such as for glaucoma associated with acute inflammatory disease of the anterior segment of the eye; for glaucomas occurring or persisting after extracapsular cataract extraction when posterior synechiae may occur; allergy to pilocarpine.

ACTIONS

An elliptically shaped unit designed for continuous release of pilocarpine following placement in the cul-de-sac of the eye. Pilocarpine is released from the system as soon as it is placed in contact with the conjunctival surfaces. Ocusert releases the drug at three times the rated value in the first hours and declines to the rated value in approximately 6 hours. The ocular hypotensive effect is fully developed within 1½ to 2 hours after placement. A satisfactory ocular response is maintained around the clock. During the first several hours after insertion, induced myopia may occur. The amount of myopia decreases after the first several hours to a low baseline level, which persists for the therapeutic life of the system.

PRECAUTIONS, WARNINGS, ADVERSE REACTIONS

See Miotics, Direct Acting.

DOSAGE

Initiation of therapy: It has been estimated that Ocusert 20 mcg is roughly equal to 1% drops and 40 mcg roughly equal to 2% drops. Ocusert reduces amount of drug necessary to achieve adequate medical control; therefore, therapy may be started with the 20 mcg system irrespective of strength of pilocarpine solution previously required. Because of patient's age, family history, and disease status or progression, therapy may be started with the 40 mcg system. The patient then returns during first week of therapy for evaluation of intraocular pressure and as often as necessary thereafter. If physician desires intraocular pressure reduction greater than that achieved with the 20 mcg system, patient is transferred to the 40 mcg system.

Placement and removal of the system: The system is readily placed in the eye by the patient. Instructions for placement and removal are provided with the drug. Because pilocarpine-induced myopia may occur during first several hours of therapy, system should be inserted H.S. By morning, the induced myopia is at a stable level. During the initial period, the unit may slip out of the conjunctival sac onto the cheek. The patient is usually aware of such movement and can replace the unit without difficulty.

In those in whom retention of the unit is a problem, superior cul-de-sac placement is often desirable. The unit can be manipulated from the lower to the upper conjunctival sac by gentle digital massage through the lid. If possible, the unit can be moved to the upper conjunctival sac before sleep for best retention. Should the unit slip out during sleep, its ocular hypotension effect following loss continues for a period of time comparable to that following instillation of eyedrops.

Remove only 1 unit from the container immediately prior to having patient insert unit.

NURSING IMPLICATIONS

HISTORY

See Appendix 4.

PHYSICAL ASSESSMENT

Evaluate patient's ability to carry out activities of daily living if vision is severely impaired.

ADMINISTRATION

See *Dosage* above.

It is recommended that system be inserted H.S.

System is inserted by patient in the inferior conjunctival cul-de-sac, but physician may recommend the superior cul-de-sac placement when retention of the unit is a problem. The unit can be manipulated from the inferior to the superior cul-de-sac by gentle digital massage through the lid.

Use normal saline (or solution prescribed by physician) to gently remove any secretions, if present, prior to having patient insert system.

Storage: Store under refrigeration (2° to 8°C).

ONGOING ASSESSMENTS AND NURSING MANAGEMENT

Evaluate drug effect by questioning patient about symptoms (especially during early weeks of therapy).

Although patient is usually aware if system has become displaced, it may be necessary in some instances to check placement of the system H.S. and on awakening in the A.M.

Check eye for signs of irritation, erythema. If these are noted, contact physician.

Gently remove secretions, when present, from lids, eyelashes, and area around eye when necessary. Use cotton ball or gauze soaked in normal saline or other cleansing solution recommended by physician.

When visual acuity is affected, patient may require assistance with ambulation or other activities. The patient's room or adjacent area should be dimly lit at night.

If patient has brought own supply of drug to hospital, label with patient's name and room number and refrigerate immediately.

Contact physician if there is an increase in severity of symptoms of glaucoma or if excessive eye irritation, erythema, or secretion of mucus is noted.

PATIENT AND FAMILY INFORMATION

NOTE: Physician or nurse must evaluate patient's ability to manage placement and removal of the system at time drug is prescribed as well as at time of first visit after initiation of therapy. Package insert instructions are also reviewed at this time.

Read package insert carefully before inserting system. Keep these directions in a safe place, separate from the drug (humid refrigerator may dampen paper). Keep drug in the refrigerator at all times; remove only one unit at a time.

The system is replaced every 7 days. Select a day most easily remembered. Replacement is best done at bedtime unless physician directs otherwise.

Check for presence of unit before retiring at night and in the morning on arising; if it becomes dislodged, it may be reinserted.

Notify physician if excessive secretions or irritation occurs.

If difficulty is encountered with the system, contact physician immediately.

Pindolol

See Beta-Adrenergic Blocking Agents.

Piperacetazine

See Antipsychotic Agents.

Piperacillin Sodium

See Penicillins.

Piperazine Rx

syrup: as citrate equivalent to 500 mg piperazine hexahydrate/5 ml	Antepar, Vermizine, _Generic_
tablets: as citrate equivalent to 250 mg piperazine hexahydrate	_Generic_
tablets: as citrate equivalent to 500 mg piperazine hexahydrate	Antepar, _Generic_

INDICATIONS
Treatment of enterobiasis (pinworm infection) and ascariasis (roundworm infection).

CONTRAINDICATIONS
Impaired renal or hepatic function; convulsive disorders; hypersensitivity.

ACTIONS
Produces hyperpolarization of the _Ascaris_ muscle by blocking its response to acetylcholine. It alters cell membrane permeability to ions responsible for maintenance of the resting potential. The paralyzed _Ascaris_ are dislodged and expelled via peristalsis. The mechanism of action against _Enterobius_ is not known. Although systemic absorption and excretion is variable, drug is readily absorbed from the GI tract; most of the dose is excreted in the urine within 24 hours.

WARNINGS
Because of potential neurotoxicity, especially in children, prolonged or repeated treatment in excess of that recommended is avoided. Safety for use in pregnancy not established.

PRECAUTIONS
If CNS, significant GI, or hypersensitivity reactions occur, drug is discontinued. Use with caution in patients with severe malnutrition, anemia, or hepatic disease.

DRUG INTERACTIONS
Piperazine may possibly exaggerate extrapyramidal effects of the **phenothiazines;** potentially fatal violent convulsions may be precipitated.

ADVERSE REACTIONS
_GI:_ Nausea, vomiting, abdominal cramps, diarrhea.

CNS: Headache, vertigo, ataxia, tremors, choreiform movements, muscular weakness, hyporeflexia, paresthesia, blurred vision, nystagmus, paralytic strabismus, convulsion, EEG abnormalities, sense of detachment, memory defect.

Ocular: Cataracts.

Hypersensitivity: Urticaria, erythema multiforme, purpura, fever, arthralgia, eczematous skin reactions, lacrimation, rhinorrhea, productive cough, bronchospasm.

DOSAGE
Ascariasis (roundworm infection)

Adults: A single daily dose of 3.5 g (hexahydrate equivalent) for 2 consecutive days.

Children: A single daily dose of 75 mg (hexahydrate equivalent)/kg/day for 2 consecutive days, with maximum dose of 3.5 g.

Severe infections: Treatment course may be repeated after a 1-week interval.

Mass therapy: When desirable to apply mass therapy as a public health measure and when repeated therapy is not practical, a single dose of 70 mg/lb up to 3 g may be used. This is successful in removing ascarids in the majority of cases but the maximum cure rate is usually obtained with the multiple-dose regimen.

Enterobiasis (pinworm infection)

Adults and children: A single daily dose of 65 mg (hexahydrate equivalent)/kg/day; maximum daily dose is 2.5 g for 7 consecutive days.

Severe infections: Treatment course may be repeated after 1-week interval.

NURSING IMPLICATIONS

HISTORY

See Appendix 4. A careful history of travel, eating habits, and sanitary facilities may be necessary to determine source of roundworm infection. Family members should also have stool examinations for roundworm. Because pinworm is easily transmitted from person to person, it is recommended that all family members be treated for complete parasite eradication.

PHYSICAL ASSESSMENT

Stool is examined for roundworm. If patient appears ill or malnourished, obtain vital signs and weight. Pinworm specimen may be collected (in early A.M. before patient gets out of bed) by means of cellophane tape wrapped sticky side out around tongue blade or fingers; press against anal area (female pinworms deposit ova at night in perianal area). Transfer tape (sticky side down) to glass slide for microscopic examination. Other laboratory tests in those with roundworm may include CBC and serum electrolytes, especially if patient shows evidence of weight loss, appears ill, or massive infection is suspected. Roundworm infections are usually reported to the public health department.

ADMINISTRATION

Use of laxatives or enema and dietary restriction are not necessary. Drug may be taken with food to minimize gastric distress.

ONGOING ASSESSMENTS AND NURSING MANAGEMENT

Isolation is rarely necessary; stool and linen precautions are usually instituted. Wash hands thoroughly before and after each patient contact, especially when disposing of urine or feces, changing bed linens.

Pinworm can be transmitted from person to person; roundworm is not passed directly from person to person.

If patient is acutely ill and is hospitalized for roundworm infection, monitor vital signs q4h.

Observe for adverse reactions; notify physician if they occur.

PATIENT AND FAMILY INFORMATION

Take prescribed doses (2 days for roundworm, 7 days for pinworm); course of therapy must be completed for drug to be effective.

If GI upset occurs, medication may be taken with food.

Notify physician or nurse if CNS, GI, or hypersensitivity reactions occur (see *Adverse Reactions*).

Wash hands thoroughly before eating and after defecation.

Pinworm: Meticulous hygiene is necessary to prevent reinfection. Change and launder undergarments, bed linens, towels, and nightclothes daily. Disinfect toilet facilities (including bathtub/shower) daily.

Clean under fingernails daily. Avoid putting fingers in mouth; nail biting must be avoided (liquid preparations that have a bitter taste and are painted on the nails and fingertips to discourage nail biting are available if child persists in biting nails).

Roundworm: Thoroughly wash all vegetables grown in contaminated soil.

Bathe daily; change undergarments and bed linens daily.

Pipobroman Rx

tablets: 25 mg   Vercyte

INDICATIONS

Treatment of polycythemia vera. Also useful in treatment of chronic granulocytic leukemia. Busulfan is the preferred agent in this form of leukemia, but pipobroman may be especially helpful in patients refractory to busulfan.

CONTRAINDICATIONS

Not administered to those with bone-marrow depression resulting from x-ray or cytotoxic chemotherapy.

ACTIONS

Has been classified as an alkylating agent, although exact mechanism of action is not known. Is readily absorbed following administration; the metabolic fate and route of excretion are unknown. See also Appendix 10.

WARNINGS

Depression of bone marrow may not occur for 4 weeks or more after treatment is initiated. Most reliable guide to bone-marrow activity is provided by the leukocyte count, but the platelet count also provides a good index to bone-marrow activity. If the leukocyte count falls to 3000 or less, or if the platelet count is reduced to 150,000 or less, drug is temporarily discontinued. Therapy may be cautiously reinstated when the leukocyte or platelet count has risen.

Dose-dependent anemia frequently develops but usually responds to blood transfusions and reduction in dosage. A rapid drop in hemoglobin, increased bilirubin levels, and reticulocytosis suggest a hemolytic process, in which case drug is discontinued.

Because of potential danger for fetal death or teratogenesis, drug is not used in women of childbearing potential (particularly during early pregnancy) unless, in the judgment of the physician, potential benefits outweigh the possible hazards. Not recommended for use in children less than 15 years because no significant clinical effect has been shown with patients in this age group.

PRECAUTIONS

Therapy is initiated in the hospital, where patient can be closely observed. Bone-marrow studies should be performed prior to treatment and again at time of maximal hematologic response. Complete blood counts should be done once or twice weekly and leukocyte counts every other day until desired response is obtained or significant toxic effects occur.

Renal- and hepatic-function tests are performed prior to therapy and at periodic intervals.

ADVERSE REACTIONS

Nausea, vomiting, abdominal cramping, diarrhea, skin rash. If persistent, these reactions may require withdrawal of drug.

DOSAGE

Given in divided daily doses. Maintenance doses are adjusted to response of patient. Therapy should be continued as long as needed to maintain satisfactory clinical response.

Polycythemia vera: Initial dose is 1 mg/kg/day. Larger doses (1.5–3 mg/kg/day) may be required in those who have been refractory to other treatment, but such doses should not be used until a dose of 1 mg/kg/day has been given for at least 30 days without improvement. Maintenance therapy usually initiated when the hematocrit has been reduced to 50% to 55%.

Chronic granulocytic leukemia: Initial doses range from 1.5 mg/kg/day to 2.5 mg/kg/day. This dosage is generally continued until a maximal clinical or hematologic response obtained. If the leukocyte count falls too rapidly, drug is discontinued until rate of decrease levels off. Maintenance ther-

apy is usually started as the leukocyte count approaches 10,000. If relapse is rapid (doubling of leukocyte count within 70 days), continuous treatment is indicated. Intermittent therapy is generally adequate if more than 70 days are required to double the leukocyte count. Maintenance doses range from about 7 mg/day to 175 mg/day.

NURSING IMPLICATIONS

HISTORY
See Appendix 4.

PHYSICAL ASSESSMENT
Obtain vital signs, weight; evaluate patient's general physical and mental status. Bone-marrow and peripheral blood studies (CBC, platelet count), renal- and hepatic-function tests are recommended prior to therapy.

ADMINISTRATION
Given in divided doses.

ONGOING ASSESSMENTS AND NURSING MANAGEMENT
Therapy is initiated in hospital, where patient can be closely observed.

Obtain vital signs q4h or as ordered; observe for adverse reactions and inform physician if they occur.

Weigh weekly or as ordered.

Bone-marrow depression may not occur for 4 weeks or more after initiation of therapy but patient should be observed for signs of bone-marrow depression (Appendix 6, section 6-8) from time of initiation of therapy.

Therapy is interrupted when platelet count is reduced to 150,000 or less or the leukocyte count falls to 3000 or less. If most recent laboratory studies show values at or less than these amounts, withhold drug and notify physician immediately.

PATIENT AND FAMILY INFORMATION
Drug may cause nausea, vomiting, abdominal cramping, diarrhea, and skin rash. Notify physician or nurse if these become pronounced.

Take drug exactly as directed. Do not omit dose unless directed to do so by the physician.

When applicable, contraceptive measures are recommended during therapy.

Piroxicam

See Nonsteroidal Anti-inflammatory Agents.

P

Plague Vaccine

See Immunizations, Active.

Plasma Protein Fractions

Albumin Human

(Normal Serum Albumin), 5%   Rx

injection: 5%	Albuminar-5, Albutein 5%, Buminate 5%, Plasbumin-5

Albumin Human

(Normal Serum Albumin), 25%   Rx

injection: 25%	Albuminar-25, Albutein 25%, Buminate 25%, Plasbumin-25

Plasma Protein Fraction   Rx

injection: 5%	Plasmanate, Plasma-Plex, Plasmatein, Protenate

INDICATIONS

Unless the condition responsible for hypoproteinemia can be corrected, albumin in any form can provide only symptomatic relief or supportive treatment.

Shock: In emergency treatment of shock due to burns, trauma, surgery, infections; in treatment of injuries of such severity that shock, although not immediately present, is likely to ensue; in other similar conditions when restoration of blood volume is urgent. For earliest treatment of shock, it may be more convenient to have 25% normal serum albumin available because it is so highly concentrated. However, the concentrated solution depends for its maximum osmotic effect on holding in the circulation additional fluids that are drawn from tissues or administered separately. If the patient is dehydrated, maximum effect cannot be obtained without additional fluids. Maximum osmotic effect is obtained with no additional fluids when normal serum albumin 5% is given.

Burns: Albumin 5% may be used in conjunction with adequate infusions of crystalloid to prevent hemoconcentration and to combat water, protein, and electrolyte losses that usually follow serious burns. Beyond 24 hours, albumin 25% can be used to maintain plasma colloid osmotic pressure.

Hypoproteinemia: For hypoproteinemia, as in the nephrotic syndrome, hepatic cirrhosis, toxemia of pregnancy; also in postoperative patients, tuberculous patients, and premature infants. These clinical situations are characterized by a low concentration of plasma protein and consequently a reduced volume of circulating blood. Administration of serum albumin IV will restore plasma proteins and relieve edema, but this is an interim measure; the cause of the condition must be corrected. Prophylactic administration of 25% Serum Albumin, 3 ml/lb to 4 ml/lb, has been found advantageous in premature infants with low serum protein levels.

Normal serum albumin 5% or plasma protein fraction 5% may be used in hypoproteinemic patients, providing sodium restriction is not a problem. If sodium restriction is imperative, 25% normal serum albumin may be used.

Adult respiratory distress syndrome (ARDS): When clinical signs are those of hypoproteinemia with a fluid volume overload, Albumin 25% together with a diuretic may be used.

Cardiopulmonary bypass: Preoperative dilution of blood using Albumin 25% and crystalloid is safe and well tolerated.

Acute liver failure: In rapid loss of liver function with or without coma, administration of albumin may serve a double purpose of supporting the colloid osmotic pressure of the plasma as well as binding excess plasma bilirubin.

Sequestration of protein-rich fluids: This occurs in conditions such as acute peritonitis, pancreatitis, mediastinitis, extensive cellulitis.

Erythrocyte resuspension: Albumin may be required to avoid excessive hypoproteinemia, during certain types of exchange transfusion, or with use of very large volumes of previously frozen or washed red cells. About 25 g of albumin/liter of erythrocytes is commonly used. Albumin 25% is added to the isotonic suspension of washed cells immediately prior to the transfusion.

Acute nephrosis: A loop diuretic and 1 dl albumin 25% repeated daily for 7 to 10 days may help control edema and the patient may then respond to treatment.

Renal dialysis: Albumin 25% may be of value in treatment of shock or hypotension in these patients. Usual volume administered is about 1 dl; fluid overload is avoided. These patients cannot tolerate substantial volumes of salt solution.

Hyperbilirubinemia and erythroblastosis fetalis: Albumin can be used in exchange transfusions for these two conditions because it reduces necessity for reexchange and increases amount of bilirubin removed with each transfusion.

CONTRAINDICATIONS

History of allergic reactions to albumin; severe anemia; cardiac failure; presence of normal or increased intravascular volume. In chronic nephrosis, serum albumin is promptly excreted by the kidneys with no relief of chronic edema or effect on the underlying renal lesion. It is of occasional use in the rapid "priming" diuresis of nephrosis. **Plasma protein fraction** is contraindicated in those on cardiopulmonary bypass.

ACTIONS

The albumin fraction of human blood has two known functions: maintainer of plasma colloid osmotic pressure and carrier of intermediate metabolites in the transport and exchange of tissue products. It comprises about 52% of the plasma proteins and provides approximately 80% of their colloid osmotic pressure. Thus, it is important in regulating the volume of circulating blood; its loss is critical, particularly in shock with hemorrhage or reduced plasma volume. When plasma volume is reduced, an adequate amount of albumin quickly restores the volume in most instances.

Twenty-five grams of albumin is the osmotic equivalent of approximately 2 units (500 ml) of fresh frozen plasma; or 1 dl of normal serum albumin 25% provides about as much plasma protein as 500 ml of plasma or 2 pt of whole blood. Normal serum albumin 5% is osmotically equivalent to an approximately equal volume of citrated plasma. The 25% albumin solution is osmotically equivalent to five times the volume of citrated plasma.

Plasma protein fraction is effective in maintenance of a normal blood volume but has not been proven effective in maintenance of oncotic pressure. When circulating blood volume has been depleted, the hemodilution following albumin administration persists for many hours. In those with normal blood volume, it usually lasts for only a few hours.

There is no indication that normal serum albumin (human) interferes with normal coagulation mechanisms.

PRECAUTIONS

Concomitant blood administration: Administration of large quantities of albumin should be supplemented with or replaced by whole blood to combat the relative anemia. Is not a substitute for blood in situations in which the oxygen-carrying capacity of whole blood is required in addition to plasma volume expansion.

Patients with marked dehydration require additional fluids, because drawing fluids from the tissues of a dehydrated patient is undesirable.

Use with caution in those with hepatic or renal failure because of the added protein load. Also use with caution in patients with low cardiac reserve or with no albumin deficiency. A rapid increase in plasma volume may cause circulatory embarrassment or pulmonary edema.

Laboratory test alterations: Infusion of normal serum albumin may result in an elevated level of alkaline phosphatase.

ADVERSE REACTIONS

Cardiovascular: Hypotension may result following rapid infusion or intra-arterial administration to those on cardiopulmonary bypass. In addition, rapid administration may result in vascular overload and pulmonary edema.

Allergic or pyrogenic reactions: Characterized primarily by fever and chills. Flushing, urticaria, low back pain, headache, rash, nausea, vomiting, increased salivation, febrile reactions, tachycardia, hypotension, and changes in respiration, pulse, and blood pressure also have been reported. If such reactions occur, discontinue the infusion and institute appropriate therapy (*e.g.,* antihistamines). If patient requires additional plasma protein fraction, use material from a different lot.

DOSAGE

ALBUMIN HUMAN (NORMAL SERUM ALBUMIN), 5%

Contains 130 mEq/liter to 160 mEq/liter sodium. Administer by IV infusion without further dilution. Depending on brand used, product is available in 50-, 250-, 500-, and 1000-ml vials.

Shock: In treatment of patient in shock with greatly reduced blood volume, may be given as rapidly as necessary to improve clinical condition and restore normal blood volume. In adults, an initial dose of 500 ml is given as rapidly as tolerated. If response within 30 minutes is inadequate, an additional 500 ml may be given. The 50-ml dosage form is appropriate for pediatric use. Therapy is guided by clinical response, blood pressure, and assessment of relative anemia. If more than 1000 ml is given, or if hemorrhage has occurred, administration of whole blood or red blood cells may be desirable.

Burns: After a burn injury (usually beyond 24 hours), there is a correlation between the amount of albumin infused and resultant increase in plasma colloid osmotic pressure. In severe burns, immediate therapy usually includes large volumes of crystalloid with lesser amounts of 5% albumin solution to maintain an adequate plasma volume. After the first 24 hours, the ratio of albumin to crystalloid may be increased to establish and maintain a plasma albumin level of about 2.5 g/dl or a total serum protein of about 5.2 g/dl. Duration of therapy decided by loss of protein from burned areas and in the urine.

Hypoproteinemia: May be used in replacing protein lost in hypoproteinemic conditions. If edema is

P

present or if large amounts of albumin are lost, albumin 25% is preferred.

ALBUMIN HUMAN (NORMAL SERUM ALBUMIN), 25%

Contains 130 mEq/liter to 160 mEq/liter sodium. Administer by IV infusion. May be given undiluted or diluted in normal saline. If sodium restriction is required, administer undiluted or diluted in a sodium-free carbohydrate solution such as 5% dextrose in water. Available in 20-, 50-, and 100-ml vials.

Hypoproteinemia with or without edema: Unless underlying pathology responsible can be corrected, IV administration is purely supportive and symptomatic. Usual daily dose for adults is 50 g to 75 g and for children 25 g. Some patients may require larger quantities. Rate of administration should not exceed 2 ml/minute; more rapid injection may precipitate circulatory embarrassment and pulmonary edema. In hepatic cirrhosis, albumin may be of value after removal of a large fluid volume (more than 1500 ml during a single paracentesis). In nephrosis initial dose of 100 ml to 200 ml may be repeated at 1- to 2-day intervals.

Burns: See albumin 5%, above; albumin 25% may also be used in treatment of burns.

Shock: Initial dose is determined by patient's condition and response to treatment. Therapy is guided by degree of venous and pulmonary congestion and hemoglobin or hematocrit measurements. In greatly reduced blood volume, administer as rapidly as desired. If initial response is inadequate, additional albumin may be given 15 to 30 minutes following the first dose. In slightly low or normal blood volume, rate of administration should be 1 ml/minute.

Hyperbilirubinemia and erythroblastosis fetalis: Administer 1 g/kg 1 to 2 hours before transfusion. In some cases it has been administered as part of the transfusion by substituting 50 ml albumin for 50 ml of plasma in the blood to be transfused.

PLASMA PROTEIN FRACTION

Contains 130 mEq/liter to 160 mEq/liter sodium. Administer by IV infusion. Is available in 50-, 250-, and 500-ml vials. Do not give more than 250 g in 48 hours.

Hypovolemic shock: Initial dose may be 250 ml to 500 ml. Rate of infusion and volume of total dose depend on patient's condition and response. Infusion rates exceeding 10 ml/minute may result in hypotension. Slow or stop infusion if sudden hypotension occurs. In infants and young children it may be used in initial therapy of shock due to dehydration or infection. Infuse a dose of 10 ml/lb to

15 ml/lb at a rate not exceeding 10 ml/minute. May be repeated, depending on patient response.

Hypoproteinemia: Daily doses of 1000 ml to 1500 ml; larger doses may be necessary. Rate of administration should not exceed 5 ml/minute to 8 ml/minute; monitor patient for signs of hypervolemia. Rate of infusion is adjusted according to response.

NURSING IMPLICATIONS

HISTORY
See Appendix 4.

PHYSICAL ASSESSMENT
Obtain vital signs, weight. Various laboratory tests (*e.g.,* hemoglobin, hematocrit, plasma albumin, total serum protein, serum electrolytes) may be ordered, depending on reason for use.

ADMINISTRATION
A CVP line may be inserted to monitor clinical response and determine future dosage.

Some of the products are supplied with an IV administration set. Consult manufacturer's directions and use the supplied materials for administration.

These preparations may be administered without regard to recipient's blood group or type.

Check expiration date on container.

Inspect contents of vial. Do not use if solution appears turbid or if a sediment is present. Do not use plasma protein fraction if it has been frozen.

Do *not* use if more than 4 hours have elapsed after container has been entered. Discard unused portion.

These preparations are ready to use without further dilution.

IV should be started with a large needle, preferably a 19 gauge to 20 gauge, as solution is moderately viscous. In children and infants, consult physician regarding needle size.

Albumin or plasma protein fraction is administered by IV piggyback or by direct IV infusion (primary line).

Obtain blood pressure, pulse, and respirations immediately prior to administration.

Physician orders infusion rate. Manufacturers recommend the following infusion rates for specific problems. For other uses, infusion rate depends on physician's clinical judgment.

ALBUMIN HUMAN, 5%
Shock: May be given as rapidly as necessary to improve clinical condition and restore normal

blood volume. Those with slightly low or normal blood volume, administer at rate of 2 ml/minute to 4 ml/minute. *Children*—¼ to ½ the adult rate.

Storage: Store at room temperature. Do not freeze.

ALBUMIN HUMAN, 25%

Shock: May be given as rapidly as necessary to improve clinical condition and restore normal blood volume. Those with slightly low or normal blood volume, administer at rate of 1 ml/minute.

Hypoproteinemia: Do not exceed 2 ml/minute.

Storage: Store at room temperature. Do not freeze.

PLASMA PROTEIN FRACTION

Hypovolemic shock: Do not exceed 10 ml/minute.

Hypoproteinemia: Do not exceed 5 ml/minute to 8 ml/minute.

Storage: Store at room temperature.

Admixture compatibility: May be given in combination with or through same administration set with the usual IV solutions of carbohydrates or saline. Certain solutions containing protein hydrolysates or alcohol must *not* be infused through the same administration set because these combinations may cause the proteins to precipitate.

ONGOING ASSESSMENTS AND NURSING MANAGEMENT

Monitor blood pressure, pulse, and respirations during time of infusion. Frequency of determinations depend on patient's condition and may range for every 5 to 15 minutes.

If the patient is dehydrated, additional IV fluids will be ordered.

CLINICAL ALERT: Observe patient closely during infusion.

Hypotension—Rapid infusion (over 10 ml/minute) may produce hypotension. If hypotension occurs, slow infusion to KVO or discontinue and run primary line; contact physician immediately.

Hypertension—Rise in blood pressure may follow rapid administration of albumin. Observe the injured patient to detect bleeding points that failed to bleed at the lower blood pressure; otherwise, new hemorrhage and shock may occur. If bleeding is noted, slow infusion rate to KVO and notify physician immediately.

Observe all patients for signs of fluid overload (Appendix 6, section 6-12) and pulmonary edema. If signs of fluid overload are apparent, slow infusion to KVO and notify physician immediately.

Observe for allergic or pyrogenic reactions (see *Adverse Reactions*). If such reactions occur, discontinue infusion, run primary line to KVO, and contact physician immediately. If preparation is being infused directly IV (primary line), slow to KVO and notify physician immediately. If reaction is severe, it may be necessary to discontinue the infusion immediately.

If CVP line is inserted, monitor CVP q15m or as ordered. Report any increase in venous pressure to physician immediately.

Measure intake and output. Notify physician if there is a change in the intake–output ratio (*e.g.,* output increased or decreased).

When used in treatment of shock, widening of the pulse pressure is correlated with an increase in stroke volume and cardiac output.

Laboratory tests to monitor clinical response may be ordered during therapy and include serum albumin, serum electrolytes, hemoglobin, hematocrit, and so on.

Plicamycin (Mithramycin) Rx

injection: 2.5 mg/vial   Mithracin

INDICATIONS

Treatment of carefully selected hospitalized patients with malignant tumors of the testis in whom successful treatment by surgery and/or radiation is impossible.

Treatment of certain symptomatic patients with hypercalcemia and hypercalciuria associated with a variety of advanced neoplasms. Because of toxicity of this drug, it should only be used for hypercalcemia and hypercalciuria *not* responsive to conventional treatment.

CONTRAINDICATIONS

Thrombocytopenia, thrombocytopathy, coagulation disorders, or increased susceptibility to bleeding due to other causes; impairment of bone-marrow function. Not recommended for use in those who are not hospitalized and cannot be observed during and after therapy, or if appropriate laboratory facilities are unavailable.

ACTIONS

Is a compound produced by *Streptomyces plicatus.* Although exact mechanism by which drug causes tumor inhibition is unknown, studies indicate this compound forms a complex with DNA and inhibits cellular RNA and enzymic RNA synthesis.

Treatment of patients with inoperable testicular tumors: May be useful in treatment of those with

P

testicular tumors resistant to other chemotherapeutic agents. Prior radiation or poor chemotherapy did not alter response rate with plicamycin. See also Appendix 10.

Treatment of patients with hypercalcemia and hypercalciuria: In a limited number of patients studied, hypercalcemia and hypercalciuria were completely reversed in all patients. In some, the primary malignancy was of nontesticular origin.

WARNINGS

Severe thrombocytopenia, hemorrhagic tendency, and even death may result from use. Although severe toxicity is more apt to occur in those with advanced disease or those considered poor risks for therapy, serious toxicity may also occur in patients in relatively good condition.

Use in pregnancy only when clearly needed and when potential benefit outweighs potential toxicity to the embryo or fetus.

PRECAUTIONS

Electrolyte imbalance (especially hypocalcemia, hypokalemia, hypophosphatemia) should be corrected prior to treatment. Use with extreme caution in those with impaired renal or hepatic function. Monitor renal function carefully. Platelet count, prothrombin and bleeding time obtained frequently during therapy and for several days after last dose. Occurrence of thrombocytopenia or a significant prolongation of prothrombin or bleeding time is indication to discontinue therapy.

ADVERSE REACTIONS

Hemorrhagic syndrome: Most important form of toxicity consists of bleeding syndrome, which usually begins with an episode of epistaxis. This syndrome may only consist of a single or several episodes of epistaxis and progress no further. It can start with an episode of hematemesis which may progress to more widespread hemorrhage in the GI tract or to a more generalized bleeding tendency. It is most likely due to abnormalities in multiple clotting factors and is dose related.

Most common: GI symptoms (anorexia, nausea, vomiting, diarrhea, stomatitis).

Less frequent: Fever, drowsiness, weakness, lethargy, malaise, headache, depression, phlebitis, facial flushing, skin rash.

Hematologic abnormalities: Depression of platelet count, white count, hemoglobin, and prothrombin content; elevation of clotting time and bleeding time; abnormal clot retraction. Thrombocytopenia may be rapid in onset and occur at any time during therapy or within several days following the last dose. With the occurrence of more severe thrombo-

cytopenia, infusion of platelet concentrates or platelet-rich plasma may be helpful. Occurrence of leukopenia is relatively uncommon. It has been uncommon for abnormalities in clotting time or clot retraction to occur prior to the onset of an overt bleeding episode noted in some patients. Performance of these tests is recommended, because abnormalities may serve as warning of impending serious toxicity.

Abnormal liver-function tests: Increased levels of SGOT, SGPT, LDH, alkaline phosphatase, serum bilirubin, ornithine carbamyl transferase, isocitric dehydrogenase.

Abnormal kidney-function tests: Increased BUN, serum creatinine; proteinuria.

Electrolyte abnormalities: Depression of serum calcium, phosphorus, potassium.

DOSAGE

Daily dose based on body weight. Ideal weight used if patient has abnormal fluid retention such as edema, hydrothorax or ascites. Administered IV only (see *Administration*).

Testicular tumors: 25 mcg/kg/day to 30 mcg/kg/day. Therapy continued for 8 to 10 days unless significant side-effects or toxicity occurs. A course of therapy consisting of more than 10 daily doses not recommended. Daily dose should not exceed 30 mcg/kg. In responsive tumors some degree of regression usually evident within 3 or 4 weeks following initial course of therapy. If tumor masses remain unchanged, additional courses at monthly intervals are warranted. When significant tumor regression is obtained, additional courses can be given at monthly intervals until complete regression or until definite tumor progression or new tumor masses occur in spite of continued therapy.

Treatment of hypercalcemia and hypercalciuria: Recommended dose is 25 mcg/kg/day for 3 to 4 days. If desired degree of reversal is not achieved with initial course of therapy, repeat at intervals of 1 week or more to achieve desired result or maintain serum and urinary calcium at normal levels. It may be possible to maintain normal calcium balance with single, weekly doses or with a schedule of two or three doses a week.

NURSING IMPLICATIONS

HISTORY

See Appendix 4. Review chart for diagnosis, recent laboratory/diagnostic studies, previous treatment modalities.

PHYSICAL ASSESSMENT

General physical and emotional status; vital signs; weight. Baseline laboratory studies include

CBC, differential, platelet count, bleeding and clotting time, prothrombin time, serum electrolytes, serum and urinary calcium, serum phosphorus, hepatic- and renal-function tests.

ADMINISTRATION

Preparation of solution: Reconstitute with 4.9 ml of Sterile Water for Injection. Each milliliter of resulting solution will then contain 500 mcg of plicamycin. Unused solution must be discarded. Fresh solutions prepared each day of therapy.

Dilute prescribed dose in 1000 ml of 5% Dextrose Injection or Sodium Chloride Injection as ordered by physician.

Manufacturer recommends administration by slow IV infusion over period of 4 to 6 hours. Physician may order this or other method of infusion. Avoid rapid direct IV injection because it may be associated with higher incidence and greater severity of GI side-effects.

Select a large vein to avoid needle displacement and extravasation; when possible avoid use of vein on back of hand. Physician may order insertion of an over-the-needle catheter (ONC) because administration of plicamycin may extend over 8 to 10 days.

A microdrip or infusion pump may be ordered.

An antiemetic may be ordered prior to infusion.

Physician may order additional (small amount) IV fluid following the infusion to flush IV tubing.

Instruct patient to mention immediately any burning or pain at injection site (may be sign of extravasation).

Storage: Store unreconstituted vial at refrigerator temperatures between 2°C and 8°C (36°F–46°F).

ONGOING ASSESSMENTS AND NURSING MANAGEMENT

Monitor IV infusion rate and infusion site q15m.

If extravasation occurs, discontinue infusion, restart in another area, and contact physician.

Application of moderate heat to extravasation site may help disperse compound and minimize discomfort and local tissue irritation. Physician may also order additional measures for extravasation.

Should thrombophlebitis or perivascular cellulitis occur, infusion should be terminated and restarted in another site and physician contacted.

An antiemetic may be ordered q4h prn to control nausea, vomiting. A liquid diet, unsalted crackers, and carbonated beverages may be offered until GI symptoms are under control.

Monitor vital signs q4h or as ordered. Report any significant changes to physician. If fever develops, physician may order antipyretic.

Measure intake and output. Contact physician immediately if there is a significant decrease in urinary output.

CLINICAL ALERT: Monitor patient q4h or more often for signs of dehydration (Appendix 6, section 6-10), especially if vomiting is severe or exceeds 600 ml to 700 ml/8 hours; signs of hematologic toxicity (see *Adverse Reactions*), especially epistaxis or any bleeding. Notify physician immediately if any of these signs or symptoms is noted.

Keep physician informed of *all* adverse reactions.

Observe for signs of hypocalcemia (Appendix 6, section 6-13), hypophosphatemia (Appendix 6, section 6-18), hypokalemia (Appendix 6, section 6-15) and report them to physician immediately.

Severe thrombocytopenia, hemorrhagic tendency, and even death may result from use of this drug.

Weigh daily. Report significant weight gain or loss to physician.

If diarrhea occurs, an antidiarrheal agent may be prescribed.

Frequent monitoring of renal and hepatic function, platelet count, prothrombin and bleeding time, and CBC are recommended during and for several days after therapy. Notify physician immediately of any abnormal laboratory reports. The occurrence of thrombocytopenia or significant prolongation of bleeding time or prothrombin time is an indication to discontinue therapy.

In patients with hypercalcemia or hypercalciuria, physician orders periodic serum and urinary calcium.

If anorexia persists for more than 2 to 3 days a high-calorie, high-protein diet may be ordered.

Give oral care q4h and/or after meals. Examine patient's oral cavity for evidence of stomatitis (patient may originally complain of burning of oral mucosa). Notify physician if erythema, ulcerative lesions noted as drug may need to be discontinued. If stomatitis occurs, begin stomatitis care (Appendix 6, section 6-22).

Physician may order a high-calcium diet if hypocalcemia occurs.

Check urine for proteinuria daily or as ordered. Inform physician if proteinuria occurs.

Pneumococcal Vaccine, Polyvalent

See Immunizations, Active.

Poliomyelitis Vaccine

See Immunizations, Active.

Poliovirus Vaccine

See Immunizations, Active.

Poloxamer 188

See Laxatives.

Polyestradiol Phosphate

See Estrogens, Antineoplastic.

Polymyxin B Sulfate

See Aminoglycosides; Antibiotics, Ophthalmic.

Polysaccharide-Iron Complex

See Iron Products, Oral.

Polythiazide

See Thiazides and Related Diuretics.

Posterior Pituitary Injection Rx

injection: 20 units/ ml   Pituitrin (S)

INDICATIONS

Control of postoperative ileus. Also used to stimulate expulsion of gas prior to pyelography. In surgery, used as an aid in achieving hemostasis. In presence of esophageal varices, may be used to promote hemostasis and as an adjunct in treatment of accompanying shock. May be useful in treatment of enuresis of diabetes insipidus, but such treatment is not curative.

CONTRAINDICATIONS

Toxemia of pregnancy; cardiac disease; hypertension; epilepsy; advanced arteriosclerosis. *Do not use as an oxytocic.* Injection before or during labor carries a high risk of inducing severe fetal distress, asphyxia neonatorum, or rupture of the uterus.

ACTIONS

Possesses oxytocic, vasopressor, and antidiuretic hormone (ADH) activity.

WARNINGS

Anaphylaxis, angioneurotic edema, and urticaria may occur. Coronary insufficiency and cardiac arrhythmias may be induced by this drug; this risk is enhanced in those under barbiturate sedation or cyclopropane anesthesia.

PRECAUTIONS

Pressor effects of this drug result from constriction of the vascular bed and increased peripheral resistance. This activity is accompanied by decreased cardiac output and diminished coronary blood flow; the underlying condition responsible for shock may be aggravated.

DRUG INTERACTIONS

Other drugs known to potentiate ADH, such as **chlorpropamide, clofibrate,** and **carbamazepine,** may potentiate the antidiuretic effects of posterior pituitary hormones.

ADVERSE REACTIONS

Facial pallor, increased GI activity, and uterine cramps are common. Tinnitus, anxiety, proteinuria, unconsciousness, eclamptic attacks, mydriasis, amaurosis (blindness), and diarrhea have been reported.

DOSAGE

Give by injection, preferably IM. The usual subcutaneous or IM dose is 10 units, with a range of 5 to 20 units.

NURSING IMPLICATIONS

HISTORY
See Appendix 4.

PHYSICAL ASSESSMENT
Obtain blood pressure, pulse, and respirations.
Postoperative ileus: Auscultate bowel sounds.

ADMINISTRATION
IM administration is recommended, but injection may be given subcutaneously.

ONGOING ASSESSMENTS AND NURSING MANAGEMENT
Monitor blood pressure, pulse, and respirations q15m or as ordered following administration.
When administering for postoperative ileus,

auscultate bowel sounds q15m. Keep physician informed of therapeutic response because other treatment modalities may be necessary if drug fails to stimulate peristalsis.

Facial pallor, increased GI activity, and uterine cramps are common side-effects; notify physician if these become severe.

Potassium Acid Phosphate Preparations

Potassium Acid Phosphate Rx

tablets: 500 mg   K-Phos Original

Potassium Acid Phosphate and Sodium Acid Phosphate Rx

tablets: 155 mg potassium acid phosphate, 350 mg sodium acid phosphate	K-Phos M.F.
tablets: 305 mg potassium acid phosphate, 700 mg sodium acid phosphate	K-Phos No. 2

INDICATIONS AND ACTIONS
Acidifies urine and lowers urinary calcium concentration. Increases antibacterial activity of methenamine mandelate, methenamine hippurate, and other drugs in which effectiveness is dependent on an acid *p*H. Eliminates odor and turbidity caused by ammoniacal urine. Lowers urinary calcium levels and increases calcification inhibitors urinary phosphate and pyrophosphate, preventing precipitation of calcium deposits in the urinary tract and in rubber goods placed in the urinary tract. Also lowers urinary calcium levels.

CONTRAINDICATIONS
Renal insufficiency, severe hepatic disease, Addison's disease, hyperkalemia.

WARNINGS (POTASSIUM ACID PHOSPHATE)
There have been reports of nonspecific small bowel lesions associated with administration of enteric-coated thiazides with potassium salts. These lesions may occur with enteric-coated potassium tablets alone or when they are used with non–enteric coated thiazides or certain other oral diuretics.

These lesions have caused obstruction, hemorrhage, and perforation. Use is discontinued immediately if abdominal pain, distention, nausea, vomiting, or GI bleeding occurs.

PRECAUTIONS (POTASSIUM ACID PHOSPHATE AND SODIUM ACID PHOSPHATE)
Caution is exercised if patient is on a sodium-restricted diet.

ADVERSE REACTIONS

POTASSIUM ACID PHOSPHATE
Some patients may experience a mild laxative effect, which usually subsides with dosage reduction. Hyperacidity and nausea may also occur.

POTASSIUM ACID PHOSPHATE AND SODIUM ACID PHOSPHATE
Nausea, vomiting, diarrhea, hyperacidity, and abdominal discomfort may occur. Laxative effect will usually subside with dosage reduction. If laxation persists, use is discontinued.

DOSAGE

POTASSIUM ACID PHOSPHATE
1 g dissolved in 180 ml to 240 ml water qid with meals and H.S.

POTASSIUM ACID PHOSPHATE AND SODIUM ACID PHOSPHATE
One to two tablets qid with a full glass of water. When urine is difficult to acidify, one tablet q2h.

NURSING IMPLICATIONS

HISTORY
See Appendix 4.

PHYSICAL ASSESSMENT
Urinalysis, urinary calcium, and other laboratory tests may be ordered, depending on reason for use.

ADMINISTRATION
POTASSIUM ACID PHOSPHATE
Dissolve dose (usually 2 tablets) in 180 ml to 240 ml water. For best results, soak in cold water for 2 to 5 minutes, then stir vigorously and administer. Drug is prepared immediately before administration.

POTASSIUM ACID PHOSPHATE AND SODIUM ACID PHOSPHATE
Give with full glass of water.

ONGOING ASSESSMENTS AND NURSING MANAGEMENT
Observe for adverse reactions. If nausea, vomiting, or diarrhea occurs, notify physician because

P

dosage reduction may be necessary. If these persist, discontinuation of drug is usually necessary.

Physician may order daily urinary *p*H measurement with reagent strips. If urine fails to maintain an acid *p*H, inform physician.

CLINICAL ALERT: If administration of **potassium acid phosphate** produces abdominal pain, distention, nausea, vomiting, or signs of GI bleeding, withhold next dose and notify physician immediately.

PATIENT AND FAMILY INFORMATION

NOTE: Physician may wish patient to check urinary *p*H daily with test strips; patient will require instructions in use of strips and interpretation of results.

POTASSIUM ACID PHOSPHATE

Soak prescribed number of tablets in 6 oz to 8 oz cold water for 2 to 5 minutes; then stir vigorously and drink. Discontinue use and contact physician immediately if abdominal pain or distention, nausea, vomiting, or black stools occur.

POTASSIUM ACID PHOSPHATE AND SODIUM ACID PHOSPHATE

Take with full glass of water.

Drug may produce a laxative effect. If this persists or diarrhea is severe, notify physician or nurse.

Potassium Citrate and Citric Acid Rx

syrup: 1100 mg potassium citrate, 334 mg citric acid/ 5 ml   Polycitra-K

INDICATIONS

A urinary alkalinizing agent useful when administration of sodium salts is undesirable or contraindicated.

CONTRAINDICATIONS

Severe renal impairment with anuria, oliguria, or azotemia; untreated Addison's disease, familial periodic paralysis; acute dehydration; heat cramps; severe myocardial damage; hyperkalemia from any cause.

PRECAUTIONS

Used with caution in those with low urinary output. Dilute with water to minimize possibility of gastrointestinal injury associated with oral ingestion of concentrated potassium salt preparations. Large doses may cause hyperkalemia and alkalosis, especially in presence of renal disease.

ADVERSE REACTIONS

Hyperkalemia or alkalosis may occur.

DOSAGE

Dilute in water, followed by additional water, if desired.

Usual dosage range: 15 ml to 20 ml qid usually maintains a urinary *p*H of 7.0 to 7.6. A dosage of 10 ml to 15 ml qid usually maintains a urinary *p*H of 6.5 to 7.4. Dose is titrated to achieve desired urinary *p*H.

Children: 5 ml to 15 ml diluted with ½ glass of water, P.C. and H.S.

NURSING IMPLICATIONS

HISTORY

See Appendix 4.

PHYSICAL ASSESSMENT

Urinalysis and other laboratory tests may be ordered, depending on reason for use.

ADMINISTRATION

Drug preferably given after meals to avoid saline laxative effect.

To minimize possibility of gastrointestinal injury associated with oral ingestion of concentrated potassium salt preparations, dilute prescribed dose with 6 oz or more cold water (cold water enhances palatability).

Have patient drink additional (chilled) water (preferably 4 oz or more) after taking medication.

ONGOING ASSESSMENTS AND NURSING MANAGEMENT

Physician may order daily urinary *p*H with reagent tests strips to monitor effect of drug on urine *p*H.

Observe for signs of hyperkalemia (Appendix 6, section 6-15).

If diarrhea occurs because of drug's possible laxative effect, notify physician.

CLINICAL ALERT: If administration produces abdominal pain, distention, nausea, vomiting, or signs of GI bleeding, withhold next dose and notify physician immediately.

Periodic serum electrolytes may be ordered for those with renal disease.

PATIENT AND FAMILY INFORMATION

NOTE: Physician may wish patient to check urinary *p*H daily with test strips; patient will require instructions in use of strips, interpreting results.

Drug must be diluted with water; 6 oz or more for adults and 4 oz for children.

Use chilled water for dilution to enhance taste. Follow with 4 oz or more of chilled water.

Notify physician or nurse immediately if abdominal distention and/or pain, nausea, vomiting, or black stools occurs, or if diarrhea occurs and persists for more than 1 day.

Potassium Citrate and Sodium Citrate Rx

tablets: 50 mg potassium citrate, 950 mg sodium citrate	Citrolith
syrup: 500 mg potassium citrate, 500 mg sodium citrate, 334 mg citric acid/ 5 ml	Polycitra, Polycitra-LC

INDICATIONS
Used to alkalinize urine in those with uric acid and cystine calculi of the GU tract. Also administered with uricosuric agents in gout therapy (urates tend to crystallize out of acid) and to correct acidosis in renal tubular disorders.

CONTRAINDICATIONS
Severe renal impairment with oliguria or azotemia; untreated Addison's disease; severe myocardial damage.

ACTIONS
Potassium and sodium citrate are absorbed and metabolized to bicarbonates, acting as systemic alkalinizers.

PRECAUTIONS
Use with caution in those with low urinary output and renal insufficiency and in those with cardiac failure, hypertension, peripheral and pulmonary edema, toxemia of pregnancy, or sodium-restricted diets.

DRUG INTERACTIONS
Concurrent administration of **potassium-containing medication, potassium-sparing diuretics,** or **cardiac glycosides** may lead to toxicity.

ADVERSE REACTIONS
Use with caution in those with abnormal renal mechanisms to avoid development of hyperkalemia or alkalosis, especially in the presence of hypocalcemia.

OVERDOSAGE
Sodium salts may cause diarrhea, nausea, vomiting, hypernoia, and convulsions. Potassium salts may cause hyperkalemia and alkalosis, especially in the presence of renal disease.

DOSAGE
Liquids: 15 ml to 20 ml qid usually maintains a urinary pH of 7.0 to 7.6 throughout 24 hours. Dosage of 10 ml to 15 ml qid will usually maintain a urinary pH of 6.5 to 7.4. _Adults_—15 ml to 30 ml diluted with water, after meals and before H.S. _Children_—5 ml to 15 ml diluted with water, after meals and before H.S.

Tablets: One to four tablets with a full glass of water, after meals and H.S.

NURSING IMPLICATIONS

HISTORY
See Appendix 4.

PHYSICAL ASSESSMENT
Urinalysis, urinary calcium, and other laboratory tests may be ordered, depending on reason for use.

ADMINISTRATION
Dilute adult liquid dose with 6 oz or more of chilled water; dilute children's dose with 3 oz to 4 oz of water.

Tablets are taken with a full glass of water.

Administer immediately after meals and with food H.S. to minimize GI upset.

ONGOING ASSESSMENTS AND NURSING MANAGEMENT
Physician may order daily urinary pH measurement with reagent tests strips to monitor effect of drug on urine pH.

Notify physician immediately if diarrhea, nausea, abdominal pain, vomiting, or signs of hyperkalemia (Appendix 6, section 6-15) or hypernatremia (Appendix 6, section 6-17) are noted.

PATIENT AND FAMILY INFORMATION
Dilute with chilled water (6 oz or more adult; 3–4 oz children).

Take immediately after meals and with food at bedtime.

Notify physician or nurse immediately if diarrhea, nausea, stomach pain, or vomiting occurs.

Potassium Iodide

See Iodine Expectorants; Iodine Thyroid Products.

P

Potassium Replacement Products, Oral Rx

Liquids

10 mEq/15 ml (5% KCl)	Generic
20 mEq/15 ml (10% KCl)	Cena-K, Kaochlor 10% (contains tartrazine), Kaochlor S-F, Kay Ciel, Klor-10%, Klorvess 10%, Potachlor 10%, Potasalan, Potassine, SK-Potassium Chloride, Generic
30 mEq/15 ml (15% KCl)	Rum-K
40 mEq/15 ml (20% KCl)	Kaon-Cl 20%, Klor-Con (contains tartrazine), Potachlor 20%, SK-Potassium Chloride, Generic
20 mEq/15 ml (as potassium gluconate)	Bayon, Kaon (contains tartrazine), Kaylixir, K-G Elixir, Generic
20 mEq/15 ml (as potassium gluconate & citrate)	Bi-K, Twin-K
15 mEq potassium & 4 mEq chloride/15 ml	Twin-K-Cl
20 mEq potassium & 3.4 mEq chloride/ 15 ml	Duo-K, Kolyum
45 mEq/15 ml potassium (from potassium acetate, bicarbonate, citrate)	Trikates, Tri-K

Powders

15 mEq KCl/packet	K-Lor
20 mEq KCl/packet	Kato, Kay Ciel, K-Lor, Klor-Con, Potage, Generic
25 mEq KCl/packet	Klor-Con/25
25 mEq KCl/dose	K-Lyte/Cl
20 mEq each potassium & chloride/ packet	Klorvess Effervescent Granules
20 mEq potassium & 3.4 mEq chloride/ packet	Kolyum

Effervescent tablets

20 mEq potassium & chloride	Kaochlor-Eff (contains tartrazine), Klorvess
25 mEq potassium & chloride	K-Lyte/Cl
50 mEq potassium & chloride	K-Lyte/Cl 50
25 mEq potassium	K-Lyte
50 mEq potassium	K-Lyte DS

Tablets (plain, unless stated otherwise)

2.5 mEq potassium gluconate	Kao-Nor
5 mEq potassium gluconate	Kaon
enteric coated: 4 mEq KCl	Generic
enteric coated: 13.4 mEq KCl	Generic
wax matrix: 6.7 mEq KCl	Kaon-Cl
wax matrix: 8 mEq KCl	Slow-K
wax matrix: 10 mEq KCl	Kaon Cl-10, Klotrix, K-Tab
chewable: 2.5 mEq potassium (from gluconate, chloride, citrate)	K-Forte Maximum Strength
chewable: 1 mEq potassium (from chloride, citrate, gluconate)	K-Forte Regular, Osto-K

Capsules

controlled release: 8 mEq potassium chloride	Micro-K

INDICATIONS

Therapeutic: Hypokalemia with or without severe or persistent metabolic alkalosis; in surgical conditions accompanied by nitrogen loss and suction drainage; in starvation and debilitation; loss of potassium due to vomiting and diarrhea; increased renal excretion of potassium due to acidosis, diuresis, or certain cases of uremia; injection of potassium-free fluids that increase extracellular fluid volume; increase glucose uptake by cells such as occurs in diabetic acidosis treated with insulin; corticosteroid therapy or adrenal cortical hyperactivity; low dietary intake of potassium after overdoses of desoxycorticosterone or ACTH therapy; cardiac arrhythmias due to digitalis intoxication; hypokalemic familial periodic paralysis. When hypokalemia is associated with alkalosis, KCl should be used. When acidosis is present, the bicarbonate, citrate, acetate, or gluconate potassium salts should be used.

Prophylactic: Prevention of potassium depletion when dietary intake is inadequate in the following: patients receiving digitalis and diuretics for CHF;

hepatic cirrhosis with ascites; states of aldosterone excess with normal renal function; potassium-losing nephropathy; certain diarrheal states. Use of potassium salts in those receiving diuretics for uncomplicated essential hypertension is often unnecessary when patient has a normal dietary pattern. Serum potassium should be checked periodically; if hypokalemia occurs, dietary supplementation with potassium-containing foods may be adequate to control milder cases. In more severe cases, supplementation with potassium salts may be needed.

Because of reports of intestinal and gastric ulceration and bleeding with slow-release KCl preparations, these drugs should be reserved for those who cannot tolerate or refuse to take liquids or effervescent potassium preparations or for those in whom there is a problem of compliance with these preparations.

CONTRAINDICATIONS

Severe renal impairment with oliguria, anuria, or azotemia; untreated Addison's disease; hyperkalemic familial periodic paralysis; acute dehydration; heat cramps. Potassium intensifies symptoms of myotonia congenita. Potassium should not be given to patients receiving potassium-sparing diuretics (spironolactone, triamterene, amiloride) or aldosterone-inhibiting agents. Contraindicated in those with hyperkalemia because further increase in potassium can produce cardiac arrest. Hyperkalemia may complicate any of the following: chronic renal failure, systemic acidosis such as diabetic acidosis, acute dehydration, extensive tissue breakdown as in severe burns, adrenal insufficiency.

Wax-matrix preparations have produced esophageal ulceration in certain cardiac patients with esophageal compression due to enlarged left atrium. All solid dosage forms of potassium supplements are contraindicated in any patients in whom there is a cause for arrest or delay in tablet passage through the GI tract. When indicated in such patients, the liquid form is recommended.

ACTIONS

Potassium ion is principal intracellular cation of most body tissues. Potassium ions participate in a number of essential physiologic processes, including maintaining intracellular tonicity, and a proper relationship with sodium across cell membranes, cellular metabolism, transmission of nerve impulses, contraction of cardiac, skeletal and smooth muscles, acid–base balance, and maintenance of normal renal function. Normal potassium serum levels range from 3.5 mEq/liter to 5.0 mEq/liter.

Potassium concentration in extracellular fluid is normally 4 mEq/liter to 5 mEq/liter; that in intracellular fluid is approximately 150 mEq/liter.

Changes in plasma potassium concentration often mirror those in cellular potassium content; plasma concentration provides a useful guide to disturbances in potassium balance. By producing large differences in the ratio of intracellular to extracellular potassium, relatively small absolute changes in extracellular concentration may have important effects on neuromuscular activity.

Despite wide variations in dietary intake of potassium, plasma potassium concentration is normally stabilized with a narrow range of 4 mEq/liter to 5 mEq/liter. Renal potassium excretion is accomplished largely by a process of potassium secretion in the distal portion of the nephron, essentially all filtered potassium is reabsorbed by the proximal tubule, and potassium that appears in the urine is added to the filtrate by a distal process of sodiumcation exchange. Fecal excretion is minimal and does not play a significant role in potassium homeostasis.

Natural potassium sources: Foods rich in potassium include beef, veal, ham, chicken, turkey, fish, shellfish, milk, bananas, dates, prunes, raisins, avocado, watermelon, molasses, beans, yams, broccoli, brussel sprouts, lentils, potatoes, and spinach.

Hypokalemia: May occur whenever rate of potassium loss through renal excretion and/or loss through the GI tract exceeds rate of potassium intake. Such depletion usually occurs slowly as a consequence of prolonged therapy with oral diuretics, primary or secondary hyperaldosteronism, diabetic ketoacidosis, severe diarrhea, especially if associated with vomiting, or inadequate replacement of potassium in patients on prolonged parenteral nutrition. Potassium deficiency due to these causes is usually accompanied by a concomitant deficiency of chloride and manifested by hypokalemia and metabolic alkalosis. See Appendix 6, section 6-15 for symptoms of hypokalemia.

Hypokalemic metabolic alkalosis: Potassium depletion is managed by correcting the fundamental causes of the deficiency when possible and administering supplemental potassium chloride; potassium-containing foods and nonchloride potassium salts are *not* effective in such cases.

Metabolic acidosis and hyperchloremia: In rare circumstances (*e.g.,* those with renal tubular acidosis), potassium depletion may be associated with metabolic acidosis and hyperchloremia. In such patients, potassium replacement should be accomplished with potassium salts other than the chloride, such as potassium bicarbonate, citrate, acetate, or gluconate.

WARNINGS

Hyperkalemia: In those with impaired mechanisms for excreting potassium, the administration of potassium salts can produce death through hyperkalemia, or cardiac depression or arrest. This occurs more commonly in patients given IV potassium but may also occur when potassium is given orally. Potentially fatal hyperkalemia can develop rapidly and be asymptomatic.

In response to a rise in concentration of body potassium, renal excretion of the ion is increased. With normal kidney function, it is difficult to produce potassium intoxication by oral administration. However, potassium supplements must be given with caution, because the amount of deficiency and corresponding daily dose is unknown. Frequent checks of the patient's clinical status and periodic ECG and/or serum potassium levels are recommended. This is particularly important in those receiving digitalis and in patients with cardiac disease. There is a hazard in giving potassium in digitalis intoxication manifested by atrioventricular conduction disturbance.

Renal impairment: Use of potassium salts in those with chronic renal disease or any other condition which impairs potassium excretion requires close monitoring of serum potassium concentration and appropriate dosage adjustment.

Gastrointestinal lesions: Potassium chloride tablets have produced stenotic and/or ulcerative lesions of the small bowel and deaths. These lesions are caused by a high localized concentration of the potassium ion in the region of the rapidly dissolving tablet, which injures the bowel wall and thereby produces obstruction, hemorrhage, and perforation. The reported frequency is much less with wax-matrix tablets than with enteric-coated tablets, but cases associated with wax-matrix tablets have been reported. Wax-matrix tablets release potassium in the stomach; there have been reports of upper GI bleeding associated with these products. Either type of tablet should be discontinued immediately and possibility of bowel obstruction or perforation considered if severe vomiting, abdominal pain, or GI bleeding occurs.

PRECAUTIONS

Hypokalemia: Diagnosis of potassium depletion is made by demonstrating hypokalemia in a patient with a clinical history suggesting some cause for potassium depletion. Acute acidosis can increase serum potassium concentration into the normal range, even in the presence of reduced total body potassium. Administration of concentrated dextrose or sodium bicarbonate may cause intracellular potassium shift, causing hypokalemia, which may lead to cardiac arrhythmias and deaths. In hypokalemic states, attention is directed toward correction of frequently associated hypochloremic alkalosis.

Tartrazine sensitivity: Some of these products contain tartrazine. See Appendix 6, section 6-23.

DRUG INTERACTIONS

Hypokalemia should not be treated by prolonged administration of potassium salts and a **potassium-sparing diuretic,** because continued administration of these agents can produce severe hyperkalemia. Caution is exercised in those receiving **aldosterone antagonists.** Concurrent administration of potassium supplements in those using **salt substitutes** may promote accumulation of potassium and lead to hyperkalemia. In digitalized patients with severe or complete heart block, concurrent use of potassium salts is not recommended with **digitalis glycosides.**

ADVERSE REACTIONS

Most common: Nausea, vomiting, diarrhea, abdominal discomfort. These symptoms are due to irritation of the GI tract and best managed by diluting the preparation further, taking dose with meals, or reducing the dose. Skin rash reported rarely.

Most severe: Hyperkalemia and GI obstruction, bleeding, or perforation.

OVERDOSAGE

Potassium intoxication may result from overdosage of potassium salts or therapeutic dosage in conditions stated under *Contraindications.* When detected, hyperkalemia must be treated immediately; lethal levels can be reached in a few hours.

Clinical manifestations

Neuromuscular: Paresthesias and weakness of extremities and flaccid paralysis, usually indistinguishable from that seen in hypokalemic paralysis, appear only in association with severe hyperkalemia; listlessness; mental confusion; weakness and heaviness of the legs; muscle weakness; hypotension; cardiac depression; cardiac arrhythmias; cardiac arrest; heart block. Death may occur from cardiac arrest before muscular weakness is evident. For this reason, the ECG is the single most important guide in appraising the threat posed by the hyperkalemia and determining therapeutic approach.

ECG effects: ECG abnormalities are the earliest and most frequent sign of disturbed membrane excitability. Changes usually appear when serum potassium concentration reaches 7 mEq/liter to 8 mEq/liter; cardiac standstill is likely to occur at a concentration of 9 mEq/liter to 10 mEq/liter. Abnormalities include early development of tall "tent-shaped" T-waves (particularly in right precordial leads); decreased amplitude of R-waves; deepening of the S-wave; P-wave widens and decreases in amplitude until it disappears; occasionally, an apparent elevation of the RS–T junction and a cove plane RS–T segment and T-wave will be noted in AVL, and later by atrial asystole. Intraventricular block, with widening of the QRS complex, may lead to development of a sine wave and ultimately to ventricular standstill.

Treatment of hyperkalemia

1. Dextrose solution, 10% or 25%, containing 10 to 50 units regular insulin per 20 g dextrose, given IV in a dose of 300 ml to 500 ml in an hour.
2. Use of sodium cycle cation-exchange resin (sodium polystyrene sulfonate) given PO, by retention enema, or by both routes to remove potassium from the body. *Caution*—Ammonium compounds are not used in those with hepatic cirrhosis.
3. To enhance potassium loss and assure rapid movement of the resin through the GI tract, administer sorbitol in quantities sufficient to induce a soft or semiliquid bowel movement every few hours. Usual dose of sorbitol 70% solution is 20 ml tid or qid. If patient is unable to take PO, administer by rectum as a retention enema of 100 g in several hundred milliliters of water.
4. Hemodialysis or peritoneal dialysis.
5. Use of potassium-containing foods and medications must be eliminated. In cases of digitalization, a too rapidly lowering plasma potassium concentration can cause digitalis toxicity.
6. Acidosis, if present, should be corrected with IV sodium bicarbonate.
7. Parenteral calcium may be used to combat the cardiotoxicity of hyperkalemia. Calcium cannot be given in the same solution with sodium bicarbonte because precipitation of the calcium ion will occur.

DOSAGE

Usual average adult dietary intake of potassium varies with dietary habits and usually ranges between 40 mEq/day and 150 mEq/day. Potassium depletion sufficient to cause hypokalemia usually requires a loss of 200 mEq or more of potassium from the total body store. Dosage must be adjusted to individual needs but is typically in the range of 16 mEq/day to 24 mEq/day for prevention of hypokalemia to 40 mEq/day to 100 mEq/day or more for treatment of potassium depletion.

NURSING IMPLICATIONS

HISTORY
See Appendix 4.

PHYSICAL ASSESSMENT
When used to correct hypokalemia, look for signs of hypokalemia (Appendix 6, section 6-15). Serum potassium is usually ordered; other baseline tests may include serum chloride, ECG, renal-function tests.

ADMINISTRATION
May cause GI upset. Administer immediately after meals or with food and with a full glass of water.

Check physician's order carefully with label of preparation because some trade names are similar (*e.g.,* Kaochlor 10%, Kaochlor S-F, Kaochlor-Eff).

Tablets: Do not crush.

Instruct patient not to chew tablet but to swallow whole immediately and take with a full glass of water.

If there is doubt whether patient is swallowing tablet immediately, check oral cavity. Tablet should not be allowed to dissolve in the mouth.

If patient has difficulty swallowing tablet, contact physician; another form (liquid, effervescent tablet, powder) may be ordered.

Liquids, soluble powders, effervescent tablets: Mix or dissolve completely in 4 oz to 8 oz of cold water, juice, or other beverage.

Effervescent tablets should stop fizzing before liquid is swallowed.

Advise patient that solution may have a salty taste.

Instruct patient to sip slowly over 5 to 10 minute period.

Some of the powders and effervescent tablets have a flavoring, which makes the solution more palatable.

If administered via nasogastric tube, dilute in same manner as for oral administration.

If patient refuses to take drug because of taste or other reason, contact physician. A more palatable form may be tried.

ONGOING ASSESSMENTS AND NURSING MANAGEMENT
Monitor blood pressure, pulse, and respirations q4h (especially during initiation of therapy) or as ordered.

CLINICAL ALERT: Potassium intoxication may result from any therapeutic dosage. When detected, hyperkalemia must be treated *immediately* because lethal levels can be reached in a few hours.

Patients likely to develop hyperkalemia include those with compromised renal function (which also includes elderly patients).

Observe for signs of hyperkalemia (Appendix 6, section 6-15), especially mental confusion, listlessness, weakness and heaviness of the extremities, muscle weakness, hypotension, and cardiac arrhythmias. Paresthesias and weakness of the extremities and flaccid paralysis (usually indistinguishable from that seen in hypokalemic paralysis) appear only when hyperkalemia is severe.

Notify physician immediately of these or any other complaints expressed by the patient. Serum potassium and ECG may be necessary to determine whether hyperkalemia is present.

Notify physician immediately if severe vomiting, abdominal pain or distention, or evidence of GI bleeding (hematemesis, tarry stools) is noted because these may be symptoms of a gastrointestinal lesion (see *Warnings*).

When patient is receiving therapeutic potassium replacement (see *Indications*), it is necessary to observe for signs of hypokalemia (Appendix 6, section 6-15) because potassium supplementation may not be sufficient to correct the deficiency.

PATIENT AND FAMILY INFORMATION

NOTE: It may be advisable that a family member of an elderly patient, when possible, be responsible for measuring/preparing and administering doses of potassium when there is a question of patient compliance.

Take exactly as directed. Do not increase the dose or skip doses except on advice of a physician.

Medication may cause GI upset (nausea, vomiting, diarrhea). Take immediately after meals or with food and a full glass of water.

Enteric-coated tablets: Do not crush or chew tablets or allow to dissolve in mouth. Tablet must be swallowed whole with a full glass of water.

Effervescent tablets: Place in 4 oz to 8 oz cold water or juice; wait until fizzing stops before drinking. Sip slowly over 5- to 10-minute period.

Oral liquids: Add to 4 oz to 8 oz cold water or juice; sip slowly over 5- to 10-minute period.

Wax-matrix tablets: Swallow whole (do not chew) with a full glass of water. The wax matrix is not absorbed and will be found in the stool.

Powders: Mix in full glass of cold water; stir thoroughly until dissolved; sip over 5- to 10-minute period.

Follow recommendation of physician about time of day when this, as well as other medications, should be taken.

Do not use salt substitutes except on advice of a physician. Do not use nonprescription drugs except on advice of physician (some may contain potassium).

If physician prescribes diet high in potassium, follow prescribed diet as to type of foods and suggested amounts. (*Note*—A list of potassium-rich foods (see *Actions,* above) may be given to the patient.)

Notify physician or nurse immediately if tingling of the hands and feet, unusual tiredness or weakness, a feeling of heaviness in the legs, severe nausea, vomiting, abdominal pain, or black stools occur.

If unable to take drug for any reason, contact physician.

Physician may order periodic laboratory tests to monitor therapy. Keep all laboratory appointments because it is important that these tests be performed at periodic intervals.

Potassium Salts, Parenteral Rx

Potassium Acetate

40 mEq/20 ml	*Generic*
120 mEq/30 ml (for additive use only after dilution)	*Generic*

Potassium Chloride

10 mEq/5 ml	*Generic*
20 mEq/10 ml	*Generic*
30 mEq/12.5 ml, 15 ml, 20 ml, or 30 ml	*Generic*
40 mEq/12.5 ml or 20 ml	*Generic*
60 mEq/30 ml or 60 ml	*Generic*
90 mEq/30 ml	*Generic*
1000 mEq/500 ml (for prescription compounding of IV admixtures)	*Generic*

INDICATIONS

When oral therapy is not feasible, parenteral therapy is indicated in prevention and correction of moderate or severe potassium deficit (see also *Indications* under Potassium Replacement Products, Oral). Also indicated in treatment of cardiac arrhythmias, especially those due to digitalis.

CONTRAINDICATIONS

Conditions predisposing the patient to increased serum levels or decreased renal excretion of potassium (see also *Contraindications* under Potassium Replacement Products, Oral).

ACTIONS

See Potassium Replacement Products, Oral.

WARNINGS

To avoid potassium intoxication, do not rapidly infuse parenteral solutions containing potassium chloride. In addition to ECG effects, irritation to veins has resulted when a potassium concentration greater than 40 mEq/liter was infused into peripheral veins or larger central veins. Concentrated solutions of potassium are for IV admixtures only and must not be used for direct injection. Direct injection may be instantaneously fatal.

When serum sodium or calcium concentration is reduced, moderate elevation of serum potassium may cause toxic effects to the heart and skeletal muscle. Weakness and later paralysis of voluntary muscles, with consequent respiratory distress and difficulty swallowing, are generally late signs, sometimes significantly preceding dangerous or even fatal cardiac toxicity.

Use of potassium chloride in renal impairment or adrenal insufficiency may cause potassium intoxication. In those with impaired mechanisms for excreting potassium, administration of potassium salts can produce hyperkalemia and cardiac arrest. Potentially fatal hyperkalemia can develop rapidly and be asymptomatic. Hypokalemia associated with metabolic acidosis is treated with an alkalinizing potassium salt (_e.g._, potassium bicarbonate, citrate, or acetate).

PRECAUTIONS

Close supervision with frequent ECGs and serum potassium determinations is recommended as guide for parenteral potassium therapy. Plasma potassium levels are not necessarily indicative of tissue potassium levels.

Potassium is used with caution in the presence of cardiac disease, particularly in digitalized patients.

High concentrations of potassium may cause death through cardiac depression, arrhythmias, or arrest.

Normal kidney function permits safe potassium therapy. Rapid infusion of an initial hydrating solution (such as 5% Dextrose in 0.2% Sodium Chloride) until diuresis is established should precede potassium administration. Temporary elevation of serum potassium level due to renal insufficiency secondary to dehydration or shock may mask an intracellular potassium deficit; potassium replacement is not attempted until renal function has been reestablished by overcoming dehydration and shock. Administration of potassium-containing solutions should be discontinued if signs of renal insufficiency develop during such infusions.

DRUG INTERACTIONS

There is a hazard in prescribing potassium in **digitalis** intoxication manifested by atrioventricular conduction disturbance. In digitalized patients with severe or complete heart block, do not use potassium salts.

Concomitant use of **potassium-sparing diuretics** (spironolactone, triamterene, or amiloride) can produce severe hyperkalemia.

ADVERSE REACTIONS

Nausea, vomiting, abdominal pain, and diarrhea have been reported. Hyperkalemia may occur. Local tissue necrosis and sloughing may result if extravasation occurs. Chemical phlebitis and venospasm have also been reported. Potassium solutions of 30 mEq/liter to 40 mEq/liter concentration may cause pain at the injection site or phlebitis. Should perivascular infiltration occur, discontinue IV administration at that site. Local infiltration of the affected area with 1% procaine HCl, to which hyaluronidase may be added, will often reduce venospasm and dilute the potassium remaining in local tissues. Local application of heat may also be helpful.

OVERDOSAGE

Symptoms: See Potassium Replacement Products, Oral.

Treatment: Terminate potassium administration. Monitor ECG. Infusion of 150 ml of 1 molar sodium lactate or combined glucose and insulin in a ratio of 5 g of glucose to 1 unit of regular insulin may be given to shift potassium into cells. Administer sodium bicarbonate 50 mEq to 100 mEq IV to reverse acidosis and also to produce an intracellular shift. Give 10 ml to 100 ml of calcium gluconate 10% to reverse ECG changes. To remove potassium from the body, use sodium polystyrene sulfonate resin, hemodialysis, or peritoneal dialysis. In digitalized patients, too-rapid lowering of serum potassium can cause digitalis toxicity.

DOSAGE

Must be diluted; administer by slow IV infusion. Usual additive dilution is 40 mEq/liter of IV fluid. A concentration of 80 mEq/liter is usually considered the maximum desirable concentration; extreme emergencies may require greater concentrations. Dosage and infusion rate depend on condition of patient and must be guided by serial ECG and serum electrolyte determinations (Table 42).

NURSING IMPLICATIONS

HISTORY
See Appendix 4.

Table 42. Recommended Dosages and Infusion Rates Based on Serum Potassium Ion Levels

Serum K+	Maximum Infusion Rate	Maximum Concentration	Maximum 24-hour Dosage
>2.5 mEq/liter	10 mEq/hour	40 mEq/liter	200 mEq
<2.0 mEq/liter	40 mEq/hour	80 mEq/liter	400 mEq

PHYSICAL ASSESSMENT

Look for signs of hypokalemia (Appendix 6, section 6-15) if used to correct potassium deficit. Baseline laboratory tests usually include serum potassium, serum chloride, ECG, and renal-function tests.

ADMINISTRATION

Check most recent serum potassium determination. If within normal range, check with physician about administration of potassium. Decision to contact physician is based on when last serum potassium was obtained, etiology of hypokalemia, amount of potassium previously administered, rationale for potassium administration (*e.g.,* therapeutic or prophylactic), and other factors. If in doubt, always check with the physician before administering potassium.

CLINICAL ALERT: Parenteral potassium preparations *must* be diluted with a large volume of parenteral solution, usually 500 ml or 1000 ml. Physician orders dose (in mEq), volume of IV solution, and rate of infusion.

Parenteral potassium is *never* given IM, subcutaneously, or by IV push. Direct IV injection (*e.g.,* undiluted) may be instantaneously fatal.

The usual additive dilution of potassium chloride is 40 mEq/1000 ml IV solution. Maximum concentration is usually 80 mEq/1000 ml, but in extreme emergencies larger concentrations may be ordered.

Generally, dextrose solutions are used for administration. In critical states, saline may be used (unless saline is contraindicated), because dextrose may lower serum potassium levels.

Gently rotate IV container to ensure even dispersion of drug.

A large vein should be used for administration. Avoid using small veins on back of hand. An IV infusion pump may be used to ensure a steady rate of infusion.

ONGOING ASSESSMENTS AND NURSING MANAGEMENT

CLINICAL ALERT: High plasma concentrations of potassium may cause death through cardiac depression, arrhythmias, or arrest. Observe for signs of hyperkalemia (Appendix 6, section 6-15); notify physician immediately if hyperkalemia or adverse reactions are apparent.

Infusion rate is ordered by physician (as drops/minute or as mEq/hour). Check infusion rate q10m to q15m (more frequently if patient is restless) and adjust as necessary to administer dosage within the prescribed time interval.

An IV containing potassium should infuse in no less than approximately 3 to 4 hours. Notify the physician immediately if the IV infusion is completed in less than the prescribed infusion time.

Measure intake and output. Report any decrease in urinary output to the physician immediately, because it may be an indication of renal insufficiency. Administration of potassium-containing solutions should be discontinued if signs of renal insufficiency develop during such infusions.

Monitor blood pressure, pulse, and respirations q½h to q1h or as ordered. Slow infusion to KVO and contact physician immediately if arrhythmia is noted. Physician may order IV discontinued and patient placed on a cardiac monitor.

Potassium-containing solutions are irritating to tissues. Check IV infusion site q10m to q15m for signs of extravasation. Local tissue necrosis and subsequent sloughing may result if extravasation occurs. If extravasation is noted, discontinue IV immediately (remove needle or catheter) and contact physician. Physician may order local infiltration of the affected area with 1% procaine HCl to which hyaluronidase has been added. Local application of heat may also be ordered.

Physician adjusts dosage and rate of infusion depending on serum potassium level and ECG. Blood for serum potassium is drawn from the arm opposite the one used for the IV infusion.

Povidone-Iodine

See Antiseptics and Germicides.

Pralidoxime Chloride (PAM) Rx

tablets: 500 mg   Protopam Chloride
injection: 1 g vial   Protopam Chloride
  (20 ml)

INDICATIONS

Antidote in treatment of poisoning due to those pesticides and chemicals of the organophosphate class that have anticholinesterase activity (dichlorvos, dioxathion, echothiophate iodide, endothion, fenthion, formothion, isoflurophate, malathion, methyl parathion, parathion, TEPP, Diazinon) and in control of overdosage by anticholinesterase drugs used in treatment of myasthenia gravis.

ACTIONS

Principal action is to reactivate cholinesterase (mainly outside the CNS) inactivated by phosphorylation due to an organophosphate pesticide or related compound. Destruction of accumulated acetylcholine can then proceed, allowing neuromuscular junctions to function normally. Also slows process of "aging" of phosphorylated cholinesterase to a nonreactive form and detoxifies certain organophosphates by direct chemical action. Drug has most critical effect in relieving paralysis of respiratory muscles. Because pralidoxime is less effective in relieving depression of the respiratory center, atropine is always required concomitantly to block the effect of accumulated acetylcholine at this site. Pralidoxime relieves muscarinic signs and symptoms (_e.g.,_ salivation, bronchospasm), but this action is relatively unimportant because atropine is adequate for this purpose. It antagonizes the effects on the neuromuscular junction of the carbamate anticholinesterases (neostigmine, pyridostigmine, ambenonium) used in treatment of myasthenia gravis. It is not nearly as effective an antidote to these drugs as it is to the organophosphates.

Pralidoxime is distributed throughout the extracellular water; it is not bound to plasma protein. It is rapidly excreted in the urine. It is relatively short acting, and repeated doses may be needed, especially where there is any evidence of continued absorption of poison.

WARNINGS

Not effective in treatment of poisoning due to phosphorus, inorganic phosphates, or organophosphates having no anticholinesterase activity. Not recommended for use in intoxication by pesticides of the carbamate class.

PRECAUTIONS

Well tolerated in most cases. A decrease in renal function will result in increased drug blood levels; dosage is reduced in the presence of renal insufficiency. Use with caution in treating organophosphate overdosage in cases of myasthenia gravis, because it may precipitate a myasthenic crisis.

DRUG INTERACTIONS

Barbiturates are potentiated by the anticholinesterases; therefore, use with caution in the treatment of convulsions. Use of **morphine, theophylline, aminophylline, succinylcholine, reserpine,** and **phenothiazines** is avoided in those with organophosphate poisoning.

ADVERSE REACTIONS

Dizziness, blurred vision, diplopia and impaired accommodation, headache, drowsiness, nausea, tachycardia, hyperventilation, muscular weakness. It is difficult to differentiate toxic effects produced by atropine or the organophosphate compounds from those of the drug. When atropine and pralidoxime are used together, signs of atropinization may occur earlier than might be expected when atropine is used alone. This is especially true if the total dose of atropine has been large and administration of pralidoxime delayed.

OVERDOSAGE

Administer artificial respiration and other supportive therapy as needed.

DOSAGE

Organophosphate poisoning

Initial measures: Removal of secretions, maintenance of a patent airway, artificial ventilation (if necessary). In absence of cyanosis, give atropine IV in doses of 2 mg to 4 mg. When cyanosis is present, give 2 mg to 4 mg atropine IM while initiating measures to improve ventilation. Repeat every 5 to 10 minutes until signs of atropine toxicity appear. Some degree of atropinization should be maintained for at least 48 hours. Pralidoxime administration should begin concomitantly with atropine.

Adults: Inject initial dose of 1 g to 2 g, preferably as an infusion in 100 ml of saline, over 15 to 30 minutes. If this is not practical or if pulmonary edema is present, give slowly by IV injection as a 5% solution in water over not less than 5 minutes. After about 1 hour, a second dose of 1 g to 2 g will be indicated if muscle weakness is not relieved. Additional doses may be given cautiously if muscle weakness persists. If IV administration is not feasible, IM or subcutaneous injection should be used.

Children: 20 mg/kg/dose to 40 mg/kg/dose given as above.

Treatment will be most effective if given within a few hours after poisoning has occurred. Usually, little will be accomplished if drug is first administered more than 48 hours after exposure, but it is still indicated in severe poisoning because patients have occasionally responded after such intervals. In severe cases, especially after ingestion of the poison, it may be desirable to monitor effect of therapy by ECG because of possibility of heart block due to anticholinesterase. When poison has been ingested, it is important to take into account the likelihood of continuing absorption from the lower bowel, because this constitutes new exposure. In such cases, additional doses may be needed q3h to q8h.

In absence of severe GI symptoms resulting from anticholinesterase intoxication, drug may be given PO in doses of 1 g to 3 g q5h. If convulsions interfere with respiration, sodium thiopental may be given IV.

Anticholinesterase overdosage

As antagonist to anticholinesterases such as neostigmine, pyridostigmine, and ambenonium, give 1 g to 2 g pralidoxime IV followed by increments of 250 mg every 5 minutes.

NURSING IMPLICATIONS

HISTORY

In those with organophosphate poisoning, it will be necessary to obtain the name or contents of the product and method of poisoning (inhaling, swallowing), and (when applicable) to approximate amount of substance ingested. In those with anticholinesterase overdosage, the dosage consumed should be determined, when possible.

PHYSICAL ASSESSMENT

Obtain blood pressure, pulse, and respirations, weight (child); check pupil size; note amount of oral secretions; auscultate lungs; look for muscular fasciculations, muscle paralysis, cyanosis; auscultate bowel sounds; look for loss of bowel or bladder control; generally survey patient for other signs and symptoms. Blood samples for cholinesterase determination may be drawn and sent to a toxicology laboratory.

ADMINISTRATION

Organophosphate poisoning: For initial measures, see *Dosage.* Oxygen may also be ordered.

If product came into contact with the skin, wash skin with copious amounts of soap and water or solution ordered by physician.

Ingested material may be removed by gastric lavage with tap water.

Obtain blood pressure, pulse, and respirations immediately prior to administration.

Initial dose of pralidoxime may be given by IV infusion. Each vial (20 ml) contains 1 g. Recommended dilution is addition of dose to 100 ml of saline, given IV over a period of 15 to 30 minutes.

When pulmonary edema is present, initial dose of pralidoxime may be given by slow IV injection as a 5% solution in water over a period of not less than 5 minutes.

Atropine is given at same time (see *Dosage*). Dose is repeated every 5 to 10 minutes until signs of atropine toxicity appear: flushed skin, dry mucous membranes, dilated pupils, rapid pulse, disorientation, restlessness.

After about 1 hour, a second dose of pralidoxime may be needed.

Drug may also be given PO in absence of severe GI symptoms.

Anticholinesterase overdosage: Initial dose given IV followed by increments of 250 mg every 5 minutes.

ONGOING ASSESSMENTS AND NURSING MANAGEMENT

Monitor blood pressure, pulse, and respirations q5m to q10m or as ordered. Less frequent intervals may be satisfactory once patient responds to therapy.

Observe for response to therapy and abolishment of symptoms. Keep physician informed of patient's response to therapy.

Physician orders subsequent doses of pralidoxime and atropine, based on patient response. Some degree of atropinization is recommended for at least 48 hours.

Measure intake and output; report any change in intake–output ratio to the physician.

When used in treatment of anticholinesterase overdosage (cholinergic crisis) in patient with myasthenia gravis, observe for myasthenic crisis (*e.g.,* extreme muscle weakness, respiratory difficulty), which may occur with overdosage of pralidoxime.

Pramoxine Hydrochloride

See Anesthetics, Local, Topical.

Prazepam

See Benzodiazepines.

Prazosin Hydrochloride Rx

capsules: 1 mg, 2 mg, 5 mg   Minipress

INDICATIONS

Treatment of hypertension. As an antihypertensive drug, it is mild to moderate in activity. Can be used as an initial agent or may be used in a general treatment program in conjunction with a diuretic or other antihypertensive drugs.

ACTIONS

Reduces peripheral resistance and blood pressure via selective blockade of postsynaptic alpha-adrenergic receptors. It dilates both resistance (arterioles) and capacitance (veins) vessels. Blood pressure is lowered in both the supine and standing positions. This effect is more pronounced on diastolic blood pressure. Unlike conventional alpha blockers, prazosin's antihypertensive action is usually not accompanied by reflex tachycardia. Tolerance to the antihypertensive effect has not been observed.

Does not appear to increase renin release as do direct-acting vasodilators; a decrease in plasma renin activity has been reported. Therapeutic lowering of blood pressure occurs without clinically significant changes in cardiac output, renal blood flow, and glomerular filtration rate. Is very effective when used in combination with a thiazide diuretic and/or a beta blocker for treating severe hypertension. Use as a single antihypertensive agent is limited by its tendency to cause sodium and water retention and increased plasma volume, which can compromise efficacy.

Following oral administration, plasma concentrations peak at about 3 hours with a plasma half-life of 2 to 3 hours. Antihypertensive effects persist for a significant period beyond plasma half-life. Drug is highly bound to plasma protein and excreted via bile and feces (more than 90%) and in the urine. Elimination is slower in those with congestive heart failure (CHF). Elimination half-life may be prolonged, protein binding decreased, and peak plasma concentrations increased in chronic renal failure.

Investigational uses: Refractory CHF. Prazosin decreases cardiac afterload (left ventricular systolic wall tension) and preload (left ventricular end-diastolic volume or pressure). By reducing aortic impedance and venous return, it helps improve reduced cardiac output and relieve pulmonary congestion. Has produced improvement in clinical symptoms, exercise tolerance, and functional class. Tolerance to these beneficial effects develops with chronic treatment.

WARNINGS

First-dose effect: May cause syncope with sudden loss of consciousness. In most cases, this is believed to be due to an excessive postural hypotensive effect, although occasionally the syncopal episode has been preceded by severe tachycardia, with a heart rate of 120 to 160/minute. Syncopal episodes have usually occurred within 30 to 90 minutes of the initial dose; occasionally they have been reported in association with rapid dosage increase or introduction of another antihypertensive drug to the regimen of a patient taking a high dose of prazosin.

The cause of this "first-dose phenomenon" is not known. Syncopal episodes are minimized by limiting the initial dose to 1 mg, increasing the dosage slowly, and introducing any additional antihypertensive drugs into the regimen with caution. Hypotension may develop in those who are also receiving a beta blocker. This effect is self-limiting and in most cases does not recur after the initial period of therapy or during subsequent dosage adjustments. More common than loss of consciousness are symptoms often associated with lowering of blood pressure (_e.g.,_ dizziness, lightheadedness).

Safety for use in pregnancy has not been established. Use only when clearly needed and when potential benefits outweigh the unknown potential hazards to the fetus.

DRUG INTERACTIONS

Because drug is highly protein bound, it may theoretically interact with **other highly bound drugs.**

ADVERSE REACTIONS

Most common: Dizziness, headache, drowsiness, lack of energy, weakness, palpitations, nausea. In most instances, side-effects disappear with continued therapy or are tolerated with no decrease in dose of drug.

The following have been associated with prazosin, some of them rarely. In some instances, exact causal relationships were not established.

_GI:_ Vomiting, diarrhea, constipation, abdominal discomfort and/or pain.

Cardiovascular: Edema, dyspnea, syncope, tachycardia, orthostatic hypotension. May aggravate preexisting angina.

CNS: Nervousness, vertigo, depression, paresthesia.

Dermatologic: Rash, pruritus, alopecia, lichen planus.

_GU:_ Urinary frequency, incontinence, impotence, priapism.

EENT: Blurred vision, reddened sclera, epistaxis, tinnitus, dry mouth, nasal congestion.

Other: Diaphoresis. A few cases of drug-induced lupus erythematosus have been reported.

OVERDOSAGE

Treatment: If hypotension occurs, it is of primary importance to support the cardiovascular system. Restore blood pressure and normalize the heart rate by keeping the patient supine. If this is inadequate, treat shock with volume expanders. If necessary, use vasopressors. Monitor and support renal function as needed. Drug is not dialyzable.

DOSAGE

Dosage is adjusted according to blood-pressure response.

Initial dose: 1 mg bid or tid. When increasing unit dosages, it is recommended to give first dose of each increment H.S. (even though total daily dose may not change). This may help reduce syncopal episodes.

Maintenance dose: Dosage may be slowly increased to a total of 20 mg/day given in divided doses. Therapeutic dosages most commonly used have ranged from 6 mg/day to 15 mg/day given in divided doses. Doses higher than 20 mg usually do not increase efficacy, but a few patients may benefit from further increases up to a dosage of 40 mg/day in divided doses. After initial dosage adjustment, some patients can be maintained on a bid dosage regimen.

Concomitant therapy: When a diuretic or another antihypertensive agent is added to regimen, dosage of prazosin is reduced to 1 mg to 2 mg tid and retitration is carried out.

NURSING IMPLICATIONS

HISTORY
See Appendix 4.

PHYSICAL ASSESSMENT
Obtain blood pressure on both arms with patient in standing and supine positions; obtain pulse and respirations, weight (if drug used as sole antihypertensive agent).

ADMINISTRATION
Initial dose: Because of first-dose phenomenon (see *Warnings*), physician may order first dose H.S. If first dose is given during daytime hours, advise patient to remain recumbent for approximately 3 to 4 hours.

Obtain blood pressure on both arms with patient in standing and supine positions, pulse immediately before administration. If a significant decrease in systolic and/or diastolic pressure or rise in pulse rate is noted, withhold drug and contact physician.

If nausea and/or vomiting occurs, check with physician about administration with food or meals.

ONGOING ASSESSMENTS AND NURSING MANAGEMENT
Obtain blood pressure on both arms with patient in standing and supine positions and pulse prior to administration of each dose as well as q4h to q8h. If blood pressure fluctuates significantly during initial dosage period, more frequent determinations may be required. Observe for ad-

verse reactions; report occurrence to physician before next dose is due.

First-dose phenomenon: May be seen 30 to 90 minutes after initial dose. Have patient remain recumbent 3 to 4 hours. Monitor blood pressure and pulse q15m to q30m; report occurrence of phenomenon to physician.

Monitor patient for the first-dose phenomenon each time drug dose is increased or another antihypertensive agent is introduced into the regimen.

Have patient seek assistance with ambulatory activities if dizziness or drowsiness occurs.

PATIENT AND FAMILY INFORMATION
Do not discontinue this drug unless directed by physician.

Take drug at prescribed times of day; do not increase or decrease dose unless instructed to do so by physician.

Do not use cough, cold, allergy, or appetite-control medications (may contain sympathomimetics) except on recommendation of physician.

May cause dizziness, drowsiness, or headache, especially during first few days of therapy. If dizziness (orthostatic hypotension) occurs, avoid sudden changes in posture, rise from a sitting or lying position slowly, and dangle legs for approximately 5 minutes before getting out of bed.

Fainting occasionally occurs after first dose. Do not drive, operate machinery, or engage in other potentially hazardous tasks for 4 hours after first dose. For this reason, physician may prescribe first dose taken at bedtime.

If nausea, vomiting, diarrhea, constipation, or other side-effects occur, notify physician or nurse.

Follow additional recommendations of physician in treatment of hypertension (*e.g.*, limiting sodium intake, weight loss).

Prednisolone

See Corticosteroids, Topical; Glucocorticoids.

Prednisolone Acetate

See Corticosteroids, Ophthalmic; Glucocorticoids.

Prednisolone Acetate and Prednisolone Sodium Phosphate

See Glucocorticoids.

Prednisolone Sodium Phosphate

See Corticosteroids, Ophthalmic; Glucocorticoids.

Prednisolone Tebutate

See Glucocorticoids.

Prednisone

See Glucocorticoids.

Prilocaine Hydrochloride

See Anesthetics, Local, Injectable.

Primaquine Phosphate Rx

tablets: 26.3 mg   *Generic*

INDICATIONS
Radical cure (prevention of relapse) of vivax malaria.

CONTRAINDICATIONS
Concomitant administration of quinacrine and primaquine. Also in the acutely ill suffering from systemic disease manifested by tendency toward granulocytopenia (*e.g.,* rheumatoid arthritis, lupus erythematosus) and during concurrent administration of other potentially hemolytic drugs or depressants of myeloid elements of the bone marrow.

ACTIONS
Primaquine is an 8-aminoquinoline compound structurally similar to the 4-aminoquinoline compounds; however, it possesses markedly different antimalarial activities. It appears to disrupt the parasite's mitochondria through a swelling. The resulting structural changes create a major disruption in the metabolic process and secondarily lead to inhibition of protein synthesis. The gametocyte and exoerythrocyte forms are inhibited; little activity is demonstrated against asexual forms. Some gametocytes are destroyed while others are rendered incapable of undergoing maturation division in the gut of the mosquito. By eliminating tissue (exoerythrocyte) infection, primaquine prevents development of blood (erythrocytic) forms responsible for relapses.

Is active against *Plasmodium vivax, P. ovale,* and the gametocytial forms of *P. falciparum.* Is effectively absorbed from the intestine to produce maximum plasma concentrations in approximately 2 hours. Drug is rapidly metabolized; only about 1% is excreted unchanged in urine.

WARNINGS
Hemolytic reactions (moderate to severe) may occur in the following groups while receiving this drug: G6PD-deficient whites; dark-skinned persons; individuals with idiosyncratic reactions; individuals with nicotinamide adenine dinucleotide (NADH) methemoglobin reductase deficiency. Safety for use during pregnancy has not been established. Use only when clearly needed and when potential benefits outweigh the unknown potential hazards to the fetus.

PRECAUTIONS
Anemia, methemoglobinemia, and leukopenia have been observed following large doses. Routine blood examinations are recommended during therapy.

DRUG INTERACTIONS
Quinacrine HCl appears to potentiate the toxicity of antimalarial compounds structurally related to primaquine. Concomitant administration of quinacrine and primaquine is contraindicated. Also, primaquine should not be administered to those who have recently received quinacrine.

ADVERSE REACTIONS
GI: Nausea, vomiting, epigastric distress, abdominal cramps.

Hematologic: Leukopenia, hemolytic anemia in G6PD individuals, and methemoglobinemia in NADH methemoglobin reductase deficient individuals.

Other: Headache, interference with visual accommodation, pruritus.

OVERDOSAGE
Symptoms: Abdominal cramps, vomiting, burning, epigastric distress, CNS and cardiovascular disturbances, cyanosis, methemoglobinemia, moderate leukocytosis or leukopenia, anemia. Most striking symptoms are granulocytopenia and acute hemolytic anemia in sensitive persons. Acute hemolysis occurs, but patient recovers completely if drug is discontinued.

DOSAGE
Primaquine phosphate 26.3 mg is equivalent to 15 mg primaquine base.

CDC-recommended treatment schedule

Take on a regular basis. Begin therapy during last 2 weeks of, or following, a course of suppression with chloroquine or a comparable drug.

P

Adults: 26.3 mg (15 mg base)/day for 14 days or 79 mg (45 mg base) once a week for 8 weeks.

Pediatric: 0.3 mg (base)/kg/day for 14 days or 0.9 mg (base)/kg/day weekly for 8 weeks.

NURSING IMPLICATIONS

HISTORY
See Appendix 4.

PHYSICAL ASSESSMENT
Base on presenting symptoms. CBC, hemoglobin may be ordered.

ADMINISTRATION
Give with food or, if prescribed by physician, an antacid.

ONGOING ASSESSMENTS AND NURSING MANAGEMENT
If nausea and vomiting persist when drug is given with meal or food, notify physician.

Routine hematologic tests (CBC, hemoglobin) and urinalysis may be ordered during therapy.

If patient is acutely ill and cannot check urine, visually check for darkening each voided sample or urine collected in a urinary drainage system.

PATIENT AND FAMILY INFORMATION
Complete full course of therapy; take until gone.

If GI upset occurs, may be taken with food or antacid. If stomach upset (nausea, vomiting, stomach pain) continues, notify physician or nurse.

Note color of urine at time of each voiding. Notify physician or nurse if a darkening of urine occurs.

Notify physician or nurse if chills, fever, chest pain, or cyanosis occurs (may be sign of hemolytic reaction).

Primidone Rx

tablets: 50 mg	Mysoline
tablets: 250 mg	Mysoline, Primoline, *Generic*
oral suspension: 250 mg/5 ml	Mysoline

INDICATIONS
Control of grand mal, psychomotor, and focal epileptic seizures, either alone or concomitantly with other anticonvulsants. May control grand mal seizures refractory to other anticonvulsant therapy.

CONTRAINDICATIONS
Porphyria; hypersensitivity to phenobarbital.

ACTIONS
Mechanism of action is not known. It has anticonvulsant activity, as do its two metabolites, phenobarbital and phenylethylmalonamide (PEMA).

Is readily absorbed from the GI tract. Peak serum concentrations occur in 3 hours after initial dose and later with continuous administration. Peak serum concentrations of PEMA occur after 7 to 8 hours. Phenobarbital appears in the plasma as a metabolite after several days of continuous therapy. Biotransformation of primidone to its active metabolites varies. PEMA is the major metabolite and is less active than primidone. Phenobarbital formation ranges from 15% to 25%. Plasma half-life of primidone is 3 to 12 or more hours. PEMA and phenobarbital have longer half-lives (24–48 hours and 2–6 days respectively) and accumulate with chronic use.

WARNINGS
Abrupt withdrawal may precipitate status epilepticus. The therapeutic efficacy of a dosage regimen takes several weeks to assess. The effects of primidone in pregnancy and nursing infants are unknown. There is evidence that the drug appears in human milk in substantial quantities.

PRECAUTIONS
Total daily dosage should not exceed 2 g. Because therapy generally extends over prolonged periods, a complete blood count and SMA-12 should be performed every 6 months.

DRUG INTERACTIONS
Few have been reported; however, all drug interactions reported with barbiturates (see p 169) should be considered when this drug is used.

ADVERSE REACTIONS
Most frequently occurring are ataxia and vertigo. These tend to disappear with continued therapy or reduction of initial dosage. Occasionally, the following have been reported: nausea, anorexia, vomiting, fatigue, hyperexcitability, emotional disturbances, sexual impotence, diplopia, nystagmus, drowsiness, and morbilliform skin eruptions. Persistent or severe side-effects may necessitate withdrawal of drug. Megaloblastic anemia may occur as a rare idiosyncrasy to this and other anticonvulsants. The anemia responds to folic acid without necessity of discontinuing medication.

DOSAGE
Adults, children over 8 yr: Patients who have received no previous treatment may be started with the following regimen: *Days 1–3*—100 mg to 125 mg H.S.; *days 4–6*—100 mg to 125 mg bid; *days 7–*

9—100 mg to 125 mg tid; *day 10–maintenance—* 250 mg tid. Usual maintenance dose is 250 mg tid or qid. If required, dosage is increased to 250 mg 5 to 6 times a day. Maximum dose is 500 mg qid.

Children under 8 yr: The following may be used to initiate therapy: *Days 1–3—*50 mg H.S.; *days 4–6—*50 mg bid; *days 7–9—*100 mg bid; *day 10–maintenance—*125 mg to 250 mg tid. Usual maintenance dose is 125 mg to 250 mg tid, or 10 mg/kg/day to 25 mg/kg/day in divided doses.

Patients already receiving other anticonvulsants: Initial dose is 100 mg to 125 mg H.S., gradually increased to maintenance level as other drug is gradually decreased. This regimen is continued until a satisfactory dosage level is achieved for the combination or the other medication is completely withdrawn. When therapy with this drug alone is the objective, the transition should not be completed in less than 2 weeks.

NURSING IMPLICATIONS

HISTORY
See Appendix 4; obtain from family, or review chart for, history of seizure disorder including average length of seizure, aura (if any), degree of impairment of consciousness, motor and psychic activity, and previous drug therapy.

PHYSICAL ASSESSMENT
Obtain vital signs; if seizures are frequent, observe and record accurate description in patient's chart. Diagnostic studies and laboratory tests may include EEG, CT scan, CBC, hemoglobin, and SMA-12.

ADMINISTRATION
If patient is unable to take tablet form, inform physician because an oral suspension is available.

If GI upset occurs, drug may be given with food or meals.

ONGOING ASSESSMENTS AND NURSING MANAGEMENT
Monitor vital signs daily; observe for adverse reactions; observe patient at frequent intervals (q1h–q2h) for occurrence of seizures, especially early in therapy and in those with a history of frequent seizures.

CLINICAL ALERT: Do *not* abruptly withdraw any anticonvulsant drug unless ordered to do so by a physician. Abrupt withdrawal may precipitate status epilepticus. Ensure continuity of prescribed therapy by notation on Kardex, informing health-team members responsible for drug administration.

Accurate observations and documentation of seizures assist physician in adjusting dosage.

Ataxia, vertigo, and drowsiness may occur, especially early in therapy. Patient may require assistance with ambulatory activities.

Notify physician immediately if skin rash, joint pain, or fever occurs.

Periodic CBC and SMA-12 are recommended. Primidone and barbiturate plasma levels may be drawn; therapeutic plasma concentrations are 5 mcg/ml to 12 mcg/ml for primidone and 15 mcg/ml to 45 mcg/ml for phenobarbital.

Neonates: If mother was or is taking primidone, observe infant for bleeding (due to a coagulation defect), especially during the first 24 hours after birth. If bleeding is noted, contact physician immediately.

Nursing newborn of primidone-treated mother is observed for undue somnolence and drowsiness. If this is noted, breast-feeding should be discontinued.

PATIENT AND FAMILY INFORMATION
NOTE: A family member should keep a record of seizures (date, time, length of seizure, severity, seizure pattern) and bring at time of each office or clinic visit.

Drowsiness, dizziness, or muscular incoordination may occur initially, but these symptoms usually disappear with continued therapy. Observe caution while driving or performing other tasks requiring alertness.

If GI upset occurs, may be taken with food.

Never discontinue medication abruptly or change dosage, except on advice of physician.

It may require several weeks before drug is effective.

Notify physician or nurse if skin rash, joint pain, or unexplained fever occurs.

Physician may require periodic laboratory tests to monitor therapy.

If pregnancy occurs or is thought to have occurred, notify physician immediately.

Carry identification such as Medic-Alert, indicating medication usage and epilepsy.

Inform other physicians and dentist of therapy with this drug.

Do not use alcohol or nonprescription drugs unless use has been approved by physician.

Probenecid Rx

tablets: 0.5 g	Benemid, Probalan, SK-Probenecid, *Generic*

INDICATIONS

Treatment of hyperuricemia associated with gout and gouty arthritis. As an adjuvant to therapy with penicillins or cephalosporins, for elevation and prolongation of plasma levels of the antibiotic.

CONTRAINDICATIONS

Hypersensitivity; children under 2 years; blood dyscrasias or uric acid kidney stones.

ACTIONS

A uricosuric and renal tubular blocking agent. It inhibits tubular reabsorption of urate, increasing urinary excretion of uric acid and decreasing serum uric acid levels. Effective uricosuria reduces the miscible urate pool, retards urate deposition and promotes resorption of urate deposits. Also inhibits tubular secretion of penicillin and cephalosporins and usually increases penicillin plasma levels by any route antibiotic is given. A twofold to fourfold elevation has been demonstrated for various penicillins.

Is well absorbed and produces peak plasma concentrations in 2 to 4 hours. It is highly protein bound to plasma albumin and has a serum half-life of 8 to 10 hours and is excreted in the urine. Probenecid is most useful in gouty arthritis in those with reduced urinary excretion of uric acid (<800 mg/day) on an unrestricted diet. Allopurinol is more appropriate for those with excessive uric acid synthesis as indicated by >800 mg uric acid urinary excretion daily on a purine-free diet.

WARNINGS

Exacerbation of gout following therapy with probenecid may occur; in such cases, colchicine therapy is advisable. Probenecid crosses the placental barrier and appears in cord blood. Use only when clearly needed and when potential benefits outweigh the unknown potential hazards to the fetus.

PRECAUTIONS

Hematuria, renal colic, costovertebral pain, and formation of urate stones associated with use in gouty patients may be prevented by alkalinization of the urine and liberal fluid intake; in these cases acid–base balance is monitored. Use with caution in those with history of peptic ulcer, acute intermittent porphyria, G6PD deficiency. Dosage requirements may be increased in renal impairment. Drug may not be effective in chronic renal insufficiency, particularly when the glomerular filtration rate is 30 ml/minute or less. Probenecid is not recommended in conjunction with penicillin in presence of known renal impairment.

DRUG INTERACTIONS

Use of **salicylates** is contraindicated because they antagonize the uricosuric action. Patients who require a mild analgesic should receive acetaminophen. The uricosuric action of probenecid is also antagonized by **pyrazinamide**. Probenecid inhibits renal excretion and may increase plasma levels of **methotrexate, sulfonamides, sulfonylureas, naproxen, indomethacin, rifampin, aminosalicylic acid, dapsone, clofibrate,** and **pantothenic acid**. To minimize potential for toxicity of drugs used concurrently, patients should be monitored closely and with appropriate dosage reductions. The tubular reabsorption of phosphorus is inhibited in hypoparathyroid, but not euparathyroid, individuals.

Drug/lab tests: A false diagnosis of glycosuria may be made because of a false-positive **Benedict's test.** Suspected glycosuria should be confirmed by using a test specific for glucose. Falsely high readings of **theophylline** have been reported when using the Schack and Waxler technique, probenecid may inhibit renal excretion of **phenolsulfonphthalein (PSP)** and **17-ketosteroids.**

ADVERSE REACTIONS

Headache; GI symptoms (anorexia, nausea, vomiting); urinary frequency; hypersensitivity reactions (including anaphylaxis, dermatitis, pruritus, fever); sore gums, flushing; dizziness; anemia; hemolytic anemia (possibly related to G6PD deficiency). Nephrotic syndrome, hepatic necrosis, and aplastic anemia occur rarely. Exacerbation of gout and uric acid stones with or without hematuria, renal colic, and/or costovertebral pain have been seen.

DOSAGE

Gout

Therapy should not be started until an acute gouty attack has subsided. If an acute attack is precipitated during therapy, probenecid may be continued and full therapeutic doses of colchicine given to control the acute attack.

Adults: Recommended dose is 0.25 g bid for 1 week, followed by 0.5 g bid thereafter. Some degree of renal impairment may be present in patients with gout; a daily dosage of 1 g may be adequate. If necessary, daily dosage may be increased by 0.5-g increments every 4 weeks within tolerance (usually not above 2 g/day) if symptoms of gouty arthritis are not controlled or the 24-hour urate excretion is not above 700 mg. It may not be effective in chronic renal insufficiency, particularly when the glomerular filtration rate is 30 ml/minute or less.

Urinary alkalinization: Urates tend to crystallize out of an acid urine; a liberal fluid intake recommended as well as sufficient sodium bicarbonate (3–

7.5 g/day) or potassium citrate (7.5 g/day) to maintain alkaline urine. Alkalinization recommended until serum uric acid level returns to normal limits and tophaceous deposits disappear. Thereafter, urinary alkalinization and usual restriction of purine-producing foods may be somewhat relaxed.

Maintenance therapy: Dosage is continued that will maintain normal serum uric acid levels. When acute attacks have been absent for 6 months or more and serum uric acid levels remain within normal limits, daily dosage may be decreased by 0.5 g every 6 months. Maintenance dose is not reduced to a point at which serum uric acid levels increase.

Penicillin or cephalosporin therapy

The PSP excretion test may be used to determine effectiveness of probenecid in retarding penicillin excretion and maintaining therapeutic levels. Renal clearance of PSP is reduced to about $\frac{1}{5}$ the normal rate when dosage of probenecid is adequate.

Adults: 2 g/day probenecid in divided doses. Dosage is reduced in older patients in whom renal impairment may be present. Not recommended in conjunction with penicillin or a cephalosporin in presence of known renal impairment.

Children (2–14 yr): Initial dose is 25 mg/kg. Maintenance dose is 40 mg/kg/day divided into four doses. _Children weighing more than 50 kg—_ Adult dosage recommended. Not used in children under 2.

Gonorrhea

Probenecid is usually given as a single 1-g dose immediately preceding penicillin administration. In children weighing less than 45 kg, probenecid dose is 24 mg/kg.

NURSING IMPLICATIONS

HISTORY
See Appendix 4.

PHYSICAL ASSESSMENT
Examine affected joints, pinna of ear for urate tophaceous deposits; describe location, appearance, size. Serum uric acid, 24-hour urine for uric acid may be ordered. If renal impairment suspected, serum creatinine or other renal-function tests may be ordered.

ADMINISTRATION
GI upset may occur. Give with meals or food. Physician may order antacid to be taken with drug.

If prescribed for gonorrhea, probenecid is usually given immediately before penicillin administration.

ONGOING ASSESSMENTS AND NURSING MANAGEMENT
If GI symptoms persist despite giving with food, notify physician before next dose is due; a reduction in dosage may be necessary.

Encourage patient to drink 10 or more glasses (8 oz each) of water/day. If patient compliance with a forced fluid regimen is questionable, measure intake and output. Urinary output should be approximately 2000 ml/day.

Physician may order alkalinization of urine with sodium bicarbonate or potassium citrate and testing of urine _p_H daily, using reagent test strips. Periodic monitoring of acid–base balance is also recommended.

Physician may order diet low in purines.

Tophaceous deposits should decrease in size during therapy.

Diabetic patient receiving a sulfonylurea: Probenecid may increase plasma levels; dosage of the sulfonylurea may require adjustment. Use Clinistix to test urine for glucose; Clinitest may produce false test results. Monitor patient closely during period of sulfonylurea dosage adjustment. Notify physician if signs of hyperglycemia or hypoglycemia (Appendix 6, section 6-14) occur.

PATIENT AND FAMILY INFORMATION
May cause GI upset; take with food or antacids (with physician approval). If GI upset (_e.g.,_ nausea, vomiting, loss of appetite) persists, notify physician or nurse.

Drink plenty of water (10 large 8 oz glasses/day) to prevent development of kidney stones.

Avoid use of aspirin or other salicylates that may antagonize the effects of this drug. If in doubt whether a product contains a salicylate, check with a pharmacist before purchase.

Follow instructions of physician regarding additional treatment modalities (_e.g.,_ weight loss, dietary restrictions).

Do not stop taking drug unless ordered to do so by physician.

Diabetic patient: May produce false test results with Clinitest; use Clinistix or other product recommended by physician for testing urine.

Probenecid and Colchicine Combinations _Rx_

tablets: 500 mg probenecid, 0.5 mg colchicine	ColBenemid, Proben-C, _Generic_

P

INDICATIONS

Treatment of chronic gouty arthritis when complicated by frequent, recurrent attacks of gout.

CONTRAINDICATIONS, ACTIONS, PRECAUTIONS, WARNINGS, DRUG INTERACTIONS, ADVERSE REACTIONS

See under separate monographs for Colchicine and Probenecid.

DOSAGE

Therapy should not be started until an acute gouty attack has subsided. If an acute attack is precipitated during therapy, additional colchicine is administered or other appropriate therapy is given to control the attack; do not alter dose of probenecid.

Initial dosage: Adults—One tablet daily for 1 week, followed by one tablet bid thereafter. Gastric intolerance may be indicative of overdose; dosage should be decreased.

Fluid intake and urinary alkalinization: See Probenecid.

Maintenance therapy: Therapy should be continued at dosage needed to maintain normal serum urate levels. When acute attacks have been absent for 6 or more months and serum urate levels remain within normal limits, daily dosage may be decreased by one tablet every 6 months. Maintenance dose should not be reduced to the point at which serum urate levels begin to rise.

Dosage in renal impairment: Some degree of renal impairment may be present in those with gout. A daily dose of two tablets may be adequate for control. If necessary, dose may be increased by one tablet every 4 weeks within tolerance (usually not more than 4 tablets/day) if symptoms are not controlled or the 24-hour urate excretion is not above 700 mg. Probenecid may not be effective in chronic renal insufficiency.

▌NURSING IMPLICATIONS

See under separate monographs for Colchicine and Probenecid.

Probucol Rx

tablets: 250 mg   Lorelco

INDICATIONS

Adjunctive therapy to diet for reduction of elevated serum cholesterol in those with primary hypercholesterolemia (elevated low-density lipoproteins) who have not responded adequately to diet, weight reduction, and control of diabetes mellitus. May be used to lower elevated cholesterol that occurs in those with combined hypercholesterolemia and hypertriglyceridemia but is not indicated when hypertriglyceridemia is the abnormality of most concern.

Response to drug is variable; it is not always possible to predict from the lipoprotein type or other factors which patients will obtain favorable results. Although antihyperlipidemic drugs have been used for many years, it is still not clear whether drug-induced lowering of serum cholesterol or lipid levels has a beneficial effect, no effect, or a detrimental effect on morbidity or mortality due to atherosclerosis or coronary heart disease.

CONTRAINDICATIONS

Hypersensitivity.

ACTIONS

May act by inhibition of earlier stages of cholesterol synthesis, increased excretion of fecal bile salts, and a slight inhibition of the absorption of dietary cholesterol. There is no increase in the cyclic precursors of cholesterol, and probucol does not affect later stages of cholesterol biosynthesis.

Absorption from GI tract is limited and variable. When given with food, peak plasma levels are higher and less variable. With continuous administration in a dosage of 500 mg bid, blood levels gradually increase over first 3 to 4 months and thereafter remain fairly constant.

WARNINGS

Cardiotoxic effects have been seen in animal studies. Until cardiotoxic effects can be evaluated in humans, probucol is discontinued in those with cardiac arrhythmias or prolongation of the Q–T interval. In those with evidence of recent or progressive myocardial damage or findings suggestive of ventricular arrhythmias, drug is used only when accompanied by periodic ECG assessment. If pronounced Q–T interval prolongation is seen, drug is not administered. Drug should not be used in those with evidence of unresponsive CHF or frequent multifocal or paired ventricular extrasystoles.

Because there are no adequate studies, use of this drug in pregnancy is not recommended. If patient wishes to become pregnant, drug is withdrawn and birth control procedures used for at least 6 months because of persistence of the drug in the body for prolonged periods. It is not known if this drug is excreted in human milk. It is recommended that nursing not be undertaken while patient is taking this drug. Safety and efficacy for use in children not established.

PRECAUTIONS

Serum cholesterol levels are recommended frequently during first few months of treatment. A favorable trend in cholesterol reduction should be evident during first 2 months of therapy. If a satisfactory reduction in serum cholesterol is not achieved within 4 months, drug is discontinued. Serum triglyceride levels are recommended periodically. If a marked sustained rise is observed during therapy, improved diet compliance, alcohol abstinence, further calorie restriction, or adjustment of carbohydrate intake is considered. Drug should not be continued if hypertriglyceridemia persists.

Oral hypoglycemic agents and oral anticoagulants do not alter the effect of probucol on serum cholesterol. Dosage of these agents is usually not modified when given with probucol.

ADVERSE REACTIONS

Are usually mild and of short duration. Most commonly affected system is the GI tract. Diarrhea occurs in about one in ten patients. Other adverse GI reactions in descending order of frequency are flatulence, abdominal pain, nausea, and vomiting. These are usually transient and seldom require that drug be discontinued.

An idiosyncratic reaction characterized by dizziness, palpitations, syncope, nausea, vomiting, and chest pain has been seen.

Other events have been reported and relationship between these complaints and probucol is not well established. Also included are events that could have been produced by the patient's state or other modes of therapy.

Most frequent: Headache, dizziness, paresthesias, eosinophilia, consistently low hemoglobin and/or hematocrit values.

Less frequent: Rash, pruritus, impotence, insomnia, conjunctivitis, tearing, blurred vision, tinnitus, diminished sense of taste and smell, enlargement of multinodular goiter, anorexia, heartburn, indigestion, GI bleeding, ecchymosis and petechiae, thrombocytopenia, nocturia, peripheral neuritis, hyperhidrosis, fetid sweat, and angioneurotic edema.

Elevated SGOT, SGPT, bilirubin, alkaline phosphatase, CPK, uric acid, BUN, and blood glucose above normal range have been seen and were transient and/or could have been related to the patient's clinical state or other modes of therapy.

DOSAGE

Recommended and maximal dose is 500 mg bid with morning and evening meals. For adult use only.

NURSING IMPLICATIONS

HISTORY
See Appendix 4.

PHYSICAL ASSESSMENT
Obtain blood pressure, pulse, respirations, weight. Baseline serum cholesterol and triglycerides are recommended. CBC and other laboratory tests may be ordered, depending on history and physical examination.

ADMINISTRATION
Give with morning and evening meal.

ONGOING ASSESSMENTS AND NURSING MANAGEMENT
Monitor blood pressure, pulse, and respirations q4h to q8h or as ordered. If cardiac arrhythmia occurs, notify physician immediately because ECG may be necessary. Prolongation of the Q–T interval usually requires discontinuation of drug.

Observe for adverse reactions. If GI or other side-effects are noted, inform physician before next dose is due.

If dizziness, palpitations, syncope, nausea, vomiting, or chest pain occurs notify physician; these may be indicative of an idiosyncratic reaction, which may require discontinuation of drug.

Appropriate dietary restrictions will also be necessary and may include calorie restriction (weight-reduction diet), low-cholesterol diet, and adjustment of carbohydrate intake.

PATIENT AND FAMILY INFORMATION
Take with meals.

May cause diarrhea, flatulence, abdominal pain, nausea, or vomiting. These effects usually disappear with continued use. Notify physician or nurse if they persist or become bothersome.

If dizziness, palpitations, syncope, or chest pain occurs, notify physician or nurse immediately.

Restriction of dietary intake of cholesterol and saturated fats and adherence to prescribed dietary regimen (which may include decrease in carbohydrate intake, calorie restriction) is an important part of therapy.

Discuss with physician alcohol intake; in some instances alcohol is not allowed or amount used is restricted.

Women of childbearing age: Birth control measures are recommended during therapy. If pregnancy is desired, birth control measures will be necessary for at least 6 months after drug is discontinued (because of prolonged action of drug).

Procainamide Hydrochloride Rx

| capsules: 250 mg | Promine, Pronestyl, Sub-Quin, *Generic* |

P

capsules: 375 mg, 500 mg	Promine, Pronestyl, *Generic*
tablets: 250 mg, 375 mg, 500 mg	Pronestyl (contains tartrazine), *Generic*
tablets, sustained release: 250 mg, 750 mg	Procan SR
tablets, sustained release: 500 mg	Procan SR, Pronestyl-SR
injection: 100 mg/ ml, 500 mg/ml	Pronestyl, *Generic*

INDICATIONS

Treatment of premature ventricular contractions and ventricular tachycardia, atrial fibrillation, and paroxysmal atrial tachycardia. Parenteral therapy is also indicated for cardiac arrhythmias associated with anesthesia and surgery.

CONTRAINDICATIONS

Patients with myasthenia gravis; hypersensitivity to drug; cross-sensitivity to procaine and related drugs; patients with complete AV block; cases of second- and third-degree AV block unless electrical pacemaker is operative.

ACTIONS

Depresses excitability of cardiac muscle to electrical stimulation and slows conduction in the atrium, the bundle of His, and the ventricle. The refractory period of the atrium is considerably more prolonged than that of the ventricle. Contractility of the heart is usually not affected and cardiac output is not decreased to any extent unless myocardial damage exists. In absence of any arrhythmias, the heart rate may occasionally be accelerated by conventional doses, suggesting the drug may have anticholinergic properties. Larger doses can induce AV block and ventricular extrasystoles, which may proceed to ventricular fibrillation. Effects on the myocardium reflected by the ECG include a widening of the QRS complex, occurring most consistently; less regularly, the P–R and Q–T intervals are prolonged, and the QRS and T-waves show some decrease in voltage.

Onset of action begins almost immediately after IM or IV administration. Plasma levels after IM injection peak in 15 to 60 minutes. Following oral administration plasma levels are 75% to 95% of those obtained parenterally and are maximal within an hour; therapeutic levels are usually attained in half that time. Between 15 and 27 hours are required to achieve steady state. Therapeutic plasma levels have been reported to be 3 mcg/ml to 10 mcg/ml, with the majority of patients in the range of 4 mcg/ml to 8 mcg/ml. Levels of 8 mcg/ml to 16 mcg/ml are potentially toxic and levels greater than 16 mcg/ml are usually associated with signs of toxicity.

Procainamide is 20% bound to plasma proteins; it is rapidly distributed to most body tissues except the brain. Plasma elimination half-life is approximately 2.5 to 4.5 hours. Approximately 25% is converted in the liver to its primary cardioactive metabolite n-acetylprocainamide (NAPA), which has a 6-hour half-life. Approximately 50% is excreted in the urine unchanged. Decreased dosages may be necessary in those with heart failure because of decreased clearance of the drug.

WARNINGS

Prolonged administration often leads to development of a positive antinuclear antibody (ANA) test with or without symptoms of lupus erythematosus–like syndrome. If a positive ANA titer develops, alternative antiarrhythmic therapy may be necessary.

PRECAUTIONS

Electrophysiological effects: Monitor for evidence of untoward myocardial responses, especially in presence of an abnormal myocardium. In atrial fibrillation or flutter, the ventricular rate may suddenly increase as the atrial rate is slowed. Adequate digitalization reduces, but does not abolish, this danger. If myocardial damage exists, ventricular tachysystole is particularly hazardous. Correction of atrial fibrillation, with resultant forceful contractions of the atrium, may cause dislodgement of mural thrombi and produce an embolic episode. In a patient who is already discharging emboli, procainmaide is more likely to stop than to aggravate the process.

Attempts to adjust the heart rate in a patient who has developed ventricular tachycardia during an occlusive coronary episode should be carried out with extreme caution. Caution also required in marked disturbances of AV conduction such as second- and third-degree AV block, bundle branch block, or severe digitalis intoxication, in which use of drug may result in additional depression of conduction and ventricular asystole or fibrillation. Because patients with severe organic heart disease and ventricular tachycardia may also have complete heart block, which is difficult to diagnose under these circumstances, this complication should always be kept in mind when treating ventricular arrhythmias with procainamide, especially parenterally. If the ventricular rate is slowed by procainamide without attainment of regular AV conduction, drug should be stopped.

In those receiving normal dosages who have both liver and kidney disease, symptoms of overdosage (principally ventricular tachycardia and severe hypotension) may occur because of drug accumulation.

Patients receiving this drug for extended periods of time should have ANA titers measured at regular intervals. If a rising titer occurs or clinical symptoms of lupus erythematosus appear, drug is discontinued. The lupus erythematous syndrome may be reversible upon discontinuation of the drug; if discontinuation does not cause remission, steroid therapy may be used concomitantly. If the syndrome develops in a patient with recurrent life-threatening arrhythmias not controllable by other antiarrhythmic agents, steroid suppressive therapy may be used concurrently with procainamide.

Tartrazine sensitivity: Some of these products contain tartrazine. See Appendix 6, section 6-23.

DRUG INTERACTIONS
The effects of **cardiotonic glycosides** may be additive with those of procainamide. Additive neurologic effects may be produced during concomitant administration of **lidocaine** and procainamide.

ADVERSE REACTIONS
Because procainamide is a peripheral vasodilator, IV administration may produce transient (but at times severe) lowering of blood pressure, particularly in conscious patients. IM injection is less likely to be accompanied by serious falls in blood pressure, and hypotension following PO administration is rare. Serious disturbances of cardiac rhythm such as ventricular asystole or fibrillation are more common with IV administration.

Large oral dosages may sometimes produce anorexia, nausea, urticaria, and/or pruritus. A syndrome resembling lupus erythematosus has been seen in those on maintenance therapy. Reactions consisting of fever and chills have been reported. Bitter taste, diarrhea, weakness, mental depression, giddiness, psychosis with hallucinations, granulomatous hepatitis, and hypersensitivity reactions such as angioneurotic edema and maculopapular rash have been reported.

Agranulocytosis has occasionally followed repeated use, and deaths have occurred. Routine blood counts are advisable during maintenance therapy. Thrombocytopenia has also been reported.

OVERDOSAGE
Dopamine, phenylephrine, or norepinephrine may be helpful in reversing severe hypotensive responses. Hemodialysis reduces serum half-life and effectively removes drug and, to a lesser degree, the active metabolite.

DOSAGE
Oral treatment is preferred for treatment of arrhythmias that do not require immediate suppression or to continue treatment after controlling serious ar-

rhythmias with parenteral procainamide or other antiarrhythmic therapy.

An initial loading dose (12 mg/kg) approximately twice the maintenance dose (6 mg/kg/3 hours) should be given upon initiation of therapy.

Oral

Ventricular tachycardia: An initial dose of 1 g followed by a maintenance dose of 50 mg/kg/day given in divided doses q3h (6 mg/kg q3h).

Premature ventricular contractions: 50 mg/kg/day in divided doses q3h. To provide 50 mg/kg/day q3h dose for those under 120 lb is 250 mg, those 120 to 200 lb, 375 mg and those over 200 lb, 500 mg.

Atrial fibrillation and paroxysmal tachycardia: An initial dose of 1.25 g may be followed in 1 hour by 0.75 g, if there are no ECG changes. A dose of 0.5 g to 1 g may then be given q2h until arrhythmia is interrupted or the limit of tolerance is reached. _Suggested maintenance dose_—0.5 g to 1 g q4h to q6h.

_IM_

This route may be preferable to PO use in those with vomiting, in those NPO before surgery, or in those in whom there is a reason to believe absorption may be unreliable. A dose of 0.5 g to 1 g may be given, repeated q4h to q8h until oral therapy is possible. For cardiac arrhythmias associated with anesthesia and surgery, 0.1 g to 0.5 g, preferably IM.

_IV_

IV use may be accompanied by a hypotensive response, sometimes marked, if dose is excessive or administration too rapid. To initiate therapy IV dose should be diluted in 5% Dextrose Injection, USP, prior to administration to facilitate control of dosage rate. Slow administration allows for some initial tissue distribution.

Direct IV: To reduce possibility of a hypotensive response, 100 mg may be administered every 5 minutes by direct slow IV injection, at a rate not exceeding 25 mg/minute to 50 mg/minute, until arrhythmia is suppressed or maximum dosage of 1 g is administered. Some effects may be seen after first 100 mg or 200 mg; it is unusual to require more than 500 mg or 600 mg to achieve satisfactory antiarrhythmic effects.

IV infusion: An alternative method of achieving and maintaining a therapeutic plasma concentration is to infuse 500 mg to 600 mg at a constant rate over a period of 25 to 30 minutes and then change to another infusion for maintenance at a rate of 2 mg/minute to 6 mg/minute.

NURSING IMPLICATIONS
HISTORY
See Appendix 4.

P.

PHYSICAL ASSESSMENT

Obtain blood pressure, pulse (apical–radial rate), respirations; arrhythmia is documented by ECG. CBC, platelet count may be ordered in maintenance therapy is planned.

ADMINISTRATION

Obtain blood pressure, pulse, and respirations immediately before administration. An apical–radial rate should be obtained, especially during initial dosage period if patient is not on cardiac monitor.

Oral

Instruct patient to swallow tablet or capsule whole and not to bite or chew preparation.

IV

Place patient in a supine position.

It is recommended a cardiac monitor be used during IV administration.

Have drugs (dopamine, phenylephrine, norepinephrine) available to treat hypotensive episodes.

Direct IV: Use 100 mg/ml dosage form.

Give at rate not to exceed 25 mg/minute to 50 mg/minute (0.25–0.5 ml/minute).

IV infusion: Physician orders IV solution (usually 5% Dextrose in Water) and infusion rate. Procainamide must be diluted before IV administration.

Physician must establish guidelines regarding discontinuation and/or slowing the infusion rate if decreased blood pressure, change in heart rate and rhythm occur.

Use a secondary line for IV infusion of procainamide. An infusion pump may be used to administer IV solution at a controlled rate.

CLINICAL ALERT: Monitor ECG continuously during IV infusion. Excessive widening of the QRS complex or prolongation of the P–R interval suggests toxicity. Discontinue infusion immediately, run primary line to KVO, and contact physician.

In atrial fibrillation or flutter, the ventricular rate may increase suddenly as the atrial rate is slowed. Observe for this phenomenon and discontinue or slow IV infusion (depending on physician's orders) if an increase in ventricular rate occurs.

Observe for *any* untoward myocardial responses such as ventricular asystole, heart block, ventricular tachycardia, ventricular fibrillation, or marked slowing of the ventricular rate without attainment of regular AV conduction. The physician should be notified of any changes in the ECG and a rhythm strip run to document observations.

Monitor blood pressure q5m to q10m during IV infusion. If fall in blood pressure exceeds 15 mm Hg, administration should be temporarily discontinued, primary line run to KVO, and physician contacted immediately.

IV therapy is usually terminated as soon as patient's basic cardiac rhythm appears to be sta-bilized. Oral therapy, if indicated, may then be instituted. A period of about 3 to 4 hours is recommended after last IV dose before administration of first oral dose.

IM

Give deep IM in gluteus muscle. Rotate injection sites; record site used.

ONGOING ASSESSMENTS AND NURSING MANAGEMENT

Obtain temperature q4h or as ordered. Notify physician if rise in temperature occurs because drug may be temporarily discontinued.

Procainamide plasma levels recommended to monitor therapy (especially parenteral administration). Keep physician informed of results. Therapeutic plasma levels are 3 mcg/ml to 10 mcg/ml. Levels of 8 mcg/ml to 16 mcg/ml are potentially toxic and levels greater than 16 mcg/ml are usually associated with signs of toxicity.

If oral therapy continued for appreciable periods, periodic ECGs are performed to monitor effects of drug and need for continued use.

Routine CBC is recommended during maintenance therapy.

CLINICAL ALERT: Observe daily for sore mouth, throat, or gums; fever; symptoms of respiratory-tract infection. If any of these occurs, notify physician immediately. If CBC indicates decrease in leukocytes, drug is discontinued immediately. Thrombocytopenia also may occur. Notify physician if bruising or evidence of easy bleeding occurs.

Control of atrial fibrillation may cause dislodgement of mural thrombi and produce an embolic episode. Observe for development of sudden chest pain, dyspnea, anxiety, cerebral changes, or any other signs or symptom that may be indicative of an embolic episode and report findings immediately.

The lupus erythematosus syndrome has been reported with maintenance therapy. Most common symptoms include polyarthralgia, arthritis, and pleuritic pain. To a lesser extent, fever, myalgia, skin lesions, pleural effusion, and pericarditis may occur. If these symptoms should occur, an ANA titer is performed.

Patients with impaired renal and hepatic function may develop symptoms of overdosage (particularly hypotension and ventricular tachycardia) because of drug accumulation. These patients are monitored closely during therapy with procainamide.

PATIENT AND FAMILY INFORMATION

NOTE: Physician may wish patient or family member to take pulse daily or before each dose. Instruction will be required in taking of pulse and which changes (recommended by physician) require either omitting a dose or contacting the physician. Physician may also utilize the 24-hour Holter ECG monitor to evaluate effects of therapy. Patient will require instruction in its use.

Take at the prescribed, evenly spaced intervals (usually q3h) around the clock. Do not increase the next dose, if a dose is missed. Do not discontinue drug unless instructed by physician.

Because drug is taken during nighttime hours, use of two alarm clocks (set at two different nighttime intervals) will ensure being awakened for night doses.

Notify physician or nurse if sore mouth, throat, or gums; unexplained fever; any symptom of upper respiratory infection; unusual bruising or bleeding; joint pain or stiffness; loss of appetite, nausea; pruritus; and/or urticaria occurs.

If lightheadedness, fainting, or dizziness occurs, contact physician immediately. Do not drive or perform potentially hazardous tasks.

Inform other physicians and dentist of therapy with this drug.

Do not use any nonprescription medication unless use has been approved by the physician.

Periodic laboratory tests, ECG may be required. Keep all physician and/or laboratory appointments, because therapy must be closely followed.

Sustained-release tablets (wax matrix): Wax matrix is not absorbed and may be found in the stool.

Procaine Hydrochloride

See Anesthetics, Local, Injectable.

Procarbazine Hydrochloride

(N-Methylhydrazine, MIH) Rx

capsules: 50 mg	Matulane

INDICATIONS
Palliative management of generalized Hodgkin's disease and in those patients resistant to other forms of therapy. Although prolongation of survival may not be evident, amelioration of disease symptoms and regression of tumors have been demonstrated. Drug should be used as an adjunct to standard modalities of therapy. See also Antineoplastic Agents.

CONTRAINDICATIONS
Hypersensitivity; inadequate marrow reserve as demonstrated by bone-marrow aspiration.

ACTIONS
Mode of cytotoxic action not clearly defined. There is evidence drug may act by inhibition of protein, RNA and DNA synthesis. No cross-resistance with other chemotherapeutic agents, radiotherapy, or steroids has been demonstrated. See also Appendix 10.

Drug rapidly equilibrates between plasma and cerebrospinal fluid after oral administration. GI absorption is excellent. Major portion of drug excreted in urine with 25% to 42% appearing during first 24 hours after administration.

WARNINGS
A phenomenon of toxicity common to many hydrazine derivatives is hemolysis and appearance of Heinz-Ehrlich inclusion bodies in erythrocytes. Use in pregnancy only when clearly needed and when potential benefits outweigh the potential hazards to the fetus.

PRECAUTIONS
Undue toxicity may occur if used in those with known impairment of renal and/or hepatic function. If radiation or a chemotherapeutic agent known to have marrow-depressant activity has been used, an interval of 1 month or longer without such therapy is recommended before starting treatment. The length of this interval may also be determined by evidence of bone-marrow recovery based on successive bone marrow studies.

DRUG INTERACTIONS
To minimize CNS depression and possible synergism, **barbiturates, antihistamines, narcotics, hypotensive agents,** or **phenothiazines** should be used with caution. **Ethyl alcohol** should not be used because there may be a disulfiramlike reaction. Concurrent administration of **tricyclic antidepressants (TCAs), monoamine oxidase (MAO) inhibitors, sympathomimetic drugs,** or **phenothiazines** and ingestion of **foods with high tyramine content** is not recommended because a sudden severe hypertensive crisis may result. TCAs are discontinued 7 days before procarbazine therapy and MAO inhibitors are discontinued 14 days prior to therapy. **Guanethidine, levodopa, methyldopa,** and **reserpine** administered concurrently with procarbazine may result in excitation and hypertension. Procarbazine may augment the hypoglycemic effects of **insulin** and **oral hypoglycemic agents. Antihypertensive agents,** particularly **thiazide diuretics,** administered concomitantly with procarbazine may enhance hypotensive effects.

ADVERSE REACTIONS
Frequent: Leukopenia, anemia, and thrombocytopenia occur frequently. Nausea and vomiting are the most commonly reported side-effects.

Less frequent

GI: Anorexia, stomatitis, dry mouth, dysphagia, diarrhea, constipation.

Hematologic: Bleeding tendencies such as petechiae, purpura, epistaxis, hemoptysis, hematemesis, melena are common.

Dermatologic: Dermatitis, pruritus, herpes, hyperpigmentation, flushing, alopecia, jaundice.

CNS: Paresthesias and neuropathies, headache, dizziness, depression, apprehension, nervousness, insomnia, hallucinations, falling, unsteadiness, ataxia, foot drop, decreased reflexes, tremors, coma, confusion, and convulsions have been less common.

Miscellaneous: Pain, including myalgia and arthralgia, chills and fever, sweating, weakness, fatigue, lethargy, and drowsiness often noted. Intercurrent infections, effusion, edema, cough, and pneumonitis symptoms have been reported.

Rare: Hoarseness, tachycardia, retinal hemorrhage, nystagmus, photophobia, photosensitivity, GU symptoms, hypotension, and fainting have been rare. Isolated instances of diplopia, inability to focus, papilledema, altered hearing, and slurred speech have occurred. Coincidental onset of leukemia during therapy has been reported rarely.

DOSAGE

Dosages based on actual weight. Estimated lean body mass (dry weight) is used if patient obese or if there has been a spurious weight gain due to edema, ascites, or other forms of abnormal fluid retention.

Adults: To minimize nausea and vomiting experienced by a high percentage of patients, single or divided doses of 2 mg/kg/day to 4 mg/kg/day (to the nearest 50 mg) for the first week is recommended. Daily dosages should then be maintained at 4 mg/kg/day to 6 mg/kg/day until WBC falls below 4000/mm^3 or platelets fall below 100,000/mm^3, or until maximum response is obtained. Upon evidence of hematologic toxicity drug should be discontinued until there is a satisfactory recovery. Treatment may then be resumed at 1 mg/kg/day to 2 mg/kg/day. When maximum response is obtained, dose may be maintained at 1 mg/kg/day to 2 mg/kg/day.

Children: Use in children is limited; close monitoring is mandatory. Toxicity, evidenced by tremors, coma, and convulsions, has occurred in a few cases. Dosage must be highly individualized. The following dosage is a guideline only: 50 mg/day recommended for first week. Daily dosage should then be maintained at 100 mg/m^2 (to nearest 50 mg) until leukopenia or thrombocytopenia occurs or maximum response obtained. Upon evidence of hematologic toxicity, drug should be discontinued until there has been a satisfactory response. Treatment may then be resumed at 50 mg/day. When maximum response is obtained, dose may be maintained at 50 mg/day.

NURSING IMPLICATIONS

HISTORY
See Appendix 4.

PHYSICAL ASSESSMENT
Obtain blood pressure, pulse, respirations, weight; general physical and emotional status. Recommended baseline studies include hemoglobin, hematocrit, WBC, differential reticulocytes, platelet count, urinalysis, renal and hepatic function studies. A bone-marrow aspiration may be performed to determine bone-marrow reserve.

ADMINISTRATION
Dosage based on weight or body surface area and calculated to nearest 50 mg.

If patient has difficulty swallowing capsule, discuss with physician. Do not open capsule and add to food without physician approval.

If nausea and vomiting persist, discuss with physician. A different time of administration such as H.S. may be tried.

ONGOING ASSESSMENTS AND NURSING MANAGEMENT
Obtain vital signs q4h or as ordered; monitor weight; observe for adverse reactions.

Use in children has been limited; close clinical observations are important.

Because a variety of adverse reactions have been associated with this drug, consider all patient complaints as potential adverse drug reactions.

If diarrhea occurs, notify physician immediately because drug may be discontinued. A nonnarcotic antidiarrheal agent may be ordered.

Measure intake and output; notify physician of any change in the intake–output ratio.

Notify physician and observe patient for signs of dehydration (Appendix 6, section 6-10) if vomiting exceeds 600 ml to 800 ml/8 hours. If vomiting is severe, an antiemetic (nonphenothiazine) may be ordered.

A diet limiting foods containing tyramine is ordered.

If anorexia occurs and persists for more than 2 days, notify physician. Small, frequent high-calorie feedings may be considered. In some instances, IV therapy or total parenteral nutrition may be necessary.

CLINICAL ALERT: Observe for signs of bone-marrow depression (Appendix 6, section 6-8), which may occur approximately 2 to 8 weeks after start of treatment.

Observe for CNS signs or symptoms such as paresthesias, neuropathies, and confusion, and report occurrence to physician immediately because drug is usually discontinued. See also *Adverse Reactions,* CNS.

Prompt cessation of therapy is recommended if any of the following occurs: CNS signs or symptoms; leukopenia (WBC < 4000/mm^3); thrombocytopenia (platelets < 100,000/mm^3); hypersensitivity reaction; stomatitis (the first small ulceration or persistent spot of soreness around the oral cavity); diarrhea (frequent bowel movements or watery stools); or hemorrhage or bleeding tendencies. The physician must be notified immediately if any of these occurs.

If drowsiness, dizziness, or blurred vision occurs, have patient seek assistance with ambulatory activities.

Begin to inspect oral cavity daily starting approximately 1 week after therapy is begun. Notify physician immediately if patient complains of soreness or burning of the mouth or one or more ulcerations noted. Begin stomatitis care (Appendix 6, section 6-21) as soon as signs/symptoms are apparent.

Dry mouth may be relieved by frequent sips of cool water, ice chips. If severe, a saliva substitute may be ordered.

If severe leukopenia occurs, protective isolation may be necessary.

Notify physician if marked increase or decrease in weight occurs.

Diabetic patient: Observe for signs of hypoglycemia (Appendix 6, section 6-14); dosage of insulin or oral hypoglycemic agent may require adjustment.

Laboratory monitoring of therapy: Hemoglobin, hematocrit, WBC, differential, reticulocytes, platelets recommended every 3 to 4 days. Urinalysis, transaminase, alkaline phosphatase, BUN recommended weekly.

PATIENT AND FAMILY INFORMATION

May produce drowsiness, dizziness, blurred vision. Observe caution when driving or performing other tasks requiring alertness.

Notify physician or nurse immediately if cough, shortness of breath, thickened bronchial secretions, fever, chills, sore throat, unusual bleeding or bruising, sores in the mouth or on the lips or burning of the mouth, vomiting of blood or black tarry stools, or skin rash occurs.

Avoid ingestion of foods containing tyramine (p 99). (*Note*—Patient should be supplied with a complete list of these foods and warned not to eat food brought or sent to the hospital without first checking with nursing personnel.)

Avoid excessive amounts of caffeine (coffee, tea, cola drinks).

Do not use nonprescription preparations unless use of a specific product approved by the physician. This includes aspirin and cold and hay fever preparations (may contain sympathomimetics and/or antihistamines).

Do not drink any alcoholic beverages (a disulfiramlike reaction may occur; some also contain tyramine).

Inform other physicians and dentist of therapy with this drug.

Medication may cause muscle or joint pain, nausea, vomiting, diarrhea, sweating, tiredness, weakness, constipation, headache, difficulty swallowing, loss of appetite. Notify physician or nurse if these become pronounced.

Avoid prolonged exposure to sunlight; photosensitivity may occur.

Loss of hair may occur. Hair will grow back, although it may be a different texture and color.

Dry mouth may be relieved by sips of cool water, ice chips, hard candy, or chewing gum.

If anorexia persists more than several days, inform physician or nurse. Frequent small, nutritious meals may help relieve appetite loss.

Weigh self weekly. Report marked weight gain or loss.

Notify physician or nurse if tingling of the hands and feet, headache, dizziness, hallucinations, mental depression, unsteady gait, staggering, foot drop, tremors, or nightmares occur. (*Note*—Some of these adverse reactions may not be noticed by the patient but will be apparent to family members.)

Frequent laboratory tests will be necessary to monitor therapy. Keep all physician and laboratory appointments.

Contraceptive measures are recommended during therapy.

Diabetic patient: Test urine at least daily or as recommended by physician. Observe for possible hypoglycemia (Appendix 6, section 6-14).

Prochlorperazine

See Antiemetic/Antivertigo Agents; Antipsychotic Agents.

Procyclidine

See Anticholinergic Antiparkinsonism Agents.

Progesterone

See Progestins.

Progestins

Hydroxyprogesterone Caproate in Oil *Rx*

injection: 125 mg/ml	Delalutin, *Generic*
injection: 250 mg/ml	Delalutin, Duralutin, Gesterol L.A., Hylutin, Hyprogest 250, Hyproval P.A., Pro-Depo, *Generic*

Medroxyprogesterone Acetate *Rx*

tablets: 2.5 mg	Provera
tablets: 10 mg	Amen, Curretab, Provera

Norethindrone *Rx*

tablets: 5 mg	Norlutin

Norethindrone Acetate *Rx*

tablets: 5 mg	Aygestin, Norlutate

Progesterone Aqueous *Rx*

injection: 25 mg/ml, 50 mg/ml, 100 mg/ml	*Generic*

Progesterone in Oil *Rx*

injection: 25 mg/ml, 100 mg/ml	Progelan In Oil, *Generic*
injection: 50 mg/ml	Femotrone In Oil, Progelan In Oil, Prostaject-50, *Generic*

INDICATIONS

Used primarily in the therapy of secondary amenorrhea and functional uterine bleeding. Also used in endometriosis. See *Dosage* for specific indications of individual agents.

Investigational uses: Medroxyprogesterone injection has been used to treat perimenopausal and menopausal symptoms. Oral medroxyprogesterone acetate has also been used to stimulate respiration in obesity–hypoventilation (pickwickian) syndrome.

CONTRAINDICATIONS

Hypersensitivity; thrombophlebitis, thromboembolic disorders, cerebral apoplexy, or past history of these conditions; markedly impaired liver function or disease; known or suspected carcinoma of the breast or genital organs; undiagnosed vaginal bleeding; missed abortion. Not indicated as a diagnostic test for pregnancy.

ACTIONS

Progesterone, a principle of the corpus luteum, is the most important endogenous progestational substance. Local reactions and pain on injection and relative inactivity of oral use have led to the synthesis of derivatives that are more effective or offer other advantages.

Progestin (progesterone and derivatives) transform the proliferative endometrium into a secretory endometrium. They inhibit (at the usual dose range) the secretion of pituitary gonadotropins, which in turn prevents follicular maturation and ovulation. They also inhibit spontaneous uterine contraction and induce secretory changes in the endometrium. Progestins may demonstrate some estrogenic, anabolic, or androgenic activity but should not be relied on for these effects. Absorption of oral and parenteral oily solutions is rapid; however, the hormone undergoes prompt hepatic transformation.

WARNINGS

Progestational agents are used beginning with the first trimester of pregnancy in an attempt to prevent habitual abortion or treat threatened abortion; however, there is no adequate evidence that such use is effective. There is evidence of potential harm to the fetus when such drugs are given during the first 4 months of pregnancy. Use of such drugs during the first 4 months is not recommended.

In the vast majority of women, the cause of abortion is a defective ovum, which progestational agents could not be expected to influence. In addition, use of these agents, with their uterine relaxant properties, in patients with fertilized defective ova may cause a delay in spontaneous abortion. Several reports suggest an association between intrauterine exposure to female sex hormones and congenital anomalies. If the patient is exposed to progestins during the first 4 months of pregnancy, she should be apprised of the potential risks to the fetus.

Ophthalmologic effects: Medication is discontinued pending examination if there is a sudden partial or complete loss of vision or if there is sudden onset of proptosis, diplopia, or migraine. If examination reveals papilledema or retinal vascular lesions, use is discontinued.

Thrombotic disorders: Because of occasional occurrence of thrombophlebitis, retinal thrombosis, and pulmonary embolism in those taking progestins, it is necessary to observe for manifestations of these disorders. If these occur, drug is discontinued immediately.

Use in pregnancy, lactation: Masculinization of the female fetus has occurred when progestins are used in pregnant women. Detectable amounts of progestins have been found in milk of mothers receiving these agents. The effect on the nursing infant has not been determined.

PRECAUTIONS

In cases of breakthrough bleeding, nonfunctional causes are considered. In cases of undiagnosed vaginal bleeding, adequate diagnostic measures are indicated.

Because these drugs may cause some degree of fluid retention, conditions that might be influenced by this factor, such as epilepsy, migraine, asthma, and cardiac or renal dysfunction, require careful observation. Patients with a history of psychic depression are observed and drug discontinued if depression recurs to a serious degree.

Progesterones have been reported to precipitate an acute attack of intermittent porphyria and used with caution in susceptible patients. The age of the patient constitutes no limiting factor, although use of progestins may mask the onset of the climacteric.

DRUG INTERACTIONS

Drug/lab tests: Laboratory tests, particularly of **hepatic** and **endocrine functions,** may be altered by progestins and/or estrogens. Tests to evaluate liver and endocrine function are considered definitive unless therapy has been discontinued for at least 60 days. A decrease in **glucose tolerance** has been seen in a small percentage of those on estrogen/progestin combination drugs. **Pregnanediol** determination may be altered by use of progestins.

ADVERSE REACTIONS

Breakthrough bleeding; spotting; change in menstrual flow; amenorrhea; edema; change in weight (increase or decrease); changes in cervical erosion and cervical secretions; cholestatic jaundice; rash (allergic) with or without pruritus; acne; melasma or chloasma; mental depression; breast changes (tenderness, secretion); alopecia; masculinization of the female fetus; hirsutism. A small percentage of patients have local reactions at the injection site.

Administration of **progesterone** is rarely accompanied by side-effects, which are usually mild. Administration of large doses (50–100 mg/day) may result in a moderate catabolic effect and a transient increase in sodium and chloride retention.

A few instances of coughing, dyspnea, constriction of the chest, and/or allergiclike reactions have occurred following **hydroxyprogesterone caproate** therapy.

DOSAGE

HYDROXYPROGESTERONE CAPROATE IN OIL
Given IM. has a 9- to 17-day duration of action.

Amenorrhea (primary, secondary); abnormal uterine bleeding due to hormonal imbalance in absence of organic pathology: 375 mg. After 4 days of desquamation, or if there is no bleeding, 21 days after administration, cyclic therapy is started. Cyclic therapy is a 28-day cycle repeated every 4 weeks as follows: 20 mg estradiol valerate on day 1 of each cycle; 2 weeks after day 1, 250 mg hydroxyprogesterone caproate and 5 mg estradiol valerate are given; 4 weeks after day 1 is day 1 of next cycle. Cyclic therapy is stopped after 4 cycles. Drug is used as a "medical D and C" to eliminate any proliferative endometrium from previous estrogenic action by conversion to secretory endometrium and desquamation. To determine onset of normal cyclic function, patient is observed for two to three cycles after cessation of therapy.

Production of secretory endometrium and desquamation: In those not on estrogen therapy, cyclic therapy (see above) is started any time and repeated every 4 weeks and stopped when cyclic therapy is no longer required. If estrogen deficiency has been prolonged, menstruation may not occur until estrogen has been given for several months. In patients currently on estrogen therapy, 375 mg hydroxyprogesterone caproate is given any time and cyclic therapy started after 4 days of desquamation, or, if there is no bleeding, 21 days after hydroxyprogesterone caproate alone. Cycle is repeated every 4 weeks and stopped when cyclic therapy is no longer required.

Adenocarcinoma of uterine corpus in advanced stage (Stage III or IV): 1 g or more at once; repeated one or more times each week (1–7 g/week) and stopped when relapse occurs or after 12 weeks with no objective response. May be used with other anticancer therapy (surgery, radiation, chemotherapy, or combination of these).

Test for endogenous estrogen production: 250 mg. For confirmation, repeat 4 weeks after first injection and stop after the second injection. In nonpregnant patients, bleeding 7 to 14 days after injection indicates endogenous estrogen.

MEDROXYPROGESTERONE ACETATE
Duration of action is prolonged and variable.

Secondary amenorrhea: 5 mg to 10 mg daily for 5 to 10 days. A dose for inducing optimum secretory transformation of an endometrium that has been adequately primed with either endogenous or exogenous estrogen is 10 mg/day for 10 days. Therapy is started any time. Withdrawal bleeding usually occurs 3 to 7 days after discontinuing therapy.

Abnormal uterine bleeding due to hormonal imbalance in absence of organic pathology: 5 mg/day to 10 mg/day for 5 to 10 days, beginning on the calculated sixteenth or twenty-first day of the menstrual cycle. To produce optimum secretory transformation of an endometrium that has been adequately primed with either endogenous or exogenous estrogen, 10 mg/day for 10 days, beginning on the sixteenth day of the cycle. Withdrawal bleeding usually occurs 3 to 7 days after discontinuing therapy. Patients with history of recurrent episodes of abnormal uterine bleeding may benefit from planned menstrual cycling with this drug.

Antineoplastic: See separate monograph, Medroxyprogesterone Acetate.

NORETHINDRONE

Amenorrhea, abnormal uterine bleeding due to hormonal imbalance in absence of organic pathology: 5 mg to 20 mg starting with the fifth and ending with the twenty-fifth day of the menstrual cycle.

Endometriosis: Initial daily dose of 10 mg for 2 weeks, increased in increments of 5 mg/day every 2 weeks until 30 mg/day is reached. Therapy may be held at this level for 6 to 9 months or until breakthrough bleeding demands temporary termination.

NORETHINDRONE ACETATE

Amenorrhea, abnormal uterine bleeding due to hormonal imbalance in absence of organic pathology: 2.5 mg to 10 mg starting with fifth day of the menstrual cycle and ending on the twenty-fifth day.

Endometriosis: Initial daily dose of 5 mg for 2 weeks. Increased in increments of 2.5 mg/day every 2 weeks until 15 mg/day is reached. Therapy may be held at this level for 6 to 9 months or until breakthrough bleeding demands temporary termination.

PROGESTERONE

For IM use.

Amenorrhea: 5 mg to 10 mg given for 6 to 8 consecutive days. If there has been sufficient ovarian activity to produce a proliferative endometrium, expect withdrawal bleeding 48 to 72 hours after last injection. This may be followed by spontaneous normal cycles.

Functional uterine bleeding: 5 mg/day to 10 mg/day for six doses. Bleeding may be expected to cease within 6 days. When estrogen is given as well, administration of progesterone is begun after 2 weeks of estrogen therapy. If menstrual flow begins during the course of injections, use is discontinued.

NURSING IMPLICATIONS

HISTORY
See Appendix 4.

PHYSICAL ASSESSMENT
Obtain blood pressure, pulse, respirations, weight. Physician's pretreatment physical examination includes special reference to breasts and pelvic organs. A Pap smear may be obtained.

ADMINISTRATION
Hydroxyprogesterone caproate and progesterone are given deep IM. Use a 20- to 21-gauge needle to withdraw and administer drug.

Local reactions at the injection site may be seen; report occurrence to physician.

Advise patient that injection may cause discomfort or pain. Rotate injection sites.

Oral preparations may be given with food to prevent GI upset.

GENERIC NAME SIMILARITIES
Norethindrone, norethindrone acetate.

TRADE NAME SIMILARITIES
Delalutin and Duralutin (both are hydroxyprogesterone caproate); Norlutin (norethindrone) and Norlutate (norethindrone acetate).

ONGOING ASSESSMENTS AND NURSING MANAGEMENT
Progestins are usually taken/administered on outpatient basis.

Obtain blood pressure and pulse at time of parenteral administration.

Weigh patient weekly to detect fluid retention. If marked increase in weight noted, check extremities for edema and inform physician of weight gain.

Question patient about development of adverse drug reactions before next parenteral dose is administered.

Label pathology specimens to indicate that patient is receiving progestin therapy.

Observe for signs of mental depression and inform physician if mental depression is apparent.

Diabetic patient: Observe for signs of hyperglycemia (Appendix 6, section 6-14); dosage of antidiabetic agent may require adjustment.

PATIENT INFORMATION
NOTE: Patient must receive full instruction in taking drug or appointments necessary for parenteral administration and should be told when breakthrough bleeding may be expected if drug is administered for amenorrhea (see *Dosage*).

Patient package insert available with product. (Not required to be dispensed to cancer patients.)

If GI upset occurs, take with food.

Avoid prolonged exposure to sunlight or any exposure to ultraviolet light. A sunscreen (with SPF above 10 or 12) should be worn on exposed areas, even on cloudy or overcast days.

Notify physician or nurse if breakthrough bleeding occurs.

Contact physician immediately if pregnancy suspected or any of the following occurs: pain in the calves accompanied by swelling, warmth, and redness; acute chest pain or sudden shortness of breath; sudden severe headache or vomiting, dizziness or fainting, visual disturbance, numbness in an arm or leg; severe depression.

Diabetic patient: Monitor urine glucose daily or as directed by physician. Report any abnormalities (*e.g.,* increase in urine glucose) to physician immediately.

Promazine Hydrochloride

See Antipsychotic Agents.

Promethazine Hydrochloride

See Antihistamines; Antiemetic/Antivertigo Agents.

Propantheline Bromide

See Gastrointestinal Anticholinergics/Antispasmodics.

Proparacaine Hydrochloride

See Anesthetics, Ophthalmic.

Propiomazine Hydrochloride Rx

injection: 20 mg/ml   Largon

INDICATIONS
Sedative for relief of restlessness and apprehension, preoperatively or during surgery. Also as an adjunct to analgesics for relief of restlessness and apprehension during labor.

CONTRAINDICATIONS
Intra-arterial injection is contraindicated because of possible occurrence of arterial or arteriolar spasm with resultant local impairment of circulation.

ACTIONS
Is a phenothiazine compound with sedative, antiemetic, and antihistamine properties. It potentiates the effects of other CNS depressants such as barbiturates, nonbarbiturate sedative–hypnotics, and narcotic analgesics. Is a premedicant of marked potency, with shorter duration of action than other agents of its type.

WARNINGS
Safety for use in first trimester of pregnancy has not been established.

PRECAUTIONS
Exercise care not to allow perivascular extravasation, because chemical irritation may occur.

DRUG INTERACTIONS
Drug enhances the effects of **CNS depressants;** the dose of **barbiturates** should be eliminated or reduced by at least one-half. Doses of **meperidine, morphine,** and other **analgesic depressants** should be reduced by one-fourth to one-half.

ADVERSE REACTIONS
Autonomic reactions are rare, and the dry mouth that may occur is usually considered desirable in patients undergoing anesthesia.

Cardiovascular effects include a moderate elevation in blood pressure and, rarely, hypotension. The moderate increase in blood pressure seen during surgical procedures is considered desirable in many instances. Tachycardia has also been reported. Among vasopressor drugs, norepinephrine appears to be most suitable if it is necessary to administer this type of drug. The pressor response to epinephrine is usually reduced and may even be reversed in the presence of propiomazine.

DOSAGE
Given IM or IV.

Adults

Preoperative medication: 20 mg propiomazine with 50 mg meperidine. Although 20 mg propiomazine is sufficient for most patients, some may require as much as 40 mg. Belladonna alkaloids may be added as required.

Sedation during surgery with local, nerve block, or spinal anesthesia: 10 mg to 20 mg.

Obstetrics: 20 mg will provide sedation and relieve apprehension in the early stages of labor. Some patients may require up to 40 mg. When labor is definitely established, give 20 mg to 40 mg of propiomazine with 25 mg to 75 mg meperidine (average dose, 50 mg). Amnesic agents may be administered as required. If average doses of both drugs are used, it is seldom necessary to repeat medication during normal labor. If necessary, additional doses may be repeated at 3-hour intervals. Neither prolongation of labor nor significant maternal or fetal depression has been observed.

Children

Used as a sedative the night before surgery and for preanesthetic and postoperative medication. For children under 60 lb, dosage is calculated on the basis of 0.25 mg/lb to 0.5 mg/lb. High dosage recommendations should be necessary only in the extremely nervous, excitable child.

NURSING IMPLICATIONS

PHYSICAL ASSESSMENT

Obtain blood pressure, pulse, and respirations immediately before drug is administered.

ADMINISTRATION

Give IM or IV.

Do not use if solution is cloudy or contains a precipitate.

IM: Give deep IM in upper outer quadrant of buttock. Aspirate syringe before administration because intra-arterial injection may result in arterial or arteriolar spasm with resultant impairment of local circulation.

IV: Because of possible occurrence of thrombophlebitis, it is important that injection be made only into a vessel previously undamaged by multiple injections or trauma. Exercise care not to allow perivascular extravasation, because chemical irritation may result.

Advise patient that dryness of the mouth may occur.

ONGOING ASSESSMENTS AND NURSING MANAGEMENT

Obtain blood pressure, pulse, and respirations 15 to 30 minutes after administration. Notify physician immediately if marked decrease in blood pressure is noted.

Drowsiness or dizziness may occur. If administered during early stages of labor and patient is allowed out of bed, assistance with ambulation will be required.

Contact physician and, when applicable, the anesthesiologist if excessive sedation is noted.

Propoxyphene Preparations

Propoxyphene Hydrochloride Rx C–IV

capsules: 32 mg	Darvon Pulvules, *Generic*
capsules: 65 mg	Darvon Pulvules, Dolene, Doxaphene, Profene 65, SK-65, *Generic*

Propoxyphene Napsylate Rx C–IV

tablets: 100 mg	Darvon-N
suspension: 10 mg/ml	Darvon-N

Combination Products Rx C–IV

tablets: 65 mg propoxyphene hydrochloride, 650 mg acetaminophen	Dolacet, Dolene AP-65, SK-65 APAP, Wygesic, *Generic*
capsules: 65 mg propoxyphene hydrochloride, 650 mg acetaminophen	*Generic*
capsules: 65 mg propoxyphene hydrochloride, 325 mg aspirin	Darvon w/A.S.A. Pulvules
capsules: 32 mg propoxyphene hydrochloride, 389 mg aspirin, 32.4 mg caffeine	Darvon Compound Pulvules
capsules: 65 mg propoxyphene hydrochloride, 389 mg aspirin, 32.4 mg caffeine	Bexophene, Darvon Compound-65 Pulvules, Dolene Compound-65, Doxaphene Compound, SK-65 Compound, *Generic*
tablets: 50 mg propoxyphene napsylate, 325 mg acetaminophen	Darvocet-N 50
tablets: 100 mg propoxyphene napsylate, 650 mg acetaminophen	Darvocet-N 100
tablets: 100 mg propoxyphene napsylate, 325 mg aspirin	Darvon-N w/A.S.A.

INDICATIONS

Relief of mild to moderate pain. Propoxyphene combinations are indicated for pain alone or pain accompanied by fever.

CONTRAINDICATIONS

Hypersensitivity.

ACTIONS

A centrally acting analgesic structurally related to methadone. It is $1/50$ to $1/25$ as potent as morphine and $^2/_3$ as potent as codeine. When given alone in usual analgesic doses (32–65 mg of the hydrochloride or 100 mg of the napsylate salt), it is no more and possibly less effective than 30 mg to 60 mg codeine sulfate or 600 mg aspirin or acetaminophen. Propoxyphene combined with other analgesics (*e.g.,* codeine, aspirin, acetaminophen) is more effective than propoxyphene or other analgesics alone.

Propoxyphene is available as two different salts. The hydrochloride is water soluble and is rapidly and completely absorbed from the GI tract; peak plasma concentrations occur in 2 to 2½ hours after dosing. The napsylate salt is only slightly soluble in water and is less rapidly absorbed; peak plasma levels occur in 3 to 4 hours. Half-life is 6 to 12 hours, and drug is metabolized by the liver and excreted in urine, primarily as metabolites.

WARNINGS

Fatalities: Propoxyphene products, either alone or in combination with other CNS depressants, including alcohol, are a major cause of drug-related deaths. In one survey, approximately 20% of the deaths occurred in the first hour and 5% occurred in 15 minutes. Because of its added depressant effects, it is prescribed with caution for those whose condition requires concomitant administration of sedatives, tranquilizers, muscle relaxants, antidepressants, or other CNS depressant drugs. Many propoxyphene-related deaths occurred in those with previous histories of emotional disturbances or suicide ideation or attempts, as well as histories of misuse of tranquilizers, alcohol, and other CNS-active drugs. Some deaths have occurred as a consequence of accidental ingestion of excessive quantities alone or in combination with other drugs.

Drug dependence: When taken in higher than recommended doses over long periods of time, propoxyphene can produce drug dependence characterized by psychic dependence and, less frequently, physical dependence and tolerance. The drug will only partially suppress the withdrawal syndrome in individuals physically dependent on other narcotics. Abuse liability is similar to that of codeine.

Safety for use in pregnancy has not been established. Withdrawal symptoms in the neonate have been reported. Use only when potential benefits outweigh the unknown potential hazards to the fetus. Low levels have been detected in human milk, but no adverse effects have been noted in breast-feeding infants.

Not recommended for use in children.

PRECAUTIONS

May impair mental or physical abilities required to perform potentially hazardous tasks.

DRUG INTERACTIONS

The CNS depressant effect is additive with other **depressants** including **barbiturate anesthetics.** The pharmacologic effects of **phenobarbital** and **tricyclic antidepressants** may be increased. **Cigarette smoke** may decrease the efficacy of propoxyphene. Concomitant administration of **carbamazepine** may increase carbamazepine levels and produce headaches, dizziness, ataxia, nausea, and fatigue. Potentiation of the hypoprothrombinemic effect of **warfarin** has been described in those receiving propoxyphene and acetaminophen. **Charcoal** decreases the GI absorption of propoxyphene.

ADVERSE REACTIONS

Most frequent: Dizziness, sedation, nausea, vomiting.

Other: Constipation, abdominal pain, skin rashes, lightheadedness, headache, weakness, euphoria, dysphoria, minor visual disturbances, hepatic dysfunction.

OVERDOSAGE

Symptoms: Patient is usually somnolent but may be stuporous or comatose and convulsing. Respiratory depression is characteristic. The ventilatory rate and/or tidal volume is decreased, resulting in cyanosis and hypoxia. Pupils, initially pinpoint, may become dilated as hypoxia increases. Cheyne-Stokes respiration and apnea may occur. Blood pressure and heart rate are usually normal initially, but blood pressure falls and cardiac performance deteriorates, which results in pulmonary edema and circulatory collapse unless respiratory depression is corrected and adequate ventilation is restored promptly. Cardiac arrhythmias and conduction delay may be present. A combined respiratory–metabolic acidosis occurs owing to retained CO_2 and to lactic acid formed during anaerobic glycolysis. Acidosis may be severe if large amounts of salicylates have also been ingested. Death may occur.

Treatment: Resuscitative measures are instituted promptly. Establish a patent airway and restore ventilation. Mechanically assisted ventilation may be required, and positive pressure respiration may be desirable if pulmonary edema is present. Naloxone will markedly reduce the degree of respiratory depression; administer promptly, preferably 0.4 mg to 0.8 mg IV, and repeat as necessary. The duration of the antagonist may be brief.

Monitor blood gases, pH, and electrolytes so that acidosis and electrolyte disturbance may be promptly corrected. Acidosis, hypoxia, and CNS depression predispose the patient to the development of cardiac arrhythmias. Ventricular fibrillation or cardiac arrest may occur. Respiratory acidosis rapidly subsides as ventilation is restored and hypercapnea is eliminated, but lactic acidosis may require IV bicarbonate for prompt correction. An anticonvulsant may be required.

General supportive measures may also include IV fluids, vasopressor-inotropic compounds, and, when infection is likely, anti-infective agents. Dialysis is of little value.

DOSAGE

PROPOXYPHENE HCl
Usual dose is 65 mg q4h as needed for pain. Maximum recommended dose is 390 mg/day.

PROPOXYPHENE NAPSYLATE
Usual dose is 100 mg q4h as needed for pain. Maximum recommended dose is 600 mg/day.

COMBINATION PRODUCTS
Average adult dose is one or two tablets or capsules q4h to q6h as needed for pain.

NURSING IMPLICATIONS

HISTORY
See Appendix 4.

PHYSICAL ASSESSMENT
Evaluate pain.

ADMINISTRATION
If nausea or vomiting occurs, drug may be given with food. Avoid freezing of the suspension.

ONGOING ASSESSMENTS AND NURSING MANAGEMENT
Question patient about relief of pain or discomfort approximately 1 hour after administration. Inform physician if drug is not effective in reducing pain or discomfort.

May cause sedation or dizziness. Assist patient with ambulatory activities as needed. If dizziness or lightheadedness persists, advise patient to remain in bed.

PATIENT AND FAMILY INFORMATION
NOTE: Patient package insert is available with product.

May cause drowsiness or lightheadedness. Observe caution while driving or performing other potentially hazardous tasks.

Cigarette smoking may reduce the effect of the drug. (*Note*—Because sedation may occur, patient should be advised not to smoke.)

Avoid alcohol and other depressants.

If GI upset occurs, take with food.

Do *not* exceed recommended dosage. If drug fails to relieve pain or discomfort, contact physician.

Propranolol Hydrochloride

See Beta-Adrenergic Blocking Agents.

Propylthiouracil

See Antithyroid Agents.

Protamine Sulfate Rx

injection: 10 mg/ml   *Generic*
powder for injection: *Generic*
  50 mg/vial, 250
  mg/vial

INDICATIONS
Treatment of heparin overdosage.

ACTIONS
Protamines are strongly basic simple proteins of low molecular weight, rich in arginine. They occur in the sperm of salmon and certain other species of fish. When administered alone, they have an anticoagulant effect, but when given in the presence of heparin (which is strongly acidic), stable salt is formed, which results in loss of anticoagulant activity of both drugs. When used with heparin, protamine sulfate's effects are almost immediate and persist for approximately 2 hours.

WARNINGS
Recurrent bleeding: Hyperheparinemia or bleeding has been reported in some patients 30 minutes to 18 hours after cardiac surgery (under cardiopulmonary bypass) in spite of complete neutralization of heparin by adequate doses of protamine sulfate at the end of the operation. Additional doses of protamine sulfate are administered if indicated by coagulation studies, such as the heparin titration test with protamine sulfate and the determination of plasma thrombin time.

Hypotensive responses: Too-rapid administration can cause severe hypotensive episodes and anaphylaticlike reactions.

Use in pregnancy: There is no adequate information as to whether this drug may affect fertility in males or females or have a teratogenic potential or other adverse effect on the fetus.

PRECAUTIONS
Because of protamine sulfate's anticoagulant effect, do not give more than 100 mg over a short period unless a larger requirement is necessary. Protamine sulfate can be inactivated by blood, and when it is used to neutralize large doses of heparin, a heparin

"rebound" may be encountered. This complication is treated by additional protamine sulfate injections as needed. Patients with an allergy to fish may develop hypersensitivity reactions.

ADVERSE REACTIONS
Administration may cause a sudden fall in blood pressure, bradycardia, dyspnea, transitory flushing, a feeling of warmth, anaphylaxis, and hypertension that may result in respiratory embarrassment. Because fatal reactions often resembling anaphylaxis have been reported, drug is given only when resuscitation techniques and measures for treatment of anaphylactoid shock are readily available.

DOSAGE
Protamine sulfate 1 mg neutralizes approximately 90 USP units of heparin activity derived from lung tissue or 115 USP units of heparin activity derived from intestinal mucosa.

Because heparin disappears from the circulation, the dose of protamine sulfate required also decreases rapidly with the time elapsed following IV injection of heparin. For example, if protamine sulfate is administered 30 minutes after heparin, one-half the usual dose may be sufficient. Blood or plasma transfusions may also be necessary; these dilute but do not neutralize the heparin.

NURSING IMPLICATIONS

HISTORY
Review chart for heparin dosage and time of administration.

PHYSICAL ASSESSMENT
Obtain blood pressure, pulse, and respirations. If bleeding due to overdosage has occurred, document symptoms (_e.g.,_ hematuria, GI bleeding). Baseline laboratory tests may include PTT, APTT, whole blood clotting time, and clot retraction time.

ADMINISTRATION
Dosage is based on degree of heparin overdosage and time elapsed since heparin was administered.

Protamine sulfate is given slowly IV. Recommended maximum rate of administration is 50 mg in a 10-minute period or 5 mg/minute.

Incompatibilities: Do not mix with other drugs without checking with pharmacist because protamine sulfate has been known to be incompatible with certain antibiotics, including several of the cephalosporins and penicillins.

Preparation of solution
Caution: The 250 mg/vial powder for injection is for single-dose use when large doses of heparin have been given during surgery.

Powder for injection: Add 5 ml of Bacteriostatic Water for Injection with Benzyl Alcohol to the vial and shake vigorously to effect a complete solution. Reconstituted solution may be kept for 24 hours if stored in a refrigerator.

Prepared solution: Is intended for use without further dilution. If further dilution is desired, Dextrose 5% in Water or normal saline may be used. Do _not_ store diluted solutions because they contain no preservative.

CLINICAL ALERT: Too-rapid administration of protamine sulfate can cause severe hypotensive and anaphylactoidlike reactions. Drugs and equipment to treat shock should be immediately available.

ONGOING ASSESSMENTS AND NURSING MANAGEMENT
Monitor blood pressure, pulse, and respirations every 15 to 30 minutes or as ordered for at least 2 or more hours (up to 18 hours after cardiac surgery) after last dose of protamine sulfate is administered.

CLINICAL ALERT: Observe patient closely after cardiac surgery under cardiopulmonary bypass. Hyperheparinemia or bleeding has been reported 30 minutes to 18 hours after surgery in spite of complete neutralization of heparin by adequate doses of protamine sulfate. Look for hematuria, GI bleeding, ecchymosis, bleeding gums or bleeding of oral mucosa, hematoma at IM injection sites, oozing from incision or IV needle insertion sites, bleeding or oozing around the site of chest tube insertion, and so on.

Additional protamine sulfate may be required and is determined by heparin titration test with protamine sulfate and plasma thrombin time. Notify physician as soon as each laboratory test is reported.

Protamine Zinc Insulin Suspension

See Insulin Preparations.

Protriptyline Hydrochloride

See Antidepressants, Tricyclic Compounds.

Pseudoephedrine Hydrochloride, Pseudoephedrine Sulfate

See Bronchodilators and Decongestants, Systemic.

Psyllium

See Laxatives.

Pyrantel Pamoate *Rx*

oral suspension: 50 mg/ml   Antiminth

INDICATIONS
Treatment of ascariasis (roundworm) and enterobiasis (pinworm).

ACTIONS
Is regarded as a drug of choice for pinworm and roundworm infections. Has demonstrated anthelmintic activity against *Enterobius vermicularis* (pinworm) and *Ascaris lumbricoides* (roundworm). Anthelmintic action is probably due to its neuromuscular blocking property. It is partially absorbed after oral dose. Plasma levels of unchanged drug are low. Peak levels are reached in 1 to 3 hours. Quantities greater than 50% of administered drug are excreted in the feces as unchanged form: only 7% or less is found in the urine as the unchanged form of the drug and its metabolites.

WARNINGS
There is no experience in pregnant women who have received this drug. Safety and efficacy for use in children under 2 not established; the relative benefit and risk should be considered in this age group.

PRECAUTIONS
Minor transient elevations of SGOT have occurred. Drug is used cautiously in those with preexisting liver dysfunction.

ADVERSE REACTIONS
The most frequently encountered adverse reactions are related to the GI tract.

   GI and hepatic: Anorexia, nausea, vomiting, gastralgia, abdominal cramps, diarrhea and tenesmus, transient elevation of SGOT.

   CNS: Headache, dizziness, drowsiness, insomnia.

   Skin: Rashes.

DOSAGE
Given as a single dose of 11 mg/kg. Maximum total dose is 1 g. This corresponds to a simplified dosage regimen of 1 ml/10 lb.

NURSING IMPLICATIONS

HISTORY
See Appendix 4. A careful history of travel, eating habits, and sanitary facilities may be necessary to determine source of roundworm infection. Family members should also have stool examinations for roundworm. Because pinworm is easily transmitted from person to person, it is recommended that all family members be treated for complete parasite eradication.

PHYSICAL ASSESSMENT
Stool is examined for roundworm. If patient is hospitalized or outpatient appears ill or malnourished, obtain vital signs and weight. Pinworm specimen may be collected (in early A.M. before patient gets out of bed) by means of cellophane tape wrapped sticky side out around tongue blade or fingers; press against anal area (female pinworms deposit ova at night in perianal area). Transfer tape (sticky side down) to glass slide for microscopic examination. Baseline laboratory tests in those with roundworm may include CBC and serum electrolytes, especially if patient shows evidence of weight loss or appears ill, or if massive infection is suspected. Roundworm infections are usually reported to the public health department.

ADMINISTRATION
Purging is not necessary prior to, during, or after therapy.

   May be administered without regard to ingestion of food or time of day.

   May be given with milk or fruit juices.

ONGOING ASSESSMENTS AND NURSING MANAGEMENT
Isolation is rarely necessary; stool and linen precautions are usually instituted. Wash hands thoroughly before and after each patient contact, especially when disposing of urine or feces, changing bed linens.

   Pinworm can be transmitted from person to person; roundworm is not passed directly from person to person.

   If patient is acutely ill and hospitalized for roundworm infection, monitor vital signs q4h.

   Observe for adverse reactions; notify physician if they occur.

PATIENT AND FAMILY INFORMATION
May be taken in milk or fruit juice, but be sure entire dose is taken.

   Take entire amount of medicine prescribed as a single dose, unless otherwise specified by physician.

   Wash hands thoroughly before eating and after defecation.

   Pinworm: Meticulous hygiene is necessary to prevent reinfection. Change and launder undergarments, bed linens, towels, and nightclothes daily. Disinfect toilet facilities (including bathtub/shower) daily.

Clean under fingernails daily. Avoid putting fingers in mouth; nail biting must be avoided (liquid preparations that have a bitter taste and are painted on the nails and fingertips to discourage nail biting are available if patient persists in biting nails).

Roundworm: Thoroughly wash all vegetables grown in contaminated soil.

Bathe daily; change undergarments and bed linens daily.

Pyrazinamide Rx

tablets: 500 mg   *Generic*

INDICATIONS
Any form of active tuberculosis when treatment with first-line drugs has failed.

CONTRAINDICATIONS
Severe hepatic damage.

ACTIONS
Is an analogue of nicotinamide and is bacteriostatic against *Mycobacterium tuberculosis*. Little is known of its mechanism. It is well absorbed from the GI tract and reaches peak plasma concentrations in 2 hours and is widely distributed throughout the body, including cerebrospinal fluid. The drug is primarily metabolized by the liver; 3% to 5% of unchanged drug is excreted in the urine. There may be some concentration in bile.

WARNINGS
Should be used only when close observation of the patient is possible and when laboratory facilities are available for performing frequent, reliable liver-function tests and blood uric acid determinations. Safety and efficacy for use in children not established. Because of its potential toxicity, use is avoided in children unless crucial to therapy.

PRECAUTIONS
Use with caution in patients with a history of gout or diabetes mellitus, because management may be more difficult. Also use with caution in patients with acute intermittent porphyria.

ADVERSE REACTIONS
Hepatotoxicity: Principal untoward effect is a hepatic reaction. This varies from a symptomless abnormality of hepatic cell function, detectable only by laboratory tests, through a mild syndrome of fever, anorexia, malaise, liver tenderness, hepatomegaly, and splenomegaly, to more serious reactions such as clinical jaundice and rare cases of fulminating acute yellow atrophy and death. Incidence of hepatotoxicity ranges from 2% to 20%; generally, the higher the dose the higher the incidence.

GI: Nausea, vomiting, diarrhea.

Miscellaneous: Active gout; sideroblastic anemia and adverse effects on the blood clotting mechanism or vascular integrity; rashes; photosensitivity.

DOSAGE
Given with at least one other effective antituberculous drug. Average adult dose is 20 mg/kg/day to 35 mg/kg/day in three or four divided doses. Maximum daily dose is 3 g.

NURSING IMPLICATIONS

HISTORY
See Appendix 4.

PHYSICAL ASSESSMENT
Obtain vital signs, weight. Recommended pretreatment laboratory tests include hepatic-function tests, serum uric acid, and culture and sensitivity tests.

ADMINISTRATION
If nausea or vomiting occurs, consult physician about giving drug with food or meals.

ONGOING ASSESSMENTS AND NURSING MANAGEMENT
Monitor vital signs daily or as ordered.

Weigh weekly.

CLINICAL ALERT: The principal untoward effect is hepatic reaction. Observe for evidence of fever, anorexia, malaise, nausea, vomiting, jaundice, skin rash, pruritus, light-colored stools, darkened urine; notify physician immediately if one or more of these are noted.

Observe for symptoms of active gout and notify physician if pain in the great toe, instep, ankle, heel, knee, or wrist occurs.

Liver-function tests (especially SGOT, SGPT) every 2 to 4 weeks and periodic serum uric acid levels are recommended during therapy.

Evidence of hepatic dysfunction or hyperuricemia accompanied by symptoms of gout requires discontinuation of therapy.

PATIENT AND FAMILY INFORMATION
Notify physician or nurse if any of the following occurs: fever; loss of appetite; malaise; nausea; vomiting; darkened urine; yellowish discoloration of the skin or eyes; severe pain in the great toe, instep, ankle, heel, wrist, or knee.

Periodic laboratory tests will be necessary to monitor therapy.

Avoid prolonged exposure to sunlight, ultraviolet light; photosensitivity may occur.

Pyridostigmine Bromide

See Muscle Stimulants, Anticholinesterase.

Pyridoxine Hydrochloride

See Vitamin B_6.

Pyrilamine Maleate

See Antihistamines.

Pyrimethamine Rx

tablets: 25 mg   Daraprim

INDICATIONS

Chemoprophylaxis of malaria due to susceptible strains of plasmodia. Fast-acting schizonticides (chloroquine, quinacrine, or quinine) are preferable for treatment of acute attacks but concurrent use of pyrimethamine will initiate transmission control and suppressive cure. Also indicated for treatment of toxoplasmosis and used concurrently with a sulfonamide because synergism exists with this combination.

ACTIONS

Is a folic acid antagonist, and therapeutic action is based on the differential requirement between host and parasite for nucleic acid precursors involved in growth, because it selectively inhibits plasmodial dihydrofolate reductase.

WARNINGS

Dosage required for treatment of toxoplasmosis is 10 to 20 times the recommended antimalarial dosage and approaches toxic level. If signs of folic or folinic acid deficiency develop, dosage is reduced or drug is discontinued according to response of the patient. Folinic acid (leucovorin) may be given in a dose of 3 mg to 9 mg IM daily for 3 days, or as required to produce a return of depressed platelet or white blood cell counts to safe levels.

Use in pregnancy, lactation: Use for confirmed acute toxoplasmosis only after weighing the possibility of teratogenic effects against the possible risks of permanent damage to the fetus from the infection. Concurrent administration of folinic acid is recommended. Safety for use in lactation not established. The drug is excreted in human milk.

PRECAUTIONS

In treatment of toxoplasmosis, semiweekly blood counts, including platelet counts, are recommended. In those with convulsive disorders, a lower initial dose for treatment of toxoplasmosis is recommended to avoid potential nervous system toxicity. Drug may precipitate hemolytic anemia in those with G6PD deficiency.

ADVERSE REACTIONS

Anorexia and vomiting may occur with large doses. Vomiting may be minimized by giving drug with meals; it usually disappears with reduction in dosage. Large doses may also produce megaloblastic anemia, leukopenia, thrombocytopenia, pancytopenia, and atrophic glossitis.

OVERDOSAGE

Acute intoxication may involve CNS stimulation including convulsions. In such cases, use of a parenteral barbiturate may be indicated followed by folinic acid (leucovorin) administration. Accidental ingestion in children has led to fatality.

DOSAGE

Chemoprophylaxis of malaria
Adults, children over 10 years: 25 mg once weekly.
Children 4–10 years: 12.5 mg once weekly.
Infants and children under 4 years: 6.25 mg once weekly. Another pediatric regimen is 0.5 mg/kg once weekly, up to a maximum adult dose of 25 mg/week.
Treatment of acute attacks: Recommended only in areas where susceptible plasmodia exist. Not recommended alone in treatment of acute attacks of malaria in nonimmune persons. Fast-acting schizonticides are indicated for treatment of acute attacks, but concomitant pyrimethamine dosage of 25 mg daily for 2 days will initiate transmission control and suppressive cure. Should circumstances arise wherein pyrimethamine must be used alone in semi-immune persons, adult dosage for an acute attack is 50 mg/day for 2 days; children 4 to 10 yrs may be given 25 mg/day for 2 days. Clinical cure is followed by the once-weekly chemoprophylactic regimen described above.
Toxoplasmosis
Young patients may tolerate higher doses than older patients.

Adults: Initially, 50 mg/day to 75 mg/day with 1 g to 4 g of sulfapyrimidine. Continue for 1 to 3 weeks, depending on response and tolerance. Dosage for each drug may then be reduced by one-half and continued for an additional 4 to 5 weeks.

Pediatric: 1 mg/kg/day divided into two equal daily doses. After 2 to 4 days, dosage is reduced to one-half and continued for approximately 1 month. Usual pediatric sulfonamide dosage is used in conjunction with pyrimethamine.

NURSING IMPLICATIONS

HISTORY
See Appendix 4.

PHYSICAL ASSESSMENT
Obtain weight. Baseline laboratory tests may include CBC, platelet count.

ADMINISTRATION
Give with food or meals.

For malaria prophylaxis, drug is taken on same day each week.

ONGOING ASSESSMENTS AND NURSING MANAGEMENT
If GI upset persists despite giving drug with food, notify physician. Dosage reduction may be necessary.

When used for treatment of toxoplasmosis, CBC and platelet counts are recommended twice weekly. Withhold next dose and notify physician if most recent blood tests show anemia, leukopenia, thrombocytopenia, or pancytopenia.

Folic acid deficiency may occur. Notify physician if sore mouth or tongue, rash, fever, fatigue, shortness of breath, palpitations, pallor, weakness, or irritability occurs.

PATIENT AND FAMILY INFORMATION
For malarial prophylaxis, take on same day each week.

May cause GI upset; take with meals or food.

Notify physician or nurse if nausea and/or vomiting persists or sore mouth or tongue, fever, rash, fatigue, shortness of breath, palpitations, weakness, or irritability occurs.

Accidental ingestion in children has led to fatality.

Pyrvinium Pamoate Rx

tablets, film coated: Povan
   50 mg

INDICATIONS
Treatment of enterobiasis (pinworm infection).

ACTIONS
A cyanine dye that inhibits oxygen uptake, resulting in respiratory inhibition in aerobes. It also interferes with absorption of exogenous glucose; the parasite's endogenous reserves are depleted, and it dies. Drug is not appreciably absorbed from the GI tract.

WARNINGS
Use in pregnancy only when clearly needed and when potential benefits outweigh the unknown potential hazards to the fetus.

ADVERSE REACTIONS
Nausea, vomiting, diarrhea, and hypersensitivity reactions (photosensitization and other allergic reactions) have been reported. The GI reactions occur most often in older children and adults who have received large doses. Isolated cases of erythema multiforme (Stevens-Johnson syndrome) have been reported.

DOSAGE
5 mg/kg as a single dose. If necessary, dose is repeated in 2 to 3 weeks. Dosage for adults need not exceed seven tablets.

NURSING IMPLICATIONS

HISTORY
See Appendix 4. Because pinworm is easily transmitted from person to person, it is recommended that all family members be treated for complete parasite eradication.

PHYSICAL ASSESSMENT
Obtain weight. Pinworm specimen may be collected (in early A.M. before patient gets out of bed) by means of cellophane tape wrapped sticky side out around tongue blade or fingers; press against anal area (female pinworms deposit ova at night in perianal area). Transfer tape (sticky side down) to glass slide for microscopic examination.

ADMINISTRATION
Drug is given as a single dose. Give with food or milk to avoid GI upset.

Caution patient not to chew tablets but to swallow whole to prevent staining of teeth.

ONGOING ASSESSMENTS AND NURSING MANAGEMENT
Stools (and vomitus) will turn red; this is normal.

P

PATIENT AND FAMILY INFORMATION

Take with food or milk to avoid stomach upset.

Swallow tablets whole to avoid staining of teeth. Take the entire amount of prescribed medication as a single dose, unless otherwise specified by physician.

Stools (and vomitus) will turn bright red.

Meticulous hygiene is necessary to prevent reinfection. Change and launder undergarments, bed linens, towels, and nightclothes daily. Disinfect toilet facilities (including bathtub/shower) daily.

Clean under fingernails daily. Avoid putting fingers in mouth; nail biting must be avoided (liquid preparations that have a bitter taste and are painted on the nails and fingertips to discourage nail biting are available if patient persists in biting nails).

Avoid excessive exposure to sunlight and ultraviolet light for several days.

QR

Q
R

Quinacrine Hydrochloride Rx

tablets: 100 mg   Atabrine HCl

INDICATIONS

Treatment and suppression of malaria and treatment of giardiasis and cestodiasis.

ACTIONS

Quinacrine couples with and fixes DNA in a double strand with a hydrogen bond so that it is unable to replicate or serve for transcription of RNA. Protein synthesis is thus decreased through ribosomal destruction. Exerts both suppressive and therapeutic action in malaria. It destroys erythrocytic asexual forms (trophozoites) of vivax, falciparum, and quartan malaria, and sexual forms of vivax and quartan malaria. Is ineffective against falciparum gametocytes and sporozoites of all forms of malaria. It also eradicates certain intestinal cestodes, for example beef tapeworm, pork tapeworm, dwarf tapeworm, and probably fish tapeworm, and eliminates *Giardia lamblia* from the intestinal tract.

Oral administration produces maximum plasma levels in 1 to 3 hours. Highly bound to tissues and plasma proteins, quinacrine persists in the body for long periods of time; excretion is slow and drug tends to accumulate. The route of metabolism is unknown. The main route of excretion is through the urine; small amounts of unchanged drug are excreted in feces, sweat, milk, saliva, and bile.

WARNINGS

Use in patients with psoriasis may precipitate a severe attack. When used in those with porphyria, the condition may be exacerbated. Not used in these conditions unless benefit to the patient outweighs the possible hazard. Use in pregnancy only when clearly needed and potential benefits outweigh the unknown potential hazards to the fetus.

Resistant strains: Certain strains of *Plasmodium falciparum* have become resistant to synthetic antimalarial compounds, including quinacrine. Treatment with quinine or other specific forms of therapy are advised for those infected with a resistant strain of parasites.

PRECAUTIONS

Periodic blood counts are recommended if patient is given prolonged therapy. If any severe blood disorder appears that is not attributable to the disease under treatment, drug is discontinued. Drug is given cautiously to those with G6PD deficiency.

DRUG INTERACTIONS

Because quinacrine increases toxicity of the antimalarial agent **primaquine,** concomitant administration is contraindicated. **Alcohol** metabolism may be inhibited and cause a minor disulfiram reaction.

ADVERSE REACTIONS

Temporarily imparts a yellow color to the urine and skin but does not cause jaundice. Following administration of normal doses, adverse reactions include the following.

Frequent: Mild and transient headache, dizziness, and GI complaints (diarrhea, anorexia, nausea, abdominal cramps, and, rarely, vomiting).

Infrequent, reversible: Pleomorphic skin eruptions, neuropsychiatric disturbances (nervousness, vertigo, irritability, emotional change, nightmares, transient psychosis).

Rarely: Episodes of convulsions and transient toxic psychosis after doses of 50 mg to 100 mg tid for a few days.

Prolonged therapy: Aplastic anemia, hepatitis, and lichen planus–like eruptions, especially after long periods of malaria-suppressive therapy.

Dermatologic: Exfoliative dermatitis can develop as a primary reaction to the drug or as a secondary response to other types of quinacrine-induced symptoms. Contact dermatitis can also occur.

CNS: Seizures reported after administration of massive doses.

Ophthalmic: Reversible corneal edema or deposits, manifested by visual halos, focusing difficulty, and blurred vision reported during long-term suppressive therapy for malaria. Retinopathy reported rarely in those receiving relatively high doses for prolonged periods.

OVERDOSAGE

Symptoms: Although extremely large doses may prove fatal, some adults in suicidal attempts have taken enormous doses and survived. Toxic effects of large doses include CNS excitation with restlessness, insomnia, psychic stimulation, and convulsions; GI disorders (nausea, vomiting, abdominal cramps, diarrhea); vascular collapse with hypotension, shock, cardiac arrhythmias or arrest; yellow pigmentation of the skin.

Treatment: Is symptomatic. Evacuate stomach by emesis or gastric lavage. Convulsions, if present, should be controlled before attempting gastric lavage. If convulsions are due to cerebral stimulation, an ultrashort-acting barbiturate may be given cautiously. Anoxia-induced convulsions should be corrected by vasopressor therapy. In vascular collapse, administer vasopressors. Because of importance of supporting respiration, tracheal intubation or tracheostomy may be advisable. A patient surviving the acute phase and who is asymptomatic should be closely observed for at least 6 hours. Fluids may be forced and ammonium chloride (8 g/day in divided doses for adults) may be administered to acidify the urine and help promote urinary excretion.

DOSAGE

Malaria

Treatment: *Adults and children over 8 years*— 200 mg with 1 g sodium bicarbonate q6h for 5 doses; then 100 mg q8h for 6 days. *Children 4–8 years*—200 mg q8h the first day; then 100 mg q12h for 6 days. *Children 1–4 years*—100 mg q8h the first day; then 100 mg once daily for 6 days.

Suppression: Therapy maintained for 1 to 3 months. *Adults*—100 mg/day. *Children*—50 mg/day.

Dwarf tapeworm

Adults: The night before the medication, give 1 tbsp sodium sulfate dissolved in water. On the first day give 900 mg on an empty stomach, in 3 portions, 20 minutes apart, with sodium sulfate purge 1½ hours later. On the following 3 days, give 100 mg tid.

Children: Administer ½ tbsp sodium sulfate the night before the medication. *Children 4–8 years*— Initial dose is 200 mg; maintenance therapy is 100 mg after breakfast for 3 days. *Children 8–10 years*—Initial dose is 300 mg; maintenance therapy is 100 mg bid for 3 days. *Children 11–14 years*— Initial dose is 400 mg; maintenance therapy is 100 mg tid for 3 days.

Tapeworm (beef, pork, fish)

Preliminary bland, semisolid, nonfat diet or milk diet on the day before the medication, with fasting following the evening meal. A saline purge or purge and cleansing enema may be given before treatment. Saline purge is given 1 to 2 hours later.

Adults: Four doses of 200 mg 10 minutes apart. Give sodium bicarbonate 600 mg with each dose.

Children: *5–10 years*—400 mg total dose; *11–14 years*—600 mg total dose. Administer in three or four divided doses 10 minutes apart. Sodium bicarbonate may be given with each dose.

Giardiasis

Adults: 100 mg tid for 5 to 7 days.

Children: 7 mg/kg/day given in three divided doses (maximum 300 mg/day) after meals for five days. Stool is examined 2 weeks later and a repeat course given if needed.

▌ *NURSING IMPLICATIONS*

HISTORY

See Appendix 4. When used for treatment of malaria, a travel history may be necessary. If used for treatment of cestodiasis or giardiasis, a thorough history of food and/or water consumption is required.

PHYSICAL ASSESSMENT

Obtain blood pressure, pulse, respirations, weight. For cestodiasis or giardiasis obtain fresh stool specimen for examination.

ADMINISTRATION

Tablets may be pulverized for administration to children. Bitter taste may be disguised in jam or honey.

When given for treatment or suppression of malaria, tablets are given after meals with a full glass of water, tea, or fruit juice.

For treatment of cestodiasis, physician orders regimen to be followed before and after administration of drug. See *Dosage* for recommended regimens.

Sodium bicarbonate is recommended with each dose to reduce tendency of nausea and vomiting.

ONGOING ASSESSMENTS AND NURSING MANAGEMENT

Save all stool specimens for laboratory examination. Consult hospital policy manual or contact laboratory regarding specimen container and directions for collection of specimen.

Provide patient with bedpan for collection of stool specimens. Toilet tissue is disposed of in a separate paper bag.

The expelled beef, pork, or fish tapeworm will be stained yellow, facilitating identification of the scolex (head).

In treatment of giardiasis the stool is examined 2 weeks after treatment with quinacrine.

Observe for adverse reactions and report occurrence to physician.

PATIENT AND FAMILY INFORMATION

NOTE: Patients with cestodiasis are most always hospitalized for treatment.

May impart a yellow color to skin and/or urine.

Promptly report any visual disturbances (blurred vision, halos around lights, difficulty focusing eyes).

Giardiasis: Take drug on an empty stomach.

Stool specimens will be necessary in approximately 2 weeks after course of therapy is completed. (*Note*—Supply patient with specimen container and instructions.)

Malaria treatment or suppression: Take after meals with a full glass of water, tea, or fruit juice.

Long-term therapy (malaria): Physician may order laboratory tests (CBC) and recommend a complete ophthalmologic examination before and periodically during therapy.

Q
R

Quinestrol

See Estrogens.

Quinethazone

See Thiazides and Related Diuretics.

Quinidine Preparations

Quinidine Gluconate Rx

tablets, sustained release: 324 mg	Quinaglute Dura-Tabs, Quinatime, Quin-Release, *Generic*
tablets, sustained release: 330 mg	Duraquin
injection: 80 mg/ml	*Generic*

Quinidine Polygalacturonate Rx

tablets: 275 mg	Cardioquin

Quinidine Sulfate Rx

tablets: 100 mg	Cin-Quin, *Generic*
tablets: 200 mg	Cin-Quin, Quinora, SK-Quinidine Sulfate, *Generic*
tablets: 300 mg	Cin-Quin, Quinora, *Generic*
tablets, sustained release: 300 mg	Quinidex Extentabs
capsules: 200 mg	Cin-Quin, *Generic*
capsules: 300 mg	Cin-Quin
injection: 200 mg/ml	*Generic*

INDICATIONS

Oral: Premature atrial and ventricular contractions; paroxysmal atrial tachycardia; paroxysmal atrioventricular (AV) junctional tachycardia; atrial flutter; paroxysmal atrial fibrillation; some cases of established atrial fibrillation; paroxysmal ventricular tachycardia when not associated with complete heart block; maintenance therapy after electrical conversion of atrial fibrillation and/or flutter.

Parenteral: When oral therapy is not feasible or when rapid therapeutic effect is required.

CONTRAINDICATIONS

Hypersensitivity or idiosyncrasy to quinidine; myasthenia gravis; history of thrombocytopenic purpura associated with previous quinidine administration; digitalis intoxication manifested by arrhythmias or AV conduction disorders; partial AV or complete heart block; complete bundle branch block or other severe intraventricular conduction defects exhibiting marked QRS widening or bizarre complexes; complete AV block with an AV nodal or idioventricular pacemaker; ectopic impulses due to escape mechanisms. Also contraindicated in renal disease resulting in significant azotemia, marked cardiac enlargement, particularly with CHF, poor renal function, and especially renal tubular acidosis.

ACTIONS

Depresses excitability, conduction velocity, and, to a lesser extent, contractility of the myocardium. Therapeutically, its most valuable action is prolonging the refractory period, thereby decreasing the excitability of heart muscle. Besides these direct effects, it exerts some indirect activity on the heart through an anticholinergic action. It decreases vagal tone and prevents cardiac slowing produced by vagal stimulation and by cholinergic drugs. Large oral doses may reduce arterial pressure by means of peripheral vasodilatation. Hypotension of a serious degree is more likely with parenteral use.

Quinidine is essentially completely absorbed after oral administration; peak plasma concentrations are achieved in 60 to 90 minutes following quinidine sulfate and in 3 to 4 hours after administration of quinidine gluconate. Activity persists for 6 to 8 or more hours. Peak serum levels are slightly lower and are achieved more slowly with the gluconate and polygalacturonate salts. It is 60% to 80% bound to plasma proteins. Metabolism is via the liver; 20% is excreted unchanged in the urine within 24 hours. Elimination half-life is approximately 6 hours. Acidification of urine facilitates quinidine excretion and alkalinization retards excretion. In those with hepatic insufficiency or CHF, the elimination half-life may be increased and the total clearance significantly decreased.

WARNINGS

Hepatotoxicity, including granulomatous hepatitis, due to quinidine hypersensitivity, has been reported. Cessation of quinidine usually results in the disappearance of toxicity.

Prior to use in atrial flutter, patient is pretreated with a digitalis preparation to block AV conduction, preventing a rapid ventricular response.

Evidence of quinidine cardiotoxicity (increased P–R and Q–T intervals, 50% widening of QRS complex, frequent ventricular ectopic beats, tachycardia) mandates immediate discontinuation of the drug and close ECG monitoring of patient.

Dangers of parenteral use are increased in the presence of atrioventricular block or in the absence of atrial activity. Administration is more hazardous in patients with extensive myocardial damage than in persons with a normal myocardium who have cardiac arrhythmia. Occasionally, a cardiac arrhythmia may have been produced by digitalis intoxication; the use of quinidine in this situation is extremely dangerous because the cardiac glycoside may already have caused serious impairment of the intracardiac conduction system. Too-rapid IV administration may cause a fall of 40 mm Hg to 50 mm Hg in arterial pressure.

Syncope may occur as a complication of long-term therapy. It is manifested by sudden loss of consciousness and ventricular arrhythmias with bizarre QRS complexes. This syndrome does not appear to be related to dose or plasma levels but occurs more often with prolonged Q–T intervals.

Use in pregnancy only when clearly needed and when potential benefits outweigh the unknown potential hazards to the fetus. Quinidine is excreted in breast milk; nursing is avoided while taking this drug.

Safety and efficacy for use in children has not been established.

PRECAUTIONS

Should be used with extreme caution when there is incomplete AV block, because complete block and asystole may result. Drug may cause unpredicatable abnormalities of rhythm in digitalized hearts and is used with caution in presence of digitalis intoxication. Use with care in patients with partial bundle branch block.

The depressant actions of quinidine on cardiac contractility and arterial blood pressure limit its use in CHF and in hypotensive states unless these conditions are due to or aggravated by the arrhythmia.

Vagolytic effects: Because quinidine antagonizes the effect of vagal excitation on the atrium and the AV node, administration of parasympathomimetic drugs or use of any other procedure to enhance vagal activity may fail to terminate paroxysmal supraventricular tachycardia in patients receiving quinidine. Quinidine is used with caution in those with poor renal function because of potential accumulation in plasma leading to toxic concentrations. The effect of quinidine is enhanced by potassium and reduced if hypokalemia is present. Periodic blood counts and liver- and renal-function tests are recommended during long-term therapy and use is discontinued if signs of hepatic disorders or blood dyscrasias occur.

DRUG INTERACTIONS

Quinidine has been reported to increase the hypoprothrombinemic effect of **oral anticoagulants** and has been implicated in the production of frank hemorrhage in patients on chronic oral anticoagulation therapy. Quinidine may potentiate the neuromuscular blocking effects in patients receiving depolarizing or nondepolarizing **neuromuscular blocking agents** (*e.g.,* decamethonium, tubocurarine, succinylcholine).

Acetazolamide, thiazide diuretics, sodium bicarbonate, antacids (calcium carbonate-glucine and aluminum and magnesium hydroxide suspensions), a **diet high in alkaline ash** (*e.g.,* milk, vegetables, citrus fruit) and other agents that alkalinize the urine may enhance tubular reabsorption of quinidine and thus could lead to increased quinidine serum levels. **Antacids** may delay absorption.

Concurrent administration of **phenobarbital, phenytoin,** or **rifampin** may induce hepatic enzymes and significantly reduce the serum half-life of quinidine. When adding or discontinuing these agents, quinidine dosage adjustment may be necessary. Concomitant administration with **digoxin** may increase serum digoxin levels, thus increasing the possibility of cardiotoxicity. Quinidine and **other antiarrhythmic agents, phenothiazines,** or **reserpine** may produce additive cardiac depressant effects when used together. Concurrent administration of quinidine and **nifedipine** may result in decreased quinidine serum concentrations. Concomitant use of quinidine and **verapamil** resulted in significant hypotension in a few patients with hypertrophic cardiomyopathy.

ADVERSE REACTIONS

Cinchonism: Ringing in the ears, headache, nausea, dizziness, fever, vertigo, lightheadedness, tremor, disturbed vision. These may appear in sensitive patients after a single dose.

Cardiovascular: Widening of the QRS complex, cardiac asystole, ventricular ectopic beats, idioventricular rhythms (including ventricular tachycardia and fibrillation), paradoxical tachycardia, arterial embolism, hypotension.

GI: Nausea, vomiting, abdominal pain, diarrhea. Reversible granulomatous hepatitis and hepatic dysfunction have been reported.

Hematologic: Acute hemolytic anemia, hypoprothrombinemia, thrombocytopenic purpura, agranulocytosis.

CNS: Headache, fever, vertigo, apprehension, excitement, confusion, delirium, syncope, and disturbed hearing (tinnitus, decreased auditory acuity).

Ophthalmic: Disturbed vision (mydriasis, blurred vision, disturbed color perception, reduced vision field, photophobia, diplopia, night blindness, scotomata), and optic neuritis.

Pulmonary: Pulmonary hemorrhage associated with thrombocytopenia.

Q R

Dermatologic: Cutaneous flushing with intense pruritus, rash, urticaria, photosensitivity.

Lupus: Has been implicated (although extremely rare) in causing systemic lupus erythematosus. Symptoms reported include arthralgia and pancytopenia.

Hypersensitivity reactions: Angioedema, acute asthma, vascular collapse, respiratory arrest, febrile reactions.

OVERDOSAGE

Cardiovascular toxicity may be treated with sodium lactate, which blocks the cellular effect of quinidine on the myocardium by decreasing plasma potassium levels and raising plasma *p*H. Adrenergic stimulants may be useful in combating hypotension and myocardial depression. In the presence of advanced AV block or ventricular asystole, temporary transvenous pacing may be used. Hemodialysis (using a hypokalemic dialysate) may be effective in removing the drug.

DOSAGE

A preliminary test dose of a single tablet or 200 mg IM is recommended to determine whether patient has an idiosyncratic reaction. Dosage is adjusted to maintain plasma concentration between 2 mcg/ml and 6 mcg/ml. Dose usually required is 10 mg/kg/day to 20 mg/kg/day in four to six divided doses.

Premature atrial and ventricular contractions: 0.2 g to 0.3 g PO tid or qid.

Paroxysmal supraventricular tachycardias: 0.4 g to 0.6 g PO every 2 or 3 hours until paroxysm is terminated.

Atrial flutter: Quinidine is administered after digitalization and dosage is individualized.

Conversion of atrial fibrillation: Various schedules have been used. One is to give 0.2 g quinidine PO every 2 or 3 hours for five to eight doses, with subsequent daily increase of the individual dose until sinus rhythm is restored or toxic effects occur. Total daily dose should not exceed 3 g to 4 g in any regimen. Prior to quinidine administration, the ventricular rate and CHF (if present) should be controlled by digitalis therapy.

Maintenance therapy: 0.2 g to 0.3 g tid or qid.

Sustained-release forms: 0.3 g to 0.6 g q8h to q12h.

Parenteral

IM: In treatment of acute tachycardia, recommended initial dose is 600 mg of quinidine gluconate. Subsequently, injection of 400 mg of quinidine gluconate can be repeated as often as q2h. The amount of each dose must be gauged by the effect of the preceding one.

IV: In many patients the arrhythmia may be terminated by 330 mg or less of quinidine gluconate or its equivalent in other salts; as much as 500 mg to 750 mg may be required in some cases.

NURSING IMPLICATIONS

HISTORY
See Appendix 4.

PHYSICAL ASSESSMENT
Obtain blood pressure, pulse, and respirations. Document pretreatment arrhythmia (if patient is on a cardiac monitor). Baseline laboratory studies may include hepatic- and renal-function tests, serum potassium, CBC.

ADMINISTRATION
Oral form may be given with food to minimize GI upset.

Oral quinidine gluconate and quinidine polygalacturonate are reported to have a lower incidence of GI irritation than quinidine sulfate.

Prior to using quinidine in atrial flutter, the patient may be pretreated with a digitalis preparation to block AV conduction, thus preventing a rapid ventricular response.

Obtain blood pressure, and pulse for 1 full minute before administration of drug, unless patient is on a continuous cardiac monitor. Withhold drug and notify the physician if there is a significant increase or decrease in the pulse rate, a change in the pulse rhythm or amplitude, or any decrease in blood pressure.

Continuous ECG monitoring is recommended when parenteral form is used and when doses of more than 2 g/day are administered.

IV administration: Dilute 10 ml of quinidine gluconate injection to 50 ml with 5% glucose. Inject slowly at a rate of 1 ml/minute unless physician orders a different rate of injection.

A preliminary test dose of a single tablet or 200 mg IM may be ordered to determine whether the patient has an idiosyncratic reaction.

ONGOING ASSESSMENTS AND NURSING MANAGEMENT

CLINICAL ALERT: Administration of quinidine is immediately discontinued when signs of cardiotoxicity occur (*i.e.,* a 50% widening of the QRS complex [25% in those with heart block, CHF, or digitalis intoxication], increased P–R and Q–T intervals, frequent ventricular ectopic beats, or tachycardia).

The ECG must be continuously observed, administration discontinued, and the physician notified if the above changes occur. In addition, observe for adverse reactions and report occurrence to the physician immediately because the appearance of adverse effects may require discontinuation of the drug.

The effect of quinidine is enhanced by potassium and reduced if hypokalemia is present. If hypokalemia is corrected by administration of potassium, observe for signs of overdosage (cardiotoxicity).

Monitor blood pressure and pulse q1h to q2h, and more frequently (q15m–q30m) if patient's condition is unstable, response to therapy is poor, or drug is administered parenterally. *Patients on maintenance therapy*—Monitor blood pressure and pulse q2h to q4h or as ordered.

Measure intake and output, especially during initial therapy and when patient is receiving parenteral form of drug. Notify physician if a change in the intake–output ratio is noted.

Observe for quinidine syncope (which may occur as a complication of long-term therapy), manifested by sudden loss of consciousness and ventricular arrhythmias that have bizarre QRS complexes.

Physician adjusts dosage to maintain plasma concentration between 2 mcg/ml and 6 mcg/ml. Quinidine plasma levels may be ordered daily or every 2 to 7 days.

If coumarin anticoagulants are given concurrently with quinidine, observe patient closely for hemorrhage (see *Drug Interactions*) *or any signs of bleeding* and notify physician immediately.

During long-term therapy, periodic CBC and renal-function tests are recommended; monitoring of hepatic function is recommended every 4 to 8 weeks. Drug is discontinued if blood dyscrasias or signs of hepatic dysfunction (unexplained fever, elevation of hepatic enzymes) occur.

PATIENT AND FAMILY INFORMATION

NOTE: Physician may wish patient or family member to monitor pulse during therapy; instruction may be necessary.

Do not discontinue therapy unless instructed by physician.

May cause GI upset; take with food.

Avoid excessive intake of citrus fruit juices (may make urine alkaline, retard quinidine excretion, and result in quinidine toxicity).

Inform other physicians of therapy with this drug.

Notify physician or nurse if any of the following occurs: persistent nausea and/or vomiting or diarrhea, ringing in the ears, visual disturbances (blurred vision, aversion to light, double vision,

difficulty seeing at night), dizziness, headache, easy bruising or bleeding, or fever.

Do not use nonprescription drugs unless use of a specific product is approved by the physician.

Follow physician's recommendations/instructions regarding rest, periods of exercise, caffeine intake (coffee, cola beverages, tea), diet, and so on.

Quinine Sulfate Rx

capsules: 130 mg, 195 mg, 325 mg	*Generic*
capsules: 200 mg, 300 mg	Quine, *Generic*
capsules: 260 mg	Strema
tablets: 260 mg	QM-260, Quinamm, Quiphile, *Generic*
tablets: 325 mg	*Generic*
suspension: 110 mg/ 5 ml	Coco-Quinine

INDICATIONS

Adjunct with pyrimethamine and sulfadiazine or tetracycline for treatment of chloroquine-resistant falciparum malaria. Also used for prevention and treatment of nocturnal recumbency leg muscle cramps, including those associated with arthritis, diabetes, varicose veins, thrombophlebitis, arteriosclerosis, and static foot deformities.

CONTRAINDICATIONS

Hypersensitivity; glucose-6-phosphate dehydrogenase (G6PD) deficiency; optic neuritis; tinnitus; history of blackwater fever and thrombocytopenic purpura (associated with previous quinine ingestion). Quinine is contraindicated in pregnancy because it has oxytocic action and passes the placental barrier. Congenital malformations (deafness, limb abnormalities, visual changes) and stillbirths have been reported, primarily with large doses for attempted abortion.

ACTIONS

Is a cinchona alkaloid generally replaced by more effective and less toxic agents. Antimalarial action is believed to be intercalation of the quinoline moiety into the DNA of the parasite, reducing effectiveness of DNA to act as a template. It depresses oxygen uptake and carbohydrate metabolism of the plasmodia. Quinine has a skeletal muscle relaxant effect and also has analgesic, antipyretic, and oxytocic effects, as well as cardiovascular effects similar to those of quinidine.

Q
R

Quinine is well absorbed, mainly from the upper part of the small intestine. Peak plasma concentrations occur within 1 to 3 hours, and half-life is 4 to 5 hours. It is widely distributed in tissues and bound to plasma protein. It is primarily metabolized by the liver with the metabolites excreted in urine, with small amounts excreted in feces, bile, gastric juice, and saliva.

WARNINGS

Repeated doses or overdosage may precipitate cinchonism. Hemolysis has been associated with a G6PD deficiency. Therapy is discontinued if evidence of hemolysis appears. Use with caution in those with cardiac arrhythmias because quinine has quinidinelike activity. Quinine is excreted in breast milk in small amounts.

PRECAUTIONS

Drug is discontinued if there is evidence of hypersensitivity.

DRUG INTERACTIONS

Increased plasma levels of **digoxin** and **digitoxin** have been seen in those taking quinidine. Because of possible similar effects from use of quinine, plasma levels for digoxin and digitoxin are recommended. Concurrent use of **aluminum-containing antacids** may delay or decrease absorption of quinine. The effects of **neuromuscular blocking agents** may be potentiated with quinine and result in respiratory difficulties.

Quinine has the potential to depress the hepatic enzyme system that synthesizes vitamin K–dependent factors. The resulting hypoprothrombinemic effect may enhance the action of **warfarin** and other **oral anticoagulants. Urinary alkalinizers** (*e.g.,* acetazolamide and sodium bicarbonate) administered concurrently with quinine may increase quinine blood levels, with potential for toxicity.

Drug/lab tests: Quinine may interfere with **17-hydroxycorticosteroid determinations** (using modification of the Rocky, Jenkins, and Thorn procedure) and elevated value for urinary **17-ketogenic steroids** (when Zimmerman method is used).

ADVERSE REACTIONS

Cinchonism (tinnitus, dizziness, headache, GI and visual disturbances) frequently occurs at full therapeutic doses but subsides rapidly upon discontinuation of the drug. With large doses or continued therapy, symptoms may become severe.

Hematologic: Active hemolysis, hemolytic anemia, thrombocytopenic purpura, agranulocytosis, hypoprothrombinemia.

Ophthalmic: Visual disturbances (disturbed color vision and perception photophobia, blurred vision with scotomata, night blindness, amblyopia, diminished visual fields, mydriasis, optic atrophy).

CNS: Tinnitus, deafness, vertigo, headache, fever, apprehension, restlessness, confusion, syncope, excitement, delirium, hypothermia, convulsions.

GI: Nausea, vomiting, epigastric pain.

Hypersensitivity: Cutaneous rashes, occasional edema of the face, asthmatic symptoms.

Cardiovascular: Anginal symptoms.

OVERDOSAGE

Symptoms: In addition to the above adverse effects, blindness, decreased blood pressure, depressed respiration, convulsions, paralysis, cardiovascular changes, coma, and death may occur.

Treatment: Perform gastric lavage or induce emesis with syrup of ipecac. Support blood pressure and use symptomatic measures to maintain renal function. Supply artifical respiration, if needed. Use sedatives, oxygen, and other supportive measures, as necessary. Maintain fluid and electrolyte balance with IV fluids. Acidification of urine will promote renal excretion. In the presence of hemoglobinuria, acidification may augment renal blockage. Drug should be dialyzable by hemoperfusion and hemodialysis procedures. Angioedema or asthma may require use of epinephrine, corticosteroids, and antihistamines. For quinine-associated blindness, vasodilators or stellate block may be used.

DOSAGE

Chloroquine-resistant malaria
Adults: 650 mg q8h for 10 to 14 days.
Children: 25 mg/kg/day q8h for 10 to 14 days.
Nocturnal leg cramps
200 mg to 300 mg H.S.

NURSING IMPLICATIONS

HISTORY

See Appendix 4. Note that drug is contraindicated in pregnancy.

PHYSICAL ASSESSMENT

Obtain weight (children).

ADMINISTRATION

Give with food or after meals to minimize GI upset.

Capsule contents should not be emptied or tablets crushed and added to food, because drug has bitter taste and is irritating to stomach. If patient has difficulty swallowing capsule or tablet, inform physician. An oral suspension is available.

ONGOING ASSESSMENTS AND NURSING MANAGEMENT

If blurred vision or dizziness occurs, assist patient with ambulatory activities.

Observe for adverse reactions and signs of cinchonism (tinnitus, dizziness, headache, diarrhea, abdominal cramps or pain, vomiting); notify physician if these occur because medication may need to be discontinued or dosage reduced.

Nocturnal leg cramps: Ask patient about relief of symptoms. If symptoms persist after a week or more of therapy, inform physician.

Malaria: Obtain vital signs q4h.

PATIENT AND FAMILY INFORMATION

Take with food or after meals to minimize GI irritation.

If tablet or capsule is difficult to swallow, inform physician. Do not break open capsule or crush tablet because drug has bitter taste and is irritating to the stomach.

May produce blurred vision or dizziness. Observe caution while driving or performing other tasks requiring alertness.

Notify physician or nurse if any of the following occurs: diarrhea, nausea, stomach cramps or pain, vomiting, ringing in the ears.

R

Rabies Prophylaxis Products

Antirabies Serum, Equine Origin *(ARS) Rx*

injection: 1000-unit vial   *Generic*

Rabies Immune Globulin, Human *(RIG) Rx*

injection: 150 IU/ml in 2-ml pediatric and 10-ml adult vial   Hyperab, Imogam

Rabies Vaccine, Human Diploid Cell Cultures *(HDCV) Rx*

injection: single-dose vial   Imovax Rabies Vaccine, WYVAC Rabies Vaccine

INDICATIONS

ANTIRABIES SERUM, EQUINE ORIGIN (ARS)

For all persons suspected of exposure to rabies. Administered as promptly as possible after exposure. Serum should be administered in all cases where this is practical, irrespective of the interval between exposure and treatment.

RABIES IMMUNE GLOBULIN, HUMAN (RIG)

Passive immunization against rabies when administered to those suspected of exposure to rabies and given as promptly as possible after exposure. If initiation of treatment is delayed for any reason, it should be given regardless of the interval between exposure and treatment.

RABIES VACCINE, HUMAN DIPLOID CELL CULTURES (HDCV)

Preexposure and postexposure treatment.

CONTRAINDICATIONS

ANTIRABIES SERUM, EQUINE ORIGIN

Positive intradermal test indicates a dangerous degree of sensitivity.

RABIES IMMUNE GLOBULIN, HUMAN

Repeated doses are contraindicated once vaccine treatment has been initiated because repeated doses may cause interference with full expression of active immunity expected from the vaccine. Also contraindicated in those known to have an allergic response to gamma globulin or thimerosal.

RABIES VACCINE, HUMAN DIPLOID CELL CULTURES

None known for postexposure treatment. Preexposure treatment not given in situations such as developing febrile illness and so on.

ACTIONS

Prophylaxis against rabies in persons exposed to rabies via animal contacts includes both passive immunization to provide immediate protection and active immunization to stimulate endogenous rabies antibody formation. There are two types of immunizing products: vaccines and globulins.

Vaccines

Induce an active immune antibody response that requires about 7 to 10 days to develop but persists for as long as a year or more.

Human diploid cell rabies vaccine (HDCV): An inactivated virus vaccine prepared from fixed rabies virus grown in human diploid cell tissue culture. High antibody titer responses has been demonstrated.

Globulins

Provide rapid immune protection that persist for a short period of time (a half-life of about 21 days).

Both globulins are effective but ARS causes serum sickness in over 40% of adult recipients; RIG rarely causes adverse reactions.

Rabies immune globulin, human (RIG): An antirabies gamma globulin. A dose of 20 IU/kg given simultaneously with the first vaccine dose results in amply detectable levels of passive rabies antibody 24 hours after injection and produces minimal, if any, interference with the response of the vaccine.

Antirabies serum, equine (ARS): A refined, concentrated serum obtained from hyperimmunized horses. Because of significantly lower incidence of adverse reaction, rabies immune globulin, human is preferred.

Rationale of treatment

Every possible exposure to rabies infection is individually evaluated. The following are considered before specific treatment is initiated:

1. *Species of biting animal*—Carnivorous animals (especially skunks, foxes, coyotes, raccoons, dogs, and cats) and bats are more likely than other animals to be infective. Bites of rabbits, hares, squirrels, rats, mice, hamsters, guinea pigs, gerbils, and other rodents seldom, if ever, call for specific rabies prophylaxis.
2. *Circumstances of biting incident*—An unprovoked attack is more likely to mean that the animal is rabid. Bites inflicted during attempts to feed or handle an apparently healthy animal should generally be regarded as provoked.
3. *Type of exposure*—Rabies is transmitted by inoculation of infectious saliva through the skin. The likelihood that rabies infection will result from exposure to a rabid animal varies with the nature and extent of exposure. Bite and nonbite exposures (scratches, abrasions, or open wounds or mucous membranes contaminated with saliva or other potentially infectious material such as the brain of a rabid animal) differs from casual contact such as that of petting the animal (without bite or nonbite exposure). Casual contact does not constitute an exposure and is not an indication for prophylaxis.
4. *Vaccination status of the biting animal*—A properly immunized animal has only minimal chance of developing rabies and transmitting the virus.
5. *Presence of rabies in the region*—If adequate laboratory and field records indicate that there is no rabies infection in a domestic species within a given region, local health officials may be justified in considering this in making recommendations on antirabies treatment.

Postexposure prophylaxis

Postexposure antirabies immunization should always include both passively administered antibody (preferably RIG) and vaccine (HDCV) with one exception: persons who have been previously immunized with rabies vaccine and have documented adequate rabies antibody titer should receive only HDVC.

Preexposure prophylaxis

The low frequency of severe reactions following HDCV has made it practical to offer preexposure immunization to persons in high-risk groups such as veterinarians, animal handlers, certain laboratory workers, persons (especially children) living in places where rabies is a constant threat, and those whose pursuits bring them into contact with potentially rabid dogs, cats, foxes, skunks, or bats.

WARNINGS

ANTIRABIES SERUM, EQUINE ORIGIN

Can cause reactions in patients with or without known sensitivity to horse serum. Immediate shock-like reactions include itching, sneezing, coughing, and asthmatic breathing. Generalized urticaria and marked hypotension may occur within minutes. Serum sickness may develop in 6 to 12 days, even with no prior history of sensitivity. Common symptoms are skin eruption, itching, lymphadenopathy, and arthralgia. In severe cases, fever, abdominal pain, malaise, and headache may be seen.

RABIES VACCINE, HUMAN DIPLOID CELL CULTURES

Pregnancy is not a contraindication to postexposure therapy. Local or systemic adverse reactions do not contraindicate continuing immunization.

DRUG INTERACTIONS

RABIES VACCINE, HUMAN DIPLOID CELL CULTURES

Corticosteroids and **immunosuppressive agents** may interfere with development of active immunity and predispose patient to developing rabies. These drugs are not administered during postexposure therapy unless essential and serum is tested for rabies antibody to ensure adequate response has developed.

ADVERSE REACTIONS

RABIES IMMUNE GLOBULIN, HUMAN

Slight soreness at injection site and slight temperature elevation may occur.

RABIES VACCINE, HUMAN DIPLOID CELL CULTURES

Local reactions include swelling, erythema, induration, itching, pain, and slight ache. Systemic reactions include mild nausea, headache, abdominal pain, muscle aches, dizziness, and malaise.

DOSAGE

ANTIRABIES SERUM, EQUINE ORIGIN (ARS)

Sensitivity testing: Intradermal test consists of intradermal injection of 0.1 ml of 1:100 or 1:1000 normal saline dilution of the antirabies serum followed by observation for 10 to 30 minutes. Redness, swelling of area, and whealing indicate a positive reaction. If desensitization is desired, schedule is given in the package insert.

Give as promptly as possible after exposure. Administer IM as a single dose of not less than 1000 units/40 lb. Part of dose is infiltrated into tissue around the wound whenever feasible.

RABIES IMMUNE GLOBULIN, HUMAN (RIG)
Single administration of 20 IU/kg (0.133 ml/kg) at time of first vaccine dose. Up to one-half of dose should be used to infiltrate the wound and the rest given IM.

RABIES VACCINE, HUMAN DIPLOID CELL CULTURES
Preexposure vaccination: Three injections of 1 ml each, on day 0, day 7, and either day 21 or 28. See package insert for recommendations for booster doses and alternative preexposure regimens.

Postexposure vaccination: Several regimens are recommended. WHO recommends six IM doses of 1 ml given on days 0, 3, 7, 14, 30, and 90 with the first dose accompanied by RIG. CDC recommends five doses and a single dose of RIG. The Immunization Practices Advisory Committee (ACIP) recommends a five-dose regimen of 1 ml on days 0, 3, 7, 14, and 28 with RIG on day 0. Individuals previously vaccinated against rabies may receive fewer injections, depending on their antibody level after vaccination. A recommended schedule is two doses, one immediately and one 3 days later. Passive immunization with RIG or ARS is not given.

NURSING IMPLICATIONS

HISTORY
An effort is made to identify the species of the biting animal and obtain information regarding the circumstances of the bite (provoked or unprovoked attack), appearance, and/or activity of the animal. If possible, the animal is captured and observed for 10 days.

PHYSICAL ASSESSMENT
Examine area of bite or area of nonbite exposure (scratches, abrasions, open wounds, mucous membranes contaminated with saliva or other potentially infectious material). Record size and appearance of wound and appearance of surrounding tissues.

ADMINISTRATION
Local wound treatment: Thoroughly cleanse area immediately with soap and water. Tetanus prophylaxis and measures to control bacterial infection may be ordered.

Have epinephrine available to counteract anaphylactoid reactions.

Injections are given IM into the deltoid region or upper, outer quadrant of the buttock (_exception_—intradermal sensitivity testing and subcutaneous desensitization with ARS or use of Imovax for preexposure vaccination following ACIP recommendations).

Sensitivity testing is recommended when ARS is to be used for passive immunization.

To prepare HDCV: Reconstitute with 1 ml of diluent supplied with the product. Gently rotate vial until completely dissolved and withdraw reconstituted vaccine by setting the vial in an upright position on the table. Remove the reconstitution needle and replace with a smaller needle for administration. (Imovax is supplied with disposable needle and syringe containing diluent and disposable needle for administration; WYVAC is not supplied with needles and syringe.)

Up to half the dose of ARS or RIG may be infiltrated around the wound and the remainder given IM.

Do not use the same syringe to administer RIG or ARS and HDVC or administer RIG or ARS and HDVC into the same site because this may result in vaccine neutralization.

ONGOING ASSESSMENTS AND NURSING MANAGEMENT
Hospitalization is usually not necessary unless multiple bites and soft-tissue injuries have occurred or patient requires close observation.

Inspect injection sites daily for local erythema, swelling, and itching and inform physician if these appear.

Obtain vital signs q4h or as ordered.

Mild local or systemic reactions may be treated with anti-inflammatory and antipyretic agents such as aspirin and antihistamines.

PATIENT AND FAMILY INFORMATION
NOTE: The vaccination schedule and the importance of adherence to the schedule are thoroughly explained. Physician may prescribe an antihistamine and/or recommend aspirin for local or systemic reactions.

Notify physician if severe itching, swelling, or pain is noted at injection site or if high fever occurs.

All injections are necessary, unless physician decides to terminate treatment.

Ranitidine Rx

tablets: 150 mg   Zantac

INDICATIONS

Short-term treatment of active duodenal ulcer. Most patients heal within 4 weeks; usefulness of further treatment has not been demonstrated. Safety in uncomplicated duodenal ulcer for periods of more than 8 weeks has not been demonstrated. In active duodenal ulcer and hypersecretory states, concomitant antacids are recommended as needed for relief of pain. Also used in treatment of pathologic hypersecretory conditions (*e.g.,* Zollinger-Ellison syndrome and systemic mastocytosis).

Unlabeled uses: Has shown some value in other pathologic states including gastric ulcer and protection against pulmonary aspiration of acid during anesthesia and reflux esophagitis.

CONTRAINDICATIONS

None known.

ACTIONS

Is a competitive, reversible inhibitor of the action of histamine at histamine H_2 receptors, including receptors on gastric cells. It does not lower serum calcium in hypercalcemic states and is not an anticholinergic agent. Ranitidine inhibits both daytime and nocturnal basal gastric acid secretion as well as gastric acid secretion stimulated by food, histamine, and pentagastrin.

Ranitidine inhibits gastric acid secretion and reduces the occurrence of diarrhea, anorexia, and pain in those with Zollinger-Ellison syndrome, systemic mastocytosis, and other pathologic hypersecretory conditions.

Ranitidine is 50% absorbed after administration, with mean peak levels occurring at 2 to 3 hours. Elimination half-life is 2 to 3 hours and duration of action is 8 to 12 hours. Absorption is not significantly impaired by food or antacids. Principal route of excretion is the urine.

WARNINGS

Use during pregnancy only if needed. Drug is excreted in human milk and caution is exercised when giving to breast-feeding mothers. Safety and efficacy for use in children have not been established.

PRECAUTIONS

Symptomatic response to therapy does not preclude the presence of gastric malignancy. Because drug is excreted primarily by the kidney, dosage is decreased in those with impaired renal function. Caution is observed in those with hepatic dysfunction because drug is metabolized in the liver.

DRUG INTERACTIONS

Use of ranitidine appears to have minimal interaction potential.

Drug/lab tests: False-positive tests for **urine protein** with Multistix may occur.

ADVERSE REACTIONS

Headache is the most frequent adverse reaction. Malaise, dizziness, constipation, nausea, abdominal pain, and rash have been reported in fewer than 1% of patients. Decreases in WBC and platelet count have been reported but did not require cessation of therapy. Some small increases in serum creatinine have also been noted. Some increases in serum transaminases and gamma-glutamyl transpeptidase have been seen. Rare cases of hepatitis have also been reported.

OVERDOSAGE

There is no experience to date with deliberate overdosage. The usual measures to remove unabsorbed material from the GI tract should be used.

DOSAGE

Duodenal ulcer: 150 mg bid. Smaller doses (100 mg bid) may also be effective.

Pathologic hypersecretory conditions: 150 mg bid. In some patients, it may be necessary to administer doses more frequently. Dosage is individualized and continued as long as indicated. Doses up to 6 g/day have been used in those with severe disease.

Impaired renal function: Recommended dose is 150 mg every 24 hours in those with a creatinine clearance under 50 ml/minute. Frequency of dosing may be cautiously increased to q12h or even further. Hemodialysis reduces the level of circulating ranitidine. Dosage timing is adjusted so that a scheduled dose coincides with the end of hemodialysis.

NURSING IMPLICATIONS

HISTORY

See Appendix 4.

PHYSICAL ASSESSMENT

Obtain vital signs, weight. If ulcer is active and bleeding, observe color of stool. Baseline laboratory/diagnostic studies may include CBC, serum creatinine, stool for occult blood, GI x-rays, and gastroscopy.

ADMINISTRATION

May be given without regard to meals or food.

ONGOING ASSESSMENTS AND NURSING MANAGEMENT

Obtain vital signs q4h or as ordered (more frequent monitoring may be necessary in those with bleeding ulcers).

Observe for signs and symptoms of hemorrhage (hematemesis, black tarry stools, signs of shock).

Antacids may be given concurrently for relief of pain.

Hematologic studies may be performed frequently if patient has active bleeding ulcer.

Therapy is usually terminated after 4 weeks, at which time GI studies may be performed.

PATIENT AND FAMILY INFORMATION

May be taken without regard to food or meals.

Follow physician's recommendations about additional treatment modalities (*e.g.,* diet, additional drugs such as antacids).

Notify physician or nurse if symptoms worsen or if severe abdominal pain, tarry stools, or vomiting occurs.

Do not use any nonprescription drug unless use is approved by physician.

Rauwolfia Derivatives

Alseroxylon *Rx*

tablets: 2 mg	Rauwiloid (contains tartrazine)

Deserpidine *Rx*

tablets: 0.1 mg (contains tartrazine), 0.25 mg	Harmonyl

Rescinnamine *Rx*

tablets: 0.25 mg, 0.5 mg	Moderil

Reserpine *Rx*

tablets: 0.1 mg	Serpalan, Serpasil, Serpate, *Generic*
tablets: 0.25 mg	Sandril, Serpalan, Serpanray, Serpasil, Serpate, SK-Reserpine, Zepine, *Generic*
tablets: 1 mg	*Generic*
capsules, timed release: 0.5 mg	Releserp-5
injection: 2.5 mg/ml	Sandril, Serpasil

Whole Root Rauwolfia *Rx*

tablets: 50 mg	Hiwolfia Tablets, Raudixin (contains tartrazine), Rauval, Rauverid, Rawfola, Wolfina, *Generic*
tablets: 100 mg	Hiwolfia Ovalets, Raudixin (contains tartrazine), Rauserpin (contains tartrazine), Rauval, Serfolia, Wolfina, *Generic*

INDICATIONS

ALSEROXYLON

Treatment of mild essential hypertension alone or as adjunctive therapy with other antihypertensive agents in more severe forms of hypertension.

DESERPIDINE

Treatment of mild essential hypertension.

RESCINNAMINE

Treatment of essential hypertension.

RESERPINE

Oral: Treatment of mild essential hypertension. May be used as adjunctive therapy with other antihypertensive agents in more severe forms of hypertension. Also indicated for relief of symptoms in agitated psychotic states, primarily in those unable to tolerate phenothiazine derivatives or those requiring antihypertensive medication.

Parenteral: Treatment of hypertensive emergencies in which it is desired to reduce blood pressure promptly. Other agents are usually preferred. This route has been used in psychiatric conditions only to initiate treatment in those unable to accept oral medication or to control symptoms of extreme agitation.

WHOLE ROOT RAUWOLFIA

Treatment of mild essential hypertension. May be used as adjunctive therapy with other antihypertensive agents in more severe forms of hypertension. Also indicated for relief of symptoms in agitated psychotic states in those unable to tolerate phenothiazine derivatives or those also requiring antihypertensive medication.

CONTRAINDICATIONS

Rauwolfia alkaloids are contraindicated in those with known hypersensitivity to these agents, a past history of bronchial asthma or allergy (may increase possibility of drug sensitivity reactions), mental depression (especially with suicidal tendencies), active peptic ulcer, ulcerative colitis, or pheochromocytoma and in those receiving electroconvulsive therapy.

ACTIONS

Rauwolfia alkaloids probably exert their antihypertensive effects by depletion of norepinephrine through inhibition of catecholamine storage in postganglionic adrenergic nerve endings. Their sedative and tranquilizing properties are thought to be related to depletion of amines in the CNS. The antihypertensive effect is often accompanied by bradycardia. There is no significant alteration in cardiac output or renal blood flow. The carotid sinus reflex is inhibited, but postural hypotension is rarely seen. Both the cardiovascular and CNS effects may persist following withdrawal of these drugs.

Onset of action is slow following oral administration; several days are required to deplete existing norepinephrine stores. Full antihypertensive effects may require up to 1 or more weeks. Effects may persist for several weeks after cessation of therapy.

The onset of antihypertensive effects produced by reserpine occurs in approximately 1 hour following a single IV dose; maximum effects are reached within 4 hours. Onset of action following IM administration is slightly longer and effects may persist up to 10 hours. Reserpine concentrates in tissues with high lipid content and crosses the placental barrier. It undergoes extensive hepatic metabolism; less than 1% is excreted unchanged in urine. Half-life ranges from 50 to 100 hours.

WARNINGS

Caution is exercised in administration to those with a history of mental depression. Drug is discontinued at first sign of despondency, early-morning insomnia, loss of appetite, impotence, or self-deprecation. Drug-induced depression may persist for several months after drug withdrawal and may be severe enough to result in suicide.

Parenteral reserpine should be used with extreme caution if patient is under treatment for hypertension with other potent drugs.

Safety for use in pregnancy not established. These drugs are used only when clearly needed and when potential benefits outweigh the unknown potential hazards to the fetus. These preparations are known to cross the placental barrier. They are also found in breast milk.

Safety for use in children not established.

PRECAUTIONS

These preparations are used with caution in those with impaired hepatic function. Rauwolfia preparations increase GI motility and secretion and are used cautiously in those with history of peptic ulcer, ulcerative colitis, or gallstones (biliary colic may be precipitated). Patients on high dosage are observed for possible reactivation of peptic ulcer. Caution is also exercised when giving these drugs to hypertensive patients with renal insufficiency because they adjust poorly to lowered blood-pressure levels.

Preoperative withdrawal of these drugs does not assure that circulatory instability will not occur. Anticholinergic and/or adrenergic drugs have been used to treat adverse vagocirculatory effects.

Some of these products contain tartrazine. See Appendix 6, section 6-23.

DRUG INTERACTIONS

These drugs are used cautiously with **digitalis** and **quinidine** because cardiac arrhythmias have occurred. Concomitant use of these preparations with **ganglionic blocking agents, guanethidine, veratrum, hydralazine, methyldopa, chlorthalidone,** or **thiazides** necessitates careful titration of dosage with each agent. **MAO inhibitors** should be avoided or used with extreme caution. Catecholamine depleting drugs (*e.g.*, reserpine) may have an additive effect when given with **beta blocking agents.** Patients treated with beta blockers plus a catecholamine depleting agent should be closely observed for hypotension and/or excessive bradycardia.

ADVERSE REACTIONS

GI: Hypersecretion; nausea and vomiting; anorexia; diarrhea; GI bleeding.

Cardiovascular: Anginalike symptoms; arrhythmias, particularly when used concurrently with digitalis or quinidine; bradycardia; syncope; fall in blood pressure; orthostatic hypotension. Rarely, water retention with edema may occur in those with hypertensive vascular disease but condition generally clears with cessation of therapy or with administration of a diuretic.

CNS: Drowsiness; depression; nervousness; paradoxical anxiety; nightmares; rare parkinsonian syndrome; CNS sensitization manifested by dull sensorium; deafness. Extrapyramidal symptoms have also occurred. These reactions are usually reversible and disappear when drug discontinued.

Ophthalmic: Glaucoma; uveitis; optic atrophy; conjunctival injection.

Dermatologic/hypersensitivity: Pruritus; rash; asthma in asthmatic patients.

Hematologic: Thrombocytopenic purpura and other hematologic reactions.

Miscellaneous: Nasal congestion is frequent. Dry mouth, dizziness, headache, dyspnea, epistaxis, impotence or decreased libido, dysuria, muscular aches, weight gain, breast engorgement, pseudolactation, and gynecomastia have been reported.

OVERDOSAGE

Symptoms: Impairment of consciousness may occur and may range from drowsiness to coma. Flushing of the skin, conjunctival injection, and pupillary constriction are to be expected. Hypotension, hypothermia, central respiratory depression, and bradycardia may develop with severe overdosage. Diarrhea may also occur.

Treatment: Evacuate stomach, taking proper precautions against aspiration and protection of the airway; instill activated charcoal slurry. Treat effects of reserpine overdosage symptomatically. If hypotension is severe enough to require treatment with a vasopressor, use one having a direct action on vascular smooth muscle (*e.g.,* phenylepinephrine, norepinephrine, metaraminol). Because reserpine is long acting, observe patient for at least 72 hours, giving treatment as required.

DOSAGE
ALSEROXYLON
Average initial dose is 2 mg/day to 4 mg/day. Usual maintenance dose is 2 mg/day.

DESERPIDINE
Mild essential hypertension: For those not receiving other antihypertensive agents, usual initial dose is 0.75 mg/day to 1 mg/day. Because 10 to 14 days are required to produce full effects, dosage is not adjusted more frequently than this. If therapeutic response is not adequate, another antihypertensive agent may be added to the regimen. *Maintenance therapy*—Dosage is reduced; a single daily dose of 0.25 mg may be adequate for some patients.

Psychiatric disorders: Average initial dose is 0.5 mg/day with a range of 0.1 mg to 1 mg. Dosage is adjusted according to patient response.

RESCINNAMINE
Average initial dose is 0.5 mg bid. Dosage is increased gradually, if necessary. Maintenance doses may vary from 0.25 mg/day to 0.5 mg/day.

RESERPINE
Hypertension: Usual initial dose is 0.5 mg/day for 1 to 2 weeks if patient is not receiving other antihypertensive agents. *Maintenance*—Dose is reduced to 0.1 mg/day to 0.25 mg/day.

Hypertensive crisis: May be given IM in short-term treatment. Because of varying responsiveness, a titration procedure is recommended. An initial dose of 0.5 mg to 1 mg IM is followed by doses of 2 mg and 4 mg at 3-hour intervals, if necessary, until blood pressure falls to the desired level. If the 4-mg dose ineffective, other antihypertensive agents should be used. An initial dose larger than 0.5 mg may induce severe hypotension, particularly in those with cerebral hemorrhage. Doses for children, adolescents, and elderly or severely debilitated patients should be proportionately lower than the adult dosage.

Psychiatric disorders: Average initial dose is 0.5 mg/day with a range of 0.1 mg to 1 mg. Dosage is adjusted to patient response.

Psychiatric emergencies: May be given IM to initiate treatment in those unable to take oral medication. Average dose is 2.5 mg to 5 mg following a small initial dose to test sensitivity.

WHOLE ROOT RAUWOLFIA
Average dose is 200 mg/day to 400 mg/day given in two divided doses. Maintenance doses vary from 50 mg/day to 300 mg/day given as a single dose or as two divided doses.

NURSING IMPLICATIONS

HISTORY
See Appendix 4.

PHYSICAL ASSESSMENT
Obtain blood pressure on both arms; obtain pulse, respirations, weight. If drug is used as a psychiatric agent, observe overt symptoms: general appearance and behavior, response to immediate environment, level of consciousness, emotional status, intellectual responses to verbal questions, and thought content.

ADMINISTRATION
Obtain blood pressure and pulse before each dose. Withhold drug and notify physician if there is a significant decrease in the systolic and/or diastolic pressure, a significant decrease in pulse rate, or a pulse rate below 60.

May be given with food or milk to minimize GI upset.

Lower doses may be prescribed for the elderly or severely debilitated patient.

ONGOING ASSESSMENTS AND NURSING MANAGEMENT
Monitor blood pressure and pulse q4h or as ordered during initial titration period.

Observe for adverse reactions.

When reserpine is administered for hypertensive crisis, monitor blood pressure and pulse q½h and keep physician informed of patient's response. Additional doses may be ordered at 3-hour intervals until desired response is obtained.

CLINICAL ALERT: Observe patient closely for signs of depression (*e.g.,* early-morning insomnia, anorexia, self-deprecation, loss of interest in surroundings, monosyllabic speech, loss of spontaneity, hypochondriasis, weeping). If one or more of these occur, withhold next dose, notify physician, and observe patient frequently (q½h) because drug-induced depression may be severe enough to result in suicide.

Q
R

When drug is used for a psychiatric disorder, observe behavior and compare to data base. If patient exhibits more disturbed behavior, notify physician immediately.

Full antihypertensive effects may require 1 or more weeks.

Drowsiness may occur, especially during first few days of therapy. Assist with ambulatory activities as needed.

Nasal congestion frequently occurs but cannot be relieved by nasal decongestants because most contain sympathomimetic agents.

Weigh two to three times a week or as ordered. If significant weight gain or loss is noted, inform physician. A diuretic agent may be necessary if weight gain is due to edema.

Dry mouth may be relieved by frequent sips of cool water, ice chips, hard candy, or chewing gum.

Dietary regimen for hypertension may consist of sodium restriction and/or calorie reduction (if weight loss is desirable).

Postural hypotension occurs rarely. If patient complains of dizziness or lightheadedness, suggest rising slowly from a sitting or lying position. If these effects persist, inform physician because a dosage reduction may be necessary.

Neonates born of mothers taking a rauwolfia alkaloid may have increased respiratory secretions, nasal congestions, cyanosis, and anorexia. Inform physician if these should occur.

When a rauwolfia derivative is discontinued prior to surgery, place a note on the front of the chart to alert the anesthesiologist to previous therapy with this agent; include date drug was discontinued.

PATIENT AND FAMILY INFORMATION

NOTE: Physician may wish patient or family member to monitor blood pressure daily or several times a week. Patient and/or family member will require instruction on this procedure.

Do not discontinue medication unless directed to do so by a physician.

Nasal congestion may occur. Do *not* use a nasal decongestant unless use of a specific agent is approved by the physician.

Do not use cough, cold, or allergy medications or nonprescription drugs available to control appetite (may contain sympathomimetics) except on professional recommendation.

May cause drowsiness, especially during first few days of therapy. Observe caution while driving or performing other potentially hazardous tasks requiring alertness.

May cause GI upset; take with food or milk.

Notify physician of any continued or severe GI pain, black tarry stools, any change in mood or sleep habits, depression.

Adhere to recommended dietary regimen and weight loss program (when applicable).

If dizziness occurs, avoid sudden changes in posture. Rise from a sitting or lying position slowly. If dizziness persists, notify physician.

Weigh self weekly. If significant (3–5 lb or more) weight gain or loss occurs or swelling in legs, ankles, or fingers is noted, contact physician.

Rauwolfia, Whole Root

See Rauwolfia Derivatives.

Rescinnamine

See Rauwolfia Derivatives.

Reserpine

See Rauwolfia Derivatives.

Rho (D) Immune Globulin

See Immunizations, Passive.

Riboflavin

See Vitamin B_2.

Rifampin Rx

capsules: 150 mg	Rifadin
capsules: 300 mg	Rifadin, Rimactane

INDICATIONS

Initial treatment and retreatment of pulmonary tuberculosis, in conjunction with at least one other antituberculous drug. Frequently used regimens include isoniazid and rifampin; ethambutol and rifampin; and isoniazid, ethambutol, and rifampin. Also used in treatment of asymptomatic carriers of *Neisseria meningitidis* to eliminate meningococci from the nasopharynx. Drug is prescribed after diagnostic laboratory procedures (serotyping and susceptibility testing); use is reserved for situations in which the risk of meningococcal meningitis is high. Because rapid emergence of resistance can occur, culture and sensitivity tests are recommended in the event of persistent positive cultures.

Unlabeled uses: Infections caused by *Staphylococcus aureus* and *S. epidermidis,* usually in combination with other drugs; gram-negative bacteremia in infancy; *Legionella* (Legionnaire's disease) not responsive to erythromycin; leprosy (in combination with dapsone); prophylaxis of meningitis due to *Haemophilus influenzae.*

CONTRAINDICATIONS

Hypersensitivity.

ACTIONS

Inhibits DNA-dependent RNA polymerase activity in susceptible cells. Specifically, it interacts with bacterial RNA polymerase but does not inhibit the mammalian enzyme. A dose of 600 mg is almost completely absorbed and achieves mean peak plasma levels within 1 to 4 hours. Food interferes with absorption. It is 75% protein bound but very lipid soluble; it penetrates and concentrates in many body tissues, including CSF. It is metabolized by the liver with about 40% excreted by the bile and undergoes enterohepatic circulation; 6% to 30% is excreted in the urine. Half-life is 1.5 to 5 hours but decreases by 40% over the first 2 weeks. Neither peritoneal nor hemodialysis removes significant amounts of rifampin from the plasma.

WARNINGS

There have been fatalities associated with jaundice in those with liver disease or patients receiving concurrent hepatotoxic drugs. The possibility of rapid emergence of resistant meningococci restricts use to short-term treatment of asymptomatic carriers. The effect of rifampin (alone or in combination with other antituberculous agents) on the fetus is unknown. It has been reported to cross the placental barrier and appear in cord blood. An increase in congenital malformations has been seen in laboratory animals; therefore, the possibility of teratogenic potential in women of childbearing age is weighed against the benefits of therapy. Rifampin is excreted in breast milk.

PRECAUTIONS

Not recommended for intermittent therapy. Urine, feces, saliva, sputum, sweat, and tears may be colored red-orange. Soft contact lenses may be permanently stained. May impart a yellow color to CSF.

DRUG INTERACTIONS

Concurrent administration of **p-aminosalicylic acid** (PAS) may decrease rifampin serum levels. Give drugs at least 8 to 12 hours apart. Severe hepatic dysfunction has been associated with concomitant **halothane** anesthesia and rifampin therapy, but causal evidence is lacking. The hepatic toxicity of **isoniazid** or rifampin may be increased and may cause one or both to be discontinued when administered concomitantly. However, evidence of synergistic hepatic toxicity requires further documentation. Predisposing factors may include female gender, large isoniazid doses, and recent general anesthesia.

Rifampin is known to induce hepatic microsomal enzymes that metabolize a wide variety of drugs. Agents that are documented to have decreased effectiveness because of this interaction are **metoprolol, propranolol, quinidine, corticosteroids, oral contraceptives, progestins, clofibrate, methadone, oral anticoagulants,** and **oral sulfonylureas** (tolbutamide, chlorpropamide). Agents with less convincing documentation include **barbiturates, benzodiazepines** (diazepam), **digitoxin,** and **dapsone.**

Drug/lab test: Therapeutic levels of rifampin inhibit standard assays for serum **folate** and **vitamin B$_{12}$.**

ADVERSE REACTIONS

Are more frequent when drug is used intermittently. A "flulike syndrome" may be seen in up to 20% to 50% of those on a high-dose (25 mg/kg once weekly) intermittent schedule but less so in commonly recommended doses.

GI (1%–2%): Heartburn, epigastric distress, anorexia, nausea, vomiting, gas, cramps, diarrhea, sore mouth and tongue, pseudomembranous colitis, pancreatitis.

Hepatic: Asymptomatic elevations of liver enzymes (up to 14%) and hepatitis (less than 1%). Hepatitis or shocklike syndrome with hepatic involvement (rare), abnormal liver-function tests, transient abnormalities in liver-function tests.

Allergic: Hypersensitivity reactions.

Dermatologic: Rash (1%–5%), pruritus, urticaria, pemphigoid reaction, flushing.

CNS: Headache, drowsiness, fatigue, dizziness, inability to concentrate, mental confusion, generalized numbness.

Hematologic: Eosinophilia, thrombocytopenia (intermittent dose), transient leukopenia, hemolytic anemia, decreased hemoglobin, hemolysis.

Musculoskeletal: Ataxia, muscular weakness, pain in extremities, osteomalacia, myopathy.

Ophthalmologic: Visual disturbances, exudative conjunctivitis.

Renal: Hemoglobinuria, hematuria, renal insufficiency, acute renal failure. These are considered hypersensitivity reactions; they have occurred during intermittent therapy or when treatment was resumed following intentional or accidental interruption and were reversible with rifampin discontinuation and appropriate therapy.

Miscellaneous: Menstrual disturbances, fever, elevations in BUN and elevated serum uric acid, possible immunosuppression, isolated reports of abnormal growth of lung tumors, reduced 25-hydroxycholecalciferol levels.

OVERDOSAGE

Signs and symptoms: Nausea, vomiting, and increased lethargy will probably occur a short time after ingestion; unconsciousness may occur with severe hepatic involvement. Reddish brown or orange discoloration of skin, urine, sweat, saliva, tears, and feces is proportional to the amount ingested. Liver enlargement, possibly with tenderness, can develop within a few hours after severe overdosage, and jaundice may develop rapidly. Hepatic involvement may be more marked in those with prior impairment of hepatic function. Other physical findings remain essentially normal. Direct and total bilirubin levels may increase rapidly with severe overdosage; hepatic enzyme levels may be affected, especially with prior impairment of hepatic function. A direct effect on the hematopoietic system, electrolyte levels, or acid–base balance is unlikely.

Treatment: Nausea and vomiting are likely to be present. Gastric lavage is probably preferable to induction of emesis. Activated charcoal slurry instilled into the stomach following evacuation of gastric contents can help absorb any remaining drug in the GI tract. Antiemetic medication may be required to control severe nausea or vomiting. Forced diuresis (with measured intake and output) will promote drug excretion. Bile drainage may be indicated in the presence of serious impairment of hepatic function lasting more than 24 to 48 hours; extracorporeal hemodialysis may be required. In those with previously adequate hepatic function, reversal of liver enlargement and impaired hepatic excretory function probably will be noted within 72 hours, with rapid return to normal thereafter.

DOSAGE

Give once daily either 1 hour A.C. or 2 hours P.C.

Pulmonary tuberculosis

Adults: 600 mg once daily.

Children: 10 mg/kg to 20 mg/kg, not to exceed 600 mg/day. Data are not available for use in children under 5 years of age.

Meningococcal carriers

Give once daily for 4 consecutive days.

Adults: 600 mg.

Children: 10 mg/kg to 20 mg/kg, not to exceed 600 mg/day.

NURSING IMPLICATIONS

HISTORY
See Appendix 4.

PHYSICAL ASSESSMENT
Obtain vital signs, weight. Baseline laboratory studies may include CBC, hepatic- and renal-function tests, urinalysis, and culture and sensitivity tests.

ADMINISTRATION
Administer on an empty stomach 1 hour A.C. or 2 hours P.C.

If PAS is given concurrently, give at least 8 to 12 hours apart. Because PAS is usually given two to four times a day, check with physician about dosage intervals.

If adult or child is unable to swallow oral capsules, check with the physician; a pharmacist can prepare an oral suspension from capsule contents.

Suspension may be prepared from the capsule by a pharmacist and must be stored under refrigeration at 2°C to 8°C (36°F–46°F) for no more than 6 weeks.

ONGOING ASSESSMENTS AND NURSING MANAGEMENT
Monitor vital signs q4h or as ordered.

Observe for adverse effects and notify physician if they occur.

Weigh weekly or as ordered.

CLINICAL ALERT: Observe for signs and symptoms of hepatotoxicity: malaise, fever, anorexia, jaundice, darkened urine, and pale stools; notify physician immediately if one or more of these are noted.

Periodic CBC and monitoring of hepatic function are recommended.

PATIENT AND FAMILY INFORMATION
Take on an empty stomach, at least 1 hour before or 2 hours after meals.

Take on a regular basis; do *not* skip a dose or discontinue therapy except on advice of a physician.

Drug may cause a reddish orange discoloration of urine, stools, saliva, tears, sweat, and sputum. This is to be expected and is not harmful.

If wearing of contact lenses is contemplated, be aware that drug may discolor the *soft* contact lens. If soft contact lenses are presently being worn, the discoloration may be undesirable; consult an ophthalmologist.

Notify physician if flulike symptoms (fever, chills, muscle and bone pain, headache), excessive tiredness or weakness, anorexia, nausea and vomiting, sore throat, unusual bleeding or bruising, yellowish discoloration of the skin or eyes, skin rash, or itching occurs.

Ritodrine Hydrochloride Rx

tablets: 10 mg   Yutopar
injection: 10 mg/ml   Yutopar

INDICATIONS
Management of preterm labor in suitable patients. Administered IV, it will decrease uterine activity and thus prolong gestation in the majority of patients. After IV ritodrine has arrested the acute episode, oral administration may help to avert relapse. Additional acute episodes may be treated by repeating the IV infusion. Successful inhibition of labor is more likely with early treatment and therapy, instituted as soon as diagnosis of preterm labor is established and contraindications are ruled out in pregnancies of 20 or more weeks of gestation. Safety and efficacy in advanced labor (cervical dilatation more than 4 cm or effacement more than 80%) have not been established.

CONTRAINDICATIONS
Before the twentieth week of pregnancy and in those conditions in which continuation of pregnancy is hazardous to the mother or fetus. Specific contraindications include antepartum hemorrhage that demands immediate delivery; eclampsia and severe preeclampsia; intrauterine fetal death; chorioamnionitis; maternal cardiac disease; pulmonary hypertension; maternal hyperthyroidism; uncontrolled maternal diabetes mellitus; and preexisting maternal medical conditions that would be seriously affected by the known properties of this drug, such as hypovolemia, cardiac arrhythmias associated with tachycardia or digitalis intoxication, uncontrolled hypertension, pheochromocytoma, bronchial asthma already treated with betamimetics or steroids, and known hypersensitivity.

ACTIONS
Is a beta-receptor agonist that has been shown to exert a preferential effect on β_2 adrenergic receptors such as those in uterine smooth muscle. Stimulation of these receptors inhibits contractility of uterine smooth muscle.

IV infusions or a single oral dose will decrease the intensity and frequency of uterine contractions. These effects are antagonized by beta-adrenergic

blocking compounds. IV administration induces an immediate dose-related elevation of heart rate. Widening of the pulse pressure is also observed. During IV infusion, transient elevations of blood glucose, insulin, and free fatty acids are also observed. Decreased serum potassium is also seen.

Ritodrine and its conjugates reach fetal circulation.

WARNINGS
Not recommended for patients with mild to moderate preeclampsia, hypertension, or diabetes unless benefits outweigh the risks.

Because cardiovascular responses are common and more pronounced during IV administration, cardiovascular effects are closely monitored.

PRECAUTIONS
When used for management of preterm labor in a patient with premature rupture of the membranes, the benefits of delaying delivery are balanced against potential risks of development of chorioamnionitis.

This drug should not be used before the twentieth week of pregnancy.

DRUG INTERACTIONS
Corticosteroids used concomitantly may lead to pulmonary edema. The effects of other **sympathomimetic amines** may be potentiated when concurrently administered and these effects may be additive. A sufficient time interval should elapse prior to administration of another sympathomimetic drug. **Beta-adrenergic blocking agents** inhibit the action of ritodrine and coadministration is avoided. When **anesthetics** are used in surgery, the possibility that hypotensive effects may be potentiated is considered.

Drug/lab tests: IV administration has been shown to elevate plasma **insulin** and **glucose** and decrease plasma **potassium concentrations;** monitoring of glucose and electrolyte levels is recommended during protracted infusions. Special attention is paid to biochemical variables when treating diabetic patients or those receiving potassium-depleting diuretics.

ADVERSE REACTIONS
IV administration

Usual effects (80%–100% of patients): Dose-related alterations in maternal and fetal heart rates and in maternal blood pressure. During studies using 0.35 mg/minute, the maximum maternal and fetal heart rates averaged, respectively, 130 (range 60–180) and 164 (range 130–200) beats per minute. The maximal maternal systolic blood pressures averaged 128 mm Hg (range 92–162 mm Hg), an average increase of 12 mm Hg from pretreatment levels. Minimum maternal diastolic blood pressures averaged 48 mm Hg (range up to 76 mm Hg), an averaged decrease of 23 mm Hg from pretreatment levels. Although more severe effects were usually managed by dosage adjustments, in fewer than 1% persistent maternal tachycardia or decreased diastolic blood pressure required withdrawal of the drug. Infusion is associated with transient elevation of blood glucose and insulin, which decreases toward normal values after 48 to 72 hours despite continued infusion.

Frequent effects: Approximately one-third of the patients experienced palpitation. Tremor, nausea, vomiting, headache, and erythema were observed in 10% to 15%.

Occasional effects: Nervousness, jitteriness, restlessness, emotional upset, anxiety, and malaise were reported in 5% to 6%.

Infrequent effects: Cardiac symptoms including chest pain or tightness (associated with ECG abnormalities) and arrhythmia were reported in 1% to 2%. Other infrequently reported maternal effects included anaphylactic shock, rash, heart murmur, epigastric distress, ileus, bloating, constipation, diarrhea, dyspnea, hyperventilation, hemolytic icterus, glycosuria, lactic acidosis, sweating, chills, drowsiness, and weakness.

Oral administration

Frequent effects: Small increases in maternal heart rate but little or no effect was found on either maternal systolic or diastolic blood pressure or fetal heart rate (FHR). Palpitation or tremor was experienced in 10% to 15%, nausea and jitteriness in 5% to 8%, and rash in 3% to 4%. Arrhythmia was infrequent (about 1%).

Neonatal effects: Infrequently reported symptoms include hypoglycemia and ileus. In addition, hypocalcemia and hypotension have been reported in neonates whose mothers were treated with other betamimetic agents.

OVERDOSAGE

Symptoms: Excessive beta-adrenergic stimulation including exaggeration of the known pharmacologic effects, the most prominent being tachycardia (maternal and fetal), palpitation, cardiac arrhythmia, hypotension, dyspnea, nervousness, tremor, nausea, and vomiting.

Treatment: Gastric lavage or induction of emesis followed by administration of activated charcoal. When symptoms of overdose occur as a result of IV administration, drug is discontinued; an appropriate beta-blocking agent may be used as an antidote. Ritodrine is dialyzable.

DOSAGE

Initial IV treatment should be followed by oral administration. Optimum dose is determined by a clinical balance of uterine response and unwanted effects. Recurrence of unwanted preterm labor may be treated with repeated infusion of ritodrine.

IV: Usual initial dose is 0.1 mg/minute (0.33 ml/minute or 20 drops/minute using a microdrip chamber at the recommended dilution) and is gradually increased according to results by 0.05 mg/minute (10 drops/minute) every 10 minutes until desired results are attained. The effective dosage usually lies between 0.15 mg/minute and 0.35 mg/minute (30–70 drops/minute). The infusion should generally be continued for at least 12 hours after uterine contractions cease.

With recommended dilution, the maximum volume of fluid that might be administered after 12 hours at the highest dose (0.35 mg/minute) will be approximately 840 ml.

Oral maintenance: 10 mg may be given approximately 30 minutes before termination of IV therapy. Usual dosage schedule for the first 24 hours of oral maintenance is 10 mg q2h. Thereafter, the usual dose is 10 mg to 20 mg q4h to q6h, the dose depending on uterine activity and unwanted effects. The usual daily dose should not exceed 120 mg.

NURSING IMPLICATIONS

HISTORY
See Appendix 4.

PHYSICAL ASSESSMENT
Obtain vital signs; frequency and intensity of uterine contractions; FHR. Baseline laboratory studies/diagnostic tests may include serum electrolytes, CBC, blood glucose, and sonography and/or amniocentesis to determine fetal maturity.

ADMINISTRATION

Preparation of IV solution: 150 mg ritodrine (3 ampules) added to 500 ml IV fluid, yielding a final concentration of 0.3 mg/ml.

Recommended IV fluids: 0.9% Sodium Chloride Solution, 5% Dextrose Solution, 10% Dextran 40 in 0.9% Sodium Chloride Solution, 10% Invert Sugar Solution. Ringer's Solution, Hartman's Solution.

Do not use IV if solution is discolored or contains any precipitate or particulate matter.

Solution should be used promptly, within 48 hours of preparation.

For appropriate control and dose titration, a controlled infusion device is recommended to adjust the rate of flow in drops/minute. An IV microdrip chamber (60 drops/ml) can provide a convenient range of infusion rates within the recommended dose range.

Ritodrine may be piggybacked into a primary line, with the primary line run to KVO if the solution is temporarily discontinued because of cardiovascular effects.

Obtain maternal blood pressure, pulse, and respirations and FHR immediately before infusion is started.

Place patient in left lateral position.

ONGOING ASSESSMENTS AND NURSING MANAGEMENT
Monitor maternal blood pressure, pulse, respirations, FHR, uterine contractions, and IV infusion rate every 15 to 30 minutes or as ordered during time of IV infusion. Keep physician informed of patient response because dosage adjustment may be necessary.

Keep patient in a left lateral position during time of IV infusion.

Measure intake and output.

CLINICAL ALERT: IV infusion almost always affects maternal blood pressure and heart rate and the FHR. Average changes given by the manufacturer include the following:
  Maternal heart rate—130 average; range of 60 to 180.
  Fetal heart rate—164 average; range of 130 to 200.
  Maternal blood pressure—Systolic, 128 mm Hg average; range of 96 to 162 mm Hg. Diastolic, 48 mm Hg average; range of up to 76 mm Hg.

Based on pretreatment maternal blood pressure and pulse and FHR, the physician establishes guidelines for slowing or temporarily discontinuing the IV infusion.

Discontinue the infusion of ritodrine and run the primary line to KVO or slow the ritodrine infusion to KVO (depending on the severity of symptoms) and notify the physician immediately if any of the following is noted: The maternal blood pressure or pulse or the FHR exceeds the established guidelines or the averages listed above; there is a sudden and significant increase in maternal or fetal heart rates or decrease in maternal blood pressure; signs of circulatory overload or pulmonary edema (early signs are dyspnea, orthopnea, cough, tachycardia) are apparent; there is cardiac arrhythmia; there is nausea and vomiting.

IV infusion is generally continued for at least 12 hours after uterine contractions cease.

Oral maintenance therapy is begun approximately 30 minutes before termination of IV therapy.

Diabetic patient: Observe for signs of hyperglycemia (Appendix 6, section 6-14). Keep physician informed of urine tests for glucose and ketone bodies.

Patient receiving potassium-depleting diuretics: Observe for signs of hypokalemia (Appendix 6, section 6-15).

Patient on oral maintenance therapy: Monitor blood pressure, pulse, and FHR q3h to q4h or as ordered. Observe for repeat onset of uterine contractions and notify physician immediately if they occur because it may be necessary to reinstitute IV administration of ritodrine.

PATIENT AND FAMILY INFORMATION
NOTE: Oral therapy may be continued after discharge from the hospital. Treatment may be continued as long as the physician considers it desirable to prolong pregnancy.

Take drug exactly as prescribed.

Do not use any nonprescription drugs unless use of a specific drug is approved by the physician.

Notify physician immediately if uterine contractions occur or if nausea, vomiting, palpitations, or shortness of breath is noted.

Frequent examinations (usually weekly) will be necessary to monitor therapy.

Rubella and Mumps Vaccine

See Immunizations, Active.

Rubella Virus Vaccine

See Immunizations, Active.

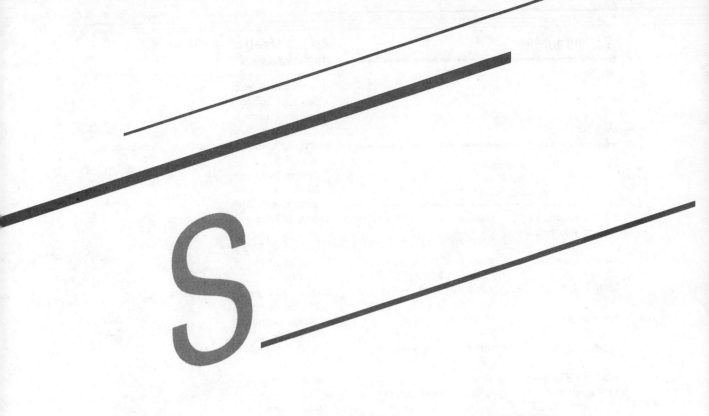

S

Salicylamide

See Salicylates.

Salicylates

Aspirin (Acetylsalicylic Acid, ASA) Rx, otc

tablets: 65 mg, 81 mg (children's aspirin) (*otc*)	*Generic*
tablets, chewable: 81 mg (*otc*)	Bayer Children's, St. Joseph Children's
tablets: 325 mg (*otc*)	A.S.A., Bayer, Empirin, Norwich, *Generic*
tablets: 487.5 mg (*otc*)	Hipirin
tablets: 500 mg (*otc*)	Norwich Extra Strength, *Generic*
tablets: 650 mg (*otc*)	*Generic*
tablets, enteric coated: 325 mg (*otc*)	A.S.A. Enseals, Cosprin, Ecotrin, *Generic*
tablets, enteric coated: 487.5 mg (*otc*)	*Generic*
tablets, enteric coated: 500 mg (*otc*)	Ecotrin Maximum Strength
tablets, enteric coated: 650 mg (*otc*)	A.S.A. Enseals, Cosprin 650, *Generic*
tablets, enteric coated: 975 mg (*Rx*)	Easprin
tablets, timed release: 650 mg (*otc*)	Arthritis Bayer, Measurin
tablets, controlled release: 800 mg (*Rx*)	ZORprin
capsules: 325 mg (*otc*)	A.S.A. Pulvules, Ecotrin
capsules: 500 mg (*otc*)	Ecotrin Maximum Strength
gum tablets: 227.5 mg (*otc*)	Aspergum
suppositories: 60 mg, 130 mg, 195 mg, 300 mg, 600 mg, 1.2 g (*otc*)	*Generic*
suppositories: 325 mg, 650 mg (*otc*)	A.S.A., *Generic*

Aspirin (Acetylsalicylic Acid), Buffered otc

effervescent tablets: 324 mg with 1.9 g sodium bicarbonate, 1 g citric acid	Alka-Seltzer
tablets: 487.5 mg with 60 mg magnesium hydroxide, 20 mg dried aluminum hydroxide	Arthritis Pain Formula
tablets: 325 mg with 75 mg magnesium hydroxide, 75 mg aluminum hydroxide	Ascriptin
tablets: 325 mg with 300 mg magnesium-aluminum hydroxide	Ascriptin A/D
tablets: 325 mg with aluminum hydroxide	Asperbuf
tablets: 324 mg with magnesium carbonate and aluminum hydroxide	Buff-A
tablets: 324 mg with 97.2 mg magnesium carbonate, 48.6 mg aluminum glycinate	Bufferin
tablets: 486 mg with 145.8 mg magnesium carbonate, 72.9 mg aluminum glycinate	Bufferin, Arthritis Strength
tablets: 500 mg with magnesium carbonate, aluminum glycinate	Bufferin Extra Strength
capsules: 500 mg with magnesium carbonate, aluminum glycinate	Bufferin Extra Strength
tablets: 324 mg with aluminum hydroxide, glycine, magnesium carbonate	Buf-Tabs
tablets: 325 mg with magnesium carbonate	Buffaprin, Buffinol
tablets: 325 mg with buffers	*Generic*

Choline Salicylate *otc*

liquid: 870 mg/5 ml	Arthropan

Magnesium Salicylate *Rx, otc*

tablets: 325 mg (*otc*)	Doan's Pills
tablets: 480 mg (*Rx*)	Durasal
tablets: 500 mg (*otc*)	Efficin
tablets: 545 mg (*Rx*)	Magan
tablets: 600 mg (*Rx*)	Mobidin
tablets: 650 mg (*Rx*)	MS-650

Salicylamide *otc*

tablets: 325 mg	*Generic*
tablets: 667 mg	Uromide

Salsalate *(Salicylsalicylic Acid)* *Rx*

tablets: 500 mg	Disalcid
tablets: 750 mg	Arthra-G, Disalcid, Mono-Gesic
capsules: 500 mg	Disalcid

Sodium Salicylate *Rx, otc*

tablets: 325 mg, 650 mg	*Generic (otc)*
tablets, enteric coated: 324 mg	Uracel 5 (*otc*)
tablets, enteric coated: 325 mg, 650 mg	*Generic (otc)*
injection: 1 g	*Generic (Rx)*

Sodium Thiosalicylate *Rx*

injection: 50 mg/ml	Arthrolate, Asproject, Jecto Sal, Nalate, Rexolate, Thiocyl, Thiodyne, Thiosol, Thiosul, Tusal, *Generic*

INDICATIONS

Mild to moderate pain; fever; various inflammatory conditions such as rheumatic fever, rheumatoid arthritis, and osteoarthritis. **Aspirin** is indicated for reducing the risk of recurrent transient ischemic attacks (TIAs) or stroke in men who have had transient ischemia of the brain because of fibrin platelet emboli. It has not been effective in women for TIAs and is of no benefit in treatment of completed strokes.

Unlabeled use: **Aspirin** in a dose of 324 mg/day was found to have a protective effect against acute myocardial infarction in men with unstable angina.

CONTRAINDICATIONS

Hypersensitivity to salicylates or nonsteroidal anti-inflammatory agents. Given with extreme caution to any patient with a history of adverse reactions to salicylates. Cross-sensitivity may exist between aspirin and other nonsteroidal anti-inflammatory agents that inhibit prostaglandin synthesis, and between aspirin and tartrazine dye. Aspirin cross-sensitivity does not appear to occur with sodium salicylate, salicylamide, or choline salicylate. Aspirin intolerance is more prevalent in those with asthma, nasal polyposis, or chronic urticaria.

Contraindicated in hemophilia, bleeding ulcers, and hemorrhagic states. **Magnesium salicylate** is contraindicated in advanced renal insufficiency. **Parenteral sodium salicylate** is contraindicated in asthmatic patients, because they may manifest asphyxial symptoms.

ACTIONS

Aspirin differs from other agents in this group in that it is a more potent inhibitor of prostaglandin synthesis and therefore has more potent anti-inflammatory effects, as well as an irreversible effect of inhibiting platelet aggregation. The acetyl group of the aspirin molecule is believed to be responsible for these differences from other salicylates.

The pharmacologic effects of these agents are qualitatively similar. The mechanism of analgesic effect is not fully understood. Salicylates lower elevated body temperature in normal doses through vasodilatation of peripheral vessels, enhancing dissipation of excess heat. The exact mechanism of the anti-inflammatory action is not fully understood, but evidence suggests that this action is mediated through inhibition of the prostaglandin synthetase enzyme complex. Aspirin inhibits the production of prostaglandins by acetylating the initial enzyme (cyclo-oxygenase) in the prostaglandin biosynthesis pathway.

Single analgesic doses of aspirin prolong bleeding time by inhibiting platelet aggregation. Platelet aggregation is inhibited by aspirin but not by other salicylates. This effect is irreversible and persists for the life of the platelet (8 days).

Aspirin has been used investigationally with some success as an antiplatelet agent in those with thromboembolic disease. Low doses will inhibit platelet aggregation and may be more effective than higher doses.

Other pharmacologic actions: Large doses (6 g or more/day) inhibit prothrombin synthesis and may prolong prothrombin time. Doses greater than 5 g/day have a uricosuric effect; low doses (less than 2 g/day) decrease uric acid secretion.

S

Salicylates are rapidly and completely absorbed following oral administration. Aspirin is partially hydrolyzed to salicylic acid during absorption. Salicylic acid is highly protein bound at therapeutic serum concentrations of 150 mcg/ml to 300 mcg/ml. Salicylic acid is conjugated with glycine to salicyluric acid and is excreted in the urine.

Aspirin has a half-life of approximately 15 minutes; salicylic acid has a half-life of 2 to 3 hours at low doses; at higher doses, the half-life may exceed 20 hours. At doses in the therapeutic anti-inflammatory range the half-life ranges from 6 to 12 hours.

WARNINGS

Reye's syndrome–salicylate association: Studies suggest that use of salicylates, especially aspirin, in children with influenza or chickenpox is associated with the development of Reye's syndrome. A rare, acute, life-threatening condition, this syndrome is characterized by vomiting and lethargy that may progress to delirium and coma. The mortality rate is 20% to 30%; permanent brain damage has been reported in survivors. A causal relationship to salicylates has not been confirmed, but use of salicylates in children with influenza and chickenpox is *not* recommended.

Otic effects: Use is discontinued if dizziness, ringing in the ears, or impaired hearing occurs.

Surgical patients: Aspirin should be avoided, if possible, for 1 week prior to surgery because of the possibility of postoperative bleeding.

Use in impaired hepatic function: Administration is avoided or carried out with caution to those with liver damage, preexisting hypoprothrombinemia, or vitamin K deficiency and to presurgical patients. Aspirin-induced hepatotoxicity has been reported following administration of therapeutic doses for rheumatoid arthritis.

Use in pregnancy, lactation: Aspirin ingestion during pregnancy may produce adverse effects in the mother: anemia, antepartum or postpartum hemorrhage, prolonged gestation, and prolonged labor. Salicylates readily cross the placenta. By inhibiting prostaglandin synthesis, salicylates may cause constriction of the ductus arteriosus and, possibly, other untoward effects on the fetus. Maternal ingestion of aspirin during the later stages of pregnancy has been associated with the following adverse fetal effects: low birth weight, increased incidence of intracranial hemorrhage in premature infants, stillbirths, and neonatal death. Salicylates are possible teratogens. Use during pregnancy, especially in the third trimester, should be avoided. Salicylates are excreted in breast milk in low concentrations.

Use in children: Safety and efficacy of **magnesium salicylate** and **salsalate** in children are not established. Administration of **aspirin** to children with acute febrile illness has been associated with the development of Reye's syndrome (see discussion above). Febrile children suffering dehydration appear more prone to salicylate intoxication.

PRECAUTIONS

Use with caution in those with chronic renal insufficiency; aspirin may cause a transient decrease in renal function. In those with renal impairment, precautions are taken when giving **magnesium salicylate.** Other drugs containing magnesium are discontinued and magnesium serum levels monitored if dosage levels of magnesium salicylate are high.

Salicylates may be cautiously tried in patients intolerant to them because of gastric irritation. Caution is observed in those with gastric ulcers, erosive gastritis, asthma, hypoprothrombinemia, or bleeding tendencies. **Salsalate** and **choline salicylate** have been reported to cause a lesser incidence of GI irritation than does aspirin. Patients developing peptic ulcers while taking salicylates for rheumatic disease have healed during treatment with cimetidine and antacids despite continued salicylate use.

Large doses of salicylates are avoided in those with clear evidence of carditis.

Periodic monitoring of plasma salicylic acid concentrations during long-term treatment is recommended to aid maintenance of therapeutically effective levels (100–300 mcg/ml). Toxic manifestations are not usually seen until plasma concentrations exceed 300 mcg/ml. Urinary *p*H should also be regularly monitored; sudden acidification, as from *p*H 6.5 to 5.5, can double the plasma level, resulting in toxicity.

The occurrence of mild "salicylism" may require dosage adjustment.

Controlled release aspirin is not recommended for antipyresis or short-term analgesia because of its relatively long onset of action. It is not recommended in children under 12, and it is contraindicated in all children with fever accompanied by dehydration.

DRUG INTERACTIONS

Caution is exercised in those on **oral anticoagulant** therapy; therapeutic doses of aspirin have an additive hypoprothrombinemic effect. A decrease in anticoagulant dosage may be necessary, as indicated by appropriate laboratory tests. Aspirin can increase the risk of bleeding in those anticoagulated with **heparin.**

The risk of GI ulceration is increased when salicylates are given with **steroids, phenylbutazone,** or **alcohol.** Ingestion of alcohol during salicylate therapy may also prolong bleeding time. Salicylates antagonize the uricosuric effect of **probenecid** and **sulfinpyrazone. Corticosteroids** increase salicylate clearance and decrease salicylate serum levels. **Urinary acidifiers** decrease salicylate excretion. **Urinary alkalinization** or **acetazolamide, methazolamide,** and **certain antacids** markedly increase renal excretion of salicylic acid. **Carbonic anhydrase inhibitors** may increase salicylate toxicity by inducing systemic acidosis, which enhances CNS penetration of salicylic acid.

Salicylates increase **methotrexate** levels and toxicity by interfering with protein binding and renal elimination of the antimetabolite.

Propranolol may decrease aspirin's anti-inflammatory action by competing for the same receptors.

Patients receiving high doses of salicylates in conjunction with **furosemide** may experience salicylate toxicity at lower doses because of competitive renal excretory sites. Aspirin may inhibit the diuretic effects of **spironolactone.**

Phenobarbital decreases aspirin efficacy by enzyme induction.

Salicylates compete with a number of substances for protein-binding sites, notably **penicillin, thiopental, thyroxine, triiodothyronine, phenytoin, sulfinpyrazone, naproxen, warfarin,** and possibly **corticosteroids. Nonsteroidal anti-inflammatory agents** may be competitively displaced from their albumin-binding sites by aspirin. This effect may ameliorate the efficacy of both drugs.

Aspirin displaces **valproic acid** from its protein-binding sites and may decrease its total body clearance.

Concurrent administration of **absorbable antacids** at therapeutic doses may increase clearance of salicylates in some individuals. Concurrent administration of **nonabsorbable antacids** may alter the rate of absorption of aspirin, resulting in a decreased acetylsalicylic acid–salicylate ratio in plasma.

Concomitant administration of **activated charcoal** decreases aspirin absorption, depending on the dose of charcoal and the time interval between the ingestions of aspirin and charcoal.

Therapeutic and toxic effects of salicylates may be increased by concurrent administration of **para-aminobenzoic acid.**

Salicylates in doses greater than 2 g/day have a hypoglycemic action, perhaps by altering pancreatic beta-cell function. They may also potentiate the glucose lowering effect of **sulfonylureas** and **exogenous insulin.**

Drug/lab tests: Salicylates compete with thyroid hormone for binding sites on thyroid-binding prealbumin and possibly thyroid-binding globulin, resulting in increases in **protein-bound iodine. Serum uric acid levels** are elevated by doses which produce salicylate levels less than 10 mg/dl and decreased by doses producing levels greater than 10 mg/dl. The combination of **phenylbutazone** and salicylates results in further decreases in uric acid excretion and may increase serum uric acid by an average of 2 mg/dl. Salicylates in moderate to large (anti-inflammatory) doses cause false-negative readings for **urine glucose** by the glucose oxidase method and false-positive readings by the copper reduction method.

Salicylates in the urine interfere with **5-HIAA** determinations (fluorescent methods). Salicylates in the urine interact with **urinary ketone** determinations by the ferric chloride method. Large doses of salicylates may decrease urinary excretion of **phenolsulfonphthalein (PSP).** Salicylates in the urine result in falsely elevated **vanillylmandelic acid (VMA)** with most tests, but falsely decrease VMA determinations by the Pisano method.

ADVERSE REACTIONS

Dyspepsia, heartburn, epigastric discomfort, anorexia, hepatotoxicity, and occult blood loss may occur. Chronic aspirin use may cause a persistent iron-deficiency anemia.

Allergic and anaphylactic reactions have been noted when hypersensitive individuals have taken aspirin. The most common allergic reaction to aspirin is induction of bronchospasm with asthmalike symptoms. Other reactions are hives, rash, and angioedema, as well as rhinitis and nasal polyps. Fatal anaphylactic shock has been reported.

Mild salicylism usually occurs after repeated administration of large doses and consists of dizziness, tinnitus, difficulty in hearing, nausea, vomiting, diarrhea, mental confusion, and lassitude.

Salicylate blood concentrations correlate with adverse effects observed (Table 43).

OVERDOSAGE

Symptoms: Respiratory alkalosis is seen initially in acute salicylate ingestions. Hyperpnea and tachypnea occur as a result of increased CO_2 production and a direct stimulatory effect of salicylate on the respiratory center. A mixed respiratory alkalosis and metabolic acidosis may develop. In young children and diabetic adults, hypoglycemia may occur (see Table 43).

Treatment: Initial treatment should include induction of emesis or gastric lavage to remove any unabsorbed drug from the gastric contents. Activated charcoal diminishes salicylate absorption if

Table 43. Correlation of Adverse Effects and Salicylate Intoxication With Serum Salicylate Concentrations

Serum Salicylate Concentration (mcg/ml)	Adverse Effects/Intoxication
~100	GI intolerance and bleeding, hypersensitivity, hemostatic defects
150–300	Mild salicylism
250–400	Nausea/vomiting, hyperventilation, salicylism, flushing, sweating, thirst, headache, diarrhea, tachycardia
>400–500	Respiratory alkalosis, hemorrhage, excitement, confusion, asterixis, pulmonary edema, convulsions, tetany, metabolic acidosis, fever, coma, cardiovascular collapse, renal and respiratory failure

given within 2 hours after ingestion. Further therapy is largely supportive and aimed at maintaining hydration and electrolyte and acid–base balance and reducing hyperthermia. Severe excitement or convulsions may be treated with a barbiturate or diazepam. Forced alkaline diuresis will enhance renal excretion. Hemodialysis is very efficient in eliminating salicylate, but is used only in those who are severely poisoned or who are at increased risk of pulmonary edema. Rarely, IV vitamin K may be indicated to correct hypoprothrombinemia.

DOSAGE

ASPIRIN (ACETYLSALICYLIC ACID)

Minor aches and pains: 325 mg to 650 mg q4h if necessary.

Arthritis and rheumatic conditions: 2.6 g/day to

Table 44. Recommended Aspirin Dosages, by Age, for Pediatric Analgesia/Antipyresis

Age (years)	Dosage (mg q4h)	Number of 81-mg Tablets q4h
<2	Not recommended	Not recommended
2–3	162	2
4–5	243	3
6–8	324	4
9–10	405	5
11	486	6
≥12	648	8

5.2 g/day in divided doses at 4- to 6-hour intervals or 3 g/m^2/24 hours in divided doses at 4- to 6-hour intervals.

Acute rheumatic fever: Up to 7.8 g/day in divided doses.

TIA in men: 1300 mg/day in divided doses (650 mg bid or 325 mg qid).

Pediatric analgesia/antipyretic dosage: 65 mg/kg/24 hours (1.5 g/m^2/24 hours) in four to six divided doses, not to exceed 3.6 g/day.

Dosage recommendations by age are given in Table 44.

CHOLINE SALICYLATE

Adults and children over 12 yrs: 870 mg. May be repeated q3h to q4h if necessary but no more than six times a day. Patients with rheumatoid arthritis may start with 0.87 g to 1.74 g up to four times a day.

MAGNESIUM SALICYLATE

Usual dose is 500 mg to 600 mg three or four times a day. May be increased to 3.6 g/day to 4.8 g/day in divided doses at intervals of 3 to 6 hours. In rheumatic fever, as much as 9.6 g/day may be required. Not recommended in children under 12.

SALICYLAMIDE

Adults: 325 mg to 650 mg three or four times a day.

SALSALATE

Usual adult dose is 3000 mg/day in divided doses.

SODIUM SALICYLATE

325 mg to 650 mg q4h to q8h.

SODIUM THIOSALICYLATE

IM administration is preferred.

Acute gout: 100 mg q3h to q4h for 2 days, then 100 mg/day.

Muscular pain and musculoskeletal disturbances: 50 mg/day to 100 mg/day or on alternate days.

Rheumatic fever: 100 mg to 150 mg q4h to q6h for 3 days; then reduce to 100 mg bid and continue until patient is asymptomatic.

NURSING IMPLICATIONS

HISTORY

For conditions other than simple analgesia, see Appendix 4.

PHYSICAL ASSESSMENT

Rheumatic fever: Obtain vital signs.

Arthritic disorders: Examine and record description of involved joints/areas, noting appearance and limitation of motion, appearance of skin over the joint; evaluate ability to carry out activities of daily living.

ADMINISTRATION

Give with a full glass of water, milk, or food (or if prescribed, with an antacid) to decrease gastric irritation.

If used as an antipyretic, check temperature immediately before administration.

Sodium thiosalicylate is given deep IM, preferably in the gluteus muscle.

ONGOING ASSESSMENTS AND NURSING MANAGEMENT

When drug is used as a simple analgesic, ask patient about relief of pain. Notify physician if drug does not relieve pain and/or discomfort.

When drug is used as an antipyretic, check temperature in 1 hour. If temperature remains elevated, contact physician because additional therapy may be required.

If the suppository form of aspirin is used, check patient in ½ hour for retention of the suppository. If it has been expelled, consult the physician because the same or a lower dose may be prescribed.

If given for arthritic conditions, observe patient response (*e.g.,* relief of pain and/or discomfort, increase in joint motion, decreased pain with motion or weight bearing).

Observe for adverse effects. If high doses are administered, observe for signs of salicylate toxicity (overdosage) *e.g.,* tinnitus, impaired hearing, dizziness, nausea, vomiting, flushing, sweating, rapid deep breathing, thirst, headache, drowsiness, tachycardia, diarrhea). If one or more of these should occur, withhold the next dose and contact the physician.

If nausea and/or vomiting or other gastric complaints persist despite giving with food, milk, or a full glass of water, consult physician; other drug therapy may be necessary.

If surgery is anticipated, salicylates are usually discontinued 1 week prior to surgery because of possibility of postoperative bleeding. If emergency surgery is necessary for a patient receiving high doses of salicylates, the patient must be closely observed during the postoperative period for bleeding tendency.

Patients on long-term therapy: Periodic monitoring of plasma salicylic acid concentrations may be ordered. Therapeutically effective levels are 100 mcg/ml to 300 mcg/ml. Dosage of a salicylate may be titrated upwards or downwards depending on patient response, serum salicylic acid levels, and occurrence of adverse effects.

PATIENT AND FAMILY INFORMATION

May cause GI upset; take with food, milk, or a full glass of water.

Notify physician or nurse if ringing in the ears, persistent GI pain, nausea, vomiting, impaired hearing, flushing, sweating, thirst, headache, diarrhea, or unusual bleeding or bruising occurs.

The ingredients of some nonprescription products contain aspirin or other salicylates (the salicylate name may not appear in the name of the drug but is listed on the label). These products should not be used while taking a salicylate, especially during high-dose or long-term salicylate therapy. If in doubt about a specific product, check with a pharmacist about product ingredients before purchase.

Use of salicylates should be avoided during pregnancy.

Salicylates, particularly aspirin, should *not* be given to children with chickenpox or influenza because these products have been associated with the development of Reye's syndrome. If an analgesic or fever-reducing agent is needed, consult a physician before using a salicylate.

Do not drink alcohol while taking salicylates.

If used to reduce fever, contact physician if temperature continues to remain elevated more than 24 hours.

Do not use salicylates consistently to treat chronic pain; seek medical advice.

Salicylates (plain or enteric coated) deteriorate with age. If these drugs have a vinegar odor, they should be discarded. Salicylates should be purchased in small amounts when used on an occasional basis. Keep the drug container tightly closed at all times because they deteriorate rapidly when exposed to air, moisture, and heat.

Patients on long-term therapy: Do not change from plain tablets to enteric-coated tablets (or the reverse) unless directed to do so by the physician. Do not use antacids with a salicylate, unless use is approved by the physician. Inform other physicians and dentist of salicylate therapy.

Saliva Substitutes otc

| solution | Moi-Stir, Orex, Salivart, Xero-Lube |

INDICATIONS

Relief of dry mouth and throat in xerostomia. These products contain electrolytes (sodium, potassium, magnesium, and calcium chlorides) in a carboxymethylcellulose base.

DOSAGE

May be used as often as needed to moisten the oral cavity. Solution may be swallowed or expectorated.

NURSING IMPLICATIONS

ADMINISTRATION

Products are available in spray cans or with pump spray. Instruct patient in use of the spray, if necessary.

Inform patient that these products may be swallowed or expectorated.

ONGOING ASSESSMENTS AND NURSING MANAGEMENT

May be kept at the bedside for use as needed.

If dry mouth is not relieved, other methods may be tried (*e.g.,* sips of cool water, hard candy, chewing gum).

PATIENT INFORMATION

NOTE: Those with cardiac or renal disease should be cautioned against overuse of these products. Expectorating the saliva substitute instead of swallowing reduces the amount of ingested electrolytes.

Salsalate

See Salicylates.

Salt Substitutes otc

97.1% potassium chloride, silicon dioxide, tartaric acid. Contains less than 10 mg sodium/100 g	Adolph's Salt Substitute
67.4% potassium chloride, silicon dioxide, tartaric acid, sugar, spices, cottonseed and soybean oil. Contains less than 20 mg sodium/100 g	Adolph's Seasoned Salt Substitute
96% potassium chloride, fumeric acid, tricalcium phosphate, monocalcium phosphate. Contains less than 0.52 mg sodium/5 g	Morton Salt Substitute
potassium chloride, glutamic acid, potassium glutamate, calcium silicate, tribasic calcium phosphate. Each 5 g contains less than 0.5 mg sodium. Each gram contains approximately 12 mEq potassium	Neocurtasal
potassium chloride, bitartrate and glutamate, adipic acid, fumaric acid, polyethylene glycol 400, disodium inosinate. Contains less than 10 mg sodium/100 g; each 2.5 g contains approximately 35 mEq potassium	NoSalt
potassium chloride, dextrose, cream of tartar. Contains less than 10 mg sodium/100 g	Nu-Salt

INDICATIONS

Use in low-sodium diets in CHF, hypertension, edema of pregnancy, and other edematous states resulting from sodium retention, obesity, cirrhosis, renal disease, or corticosteroid therapy.

CONTRAINDICATIONS

Oliguria and severe kidney disease.

CAUTION

Excessive sodium depletion may lead to symptoms such as weakness, nausea, and muscle cramps; in severe cases, uremia may follow. On the appearance of early symptoms, sodium intake must be liberalized.

Salt substitutes contain a significant amount of potassium and electrolytes other than sodium. The potassium content of these products averages between 10 mEq/g and 13 mEq/g (50–60 mEq potassium/level teaspoon). Excessive use could result in hyperkalemia.

NURSING IMPLICATIONS

ONGOING ASSESSMENTS AND NURSING MANAGEMENT

If used in large quantities, observe for hyperkalemia (Appendix 6, section 6-15).

Patients on low-sodium diets and using a salt substitute are observed for hyponatremia (Appendix 6, section 6-17).

PATIENT INFORMATION

Restriction of sodium may lead to depletion of this electrolyte and weakness, nausea, and muscle cramps may occur. The use of a small amount of table salt should relieve these symptoms, but the physician should be made aware of this problem.

Salt substitutes should be used in moderation.

Scopolamine Hydrobromide

See Antiemetic/Antivertigo Agents; Gastrointestinal Anticholinergics/Antispasmodics; Mydriatics, Cycloplegic.

Scopolamine Transdermal

See Antiemetic/Antivertigo Agents.

Secobarbital and Secobarbital Sodium

See Barbiturates.

Senna

See Laxatives.

Silver Nitrate

See Antiseptics and Germicides.

Silver Protein, Mild

See Antiseptics and Germicides.

Silver Sulfadiazine Rx

cream: 10 mg/g   Silvadene, *Generic*

INDICATIONS

Prevention and treatment of sepsis in second- and third-degree burns.

CONTRAINDICATIONS

Because sulfonamide therapy is known to increase the possibility of kernicterus, do not use in pregnancy at term, on premature infants, or on newborn infants during the first month of life.

ACTIONS

Acts only on the cell membrane and cell wall to produce its bactericidal effect. It is not a carbonic anhydrase inhibitor and acidosis has not been reported; it may be of particular value in treating pediatric burn patients. It has broad antimicrobial activity and is bactericidal for many gram-negative and gram-positive bacteria and is also effective against yeast. Silver sulfadiazine will inhibit bacteria that are resistant to other microbial agents and is superior to sulfadiazine.

WARNINGS

Administer with caution to patients with history of hypersensitivity. It is now known whether there is cross-sensitivity to other sulfonamides. If allergic reactions attributable to treatment with this drug occur, consideration is given to discontinuing drug.

Use in G6PD-deficient individuals may cause hemolysis. Fungal colonization in and below the eschar may occur concomitantly with reduction of bacterial growth, but fungal dissemination is rare.

In treatment of burns involving extensive areas of the body, the serum sulfonamide concentration may approach adult therapeutic levels (8–12 mg/dl). In these patient, monitoring of serum sulfa concentrations is recommended.

Safety for use in pregnancy is not established. Not recommended in women of childbearing potential unless the burned area covers more than 20% of the total body surface area or the need for therapeutic benefit is greater than the possible risk to the fetus.

PRECAUTIONS

If hepatic or renal functions become impaired and elimination of drug decreases, accumulation may occur. Discontinuation is weighed against the therapeutic benefit being achieved.

DRUG INTERACTIONS

In considering topical use of **proteolytic enzymes** with this drug, note that there is a possibility that silver may inactivate such enzymes.

S

ADVERSE REACTIONS

It is frequently difficult to distinguish between an adverse reaction due to silver sulfadiazine and reactions that may occur due to concomitant use of other therapeutic agents in treatment of severe burn wounds. Possible adverse reactions include burning, rash, and itching. Because significant quantities of the drug are absorbed, it is possible that any of the adverse reactions attributable to sulfonamides (p 990) may occur.

DOSAGE

Apply once or twice a day to a thickness of approximately $\frac{1}{16}$ inch. Treatment is continued until satisfactory healing has occurred or until the burn site is ready for grafting. Drug is not withdrawn from the therapeutic regimen while possibility of infection remains, unless a significant adverse reaction occurs.

NURSING IMPLICATIONS

HISTORY AND PHYSICAL ASSESSMENT

Prompt institution of appropriate measures to control shock and pain is of prime importance. If initial treatment has been given, review chart for type and extent of burns, recent laboratory tests. See also Appendix 4.

ADMINISTRATION

Physician may order an analgesic or tranquilizer to be given prior to application when burns are extensive or deep. The drug should be given 30 to 60 minutes before application of silver sulfadiazine.

Apply with a sterile gloved hand. Cover burn areas to a thickness of approximately $\frac{1}{16}$ inch.

Whenever necessary, reapply the cream to any areas from which it has been removed by patient activity.

Dressings are normally not required, but individual patient requirements may make dressings necessary.

ONGOING ASSESSMENTS AND NURSING MANAGEMENT

When feasible, patient is bathed daily; this is an aid to debridement. A whirlpool bath may be ordered, but patient may also be bathed in bed or in a shower.

Inspect burned area q1h to q2h, especially when patient is restless, because area must be covered with cream at all times.

If rash or itching occurs, especially in unburned areas, notify physician. These symptoms may be indicative of hypersensitivity.

Monitor vital signs q1h to q4h, depending on patient's condition and extent of burns. Notify physician immediately of any changes in vital signs.

Note and record appearance of burned area after bathing (cream is in a water-miscible base and may be removed with water) and before cream is reapplied.

Monitor intake and output; notify physician immediately of any decrease in urinary output.

Renal- and hepatic-function tests, urine tests for sulfa crystals, and serum sulfa levels may be performed on those with burns involving extensive areas of the body. The serum sulfa concentration may approach adult therapeutic levels (8–12 mg/dl) in those with extensive burns.

Because significant quantities of the drug are absorbed, observe patient for adverse reactions attributable to sulfonamides (p 990).

Simethicone otc

tablets: 50 mg	Silain
tablets, chewable: 40 mg	Mylicon
tablets, chewable: 80 mg	Gas-X, Mylicon-80
drops: 40 mg/0.6 ml	Mylicon

INDICATIONS

Relief of painful symptoms of excess gas in the digestive tract. Used as an adjunct in treatment of many conditions in which gas retention may be a problem, such as postoperative gaseous distention, air swallowing, functional dyspepsia, peptic ulcer, spastic or irritable colon, or diverticulitis.

ACTIONS

The defoaming action relieves flatulence by dispersing and preventing the formation of mucus-surrounded gas pockets in the GI tract. It acts in the stomach and intestines to change the surface tension of gas bubbles, enabling them to coalesce. The gas is then freed and eliminated more easily by belching or passing flatus.

DOSAGE

Tablets: 40 mg to 80 mg qid after each meal and H.S.

Drops: 40 mg qid after meals and H.S.

NURSING IMPLICATIONS

ADMINISTRATION

Instruct patient to chew tablets thoroughly.

Shake liquid preparation well before dispensing.

ONGOING ASSESSMENTS AND NURSING MANAGEMENT
If excess gas is not relieved, inform physician.

PATIENT AND FAMILY INFORMATION
If excess gas persists or other GI complaints occur, consult a physician.

Sodium Ascorbate

See Vitamin C.

Sodium Bicarbonate, Oral otc

tablets: 325 mg,   *Generic*
  650 mg
powder: 120, 240,   *Generic*
  and 300 g; 1 lb

INDICATIONS
A gastric (see Antacids), systemic, and urinary alkalinizer. Used as a urinary alkalinizer, sodium bicarbonate corrects acidosis in renal tubular disorders and is an adjunct to uricosuric agents in gout (minimizes uric acid crystallization). See also Sodium Bicarbonate, Parenteral.

PRECAUTIONS
Use cautiously in those with edematous sodium retaining states, CHF, cirrhosis of the liver, toxemia of pregnancy, or renal impairment. Prolonged therapy may lead to systemic alkalosis.

DOSAGE
Usual dose is 325 mg to 2 g up to four times a day. Total daily dose should not exceed 16 g.

NURSING IMPLICATIONS

HISTORY
See Appendix 4.

PHYSICAL ASSESSMENT
Baseline laboratory studies may include urinary *p*H.

ADMINISTRATION
Give tablets with full glass of water. Dissolve powder form in full glass of water.

ONGOING ASSESSMENTS AND NURSING MANAGEMENT
If used as a urinary alkalinizer, using nitrazine paper, check urinary *p*H two to three times/day or as ordered. If urine is acidic, notify physician because dosage adjustment may be necessary.

PATIENT AND FAMILY INFORMATION
Use as directed. Do not increase dose unless advised to do so by physician.

Excessive sodium bicarbonate (baking soda), except on advice of a physician, may disguise a more serious illness or lead to an excess of sodium, with fluid retention and other serious problems.

Sodium Bicarbonate, Parenteral Rx

solution: 4%   Neut
solution: 4.2%, 5%,   *Generic*
  7.5%, 8.4%

INDICATIONS
Metabolic acidosis: In severe renal disease, uncontrolled diabetes, circulatory insufficiency due to shock or severe dehydration, extracorporeal circulation of blood, cardiac arrest, and severe primary lactic acidosis. Treatment of metabolic acidosis should be used in addition to measures designed to control the cause of acidosis.

Urinary alkalinization: In the treatment of certain drug intoxications (*i.e.,* barbiturates, salicylates, lithium, methyl alcohol) and in hemolytic reactions requiring alkalinization of the urine to diminish nephrotoxicity of blood pigments. Urinary alkalinization is also used in methotrexate therapy to prevent nephrotoxicity.

Severe diarrhea: In severe diarrhea, which is often accompanied by a significant loss of bicarbonate.

For oral uses, see Antacids; Sodium Bicarbonate, Oral.

CONTRAINDICATIONS
Contraindicated in patients losing chloride by vomiting or from continuous gastrointestinal suction, receiving diuretics known to produce hypochloremic alkalosis, with metabolic and respiratory alkalosis, and with hypocalcemia, in which alkalosis may produce tetany.

ACTIONS
Increases plasma bicarbonate; buffers excess hydrogen ion concentration; raises blood *p*H; reverses clinical manifestations of acidosis.

S

WARNINGS

Neonates and children: Rapid injection (10 ml/minute) of hypertonic sodium bicarbonate solutions into neonates and children under 2 years of age may produce hypernatremia, a decrease in CSF pressure, and possible intracranial hemorrhage.

In emergencies such as cardiac arrest, the risk of rapid infusion may be necessary because of the potential for fatality due to acidosis.

Electrolyte/solute overload: The risk of dilutional states is inversely proportional to the electrolyte concentrations of administered parenteral solutions. The risk of solute overload causing congested states with peripheral and pulmonary edema is directly proportional to the electrolyte concentrations of such solutions.

Use in impaired renal function: Administration of solutions containing sodium ions may result in sodium retention.

Use in pregnancy: Safe use not established. Use only if clearly needed.

PRECAUTIONS

Overdosage and alkalosis are avoided by giving repeated small doses and by periodic monitoring by appropriate laboratory tests.

CHF: Because sodium accompanies bicarbonate, caution is exercised in those with CHF or other edematous or sodium-retaining states, as well as in patients with oliguria or anuria. Potassium depletion may predispose the patient to metabolic alkalosis, and coexistent hypocalcemia may be associated with carpopedal spasm as the plasma pH rises. These dangers can be minimized if such electrolyte imbalances are appropriately treated prior to or concomitantly with bicarbonate infusion.

Excessive administration can cause a shift of potassium in the intracellular pool, inducing clinical hypokalemia and predisposing the patient to cardiac arrhythmias. Patients losing chloride by vomiting or gastrointestinal intubation are more susceptible to development of severe alkalosis if given alkalinizing agents.

DRUG INTERACTIONS

Addition of sodium bicarbonate to parenteral solutions containing **calcium** should be avoided, except when compatibility has been previously established; precipitation or haze may result.

Use with caution when giving parenteral fluids, especially those containing sodium ions, to patients receiving **corticosteroids** or **corticotropin.**

Increased half-lives and duration of action of **quinidine, amphetamines, ephedrine,** and **pseudoephedrine** may occur with urinary alkalinization by sodium bicarbonate. Sodium bicarbonate, by producing alkaline urine, increases the renal clearance of **tetracyclines,** especially **doxycycline.**

OVERDOSAGE

Symptoms: Excessive or too-rapid administration may produce alkalosis. Severe alkalosis may be accompanied by hyperirritability or tetany.

Treatment: If clinical evidence of alkalosis develops, symptoms may be readily controlled by rebreathing expired air from a paper bag or mask or, if severe, by parenteral injection of calcium gluconate. Severe alkalosis, inadvertently produced, can be corrected by IV infusion of 2.14% ammonium chloride solution, except in those with hepatic disease, in whom ammonia administration is contraindicated. Discontinue sodium bicarbonate; sodium chloride 0.9% IV or potassium chloride may be indicated if there is severe hypokalemia. Administer calcium gluconate to control tetany.

DOSAGE

Administer by IV route.

Cardiac arrest: Administer according to results of arterial blood pH and $PaCO_2$ and calculation of base deficit.

Adults: Initial dose of 1 mEq/kg followed by 0.5 mEq/kg every 10 minutes of arrest, depending on arterial blood gases. Caution is observed when rapid infusion of large quantities of sodium bicarbonate is indicated because these solutions are hypertonic and may produce an undesirable rise in plasma sodium concentration. In cardiac arrest, the risks from acidosis exceed those of hypernatremia.

Infants (up to 2 years): 4.2% solution is recommended for IV administration, at a rate not to exceed 8 mEq/kg/day. This dosage is recommended for neonates to guard against possibility of producing hypernatremia, decreasing CSF pressure, and inducing intracranial hemorrhage. Initial dose of 1 mEq/kg to 2 mEq/kg is given over 1 to 2 minutes, followed by 1 mEq/kg every 10 minutes of arrest. If only 7.5% or 8.4% is available, dilute 1:1 with 5% dextrose in water before administration.

Less urgent forms of metabolic acidosis: Sodium bicarbonate may be added to other IV fluids. The amount given to older children and adults over a 4- to 8-hour period is approximately 2 mEq/kg to 5 mEq/kg, depending on the severity of the acidosis judged by the lowering of total CO_2 content, blood pH, and patient's clinical condition. Initially, infusion of 2 mEq/kg to 5 mEq/kg over a period of 4 to 8 hours will produce a measurable improvement in the abnormal acid–base status of the blood.

NURSING IMPLICATIONS

HISTORY
See Appendix 4.

PHYSICAL ASSESSMENT
Obtain blood pressure, pulse, and respirations. Observe for signs of metabolic acidosis (Appendix 6, section 6-1). Baseline laboratory tests may include blood pH, CO_2 content, serum electrolytes, urine pH, plasma bicarbonate, pCO_2.

ADMINISTRATION
Sodium bicarbonate is available in fliptop and pintop vials, ampules, and disposable syringes. The 5% solution is available only in the 500-ml size and is used for IV infusion of sodium bicarbonate.

Solutions available are listed in Table 45.

The 500-ml 5% solution is given by IV piggyback. The 4%, 4.2%, 7.5%, and 8.4% solutions are administered by direct IV or are added to other IV fluids.

In cardiac arrest, initial and subsequent doses are given by IV push until patient's condition is stabilized. Flush lines before and after use.

Dosage is based on degree of metabolic acidosis, response of patient, initial cause of the metabolic acidosis, and age of patient.

In treatment of cardiac arrest, initial recommended dose is 200 mEq to 300 mEq, followed by repeat doses (usually at 5- to 10-minute intervals) until cardiac function is restored and blood gas studies indicate a normal blood pH.

Have available a rebreathing bag or a paper bag, calcium gluconate, 2.14% ammonium chloride for treatment of overdosage (metabolic alkalosis), and KCl for treatment of possible hypokalemia.

ONGOING ASSESSMENTS AND NURSING MANAGEMENT
Monitor blood pressure, pulse, and respirations q1h to q2h (more frequent determinations may be performed during and immediately following treatment of cardiac arrest).

Extravasation (IV infusion or IV push) requires discontinuation of IV (drug is irritating to tissues) and selection of an alternate IV site.

Measure intake and output. Notify physician of any change in the intake–output ratio because dosage may need to be decreased.

CLINICAL ALERT: Because dosage is individualized, overdosage may occur. Observe for signs of overdosage: metabolic alkalosis (Appendix 6, section 6-4) and fluid overload (Appendix 6, section 6-12); report occurrence immediately.

Observe for signs of clinical improvement (*e.g.,* decrease in symptoms of metabolic acidosis). Keep physician informed of patient's response to administration of sodium bicarbonate.

Frequent monitoring of blood pH, blood gases, and serum electrolytes is performed to determine dosage. Drug is discontinued when symptoms of metabolic acidosis (Appendix 6, section 6-1) are relieved and laboratory studies (blood pH, pCO_2) are normal or near normal.

Continue to observe the patient treated for metabolic acidosis for recurrence of symptoms.

Sodium Cellulose Phosphate Rx

powder: 2.5 g/sachet   Calcibind

INDICATIONS
Absorptive hypercalciuria Type I with recurrent calcium oxalate or calcium phosphate nephrolithiasis. Appropriate use substantially reduces the incidence of new stone formation in these cases. Causes of hypercalciuria other than hyperabsorption cannot be expected to respond to this drug.

CONTRAINDICATIONS
Primary or secondary hyperparathyroidism, including renal hypercalciuria (renal calcium leak); hypomagnesemic states; bone disease; hypocalcemic states; normal or low intestinal absorption and renal excretion of calcium; and enteric hyperoxaluria.

ACTIONS
Is a synthetic compound insoluble in water and nonabsorbable. It has excellent ion-exchange properties, the sodium ion exchanging for calcium.

Table 45. Percentages and Total mEq per Container of Sodium Bicarbonate Solutions

Percentage	mEq/ml	Total mEq per Vial, Ampule, Syringe, IV Solution
4	0.48	5 ml = 2.4 mEq
4.2	0.5	10 ml = 5 mEq
5	0.595	500 ml = 297.5 mEq
7.5	0.892	10 ml = 8.9 mEq 50 ml = 44.6 mEq
8.4	1.0	10 ml = 10 mEq 50 ml = 50 mEq

When taken orally, it binds calcium. The complex of calcium and cellulose phosphate is excreted in the feces.

When given orally with meals, sodium cellulose phosphate (SCP) binds dietary and secreted calcium and reduces urinary calcium. It also binds dietary magnesium and lowers urinary magnesium.

WARNINGS

The sodium contained in SCP (25–50 mEq/15 g) may represent a hazard in those with congestive heart failure or ascites. Safety for use in pregnancy has not been established. Because of the increased dietary calcium requirement in pregnant women, SCP is used only when clearly needed and when potential benefits outweigh the unknown potential hazards to the fetus. Because of the increased requirement for dietary calcium in growing children, use of SCP in children under 16 years of age is not recommended.

PRECAUTIONS

By inhibiting calcium absorption, SCP may stimulate parathyroid function, leading to hyperparathyroid bone disease. It is necessary to monitor parathyroid hormone levels. SCP treatment has been shown to maintain parathyroid function within normal limits if used only in those with absorptive hypercalciuria Type I at a dosage sufficient to restore normal calcium absorption.

Additional complications may potentially develop during long-term use: hyperoxaluria and hypomagnesiuria, which would negate the beneficial effect of hypocalciuria on new stone formation; magnesium depletion; depletion of trace metals (copper, zinc, iron). Effects may be minimized by restricting use of SCP to absorptive hypercalciuria Type I and by monitoring serum calcium, magnesium, copper, zinc, iron, parathyroid hormone, and complete blood count every 3 to 6 months.

ADVERSE REACTIONS

Unpleasant taste of the drug; loose bowel movements; diarrhea; dyspepsia.

DOSAGE

Recommended initial dose is 15 g/day (5 g with each meal) in those with urinary calcium greater than 300 mg/day (on moderate calcium-restricted diet). When urinary calcium declines to less than 150 mg/day, dosage should be reduced to 10 g/day (5 g with supper, 2.5 g with each remaining meal). Those with controlled urinary calcium on moderate calcium-restricted diet of less than 300 mg/day but greater than 200 mg/day should begin on SCP 10 g/day.

Concomitant magnesium supplements: The dose of oral magnesium, given as magnesium gluconate, depends on the dose of SCP. Those receiving 15 g of SCP/day should take 1.5 g of magnesium gluconate A.C. breakfast and again H.S. (separately from the SCP). Those taking 10 g of SCP/day should take 1 g of magnesium gluconate bid. To avoid binding of magnesium by SCP, supplemental magnesium is given at least 1 hour before or after a dose of SCP.

NURSING IMPLICATIONS

HISTORY
See Appendix 4.

PHYSICAL ASSESSMENT
Baseline laboratory tests may include 24-hour urinary calcium; CBC; urinalysis; serum magnesium, zinc, copper, iron; serum parathyroid hormone.

ADMINISTRATION
SCP is given within 30 minutes of each meal. Giving the drug more than 1 hour after a meal reduces drug effectiveness.

Suspend each dose in a glass of water, soft drink, or fruit juice; stir thoroughly.

Magnesium supplements are usually ordered and are given at least 1 hour before or after administration of SCP.

ONGOING ASSESSMENTS AND NURSING MANAGEMENT
The drug has an unpleasant taste, which may interfere with patient compliance.

Recommended dietary restrictions include moderate intake of calcium with avoidance of dairy products; moderate restriction of dietary oxalate (avoiding spinach and similar dark greens, rhubarb, chocolate, brewed tea); a sodium intake of less than 150 mEq/day.

Encourage a fluid intake so that urine output is 2 liters/day. During initial therapy, measure intake and output to ensure patient compliance with recommended increase of fluid intake.

Initial and maintenance doses of SCP are based on measurements of 24-hour urinary calcium excretion.

Notify physician if patient refuses the drug, if fluid intake is below the desired levels, or if diarrhea occurs.

PATIENT AND FAMILY INFORMATION
NOTE: Supply patient with a list of foods high in calcium, oxalate, and sodium as well as a list

of foods to be avoided (mainly dairy products) or taken in moderate amounts.

Mix prescribed dose (1–2 sachets) in a large glass of water, soft drink, or fruit juice; stir thoroughly.

For drug to be effective, it must be taken within 30 minutes of eating a meal.

Take magnesium supplement at least 1 hour before or after dose of SCP.

Do not take vitamin C (separately or in multivitamin preparations) unless use is approved by physician.

Dietary restrictions are an important part of therapy. Use of this drug does not eliminate the necessity of restricting calcium, oxalate, and sodium intake.

Sodium Chloride, Oral *otc*

tablets: 650 mg, 1 g, 2.25 g	*Generic*
tablets, enteric coated: 1 g	*Generic*
tablets, wax matrix: 600 mg	Slo-Salt
tablets: NaCl w/dextrose	*Generic*
tablets: NaCl w/dextrose, vitamin B$_1$	*Generic*
tablets: 450 mg NaCl, 30 mg KCl, 18 mg calcium carbonate, 200 mg dextrose	Thermotabs
tablets: 635 mg NaCl, 40.6 mg KCl, 31.5 mg calcium phosphate tribasic, 9.1 mg magnesium carbonate	Heatrol

INDICATIONS

May be used to treat deficiencies of sodium and chloride ions lost from the body and to prevent muscle cramps and heat prostration due to excessive perspiration during exposure to high temperature. Also used to treat deficiencies of sodium and chloride due to excessive diuresis or excessive salt restriction. Individuals with adequate dietary sodium intake and normal renal function should not require sodium chloride supplementation. Use of balance electrolyte supplements may be preferred to prevent hypokalemia.

PRECAUTIONS

Used with caution in presence of CHF, circulatory insufficiency, kidney dysfunction, hypoproteinemia.

OVERDOSAGE

May cause serious electrolyte disturbances. Signs of salt overdose include diarrhea and muscle twitching.

DOSAGE

For prevention of diarrhea and heat cramps due to prolonged exposure to high temperature, 0.5 g to 1 g with every drink of water (5–10 times daily).

NURSING IMPLICATIONS

PATIENT INFORMATION

Those with a normal dietary intake and normal kidney function should not require salt tablets, unless use is recommended by a physician.

Do not use in the presence of heart or kidney problems or poor circulation, or when eating a protein-restricted diet.

Avoid excessive use as serious electrolyte disturbances (excess salt) may occur. Discontinue use if diarrhea or muscle twitching occurs.

Sodium Chloride, Parenteral *Rx*

	Na$^+$ (mEq/liter)	Cl$^-$ (mEq/liter)	Osmolarity (mOsm/ liter)
0.45% sodium chloride (1/2 normal saline)	77	77	155
0.9% sodium chloride (normal saline)	154	154	310
3% sodium chloride	513	513	1025
5% sodium chloride	855	855	1710

INDICATIONS

0.45% SODIUM CHLORIDE (HYPOTONIC)

Provides fluid replacement when fluid losses exceed electrolyte depletion.

0.9% SODIUM CHLORIDE (ISOTONIC)

Restores both water and sodium chloride losses.

3% or 5% SODIUM CHLORIDE (HYPERTONIC)

Used in hyponatremia and hypochloremia due to electrolyte losses, drastic dilution of body water following excessive water intake, and emergency treatment of severe salt depletion.

Administered IV in varying proportions, as a source of water and electrolytes.

S

CONTRAINDICATIONS

3% and 5% sodium chloride solutions are contraindicated in the presence of elevated, normal, or only slightly decreased plasma sodium and chloride concentrations.

ACTIONS

Normal osmolarity of the extracellular fluid ranges between 280 mOsm/liter and 300 mOsm/liter; it is primarily a function of sodium and its accompanying ions, chloride and bicarbonate. Sodium chloride is the principal salt involved in maintenance of plasma tonicity. One gram of sodium chloride provides 17.1 mEq of sodium and 17.1 mEq of chloride.

WARNINGS

Give with caution to those with CHF or severe renal insufficiency and when edema exists with sodium retention. In those with impaired renal function, administration may result in excessive sodium retention.

Fluid/solute overload: Administration of IV solutions can cause fluid or solute overload resulting in dilution of serum electrolyte concentrations, overhydration, congested states, or pulmonary edema. The risk of dilutional states is inversely proportional to the electrolyte concentration. The risk of solution overload's causing congested states with peripheral and pulmonary edema is directly proportional to the electrolyte concentration. Infusion of more than 1 liter of isotonic (0.9%) sodium chloride may supply more sodium and chloride than normally found in serum, resulting in hypernatremia; this may cause loss of bicarbonate ions, resulting in an acidifying effect. Infusion of isotonic sodium chloride during or immediately after surgery may result in excessive sodium retention.

Use in pregnancy: Safe use not established. Use only when clearly needed.

PRECAUTIONS

Administered cautiously to those with decompensated cardiovascular, cirrhotic, and nephrotic disease and to those receiving corticosteroids or corticotropin. The 3% and 5% solutions are infused very slowly and used with caution to avoid pulmonary edema.

Clinical evaluation and periodic laboratory determinations are necessary to monitor changes in fluid balance, electrolyte concentrations, and acid–base balance.

Extraordinary electrolyte losses such as may occur during protracted nasogastric suction, vomiting, diarrhea, or GI fistula drainage may necessitate additional electrolyte supplementation.

ADVERSE REACTIONS

Reactions that may occur because of the solution or the technique of administration include febrile response, infection of the injection site, venous thrombosis or phlebitis extending from the injection site, extravasation, and hypervolemia. Hypernatremia may be associated with edema and exacerbation of CHF due to retention of water, resulting in expanded extracellular fluid volume. If infused in large amounts, chloride ions may cause a loss of bicarbonate ions, resulting in an acidifying effect.

DOSAGE

Dosage is individualized.

3% or 5% solutions: Calculate sodium deficit:

$$(140 \text{ mEq/liter} - \text{patient's serum Na})$$
$$\times \text{(total body water in liters)} = \text{mEq Na}$$

Administer one-half over 8 hours. Do not exceed a maximum of 100 ml/hour. Treatment continued until serum Na is 130 mEq/liter or neurologic symptoms improve. Remainder of deficit can be replaced slowly over several days. Replacement seldom requires more than one-half the calculated deficit.

NURSING IMPLICATIONS

HISTORY
See Appendix 4.

PHYSICAL ASSESSMENT
Obtain blood pressure, pulse, and respirations. Baseline laboratory studies may include serum electrolytes, bicarbonate concentration, and other arterial blood gas studies.

ADMINISTRATION
Use only if solution is clear.

Administer 3% or 5% sodium chloride solution by IV piggyback.

Rate of infusion (as drops/minute or ml/hour) is ordered by the physician.

Maximum rate of infusion of the 3% or 5% sodium chloride solution is 100 ml/hour.

Stability and storage: Protect from freezing; store below 40°C.

ONGOING ASSESSMENTS AND NURSING MANAGEMENT

CLINICAL ALERT: Patient receiving 3% or 5% solution is observed closely for signs of pulmonary edema (*i.e.,* dyspnea, cough, restlessness, tachycardia). If one or more of these are apparent, discontinue infusion, run primary line to KVO, and notify the physician.

Observe patient for hypokalemia (Appendix 6, section 6-15), which may result from excessive administration of potassium-free solutions.

Check IV infusion site and rate of infusion q15m. Adjust infusion rate as necessary.

Check IV infusion site for evidence of infection, venous thrombosis or phlebitis, or extravasation. If one or more of these are apparent, select a different administration site and notify the physician immediately.

Periodic determinations of serum electrolytes are recommended. Keep physician informed of most recent laboratory values, especially when patient is receiving the 3% or 5% solution.

If patient is receiving a 3% or 5% sodium chloride infusion and the most recent serum sodium and chlorides are normal or only slightly decreased, slow the infusion to KVO and notify the physician. These concentrations are contraindicated in presence of normal or only slightly decreased sodium and chloride concentrations.

Replace the IV administration apparatus at least once every 24 hours.

Sodium Chloride 20% Rx

solution for injection: *Generic*
   20%

INDICATIONS
For transabdominal intra-amniotic injection to induce abortion in appropriately selected pregnant patients during the second trimester (preferably between 16 and 22 weeks of gestation). Hypertonic saline generally causes fewer side-effects than prostaglandins; however, the induction interval is much longer.

CONTRAINDICATIONS
Pregnancies of less than 15 weeks or more than 24 weeks of gestation; increased intra-amniotic pressure, as in an actively contracting or hypertonic uterus; patients with major systemic disorders (including diabetes mellitus, renal, hepatic, or sickle cell disease); a history of prior uterine surgery (including surgery of the cervix); and pelvic adhesions.

ACTIONS
Transabdominal intra-amniotic injection of hypertonic salt solution induces fetal death and abortion. The mechanism of its abortifacient actions, which results in rapid and generally complete emptying of the gravid uterus, remains unknown. Intra-amniotic injection of hypertonic saline may be associated with a temporary rise in serum sodium and chloride.

WARNINGS
Care is exercised to avoid extra-amniotic injection. Inadvertent, direct intravascular injection into the vasculature of the uterus and placenta is avoided, because this may result in severe, sudden hypernatremia.

The following complications have been reported and occur more frequently when hypertonic saline is augmented with IV oxytocin: disseminated intravascular clotting (DIC) with occasional fatal consequences, cervical lacerations (some of major degree) and cervical fistula, excessive blood loss.

PRECAUTIONS
During intra-amniotic instillation, patient is observed for symptoms of intravascular injection. To ensure that patient remains alert and able to report any untoward reactions, general anesthesia or sedation should not be used. Should intravascular injection occur, discontinue administration immediately, infuse IV Dextrose 5% in Water rapidly, and, if indicated, give additional supportive care for hypernatremia.

If the volume of solution instilled exceeds the volume of amniotic fluid removed, positive pressure within the cavity may occur. A "reverse dialysis" may then be created intraperitoneally, resulting in ascites, severe electrolyte disturbances, hypervolemia, and circulatory failure.

ADVERSE REACTIONS
Inadvertent intravascular injection, febrile response, flushing, water intoxication, pulmonary embolus, pneumonia, changes in the coagulation mechanism with resultant severe hemorrhage, and significant infection at the site of needle entry. In addition, intra-amniotic instillation has reportedly caused necrosis of uterine musculature as a result of backflow along the needle track when increased intra-amniotic pressure is present. Retention of placental tissue may occur.

The severe, sudden hypernatremia resulting from inadvertent intravascular injection has produced complications such as cardiovascular shock, extensive hemolysis, and cortical necrosis of the kidney. This may be preceded by such signs or symptoms as mental confusion, hypotension, vague distress, pelvic or abdominal pain, headache, numbness of fingertips, tinnitus, salty taste, and dryness of the mouth.

DOSAGE
Approximately 250 ml is considered the maximum dose. Solution is instilled, preferably through a

S

three-way stopcock, with the needle or polyethylene catheter inserted into the amniotic cavity. Careful placement and fixation are important to prevent dislocation.

Amniotic fluid is aspirated and hypertonic saline solution replaced at a relatively slow rate. Fluid samples are taken at regular intervals to be sure needle is within the amniotic cavity.

NURSING IMPLICATIONS

HISTORY
See Appendix 4.

PHYSICAL ASSESSMENT
Obtain vital signs, weight.

ADMINISTRATION
It is recommended that this procedure be performed in a medical unit with intensive care facilities available.

The assistance of a supportive individual before and during the procedure is essential.

Surgical preparation (shaving, cleansing) of abdomen is recommended.

Have available 20% sodium chloride solution, local anesthetic, and equipment for administration of abortifacient.

Obtain vital signs immediately before procedure.

ONGOING ASSESSMENTS AND NURSING MANAGEMENT
Monitor blood pressure, pulse, and respirations continuously during instillation and q1h to q2h following instillation and until patient is discharged.

Oxytocin (p 825) may be administered as an adjunctive uterine stimulant to shorten the abortifacient-to-abortion interval. It is administered with 5% Dextrose and Water to offset the antidiuretic effect of sodium chloride and avoid water intoxication.

During the infusion, observe the patient closely for adverse reactions due to inadvertent injection of sodium chloride 20%. Early signs and symptoms may include mental confusion, hypotension, vague complaints, pelvic or abdominal pain, headache, numbness of fingertips, tinnitus, and salty taste or dryness in the mouth.

Unless ordered otherwise, patient is encouraged to drink at least 2 qt of water the day of the procedure to assist in salt excretion.

Labor can be expected to begin in 8 to 48 hours.

Depending on hospital policy, patient may be discharged following the procedure and in-structed to return when labor begins. Patients receiving oxytocin and those developing complications remain hospitalized.

PATIENT INFORMATION
NOTE: Instructions regarding return to the hospital may vary according to hospital policy or physician preference.

Labor can be expected in 8 to 48 hours. Return to the hospital when labor contractions begin, if excessive bleeding is noted, or if passage of the fetus occurs.

Continue to drink extra amounts of water for the remainder of the day.

Sodium Citrate and Citric Acid Solution Rx

liquid: 500 mg sodium citrate, 334 mg citric acid/ 5 ml	Bicitra

Sodium citrate and citric acid solution is also known as modified Shohl's solution.

INDICATIONS
A urinary alkalinizing agent useful when administration of potassium salts is undesirable or contraindicated. Also useful in treatment of chronic metabolic acidosis as seen in chronic renal insufficiency or renal tubular acidosis. Also useful for neutralizing gastric hydrochloric acid.

CONTRAINDICATIONS
Patients on sodium-restricted diet or with severe renal impairment.

ACTIONS
Is absorbed and metabolized to sodium bicarbonate, acting as a systemic alkalinizer.

PRECAUTIONS
Use with caution in those with low urinary output, cardiac failure, hypertension, impaired renal function, peripheral and pulmonary edema, and toxemia of pregnancy.

ADVERSE REACTIONS
Use with caution in those with abnormal renal mechanisms to avoid development of alkalosis, especially in the presence of hypocalcemia.

OVERDOSAGE
Symptoms include diarrhea, nausea and vomiting, hypernoia, and convulsions.

DOSAGE

Adults: 10 ml to 30 ml diluted in 30 ml to 90 ml water, P.C. and H.S.

Children: 5 ml to 15 ml diluted in 30 ml to 90 ml water, P.C. and H.S.

NURSING IMPLICATIONS

HISTORY
See Appendix 4.

PHYSICAL ASSESSMENT
Baseline laboratory tests may include urinalysis, serum electrolytes, and serum bicarbonate.

ADMINISTRATION
Best administered after meals to avoid saline laxative effect.

Palatability is enhanced if solution is chilled before administration.

Add prescribed dose to 30 ml or more of cold water.

Instruct patient to drink water, if desired, to relieve aftertaste.

ONGOING ASSESSMENTS AND NURSING MANAGEMENT
Check urine pH daily to bid, or as ordered, with nitrazine paper.

Inform physician if urine becomes acidic, because an increase in dose or other measures may be necessary.

If diarrhea, nausea, or vomiting occurs, notify physician before next dose is due. Drug may need to be temporarily discontinued or dosage reduced.

PATIENT AND FAMILY INFORMATION
Drug is more palatable if kept chilled (may be kept in the refrigerator).

Add prescribed dose to 1 oz to 3 oz of chilled water. This may be followed by additional water, if desired.

If diarrhea, nausea, or vomiting occurs, notify physician or nurse.

Sodium Iodide

See Iodine Thyroid Products.

Sodium Iodide ¹³¹I _Rx_

capsules: radioactivity ranging from 1 mCi to 50 mCi   Iodotope

per capsule at time of calibration

oral solution: radioactivity concentration of 7.05 mCi/ml at time of calibration

capsules: radioactivity ranging from 0.8 mCi to 100 mCi per capsule   Sodium Iodide I 131

oral solution: radioactivity ranging from 3.5 mCi to 150 mCi per vial

INDICATIONS
Treatment of hyperthyroidism and selected cases of carcinoma of the thyroid. Palliative effects may be seen in patients with papillary or follicular carcinoma of the thyroid. Stimulation of radioiodide uptake may be achieved by administration of thyrotropin. Radioiodide will not be taken up by giant cell and spindle cell carcinoma of the thyroid or by amyloid solid carcinomas.

CONTRAINDICATIONS
Preexisting vomiting or diarrhea.

ACTIONS
Readily absorbed from the GI tract. Following absorption, the iodide is distributed primarily within the extracellular fluid of the body. It is trapped and rapidly converted to protein-bound iodine by the thyroid; it is concentrated, but not protein bound, by the stomach and salivary glands. It is also promptly excreted by the kidneys. About 90% of the local radiation is caused by beta radiation and 10% by gamma radiation.

WARNINGS
Sodium iodide ¹³¹I is not usually used for treatment of hyperthyroidism in patients under 30 unless circumstances preclude other treatment. Not administered to patients who are pregnant or may become pregnant, or during lactation unless indications are exceptional and the need outweighs the possible potential risks from the radiation exposure involved. Iodine is excreted in milk during lactation; formula feedings should be substituted for breast-feeding.

DRUG INTERACTIONS
Uptake of ¹³¹I will be affected by recent intake of **stable iodine** in any form or by use of thyroid, antithyroid, and certain other drugs. Patient must be carefully questioned about previous medication and procedures involving radiographic contrast media.

PRECAUTIONS
Antithyroid therapy of a severely hyperthyroid patient is usually discontinued 3 to 4 days before administration of radioiodide.

ADVERSE REACTIONS
Immediate reactions are usually mild. Following larger doses used in treating thyroid carcinoma, adverse reactions may be more severe and may present special problems.

Untoward effects include depression of the hematopoietic system when large doses are used, radiation sickness (some degree of nausea, vomiting), increase in clinical symptoms, bone-marrow depression, severe sialoadenitis, acute leukemia, anemia, chromosomal abnormalities, acute thyroid crisis, blood dyscrasia, leukopenia, and thrombocytopenia.

Tenderness and swelling of the neck, pain on swallowing, sore throat, and cough may occur around the third day after treatment and are usually relieved by analgesics. Temporary thinning of the hair may occur 2 to 3 months after treatment.

DOSAGE
Dose is measured by radioactivity calibration immediately prior to administration.

Hyperthyroidism: Amount needed to achieve clinical remission without destruction of the entire thyroid varies widely. Usual dose range is 4 mCi to 10 mCi. Toxic nodular goiter and other special situations require larger doses.

Carcinoma of the thyroid: Dosage is individualized. Usual dose for ablation of normal thyroid tissue is 50 mCi, with subsequent therapeutic doses usually 100 mCi to 150 mCi.

Physical characteristics: ^{131}I decays by beta and gamma emissions with a physical half-life of 8.06 days.

NURSING IMPLICATIONS

HISTORY
See Appendix 4. Determination of allergy to iodine is important. Obtain a thorough history about any x-rays (x-rays using radiographic contrast media may interfere with radioiodide uptake). Question patient about recent consumption of large quantities of seafood or health foods or products, especially those with a high iodine content.

PHYSICAL ASSESSMENT
Hyperthyroidism: Obtain vital signs, weight; note presence of overt signs of hyperthyroidism (*e.g.*, nervousness, fine tremor of hands, visible enlargment in the thyroid area, skin changes [usually warm, moist, flushed], eyes [exophthalmos]); review previous laboratory and diagnostic tests (if available). Laboratory tests include T_3 and T_4 uptake, serum cholesterol, CBC, and so on; diagnostic tests include radioactive iodine uptake and thyroid ultrasonography.

Carcinoma of thyroid: Obtain vital signs, weight; evaluate patient's physical and emotional status.

ADMINISTRATION
Sodium Iodide ^{131}I is usually administered by the department of nuclear medicine. In certain instances, nursing personnel may be responsible for administration of low-dose capsule form or oral solution.

Patient is usually kept NPO from midnight before administration (food delays absorption).

If antithyroid medication had been prescribed, check to be sure patient has *not* received the drug 3 to 4 days prior to administration of sodium iodide ^{131}I.

The physician should explain the procedure and possible after-effects. Required restrictions should be reviewed for the patient and his family the evening before or the day of radioiodide administration.

If nursing personnel administer the capsule form, have patient remove capsule from the cup and swallow with water. Have several glasses of water available in case extra fluid is required to swallow the capsule. Record the exact time capsule is administered.

Solution form is administered in a glass or plastic container. Following ingestion, water is added to the empty container two to three times and the patient is asked to drink the water in the container. This ensures proper delivery of the calculated doses.

If any of the solution is spilled before or at the time of administration, the radiation safety officer or the department of nuclear medicine must be notified immediately.

ONGOING ASSESSMENTS AND NURSING MANAGEMENT
The nurse must be familiar with patient management guidelines established by the hospital's department of nuclear medicine. Precautionary measures for safety of the patient, visitors, and hospital personnel may vary.

High dosage for the destruction of thyroid tissue in thyroid carcinoma usually requires some or all of the following: a private room, limitation or exclusion of visitors, limitation of the time nursing personnel spend in the room, saving of urine for separate disposal, special handling of bed linen, posting of a radiation warning sign on door, disposable eating utensils, special handling of all disposable materials (*e.g.,* tissues, eating utensils), wearing of hospital gown rather than own clothing, use of radiation exposure badges by nursing personnel, and radiation survey of the room, furniture, bedding, and utensils when treatment is concluded. Lower dosage in treatment of hyperthyroidism usually requires less stringent precautionary measures.

With high dosage, *all* patient-care activities must be carefully planned and implemented; the amount of time spent in the patient's room is often limited to 15 to 30 minutes per person per day. The radiation safety officer or department of nuclear medicine should supply exposure guidelines for nursing personnel. Lower dosage for treatment of hyperthyroidism usually allows longer exposure periods.

Monitor vital signs q4h or as ordered.

Sodium iodide ^{131}I is promptly excreted by the kidneys. A push of fluids may be ordered to dilute urine and decrease amount of radiation to gonads. The patient should be urged to void frequently.

Observe patient for adverse reactions: tenderness and swelling of neck, pain on swallowing, sore throat, and cough, which may occur on the third day after treatment. Physician may order analgesics to relieve discomfort. If symptoms become severe, notify the physician promptly.

Following treatment for hyperthyroidism, the physician will continue to monitor the patient's thyroid activity at frequent intervals for several months. Repeat treatment may be necessary to obtain a euthyroid state.

Following treatment for thyroid carcinoma, the patient will be closely monitored for response to therapy. Subsequent treatments may be necessary for ablation of thyroid tissue. Monitoring of the hematopoietic system by blood counts at periodic intervals will also be necessary.

PATIENT AND FAMILY INFORMATION

Notify physician or nurse promptly if fever, sore throat, unusual bleeding or bruising, headache, or general malaise occurs.

Record weight twice a week or as directed by physician. Take pulse daily (patient may need instruction) and record. Bring record of weight and pulse rate to each physician's office or clinic visit.

Avoid use of nonprescription drugs unless use is approved by physician.

Sodium Lactate Rx

167 mEq/liter each of sodium and lactate ions	$\frac{1}{6}$ molar sodium lactate
50 mEq in 10 ml (5 mEq/ml)	sodium lactate injection

INDICATIONS

Treatment of metabolic acidosis.

ACTIONS

One liter of $\frac{1}{6}$ molar sodium lactate administered IV provides 167 mEq each of sodium and lactate ions and is potentially equivalent in alkalinizing effect to approximately 280 ml of 5% sodium bicarbonate.

Sodium lactate is metabolized to bicarbonate in the liver. The alkalinizing effects of sodium lactate are provided from the simultaneous removal of lactate and hydrogen ions. Lactate is metabolized to glycogen and ultimately converted to carbon dioxide and water via oxidation in the liver. The conversion of sodium lactate to bicarbonate requires 1 to 2 hours; therefore, sodium bicarbonate is used if an immediate effect is desired.

WARNINGS

The conversion of lactate to bicarbonate may be impaired in the severely ill and in persons with hepatic disease. Not used to treat lactic acidosis; lactic metabolism is impaired and bicarbonate is not formed.

NURSING IMPLICATIONS

HISTORY
See Appendix 4.

PHYSICAL ASSESSMENT
Note and record signs of metabolic acidosis (Appendix 6, section 6-1). Baseline laboratory tests may include serum potassium, blood glucose, arterial blood gas studies, urinalysis, and determination of anion gap (Delta).

ADMINISTRATION
Have sodium bicarbonate available because it may be used, when necessary, for its immediate effect.

Rate of infusion is individualized.

ONGOING ASSESSMENTS AND NURSING MANAGEMENT
Observe for decrease in symptoms.

Frequent laboratory tests may be ordered if

S

acidosis is severe. Keep physician informed of most recent laboratory values.

Monitor IV infusion rate and check infusion site for signs of extravasation every 15 to 30 minutes.

Sodium Phosphate

See Laxatives.

Sodium Phosphate P 32 Rx

injection: 0.67   *Generic*
    mCi/ml

INDICATIONS
Principal use is for treatment of polycythemia vera; also effective for treatment of chronic myelocytic leukemia and chronic lymphocytic leukemia. Also used in the palliative management of selected patients with multiple areas of skeletal metastases.

CONTRAINDICATIONS
Not used as part of sequential treatment with a chemotherapeutic agent. Should not be administered in polycythemia vera when the leukocyte count is below 5000/mm³ or platelet count is below 150,000/mm³.

Not used in chronic myelocytic leukemia when the leukocyte count is below 20,000/mm³. Usually not administered in skeletal metastases when the leukocyte count is below 5000/mm³ and the platelet count is below 100,000/mm³. Should not be given for therapeutic purposes to patients who are pregnant or to nursing mothers.

ACTIONS
Phosphorus is necessary to the metabolic and proliferative activity of cells. Radioactive phosphorus concentrates to a very high degree in rapidly proliferating tissue. Has a half-life of 14.3 days.

WARNINGS
Not intended for intracavitary injection. Safety for use in pregnancy is not established. Drug is administered to pregnant women only when potential benefits outweigh the possible risks. It is not known whether sodium phosphate is excreted in human milk; breast-feeding should be discontinued during therapy. Safety and efficacy for use in children are not established.

ADVERSE REACTIONS
Some patients with polycythemia vera treated with sodium phosphate have subsequently developed myeloid leukemia.

OVERDOSAGE
May produce serious effects on the hematopoietic system including leukopenia, thrombocytopenia, and anemia.

DOSAGE
Can be given orally or intravenously. Oral doses are incompletely absorbed. The equivalent IV dose is approximately 75% of the oral dose. However, oral administration in the fasting state may be equal to IV administration.

Polycythemia vera: IV dose ranges from 1 mCi to 8 mCi depending on the stage of disease and the size of the patient. Repeat doses are titrated to individual needs.

Chronic leukemia: Individual dose is 6 mCi to 15 mCi.

NURSING IMPLICATIONS

HISTORY
See Appendix 4.

PHYSICAL ASSESSMENT
Obtain vital signs, weight. Evaluate patient's physical and emotional status. Baseline laboratory tests and diagnostic studies may include bone-marrow aspiration, CBC, hematocrit, hemoglobin, and platelet count.

ADMINISTRATION
If given orally, fasting from midnight may be ordered.

Dose is measured and administered by the department of nuclear medicine.

ONGOING ASSESSMENTS AND NURSING MANAGEMENT
Review protocol established by the radiation officer for procedures and policies relevant to care of patient receiving this radiopharmaceutical. These policies should include patient isolation (usually not necessary with sodium phosphate); disposal of linens, feces, vomitus, urine, and dressings; and a recommended length of bedside exposure time for hospital personnel.

CLINICAL ALERT: Observe patient for signs of bone-marrow depression (Appendix 6, section 6-8) or evidence of radiation sickness (*e.g.,* fever, malaise, nausea, vomiting, diarrhea).

Wear a film badge or exposure meter when giving care to a patient receiving sodium phosphate. Pregnant nurses should not be assigned to patients receiving this radiopharmaceutical.

Laboratory tests are performed at regular intervals following therapy and usually include CBC, hemoglobin, hematocrit, platelet counts, and in some instances bone-marrow aspiration.

PATIENT AND FAMILY INFORMATION

Laboratory tests at periodic intervals will be necessary to monitor the results of therapy.

Sodium Polystyrene Sulfonate Rx

powder
suspension: 1.25 g/
  5 ml

Kayexalate
SPS

INDICATIONS

Treatment of hyperkalemia.

ACTIONS

An ion-exchange resin for reduction of elevated potassium levels. As the resin passes along the intestine or is retained in the colon after administration by enema, sodium ions are partially released and replaced by potassium ions. This action occurs mainly in the large intestine, which excretes potassium ions to a greater degree than does the small intestine. Efficacy of this product is limited and unpredictably variable. It commonly approximates the order of 33% (1 mEq potassium/g), but the range is so large that electrolyte balance must be monitored. Sodium content is approximately 100 mg/g.

WARNINGS

Because effective lowering of serum potassium may take hours to days, treatment with this drug alone may be insufficient to rapidly correct severe hyperkalemia associated with states of rapid tissue breakdown (*e.g.,* burns, renal failure) or hyperkalemia so marked as to constitute a medical emergency. Other definitive measures, including use of IV calcium to antagonize the effects of hyperkalemia on the heart, IV sodium bicarbonate or glucose and insulin to cause an intracellular shift of potassium, or dialysis, may be necessary.

Serious potassium deficiency can occur from therapy. Frequent serum potassium levels are recommended. The level at which treatment is discontinued is determined on an individual basis. Important aids in making this determination are the patient's clinical condition and the ECG.

Like all cation-exchange resins, sodium polystyrene sulfonate is not totally selective for potassium; small amounts of other cations such as magnesium and calcium can also be lost during treatment.

PRECAUTIONS

Caution is advised when giving to patients who cannot tolerate even a small increase in sodium loads (*e.g.,* in severe CHF, severe hypertension, or marked edema). In such instances, compensatory restriction of sodium intake from other sources may be indicated. If constipation occurs, patient may be given 10 ml to 20 ml of 70% sorbitol q2h or as needed to produce one or two loose watery stools a day. This measure also reduces any tendency toward fecal impaction.

DRUG INTERACTIONS

Systemic alkalosis has been reported after cation-exchange resins were administered orally in combination with **nonabsorbable cation-donating antacids and laxatives,** including **aluminum carbonate, glycinate, hydroxide, phosphate; calcium carbonate; dihydroxyaluminum sodium carbonate; magaldrate; magnesium carbonate, hydroxide, oxide, trisilicate; sodium bicarbonate. Glucose insulin infusions** are used with caution to avoid hypokalemia.

ADVERSE REACTIONS

GI: May cause some degree of gastric irritation. Anorexia, nausea, vomiting, and constipation may occur, especially if high doses are given. Occasionally, diarrhea develops. Large doses in elderly patients can cause fecal impaction. This effect may be obviated through use of the resin in enemas. Intestinal obstruction, due to concretions of aluminum hydroxide when used in combination with polystyrene sulfonate, has been reported.

Electrolyte imbalance: Hypokalemia, hypocalcemia, and significant sodium retention have been reported.

DOSAGE

Intensity and duration of therapy depend on the severity and resistance of hyperkalemia.

Adults: Average daily dose is 15 g to 60 g. This is best provided by administering 15 g (approximately 4 level teaspoons of the powder) 1 to 4 times a day. One gram of powder contains approximately 4.1 mEq of sodium; 1 level teaspoon contains approximately 3.5 g of sodium polystyrene sulfonate and 15 mEq sodium. A heaping teaspoon may contain as much as 10 g to 12 g of sodium polystyrene sulfonate.

Children: In smaller children and infants, lower

S

doses are employed by using a rate of 1 mEq of potassium per gram of resin as the basis for calculation.

Enema: Results are less effective. Dosage for adults is 30 g to 50 g q6h. Retention time is 30 to 60 minutes to several hours.

NURSING IMPLICATIONS

HISTORY
See Appendix 4.

PHYSICAL ASSESSMENT
Obtain blood pressure, pulse, and respirations. Baseline laboratory studies and diagnostic tests may include serum electrolytes (especially potassium, calcium, magnesium, sodium), renal-function studies, and ECG.

ADMINISTRATION
Oral: Add prescribed dose of powder to a small quantity of water to make a suspension. Usually 3 ml to 4 ml of water is used per gram of resin, but physician may order other dilutions.

To improve palatability, syrup instead of water may be used to make the suspension.

When ordered, the oral suspension may be administered via a nasogastric tube and may also be mixed with a diet appropriate for a patient in renal failure.

Enema: Prior to administration of the resin, give a cleansing enema.

Add dose of powder to 100 ml of the prescribed solution, which should be warmed to body temperature; sorbitol or 20% dextrose in water is recommended. Agitate gently to mix.

Place patient in the left lateral position.

Use a large-sized, soft rubber or plastic tube; lubricate with water-soluble lubricant, insert in the sigmoid colon about 20 cm, and tape in place.

Introduce solution by gravity, with particles kept in suspension by gentle stirring or agitation.

Flush the suspension with 50 ml or 100 ml of fluid (to make a total fluid of 150–200 ml); clamp the tube and leave in place.

If back leakage occurs, elevate the patient's hips on pillows or have the patient assume a knee–chest position for a few minutes or as tolerated.

The suspension is kept in the sigmoid colon for several hours, if possible. Retention times of 30 to 60 minutes have also been recommended.

Following the designated retention time, the colon is irrigated to remove the resin:

Use up to 2 qt of the prescribed non–sodium containing solution warmed to body temperature.

Instruct the patient to assume a left lateral position.

Place a Y-connector on the end of the rectal tube. Insert a long drainage tube into one part of the Y and place below the level of the bed in a collection container. Use the other part of the Y to administer the 1 to 2 qt of irrigating solution, which is allowed to drain in by gravity.

The returns are drained constantly through the drainage tube connected to the Y-connector.

Preparation and storage: Suspension should be freshly prepared and not stored beyond 24 hours. Do not heat because this may alter the exchange properties of the resin.

ONGOING ASSESSMENTS AND NURSING MANAGEMENT
Check patient every 15 to 30 minutes for retention of fluid if given rectally. If there is difficulty retaining fluid, inform physician.

Monitor blood pressure, pulse, and respirations q2h to q4h.

Observe for adverse reactions and inform physician of occurrence.

Observe for signs of electrolyte imbalance, principally hypokalemia (Appendix 6, section 6-15), hypernatremia (Appendix 6, section 6-17), hypomagnesemia (Appendix 6, section 6-16), hypocalcemia (Appendix 6, section 6-13). Daily monitoring of serum electrolytes is recommended. Keep physician informed of all abnormal laboratory values.

Withhold next dose and notify physician if most recent serum potassium level is within or close to the normal range.

An ECG may also be ordered to detect hypokalemia. Severe hypokalemia is often associated with a lengthened Q–T interval; widening, flattening, or inversion of the T wave; and prominent U waves. Cardiac arrhythmias may occur, such as premature atrial, nodal, or ventricular contractions and supraventricular and ventricular tachycardias.

Constipation may be corrected by use of a stool-softening laxative or 70% sorbitol.

If the patient cannot tolerate even a small increase in sodium loads (*e.g.,* in severe CHF, severe hypertension, or marked edema), dietary sodium restriction may be necessary.

Sodium Salicylate

See Salicylates.

Sodium Sulfacetamide

See Sulfonamides, Ophthalmic.

Sodium Thiosalicylate

See Salicylates.

Somatropin *(Somatotropin)* Rx

powder for injection: Asellacrin
2 IU/vial, 10 IU/
vial
powder for injection: Crescormon
4 IU/vial

INDICATIONS

Growth failure due to a deficiency of pituitary
growth hormone in children.

Criteria for treatment: Patient must show significant short stature or retarded growth rate. Those
with congenital growth hormone deficiency should
be below the third percentile for height and growing
at a rate of less than 5 cm/year over at least 1 year
of continuous observation. Height is compared to
appropriate standards for age (*i.e.,* those of the National Center for Health Statistics). Patients with acquired growth hormone deficiency should also have
grown less than 5 cm/year and should have been
observed for at least 1 year.

Skeletal maturation should be compatible with a
beneficial response to therapy. Epiphyseal maturation should be incomplete. In general, response to
therapy is diminished when bone age is advanced
beyond 13 to 14 years.

Diagnosis of growth hormone deficiency is confirmed by objective tests of growth hormone function. There must be a failure to increase the serum
concentration of growth hormone above 5 ng/ml to
7 ng/ml in response in two standard stimuli.

Deficiency of thyrotropin is treated before testing
for growth hormone deficiency; patient must be euthyroid for 4 to 8 weeks prior to testing and must
be observed for at least 6 months while euthyroid to
determine if growth rate meets treatment criteria.
Corticotropin deficiency and any deficiency of antidiuretic hormone are also treated. Gonadotropin
deficiency may be treated concomitantly with somatropin, but this may rapidly advance epiphyseal
maturation.

CONTRAINDICATIONS

Closed epiphyses; any progression of an underlying
or actively growing intracranial lesion, especially in

hypopituitary children. Intracranial lesions must be
inactive for 1 year prior to therapy. Therapy is discontinued if recurrent activity is evident.

ACTIONS

A purified polypeptide hormone extracted from the
anterior lobe of human pituitary glands, somatropin
stimulates linear growth in those with pituitary
growth hormone deficiency. Somatropin increases
skeletal muscle mass; affects cartilaginous growth
areas of long bones; influences the size of internal
organs; increases red cell mass through erythropoie-
tin stimulation; increases cellular protein synthesis;
has diabetogenic activity; stimulates intracellular lipolysis and oxidation of fatty acids and increases
the plasma concentration of free fatty acids, resulting in fat mobilization; stimulates synthesis of chon-
droitin sulfate and collagen and urinary excretion of
hydroxyproline; induces net retention of phosphorus and potassium, sodium-increased intestinal absorption of calcium, and increased renal tubular
reabsorption of phosphorus; increases calcium excretion in the urine (but there is a simultaneous increase in calcium absorption in the intestine).

WARNINGS

The possibility of hypothyroidism during therapy
must not go undiagnosed, because this would jeop-
ardize the response to growth hormone. The risk of
transmitting hepatitis cannot be excluded but is extremely small; no cases have been reported.

PRECAUTIONS

Hyperglycemic effects: Because of its diabetogenic
actions, which include the induction of hyperglycemia and ketosis, somatropin is used with caution
in those with diabetes mellitus or family history of
diabetes mellitus. Monitoring of urine for glycosuria
is recommended.

Hypothyroidism: Hypothyroidism of pituitary or
hypothalamic origin may develop. Patients should
have periodic thyroid-function tests and be treated
with thyroid hormone, when indicated.

Subcutaneous administration: Subcutaneous administration may lead to local lipoatrophy or lipodystrophy and may enhance development of neutralizing antibodies.

Bone age: Bone age is monitored annually, especially in those who are pubertal or who are receiving concomitant thyroid replacement therapy. Under these circumstances, epiphyseal maturation may
progress rapidly to closure.

Intracranial lesion: Those with growth hormone
deficiency secondary to an intracranial lesion are
examined frequently for progression or recurrence
of the underlying disease process.

S

DRUG INTERACTIONS
Concomitant **glucocorticoid** therapy may inhibit response to somatropin and should not exceed 10 mg/m^2 to 15 mg/m^2 hydrocortisone equivalent.

ADVERSE REACTIONS
Antibodies to somatropin are formed in 30% to 40% of patients who receive the drug prepared by similar methods. In general, these antibodies are not neutralizing and do not interfere with response to the hormone; however, 5% of patients fail to respond. Test for antisomatropin antibodies is recommended in any patient who fails to respond to therapy.

DOSAGE
For IM use only. Give an initial dose of 2 IU three times a week with at least 48 hours between injections. Maximum growth rate occurs at or near a dosage of 0.3 IU/kg/week. It may be necessary to increase the dosage in older hypopituitary children, particularly if sexual maturation has not occurred. After long periods of therapy (2 or more years), growth rate may decline in spite of therapy. Withdrawal for several months may result in a renewal of growth response upon resumption of treatment.

If, at any time during continuous administration, the growth rate does not exceed 2.5 cm (1 inch) in a 6-month period, the dose may be doubled for the next 6 months. If there is still no satisfactory response, treatment is discontinued and diagnosis reevaluated.

Treatment is discontinued when patient has reached a satisfactory adult height, when epiphyses have fused, or when patient fails to respond to administration.

▌NURSING IMPLICATIONS

HISTORY
See Appendix 4.

PHYSICAL ASSESSMENT
Obtain height, weight. Baseline laboratory studies (other than diagnostic) may include CBC, urinalysis, fasting blood sugar, serum electrolytes, thyroid-function tests.

ADMINISTRATION
Both products are supplied with a diluent. Record date of reconstitution on vial.

Store reconstituted vial under refrigeration and use within 1 month. Unreconstituted vials may be stored at room temperature.

Administer IM only.

Injections are given three times a week over a possible period of 2 or more years. Formulate a systematic plan for rotation of injection sites and keep it with the patient's record.

Prior to each injection, inspect previous injection sites for evidence of lipoatrophy or lipodystrophy (*e.g.,* dimpling of skin, pitting of subcutaneous fat, extreme firmness of subcutaneous tissue).

ONGOING ASSESSMENTS AND NURSING MANAGEMENT
Measure height and weigh patient every month or as ordered.

Periodic laboratory tests may include CBC; urine for glucose, ketones; blood glucose; urinary calcium; serum electrolytes.

Bone surveys are usually performed yearly to monitor effect of therapy and detect epiphyseal closure.

FAMILY INFORMATION
Keep all appointments for injections because continuity of treatment is important.

Periodic laboratory tests will be required and a yearly x-ray examination of the bones will be performed.

Inform physician or nurse if soreness or redness at an injection site persists, if child complains of abdominal or flank pain, or if chills or fever occurs.

Soy Protein Complex

See Iron Products, Oral.

Spectinomycin Hydrochloride Rx

powder for injection: Trobicin
400 mg/ml when
reconstituted

INDICATIONS
Treatment of acute gonorrheal urethritis and proctitis in the male and acute gonorrheal cervicitis and proctitis in the female when due to susceptible strains of *Neisseria gonorrhoeae*. Men and women with known recent exposure to gonorrhea should be treated as those known to have gonorrhea.

CONTRAINDICATIONS
Hypersensitivity.

ACTIONS
An antibiotic that is an inhibitor of protein synthesis in the bacterial cell. It is active against most

strains of *N. gonorrhoeae.* It is rapidly absorbed after IM injection. A single injection produces peak serum concentrations in 1 hour. The majority of the drug is excreted in the urine.

WARNINGS

Not effective in the treatment of syphilis. Antibiotics used in high doses for short periods of time to treat gonorrhea may mask or delay symptoms of incubating syphilis. Because treatment of syphilis demands prolonged therapy with any effective antibiotic, patients being treated for gonorrhea should be observed clinically. All those with gonorrhea should have a serologic test for syphilis at the time of diagnosis and a follow-up test in 3 months.

Safety for use in pregnancy and children is not established.

PRECAUTIONS

The usual precautions should be observed with allergic individuals. The clinical effectiveness of spectinomycin should be monitored to detect evidence of development of resistance by *N. gonorrhoeae.*

ADVERSE REACTIONS

The following have been reported after single doses: soreness at injection site, urticaria, dizziness, nausea, chills, fever, and insomnia. The following have been reported after multiple doses: decrease in hemoglobin, hematocrit, and creatinine clearance; elevation of alkaline phosphatase, BUN, and SGPT. A reduction in urine output has been noted, but no consistent changes indicative of renal toxicity have been demonstrated.

DOSAGE

Inject 5 ml IM for a 2-g dose. This dose is also recommended for those being treated after failure of previous antibiotic therapy. In geographic areas where antibiotic resistance is known to be prevalent, initial treatment with 4 g (10 ml) IM is preferred, divided between two gluteal region sites.

CDC-recommended treatment schedules for gonorrhea

Uncomplicated gonococcal infections in adults: For penicillin-allergic patients or those who cannot tolerate tetracycline, 2 g IM in a single injection.

Penicillinase-producing **N. gonorrhoeae** *(PPNG):* For patients with uncomplicated PPNG infections and their sexual contacts, 2 g IM in a single injection. Because gonococci are very rarely resistant to spectinomycin and reinfection is the most common cause of treatment failure, patients with positive cultures after therapy should be retreated with the same dose.

Disseminated gonococcal infection: 2 g IM bid for 3 days (the treatment of choice for disseminated infections caused by PPNG).

Children less than 100 pounds (45 kg): 40 mg/kg IM.

NURSING IMPLICATIONS

HISTORY
See Appendix 4.

PHYSICAL ASSESSMENT
Baseline laboratory studies include smear for *N. gonorrhoeae,* serologic test for syphilis. Culture and sensitivity tests may also be performed.

ADMINISTRATION
Diluent is supplied with product and supplies 400 mg/ml.

Shake vial vigorously after adding diluent.

Advise patient that soreness at injection site may be noted.

Use a 20-gauge needle for injection.

Inject IM into the upper outer quadrant of the gluteus. If 4 g is ordered (10 ml), divide dose and give in two gluteal injection sites.

Reconstituted drug is stable at room temperature for 24 hours; do *not* refrigerate or freeze.

ONGOING ASSESSMENTS AND NURSING MANAGEMENT
If giving for disseminated gonococcal infection, monitor vital signs q4h.

Repeat culture and sensitivity tests or smears for *N. gonorrhoeae* may be ordered.

PATIENT INFORMATION
All sexual contacts should be treated.

Notify physician or nurse if hives, dizziness, nausea, chills, or fever occurs.

A repeat culture (or smear) will be necessary to ensure that infection has been controlled.

S

Spironolactone Preparations

Spironolactone *Rx*

tablets: 25 mg	Aldactone, Spiractone, *Generic*
tablets: 50 mg, 100 mg	Aldactone

Spironolactone With Hydrochlorothiazide Rx

tablets: 25 mg spironolactone, 25 mg hydrochlorothiazide	Alazide, Aldactazide, Spiractazide, Spironazide, Spirozide, *Generic*
tablets: 50 mg spironolactone, 50 mg hydrochlorothiazide	Aldactazide 50/50

INDICATIONS

SPIRONOLACTONE

Primary hyperaldosteronism

Is used in establishing diagnosis of primary hyperaldosteronism by therapeutic trial. It is used in the short-term treatment of those with primary hyperaldosteronism, in long-term maintenance therapy for patients with aldosterone-producing adrenal adenomas who are judged poor operative risks or who decline surgery, and in long-term maintenance therapy for those with bilateral micro- or macronodular adrenal hyperplasia.

Edematous conditions

CHF: Used for management of edema and sodium retention when the patient is only partially responsive to, or is intolerant of, other measures. It may be used with digitalis when other therapies are inappropriate.

Cirrhosis of the liver with edema and/or ascites: Aldosterone levels may be exceptionally high in this condition. Spironolactone is indicated for maintenance therapy in conjunction with bedrest and restriction of fluid and sodium.

Nephrotic syndrome: Used for nephrotic patients when treatment of the underlying disease, restriction of fluid and sodium intake, and use of other diuretics do not provide adequate response.

Essential hypertension

Usually in combination with other drugs, spironolactone is indicated for those who cannot be treated adequately with other agents or for whom other agents are considered inappropriate.

Hypokalemia

For treatment of hypokalemia when other measures are considered inappropriate or inadequate. Also indicated for prophylaxis of hypokalemia in those taking digitalis when other measures are considered inadequate or inappropriate.

SPIRONOLACTONE WITH HYDROCHLOROTHIAZIDE

Management of edema or hypertension. Not indicated for initial therapy. If the fixed combination represents the dosage determined by titration to the individual patient, its use may be more convenient in patient management.

CONTRAINDICATIONS

Anuria, acute renal insufficiency, significant impairment of renal function, hyperkalemia. See also Thiazides and Related Diuretics.

ACTIONS

Spironolactone is a specific antagonist of aldosterone, acting through competitive binding at the aldosterone receptor in the nuclei of distal renal tubular cells. Resultant alterations in nuclear protein synthesis affect sodium and potassium exchange in the distal renal tubule. Spironolactone increases the amount of sodium and water excreted, while potassium is retained. In addition, antagonism of aldosterone may inhibit hydrogen-ion excretion. The drug acts both as a diuretic and as an antihypertensive. It may be given alone or in combination with other diuretic agents that act more proximally in the renal tubule.

Spironolactone is effective in lowering systolic and diastolic blood pressure in primary hyperaldosteronism. It is also effective in most cases of essential hypertension, despite the fact that aldosterone secretion may be normal in benign essential hypertension. It does not elevate serum uric acid, precipitate gout, or alter carbohydrate metabolism as do the thiazides.

Spironolactone is rapidly metabolized; the primary metabolite is canrenone, which reaches peak plasma levels in 2 to 4 hours. The metabolites are excreted primarily in the urine but also in bile.

When the combination of spironolactone and hydrochlorothiazide is given, the action of the thiazide must also be considered.

WARNINGS

Spironolactone and its metabolites may cross the placental barrier. Use in pregnant women requires that the anticipated benefit be weighed against the possible hazard to the fetus. Canrenone (metabolite of spironolactone) is found in breast milk. If use of spironolactone is essential, an alternate method of infant feeding is instituted.

The use of diuretics during pregnancy is inappropriate and exposes the mother and fetus to unnecessary hazards. Diuretics do not prevent development of toxemia of pregnancy, and there is no evidence that they are useful in treating toxemia of pregnancy. Diuretics are indicated in pregnancy when edema is due to pathologic causes, just as it is in the absence of pregnancy.

PRECAUTIONS

Hyperkalemia: Because of the diuretic action of spironolactone, patients should be carefully evaluated for possible fluid and electrolyte imbalances. Hyperkalemia may occur in those with impaired renal function or excessive potassium intake and can cause cardiac irregularities that may be fatal. No potassium supplement should ordinarily be given with spironolactone. Hyperkalemia may be treated promptly by rapid IV administration of 20% to 50% glucose and regular insulin, using 0.25 units/g to 0.5 units/g of glucose. This is a temporary measure to be repeated as needed. Treatment of hyperkalemia may also include use of IV calcium to antagonize effects on the heart, use of bicarbonate if patient is acidotic, and/or use of sodium polystyrene sulfonate exchange resin to remove potassium. Use of spironolactone is discontinued and potassium intake (including dietary) is restricted.

Hyponatremia: May be caused or aggravated by spironolactone, especially when drug is given in combination with other diuretics. Diagnosis is confirmed by low serum sodium level.

Gynecomastia: Development appears to be related to both dosage and duration of therapy and is normally reversible when treatment is discontinued. In rare instances, breast enlargement may persist.

Use in impaired renal function: Spironolactone therapy may cause a transient elevation of BUN, especially in patients with preexisting renal impairment. The drug may cause mild acidosis.

DRUG INTERACTIONS

Potassium supplementation, in the form of either medication or a diet rich in potassium, should not ordinarily be given in association with spironolactone therapy. Excessive potassium intake may cause hyperkalemia.

Do not administer concurrently with **other potassium-sparing diuretics. Lithium** generally should not be given with diuretics because diuretics reduce renal clearance and increase the risk of lithium toxicity. Concomitant use with **other diuretics** or **antihypertensive agents** may result in additive effects. Dosage of such drugs, particularly the **ganglionic blocking agents,** should be reduced by at least 50% when spironolactone is added to the regimen.

Unexpected increases in serum levels of **digitalis glycosides** may occur with spironolactone. Potassium retention caused by spironolactone may reduce cardiac effects of digitalis glycosides.

Spironolactone reduces the vascular responsiveness to **norepinephrine** and is used with caution in management of patients subjected to regional or general anesthesia. Diuretic-induced hemoconcentration with subsequent concentration of clotting factors has been reported to decrease the effect of **oral anticoagulants.**

ADVERSE REACTIONS

Are usually reversible upon discontinuation of the drug. Gynecomastia has been seen. Other adverse reactions include the following.

GI: Cramping, diarrhea.

CNS: Drowsiness, lethargy, headache, mental confusion, ataxia.

Endocrine: Inability to achieve or maintain erection, irregular menses or amenorrhea, postmenopausal bleeding, hirsutism, deepening of the voice, hyperchloremic acidosis in cirrhosis.

Other: Maculopapular or erythematous cutaneous eruptions, urticaria, and drug fever. Carcinoma of the breast has been reported in patients taking spironolactone, but a cause-and-effect relationship has not been established.

DOSAGE

SPIRONOLACTONE

May be given in single or divided doses.

Diagnosis of primary hyperaldosteronism: May be used as an initial diagnostic measure to provide presumptive evidence of primary hyperaldosteronism in patients on normal diets, as follows:

Long test—400 mg/day for 3 to 4 weeks. Correction of hypokalemia and hypertension provides presumptive evidence for diagnosis.

Short test—400 mg/day for 4 days. If serum potassium increases during this time but drops when spironolactone is discontinued, a presumptive diagnosis is considered.

Maintenance of hyperaldosteronism: After diagnosis has been made by more definitive testing procedures, 100 mg/day to 400 mg/day is given in preparation for surgery. For those unsuitable for surgery, drug may be used for long-term maintenance at lowest effective dose.

Edema: For adults, an initial dose of 100 mg/day is recommended but may range from 25 mg/day to 200 mg/day. When given as sole agent for diuresis, continue for at least 5 days at the initial dosage level. If after 5 days an adequate diuretic response has not occurred, a second diuretic that acts more proximally in the renal tubule may be added. Because of the additive effect of spironolactone when administered concurrently with such diuretics, an enhanced diuresis usually begins on the first day of combined treatment. Combined therapy is indicated when more rapid diuresis is desired. The dosage of spironolactone should remain unchanged when other diuretic therapy is added.

For children, daily dosage should provide 1.5 mg of spironolactone/lb.

Essential hypertension: For adults, 50 mg/day to 100 mg/day. May also be combined with other diuretics that act more proximally with other antihypertensive agents. Treatment is continued for at least 2 weeks because maximal response may not occur sooner. Subsequent dosage is adjusted according to patient response.

Hypokalemia: 25 mg/day to 100 mg/day to treat diuretic-induced hypokalemia when oral potassium supplements or other potassium-sparing regimens are inappropriate.

SPIRONOLACTONE 25 MG WITH HYDROCHLOROTHIAZIDE 25 MG
Two to four tablets a day.

SPIRONOLACTONE 50 MG WITH HYDROCHLOROTHIAZIDE 50 MG
One to two tablets a day.

NURSING IMPLICATIONS

HISTORY
See Appendix 4.

PHYSICAL ASSESSMENT
Obtain blood pressure on both arms with patient in sitting and supine positions; obtain pulse, weight. When using to treat edematous condition, examine extremities for edema and record extent and severity. When using to diagnose or treat primary hyperaldosteronism, look for signs of hypokalemia (Appendix 6, section 6-15). If using in treatment of ascites, measure abdominal girth. Baseline laboratory tests may include serum electrolytes, renal-function studies.

ADMINISTRATION
Spironolactone may be given in single or divided doses. If single dose is prescribed and drug is used for edematous states, give early in morning.

If prescribed for hypertension, obtain blood pressure immediately before administration. Withhold drug and contact physician if a significant decrease in the systolic or diastolic pressure has occurred.

ONGOING ASSESSMENTS AND NURSING MANAGEMENT
Monitor blood pressure daily to q4h or as ordered, depending on reason for use, amount of diuresis, and general condition of patient.

Weigh daily. Withhold drug and notify physician if a significant weight loss (3–4 lb over 3–5 days) has occurred.

Frequent urination may occur in several days. When spironolactone and another diuretic are given, diuresis usually begins on the first day of combined treatment.

Measure intake and output, especially during initial therapy.

In edematous conditions, check extremities daily and compare to data base; record findings.

In ascites, measure abdominal girth daily.

Observe for adverse reactions; notify physician if one or more occur.

Observe for signs of hyperkalemia (Appendix 6, section 6-15) and hyponatremia (Appendix 6, section 6-17). If excessive diuresis has occurred, observe for signs of dehydration (Appendix 6, section 6-10). Withhold next dose and notify physician if one or more signs or symptoms are apparent.

If drowsiness occurs, provide assistance with ambulation.

Serum electrolytes are monitored, especially during initial treatment phase. Serum potassium is obtained following the short or long test for diagnosis of primary hyperaldosteronism.

Potassium supplementation (as medication or dietary supplementation) is usually not indicated during therapy with spironolactone.

Patients receiving oral anticoagulants: Dosage adjustment of the oral anticoagulant may be necessary. Observe patient closely for signs of bleeding, especially during the adjustment period.

When spironolactone is given with a thiazide diuretic, see p 1037.

PATIENT AND FAMILY INFORMATION
NOTE: Physician may wish patient with hypertension to monitor his own blood pressure. Patient or family member will require instruction.

May produce drowsiness, ataxia, and mental confusion; observe caution while driving or performing other tasks requiring alertness.

May cause abdominal cramping, diarrhea, lethargy, thirst, headache, skin rash, deepening of the voice, or breast enlargement. Notify physician or nurse if any of these occurs.

Frequent urination may occur in several days (with spironolactone and another diuretic, frequent urination may begin on the first day of therapy).

Female patient: If menstrual abnormalities occur, notify physician.

Male patient: If inability to achieve or maintain an erection occurs, discuss with physician.

Stanozolol

See Anabolic Hormones.

Streptomycin Sulfate

See Aminoglycosides, Parenteral.

Streptozocin Rx

powder for injection: Zanosar
  100 mg/ml when
  reconstituted

INDICATIONS

Treatment of metastatic islet cell carcinoma of the pancreas. Responses have been obtained with both functional and nonfunctional carcinomas.

ACTIONS

Inhibits DNA synthesis in bacterial and mammalian cells. The biochemical mechanism leading to mammalian cell death has not been definitely established. No specific phase of the cell cycle is particularly sensitive to its lethal effects.

WARNINGS

Renal toxicity: Many patients treated with this drug experienced renal toxicity as evidenced by azotemia, anuria, hypophosphatemia, glycosuria, and renal tubular acidosis. _Such toxicity is dose related and cumulative and may be severe or fatal._ Renal function is monitored before and after each course of therapy. Use in those with preexisting renal disease requires judgment by the physician of potential benefits as opposed to the known risk of serious renal damage. This drug should not be used in combination with or concomitantly with other potential nephrotoxins.

Mutagenesis, carcinogenesis, impairment of fertility: Streptozocin is mutagenic in bacteria, plants, and mammalian cells. Renal, liver, and other tumors have occurred in animals. It has also been shown to be carcinogenic and to affect fertility adversely in some animals.

Use in pregnancy, lactation: There have been no studies in pregnant women. Drug is used during pregnancy only if potential benefit outweighs the potential risks. It is not known whether drug is excreted in human milk. Because of the potential for serious adverse reactions in nursing infants, nursing should be discontinued in patients receiving this drug.

PRECAUTIONS

Patient monitoring: Close patient monitoring, especially for evidence of renal, hepatic, and hematopoietic function, is recommended.

Topical exposure: Streptozocin may pose a carcinogenic hazard following topical exposure if not handled properly.

ADVERSE REACTIONS

Renal: See _Warnings._

GI: Most patients experience severe nausea and vomiting, occasionally requiring discontinuation of therapy. Some experience diarrhea. Hepatic toxicity, as characterized by elevated liver enzyme (SGOT, LDH) and hypoalbuminemia have been reported.

Hematologic: Toxicity has been rare, most often involving mild decreases in hematocrit values. _Fatal hematologic toxicity with substantial reduction in leukocyte and platelet count has been seen._

Metabolic: Mild to moderate abnormalities of glucose tolerance have been noted in some patients. These have generally been reversible, but insulin shock with hypoglycemia has occurred.

CNS: Confusion, lethargy, and depression have been reported in regimens using 5-day continuous infusions.

OVERDOSAGE

No specific antidote is known.

DOSAGE

Administer IV. Streptozocin is not active orally. Intra-arterial administration is not recommended pending further evaluation of the possibility that adverse renal effects may be evoked more rapidly by this route.

The following dosage schedules have been used:

Daily schedule: Recommended dose for daily IV administration is 500 mg/m^2 for 5 consecutive days every 6 weeks until maximum benefit or treatment-limiting toxicity is observed. Escalation of this dosage schedule is not recommended.

Weekly schedule: Recommended initial dose is 1000 mg/m^2 at weekly intervals for the first two courses (_i.e.,_ 2 weeks). In subsequent courses, drug doses may be escalated in those who have not achieved a therapeutic response and who have not experienced significant toxicity with the previous course of treatment. Exceeding a dose of 1500 mg/m^2 is not recommended. When drug is administered on this schedule, the median time to onset of response is about 17 days and the median time to maximum response is about 35 days. The median total dose to onset of response is about 2000 mg/m^2

S

and the median total dose to maximum response is about 4000 mg/m^2.

The ideal duration of maintenance therapy has not been established for either of the above schedules.

NURSING IMPLICATIONS

HISTORY
See Appendix 4.

PHYSICAL ASSESSMENT
Obtain vital signs, weight; evaluate patient's physical and emotional status. Baseline laboratory studies may include CBC, differential, platelet count, hemoglobin, hematocrit, FBS, BUN, serum creatinine, creatinine clearance, SGOT, SGPT, serum bilirubin, alkaline phosphatase, fasting insulin level, and serum electrolytes.

ADMINISTRATION
Caution: Wear plastic disposable gloves when preparing and administering streptozocin. If powder or solution contacts the skin or mucosae, immediately wash the area thoroughly with soap and water, and rinse under running water.

Reconstitute with 9.5 ml of Dextrose Injection, USP, or 0.9% Sodium Chloride Injection, USP. The resulting pale gold solution will contain 100 mg streptozocin and 22 mg citric acid/ml.

Drug must be used within 12 hours of reconstitution because it contains no preservative. It is not intended as a multiple-dose vial.

Physician orders further dilution of the prescribed dose (usually in 50–150 or more ml of 5% Dextrose in Water or 0.9% Sodium Chloride).

Time of infusion is ordered by the physician. Average time is 15 to 60 minutes.

An antiemetic may be ordered to be given before administration of streptozocin.

Storage: Store unopened vials under refrigeration at 2°C to 8°C and protect from light.

ONGOING ASSESSMENTS AND NURSING MANAGEMENT
Obtain vital signs q4h or as ordered. Notify physician if fever occurs or if a significant decrease in blood pressure or rise in pulse occurs.

Nausea and vomiting may be moderate to severe and may begin 30 minutes to 2 to 3 or more hours after administration. An antiemetic is usually prescribed.

CLINICAL ALERT: Measure intake and output. Because of drug's potential for renal toxicity, notify physician immediately if there is any decrease in urinary output.

Physician may order urine tested for glucose and proteinuria q8h to once daily. Inform physician immediately if urine is positive for protein or glucose. A 24-hour urine sample may be ordered if urine is positive for protein, because proteinuria is one of the first signs of renal toxicity.

Observe patient for signs of hypoglycemia (Appendix 6, section 6-14), and if they are noted give a food or liquid containing sugar and notify physician. Because vomiting may also be present and patient may be unable to retain oral glucose, have parenteral glucose immediately available.

Bone-marrow toxicity, although rare, has occurred. Observe for signs of bone-marrow depression (Appendix 6, section 6-8) and notify physician immediately if one or more signs or symptoms are apparent.

Notify physician if vomiting exceeds 600 ml to 800 ml/8 hours.

Observe patient for signs of dehydration (Appendix 6, section 6-10), especially if vomiting is severe.

Offer clear liquids at frequent intervals until nausea and vomiting subside. Dry toast and unsalted crackers may also be given.

Weigh patient daily. Inform physician if significant weight loss occurs.

Anorexia may occur. If it persists for more than 2 days, inform physician. A high-protein, high-calorie diet in small frequent feedings may be ordered.

If diarrhea occurs, inform physician. An antidiarrheal agent may be necessary.

CBC, platelet count, and liver- and renal-function tests are recommended weekly. To determine response to therapy, fasting insulin levels may also be ordered for those with functional tumors.

PATIENT AND FAMILY INFORMATION
NOTE: Streptozocin may be given on an outpatient basis when laboratory and supportive resources are sufficient to monitor drug tolerance and to protect and maintain a patient compromised by drug toxicity. An antiemetic may be prescribed to be taken approximately ½ hour before administration of the drug or may be given, in the physician's office or clinic, immediately before the start of the infusion.

Frequent laboratory tests will be required to monitor results of therapy.

Nausea and vomiting may occur and may be severe. Take the prescribed antiemetic as directed. If severe vomiting persists and is not relieved by the drug, notify physician or nurse.

To prevent dehydration, take liquids in frequent and small amounts. Dry toast and unsalted crackers may be tried between liquids.

Once nausea and vomiting have subsided, eat small frequent meals instead of three large meals each day.

If loss of appetite occurs and persists for more than 2 days, inform physician.

Notify physician or nurse immediately if any of the following occurs: severe, persistent diarrhea; easy bleeding or bruising; fever; decrease in urinary output or failure to urinate every 4 to 6 hours; extreme fatigue; sore throat or other signs of a respiratory infection; burning or stinging sensation of, or sores in, the mouth; yellowing of the skin or sclera, pruritus, darkly colored urine.

A decrease in blood sugar may occur; signs are weakness, tremulousness, hunger, perspiration, headache, flushed feeling, lightheadedness, and personality changes. If these occur, take orange juice or candy and notify physician immediately.

Inform other physicians and dentist of therapy with this drug.

Strong Iodine Solution

See Iodine Thyroid Products.

Succinylcholine Chloride Rx

injection: 20 mg/ml	Anectine, Quelicin, Sucostrin
injection: 50 mg/ml	Quelicin
injection: 100 mg/ml	Quelicin, Sucostrin
powder for injection	Succinylcholine Chloride Min-i-Mix
powder for infusion: 500 mg/vial	Anectine Flo-Pack

INDICATIONS

Muscle relaxant used as an adjunct to general anesthesia to facilitate endotracheal intubation and to induce skeletal muscle relaxation during surgery or mechanical ventilation. May be employed to reduce intensity of muscle contractions of pharmacologically or electrically induced convulsions.

CONTRAINDICATIONS

Those with genetically determined disorders of plasma pseudocholinesterase; personal or familial history of malignant hyperthermia; myopathies associated with elevated CPK values; acute narrow-angle glaucoma; penetrating eye injuries; or hypersensitivity.

ACTIONS

An ultra-short-acting depolarizing muscle relaxant. Like acetylcholine, it combines with cholinergic receptors of the motor endplate to produce depolarization followed by an initial muscle contraction often visible as fasciculations. Neuromuscular transmission is then inhibited and remains so as long as an adequate concentration of succinylcholine remains at the receptor site. Neuromuscular blockade results in flaccid paralysis.

Has no known effect on consciousness, pain threshold, or cerebration. Has no direct effect on the myocardium. Initially, a transient bradycardia with hypotension, arrhythmias, and even sinus arrest may occur owing to increased vagal tone. This is noted particularly in children, or from potassium-mediated alterations in electrical conductivity, and is more apparent after repeated administration.

Following IV administration, complete muscular relaxation occurs within 1 minute and lasts approximately 4 to 6 minutes. Following IM injection, onset of action may be delayed up to 3 minutes. Drug is excreted in the urine.

WARNINGS

Use only when facilities are instantly available for endotracheal intubation and for providing adequate ventilation of the patient, including the administration of oxygen under positive pressure and the elimination of carbon dioxide.

Malignant hyperthermia: Administration has been associated with malignant hyperthermic crisis. Early signs include jaw muscle spasm, lack of laryngeal relaxation, generalized rigidity, increased oxygen demand, tachycardia, tachypnea, and profound hyperpyrexia. Successful outcome depends on recognition of early signs, such as jaw muscle spasm, lack of laryngeal relaxation, or generalized rigidity to initial administration of drug or failure of tachycardia to respond to deepening anesthesia. Recognition of the syndrome is cause for discontinuing anesthesia. Dantrolene IV is recommended as an adjunct to supportive measures in management of this problem.

Use in pregnancy: Safety not established. Use in women of childbearing potential only when clearly needed and when potential benefits outweigh unknown potential hazards.

Use in labor and delivery: Used to provide muscle relaxation during delivery by cesarean section. Small amounts cross the placental barrier. Under normal conditions, the quantity of drug entering fetal circulation after a dose of 1 mg/kg to the mother will not endanger the fetus. However, the amount that crosses the placental barrier depends on the concentration gradient between maternal and fetal circulations, and residual neuromuscular blockade (apnea, flaccidity) may occur in the neonate after repeated high doses to, or in presence of, atypical pseudocholinesterase in the mother.

PRECAUTIONS

Use with caution in cardiovascular, hepatic, pulmonary, metabolic, or renal disorders. Also used with caution in those with severe burns or electrolyte imbalance, those receiving quinidine, those who are digitalized or may have digitalis toxicity, or those recovering from severe trauma, because serious cardiac arrhythmias or cardiac arrest may result. Caution is also observed in those with preexisting hyperkalemia or those who are paraplegic, who have suffered spinal cord injury, or who have degenerative or dystrophic neuromuscular disease, because such patients tend to become severely hyperkalemic when this drug is given.

IM or IV injections (single or repeated) have been associated with myoglobinemia and myoglobinuria, especially in children. Use of small doses of nondepolarizing agents such as tubocurarine before injection of succinylcholine reduces severity of muscular fasciculations and decreases incidence of myoglobinuria.

Respiratory depression or prolonged apnea may occur if given in amounts greater than recommended, and also when normal amounts are given to those who are genetically susceptible.

Drug should not be used when an open eye injury is present and is used with caution, if at all, during intraocular surgery and in those with glaucoma. Use with caution in those with fractures because muscle fasciculations may cause additional trauma.

Muscle fasciculations and hyperkalemia can be reduced by administration of a small dose of a nondepolarizing relaxant prior to succinylcholine.

DRUG INTERACTIONS

Duration of action of neuromuscular blockade may be reduced following administration of **diazepam**. Neuromuscular blocking action may be enhanced by **phenelzine, promazine, oxytocin,** certain **nonpenicillin antibiotics, quinidine, beta-adrenergic blocking agents, procainamide, lidocaine, trimethaphan, lithium carbonate, magnesium salts, quinine, chloroquine,** and **isoflurane.** Drug's action may be altered by **acetylcholine, anticholinesterases,** administration of other **nondepolarizing** or **depolarizing relaxants, antibiotics** other than the penicillin group, and **procaine-type local anesthetics. Furosemide** may potentiate action of succinylcholine.

ADVERSE REACTIONS

Consist primarily of an extension of drug's pharmacologic actions. Profound and prolonged muscle relaxation may occur, resulting in respiratory depression to the point of apnea. Rarely, hypersensitivity to drug may exist. Bradycardia, tachycardia, hypertension, hypotension, cardiac arrest, arrhythmias, respiratory depression or apnea, hyperthermia or malignant hyperthermia, increased intraocular pressure, muscle fasciculation, postoperative muscle pain, excessive salivation, hyperkalemia, rash, myoglobinemia, and anaphylactoid reactions may also occur.

DOSAGE

Usually given IV; may be given IM to infants, older children, or adults when a suitable vein is inaccessible. A dose of up to 2.5 mg/kg to 4 mg/kg is given. No more than 150 mg total dose is recommended. To avoid distress to patient, administer only after unconsciousness has been induced.

NURSING IMPLICATIONS

HISTORY

Alert anesthesiologist to current drug therapy and history of allergies; history (family, patient) of malignant hyperthermia. Notification may be made by attaching note to cover of chart prior to transporting patient to surgery.

ADMINISTRATION

Drug is administered by anesthesia department.

ONGOING ASSESSMENTS AND NURSING MANAGEMENT

CLINICAL ALERT: Patient must not be left unattended until recovered fully from anesthesia. This includes a partially awake patient with adequate respiratory exchange, movement in the extremities, return of swallowing and gag reflexes, and adequate circulation (arterial blood pressure returns to preanesthetic level).

Postanesthesia: Monitor blood pressure, pulse, and respirations q15m (or as ordered) until full recovery from anesthesia.

Maintain patent airway until patient is able to swallow or speak or until gag reflex returns.

Check for movement in the extremities, chest muscles (on inspiration and expiration), jaw and neck muscles, swallowing and gag reflexes.

Notify anesthesia department immediately if any of the following occurs: profound and prolonged muscle paralysis, respiratory depression, apnea, bronchospasm, change in heart rate or rhythm, hyperthermia, change in blood pressure, eye pain.

Additional nursing management is based on individual factors, such as type of surgery, condition of patient, complications during surgery (*e.g.,* prolonged procedure, hemorrhage, episodes of hypotension, development of a cardiac arrhythmia), additional medical problems present prior to surgery (*e.g.,* diabetes mellitus, COPD), and patient's age.

Neonates whose mothers received succinylcholine should be observed for evidence of apnea and muscle flaccidity. If these are noted, notify physician immediately.

Sucralfate Rx

tablets: 1 g   Carafate

INDICATIONS
Short-term treatment of duodenal ulcer.

CONTRAINDICATIONS
None known.

ACTIONS
Sucralfate is only minimally absorbed from the GI tract. The small amounts that are absorbed are excreted primarily in urine. Although the mechanism of the drug's ability to accelerate healing of duodenal ulcers remains to be fully defined, it is known that it exerts its effect through a local, rather than systemic, action. Studies have shown that sucralfate forms an ulcer-adherent complex with proteinaceous exudate at the ulcer site. In doses recommended for ulcer therapy, it inhibits pepsin activity in gastric juice by 32%. It is suggested that sucralfate's anti-ulcer activity is the result of formation of an ulcer-adherent complex that covers the ulcer and protects it against further attack by acid, pepsin, and bile salts. Sucralfate has negligible acid-neutralizing capacity, and its anti-ulcer activity cannot be attributed to neutralization of gastric acid.

WARNINGS
There are no adequate and well-controlled studies in pregnant women; this drug should be used during pregnancy only if clearly needed. It is not known whether this drug is excreted in human milk. Caution should be exercised when administering to a nursing woman. Safety and efficacy for use in children are not established.

PRECAUTIONS
Duodenal ulcer is a chronic disease. Although short-term sucralfate treatment can result in complete healing, a successful course of treatment should not be expected to alter the post-healing frequency or severity of duodenal ulceration.

DRUG INTERACTIONS
Because sucralfate is an aluminum salt of a sulfated disaccharide, it may prevent absorption of **tetracycline.**

ADVERSE REACTIONS
Constipation is the most frequent complaint (2.2%). Other adverse effects are diarrhea, nausea, gastric discomfort, indigestion, dry mouth, rash, pruritus, back pain, dizziness, sleepiness, and vertigo.

DOSAGE
1 g qid on an empty stomach 1 hour before each meal and H.S. Antacids may be prescribed as needed for relief of pain but should not be taken within ½ hour before or after sucralfate.

NURSING IMPLICATIONS

HISTORY
See Appendix 4.

ADMINISTRATION
See *Dosage.* If an H.S. feeding is part of the dietary management, the drug must be administered ½ hour before eating.

If patient has an antacid at the bedside to be taken at regular intervals or prn, instruct patient to wait ½ hour after medication is administered before taking the antacid.

ONGOING ASSESSMENTS AND NURSING MANAGEMENT
Obtain vital signs daily or as ordered.

Assess daily for reduction of signs and symptoms and compare with data base. Notify physician if pain becomes more severe or GI bleeding is noted.

Constipation may occur. Keep a record of daily bowel movements; notify physician if constipation occurs. A stool softener or other methods of relieving constipation may be necessary.

Adverse reactions are usually mild and rarely require discontinuation of therapy.

PATIENT AND FAMILY INFORMATION
Drug must be taken on an empty stomach 1 hour before each meal and at bedtime.

S

If antacids are being taken, do not take the antacid within ½ hour before or after taking sucralfate.

Notify physician or nurse if any of the following occurs: increase in the severity of symptoms of the ulcer, constipation, diarrhea, nausea, or any other GI symptoms. Do not self-medicate for constipation unless use of a specific drug is approved by the physician.

Sulfacytine

See Sulfonamides.

Sulfadiazine

See Sulfonamides.

Sulfadoxine and Pyrimethamine Rx

tablets: 500 mg sulfa-   Fansidar
doxine, 25 mg py-
rimethamine

INDICATIONS

Treatment of malaria due to susceptible strains of plasmodia that are resistant to chloroquine. Susceptibility of plasmodia may vary by locations and time. For prophylaxis using a weekly or biweekly regimen. Sulfadoxine and pyrimethamine are compatible with other antimalarial drugs, particularly quinine, and with antibiotics. They do not interfere with antidiabetic agents.

CONTRAINDICATIONS

Hypersensitivity to pyrimethamine or sulfonamides; patients with documented megaloblastic anemia due to folate deficiency; infants less than 2 months of age.

Use in pregnancy: Pregnancy at term and during the nursing period because sulfonamides pass the placenta and are excreted in the milk and may cause kernicterus.

ACTIONS

An antimalarial agent that acts by reciprocal potentiation of its two components, achieved by a sequential blockade of two enzymes involved in the biosynthesis of folinic acid within the parasites. Both sulfadoxine and pyrimethamine are absorbed orally and excreted mainly by the kidney. Peak plasma concentrations of sulfadoxine are achieved in 2.5 to 6 hours and pyrimethamine peak plasma concentrations are achieved in 1.5 to 8 hours.

WARNINGS

Hematologic effects: Deaths associated with administration of sulfonamides have been reported from hypersensitivity reactions, agranulocytosis, aplastic anemia, and other blood dyscrasias. Drug is discontinued if a significant reduction in the count of any formed blood element is noted or at the occurrence of active bacterial or fungal infections. The prophylactic regimen has been reported to cause leukopenia during treatment of 2 months or longer. This leukopenia is generally mild and reversible.

Use in pregnancy, lactation: There are no adequate well-controlled studies in pregnant women. Because both drugs may interfere with folic acid metabolism, they are used during pregnancy only if the potential benefit justifies the potential risk to the fetus. Both drugs appear in the breast milk of nursing mothers.

Use in children: Do not give to infants under 2 months of age because of inadequate development of the glucuronide-forming enzyme system.

PRECAUTIONS

Administer with caution to those with impaired renal or hepatic function, to those with possible folate deficiency, and to those with severe allergy or bronchial asthma. As with some sulfonamide drugs, hemolysis may occur in G6PD-deficient individuals. If signs of folic acid deficiency develop, drug is discontinued. Folinic acid (leucovorin) may be given in doses of 3 mg to 9 mg IM daily, for 3 days or longer, for depressed platelet or white blood cell counts in those with drug-induced folic acid deficiency when recovery is slow.

DRUG INTERACTIONS

Antifolic drugs such as **sulfonamides** or **trimethoprim-sulfamethoxazole combinations** should not be used while patient is receiving this drug for antimalarial purposes.

ADVERSE REACTIONS

All major reactions to sulfonamides and pyrimethamine are included below, even though they may not have been reported with this combination.

Hematologic: Agranulocytosis, aplastic anemia, megaloblastic anemia, thrombopenia, leukopenia, hemolytic anemia, purpura, hypoprothrombinemia, methemoglobinemia.

Hypersensitivity: Erythema multiforme, Stevens-Johnson syndrome, generalized skin eruptions, epidermal necrolysis, urticaria, serum sickness, pruritus, exfoliative dermatitis, anaphylactoid reactions, periorbital edema, conjunctival and scleral injection, photosensitization, arthralgia, allergic myocarditis.

GI: Glossitis, stomatitis, nausea, emesis, abdominal pains, hepatitis, diarrhea, pancreatitis.

CNS: Headache, peripheral neuritis, mental depression, convulsions, ataxia, hallucinations, tinnitus, vertigo, insomnia, apathy, fatigue, muscle weakness, nervousness.

Miscellaneous: Drug fever, chills, toxic nephrosis with oliguria and anuria. Periarteritis nodosa and LE phenomena have occurred.

The sulfonamides bear certain chemical similarities to some goitrogens, diuretics (acetazolamide, the thiazides), and oral hypoglycemic agents. Diuresis and hypoglycemia have occurred rarely in those receiving sulfonamides. Cross-sensitivity may exist with these agents.

OVERDOSAGE

Symptoms: Acute intoxication may be manifested by anorexia, vomiting, and CNS stimulation (including convulsions), followed by megaloblastic anemia, leukopenia, thrombocytopenia, glossitis, and crystalluria.

Treatment: In acute intoxication, emesis and gastric lavage followed by purges may be of benefit. Adequately hydrate the patient to prevent renal damage. Monitor renal and hematopoietic systems for at least 1 month after an overdosage. If patient is having convulsions, use of a parenteral barbiturate is indicated. For depressed platelet or white blood cell count, give folinic acid (leucovorin) in a dosage of 3 mg to 9 mg IM daily for 3 days or longer.

DOSAGE

Acute attack: Administer with a single dose, either alone or in sequence with quinine or primaquine. *Adults*—2 to 3 tablets. *Children*—9–14 yr, 2 tablets; 4–8 yr, 1 tablet; under 4 yr, ½ tablet.

Prophylaxis: This combination may be used alone either once a week or once every 2 weeks, according to the dosage schedule in Table 46. Take the first dose 1 or 2 days before departure to an endemic area; continue drug during the stay and for 4

Table 46. Recommended Weekly and Biweekly Dosage Schedules for Malaria Prophylaxis With Sulfadoxine and Pyrimethamine

Age of Patient	Weekly Dose (tablets)	Biweekly Dose (tablets)
Adult	1	2
Child		
9–14 years	¾	1½
4–8 years	½	1
<4 years	¼	½

to 6 weeks after return; follow with a regimen of primaquine.

Acute attacks of malaria due to **Plasmodium vivax** *and* **P. malaria:** A single dose, followed by primaquine for 2 weeks to prevent relapse.

NURSING IMPLICATIONS

HISTORY
See Appendix 4.

PHYSICAL ASSESSMENT
Obtain vital signs. Baseline laboratory tests may include urinalysis, CBC and differential, and renal-function tests.

ADMINISTRATION
Tablets are scored.
Give with a full glass of water.

ONGOING ASSESSMENTS AND NURSING MANAGEMENT
Acute attack: Obtain vital signs q4h or as ordered.

Encourage high fluid intake (2000 ml or more a day) to prevent crystalluria and stone formation. Measure intake and output. If patient fails to take 2000 ml or more the day of medication, inform physician. Extra fluid intake should continue for 2 to 3 days after taking the single dose.

Observe for adverse effects. Withhold next dose and notify physician if rash or other skin manifestations, nausea, vomiting, or other adverse reactions occur.

Prolonged prophylaxis: Periodic blood counts and analysis of urine for crystalluria are recommended.

Patients with impaired renal function: Urinalysis with microscopic examination and renal-function tests are recommended during therapy.

PATIENT AND FAMILY INFORMATION
Take the prescribed number of tablets on same day of the week each time. Begin therapy as directed on the prescription container (*e.g.,* 1 or 2 days before departure). Continue taking medication during the stay, and continue taking the drug for 4 to 6 weeks after return.

Maintain adequate fluid intake to prevent crystalluria and stone formation. Drink 8 to 10 large (8 oz) glasses of fluid each day.

Notify physician or nurse if any of the following occurs: sore throat, fever, pallor, purple skin discolorations, yellowing of skin or sclera, tongue inflammation.

S

Contraceptive measures are recommended to avoid pregnancy during therapy.

Avoid breast-feeding while taking this drug.

Sulfamethizole

See Sulfonamides.

Sulfamethoxazole

See Sulfonamides.

Sulfapyridine

See Sulfonamides.

Sulfasalazine

See Sulfonamides.

Sulfinpyrazone Rx

tablets: 100 mg   Anturane
capsules: 200 mg   Anturane

INDICATIONS

Treatment of chronic gouty arthritis and intermittent gouty arthritis. Because of its potency, it is often effective in those refractory to other uricosuric agents. May be used with caution in patients who have diminished renal function, whether secondary to gout or from coexisting renal disease.

Investigational uses: Current data suggest that antiplatelet drug therapy may decrease the incidence of sudden death during the first year after a myocardial infarction. Sulfinpyrazone, a reversible inhibitor of platelet prostaglandin synthetase, impairs platelet release, reduces platelet aggregation, and increases platelet survival time at doses of 600 mg/day to 800 mg/day.

CONTRAINDICATIONS

Active peptic ulcer or symptoms of GI inflammation or ulceration; when there is history or presence of hypersensitivity to phenylbutazone or other pyrazoles; and in blood dyscrasias.

ACTIONS

Sulfinpyrazone, a pyrazoline derivative, is a potent uricosuric agent that also has antithrombotic and platelet inhibitory effects. Anti-inflammatory and analgesic activity are minimal.

Sulfinpyrazone inhibits tubular reabsorption of uric acid. It reduces renal tubular secretion of other organic anions (PAH, salicylic acid) and displaces other organic anions bound extensively to plasma proteins (sulfonamides, salicylates). It has been shown to inhibit competitively prostaglandin synthesis, which prevents platelet aggregation.

Drug is well absorbed after administration with 98% to 99% bound to plasma proteins. In most patients, it rapidly reduces the serum uric acid levels to normal, usually below 6 mg/dl. This not only prevents the formation of new tophaceous deposits, but also mobilizes and promotes excretion of uric acid already present in tissues. The reduction of tophi and periarticular crystals results in greater mobility of joints, aiding in patient rehabilitation. It has minimal anti-inflammatory effects and is not intended for relief of an acute attack of gout. By controlling the serum urate level, sulfinpyrazone materially reduces or eliminates the number and severity of acute attacks in both chronic tophaceous and acute intermittent gout.

WARNINGS

There have been no reported cases of human congenital malformation due to use of the drug. Sulfinpyrazone is used during pregnancy only when clearly needed and when potential benefits outweigh the unknown potential hazards to the fetus.

PRECAUTIONS

Patient should be kept under close medical supervision; periodic blood counts are recommended. It may be given with care to patients with a history of healed peptic ulcer. Because of its potent uricosuric effect, sulfinpyrazone may precipitate acute gouty arthritis, urolithiasis, and renal colic, especially in the initial stages of therapy. Adequate fluid intake and alkalinization of the urine are recommended. In cases of significant renal impairment, periodic assessment of renal function is indicated. Occasional cases of renal failure have been reported, but a cause-and-effect relationship has not always been clearly established.

DRUG INTERACTIONS

Salicylates antagonize the action of sulfinpyrazone and are contraindicated. Sulfinpyrazone potentiates the action of certain **sulfonamides,** such as sulfadiazine and sulfisoxazole. In addition, other pyrazoline compounds (phenylbutazone) have been observed to potentiate the **hypoglycemic sulfonylurea agents,** as well as **insulin.** Use with caution in conjunction with sulfa drugs, the sulfonylurea hypoglycemic agents, and insulin.

Sulfinpyrazone may accentuate the action of **cou-**

marin-type anticoagulants by displacement of the coumarins from the albumin-binding sites. As a result, prothrombin activity is further depressed when these drugs are given concurrently.

ADVERSE REACTIONS

Most frequent: Upper GI disturbances. It is advisable to administer drug with food, milk, or antacids; despite this precaution, drug may aggravate or reactivate peptic ulcer.

Less frequent: Rash has been reported, but in most instances, this reaction did not necessitate discontinuance of therapy. In general drug has not been observed to affect electrolyte balance. Blood dyscrasias (anemia, leukopenia, agranulocytosis, thrombocytopenia, aplastic anemia) have been reported. A few instances of bronchoconstriction in those with aspirin-induced asthma have been reported. Reversible renal dysfunction has been reported following administration of this drug.

OVERDOSAGE

Symptoms: Nausea, vomiting, diarrhea, epigastric pain, ataxia, labored respiration, convulsions, coma. Possible symptoms, seen after overdosage with other pyrazoline derivatives: anemia, jaundice, and ulceration.

Treatment: No specific antidote. Induce emesis, gastric lavage, and supportive treatment (IV glucose infusions, analeptics).

DOSAGE

Initial: 200 mg/day to 400 mg/day in two divided doses, with meals or milk, gradually increasing when necessary to full maintenance dosage in 1 week.

Maintenance: 400 mg/day in two divided doses; may be increased to 800 mg/day or reduced to as low as 200 mg/day after blood urate level is controlled. Treatment should be continued without interruption, even in the presence of acute exacerbations, which can be concomitantly treated with phenylbutazone or colchicine. Patients previously controlled with other uricosuric therapy may be transferred to sulfinpyrazone at full maintenance dosage.

NURSING IMPLICATIONS

HISTORY
See Appendix 4.

PHYSICAL ASSESSMENT
Obtain vital signs; examine involved joints for swelling and tophaceous deposits (tophi); note mobility of involved joints. Baseline laboratory studies may include serum uric acid, CBC, urinalysis.

ADMINISTRATION
Administer with food, milk, or (if ordered) an antacid to prevent GI distress.

ONGOING ASSESSMENTS AND NURSING MANAGEMENT
An adequate daily fluid intake (2000–3000 ml) is necessary to prevent urolithiasis and renal colic. If there is a question about patient compliance with increasing the fluid intake, measure intake and output. Urinary output should be approximately 2000 ml/day.

Alkalinization of the urine is recommended to prevent urolithiasis and renal colic. Physician may order sodium bicarbonate or potassium citrate and sodium citrate. Check urine pH with nitrazine paper daily or as ordered. Notify physician if urine is acidic.

CLINICAL ALERT: Because of its potent uricosuric effect, drug may precipitate an attack of acute gouty arthritis, urolithiasis, and renal colic, especially early in therapy. Observe for fever; acute joint pain; hot, inflamed, tender joints; back or flank pain; difficulty in urinating. Notify physician immediately if any of these should occur.

Colchicine may be prescribed concurrently to prevent attacks of acute gouty arthritis.

Drug therapy usually produces a reduction of tophi and periarticular crystals, which in turn results in greater joint mobility. Assess patient daily for improvement in joint mobility and compare to data base.

If GI distress occurs despite giving with food, milk, or antacid, inform physician.

Dosage is adjusted according to serum uric acid levels.

Periodic blood counts are recommended during therapy.

Patients taking oral sulfonylureas, insulin, or oral anticoagulants: Dosage adjustment of these drugs may be required during therapy with sulfinpyrazone.

PATIENT AND FAMILY INFORMATION
Take exactly as prescribed. Do not increase or decrease the dose except when recommended by the physician.

May cause GI upset; take with food, milk, or (if recommended by physician) antacids.

The use of aspirin and other products containing salicylates must be avoided because salicylates may antagonize the action of this drug. If

S

there is a question about the ingredients in a nonprescription drug, always consult a pharmacist before purchase.

Drink at least 10 to 12 glasses (8 oz each) of fluid each day.

Do not use vitamin C preparations because large doses may acidify the urine and increase the possibility of kidney stone formation. If any vitamin therapy (including multivitamin preparations) is desirable, consult the physician about dose and product.

Notify physician or nurse if GI distress persists despite taking drug with food or milk; rash or other skin manifestations are noted; easy bruising or bleeding, fever, sore throat, or extreme fatigue occurs.

If an acute attack of gout occurs, continue taking the medication and contact the physician, because additional medication may be required.

Sulfisoxazole

See Sulfonamides; Sulfonamides, Ophthalmic.

Sulfonamides*

Sulfacytine Rx

tablets: 250 mg	Renoquid

Sulfadiazine Rx

tablets: 500 mg	Microsulfon, *Generic*

Sulfamethizole Rx

tablets: 250 mg	Thiosulfil
tablets: 500 mg	Microsul, Proklar, Thiosulfil Forte, Urifon
tablets: 1 g	Microsul

Sulfamethoxazole Rx

tablets: 500 mg	Gantanol, Urobak, *Generic*
tablets: 1 g	Gantanol DS, *Generic*
oral suspension: 500 mg/5 ml	Gantanol

Sulfapyridine Rx

tablets: 500 mg	*Generic*

* Ophthalmic sulfonamides are discussed in the following monograph.

Sulfasalazine Rx

tablets: 500 mg	Azulfidine, S.A.S.-500, Sulfadyne, *Generic*
tablets: enteric coated: 500 mg	Azulfidine EN-tabs
oral suspension: 250 mg/5 ml	Azulfidine

Sulfisoxazole Rx

tablets: 500 mg	Gantrisin, SK-Soxazole, Sulfizin, *Generic*
syrup: 500 mg/5 ml	Gantrisin
pediatric suspension: 500 mg/5 ml	Gantrisin
emulsion, long acting: 1 g/5 ml	Lipo Gantrisin
injection: 400 mg/ml	Gantrisin

Multiple Sulfonamide Preparations Rx

tablets and suspension: 167 mg sulfadiazine, 167 mg sulfamerazine, 167 mg sulfamethazine/tablet or 5 ml	Neotrizine, Sulfaloid (contains tartrazine), Terfonyl, Triple Sulfa
tablets: 162 mg sulfadiazine, 162 mg sulfamerazine, 162 mg sulfamethazine/tablet	Sul-Trio MM #2, Triple Sulfa No. 2

INDICATIONS

Urinary-tract infections when caused by *Escherichia coli, Staphylococcus aureus, Klebsiella-Enterobacter, Proteus mirabilis, P. vulgaris* (**sulfacytine, sulfadiazine, sulfamethizole, sulfamethoxazole, sulfisoxazole, multiple sulfonamides**).

Chancroid, inclusion conjunctivitis, trachoma, nocardiosis, toxoplasmosis (with pyrimethamine), malaria (as adjunctive therapy due to chloroquine-resistant strains of *Plasmodium falciparum*), acute otitis media (due to *Haemophilus influenzae* when used with penicillin or erythromycin) (**sulfadiazine, sulfamethoxazole, sulfisoxazole, multiple sulfonamides**).

H. influenzae meningitis (with streptomycin) (**sulfadiazine, sulfisoxazole, multiple sulfonamides**).

Meningococcal meningitis (when the organism is susceptible and for prophylaxis when sulfonamide-sensitive group A strains are known to prevail) (**sulfadiazine, sulfamethoxazole, sulfisoxazole, multiple sulfonamides**).

Rheumatic fever (**sulfadiazine**).

Ulcerative colitis (**sulfasalazine**).
Dermatitis herpetiformis (**sulfapyridine**).

CONTRAINDICATIONS

Hypersensitivity to sulfonamides or chemically related drugs (*i.e.,* sulfonylureas and thiazides). **Sulfasalazine** also is contraindicated in those sensitive to salicylates. In pregnancy at term and in lactation, because sulfonamides compete with bilirubin for binding sites on plasma proteins, cross the placenta, are excreted in breast milk, and may cause kernicterus. Also contraindicated in infants under 2 months of age (except in treatment of congenital toxoplasmosis as adjunctive therapy with pyrimethamine). **Sulfasalazine** is contraindicated in infants under 2 years of age. Sulfonamides are contraindicated in those with porphyria because these drugs have been reported to precipitate an acute attack. **Sulfasalazine** is contraindicated in intestinal and urinary obstruction.

ACTIONS

The mechanism of sulfonamide bacteriostatic action is competitive antagonism of para-aminobenzoic acid (PABA), an essential component in folic acid synthesis. Microorganisms that require exogenous folic acid and do not synthesize folic acid are not susceptible to the action of sulfonamides.

Sulfonamides have a broad antibacterial spectrum that includes both gram-positive and gram-negative organisms. Resistance develops in organisms that produce excessive amounts of PABA; resistance may also be due to destruction of the sulfonamide molecule. The increasing frequency of resistant organisms is a limitation to the usefulness of these drugs, especially in treatment of chronic and recurrent urinary-tract infections. Once resistance develops, cross-resistance between sulfonamides is common. Resistance is minimized by initiating treatment promptly with adequate doses, with treatment continued for a sufficient period. Sensitivity tests are not always reliable, and sensitivity tests are coordinated with bacteriologic and clinical response. When patient is taking sulfonamides, follow-up cultures should have aminobenzoic acid added to the culture media.

The systemic sulfonamides are readily absorbed from the GI tract; food may delay absorption but should not significantly affect the total amount of drug absorbed. These agents are widely distributed into body fluids, including cerebrospinal fluid, pleura, synovial fluids, the eye, placenta, and the fetus. Sulfonamides are bound to plasma proteins in varying degrees. The duration of antibacterial activity depends on the rate of metabolism and renal excretion. Metabolism occurs in the liver; renal excretion is mainly by glomerular filtration, with tubular absorption occurring in varying degrees. Urinary solubility of these compounds is *p*H dependent. To prevent the possibility of crystalluria, alkalinization of the urine by concomitant administration of bicarbonate is recommended when using the less soluble sulfonamides (*e.g.,* **sulfadiazine** and **sulfapyridine**).

WARNINGS

Do not use for treatment of group A beta-hemolytic streptococcal infections. In an established infection, they will not eradicate the streptococcus and will not prevent sequelae, such as rheumatic fever and glomerulonephritis.

Administration of sulfonamides has been associated with deaths from hypersensitivity reactions, agranulocytosis, aplastic anemia, other blood dyscrasias, and renal and hepatic damage. Administration has also been associated with irreversible neuromuscular and CNS changes and fibrosing alveolitis. Occasional severe systemic reactions may follow rapid IV administration. The presence of clinical signs such as sore throat, fever, pallor, purpura, and jaundice may be early signs of serious blood disorders.

Use with caution in impaired renal or hepatic function. The frequency of renal complications is considerably lower in those receiving the more soluble sulfonamides (**sulfisoxazole** and **sulfamethizole**).

Photosensitization (photoallergy and/or phototoxicity) may occur, and protective measures should be taken to avoid exposure to sunlight and ultraviolet light.

Safety for use in pregnancy is not established. **Sulfacytine** is not recommended for use in children under age 14. At present there are insufficient clinical data on prolonged or recurrent therapy with **sulfamethoxazole** in chronic renal diseases in children under 6 years.

PRECAUTIONS

Oligospermia and infertility have been described in men treated with **sulfasalazine;** withdrawal of the drug appears to reverse these effects. Sulfonamides are given with caution to those with severe allergy or bronchial asthma. Hemolytic anemia, frequently dose related, may occur in G6PD-deficient individuals.

Sulfasalazine enteric-coated tablets have passed undisintegrated in isolated instances. This may be because of lack of intestinal esterases in some patients. If this occurs, drug is discontinued.

Some of these products contain tartrazine. See Appendix 6, section 6-23.

S

DRUG INTERACTIONS

The sulfonamides may displace or be displaced by other highly protein-bound drugs. Such interactions may occur with **tolbutamide, methotrexate, warfarin, phenylbutazone, salicylates, probenecid,** and **phenytoin.** The clinical significance of such interactions is not well documented. It is possible that an increase in serum levels due to displacement will be compensated for by an increase in clearance. Monitor patients for increased effects of highly bound drugs when sulfonamides are added to therapy.

The bioavailability of **digoxin** appears to be decreased during concomitant administration of sulfasalazine; therefore, patient is monitored for an altered digoxin effect. Sulfonamides also compete with **tolbutamide** and **methotrexate** for renal tubular excretion. Sulfamethizole inhibits hepatic biotransformation of **tolbutamide, chlorpropamide,** and **phenytoin,** extending the half-life and increasing the potential for hypoglycemia and phenytoin toxicity.

Antibiotics that decrease intestinal flora alter distribution of sulfasalazine and its possibly active metabolites. The clinical implications are undetermined. Concomitant administration of **ferrous sulfate** and sulfasalazine results in decreased blood level of sulfasalazine. **Folic acid** absorption is inhibited and pharmacologic effects may be decreased by sulfasalazine.

PABA, and possibly **local anesthetics** that are PABA derivatives, may antagonize the effect of sulfonamides. Concomitant administration of the less soluble sulfonamides with **methenamine** is avoided because crystalluria may result.

Drug/lab tests: Sulfonamides frequently produce false-positive **urinary glucose tests** when Benedict's solution is used. Sulfisoxazole may interfere with the **Urobilistix test** and may produce false-positive results with sulfosalicylic acid tests for urinary protein.

ADVERSE REACTIONS

Hematologic: Agranulocytosis, aplastic anemia, thrombocytopenia, leukopenia, hemolytic anemia, purpura, hypoprothrombinemia, cyanosis, methemoglobinemia, megaloblastic anemia, Heinz body anemia, petechiae.

Hypersensitivity: Erythema multiforme (Stevens-Johnson syndrome); parapsoriasis varioliformis acuta (Mucha-Habermann syndrome); generalized skin eruptions; epidermal necrolysis with or without corneal damage; urticaria; serum sickness; pruritus; exfoliative dermatitis; anaphylactoid reactions; periorbital edema; conjunctival and scleral injection; photosensitization; arthralgia; allergic myocarditis; transient pulmonary changes with eosinophilia, decreased pulmonary function, and eosinophilic pneumonia.

GI: Nausea, emesis, abdominal pains, diarrhea, bloody diarrhea, anorexia, pancreatitis, stomatitis, impaired folic acid absorption.

Hepatic: Hepatitis.

CNS: Headache, peripheral neuritis, peripheral neuropathy, mental depression, convulsions, ataxia, hallucinations, tinnitus, vertigo, insomnia, hearing loss, drowsiness, transient lesions of posterior spinal column, transverse myelitis.

Renal: Crystalluria, hematuria, proteinuria, nephrotic syndrome, toxic nephrosis with oliguria and anuria.

Miscellaneous: Drug fever, chills, alopecia, oligospermia, infertility, periarteritis nodosum, LE phenomenon. Local reaction may occur with IM injection. The sulfonamides bear chemical similarities to some goitrogens, diuretics (acetazolamide and the thiazides), oral hypoglycemic agents, and probenecid. Goiter production, diuresis, and hypoglycemia have occurred rarely in those receiving sulfonamides. Cross-sensitivity may exist with these agents. **Sulfasalazine** produces an orange-yellow urine when the urine is alkaline. Similar skin discoloration has also been reported.

OVERDOSAGE

Therapeutic doses of 2 g/day to 5 g/day may produce toxicity or fatalities. The aniline radical is largely responsible for the effects on the blood or hematopoietic system.

Symptoms: Within 1 to 2 days after discontinuation of the drug, the less serious symptoms disappear; grave symptoms require 1 to 3 weeks for remission.

GI: Anorexia, colic, nausea, vomiting.

CNS: Dizziness, headache, drowsiness, unconsciousness.

Toxic fever: Precedes serious manifestations and may develop 1 or more days after the fever due to infection has subsided.

Serious manifestations: Acidosis, acute hemolytic anemia, agranulocytosis, sensitivity reactions, dermatitis (maculopapular), toxic neuritis, hepatic jaundice, death (occurring several days after first dose).

Treatment: Discontinue drug immediately. Administer an emetic or perform gastric lavage if large doses are ingested. Alkalinize the urine with sodium lactate or sodium bicarbonate to enhance solubility and excretion. Force fluids if kidney function is normal, up to 4 liters/day to increase excretion. If anuria is present, restrict fluids and salt and treat for renal failure. Catheterization of the ureters may be indicated for complete blockage by crystals. For agranulocytosis, give antibiotic therapy to combat infection; for severe anemia or thrombocytopenia, give blood or platelet transfusions. Urticaria, other skin rashes, and serum sickness–like reactions may be controlled with antihistamines and, if necessary, systemic corticosteroids.

DOSAGE

SULFACYTINE

Give a loading dose of 500 mg. Maintenance dose is 250 mg qid for 10 days. Not recommended for children under 14 years.

SULFADIAZINE

Adults: Give a loading dose of 2 g to 4 g; maintenance dose is 2 g/day to 4 g/day in three to six divided doses.

Children over 2 months: Give a loading dose of 75 mg/kg; maintenance dose is 150 mg/kg/day in four to six divided doses. Do not exceed a maximum dose of 6 g/day.

Prevention of recurrent attacks of rheumatic fever (not recommended for initial treatment of streptococcal infections): _Patients over 30 kg_—1 g/day. _Patients under 30 kg_—0.5 g/day.

SULFAMETHIZOLE

Adults: 0.5 g to 1 g three or four times a day.

Children and infants over 2 months: 30 mg/kg/day to 45 mg/kg/day in four divided doses.

SULFAMETHOXAZOLE

Adults: _Mild to moderate infections_—2 g initially; maintenance dose is 1 g morning and evening thereafter. _Severe infections_—2 g initially, then 1 g tid.

Children or infants over 2 months: 50 mg/kg to 60 mg/kg initially; maintenance dose is 25 mg/kg to 30 mg/kg morning and evening. Do not exceed 75 mg/kg/day.

SULFAPYRIDINE

500 mg qid until improvement is noted; then reduce by 500 mg/day at 3-day intervals until symptom-free maintenance is achieved. Maintenance dose should not exceed the minimum effective dose. Increased dosage may be required with recurrences.

SULFASALAZINE

About one-third of an oral dose is absorbed from the small intestine. The remaining two-thirds passes to the colon, where it is split into 5-aminosalicylic acid and sulfapyridine. Most of the sulfapyridine is absorbed, whereas only about one-third of the 5-aminosalicylic acid is absorbed, the remainder being excreted in the feces. Dosage is adjusted to patient response and tolerance. Drug is given in divided doses over each 24-hour period; intervals between nighttime doses should not exceed 8 hours. Give after meals when feasible. Four grams or more per day tends to increase adverse reactions. It is often necessary to continue medication even when clinical symptoms, including diarrhea, have been controlled. When endoscopic examination confirms satisfactory improvement, dosage is reduced to maintenance level. If diarrhea recurs, dosage is increased to previously effective levels.

Symptoms of gastric intolerance (_e.g.,_ anorexia, nausea, vomiting) after the first few doses are probably due to mucosal irritation and may be relieved by distributing the total daily dose more evenly or by giving enteric-coated tablets. If such symptoms occur after the first few days of treatment, they are probably due to increased serum levels of total sulfapyridine and may be alleviated by halving the dose and subsequently increasing it gradually over several days. If symptoms continue, drug is stopped for 5 to 7 days and then reinstituted at a lower daily dose.

Initial therapy: _Adults_—3 g/day to 4 g/day in evenly divided doses. Initial doses of 1 g/day to 2 g/day may lessen GI side-effects. If doses up to 8 g/day are required, the risk of toxicity increases. _Children_—40 mg/kg/24 hours to 60 mg/kg/24 hours in three to six divided doses.

Maintenance therapy: _Adults_—2 g/day (500 mg qid). _Children_—30 mg/kg/24 hours in four divided doses.

SULFISOXAZOLE

Oral: Give a loading dose of 2 g to 4 g; maintenance dose is 4 g to 8 g/day in four to six divided doses. _Children and infants over 2 months_—Initial dose is 75 mg/kg. Maintenance dose is 150 mg/kg/day in four to six divided doses with a maximum of 6 g/day.

Parenteral: Use only when oral administration is impractical. Initially, give 50 mg/kg; maintenance dose is 100 mg/kg/day in a 5% solution. _Subcutaneous_—Divide into three doses a day. _IV_—Divide into four doses a day. Give by slow injection or IV drip. _IM_—Divide into two or three doses a day. Up to 10 ml can be given, but no more than 5 ml in any one site. For children, the volume given IM in any one site should be less than in adults.

MULTIPLE SULFONAMIDES

Use of multiple sulfonamides provides a therapeutic effect of the total sulfonamide content but reduces

S

the chance of precipitation in the kidneys, because solubility of each sulfonamide is independent of the presence of others.

Adults: 2 g to 4 g initially, then 2 g/day to 4 g/day in three to six divided doses.

Children or infants over 2 months: 75 mg/kg initially, then 150 mg/kg/day in four to six divided doses. Do not exceed 6 g/day.

NURSING IMPLICATIONS

HISTORY
See Appendix 4.

PHYSICAL ASSESSMENT
Obtain vital signs, weight (children, infants, acutely ill patient, patient with ulcerative colitis). Baseline laboratory tests may include urinalysis, CBC, urine culture (sensitivity tests are not always reliable), microscopic examination of the urine, renal- and hepatic-function tests.

ADMINISTRATION
Give on an empty stomach at least 1 hour before or 2 hours after meals unless physician orders otherwise.

Have patient drink a full glass of water with drug.

Sulfasalazine may be given with food or immediately after meals.

SULFISOXAZOLE
IM: Up to 10 ml may be prescribed. Give in divided doses of not more than 5 ml in any one site. May be given without dilution.

IV, subcutaneous: The 40% solution must be diluted to a 5% solution by combining the 5-ml ampule with 35 ml of water for injection (the use of diluents other than water may cause precipitation).

Administration in combination with parenteral fluids is not recommended.

IV administration is by slow injection or by IV drip by means of an IV additive set. Physician orders rate of infusion.

ONGOING ASSESSMENTS AND NURSING MANAGEMENT
Monitor vital signs q4h or as ordered. If fever suddenly increases or if temperature was normal and suddenly rises, inform physician immediately as this may be a sign of sensitization.

Observe for adverse effects. If one or more adverse reactions are noted, withhold next dose and notify physician immediately.

CLINICAL ALERT: Hypersensitivity may be denoted by skin manifestations such as rash, urticaria, symmetric skin lesions that are vivid red, and pruritus. Inspect oral mucosa for oral lesions (blisters, erosions) and inspect the skin daily. If rash or other skin or oral lesions occur, notify the physician immediately. Do not administer further doses until the patient is seen by a physician.

Force fluids to 2000 ml or more per day to prevent crystalluria and stone formation. Monitor intake and output. Notify physician if urinary output decreases or patient fails to increase oral intake. Check with physician regarding oral fluids for pediatric patients.

Observe and record patient response to therapy (*e.g.,* relief of symptoms, decrease in temperature [if elevation present]).

Physician may prescribe sodium bicarbonate or other urinary alkalinizer when sulfadiazine or sulfapyridine is prescribed. Using nitrazine paper, monitor urinary pH daily or as ordered. Notify physician if urine becomes acidic.

Enteric-coated sulfasalazine tablets have been known to pass undisintegrated in the stool. Patients receiving the enteric-coated form of this drug should have their stool inspected the first several days of therapy for undisintegrated tablets. If tablets are seen, notify physician because drug should be discontinued.

Patients receiving tolbutamide or chlorpropamide (oral hypoglycemic agents) are observed for hypoglycemic reactions (Appendix 6, section 6-14). More frequent determinations of blood glucose levels may be necessary during sulfonamide therapy.

Patients receiving phenytoin are observed for toxicity. Dosage adjustment of phenytoin may be necessary.

Microscopic examination of the urine is recommended weekly when patient is treated for longer than 2 weeks, and at approximate intervals thereafter.

Periodic renal- and hepatic-function tests are recommended during long-term treatment.

If follow-up urine cultures are ordered, label laboratory slips with sulfonamide being taken because aminobenzoic acid must be added to the culture media.

PATIENT AND FAMILY INFORMATION
Take as prescribed on the prescription container. Do not lengthen time between doses unless advised to do so by the physician. Complete full course of therapy, even if symptoms are relieved.

Drink 8 to 10 or more glasses (8 oz) of fluid every day while taking this drug.

Take on an empty stomach at least 1 hour before or 2 hours after meals with a full glass of water. (*Exception*—Take **sulfasalazine** with food or immediately after meals.)

Notify physician or nurse immediately if skin rash or other skin manifestations, nausea, vomiting, easy bleeding or bruising, sore throat, extreme fatigue, chills, fever, or any other reactions occur.

Avoid prolonged exposure to sunlight or ultraviolet light; photosensitivity may occur.

SULFASALAZINE

Drug may cause an orange-yellow discoloration of the urine; this is not abnormal. Avoid drugs containing iron unless use has been approved by the physician.

SULFADIAZINE, SULFAPYRIDINE

A drug to make urine alkaline may be ordered. Avoid use of nonprescription drugs (some, such as vitamin C, may make the urine acidic) unless use of a specific product and dose are approved by the physician.

Sulfonamides, Ophthalmic

solution: 10% sodium sulfacetamide	AK-Sulf, Bleph-10 Liquifilm, Opthacet, Sodium Sulamyd 10%, Sulf-10, Sulten-10, *Generic*
solution: 15% sodium sulfacetamide	AK-Sulf, Isopto Cetamide, Sulfacel-15, *Generic*
solution: 30% sodium sulfacetamide	Ak-Sulf Forte, Sodium Sulamyd 30%, *Generic*
solution: 4% sulfisoxazole	Gantrisin
ointment: 10% sodium sulfacetamide	AK-Sulf, Cetamide, Sodium Sulamyd, *Generic*
ointment: 4% sulfisoxazole	Gantrisin

INDICATIONS

Treatment of conjunctivitis, corneal ulcer, and other superficial ocular infections due to susceptible microorganisms; adjunctive treatment in systemic sulfonamide therapy of trachoma.

CONTRAINDICATIONS

Hypersensitivity to sulfonamides or components.

ACTIONS

Exert a bacteriostatic effect against a wide range of susceptible gram-positive and gram-negative organisms. Through competition with para-aminobenzoic acid (PABA), they restrict synthesis of folic acid, which bacteria need for growth. See also Sulfonamides.

PRECAUTIONS

Solutions are incompatible with silver preparations. Ophthalmic ointments may retard corneal healing. Nonsusceptible organisms, including fungi, may proliferate with use of these preparations. Sulfonamides are inactivated by the PABA present in purulent exudates. Sensitization may recur when a sulfonamide preparation is readministered regardless of the route of administration, and cross-sensitivity between different sulfonamides may occur. If signs of sensitivity or untoward reactions occur, use discontinued.

ADVERSE REACTIONS

May cause local irritation; transient stinging or burning has been reported with 30% solution.

DOSAGE

Solutions: Instill one or two drops into conjunctival sac every 1 to 2 hours initially, increasing time interval as condition responds.

Ointments: Apply small amount in the conjunctival sac one to three times a day and H.S.

NURSING IMPLICATIONS

HISTORY

See Appendix 4.

PHYSICAL ASSESSMENT

Examine external eye structures, noting if inflammation is present. Culture and sensitivity test may be ordered.

ADMINISTRATION

Do not use if solution is discolored dark brown.

Place patient in upright position; tilt head back.

Instill in conjunctival sac.

Apply light pressure to lacrimal sac for 1 minute after instillation of drops.

ONGOING ASSESSMENTS AND NURSING MANAGEMENT

Inspect eye when applying drug. Notify physician if irritation is apparent, if condition worsens, or if no improvement is seen in 3 days.

S

NOTE: Explain proper instillation technique. If patient is a child, demonstrate safe restraining techniques.

Take care not to contaminate tip of tube or dropper.

Do not use if solution is discolored dark brown.

Apply light finger pressure to lacrimal sac for 1 minute after instillation of drops.

Transient stinging may occur for first few minutes after instillation of drops.

Ointment may produce a transient visual haze; do not attempt to drive or engage in potentially hazardous tasks while vision is impaired.

Notify physician or nurse if improvement is not seen after 3 days, if condition worsens, or if irritation occurs.

Sulfonylureas

First Generation

Acetohexamide Rx

tablets: 250 mg, 500 mg	Dymelor

Chlorpropamide Rx

tablets: 100 mg, 250 mg	Diabinese, *Generic*

Tolazamide Rx

tablets: 100 mg, 250 mg, 500 mg	Tolinase

Tolbutamide Rx

tablets: 250 mg	Orinase
tablets: 500 mg	Oramide, Orinase, SK-Tolbutamide, *Generic*

Second Generation

Glipizide Rx

tablets: 5 mg, 10 mg	Glucotrol

Glyburide Rx

tablets: 1.25 mg, 2.5 mg, 5 mg	DiaBeta (5 mg contains tartrazine), Micronase

INDICATIONS

As an adjunct to lower the blood glucose in patients with non–insulin dependent diabetes mellitus (Type II) whose hypoglycemia cannot be controlled on diet alone. Also used as an adjunct to insulin therapy in the stabilization of insulin-dependent maturity-onset diabetes, resulting in a reduction of insulin requirement and a lesser chance of hypoglycemic reactions.

Unlabeled uses: Chlorpropamide in doses of 125 mg/day to 250 mg/day has been used in the treatment of neurogenic diabetes insipidus.

CONTRAINDICATIONS

Known hypersensitivity to sulfonylureas; diabetes complicated by fever, severe infections, severe trauma or major surgery, ketosis, acidosis, or coma. Not indicated for therapy of juvenile or labile (brittle, Type I) diabetes. Contraindicated in those with serious impairment of hepatic, renal, thyroid, or endocrine function, and in those with uremia. Contraindicated in patients with hyperglycemia and glycosuria associated with primary renal disease. Also contraindicated during pregnancy. See *Warnings.*

ACTIONS

The sulfonylurea hypoglycemic agents are sulfonamide derivatives but are devoid of antibacterial effects. They appear to lower blood glucose acutely by stimulating insulin release from the pancreas, an effect dependent on functioning beta cells in the pancreatic islets. These agents will not lower blood glucose in the patient lacking functional pancreatic beta cells and are only effective in those with some capacity for endogenous insulin production. They are useful in maturity-onset diabetes with little or no tendency toward ketoacidosis. These agents may improve the binding between insulin and insulin receptors or increase the number of insulin receptors. Hypoglycemic effects seem to be due to improved beta cell sensitivity or extrahepatic effects occurring in the liver, and on insulin sensitivity of peripheral tissues. Prolonged administration lowers blood glucose, but plasma insulin levels are unchanged or tend to decline.

Although mechanisms of action are similar, the second- and first-generation sulfonylureas differ: second-generation compounds possess a more nonpolar or lipophilic side chain. Therapeutically effective doses and serum concentrations of second-generation sulfonylureas are lower owing to their higher intrinsic potency.

Other pharmacologic activity: Tolazamide, acetohexamide, glyburide, and glipizide may produce a mild diuresis; chlorpropamide can potentiate the effect of antidiuretic hormone (ADH); acetohexamide has significant uricosuric activity.

Sulfonylureas are well absorbed after oral administration. Tolazamide is absorbed more slowly than other sulfonylureas. They are metabolized in the liver to active and inactive metabolites and are excreted primarily in urine. They are bound to plasma proteins (primarily albumin). The hypoglycemic effects of sulfonylureas may be prolonged in severe liver disease. Glyburide is excreted as metabolites in the bile and urine.

Differences exist among the sulfonylureas in the duration of hypoglycemic effects as shown in Table 47. Tolbutamide is short acting and may be useful in those with kidney disease.

WARNINGS

Administration of oral hypoglycemic drugs has been associated with increased cardiovascular mortality as compared with treatment with diet alone or diet plus insulin. Patients treated for 5 to 8 years with diet plus tolbutamide (1.5 g/day) had a rate of cardiovascular mortality approximately 2½ times that of patients treated with diet alone. A significant increase in total mortality was not observed.

Although sulfonylureas given alone have controlled some patients with mild Type II diabetes during the stress of mild infection or minor surgery, insulin therapy is generally essential during intercurrent complications (_e.g.,_ ketoacidosis, severe trauma, major surgical procedures, severe infections, severe diarrhea, nausea, and vomiting). The severity of diabetes, the nature of the complication, and availability of laboratory facilities determine whether therapy can be continued or should be withheld while insulin is being used.

Use in pregnancy: Use during pregnancy only when clearly needed. In general, use of these agents should be avoided in pregnancy because they will not provide good control in patients whose diabetes cannot be controlled by diet alone. Because abnormal blood glucose levels during pregnancy may be associated with a higher incidence of congenital abnormalities, insulin is recommended during pregnancy to maintain blood glucose levels as close to normal as possible.

Use in labor: Prolonged severe hypoglycemia (4–10 days) has been reported in neonates born to mothers who were receiving a sulfonylurea at the time of delivery. This has been reported more frequently with use of agents with prolonged half-lives. If sulfonylureas are used during pregnancy, they are discontinued at least 48 hours (_glipizide_—one month) before the expected delivery date.

Use in lactation: Chlorpropamide and tolbutamide are excreted in breast milk. Data on other sulfonylureas are unknown. Because of the potential for hypoglycemia in nursing infants, a decision whether to discontinue nursing or discontinue the drug must be made.

Use in children: Safety and efficacy in children have not been established.

PRECAUTIONS

These agents are not oral insulin or a substitute for insulin. They have no blood glucose lowering effects in the absence of pancreatic beta cells and must not be used as sole therapeutic agents in Type I (juvenile type) diabetes. These agents are of no value in diabetes complicated by acidosis and coma, in which case insulin is essential.

Diet and exercise remain the primary considerations of diabetes management. Calorie restriction and weight loss are essential in the obese diabetic. These drugs are an adjunct to, not a substitute for, dietary regulation.

Tolazamide is effective in some patients with a history of ketoacidosis or coma. Such patients are observed closely, particularly during the transitional period.

Monitoring therapy: Patients are kept under continuous medical supervision. During the initial period, the patient should communicate with the physician daily and report at least weekly for the first month for physical examination and evaluation of diabetes control. After the first month, the patient

Table 47. Pharmacokinetic Parameters of the Sulfonylureas

Sulfonylurea	Equivalent Doses (mg)	Doses/Day	Serum Half-Life (hr)	Onset (hr)	Duration (hr)
First Generation					
Acetohexamide	500	1–2	6–8	1	12–24
Chlorpropamide	250	1	36	1	Up to 60
Tolazamide	250	1–2	7	4–6	10–16
Tolbutamide	1000	2–3	4–5	1	6–12
Second Generation					
Glipizide	5	1–2	2–4	1–1.5	10–24
Glyburide	5	1–2	10	2–4	24

should be examined at monthly intervals or as indicated. Uncooperative patients may be unsuitable for treatment with oral agents. When oral agents are given as sole therapy to those previously requiring combination therapy with insulin, careful patient observation is mandatory, especially during transition. If significant ketonuria develops or hyperglycemia persists, the oral agent is discontinued and insulin therapy is instituted. During the transition period, the urine is tested for glucose and acetone at least three times a day and the results reviewed by the physician at least once a week. Measurement of glycosylated hemoglobin may also be useful.

Hypoglycemia: All sulfonylureas may produce severe hypoglycemia. Proper patient selection, dosage, and instructions are important to avoid hypoglycemic episodes. Renal or hepatic insufficiency may elevate drug blood levels and the latter may also diminish gluconeogenic capacity, both of which increase the risk of serious hypoglycemic reactions. Elderly, debilitated, or malnourished patients and those with adrenal or pituitary insufficiency are particularly unsuitable to the hypoglycemic action of glucose-lowering drugs. Hypoglycemia may be difficult to recognize in the elderly and in those who are taking beta-adrenergic blocking drugs. Hypoglycemia is more likely to occur when calorie intake is deficient, after severe or prolonged exercise, when alcohol is ingested, or when more than one glucose-lowering agent is used. Because of the prolonged half-life of **chlorpropamide,** patients who become hypoglycemic during therapy may require careful supervision of the dose and frequent feedings for at least 3 to 5 days. Hospitalization and IV glucose may be necessary.

Loss of blood glucose control: When a patient stabilized on any diabetic regimen is exposed to stress such as fever, trauma, infection, or surgery, loss of diabetes control may occur. At such times it may be necessary to discontinue the drug and administer insulin. The effectiveness of any oral hypoglycemic in lowering blood glucose to a desired level decreases in many patients over time (secondary failure); this may be because of progression of the severity of diabetes or diminished drug responsiveness. Primary failure occurs when the drug is ineffective in a patient when first given. Certain patients who demonstrate an inadequate response or true primary or secondary failure to one sulfonylurea may benefit from a transfer to another sulfonylurea.

Hepatic effects: Hepatic function is monitored frequently. Toxicity manifested by alterations in hepatic-function tests and by cholestatic jaundice has occasionally been associated with therapy. Jaundice is usually reversible on discontinuance of therapy.

Transient minor alterations, particularly of cephalin flocculation, thymol turbidity, and serum alkaline phosphatase levels are not unusual and are probably of no clinical significance. A progressive rise in alkaline phosphatase indicates the possibility of incipient biliary stasis and jaundice, and therapy is discontinued promptly. These drugs may aggravate hepatic prophyria.

Tartrazine sensitivity: Some products contain tartrazine (see Appendix 6, section 6-23).

DRUG INTERACTIONS

Oral hypoglycemic agents may increase metabolism of **digitoxin** by hepatic microsomal enzyme reduction. Certain drugs may prolong or enhance the action of sulfonylureas and thereby increase the risk of hypoglycemia. These include **insulin, sulfonamides, chloramphenicol, fenfluramine, oxyphenbutazone, phenylbutazone, salicylates, nonsteroidal anti-inflammatory agents, probenecid, monoamine oxidase inhibitors, clofibrate,** and **dicumarol.**

The pharmacologic effect of sulfonylureas may be decreased by **beta-adrenergic blocking agents.** The clinical manifestations of hypoglycemia may also be blunted. When sulfonylureas are given with **diazoxide,** the pharmacologic effects of both drugs may be decreased owing to their antagonist activities. Diazoxide has been used in the treatment of chlorpropamide-induced hypoglycemia.

Certain drugs tend to produce hyperglycemia and may lead to loss of control. These drugs include the **thiazides** and **other diuretics, corticosteroids, phenothiazines, thyroid products, estrogens, oral contraceptives, phenytoin, nicotinic acid, sympathomimetics, calcium channel blockers,** and **isoniazid.**

Both hypoglycemia and hyperglycemia have occurred during combined treatment with **ethanol** and sulfonylureas. Acute alcohol intolerance ("disulfiram reaction") may also occur. Alcohol possesses intrinsic hypoglycemic activity and may augment the hypoglycemic effects of sulfonylureas. Conversely, prolonged use of large amounts of ethanol may stimulate hepatic metabolism of sulfonylureas, decreasing therapeutic effectiveness. Photosensitivity reactions after ingestion of **alcohol** have been reported occasionally in those taking **tolazamide** and **tolbutamide.**

Rifampin may stimulate the metabolism of chlorpropamide and tolbutamide by hepatic microsomal enzymes, reducing the hypoglycemic activity of the sulfonylurea.

Drug/lab tests: A metabolite of tolbutamide in the urine may give a false-positive reaction for **albumin** if measured by the acidification-after-boiling test.

ADVERSE REACTIONS

Dose-related side-effects are generally transient and not serious. These effects include anorexia, nausea, vomiting, epigastric discomfort, heartburn, and various vague neurologic symptoms, particularly weakness and paresthesias. They are reversible with reduction of daily dosage or, if necessary, by withdrawal of the medication. Drug administration in divided doses is sometimes effective in relieving symptoms of GI intolerance.

Hypoglycemia: See *Precautions.*

GI: Cholestatic jaundice (rare); drug is discontinued if this occurs. GI disturbances (*e.g.,* nausea, epigastric fullness, heartburn) are most common reactions. They tend to be dose related and may disappear when dosage is reduced. Diarrhea has been reported with glipizide.

Dermatologic: Allergic skin reactions, eczema, pruritus, erythema, urticaria, and morbilliform or maculopapular eruptions. These may be transient and may disappear despite continued use of the drug. If skin reactions persist, drug is discontinued. Porphyria cutanea tarda and photosensitivity reactions have been reported.

Hematopoietic: Leukopenia, thrombocytopenia, and mild anemia, which occur occasionally, are generally benign and revert to normal following discontinuation. Mild leukopenia, not associated with a shift in the differential count, may be transient and frequently reverts to normal even while the drug is continued. Aplastic anemia, agranulocytosis, hemolytic anemia, pancytopenia, and hepatic porphyria have been reported.

Hypersensitivity: Hematologic and allergic reactions as manifested by urticaria and rash have been reported occasionally. Some hypersensitivity side-effects may be severe; deaths have been reported. Chlorpropamide has a higher incidence of side-effects than tolbutamide.

Untoward reactions associated with idiosyncrasy or hypersensitivity, including jaundice, skin eruptions rarely progressing to erythema multiforme and exfoliative dermatitis, and probably depression of formed elements of the blood, show no direct relationship to dose size. They occur characteristically during the first 6 weeks of therapy. These manifestations are mild and readily reversible on withdrawal of the drug.

Low-grade fever and eosinophilia may also occur in association with, or preceding the development of, clinical jaundice. Rarely, severe diarrhea, sometimes accompanied by bleeding into the lower bowel and due to nonspecific proctocolitis, has been associated with other hypersensitivity manifestations, particularly jaundice, skin rash, or both. Occurrence of any of these is an indication for prompt termination of the drug. More severe manifestations may require other therapeutic measures, including corticosteroid therapy.

Miscellaneous: Weakness, fatigue, dizziness, vertigo, malaise, and headache (infrequent). Occasional mild to moderate elevations in BUN and serum creatinine. **Chlorpropamide** has caused a reaction identical to the syndrome of inappropriate antidiuretic hormone secretion (SIADH); it appears to augment the action of ADH on the renal distal tubule, resulting in excessive water retention, hyponatremia, low serum osmolality, and high urine osmolality. **Tolbutamide** is mildly goitrogenic and has caused a reduction of radioactive iodine uptake after long-term use without producing clinical hypothyroidism or thyroid enlargement.

OVERDOSAGE

Symptoms: Overdosage can produce hypoglycemia. In order of general appearance, the signs and symptoms associated with hypoglycemia include tingling of the lips and tongue, air hunger, nausea, diminished cerebral function (lethargy, yawning, confusion, agitation, nervousness), increased sympathetic activity (tachycardia, sweating, tremor), and ultimately convulsions, stupor, and coma.

Treatment: Treat mild hypoglycemia, without loss of consciousness or neurologic findings, aggressively with oral glucose and adjustments in drug dosage or meal patterns. Continue close monitoring until patient is out of danger. Severe hypoglycemic reactions occur infrequently but require immediate hospitalization. If hypoglycemic coma is suspected, rapidly inject concentrated (50%) dextrose IV. Follow by a continuous infusion of more dilute (10%) dextrose at a rate that will maintain blood glucose at a level above 100 mg/dl. Closely monitor for a minimum of 24 hours to 48 hours because hypoglycemia may recur after apparent clinical recovery. Because of the prolonged hypoglycemic action of **chlorpropamide,** patients who have become hypoglycemic from this drug require close supervision for a minimum of 3 to 5 days.

DOSAGE

Institution of therapy: There is no fixed dosage regimen and dosage is individualized.

Replacement therapy

Oral hypoglycemic agents: When transferring patient from one oral hypoglycemic agent to another, no transitional period and no initial or priming dose are necessary. When transferring patients from **chlorpropamide,** care is exercised during the first 2 weeks because the prolonged retention of chlorpropamide in the body and subsequent overlapping drug effects may provoke hypoglycemia.

S

Insulin: During insulin withdrawal period, test urine for glucose and ketones three times a day and report results to the physician daily. Table 48 may be used as a guide.

Elderly patients: May be hyperresponsive and may be started with a lower initial dose before breakfast with a check of blood and urine glucose during the first 24 hours of therapy. If control is satisfactory, the dose may be continued on a daily basis or gradually increased. If there is a tendency toward hypoglycemia, dosage is reduced or drug is discontinued.

Concomitant insulin therapy: Use of sulfonylureas as a supplement to insulin therapy in insulin-dependent diabetics with maturity-onset or growth-onset diabetes may decrease insulin requirement and provide easier regulation and stabilization of the diabetes. The daily insulin requirement may be reduced 10% to 70% in certain stable patients and 10% to 50% in certain labile patients. In insulin-resistant patients, use of the combination may be warranted in an effort to reduce insulin requirement.

Acute complications: During the course of intercurrent complications (*e.g.,* ketoacidosis, severe trauma, major surgery, infections, severe diarrhea, or nausea and vomiting), supportive therapy with insulin may be necessary. Sulfonylurea therapy may be continued or withdrawn while insulin is used. Insulin is indispensable in managing acute complications, and all diabetics should be carefully instructed in its use.

ACETOHEXAMIDE

Dosage may range between 250 mg/day and 1.5 g/day. Patients on 1 g/day or less can be controlled with once-daily dosage. Those receiving 1.5 g/day usually benefit from twice-daily dosage before morning and evening meals. Dosages in excess of 1.5 g/day are not recommended.

Table 48. Recommendations for Insulin Replacement Therapy with Sulfonylureas

Daily Insulin Requirements (units)	Recommended Replacement Therapy
≤20	Start directly on oral agent; insulin discontinued abruptly
20–40	Oral therapy initiated with concurrent 30% to 50% reduction in insulin dose; insulin dose further reduced as response is observed
>40	Oral therapy initiated with concurrent 20% reduction in insulin dose; insulin dose further reduced as response is observed

CHLORPROPAMIDE

Initial therapy: 250 mg/day in the mild to moderately severe, middle-aged, stable diabetic patient; use 100 mg to 125 mg in older patients.

Maintenance therapy: 100 mg/day to 250 mg/day. Severe diabetes may require 500 mg/day. Dosages above 750 mg/day should be avoided.

GLIPIZIDE

Give approximately 30 minutes before a meal to achieve the greatest reduction in postprandial hyperglycemia. Initial dose: 5 mg before breakfast. Geriatric patients or those with liver disease may be started on 2.5 mg. Dosage is adjusted in increments of 2.5 mg to 5 mg, as determined by blood glucose response. At least several days should elapse between titration steps. If response to a single dose is not satisfactory, dividing the dose may prove effective. The maximum recommended once-daily dose is 15 mg. Doses above 15 mg should be divided and given before meals of adequate calorie content. The maximum recommended total daily dose is 40 mg.

GLYBURIDE

Initial dose: 2.5 mg to 5 mg daily, administered with breakfast or the first main meal. For those who may be more sensitive to hypoglycemic drugs, start at 1.25 mg daily.

Maintenance dose: 1.25 mg/day to 20 mg/day. Give as a single dose or in divided doses. Increase in increments of no more than 2.5 mg at weekly intervals based on the patient's blood glucose response.

TOLAZAMIDE

Suggested initial dose is 100 mg/day if fasting blood glucose is less than 200 mg/dl, or 250 mg/day if fasting blood glucose is greater than 200 mg/dl. Dosage is adjusted to response. If more than 500 mg/day is required, give in divided doses twice daily. Doses larger than 1 g/day are not likely to improve control.

TOLBUTAMIDE

Average starting dose is 1 g/day to 2 g/day (range 0.25–3 g). Maintenance dose over 2 g/day is seldom required. Total dose may be taken in the morning, but divided doses may be preferred from the standpoint of GI tolerance.

NURSING IMPLICATIONS

HISTORY
See Appendix 4. Unless patient is newly diabetic, history must also include type of dietary man-

agement, name of hypoglycemic agent and dose, and method used to test urine.

PHYSICAL ASSESSMENT

Obtain vital signs, weight; identify problem areas (if present) that may be related to or due to diabetes, such as skin ulcers or other changes, poor circulation in the extremities, eye changes, and so on. Baseline laboratory tests may include FBS, CBC, urinalysis, postprandial blood glucose, and hepatic-function tests.

ADMINISTRATION

Elderly patients are usually given a lower initial dose.

Acetohexamide, chlorpropamide, tolazamide, and tolbutamide may be given with food to prevent GI upset.

Glipizide is given 30 minutes before a meal.

Glyburide is given with breakfast or the first main meal. The physician orders the meal with which the drug is given.

Physician may order drug given in single or divided doses.

When patient is transferred from one oral hypoglycemic agent to another, no transitional period and no initial priming dose are necessary.

When giving during the insulin withdrawal period, see _Administration_ for recommended guidelines.

See also Insulin if patient is receiving this drug concurrently.

ONGOING ASSESSMENTS AND NURSING MANAGEMENT

Monitor vital signs daily or as ordered. If elevation in temperature occurs, notify physician. Temperature elevation may indicate infection or development of clinical jaundice. Infection may require adjustment of dosage or addition of insulin to therapeutic regimen; jaundice may require discontinuation of the drug.

Observe for adverse drug effects, especially during the initial dosage period.

Test urine for glucose and ketones (acetone) qid (A.C. and H.S.). Keep physician informed of test results. If there is a sudden increase in urine glucose or the urine is positive for ketones, notify physician immediately.

Elderly patients may be hyperresponsive and require close observation, especially during initial therapy.

Diabetics taking sulfonylureas who are admitted to the hospital with severe infection, trauma, vomiting, or diarrhea require close monitoring of their urine for glucose or ketones. Notify the physician immediately if urine glucose increases

or test for ketones is positive because insulin administration may be necessary.

CLINICAL ALERT: Observe for signs of hyperglycemia (Appendix 6, section 6-14) and ketoacidosis (Appendix 6, section 6-11) and notify physician immediately if they occur; insulin administration may be necessary.

Observe for signs of hypoglycemia (Appendix 6, section 6-14), especially during the initial dosage adjustment period and if the patient is elderly, debilitated, malnourished, semistarved, or receiving concurrent insulin. Early signs and symptoms of hypoglycemia may be vague. Always investigate any unusual behavior change or patient complaint. Assess patient q15m for additional changes or complaints. If possible, obtain a urine sample and test for glucose.

Although severe hypoglycemic episodes are uncommon, they may occur. Hypoglycemic episodes are terminated immediately by administration of glucose such as in 4 oz of orange juice, 2 teaspoons of honey, ginger ale, hard candy, and so on. _Do not_ administer an oral carbohydrate if patient is semiconscious or has difficulty in swallowing; contact the physician immediately because IV glucose administration may be necessary.

Hospital policy or the physician's preference may determine protocol for treatment of hypoglycemia (_i.e.,_ type and amount of carbohydrate administered and obtaining a venous blood sample for glucose). Notify the physician immediately of a hypoglycemic reaction because adjustment in dosage or diet may be necessary. Continue to observe patient q15m to q30m following termination of a hypoglycemic reaction.

See also _Overdosage._

Certain drugs (see _Drug Interactions_) prolong or enhance the effects of sulfonylureas and thereby increase the risk of hypoglycemia. Certain drugs (see _Drug Interactions_) tend to produce hyperglycemia and may lead to loss of control. Patients receiving these drugs are assessed at more frequent intervals for signs of hypoglycemia or hyperglycemia; record this fact as a potential problem on the Kardex.

**Patients receiving beta-adrenergic agents:** The clinical manifestations of hypoglycemia may be blunted and therefore difficult to identify. These patients are carefully assessed and examined any time a hypoglycemic reaction is suspected.

Weigh daily or as ordered. Notify physician if there is a significant increase or decrease in weight.

Monitor patient's dietary intake. The dietary department usually estimates and provides replacement for uneaten food.

If diabetes is difficult to control, investigate factors that may be the cause (_e.g.,_ eating more than allowed or eating foods not permitted [visitors may be bringing in food], hiding or discarding uneaten food, patient or family misunderstanding of the dietary regimen).

S

Institution of sulfonylurea administration as a means to reduce daily insulin dosage requires frequent assessment during the transitional period. Observe for signs of hyperglycemia (Appendix 6, section 6-14) and ketoacidosis (Appendix 6, section 6-11). Contact physician if urinary glucose increases or urine is positive for ketones.

Check with physician about drug administration if diagnostic tests or laboratory studies require a prolonged fasting state.

Periodic hepatic-function tests may be ordered.

PATIENT AND FAMILY INFORMATION

NOTE: For the newly diabetic patient and his family, the nature of diabetes and its treatment should become part of the teaching plan as soon as the physician has explained the diagnosis. Patients taking oral hypoglycemic agents must receive full and complete instructions about the nature of the disease, how the drug works, what must be done to prevent and detect complications, and how to control this condition. Insulin is indispensable in managing acute complications of diabetes. Patients prescribed an oral hypoglycemic agent should be carefully instructed in its use.

This drug is *not* oral insulin.

Take the drug with food unless the physician directs otherwise.

Do not discontinue this medication or increase or decrease the dosage except on advice of the physician.

Take this drug at the same time each day, as directed on the prescription container.

Adherence to diet and maintenance of ideal body weight is extremely important in controlling diabetes. Oral hypoglycemic agents are an adjunct to, not a substitute for, dietary regulation.

Meals should be eaten at approximately the same time each day. Erratic meal patterns or skipped meals may result in difficulty in achieving balance between the correct diet and therapeutic drug dose.

Weigh self weekly. Inform physician of any significant (3–4 lb) increase or decrease in weight.

Avoid dieting or commercial weight-loss programs and strenuous exercise programs unless approved by a physician.

Test urine for glucose and ketones (acetone) as directed. Keep a record of urine testing and bring to the physician's office.

Avoid alcohol except on professional advice.

Even small amounts of alcohol may result in sweating, flushing, nausea, vomiting, headache, slurred speech, abdominal cramps (disulfiram reaction) and hypoglycemia. These signs and symptoms may be misinterpreted as signs of inebriation.

Notify physician or nurse immediately if any of the following occurs:

Hypoglycemia—Fatigue, excessive hunger, profuse sweating, numbness in the extremities, personality changes.

Hyperglycemia—Excessive thirst and/or urination, urine positive for glucose and/or ketones.

Other—Fever, sore throat, unusual bleeding or bruising, diarrhea, rash, itching, yellowing of skin or sclera, dark urine, light-colored stools.

Female patient: If pregnancy is suspected or confirmed, notify the physician immediately.

Avoid use of nonprescription products (especially salicylates) unless use has been approved by the physician.

Notify the physician immediately of any injury, or if severe illness such as high fever, severe and/or prolonged nausea, vomiting, or diarrhea occurs. Severe illness, injury, or surgery may require temporary administration of insulin.

Periodic laboratory tests will be necessary to monitor therapy.

A planned program of exercise is important. Avoid strenuous exercise as well as erratic periods of exercise.

Good skin care and foot care, routine ophthalmologic examinations, and frequent dental checkups are an important part of managing diabetes.

Wear identification such as Medic-Alert to inform medical personnel of diabetes and current treatment.

Patient using oral contraceptives: A different method of birth control is advisable.

Sulindac

See Nonsteroidal Anti-inflammatory Agents.

Sutilains Rx

ointment: 82,000 casein units/g	Travase

INDICATIONS

Adjunct to established methods of wound care for biochemical debridement of the following: second-

and third-degree burns; decubitus ulcers; incisional, traumatic, and pyogenic wounds; ulcers secondary to peripheral vascular disease.

CONTRAINDICATIONS
Not used on wounds communicating with major body cavities, wounds containing exposed major nerves or nerve tissue, or fungating neoplastic ulcers. Contraindicated in pregnancy because of lack of studies on the developing fetus.

ACTIONS
Selectively digests necrotic soft tissues by proteolytic action. It dissolves and facilitates removal of necrotic tissues and purulent exudates that otherwise impair formation of granulation tissue and delay wound healing.

WARNINGS
Do not permit ointment to come into contact with the eyes. If this inadvertently occurs, rinse immediately with copious amounts of sterile water.

PRECAUTIONS
A moist environment is essential for optimal activity of this enzyme. In cases in which there is existent or threatened invasive infection, systemic antibiotics may be ordered. Although there have been no reports of systemic allergic reactions, studies have shown that there may be an antibody response to the absorbed enzyme.

DRUG INTERACTIONS
Enzyme activity may be impaired by certain agents. Several detergents and antiseptics (**benzalkonium chloride, hexachlorophene, iodine, nitrofurazone**) render the substrate indifferent to the action of this enzyme. Compounds such as **thimerosal** that contain metallic ions interfere directly with enzyme activity to a slight degree, whereas **neomycin, streptomycin,** and **penicillin** do not affect enzyme activity. In cases in which adjunctive topical therapy has been used and no dissolution of slough occurs after treatment for 24 to 48 hours, further application, because of interference by adjunctive agents, is unlikely to be successful.

ADVERSE REACTIONS
Consist of mild, transient pain, paresthesias, bleeding, and transient dermatitis. If bleeding or dermatitis occurs, therapy is discontinued. Pain can usually be controlled by administration of mild analgesics. Side-effects severe enough to warrant discontinuation of therapy have occasionally occurred. No systemic toxicity has been observed as a result of topical application.

DOSAGE
See *Administration.*

NURSING IMPLICATIONS

HISTORY
See Appendix 4.

PHYSICAL ASSESSMENT
Examine involved area, noting location and size of lesion, presence or absence of purulent exudate, odor of drainage (if any), appearance of tissue, skin changes adjacent to the lesion, and presence or absence of eschar. Baseline laboratory tests may include culture and sensitivity tests of the exudate.

ADMINISTRATION
Unless physician orders otherwise, thoroughly cleanse and irrigate the wound area using the prescribed solution (usually sodium chloride or water).

The wound *must* be cleansed of antiseptics or heavy-metal antibacterials, which may denature the enzyme or alter substrate characteristics (*e.g.,* hexachlorophene, silver nitrate, benzalkonium chloride, nitrofurazone).

Thoroughly moisten wound area by means of tubbing, showering, or wet soaks (*e.g.,* sodium chloride or water solutions, as ordered).

Apply ointment in a thin layer, assuring intimate contact with necrotic tissue and complete wound coverage extending ¼ inch to ½ inch beyond area to be debrided. Apply loose wet dressings.

Repeat cleansing procedure and application three to four times a day.

Avoid contact with the eyes. If this inadvertently occurs, rinse immediately with copious amounts of sterile water.

ONGOING ASSESSMENTS AND NURSING MANAGEMENT
Inspect lesions each time ointment is applied and compare to data base.

S

Inform physician and withhold next application if bleeding or dermatitis occurs because drug may be discontinued.

If mild transient pain occurs with application, inform physician. An analgesic may be ordered.

A moist environment is *essential* for optimal activity of the enzyme. The loose wet dressing applied following application of the ointment must be kept wet at all times. Depending on the speed of evaporation, reapplication of solution to keep the dressings moist may be necessary every ½ hour. Wrapping or covering the area with disposable plastic-backed pads slows evaporation of the solution.

The bedding beneath the lesion should be protected with plastic or waterproof padding to prevent soaking of bed linens following application of solution to the dressings. Inspect the bedding hourly and change as necessary.

Inform physician if any of the following is noted: increase in exudate, change in odor of the exudate, maceration of surrounding tissues.

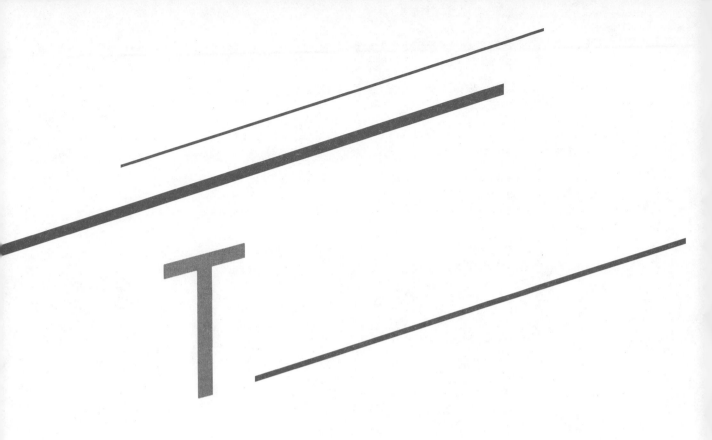

T

Talbutal

See Barbiturates.

Tamoxifen Rx

tablets: 10 mg   Nolvadex

INDICATIONS

Palliative treatment of advanced breast cancer in postmenopausal women. Patients who have had a recent negative estrogen receptor assay are unlikely to respond.

CONTRAINDICATIONS

None known.

ACTIONS

A nonsteroidal agent that has demonstrated potent antiestrogenic properties. The antiestrogenic effects may be related to its ability to compete with estrogen for binding sites in target tissues such as the breast. The drug is apparently slowly excreted in the feces; only small amounts appear in the urine.

WARNINGS

Ophthalmologic effects: Ocular changes have been reported in a few patients treated for periods greater than 1 year at dosages at least four times the highest recommended daily dosage. Changes consist of retinopathy, corneal changes, and decreased visual acuity. Ophthalmologic examinations of patients receiving long-term therapy at recommended doses have not detected any ocular pathology.

Hypercalcemia: Has been reported in some breast cancer patients with bone metastasis. If hypercalcemia does occur, appropriate measures are taken and, if they are severe, drug is discontinued.

Carcinogenicity: The possibility of this potential should be considered.

Use in pregnancy: Safety for use is not established.

PRECAUTIONS

Use cautiously in those with leukopenia or thrombocytopenia. Transient decreases in platelet counts (usually to 50,000–100,000/mm^3) have been seen. No hemorrhagic tendency has been recorded, and platelet counts returned to normal even though treatment was continued.

DRUG INTERACTIONS

Drug/lab tests: Tamoxifen may produce a transient increase in **serum calcium.**

ADVERSE REACTIONS

Most frequent: Hot flashes, nausea, and vomiting may occur in up to 25% of patients but have rarely been severe enough to warrant discontinuation of treatment.

Less frequent: Vaginal bleeding, vaginal discharge, menstrual irregularities, skin rash. Usually these reactions have not been severe enough to require dosage reduction or discontinuation of treatment.

Infrequent: Hypercalcemia, peripheral edema, distaste for food, pruritus vulvae, depression, dizziness, lightheadedness, headache.

Increased bone and tumor pain and local disease flare have occurred, which are sometimes associated with a good tumor response. Patients with increased bone pain may require additional analgesics. Patients with soft-tissue disease may have sudden increases in size of preexisting lesions, sometimes associated with marked erythema within and surrounding the lesions, or development of new lesions. When they occur, bone pain and disease flare are seen shortly after starting tamoxifen and generally subside rapidly.

If adverse reactions are severe, it is sometimes possible to control them by a reduction of dosage without losing control of the disease.

DOSAGE

10 mg to 20 mg bid (morning and evening).

NURSING IMPLICATIONS

HISTORY

See Appendix 4.

PHYSICAL ASSESSMENT

Obtain vital signs, weight. Evaluate patient's general physical and emotional status. Baseline laboratory tests may include CBC, platelet count, serum calcium, estrogen receptor assay.

ADMINISTRATION

Give drug bid in the morning and evening.

ONGOING ASSESSMENTS AND NURSING MANAGEMENT

Obtain vital signs q8h or as ordered.

If nausea or vomiting occurs, notify physician; an antiemetic may be ordered.

Dry toast, unsalted crackers, or carbonated beverages may help relieve nausea.

If soft-tissue lesions are present, examine areas daily, noting changes in size and color of the lesions and appearance of new lesions. Compare findings with data base and record on patient's chart.

Weigh daily or as ordered. If significant weight gain or loss occurs, inform physician.

Observe for adverse effects, especially marked weakness, mental confusion, pain or swelling in the extremities, shortness of breath, anorexia, headache, skin rash, visual changes, and vaginal bleeding. Report occurrence to the physician because dosage adjustment may be considered.

If weakness or lightheadedness occurs, assist with ambulatory activities.

Periodic CBC, platelet count, and serum calcium are recommended.

If the serum calcium rises, observe for signs of hypercalcemia (Appendix 6, section 6-13) and report occurrence to physician immediately.

PATIENT AND FAMILY INFORMATION

Take prescribed dose in the morning and evening. Doses should be approximately 12 hours apart.

Medication may cause bone pain shortly after beginning of therapy; this generally subsides rapidly. If bone pain occurs, notify physician or nurse, because additional analgesics may be prescribed.

Patient with soft-tissue lesions: An increase in the size of the lesions associated with marked redness within and surrounding the lesion, as well as the development of new lesions, may occur shortly after therapy is started; these symptoms generally subside rapidly.

Nausea or vomiting may occur. If these are severe, notify physician or nurse, because an antiemetic may be necessary.

Weigh self weekly. Inform physician if significant weight gain or loss (more than 3 lb/week) occurs.

Weight gain, menstrual irregularities, vaginal bleeding or discharge, dizziness, loss of appetite, skin rash, and headache may occur. Notify physician or nurse if these become pronounced. Also report marked weakness, sleepiness, mental confusion, pain or swelling of the legs, or shortness of breath.

Notify physician or nurse immediately of any visual changes such as blurred vision or difficulty seeing at night.

Avoid prolonged exposure to sunlight; photosensitivity may occur.

Periodic laboratory examinations and eye examinations may be necessary.

Temazepam Rx C-IV

capsules: 15 mg, 30 mg   Restoril

INDICATIONS

Relief of insomnia associated with difficulty in falling asleep, frequent nocturnal awakenings, or early morning awakenings. Insomnia is often transient and intermittent; prolonged administration is not recommended. Because insomnia may be a symptom of other disorders, the possibility that the complaint may be related to a condition for which there is more specific treatment should be considered.

CONTRAINDICATIONS

Drug is contraindicated in pregnancy. If there is a likelihood that the patient may become pregnant while receiving temazepam, she is warned of the potential risk to the fetus. Patient should discontinue drug before becoming pregnant. The possibility that a woman of childbearing potential may be pregnant when therapy is instituted must be considered. Temazepam is a benzodiazepine. Benzodiazepines may cause fetal damage when given during pregnancy. An increased risk of congenital malformations associated with the use of diazepam and chlordiazepoxide (both are benzodiazepines) during the first trimester of pregnancy has been suggested. Transplacental distribution results in neonatal CNS depression following ingestion of therapeutic doses of a benzodiazepine hypnotic during the last weeks of pregnancy.

ACTIONS

Is a benzodiazepine derivative useful as a hypnotic. Absorption is complete and detectable blood levels are achieved at 20 to 40 minutes; peak concentrations are reached in 2 to 3 hours. The unchanged drug is 96% bound to plasma proteins. Temazepam is completely degraded to inactive metabolites prior to excretion in the urine.

Temazepam significantly improves sleep maintenance parameters (*i.e.,* wake time after sleep onset, total sleep time, and number of nocturnal awakenings) without significant reduction in sleep latency. Residual medication effects (hangover) are essentially absent, and early morning awakening, a particular problem in geriatric patients, is reduced. REM sleep is essentially unchanged, slow wave sleep is decreased, and no rebound effects occur in these sleep stages. Transient sleep disturbances, mainly on the first night, occur after withdrawal of the drug. In studies, there was no evidence of tolerance when patients were given the drug nightly for approximately 1 month.

WARNINGS

The risk of oversedation, dizziness, confusion, and ataxia increases substantially with larger doses of benzodiazepines in elderly and debilitated patients; 15 mg is the recommended initial dosage. Abnormal hepatic-function tests as well as blood dyscrasias have been reported with benzodiazepines. Safety for use in the nursing mother and children under 18 is not established.

PRECAUTIONS

May produce drowsiness. Disturbed nocturnal sleep may occur for the first or second night after discontinuing use. Temazepam is given with caution in severely depressed patients or in those in whom there is evidence of latent depression; suicidal tendencies may be present and protective measures may be necessary.

Abuse and dependence: Withdrawal symptoms following abrupt discontinuation of benzodiazepines have been reported in patients receiving excessive doses over extended periods of time. These symptoms (including convulsions) are similar to those seen after barbiturate withdrawal. Although infrequently seen, milder withdrawal symptoms have been reported following abrupt discontinuance of benzodiazepines taken continuously, generally at higher therapeutic levels, for at least several months. Caution is exercised in giving temazepam to individuals known to be addiction prone or those whose history suggests they may increase the dosage on their own initiative. It is recommended that repeat prescriptions have adequate medical supervision.

DRUG INTERACTIONS

Possible additive effects may occur with concomitant use of **alcohol** or other **CNS depressants.**

ADVERSE REACTIONS

Drug is well tolerated, and side-effects are usually mild and transient.

Neuropsychiatric: Drowsiness (17%); dizziness (7%); lethargy (5%); confusion, euphoria, relaxed feeling (2%–3%); weakness (1%–2%); tremor, ataxia, lack of concentration, loss of equilibrium (<1%). Hallucinations, horizontal nystagmus, and paradoxical reactions including excitement, stimulation, and hyperactivity are rare.

GI: Anorexia, diarrhea (1%–2%).

Cardiac: Palpitations (<1%).

OVERDOSAGE

Symptoms: Somnolence, confusion, and coma, with reduced or absent reflexes, respiratory depression, and hypotension.

Treatment: If patient is conscious, induce vomiting mechanically or with emetics. If patient is unconscious, employ gastric lavage using a cuffed endotracheal tube to prevent aspiration and pulmonary complications. Maintenance of adequate pulmonary ventilation is essential. IV pressor agents may be necessary to combat hypotension. IV fluids are recommended to encourage diuresis. The value of dialysis has not been determined. If excitation occurs, do not use barbiturates. The possibility that multiple agents may have been ingested should be considered.

DOSAGE

Dosage is individualized. Usual adult dose is 30 mg before retiring, but 15 mg may be sufficient.

Elderly or debilitated patients: Therapy is initiated with 15 mg until individual responses are determined.

NURSING IMPLICATIONS

HISTORY
See Appendix 4.

PHYSICAL ASSESSMENT
Determine whether specific factors that may be controlled or eliminated may be interfering with sleep. Factors may include noise, bright lights, pain, and discomfort.

ADMINISTRATION
Do not administer this drug if the patient has pain, which should be controlled with an analgesic.

Do not administer this drug shortly before or after administration of a narcotic or another CNS depressant. If the patient has an order for a narcotic (or another CNS depressant) and a hypnotic, check with physician about time interval between administration of these agents. Usually 2 or more hours should elapse between administration of this drug and other CNS depressants, but interval may vary with a specific CNS depressant and the dose administered.

Following administration, raise the siderails and advise patient to remain in bed and to call for assistance if it is necessary to get out of bed.

T

ONGOING ASSESSMENTS AND NURSING MANAGEMENT

Observe patient 1 to 2 hours after administration to evaluate effect of the drug.

Notify physician if drug fails to produce sleep; sleep is interrupted during the night; excitement, hyperactivity, or stimulation (paradoxical effects) is noted; or patient is sleepy during the morning hours.

The occurrence of a paradoxical reaction requires more frequent observation of the patient (as often as every 5–10 minutes may be necessary) for the duration of the reaction.

Observe for adverse reactions and inform physician before next dose is due.

CLINICAL ALERT: Abrupt discontinuation in those on prolonged therapy with high doses may result in withdrawal symptoms similar to those seen with barbiturates (p 170).

PATIENT AND FAMILY INFORMATION

May cause drowsiness. Take drug immediately before retiring.

Alcohol and other CNS depressants must not be taken.

Do not exceed the prescribed dosage. If drug fails to produce sleep after several nights' use, inform physician or nurse.

Sleep disturbances may be noted for the first or second night after drug is discontinued.

Terbutaline Sulfate

See Bronchodilators and Decongestants, Systemic.

Testolactone Rx

tablets: 50 mg   Teslac

INDICATIONS

Adjunctive therapy in the palliative management of advanced or disseminated breast cancer in post-menopausal women when hormonal therapy is indicated. May also be used in women diagnosed as having disseminated breast carcinoma when pre-menopausal, in whom ovarian function has been subsequently terminated.

CONTRAINDICATIONS

Treatment of breast cancer in men; premenopausal women.

ACTIONS

The precise mechanism by which testolactone produces its clinical antineoplastic effects is unknown.

Although chemical configuration of testolactone is similar to that of other androgenic hormones, it is devoid of androgenic activity in the doses commonly used. It was found to be effective in approximately 15% of patients with advanced or disseminated breast cancer.

WARNINGS

Safety for use in pregnancy is not established; drug should not be used during pregnancy.

PRECAUTIONS

Plasma calcium levels should be routinely determined in any patient receiving therapy for mammary cancer, particularly during periods of active remission of bony metastases. If hypercalcemia occurs, appropriate measures are instituted.

DRUG INTERACTIONS

May increase the effects of **oral anticoagulants;** monitor and adjust dosage accordingly.

ADVERSE REACTIONS

It is often impossible to determine the relationships of the underlying disease and drug administration to reported reactions. Signs and symptoms reported include maculopapular erythema, increase in blood pressure, paresthesia, aches and edema of the extremities, glossitis, anorexia, nausea, and vomiting. Alopecia, alone and with associated nail growth disturbance, has been reported rarely; this side-effect subsided without interruption of therapy.

DOSAGE

Recommended oral dose is 250 mg qid. In order to evaluate response, therapy is continued for a minimum of 3 months unless there is active progression of the disease.

NURSING IMPLICATIONS

HISTORY

See Appendix 4.

PHYSICAL ASSESSMENT

Obtain vital signs, weight. Evaluate patient's general physical and emotional status. Baseline laboratory studies may include CBC, urinalysis, hepatic-function tests, plasma calcium level. Diagnostic studies may include skeletal survey for bone metastasis.

ADMINISTRATION

Give without regard to meals. If nausea and vomiting occur, consult physician about giving drug with meals or food.

ONGOING ASSESSMENTS AND NURSING MANAGEMENT

Monitor vital signs daily or as ordered.

Weigh weekly or as ordered. Inform physician if significant weight loss (more than 3–4 lb/week) is noted.

Observe for adverse effects and notify physician if they occur. Usually, treatment is not discontinued unless reactions become severe.

Observe for signs of hypercalcemia (Appendix 6, section 6-13) and flank or abdominal pain and fever (which may be indicative of calcium stone formation).

Encourage a high fluid intake to prevent calcium stone formation.

Encourage patient to ambulate, if possible. If ambulation is not possible, institute passive exercises q2h to q4h.

Plasma calcium levels are recommended periodically, particularly during periods of active remission.

Clinical response is evaluated after 2 to 3 months of therapy according to the following criteria: measurable decrease in size of all demonstrable tumor masses; decrease in size of more than 50% of nonosseus lesions although all bone lesions remain static; improvement in more than 50% of total lesions while the remainder are static.

PATIENT AND FAMILY INFORMATION

Notify physician if any of the following occurs: numbness or tingling of the fingers, toes, or face; diarrhea; loss of appetite; nausea, vomiting; loss of hair; edema; swelling or redness of the tongue; flank or abdominal pain; fever.

Periodic laboratory and x-ray tests will be necessary to monitor therapy.

Testosterone

See Androgens.

Testosterone Cypionate

See Androgens.

Testosterone Enanthate

See Androgens.

Testosterone Propionate

See Androgens.

Tetanus Antitoxin

See Antitoxins and Antivenins.

Tetanus Immune Globulin

See Immunizations, Passive.

Tetanus Toxoid

See Immunizations, Active.

Tetracaine

See Anesthetics, Local, Injectable; Anesthetics, Local, Topical; Anesthetics, Ophthalmic.

Tetracycline Hydrochloride

See Tetracyclines.

Tetracycline Hydrochloride and Amphotericin B

See Tetracyclines.

Tetracycline Phosphate Complex

See Tetracyclines.

Tetracyclines

Demeclocycline Hydrochloride Rx

capsules: 150 mg	Declomycin
tablets: 150 mg, 300 mg	Declomycin

Doxycycline Rx

tablets: 100 mg (as hyclate)	Doxy-Tabs, Vibra Tabs, *Generic*
capsules: 50 mg (as hyclate)	Doxychel Hyclate, Vibramycin, *Generic*
capsules: 100 mg (as hyclate)	Doxychel Hyclate, Doxy-Lemmon, Vibramycin, *Generic*
powder for oral suspension: 25 mg/5	Vibramycin

T

ml (as monohy-
drate)

syrup: 50 mg/5 ml (as calcium salt)	Vibramycin
powder for injection: 100 mg/vial, 200 mg/vial (as hy-clate)	Doxy 100, Doxy 200, Vibramycin IV

Methacycline Hydrochloride *Rx*

capsules: 150 mg, 300 mg	Rondomycin

Minocycline Hydrochloride *Rx*

tablets: 50 mg, 100 mg	Minocin
capsules: 50 mg, 100 mg	Minocin
oral suspension: 50 mg/5 ml	Minocin
powder for injection: 100 mg/vial	Minocin IV

Oxytetracycline *Rx*

tablets: 250 mg	Terramycin
capsules: 125 mg	Terramycin
capsules: 250 mg	E.P. Mycin, Terramycin, Uri-Tet, *Generic*
injection: 50 mg/ml with 2% lidocaine	Oxymycin, Terramycin IM
injection: 125 mg/ml with 2% lidocaine	Terramycin
powder for injection: 250 mg/vial, 500 mg/vial	Terramycin IV

Tetracycline Hydrochloride *Rx*

tablets: 250 mg	Sumycin '250,' *Generic*
tablets: 500 mg	Sumycin '500'
capsules: 100 mg	*Generic*
capsules: 250 mg	Achromycin V, Cycline-250, Cyclopar, Deltamycin, Nor-Tet, Panmycin, Retet, Robitet '250' Robicaps, SK-Tetracycline, Sumycin '250,' Tetra-C, Tetracap, Tetrachel, Tetracyn, Tetralan-250, Tetram, *Generic*
capsules: 500 mg	Achromycin V, Cyclopar 500, Nor-Tet, Retet-500, Robitet '500' Robicaps, SK-Tetracycline, Sumycin

	'500,' Tetrachel 500, Tetracyn, Tetralan-500, *Generic* Achromycin V, SK-Tetracycline Syrup, Sumycin Syrup, *Generic*
oral suspension: 125 mg/5 ml	Achromycin V, SK-Tetracycline Syrup, Sumycin Syrup, *Generic*
powder for injection: 100 mg with 40 mg procaine HCl/vial, 250 mg with 40 mg procaine HCl/vial	Achromycin IM
powder for injection: 250 mg/vial, 500 mg/vial	Achromycin IV

Tetracycline Hydrochloride and Amphotericin B *Rx*

capsules: 250 mg tetracycline HCl and 50 mg amphotericin B	Mysteclin-F
syrup: 125 mg tetracycline HCl and 25 mg amphotericin B/5 ml	Mysteclin-F

Tetracycline Phosphate Complex *Rx*

capsules: 250 mg	Tetrex
capsules: 500 mg	Tetrex bidCAPS

Tetracyclines and Nystatin *Rx*

capsules: 250 mg tetracycline HCl and 250,000 units nystatin	Tetrastatin
capsules: 250 mg oxytetracycline and 250,000 units nystatin	Terrastatin

INDICATIONS

Infections caused by the following microorganisms: Rickettsiae (Rocky Mountain spotted fever, typhus fever and the typhus group, Q fever, rickettsial pox, tick fever); *Mycoplasma pneumoniae* (PPLO, Eaton agent); agents of psittacosis and ornithosis; agents of lymphogranuloma venereum and granuloma inguinale; the spirochetal agent of relapsing fever (*Borrelia recurrentis*).

Infections caused by the following gram-negative microorganisms: Haemophilus ducreyi (chancroid);

Pasturella pestis and _P. tularensis; Bartonella bacil-_
liformis; Bacteroides species; _Vibrio comma_ and _V._
fetus; Brucella species (in conjunction with streptomycin).

Tetracycline is indicated for treatment of infections caused by the following microorganisms when
bacteriologic testing indicates appropriate susceptibility to the drug:

Gram-negative: Escherichia coli; Enterobacter
aerogenes; Shigella species; _Acinetobacter calcoaceti-_
cus; H. influenzae; Klebsiella species (respiratory
and urinary infections).

Gram-positive: Streptococcus pneumoniae.

When penicillin is contraindicated, tetracyclines
are alternative drugs in treatment of infections due
to _Neisseria gonorrhoeae; Treponema pallidum_ and
T. pertenue (syphilis and yaws); _Listeria monocyto-_
genes; Clostridium species; _Bacillus anthracis; Fuso-_
bacterium fusiforme (Vincent's infection); _Actino-_
myces species; _N. meningitidis_ (IV only).

In acute intestinal amebiasis, the tetracyclines
may be a useful adjunct to amebicides.

Tetracyclines are indicated in treatment of trachoma, although the infectious agent is not always
eliminated.

In addition, oral therapy is indicated in severe
acne, in which it may be useful as adjunctive therapy, and inclusion conjunctivitis, which may be
treated with oral tetracyclines or with a combination of oral and topical agents.

Oral minocycline is also indicated in treatment of
asymptomatic carriers of _N. meningitidis_ to eliminate meningococci from the nasopharynx. It also
has been used in treatment of infections caused by
Mycobacterium marinum. Minocycline is indicated
for the treatment of uncomplicated urethral, endocervical, or rectal infections in adults caused by
Ureaplasma urealyticum; uncomplicated gonococcal
urethritis in men due to _N. gonorrhoeae;_ as an alternative drug (when penicillin is contraindicated) for
N. gonorrhoeae in women.

Unlabeled uses: **Demeclocycline** has been used
successfully in management of the chronic form of
the syndrome of inappropriate antidiuretic hormone
(SIADH) secretion. **Doxycycline** has been used
to prevent traveler's diarrhea commonly caused by
enterotoxigenic _E. coli._

Minocycline has been used as an alternative to
sulfonamides in the treatment of nocardiosis.

Tetracycline instilled through a chest tube is employed as a pleural sclerosing agent in malignant
pleural effusions.

CONTRAINDICATIONS

Hypersensitivity to any of the tetracyclines.

ACTIONS

Tetracyclines are readily absorbed in children and
adults, but absorption in infants is poor when they
are administered orally. Achlorhydria has no effect
on absorption, but food will decrease absorption
(except with **doxycycline** and **minocycline,** which
should be taken with food).

Doxycycline and minocycline are highly lipid soluble and readily penetrate into cerebrospinal fluid,
the eye, and the prostate. In addition, minocycline
displays good penetration of the saliva, making it
useful in eliminating meningococci from the nasopharynx of asymptomatic carriers. Tetracycline and
demeclocycline are intermediate in terms of lipid
solubility; oxytetracycline is the least lipid-soluble
derivative. Hemodialysis removes 20% to 30% of
tetracycline but has little effect on doxycycline or
minocycline. Peritoneal dialysis has no effect on the
tetracyclines.

The tetracyclines are concentrated by the liver in
the bile and excreted in urine and feces, largely unchanged. Appropriate dosage adjustments are made
in those with impaired renal function. Conventional
tetracyclines are contraindicated in anuria. Doxycycline and minocycline are excreted largely by nonrenal routes and their serum half-lives do not increase to a significant degree in renal impairment.
Doxycycline is secreted in inactive form into the intestinal lumen and eliminated in the feces; hence its
half-life is largely independent of renal or hepatic
function. Minocycline is metabolized and its half-
life prolonged in oliguria.

The tetracyclines are bacteriostatic at recommended dosages. They exert their antimicrobial effect by inhibition of protein synthesis. Tetracyclines
are active against a wide range of gram-negative and
gram-positive organisms. Drugs in the tetracycline
class have closely similar antimicrobial spectra, and
cross-resistance among them is common.

WARNINGS

Use in children: Tetracyclines should not generally be used in children under 8 years of age unless
other drugs are not likely to be effective or are contraindicated. The use of tetracyclines during the period of tooth development (from the last half of
pregnancy through the eighth year) may cause permanent discoloration (yellow-gray-brown) and inadequate calcification of the deciduous and permanent
teeth. This adverse reaction is more common during long-term use of the drugs but has been observed following repeated short-term courses.
Enamel hypoplasia has also been reported. Doxycycline is less likely to affect teeth.

Tetracycline forms a stable calcium complex in

T

any bone-forming tissue. A decrease in fibular growth rate has been observed in premature infants given oral tetracycline in doses of 25 mg/kg q6h. This reaction was reversible when drug was discontinued.

Use in renal impairment: If renal impairment exists, even usual doses may lead to excessive systematic accumulation of tetracyclines (with the exception of doxycycline and minocycline) and possible liver toxicity. Lower than usual doses are indicated and, if therapy is prolonged, serum level determinations of the drug are recommended. Total dosage is decreased by reduction of individual doses or by extending the time intervals between doses. The hazard that even usual doses may lead to accumulation and liver toxicity is of particular importance in parenteral administration to pregnant or postpartum patients with pyelonephritis.

The antianabolic action of tetracyclines may cause an increase in BUN. In patients with significantly impaired renal function, higher serum levels of tetracycline may lead to azotemia, hyperphosphatemia, and acidosis. This does not occur with doxycycline.

Photosensitivity: In those taking **demeclocycline,** exaggerated sunburn reactions are characterized by severe burns of exposed surfaces, resulting from direct exposure to sunlight during therapy with moderate or large doses. Phototoxic reactions are most frequent with demeclocycline, tetracycline, and oxytetracycline and are minimal with methacycline and minocycline.

Parenteral therapy: Parenteral route is reserved for situations in which oral therapy is not adequate or is not tolerated. Oral therapy is instituted as soon as possible. If IV therapy is given over prolonged periods of time, thrombophlebitis may result. IM administration produces lower blood levels than does oral administration in recommended dosages. If rapid, high blood levels are needed, drug is given IV.

Hepatic effects: IV doses in excess of 2 g/day can be extremely dangerous. In the presence of renal dysfunction, and particularly in pregnancy, IV tetracycline therapy in daily doses exceeding 2 g has been associated with death secondary to liver failure. When the need for intensive treatment outweighs the potential dangers (mostly during pregnancy or in those with known or suspected renal and hepatic impairment), renal- and hepatic-function tests are monitored. Serum tetracycline concentrations should not exceed 15 mcg/ml. Other potentially hepatotoxic drugs should not be given concomitantly.

SIADH: Administration of **demeclocycline** has resulted in appearance of diabetes insipidus syndrome (polyuria, polydipsia, weakness) in some patients on long-term therapy. The syndrome has been shown to be nephrogenic, dose dependent, and reversible on discontinuation of therapy.

CNS effects: Vestibular side-effects including lightheadedness, dizziness, and vertigo have been reported with **minocycline.** These symptoms may disappear during therapy and always disappear rapidly when drug is discontinued.

Use in pregnancy, lactation: Tetracyclines should not be used in pregnancy. Results of studies indicate tetracyclines readily cross the placental barrier, are found in fetal tissues, and can have toxic effects on the developing fetus (often related to skeletal development). Tetracyclines are excreted in breast milk. See also *Warnings* about use during tooth development in children.

PRECAUTIONS

Superinfections: Use of antibiotics, especially prolonged or repeated therapy, may result in bacterial or fungal overgrowth of nonsuceptible organisms. Such overgrowth may lead to a secondary infection. Appropriate measures should be taken if superinfection occurs. Superinfection of the bowel by staphylococci may be life threatening.

Laboratory tests: In venereal diseases when coexistent syphilis is suspected, darkfield examination should be done before treatment is started and blood serology should be repeated monthly for at least 4 months. In long-term therapy, periodic laboratory evaluation of organ systems, including hematopoietic, renal, and hepatic studies, should be performed.

Outdated products: Should never be administered because degradation products of tetracyclines are highly nephrotoxic and have, on occasion, produced a Fanconilike syndrome.

Tartrazine sensitivity: Some of these products contain tartrazine. See Appendix 6, section 6-23.

DRUG INTERACTIONS

Bacteriostatic drugs may interfere with the bactericidal action of **penicillin;** concomitant use of tetracycline and penicillin is avoided.

Antacids containing aluminum, calcium, zinc, bismuth, or magnesium and other **divalent** and **trivalent cations** impair absorption and should not be given to patients taking oral tetracyclines. Concurrent ingestion of **iron** will inhibit tetracycline absorption. **Alkali** (*e.g.,* sodium bicarbonate) has been reported to inhibit tetracycline absorption by alteration of the gastric *p*H.

Food and **some dairy products** also interfere with absorption. Administer oral tetracycline 1 hour before or 2 hours after meals. Doxycycline has a low affinity for calcium binding. Gastrointestinal absorption of minocycline and doxycycline is not significantly affected by food or milk.

Tetracyclines may increase the bioavailability of **digoxin;** this could lead to digoxin toxicity. These effects may last for months after tetracycline administration is discontinued.

Tetracyclines depress plasma prothrombin activity; concomitant **anticoagulant** therapy may require downward adjustment of the anticoagulant dose.

Barbiturates, carbamazepine, and **phenytoin** may increase the rate of metabolism, and therefore decrease the half-life, of doxycycline.

Tetracyclines may enhance **methoxyflurane**-induced nephrotoxicity; avoid concurrent use.

Concomitant use of **oral contraceptives** and tetracyclines may decrease the pharmacologic effects of oral contraceptives; breakthrough bleeding or pregnancy may occur.

Concomitant administration of **theophylline** and tetracyclines may increase the incidence of GI side-effects.

Drug/lab test interactions: Following a course of therapy, persistence for several days in both urine and blood of bacteriosuppressive levels of **demeclocycline** may interfere with culture studies.

ADVERSE REACTIONS

GI: Oral and parenteral administration—Anorexia, nausea, vomiting, diarrhea, epigastric distress; bulky loose stools, stomatitis; sore throat; glossitis, hoarseness; black hairy tongue, dysphagia, enterocolitis, steatorrhea, and inflammatory lesions (with monilial overgrowth) in the anogenital region. *Oral administration*—Esophageal ulcers, most commonly in those with esophageal obstructive element or hiatal hernia. Taking the drug with a full glass of water and at least 1 hour before going to bed may minimize this problem.

Skin: Maculopapular and erythematous rashes; exfoliative dermatitis (uncommon). Photosensitivity (see *Warnings*). Onycholysis and discoloration of the nails have been reported rarely. Onycholysis has been reported in up to 25% of patients experiencing phototoxic reactions to tetracyclines. This may also occur without phototoxicity. Blue-gray pigmentation of the skin and mucous membranes has been reported, primarily with minocycline.

Renal toxicity: Rise in BUN (dose related).

Hepatic toxicity: Fatty liver. Hepatic cholestasis has been reported rarely and is usually associated with high dosage levels.

CNS: Vestibular disturbances have been reported in a large percentage of patients treated with minocycline. These may include ataxia, vertigo, nausea, and vomiting. These symptoms are rapidly revers-

ible on discontinuation of the drug. Transient myopathy also reported.

Hypersensitivity: Urticaria, angioneurotic edema, anaphylaxis, anaphylactoid purpura, pericarditis, exacerbation of systemic lupus erythematosus, and serum sickness–like reactions, such as fever, rash, and arthralgia. Increased intracranial pressure and bulging fontanelles (pseudomotor cerebri) have been reported most frequently in young infants following full therapeutic dosage. Severe headache, impairment of vision, and papilledema may result. Benign intracranial hemorrhage has been reported in adults receiving full therapeutic dosages. Symptoms include vomiting, headache, and sixth cranial nerve palsy. These signs disappeared rapidly when drug was discontinued.

Hematologic: Hemolytic anemia, thrombocytopenia, thrombocytopenic purpura, neutropenia, eosinophilia, leukocytosis, leukopenia.

Miscellaneous: Nephrogenic diabetes insipidus has been reported with **demeclocycline.** When given over prolonged periods, tetracyclines have been reported to produce brown-black microscopic and apparently innocuous discoloration of the thyroid glands. No abnormalities of thyroid-function studies are known to occur. Drug disposition in the eye may produce abnormal pigmentation of the conjunctiva.

Local: Irritation may occur with IM administration.

DOSAGE

DEMECLOCYCLINE

Oral

Adults: Usual daily dosage is four divided doses of 150 mg each or two divided doses of 300 mg each.

Children over 8 years: Usual daily dosage is 3 mg/lb to 6 mg/lb (6–12 mg/kg) depending on the severity of the illness, divided into two or four doses.

Gonorrhea patients sensitive to penicillin: Initially 600 mg, followed by 300 mg q12h for 4 days to a total of 3 g.

DOXYCYCLINE

The therapeutic antibacterial serum activity will usually persist for 24 hours following recommended dosage.

Oral

Adults: Usual dosage is 200 mg on first day of treatment (given as 100 mg q12h), followed by a maintenance dosage of 100 mg/day. The maintenance dosage may be administered as a single dose or as 50 mg q12h. In management of more severe

T

infections (particularly chronic infections of the urinary tract), 100 mg q12h is recommended.

Children over 8 years: Recommended dosage schedule for children weighing 100 lb or less is 2 mg/lb (4.4 mg/kg) divided into two doses on the first day of treatment, followed by 1 mg/lb (2.2 mg/kg) given as a single daily dose or divided into two doses on subsequent days. For more severe infections, up to 2 mg/lb may be used. For children over 100 pounds, usual adult dosage should be used.

Traveler's diarrhea: 100 mg/day.

CDC recommended treatment schedule for sexually transmitted diseases

Chlamydia trachomatis—Uncomplicated urethral, endocervical, or rectal infections in adults, 100 mg bid for at least 7 days.

Gonococcal infections—Uncomplicated infections in adults, 100 mg bid for 7 days.

Nongonococcal urethritis—100 mg bid for at least 7 days.

Acute pelvic inflammatory disease—For ambulatory treatment, 2 g cefoxitin IM or 3 g oral amoxicillin, or 3.5 g ampicillin, or 4.8 million units aqueous procaine penicillin G, IM at two sites; each along with 1 g oral probenecid. Follow with doxycycline 100 mg bid for 10 to 14 days.

Sexually transmitted epididymo-orchitis—100 mg bid for at least 10 days.

Lymphogranuloma venereum—For genital, inguinal, or anorectal infections, 100 mg bid for at least 2 weeks.

Rape victims—For prophylaxis, 100 mg bid for at least 7 days.

IV

Studies indicate that use at recommended doses does not lead to excessive accumulation in those with renal impairment.

Adults: Usual dosage is 200 mg on first day of treatment, administered in one or two infusions. Subsequent daily dosage is 100 mg to 200 mg, depending on the severity of the infection, with 200 mg administered in one or two infusions. In the treatment of primary and secondary syphilis, recommended dosage is 300 mg/day for at least 10 days.

Children over 8 years: For children weighing 100 lb or less, give 2 mg/lb on the first day of treatment, in one or two infusions. Subsequent daily dosage is 1 mg/lb to 2 mg/lb given as one or two infusions, depending on the severity of the infection. For children over 100 lb, use the usual adult dose.

Children under 8 years: Use is not recommended because safety is not established.

CDC recommended treatment schedule for acute pelvic inflammatory disease

Endometritis, salpingitis, parametritis, and/or

peritonitis—100 mg IV twice a day and 2 g cefoxitin IV four times a day. Alternatively, 100 mg doxycycline IV twice a day and 1 g metronidazole IV twice a day. Continue IV drugs for at least 4 days and for at least 48 hours after patient defervesces.

METHACYCLINE HYDROCHLORIDE

Oral

Adults: Usual dosage is 600 mg/day. This may be given in four divided doses of 150 mg each or two divided doses of 300 mg each. An initial dose of 300 mg is followed by 150 mg q6h, or 300 mg q12h may be used in more severe infections.

Children over 8 years: Recommended dosage schedule is 3 mg/lb/day to 6 mg/lb/day (6–12 mg/kg/day) divided into two or four equally spaced doses.

Uncomplicated gonorrhea when penicillin is contraindicated: 900 mg initially, followed by 300 mg qid for a total of 5.4 g.

Syphilis when penicillin is contraindicated: Give a total of 18 g to 24 g in equally divided doses over a period of 10 to 15 days. Close followup, including laboratory tests, is recommended.

Eaton agent (PPLO) pneumonia: 900 mg/day for 6 days.

MINOCYCLINE

Oral

Adults: Usual dosage is 200 mg initially, followed by 100 mg q12h. Alternatively, if more frequent doses are preferred, 100 mg to 200 mg may be given initially followed by 50 mg qid.

Children over 8 years: Usual dosage is 4 mg/kg initially, followed by 2 mg/kg q12h.

Syphilis: Give usual dosage over a period of 10 to 15 days. Close followup, including laboratory tests, is recommended.

Gonorrhea: Patients sensitive to penicillin may be treated with minocycline, given as 200 mg initially, followed by 100 mg q12h for a minimum of 4 days, with post-therapy cultures within 2 to 3 days.

Meningococcal carrier state: Recommended dosage is 100 mg q12h for 5 days.

Mycobacterium marinum *infections:* Although optimal dosage is not established, 100 mg bid for 6 to 8 weeks has been used.

IV

Adults: 200 mg, followed by 100 mg q12h; do not exceed 400 mg in 24 hours.

Children over 8 years: Usual dosage is 4 mg/kg, followed by 2 mg/kg q12h.

OXYTETRACYCLINE HYDROCHLORIDE

Oral

See Tetracycline Hydrochloride.

IM
Adults: Usual daily dosage is 250 mg given once every 24 hours or 300 mg given in divided doses at 8- to 12-hour intervals.

Children over 8 years: 15 mg/kg to 25 mg/kg, up to a maximum of 250 mg per single daily injection. Dosage may be divided and given at 8- to 12-hour intervals.

IV
Adults: 250 mg to 500 mg q12h; do not exceed 500 mg q6h.

Children over 8 years: 12 mg/kg/day, divided into two doses; from 10 mg/kg/day to 20 mg/kg/day may be given, depending on the severity of the infection.

TETRACYCLINE HYDROCHLORIDE
Oral
Adults: Usual dose is 1 g/day to 2 g/day in two to four equal doses, depending on severity of the infection.

Children over 8 years: Daily dose is 10 mg/lb to 20 mg/lb (25–50 mg/kg) in two to four equal doses.

Brucellosis: 500 mg four times a day for 3 weeks, accompanied by 1 g streptomycin IM twice a day the first week and once daily the second week.

Severe acne (long-term therapy): Initially, 1 g/day in divided doses. For maintenance, 125 mg/day to 500 mg/day.

CDC recommended treatment schedules for sexually transmitted diseases

Chlamydia trachomatis—Uncomplicated urethral, endocervical, or rectal infection in adults, 500 mg qid for 7 days.

Gonococcal infections—Uncomplicated gonococcal infections in adults, 500 mg qid for 7 days (total dose 14 g). In children over 8 years who are allergic to penicillin, 40 mg/kg/day in four divided doses for 5 days.

Disseminated gonococcal infections—500 mg qid for at least 7 days.

Nongonococcal urethritis—500 mg four times a day for at least 7 days.

Acute pelvic inflammatory disease—For ambulatory treatment, give 2 g cefoxitin IM, or 3 g oral amoxicillin, or 3.5 g oral ampicillin, or 4.8 million units aqueous procaine penicillin IM at 2 sites; each along with 1 g oral probenecid. Follow with 500 mg tetracycline four times a day.

Sexually transmitted epididymo-orchitis—500 mg four times a day for at least 10 days.

Syphilis in penicillin-allergic patients—For early syphilis, 500 mg four times a day for 15 days. For syphilis of more than 1 year's duration, 500 mg four times a day for 30 days.

Lymphogranuloma venereum—For genital, inguinal, or anorectal infections, 500 mg four times a day for at least 2 weeks.

Rape victims—For prophylaxis, 500 mg four times a day for at least 7 days.

IM
Adults: Usual daily dose is 250 mg once every 24 hours or 300 mg given in divided doses at 8- to 12-hour intervals.

Children over 8 years: 15 mg/kg to 25 mg/kg up to a maximum of 250 mg per single daily injection. Dosage may be divided and given at 8- to 12-hour intervals.

IV
Adults: 250 mg to 500 mg q12h; do not exceed 500 mg q6h.

Children over 8 years: 12 mg/kg/day divided into two doses; from 10 mg/kg/day to 20 mg/kg/day may be given, depending on the severity of the infection.

TETRACYCLINE HYDROCHLORIDE AND AMPHOTERICIN B
See Tetracycline.

TETRACYCLINE PHOSPHATE COMPLEX
See Tetracycline.

TETRACYCLINES AND NYSTATIN
See Tetracycline.

NURSING IMPLICATIONS

HISTORY
See Appendix 4.

PHYSICAL ASSESSMENT
Obtain vital signs, weight; record overt signs of infection; assess patient's general status, especially if patient is severely ill. Baseline laboratory tests may include culture and sensitivity tests, renal- and hepatic-function tests, darkfield examination and serology (if syphilis suspected), CBC.

ADMINISTRATION
Check expiration date on container or package. Do not use outdated products because the degradation products of tetracyclines are highly nephrotoxic.

Oral: Oral tetracyclines are given on an empty stomach, 1 hour before or 2 hours after meals. **Doxycycline** and **minocycline** may be given with food or milk.

Give with a full glass (8 oz) of water.

Simultaneous administration of tetracyclines and iron-containing products or laxatives is avoided. If these drugs are prescribed, schedule administration at least 2 hours before or after administration of a tetracycline.

T

Antacids are not administered before or with a tetracycline. If an antacid is prescribed, it must be given 3 hours after administration of a tetracycline.

IM: Oxytetracycline and tetracycline HCl are available for IM administration.

Inject deeply into a large muscle mass such as the gluteal region; take care not to injure the sciatic nerve or to inject intravascularly.

Rotate injection sites and record site used.

Inadvertent injection into subcutaneous or fat layers may cause pain and induration.

To decrease pain on injection, oxytetracycline and tetracycline contain lidocaine HCl or procaine HCl respectively.

Tetracycline—Add 2 ml of Sterile Water for Injection or Sodium Chloride Injection to the 100-mg or 250-mg vial. Store resulting solution at room temperature; do not use after 24 hours.

IV: Doxycycline, minocycline HCl, oxytetracycline HCl, and tetracycline HCl are available for IV administration.

Solutions stored under refrigeration are warmed to room temperature before administration.

Select a large vein, when possible, for IV infusion.

Rapid administration of these drugs is avoided. Physician must order rate of infusion.

DOXYCYCLINE

To prepare solution containing 10 mg/ml, reconstitute contents of the vial with 10 ml (for 100 mg/vial container) or 20 ml (for 200 mg/vial container) of Sterile Water for Injection or any of the IV solutions listed below. Dilute further with 100 ml to 1000 ml (200–2000 ml for 200-mg vial) of the following IV solutions:

Sodium Chloride Injection	5% Dextrose in Lactated Ringer's
5% Dextrose Injection	Normosol-M in D5-W
Ringer's Injection	Normosol-R in D5-W
10% Invert Sugar in Water	Plasma-Lyte 56 in 5% Dextrose
Lactated Ringer's Injection	Plasma-Lyte 148 in 5% Dextrose

This will result in desired concentrations of 0.1 mg/ml to 1 mg/ml. Concentrations less than 0.1 mg/ml or greater than 1 mg/ml are not recommended.

Infusion must be completed in 6 hours after reconstitution when drug is diluted with Lactated Ringer's or 5% Dextrose in Lactated Ringer's.

Infusion must be completed within 12 hours after reconstitution when drug is diluted with any other of the solutions listed above.

Reconstituted solutions may also be stored up to 72 hours prior to the start of the infusion if refrigerated and protected from sunlight and artificial light.

The duration of infusion may vary with the dose (100–200 mg/day) but is usually 1 to 4 hours. Physician must order IV solution for dilution and rate of infusion.

MINOCYCLINE

Drug is initially dissolved and then further diluted to 500 ml to 1000 ml with either Sodium Chloride Injection, Dextrose Injection, Dextrose and Sodium Chloride Injection, Ringer's Injection, or Lactated Ringer's Injection, but not in other solutions containing calcium because a precipitate may form.

Reconstituted solutions are stable at room temperature for 24 hours without significant loss of potency. Discard unused portions after that period. The final dilution for administration should be administered immediately.

Physician must order solution for dilution, volume of the diluent, and rate of infusion.

OXYTETRACYCLINE

Dissolve powder in 10 ml of Sterile Water for Injection or 5% Dextrose Injection. Then redilute to make at least 100 ml of 5% Dextrose in Water. Isotonic Sodium Chloride or Ringer's Solution may also be used.

Physician must order solution for dilution, volume of diluent and rate of infusion.

TETRACYCLINE HCl

Reconstitute 250-mg and 500-mg vials by adding 5 ml or 10 ml, respectively, of Sterile Water for Injection. Further dilute, prior to administration, to at least 100 ml (up to 1000 ml) with any of the following: Ringer's Injection; Sodium Chloride Injection; 5% Dextrose in Water for Injection; Dextrose and Sodium Chloride Injection (5% Sodium Chloride Injection); Lactated Ringer's Injection. Avoid use of solutions containing calcium because these tend to form precipitates (especially in neutral to alkaline solution). Ringer's and Lactated Ringer's can be used with caution because the calcium ion content in these diluents does not normally precipitate tetracycline in an acid medium.

The initial reconstituted solutions are stable at room temperature for 12 hours without significant loss of potency. Administer the final dilution immediately.

Achromycin IM and Achromycin IV; Terramycin IM and Terramycin IV.

ONGOING ASSESSMENTS AND NURSING MANAGEMENT
Monitor vital signs q4h or as ordered.

Observe for adverse reactions.

Observe for therapeutic drug effects (*e.g.,* decrease in temperature and other signs of infection).

Measure intake and output if patient has known renal or hepatic impairment, is febrile, or is acutely ill. Report any change in the intake–output ratio to the physician.

CLINICAL ALERT: Observe daily for signs of superinfection (Appendix 6, section 6-22): Inspect the oral cavity for black, hairy appearance of tongue and stomatitis; inspect anogenital region for inflammatory lesions; ask patient about itching in the vaginal or anogenital area. Notify physician immediately if one or more signs or symptoms are noted because appropriate measures (discontinuation of drug or institution of antifungal therapy) are usually necessary.

Diarrhea may be indicative of superinfection of the bowel by staphylococci, which may be life threatening. Notify the physician immediately if diarrhea occurs, because it will be necessary to distinguish between a staphylococcal infection and diarrhea due to other causes. A stool culture may be ordered.

Prolonged IV administration may result in thrombophlebitis. Inspect site of needle insertion and vein pathway daily for redness, tenderness, swelling, and induration; notify the physician if these occur and change IV site to a different extremity.

Ataxia, vertigo, nausea, and vomiting have occurred in a large percentage of patients receiving **minocycline.** If vestibular disturbances are noted, inform physician and assist patient with ambulatory activities.

Renal- and hepatic-function tests may be monitored during intensive IV treatment. Serum tetracycline concentrations may also be obtained and should not exceed 15 mcg/ml.

Administration of a tetracycline is usually continued for 24 to 72 hours after fever and other symptoms of infection have subsided.

PATIENT AND FAMILY INFORMATION
Complete the full course of therapy. Do not stop taking the drug, even if symptoms have improved, unless advised to do so by the physician.

Take on an empty stomach at least 1 hour before or 2 hours after meals. Doxycycline and minocycline may be taken with food or milk.

Take each dose with a full glass (8 oz) of water.

Avoid simultaneous ingestion of dairy products (milk, cheese), antacids, laxatives, or iron-containing products. If a laxative or iron-containing product (including multivitamins, iron tablets) has been prescribed or recommended, take it at least 2 hours before or after taking this drug. If an antacid has been prescribed or recommended, take it at least 3 hours after taking this drug.

Minocycline may cause vertigo or ataxia. Observe caution while driving or performing other potentially hazardous tasks.

Notify the physician immediately if any of the following occurs: nausea, vomiting, diarrhea, skin manifestations (*e.g.,* rash, itching, hives), sore mouth or throat, black hairy tongue, vaginal or rectal itching.

Avoid prolonged exposure to sunlight and ultraviolet light because drug (especially demeclocycline) may cause a photosensitivity reaction.

If a portion of the prescription is left over, discard the tablets, capsules, or liquid because the tetracyclines deteriorate with time and use may result in renal damage.

Tetracyclines and Nystatin

See Tetracyclines.

Tetrahydrozoline Hydrochloride

See Decongestants, Nasal, Topical; Mydriatics/Ophthalmic Vasoconstrictors.

Theophylline

See Bronchodilators and Decongestants, Systemic.

Theophylline Sodium Glycinate

See Bronchodilators and Decongestants, Systemic.

Thiabendazole Rx

tablets, chewable: 500 mg	Mintezol
oral suspension: 500 mg/5 ml	Mintezol

T

INDICATIONS

Treatment of enterobiasis (pinworm infection), strongyloidiasis (threadworm infection), ascariasis (roundworm infection), uncinariasis (hookworm infection), trichuriasis (whipworm infection), and cutaneous larva migrans (creeping eruption). Therapeutic effect of this drug in trichuriasis is limited. Also indicated for alleviating symptoms of trichinosis during the invasive phase of the disease.

CONTRAINDICATIONS

Hypersensitivity.

ACTIONS

Is vermicidal against *Enterobius vermicularis* (pinworm), *Ascariasis lumbricoides* (roundworm), *Strongyloides stercoralis* (threadworm), *Necator americanus* and *Ancylostoma duodenale* (hookworm), *Trichuris trichuria* (whipworm), and *Ancylostoma braziliense* (dog and cat hookworm). Its effect on larvae of *Trichinella spiralis* that have migrated to muscle is questionable. Also suppresses egg and/or larval production and may inhibit subsequent development of those eggs or larvae that are passed in the feces. Although the exact mechanism is unknown, the drug has been shown to inhibit the helmintic-specific enzyme fumarate reductase. The anthelmintic activity against *Trichuris trichuria* (whipworm) is least predictable.

The drug is rapidly absorbed and peak plasma concentration is reached 1 to 2 hours after the dose. It is metabolized almost completely and excreted mainly in the urine, with a small amount excreted in feces. Most is excreted in the first 24 hours.

WARNINGS

If hypersensitivity reactions occur, drug is discontinued immediately. Erythema multiforme has been associated with therapy; in severe cases (*i.e.,* Stevens-Johnson syndrome), fatalities have occurred. Safety for use in pregnancy and lactation is not established.

PRECAUTIONS

Supportive therapy is indicated for anemic, dehydrated, or malnourished patients before initiation of therapy. In the presence of hepatic or renal dysfunction, patient is monitored closely.

ADVERSE REACTIONS

Most frequent: Anorexia, nausea, vomiting, dizziness.

Less frequent: Diarrhea, epigastric distress, pruritus, fatigue, weariness, drowsiness, giddiness, headache.

Rare: Tinnitus; hyperirritability; numbness; abnormal sensation in the eyes, blurred vision, xanthopsia; bradycardia; hypotension; collapse; enuresis; transient rise in SGOT; jaundice, cholestasis, and parenchymal liver damage; hyperglycemia; transient leukopenia; perianal rash; malodor of the urine, crystalluria, hematuria; appearance of live *Ascaris* in the mouth and nose.

Hypersensitivity: Fever, facial flush, chills, conjunctival injection, angioedema, anaphylaxis, skin rashes, erythema multiforme (including Stevens-Johnson syndrome), lymphadenopathy.

DOSAGE

Size of the dose is determined by the patient's weight. For patients weighing less than 150 lb, give 10 mg/lb. For patients weighing more than 150 lb, give 1.5 g.

The dosage regimen for each indication is given in Table 49.

NURSING IMPLICATIONS

HISTORY

See Appendix 4. A careful history of travel, eating habits, and sanitary facilities may be necessary to determine source of roundworm, thread-

Table 49. Dosage Regimens of Thiabendazole Based on Indication for Use

Indication	Regimen	Comments
Intestinal parasitosis Enterobiasis (pinworm infection)	2 doses/day for 1 day; repeated in 7 days	If impractical, give 2 doses/day for 2 successive days
Strongyloidiasis Ascariasis Uncinariasis Trichuriasis	2 doses/day for 2 successive days	Single dose of 20 mg/lb may also be used, but higher incidence of side-effects should be expected
Cutaneous larva migrans	2 doses/day for 2 successive days	If active lesions still present 2 days after end of therapy, a second course is recommended
Trichinosis	2 doses/day for 2 to 4 successive days according to patient response	Optimal dosage not established

worm, hookworm, whipworm, or trichinosis infection. A history of animal (cat, dog) handling or contact is necessary for dog and cat hookworm and cutaneous larva migrans. Because pinworms are easily transmitted from person to person it is recommended that all members of the family be treated for complete parasite eradication.

PHYSICAL ASSESSMENT

Obtain weight. For severe infections, obtain vital signs and evaluate patient's general physical status. Stool is examined for roundworm, threadworm, hookworm, whipworm. Pinworm specimen may be collected (in early A.M. before patient gets out of bed) by means of a cellophane tape wrapped sticky side out around a tongue blade; press against the anal area (female pinworms deposit ova at night in the perianal area). Transfer tape (sticky side down) to glass slide for microscopic examination. For cutaneous larva migrans, examine and describe skin lesions (tunnel-like meandering or linear red lines). Look for crusting and signs of a secondary infection. In severe infections or the acutely ill patient, baseline laboratory tests may include CBC, serum electrolytes.

ADMINISTRATION

Dietary restriction, complementary medications, and cleansing enemas are not necessary.

Give with food to minimize GI distress.

Instruct patient to chew tablets thoroughly before swallowing.

For young children and those unable to chew tablets properly, an oral suspension is available.

ONGOING ASSESSMENTS AND NURSING MANAGEMENT

If patient is acutely ill or has a severe infection, obtain vital signs q4h or as ordered.

Isolation is usually not necessary; stool and linen precautions are usually instituted. Wash hands thoroughly before and after each patient contact, especially when disposing of urine or feces or changing bed linens.

Observe for adverse reactions (nausea, vomiting, anorexia, and dizziness are most common adverse effects) and, if they are severe, notify physician.

May produce drowsiness or dizziness. Patient may require assistance with ambulatory activities.

Patient with cutaneous larva migrans may experience severe itching.

Patient with threadworm may be acutely ill. Measure intake and output and notify physician of any change in the intake–output ratio. IV fluids, blood transfusion (for anemia), and a high-protein diet may also be ordered.

PATIENT AND FAMILY INFORMATION

May cause GI upset; take with food.

Chew tablets thoroughly before swallowing.

May produce drowsiness or dizziness; observe caution while driving or performing other tasks requiring alertness.

Follow-up examinations of stool may be necessary (*exceptions*—pinworm, cutaneous larva migrans, and trichinosis).

Wash hands thoroughly before eating and after defecation.

Pinworm: Meticulous hygiene is necessary to prevent reinfection. Change and launder undergarments, bed linens, towels, and nightclothes daily. Disinfect toilet facilities (including bathtub/shower) daily.

Clean fingernails daily. Avoid putting fingers in mouth; nail biting must be avoided (liquid preparations that have a bitter taste and are painted on the nails and fingertips to discourage nail biting are available if patient persists in biting nails).

Roundworm: Thoroughly wash all vegetables grown in contaminated soil.

Bathe daily; change undergarments and bed linens daily.

Threadworm and hookworm: Wear shoes when outdoors (in endemic areas).

Dispose of contaminated feces properly.

Whipworm: Dispose of contaminated feces properly.

Avoid handling contaminated soil, when possible. Keep small children away from areas with contaminated soil.

Trichinosis: Cook all pork, pork products, and meat from carnivores thoroughly.

Avoid eating pork in known endemic areas.

Larva migrans: Household pets should be checked yearly (or as recommended by the veterinarian) for intestinal parasites.

Wear shoes in areas of possible contamination with dog and cat feces.

Thiamine Hydrochloride

See Vitamin B_1.

Thiamylal Sodium

See Anesthetics, General, Barbiturates.

Thiazides and Related Diuretics

Bendroflumethiazide Rx

tablets: 2.5 mg, 5 mg, 10 mg	Naturetin (contains tartrazine)

Benzthiazide Rx

tablets: 25 mg	Aquatag
tablets: 50 mg	Aquatag (contains tartrazine), Exna (contains tartrazine), Hydrex, Marazide, Proaqua (contains tartrazine), Generic

Chlorothiazide Rx

tablets: 250 mg	Diachlor, SK-Chlorothiazide, Generic
tablets: 500 mg	Diachlor, Diuril, SK-Chlorothiazide, Generic
oral suspension: 250 mg/5 ml	Diuril
powder for injection: 500 mg (as sodium) per 20-ml vial	Diuril

Chlorthalidone Rx

tablets: 25 mg	Hygroton, Hylidone, Thalitone, Generic
tablets: 50 mg, 100 mg	Hygroton, Hylidone, Generic

Cyclothiazide Rx

tablets: 2 mg	Anhydron, Fluidil

Hydrochlorothiazide Rx

tablets: 25 mg	Esidrix, HydroDiuril, Hydro-T, Oretic, SK-Hydrochlorothiazide, Thiuretic, Generic
tablets: 50 mg	Aquazide H, Chlorzide, Diaqua, Diu-Scrip, Esidrix, Hydro-Chlor, HydroDiuril, Hydromal, Hydro-T, Hydro-Z-50, Mictrin, Oretic, SK-Hydrochlorothiazide, Thiuretic, Zide, Generic

tablets: 100 mg	Esidrix, HydroDiuril, Hydro-T, Generic

Hydroflumethiazide Rx

tablets: 50 mg	Diucardin, Saluron, Generic

Indapamide Rx

tablets: 2.5 mg	Lozol

Methyclothiazide Rx

tablets: 2.5 mg	Enduron, Ethon, Generic
tablets: 5 mg	Aquatensen, Enduron, Ethon, Generic

Metolazone Rx

tablets: 2.5 mg, 5 mg, 10 mg	Diulo, Zaroxolyn

Polythiazide Rx

tablets: 1 mg, 2 mg, 4 mg	Renese

Quinethazone Rx

tablets: 50 mg	Hydromox

Trichlormethiazide Rx

tablets: 2 mg	Metahydrin, Naqua, Generic
tablets: 4 mg	Aquazide, Diurese, Metahydrin, Mono-Press, Naqua, Niazide, Trichlorex, Generic

INDICATIONS

Edema: Adjunctive therapy in edema associated with congestive heart failure (CHF), hepatic cirrhosis, and corticosteroid and estrogen therapy. Useful in edema due to renal dysfunction (*i.e.,* nephrotic syndrome, acute glomerulonephritis, and chronic renal failure). **Indapamide** is indicated for edema associated with CHF.

Hypertension: Either as the sole therapeutic agent or to enhance other antihypertensive drugs.

Unlabeled uses: Thiazide diuretics have been used (alone and in combination with amiloride and allopurinol) to prevent formation and recurrence of calcium stones in hypercalciuric and normally calciuric patients. The thiazides correct hypercalciuria, reduce urinary saturation, enhance inhibitor activity against spontaneous nucleation of both calcium oxalate and brushite, and restore normal parathyroid function and intestinal calcium absorption. Doses used have been hydrochlorothiazide 50 mg, one or two times a day; trichloromethiazide 4 mg/day; chlorthalidone 50 mg/day; and metolazone 2.5 mg/ day to 10 mg/day. In diabetes insipidus, thiazide diuretics reduce urine volume by 30% to 50%. Although these agents play an adjuvant role in neurogenic diabetes insipidus, they are the only drug therapy available for nephrogenic diabetes insipidus.

CONTRAINDICATIONS

Anuria, renal decompensation, hypersensitivity to thiazides or sulfonamides. Metolazone is contraindicated in those with hepatic coma or precoma.

ACTIONS

Thiazide diuretics increase the renal excretion of sodium and chloride. They inhibit tubular reabsorption of sodium and chloride by direct action on the distal segment. All of these compounds possess some degree of carbonic anhydrase inhibition activity because of the sulfonamide moiety. Other common actions include increased potassium excretion, decreased calcium excretion, and uric acid retention. At maximal therapeutic doses all thiazides are approximately equal in their diuretic efficacy, except that metolazone may be more effective in those with impaired renal function. Metolazone, quinethazone, chlorthalidone, and indapamide are not thiazide derivatives but are included here because of their structural and pharmacologic similarity to the thiazides.

The exact mechanism of the antihypertensive action of the thiazides is unknown, although it may result from an altered sodium balance. During initial therapy, cardiac output decreases and blood volume diminishes. With chronic therapy, cardiac output normalizes, peripheral vascular resistance falls, and there is a persistent small reduction in extracellular water and plasma volume.

In hypertensive patients, daily doses of indapamide have no appreciable cardiac inotropic or chronotropic effect and little or no effect on glomerular filtration rate or renal plasma flow. The drug decreases peripheral resistance, with little or no effect on cardiac output, rate, or rhythm. Vascular action may also be due to an alteration of transmembrane calcium currents. Indapamide had an antihypertensive effect in patients with varying degrees of renal impairment, although in general, diuretic effects declined as renal function decreased.

The onset, peak, and duration of diuretic action for each thiazide are given in Table 50. The antihypertensive action requires several days to produce effects. Administration for up to 3 to 4 weeks is usually required for optimal therapeutic effect. The duration of the antihypertensive effect of the thiazides

Table 50. Onset, Peak, and Duration of Diuretic Action of the Thiazides and Related Diuretics

Agent	Onset (hr)	Peak (hr)	Duration (hr)
Bendroflumethiazide	2	4	6–12
Benzthiazide	2	4–6	6–12
Chlorothiazide	1–2	4	6–12
Chlorthalidone	2	2–6	24–72
Cyclothiazide	Within 6	7–12	18–24
Hydrochlorothiazide	2	4–6	6–12
Hydroflumethiazide	2	4	6–12
Indapamide	1–2	Within 2	Up to 36
Methyclothiazide	2	6	24
Metolazone	1	2	12–24
Polythiazide	2	6	24–48
Quinethazone	2	6	18–24
Trichlormethiazide	2	6	24

is sufficiently long to provide adequate control of blood pressure with a single daily dose.

WARNINGS

Parenteral use: IV **chlorothiazide** is used only when patient is unable to take oral medication or in emergency situations. IV use in infants and children has been limited and is not recommended.

Impaired renal function: Use with caution in severe renal disease because thiazides may precipitate azotemia. Cumulative effects may develop in those with impaired renal function. If progressive renal impairment becomes evident, as indicated by a rising nonprotein nitrogen (NPN) or BUN, drug may be withheld or therapy discontinued.

Impaired hepatic function: Use with caution in those with impaired hepatic function or progressive liver disease, because minor alterations of fluid and electrolyte balance may precipitate hepatic coma.

Hypersensitivity reactions may occur in those with a history of allergy or bronchial asthma. Cross-sensitivity with sulfonamides may also occur.

Lupus: Exacerbation or activation of systemic lupus erythematosus has been reported.

Pregnancy: Routine use during normal pregnancy is inappropriate and exposes the mother and fetus to unnecessary hazards. Thiazides cross the placental barrier and appear in cord blood. These drugs are used only when clearly needed and when potential benefits outweigh the unknown potential hazards to the fetus. These hazards include fetal or neonatal jaundice, thrombocytopenia, altered carbohydrate metabolism, and possibly other adverse reactions that have occurred in the adult. Thiazides are indicated in pregnancy when edema is due to pathologic causes.

Lactation: Thiazides appear in breast milk. If use

T

of drug is deemed essential, the patient should stop nursing.

Use in children: Until additional data are obtained, **metolazone** is not recommended for use in children.

PRECAUTIONS

Fluid and electrolyte status: Periodic determinations of serum electrolytes, BUN, uric acid, and glucose levels are recommended. Serum and urine electrolyte determinations are particularly important when patient is vomiting excessively or receiving parenteral fluids. Medication such as **digitalis** may also influence serum electrolytes.

Hypokalemia: May develop, especially with brisk diuresis, when severe cirrhosis is present, during concomitant use of **corticosteroids** or **ACTH,** or after prolonged therapy. Inadequate oral electrolyte intake will also contribute to hypokalemia. Hypokalemia can sensitize or exaggerate the response of the heart to the toxic effects of **digitalis** (*e.g.,* increased ventricular irritability). Ventricular arrhythmias may also develop in nondigitalized patients. Hypokalemia is avoided or treated with potassium-sparing diuretics, potassium supplements, or foods high in potassium content.

Sodium and chloride: A chloride deficit is generally mild and usually does not require specific treatment except under extraordinary circumstances (as in liver or renal disease). However, treatment of metabolic or hypochloremic alkalosis may require chloride replacement. Dilutional hyponatremia may occur in edematous patients in hot weather; appropriate therapy is water restriction, rather than administration of salt, except in rare instances when the hyponatremia is life threatening. In actual salt depletion, appropriate replacement is the therapy of choice.

Calcium: Calcium excretion is decreased by thiazides. Thiazides may cause intermittent and slight elevation of serum calcium in the absence of disorders of calcium metabolism. Values return to normal when the medication is stopped. Common complications of hyperparathyroidism such as renal lithiasis, bone resorption, and peptic ulceration have not been seen.

Hypercalcemia induced by thiazides has aggravated manic-depressive episodes previously controlled with lithium.

Hyperuricemia: Hyperuricemia may occur or frank gout may be precipitated in certain individuals receiving thiazide therapy.

Glucose tolerance: Insulin requirements in diabetic patients may be increased, decreased, or unchanged. Latent diabetes mellitus may become manifest during thiazide administration; diabetic

complications, such as reversible oculomotor paresis, may occur.

Tartrazine sensitivity: Some of these products contain tartrazine. See Appendix 6, section 6-23.

Antihypertensive effects may be enhanced in the postsympathectomy patient.

DRUG INTERACTIONS

Thiazides may add to or potentiate the action of **other antihypertensive drugs.** Orthostatic hypotension may be aggravated by **alcohol, barbiturates,** or **narcotics.** Potentiation occurs with **ganglionic** or **peripheral adrenergic blocking agents.**

Indomethacin may attenuate the hypotensive response to thiazide diuretics. **Cholestyramine** and **colestipol** decrease the absorption of thiazides.

Hypokalemia is more likely to develop during concomitant use of **corticosteroids** or **ACTH.** Diuretic-induced hypokalemia may precipitate **digitalis** toxicity. Thiazides may increase the responsiveness to **tubocurarine.** Thiazides may decrease arterial responsiveness to **norepinephrine,** but not enough to preclude effectiveness of the pressor agent for therapeutic use.

Dosage adjustment of **antidiabetic agents** is frequently indicated during thiazide therapy. Generally, **lithium** is not given with diuretics because diuretics reduce lithium renal clearance and add a high risk of lithium toxicity.

Concomitant administration of hydrochlorothiazide and **calcium carbonate** has been associated with hypercalcemia. Unusually large or prolonged effects on volume and electrolytes may result when **metolazone** and **furosemide** are administered concurrently. **Quinidine,** a weak base, may have its half-life prolonged by concomitant administration of thiazide diuretics, which alkalinize the urine. **Sulfonamides** may potentiate the action of thiazides, possibly by displacement from binding sites on plasma albumin. The effects of antihypertensive agents, including the thiazide diuretics, may be potentiated by **fenfluramine.**

Laboratory test alterations: Thiazides may alter various laboratory test results. These include all electrolytes, particularly potassium, BUN, uric acid, glucose, and protein-bound iodine (PBI). Thiazides may decrease serum PBI levels without signs of thyroid disturbance.

ADVERSE REACTIONS

GI: Anorexia, gastric irritation, nausea, vomiting, cramping, abdominal bloating, diarrhea, constipation, jaundice (intrahepatic and cholestatic), pancreatitis, sialadenitis, hepatitis, dry mouth.

GU: Frequent urination, nocturia, polyuria.

Acute interstitial nephritis (rare), impotence, reduced libido.

CNS: Dizziness, vertigo, headache, paresthesias, xanthopsia, weakness, restlessness sometimes resulting in insomnia, syncope, drowsiness, fatigue. **Indapamide**—Greater than 5%, headache, dizziness, fatigue, weakness, loss of energy, lethargy, tiredness, malaise, anxiety, irritability, agitation; less than 5%, lightheadedness, drowsiness, vertigo, insomnia, depression, blurred vision, tingling of the extremities.

Hematologic: Leukopenia, thrombocytopenia, agranulocytosis, aplastic anemia, hemolytic anemia, neutropenia.

Cardiovascular: Orthostatic hypotension (may be aggravated by alcohol, barbiturates, or narcotics), venous thrombosis, excessive volume depletion, hemoconcentration, palpitation, chest pain, premature ventricular contractions, irregular heartbeat.

Hypersensitivity: Purpura, photosensitivity, rash, urticaria, necrotizing angiitis (vasculitis, cutaneous vasculitis), toxic epidermal necrolysis, Stevens-Johnson syndrome, fever, respiratory distress including pneumonitis and pulmonary edema, anaphylactic reactions, allergic glomerulonephritis, hives, pruritus.

Musculoskeletal: Muscle cramps or spasm.

Miscellaneous: Acute gouty attacks, transient blurred vision, chills, rhinorrhea, flushing, weight loss.

Clinical laboratory test findings: Hypercalcemia, metabolic acidosis in diabetic patients, symptomatic and asymptomatic hypokalemia, hyponatremia, hypochloremia, hypochloremic alkalosis, hypophosphatemia, hyperuricemia, increase in BUN, elevation of creatinine, hyperglycemia, glycosuria, decreased PBI levels. Increases in plasma levels of total cholesterol, triglycerides and LDL cholesterol (but not HDL cholesterol) has been seen with **chlorthalidone** therapy. Clinical hypokalemia occurred in 3% and 7% of those given **indapamide** 2.5 mg and 5 mg respectively.

Fluid/electrolyte imbalance: There have been isolated reports that certain nonedematous individuals developed severe fluid and electrolyte derangements after only brief exposure to normal doses of thiazide and nonthiazide diuretics. This is usually manifested as severe dilutional hyponatremia, hypokalemia, and hypochloremia. It has been reported to be due to inappropriately increased ADH secretion and appears to be idiosyncratic. Potassium replacement is apparently the most important therapy in treatment, along with removal of the offending drug.

The adverse reactions associated with **indapamide** occurred in fewer than 5% of patients, except as indicated above.

OVERDOSAGE

Symptoms: Electrolyte imbalance, signs of potassium deficiency, nausea. In severe cases, hypotension and depressed respiration may occur. Lethargy of varying degrees may progress to coma within a few hours, with minimal depression of respiration and cardiovascular function and without significant serum electrolyte changes or dehydration. Temporary BUN elevations and seizures have also been reported.

Treatment: Perform gastric lavage or induce emesis; give activated charcoal. Prevent aspiration. GI effects are usually of short duration but may require symptomatic treatment. Maintain hydration, electrolyte balance, respiration, and cardiovascular–renal function. Asymptomatic hyperuricemia usually responds to fluids, but if clinical gout is suspected, indomethacin may be given. Support respiration and cardiac circulation if hypotension and depressed respiration occur.

DOSAGE

Therapy is individualized according to patient response. Dosage is titrated to gain maximal therapeutic response at the minimal dose possible.

Edema: Intermittent therapy may be advantageous in many patients. By giving the drug every other day, or on a 3 to 5 day/week schedule, electrolyte imbalance is less likely to occur.

Hypertension: To prevent excessive hypotension, dosage of other agents is reduced by at least 50% as soon as thiazides are added to the regimen. As blood pressure falls, a further reduction in dosage or even discontinuation of other agents may be necessary.

Renal impairment: Metolazone is the only thiazidelike diuretic that may have significant activity if the serum creatinine is greater than 2 mg/dl. In such instances, a loop diuretic would be more effective.

BENDROFLUMETHIAZIDE

Edema: 5 mg once daily, preferably in the morning. To initiate therapy, up to 20 mg may be given once daily or divided into two doses. A single daily dose of 2.5 mg to 5 mg should be sufficient for maintenance.

Hypertension: Initial dosage is 5 mg/day to 20 mg/day. Maintenance dosage ranges from 2.5 mg/day to 15 mg/day.

BENZTHIAZIDE

Edema

Initiation of diuresis: 50 mg to 200 mg daily for several days or until dry weight is attained. When dosages exceed 100 mg daily, it is preferable to give in two doses, following morning and evening meals.

Maintenance: 50 mg/day to 150 mg/day.

Hypertension

Initiation of therapy: 50 mg to 100 mg daily. It may be given in two doses of 25 mg or 50 mg each, after breakfast and after lunch. This dosage may be continued until a therapeutic drop in blood pressure occurs.

Maintenance: Dosage is adjusted according to response. Maximal effective dose is 200 mg/day.

CHLOROTHIAZIDE

Bioavailability studies demonstrate that a saturable absorption of chlorothiazide occurs. Doses greater than 250 mg do not produce an increased effect. Chlorothiazide, 250 mg once every 6 to 12 hours produces a greater diuresis than doses greater than 250 mg administered at one time.

Edema: Usual adult dosage is 0.5 g to 2 g once or twice a day, PO or IV. IV therapy is reserved for patients unable to take oral medication or for emergency situations.

Hypertension (oral forms only): Usual adult starting dose is 0.5 g/day to 2 g/day as a single or divided dose. Dosage is adjusted according to blood pressure response. Rarely, some patients may require up to 2 g/day in divided doses.

Infants and children: IV use in children and infants is not generally recommended. Usual oral pediatric dose is based on 10 mg/lb/day in two doses. Infants under 6 months may require up to 15 mg/lb/day in two doses. On this basis, infants up to 2 years may be given 125 mg/day to 375 mg/day in two doses. Children from 2 to 12 years may be given 375 mg/day to 1 g/day in two doses.

CHLORTHALIDONE

Give a single dose with food in the morning.

Edema: Therapy is initiated with 50 mg/day to 100 mg/day, or 100 mg on alternate days. Some patients may require 150 mg to 200 mg at these intervals, or up to 200 mg/day. Doses above this level do not usually produce greater response.

Hypertension: Therapy is instituted with a single dose of 25 mg/day. If response is insufficient after a suitable trial, dosage is increased to 50 mg. If additional control is required, dosage is increased to 100 mg once a day or a second antihypertensive agent is added. Dosage above 100 mg/day does not usually increase effectiveness. Increases in serum uric acid and decreases in serum potassium are dose related over the 25 mg/day to 100 mg/day range.

CYCLOTHIAZIDE

Edema: Usual adult dosage is 1 mg or 2 mg once a day, preferably in the morning. After edema is

eliminated, dosage is reduced according to patient's need. *Maintenance therapy*—1 mg to 2 mg given on alternate days or 2 to 3 times a week may be sufficient.

Hypertension: 2 mg once a day; occasionally 4 mg to 6 mg may be necessary.

HYDROCHLOROTHIAZIDE

Edema: Initially, 25 mg to 200 mg daily for several days, or until dry weight is attained. *Maintenance*—25 mg to 100 mg daily or intermittently. Refractory cases may require up to 200 mg daily.

Hypertension: Initially, 50 mg to 100 mg daily as a single or divided dose. Maintenance may range from 25 mg to 100 mg daily. Rarely, some patients may require up to 200 mg daily in divided doses.

Infants and children: Usual dose is based on 1 mg/lb daily in two doses. Infants under 6 months may require up to 1.5 mg/lb daily in two doses. Infants up to 2 years may be given 12.5 mg to 37.5 mg daily in two doses. Children 2 to 12 years may be given 37.5 mg to 100 mg daily in two doses.

HYDROFLUMETHIAZIDE

Edema: Initial dose is 50 mg once or twice a day. *Maintenance dose*—25 mg/day to 200 mg/day. Give in divided doses when dosages exceed 100 mg/day.

Hypertension: Initial dose is 50 mg bid. *Maintenance*—50 mg/day to 100 mg/day. Dosage should not exceed 200 mg/day.

INDAPAMIDE

Hypertension and edema of congestive heart failure for adults: 2.5 mg as a single daily dose taken in the morning. If response is not satisfactory after 1 (edema) to 4 (hypertension) weeks, daily dosage may be increased to 5 mg once daily. If the antihypertensive response is insufficient, indapamide may be given with other antihypertensives. The usual dose of other agents is reduced by 50% during initial combination therapy. Further dosage adjustments may be necessary. In general, doses of 5 mg and greater have not provided additional effects on blood pressure or heart failure but are associated with a greater degree of hypokalemia.

METHYCLOTHIAZIDE

Edema: Usual adult dose ranges from 2.5 mg to 10 mg once daily. Maximum effective single dose is 10 mg.

Hypertension: Usual adult dose ranges from 2.5 mg to 5 mg once daily. If control of blood pressure is not satisfactory after 8 to 12 weeks with 5 mg once daily, another antihypertensive drug should be added.

METOLAZONE
Edema of cardiac failure: 5 mg to 10 mg once daily.
Edema of renal disease: 5 mg to 20 mg once daily.
Mild to moderate essential hypertension: 2.5 mg to 5 mg once daily.

For those with cardiac failure who tend to experience paroxysmal nocturnal dyspnea, it is usually advisable to employ a dosage near the upper end of the range to ensure prolongation of diuresis and saluresis for a full 24-hour period.

POLYTHIAZIDE
Edema: 1 mg to 4 mg daily.
Hypertension: 2 mg to 4 mg daily.

QUINETHAZONE
For use in adults. 50 mg to 100 mg once daily. Occasionally, 150 mg to 200 mg daily may be necessary.

TRICHLORMETHIAZIDE
Edema: 1 mg to 4 mg daily.
Hypertension: 2 mg to 4 mg daily.

NURSING IMPLICATIONS

HISTORY
See Appendix 4.

PHYSICAL ASSESSMENT
Obtain blood pressure in both arms with patient in sitting and supine positions; obtain pulse, respiratory rate, weight. If patient has edema, identify areas involved and determine degree and extent of edema. Baseline laboratory studies may include serum electrolytes, serum uric acid, renal- and hepatic-function studies, CBC. Urine electrolyte determinations may be performed if patient is vomiting excessively or receiving parenteral fluids.

ADMINISTRATION
Give with food or milk to prevent GI distress.

Daily doses are given in the morning (usually with or immediately after breakfast) so that the diuretic effect occurs during waking hours.

Before therapy is initiated, advise patient that frequent urination usually occurs. For expected onset of diuresis, see Table 50.

If used as an antihypertensive agent, obtain blood pressure and pulse immediately before administration. Withhold drug and notify physician if there is a significant decrease in the systolic or diastolic pressure.

CHLOROTHIAZIDE
Parenteral solution is prepared by adding 18 ml of Sterile Water for Injection to the vial to form an isotonic solution for IV injection. Never add less than 18 ml. The resulting total volume in the vial will be 20 ml (25 mg/ml).

Unused solution may be stored at room temperature for 24 hours, after which it must be discarded.

The solution is compatible with dextrose or sodium chloride solution for IV infusion.

Physician must order rate of IV infusion.

Avoid administration with whole blood or its derivatives.

Do not give IM or subcutaneously.

Check needle site q15m because extravasation must be avoided.

Diuresis usually begins in approximately 15 minutes.

Measure and record intake and output q15m to q30m or as ordered. Notify physician if diuresis fails to occur. The acutely ill patient may require an indwelling catheter inserted prior to administration of the IV infusion.

ONGOING ASSESSMENTS AND NURSING MANAGEMENT
Obtain blood pressure and pulse daily to q4h depending on reason for use. Use same arm and same position each time blood pressure is obtained.

Body weight is a useful guide in adjusting dosage for edema.

Weigh daily, preferably early in the morning before breakfast. Notify physician before next dose is due if there is a significant decrease in weight (_i.e.,_ more than 1 lb/day). In some instances, a weight loss of more than 1 lb/day may be desirable.

Measure intake and output, especially during initial therapy. Notify physician if there is a decrease in urinary output or if there is any change in the intake–output ratio.

Provide patient on bedrest with a call light and, when necessary, a bedpan or urinal.

If orthostatic hypotension occurs, some ambulatory patients may require assistance getting out of bed or walking, especially early in therapy.

Check areas of edema daily and compare with data base. Record findings.

Observe for adverse effects and report occurrence to the physician. Whenever adverse reactions are moderate to severe, dosage is usually reduced or drug discontinued.

Be sure patient (especially the elderly) has an adequate fluid intake and fluids are readily accessible and within reach.

CLINICAL ALERT: Observe for clinical signs of fluid or electrolyte imbalance: hypokalemia (Appendix 6, section 6-15), hyponatremia (Appendix 6, section 6-17), hypochloremic alkalosis, hypomagnesemia (Appendix 6, section 6-16), and dehydration (Appendix 6, section 6-10). Warning signs of imbalance, irrespective of cause, are dry mouth, thirst, weakness, lethargy, drowsiness, restlessness, muscle pains or cramps, muscular fatigue, hypotension, oliguria, tachycardia, and GI disturbances. Notify physician immediately if one or more signs of fluid or electrolyte imbalance are apparent.

Patients receiving concomitant **digitalis preparations** are observed for signs of digitalis toxicity (p 248) (*e.g.,* increased ventricular irritability). Ventricular arrhythmias may also occur in nondigitalized patients.

Hypokalemia may occur with brisk diuresis, when severe cirrhosis is present, during concomitant use of **corticosteroids** or **ACTH,** or after prolonged therapy.

Thiazide-induced hyponatremia has been associated with death and neurologic damage in elderly patients. CNS manifestations include seizures, coma, and extensor plantar response. The elderly patient must be observed closely, especially during initial therapy or when brisk diuresis occurs.

Report excessive vomiting to physician immediately because serum electrolyte determinations may be necessary.

Adequate intake of potassium either by diet or by potassium supplements is usually necessary to prevent hypokalemia. Inform physician if patient's dietary intake is poor. This is especially important in those experiencing brisk diuresis and those who have not attained dry weight.

When another antihypertensive agent is added to the therapeutic regimen, monitor blood pressure q4h or as ordered during initial therapy.

Monitor current serum electrolyte determinations; report abnormal values to physician immediately.

The antihypertensive effect of these agents requires several days before effects are noted. Administration for 3 to 4 weeks is usually required for optimal therapeutic effect.

The serum uric acid level may be increased. Those with a history of gout may have an acute flare-up of the disease.

Thiazide diuretics are discontinued before performing tests for parathyroid function.

Diabetic patient: Notify physician if glycosuria or ketonuria occurs because insulin dosage may require adjustment.

PATIENT AND FAMILY INFORMATION

NOTE: If drug is used as an antihypertensive, physician may wish the patient or a family member to monitor the blood pressure and pulse. Instruction in the proper technique will be required.

May cause GI upset; take with food or milk or immediately after meals.

Drug will increase urination; take early in the morning (*exception*—when prescribed bid after breakfast and evening meal).

Notify physician or nurse if muscle weakness or cramps, nausea, vomiting, dizziness, dry mouth, thirst, general weakness, rapid pulse, or GI distress occurs.

May cause orthostatic hypotension, especially during early therapy. Rise from a sitting or lying position slowly and avoid tasks that are potentially hazardous if dizziness occurs.

Weigh self weekly (or as recommended by the physician) in the morning immediately after arising. Keep a record of weight and bring to physician's office or clinic. Notify physician if weight loss exceeds 3 to 4 lb/week.

Inform other physicians of therapy with this drug.

Periodic laboratory tests are usually necessary to monitor therapy.

Diabetic patient: Check urine more frequently (at least daily), especially early in therapy. If an increase in glucose in the urine occurs, notify physician immediately. Hypoglycemic reactions are also brought to the immediate attention of the physician.

Thiethylperazine Maleate

See Antiemetic/Antivertigo Agents.

Thimerosal

See Antiseptics and Germicides.

Thioguanine (TG, 6-Thioguanine) Rx

tablets: 40 mg   Generic

INDICATIONS

Acute leukemias: Remission induction and consolidation and maintenance therapy of acute leukemias. Response depends on the particular subclassification of the leukemia (lymphatic, myelogenous, undifferentiated), age of patient (child or adult), and previous treatment. Thioguanine alone induces complete remission in approximately 50% of previously untreated children with acute leukemia. These results can be improved by using multiple agents in combination. Reliance on this drug alone is seldom justified for initial remission induction in children with acute leukemia. Duration of complete remission is brief; maintenance therapy is essential following successful remission induction.

In adults, thioguanine has most frequently been used in combination with other agents (particularly cytosine arabinoside) for treatment of acute myelogenous (granulocytic) leukemia and acute lymphatic (lymphocytic, lymphoblastic) leukemia. The incidence of complete remission varies widely, depending on agents used, the type of leukemia (lymphatic generally responding better than myelogenous), and patient age (younger patients faring better than older). Because of the brief duration of "unmaintained" complete remission following induction, most therapy for adults uses some form of maintenance chemotherapy.

Chronic myelogenous (granulocytic) leukemia: Thioguanine is one of several agents with demonstrated efficacy; approximately 50% of patients have an objective response. This is less than the response to busulfan, which is usually preferred for initial therapy.

Thioguanine is not effective for prophylaxis or treatment of CNS leukemia. It is also not effective in chronic lymphatic leukemia, the lymphomas (including Hodgkin's disease), multiple myeloma, or solid tumors.

CONTRAINDICATIONS

Patients whose disease has demonstrated prior resistance to this drug. There is usually complete cross-resistance between mercaptopurine and thioguanine.

ACTIONS

Is an antimetabolite that is closely related structurally and functionally to 6-mercaptopurine. Thioguanine has multiple metabolic effects; it is not possible to designate one major site of action. Its tumor inhibitory properties may be due to one or more of its effects on feedback inhibition of purine synthesis, inhibition of purine nucleotide interconversions, and incorporation into DNA and RNA. The net consequence of its actions is a sequential blockade of synthesis and utilization of purine nucleotides.

Oral absorption is incomplete and variable. Thioguanine is incorporated into DNA and RNA of human bone-marrow cells. Only trace quantities of the parent drug are excreted in the urine. See also Appendix 10.

WARNINGS

Thioguanine is a potent drug. Although it may be used in those with anemia, thrombocytopenia, and granulocytopenia secondary to leukemia, these same abnormalities may be produced as a result of a direct myelotoxic effect of the drug. Evaluation of response to therapy requires weekly examination of peripheral blood for changes in the formed elements. Bone-marrow aspiration or biopsy may be used to distinguish among resistance to therapy, progression of leukemia, and marrow hypoplasia induced by therapy.

The most consistent dose-related toxicity is bone-marrow suppression. This may be manifested by anemia, leukopenia, thrombocytopenia, or any combination of these. Any of these findings may also reflect progression of the underlying disease. Because thioguanine may have a delayed effect, it is withdrawn temporarily at the first sign of an abnormally large fall in any of the formed elements of the blood. If subsequently the leukocyte or platelet count remains constant for 2 or 3 days, or rises, treatment may be resumed.

The decision to increase, continue, or decrease a given dosage is based not only on absolute hematologic values, but also on the rate at which changes are occurring. The dosage may need to be reduced when thioguanine is combined with other drugs whose primary toxicity is myelosuppression.

Myelosuppression is often unavoidable during the induction phase of adult acute leukemia if remission response is to be successful. Whether this demands modification or cessation of dosage depends both on the response of the underlying disease and on consideration of supportive facilities (granulocyte and platelet transfusions). Life-threatening infections and bleeding have been seen as a consequence of thioguanine-induced granulocytopenia and thrombocytopenia.

Carcinogenic potential exists in humans, but the extent of the risk is unknown. The effect of thioguanine on the immunocompetence of patients is unknown. Drugs such as thioguanine are potential mutagens and teratogens. Because of the possibility of fetal damage, thioguanine is used during pregnancy only if the benefit clearly justifies the risk to the fetus. Whenever possible, use should be deferred until after the first trimester of pregnancy. The effects on fertility in both males and females and potential hazards to the fetus are unknown.

PRECAUTIONS

A few cases of jaundice have been reported in patients with leukemia receiving thioguanine. Monitoring of hepatic-function tests is recommended at weekly intervals when beginning therapy and at monthly intervals thereafter. More frequent hepatic-function tests may be advisable in those with preexisting liver disease or who are receiving other hepatotoxic drugs.

DRUG INTERACTIONS

Drug/lab tests: Uric acid levels in blood and urine may be increased.

ADVERSE REACTIONS

Bone marrow and hepatic toxicity: See *Warnings* and *Precautions.*

GI: Nausea, vomiting, and stomatitis may occur, particularly with overdosage.

Hyperuricemia: Frequently occurs as a consequence of rapid cell lysis accompanying the antineoplastic effects of the drug. Adverse effects can be minimized by increased hydration, urine alkalinization, and prophylactic administration of a xanthine oxidase inhibitor such as allopurinol.

OVERDOSAGE

There is no known pharmacologic antagonist of thioguanine. Treatment is discontinued immediately if unintended toxicity occurs during treatment. Severe hematologic toxicity may require supportive therapy with platelet transfusions for bleeding and granulocytic transfusions and antibiotics if sepsis is documented. If the patient is seen immediately following an overdosage, induced emesis may be useful. Hemodialysis is thought to be of marginal value.

DOSAGE

The dosage that will be tolerated or that will be effective varies. Careful dose titration is necessary to obtain optimum therapeutic effect without incurring excessive, unintended toxicity.

Usual initial dosage for children and adults is approximately 2 mg/kg/day. If, after 4 weeks on this dosage, there is no clinical improvement and no leukocyte or platelet depression, dosage may be increased to 3 mg/kg/day. The total daily dosage may be given at one time. It is usually calculated to the closest multiple of 20 mg.

The dosage of thioguanine does not depend on whether the patient is receiving allopurinol. This is in contradistinction to dosage reduction, which is mandatory when mercaptopurine or azathioprine is used simultaneously with allopurinol.

If complete hematologic remission is obtained, either with thioguanine alone or with thioguanine in combination with other agents, maintenance therapy should be instituted. Maintenance doses will vary depending on the regimen used.

NURSING IMPLICATIONS

HISTORY
See Appendix 4.

PHYSICAL ASSESSMENT
Obtain vital signs, weight. Evaluate patient's general physical and emotional status. Baseline laboratory tests and diagnostic studies may include CBC, differential, platelet count, hepatic-function tests (bilirubin, alkaline phosphatase, serum transaminases), BUN, urinalysis, serum uric acid, and bone-marrow aspiration and/or biopsy.

ADMINISTRATION
May be ordered once daily or in divided doses.

Tablets are scored and dosage is calculated to the closest multiple of 20 mg.

Allopurinol may be prescribed to prevent hyperuricemia.

ONGOING ASSESSMENTS AND NURSING MANAGEMENT

CLINICAL ALERT: The most consistent dose-related toxicity is bone-marrow suppression (myelosuppression). Life-threatening infections and bleeding have occurred as a consequence of therapy with this drug.

Drug effect occurs slowly, over a period of 2 to 4 weeks. Occasionally there may be a rapid fall in leukocyte count in 1 to 2 weeks. This may occur in some adults with acute leukemia and high leukocyte counts, as well as in certain adults with chronic granulocytic leukemia.

Begin to observe closely for signs of bone-marrow depression (Appendix 6, section 6-8) in both children and adults beginning with the first week of therapy. The physician is notified immediately if one or more signs of bone-marrow suppression occur.

Observe patient for signs of hepatic toxicity (*e.g.,* jaundice, tenderness in the right upper quadrant, light-colored stools, dark urine, swelling of the feet or legs). Notify physician immediately if hepatic toxicity is suspected because drug may be discontinued until etiology of symptoms is determined.

Monitor vital signs q4h to q8h or as ordered. Notify physician immediately of any elevation in temperature.

Measure intake and output. Report any change in the intake–output ratio to the physician.

Hyperuricemia frequently occurs as a response to lysis of cells. Encourage a fluid intake of at least 2000 ml/day for adults. For children, discuss the amount of fluid intake desired with the physician. Also observe for occurrence of abdominal, flank, or joint pain, which may be indicative of uric acid stone formation.

If patient's oral fluid intake is inadequate, discuss this problem with the physician.

Weigh twice weekly or as ordered. Inform physician if a significant weight gain or loss is noted.

If severe leukopenia occurs, protective (reverse) isolation may be necessary. Granulocyte transfusions may be necessary.

Development of thrombocytopenia requires protection of patient from injury by padding of the siderails, prolonged pressure on parenteral administration and venipuncture sites, care in moving and lifting the patient, soft diet, gentle oral care with mouth rinses and cotton-tipped applicators, and so on. Platelet transfusions may be necessary.

If stomatitis develops, see Appendix 6, section 6-21.

Nausea and vomiting may occur; an antiemetic may be necessary to relieve symptoms. Dry toast, unsalted crackers, or carbonated beverages may help relieve nausea and provide some nourishment and fluid. Frequent small feedings, instead of three meals a day, may be offered.

If anorexia develops and persists more than 2 days, notify physician.

Peripheral blood studies, bone-marrow aspiration or biopsy, and hepatic-function tests are recommended (see _Warnings, Precautions_).

PATIENT AND FAMILY INFORMATION

Take drug exactly as prescribed.

It is extremely important to drink eight to ten (8-oz) glasses of fluid each day (children should drink proportionately less, depending on age and/or weight).

Notify physician or nurse immediately if fever; chills; sore throat; sores in the mouth; unusual bleeding or bruising; yellow discoloration of the skin or eyes; swelling of the feet or legs; or flank, stomach, or joint pain occurs.

Adults (male and female): Contraceptive measures are recommended during therapy.

Inform other physicians and dentist of therapy with this drug.

Weigh self weekly. Report a weight increase or decrease of more than 3 to 4 lb.

Report occurrence of nausea and vomiting. An antiemetic will be prescribed.

Nausea may be relieved by dry toast, unsalted crackers, or carbonated beverages. Eat small frequent meals rather than three large meals a day.

Frequent laboratory tests will be necessary. It is important to report for these tests, because drug dosage is determined on the basis of these results.

Thiopental Sodium

See Anesthetics, General, Barbiturates.

Thioridazine Hydrochloride

See Antipsychotic Agents.

Thiothixene

See Antipsychotic Agents.

Thiphenamil Hydrochloride

See Gastrointestinal Anticholinergics/Antispasmodics.

Thrombin, Topical Rx

| powder: 1000-, 5000-, 10,000-unit vials | Thrombinar, Thrombostat |
| powder: 20,000-unit vials | Thrombostat |

INDICATIONS

Aid in hemostasis whenever oozing blood from capillaries and small venules is accessible. In various types of surgery, solutions of thrombin may be used in conjunction with absorbable gelatin sponges for hemostasis.

CONTRAINDICATIONS

Known sensitivity to any of its components or to material of bovine origin.

ACTIONS

Directly catalyzes the conversion of fibrinogen to fibrin. Commercially available thrombin is derived from bovine sources. Blood fails to clot in rare cases in which the primary clotting defect is absence of fibrinogen itself. The speed with which thrombin clots blood depends on its concentration.

WARNINGS

Because of its action in the clotting mechanism, thrombin must not be injected or otherwise allowed to enter large blood vessels. Extensive intravascular clotting and even death may result.

Safety for use in pregnancy is not established. Thrombin is used in pregnant women only when clearly needed and when potential benefits outweigh the unknown potential hazards to the fetus. Safety and efficacy for use in children are not established.

ADVERSE REACTIONS

An allergic-type reaction following use for treatment of epistaxis has been reported. Febrile reactions have also been observed.

DOSAGE

For general use in plastic surgery, dental extractions, skin grafting, neurosurgery, and so on, solu-

T

tions containing 100 units/ml are frequently used. Where bleeding is profuse, as from cut surfaces of the liver or spleen, concentrations as high as 1000 units/ml or 2000 units/ml may be required. The intended use determines strength of the solution. Thrombin may also be applied in dry form on oozing surfaces.

NURSING IMPLICATIONS

HISTORY
When appropriate, obtain allergy history and cause of bleeding (*i.e.,* type of injury or trauma).

PHYSICAL ASSESSMENT
When appropriate, note amount of bleeding and size and depth of wound.

ADMINISTRATION
Preparation of solution: Prepare in Sterile Distilled Water or Isotonic Saline. Physician orders strength of solution.

Topical use: The recipient surface should be sponged (not wiped) free of blood before thrombin is applied. A spray may be used or the surface may be flooded using a sterile syringe and a small-gauge needle. The most effective hemostasis results when the thrombin mixes freely with the blood as soon as it reaches the surface. In instances in which thrombin in dry form is needed, the vial is opened and the dried thrombin is then broken up into powder. Sponging of treated surfaces is avoided to ensure that the clot remains securely in place.

Use in conjunction with gelatin sponge: Immerse sponge strips in the thrombin solution. Knead sponge strips vigorously to remove trapped air. Saturated sponge is applied to bleeding area and held in place 10 to 15 seconds with a pledget of cotton or a small gauze sponge.

Stability and storage: Use solutions on the day they are prepared. If several hours are to elapse, solution should be refrigerated or, preferably, frozen. Solutions with preservatives should not be used after 48 hours. Preservative-free solutions should not be used after 4 hours.

ONGOING ASSESSMENTS AND NURSING MANAGEMENT
Superficial application: Observe area for continued bleeding; inform physician if bleeding continues.

Application during a surgical procedure: Observe for febrile reaction; report temperature elevation (which may also be due to other causes) to physician.

Use for treatment of epistaxis: Observe for an allergic-type reaction, which may include sneezing and urticaria.

PATIENT AND FAMILY INFORMATION
Epistaxis: Do not blow nose or try to remove packing or other material placed in the nose. If sneezing or itching occurs, notify physician or nurse.

Superficial application: Do not remove dressing, and do not allow dressing to become wet. If bleeding recurs, notify physician or nurse.

Thyroglobulin

See Thyroid Hormones.

Thyroid Desiccated

See Thyroid Hormones.

Thyroid Hormones

Levothyroxine Sodium (T₄, L-Thyroxine) Rx

tablets: 0.025 mg, 0.05 mg, 0.1 mg, 0.125 mg, 0.15 mg, 0.3 mg	Levothroid, Synthroid (0.1 mg, 0.3 mg contain tartrazine)
tablets: 0.075 mg	Synthroid
tablets: 0.175 mg	Levothroid
tablets: 0.2 mg	Levothroid, Noroxine, Synthroid
injection: 100 mcg/ vial	Synthroid
injection: 200 mcg/ vial	Levothroid, Synthroid
injection: 500 mcg/ vial	Levothroid, Noroxine, Synthroid

Liothyronine Sodium (T₃) Rx

tablets: 5 mcg, 25 mcg, 50 mcg	Cytomel

Liotrix Rx

tablets: 30 mcg T₄, 7.5 mcg T₃ (30 mg thyroid equivalent)	Euthroid-½
tablets: 60 mcg T₄, 15 mcg T₃ (60 mg thyroid equivalent)	Euthroid-1

tablets: 120 mcg T_4, 30 mcg T_3 (120 mg thyroid equivalent)	Euthroid-2
tablets: 180 mcg T_4, 45 mcg T_3 (180 mg thyroid equivalent)	Euthroid-3
tablets: 12.5 mcg T_4, 3.1 mcg T_3 (15 mg thyroid equivalent)	Thyrolar-¼
tablets: 25 mcg T_4, 6.25 mcg T_3 (30 mg thyroid equivalent)	Thyrolar-½
tablets: 50 mcg T_4, 12.5 mcg T_3 (60 mg thyroid equivalent)	Thyrolar-1
tablets: 100 mcg T_4, 25 mcg T_3 (120 mg thyroid equivalent)	Thyrolar-2
tablets: 150 mcg T_4, 37.5 mcg T_3 (180 mg thyroid equivalent)	Thyrolar-3

Thyroglobulin Rx

tablets: 32 mg, 65 mg, 100 mg, 130 mg, 200 mg	Proloid

Thyroid Desiccated (Thyroid USP) Rx

tablets: 16 mg	Armour Thyroid, Westhroid ¼ A, *Generic*
tablets: 32 mg	Armour Thyroid, Westhroid ½, *Generic*
tablets: 65 mg	Armour Thyroid, Thyro-Teric, Westhroid 1, *Generic*
tablets: 98 mg	Armour Thyroid
tablets: 130 mg	Armour Thyroid, Westhroid 2, *Generic*
tablets: 195 mg	Armour Thyroid, Westhroid 3, *Generic*
tablets: 260 mg	Armour Thyroid, Westhroid 4
tablets: 325 mg	Armour Thyroid, Westhroid 5, *Generic*
tablets, enteric coated: 65 mg, 130 mg, 195 mg	*Generic*
tablets: 32 mg, 65 mg, 130 mg (50% stronger than Thyroid USP)	Thyroid Strong
tablets, sugar coated: 32 mg, 65 mg, 130 mg, 195 mg (50% stronger than Thyroid USP)	Thyroid Strong
tablets, bovine thyroid: 32 mg, 65 mg, 130 mg	Thyrar
capsules (pork thyroid in soybean oil): 65 mg, 130 mg, 195 mg, 325 mg	S-P-T

INDICATIONS

Hypothyroidism: As replacement or supplemental therapy in hypothyroidism of any etiology, except transient hypothyroidism during the recovery phase of subacute thyroiditis. This category includes cretinism, myxedema, and ordinary hypothyroidism in patients of any age (children, adults, elderly) or state (including pregnancy); primary hypothyroidism resulting from functional deficiency, primary atrophy, partial or total absence of thyroid gland, or the effects of surgery, radiation, or drugs, with or without the presence of goiter; secondary (pituitary) or tertiary (hypothalamic) hypothyroidism.

Pituitary thyroid-stimulating hormone (TSH) suppressants: In treatment or prevention of various types of euthyroid goiters, including thyroid nodules, subacute or chronic lymphocytic thyroiditis (Hashimoto's), and multinodular goiter, and in management of thyroid cancer.

Thyrotoxicosis: Thyroid hormones may be used with antithyroid drugs. This combination has been used to prevent goitrogenesis and hypothyroidism and may be useful in management of thyrotoxicosis during pregnancy.

Diagnostic use: **Liothyronine sodium** is used in the T_3 suppression test to differentiate suspected hyperthyroidism from euthyroidism.

CONTRAINDICATIONS

Presence of thyrotoxicosis or cardiovascular conditions (*e.g.,* acute MI, angina pectoris, hypertension) uncomplicated by hypothyroidism. When hypothyroidism is a complicating factor in MI or heart disease, small doses may be used. When hypothyroidism and Addison's disease coexist, thyroid hormones are contraindicated unless treatment of hypoadrenalism with adrenocortical steroids precedes initiation of thyroid therapy. Also contraindicated in apparent hypersensitivity to active or extraneous constituents.

T

ACTIONS

Thyroid hormones include both natural and synthetic derivatives. The natural products, desiccated thyroid and thyroglobulin, are derived from beef or swine. Although these preparations are most economical, standardization by iodine content or bioassay is very inexact. Synthetic derivatives are generally preferred because of more uniform standardization of potency. Commercially available synthetic products include levothyroxine (T_4), liothyronine (T_3), and liotrix (a 4:1 mixture of T_4 and T_3).

The mechanisms by which thyroid hormones exert their physiological action are not well understood. The principal effect of thyroid hormones is to increase the metabolic rate of tissues. This effect may be noted by increases in the following: oxygen consumption; respiratory rate; body temperature; cardiac output; heart rate; blood volume; rate of fat, protein, and carbohydrate metabolism; enzyme system activity; and growth and maturation. Thyroid hormones exert a prolonged influence on every organ system in the body and in growth and development of the brain.

Thyroid hormones are also concerned with growth and differentiation of tissues. In deficiency states in the young there is retardation of growth and failure of maturation of skeletal and other body systems, especially in failure of ossification in the epiphyses and in growth and development of the brain.

The synthesis of thyroid hormones is controlled by thyrotropin (thyroid-stimulating hormone, TSH) secreted by the anterior pituitary. This hormone's secretion is in turn controlled by a feedback mechanism effected by the thyroid hormones themselves and by thyrotropin-releasing hormone (TRH), a tripeptide of hypothalamic origin. Endogenous thyroid hormone secretion is suppressed when exogenous thyroid hormones are administered to euthyroid individuals in excess of the normal gland's secretion.

Thyroid administration increases the basal metabolic rate, increases the protein-bound iodine (PBI), and lowers the level of cholesterol. The effect develops slowly but is prolonged. It begins within 48 hours and reaches a maximum in 8 to 10 days, although the full effect of continued administration may not be evident for several weeks.

Triiodothyronine (T_3) level is low in the fetus and newborn, in old age, in chronic calorie deprivation, in hepatic cirrhosis, in renal failure, in surgical stress, and in chronic illness.

T_4 is only partially absorbed from the GI tract. Absorption varies from 48% to 79%; fasting increases absorption. T_3 is 95% absorbed in 4 hours. Hormones contained in natural preparations are absorbed in a manner similar to that of synthetic hormones.

Under normal circumstances, the ratio of T_4 to T_3 that is released from the thyroid gland is 20:1. Approximately 35% of T_4 is converted in the periphery to T_3. The primary effect of the thyroid hormones is the result of T_3 activity.

WARNINGS

Obesity: Drugs with thyroid hormone activity have been used for treatment of obesity. Small doses do not produce an increase in metabolic rate; hormonal replacement doses are ineffective for weight reduction. Larger doses may produce serious or even life-threatening toxicity, particularly when given with sympathomimetic amines such as those used as anorexiants.

Infertility: Thyroid hormone therapy is unjustified for treatment of male or female infertility unless the condition is accompanied by hypothyroidism.

Cardiovascular disease: Caution is used when integrity of the cardiovascular system, particularly the coronary arteries, is suspect. This includes patients with angina pectoris and the elderly, in whom there is a greater likelihood of occult cardiac disease. In these patients, therapy is initiated with low doses. Patients with cardiac disease should be observed during surgery, because the possibility of precipitating cardiac arrhythmias may be greater in those treated with thyroid hormones.

Endocrine disorders: The signs and symptoms of diabetes mellitus, Addison's disease, hypopituitarism, and diabetes insipidus may be diminished in severity or obscured by hypothyroidism. Thyroid hormone therapy in those with diabetes mellitus or insipidus or Addison's disease aggravates the intensity of symptoms. Adjustments of the various therapeutic measures directed at these concomitant endocrine diseases are required. Severe, prolonged hypothyroidism can lead to a decreased level of adrenocortical activity. When thyroid replacement therapy is given, metabolism increases at a greater rate than does adrenocortical activity, and this can precipitate adrenocortical insufficiency. Supplemental adrenocortical steroids may be necessary. Therapy of myxedema coma requires simultaneous administration of glucocorticoids. In those whose hypothyroidism is secondary to hypopituitarism, adrenal insufficiency will probably be present and should be corrected by corticosteroids before thyroid hormones are administered.

Hypothyroidism: Patients with hypothyroidism (particularly myxedema) are particularly sensitive to thyroid preparations. Treatment is begun with small doses and increments are gradual.

Use in pregnancy, lactation: Thyroid hormones do not readily cross the placental barrier. Experience does not indicate any adverse effect on fetuses when thyroid hormones are administered to pregnant women. Thyroid replacement to hypothyroid women should not be discontinued during pregnancy. Minimal amounts of hormones are excreted in human milk. Caution should be exercised when thyroid is administered to nursing women.

Congenital hypothyroidism: Pregnant women provide little or no thyroid hormone to the fetus. Treatment is initiated immediately upon diagnosis and maintained for life unless transient hypothyroidism is suspected, in which case therapy may be interrupted for 2 to 8 weeks after age 3 to reassess the condition. In infants, excessive doses of thyroid hormone may produce craniosynostosis. In children, partial loss of hair may be seen in the first few months of thyroid therapy; this is usually transient.

Laboratory tests: Treatment with thyroid hormones requires periodic assessment of thyroid status. Persistent clinical and laboratory evidence of hypothyroidism in spite of adequate dosing indicates either poor patient compliance, poor absorption, excessive fetal loss, or inactivity of the preparation. Intracellular resistance to thyroid hormone is rare.

Tartrazine sensitivity: Some of these products contain tartrazine. See Appendix 6, section 6-23.

DRUG INTERACTIONS

Injection of **epinephrine** in patients with coronary artery disease may precipitate an episode of coronary insufficiency. This may be enhanced in those receiving thyroid preparations. Careful observation is required if **catecholamines** are administered.

Thyroid hormones appear to increase catabolism of vitamin K–dependent clotting factors. If **oral anticoagulants** are also being given, compensatory increases in clotting factor synthesis are impaired. Thyroid replacement may potentiate anticoagulant effects with agents such as **warfarin** or **bishydroxycoumarin.** Anticoagulant dosage is reduced by one-third upon initiation of thyroid therapy, and subsequent anticoagulant dosage adjustments are made on the basis of prothrombin time determinations. No special precautions appear necessary when anticoagulant therapy is begun in patients stabilized on maintenance thyroid therapy.

In those with diabetes mellitus, addition of thyroid hormone therapy may cause an increase in the required dosage of **insulin** or **oral hypoglycemic agents.** Conversely, decreasing the dose of thyroid hormone may cause hypoglycemic reactions if the dosage of insulin or oral hypoglycemic agent is not adjusted.

Cholestyramine binds both T_4 and T_3 in the intestine, impairing absorption. Four to five hours should elapse between administration of cholestyramine and thyroid hormone.

Estrogens tend to increase serum thyroxine-binding globulin. Patients without a functioning thyroid gland who are on thyroid replacement therapy may need to increase their thyroid dose if estrogens are given.

Cardiotonic glycosides are given with caution to those receiving thyroid; such preparations increase the susceptibility to toxic effects of the glycosides.

Drug/lab tests: Medicinal or dietary iodine interferes with all tests of radioiodine uptake, producing low uptakes that may not be reflective of a true decrease in hormone synthesis. Table 51 shows interactions of various drugs with thyroid function tests.

ADVERSE REACTIONS

Adverse reactions, other than those indicative of hyperthyroidism because of therapeutic overdosage, either initially or during the maintenance period, are rare. If symptoms of excessive dosage occur, medication is discontinued for several days and reinstituted at a lower dosage. Symptoms of overdosage or too rapid increase in dosage include the following.

Cardiac: Palpitation, elevated pulse pressure, tachycardia, cardiac arrhythmias, angina pectoris, cardiac arrest.

CNS: Tremors, headache, nervousness, nausea, insomnia.

_GI:_ Abdominal cramps, changes in appetite, diarrhea. Gastric intolerance may occur rarely in those highly sensitive to beef or pork products or corn.

Hypersensitivity: Allergic skin reactions.

Miscellaneous: Weight loss, menstrual irregularities, sweating, intolerance to heat, fever.

OVERDOSAGE

Chronic excessive overdosage: Will produce signs and symptoms of hyperthyroidism (headache, irritability, nervousness, sweating, tachycardia, increased bowel motility, menstrual irregularities). Chronic overdosage may result in emaciation. Angina pectoris or congestive heart failure (CHF) may be induced or aggravated. Shock may develop. Complications as a result of the induced hypermetabolic state may include cardiac failure and arrhythmia, which could be fatal. Massive overdosage may result in symptoms resembling thyroid storm. Dosage is reduced or drug temporarily discontinued if signs of overdosage appear; treatment is reinstituted at lower dosages.

Acute massive overdosage: Treatment is aimed at reducing GI absorption of the drug and counteracting central and peripheral effects, mainly those of increased sympathetic activity. Vomiting may be induced initially if further GI absorption can reasonably be prevented, barring contraindications such as coma, convulsions, or loss of gag reflex. Treatment

Table 51. Effects of Drugs on Thyroid Function Tests

Drug	Thyroid Function Test				
	Serum T_4	T_3 Uptake Resin (RT$_3$U)	Free Thyroxine Index (FTI)	Serum T_3	Serum TSH
p-Aminosalicylic acid	↓		↓		
Aminoglutethimide	↓				↑
Anabolic steroids/androgens	↓	↑	0	↓/0	
Antithyroid (PTU, methimazole)	↓	↓	↓	↓	0/↑
Asparaginase	↓	↑			
Barbiturates	↓		↓	0/⇓	
Contraceptives, oral	↑	↓	0	↑	0
Corticosteroids	0/↓	0/↑	0/↓	↓	↓
Danazol	↓	↑	0/⇑	0/↓	↓
Diazepam	↓		⇓		
Estrogens	↑	↓	0/⇑	↑	0
Ethionamide	↓				
Fluorouracil	↑	↓	0	↑	0
Heparin (IV)	↓	0/↑	↑	0	
Insulin	↑				
Lithium carbonate	0/↓	0/↓	0/↓	0/↓	0/↑
Methadone	↑	↓	0	↑	0
Mitotane	↓	0			
Nitroprusside	↓				
Oxyphenbutazone/ phenylbutazone	0/↓	↑	↓		
Perphenazine	↑	↓	↓	↑	
Phenytoin	↓	0/⇑	0/⇓	↓	0
Propranolol	0		⇑	↓	0
Resorcinol (excessive topical use)	↓	↓	↓	↓	↑
Salicylates (large doses)	↓	⇑		↓	
Sulfonylureas	↓	0	0		
Thiazides	0			↑	

Adapted from Medical Letter on Drugs and Therapeutics 1981;23:30–32 with permission from the Medical Letter, Inc.

↑ Increased
⇑ Slightly increased
↓ Decreased
⇓ Slightly decreased
0 No effect
Blank spaces signifies no data

is symptomatic and supportive. Administer oxygen and maintain ventilation. Cardiac glycosides may be given if CHF develops. Institute measures to control fever, hypoglycemia, or fluid loss, if needed. Antiadrenergic agents, particularly propranolol, have been used in treatment of increased sympathetic activity. Propranolol may be given IV at a dosage of 1 mg to 3 mg over a 10-minute period, or orally, 80 mg/day to 160 mg/day, especially when no contraindications exist for its use. Treatment of unrecognized adrenal insufficiency should be considered.

DOSAGE

Individualized to approximate the defect in the patient's thyroid secretion. Patient response is determined by clinical judgement and laboratory findings. Generally, therapy is instituted at low doses and increased in small increments until desired response is obtained. Thyroid is given as a single daily dose, preferably before breakfast.

Under most circumstances T_4 is the treatment of choice of hypothyroidism because of its purity and prolonged duration of action. It has a slow onset of action and its effects are cumulative over a period of 3 to 4 weeks. The rapid onset and dissipation of action of T_3 as compared with those of T_4 may be preferred for use in those more susceptible to the untoward effects of thyroid medication. The wide swings in T_3 levels following administration and the possibility of more pronounced cardiovascular side-effects tend to counterbalance the stated advantages. If there is a need for rapidly correcting the hypothyroid state, T_3 is preferable because of its rapid onset and dissipation of action.

Laboratory tests useful in diagnosis and evaluation of thyroid function are free T_4 (unbound), total T_4, serum T_3, T_3 resin uptake (RT_3U), free thyroxine index, TSH. In primary hypothyroidism all values are decreased except the TSH, which is increased. In secondary hypothyroidism all values are decreased. In hyperthyroidism all values are increased except the TSH, which is normal.

Serum T_4 and RT_3U values are usually sufficient to diagnose hypothyroidism. Maintenance dose adjustments can be based on T_4 and RT_3U values and clinical judgment, except in patients being treated with T_3. If available, TSH suppression into the normal range is an accurate indication of therapy in primary hypothyroidism but is of no value in determining if dosage is too large or in secondary hypothyroidism. Thyrotropin may be used to determine subclinical hypothyroidism and to differentiate primary and secondary hypothyroidism. Protirelin (thyrotropin-releasing hormone) may be useful in differentiation of primary, secondary, and tertiary hypothyroidism.

LEVOTHYROXINE SODIUM (T₄)

Is an active principle of the thyroid gland prepared synthetically in pure crystalline form.

Dosage equivalence: 0.1 mg equals approximately 65 mg of thyroid.

Bioavailability: Bioequivalence problems have been documented for products marketed by different manufacturers. Brand name interchange is not recommended unless comparative bioavailability data that provide evidence of therapeutic equivalence are available.

Oral

Adults: In healthy patients with a relatively recent onset of hypothyroidism, a full replacement dose of 0.15 mg or 0.2 mg may be instituted immediately. The age, general physical condition, and severity and duration of hypothyroid symptoms determine the starting dosage and rate of increase leading to final maintenance dosage. For some, the starting dose may be as little as 0.025 mg/day with further incremental increases of 0.025 mg/day at 3- to 4-week intervals. Otherwise healthy adults may be started at a higher daily dosage and raised to the full replacement dosage in 2 to 3 weeks.

Concomitant appearance of other diseases, especially cardiovascular diseases, usually requires a replacement regimen with initial doses smaller than 0.1 mg/day.

For most, a final dose of 0.1 mg/day to 0.2 mg/day will provide normal thyroid function; occasionally patients will require large doses. Failure to respond adequately to 0.4 mg/day is rare.

Children: In infants and children, there is a great urgency to achieve full thyroid replacement because of importance of the hormone in sustaining growth and maturation. Despite smaller body size, the dosage needed to sustain a full rate of growth and development and to thrive is higher in the child than in the adult. Recommended daily replacement dosage is given in Table 52.

In cretinism or severe hypothyroidism, initial dosage should be 0.025 mg to 0.05 mg, with increases of 0.05 mg to 0.1 mg at 2-week intervals until child is clinically euthyroid and laboratory values are in the normal range. In growing children, usual maintenance dose may be as high as 0.3 mg/day to 0.4 mg/day.

Parenteral

IV administration can be substituted for oral dosage when oral ingestion is precluded for long periods of time.

Myxedema coma or stupor without concomitant heart disease: 0.2 mg to 0.5 mg IV as a solution containing 0.1 mg/ml. *Do not* add to other IV fluids. Although patient may show responsiveness in 6 to 8 hours, full therapeutic effect may not be evident until the following day. An additional 0.1 mg to 0.3 mg or more may be given on the second day. Continued IV administration of lesser amounts should be maintained until patient is capable of taking oral form.

Myxedema coma or stupor with concomitant heart disease: Sudden administration of large IV doses has cardiovascular risks. IV therapy is not undertaken without weighing the alternative risks.

LIOTHYRONINE SODIUM (T₃)

A synthetic form of a natural thyroid hormone with all pharmacologic activities of the natural substance. Has a shorter duration of activity, which permits quick dosage adjustment and facilitates control of overdosage. Can be used in those allergic to desiccated thyroid or thyroid extract derived from pork or beef.

Dosage equivalents: 25 mcg equals approximately 65 mg desiccated thyroid.

Mild hypothyroidism: Recommended starting

Table 52. Recommended Pediatric Dosage of Levothyroxine Sodium for Congenital Hypothyroidism

Age	Doses/day (mcg)	Daily Doses/kg (mcg)
0–6 months	25–50	8–10
6–12 months	50–75	6–8
1–5 years	75–100	5–6
6–12 years	100–150	4–5
>12 years	>150	2–3

dose is 25 mcg/day. Daily dosage may be increased by 12.5 mcg or 25 mcg every 1 to 2 weeks. Usual maintenance dose is 25 mcg/day to 75 mcg/day. Smaller doses may be effective in some patients, while a dosage of 100 mcg/day may be required in others.

Myxedema: Recommended starting dose is 5 mcg/day. This may be increased by 5 mcg/day to 10 mcg/day every 1 to 2 weeks. When 25 mcg/day is reached, dosage may often be increased by 12.5 mcg to 25 mcg every 1 to 2 weeks. Usual maintenance dose is 50 mcg/day to 100 mcg/day.

Cretinism: Recommended starting dose is 5 mcg/day, with a 5-mcg increment every 3 to 4 days until desired response is achieved. Infants a few months old may require only 20 mcg/day for maintenance. At 1 year, 50 mcg/day may be needed. Above 3 years, full adult dose may be necessary.

Simple (nontoxic) goiter: Recommended starting dose is 5 mcg/day. Dosage may be increased every week or two by 12.5 mcg to 25 mcg. Usual maintenance dose is 75 mcg/day.

T₃ suppression test: When ^{131}I thyroid uptake is in the borderline high range, 75 mcg to 100 mcg is given daily for 7 days; then a repeat of the ^{131}I thyroid uptake is performed. In the hyperthyroid patient, 24-hour ^{131}I thyroid uptake will not be significantly affected. In the euthyroid patient, 24-hour ^{131}I thyroid uptake will drop to less than 20%.

The elderly or children: Therapy is started with 5 mcg/day and increased by 5-mcg increments at recommended intervals.

Exchange therapy: When patient is changed to liothyronine sodium from thyroid, L-thyroxine or thyroglobulin, the other medication is discontinued and liothyronine sodium started at a low dosage and increased gradually according to patient response.

LIOTRIX

A uniform mixture of synthetic levothyroxine (T₄) and liothyronine sodium (T₃) in a 4:1 ratio by weight.

Dosage equivalents: Manufacturers of liotrix differ on approximate equivalents to 65 mg of thyroid. In patients previously rendered euthyroid with another thyroid product, each 60-mg liotrix tablet will usually replace 65 mg of desiccated thyroid, 0.1 mg levothyroxine sodium, or 25 mcg liothyronine sodium. Dosage adjustments other than those routinely necessary with any thyroid therapy are seldom necessary.

Dosage of liotrix is given in thyroid equivalents (60 mg = 1 grain or 65 mg of thyroid).

Hypothyroidism newly diagnosed or untreated: Therapy is initiated with a 15-mg or 30-mg tablet each day and increased gradually every 1 to 2 weeks. In children, increments in dosage should be made every 2 weeks.

THYROGLOBULIN

Contains levothyroxine (T₄) and liothyronine (T₃) and conforms to USP specifications for desiccated thyroid. The ratio of T₄ to T₃ is approximately 2.5:1.

Initial dose: 32 mg, increased gradually by increments at intervals of 1 to 2 weeks.

Maintenance: 32 mg/day to 200 mg/day.

THYROID DESICCATED (THYROID USP)

Thyroid USP is composed of desiccated animal thyroid glands. The active thyroid hormones (T₄, T₃) are available in the natural state and ratio.

Adult myxedema: 16 mg/day for 2 weeks, increased to 32 mg/day for 2 more weeks and then to 65 mg/day. Patient is examined after first and second months of treatment with 65-mg dose. If necessary, dosage may be increased to 130 mg/day for 2 months and examination repeated. If laboratory values are low or clinical response is inadequate, dosage is increased to 195 mg/day. Further increases in increments of 32 mg/day or 65 mg/day may be made. *Maintenance dosage*—Usual dose is 65 mg/day to 195 mg/day.

Adult hypothyroidism without myxedema: Initial dosage is 65 mg/day, increased by 65 mg every 30 days until desired result is obtained. Some patients may be severely hypothyroid without manifesting typical appearance of myxedema. Such patients could be harmed by the initial dosage of 65 mg/day. Clinical examination monthly and laboratory evaluation every 3 months may be desirable. *Maintenance dosage*—65 mg/day to 195 mg/day.

Children (cretinism or severe hypothyroidism): Dosage is as for adults with myxedema, with each dosage increment made at intervals of 2 weeks. Final maintenance dose may be greater in the growing child than in the adult.

NURSING IMPLICATIONS

HISTORY
See Appendix 4. If radioiodine uptake tests are scheduled, it is important to know if patient has ingested any foods high in iodine or taken drugs containing iodine within the past 3 months.

PHYSICAL ASSESSMENT
Obtain basal temperature (taken before rising); pulse (including a sleeping pulse); respiratory rate; blood pressure; weight; height (child) or length (infant). Observe for signs of hypothyroid-

ism, cretinism (infant, child), or myxedema. Baseline laboratory tests and diagnostic studies may include free T_4 (unbound), total T_4, serum T_3, TSH, RT_3U, free thyroxine index, CBC, serum cholesterol, triglycerides, and ECG.

ADMINISTRATION

Give as single dose early in the morning, preferably before breakfast; fasting increases absorption.

For administration to infants, tablets may be crushed and added to a small amount of liquid.

Prior to each administration, assess patient for signs of overdosage (p 1035). Withhold drug and contact physician if overdosage is apparent.

Preparation of parenteral solution of levothyroxine: Prepare immediately before use.

To the 500-mcg vial, add 5 ml of 0.9% Sodium Chloride Injection, USP.

To the 200-mcg vial, brand name Levothroid, add 2 ml of 0.9% Sodium Chloride Injection, USP. To the 200-mcg vial, brand name Synthroid, add 5 ml of 0.9% Sodium chloride Injection, USP.

To the 100-mcg vial, add 5 ml of 0.9% Sodium Chloride Injection, USP.

The manufacturer of Levothroid recommends use of 0.9% Sodium Chloride, USP only. The manufacturer of Synthroid recommends use of 0.9% Sodium Chloride Injection, USP or Bacteriostatic Sodium Chloride Injection, USP with Benzyl Alcohol only.

Drug is administered IV. Do *not* add to other IV fluids.

ONGOING ASSESSMENTS AND NURSING MANAGEMENT

Full effects of thyroid administration may take several weeks, but early effects may be seen in 48 hours.

Monitor vital signs daily or as ordered.

A sleeping pulse and basal temperature may be ordered during initial therapy.

Observe for signs of overdosage and report findings to physician because dosage adjustment may be necessary.

CLINICAL ALERT: Observe for adverse reactions and signs of overdosage (p 1035). More serious signs of overdosage include cardiac arrhythmias, increased pulse pressure, and palpitations. Occurrence of adverse reactions may require discontinuation of drug or reduction of dosage.

Weigh daily or as ordered.

Measure intake and output during initial therapy.

Signs of a therapeutic response in adults include gradual weight loss; mild diuresis; sense of well-being; increased appetite; decreased puffiness of face, hands, and feet; increased pulse rate; increased mental activity; and decrease in constipation.

Signs of therapeutic response in infants and children include increased alertness; decreased sleeping time; increased appetite; increased crying episodes (infants); decreased puffiness of face, hands, and feet; increased skin warmth; increased pulse; increased basal temperature; and increased growth rate (height or length). Partial loss of hair may be seen in children during the first few months of therapy.

Patients with myxedema are particularly sensitive to thyroid preparations. Treatment is begun with small doses, dosage increments are gradual, and patient is monitored closely for signs of overdosage as well as lack of clinical response.

Inadequate dosage results in continuation of symptoms of hypothyroidism.

Thyroid hormone therapy in those with diabetes mellitus or insipidus or Addison's disease aggravates the intensity of symptoms. Appropriate adjustments may be necessary in the therapeutic regimen of these disorders.

Patient with diabetes mellitus: Closely monitor patient, especially during early therapy, for signs of hyperglycemia (Appendix 6, section 6-14). Notify physician if urine is positive for glucose or ketones. An increase in dosage of insulin or oral hypoglycemic agent may be necessary.

Patient receiving an oral anticoagulant: Thyroid hormones may potentiate anticoagulant effects and a decrease in dosage may be required. Observe patient for episodes of bleeding. Monitor prothrombin times. See also Anticoagulants.

Pediatric patients: Serial height or length measures are taken, usually at monthly intervals.

Periodic laboratory tests are performed to monitor results of therapy and may include TSH suppression test, serum T_4 levels (except for those receiving liothyronine), free T_4 (unbound).

PATIENT AND FAMILY INFORMATION

Replacement therapy is taken for life (*exceptions*—transient hypothyroidism usually associated with thyroiditis and in those receiving a trial of the drug).

Do not increase or decrease the dose or stop taking the medication, even if symptoms improve, except on the advice of the physician.

Notify physician or nurse if any of the following occurs: headache, nervousness, diarrhea, excessive sweating, heat intolerance, chest pain, increased pulse rate, or palpitations (symptoms of hyperthyroidism), or if any unusual event occurs.

Dosage changes are based on response to therapy.

In children, partial loss of hair in the first few months of therapy may occur; this is usually transient and normal hair growth usually occurs after several months.

Weigh self (or child) weekly. Report any significant weight loss or gain to the physician.

Measure child's height (in infants, length) monthly. Keep a record of measurements.

Therapy will be evaluated at periodic intervals and may vary from every 2 weeks during the beginning of therapy to every 6 to 12 months once symptoms are controlled.

Patient taking concomitant oral anticoagulants: Dosage adjustments and frequent prothrombin time determinations may be necessary. Notify physician immediately of any signs of bleeding tendencies or easy bruising.

Thyrotropin

(Thyroid-Stimulating Hormone, TSH)   Rx

powder for injection: Thytropar
   10 IU thyrotropic
   activity/vial

INDICATIONS
As a diagnostic agent to differentiate thyroid failure and to establish a diagnosis of decreased thyroid reserve. Can also be used for protein-bound iodine (PBI) or ^{131}I uptake determinations.

CONTRAINDICATIONS
Hypersensitivity to thyrotropin; coronary thrombosis; untreated Addison's disease.

ACTIONS
Thyrotropin produces increased uptake of iodine by the thyroid, increased formation of thyroid hormone, increased release of thyroid hormone, and cellular hyperplasia of the thyroid on prolonged stimulation. After injection, the effect on the thyroid in normal individuals is evident within 8 hours, reaching a maximum in 24 hours to 48 hours.

WARNINGS
Anaphylactic reactions have occurred with repeated administration.

Use in pregnancy and lactation: Safety for use during pregnancy and lactation has not been established.

Use in children: Safety and efficacy for use in children have not been established.

PRECAUTIONS
Thyrotropin can stimulate thyroid secretion; use cautiously in those with cardiac disease who are unable to tolerate additional stress.

ADVERSE REACTIONS
Most common: Nausea, vomiting, headache, urticaria.

Cardiovascular: Transitory hypotension, tachycardia (probably related to sensitivity reaction).

Other: Anaphylactic reactions with patient collapse, thyroid gland swelling.

OVERDOSAGE
Symptoms: Headache, irritability, nervousness, sweating, tachycardia, increased bowel motility, menstrual irregularities. Angina pectoris or congestive heart failure may be induced or aggravated. Shock may also develop. Excessive doses may result in symptoms resembling thyroid storm. Chronic overdosage will produce signs and symptoms of hyperthyroidism.

Treatment: In shock, supportive measures and treatment of unrecognized adrenal insufficiency are considered. Drug is discontinued.

DOSAGE
Give IM or subcutaneously.

Usual dose: 10 IU for 1 to 3 days. Follow by a radioiodine study 24 hours after the last injection. No response will occur in thyroid failure, but substantial response will occur in pituitary failure.

NURSING IMPLICATIONS

HISTORY
See Appendix 4.

PHYSICAL ASSESSMENT
Obtain vital signs; assess for symptoms of hyperthyroidism or hypothyroidism. Baseline laboratory tests may include serum T_4 levels and serum TSH levels if thyrotropin is used in differential diagnosis of primary or secondary hypothyroidism or if patient is receiving thyroid medication.

ADMINISTRATION
If patient is receiving thyroid hormone, it is usually not discontinued when testing for thyroid status.

Diluent is supplied with product.

Dissolve the powder for injection with entire

amount (2 ml) of diluent (sterile physiologic saline) to produce a ratio of 10 IU/2 ml.

Give subcutaneously or IM. Rotate injection sites.

Storage: After reconstitution, store between 2°C and 8°C (36°F–46°F), for no longer than 2 weeks.

ONGOING ASSESSMENTS AND NURSING MANAGEMENT

Monitor vital signs qid or as ordered. Notify physician if fever, hypotension, tachycardia, or cardiac arrhythmia is noted.

Postadministration laboratory studies may include TSH levels, ^{131}I uptake determination, and serum T_4.

In normal individuals, the ^{131}I uptake and serum T_4 are increased. In those with diminished thyroid reserve or primary hypothyroidism, there is no response to administration of TSH. In those with secondary hypothyroidism, ^{131}I uptake and serum T_4 are increased.

Ticarcillin Disodium

See Penicillins.

Timolol Maleate Rx

solution: 0.25%, 0.5%   Timoptic

INDICATIONS

Effective in lowering intraocular pressure and may be used in patients with chronic open-angle glaucoma; aphakic patients with glaucoma; some patients with secondary glaucoma; patients with elevated intraocular pressure who are at sufficient risk to require lowering of ocular pressure. Clinical trials have shown that in patients who respond inadequately to multiple antiglaucoma drug therapy, addition of timolol may produce a further reduction of intraocular pressure. See also Beta-Adrenergic Blocking Agents for oral use in the management of hypertension and myocardial infarction.

CONTRAINDICATIONS

Hypersensitivity; bronchospasm, including bronchial asthma or severe chronic obstructive disease; uncontrolled cardiac failure.

ACTIONS

A nonselective beta-adrenergic receptor blocking agent that does not have significant intrinsic sympathomimetic, direct myocardial depressant, or local anesthetic activity. When applied topically in the eye, timolol acts to reduce elevated as well as normal intraocular pressure, whether or not accompanied by glaucoma. The precise mechanism of action is not clearly established. Its predominant action may be related to reduced aqueous formation. A slight increase in outflow has also been seen.

Unlike miotics, timolol reduces intraocular pressure with little or no effect on pupil size or visual acuity due to increased accommodation. Dim or blurred vision and night blindness produced by miotics are not evident. In cataract patients, the inability to see around lenticular opacities when the pupil is constricted is avoided. Timolol is generally well tolerated and produces fewer and less severe side-effects than either pilocarpine or epinephrine.

The onset of reduction in intraocular pressure following administration can be detected within ½ hour after a single dose. The maximum effect occurs in 1 to 2 hours. Significant lowering of intraocular pressure can be maintained for periods as long as 24 hours with a single dose.

WARNINGS

As with other topical ophthalmic agents, timolol may be absorbed systemically. Safety for use in pregnancy is not established. Timolol is used only when clearly needed and when potential benefits outweigh the unknown potential hazards to the fetus. Safety and efficacy for use in children are not established.

PRECAUTIONS

Use with caution in those with known contraindications to systemic use of beta-adrenergic receptor blocking agents. These include sinus bradycardia and greater than first-degree heart block; cardiogenic shock; diabetes, especially labile diabetes; concomitant use with adrenergic-augmenting psychotropic drugs. Cardiac failure should be adequately controlled before beginning therapy. In those with a history of severe cardiac disease, watch for signs of cardiac failure and monitor pulse rates. When used to reduce elevated intraocular pressure in angle-closure glaucoma, timolol is used with a miotic and not used alone.

Diminished responsiveness after prolonged therapy has been reported in some patients.

DRUG INTERACTIONS

Patients receiving an oral **beta-adrenergic blocking agent** and timolol should be observed for a potential additive effect either on intraocular pressure or on the known systemic effects of beta blockade. Although timolol alone has little or no effect on pupil size, mydriasis resulting from concomitant therapy with **epinephrine** has occasionally been reported.

ADVERSE REACTIONS

Ophthalmic: Signs and symptoms of mild ocular irritation, including conjunctivitis, blepharitis, and keratitis. Visual disturbances, including refractive changes (due to withdrawal of miotic therapy in some cases) have been infrequently associated with therapy. Rarely, aphakic cystoid macular edema has been reported, but a causal relationship has not been established. Corneal anesthesia and blepharoptosis have been reported.

Systemic effects: Aggravation or precipitation of certain cardiovascular, pulmonary, and other disorders, presumably related to effect of systemic beta blockade, have been reported. These include bradyarrhythmia, hypotension, syncope, and bronchospasm (predominantly in those with preexisting bronchospastic disease). Respiratory failure, CHF, and masked symptoms of hypoglycemia in insulin-dependent diabetics have been reported rarely.

Hypersensitivity reactions: Localized and generalized rash and urticaria (rare).

Rare (causal relationship unknown): Headache, dry mouth, anorexia, dyspepsia, nausea, dizziness, CNS effects (*e.g.,* fatigue, confusion, depression, somnolence, anxiety), palpitations, and hypertension.

Brown discoloration of fingernails and toenails has also been reported.

DOSAGE

Initial therapy: One drop of 0.25% in the eye bid. If clinical response is not adequate, dosage is changed to one drop of 0.5% solution in eye bid. If intraocular pressure is maintained at satisfactory levels, the dosage schedule may be changed to one drop once a day. Because of diurnal variation in intraocular pressure, satisfactory response to the once-a-day dose is determined by measuring intraocular pressure at different times during the day.

Replacement therapy: When transferring from another antiglaucoma agent, on the first day the agent already being used is continued and one drop of 0.25% timolol in the eye bid is added. On the following day, the previously used agent is discontinued completely and timolol is continued. If a higher dosage is required, one drop of the 0.5% solution bid may be substituted.

Concomitant therapy: Dosages above one drop of 0.5% solution bid have not been shown to produce further reduction in intraocular pressure. If intraocular pressure is still not at a satisfactory level on this regimen, concomitant therapy with pilocarpine or other miotics and/or epinephrine and/or systemically administered carbonic anhydrase inhibitors such as acetazolamide may be given. In concomitant therapy, administer 0.25% solution in each eye bid. If higher dosage is required, one drop of 0.5% may be used.

NURSING IMPLICATIONS

HISTORY
See Appendix 4.

PHYSICAL ASSESSMENT
Obtain blood pressure, pulse, and respirations. Baseline diagnostic studies may include measurement of intraocular pressure.

ADMINISTRATION
Timolol can be used in patients wearing conventional (PMMA) hard contact lenses.

In angle-closure glaucoma, a miotic is also prescribed.

Take pulse prior to administration. If pulse is decreased significantly below pretreatment level, withhold drug and notify physician.

Mild ocular irritation may occur. Inspect eyes and eyelids for signs of irritation (*i.e.,* redness and discharge). If these are present, inform physician.

Instill one drop of the prescribed solution (0.25% or 0.5%) in the lower conjunctival sac.

Apply digital pressure on the lacrimal sac for 1 minute following instillation to lessen possibility of systemic absorption.

ONGOING ASSESSMENTS AND NURSING MANAGEMENT
Obtain blood pressure and pulse daily or as ordered. Withhold next dose and notify physician if hypotension, significant decrease in pulse, or other systemic adverse reactions are noted.

Observe for relief of symptoms of glaucoma. The onset of reduction of intraocular pressure can be detected in ½ hour and maximum effect occurs in 1 to 2 hours. In some patients, the pressure-lowering response may require a few weeks to stabilize.

In patients with a history of severe heart disease, observe for signs of cardiac failure (CHF).

In diabetic patients, systemic absorption may result in a masking of signs of hypoglycemia (Appendix 6, section 6-14).

If epinephrine is administered concomitantly, mydriasis may occasionally occur with resultant aversion to bright lights.

Intraocular pressure is measured approximately 4 weeks after initiation of treatment. In some instances, more frequent measurements may be necessary. Normal intraocular pressure is 12 mm Hg to 20 mm Hg and tends to be highest in the early morning upon waking and lowest in the evening. Measurement of intraocular pressure may be scheduled at different times during the day because of diurnal variation.

Diminished responsiveness to timolol after prolonged therapy may occur.

PATIENT AND FAMILY INFORMATION

NOTE: Patient may require instructions in instillation of drug and applying pressure on the lacrimal sac.

Instill drug in lower conjunctival sac. Apply light finger pressure on the lacrimal sac for 1 minute following instillation.

Do not increase or decrease the prescribed number of applications or the amount used, except on advice of the physician.

Notify physician or nurse immediately if any of the following occurs: sudden eye pain, difficulty breathing, irritation or redness of the eye, visual disturbances, rash or hives, dizziness, or worsening of symptoms of glaucoma.

Follow-up examinations are an important part of therapy.

Tobramycin Sulfate

See Aminoglycosides, Parenteral.

Tolazamide

See Sulfonylureas.

Tolazoline Hydrochloride Rx

injection: 25 mg/ml   Priscoline

INDICATIONS

"Possibly effective" for spastic peripheral vascular disorders associated with acrocyanosis, acroparesthesia, arteriosclerosis obliterans, thromboangiitis obliterans (Buerger's disease), causalgia, diabetic arteriosclerosis, gangrene, endarteritis, frostbite (sequelae), post-thrombotic conditions (thrombophlebitis), Raynaud's disease, and scleroderma.

Investigational uses: Used as a pulmonary vasodilator in infants (with or without congenital heart disease) with acutely increased pulmonary vascular resistance.

CONTRAINDICATIONS

Following a cerebrovascular accident; known or suspected coronary artery disease; hypersensitivity.

ACTIONS

A peripheral vasodilator with alpha-adrenergic blocking and histaminelike actions. With usual doses, it produces an incomplete and transient alpha-adrenergic blockade. Vasodilatation results primarily from direct action on vascular smooth muscle. Cutaneous blood flow is increased. Also causes cardiac and GI stimulation. Tolazoline is slowly absorbed following parenteral administration. It is excreted primarily unchanged in the urine.

WARNINGS

Use in peptic ulcer disease: Stimulates gastric secretion and may activate peptic ulcers. Use cautiously in those with gastritis or known or suspected peptic ulcer.

Use in mitral stenosis: Administration may produce either a fall or rise in pulmonary artery pressure and total pulmonary resistance. Use with caution in known or suspected mitral stenosis.

Use in pregnancy, lactation: Safety for use during pregnancy or lactation is not established. Use only when clearly needed and when potential benefits outweigh the unknown potential hazards to the fetus.

DRUG INTERACTIONS

Concomitant ingestion of **alcohol** and tolazoline may theoretically result in a disulfiramlike reaction. Do not use **epinephrine** or **norepinephrine** because large doses of tolazoline may cause "epinephrine reversal" (further reduction of blood pressure followed by exaggerated rebound).

ADVERSE REACTIONS

Cardiovascular: Arrhythmias, tachycardia, anginal pains, marked hypertension, slight rise or fall in blood pressure. Tolazoline has been implicated as a precipitating factor in myocardial infarction.

GI: Exacerbations of peptic ulcer; nausea; vomiting; diarrhea; epigastric discomfort; duodenal perforation; rarely, hepatitis.

Hematologic: Rarely, thrombocytopenia and leukopenia.

CNS: Apprehension. Psychiatric reactions characterized by confusion or hallucinations have been rarely reported.

GU: Rarely, hematuria and oliguria.

Miscellaneous: Flushing; increased pilomotor activity with tingling or chilliness, rash, and edema.

Intra-arterial administration may produce a feeling of warmth or a burning sensation in the injected extremity, transient weakness, transient postural vertigo, palpitations, formication, and apprehension. Rarely, a paradoxical response (further decrease in an already impaired blood supply) may

T

occur in the seriously damaged limb with incipient or established gangrene. This usually disappears with continued treatment and may be prevented by administration of histamine.

OVERDOSAGE

Symptoms: Increased pilomotor activity, peripheral vasodilatation, and skin flushing; in rare instances, hypotension to shock levels.

Treatment: In treating hypotension, place patient in the head-low position and administer IV fluids. If a vasopressor is necessary, one having both central and peripheral action (*e.g.,* ephedrine) may be used. Do not use epinephrine or norepinephrine because large doses may cause epinephrine reversal (see *Drug Interactions*).

DOSAGE

Individualized according to condition treated and patient response.

Subcutaneous, IV, or IM: 10 mg to 50 mg qid. Patient is kept under close observation and started with low doses, increasing until optimal dosage (determined by appearance of flushing) is established.

Intra-arterial: Because of the risks involved, the special technique, and the strict aseptic precautions required, intra-arterial injection is used only in a hospital or clinic facility. Initially, 25 mg is given slowly as a test dose to determine response. Subsequently, the average single dose may be 50 mg to 75 mg per injection, depending on response. One or two injections daily are usually required initially to achieve maximum response. For maintenance, two or three injections a week may be enough to sustain improved circulation, but more may be needed.

█ NURSING IMPLICATIONS

HISTORY
See Appendix 4.

PHYSICAL ASSESSMENT
Obtain vital signs. Examine affected extremity, noting color and skin temperature. Palpate peripheral pulses, noting amplitude and rate. Pretreatment diagnostic tests may include ECG, Doppler ultrasonography, plethysmography, and arteriography.

ADMINISTRATION
Give subcutaneously, IM, or IV. Rotate injection sites; record site used.

Before giving each dose, examine the affected extremity for flushing, warmth, increased pilomotor activity (gooseflesh); if these are present, withhold next dose and notify the physician. Op-

timal dose is determined by the appearance of these signs and symptoms generally or in the affected extremity.

Intra-arterial injection is administered by a physician.

Prior to intra-arterial injection, patient is placed in the supine position. Histamine may be given prior to injection.

Monitor blood pressure and pulse during and after intra-arterial injection.

ONGOING ASSESSMENTS AND NURSING MANAGEMENT
Keep patient recumbent approximately 30 minutes after administration unless physician directs otherwise.

Obtain vital signs qid or as ordered.

Keeping patient warm will often increase the effectiveness of the drug.

Adverse reactions are usually mild and may decrease progressively during therapy. If adverse reactions occur, keep physician informed. Notify the physician immediately if any adverse reaction becomes severe, if the patient complains of chest pain, or if psychiatric reactions are noted.

PATIENT AND FAMILY INFORMATION
Teaching is directed toward general care of the affected extremity and should include avoiding extreme temperature changes, especially cold weather; avoiding use of heating pads or other thermal devices on the affected extremity; avoiding smoking; being aware of the importance of properly fitting shoes; avoiding tight fitting clothes; following physician's instructions about exercise; maintaining proper skin care; avoiding alcohol unless use is approved by the physician; and avoiding positions that may impair circulation to the extremity.

Tolbutamide

See Sulfonylureas.

Tolmetin Sodium

See Nonsteroidal Anti-inflammatory Agents.

Tolnaftate otc

cream 1%; powder 1% (with corn-starch and talc); powder, aerosol 1% (with talc); liq-	Tinactin

uid, aerosol 1%;
solution 1%

gel 1%; powder 1%;   Aftate for Athlete's Foot
powder, aerosol
1%; liquid, aerosol
1%; liquid, pump
spray 1%

gel 1%; powder 1%;   Aftate for Jock Itch
powder, aerosol
1%

INDICATIONS

Topical treatment of tinea pedis, tinea cruris, tinea corporis, and tinea manuum due to infection with *Trichophyton rubrum, T. mentagrophytes, T. tonsurans, Microsporum canis, M. audouini,* and *Epidermophyton floccosum* and of tinea versicolor due to *Malassezia furfur.*

An oral antifungal agent, such as griseofulvin, is required in onychomycosis; chronic infections of the scalp in which fungi are numerous and widely distributed in the skin and hair follicles; where kerion formation has occurred. An oral antifungal agent may be required in chronic refractory fungus infections of the palms and soles that have not responded to tolnaftate. May also be used concurrently for adjunctive local benefit in the treatment of these lesions.

Cream, gel, or solution: Good results can be anticipated in those with recent fungus infection of the scalp.

Powder and powder aerosol: Recommended for adjunctive use in fungus infections of intertriginous and other naturally moist areas in which drying may enhance the therapeutic response. May also be used alone in simple cases of mild infection that responds to treatment with antifungal powder and measures to promote skin hygiene. Powder is also helpful in preventing reinfection.

WARNINGS

In case of sensitization, discontinue use. Not recommended for nail or scalp infection. If symptoms do not improve in 10 days, use may be discontinued.

PRECAUTIONS

If no improvement is seen in 4 weeks, diagnosis is reevaluated. In mixed infections in which bacteria or nonsusceptible fungi (such as *Candida albicans*) are present, supplementary topical or systemic therapy is indicated.

ADVERSE REACTIONS

Is essentially nonsensitizing and does not sting or irritate intact or broken skin in either exposed or intertriginous areas. A few cases of sensitization have been reported. Mild irritation has also been reported rarely.

DOSAGE

Apply bid for 2 to 3 weeks; treatment for 4 to 6 weeks may be required. Treatment can be continued to help maintain remission in those susceptible to tinea.

In general, powders are used only as adjunctive therapy with ointments, creams, and liquids as primary therapy in very mild conditions or as prophylactic agents, especially in inherently moist areas. Liquids or solutions are generally preferred for primary therapy or if the affected area is hairy. Powders with a cornstarch base may be preferred over those with a talc base.

NURSING IMPLICATIONS

HISTORY

Record description and duration of symptoms, location of lesions.

PHYSICAL ASSESSMENT

Examine lesions.

ADMINISTRATION

Cleanse area prior to application with soap and water, rinse thoroughly, and pat dry.

Apply in small quantities or as directed by physician.

Do not use an occlusive dressing.

ONGOING ASSESSMENTS AND NURSING MANAGEMENT

Inspect affected area at time of each application. If redness or irritation is noted or patient complains of itching, do not apply next dose and contact physician.

If patient shows no clinical improvement after 3 to 4 weeks, inform physician.

PATIENT AND FAMILY INFORMATION

Clean area with soap and water, rinse thoroughly, and pat dry before each application.

Do not apply a dressing over the area.

If condition persists more than 3 to 4 weeks, becomes worse, or spreads to other areas, see a physician.

Tinea infections

Keep towels, face cloths, and bedding separate from those of other members of the family. Launder clothing and linens daily; use hot water and detergent. Do not wash clothes or bedding used by other members of the family at same time.

Tinea corporis, cruris: Change clothing contacting the infected area after each application.

Tinea pedis: Keep feet dry; change socks daily or whenever damp or wet. Expose feet to air as much as possible. Wear loosely fitting shoes and avoid shoes made of plastic or with a plastic (waterproofing) coating.

Tranylcypromine Sulfate

See Antidepressants, Monoamine Oxidase Inhibitors.

Trazodone

See Antidepressants.

Triacetin (Glyceryl Triacetate) Rx, otc

cream: 250 mg/g	Enzactin (*otc*)
ointment: 25%	Fungacetin (*otc*)
liquid: triacetin, cetylpyridinium chloride, chloroxylenol	Fungoid Tincture (*Rx*)
solution: triacetin, cetylpyridinium chloride, chloroxylenol	Fungoid (*Rx*)
cream: triacetin, cetylpyridinium chloride, chloroxylenol	Fungoid Cream (*Rx*)

INDICATIONS
A fungistat for athlete's foot (tinea pedis) and other superficial fungus infections.

DOSAGE
Apply bid. Continue use for 1 week after symptoms have disappeared.

NURSING IMPLICATIONS

HISTORY
Record description and duration of symptoms; location of lesions.

PHYSICAL ASSESSMENT
Examine involved area.

ADMINISTRATION
Cleanse affected areas as directed by physician (manufacturers recommend dilute alcohol or mild soap and water), rinse thoroughly, and pat dry.

Cream, ointment: Apply in thin layer or as directed by the physician.

Powder: Lightly dust affected area.

Liquid, solution: Apply with cotton-tipped applicator.

Prevent contact with rayon fabrics by covering treated area on body with clean cloth or bandage, unless physician directs otherwise.

ONGOING ASSESSMENTS AND NURSING MANAGEMENT
Examine affected area at time of each application. If redness or irritation is noted, contact physician.

If patient shows no clinical improvement after 2 weeks, inform physician.

PATIENT AND FAMILY INFORMATION
If condition persists more than 2 weeks, becomes worse, or spreads to other areas, contact physician.

If affected area is on the body, cover with clean cloth or bandage to prevent contact with rayon fabrics.

Clean area with *dilute* alcohol or soap and water, rinse thoroughly, and pat dry before each application.

Keep towels, face cloths, and bedding separate from those of other members of the family. Launder clothing and linens daily; use hot water and detergent. Do not wash clothes or bedding used by other members of the family at the same time.

Change clothing contacting the infected area after each application.

Athlete's foot: Keep feet dry; change socks daily or whenever damp or wet. Expose feet to air as much as possible. Wear loosely fitting shoes and avoid shoes made of plastic or with a plastic (waterproofing) coating.

Triamcinolone

See Glucocorticoids.

Triamcinolone Acetonide

See Corticosteroids, Topical; Glucocorticoids.

Triamcinolone Diacetate

See Glucocorticoids.

Triamcinolone Hexacetonide

See Glucocorticoids.

Triamterene Preparations

Triamterene *Rx*

capsules: 50 mg, Dyrenium
   100 mg

Triamterene With Hydrochlorothiazide *Rx*

capsules: 50 mg Dyazide
   triamterene, 25 mg
   hydrochloro-
   thiazide

INDICATIONS

TRIAMTERENE

Treatment of edema associated with CHF, cirrhosis of the liver, and the nephrotic syndrome; also in steroid-induced edema, idiopathic edema, and edema due to secondary hyperaldosteronism. It may be used alone or with other diuretics either for its added diuretic effect or for its potassium-conserving potential. It also promotes increased diuresis when cases prove resistant or only partially responsive to thiazides or other diuretics because of secondary hyperaldosteronism.

TRIAMTERENE WITH HYDROCHLOROTHIAZIDE

Indicated primarily in treatment of edema. Usefulness of this combination in hypertension is derived from the potassium-sparing effect of triamterene. It is indicated as adjunctive therapy in edema associated with CHF, hepatic cirrhosis, and the nephrotic syndrome. It also is used in corticosteroid- and estrogen-induced edema and idiopathic edema.

CONTRAINDICATIONS

Not given to those receiving other potassium-sparing agents such as spironolactone or amiloride. Also not given in anuria; severe hepatic disease; hyperkalemia; hypersensitivity to triamterene; or severe or progressive kidney disease or dysfunction, with the possible exception of nephrosis.

For triamterene with hydrochlorothiazide, see also Thiazides and Related Diuretics.

ACTIONS

Triamterene inhibits the reabsorption of sodium ions in exchange for potassium and hydrogen ions at that segment of the distal tubule under the control of adrenal mineralocorticoids (especially aldosterone). This is the result of a direct effect on the renal tubule and not through competitive aldosterone antagonism. It is 30% to 70% absorbed. Onset of action is 2 to 4 hours. Most patients respond on the first day of treatment, but maximum therapeutic effect may not be seen for several days. Duration of diuresis depends on several factors, especially renal function; it generally tapers off 7 to 9 hours after administration. It is metabolized primarily in the liver; about 3% to 5% is excreted unchanged in the urine.

For triamterene with hydrochlorothiazide, see also Thiazides and Related Diuretics.

WARNINGS

Patient is monitored regularly for occurrence of blood dyscrasias, liver damage, or other idiosyncratic reactions.

Use in impaired renal function: Periodic BUN and serum potassium determinations are recommended to check kidney function, especially in those with suspected or confirmed renal insufficiency and in elderly and diabetic patients.

Use in pregnancy and lactation: Triamterene may cross the placental barrier and appear in cord blood. No congenital defects have been noted when used during pregnancy. Drug is used only when clearly needed and when potential benefits outweigh the unknown potential hazards to the fetus. Triamterene may appear in human milk. If the drug is deemed essential, the woman should stop nursing. Routine use of diuretics during pregnancy is inappropriate and exposes mother and fetus to unnecessary hazards. Diuretics do not prevent development of toxemia and are not useful in treatment of developed toxemia. Diuretics are indicated during pregnancy when edema is due to pathologic causes.

Triamterene with hydrochlorothiazide is not indicated for initial therapy of edema or hypertension. See also Thiazides and Related Diuretics.

PRECAUTIONS

Hyperkalemia: Triamterene tends to conserve potassium and can increase serum potassium, which may result in hyperkalemia, especially in those with renal insufficiency, in those receiving potassium supplements, and in those with diabetic nephropathy. Hyperkalemia has been associated with cardiac irregularities. Hyperkalemia rarely occurs in those with adequate renal output, but it is a possibility if large doses are used for considerable periods of time. If it occurs, drug is discontinued. When triamterene is added to other diuretic therapy, or

T

when patients are switched to triamterene from other diuretics, potassium supplementation is discontinued.

Electrolyte imbalance: In CHF, renal disease, or cirrhosis, electrolyte imbalance may be aggravated or caused independently by diuretic agents. The use of a full dose of a diuretic when salt intake is restricted can result in a low salt syndrome. Triamterene can cause mild nitrogen retention, which is reversible upon withdrawal; this is seldom observed during intermittent therapy.

Renal stones: Triamterene has been found in renal stones with other usual calculus components, and it is therefore used cautiously in those with a history of stone formation.

Triamterene is a weak folic acid antagonist. Because cirrhotics with splenomegaly may have marked variations in hematologic status, it may contribute to the appearance of megaloblastosis in those in whom folic acid stores have been depleted. Periodic blood counts are performed on these patients.

For triamterene with hydrochlorothiazide, see also Thiazides and Related Diuretics.

DRUG INTERACTIONS

Although triamterene is not a consistent antihypertensive agent, a possible lowering of blood pressure may occur. Concomitant use with **antihypertensive drugs** may result in an additive effect. Triamterene may cause a decreasing alkali reserve with the possibility of metabolic acidosis. Triamterene used concomitantly with other potassium-sparing diuretics (**spironolactone, amiloride**) or **potassium preparations** may result in hyperkalemia.

Because **captopril** decreases aldosterone production, elevation of serum potassium may occur. Potassium-sparing diuretics or potassium supplements should be given only for documented hypokalemia, and then with caution, because they may lead to a significant increase in serum potassium. Unexpected increases in serum levels of **digitalis glycosides** may occur with triamterene. Potassium retention caused by triamterene may reduce the cardiac effects of digitalis glycosides.

A possible interaction resulting in acute renal failure has been reported when **indomethacin** was given with triamterene. **Nonsteroidal anti-inflammatory agents** are given cautiously with triamterene.

Lithium generally should not be given with diuretics because diuretics reduce the renal clearance of lithium and increase the risk of lithium toxicity.

Drug/lab tests: Triamterene will interfere with the fluorescent measurement of quinidine serum levels.

For triamterene with hydrochlorothiazide, see also Thiazides and Related Diuretics.

ADVERSE REACTIONS

GI: There have been occasional reports of diarrhea, nausea, vomiting, and other GI disturbances. Symptoms of nausea and vomiting are also symptoms of electrolyte imbalance.

Renal: Triamterene has been found in renal stones. Rare occurrences of acute interstitial nephritis have been reported in those receiving triamterene or a triamterene/hydrochlorothiazide combination. Onset was immediate to 10 weeks after initiation of therapy; resolution began upon discontinuation of the drug. Triamterene normally has little or no effect on serum uric acid levels or carbohydrate metabolism, but in those predisposed to gouty arthritis serum uric acid levels may increase.

Electrolyte imbalance and hyperkalemia: See *Precautions.*

Miscellaneous: Weakness, headache, dry mouth, anaphylaxis, photosensitivity, and rash have also been reported. Only rarely has it been necessary to discontinue therapy because of these side-effects.

For triamterene with hydrochlorothiazide, see also Thiazides and Related Diuretics.

OVERDOSAGE

Symptoms: Electrolyte imbalance is the major concern, with particular attention to possible hyperkalemia. Other symptoms may include nausea, vomiting, other GI disturbances, and weakness. Hypotension may occur.

Treatment: There is no specific antidote. Induce immediate evacuation of the stomach through emesis and gastric lavage. Make careful evaluation of the electrolyte pattern and fluid balance. Although triamterene is highly protein bound, dialysis may be of some benefit.

For triamterene with hydrochlorothiazide, see also Thiazides and Related Diuretics.

DOSAGE

TRIAMTERENE

Dosage is individualized. When used alone, usual starting dose is 100 mg bid, P.C. When combined with another diuretic, the total daily dosage of each agent is decreased initially, and then dosage is adjusted to patient's needs. Total daily dosage should not exceed 300 mg.

TRIAMTERENE WITH HYDROCHLOROTHIAZIDE

One or two capsules bid, P.C.

NURSING IMPLICATIONS

HISTORY
See Appendix 4.

PHYSICAL ASSESSMENT
Obtain blood pressure in both arms with patient in sitting, standing, and lying positions; obtain pulse, respirations, weight; examine extremities for edema. Baseline laboratory tests may include serum electrolytes, CBC, and hepatic-function tests.

ADMINISTRATION
Give after meals to prevent GI upset.

Obtain blood pressure and pulse before administration. Use same arm and same patient position each time blood pressure is measured. If a significant decrease has occurred, withhold next dose and notify physician.

ONGOING ASSESSMENTS AND NURSING MANAGEMENT
Monitor blood pressure and pulse q4h or as ordered. Notify physician of significant increases or decreases in blood pressure and pulse.

CLINICAL ALERT: Observe for signs of hyperkalemia (Appendix 6, section 6-15) and notify physician if they occur. This is especially important in elderly or diabetic patients and in those with known renal insufficiency. Diabetic patients with nephropathy are especially prone to develop hyperkalemia.

Patients with CHF, renal disease, or cirrhosis are observed closely for signs of electrolyte imbalance, which may be aggravated or caused by diuretic agents.

Hyperkalemia rarely occurs in those with adequate urinary output. Check with physician about any increase in oral intake, especially if the patient has CHF or cirrhosis.

Measure intake and output, especially during early therapy. Report any changes in the intake–output ratio to the physician.

Weigh daily, preferably before breakfast, during initial dosage period. Notify physician if significant weight loss (1 lb/day or more) occurs.

If edema was present before institution of therapy, examine extremities daily and compare findings with data base.

Observe for adverse effects.

Most patients respond during the first day of treatment, but maximum therapeutic effect may not be seen for several days.

Periodic serum electrolytes, CBC, and hepatic-function tests may be ordered.

Potassium supplements or a diet high in potassium is usually not necessary. Restriction of sodium intake is usually not necessary because of the possibility of a low salt syndrome, which may occur with full doses of a diuretic.

Patients receiving a digitalis glycoside are observed for digitalis toxicity.

Renal stones have occurred in those with histories of stone formation. Notify physician if flank or abdominal pain, fever, or signs of a urinary-tract infection occur.

For triamterene with hydrochlorothiazide, see also Thiazide and Related Diuretics.

PATIENT AND FAMILY INFORMATION
NOTE: If drug is given for hypertension, physician may wish patient or family member to monitor blood pressure. Instruction will be necessary.

May cause GI upset; take after meals.

May cause skin rash, weakness, headache, nausea, vomiting, and dry mouth; notify physician or nurse if these become severe or persistent.

Dry mouth may be relieved by frequent sips of water, chewing gum, or hard candy.

Notify physician or nurse if fever, sore throat, mouth sores, or unusual bleeding or bruising occurs.

Avoid prolonged exposure to sunlight; photosensitivity may occur.

Triazolam Rx C-IV

tablets: 0.25 mg, 0.5   Halcion
   mg

INDICATIONS
Short-term management of insomnia characterized by difficulty in falling asleep, frequent nocturnal awakenings, and/or early morning awakenings.

CONTRAINDICATIONS
Hypersensitivity to triazolam or other benzodiazepines. Contraindicated in pregnancy. If there is a likelihood that the patient may become pregnant while receiving triazolam, patient is warned of potential risk to the fetus. The possibility that the patient may be pregnant at the time therapy is instituted is considered. Benzodiazepines may cause fetal damage when given during pregnancy. An increased risk of congenital malformations associated with use of diazepam and chlordiazepoxide during the first trimester has been suggested. Trans-

placental distribution results in neonatal CNS depression following therapeutic doses of a benzodiazepine hypnotic during the last weeks of pregnancy.

ACTIONS

Is a triazolobenzodiazepine hypnotic. It is readily absorbed. Mean peak concentration occurs 1.3 hours following a single dose. Triazolam has a short mean plasma half-life of 2.3 hours, with a range of 1.7 to 3 hours. Triazolam and its metabolites are excreted primarily in the urine. It decreases sleep latency, increases the duration of sleep, decreases the number of nocturnal awakenings, and after 2 weeks of consecutive nightly administration decreases total wake time.

WARNINGS

It is recommended that drug not be prescribed in quantities exceeding a 1-month supply. In elderly or debilitated patients, a lower initial dosage is used to decrease possibility of oversedation, dizziness, or impaired coordination.

Anterograde amnesia of varying severity and paradoxical reactions have been reported.

A child born of a mother who is on benzodiazepines may be at some risk for withdrawal symptoms from the drug during the postnatal period. Administration to nursing mothers not recommended. Safety and efficacy for use in children under 18 are not established.

PRECAUTIONS

Signs or symptoms of depression may be intensified by hypnotic drugs. Suicidal tendencies may be present and protective measures may be required.

Abuse and dependence: Withdrawal symptoms similar to those noted with barbiturates and alcohol have occurred following abrupt discontinuance. These range from mild dysphoria to a major syndrome, which may include abdominal and muscle cramps, vomiting, sweating, tremor, and convulsions. Patients with a history of seizures should not be abruptly withdrawn from any CNS depressant agent. Caution is exercised in giving to addiction-prone individuals because of the predisposition of such patients to habituation and dependence.

Usual precautions are observed when using in impaired renal or hepatic function and chronic pulmonary insufficiency.

Laboratory tests: When triazolam treatment is protracted, periodic blood counts, urinalysis, and blood chemistries are recommended.

DRUG INTERACTIONS

Possible additive CNS depressant effects may occur when coadministered with other **psychotropic medi-** cations, anticonvulsants, antihistamines, alcohol, ethanol, and other **CNS depressant** drugs.

ADVERSE REACTIONS

Common: Drowsiness (14%), headache (9.7%), dizziness (7.8%), nervousness (5.2%), lightheadedness (4.9%), coordination disorders/ataxia (4.6%), nausea/vomiting (4.6%).

Less frequent: Euphoria, tachycardia, tiredness, confusional states/memory impairment, cramps/pain, depression, visual disturbances.

Rare: Constipation, taste alterations, diarrhea, dry mouth, dermatitis/allergy, dreaming/nightmares, insomnia, paresthesia, tinnitus, dysesthesia, weakness, congestion. See also Antianxiety Agents, Benzodiazepines for additional adverse reactions reported with all benzodiazepines.

OVERDOSAGE

Symptoms: Somnolence, confusion, impaired coordination, slurred speech, and, ultimately, coma. Overdosage may occur at 2 mg, four times the recommended maximum dose.

Treatment: Monitor respiration, pulse, and blood pressure. Support by general measures; perform immediate gastric lavage and maintain an adequate airway. IV fluids may be given. Hemodialysis and forced diuresis are of little value. The ingestion of multiple agents should be considered.

DOSAGE

Range for adults is 0.25 mg to 0.5 mg H.S. In geriatric or debilitated patients, the range is 0.125 mg to 0.25 mg. Initiate therapy at 0.125 mg until individual response is determined.

NURSING IMPLICATIONS

HISTORY

See Appendix 4.

PHYSICAL ASSESSMENT

Obtain blood pressure, pulse, and respirations. Determine whether specific factors that may be controlled or eliminated may be interfering with sedation or sleep. Factors may include noise, bright lights, pain, and discomfort.

ADMINISTRATION

Do not administer if the patient has pain, which should be controlled with an analgesic.

Do not administer shortly before or after administration of a narcotic analgesic or other CNS depressant. If patient has an order for a narcotic analgesic (or other CNS depressant) and a hypnotic, check with physician about time interval between administration of these agents. Usually 2 or more hours should elapse between administration of this drug and other CNS depressants, but interval may vary with a specific CNS depressant and the dose administered.

Dosage should be reduced in elderly or debilitated patients because these patients may be more sensitive to this drug.

Following administration, raise the siderails and advise patient to remain in bed and call for assistance if it is necessary to get out of bed.

ONGOING ASSESSMENTS AND NURSING MANAGEMENT

Observe patient in 1 to 2 hours after administration to evaluate effect of the drug.

If patient awakens during the night or early morning hours, inform physician. A different hypnotic may be necessary.

Observe for adverse reactions.

Observe patient, especially the elderly or debilitated, for oversedation and confusional states. If these occur, observe at frequent intervals (as often as every 5–10 minutes may be necessary) for duration of these adverse effects. Inform physician of problem because a different drug may be necessary.

Due to its short half-life, triazolam may pose fewer problems (*e.g.,* daytime sedation, CNS depression) due to accumulation but may cause increased wakefulness during the last third of the night or increased daytime anxiety.

CLINICAL ALERT: Withdrawal symptoms similar in character to those noted with barbiturates have occurred following abrupt discontinuance. Patients with a history of seizures should also not be abruptly withdrawn from this drug.

Signs or symptoms of depression may be intensified. Suicidal tendencies may be present and protective measures may be required.

When drug is given for a prolonged period of time, periodic blood counts, urinalysis, and blood chemistries are recommended.

If a mother has been taking this drug prior to delivery, closely observe the neonate for flaccidity.

On the first night after the drug is discontinued, insomnia may occur.

PATIENT AND FAMILY INFORMATION

Avoid alcohol and other CNS depressants while taking this drug.

Do not exceed prescribed dosage. If drug fails to produce sleep, contact physician.

Do not discontinue medication abruptly after prolonged therapy.

May cause drowsiness or dizziness. This drug should be taken immediately before retiring. Do not attempt to drive or perform other potentially hazardous tasks after taking this drug.

Notify physician or nurse if nausea, vomiting, headache, confusion, or visual disturbances occur.

Accidental overdose has occurred when an individual awakens during the night and has forgotten use of a "sleeping pill" that may have been ingested only a short time earlier. To avoid accidental overdose, keep this medication in an area other than the bedroom or bathroom.

Trichlormethiazide

See Thiazides and Related Diuretics.

Triclofos Sodium

See Chloral Derivatives.

Triethylenethiophosphoramide

(TSPA, TESPA) Rx

powder for injection: Thiotepa
15 mg/vial

INDICATIONS

Adenocarcinoma of the breast or ovary; control of intracavitary effusions secondary to diffuse or localized neoplastic disease of various serosal cavities; treatment of superficial papillary carcinoma of the urinary bladder. Although now superseded by other treatments, this drug has been effective against lymphomas, such as lymphosarcoma and Hodgkin's disease.

Investigational uses: Has been used for prevention of pterygium recurrences following surgery.

CONTRAINDICATIONS

Known hypersensitivity; existing hepatic, renal, or bone-marrow damage. If benefits outweigh the potential risks, drug is used in low doses and hepatic, renal, and hematopoietic functions are monitored.

ACTIONS

A cell cycle nonspecific alkylating agent related to nitrogen mustard. It is not a vesicant, like nitrogen mustard, and causes less tissue necrosis at the administration site, which makes it suitable for intracavity administration.

Its radiomimetic action is believed to occur

through release of ethylenimine radicals, which disrupt the bonds of DNA. The drug has no differential affinity for neoplasms. It is rapidly cleared from plasma following IV administration. About 85% is excreted unchanged in the urine. See also Appendix 10.

WARNINGS

This drug is highly toxic to the hematopoietic system. A rapidly falling WBC or platelet count indicates the necessity for discontinuing or reducing dosage. Weekly blood and platelet counts are recommended during therapy and for at least 3 weeks after therapy has been discontinued.

The most serious complication of excessive therapy or sensitivity is bone-marrow depression. The drug may cause leukopenia, thrombocytopenia, and anemia. Death from septicemia and hemorrhage has occurred as a result of hematopoietic depression.

If the WBC falls to 3000 or less, or the platelet count falls to 150,000, therapy is discontinued. The red blood cell count is a less accurate indicator of toxicity.

Like all alkylating agents, this drug is carcinogenic; strong circumstantial evidence suggests carcinogenicity in humans.

This drug is not recommended in pregnancy unless potential benefits outweigh the risk of teratogenicity.

PRECAUTIONS

It is not advisable to combine therapeutic modalities having the same mechanism of action. This drug, combined with other alkylating agents or with irradiation, would intensify toxicity rather than enhance therapeutic response. If these agents must follow each other, it is important that recovery from the first, as indicated by WBC count, be complete before therapy with the second agent is instituted.

DRUG INTERACTIONS

Other drugs known to produce bone-marrow depression are avoided.

ADVERSE REACTIONS

Apart from its effect on blood-forming elements, this drug may cause other adverse reactions including pain at the injection site, nausea, vomiting, dizziness, headache, amenorrhea, anorexia, and interference with spermatogenesis. Febrile reactions and weeping from a subcutaneous lesion may occur owing to breakdown of tumor. Allergic reactions are rare, but hives and skin rash have been seen occasionally.

DOSAGE

Is carefully individualized. A slow response may be deceptive and may lead to unwarranted frequency of administration with subsequent toxicity. After maximum benefit is obtained by initial therapy, it is necessary to continue the patient on maintenance therapy (1- to 4-week intervals).

Initial and maintenance doses: Usually the higher dose in the given range is administered initially. The maintenance dose is adjusted weekly based on pretreatment control blood counts and subsequent blood counts.

IV administration: May be given by rapid administration in doses of 0.3 mg/kg to 0.4 mg/kg. Doses should be given at 1- to 4-week intervals.

Intratumor administration: Initial doses of 0.6 mg/kg to 0.8 mg/kg may be injected directly into a tumor. Maintenance doses at 1- to 4-week intervals range from 0.07 mg/kg to 0.8 mg/kg.

Intracavitary administration: Recommended dosage is 0.6 mg/kg to 0.8 mg/kg.

Intravesical administration: Patients with papillary carcinoma of the bladder are dehydrated for 8 to 12 hours prior to treatment. Then 60 mg in 30 ml to 60 ml of distilled water is instilled into the bladder by catheter. For maximum effect, the solution should be retained for 2 hours. If the patient finds it impossible to retain 60 ml for 2 hours, the dose may be given in a volume of 30 ml. The usual course of treatment is once a week for 4 weeks. The course may be repeated if necessary, but second and third courses are given with caution, because bone-marrow depression may be increased. Deaths have occurred after intravesical administration, caused by bone-marrow depression from systemic absorption of the drug.

NURSING IMPLICATIONS

HISTORY
See Appendix 4.

PHYSICAL ASSESSMENT
Obtain vital signs, weight; evaluate patient's general physical and emotional status. Baseline laboratory studies may include CBC, differential, platelet count, renal- and hepatic-function studies.

ADMINISTRATION
Preparation of solution: Powder is reconstituted with Sterile Water for Injection. Unless physician orders otherwise, dilute with 1.5 ml,

resulting in a drug concentration of 5 mg/0.5 ml of solution. Larger volumes are usually used for intracavitary use, IV drip, or perfusion therapy.

The reconstituted preparation may be added to larger volumes of other diluents: Sodium Chloride Injection USP, Dextrose Injection USP, Dextrose and Sodium Chloride Injection USP, or Lactated Ringer's Injection USP. Physician orders type and volume of diluent.

The reconstituted solution should be clear to slightly opaque. Solutions that are grossly opaque or contain a precipitate should not be used.

Sterile Water for Injection produces an isotonic solution. The addition of other diluents may result in hypertonic solutions, which may cause mild to moderate discomfort on injection.

For local use into single or multiple sites, this drug may be mixed with 2% procaine HCl, 1:1000 epinephrine HCl, or both.

Prior to administration, obtain vital signs and advise patient that pain may occur at the injection site.

Storage: Store original powder and reconstituted solution in the refrigerator at 2° to 8°C (36°F to 46°F). Reconstituted solutions are stable for 5 days when kept under refrigeration.

IV administration: Physician orders method of administration (*i.e.,* direct IV or IV infusion). If given by IV infusion, physician orders rate of infusion.

May be given by rapid IV administration as drug is a nonvesciant.

Intratumor infusion: Obtain necessary materials for administration (*e.g.,* local anesthetic, gloves, syringes, needles).

Physician orders type and volume of diluent. Usually, the drug is diluted in sterile water to 10 mg/ml.

A small amount of local anesthetic is injected first; then the syringe is removed and the drug is injected through the same needle.

Intracavitary administration: Physician orders type and volume of diluent.

Administration is usually effected through the same tubing used to remove fluid from the cavity.

Intravesical administration: Patient is dehydrated 8 to 12 hours prior to administration, usually by being kept NPO for this period of time.

Sixty milligrams is diluted in either 30 ml or 60 ml of water, depending on physician preference.

Solution is instilled into the bladder by means of a catheter.

Following instillation, the catheter is usually removed.

ONGOING ASSESSMENTS AND NURSING MANAGEMENT

When drug is instilled into the bladder, the physician may order the patient repositioned every 15 minutes for approximately 2 hours to ensure maximum area contact.

Monitor vital signs q4h or as ordered.

Measure intake and output. If oral intake is low or there is any change in the intake–output ratio, notify physician.

Observe for adverse reactions. Skin rash and urticaria are reported to the physician immediately.

CLINICAL ALERT: This drug is highly toxic to the hematopoietic system. This drug may cause leukopenia, thrombocytopenia, and anemia. Initial effects of this drug on the bone marrow may not be evident for up to 30 days.

Observe patient closely for signs of bone-marrow depression (Appendix 6, section 6-8) beginning with the first week of therapy. If one or more signs or symptoms are apparent, notify the physician immediately.

Monitor blood and platelet counts; notify physician of any decrease in WBC, hemoglobin, or platelet count.

If leukopenia occurs, protective (reverse) isolation may be necessary.

If thrombocytopenia occurs, assess for evidence of bleeding q4h. Look for bleeding gums; hematemesis; black, tarry stools; rectal bleeding; ecchymosis; epistaxis; hematuria. Report occurrence of bleeding immediately. Use prolonged pressure on IM and venipuncture sites. Exercise care in applying blood-pressure cuff to avoid bruising of the area. Rectal temperatures are usually avoided. Use a soft toothbrush and frequent mouth rinses with warm water for oral care.

Weigh weekly or as ordered. Inform physician if a significant weight loss occurs.

If patient has experienced nausea and vomiting with a prior dose, inform physician; an antiemetic may be necessary.

If nausea and vomiting are severe, a liquid diet, carbonated beverages, dry toast, or unsalted crackers may be offered.

If anorexia persists for more than 2 days, inform physician. A high-calorie, high-protein diet in small frequent feedings or other methods of providing calories may be necessary.

Febrile reactions and weeping from subcutaneous lesions may occur because of breakdown of the tumor. Meticulous skin care and prevention of infection will be essential.

Notify physician or nurse immediately if any of the following occurs: fever, upper respiratory illness (*e.g.,* cold, cough), abscess formation, easy bleeding or bruising, severe nausea and vomiting, extreme fatigue, skin rash, or hives.

If nausea and vomiting occur, contact the physician. An antiemetic may be ordered.

If anorexia occurs, eat small frequent meals.

Mild nausea and vomiting may be relieved by carbonated beverages, dry toast, or unsalted crackers.

A change in the menstrual pattern (amenorrhea) may occur.

Interference with spermatogenesis may occur.

Inform other physicians and dentist of therapy with this drug.

Trifluoperazine

See Antipsychotic Agents.

Triflupromazine Hydrochloride

See Antiemetic/Antivertigo Agents; Antipsychotic Agents.

Trifluridine Rx

ophthalmic solu-   Viroptic
   tion: 1%

INDICATIONS
Treatment of primary keratoconjunctivitis and recurrent epithelial keratitis due to herpes simplex virus, types 1 and 2. Also effective in treatment of epithelial keratitis that has not responded to topical administration of idoxuridine or when ocular toxicity or hypersensitivity to idoxuridine has occurred. In a smaller number of patients found to be resistant to vidarabine, trifluridine was also effective.

CONTRAINDICATIONS
Hypersensitivity reactions or chemical intolerance to trifluridine.

ACTIONS
Has activity against herpes simplex virus, types 1 and 2, and vaccinia virus. Some strains of adenovirus are also inhibited. Its antiviral mechanism of action is not completely understood.

Intraocular penetration occurs after topical instillation. Decreased corneal integrity or stromal or uveal inflammation may enhance penetration into the aqueous humor. Systemic absorption appears to be negligible.

WARNINGS
Has been shown to exert mutagenic, DNA-damaging, and cell-transforming activities in various standard *in vitro* tests. The significance of these test results is not clear. The possibility exists that mutagenic agents may cause genetic damage in humans. The oncogenic potential is unknown. Safety for use in pregnancy is not established. Drug is used only when clearly needed and when potential benefits outweigh the unknown potential hazards to the fetus.

It is unlikely that this drug is excreted in human milk after ophthalmic instillation; however, it is not recommended for nursing mothers unless the potential benefits outweigh the potential risks.

PRECAUTIONS
The diagnosis of herpetic keratitis should be established prior to use. Trifluridine may cause mild local irritation of the conjunctiva and cornea when instilled, but these effects are usually transient.

ADVERSE REACTIONS
Most frequent were mild, transient burning or stinging upon instillation (4.6%) and palpebral edema (2.8%). Other adverse reactions in decreasing order of frequency were superficial punctate keratopathy, epithelial keratopathy, hypersensitivity reaction, stromal edema, irritation, keratitis sicca, hyperemia, and increased intraocular pressure.

DOSAGE
One drop instilled onto the cornea of the affected eye every 2 hours while awake for a maximum daily dosage of nine drops until the corneal ulcer has completely reepithelialized. Following reepithelialization, continue treatment for an additional 7 days of one drop q4h while awake for a minimum daily dosage of five drops.

If there are no signs of improvement after 7 days or complete reepithelialization has not occurred after 14 days, other forms of therapy are considered. Continuous administration for periods exceeding 21 days is avoided because of potential ocular toxicity.

NURSING IMPLICATIONS

HISTORY
See Appendix 4.

PHYSICAL ASSESSMENT
Examine adjacent structures of the eye for signs of inflammation and infection.

ADMINISTRATION
Instill one drop in the lower conjunctival sac.

Apply light finger pressure on lacrimal sac for approximately 1 minute.

Storage: Prior to dispensing, product is stored under refrigeration at 2°C to 8°C (36°F to 46°F). Elevated temperatures accelerate degradation of the drug.

ONGOING ASSESSMENTS AND NURSING MANAGEMENT
Inspect eye daily for evidence of irritation or secondary infection.

If improvement is not noted within 7 days, inform physician.

PATIENT AND FAMILY INFORMATION
NOTE: Proper instillation technique is explained to patient or family member.

Transient stinging or burning may occur upon instillation.

Use exactly as prescribed. Do not increase or decrease the dose or the intervals between doses.

Take care not to contaminate tip of dropper. Replace dropper in bottle immediately after instilling medicine.

Apply light finger pressure to lacrimal sac for 1 minute following instillation.

Do not discontinue use without consulting physician.

Notify physician or nurse if improvement is not seen after 7 days, if condition worsens, or if irritation occurs.

Trihexyphenidyl Hydrochloride

See Anticholinergic Antiparkinsonism Agents.

Trimeprazine

See Antihistamines.

Trimethadione

See Anticonvulsants, Oxazolidinediones.

Trimethaphan Camsylate Rx

injection: 50 mg/ml   Arfonad

INDICATIONS
Production of controlled hypotension during surgery; short-term control of blood pressure in hypertensive emergencies; emergency treatment of pulmonary edema in those with pulmonary hypertension associated with systemic hypertension.

Investigational use: Has been used in patients with dissecting aortic aneurysm or in ischemic heart disease when other agents cannot be used.

CONTRAINDICATIONS
When hypotension may subject patient to undue risk (*e.g.,* uncorrected anemia, hypovolemia, shock [both incipient and frank], asphyxia, or uncorrected respiratory insufficiency). Inadequate availability of fluids and inability to replace blood for technical reasons may also be a contraindication.

ACTIONS
A short-acting ganglionic blocking agent. Blocks transmission in autonomic (both sympathetic and parasympathetic) ganglia without producing any preceding or concomitant change in membrane potentials. Does not modify conduction of impulses in preganglionic or postganglionic neurons and does not prevent release of acetylcholine by preganglionic impulse. Produces ganglionic blockade by occupying ganglion receptors and by stabilizing postsynaptic membranes against the action of acetylcholine from the presynaptic nerve endings. In addition, it may also exert a direct peripheral vasodilator effect. It causes pooling of blood in the dependent periphery and the splanchnic system, resulting in lowering of blood pressure. The drug liberates histamine.

Has an immediate onset and brief duration of action after IV infusion. Tachyphylaxis may occur, requiring increasing doses to maintain effect.

WARNINGS
Adequate oxygenation must be assured during treatment, especially in regard to coronary and cerebral circulation. Extreme caution is used in those with arteriosclerosis, cardiac disease, hepatic or renal disease, degenerative disease of the CNS, Addison's disease, or diabetes and in patients under treatment with steroids.

Use in pregnancy: Induced hypotension may have serious consequences to the fetus.

PRECAUTIONS
Use with great caution in elderly or debilitated patients and in children. Because this drug liberates histamine, it is used with caution in allergic individuals.

Pupillary dilatation does not necessarily indicate anoxia or the depth of anesthesia, because the drug appears to have a specific effect on the pupil.

Rare cases of respiratory arrest due to aggressive dosage may occur, although a causal relationship has not been established.

DRUG INTERACTIONS

Use with care in those receiving **other antihypertensive drugs** and **diuretics,** because an additive effect may occur. Use with caution with **anesthetic agents,** especially spinal anesthetics, which may produce hypotension. Concomitant therapy with other drugs can modify the dose necessary to achieve a desired response.

OVERDOSAGE

Vasopressor agents may be used to correct undesirable low pressures during surgery or to effect a more rapid return to normotensive levels. Phenylephrine HCl or mephentermine sulfate should be tried initially. Norepinephrine is reserved for refractory cases.

DOSAGE

Administer by IV drip. Rates from 0.3 ml to 6 ml/minute of a solution containing 1 mg/ml have been found necessary.

Surgical use: Administration is stopped prior to wound closure to permit blood pressure to return to normal. A systolic pressure of 100 mm Hg will usually be attained within 10 minutes after discontinuation.

NURSING IMPLICATIONS

HISTORY

See Appendix 4. A history of allergy to any substance is extremely important because this drug is given with caution to those with an allergy history.

PHYSICAL ASSESSMENT

Obtain blood pressure, pulse, and respirations; evaluate patient's general physical status (*i.e.,* skin color, level of consciousness, presence of focal neurologic signs). If pulmonary edema is present, auscultate lungs; note presence of neck vein distention and character of sputum.

ADMINISTRATION

Have available oxygen, equipment for resuscitation and ventilation, and vasopressor agents (*e.g.,* phenylephrine HCl, mephentermine sulfate, and norepinephrine) to counteract hypotensive episodes.

This drug is a powerful hypotensive agent and *must* be diluted before use.

Prepare solution immediately before use; discard any unused portion.

Dilute 10 ml (500 mg or one 10-ml ampule) of trimethaphan to 500 ml in 5% Dextrose Injection. Other diluents are *not* recommended.

This dilution will give 1 mg/ml.

Do *not* use this infusion fluid as a vehicle for administration of other drugs.

Use an infusion pump or microdrip regulator for precise administration of drug.

Obtain blood pressure, pulse, and respirations immediately before start of the infusion.

Use a large vein to start IV infusion.

Unless physician orders otherwise, place patient in a position to prevent cerebral anoxia (*e.g.,* a head-down [Trendelenburg] or supine position). Action of the drug is enhanced by placing patient in a reversed Trendelenburg position.

Physician orders infusion rate as milligrams per minute or drops per minute. Recommended initial infusion rate is 3 ml/minute to 4 ml/minute (Table 53).

ONGOING ASSESSMENTS AND NURSING MANAGEMENT

CLINICAL ALERT: Monitor blood pressure, pulse, and respirations every 1 to 2 minutes or as ordered by the physician. Use a flow sheet to record vital signs and rate of IV infusion.

Monitor patient's respiratory status closely. Although rare, respiratory arrest has occurred.

Physician establishes parameters for maintenance of blood pressure. Adjust rate of infusion to maintain desired blood-pressure level.

If pressure fails to drop, slowly raise head of bed to enhance effect of the drug.

Measure intake and output. Notify physician if there is a change in the intake–output ratio. If patient does not have an indwelling catheter, palpate lower abdomen for bladder distention q2h.

If patient had pulmonary edema or neurologic symptoms prior to initiation of therapy, observe for alleviation of symptoms. Continue assessments (see *Physical Assessment,* above) q15m to q30m and record findings.

Drug has a specific effect on the pupil, causing pupillary dilatation. Pupil size cannot be used to determine presence of anoxia.

Resistance to drug (tachyphylaxis) may de-

Table 53. Recommended Infusion Rates for 0.1% (1 mg/ml) Concentration of Trimethaphan

Delivery System (drops/ml)	Drops/Minute to Obtain 3–4 ml (3–4 mg)
10	30–40
15	45–60
60	180–240

velop. Notify the physician immediately if the blood pressure fails to remain below the desired level; dosage increases may be necessary.

Treatment may be terminated slowly. Monitor blood pressure, pulse, and respirations every 5 to 10 minutes after IV infusion is discontinued because drug has a brief duration of action. If the blood pressure stabilizes, continue to monitor these vital signs q½h or as ordered.

Following termination of trimethaphan, another antihypertensive agent is usually ordered to maintain the blood pressure at the desired level.

Trimethobenzamide Hydrochloride

See Antiemetic/Antivertigo Agents.

Trimethoprim Preparations

Trimethoprim *(TMP)* Rx

| tablets: 100 mg | Proloprim, Trimpex, *Generic* |
| tablets: 200 mg | Proloprim |

Trimethoprim and Sulfamethoxazole

(Co-Trimoxazole, TMP-SMZ) *Rx*

tablets: 80 mg trimethoprim, 400 mg sulfamethoxazole	Bactrim, Bethaprim SS, Cotrim, Septra, Sulfatrim, *Generic*
tablets, double strength: 160 mg trimethoprim, 800 mg sulfamethoxazole	Bactrim DS, Bethaprim DS, Cotrim DS, Septra DS, Sulfatrim DS, *Generic*
oral suspension: 40 mg trimethoprim, 200 mg sulfamethoxazole/5 ml	Bactrim, Bethaprim, Septra, SMZ-TMP, Sulfatrim
infusion: 80 mg trimethoprim, 400 mg sulfamethoxazole/5 ml	Bactrim I.V., Septra I.V.

INDICATIONS
TRIMETHOPRIM

Treatment of initial episodes of uncomplicated urinary-tract infections (UTIs) due to susceptible strains including *Escherichia coli, Proteus mirabilis, Klebsiella pneumoniae, Enterobacter* species, and coagulase-negative *Staphylococcus* species, including *S. saprophyticus.*

TRIMETHOPRIM AND SULFAMETHOXAZOLE

UTIs: Due to susceptible strains of *E. coli, Klebsiella-Enterobacter, P. mirabilis, P. vulgaris,* and *P. morganii.* Initial episodes of uncomplicated UTI should be treated with a single antibacterial agent rather than with this combination.

Acute otitis media in children: Due to susceptible strains of *Haemophilus influenzae* or *Streptococcus pneumoniae.* There are limited data on use in children under 2 years. Not indicated for prophylactic use or prolonged administration.

Acute exacerbation of chronic bronchitis in adults: Due to susceptible strains of *H. influenzae* and *S. pneumoniae.*

Shigellosis: Treatment of enteritis caused by susceptible strains of *Shigella flexneri* and *S. sonnei* when antibacterial therapy is indicated.

Pneumocystis carnii *pneumonitis:* In children and adults.

Unlabeled uses: Treatment of cholera and salmonella-type infections. Forty milligrams trimethoprim and 200 mg sulfamethoxazole daily H.S. or a minimum of three times a week has been used to prevent recurrent UTIs in females. Also used in treatment of nocardiosis, prevention of traveler's diarrhea, and prophylaxis in granulocytopenic patients.

CONTRAINDICATIONS
TRIMETHOPRIM

Hypersensitivity; documented megaloblastic anemia due to folate deficiency.

TRIMETHOPRIM AND SULFAMETHOXAZOLE

Hypersensitivity; documented megaloblastic anemia due to folate deficiency. Contraindicated during pregnancy at term and in the nursing period because sulfonamides pass the placenta and are excreted in the milk and may cause kernicterus. Contraindicated in infants less than 2 months of age.

ACTIONS
TRIMETHOPRIM

Blocks production of tetrahydrofolic acid from dihydrofolic acid by binding to and reversibly inhibiting the enzyme dihydrofolate reductase. This binding is much stronger for the bacterial enzyme than for the corresponding mammalian enzyme. Selectively interferes with bacterial biosynthesis of nucleic aids and proteins. Trimethoprim is rapidly and completely absorbed following oral administration. Mean peak serum levels occur 1 to 4 hours after oral administration. Approximately 44% is protein bound in the blood. Half-life is 8 to 16 hours. Elimination is delayed and half-life is prolonged in those with renal failure. Excretion is chiefly by the kidneys through glomerular filtration and tubular se-

T

cretion. After oral administration, 50% to 60% is excreted in the urine in 24 hours.

TRIMETHOPRIM AND SULFAMETHOXAZOLE

Sulfamethoxazole inhibits bacterial synthesis of dihydrofolic acid by competing with para-aminobenzoic acid. When combined with trimethoprim, the combination blocks two consecutive steps in the biosynthesis of nucleic acids and proteins essential to many bacteria. Studies show that bacterial resistance develops more slowly with the combination of trimethoprim and sulfamethoxazole.

The trimethoprim and sulfamethoxazole combination is rapidly and completely absorbed following oral administration. Peak plasma levels occur in 1 to 4 hours. Following oral administration, the half-lives of both drugs are similar (average 10 hours). Following IV administration, detectable amounts of both drugs are present in the blood 24 hours after administration. Excretion of the drugs is chiefly by the kidneys.

WARNINGS

TRIMETHOPRIM

Hematologic effects: Has been reported rarely to interfere with hematopoiesis, especially in large doses or for prolonged periods.

Use in pregnancy, lactation: There are no well-controlled studies in pregnant women. Drug is used only when the potential benefits outweigh the potential hazards to the fetus. Drug is excreted in human milk. Because trimethoprim may interfere with folic acid metabolism, caution is used when giving to nursing women.

Use in children: Safety for use in infants under 2 months is not established. Efficacy for use in children under 12 is not established.

TRIMETHOPRIM AND SULFAMETHOXAZOLE

Not used in treatment of streptococcal pharyngitis. Patients with group A beta-hemolytic streptococcal tonsillopharyngitis have a greater incidence of bacteriologic failure with this combination than with penicillin.

Hematologic effects: Deaths associated with sulfonamides have been reported because of hypersensitivity reactions, agranulocytosis, aplastic anemia, and other blood dyscrasias. In elderly patients receiving certain diuretics, particularly thiazides, an increased incidence of thrombocytopenia with purpura has been reported. IV use at high doses or for extended periods of time may cause bone-marrow depression, manifested as thrombocytopenia, leukopenia, or megaloblastic anemia. If signs of bone-marrow depression occur, leucovorin 3 mg to 6 mg IM daily for 3 days or as required to restore normal

hematopoiesis is recommended. See also Trimethoprim, above.

Use in pregnancy: Use during pregnancy only if potential benefits outweigh the potential risks.

PRECAUTIONS

TRIMETHOPRIM

Give with caution to those with possible folate deficiency. Folates may be given concomitantly without interfering with antibacterial action. Also give with caution to patients with impaired renal or hepatic function.

TRIMETHOPRIM AND SULFAMETHOXAZOLE

Give with caution to those with impaired hepatic function, possible folate deficiency, severe allergy, or bronchial asthma. In G6PD-deficient individuals, hemolysis may occur. This reaction is frequently dose related. Use with caution in impaired renal function. Adequate fluid intake must be maintained to prevent crystalluria and stone formation. Urinalysis and renal-function tests are recommended during therapy, particularly in those with impaired renal function.

DRUG INTERACTIONS

TRIMETHOPRIM

Pharmacologic effects of **phenytoin** may be increased by concurrent administration of trimethoprim.

TRIMETHOPRIM AND SULFAMETHOXAZOLE

May prolong prothrombin time of those receiving **warfarin.** Coagulation tests are monitored and dosage adjustments made as required. The hypoglycemic response to **sulfonylurea** agents may be increased because of displacement from protein-binding sites. Renal excretion of **methotrexate** may be impaired. Hepatic clearance of **phenytoin** may be decreased and the biological half-life prolonged.

Drug/lab tests: May produce elevated serum creatinine, bilirubin, and alkaline phosphatase.

ADVERSE REACTIONS

TRIMETHOPRIM

Dermatologic: Rash (3%–7%), pruritus, exfoliative dermatitis. In high-dose studies, an increased incidence of maculopapular, morbilliform, and pruritic rashes occurred and were generally mild to moderate, appearing 7 to 14 days after initiation of therapy.

GI: Epigastric distress, nausea, vomiting, glossitis.

Hematologic: Thrombocytopenia, leukopenia, neutropenia, megaloblastic anemia, methemoglobinemia.

Miscellaneous: Fever, elevation of serum transaminase and bilirubin, increases in BUN and serum creatinine levels.

TRIMETHOPRIM AND SULFAMETHOXAZOLE

Blood dyscrasias: Agranulocytosis, aplastic and megaloblastic anemia, thrombocytopenia, leukopenia, hemolytic anemia, purpura, hypoprothrombinemia, methemoglobinemia.

Allergic: Erythema multiforme, Stevens-Johnson syndrome, generalized skin eruptions, epidermal necrolysis, urticaria, serum sickness, pruritus, exfoliative dermatitis, anaphylactoid reactions, periorbital edema, conjunctival and scleral injection, photosensitization, arthralgia, allergic myocarditis.

GI: Glossitis, stomatitis, nausea, emesis, abdominal pain, hepatitis, jaundice, diarrhea, pseudomembranous colitis, pancreatitis. Tablets lodged in the esophagus following administration without food or water have been reported to produce esophageal ulcers.

CNS: Headache, peripheral neuritis, mental depression, convulsions, ataxia, hallucinations, tinnitus, vertigo, insomnia, apathy, fatigue, muscle weakness, nervousness.

Miscellaneous: Drug fever, chills, and toxic necrosis with oliguria and anuria. Periarteritis nodosa and lupus erythematosus phenomenon have occurred. The sulfonamides bear certain chemical similarities to some goitrogens, diuretics (acetazolamide and the thiazides), and oral hypoglycemic agents. Goiter production, diuresis, and hypoglycemia occur rarely in those receiving sulfonamides. Cross-sensitivity may exist with these agents.

Parenteral therapy: Most frequent effects are nausea, vomiting, thrombocytopenia, and rash. These occur in fewer than 5% of patients. Local reactions, pain, and slight irritation on IV administration are infrequent. Thrombophlebitis has been observed rarely.

OVERDOSAGE

TRIMETHOPRIM

Acute: Signs may appear following ingestion of 1 g or more and include nausea, vomiting, dizziness, headaches, mental depression, confusion, and bone-marrow depression (see Overdosage, Chronic, below). Treatment includes gastric lavage and general supportive measures. Acidification of the urine increases renal elimination. Peritoneal dialysis is not effective and hemodialysis is only moderately effective in eliminating the drug.

Chronic: Symptoms occurring after use of high doses over extended periods may cause bone-marrow depression manifested by thrombocytopenia, leukopenia, and/or megaloblastic anemia. Treatment includes discontinuation of drug and administration of leucovorin, 3 mg to 6 mg IM daily for 3 days or as required to restore normal hematopoiesis.

TRIMETHOPRIM AND SULFAMETHOXAZOLE

Symptoms noted in animal studies following high IV doses included ataxia, decreased motor activity, loss of righting reflex, tremors or convulsions, and respiratory depression. There has been no extensive experience in humans with high single-infusion doses, and the maximum tolerated dose in humans is unknown. Peritoneal dialysis is not effective, and hemodialysis is only moderately effective, in removing the drug.

DOSAGE

TRIMETHOPRIM

Adults: 100 mg q12h or 200 mg q24h, each for 10 days.

Renal impairment: If creatinine clearance is less than 15 ml/minute, use is not recommended. If creatinine clearance is 15 ml/minute to 30 ml/minute, 50 mg q12h.

Children (under 12): Effectiveness not established.

TRIMETHOPRIM AND SULFAMETHOXAZOLE

UTIs, shigellosis, and acute otitis media

Adults: 160 mg trimethoprim/800 mg sulfamethoxazole q12h for 10 to 14 days in UTIs and 5 days for shigellosis.

Children: 8 mg/kg trimethoprim and 40 mg/kg sulfamethoxazole per 24 hours, given in two divided doses q12h for 10 days in UTIs and acute otitis media and for 5 days in shigellosis. In children weighing 88 lb (40 kg) or more, 160 mg trimethoprim and 800 mg sulfamethoxazole q12h for 10 days.

IV infusion: 8 mg/kg/day to 10 mg/kg/day (based on the trimethoprim component), in two to four divided doses every 6, 8, or 12 hours for up to 14 days for UTIs; 5 days for shigellosis.

Acute exacerbations of chronic bronchitis in adults

160 mg trimethoprim/800 mg sulfamethoxazole q12h for 14 days.

Pneumocystis carinii *pneumonitis*

Adults and children: 20 mg/kg trimethoprim and 100 mg/kg sulfamethoxazole per 24 hours, in equally divided doses q6h for 14 days.

IV infusion: 15 mg/kg/day to 20 mg/kg/day (based on the trimethoprim component) in three to four divided doses q6h to q8h for up to 14 days.

CDC recommended treatment schedules for sexually transmitted diseases

Penicillinase producing **Neisseria gonorrhoeae:** For pharyngeal infections, a single daily dose of nine tablets (80 mg trimethoprim/400 mg sulfameth-oxazole) for 5 days.

H. ducreyi *infection (chancroid):* 160 mg tri-methoprim/800 mg sulfamethoxazole bid for a min-imum of 10 days until ulcers or lymph nodes have healed.

Shigella: 160 mg trimethoprim/800 mg sulfa-methoxazole bid for 7 days.

Use in impaired renal function

When creatinine clearance is above 30 ml/min-ute, standard dose regimen is used. When the creat-inine clearance is 15 ml/minute to 30 ml/minute, one-half the usual dosage is used. Drug is not rec-ommended if the creatinine clearance is below 15 ml/minute.

NURSING IMPLICATIONS

HISTORY
See Appendix 4.

PHYSICAL ASSESSMENT
Obtain vital signs, weight (if dosage is deter-mined by weight). Baseline laboratory studies may include culture and sensitivity testing, CBC, and renal- and hepatic-function tests.

ADMINISTRATION
Therapy may be instituted prior to obtaining re-sults of culture and sensitivity tests.

Oral: Give with a full glass of water.

If patient has difficulty swallowing tablet or fails to take sufficient amount of fluid with the tablet, contact the physician. An oral suspension is available for trimethoprim and sulfamethoxa-zole.

Parenteral (trimethoprim and sulfamethoxa-zole): Infusion must be diluted.

Add each 5 ml ampule to 125 ml of 5% Dex-trose in Water. After diluting, use within 6 hours; do not refrigerate.

When fluid restriction is desirable, each am-pule may be added to 75 ml of 5% Dextrose in Water. Mix solution just prior to use and admin-ister within 2 hours.

If solution is cloudy or contains a precipitate after mixing, discard and prepare a fresh solu-tion.

Do not mix with other drugs or solutions.

Administer by IV drip over 60 to 90 minutes. Rapid infusion or bolus injection is avoided. Do not give IM.

A volume control set may be used for admin-istration.

When administering by an infusion device, thoroughly flush all lines used to remove any re-sidual drug.

Storage: Store in a cool, dry place. *Trimetho-prim*—Protect the 200-mg tablets from light.

ONGOING ASSESSMENTS AND NURSING MANAGEMENT
Check IV infusion site q5m to q10m for signs of local irritation and inflammation due to extra-vascular infiltration. If extravasation is apparent, discontinue the infusion and restart at another site.

Rarely, local reaction, pain, and slight irrita-tion on IV administration may occur. Notify physician if these symptoms become severe.

Monitor vital signs q4h or as ordered.

CLINICAL ALERT: The presence of sore throat, fever, pal-lor, purpura, or jaundice may be an early indication of a serious blood disorder. Notify physician immediately if one or more of these occur. A CBC may be ordered. A signifi-cant reduction in the count of any formed blood element may require discontinuation of therapy.

Observe for adverse reactions.

Monitor intake and output. Notify physician of any change in the intake–output ratio.

Unless physician directs otherwise or patient's fluid intake is restricted, encourage fluid intake of 2500 ml to 3000 ml per day to prevent crys-talluria and stone formation. This is especially necessary with the combination of trimethoprim and sulfamethoxazole.

Observe for relief of symptoms of infection. Notify physician if symptoms do not improve in 3 to 4 days or become worse.

Periodic blood counts are recommended dur-ing prolonged therapy.

Patients receiving trimethoprim and sulfa-methoxazole combination and warfarin may re-quire dosage adjustments. Observe such patients for evidence of easy bleeding or bruising.

PATIENT AND FAMILY INFORMATION
Complete full course of therapy. Do not discon-tinue drug even though symptoms may be re-lieved.

Take each dose with a full glass of water.

Drink 8 to 10 glasses (8 oz each) of water each day unless physician directs otherwise.

Notify physician or nurse if skin rash, sore throat, fever, mouth sores, or unusual bruising or bleeding occurs, or if symptoms do not im-prove in 3 to 4 days or become worse.

Trimipramine Maleate

See Antidepressants, Tricyclic Compounds.

Tripelennamine Hydrochloride

See Antihistamines.

Triprolidine Hydrochloride

See Antihistamines.

Troleandomycin (Triacetyloleandomycin) Rx

capsules: 250 mg   Tao
suspension: 125 mg/   Tao
   5 ml

INDICATIONS
Infection caused by the following microorganisms:

Streptococcus pneumoniae: Pneumococcal pneumonia due to susceptible strains.

S. pyogenes: Group A beta-hemolytic streptococcal infections of the upper respiratory tract.

CONTRAINDICATIONS
Hypersensitivity.

ACTIONS
An antibiotic of the macrolide group shown to be active against the gram-positive organisms _S. pyogenes_ and _S. pneumoniae._

WARNINGS
Hepatic effects: Administration has been associated with an allergic type of cholestatic hepatitis. Some patients receiving this drug for more than 2 weeks or in repeated courses have shown jaundice accompanied by right upper quadrant pain, fever, nausea, vomiting, eosinophilia, and leukocytosis. The changes have been reversible on discontinuance of the drug. Monitoring of hepatic-function tests is recommended in patients on such dosage, and drug is discontinued if abnormalities develop.

Safety for use in pregnancy has not been established.

PRECAUTIONS
Superinfection: Use of antibiotics (especially prolonged or repeated therapy) may result in bacterial or fungal overgrowth of nonsusceptible organisms. Such overgrowth may lead to a secondary infection.

Use in impaired hepatic function: Drug is principally excreted by the liver. Caution is advised in giving to patients with impaired hepatic function.

DRUG INTERACTIONS
Reports suggest that concurrent use of **ergotamine-containing drugs** and troleandomycin may induce ischemic reactions. Concomitant administration of troleandomycin and **oral contraceptives** has been reported to produce marked cholestatic jaundice. Troleandomycin may inhibit hepatic metabolism of **theophylline** (except dyphylline), **carbamazepine,** and **corticosteroids,** resulting in increased plasma levels and pharmacologic/toxic effects.

ADVERSE REACTIONS
Most frequent dose-related side-effects are GI, such as abdominal cramping and discomfort. Nausea, vomiting, and diarrhea occur infrequently. Mild allergic reactions, such as urticaria and other skin rashes, have occurred. Serious allergic reactions, including anaphylaxis, have been reported.

DOSAGE
Adults: 250 mg to 500 mg four times a day.
Children: 125 mg to 250 mg (6.6–11 mg/kg) q6h.

When used in streptococcal infection, therapy should be continued for 10 days.

NURSING IMPLICATIONS

HISTORY
See Appendix 4.

PHYSICAL ASSESSMENT
Obtain vital signs; record overt signs of infection; assess patient's general status, especially if severely ill. Baseline laboratory studies may include culture and sensitivity studies, hepatic-function studies, and CBC.

ADMINISTRATION
Obtain culture and sensitivity _before_ administration of first dose.

Give on an empty stomach at least 1 hour before or 2 hours after meals.

Give drug at evenly spaced intervals, preferably around the clock.

ONGOING ASSESSMENTS AND NURSING MANAGEMENT
Obtain vital signs q4h or as ordered.

Observe for adverse reactions.

CLINICAL ALERT: Observe for signs of superinfection (Appendix 6, section 6-22). If these are noted, inform physician before next dose is due because drug may be discontinued.

If patient is receiving drug for more than 2 weeks or is receiving a repeat course of troleandomycin, observe for jaundice, right upper quadrant pain, fever, nausea, and vomiting. Notify physician immediately if one or more of these are apparent because drug is usually discontinued if hepatic effects occur. Hepatic effects are usually reversible when drug is discontinued.

T

Hepatic-function tests are recommended during prolonged therapy (more than 10 days) or repeated courses of therapy.

Observe for relief of symptoms of infection. If symptoms become worse, inform physician.

PATIENT AND FAMILY INFORMATION

Take on an empty stomach 1 hour before or 2 hours after meals.

Take at evenly spaced intervals, preferably around the clock.

Complete full course of therapy unless physician directs otherwise.

Notify physician or nurse immediately if any of the following occurs: sores in mouth, vaginal or rectal itching, diarrhea, back furry tongue, jaundice, dark urine, light-colored stools.

Inform other physicians and dentist of therapy with this antibiotic.

Tropicamide

See Mydriatics, Cycloplegic.

Trypsin Rx

aerosol   Granulex

INDICATIONS

Treatment of decubitus ulcers and varicose ulcers and debridement of eschar, dehiscent wounds, and sunburn.

ACTIONS

Is intended for debridement of eschar and other necrotic tissue. It appears that, in many instances, removal of wound debris strengthens humoral defense mechanisms sufficiently to retard proliferation of local pathogens. Contents of product are trypsin, balsam Peru, and castor oil. Balsum Peru is an effective capillary bed stimulant used to increase circulation in the wound site area. It also has mild

bactericidal action. Castor oil is used to improve epithelization by reducing premature epithelial desiccation and cornification. It also acts as a protective covering, aiding in reduction of pain.

WARNINGS

Do not spray onto fresh arterial clots. Avoid spraying into eyes.

DOSAGE

Apply bid or as often as necessary.

NURSING IMPLICATIONS

HISTORY

See Appendix 4.

PHYSICAL ASSESSMENT

Note and record size and appearance of lesions, type and amount of drainage (if any).

ADMINISTRATION

Clean area, as directed by physician, prior to application.

Coat wound rapidly but not excessively.

Avoid getting spray into eyes.

ONGOING ASSESSMENTS AND NURSING MANAGEMENT

Note appearance of lesion each time drug is applied; compare with data base.

Notify physician if drainage increases, becomes more purulent, or develops a different odor or if lesions enlarge; other therapy may be necessary.

Tubocurarine Chloride

See Curare Preparations.

Typhoid Vaccine

See Immunizations, Active.

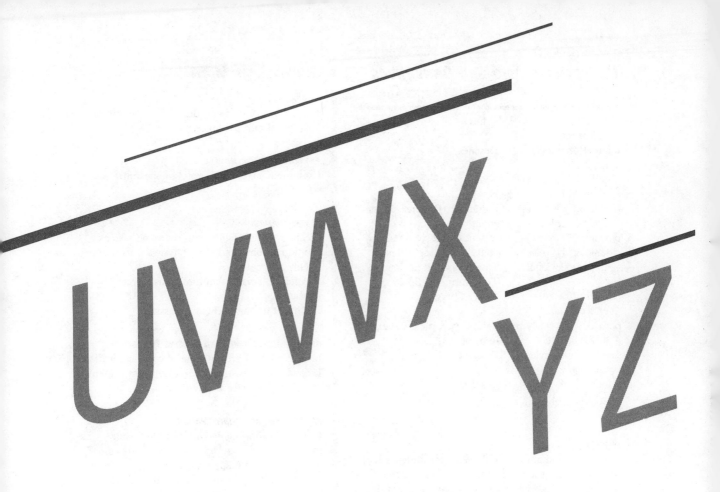

UVWXYZ

U
V
W
X
Y
Z

Undecylenic Acid and Derivatives

otc

cream: 20% zinc undecylenate	Cruex
foam: 10% undecylenic acid	Desenex
liquid: 10% undecylenic acid	NP-27
ointment: 5% undecylenic acid	Merlenate, Desenex, Undoguent
powder: 2% undecylenic acid, 20% zinc undecylenate	Desenex Aerosol, Desenex Shaker, Quinsana Plus, Ting Improved Shaker, Ting Improved Spray
powder: 20% zinc undecylenate	NP-27 Spray
powder: 10% calcium undecylenate	Caldesene, Cruex, Cruex Aerosol
soap: 2% undecylenic acid	Desenex
solution: 10% undecylenic acid	Desenex

INDICATIONS

Fungistatic and antibacterial agents for athlete's foot and ringworm, exclusive of nails and hairy areas. Also recommended for relief and prevention of diaper rash; itching, burning, and chafing; prickly heat; minor skin irritations and burns; jock itch (tinea cruris); excessive prespiration; and irritation in the groin area.

The above products may contain additional ingredients and are listed only according to the undecylenic acid and derivatives contents.

WARNINGS

Avoid inhalation and contact with the eyes or other mucous membranes. Do not use if skin is pustular or severely broken. Individuals with impaired circulation, including diabetics, should consult a physician before using.

DOSAGE

Apply as needed. In general, powders are used only as adjunctive therapy with ointments, creams, and liquids in primary therapy in very mild conditions or as prophylactic agents, especially in inherently moist areas. Liquids and solutions are generally preferred for primary therapy or if the affected area is hairy. In addition, powders with a cornstarch base may be preferable to those with a talc base.

NURSING IMPLICATIONS

HISTORY

Record description and duration of symptoms, location of affected areas.

PHYSICAL ASSESSMENT

Examine affected area, noting appearance and size of lesion.

ADMINISTRATION

Clean area thoroughly with soap and water or solution recommended by physician; rinse thoroughly and pat dry.

Apply in small quantities or as directed by physician.

Do not use an occlusive dressing.

ONGOING ASSESSMENTS AND NURSING MANAGEMENT

Inspect affected area at time of each application. If condition persists or shows no improvement after 3 weeks, inform physician.

PATIENT AND FAMILY INFORMATION

Clean area thoroughly with soap and water, rinse thoroughly, and pat dry. Be sure area is completely dry before application.

If condition persists for more than 3 weeks, becomes worse, or spreads to other areas, see a physician.

Ringworm: Keep towels, face cloths, and bedding separate from those of other members of the family. Launder clothing and linens daily; use hot water and detergent. Do not wash clothes or bedding used by other members of the family at the same time.

Athlete's foot: Keep feet dry; change socks daily or whenever damp or wet. Expose feet to air as much as possible. Wear loosely fitting shoes and avoid shoes made of plastic or with a plastic (waterproofing) coating.

Uracil Mustard Rx

capsules: 1 mg	*Generic* (contains tartrazine)

INDICATIONS

Chronic lymphocytic leukemia: Usually effective in palliative treatment of symptomatic chronic lymphocytic leukemia.

Non-Hodgkin's lymphomas: Effective for palliative treatment of lymphomas of the histiocytic or lymphocytic type.

Chronic myelogenous leukemia: May be effective in palliative treatment. It is not effective in acute blastic crisis or in acute leukemia.

Other conditions: May be effective in palliative treatment of early stages of polycythemia vera before development of leukemia or myelofibrosis. May also be beneficial as palliative therapy in mycosis fungoides.

CONTRAINDICATIONS
Severe leukopenia or thrombocytopenia.

ACTIONS
An orally active alkylating agent belonging to the class of substances known as nitrogen mustards. It has clinically been found to be of value in palliative treatment of certain neoplasms affecting the reticuloendothelial system. It is readily absorbed following oral administration.

WARNINGS
Uracil mustard has a cumulative effect against the hematopoietic system. It is used during pregnancy only when clearly needed and when potential benefits outweigh the unknown potential hazards to the fetus.

PRECAUTIONS
Hematopoietic toxicity: Patient is monitored to avoid irreversible damage to the bone marrow. If severe bone-marrow depression occurs, as indicated by sharp drop in any of the formed blood elements, therapy is discontinued. Although therapy need not be discontinued following initial depression of blood counts, it should be understood that maximum depression of bone-marrow function may not occur until 2 to 4 weeks after discontinuing the drug and that as the total accumulated doses approach 1 mg/kg, there is a real danger of producing irreversible bone-marrow damage. Although there is no specific therapy for severe bone-marrow depression, frequent blood and blood-component transfusions with antibiotics to combat secondary infection may sustain the patient until recovery has occurred.

Carcinogenesis: Alkylating agents are suspected carcinogens in humans. Their possible effect on fertility should be considered; amenorrhea and impaired spermatogenesis have been reported following therapy with alkylating compounds.

Uric acid: Uracil mustard may increase serum uric acid levels in blood and urine and are used with caution in those with a history of gout or urate renal stones.

Tartrazine sensitivity: See Appendix 6, section 6-23.

DRUG INTERACTIONS
Uracil mustard may raise serum uric acid levels; an upward adjustment in dosage of **antigout medications** may be required to control hyperuricemia and gout. Uracil mustard can cause immunosuppression; immunization with **smallpox vaccine** may result in generalized vaccinia.

ADVERSE REACTIONS
Uracil mustard produces toxic effects characteristic of nitrogen mustards. These effects include depression of the hematopoietic system as indicated initially by severe thrombocytopenia and granulocytic and lymphocytic leukopenia and later by depression of the erythrocyte count and hemoglobin values.

In addition to toxic effects on the hematopoietic system, evidence of toxicity may be manifested by nausea, vomiting, or diarrhea of varying degrees of severity. These are dose related; the greater the dose, the more severe the symptoms.

Hepatotoxicity has been reported rarely. Amenorrhea or azoospermia may occur. Other adverse reactions include nervousness, irritability, or depression and various skin reactions such as pruritus, dermatitis, and hair loss. Some of these may not be drug related. Frank alopecia has not been reported.

DOSAGE
Not administered until about 2 to 3 weeks after maximum effect of any previous x-ray or cytotoxic drug therapy of the bone marrow has been obtained. An increasing WBC count is probably the best criterion for determining that such maximum effect has subsided. Some investigators prefer to wait until the blood count has returned to normal before beginning a new course of therapy. Not administered in the presence of pronounced leukopenia, thrombocytopenia, or aplastic anemia. In the presence of bone marrow infiltrated with malignant cells, hematopoietic toxicity may be increased.

Suggested dosage schedules

Adults: A single weekly dose of 0.15 mg/kg should be given for 4 weeks to provide an adequate trial.

Children: A single weekly dose of 0.30 mg/kg should be given for 4 weeks to provide an adequate trial.

If response occurs, the same dose may be continued weekly until relapse. These dosages must be carefully individualized and reduced or discontinued in accordance with the severity of depression of bone-marrow function.

U
V
W
X
Y
Z

NURSING IMPLICATIONS

HISTORY
See Appendix 4.

PHYSICAL ASSESSMENT
Obtain vital signs, weight; evaluate patient's general physical and emotional status. Baseline laboratory studies may include CBC and differential, platelet count, hemoglobin, serum uric acid, and hepatic-function studies.

ADMINISTRATION
Drug is administered once a week.

May be given after a meal to decrease GI distress.

ONGOING ASSESSMENTS AND NURSING MANAGEMENT

CLINICAL ALERT: Bone-marrow depression is the most serious adverse effect. Although bone-marrow depression may not occur until 2 to 4 weeks after drug is discontinued, observe patient daily for signs of bone-marrow depression (Appendix 6, section 6-8); inform physician immediately if one or more symptoms are noted.

Monitor signs q4h or as ordered.

Observe for adverse drug reactions.

Measure intake and output. Notify physician if there is any change in the intake–output ratio.

Encourage a high fluid intake of 2500 ml to 3000 ml per day and encourage frequent urination to prevent uric acid stone formation. If patient fails to increase fluid intake, discuss with physician.

Weigh weekly or as ordered. Inform physician if a significant increase or decrease in weight occurs.

CBC and platelet count are recommended once or twice weekly. Periodic serum uric acid levels may also be ordered.

If nausea, vomiting, or diarrhea occurs, inform physician; an antiemetic or reduction of dosage may be necessary. If vomiting or diarrhea is persistent and severe, drug may be discontinued.

Small frequent feedings, as well as dry toast, carbonated beverages, or unsalted crackers, may be used to relieve nausea.

An antigout agent may be necessary when serum uric acid level is elevated. Notify physician if patient complains of flank, stomach, or joint pain.

Check extremities daily. If swelling of the feet or legs occurs, notify the physician.

PATIENT AND FAMILY INFORMATION
Drink 10 or more glasses (8 oz each) of water each day and urinate frequently while taking this medication.

May cause nausea, vomiting, or diarrhea. Notify physician or nurse if these effects persist.

Notify physician or nurse immediately if fever, chills, sore throat, unusual bleeding or bruising, flank or stomach pain, joint pain, or swelling of the feet or legs occurs.

Frequent (1–2 times a week) laboratory tests will be necessary to monitor therapy.

Some hair loss may occur.

Urea Rx

injection: 40 g/   Ureaphil
150 ml

INDICATIONS
The 30% solution is used to reduce intracranial pressure (in the control of cerebral edema) and intraocular pressure.

CONTRAINDICATIONS
Not used in patients with severely impaired renal function, active intracranial bleeding, or marked dehydration. Frank liver failure is also a contraindication for use.

ACTIONS
An osmotic dehydrating and diuretic agent for IV administration. When an osmotic diuretic is indicated, mannitol is usually preferred.

The reduction of intracranial edema and abnormally elevated CSF pressure following IV administration of hypertonic urea solutions depends on osmotic pressure gradients between the blood, extracellular, and intracellular fluid compartments. The primary mechanism of action appears to be physical. Hypertonic urea rapidly increases blood tonicity, effecting a greater urea concentration gradient in the blood than in the extravascular fluid. This results in transudation of fluid from tissues, including the brain and CSF, into the blood. As the concentration of urea in the glomerular filtrate increases, this prevents reabsorption of a proportional amount of water. Such retardation of proximal tubular reabsorption increases the rate and volume of urine flow.

WARNINGS
Electrolyte imbalance: Urea may cause depletion of electrolytes, which can result in hyponatremia

and hypokalemia. Early signs of such depletion may indicate the need for supplementation before serum levels are reduced.

Extravasation: Extreme care is essential to prevent accidental extravasation of the solution at the site of injection because this may cause local reactions ranging from mild irritation to tissue necrosis.

Use in hepatic impairment: If used, administer with caution because there may be a significant rise in blood ammonia levels.

Use in pregnancy, lactation: The use of any drug in pregnancy or lactation or in the childbearing years requires that potential benefits of the drug be weighed against the possible hazards to the mother and child.

PRECAUTIONS
Rapid IV administration may be associated with hemolysis as well as a direct effect in the cerebral vasomotor centers, which may result in increased capillary bleeding. These effects can usually be avoided by not exceeding an infusion rate of 4 ml/minute.

Intracranial bleeding: Arterial oozing has been reported when intracranial surgery is performed on patients following treatment with urea. Sterile urea should *not* be used in the presence of active intracranial bleeding unless such use is preliminary to prompt surgical intervention to control hemorrhage. Reduction of brain edema induced by urea may result in reactivation of intracranial bleeding.

Use in renal impairment: Give with caution in the presence of renal impairment. Mild elevation of BUN does not preclude use of urea, but frequent laboratory studies should be made to determine whether kidney function is adequate to eliminate the infused urea as well as that produced endogenously. Patients exhibiting a temporary reduction in urine volume are generally able to maintain a satisfactory elimination of urea. If diuresis does not follow the injection of urea to such patients within 6 to 12 hours, drug is withdrawn pending further evaluation of renal function.

As with other infused solutions, urea may temporarily maintain circulatory volume and blood pressure in spite of considerable blood loss. When excessive blood loss occurs within a short period of time, blood replacement should be adequate and simultaneous with the infusion of urea. Hypothermia, when used with the urea infusion, may increase the risk of venous thrombosis and hemoglobinuria.

ADVERSE REACTIONS
Headaches (reported to be similar to those that occur in some patients following lumbar puncture),

nausea and vomiting, and occasionally syncope and disorientation have occurred. Less often reported is a transient agitated confusional state. No serious reactions have been reported when solutions have been infused slowly, provided renal function is not seriously impaired and there is no evidence of active intracranial bleeding. Chemical phlebitis and thrombosis near the site of injection have been reported infrequently.

DOSAGE
Administer as a 30% solution by slow IV infusion at a rate not to exceed 4 ml/minute. The amount administered is estimated on the basis of grams per kilogram of body weight. Dosage must also take into account the clinical condition of the patient, especially the state of hydration, electrolyte balance, and integrity of renal function. The total daily dose should not exceed 120 g.

Reduction of increased intracranial or intraocular pressure

Adults: Dosage ranges from 1 g/kg to 1.5 g/kg.

Children: Dosage ranges from 0.5 g/kg to 1.5 g/kg. In young children (up to 2 years), as little as 0.1 g/kg may be adequate.

NURSING IMPLICATIONS

HISTORY
See Appendix 4.

PHYSICAL ASSESSMENT
Obtain vital signs; evaluate mental status. For patient with increased intracranial pressure, evaluate neurologic status (*e.g.*, level of consciousness, motor and sensory status, reflexes). Baseline laboratory studies may include CBC, serum electrolytes, and renal- and hepatic-function tests.

ADMINISTRATION
Select a large vein for infusion. Do not infuse into veins of lower extremities of elderly patients because phlebitis and thrombosis of superficial and deep veins may occur.

Do not administer through the same administration set through which blood is being infused.

An infusion pump may be used to control infusion rate if a rate of less than 200 ml/hour is ordered.

To ensure bladder emptying, an indwelling catheter is usually ordered for comatose patients.

Physician orders rate of infusion. It is recom-

U
V
W
X
Y
Z

mended that the infusion rate not exceed 4 ml/minute.

Preparation of solution: Prepare immediately before use.

Use 5% or 10% Dextrose Injection or 10% Invert Sugar in Water.

For 135 ml of 30% solution, mix contents of one vial (40 g) with 105 ml of the diluent.

Each milliliter of the 30% solution provides 300 mg of urea.

Discard any unused solution.

ONGOING ASSESSMENTS AND NURSING MANAGEMENT

Check infusion rate q5m to q10m; adjust as necessary. If an infusion pump is used, monitor flow rate and adjust as needed.

CLINICAL ALERT: Check infusion site q5m to q15m. Extravasation must be avoided; accidental extravasation may result in local reactions ranging from mild irritation to tissue necrosis.

Observe for signs and symptoms of hyponatremia (Appendix 6, section 6-17), hypokalemia (Appendix 6, section 6-15), dehydration due to brisk diuresis (Appendix 6, section 6-10) and fluid overload (Appendix 6, section 6-12). Notify physician if one or more are apparent. Early signs of electrolyte or fluid depletion may indicate the need for supplementation.

Measure urinary output hourly or as ordered. Inform physician of any significant decrease in urine output.

Inspect IV infusion site for signs of inflammation (*e.g.,* swelling, heat, redness, pain). If inflammation is apparent, IV infusion is stopped and is restarted in the opposite extremity.

Monitor mental and neurologic status (especially in those with cerebral edema) q15m to q30m. Inform physician immediately of any deterioration in mental status or level of consciousness or of any neurologic changes.

Frequent serum electrolyte determinations may be ordered. Those with renal impairment may require frequent determinations of renal function to determine if function is adequate to eliminate the infused area as well as that produced endogenously. In patients with impaired renal function, if diuresis does not occur in 6 to 12 hours, drug may be discontinued pending further evaluation.

If urea is administered prior to intracranial surgery to control hemorrhage, observe patient closely during the postoperative period for reactivation of intracranial bleeding.

Patient with increased intraocular pressure: Observe for relief of symptoms (*e.g.,* decrease in pain, increase in visual acuity, relief of nausea and vomiting).

V

Valproic Acid Rx

capsules: 250 mg	Depakene
syrup: 250 mg/5 ml	Depakene
tablets, enteric coated: 250 mg, 500 mg	Depakote

INDICATIONS

Sole and adjunctive therapy in treatment of simple (petit mal) and complex absence seizures. May also be used adjunctively in those with multiple seizure types that include absence seizures.

Unlabeled uses: Investigational trials suggest effectiveness alone or in combination in treatment of atypical absence, myoclonic, and grand mal seizures, and possible effectiveness against atonic, complex partial, elementary partial, and infantile spasm seizures. It has been used prophylactically in preventing recurrent febrile seizures in children.

CONTRAINDICATIONS

Hepatic disease or significant hypersensitivity to valproic acid.

ACTIONS

An anticonvulsant chemically unrelated to other drugs. The mechanism of action has not been established. It has been suggested that its activity is related to increased brain levels of gamma-aminobutyric acid (GABA). It is rapidly absorbed. Peak serum levels occur approximately 1 to 4 hours after a single dose. Absorption is more rapid from the syrup, with peak levels in 15 minutes to 2 hours. A slight delay in absorption occurs when administered with meals, but this does not affect total absorption.

The drug is primarily metabolized by the liver; elimination of valproic acid and its metabolites occurs principally in the urine, with minor amounts in feces and expired air. Serum half-life is 6 to 16 hours, which may be increased in children under 18 months and in those with cirrhosis or acute hepatitis (up to 25 hours).

WARNINGS

Hepatic failure resulting in fatalities has occurred, usually during the first 6 months of treatment. Drug is used with caution in those with a history of hepatic disease. Patients with various unusual congenital disorders, those with severe seizure disorders accompanied by mental retardation, and those with organic brain disease may be at particular risk. Drug is discontinued immediately in the presence of significant hepatic dysfunction, suspected or apparent. In some cases hepatic dysfunction has progressed in spite of drug discontinuation. The frequency of elevated liver enzymes may be dose related.

Use in pregnancy: Valproic acid may produce teratogenicity in the offspring of women receiving the drug during pregnancy. Antiepileptic drugs are given to women of childbearing potential only if essential in management of their seizures. Do not discontinue antiepileptic drugs given to prevent major seizures because of the strong possibility of precipitating status epilepticus with attendant hypoxia and threat to life. In cases in which severity and frequency of the seizure disorder are such that removal of medication does not pose a serious threat to the patient, discontinuation of the drug prior to and during pregnancy may be considered, although minor seizures do pose some hazard to the developing embryo or fetus.

Use in lactation: Drug is excreted in breast milk. It is not known what effect this has on a nursing infant. Caution is exercised when administering to a nursing woman.

PRECAUTIONS

Hematologic effects: Thrombocytopenia and platelet aggregation dysfunction have been reported. Hemorrhage, bruising, or a disorder of hemostasis/coagulation is an indication for reduction of dosage or withdrawal of therapy.

Hyperammonemia: May occur with or without lethargy and coma in the absence of abnormal hepatic-function tests. If elevation occurs, drug is discontinued.

Concomitant anticonvulsant use: Valproic acid may interact with concurrently administered anticonvulsant drugs. Periodic serum level determinations of concomitant anticonvulsant drugs are recommended during early course of therapy.

DRUG INTERACTIONS

Valproic acid may potentiate the CNS depressant activity of **alcohol** and other **CNS depressants.** Valproic acid may increase serum **phenobarbital** levels by impairment of nonrenal clearance; this may result in severe CNS depression. The combination of valproic acid and phenobarbital has been reported

to produce CNS depression without significant elevations of barbiturate or valproate serum levels. Monitor patients receiving concomitant therapy for neurotoxicity. Obtain serum barbiturate levels, if possible, and decrease barbiturate dosage, if needed. **Primidone** is metabolized into a barbiturate and therefore may interact.

Breakthrough seizures occur with the combination of valproic acid and **phenytoin.** Most reports have noted a decrease in plasma phenytoin concentration, but increases, as well as an initial fall with subsequent increase, have been reported. The dosage of phenytoin should be adjusted as needed. Concomitant use of valproic acid and **clonazepam** may produce absence status (petit mal). Conversely, excellent control of absence seizures has been reported with this combination.

Valproic acid inhibits the secondary phase of platelet aggregation; use with caution when giving with **drugs affecting coagulation** (*e.g.,* aspirin, warfarin). **Salicylates** may elevate valproic acid plasma levels by protein displacement and decreased clearance, possibly increasing toxicity. Valproic acid dosage may need to be reduced.

Drug/lab tests: A false interpretation of the **urine ketone test** may be seen. There have been reports of altered **thyroid-function tests** associated with valproic acid.

ADVERSE REACTIONS

Because the drug is used with other anticonvulsants, it is not possible to determine whether the adverse reactions can be ascribed to valproic acid alone or the combination of drugs.

GI: Most common initial side-effects are nausea, vomiting, and indigestion. These are usually transient and rarely require discontinuation of therapy. Diarrhea, abdominal cramps, and constipation have been reported, as have anorexia with weight loss and increased appetite with weight gain.

CNS: Sedative effects have been seen in patients receiving valproic acid alone but are found more often in those receiving combination therapy. Sedation usually disappears upon reduction of the other anticonvulsant drug. Other rare effects include ataxia, headache, nystagmus, diplopia, asterixis, "spots before eyes," tremor, dysarthria, dizziness, incoordination, and insomnia; coma has been noted with valproic acid alone or in conjunction with phenobarbital.

Dermatologic: Transient increases in hair loss, skin rash, petechiae.

Psychiatric: Emotional upset, depression, psychosis, aggression, hyperactivity, behavioral deterioration.

Musculoskeletal: Weakness.

Hematopoietic: Altered bleeding time, thrombocytopenia, bruising, hematoma formation, frank hemorrhage, relative leukocytosis, hypofibrinogenemia, leukopenia, eosinophilia, anemia, bone-marrow suppression.

Hepatic: Minor elevations of transaminase (SGOT, SGPT) and LDH are frequent and appear to be dose related. Occasionally, laboratory test results include increases in serum bilirubin and abnormal changes in hepatic-function tests. Severe hepatotoxicity and death may occur.

Endocrine: Irregular menses, secondary amenorrhea, abnormal thyroid-function tests.

Pancreatic: Acute pancreatitis.

Metabolic: Hyperammonemia.

OVERDOSAGE

Symptoms: Overdosage may result in deep coma. Massive pulmonary edema, coma, and death have been reported to occur 6 days after initiation of treatment with larger than recommended doses in a patient receiving concomitant phenobarbital and phenytoin.

Treatment: Because drug is absorbed rapidly, the efficacy of gastric lavage will vary with the time since ingestion. General supportive measures should be applied with particular attention to maintaining adequate urinary output. Naloxone has been reported to reverse CNS depressant effects. Because naloxone could theoretically also reverse the anticonvulsant effects, use with caution.

DOSAGE

Recommended initial dose is 15 mg/kg/day, increasing at 1-week intervals by 5 mg/kg/day to 10 mg/kg/day until seizures are controlled or side-effects preclude further increases. Maximum recommended dosage is 60 mg/kg/day. If total dose exceeds 250 mg/day, give in divided doses.

NURSING IMPLICATIONS

HISTORY
See Appendix 4.

PHYSICAL ASSESSMENT
Obtain vital signs. If seizures are frequent, observe and enter accurate description in patient's chart. Baseline laboratory studies may include hepatic-function tests, CBC, hemoglobin, hematocrit, platelet count, and bleeding time determination.

ADMINISTRATION
H.S. administration may minimize CNS effects.

If GI upset occurs, may be given with food.

Instruct patient to swallow capsules without chewing to avoid local irritation of the mouth and throat.

ONGOING ASSESSMENTS AND NURSING MANAGEMENT

CLINICAL ALERT: Serious or fatal hepatotoxicity may occur and may be preceded by nonspecific symptoms such as loss of seizure control, malaise, weakness, lethargy, anorexia, and vomiting. If these or other nonspecific symptoms occur, inform physician immediately because drug may be discontinued. If drug must be discontinued for this reason, observe patient closely for loss of seizure control.

Look for signs of easy bruising and evidence of bleeding, including bleeding of gums after oral care, blood in the urine or stool, hematemesis, epistaxis, and hematoma formation. If any of these is noted, inform physician.

Monitor vital signs q4h to q8h or as ordered.

Observe for therapeutic drug action (*i.e.,* decrease in frequency or intensity of seizures). The dosage of anticonvulsants is adjusted to individual needs and patient response to therapy. For those with frequent seizures, accurate observation and documentation assists physician in adjusting dosage.

Observe for adverse reactions. When dosage is titrated upward, observe for an increase in adverse drug reactions.

Drug may cause sedation, which may require reduction in dosage. If sedation or other CNS side-effects occur, assist patient with ambulatory activities.

Patients receiving concomitant therapy with phenobarbital are observed closely for signs of CNS depression (*e.g.,* sedation).

Valproic acid serum levels may be drawn. Therapeutic serum levels for most patients will range from 50 mcg/ml to 100 mcg/ml. Plasma levels of anticonvulsants given concomitantly may also be obtained.

Periodic hepatic-function tests are recommended during the first 6 months of therapy.

Periodic CBC, platelet count, hemoglobin, and bleeding time determination may be performed during therapy.

Diabetic patient: A false-positive test for ketones in urine may occur. If urine is positive for ketones, inform physician because blood glucose determination or other tests may be necessary.

PATIENT AND FAMILY INFORMATION
Do not discontinue this or other medications for epilepsy unless instructed to do so by the physi-

cian. Abrupt discontinuation may result in status epilepticus.

If GI upset occurs, may be taken with food. Take at bedtime to minimize drowsiness.

Do not chew capsules; swallow whole to avoid local irritation of mouth and throat. If capsule is difficult to swallow, contact physician.

May cause drowsiness. Observe caution while driving or performing other tasks requiring alertness.

Do not drink alcohol or take other CNS depressants while taking this drug. Avoid use of all nonprescription drugs, unless use is approved by the physician. Some nonprescription preparations may contain a depressant; others, such as aspirin, may increase bleeding tendencies.

Notify physician or nurse immediately if any of the following occurs: bleeding tendencies, bruising, hematoma formation, malaise, weakness, lethargy, anorexia, vomiting, sore throat or other infection, or an increase in frequency or severity of seizures.

Inform other physicians and dentist of therapy with this drug.

Frequent laboratory tests are necessary to monitor therapy.

Carry identification such as Medic-Alert indicating medication usage and epilepsy.

Female patient: If pregnancy occurs or a pregnancy is planned, inform physician.

Diabetic patient: Medication may interfere with urine test for ketones. If ketones are positive, inform physician because blood tests may be necessary.

Vancomycin Rx

powder for injection: 500 mg (as HCl)/ 10 ml vial	Vancocin
powder for oral solution: 10 g	Vancocin

INDICATIONS

Parenteral: Potentially life-threatening infections that cannot be treated with another effective, less toxic antimicrobial, including the penicillins and cephalosporins. It is useful in therapy of severe staphylococcal infections in those who cannot receive or who have failed to respond to the penicillins or cephalosporins or who have infections with staphylococci that are resistant to other antibiotics. It has been used successfully alone in treatment of staphylococcal endocarditis. Is effective in other staphylococcal infections including osteomyelitis,

pneumonia, septicemia, and soft-tissue infections. When staphylococcal infections are localized and purulent, antibiotics are used as adjuncts to appropriate surgical measures. Concomitant administration of the oral solution and parenteral form may be used for treatment of staphylococcal enterocolitis.

Oral: Treatment of staphylococcal enterocolitis. Not effective for systemic types of infection.

Investigational uses: Oral form, 1 g/day to 2 g/day in divided doses for 5 to 6 days has been used in treatment of antibiotic-induced pseudomembranous colitis caused by an exotoxin of *Clostridium difficile.* Relapse of colitis has occurred after discontinuation of oral vancomycin.

CONTRAINDICATIONS

Known hypersensitivity.

ACTIONS

A glycopeptide antibiotic derived from *Streptomyces orientalis* that exerts its effect by inhibiting synthesis of components of the bacterial cell wall. It is bactericidal against many strains of bacteria. It is poorly absorbed by mouth. Clinically effective concentrations in the blood are achieved and maintained by IV administration. Inhibitory concentrations can be demonstrated in pleural, pericardial, ascitic, and synovial fluids and in urine. It does not readily diffuse across normal meninges into spinal fluid, but when meninges are inflamed as a result of infection, the drug penetrates into spinal fluid.

About 80% of injected vancomycin is excreted by the kidneys; concentrations are high in urine. Its half-life in the circulation is approximately 6 hours. Renal impairment results in delayed excretion and in high blood levels associated with an increase in drug toxicity.

WARNINGS

Use in renal impairment: Because of its ototoxicity and nephrotoxicity, use is avoided in renal insufficiency. Toxicity is appreciably increased by high serum levels concentrations or prolonged therapy. If necessary to use vancomycin, dosages of less than 2 g/day usually will provide satisfactory serum levels.

Ototoxicity: Use in patients with a hearing loss is avoided. If used, dosage is regulated by periodic determination of drug serum levels. Deafness may be preceded by tinnitus. The elderly are more susceptible to auditory damage. Deafness may be progressive despite cessation of treatment.

Superinfection: Use of antibiotics, especially prolonged or repeated therapy, may result in bacterial or fungal overgrowth. Such overgrowth may lead to a secondary infection.

U V W X Y Z

PRECAUTIONS

Patients with borderline renal function and those over age 60 should be given serial tests for auditory function and vancomycin serum levels. Periodic hematologic studies, urinalysis, and renal-function tests are recommended in all patients.

For IV administration only. IM injection causes tissue irritation and necrosis. Pain and thrombophlebitis occur and are occasionally severe. The frequency and severity of thrombophlebitis can be minimized by giving the drug in a volume of at least 200 ml of glucose or saline solution and by rotation of injection sites. Rapid administration may produce a sudden drop in blood pressure. To avoid hypotension, drug is given in a dilute solution over 30 minutes.

DRUG INTERACTIONS

Concurrent or sequential use of other neurotoxic or nephrotoxic antibiotics, particularly **streptomycin, neomycin, kanamycin, gentamicin, paromomycin, polymyxin B, colistin,** and **tobramycin,** is avoided.

ADVERSE REACTIONS

Nausea, chills, fever, urticaria, macular rashes, eosinophilia, and anaphylactoid reactions. Several cases of reversible neutropenia have been reported. Ototoxicity and nephrotoxicity may occur.

DOSAGE

Oral: Usual dose is 500 mg q6h or 1 g q12h.

Children: A total daily dose of 20 mg/lb in divided doses.

Parenteral

Adults: Usual IV dose is 500 mg q6h or 1 g q12h in 0.9% Sodium Chloride Injection or 5% Dextrose in Water.

Children: Total daily dose of 44 mg/kg/day in divided doses. Drug can be added to the child's 24-hour fluid replacement.

Prevention of bacterial endocarditis in penicillin-allergic patients undergoing dental procedures or upper respiratory tract surgery or instrumentation: *Adults*—1 g vancomycin IV over 30 to 60 minutes, beginning 30 to 60 minutes prior to the procedure; then oral erythromycin 500 mg q6h for 8 doses. *Children*—20 mg/kg vancomycin IV over 30 to 60 minutes. Timing of doses is the same as for adults. Erythromycin dosage is 10 mg/kg q6h for 8 doses.

Prevention of bacterial endocarditis in penicillin-allergic patients undergoing GI or GU surgery and instrumentation: *Adults*—1 g vancomycin IV over 30 to 60 minutes plus 1 g streptomycin IM 30 to 60 minutes prior to procedure. In prolonged proce-

dures or delayed healing, these doses are repeated in 12 hours. *Children*—Vancomycin and streptomycin 20 mg/kg each. Timing of doses is same as for adults. Pediatric doses should not exceed the recommended single dose or 24-hour dose for adults.

NURSING IMPLICATIONS

HISTORY

See Appendix 4.

PHYSICAL ASSESSMENT

Obtain vital signs. Baseline laboratory tests may include culture and sensitivity, CBC and differential, hemoglobin, urinalysis, and hepatic- and renal-function tests.

ADMINISTRATION

Preparation of oral solution

Powder for oral solution: Usually mixed by a pharmacist. When mixed as recommended, each 6 ml of solution will contain approximately 500 mg.

Alternatively, the contents of one 500-mg vial for injection may be diluted in 1 oz of water for oral or nasogastric tube administration.

Preparation of parenteral solution

Reconstitute powder for injection with 10 ml of Sterile Water for Injection to yield a concentration of 500 mg/10 ml. Further dilution is required as follows:

Intermittent infusion (preferred method of administration): Add the reconstituted solution to 100 ml to 200 ml of 0.9% Sodium Chloride or 5% Dextrose in Water; 200 ml is recommended to prevent thrombophlebitis.

Continuous infusion (used when intermittent infusion is not feasible): Add two to four vials (1–2 g) of reconstituted solution to a sufficiently large volume of 0.9% Sodium Chloride Injection or 5% Dextrose in Water to permit slow IV drip administration of the desired dose over a 24-hour period. Apply a timing label.

Physician orders method of administration (intermittent or continuous infusion) and parenteral solution used for administration. When giving by intermittent or continuous infusion, physician orders volume of final dilution.

Obtain baseline blood pressure, pulse, and respirations immediately prior to administration.

Intermittent infusion: Infuse over a period of 20 to 30 minutes or as ordered.

Continuous infusion: Calculate rate of infusion according to volume used (usually 1000 ml over a 24-hour period).

Stability and storage: Oral solution is stable for 14 days in refrigerator after initial dilution. Parenteral solution is stable for 96 hours under refrigeration after reconstitution.

ONGOING ASSESSMENTS AND NURSING MANAGEMENT

CLINICAL ALERT: Rapid infusion may produce a sudden drop in blood pressure. Monitor blood pressure, pulse, and infusion rate every 5 minutes during administration by intermittent infusion. Monitor blood pressure, pulse, and rate of infusion q½h during continuous infusion.

If hypotension occurs slow rate of infusion to KVO, elevate the patient's legs and notify the physician. Continue to monitor the blood pressure and pulse every 3 to 5 minutes.

Drug is ototoxic and nephrotoxic.

Check infusion site each time blood pressure is taken. Extravasation must be avoided because tissue irritation and necrosis may result. If extravasation occurs, discontinue IV, restart in the opposite extremity, and notify the physician.

Take temperature q4h or as ordered.

Measure intake and output. Notify physician of any change in the intake–output ratio. A decrease in urine output when fluid intake is adequate, cloudy urine, or hematuria may indicate nephrotoxicity.

Observe for adverse drug reactions.

Tinnitus often produces hearing loss. Ask patient about any changes in hearing or other sensations such as ringing or buzzing in the ears. An acutely ill patient may not notice tinnitus. Elderly patients are more susceptible to auditory damage.

Periodic hematologic studies, urinalysis, and hepatic- and renal-function tests are recommended. Serum drug levels may also be obtained.

When giving orally for pseudomembranous colitis, note and record appearance and consistency of each bowel movement, and observe patient for signs of dehydration (Appendix 6, section 6-10), hypokalemia (Appendix 6, section 6-15) and hyponatremia (Appendix 6, section 6-17).

Varicella-Zoster Immune Globulin

See Immunizations, Passive.

Vasopressin Preparations

Vasopressin Rx

injection: 20 pressor units/ml — Pitressin Synthetic

Vasopressin Tannate Rx

injection: 5 pressor units/ml — Pitressin Tannate In Oil

INDICATIONS
VASOPRESSIN

Diabetes insipidus; prevention and treatment of postoperative abdominal distention; in abdominal roentgenography to dispel interfering gas shadows.

VASOPRESSIN TANNATE

Control or prevention of symptoms and complications of diabetes insipidus due to a deficiency of endogenous posterior pituitary antidiuretic hormone (ADH).

CONTRAINDICATIONS
Anaphylaxis or hypersensitivity.

ACTIONS
Possesses vasopressor and ADH activity.

WARNINGS
Not used in patients with vascular disease, especially of the coronary arteries, except with extreme caution. In such patients, even small doses may precipitate anginal pain, and with larger doses, the possibility of myocardial infarction is considered. May produce water intoxication.

PRECAUTIONS
Use cautiously in presence of epilepsy, migraine, asthma, heart failure, or any state in which a rapid addition to extracellular water may produce a hazard for an already overloaded system. Chronic nephritis with nitrogen retention contraindicates use until reasonable nitrogen blood levels are attained.

DRUG INTERACTIONS
Other drugs known to potentiate ADH, such as **chlorpropamide, clofibrate,** and **carbamazepine,** may potentiate the antidiuretic effect of vasopressin.

ADVERSE REACTIONS
Local or systemic reactions may occur in hypersensitive individuals. The following have been reported: tremor, sweating, vertigo, circumoral pallor, "pounding" in head, abdominal cramps, passage of gas, nausea, vomiting, urticaria, and bronchial con-

U V W X Y Z

striction. Anaphylaxis (cardiac arrest and/or shock) has been observed shortly after injection.

DOSAGE

VASOPRESSIN

May be given subcutaneously or IM. Ten units usually will produce a response in adults; 5 units is adequate in many cases. Should be given IM at 3- to 4-hour intervals as needed. Dosage is reduced proportionately for children. It is desirable to give a dose not much larger than is sufficient to elicit the desired physiological response.

Diabetes insipidus: May be given by injection or administered intranasally on cotton pledgets, by nasal spray or by dropper. Injectable dose is 5 to 10 units repeated two or three times daily as needed. Intranasal dose is based on individual response.

Abdominal distention: 5 units, increased to 10 units at subsequent injections if necessary. Give IM at 3- or 4-hour intervals. Dosage is reduced proportionately for children.

Abdominal roentgenography: Give two injections of 10 units each. These should be given 2 hours and ½ hour before films are exposed.

VASOPRESSIN TANNATE

0.3 ml to 1 ml IM; repeat as required. Duration of action varies with the patient and his condition and may be as prolonged as 48 to 96 hours.

NURSING IMPLICATIONS

HISTORY

See Appendix 4.

PHYSICAL ASSESSMENT

Obtain blood pressure, pulse, respirations, and weight. Baseline laboratory studies may include serum electrolytes if patient has diabetes insipidus.

ADMINISTRATION

Vasopressin may be given IM, subcutaneously, or intranasally.

If giving for abdominal distention, auscultate abdomen for peristaltic sounds and measure abdominal girth prior to administration.

If giving for abdominal roentgenography, an enema may be ordered prior to first dose.

Vasopressin tannate is given IM. Injection can cause pain. Advise patient of this prior to injection.

Prior to administration of vasopressin tannate (which is in peanut oil), warm ampule to body temperature and shake vigorously to disperse drug.

Unless ordered otherwise, one or two glasses of water may be given at time of administration to reduce side-effects.

Intranasal administration of vasopressin

Use technique (spray, dropper, cotton pledget) ordered by physician.

Prior to administration, inspect nares for nasal congestion (which may impair absorption); if apparent, notify physician because a different route of administration may be necessary.

Instillation by dropper: Place patient in an upright position with head tilted back. Instill in one or both nares, as directed by physician.

Instillation by spray: Obtain nasal spray and add prescribed amount to container. Place patient in an upright position, with head upright. Spray in one or both nares, as directed by physician.

Instillation by cotton pledget: Administer as directed by physician. With small forceps, a cotton pledget may be soaked with vasopressin and inserted gently into nares or a dry cotton pledget may be inserted in the nares and a dropper used to soak the cotton with the prescribed dose. Exercise care when inserting the cotton pledget into the anterior portion of the nares.

ONGOING ASSESSMENTS AND NURSING MANAGEMENT

Following administration, observe patient every 10 to 15 minutes for signs of excessive dosage. This may cause undesirable side-effects (blanching of the skin, abdominal cramps, nausea), which may be alarming to the patient. Reassure patient that recovery from these effects will occur in a few minutes. If signs of excessive dosage occur, notify physician before next dose is due; a reduction in dosage may be necessary. Administration of one to two glasses of water at time of administration may minimize these side-effects.

CLINICAL ALERT: Vasopressin may produce water intoxication. Observe for drowsiness, listlessness, confusion, and headache. Notify physician immediately if one or more of these are noted because water intoxication, if undetected, can proceed to coma and convulsions. Treatment of water intoxication includes restriction of fluids and administration of a diuretic.

Measure intake and output. In diabetes insipidus, urinary output and specific gravity may be measured hourly until optimal dosage is established. Notify physician of any change in the intake–output ratio, because dosage adjustment may be necessary.

Obtain blood pressure, pulse, and respirations q4h or as ordered. Notify physician of any changes because dosage adjustment may be necessary.

Observe for local or systemic reactions, which may occur in hypersensitive individuals. Notify physician immediately if any adverse reaction occurs.

Following use to relieve abdominal distention, a rectal tube may be ordered. Insert a lubricated rectal tube past the anal spinchter, tape and leave in place for 1 hour or as ordered. Auscultate abdomen for peristaltic activity at 15-minute intervals; measure abdominal girth q1h to q2h; ask patient about passage of gas.

With vasopressin tannate, check previous injection sites for inflammation, development of sterile abscess.

PATIENT AND FAMILY INFORMATION

NOTE: If drug has been prescribed for self-administration, patient or family member will require instruction in preparation and administration of drug and measurement of urine specific gravity.

Drink one to two glasses of water immediately before injection of drug.

Measure fluid intake; measure urinary output at time of each voiding. Keep a record of total daily intake and output and bring to physician each visit.

Rotate injection sites.

Immediately report occurrence of the following: significant increase or decrease in urinary output; abdominal cramps, blanching of the skin, nausea (signs of overdosage); inflammation or signs of infection at injection sites; drowsiness, lethargy, confusion, headache (signs of water intoxication).

Verapamil Hydrochloride _Rx_

tablets: 80 mg, 120 mg	Calan, Isoptin
injection: 5 mg/2 ml	Calan, Isoptin

INDICATIONS

Oral: Treatment of angina pectoris including angina at rest, including vasospastic (Prinzmetal's variant) and unstable (crescendo, preinfarction) angina; chronic stable angina (classic effort-associated angina)

Parenteral: Treatment of supraventricular tachyarrhythmias including rapid conversion to sinus rhythm of paroxysmal supraventricular tachycardias, including those associated with accessory bypass tracts such as Wolff-Parkinson-White and Lown-Ganong-Levine syndromes. When clinically advisable, attempt appropriate vagal maneuvers (_e.g.,_ Valsalva's maneuver) prior to administration. Also used for temporary control of rapid ventricular rate in atrial flutter or atrial fibrillation.

Investigational use: Orally, 80 mg to 160 mg tid has been evaluated for use in paroxysmal supraventricular tachycardia.

CONTRAINDICATIONS

Severe hypotension or cardiogenic shock; second- or third-degree AV block; sick sinus syndrome (except in those with a ventricular pacemaker); severe CHF, unless secondary to a supraventricular tachycardia amenable to verapamil therapy.

Patients receiving IV beta-adrenergic blocking agents (_e.g.,_ propranolol): Do not administer IV verapamil and IV beta-adrenergic blocking agents concomitantly (within a few hours of one another) because both may depress myocardial contractility and AV conduction.

ACTIONS

Inhibits calcium ion (and possibly sodium ion) influx through slow channels into conductile and contractile myocardial cells and vascular smooth muscle cells. In contrast to beta blockers, it does not induce bronchoconstriction or peripheral arterial spasm. The antiarrhythmic effect appears to be due to its effect on the slow channel cells of the cardiac conductile system.

By inhibiting calcium influx, verapamil slows AV conduction and prolongs the effective refractory period within the AV node in a rate-related manner, reducing elevated ventricular rate in supraventricular tachycardia due to atrial flutter and/or atrial fibrillation. By interrupting reentry at the AV node, it can restore normal sinus rhythm in those with paroxysmal supraventricular tachycardia, including Wolff-Parkinson-White syndrome. It can interfere with sinus node impulse generation and induce sinus arrest in patients with sick sinus syndrome and also can induce atrioventricular block, although this has been seen rarely. Verapamil may shorten the antegrade effective refractory period of the accessory bypass tracts. It does not alter the normal atrial action potential or intraventricular conduction time, but depresses amplitude, velocity of depolarization, and conduction in depressed atrial fibers.

Antianginal effects: Precise mechanism of action of oral verapamil as an antianginal agent remains to be determined but includes relaxation and preven-

U V W X Y Z

tion of coronary artery spasm and reduction of oxygen utilization.

More than 90% of the oral dose is absorbed. The mean elimination half-life in single-dose studies ranged from 2.8 to 7.4 hours. After repetitive dosing, half-life increased to 4.5 to 12 hours. Following IV infusion, verapamil is eliminated bi-exponentially, with an elimination phase half-life of 2 to 5 hours. Verapamil is excreted in the urine and feces.

WARNINGS

Hypotension: IV verapamil often produces a decrease in blood pressure. This is usually transient and asymptomatic but may result in dizziness. Systolic pressure less than 90 mm Hg or diastolic pressure less than 60 mm Hg was seen in 5% to 10% of those with supraventricular tachycardia and in about 10% of those with atrial flutter/fibrillation. The incidence of symptomatic hypotension is approximately 1.5% and may require pharmacologic treatment (IV use of norepinephrine, metaraminol, or calcium gluconate). Occasionally, the oral form may produce a decrease in blood pressure, which may result in dizziness or symptomatic hypotension. Hypotension is usually asymptomatic, orthostatic, and mild and can be controlled by a decrease in dose.

Rapid ventricular response: Patients with atrial flutter/fibrillation and an accessory AV pathway may develop increased antegrade conduction across the aberrant pathway, producing a very rapid ventricular response after verapamil (or digitalis). Treatment is usually DC conversion, which has been used safely and effectively.

Premature ventricular contractions: During conversion or marked reduction in ventricular rate, benign complexes of unusual appearance (sometimes resembling premature ventricular contractions) may be seen after IV verapamil and appear to have no clinical significance.

Heart block/extreme bradycardia/asystole: IV verapamil slows AV nodal conduction and rarely produces second- or third-degree AV block, bradycardia, and, in extreme cases, asystole. This is more likely to occur in those with sick sinus syndrome. Asystole in patients other than those with sick sinus syndrome is usually of short duration (few seconds or less), with spontaneous return to AV nodal or normal sinus rhythm. If return does not occur, treatment is initiated immediately. The effect of oral verapamil on AV conduction and SA node leads to first-degree AV block and transient bradycardia, sometimes accompanied by nodal escape rhythms, fairly common during peaks of serum concentration. Higher degrees of AV block are infrequent. Marked first-degree block or progressive develop-

ment of second- or third-degree AV block or unifascicular, bifascicular, or trifascicular bundle branch block requires reduction in dose or discontinuation of drug.

Patients with hypertrophic cardiomyopathy: Various serious adverse effects have been seen and include pulmonary edema, pulmonary edema and/or severe hypotension, sinus bradycardia, second-degree AV block, and sinus arrest. Most adverse effects respond well to dosage reduction; only rarely does verapamil have to be discontinued.

Heart failure: When heart failure is not severe or rate related, control with digitalis and diuretics, as appropriate, before verapamil is used. In moderately severe to severe cardiac dysfunction, acute worsening of heart failure may be seen.

Hepatic and renal failure: Significant hepatic and renal failure should not increase the effects of a single IV dose of verapamil but may prolong its duration. Repeated IV injections may lead to accumulation and an excessive pharmacologic effect. Severe liver dysfunction prolongs elimination half-life to about 14 to 16 hours; therefore, approximately 30% of dose given to patients with normal liver function is recommended. About 70% of a dose of verapamil is excreted as metabolites in urine, and drug is given cautiously to those with impaired renal function.

Elevated liver enzymes: Occasional elevations of transaminase and alkaline phosphatase have been reported. Because the potential exists for hepatocellular injury, periodic monitoring of liver enzymes is recommended.

Use in pregnancy, lactation: Use in pregnancy only when clearly needed and when potential benefits outweigh the unknown potential hazards to the etus. It is not known whether drug is excreted in human milk. Because of the potential for adverse reactions in nursing infants, discontinue nursing during therapy.

Use in children: Results of treatment are similar to those in adults.

DRUG INTERACTIONS

IV verapamil has been used with **other cardioactive drugs** (especially digitalis and quinidine) without evidence of serious drug interactions, except, in rare instances, when patients with severe cardiomyopathy, CHF, or recent MI were given IV **beta-adrenergic blocking agents** or **disopyramide.** Controlled studies suggest that concomitant use of oral verapamil and **beta-adrenergic blocking agents** may be beneficial in those with chronic stable angina, but available information is not sufficient to predict the effects of concurrent treatment, especially in those with left ventricular dysfunction or cardiac conduction abnormalities, in whom combined therapy should usually be avoided. The combination can have adverse effects on cardiac function; thus it is preferable that verapamil be used alone. If combined therapy is used, patient is monitored closely. IV verapamil has been given to patients receiving oral **beta-adrenergic blocking agents** without serious adverse effects. Because both drugs may depress myocardial contractibility or AV conduction, the possibility for untoward response is considered.

Until data on possible interactions between verapamil and **disopyramide** are obtained, do not administer disopyramide within 48 hours before or 24 hours after verapamil administration.

Chronic verapamil treatment increases serum **digoxin** levels by 50% to 70% during the first week of therapy. Maintenance doses of digoxin are reduced when verapamil is administered, and patient is closely monitored. IV verapamil has been used concomitantly with **digitalis** preparations without serious adverse effects. Because both drugs slow AV conduction, patient is monitored for AV block or excessive bradycardia.

Verapamil administered concomitantly with **oral antihypertensive agents** (*e.g.,* vasodilators, diuretics) may have an additive effect in lowering blood pressure. In patients who have recently received **methyldopa,** which attenuates alpha-adrenergic response, combined therapy with verapamil and propranolol should probably be avoided because severe hypotension may occur.

In a small number of patients with hypertrophic cardiomyopathy, concomitant use of oral verapamil and **quinidine** resulted in significant hypotension. Until further data are available, combined therapy should be avoided.

Because verapamil is highly protein bound to plasma proteins, drug is given with caution to those receiving other **highly protein-bound drugs** (*e.g.,* warfarin, oral hypoglycemics).

Because of the potential for antagonism of the beneficial effects of verapamil, **calcium** administration is avoided or done with extreme caution to avoid significant increases in serum calcium levels.

ADVERSE REACTIONS
Oral therapy
Serious reactions are rare when therapy is initiated with upward dose titration within recommended single and total daily dose.

Cardiovascular: Hypotension (2.9%); peripheral edema (1.7%); AV block: third degree (0.8%); bradycardia: heart rate less than 50/min. (1.1%); CHF or pulmonary edema (0.9%).

CNS: Dizziness (3.6%); headache (1.8%); fatigue (1.1%).

GI: Constipation (6.3%); nausea (1.6%).
Hepatic: Hepatotoxicity; hepatitis.
Causal relationship unknown (less than 0.5%): Confusion, paresthesia, insomnia, somnolence, equilibrium disorders, blurred vision, syncope, muscle cramps, shakiness, claudication, hair loss, maculae, spotty menstruation.

IV therapy
Cardiovascular: Symptomatic hypotension (1.5%); bradycardia (1.2%); severe tachycardia (1%).
CNS: Dizziness (1.2%); headache (1.2%).
GI: Nausea (0.9%); abdominal discomfort (0.6%).

OVERDOSAGE
Treatment is supportive. Beta-adrenergic stimulation or parenteral administration of calcium may increase calcium ion flux across the slow channel and has been used effectively. Clinically significant hypotensive reactions or fixed high-degree AV block is treated with vasopressor agents or cardiac pacing respectively. Asystole is treated by usual measures including isoproterenol, other vasopressor agents, and cardiopulmonary resuscitation.

DOSAGE
Oral (angina at rest and chronic stable angina): Dosage is individualized by titration. Usual initial dose is 80 mg three or four times a day. Dosage may be increased daily (*e.g.,* patients with unstable angina) or weekly intervals until optimal clinical response obtained. Total daily dose ranges from 240 mg to 480 mg. The optimum daily dose for most patients ranges from 320 mg to 480 mg. Usefulness and safety of dosages exceeding 480 mg/day in angina pectoris are not established.

Parenteral (supraventricular tachyarrhythmias): For IV use only. Give as a slow IV injection over at least 2 minutes.

Initial dose—5 mg to 10 mg (0.075–0.15 mg/kg) as an IV bolus over 2 minutes.

Repeat dose—10 mg (0.15 mg/kg) 30 minutes after first dose if initial response is not adequate.

Older patients—Give dose over at least 3 minutes to minimize risk of untoward drug effects.

Children—0 to 1 year, 0.1 mg/kg to 0.2 mg/kg (usual dose range is 0.75–2 mg) as an IV bolus over 2 minutes under continuous ECG monitoring; 1 to 15 years, 0.1 mg/kg to 0.3 mg/kg (usual dose range is 2–5 mg) as an IV bolus over 2 minutes. Do not exceed 5 mg. Repeat dose—Repeat these doses 30 minutes after first dose if initial response is not adequate (under continuous ECG monitoring).

NURSING IMPLICATIONS

HISTORY
See Appendix 4.

U
V
W
X
Y
Z

PHYSICAL ASSESSMENT

Obtain blood pressure, pulse, and respiration. Baseline laboratory tests may include renal- and hepatic-function tests, serum digoxin levels (when applicable). Baseline diagnostic tests may include ECG, stress testing (when applicable).

ADMINISTRATION

Oral: Dosage is titrated upward at daily or weekly intervals until maximum response is obtained.

Obtain blood pressure, pulse, and respirations immediately before administration. If there is significant decrease in blood pressure or pulse from baseline values, withhold drug and notify physician.

Parenteral: ECG monitoring is recommended because a small fraction (less than 1%) of patients may have life-threatening adverse reactions (rapid ventricular rate in atrial flutter/fibrillation, marked hypotension, or extreme bradycardia/asystole).

Have available drugs for treatment of acute cardiovascular reactions. The following are recommended:

Symptomatic hypotension requiring treatment— Norepinephrine, metaraminol, isoproterenol, calcium gluconate 10% solution.
*Bradycardia, AV block, asystole—*Isoproterenol, norepinephrine, atropine sulfate, calcium gluconate 10% solution.
*Rapid ventricular rate—*Procainamide, lidocaine.

Equipment and facilities for cardioversion and cardiac pacing are recommended for treatment of acute cardiovascular reactions. Cardiac pacing is recommended for bradycardia, AV block, or asystole. Cardioversion is recommended for rapid ventricular rate.

Place patient in a recumbent position, unless physician directs otherwise.

Obtain blood pressure, pulse, and respirations immediately before administration.

Given IV only as a bolus over a period of 2 or more minutes (elderly patients 3 or more minutes).

Storage: Store at 15°C to 30°C (59°–86°F) and protect IV solution from light.

ONGOING ASSESSMENTS AND NURSING MANAGEMENT

Oral administration for angina pectoris: Expected therapeutic response is a decrease in frequency and/or severity of anginal pain, decrease in use of nitroglycerin or other antianginal agent, and increased exercise tolerance.

Record all anginal episodes (*i.e.,* time of occurrence, duration of attack, severity, possible precipitating factors such as ambulation or emotional stress). This assists physician in determining optimal therapeutic dosage.

Observe for adverse reactions. Notify physician of the occurrence of an adverse reaction because dosage adjustment may be necessary.

Inform physician if orthostatic hypotension persists or is severe; a dosage reduction may be necessary.

Provide assistance with ambulation if dizziness occurs.

Periodic hepatic-function tests may be performed. Elevation of hepatic enzymes may indicate hepatotoxicity, requiring discontinuation of the drug.

If patient is receiving digoxin, chronic verapamil therapy increases serum digoxin levels during the first week of therapy. Maintenance doses of digoxin are reduced and periodic digoxin serum levels may be drawn. Observe for signs of digitalis toxicity (p 248).

Parenteral administration for treatment of supraventricular tachyarrhythmias: Observe ECG monitor before, during, and following administration. If a rapid ventricular rate, extreme bradycardia, heart block, or asystole occurs, notify physician immediately because emergency treatment of the acute cardiovascular reaction is usually necessary (see *Administration,* above).

During conversion or marked reduction in ventricular rate, benign complexes of unusual appearances (sometimes resembling premature ventricular contractions) may be seen. These complexes appear to have no clinical significance.

Monitor blood pressure every 5 to 10 minutes or as ordered. If hypotension occurs, notify physician immediately. Transient, asymptomatic hypotension may not require treatment. Transient symptomatic hypotension usually requires pharmacologic treatment (see *Administration,* above).

Keep patient recumbent following IV administration for at least 1 hour, unless physician orders otherwise.

Measure intake and output. Notify physician of any change in the intake–output ratio. If urinary output is decreased despite adequate intake, renal-function studies may be ordered.

PATIENT AND FAMILY INFORMATION

Make position changes slowly to avoid orthostatic hypotension and dizziness.

May cause dizziness. Do not drive or engage in other potentially hazardous tasks until response to drug is known.

Take drug exactly as prescribed and increase doses at the recommended intervals. Do not exceed the prescribed dose or change the intervals between doses.

Report occurrence of any of the following: irregular or slow heartbeat, shortness of breath, swelling of the hands and feet, or pronounced dizziness, constipation, or nausea.

Notify physician or nurse immediately if anginal pain increases in severity or occurs at more frequent intervals.

Follow the guidelines established by the physician about exercise. Do not increase physical activities once the anginal pain is controlled, unless an increase is approved by the physician.

Beginning with the first dose, record time, duration, and severity of each anginal attack. Bring this record to each physician's office or clinic visit. This will aid the physician in evaluating the drug and adjusting the dosage.

Periodic evaluation of drug's therapeutic effect will be necessary.

Vidarabine (Adenine Arabinoside, ARA-A) Rx

ophthalmic oint-	Vira-A
ment: 3%	
injection: 200 mg/ml	Vira-A

INDICATIONS
Ophthalmic ointment: Treatment of acute keratoconjunctivitis and recurrent epithelial keratitis due to herpes simplex virus types 1 and 2. Is also effective in superficial keratitis caused by herpes simplex virus not responding to topical idoxuridine or when toxic or hypersensitivity reactions to idoxuridine have occurred. Topical antibiotics or topical steroids have been administered concurrently with vidarabine without an increase in adverse reactions.

Injection: Herpes simplex virus encephalitis. Vidarabine will reduce the mortality caused by herpes simplex virus encephalitis; it does not appear to alter morbidity and resulting serious neurologic sequelae in the comatose patient. Therefore, early diagnosis and treatment are essential.

CONTRAINDICATIONS
Hypersensitivity.

ACTIONS
Possesses antiviral activity against herpes simplex virus types 1 and 2. The antiviral mechanism has not been established, but it appears to interfere with the early steps of viral DNA synthesis. Excretion of the injectable form is probably via the kidneys.

WARNINGS
Ophthalmic ointment: Use in pregnancy only when clearly indicated. It is not known if drug is excreted in human milk. However, excretion is unlikely as drug is rapidly deaminated in the GI tract.

Injection: Do not administer IM or subcutaneously because of low solubility and poor absorption. Safety for use in pregnancy and lactation is not established. Use should be limited to life-threatening illnesses in which possible benefits outweigh the potential risks involved.

PRECAUTIONS
Ophthalmic ointment: Although viral resistance to vidarabine has not been demonstrated, this possibility may exist.

Injection: Care is exercised when administering to patients susceptible to fluid overloading or cerebral edema (*e.g.,* patients with CNS infections or impaired renal function). Patients with impaired renal function may have a slower rate of excretion; dosage may require adjustment according to severity of impairment. Patients with impaired hepatic function should be observed for possible adverse effects. A mutagenic and oncogenic potential has been demonstrated in laboratory animals.

DRUG INTERACTIONS
Injection: Studies indicate that **allopurinol** may interfere with vidarabine metabolism. Caution is advised when administering these two drugs concomitantly.

ADVERSE REACTIONS
Ophthalmic ointment

Lacrimation, foreign body sensation, conjunctival injection, burning, irritation, superficial punctate keratitis, pain, photophobia, punctal occlusion, and sensitivity. The following have been reported, but appear disease related: uveitis, stromal edema, secondary glaucoma, trophic defects, corneal vascularization, hyphema.

Injection

GI: Anorexia, nausea, vomiting, hematemesis, diarrhea. These reactions are mild to moderate and seldom require termination of therapy.

CNS: Tremor, dizziness, hallucinations, confusion, psychosis, ataxia, fatal metabolic encephalopathy.

Hematologic: Decrease in reticulocyte count. Clinical laboratory changes noted were a decrease in hemoglobin or hematocrit, white blood cell count, and platelet count.

Miscellaneous: Weight loss, malaise, pruritus, rash, pain at injection site, elevated total bilirubin, SGOT elevation.

U
V
W
X
Y
Z

OVERDOSAGE

Ophthalmic ointment: Overdosage by ocular instillation is unlikely because any excess should be quickly expelled from the conjunctival sac. Too-frequent administration should be avoided.

Injection: Acute massive overdose has been reported without any serious evidence of adverse effect. Acute water overloading would pose a greater threat than would vidarabine overdosage, because of vidarabine's low solubility. Doses over 20 mg/kg/day can produce bone-marrow depression with concomitant thrombocytopenia and leukopenia. If a massive overdose occurs, monitor hematologic, hepatic, and renal functions.

DOSAGE

Ophthalmic ointment: One-half inch of ointment into lower conjunctival sac five times daily at 3-hour intervals. If there are no signs of improvement after 7 days, or if complete reepithelialization has not occurred in 21 days, other forms of therapy may be considered. Some severe cases may require longer treatment. After reepithelialization has occurred, treatment for an additional 7 days at a reduced dosage (such as bid) is recommended in order to prevent recurrence.

Injection: 15 mg/kg/day for 10 days. Slowly infuse the total daily dose by IV infusion at a constant rate over 12 to 24 hours.

NURSING IMPLICATIONS

HISTORY
See Appendix 4.

PHYSICAL ASSESSMENT

Herpes simplex virus encephalitis: Obtain vital signs, weight; document neurologic symptoms. Baseline laboratory studies may include hemoglobin, hematocrit, WBC count, platelet count. Diagnostic tests may include examination of CSF, brain scan, EEG, CT scan.

Keratoconjunctivitis or recurrent epithelial keratitis: Examine external structures of the eye. Look for signs of inflammation, excessive lacrimation, presence of a purulent exudate, signs of conjunctivitis.

ADMINISTRATION

Ophthalmic ointment

Place patient in sitting position with head tilted back.

Instill prescribed amount (usually approximately ½ inch of ointment) in the lower conjunctival sac.

Injection

Preparation: Dilute just prior to administration and use within 48 hours. Do not refrigerate the dilution.

Solubility in IV fluids is limited. Each milligram requires 2.22 ml of IV infusion fluid for complete solubilization. Each liter of IV fluid will solubilize a maximum of 450 mg of vidarabine. If more than 450 mg/day is ordered, more than 1 liter of IV fluid will be necessary.

Any appropriate IV solution is suitable for use as a diluent *except* biological or colloidal fluids (*e.g.,* blood products, protein solutions).

Shake vial well to obtain a homogeneous suspension before measuring and transferring to the IV solution.

Aseptically transfer the dose into the IV solution ordered by the physician. The IV solution may be prewarmed to 35°C to 40°C (95°F–100°F) to facilitate solution of the drug following transference.

Thoroughly agitate the prepared admixture until completely clear. Complete solubilization is indicated by a completely clear solution.

Final filtration with an in-line membrane filter (0.45 micron pore size or smaller) is necessary.

An IV infusion pump and an over-the-needle catheter (ONC) or inside-the-needle catheter (INC) may be used for administration.

Administration: Give as an IV infusion, at a constant rate, over a period of 12 to 24 hours. Physician orders rate of IV infusion or IV infusion rate may be calculated according to the total volume of IV fluid to be administered in 12 or 24 hours.

A timing label may be applied if an IV infusion pump is not used for administration.

ONGOING ASSESSMENTS AND NURSING MANAGEMENT

Ophthalmic ointment: Inspect eye each time ointment is instilled and compare with data base. If symptoms appear to worsen, if there is an increase in exudate or signs of inflammation, or if patient complains of pain or burning, notify physician.

Keep room dimly lit because drug may cause sensitivity to bright light. Patient may prefer to wear sunglasses rather than have a darkened room.

If there are no signs of improvement after 7 days, or if reepithelialization has not occurred in 21 days, other forms of therapy may be considered.

Injection: Monitor vital signs q4h or as ordered.

Evaluate neurologic status q2h to q4h and compare with data base.

Check IV infusion rate and every 15 to 30 minutes. If infusion pump is used, check the flow rate q1h to q2h, and adjust as needed.

Check the IV infusion site q½h or more frequently if patient is restless.

Observe for adverse reactions, signs of fluid overload (Appendix 6, section 6-12), and signs of cerebral edema.

Periodic hemoglobin, hematocrit, WBC count, and platelet count are recommended during therapy.

PATIENT AND FAMILY INFORMATION
Ophthalmic ointment
NOTE: Explain proper technique of instillation and importance of not contaminating the tip of the ointment tube.

Ointment may produce a temporary visual haze. Do not attempt to drive following instillation of ointment, until vision has cleared.

May cause a sensitivity to bright light; this may be minimized by wearing sunglasses.

Do not discontinue use without consulting physician.

Notify physician if improvement is not seen after 7 days, if condition worsens, or if pain, burning, or irritation of the eye occurs.

Vinblastine Sulfate (VLB) Rx

injection: 10 mg/vial   Velban

INDICATIONS
Palliative treatment of the following
Frequently responsive malignancies: Generalized Hodgkin's disease (stages III and IV); lymphocytic lymphoma; histiocytic lymphoma; mycosis fungoides (advanced stages); advanced carcinoma of the testis; Kaposi's sarcoma and Letterer-Siwe disease.

Less frequently responsive malignancies: Choriocarcinoma resistant to other chemotherapeutic agents; carcinoma of the breast unresponsive to appropriate surgery and hormonal therapy.

Multiple drug protocols
Is effective as a single agent but is usually administered concomitantly with other antineoplastic drugs. Combination therapy produces an enhanced therapeutic effect without additive toxicity when agents with different dose-limiting clinical toxicities and different mechanisms of action are selected.

Hodgkin's disease
Has been shown to be one of the most effective single agents for treatment. Advanced Hodgkin's disease has also been successfully treated with several multiple-drug regimens that included vinblastine. Patients who suffered relapses after treatment with the MOPP program have responded to combination drug therapy that included vinblastine. A protocol using cyclophosphamide in place of nitrogen mustard and vinblastine instead of vincristine is an alternative therapy for previously untreated patients with advanced Hodgkin's disease.

Advanced testicular germinal cell cancers (embryonal carcinoma, teratocarcinoma, and choriocarcinoma)
Are sensitive to vinblastine alone, but better clinical results are achieved when administered concomitantly with other antineoplastic agents. The effect of bleomycin is significantly enhanced if vinblastine is given 6 to 8 hours prior to administration of bleomycin.

CONTRAINDICATIONS
Patients who are leukopenic. Presence of bacterial infection; infections must be brought under control prior to initiation of therapy.

ACTIONS
Is an alkaloid extracted from *Vinca rosea* Linn. Studies suggest an interference with metabolic pathways of amino acids leading from glutamic acid to the citric acid cycle and urea. Other studies indicate that vinblastine has an effect on cell-energy production required for mitosis and interferes with nucleic acid synthesis.

WARNINGS
Clinically, leukopenia is an expected effect of vinblastine; the level of the leukocyte count is an important guide to therapy. In general, the larger the dose used, the more profound and longer lasting leukopenia will be. The fact that the WBC count returns to normal levels after drug-induced leukopenia is an indication that the white cell–producing mechanism is not permanently depressed.

Although the thrombocyte (platelet) count ordinarily is not significantly lowered by therapy, patients whose bone marrow has been recently impaired by prior therapy with radiation or with oncolytic drugs may show thrombocytopenia (less than 200,000/cu mm). When other chemotherapy or radiation has not been used previously, thrombocyte reduction is rarely encountered, even when significant leukopenia occurs.

The effect on the RBC count and hemoglobin is

UVWXYZ

usually insignificant when other therapy does not complicate the picture. However, patients with malignant disease may exhibit anemia in the absence of any therapy.

Aspermia has been reported in man. Information on use in pregnancy is limited. Animal studies suggest that teratogenic effects may occur.

PRECAUTIONS

If leukopenia with less than 2000 WBC/cu mm occurs following a dose, patient is watched carefully for evidence of infection until the WBC has returned to a safe level. When cachexia or ulcerated areas of the skin surface are present, there may be a more profound leukopenic response; use is avoided in older persons suffering from these conditions.

In those with malignant cell infiltration of bone marrow, the leukocyte and platelet counts have sometimes fallen precipitously after moderate doses. Further use of the drug in such patients is inadvisable.

DRUG INTERACTIONS

There are isolated reports of Raynaud's phenomenon occurring in those with testicular carcinoma treated with a combination of **bleomycin sulfate** and vinblastine.

ADVERSE REACTIONS

Incidence of adverse effects appears to be dose related. With the exception of epilation, leukopenia, and neurologic side-effects, adverse reactions have usually not persisted for longer than 24 hours. Neurologic side-effects are not common, but when they do occur they often last for more than 24 hours. Leukopenia, the most common adverse reaction, is usually the dose-limiting factor.

GI: Nausea; vomiting; constipation; vesiculation of the mouth; ileus; diarrhea; anorexia; abdominal pain; rectal bleeding; pharyngitis; hemorrhagic enterocolitis; bleeding from an old peptic ulcer.

Neurologic: Numbness; paresthesias; peripheral neuritis; mental depression; loss of deep tendon reflexes; headache; convulsions.

Miscellaneous: Malaise; weakness; dizziness; pain in tumor site; vesiculation of the skin. When epilation develops, it frequently is not total, and in some cases hair regrows while maintenance therapy continues. Extravasation during IV injection may lead to cellulitis and phlebitis. If the amount of extravasation is great, sloughing may occur.

DOSAGE

Drug is administered not more than once every 7 days. Therapy is initiated in adults with a single IV dose of 3.7 mg/m². Thereafter, WBC counts are

Table 54. An Incremental Approach to Vinblastine Dosage at Weekly Intervals

	Adult Dose (mg/m²)	Children's Dose (mg/m²)
First dose	3.7	2.5
Second dose	5.5	3.75
Third dose	7.4	5.0
Fourth dose	9.25	6.25
Fifth dose	11.1	7.5

made to determine patient's sensitivity. Table 54 presents an incremental approach to dosage at weekly intervals.

The same increments are used until a maximum dose (not exceeding 18.5 mg/m² for adults and 12.5 mg/m² for children) is reached. Dose is not increased after WBC count is reduced to approximately 3000 cells/cu mm.

When the dose that produces the above degree of leukopenia has been established, a dose one increment smaller should be given at weekly intervals for maintenance. Even if 7 days have elapsed, the next dose is not given until the WBC count has returned to at least 4000/cu mm.

The duration of maintenance therapy varies according to the disease being treated and the combination of antineoplastic agents being used. There are differences of opinion regarding the duration of maintenance therapy with the same protocol for a particular disease.

NURSING IMPLICATIONS

HISTORY
See Appendix 4.

PHYSICAL ASSESSMENT
Obtain vital signs, weight; evaluate patient's general physical and emotional status. Baseline laboratory tests may include CBC, differential, platelet count, and renal- and hepatic-function tests.

ADMINISTRATION
Preparation of solution

CLINICAL ALERT: Take care to avoid accidental contact of the solution with the eyes when preparing the solution because severe irritation (or, if the drug was delivered under pressure, even corneal ulceration) may result. If accidental contact does occur, wash the eyes with water immediately and thoroughly.

To prepare a solution containing 1 mg/ml, add 10 ml of Sodium Chloride Injection preserved with phenol or benzyl alcohol to the vial.

Other solutions for dilution are not recommended.

The drug dissolves instantly to give a clear solution.

After solution has been made and a portion removed from the vial, the remainder may be refrigerated for 30 days without loss of potency. Label bottle with date of reconstitution.

Have available drugs for treatment of extravasation. Hyaluronidase is recommended.

A Kold Kap or scalp tourniquet may be used to prevent alopecia. The scalp tourniquet remains in place during and approximately 15 minutes after IV administration; the Kold Kap remains in place during and for approximately 1 hour after injection.

Administration

Physician may prescribe an antiemetic to be given immediately before drug is administered.

Tell patient that pain in the tumor site may occur shortly after the injection is completed. If the pain is severe, an analgesic may be necessary.

Select a large vein, such as in the forearm.

Vinblastine may be given into the tubing of a running IV solution or directly into a vein. The physician selects the method of administration. The dose should not be diluted in large volumes of diluent (*i.e.,* 100–250 ml) or given IV for prolonged periods (30–60 minutes or more), because this frequently results in irritation of the vein and increases chances of extravasation.

CLINICAL ALERT: Extravasation during IV injection may lead to cellulitis and phlebitis. If the amount of extravasation is great, sloughing may occur. Care must be taken to be sure needle is securely within the vein.

Check for blood return during administration. Advise patient to mention immediately any burning or pain felt at the injection site. If extravasation occurs during IV administration, the injection is discontinued immediately and any remaining portion of the dose is given in another vein.

The injection may be completed in about 1 minute.

Following completion of the injection, the syringe and needle are rinsed with venous blood before withdrawal of the needle.

Treatment of extravasation

Local injection of hyaluronidase and the application of moderate heat to the area of leakage help to disperse the drug and minimize discomfort and the possibility of cellulitis.

ONGOING ASSESSMENTS AND NURSING MANAGEMENT

Monitor vital signs q4h or as ordered. If patient is acutely ill, monitor blood pressure, pulse, and respirations q1h to q2h.

Measure intake and output. Notify physician if oral intake is inadequate, if there is any change in the intake–output ratio, or if urinary output decreases.

Observe for adverse reactions; notify physician immediately if any one or more adverse reactions occur.

CLINICAL ALERT: Hematologic response includes a decrease in WBC count. If the WBC is less than 2000/cu mm, observe patient closely for evidence of infection until WBC count has returned to a safe level. Signs of infection may include fever, chills, signs of a urinary or upper respiratory tract infection, malaise, headache, abscess formation, or ulceration.

Patients whose bone marrow has been recently impaired by prior therapy with radiation or antineoplastic drugs and those who have malignant cell infiltration of the bone marrow are more likely to develop thrombocytopenia. Observe these patients closely for signs of easy bleeding and bruising, petechiae, purpura, bleeding gums, and blood in the urine, stool, or vomitus.

Neurotoxicity may be manifested by numbness, paresthesias, peripheral neuritis, mental depression, loss of deep tendon reflexes, and convulsions.

An antiemetic may be ordered for nausea and vomiting (which usually subside in 24 hours).

A liquid diet or dry toast, carbonated beverages, and unsalted crackers may be offered during the period of nausea and vomiting. If vomiting is severe, observe for signs of dehydration (Appendix 6, section 6-10).

Following therapy, the nadir in WBC count may be expected to occur 5 to 10 days after the last dose of the drug is given. Recovery of the WBC count is fairly rapid thereafter and is usually complete within 7 to 14 days.

With smaller doses employed for maintenance therapy, leukopenia may not occur.

If severe leukopenia occurs, protective or reverse isolation may be necessary until the WBC has returned to a safe level.

If severe thrombocytopenia develops, use methods to protect patient from injury (*e.g.,* padding of the siderails if patient is restless, prolonged pressure on parenteral administration sites).

Monitor bowel elimination pattern because constipation may occur. A stool softener may be necessary.

If neurotoxicity occurs, patient may require assistance with ambulatory activities. If patient is not ambulatory, take measures to prevent footdrop, wristdrop, and loss of muscle tone. Passive exercises may be necessary.

Weigh weekly or as ordered. Inform physician of any significant increase or decrease in weight.

U V W X Y Z

If patient is not ambulatory, inspect skin over pressure points for signs of skin breakdown. Turn patient q2h and massage pressure points. Inform physician immediately if skin breakdown is noted because patient with this condition may have a more profound leukopenic response to the drug.

PATIENT AND FAMILY INFORMATION

NOTE: Diagnosis, chemotherapeutic regimen, and anticipated adverse effects should be discussed with the patient and/or family.

Immediately report the occurrence of any of the following: fever, chills, malaise, upper respiratory infection, pain/burning on urination, bleeding tendency, easy bruising, blood in the urine or stool, numbness, paresthesias, headache, mental depression.

Follow physician's recommendations about physical activity. Avoid exposure to infection.

If nausea and vomiting occur, an antiemetic will be prescribed. A liquid diet or dry toast, unsalted crackers, and carbonated beverages may help relieve nausea.

Hair loss may occur. A wig, scarf, or cap can be used. Hair loss may be complete or partial; hair will grow back but may be a different color or texture.

Inform other physicians and dentist of therapy with this drug.

Frequent laboratory tests will be necessary to monitor results of therapy.

Vincristine Sulfate (VCR) Rx

injection: 1 mg/ml in Oncovin
1-, 2-, and 5-ml
vials

INDICATIONS

Acute leukemia. Also used in combination therapy in Hodgkin's disease, lymphosarcoma, reticulum-cell sarcoma, rhabdomyosarcoma, neuroblastoma, and Wilms' tumor.

ACTIONS

Is an alkaloid obtained from *Vinca rosea* Linn. The mode of action is unknown. Treatment of neoplastic cells demonstrates that it causes an arrest of mitotic division at the stage of metaphase. Central nervous system leukemia has been reported in patients undergoing otherwise successful therapy with vincristine. This suggests that vincristine does not penetrate well into cerebrospinal fluid.

WARNINGS

There is insufficient information as to whether this drug affects fertility or has teratogenic or other adverse effects on the fetus.

PRECAUTIONS

Acute uric acid nephropathy has been reported. In the presence of leukopenia or complicating infection, administration of the next dose requires careful consideration. If CNS leukemia is diagnosed, additional agents and routes of administration may be required, because the drug does not cross the blood–brain barrier in adequate amounts. Particular attention should be given to dosage and neurologic side-effects, if given to patients with preexisting neuromuscular disease or when other drugs with neurotoxic potential are administered.

ADVERSE REACTIONS

In general, adverse reactions are dose related and reversible. The most common is hair loss; the most troublesome adverse reactions are neuromuscular.

With single weekly doses, leukopenia, neuritic pain, constipation, and difficulty walking occur and are usually of short duration (*i.e.,* less than 7 days). When dosage is reduced, these reactions may lessen or disappear, and they seem to be increased when drug is given in divided doses. Other adverse reactions, such as hair loss, sensory loss, paresthesia, slapping gait, loss of deep tendon reflexes, and muscle wasting, may persist for the duration of therapy. In most instances, they have disappeared by about the sixth week after treatment is discontinued, but in some patients neuromuscular difficulties may persist for longer periods.

Neurologic: Ataxia; cranial nerve manifestations; footdrop; headache; convulsions, frequently with hypertension; bladder neuropathy. Frequently, there is a sequence in the development of neuromuscular side-effects. Initially, only sensory impairment and paresthesia may be encountered. With continued treatment, neuritic pain may appear and, later, motor difficulties.

Rare instances of the syndrome attributed to inappropriate antidiuretic hormone secretion have been seen. The syndrome has been described in association with several disease states. There is high urinary sodium excretion in the presence of hyponatremia; renal or adrenal disease, hypotension, dehydration, azotemia, and clinical edema are absent. With fluid deprivation, improvement occurs in hyponatremia and in renal sodium loss.

GI: Oral ulceration, abdominal cramps, vomiting, diarrhea, intestinal necrosis or perforation. Constipation may take the form of upper-colon impaction, and the rectum may be found empty. Colicky abdominal pain coupled with an empty rectum may be misleading. A flat film of the abdomen is useful in demonstrating this condition. Cases respond to high enemas and laxatives. Paralytic ileus may occur, particularly in young children. The ileus will reverse itself upon temporary discontinuation of vincristine and with symptomatic care.

Hematologic: This drug does not appear to have any constant or significant effect on the platelets or red blood cells. Thrombocytopenia, if present when therapy is begun, may actually improve before the appearance of marrow remission.

Ophthalmic: Optic atrophy with blindness, transient cortical blindness, ptosis, diplopia, photophobia.

Other: Weight loss, fever, polyuria, dysuria.

DOSAGE

Usual dosage for adults is 1.4 mg/m^2 and for children 2 mg/m^2. Drug is given IV at weekly intervals.

NURSING IMPLICATIONS

HISTORY
See Appendix 4.

PHYSICAL ASSESSMENT
Obtain vital signs, weight; evaluate patient's general physical and emotional status. Baseline laboratory tests may include CBC, differential, platelet count, serum uric acid, and renal- and hepatic-function tests.

ADMINISTRATION
Have available drugs for treatment of extravasation. Hyaluronidase is recommended.

A Kold Kap or scalp tourniquet may be used to prevent alopecia. The scalp tourniquet remains in place during and approximately 15 minutes after IV administration; the Kold Kap remains in place during and for approximately 1 hour after injection.

May be injected either directly into a vein or into tubing of a running IV infusion. The physician selects method of administration.

Use a large vein, preferably on the forearm, for injection.

CLINICAL ALERT: It is extremely important that the needle be properly positioned in the vein before vincristine is injected. If leakage into surrounding tissue should occur during IV administration, it may cause considerable irritation.

Check for blood return during administration. Advise patient to immediately mention any burning or pain felt at the injection site. If extravasation occurs during IV administration, the injection is discontinued immediately and any remaining portion of the dose is given in another vein.

The injection may be completed in about 1 minute.

Treatment of extravasation: Local injection of hyaluronidase and the application of moderate heat to the area of leakage help to disperse the drug and minimize discomfort and the possibility of cellulitis.

Storage: This product should be refrigerated.

ONGOING ASSESSMENTS AND NURSING MANAGEMENT
Monitor vital signs q4h or as ordered. If patient is acutely ill, monitor blood pressure, pulse, and respirations q1h to q2h.

Measure intake and output. Notify physician if oral intake is inadequate, if there is any change in the intake–output ratio, or if urinary output decreases.

Observe for adverse reactions; notify physician immediately if any one or more adverse reactions occur.

CLINICAL ALERT: Observe for signs of neurotoxicity. Initial signs may include sensory impairment and paresthesias; therefore, question patient about the development of these symptoms. With continued treatment, neuritic pain may occur; later, motor difficulties may occur including difficulty in walking, climbing stairs, and so on. Notify the physician at the first sign of neurologic involvement because dose reduction may be necessary.

Leukopenia occasionally occurs. Observe for signs of infection (*i.e.,* chills, fever, sore throat, signs of urinary or upper respiratory tract infection, malaise, headache, abscess formation, or ulceration).

Monitor bowel elimination pattern because constipation may occur.

If patient complains of colicky abdominal pain, auscultate bowel sounds. Notify the physician of the problem. An abdominal film may be ordered.

Patient (especially young children) should be observed for signs of paralytic ileus (*i.e.,* absent or diminished bowel sounds, abdominal distention and pain, and possibly vomiting).

A routine prophylactic regimen against constipation is recommended. Physician may order a stool softener or other laxative and a diet high in roughage. Extra fluids should be encouraged.

Weigh weekly or as ordered. Inform physician of any significant increase or decrease in weight.

If neurotoxicity occurs, patient may require assistance with ambulatory activities. If patient is not ambulatory, take measures to prevent foot-

U
V
W
X
Y
Z

drop, wristdrop, and loss of muscle tone. Passive exercises may be necessary.

Serum uric acid levels may increase due to rapid lysis of tumor cells. Encourage an increased fluid intake.

Laboratory tests prior to each weekly injection may include CBC, differential, hemoglobin, and platelet count. Serum uric acid, serum electrolytes, and renal-, and hepatic-function tests may be ordered periodically.

Rarely, a syndrome attributed to inappropriate antidiuretic hormone secretion may occur and may be evidenced by signs of hyponatremia (Appendix 6, section 6-17). If this syndrome is confirmed, the physician may order a limitation of fluid intake until condition is corrected.

PATIENT AND FAMILY INFORMATION

NOTE: Diagnosis, chemotherapeutic regimen, and anticipated adverse effects should be discussed with the patient and/or family.

Immediately report the occurrence of any of the following: numbness or tingling in one or more extremities, difficulty walking or climbing stairs, constipation, abdominal cramps or pain, fever, chills, signs of a urinary or upper respiratory tract infection.

Drink plenty of fluids during daytime hours.

Take the prescribed laxative. If diarrhea occurs, contact physician.

Hair loss may occur. A wig, scarf or cap can be used. Hair loss may be complete or partial; hair will grow back but may be a different color or texture.

Inform other physicians and dentist of therapy with this drug.

Frequent laboratory tests will be necessary to monitor therapy with this drug.

Vitamin A Rx, otc

drops: 5000 IU/0.1 ml (otc)	Aquasol A
tablets, chewable: 25,000 IU (otc)	Generic
capsules: 10,000 IU (otc)	Generic
capsules: 25,000 IU (Rx)	Aquasol A, Generic
capsules: 50,000 IU (Rx)	Alphalin Gelseals, Aquasol A, Generic
injection: 50,000 IU/ ml (Rx)	Aquasol A

INDICATIONS

Treatment of vitamin A deficiency. Conditions that may cause deficiency include biliary tract or pancreatic disease, sprue, colitis, hepatic cirrhosis, celiac disease, regional enteritis, extreme dietary inadequacy, and portal gastrostomy. Deficiency is rare in well-nourished individuals.

CONTRAINDICATIONS

Hypervitaminosis A; oral administration in malabsorption syndrome; sensitivity to any ingredient; IV administration.

ACTIONS

One IU vitamin A is equal to 0.3 mcg of retinol or 0.6 mcg of beta-carotene. Beta-carotene, known as provitamin A, yields retinol after absorption from the intestinal tract. Retinol combines with opsin, the red pigment in the retina, to form rhodopsin, which is necessary for visual adaption to darkness. Vitamin A prevents retardation of growth and preserves the integrity of the epitheleal cells. Deficiency is characterized by nyctalopia (night blindness), keratomalacia (necrosis of the cornea), keratinization and drying of the skin, lowered resistance to infection, retardation of growth, thickening of bone, diminished production of cortical steroids, and fetal malformations.

Because vitamin A is fat soluble, absorption requires bile salts, pancreatic lipase, and dietary fat. The vitamin is stored in the Kupffer cells of the liver. Normal adult liver stores are sufficient to provide 2 years' requirements of vitamin A.

WARNINGS

Safety of amounts exceeding 6000 IU daily during pregnancy is not established. Use of vitamin A in excess of the RDA during normal pregnancy should be avoided. Vitamin A toxicity and elevated plasma calcium and alkaline phosphatase concentrations have been reported in chronic renal failure patients undergoing hemodialysis.

PRECAUTIONS

Prolonged daily administration over 25,000 IU should be under close supervision.

DRUG INTERACTIONS

Oral contraceptives significantly increase plasma vitamin A levels. Prolonged use of **mineral oil** may interfere with intestinal absorption of vitamin A.

ADVERSE REACTIONS

See *Overdosage.* Anaphylactic shock and death have been reported after IV use.

OVERDOSAGE

The following amounts have been found to be toxic. Toxicity manifestations depend on age of patient, dose, and duration of administration.

Acute toxicity: Single dose of 25,000 IU/kg. *Infants*—75,000 IU. *Adults*—Over 2 million IU.

Chronic toxicity: 4000 IU/kg administered for 6 to 15 months. *Infants (3–6 months)*—18,500 IU (water dispersed) daily for 1 to 3 months. *Adults*—1 million IU daily for 3 days, 50,000 IU daily for longer than 18 months, or 500,000 IU daily for 2 months.

Hypervitaminosis A syndrome

General: Fatigue, malaise, lethargy, night sweats, abdominal discomfort, anorexia, vomiting.

Skeletal: Slow growth, hard tender cortical thickening over radius and tibia, migratory arthralgia, premature closure of epiphysis, bone pain.

CNS: Irritability; headache; vertigo; increased intracranial pressure as manifested by bulging fontanels, papilledema, and exophthalmos.

Dermatologic: Fissures of the lips; drying and cracking of the skin; alopecia; scaling; massive desquamation; increased pigmentation; generalized pruritus; erythema; inflammation of the tongue, lips, and gums.

Systemic: Hypomenorrhea, hepatosplenomegaly, jaundice, edema of the lower extremities, leukopenia, vitamin A plasma level over 1200 IU/dl.

Treatment: Immediate withdrawal of the vitamin along with symptomatic and supportive treatment.

DOSAGE

Recommended Dietary Allowances (RDAs)

Adult males: 5000 IU.

Adult females: 4000 IU.

Treatment of severe deficiency states in adults and children over 8 years

Severe deficiency with xeropthalmia: 500,000 IU/day for 3 days, followed by 50,000 IU/day for 2 weeks.

Severe deficiency: 100,000 IU/day for 3 days, followed by 50,000 IU/day for 2 weeks.

Follow-up therapy: 10,000 to 20,000 IU/day for 2 months.

Parenteral (IM): *Adults*—100,000 IU/day for 3 days followed by 50,000 IU/day for 2 weeks. *Children (1–8 yr)*—17,500 to 35,000 IU/day for 10 days. *Infants*—7500 to 15,000 IU/day for 10 days.

NURSING IMPLICATIONS

HISTORY

See Appendix 4. A thorough dietary history is important.

PHYSICAL ASSESSMENT

Obtain vital signs, weight, height or length (children, infants); look for overt signs of vitamin A deficiency (*e.g.,* dry scaly skin, drying of the conjunctiva, changes such as shrinking and hardening in mucous membranes, evidence of failure to thrive [infants]). Because vitamin A deficiency may be associated with protein and other vitamin deficiencies, signs and symptoms of these deficiencies may also be present.

ADMINISTRATION

Give with or after meals. For infants, vitamin A drops may be added to the infant formula.

Liquid (drops) is supplied with a dropper measuring 5000 IU/0.1 ml.

Parenteral form is administered IM only. Give deep IM; rotate injection sites.

ONGOING ASSESSMENTS AND NURSING MANAGEMENT

A diet high in foods containing vitamin A may be ordered.

Weigh daily or as ordered.

Monitor dietary intake. Inform physician if patient is unable to, or refuses to, take diet.

PATIENT AND FAMILY INFORMATION

NOTE: Give patient or family member a list of foods high in vitamin A (*e.g.,* milk products, foods fortified with vitamin A, carrots, corn, spinach, sweet potatoes, beet greens, liver, swordfish or whitefish, apricots, orange juice, peaches, prunes, cornbread). The nurse or dietitian must provide nutritional counseling. Referral to a community agency may be necessary if the patient or family is unable to purchase foods required for an adequate and balanced nutritional intake.

Avoid prolonged use of mineral oil while taking this drug. If a laxative is necessary, consult physician.

Do not exceed recommended dosage.

Immediately report occurrence of signs of overdosage (nausea, vomiting, anorexia, malaise, drying or cracking of skin or lips, irritability, headache, loss of hair).

Vitamin B₁ (Thiamine Hydrochloride) Rx, otc

tablets: 5 mg, 250 mg, 500 mg (*otc*)	*Generic*
tablets: 10 mg, 25 mg, 50 mg, 100 mg (*otc*)	Betalin S, *Generic*

UVWXYZ

elixir: 1 mg/5 ml   *Generic*
  (*otc*)
elixir: 2.25 mg/5 ml   Betalin S
  (*otc*)
injection: 100 mg/ml   Betalin S, Biamine, *Generic*
  (*Rx*)

INDICATIONS

Treatment of thiamine deficiency. The deficiency state beriberi is characterized by GI manifestations, peripheral neurologic changes, cerebral deficits, and cardiovascular complications. Single vitamin B₁ deficiency is rare. Multiple vitamin deficiencies should be suspected in any case of dietary inadequacy.

Parenteral route is used when oral route is not feasible (*e.g.,* in anorexia, nausea, vomiting, preoperative and postoperative conditions) and in impaired GI absorption in malabsorption syndromes.

CONTRAINDICATIONS

Hypersensitivity.

ACTIONS

Thiamine combines with adenosine triphosphate (ATP) to form thiamine pyrophosphate, a coenzyme. Its role in carbohydrate metabolism is the decarboxylation of pyruvic and alpha keto acids. An increase in serum pyruvic acid is one sign of a deficiency state. The need for thiamine is greater when the carbohydrate content of the diet is high. Significant B₁ depletion can occur in 3 weeks of total thiamine dietary absence. Oral absorption is 8 mg to 15 mg daily. Tissue stores are saturated when intake exceeds the minimal daily requirement; excess thiamine is excreted in the urine.

WARNINGS

Serious sensitivity reactions can occur. Deaths have resulted from IV use. An intradermal test dose is recommended in patients with suspected sensitivity. Thiamine-deficient patients may experience a sudden onset or worsening of Wernicke's encephalopathy (characterized by nystagmus, bilateral sixth cranial nerve palsy, ataxia, and confusion) following IV glucose administration; in suspected thiamine deficiency, give thiamine before a glucose load is given.

DRUG INTERACTIONS

Thiamine is unstable in neutral or alkaline solutions; do not use in combination with alkaline solutions (*e.g.,* **carbonates, citrates, barbiturates**).

ADVERSE REACTIONS

Feeling of warmth, pruritus, urticaria, weakness, sweating, nausea, restlessness, tightness of the throat, angioneurotic edema, cyanosis, pulmonary edema, hemorrhage into the GI tract, cardiovascular collapse, and death have been reported.

DOSAGE

Recommended Dietary Allowances (RDAs): Adult males, 1.4 mg; adult females, 1 mg. Thiamine is recommended at 0.5 mg/1000 kcal intake.

Dietary supplement dosage: Usual adult dose is 5 mg/day to 30 mg/day PO.

Wet beriberi with myocardial failure: Myocardial failure must be treated as an emergency cardiac condition. Give IV doses up to 30 mg tid to correct the condition.

Beriberi: 10 mg to 20 mg IM tid for 2 weeks. An oral therapeutic multivitamin preparation containing 5 mg to 10 mg thiamine administered daily for 1 month is recommended to achieve body-tissue saturation.

NURSING IMPLICATIONS

HISTORY

See Appendix 4. A thorough dietary and alcohol-intake history is important.

PHYSICAL ASSESSMENT

Obtain vital signs, weight, height or length (infants). Look for signs of deficiency (*e.g.,* edema, pallor, emaciation, cardiac failure, nystagmus, ataxia, peripheral neuropathy, tachycardia). Because vitamin B₁ deficiency may be associated with other vitamin deficiencies, signs and symptoms of those deficiencies may also be present.

ADMINISTRATION

Intradermal test is recommended in patients with suspected sensitivity before IV administration (IV route rarely used).

IM administration may be painful. Advise patient that injection may cause discomfort. Rotate injection sites. Application of cold may relieve pain from injection.

ONGOING ASSESSMENTS AND NURSING MANAGEMENT

A diet high in protein and adequate calories plus foods high in thiamine (pork, liver, whole grains, wheat, peas and other vegetables) may be ordered.

If giving IM, inspect previous injection sites for signs of irritation.

Observe for adverse reactions and inform physician if they occur because dose reduction may be necessary.

Therapeutic effectiveness of treatment includes relief of symptoms, weight gain, and improvement in general well-being.

PATIENT AND FAMILY INFORMATION

NOTE: Give patient or family member a list of foods high in vitamin B_1. The nurse or dietitian must provide nutritional counseling. Referral to a community agency may be necessary if the patient or family is unable to purchase foods required for an adequate and balanced nutritional intake.

Take as directed by physician or recommended on the label of the product. Do not exceed recommended dose.

A well-balanced diet containing thiamine-rich foods is an important part of therapy.

Vitamin B₂ (Riboflavin) Rx, otc

tablets: 5 mg, 10 mg,   *Generic*
    25 mg, 50 mg, 100
    mg
injection: 50 mg/ml   Riobin-50

INDICATIONS

Treatment and prevention of riboflavin deficiency. Symptoms include vascularization of the cornea, cheilosis, glossitis, and seborrheic dermatitis, especially in skin folds. Corneal vascularization is usually accompanied by itching, burning, and roughness of the eyelids, blepharospasm, and photophobia. Riboflavin deficiency seldom occurs alone and is often associated with deficiency states of other B vitamins and protein.

ACTIONS

Riboflavin functions in the body as a coenzyme in the forms of flavin adenine dinucleotide (FAD) and flavin mononucleotide (FMN), which play a vital metabolic role in numerous tissue respiration systems.

DOSAGE

Recommended Dietary Allowances (RDAs): Adult males, 1.6 mg; adult females, 1.2 mg.

Dietary supplement dosage: *Adults and children over 12*—5 mg/day to 10 mg/day PO.

Treatment of deficiency states: Usual dose is 50 mg IM.

NURSING IMPLICATIONS

HISTORY

See Appendix 4. A thorough dietary history is essential.

PHYSICAL ASSESSMENT

Obtain vital signs. In severe deficiency in children, measure height, obtain weight; in an infant, measure length, obtain weight. Look for signs of deficiency (*e.g.,* cheilosis; glossitis; seborrheic dermatitis, especially in skin folds). Examine eyes for evidence of inflammation (patient may complain of photophobia, burning, itching of the eyes), tearing, roughness of the eyelids, blepharospasm. Because vitamin B_2 deficiency may be associated with protein and other vitamin B deficiencies, signs and symptoms of these deficiencies may also be present.

ADMINISTRATION

Riboflavin may be administered alone or in combination with other B vitamins.

Severe deficiency state may require parenteral administration. Give deep IM; rotate injection sites.

ONGOING ASSESSMENTS AND NURSING MANAGEMENT

A diet high in protein and adequate calories plus foods high in riboflavin (meats, green leafy vegetables, eggs, cereal, milk, and dairy products) may be ordered.

If given IM, inspect previous injection sites for signs of irritation.

Therapeutic effectiveness of treatment includes relief of symptoms and improvement in general well-being.

PATIENT AND FAMILY INFORMATION

NOTE: Give patient or family member a list of foods high in vitamin B_2. The nurse or dietitian must provide nutritional counseling. Referral to a community agency may be necessary if the patient or family is unable to purchase foods required for an adequate and balanced nutritional intake.

Take as directed by physician or recommended on the label of the product. Do not exceed recommended dose.

A well-balanced diet containing foods high in riboflavin is an important part of therapy.

Riboflavin may cause a yellow discoloration of the urine.

U
V
W
X
Y
Z

Vitamin B₅ (Calcium Pantothenate) otc

tablets: 10 mg   Pantholin
tablets: 10 mg with   Durasil
    200 mg aluminum
    hydroxide, 200 mg

magnesium trisili-
cate
tablets: 30 mg, 100   *Generic*
    mg, 218 mg

INDICATIONS

A spontaneously occurring deficiency of this vitamin in humans on a natural diet has not been recognized. However, weakness, fatigue, mood
changes, dizziness, psychoses, unsteady gait, and
torpor develop in individuals when a diet low in
this vitamin is given in conjunction with a pantothenic antagonist. The burning-foot or electric-
foot syndrome is reported to be improved by administration of pantothenic acid. It is inferred from
these and other studies that pantothenic acid is essential for humans. The daily requirement is not
definitely known but a dosage of 10 mg/day is
probably adequate to satisfy human requirements.

ACTIONS

Pantothenic acid is an essential element in cellular
metabolism. It functions as a part of coenzyme A,
which is vital in a variety of metabolic reactions involving transfer of acetyl groups. It is associated
with release of energy from utilization of carbohydrate and seems to be necessary for synthesis and
degradation of fatty acids, sterols, and steroid hormones.

DOSAGE

Although 10 mg will provide the approximate daily
allowance, doses of 20 mg to 100 mg have been
used for experimental and therapeutic purposes.

NURSING IMPLICATIONS

Vitamin B₅ is found in many animal and vegetable foods. This vitamin may be given, either
alone or in a multivitamin preparation, when
other vitamin deficiencies exist.

Vitamin B₆ *(Pyridoxine Hydrochloride)* Rx, otc

tablets: 5 mg, 100   *Generic*
    mg, 200 mg, 250
    mg, 500 mg (*otc*)
tablets: 10 mg, 25   Hexa-Betalin, *Generic*
    mg, 50 mg (*otc*)
capsules, timed re-   TexSixT.R.
    lease: 100 mg (*otc*)
injection: 100 mg/ml   Beesix, Hexa-Betalin, Py-
    (*Rx*)   roxine, *Generic*

INDICATIONS

Treatment of pyridoxine deficiency states including
inadequate dietary intake; drug-induced deficiency
(from isoniazid [INH] or oral contraceptives); in-
born errors of metabolism (*e.g.,* B₆-dependent convulsions or B₆-responsive anemia). The parenteral
route is indicated when oral use is not feasible, as in
anorexia, nausea, vomiting, and preoperative and
postoperative conditions. Also indicated when GI
absorption is impaired.

Investigational uses: Pyridoxine has been used in
hydrazine poisoning. Although experience is limited, reversal of neurologic symptoms and CNS
depression has been reported.

CONTRAINDICATIONS

Sensitivity to pyridoxine.

ACTIONS

Vitamin B₆ acts as a coenzyme in the metabolism
of protein, carbohydrate, and fat. In protein metabolism, it participates in the decarboxylation of
amino acids, conversion of trytophan to niacin or
serotonin, and deamination transamination and
transulfuration of amino acids. In carbohydrate metabolism, it is responsible for the breakdown of glycogen to glucose-1-phosphate. The total adult body
pool consists of 16 mg to 25 mg of pyridoxine. The
need for pyridoxine increases with the amount of
protein in the diet. Its half-life appears to be 15 to
20 days. It is degraded to 4-pyridoxic acid in the
liver; this metabolite is excreted in the urine.

WARNINGS

Pyridoxine may inhibit lactation by suppression of
prolactin.

PRECAUTIONS

Single deficiency of pyridoxine alone is rare. Multiple vitamin deficiency is to be expected in any inadequate diet.

DRUG INTERACTIONS

Patients treated with **levodopa** should avoid supplemental vitamins that contain more than 5 mg of
pyridoxine in the daily dose. Pyridoxine reverses the
therapeutic effect of levodopa by stimulating the decarboxylation of dopa to dopamine in peripheral
tissues. The antagonistic effect of pyridoxine does
not occur when patients are taking the decarboxylase inhibitor carbidopa and levodopa concomitantly.

INH, cycloserine, penicillamine, hydralazine, and
oral contraceptives may increase pyridoxine requirements.

ADVERSE REACTIONS
Paresthesia, somnolence, and low serum folic acid levels.

OVERDOSAGE
In humans, a dose of 25 mg/kg is well tolerated. Vitamin B_6 dependency has been induced in normal human adults on intakes of 200 mg/day for 33 days on normal diets.

DOSAGE
Recommended dietary allowances (RDAs): Adult males, 2.2 mg; adult females, 2 mg. Requirements are more in those having certain genetic defects or those being treated with INH or oral contraceptives.

Dietary deficiency: 10 mg to 20 mg daily for 3 weeks. Follow-up treatment is recommended daily for several weeks with an oral therapeutic multivitamin preparation containing 2 mg to 5 mg of pyridoxine.

Vitamin B_6 dependency syndrome: May require a therapeutic dosage of as much as 600 mg/day and an intake of 50 mg/day for life.

Deficiencies due to INH: 100 mg/day for 3 weeks followed by 50 mg/day maintenance dose. In poisoning caused by ingestion of more than 10 g of INH, an equal amount of pyridoxine should be given: 1 g IV followed by 1 g IM every 30 minutes. In patients on INH therapy at increased risk for pyridoxine deficiency (the malnourished, alcoholics, diabetics, epileptics, or slow acetylators), a prophylactic dose of 10 mg/day of pyridoxine is sufficient.

NURSING IMPLICATIONS

HISTORY
See Appendix 4. A thorough dietary history is important.

PHYSICAL ASSESSMENT
Obtain vital signs, weight. A frank deficiency in adults is rare, with the exception of those receiving INH, penicillamine, hydralazine, cycloserine, or oral contraceptives. Deficiency may be seen in infants. Look for signs of vitamin B_6 deficiency (*e.g.,* nausea, vomiting, abdominal distress, cheilosis, ataxia, convulsions). Because vitamin B_6 deficiency may be associated with other vitamin deficiencies, signs and symptoms of these deficiencies may also be present.

ADMINISTRATION
When administered IV for convulsions or poisoning caused by ingestion of more than 10 g of INH, drug is usually given by slow IV injection.

ONGOING ASSESSMENTS AND NURSING MANAGEMENT
A diet high in protein and adequate calories plus foods high in pyridoxine (pork, lamb, veal, glandular meats, legumes, potatoes, bananas, oatmeal, wheat germ) may be ordered.

Therapeutic effectiveness of treatment includes relief of symptoms and improvement in general well-being.

PATIENT AND FAMILY INFORMATION
NOTE: Give patient or family member a list of foods high in vitamin B_6. The nurse or dietitian must provide nutritional counseling. Referral to a community agency may be necessary if the patient or family is unable to purchase foods required for an adequate and balanced nutritional intake.

Take as directed by physician or recommended on the label of the product. Do not exceed recommended dose.

A well-balanced diet containing foods high in pyridoxine is an important part of therapy.

Vitamin B₁₂ Preparations

Cyanocobalamin otc

tablets: 25 mcg, 50 mcg, 100 mcg, 250 mcg	Generic
tablets, soluble: 25 mcg, 50 mcg	Generic
tablets, soluble: 100 mcg	Generic
capsules: 25 mcg	Generic

Cyanocobalamin Crystalline Rx, otc

tablets: 500 mcg (*otc*)	Generic
tablets: 1000 mcg (*otc*)	Generic
injection: 30 mcg/ml (*Rx*)	Generic
injection: 100 mcg/ml (*Rx*)	Betalin 12, Rubramin PC, Generic
injection: 120 mcg/ml (*Rx*)	Generic
injection: 1000 mcg/ml (*Rx*)	Berubigen, Betalin 12, Cabadon-M, Crystimin-1000, Cyanoject, Cyomin, Kaybovite-1000, Pernavit, Redisol, Rubesol 1000, Rubramin PC, Ruvite 1000, Vi-Twel, *Generic*

U V W X Y Z

Hydroxocobalamin, Crystalline Rx

injection: 1000 mcg/ ml	Alphamin, AlphaRedisol, Alpha-Ruvite, Codroxomin, Droxomin, Hydrobexan, Hydro-Cobex, Hydroxo-12, LA-12, *Generic*

INDICATIONS

Vitamin B₁₂ deficiency due to malabsorption syndrome as seen in pernicious anemia; GI pathology, dysfunction, or surgery; fish tapeworm infestation; gluten enteropathy, sprue, and accompanying folic acid deficiency.

Increased requirements associated with pregnancy, thyrotoxicosis, hemolytic anemia, hemorrhage, malignancy, and hepatic and renal disease.

Also indicated for the vitamin B₁₂ absorption test (Schilling test).

Oral preparations containing less than 500 mcg are used only as nutritional supplements.

CONTRAINDICATIONS

Sensitivity to cobalt or vitamin B₁₂.

ACTIONS

Is essential to growth, cell reproduction, hematopoiesis, and nucleoprotein and myelin synthesis. In general, oral absorption is inadequate in pernicious anemia (unless intrinsic factor is simultaneously given) and in the presence of malabsorption states. Oral route is not recommended under most indications.

Cyanocobalamin is readily absorbed from IM and subcutaneous injection sites; the plasma level reaches its peak within 1 hour. Vitamin B₁₂ is transported via the bloodstream to the liver, the main organ for vitamin B₁₂ storage. Within 48 hours after injection of 100 mcg to 1000 mcg from 50% to 98% of the injected dose may appear in the urine. The major portion is excreted within the first 8 hours.

WARNINGS

Parenteral administration is preferred for pernicious anemia. The IV route is avoided. Blunted or impeded therapeutic response may be due to infection, uremia, drugs (such as chloramphenicol) having bone-marrow suppressant properties, concurrent iron or folic acid deficiency, or misdiagnosis.

Vitamin B₁₂ deficiency that is allowed to progress for 3 months or longer may produce *permanent* degenerative lesions of the spinal cord. Patients with early Leber's disease (hereditary optic nerve atrophy) treated with cyanocobalamin have been found to suffer severe and swift optic atrophy. Fatal hypokalemia could occur upon conversion of megaloblastic to normal erythropoiesis with vitamin B₁₂ therapy as a result of increased erythrocyte potassium needs.

Studies in pregnant women have not shown that cyanocobalamin increases the risk of fetal abnormalities if administered during pregnancy. Use during pregnancy only if clearly needed, because studies cannot rule out the possibility of harm. Safety for use in lactation has not been established. Safety and efficacy for use in children have not been established.

PRECAUTIONS

An intradermal test dose is recommended before cyanocobalamin crystalline and hydroxocobalamin are administered to patients sensitive to the cobalamins. Patients taking most antibiotics, methotrexate, and pyrimethamine will not have valid folic acid and vitamin B₁₂ diagnostic blood assays.

Doses exceeding 10 mcg/day may produce hematologic response in those with folate deficiency. Indiscriminate administration may mask the true diagnosis. Single deficiency of vitamin B₁₂ alone is rare. Multiple vitamin deficiency is expected in any dietary deficiency. Vitamin B₁₂ deficiency may suppress the signs of polycythemia vera. Treatment with vitamin B₁₂ may unmask the condition.

DRUG INTERACTIONS

GI absorption of cyanocobalamin may be impaired by administration of **aminosalicylic acid, neomycin,** or **alcohol. Colchicine** appears to enhance the neomycin-induced malabsorption. Colchicine, aminosalicylic acid, and heavy alcohol intake for periods exceeding 2 weeks may produce malabsorption of vitamin B₁₂. Concurrent administration of **chloramphenicol** may cause a poor response to B₁₂ therapy in those with pernicious anemia; this effect is thought to be due to interference with erythrocyte maturation by chloramphenicol.

ADVERSE REACTIONS

CYANOCOBALAMIN CRYSTALLINE AND HYDROXOCOBALAMIN, CRYSTALLINE

Mild transitory diarrhea, polycythemia vera, peripheral vascular thrombosis, itching, acne, transitory exanthema, feeling of swelling of the entire body, pulmonary edema, CHF in early treatment, anaphylactic shock, and death have been reported. A few patients may experience pain at the injection site.

DOSAGE

CYANOCOBALAMIN

Recommended dietary allowances (RDAs) are 3 mcg for adults. For nutritional deficiency, 25 mcg/day to 250 mcg/day PO.

CYANOCOBALAMIN CRYSTALLINE

Parenteral therapy is recommended in addisonian pernicious anemia; it will be required for the rest of the patient's life. Oral therapy is not dependable. In others with vitamin B$_{12}$ deficiency, the duration of therapy and route of administration will depend on the causes and on whether it is reversible. In seriously ill patients, both vitamin B$_{12}$ and folic acid may be given while awaiting results of distinguishing laboratory tests. Folic acid should be coadministered early in the treatment of sprue. Poor dietary habits and malabsorption should be corrected. Serum potassium should be closely observed the first 48 hours and potassium administered if necessary.

Vitamin B$_{12}$ deficiency

Oral: 1000 mcg/day. Patients with normal intestinal absorption may receive a daily oral multivitamin preparation containing 15 mcg of vitamin B$_{12}$.

IM or subcutaneous: 30 mcg/day for 5 to 10 days, followed by 100 mcg to 200 mcg monthly. If patient is critically ill or has neurologic disease, an infectious disease, or hyperthyroidism, considerably higher doses may be indicated. Current data indicate that the optimum obtainable neurologic response may be expected with a dosage sufficient to produce good hematologic response.

Schilling test: The flushing dose is 1000 mcg IM.

HYDROXOCOBALAMIN, CRYSTALLINE

Give IM only. Recommended dosage is 30 mcg/day for 5 to 10 days, followed by 100 mcg to 200 mcg monthly. Concurrent folic acid therapy should be instituted early in the treatment, if needed.

NURSING IMPLICATIONS

HISTORY

See Appendix 4. In those eating a diet that includes meat, deficiency of vitamin B$_{12}$ is rare, but this deficiency may be seen in vegetarians and their breast-fed infants.

PHYSICAL ASSESSMENT

Obtain vital signs, weight. In pernicious anemia, identify neurologic symptoms if present (_e.g.,_ ataxia, disturbed position sense, paresthesias, numbness, weakness in the extremities, lack of coordination, visual disturbances, poor memory, loss of bowel and bladder control, depression, impairment of fine finger movement). Other symptoms may include glossitis, nausea, vomiting, weight loss, bleeding of the gingiva, anorexia, constipation, and diarrhea. Baseline laboratory tests may include hemoglobin, hematocrit, RBC, WBC, platelet count, reticulocyte count, vitamin B$_{12}$ and folic acid plasma levels, serum potassium, and Schilling test. A gastric analysis may be performed. Because a vitamin B$_{12}$ nutritional deficiency may be associated with other vitamin deficiencies, signs and symptoms of these deficiencies may also be present.

ADMINISTRATION

An intradermal test dose may be administered if patient is suspected to be sensitive to cobalamins.

In those with pernicious anemia, the parenteral route is preferred because oral absorption is inadequate. The parenteral route may also be used in those with inadequate intestinal absorption.

Hydroxocobalamin, crystalline is administered IM only; **cyanocobalamin crystalline** may be administered IM or subcutaneously.

Advise patient that discomfort at the injection site may be experienced.

The Schilling test for absorption of vitamin B$_{12}$ may be performed for diagnosis of pernicious anemia. Patient fasts 12 hours before test. Vitamin B$_{12}$ tagged with radioactive cobalt is given PO. After 2 hours, 1000 mcg of nonradioactive vitamin B$_{12}$ is given IM to saturate tissue-binding sites. Consult hospital procedure manual for collection of urine specimens (usually for 24 hours).

ONGOING ASSESSMENTS AND NURSING MANAGEMENT

Deficiency of vitamin B$_{12}$ (other than pernicious anemia): A well-balanced diet containing foods high in vitamin B$_{12}$ is ordered.

Monitor bowel movements daily. Constipation or diarrhea may interfere with absorption if the oral preparation is administered.

Periodic hemoglobin, hematocrit, RBC, and reticulocyte count may be ordered.

Effectiveness of therapy is determined by improvement in symptoms associated with the deficiency.

Pernicious anemia: Monitor vital signs daily to q4h, depending on severity of disorder.

Evaluate patient's symptoms daily; compare with data base. Response to vitamin B$_{12}$ may be dramatic, with some symptoms relieved in 2 to 3 days. Vitamin B$_{12}$ deficiency that is allowed to progress for 3 or more months may produce permanent degenerative lesions of the spinal cord; thus, not all neurologic symptoms may be relieved by therapy.

Periodic hemoglobin, hematocrit, RBC, and

U
V
W
X
Y
Z

reticulocyte count are recommended. Vitamin B_{12} and serum folic acid levels are recommended between the fifth and seventh days of treatment.

Effectiveness of therapy is determined by improvement in symptoms and improvement in laboratory tests (*i.e.,* a rise of the laboratory values to normal).

Observe for adverse reactions, especially pulmonary edema or congestive heart failure, which may occur early in treatment.

Monitoring of serum potassium levels is recommended because fatal hypokalemia could occur. Observe for signs of hypokalemia (Appendix 6, section 6-15); notify physician immediately if they occur because potassium supplements may be necessary.

Weigh weekly or as ordered. Inform physician if any significant weight loss has occurred.

A well-balanced diet, including foods high in vitamin B_{12}, is ordered. If anorexia is severe, small feedings as well as between-meal snacks may be necessary.

PATIENT AND FAMILY INFORMATION

NOTE: Provide patient with a list of foods that are high in vitamin B_{12}. If parenteral vitamin B_{12} is to be administered by the patient or a family member, instruction in administration will be necessary.

Deficiency of vitamin B_{12} (other than pernicious anemia): Eat a well-balanced diet, including seafood, meats, eggs, and dairy products.

If taking oral vitamin B_{12}, bowel regularity is important. Inform physician or nurse if persistent constipation or diarrhea occurs.

Periodic laboratory tests may be necessary to monitor therapy.

Do not stop taking the vitamin, even if symptoms have improved, unless advised to do so by the physician.

Pernicious anemia: Lifetime therapy with vitamin B_{12} will be necessary.

Eat a well-balanced diet, including seafood, meats, eggs, and dairy products. Eating a proper diet is an important part of therapy.

Periodic laboratory tests will be necessary to monitor therapy.

Inform physician or nurse if symptoms recur or do not improve (in some instances, neurologic symptoms may be permanent).

Avoid contact with those with infections (*e.g.,* upper respiratory, communicable diseases). Report any signs of infection promptly because an increase in dosage or other medication may be necessary.

Vitamin C Preparations

Ascorbic Acid Rx, otc

tablets: 25 mg, 50 mg	Vitacee, *Generic (otc)*
tablets: 100 mg, 250 mg	Cevalin, Vitacee, *Generic (otc)*
tablets: 500 mg	Cevalin, Cevita, Vitacee, *Generic (otc)*
tablets: 1000 mg	*Generic (otc)*
tablets, chewable: 100 mg, 250 mg	Flavorcee, *Generic (otc)*
tablets, chewable: 500 mg, 1000 mg	*Generic (otc)*
tablets, timed release: 250 mg, 500 mg	Cemill (*otc*)
tablets, timed release: 750 mg	Arco-Cee (*otc*)
capsules, timed release: 500 mg	Ascorbicap, Best-C, Cetane, Cevi-Bid, Cevita, C-Long Granucaps, C-Span, *Generic (otc)*
drops: 35 mg/0.6 ml	Ce-Vi-Sol (*otc*)
drops: 100 mg/ml	Cecon (*otc*)
syrup: 20 mg/ml	*Generic (otc)*
injection: 50 mg/ml, 500 mg/ml	Cevalin (*Rx*)
injection: 100 mg/ml	Cevalin, *Generic (Rx)*
injection: 200 mg/ml, 250 mg/ml	*Generic (Rx)*

Sodium Ascorbate Rx

injection: 250 mg/ml	Cevita, *Generic*
injection: 562.5 mg/ml (equivalent to 500 mg/ml ascorbic acid)	Cenolate

INDICATIONS

Recommended for prevention and treatment of scurvy. Parenteral administration is desirable for those with an acute deficiency or those whose absorption of orally ingested ascorbic acid is uncertain.

Symptoms of mild vitamin C deficiency may include faulty bone and tooth development, gingivitis, bleeding gums, and loosened teeth. Febrile states, chronic illness, and infection increase the need for ascorbic acid. Premature and immature infants require relatively large amounts of the vitamin. Hemovascular disorders, burns, and delayed fracture and wound healing are indications for an increase in the daily intake.

CONTRAINDICATIONS

None known. Too-rapid IV injection is to be avoided. **Sodium ascorbate** should not be given to those on a sodium-restricted diet.

ACTIONS

Ascorbic acid is an essential vitamin in humans but its exact biological functions are not fully understood. Ascorbic acid and its reversibly oxidizable form, dehydroascorbic acid, are believed to play an important role in biological oxidations and reductions used in cellular respiration. It is essential for the formation and maintenance of intercellular ground substance and collagen. The ascorbic acid deficiency state (scurvy) is characterized by degenerative changes in the capillaries, bone, and connective tissues.

Vitamin C may be used as a urinary acidifier in conjunction with methenamine therapy. Failure of vitamin C to lower urine *p*H significantly may be attributed to inadequate dosage.

WARNINGS

Dosage of ascorbic acid in excess of the amount needed for treatment should not be administered to pregnant women. The possibility that the fetus may adapt to high levels of the vitamin could result in a scorbutic condition after birth, when the intake of the vitamin drops to normal levels.

PRECAUTIONS

Ascorbic acid is chemically incompatible with **potassium penicillin G** and should not be used in the same syringe or parenteral solution. Ascorbic acid and penicillin may be administered concurrently provided they are not mixed together prior to injection.

DRUG INTERACTIONS

Large doses (over 2 g/day) of ascorbic acid (but not sodium ascorbate) may lower urine *p*H and therefore may cause unexpected renal tubular reabsorption of **acidic drugs,** causing an exaggerated response. Conversely, **basic drugs** (*e.g.,* amphetamines, tricyclic antidepressants) may exhibit decreased reabsorption and therefore a decreased therapeutic effect. When given concurrently with **sulfonamides,** crystallization may occur.

Limited evidence suggests that ascorbic acid may influence the intensity and duration of action of **dicumarol.** It also has been reported to inhibit the anticoagulant response of **warfarin** (*i.e.,* decrease prothrombin time response).

Because ascorbic acid has occasionally been used as a specific antidote for symptoms resulting from interaction between ethanol and **disulfiram,** concurrent administration of ascorbic acid may interfere with the effectiveness of disulfiram used as an antialcoholic.

Concomitant administration of ethinyl estradiol and ascorbic acid may elevate plasma concentrations of ethinyl estradiol; intermittent administration of ascorbic acid may increase the risk of contraceptive failure.

Smoking decreases ascorbic acid serum levels and may increase ascorbic acid requirements.

Drug/lab tests: Large doses may cause false-negative urine glucose determinations using the glucose oxidase method, or false-positive results when using the copper reduction method or Benedict's solution.

ADVERSE REACTIONS

Large doses may cause significant diarrhea and may cause precipitation of oxalate or urate renal stones if the urine becomes acidic during therapy. Transient soreness may occur at the site of IM or subcutaneous injection. Too-rapid IV administration may cause temporary faintness or dizziness.

OVERDOSAGE

Because of loss in the urine, excessively high doses of parenterally administered ascorbic acid are wasteful after saturation of body tissues. Serious toxicity is very uncommon. In the event of severe or unusual untoward effects, ascorbic acid therapy should be terminated, pending further evaluation.

DOSAGE

Recommended dietary allowances (RDAs): Adults, 60 mg.

Oral: Prophylactic—50 mg to 100 mg. *Therapeutic*—100 mg or more as needed.

When used for urine acidification, only ascorbic acid (not sodium ascorbate) should be used; 4 g/day to 12 g/day given in divided doses q4h around the clock is recommended. It is advisable to monitor urinary *p*H to assure adequate dosage.

When extensive injuries are treated, ascorbic acid may be given if any doubt exists about previous nutrition with the vitamin. Patients with deep and extensive burns may require 200 mg/day to 500 mg/day to maintain measurable blood concentrations. Doses of 1 g/day to 4 g/day for 4 to 7 days may be given before surgery in gastrectomy patients. Similar doses have also been used postoperatively to aid wound healing following extensive surgical procedures.

Parenteral: Usual therapeutic parenteral dose ranges from 100 mg to 250 mg, once or twice daily. If the deficiency is extreme, 1 g to 2 g may be

U
V
W
X
Y
Z

given. There is no appreciable danger from excessive dosage because superfluous amounts of the vitamin are rapidly excreted in the urine.

NURSING IMPLICATIONS

HISTORY
See Appendix 4. A thorough dietary history is important if a vitamin C deficiency exists.

PHYSICAL ASSESSMENT
If rationale for administration is a dietary deficiency, look for signs of vitamin C deficiency (gingivitis, bleeding gums, loosened teeth, ecchymosis, follicular hyperkeratosis, joint pain [especially in the knees], lethargy, depression, poor wound healing, insomnia). Signs and symptoms of other vitamin deficiencies may also be present if patient has an inadequate dietary intake.

ADMINISTRATION
Avoid rapid IV injection because temporary faintness or dizziness may result.

When giving IM or subcutaneously, advise patient that transient mild soreness may be noted at the injection site.

When used for urinary acidification, administration q4h around the clock is recommended.

May be administered parenterally in combination with vitamin B complex and added to IV solutions.

ONGOING ASSESSMENTS AND NURSING MANAGEMENT
When administering for dietary deficiency, observe patient for relief of symptoms.

A well-balanced diet with foods high in vitamin C (citrus fruits, berries, cabbage, tomatoes, broccoli, spinach) may be ordered.

The blood level of ascorbic acid in normal individuals ranges from 0.4 mg/dl to 1.5 mg/dl.

If used for acidification of the urine, check urinary *p*H three to four times a day or as ordered. If urine does not remain acidic, inform physician because an increase in the dose of vitamin C may be necessary.

If diarrhea occurs, inform physician. A reduction in dosage may be necessary.

Urine testing: False-negative results may occur if the glucose oxidase method (Chemstrip G strips, Clinistix, Diastix, Tes-Tape) is used and the patient is receiving large doses of vitamin C. False-positive results may be seen with Benedict's solution or the copper sulfate reduction method (Clinitest, Clinitest 2 Drop Method).

PATIENT AND FAMILY INFORMATION
NOTE: Give patient or family member a list of foods high in vitamin C. The nurse or dietitian must provide nutritional counseling. Referral to a community agency may be necessary if the patient or family is unable to purchase foods required for an adequate and balanced nutritional intake.

Take as directed by the physician or manufacturer.

If pregnant, do not exceed dose recommended by the physician.

Do not take vitamin C if taking an anticoagulant, unless use is approved by the physician.

Tablets may discolor slightly with age; this apparently does not affect potency.

Acidification of urine: Take as directed by the physician (usually q4h around the clock). If checking urinary *p*H is recommended, contact physician if urine does not remain acidic.

Diabetic patient: False-positive or false-negative results may be obtained with testing materials when large doses of vitamin C are taken. If vitamin C supplementation is necessary, follow physician's recommended dose.

Vitamin D Preparations

Calcifediol Rx

capsules: 20 mcg, 50 mcg	Calderol

Calcitriol Rx

capsules: 0.25 mcg, 0.5 mcg	Rocaltrol

Dihydrotachysterol Rx

tablets: 0.125 mg, 0.2 mg, 0.4 mg	*Generic*
capsules: 0.125 mg	Hytakerol
solution: 0.25 mg/ml in oil	Hytakerol

Ergocalciferol (Vitamin D₂) Rx

capsules: 25,000 IU, 50,000 IU	*Generic*
capsules: 50,000 IU D₂	Deltalin Gelseals, Drisdol
tablets: 50,000 IU D₂	Calciferol

liquid: 8000 IU   Drisdol
  D_2/ml

injection: 500,000 IU   Calciferol
  D_2/ml

drops: 200 IU D_2/   Calciferol
  drop

INDICATIONS

CALCIFEDIOL

Management of metabolic bone disease or hypocalcemia in patients on chronic renal dialysis. Has been shown to increase serum calcium levels and to decrease alkaline phosphatase, parathyroid hormone levels, subperiosteal bone resorption, histologic signs of hyperparathyroid bone disease, and mineralization defects in some patients.

CALCITRIOL

Management of hypocalcemia in patients on chronic renal dialysis. Has been shown to reduce elevated parathyroid hormone levels in some of these patients.

DIHYDROTACHYSTEROL

Treatment of acute, chronic, and latent forms of postoperative tetany, idiopathic tetany, and hypoparathyroidism.

ERGOCALCIFEROL

Treatment of refractory rickets (also known as vitamin D–resistant rickets), familial hypophosphatemia, and hypoparathyroidism.

CONTRAINDICATIONS

Hypercalcemia; evidence of vitamin D toxicity; hypervitaminosis D; abnormal sensitivity to the effects of vitamin D.

ACTIONS

Vitamin D is a fat-soluble vitamin derived from natural sources such as fish liver oils and from conversion of provitamins derived from foods. Vitamin D_2 is the form used in fortified milk, bread, and cereals. Natural supplies of vitamin D depend on ultraviolet light for conversion of 7-dehydrocholesterol to vitamin D_3 (cholecalciferol). Vitamin D_3 is transformed by hepatic microsomal enzymes to calcifediol, which is the major transport form of vitamin D_3 and can be monitored in the serum. Calcifediol possesses intrinsic vitamin D activity but is further metabolized in the mitochondria of the kidney to calcitriol, the active form of vitamin D_3, and 24,25-dihydroxycholecalciferol. The physiological role of the latter has not been clearly established. It has been suggested that a vitamin D–resistant state

exists in uremic patients because of failure of the kidney to convert vitamin D precursors adequately to the active form, calcitriol. Enzyme activity is stimulated by endocrine levels (parathyroid hormone, prolactin, estrogen) and increased by dietary deficiencies (vitamin D, calcium, phosphate). Low calcium and phosphate levels stimulate parathyroid secretion, which in turn enhances activity of the enzyme.

Dihydrotachysterol is an analogue of vitamin D. When activated by the liver to produce 25-hydroxydihydrotachysterol, it is effective in raising serum calcium by stimulation of intestinal calcium absorption and bone calcium mobilization in the absence of parathyroid hormone and functioning renal tissue.

Vitamin D is now frequently considered to be a hormone. In healthy individuals, the biological effects of the various forms of vitamin D are equivalent. Vitamin D, in conjunction with parathyroid hormone and calcitonin, regulates calcium metabolism. Vitamin D metabolites promote the active absorption of calcium and phosphorus by the midjejunum intestinal mucosa. They increase the rate of accretion and resorption of minerals in bone and promote the resorption of phosphate by renal tubules. The action on calcium and phosphate metabolism is similar to that of parathyroid hormone. Vitamin D is also involved in magnesium metabolism.

Vitamin D deficiency leads to rickets in children and osteomalacia in adults. Administration of vitamin D completely reverses the symptoms of nutritional rickets or osteomalacia unless permanent deformities have occurred. Individual response to vitamin D varies.

Vitamin D is readily absorbed from the intestine. Vitamin D_3 may be absorbed more rapidly and more completely than vitamin D_2. Intestinal absorption is dependent on an adequate amount of bile. Absorption is reduced in patients with liver disease and intestinal malabsorption syndrome.

Vitamin D is stored chiefly in the liver but is also found in fat, muscle, skin, brain, spleen, and bones. In plasma it is bound to alpha globulins and albumin. Serum half-life of calcifediol is approximately 16 days, with duration of pharmacologic activity of 15 to 20 days following oral administration. In renal failure it is prolonged two- to threefold. Serum half-life of calcitriol is 7 to 12 hours; pharmacologic activity persists for 3 to 5 days following oral administration. Dihydrotachysterol is faster acting and less persistent after cessation of treatment. With natural forms of vitamin D there is a lag of 12 to 24 hours between administration and initiation of action in the body.

U
V
W
X
Y
Z

WARNINGS

Hypersensitivity to vitamin D may be one etiologic factor in infants with idiopathic hypercalcemia. In these cases, vitamin D must be severely restricted.

Dosage is readjusted as soon as there is clinical improvement. Dosage is individualized to prevent serious effects. In vitamin D–resistant rickets, the range between the therapeutic and toxic doses is narrow.

The product of serum calcium times phosphate (Ca × P) should not exceed 70; exceeding the solubility product will result in precipitation of calcium phosphate. Progressive hypercalcemia due to overdosage may be so severe as to require emergency attention. Chronic hypercalcemia can lead to generalized vascular calcification, nephrocalcinosis, and other soft-tissue calcification. Radiographic or slit lamp evaluation of suspect anatomic regions may be useful in early detection of hypercalcemia. A fall in serum phosphatase levels usually precedes hypercalcemia and may be an indication of impending hypercalcemia. Should hypercalcemia develop, drug is discontinued immediately. After normocalcemia is achieved, the drug may be readministered at a lower dosage.

Safety of amounts in excess of 400 IU/day in pregnancy is not established. Doses greater than the RDA during a normal pregnancy should be avoided. Use during pregnancy only if potential benefit justifies the potential risk to the fetus. These drugs are excreted in human milk. Caution is exercised when administering to nursing women. Safety and efficacy in children in doses in excess of the RDA have not been established.

PRECAUTIONS

The amount of vitamin D ingested in fortified foods, dietary supplements, and other concomitantly administered drugs should be evaluated. In treatment of hypoparathyroidism, calcium, parathyroid hormone, and/or dihydrotachysterol may be required. Because of the effect on serum calcium, vitamin D is given to patients with renal stones only when potential benefits outweigh possible hazards.

DRUG INTERACTIONS

Use of **magnesium-containing antacids** may lead to development of hypermagnesemia. **Cholestyramine** has been reported to reduce intestinal absorption of fat-soluble vitamins. Prolonged use of **mineral oil** interferes with absorption of fat-soluble vitamins. Vitamin D is given cautiously to those on **digitalis** because hypercalcemia in such patients may precipitate cardiac arrhythmias. Administration of **thiazide diuretics** to hypoparathyroid patients concurrently treated with vitamin D may cause hypercalcemia.

Phenytoin and **barbiturates** may increase metabolic inactivation of vitamin D and decrease its half-life, possibly resulting in hypocalcemia and clinical osteomalacia or rickets.

ADVERSE REACTIONS

Early: Weakness, headache, somnolence, nausea, vomiting, dry mouth, constipation, muscle pain, bone pain, metallic taste.

Late: Polyuria, polydipsia, anorexia, irritability, weight loss, nocturia, conjunctivitis (calcific), pancreatitis, photophobia, rhinorrhea, pruritus, hyperthermia, decreased libido, elevated BUN, proteinuria, hypercholesterolemia, elevated SGOT and SGPT, ectopic calcification, hypertension, cardiac arrhythmias, and, rarely, overt psychosis.

OVERDOSAGE

Symptoms: Administration in excess of daily requirements can cause hypercalcemia, hypercalciuria, and hyperphosphatemia. Concomitant high intake of calcium and phosphate may lead to similar abnormalities.

Hypercalcemia leads to anorexia, nausea, weakness, weight loss, vague aches and stiffness, constipation, diarrhea, convulsions, mental retardation, anemia, and mild acidosis. Impairment of renal function may result in polyuria, nocturia, polydipsia, hypercalciuria, reversible azotemia, hypertension, nephrocalcinosis, generalized vascular calcification, irreversible renal insufficiency that may result in death, proteinuria, or urinary casts. Widespread calcification of soft tissues, including the heart, blood vessels, renal tubules, and lungs, can occur. Bone demineralization (osteoporosis) may occur in adults; decline in average rate of linear growth and increased mineralization of bones may occur in infants and children (dwarfism). Effects can persist for 2 or more months after treatment with ergocalciferol and cholecalciferol, 1 month after cessation of therapy with dihydrotachysterol, 2 to 7 days for calcitriol, and 2 to 4 weeks for calcifediol. Death can result from cardiovascular or renal failure.

Treatment of hypervitaminosis D with hypercalcemia: Immediate withdrawal of the vitamin, low-calcium diet, generous intake of fluids, and acidification of the urine along with symptomatic and supportive treatment. Hypercalcemic crisis with dehydration, stupor, coma, and azotemia requires more vigorous treatment. The first step should be hydration; IV saline may quickly and significantly increase urinary calcium excretion. A loop diuretic (furosemide, ethacrynic acid) may be given with saline infusion to further increase renal calcium excretion. Other therapeutic measures include dialysis or administration of citrates, sulfate, phosphates, corticosteroids, EDTA, and plicamycin (mithramycin). Persistent or markedly elevated serum calcium levels may be corrected by dialysis. With appropriate therapy, recovery is the usual outcome when no permanent damage has occurred.

Treatment of accidental overdosage: General supportive measures are indicated. If ingestion is discovered within a short time, emesis or gastric lavage may be of benefit. Mineral oil may promote fecal elimination. Hypercalcemia is treated in the same manner as hypervitaminosis D (above).

DOSAGE

The optimal daily dosage is individualized for each patient. Effectiveness of therapy is predicated on adequate daily intake of calcium. The RDA for calcium in adults is 1000 mg.

CALCIFEDIOL

Recommended initial dose is 300 mcg/week to 350 mcg/week, administered on a daily or alternate-day schedule. If satisfactory response is not obtained, dosage may be increased at 4-week intervals. During this period, serum calcium levels are recommended weekly; if hypercalcemia is noted, drug is discontinued until normocalcemia ensues. Some patients with normal serum calcium levels may respond to doses of 20 mcg every other day. Most patients respond to doses between 50 mcg/day and 100 mcg/day or between 100 mcg and 200 mcg on alternate days.

CALCITRIOL

Recommended initial dosage is 0.25 mcg/day. If a satisfactory response is not seen, dosage may be increased by 0.25 mcg/day at 2- to 4-week intervals. During this titration period, serum calcium levels are recommended twice weekly; if hypercalcemia is noted, use is discontinued until normocalcemia ensues. Patients with normal or only slightly reduced serum calcium levels may respond to doses of 0.25 mcg every other day. Most patients undergoing hemodialysis respond to doses between 0.5 mcg/day and 1 mcg/day.

DIHYDROTACHYSTEROL

Initial dose is 0.75 mg/day to 2.5 mg/day for several days. Maintenance dose is 0.2 mg/day to 1 mg/day as required for normal serum calcium levels. Average dose is 0.6 mg/day. May be supplemented with oral calcium.

ERGOCALCIFEROL

1 mg provides 40,000 units of vitamin D activity. RDA for adults is 200 IU. A daily dosage of 400 IU satisfies requirements for all age groups, unless there has been exposure to ultraviolet radiation. Dosage is individualized and calcium intake must be adequate. One USP unit of vitamin D activity is equal to 0.025 mcg of ergocalciferol (1 mg = 40,000 units). 1 USP unit = 1 IU.

Vitamin D–resistant rickets: 50,000 to 500,000 units daily. Normal serum calcium and phosphate levels may be seen after 2 weeks of therapy; evidence of bone healing may be seen in 4 weeks. Carefully adjust dose to avoid hypercalcemia.

Hypoparathyroidism: 50,000 to 400,000 IU vitamin D daily plus 4 g of calcium lactate, administered six times a day.

IM therapy: Patients with GI, liver, or biliary disease associated with malabsorption of vitamin D require IM administration.

NURSING IMPLICATIONS

HISTORY

See Appendix 4. A thorough dietary history is important because dosage may be based on concomitant vitamin D intake in fortified foods.

PHYSICAL ASSESSMENT

Obtain vital signs, weight. *Infants and children*— measure length or height. Assess for signs of hypovitaminosis D (*e.g.,* bone malformations, beading of ends of ribs, pigeon breast, skull softening, delayed closing of fontanelles in infants, bulging forehead, enlargement of wrists and ankles, enlarged abdomen, tetany [infants], pain in legs and lower back, difficulty walking, multiple fractures). Early symptoms of deficiency may include restlessness, irritability, and profuse sweating. Baseline laboratory tests may include serum calcium, serum alkaline phosphatase, serum potassium, serum magnesium, vitamin D levels, serum calcium, serum phosphorus, CBC, hemoglobin, BUN, 24-hour urinary calcium and phosphorus, and urinalysis. Bone x-ray examinations may be performed for diagnosis.

ADMINISTRATION

May be given daily or on an alternate-day schedule.

IM administration (ergocalciferol): Give deep IM, preferably in the gluteus muscle. Rotate injection sites.

Supplemental calcium may be ordered.

ONGOING ASSESSMENTS AND NURSING MANAGEMENT

Vitamin D levels below 50 IU/dl (normal range is 50–135 IU/dl) and low serum levels of calcium and phosphorus and elevated serum alkaline phosphatase indicate vitamin D deficiency.

Periodic serum calcium levels are ordered. Early in therapy, these may be determined weekly or twice weekly. Serum calcium concentration should be kept between 9 mg/dl and 10 mg/dl. Periodic serum phosphorus and magnesium and alkaline phosphatase and 24-hour urinary calcium and phosphorus are also recommended.

When high doses are given, frequent serum and urinary calcium, potassium, and urea nitrogen levels are ordered.

Assess for relief of symptoms of hypovitaminosis D; record findings. Physician adjusts dosage according to response to therapy.

CLINICAL ALERT: Patient should be observed for signs and symptoms of hypervitaminosis D. Look for signs of hypercalcemia, hypercalciuria, and hyperphosphatemia (see *Overdosage*). Contact physician immediately if any of these occurs, because drug will be discontinued and a low-calcium diet instituted. Acidification of the urine and a generous intake of fluids may also be necessary.

Adequate dietary calcium is necessary for clinical response to vitamin D therapy. If anorexia occurs, inform physician.

Weigh patient weekly or as ordered.

Measure length or height monthly in infants and children.

Patients with hyperphosphatemia or renal osteodystrophy accompanied by hypophosphatemia may be prescribed a diet low in phosphate as well as be given aluminum gels as intestinal phosphate binders to prevent metastatic calcification.

Notify physician of any decrease in serum alkaline phosphate levels because a fall in alkaline phosphatase usually precedes hypercalcemia and may be an indication of impending hypercalcemia.

PATIENT AND FAMILY INFORMATION

NOTE: Physician may recommend a diet high in vitamin D. Patient should be instructed about foods containing vitamin D (*e.g.,* vitamin D–fortified foods such as milk and cereals [lesser amounts are found in cream, butter, eggs, and liver]), and foods containing calcium (*e.g.,* milk, yogurt, cheese, eggs, lean meat, beans, peanut butter, oranges, broccoli, carrots, apples, peaches, pears, white or whole wheat bread, macaroni, noodles, spaghetti).

Do *not* exceed prescribed dose; take only as directed.

Take calcium supplement (if ordered) as directed.

Eat diet recommended by the physician.

Report the occurrence of any of the following: weakness, lethargy, headache, anorexia, weight loss, nausea, vomiting, abdominal cramps, diarrhea, constipation, vertigo, excessive thirst, passage of large volumes of urine, dry mouth, or muscle or bone pain.

Avoid use of mineral oil, magnesium-containing antacids/laxatives, and multivitamin preparations (unless recommended by the physician) while taking vitamin D.

Close medical supervision and periodic laboratory tests will be necessary.

Vitamin E Rx, otc

tablets: 100 IU, 200 IU, 400 IU, 1000 IU (*otc*)	*Generic*
tablets: 100 IU, 400 IU (as d-alpha tocopheryl succinate) (*otc*)	Pheryl-E
tablets, chewable: 200 IU, 400 IU (*otc*)	*Generic*
capsules: 50 IU, 100 IU, 200 IU, 400 IU, 600 IU, 800 IU, 1000 IU (*otc*)	*Generic*
capsules: 50 IU (as dl-alpha tocopheryl acetate) (*otc*)	Eprolin Gelseals
capsules: 100 IU (as dl-alpha tocopheryl acetate) (*otc*)	Eprolin Gelseals, Viterra E
capsules: 100 IU (as d-alpha tocopheryl acetate) (*otc*)	Aquasol E, CEN-E, D-Alpha-E, Epsilan-M
capsules: 200 IU, 400 IU, 600 IU (as dl-alpha tocopheryl acetate) (*otc*)	Viterra E
capsules: 200 IU (as d-alpha tocopheryl acetate) (*otc*)	CEN-E
capsules: 200 IU, 400 IU (as d-alpha tocopheryl succinate) (*otc*)	E-Ferol Succinate
capsules: 400 IU (as d-alpha tocopheryl acetate) (*otc*)	Aquasol E, CEN-E, Vita-Plus E
injection: 200 IU/ml (*Rx*)	*Generic*

INDICATIONS

Although many uses for vitamin E have been advanced, its only established use is for treatment or prevention of vitamin E deficiency.

Investigational use: Has been used in certain premature infants to reduce toxic effects of oxygen therapy on lung parenchyma (bronchopulmonary dysplasia) and the retina (retrolental fibroplasia). It has also been used to decrease the severity of hemolytic anemia in infants.

ACTIONS

Although the exact biochemical mechanisms for function of vitamin E in the body are unclear, it is considered an essential element in human nutrition. Many actions of vitamin E are related to its antioxidant properties. In humans, vitamin E is thought to stabilize cell membranes by protecting against peroxidative cleavage of unsaturated bonds. Vitamin E preserves the integrity of red blood cell walls and protects them against hemolysis. Vitamin E may also act as a cofactor in enzyme systems. Enhancement of vitamin A utilization and suppression of platelet aggregation have also been attributed to vitamin E.

Clinical deficiency is rare, because adequate amounts are supplied in the usual diet. Low plasma levels have been noted in premature and some full-term infants; severe protein-calorie malnourished infants with macrocytic megaloblastic anemia; some patients with prolonged fat malabsorption (as in cystic fibrosis, hepatic cirrhosis, sprue, celiac disease, biliary atresia); and patients with acanthocytosis. Vitamin E deficiency may result in hemolysis, muscle necrosis, creatinuria, and deposition of ceroid pigment in muscle. Hematologic abnormalities and creatinuria are generally responsive to vitamin E administration.

Vitamin E requirements: Absolute daily requirements in humans are not established, but they appear to be directly related to the amount of polyunsaturated fatty acids (PUFA) in the diet. Vitamin E requirements may be increased in patients taking large doses of iron; diets containing selenium, sulfur-amino acids, or antioxidants may decrease the daily requirement. Vitamin E supplementation has been shown to be effective in correcting hemolytic anemia and relieving edema and skin lesions (flaky dermatitis) that develop in low–birth weight premature infants fed artificial formulas containing iron and high concentrations of PUFA. Infant formulas are supplemented with vitamin E in proportion to their PUFA content.

DOSAGE

Recommended dietary allowances (RDAs): Adult males, 15 IU; adult females, 12 IU. The dosages of the several forms of vitamin E vary; dosage is usually standardized in International Units (IU), based on activity.

NURSING IMPLICATIONS

HISTORY

Vitamin E deficiency is rare and may be difficult to recognize. A deficiency may be seen in premature low–birth weight infants fed artificial formulas containing iron and high concentrations of PUFA.

PHYSICAL ASSESSMENT

In infants, look for edema, skin lesions (flaky dermatitis), signs of hemolytic anemia. Baseline laboratory tests may include CBC and 24-hour urine creatinine. Because vitamin E deficiency may be associated with other vitamin deficiencies, signs and symptoms of those deficiencies may also be present.

ADMINISTRATION

For infants, formula with vitamin E added may be ordered. May also be given as drops (added to feeding or orally) or by injection if deficiency is severe.

Many multivitamin preparations contain vitamin E. Physician may order vitamin E supplementation as a single vitamin or as a multivitamin preparation.

ONGOING ASSESSMENTS AND NURSING MANAGEMENT

A diet high in vitamin E may be ordered. Foods containing large amounts of this vitamin include vegetable oils, vegetable shortening, margarine, leafy vegetables, whole grains, wheat germ, milk, eggs, and meat.

Infants: Look for relief of symptoms of deficiency (*e.g.,* improvement in skin lesions and decrease in edema).

PATIENT AND FAMILY INFORMATION

Take as directed by physician.

Drops are supplied with a dropper. Vitamin may be added to the infant formula.

Eat foods high in vitamin E: Margarine, leafy vegetables, whole grains, milk, eggs, meat, liver, wheat germ. Vegetable oils and shortening also contain large high amounts of vitamin E.

Vitamin K Preparations

Menadiol Sodium Diphosphate (K₄) Rx

tablets: 5 mg	Synkayvite
injection: 5 mg/ml, 10 mg/ml, 37.5 mg/ml	Synkayvite

U
V
W
X
Y
Z

Menadione *(K₃)* Rx

tablets: 5 mg   *Generic*

Phytonadione

(K₁, Phylloquinone, Methylphytyl Naphthoquinone) Rx

tablets: 5 mg   Mephyton
injection, aqueous   AquaMEPHYTON
  colloidal solution:
  2 mg/ml, 5 mg/ml
injection, aqueous   Konakion
  dispersion: 2 mg/
  ml, 10 mg/ml (for
  IM use only)

INDICATIONS

Useful in the following coagulation disorders that are due to faulty formation of factors II, VII, IX, and X when caused by vitamin K deficiency or interference with vitamin K activity.

Oral: Vitamin K deficiency secondary to administration of antibacterial therapy; hypoprothrombinemia secondary to administration of salicylates; hypoprothrombinemia secondary to obstructive jaundice and biliary fistulas, but only if bile salts are administered concomitantly with phytonadione, which is ineffective when given alone. The menadiol sodium diphosphate may be effective alone.

Parenteral: Hypoprothrombinemia secondary to conditions limiting absorption or synthesis of vitamin K (*e.g.,* obstructive jaundice, biliary fistulas, sprue, ulcerative colitis, celiac disease, intestinal resection, cystic fibrosis of the pancreas, regional enteritis, antibacterial therapy, and other drug-induced hypoprothrombinemia due to interference with vitamin K metabolism [*e.g.,* salicylates]).

Phytonadione is also indicated for oral anticoagulant–induced prothrombin deficiency and for prophylaxis and therapy of hemorrhagic disease of the newborn.

CONTRAINDICATIONS

Hypersensitivity. **Menadione and menadiol sodium diphosphate** should not be given to women during the last 4 weeks of pregnancy or during labor as a prophylactic measure against physiological hypoprothrombinemia or hemorrhagic disease of the newborn and are not intended for administration to infants.

ACTIONS

Vitamin K is necessary for hepatic synthesis of active prothrombin (factor II), proconvertin (factor VII), plasma thromboplastin component (factor IX), and Stuart factor (factor X). The prothrombin test is sensitive to levels of factors II, VII, and X. The mechanisms by which vitamin K promotes formation of these clotting factors in the liver is not known.

Phytonadione (vitamin K₁) and menadione (vitamin K₃) are lipid soluble synthetic analogs of vitamin K. Menadiol sodium diphosphate (vitamin K₄) is a water-soluble derivative that is converted to menadione *in vivo*. Phytonadione possesses essentially the same type and degree of activity as naturally occurring vitamin K. Phytonadione has a more rapid and prolonged effect than does menadione or menadiol sodium diphosphate and is generally more effective, particularly in treatment of oral anticoagulant–induced hypoprothrombinemia. Menadiol sodium diphosphate is approximately one-half as potent as menadione. In prophylaxis and treatment of hemorrhagic disease of the newborn, phytonadione has demonstrated a greater margin of safety than menadiol sodium diphosphate.

Phytonadione is absorbed from the GI tract via intestinal lymphatics only in the presence of bile salts. Menadione and menadiol sodium diphosphate enter the bloodstream directly and are absorbed in the absence of bile. Although initially concentrated in the liver, vitamin K is rapidly metabolized and very little tissue accumulation occurs.

The action of parenteral phytonadione is generally detectable within an hour or two, and hemorrhage is usually controlled within 3 to 6 hours. A normal prothrombin level may often be obtained in 12 to 14 hours. Oral phytonadione exerts its effect within 6 to 12 hours. Response to parenteral menadiol sodium diphosphate may require 8 to 24 hours.

Minimum daily requirements (MDRs): The human MDRs for vitamin K have not been officially established but have been estimated to be 1 mcg/kg to 5 mcg/kg for infants and 0.03 mcg/kg for adults. Usually, the dietary abundance of vitamin K will satisfy these requirements, except during the first 5 to 8 days of the neonatal period.

WARNINGS

Because the liver is the site of prothrombin synthesis, hypoprothrombinemia resulting from hepatocellular damage is not corrected by administration of vitamin K. Repeated large doses of vitamin K are not warranted in liver disease if response to initial use of the vitamin is unsatisfactory. Failure to respond to vitamin K may indicate the presence of a coagulation defect or that the condition being treated is unresponsive to vitamin K. In those with hepatic disease, large doses may further depress liver function.

For treatment of hemorrhage due to oral anticoagulant–induced hypoprothrombinemia, vitamin K_1 is preferred to menadione or its derivative. Vitamin K will *not* counteract the action of heparin.

Vitamin K_1 promotes synthesis of prothrombin by the liver but does not directly counteract the effects of the oral anticoagulants. Immediate coagulant effect should not be expected. It takes a minimum of 1 to 2 hours for a measurable improvement in the prothrombin time.

When vitamin K_1 is used to correct excessive anticoagulant-induced hypoprothrombinemia and anticoagulant therapy is still being indicated, the patient is again faced with the clotting hazards existing prior to starting anticoagulant therapy. Phytonadione is not a clotting agent, but overzealous therapy with vitamin K_1 may restore conditions that originally permitted thromboembolic phenomena. Dosage should be kept as low as possible and prothrombin time checked as clinical conditions indicate.

In the prophylaxis and treatment of hemorrhagic disease of the newborn, menadione and menadiol sodium diphosphate analogues are not as safe as phytonadione. In infants, particularly those who are premature, excessive doses of vitamin K analogues may cause increased bilirubinemia during the first few days of life. Severe hemolytic anemia, hemoglobinuria, kernicterus, brain damage, and death in newborn infants may also occur. Administration of these drugs to the mother during the last few weeks of pregnancy may also induce these toxic reactions in the newborn infant; pregnant women and newborn infants should not be given menadione or menadione derivatives.

Vitamin K crosses the placenta. Effects on reproduction have not been studied. There is no adequate information on whether this drug may affect fertility in humans or have a teratogenic potential or other adverse effects on the fetus.

DRUG INTERACTIONS

Vitamin K_1, menadione, and menadiol sodium diphosphate antagonize the anticoagulant effects of **coumarins** and **indandiones.** Temporary resistance to **prothrombin-depressing anticoagulants** may result, especially when larger doses are used. If relatively large doses have been employed, it may be necessary when reinstituting anticoagulant therapy to use larger doses of the prothrombin-depressing anticoagulant, or to use one that acts on a different principle, such as heparin. Phytonadione and menadione are oil-soluble vitamins. Concurrent administration with **mineral oil** or **cholestyramine** may decrease absorption of vitamin K.

Drug/lab tests: Prolongation of prothrombin time has been reported with maximum doses of phytonadione, menadione, and menadione derivatives.

ADVERSE REACTIONS

Phytonadione: Severe reactions, including fatalities, have occurred during and immediately after IV injection of AquaMEPHYTON (brand of phytonadione), even when precautions have been taken to dilute the injection and to avoid rapid infusion. Typically, these reactions have resembled hypersensitivity or anaphylaxis, including shock and cardiac and respiratory arrest. Some patients have exhibited these severe reactions on receiving vitamin K for the first time. The IV route should be restricted to those situations in which other routes are not feasible and the serious risk is considered justified.

Allergic reactions: Allergic sensitivity, including anaphylactoid reactions, is a possibility. Occasional allergic reactions such as rash and urticaria have been reported.

GI: Gastric upset with nausea, vomiting, and headache have also occurred after oral dosage.

Parenteral administration: Pain, swelling, and tenderness at the injection site may occur. Rarely, after repeated injections, reactions resembling erythema perstans have been reported. Delayed cutaneous reactions (pruritic erythematous placques) at the site of IM injection have been reported.

Miscellaneous: Other reactions include transient "flushing sensations" and "peculiar" sensations of taste; rarely, dizziness, rapid and weak pulse, profuse sweating, brief hypotension, dyspnea, and cyanosis.

G6PD deficiency: Menadione and menadiol sodium diphosphate can induce erythrocyte hemolysis in patients having a genetic deficiency of G6PD.

Hyperbilirubinemia: Hyperbilirubinemia has been reported in newborns, particularly prematures, following parenteral administration. This, in turn, may result in kernicterus, which can lead to brain damage or even death. Immaturity is apparently an important factor in the development of toxic reactions to vitamin K analogues, because full-term and larger premature infants show greater tolerance than do smaller premature infants. These effects are more frequent with menadione and its soluble derivatives.

DOSAGE

MENADIOL SODIUM DIPHOSPHATE

Oral: Hypoprothrombinemia secondary to obstructive jaundice and biliary fistulas—5 mg/day. *Hypoprothrombinemia secondary to administration of antibacterials or salicylates*—5 mg/day to 10 mg/day.

Parenteral: Adults, 5 mg to 15 mg once or twice

U
V
W
X
Y
Z

daily. Children, 5 mg to 10 mg once or twice daily. May be given subcutaneously, IM, or IV. Response after IV administration may be more prompt, but more sustained action follows IM or subcutaneous use. In absence of impaired liver function, a single dose usually completely corrects hypoprothrombinemia in 8 to 24 hours. Injection is repeated in 12 hours if tests at this time show no evidence of improvement.

MENADIONE

5 mg/day to 10 mg/day. Not for administration to infants.

PHYTONADIONE

When possible, give subcutaneously or IM. When IV administration is unavoidable, inject very slowly, not exceeding 1 mg/minute.

Anticoagulant-induced prothrombin deficiency

To correct excessively prolonged prothrombin time caused by oral anticoagulant therapy, 2.5 mg to 10 mg or up to 25 mg (rarely, 50 mg) initially. Frequency and amount of subsequent doses are determined by prothrombin time response or clinical condition. If, 6 to 8 hours after parenteral administration (or 12–48 hours after oral administration), the prothrombin time has not been shortened satisfactorily, repeat dose. In the event of shock or excessive blood loss, the use of whole blood or component therapy is indicated. Smaller doses are used for patients being treated with the shorter-acting anticoagulants and for those in need of continued anticoagulant therapy, and to avoid lowering the prothrombin time too far below that indicating an effective level of anticoagulant therapy. Larger doses are used on patients on longer-acting anticoagulants, those with severe bleeding, and those not needing further anticoagulant therapy. Although more than 25 mg may be needed and a dose may need to be repeated, these courses of action are indicated only rarely.

Prophylaxis and treatment of hemorrhagic disease of the newborn

Prophylaxis: Single IM dose of 0.5 mg to 2 mg. Although less desirable, 1 mg to 5 mg may be given to the mother 12 to 24 hours before delivery.

Treatment: 1 mg to 2 mg subcutaneously or IM daily. Higher doses may be necessary if the mother has been receiving oral anticoagulants. Empiric administration of vitamin K_1 should not replace proper laboratory evaluation of the coagulation mechanism. A prompt response (shortening of the prothrombin time in 2–4 hours) following administration is usually diagnostic of hemorrhagic disease of the newborn; failure to respond indicates another diagnosis or coagulation disorder. Whole blood or component therapy may be indicated if bleeding is excessive. This therapy does not correct the underlying disorder, and phytonadione should be given concurrently.

Hypoprothrombinemia due to other causes

2 mg to 25 mg or more (rarely up to 50 mg); amount and route of administration depend on the severity of the condition and response obtained. Avoid oral route when clinical disorder would prevent proper absorption. Give bile salt tablets when endogenous supply of bile to GI tract is deficient.

If possible, discontinuation or reduction of dosage of drugs interfering with coagulation mechanisms (such as salicylates, antibiotics) is an alternative to administration of phytonadione. The severity of the coagulation disorder determines whether the immediate administration of phytonadione is required in addition to discontinuation or reduction of interfering drugs.

NURSING IMPLICATIONS

HISTORY
See Appendix 4.

PHYSICAL ASSESSMENT
Obtain blood pressure, pulse, and respirations. Look for evidence of bleeding (*e.g.*, skin [ecchymosis, petechiae], oral mucous membranes, gums, urine, stool, emesis). Laboratory tests may include prothrombin time, bleeding time, CBC, hemoglobin.

ADMINISTRATION
Advise patient that IM or subcutaneous injection may produce discomfort. Pain, swelling, and tenderness at the injection site may occur.

MENADIOL SODIUM PHOSPHATE

May be given PO, subcutaneously, IM, or IV.

Is approximately one-half as potent as menadione.

IM: Inject deep into large muscle mass.

IV: Inject slowly IV over a period of 1 or more minutes or as ordered.

MENADIONE

Give PO only. Not indicated for administration to infants. Bile salts are required for absorption from the GI tract and are ordered when the endogenous supply of bile to the GI tract is deficient.

PHYTONADIONE

AquaMEPHYTON may be given PO, subcutaneously, IM, or IV. IV administration is reserved for those instances in which other routes are not feasible.

Konakion is for IM use only.

Phytonadione is the drug of choice for administration of vitamin K to newborns.

Oral: Bile salts (oral) are ordered with oral phytonadione when the endogenous supply of bile to the GI tract is deficient.

IM: Inject deep into muscle mass to avoid sciatic nerve paralysis. In older children and adults, use upper outer quadrant of the buttocks. In infants and young children, the anterolateral aspect of the thigh or the deltoid region is preferred.

IV (AquaMEPHYTON): May be diluted with 0.9% Sodium Chloride Injection, 5% Dextrose Injection, or 5% Dextrose and Sodium Chloride Injection. Do *not* use a diluent containing a preservative because benzyl alcohol (as a preservative) has been associated with toxicity in newborns. Use immediately after dilution and discard unused portions. Inject very slowly; do not exceed 1 mg/minute. If IV infusion is ordered, dilute as for IV injection (above) and add to prescribed IV solution, discarding any unused portion. Protect the IV infusion bottle from light by covering with aluminum foil or other opaque material because drug is photosensitive and deteriorates in the presence of light. Administer immediately after adding to the IV solution.

CLINICAL ALERT: Patient receiving IV injection or infusion is *monitored continuously* during and immediately following administration of phytonadione. Severe reactions, including death, have occurred. These reactions have resembled hypersensitivity reactions or anaphylaxis, including shock and cardiac or respiratory arrest. Resuscitation equipment should be immediately available. Monitor blood pressure and pulse and respiratory rates every 1 to 2 minutes during injection, every 5 minutes during infusion, and every 10 to 15 minutes following injection or infusion for at least 1 hour.

ONGOING ASSESSMENTS AND NURSING MANAGEMENT

Observe patient with hypoprothrombinemia for response to therapy.

Times for expected response to therapy are as follows.

MENADIONE

Onset and duration of action are not reported in the literature.

MENADIOL SODIUM DIPHOSPHATE

Onset and duration of action of oral form are not reported in the literature. After IM or subcutaneous administration, bleeding may be controlled in 1 to 2 hours; the prothrombin time may return to normal in 8 to 24 hours.

PHYTONADIONE

With oral administration blood coagulation factors increase in 6 to 12 hours; the prothrombin time is usually shortened in 12 to 48 hours. After parenteral administration, bleeding is usually controlled within 3 to 8 hours; the prothrombin time may be shortened in 6 to 8 hours and a normal prothrombin time obtained in 12 to 14 hours.

The normal prothrombin time is 12 to 14 seconds.

Keep physician informed of response to therapy (*e.g.,* a decrease in amount of bleeding and current prothrombin times).

Fresh blood transfusions, frozen plasma, or other therapy may be required for severe blood loss or lack of response to vitamin K.

If anticoagulant therapy is reinstituted, larger doses of the anticoagulant may be necessary because temporary resistance to prothrombin-depressing anticoagulants may follow vitamin K administration. Heparin, instead of an oral anticoagulant, may be prescribed because heparin acts on a different principle.

Routine administration of phytonadione is recommended as prophylaxis against hemorrhagic disease of the newborn. The neonate is unable to utilize vitamin K for hepatic synthesis of prothrombin for the first 5 to 8 days following birth.

Observe newborns, particularly prematures, for hyperbilirubinemia, which may result in kernicterus. Notify physician immediately of any signs of jaundice.

PATIENT AND FAMILY INFORMATION

NOTE: When oral vitamin K is prescribed for dietary vitamin K deficiency, patient will require a list of foods high in vitamin K (*e.g.,* green leafy vegetables, cheese, eggs [yolks], liver, tomatoes, cauliflower).

Take as prescribed.

Follow dietary plan recommended by the physician.

Avoid use of mineral oil, which decreases absorption of vitamin K.

Do not take multivitamin preparations containing vitamin K unless use is approved by the physician.

U
V
W
X
Y
Z

W

Warfarin Potassium, Sodium

See Coumarin and Indandione Derivatives.

Wet Dressings and Soaks

Aluminum Acetate Solution

(Burow's Solution) *otc*

aluminum acetate solution (Burow's solution)	*Generic*
Burow's solution w/ benzethonium chloride	Buro-Sol Powder

Modified Burow's Solution *otc*

aluminum sulfate, calcium acetate	Bluboro Powder, Domeboro Powder, Domeboro Tablets, Pedi-Boro Soak Paks

INDICATIONS

Astringent wet dressing for relief of inflammatory conditions of the skin, such as insect bites, poison ivy, swellings and bruises, athlete's foot, and allergic or environmental skin conditions.

PRECAUTIONS

For external use only. Keep away from the eyes and nose. Discontinue use if irritation occurs or persists.

DOSAGE

See *Administration.*

NURSING IMPLICATIONS

PHYSICAL ASSESSMENT

Inspect involved areas, noting location, size, and appearance of lesions.

ADMINISTRATION

Preparation of solution

Buro-Sol Powder: Dissolve 1 packet in 1 pint of solution. This produces a 1:15 clear Burow's solution with benzethonium chloride.

Bluboro Powder, Domeboro Powder or Tablets: Dissolve one packet or tablet in 1 pint of water. This produces a modified 1:40 Burow's solution.

Pedi-Boro: Dissolve one or two packets (as prescribed by the physician) in 1 pint of water.

Administration

Apply a loose bandage or compresses (which may be loosely bandaged to keep in place, when necessary). Soak the dressing with the prepared solution. Do *not* use plastic or other impervious material to prevent evaporation.

Burow's solution: Apply for 15 to 30 minutes several times a day (or as directed by the physician) to compresses or bandage over site of application.

Bluboro, Domeboro: Pour solution on bandage every 15 to 30 minutes to keep dressing moist. Continue for 4 to 8 hours unless otherwise directed by physician.

Pedi-Boro: Apply every 15 to 30 minutes for 4 to 8 hours.

ONGOING ASSESSMENTS AND NURSING MANAGEMENT

If application is for more than 4 hours, change dressings, compresses, or bandages q4h or as necessary.

PATIENT AND FAMILY INFORMATION

Mix packet, powder, or tablet in 1 pint of water or as directed by the physician. Stir thoroughly.

Apply as directed by the physician or as stated on the container to a loosely applied dressing or compress. If needed, the dressing or compress may be held in place with a lightly applied bandage.

Keep away from the eyes and nose.

Do not cover area with plastic.

Discontinue use and notify the physician if condition worsens, irritation occurs, or there is an extension of the inflammatory area.

Whole Root Rauwolfia

See Rauwolfia Derivatives.

X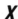

Xylometazoline Hydrochloride

See Decongestants, Nasal, Topical.

Z

Zinc Oxide *otc*

ointment: 20%, 25%	*Generic*
paste: 25% zinc oxide, 25% starch	*Generic*

INDICATIONS

For use on small cuts or fissures, minor skin irritations, abrasions, chafed skin, and diaper rash.

DOSAGE

Apply to affected areas as required.

NURSING IMPLICATIONS

PHYSICAL ASSESSMENT

Inspect involved areas, noting location, size, and appearance of lesions.

ADMINISTRATION

Cleanse skin gently to remove previous application of zinc oxide. If ointment has a lanolin base, check with physician about appropriate vehicle for removal. Thoroughly dry the skin before application.

Apply in a thin layer unless physician orders otherwise.

Check skin for signs of maceration, folliculitis (especially if applied around hairy areas), infection, or other skin changes. Discontinue use if these occur and notify physician.

PATIENT AND FAMILY INFORMATION

Remove previous application with soap and water or other vehicle recommended by the physician; pat dry.

Apply in a thin layer unless physician directs otherwise.

If excessive wrinkling or other skin changes occur, discontinue use. Contact physician if other skin problems occur, because a different product may be necessary.

Zinc Sulfate (23% Zinc) Rx, otc

tablets: 66 mg (15 mg zinc)	*Generic (otc)*
tablets: 110 mg (25 mg zinc)	Zinc 25 *(otc)*
tablets: 200 mg (45 mg zinc)	*Generic (Rx)*
tablets: 220 mg (50 mg zinc)	Medizinc *(Rx)*
capsules: 110 mg (25 mg zinc)	Orazinc *(otc)*, Zincate *(otc)*, Zinkaps-110 *(otc)*
capsules: 220 mg (50 mg zinc)	Orazinc *(otc)*, Scrip Zinc *(Rx)*, Verazinc *(otc)*, Zincate *(Rx)*, Zinkaps-220 *(otc)*, *Generic (Rx)*
capsules: 220 mg (55 mg zinc)	Zinc-220 *(otc)*

INDICATIONS

Dietary supplement. Recommended for deficiencies or the prevention of deficiencies of zinc. Zinc deficiency may be caused by inadequate dietary intake, malabsorption, increased body losses, and intravenous feeding. Manifestations of deficiency include anorexia, growth retardation, impaired taste and olfactory sensation, and mood alteration.

Investigational uses: Acrodermatitis enteropathica and delayed wound healing, which are believed to be associated with zinc deficiency. Mental and skin diseases responsive to zinc have been associated with extensive bowel surgery, which may induce malabsorption syndrome. Doses of 220 mg tid are used. Zinc sulfate has also been used investigationally to treat acne and rheumatoid arthritis, to delay the onset of dementia in patients genetically at risk, and to improve immune response in the elderly. Data are insufficient to recommend these uses.

ACTIONS

Normal growth and tissue repair are directly dependent on an adequate supply of zinc in the diet. Zinc functions as an integral part of a number of enzymes important to protein and carbohydrate metabolism.

PRECAUTIONS

Do not exceed prescribed dosage; severe vomiting, dehydration, and restlessness may occur. Will cause an emetic effect if administered in single 2-g doses.

DRUG INTERACTIONS

Zinc will impair the absorption of **tetracycline derivatives. Bran products** (including brown bread) and **dairy products** will decrease absorption of zinc.

ADVERSE REACTIONS

Most common are GI (nausea, vomiting); gastric ulceration has been reported.

OVERDOSAGE

Nausea, mild diarrhea, rash, severe vomiting, dehydration, and restlessness may occur. Reduce dosage or discontinue drug to control symptoms.

DOSAGE

Recommended dietary allowances (RDAs): Adults, 15 mg.

Dietary supplement: Average adult dose is 15

mg/day to 55 mg/day. It is recommended that zinc be taken with milk or meals to avoid gastric distress; however, some studies indicate that ingestion with some foods may inhibit zinc absorption.

NURSING IMPLICATIONS

HISTORY
See Appendix 4. A thorough dietary history is important.

PHYSICAL ASSESSMENT
Look for signs and symptoms of zinc deficiency (*e.g.,* anorexia, mood alteration, poor wound healing, sparse hair growth, growth retardation, and patient complaints of impaired taste and olfactory sensation). Zinc deficiency may be accompanied by other nutritional deficiencies; symptoms of these deficiencies may also be present.

ADMINISTRATION
If GI distress occurs, drug may be given with meals or milk.

ONGOING ASSESSMENTS AND NURSING MANAGEMENT
If gastric distress occurs despite giving drug with meals or milk, notify physician.

Observe for relief of symptoms of deficiency.

Gastric ulceration has been reported. If epigastric pain, hematemesis, or tarry stools occur, notify physician.

PATIENT AND FAMILY INFORMATION
If GI upset occurs, take with food or milk. If GI upset persists, discontinue use and notify the physician.

Do not exceed recommended or prescribed dose.

Avoid consumption of excess amounts of bran products and dairy products because they may decrease the absorption of zinc.

Immediately report occurrence of nausea, diarrhea, rash, severe vomiting, or restlessness.

Appendix 1
General Principles Applicable to the Administration of Pharmacologic Agents

The following general principles apply to the administration of pharmacologic agents.

Transcribe the physician's orders clearly. Handwriting or printing should be legible; poor handwriting by physicians and nurses can lead to errors in drug dosage.

Avoid the use of unofficial abbreviations in transcribing the physician's orders, writing medicine cards, or entering drugs on the Kardex or chart. Hospitals are required to provide a list of approved abbreviations for use by members of the health team; *official* abbreviations should be used and others avoided.

Always question written orders that appear unclear or do not specify exact administration techniques.

The patient has the right to know the name or type of drug being administered and the reason for its use, unless the physician specifically orders this information to be withheld.

The maximum or highest recommended dose is normally not exceeded, except in unusual circumstances. Always question an order and check with the physician if the prescribed dose exceeds the recommended dosage. If there is still doubt, check with a pharmacist.

Use caution when handling antineoplastic agents. These agents should be prepared carefully, avoiding skin contact and inhalation of drug particles. The use of long-sleeved gowns, disposable gloves, masks, and safety glasses is recommended. Disposable syringes and related equipment should be discarded in special containers, sealed, and labeled as contaminated before final disposal. Pregnant women should not prepare or administer antineoplastic agents because of a potential hazard to the fetus.

The patient receiving chemotherapy for a malignancy will experience a variety of emotional as well as physical effects. The nurse must establish rapport with the patient, evaluate his physical and emotional status, identify his needs, and develop a plan to meet the identified needs. The patient and his family must receive emotional support from all members of the health team and must be allowed to work through the emotional responses to his diagnosis and treatment.

When checking drug references, note whether a drug has cross-allergenicity with another drug. If so, this means that of the two drugs mentioned, a patient who is allergic or hypersensitive to one of the two drugs may also be allergic to the other drug.

When the dosage of a drug is expressed in kilograms (kg) in drug references or package inserts, the patient's weight should be converted from pounds to kilograms, if necessary, and entered on the Kardex. In critical care areas, each patient's weight in pounds and kilograms should be posted in medicine preparation areas.

The dosage for some drugs may be determined by square meters (m^2) of body surface.

Impaired renal or hepatic function may be taken into consideration when dosages are calculated by the physician.

Because some drugs interfere with specific laboratory tests, enter current drug therapy on all laboratory request slips.

Store all medications in a dry place and at room temperature unless the manufacturer directs otherwise. Firmly replace caps or lids immediately after removing the drug from the container.

Drugs are always given by the manufacturer's recommended route.

Always check the patient's identification band before administration of any drug.

In order to attain and maintain therapeutic blood levels, drugs must be administered at the time intervals ordered.

There has been a marked increase in nosocomial infections. Health-team members must practice good handwashing technique when preparing and administering all medications.

Good lighting is essential in preparing drugs for administration.

Avoid talking to others when preparing drugs for administration; distractions can lead to errors.

Always check labels and outer packages of drugs for an expiration date. Do not use an outdated drug.

Before administration of the first dose of a drug, always question the patient about drug allergies as well as allergies to other substances (*e.g.,* dust, pollen, grasses), even if an allergy history has been obtained. If the patient has a history of allergy to one or more substances, check with the physician before administering the first dose of any drug.

Never administer a drug to an individual with a known hypersensitivity (allergy) to the drug.

Administer a drug with caution to an individual who may be hypersensitive to it.

Some drugs are capable of causing many adverse reactions. Some of these reactions may be obvious, whereas others are vague and obscure. Consider every patient problem as a *potential* adverse reaction or part of the clinical picture of the disease until proven otherwise.

The patient must have absolutely uninterrupted privacy when a drug is administered by the vaginal or rectal route; applied or administered to areas such as the breasts, buttocks, inguinal area, or abdomen; or administered to an area that is disfigured or mutilated or has an odor.

Those receiving a preoperative medication are advised to remain in bed; the siderails are raised immediately after administration of the drug.

When repeat parenteral injections are necessary, develop and implement a plan for rotation of injection sites. Record sites used following each administration.

Observe for patient hoarding of drugs, especially drugs classified as controlled substances.

When administering narcotics or prn medications, always record the drug, dosage, and other pertinent information (*e.g.,* vital signs, location and type of pain) in the patient's chart immediately after giving the drug. This prevents inadvertent readministration by another member of the health team.

Almost all systemic drugs, and some topical drugs, are generally considered to pose a potential hazard to the fetus and are therefore not considered safe for use during pregnancy.

Do not leave drugs unattended, even for a few minutes, on carts or trays in areas accessible to visitors and patients. Never leave empty needles or syringes at the bedside.

Appendix 2
The Geriatric Patient: Special Considerations

Erratic drug response, drug toxicity, adverse drug reactions, prolonged drug effects, and diminished therapeutic response may be seen at any age but sometimes tend to be more prominent in the elderly because of the effects of aging on various organs and body systems. In some instances, alterations in the absorption, distribution, metabolism, or excretion of a drug may require modification of drug dosage. In addition, many elderly patients have multiple disease entities being treated with several different drugs; drug interactions or incompatibilities are especially likely to occur in these patients.

General nursing implications in geriatric pharmacology include the following:

Encourage a liberal fluid intake throughout the waking hours. Dehydration, a common problem in the elderly, can lead to electrolyte imbalance and renal impairment (as well as other problems), which in turn may affect drug activity, increase the possibility of drug toxicity, or decrease a drug's rate of excretion.

When a drug is known to be nephrotoxic, monitor the intake and output closely. Any change in the intake–output ratio is reported to the physician immediately.

CNS depressants, narcotics, and psychotropic agents may produce idiosyncratic or unfavorable adverse reactions. Observe the patient at frequent intervals for adverse reactions. Oversedation, postural hypotension, confusion, ataxia, restlessness,

urinary retention, extrapyramidal reactions, tardive dyskinesia, respiratory depression, circulatory collapse, and so on can have serious and even fatal consequences. Medical or nursing management will depend on the reaction.

Occasionally, a patient may refuse to take a prescribed drug or take less of the drug than prescribed. This may be difficult to detect but should be considered a possibility when the patient complains that the drug does not help or when it is apparent that the expected therapeutic response is not attained.

Take time to listen to the patient's complaints about his medication. Adverse drug effects, failure of the drug to produce a therapeutic response, and patient noncompliance can often be detected during what may seem to be an irrelevant or rambling discussion.

ORAL PREPARATIONS

Because of poor vision, arthritis, parkinsonism, or another neurologic deficit, the patient may require assistance in removing drugs from a medicine cup, placing drugs in the mouth, or holding a glass of water.

Rinsing the mouth with water or swallowing a few sips of water before taking a medication often facilitates the swallowing of tablets or capsules, especially when the oral mucosa is dry.

The elderly patient may become agitated when rushed to swallow several medications at one time.

Do not rush the patient, and allow sufficient time for the patient to swallow the drug and water before offering the next drug.

If the patient complains that the tablet or capsule does not go "all the way down," offer a few sips of warm water. If warm water fails to help or if the problem is repeated each time a tablet or capsule is administered, contact the physician.

Tablets or capsules are not to be given to those experiencing difficulty in swallowing food other than liquids or soft foods. If difficulty in swallowing solid foods is noted, withhold the drug and check approved references or check with a pharmacist to see if the drug is available in liquid form. Consult the physician about a change to a liquid drug (if available) or a change to a drug available in liquid form.

In some patients it will be necessary to inspect the oral cavity visually, especially the buccal areas, to be sure a tablet or capsule has been swallowed.

Drugs in granular form have a tendency to become lodged in patients' dentures, decreasing the amount of drug swallowed, becoming a source of irritation and discomfort of gum tissue under the denture, and possibly irritating the oral mucosa.

Take time to answer the patient's questions about his drug, even if the information has been given on previous occasions.

PARENTERAL ADMINISTRATION

Muscle mass of the elderly tends to be smaller, and administration of intramuscular injections may be more difficult. The normal volume of an intramuscular injection for an adult may be too great for the elderly, in which case the dosage is divided and given in two injections.

Because of a decrease in circulation, a drug may take longer to be absorbed from muscle or adipose tissue, lengthening the time for an expected drug response.

The confused patient, unable to comprehend the importance of an intramuscular or subcutaneous medication, may require gentle restraining measures while the drug is administered.

Veins are often fragile. Use the smallest possible needle for the administration of an intravenous preparation.

The skin of the elderly is usually fragile. Exercise care in applying tape to anchor intravenous needles or catheters. Extra padding of the tape with cotton or gauze and minimal tape contact with the skin may prevent irritation. When the IV is terminated, remove the tape carefully to prevent damage to the skin.

The confused patient requires frequent observation when an intravenous infusion is administered. If restraining measures are necessary to prevent dislodgement or removal of the needle, check the restrained extremity every 30 minutes for blanching, cyanosis, absence of a pulse, or a decrease in pulse amplitude. Any skin or pulse change requires loosening or reapplication of the restraint.

The elderly patient is especially prone to fluid overload (water intoxication) if an intravenous infusion is given at too rapid a rate.

Exercise care in removing intravenous needles and catheters from veins. Apply firm pressure over the site until there is no blood or oozing from the vein.

Check previous intramuscular and subcutaneous injection sites for signs of redness, induration, abscess formation, or skin breakdown. The elderly patient, who is relatively immobile, is often more prone to complications of parenteral administration of drugs.

TEACHING THE PATIENT

More time than usual must be assigned for teaching the elderly patient. Information is best given in small increments, allowing the patient time to think about the material and ask questions.

Patient teaching may be difficult because of impairment of memory, hearing, and vision and a limited attention span. This, in turn, results in poor patient compliance; these facts are taken into consideration when planning and implementing patient teaching. Whenver possible, enlist the help of a family member, relative, or friend when the patient is unable to assume full responsibility for his drug therapy.

The elderly are more likely to miss doses, fail to take a prescribed medication, or overuse some non-prescription drugs.

Whenever possible, family members, a relative, or a friend is made aware of the patient's drug regimen, adverse drug reactions, and specific instructions for each drug (e.g., drink extra fluids, take with milk or food, take on an empty stomach).

Because it may be viewed as a failure to exert full control over activities, a patient may not admit to difficulty in seeing or hearing. Oral instructions are often misinterpreted or not heard at all, and written instructions may not be read or followed. Speaking slowly and clearly, avoiding lengthy discussions, and giving written instructions printed in large letters on a card may improve patient compliance and reduce embarrassment over failure to read or hear instructions.

Using clear, understandable terms, explain the purpose of the drug. Terms such as "blood pressure pill," "heart medication," "water pill," and "stomach pill" label the general purpose of each drug. Discuss when the drug's effect will be noted, what adverse effects may occur, how long the patient will take the drug, how the drug is stored, and what to do if adverse effects occur.

Many patients visit more than one physician; instructions given by several physicians and nurses often become a source of confusion. Advise the patient to carry a list of all drugs (prescription and nonprescription) taken on a regular or occasional basis and to give this list to every physician each time a drug is prescribed.

Advise the patient to purchase all drugs at the same pharmacy, especially when the patient sees more than one physician. Some pharmacies keep patient profiles and alert physicians when combinations of drugs may produce unfavorable reactions or when a drug is prescribed for a specific disorder by two different physicians.

Difficulty in reading the small label of a prescription container may result in inaccurate dosing. Giving the patient a card identifying each drug prescribed, with dosage directions typed or printed in large letters, may help the visually impaired to adhere to a dosage regimen.

The patient may encounter difficulty in understanding or following the dosage schedule when more than one drug is prescribed. A written schedule for medications (_e.g.,_ what drug is taken after breakfast or which two drugs are taken in the middle of the afternoon) often helps the patient correctly follow a dosage schedule.

A drug scheduled to be taken after the patient's usual time for sleep may be missed because the patient fails to set (or hear) an alarm clock or does not wish to be disturbed during sleep. Whenever possible, drugs are scheduled to be taken during waking hours.

In order to facilitate taking a medication, the patient may break or crush a tablet or open a capsule. However, certain tablets should not be crushed or broken, and some capsules should not be opened. Inform the patient not to break or crush tablets or open capsules without consulting a physician or pharmacist.

The expense of some drugs may place an added drain on the limited retirement income of some patients. This may cause the patient not to have a prescription filled or to take less of the drug than prescribed in order to save money. An inquiry into the ability to pay for a drug may not always result in a correct response. In some instances, discussion with a family member may identify the problem. Appropriate agencies are contacted when the patient is unable to pay for health care.

Appendix 3
The Pediatric Patient: Special Considerations

In children, immaturity of physiological processes can cause variations in the absorption, distribution, biotransformation, or excretion of drugs. These factors may alter the effect of a drug and influence the dose required for a therapeutic response. For most drugs, dosage ranges are not standardized for children as they are for adults. Therefore, dosages are usually based on weight, body surface area (BSA, m^2), or age.

General nursing implications in pediatric pharmacology include the following:

When possible, provide an explanation of the drug therapy according to the child's level of understanding. Subjects that may be included are the reason for the medication, how it will be administered, the position to be assumed, and the sensations that may be felt (*e.g.,* taste of a liquid medication, blurring of vision with an ophthalmic drug).

Visual materials can be used to enhance understanding of some procedures. These include demonstration of the procedure on a stuffed animal or doll and use of coloring or comic books containing descriptive pictures and text.

Allow the child to participate as much as possible when a drug is to be administered. For example, the cooperative toddler may wish to hold his own medicine cup; an older child may be able to self-administer a nasal spray with supervision.

Restraining, with or without assistance from a second person, is often necessary. Restrain the child firmly but gently; forcible restraint leads to further anxiety and possible patient injury.

To reduce anxiety, keep drugs and equipment, especially trays with needles, syringes, and skin preparation materials, out of the child's line of vision until ready to administer the drug.

Do not scold or threaten the child for crying or resisting. Praise and comfort the child after the medication has been administered, regardless of his behavior.

Do not try to administer a liquid medication to a crying or resisting infant or small child, or try to force an uncooperative child to swallow a tablet or capsule, because of the danger of aspiration.

The child may be promised a small amount of juice or carbonated beverage as a reward for taking the medication. (Avoid giving milk or milk products with oral medications, because they may interfere with the absorption of some drugs.)

Notify the physician if the patient experiences difficulty in swallowing all of an oral drug, refuses the drug, or persists in spitting out the drug.

To give liquid medication to an infant, place the patient in a semireclining position, support the head, and lightly restrain the infant's hands and arms. To open his mouth, depress his chin downward with the thumb. Place the liquid along the side of the tongue, and administer in small amounts to give the infant time to swallow.

When necessary, a liquid drug may be diluted with a small amount of water. (_Exception_—elixirs should not be diluted.)

Avoid use of regular dietary foods (_e.g.,_ cereal, juices) to disguise a medication, because the child may later refuse to eat these foods.

Do not add a drug to a feeding formula, unless prescribed by the physician.

With some drugs, unpleasant taste may be disguised with flavored syrup, honey, or jam. (Check with the pharmacist before using a vehicle to disguise taste, because some vehicles may interfere with the drug's action. In addition, the diagnosis may contraindicate use of a product containing sugar.)

Frozen fruit popsicles or ice chips may be used to disguise an unpleasant aftertaste.

The toddler or small child may be able to swallow a whole tablet if its size is small.

Scored tablets may be carefully broken in half to facilitate administration.

Some tablets can be crushed using two spoons or a mortar and pestle; make sure all crushed particles are collected. Avoid using a glass, because small chips may be broken off the rim.

Crushed tablets may be mixed with a small amount of water, juice, honey, jam, or flavored syrup. It is best to check with the pharmacist before adding crushed tablets to any vehicle. Some drugs may dissolve poorly in water and therefore are difficult to administer. There are also some drugs that are not to be given in an acid vehicle (_e.g.,_ some fruit juices).

Tablets _not_ to be crushed include enteric-coated tablets, those with special coatings that provide immediate and delayed action, uncoated tablets impregnated with beads, tablets within tablets, and sublingual or buccal tablets. Check with a pharmacist if there is a question about a specific product.

Capsules are usually given whole, but in some instances the contents may be emptied into water, juice, honey, jam, or flavored syrup. Check with the physician or pharmacist regarding the feasibility of emptying a capsule into another vehicle. Capsules are never crushed.

With tablets or capsules, check the oral cavity to be sure that the drug has been swallowed.

Warm eye and ear drops to body temperature by holding the bottle in the hand for a few minutes. Also warm irrigating solutions to body temperature.

With ophthalmic products, great care must be exercised; injury to the eye may occur, especially if the child is uncooperative. Even the apparently cooperative child can suddenly become frightened and push or grab the nurse's hand. As a precautionary measure, have a second person lightly hold the hands of all patients.

For instillation of ear drops in children younger than 3 years, gently pull the pinna downward and straight back. In children older than 3 years, gently pull the pinna upward and back. Direct the liquid along the side of the auditory canal.

For ear irrigations, gently retract the pinna as for ear drops. Direct the irrigating fluid toward the top of the external auditory canal. Do not use force in instilling irrigation fluid. Allow the liquid return to flow into emesis basin.

For nasal instillations, check labels carefully; only aqueous solutions are used for pediatric patients. Oily solutions are not used because they may be aspirated, resulting in lipid pulmonary conditions.

Avoid use of stock nasal solutions, because sterility cannot be assured. Each child should have his own nasal medication. If a stock solution is used, sterile disposable droppers are necessary.

Avoid dividing a suppository to obtain a smaller dose, because the drug may not be evenly distributed throughout the product.

Intramuscular injection sites in infants are the ventrogluteal and vastus lateralis muscles; in toddlers and school-age children, the ventrogluteal, deltoid, vastus lateralis, and rectus femoris muscles; and in older children and adolescents, the same sites as for adults (posterior gluteal, ventrogluteal, rectus femoris, deltoid, and vastus lateralis).

Sites of administration for IV infusions in infants and toddlers are a scalp vein, any superficial vein in the arm, hand, or foot, or a cut-down.

Restraints during infusions include gentle physical restraint when the infusion is being started and restraint of the extremity during the time of the infusion. (Arm boards, sand bags, straps, and commercially available restraints may be selected on the basis of the patient's needs.)

For protection, plastic or paper cups may be cut and taped over the IV infusion site.

GENERAL PARENT INFORMATION

The nurse should explain the dosage regimen, demonstrate the method of administration, and discuss adverse drug effects. When necessary, restraining methods can also be demonstrated or explained.

General instructions for parents include the following:

Notify the physician or nurse if difficulty is encountered in administration or if the condition being treated becomes worse or does not improve.

Avoid contamination of droppers and caps. Return them to the container immediately after use.

To avoid injury to the eye, care must be taken when instilling ophthalmic drops or ointment. If necessary, have a second person assist in administration of the drug.

Visually inspect solutions prior to each use. Do not use a solution if it has turned cloudy or changes color.

Do not place a cotton plug in the ear following administration of an otic drug unless ordered by the physician. If ordered, keep the cotton plug saturated with the drug. Remove the plug and replace with new cotton each time the drug is administered or if the plug falls out of the ear.

Some topical drugs may stain clothing. Do not cover with a dressing (unless physician orders a dressing) to protect clothing. Have the child wear old clothing, clothing that will not show a stain, or clothing that can be discarded after treatment.

Appendix 4
The Patient History

The patient history may be obtained from the chart, the patient, or the patient's family, or, in some cases, friends. Before a drug is administered for the first time, the nurse must review the patient history and obtain additional information as necessary.

It is important to stress to the patient that complete honesty is absolutely essential in answering questions, because certain circumstances (*e.g.,* use of nonprescription drugs, dietary restrictions, drug abuse, exposure to communicable disease, traveling) may be relevant to diagnosis and treatment (including administration of pharmacologic agents). In a few instances, failure to answer questions honestly can have serious and even potentially fatal consequences.

The following information is relevant to administration of pharmacologic preparations and/or preparing a plan of patient teaching. Not all the information listed below may be applicable to every drug.

PERSONAL AND SOCIAL HISTORY

Occupational history: Exposure to toxic chemicals, dust, carcinogens, infectious diseases, physical danger, or other hazards.

Language: English speaking (including fluency); non–English speaking, including languages spoken and accessibility of a translator.

Exercise: Limitations imposed by health problems, accidents, birth injuries or defects; limitations recommended by a physician.

Sleep pattern.
Hobbies.

Diet: Normal; medically restricted (*e.g.,* low sodium, diabetic diet); calorie restrictions (including weight-loss diet plans); vegetarian diet including type (*e.g.,* full vegetarian, lacto-vegetarian [eats dairy products], ovo-lacto-vegetarian [eats eggs and dairy products]); health foods as main source of dietary intake (including foods usually eaten); macrobiotic diet; religious food patterns (kosher, Islamic, Hindu); ethnic eating habits; intake of coffee, tea, cola, or other beverages containing caffeine.

Smoking history.

Living pattern: Resides alone or with others; proximity or availability of family members, relatives, friends; institutionalized; lives in supervised housing (*e.g.,* elderly, mentally retarded); ability to purchase food and drugs at nearby shopping areas.

Travel history: Foreign countries; vaccinations required for travel; history of service and travel in the armed forces.

FAMILY HISTORY

Current and past diseases and disorders of living family members (including current treatment of each):

Alcohol/drug abuse
Allergies
Anemia
Arthritis
Asthma

Birth defects
Bleeding disorders
C53cer
Diabetes
Emphysema
Epilepsy
Gout
Heart attack, angina
History of mother given DES
Hypertension
Hypotension
Infectious diseases
Inherited diseases and disorders
Kidney disease
Neurologic disorders (acute, chronic)
Psychiatric disorders
Rheumatic fever
Sexually transmitted diseases
Stroke

Diseases and disorders of deceased family members (including cause of death): Mother, father, spouse, children, siblings.

MEDICAL HISTORY

Childhood diseases: Age; sequelae.
Immunizations: Type; date.
Surgeries: Type; date; length of hospitalization; length of time for recovery; sequelae.
Medical disorders: Type; treatment (including hospitalizations, medications, physical therapy, diet).
Injuries: Home; occupational; automobile; treatment of each.
X-rays (within past 5 years): Diagnostic; dental. History of irradiation therapy at any time during life (including childhood).
Blood transfusions: Date; reason for transfusion; blood type (if known).
Allergies: Known or suspected drug allergies; allergies to environmental substances (*e.g.,* dust, feathers, animals, trees, grasses, flowers); food allergies or food intolerances; treatment (if any) for allergy, including use of nonprescription preparations.
Drug history: Prescription drugs used currently (on a regular or prn basis); prescription drugs used in the past; nonprescription drugs used on a regular basis; nonprescription drugs used occasionally; problems encountered with use of any prescription or nonprescription drug in the past (*e.g.,* allergy, side-effects); history of drug abuse (including prescription drugs, illegal substances) or drug dependence (may not always be reliable); treatment for drug abuse or dependence.

Alcohol intake (may not always be reliable): Type and amount consumed; treatment for alcoholism (including type of treatment).

Pregnancy history: Date of last (normal) menstrual period; average number of days of menstrual cycle; previous pregnancies; number of live births and method of delivery; problems encountered with delivery; number of stillbirths; number of miscarriages; previous abortions, including method used for abortion.

Prosthesis: Type; normal care of prosthetic device; replacement schedule (when applicable).

Vision: Wearing of glasses; reason for glasses (reading, distance, cataract surgery); use of contact lenses, type and care of lenses, removal of lenses (some cataract lenses are removed, cleaned, and replaced only by an ophthalmologist).

Hearing: Use of a hearing aid, type used, maintenance (including battery replacement). If patient has a hearing impairment but a hearing aid is not used, determine degree of impairment and methods used to understand the spoken word such as lip reading or signing.

Dentures: Full; partial; permanent bridges.

CURRENT ILLNESS OR CHIEF COMPLAINT

Description of symptoms: Intensity; degree; location; frequency; factors that precipitate, aggravate, or alleviate symptoms; degree of impairment (if any) resulting from problem.

Chronological progression of symptoms up to time professional help is sought (hospitalization, visit to physician's office, clinic, or emergency department).

Injury: Document all overt symptoms and patient's description of the injury (or events leading to the injury), because legal action may be involved.

Appendix 5
Patient Teaching Related to Drug Therapy

The following are general points of information that apply to almost all drugs. In teaching patients and their families, the nurse must select information relevant to a specific drug.

The medical terminology given in the drug monographs under *Patient and Family Information,* as well as in this section, must be adapted to the patient's level of understanding.

PURCHASE OF PRESCRIPTION DRUGS

It is good practice to purchase all prescriptions from the same pharmacy. Many pharmacies keep patient profile records (lists of current prescriptions, physicians, medical history). Thus, if a newly prescribed drug would interfere with a drug currently being taken, the pharmacist will alert the physician. This is especially important when you are seeing more than one physician.

Before selecting a pharmacy for filling a prescription, check whether a prescription can be delivered to the home, if necessary. This is especially important when illness may prevent traveling to the pharmacy for a new prescription or a refill.

If the drug in a refill prescription differs in size, color, or shape from the drug originally received, question the pharmacist about this change before leaving the pharmacy. If the difference is not noted until the prescription container is opened at home, call the pharmacist before removing any medication from the container.

Anticipate emergencies and other events (*e.g.,* bad weather, holidays) that prevent obtaining a prescription refill. Keep an adequate supply of all medications by having prescriptions refilled (when a refill is prescribed) before the last several doses are taken. It is good practice to have a prescription refilled when a 4- to 5-day supply of the drug remains in the prescription container.

THE DRUG, THE DRUG CONTAINER, AND STORAGE OF DRUGS

The term *drug* applies to nonprescription as well as prescription drugs.

A drug should always remain in the container in which it was dispensed or purchased. Some drugs require special containers, such as light-resistant (brown) bottles to prevent deterioration, which may occur on exposure to light.

If any drug changes color or develops a new odor, ask a pharmacist about continued use of the drug. If possible, take the drug in its original container to the pharmacist for inspection.

Never remove the original label on a prescription container while it is used to hold the drug.

If the label on a prescription bottle becomes difficult to read, ask the pharmacist for a new label or a new container and label, even if a refill of the prescription is not necessary.

Two or more different drugs should never be mixed in one container, even for a brief period of time, because one drug may chemically affect another. Mixing drugs can also lead to mistaking one drug for another, especially when the size and color are similar.

Replace the lid or cap immediately after removing a drug from the container. The lid or cap should be firmly snapped or screwed in place. Exposure to air and moisture shortens the life of many drugs.

If difficulty is experienced in removing child-proof caps or tape on a prescription drug container, request a non–child-proof cap or lid at the time the prescription is filled. If a family member is having a prescription filled for you, remind him or her to ask the pharmacist for regular caps or lids.

Drugs requiring refrigeration will be so labeled. Return the container to the refrigerator immediately after removing the medication from the container.

Keep *all* drugs out of the reach of children, preferably in a locked drawer or cabinet.

Unless otherwise directed, drugs should be stored in a cool, dry place.

No drug should be exposed, even for a short time, to excessive heat, sunlight, cold, or moisture, because deterioration may occur. This includes areas such as car seats or glove compartments, on windowsills or near a sunny window, near or on radiators, and in bathroom medicine chests.

Cotton plugs inserted in some drug containers should be removed and discarded when the container is opened for the first time.

Before purchasing a nonprescription drug, check the package or container for signs of tampering. If a package appears to have been opened or the seal broken, alert the pharmacist or clerk.

In some instances, especially when ointments or liquids are prescribed, there may be some medication remaining after it is used or taken the prescribed number of times. Some drugs have a short life (a few weeks to a few months) and may deteriorate or change chemically after a period of time. Using or taking drugs that have deteriorated or changed chemically can be potentially dangerous. *Never* save any prescription for use at a later time unless instructed to do so by a physician.

When purchasing nonprescription drugs, write the date of purchase on the label. If some drug remains after 6 months, ask the pharmacist whether the drug may still be used.

DIRECTIONS AND WARNINGS ON THE LABEL AND PATIENT INFORMATION INSERTS

Always read the entire label, including warnings, on the container of a nonprescription drug.

If there is any question about warnings on a nonprescription drug label, a physician or pharmacist should be consulted.

Follow all directions printed on a label (*e.g.,* "shake well before using," "keep refrigerated," "take before meals").

Any question or doubt about how or when to take a drug should be brought to the attention of the physician or pharmacist.

Follow the directions for taking a drug exactly as printed on the container, and in some instances as suggested by the physician or pharmacist. Failure to follow directions could result in serious consequences.

Some drugs are supplied with patient information inserts. Read these inserts carefully. If any material is unclear, check with the physician or a pharmacist.

THE DOSAGE REGIMEN

Use water to take a tablet or capsule unless the physician or pharmacist directs otherwise (*e.g.,* taking with food, milk, or an antacid). Some liquids (coffee, tea, fruit juice, carbonated beverages) may interfere with the action of some drugs.

Drink a full glass of water when taking an oral medication. In some instances it may be necessary to drink extra fluids during the day while taking certain medications.

If difficulty is encountered in swallowing a capsule or tablet, discuss this problem with the physician as soon as possible, because a liquid form of the drug may be available, or the tablet may be broken or crushed to facilitate swallowing. Because not all tablets can be crushed (owing to special coatings on some tablets), check with a physician or pharmacist before crushing a tablet.

Do not chew capsules before swallowing; they must be swallowed whole. Chewing a capsule may result in injury to the mouth and interfere with drug action.

At times, other drugs, alcoholic beverages, certain foods, and liquids such as milk, juices, and coffee can interfere with a drug's action. It is best at the time a drug is prescribed to ask the physician or a pharmacist if there are any restrictions or limitations regarding food, alcohol, or other prescription or nonprescription drugs.

If difficulty is experienced in taking a drug because of its unpleasant taste, discuss this problem with the physician or a pharmacist. In some instances, disguising the taste by adding juice or flavoring may be allowed.

Never increase or decrease the dose or the time intervals between doses unless directed to do so by a physician.

A prescription drug or a physician-recommended nonprescription drug is not stopped or omitted except on advice of a physician.

Unless advised to do so by a physician, do not stop taking a prescribed drug even if feeling better or take more than the prescribed amount even if feeling worse.

If the symptoms for which the drug was prescribed do not improve, or if symptoms become worse, contact the physician, because a change in dosage or a different drug may be necessary.

Sometimes a drug may not produce noticeable effects (*e.g.,* a drug prescribed for hypertension). Do not stop taking the drug, even if no appreciable changes are noted, unless the physician directs doing so.

Some drugs may take days or even weeks to produce results (*e.g.,* antidepressants). If a drug does not appear to be producing the expected results, discuss this with the physician.

Use a calendar as a reminder when taking a drug on other than a daily basis (*e.g.,* every other day, three times a week).

If a dose of a drug is omitted or forgotten, do *not* double the next dose or take the next dose or two at more frequent intervals unless advised to do so by a physician.

All drug doses should be accurate. For a liquid preparation that has a dose prescribed and written as a "teaspoon," a calibrated spoon for measuring the drug can be purchased at many pharmacies. Use of a calibrated spoon is recommended for giving a liquid drug to children.

Always inform other physicians, nurses, dentists, and other health personnel (*e.g.,* physical therapists, dietitian) of all drugs (prescription and nonprescription) currently being taken on a regular or irregular basis.

Keep the exact names of all prescription and nonprescription drugs currently being taken in a wallet or purse for instant reference when seeing a physician or dentist.

When taking a drug for a period of time, especially drugs such as anticoagulants, steroids, oral hypoglycemic agents, insulin, or digitalis, wear a Medic-Alert or other type of identification. In case of an emergency, this will ensure that medical personnel will be aware of health problems and current drug therapy.

ADVERSE DRUG EFFECTS

Some drugs may cause adverse reactions. There are a wide variety of these reactions. Some of the more common adverse reactions include nausea, vomiting, diarrhea, constipation, skin rash, dizziness, drowsiness, and dry mouth. Some may be potentially serious, whereas others are mild and disappear when the physician adjusts the dosage. In some instances, mild reactions (*e.g.,* dry mouth) may have to be tolerated.

If *any* drug reaction occurs during or after a course of drug therapy, the physician should be made aware of the problem as soon as possible. If you are unable to contact the physician before the next dose is due, a pharmacist should be contacted.

If allergic to any drug, always tell medical personnel of the allergy *before* any treatment or drug is given.

At times, the physician may give instructions to avoid the use of alcohol while taking a drug. This is important, because use of alcohol in any form while taking some drugs may cause excessive sedation, nausea, vomiting, or a drop in blood pressure. In some instances the ingestion of alcohol with certain drugs, such as barbiturates, may cause death.

When told that a drug is capable of causing a photosensitivity reaction, avoid exposure to sunlight and ultraviolet light. Sunlamps and commercial tanning booths use ultraviolet light and their use must be avoided in these instances.

FAMILY MEMBERS

Family members or relatives should be made aware of all drugs, prescription and nonprescription, that are currently being taken.

Never give a drug prescribed for one family member to another family member, relative, or friend, unless directed to do so by a physician.

TRAVELING

When traveling, do not place prescription drugs in checked baggage (which can be lost). Carry drugs in a pocket, purse, or carry-on luggage.

Do not leave prescription drugs in the open in a hotel or motel room; they should be locked in luggage or taken with you when leaving the room.

Carry a written prescription for each drug being taken in case the drug is lost. If traveling to a foreign country, ask your physician or pharmacist to check whether the drug is available in the country being visited.

Place necessary drugs in two separate containers and carry them separately, in case one is lost or stolen.

Appendix 6
Signs and Symptoms of Adverse Reactions Related to Drug Administration

6-1. ACIDOSIS, METABOLIC
(Primary Base Bicarbonate Deficit)

Signs and symptoms: Disorientation; weakness; hyperventilation; headache; nausea, vomiting; diarrhea. *Laboratory findings:* Arterial blood pH below 7.35; PCO_2 below 40 mm Hg; urine pH may be below 6; plasma bicarbonate less than 24 mEq/liter.

6-2. ACIDOSIS, RESPIRATORY
(Primary Carbonic Acid Excess)

Signs and symptoms: Disorientation; apprehension; headache; weakness; rapid pulse; dyspnea; tachypnea; cardiovascular abnormalities (tachycardia), hypertension (in severe acidosis, hypotension and vasodilatation), arrhythmias; asterixis (flapping tremors); cyanosis (later stages); coma. *Laboratory findings:* Arterial blood pH below 7.35; PCO_2 above 40 mm Hg; urine pH below 6; plasma bicarbonate above 24 mEq/liter.

6-3. ADRENAL INSUFFICIENCY

Adrenal insufficiency may occur when the dosage of a glucocorticoid is omitted or is insufficient to meet the patient's requirement for glucocorticoid replacement.

Signs and symptoms of adrenal insufficiency: Nausea; fatigue; anorexia; vomiting; dyspnea; hypotension; hypoglycemia; myalgia; arthralgia; weight loss; hyperpigmentation of skin; mental or behavioral changes.

Signs and symptoms of addisonian crisis (acute adrenal insufficiency): Hypotension; hyperkalemia; dehydration; nausea, vomiting; muscular weakness; hypoglycemia; vascular collapse.

6-4. ALKALOSIS, METABOLIC
(Primary Base Bicarbonate Excess)

Signs and symptoms: Irritability; twitching; confusion; picking at the bedclothes (carphology); numbness, tingling of extremities; cyanosis; slow, shallow respirations with periods of apnea; tetany; muscle hypertonicity. *Laboratory findings:* Arterial blood pH above 7.45; PCO_2 above 40 mm Hg; urine pH 7 (sometimes above 7); plasma bicarbonate above 24 mEq/liter.

6-5. ALKALOSIS, RESPIRATORY
(Primary Carbonic Deficit)

Signs and symptoms: Hyperventilation; paresthesia; circumoral numbness; blurred vision; tinnitus; sweating; anxiety; tetany; dry mouth; coma. *Laboratory findings:* Arterial blood pH above 7.45; PCO_2 below 40 mm Hg; urine pH above 7; plasma bicarbonate below 24 mEq/liter.

6-6. ANAPHYLACTOID SHOCK (Anaphylaxis)

Signs and symptoms: Early signs may include apprehension; burning and warm sensation of the skin; itching; urticaria; tight feeling in the chest; difficulty in breathing. These may suddenly progress to rapid circulatory collapse with a rapid fall in blood pressure, rise in pulse rate (pulse may be weak, difficult to obtain), edema of the respiratory passages resulting in bronchospasm, and laryngeal edema. Death can occur in a few minutes unless appropriate treatment is instituted.

6-7. ANEMIA

A decrease in erythrocytes may occur with administration of antineoplastic agents but may also be seen with the administration of other drugs, as well as part of a disease process.

Nursing management: Fatigue, ranging from mild to severe, is the most common sign of anemia.

Monitor vital signs every 4 to 8 hours. An increase in the respiratory rate may require the administration of oxygen.

Assess the patient's ability to carry out the activities of daily living (ADL); then develop a plan of care based on an assessment of the patient's needs. Depending on the degree of fatigue, the following may be necessary:

Allow sufficient time for bathing, dressing, and grooming.
Provide frequent rest periods between activities.
Keep the head of the bed raised; dyspnea is a common symptom of anemia.
Assist with ambulatory activities. Avoid overexertion.
Keep personal articles (*e.g.,* water, tissues, chair, slippers) within easy reach.
Blood transfusions may be necessary when the anemia is severe. Packed cells or whole blood may be ordered.

6-8. BONE-MARROW DEPRESSION (Myelosuppression)

Bone-marrow depression (myelosuppression) may occur during or following the administration of antineoplastic agents as well as other pharmacologic agents, and may result in stomatitis, leukopenia, thrombocytopenia, or anemia.

Signs and symptoms: Fever; chills; fatigue; easy bruising; petechiae; easy bleeding (especially from gums, venipuncture sites, intramuscular or subcutaneous injection sites, small cuts); sore throat; sores in the mouth or on the lips; ulceration or abscess formation; symptoms of a common cold; symptoms of a urinary tract infection (burning on urination, foul odor to urine, frequent urination).

6-9. CONGESTIVE HEART FAILURE (CHF) AND PULMONARY EDEMA

Signs and symptoms of congestive heart failure: Dyspnea; orthopnea; cough; dizziness; fatigue; weight gain; peripheral edema; distended neck veins; rales at the base of the lungs; cool extremities; oliguria.

Signs and symptoms of pulmonary edema: Severe dyspnea; orthopnea; severe anxiety; extreme restlessness; confusion; distended neck veins; weak, rapid pulse; hypotension; cold, cyanotic, mottled extremities; cyanosis of the nail beds, lips; cough; copious frothy, blood-tinged sputum; stupor.

6-10. DEHYDRATION

Signs and symptoms: Poor skin turgor; dry mucous membranes; oliguria or anuria; increased urine specific gravity; restlessness; irritability; rapid respirations; depressed fontanel (infant); difficulty speaking, swallowing food; longitudinal furrows in tongue; weight loss; increase in pulse rate; decreased central venous pressure (CVP); decreased tearing, salivation.

6-11. DIABETIC KETOACIDOSIS (DKA)

Diabetic ketoacidosis may be present prior to the administration of insulin.

Signs and symptoms: Drowsiness; dim vision; thirst; Kussmaul breathing; air hunger; dry mouth; fruity (acetone) odor to breath; nausea; vomiting; abdominal pain; dry, flushed skin; rapid pulse; softening of the eyeballs.

6-12. FLUID OVERLOAD (Water Intoxication)

Signs and symptoms: Headache; weakness; blurred vision; behavioral changes (confusion, disorientation, delirium, drowsiness); weight gain; incoordination; isolated muscle twitching; rise in intracranial pressure with rise in blood pressure and decrease in pulse rate; convulsions; hyponatremia. Cardiac symptoms may include rapid breathing; rales, wheezing, coughing; rise in blood pressure; distended neck veins; elevated central venous pressure (CVP).

6-13. HYPOCALCEMIA AND HYPERCALCEMIA
Normal Laboratory Values (Total): 4.5 to 5.3 mEq/liter or 9 to 11 mg/dl*

Signs and symptoms of hypocalcemia: Hyperactive reflexes; carpopedal spasm; perioral paresthesias; positive Trousseau's sign; positive Chvostek's sign; muscle twitching; muscle cramps; tetany; laryngospasm; cardiac arrhythmias; nausea, vomiting; confusion, anxiety, emotional lability; convulsions; pathologic fractures (seen in long-standing hypocalcemia). *Laboratory findings:* Serum calcium decreased.

Signs and symptoms of hypercalcemia: Anorexia, nausea, vomiting; lethargy; bone tenderness or pain; polyuria; polydipsia; constipation; dehydration; muscle weakness and atrophy; stupor; coma; cardiac arrest. *Laboratory findings:* Serum calcium increased, BUN elevated. Generalized osteoporosis may be seen on x-ray examination.

6-14. HYPOGLYCEMIA AND HYPERGLYCEMIA
Normal Glucose Laboratory Values: 70 to 100 mg/dl (fasting serum); 60 to 100 mg/dl (fasting whole blood)*

Signs and symptoms of hypoglycemia (hyperinsulinism): Fatigue; weakness; confusion; headache; diplopia; psychosis; personality changes; rapid, shallow respirations; numbness of the mouth, lips, tongue; hunger; nausea; tingling; pulse rate may be normal or abnormal; pallor; slurred speech; staggering gait; tremors; diaphoresis; slow cerebration; lack of coordination; dizziness; convulsions; coma.

Signs and symptoms of hyperglycemia (hypoinsulinism): Polyphagia; polyuria; polydipsia; dehydration; glucosuria; ketonuria; blurred vision, changes in vision; weight loss; hypovolemia; recurrent or persistent infections; weakness; fatigue; muscle wasting; muscle cramps.

6-15. HYPOKALEMIA AND HYPERKALEMIA
Normal Laboratory Values: 3.5 to 5.0 mEq/liter*

Signs and symptoms of hypokalemia: Anorexia, nausea, vomiting; mental depression, confusion, delayed or impaired thought processes, drowsiness; abdominal distention, decreased bowel sounds, paralytic ileus; muscle weakness or fatigue, flaccid paral-

ysis; absent or diminished deep tendon reflexes; hypotension; weak, irregular pulse; paresthesias; leg cramps. *ECG changes:* Flattened or depressed T-waves, elevated U-waves, depressed S–T segment. *Laboratory findings:* Decreased serum potassium.

Signs and symptoms of hyperkalemia: Irritability, anxiety, listlessness, mental confusion; nausea, diarrhea, abdominal distress, gastrointestinal hyperactivity; paresthesias, weakness of the extremities, weakness and heaviness of the legs, flaccid paralysis (usually indistinguishable from that seen in hypokalemia); hypotension; cardiac arrhythmia, heart block, cardiac depression, cardiac arrest. *ECG changes:* Elevated T-waves, widened QRS complex, flat or absent P-waves, depressed S–T segment, prolonged Q–T interval. *Laboratory findings:* Increased serum potassium.

CLINICAL ALERT: When blood is drawn for analysis of potassium levels, it is important to recognize that artificial elevations do occur after repeated clenching of the fist to make the veins more prominent following application of a tourniquet.

6-16. HYPOMAGNESEMIA AND HYPERMAGNESEMIA
Normal Laboratory Values: 1.5 to 2.5 mEq/liter or 1.8 to 3.0 mg/dl*

Signs and symptoms of hypomagnesemia: Leg and foot cramps; hypertension; tachycardia; neuromuscular irritability; tremor; hyperactive deep tendon reflexes; confusion, disorientation, visual and/or auditory hallucinations; painful paresthesias; positive Trousseau's sign; positive Chvostek's sign; convulsions. *Laboratory findings:* Serum magnesium decreased; serum potassium may be decreased.

Signs and symptoms of hypermagnesemia: Lethargy; drowsiness; impaired respiration; flushing; sweating; hypotension; weak to absent deep tendon reflexes. *Laboratory findings:* Serum magnesium increased. ECG may show premature ventricular contractions, prolonged P–R and QRS intervals, tall T-waves, or AV block.

6-17. HYPONATREMIA AND HYPERNATREMIA
Normal Laboratory Values: 132 to 145 mEq/liter*

Signs and symptoms of hyponatremia: Cold clammy skin, decreased skin turgor; apprehension, confu-

---

* The laboratory values given may not concur with the normal range of values in all hospital or independent laboratories, because such values vary from lab to lab. The hospital policy manual or laboratory values sheet should be consulted for the normal ranges of all laboratory tests for each facility.

sion, irritability, anxiety; hypotension, postural hypotension; tachycardia; headache; tremors, convulsions; abdominal cramps, nausea, vomiting, diarrhea. *Laboratory findings:* Decreased serum sodium.

Signs and symptoms of hypernatremia: Fever; hot flushed dry skin; dry sticky mucous membranes; rough, dry, red tongue; edema; weight gain; intense thirst; excitement, restlessness, agitation; oliguria or anuria. *Laboratory findings:* Increased serum sodium.

6-18. HYPOPHOSPHATEMIA AND HYPERPHOSPHATEMIA
Normal Laboratory Values (Serum Phosphate/Inorganic Phosphorus): Adults—2.5 to 4.8 mg/dl; Children—3.5 to 5.8 mg/dl*

Signs and symptoms of hypophosphatemia: Anorexia; weakness; pathologic fractures (chronic deficit); circumoral paresthesia; hyperventilation. *Laboratory findings:* Hemolytic anemia; increased urinary concentration of bicarbonate, calcium, and magnesium; normal serum calcium levels; decreased serum phosphate levels.

Signs and symptoms of hyperphosphatemia: Signs of hypocalcemia may be present. *Laboratory findings:* Decrease in serum calcium levels; increased serum phosphate levels.

6-19. LEUKOPENIA

Most antineoplastic drugs or high doses of radiation to functioning bone marrow are capable of causing leukopenia. Although other drugs are also capable of causing leukopenia, this hematologic manifestation is usually most severe when antineoplastic agents are administered.

Nursing management: Protective (or reverse) isolation may be instituted to reduce contact with microorganisms carried by others. The reason for this procedure is explained to the patient. A private room is necessary. All equipment necessary for patient care (*e.g.,* sphygmomanometer, stethoscope, thermometer, bathing utensils, bedpan) remains in the room until isolation technique is discontinued. Masks and gowns are worn in the room, and gloves worn if there is physical contact with the patient. Health-team members and visitors with upper respiratory infections should not enter the room. The

patient wears a mask and gown when leaving the room. Strict handwashing technique when entering and leaving the room is essential.

Obtain vital signs every 4 to 8 hours or as ordered.

Observe for signs of urinary tract infection; upper respiratory infection; septicemia; phlebitis.

Change the patient's position every 2 hours and encourage deep breathing and coughing. Check bony prominences for signs of skin breakdown.

Encourage an adequate dietary and fluid intake. Food may be offered in small, frequent feedings or meals. Offer water and other fluids hourly.

Monitor intake and output. Report any change in the intake–output ratio to the physician immediately.

Assess the patient's mental status; observe for signs of depression, detachment, or other behavioral changes.

Inspect the patient's oral cavity daily. Stomatitis care is instituted at the first sign of oral erythema or burning.

Avoid trauma to the skin. Injections are avoided when possible.

Diversional therapy will be necessary and may include books, newspapers, magazines, television, and radio (when available). Spend as much time as possible with the patient.

6-20. STEVENS-JOHNSON SYNDROME

A prodromal period characterized by fever, cough, malaise, sore throat, head cold, muscular aches, arthralgia, and vomiting may be seen in some patients. This is followed by development of skin and mucous membrane lesions or eruptions, usually red or purple macules, wheals, vesicles, bullae, or papules. Hemorrhage into the affected areas may be seen. This syndrome may be life threatening when large areas of the skin slough off. The skin lesions may be the first and only manifestations of the syndrome. The Stevens-Johnson syndrome is also known as erythema multiforme (major).

6-21. STOMATITIS

Early symptoms of stomatitis (mucositis) include erythema of mucous membranes, dry mouth, burning of the oral mucosa, and difficulty in swallowing. This is followed in several days by the appearance of isolated, small ulcerations, later progressing to generalized ulcerations of the oral mucosa. Hemorrhagic ulceration may also be seen.

Nursing management: Give care every 4 hours around the clock.

Solutions that may be used include the following:

---

* The laboratory values given may not concur with the normal range of values in all hospital or independent laboratories, because such values vary from lab to lab. The hospital policy manual or laboratory values sheet should be consulted for the normal ranges of all laboratory tests for each facility.

Warm-water mouth rinses.
Hydrogen peroxide (H_2O_2) solution (equal parts hydrogen peroxide and water).
Milk of magnesia: Allow to stand 2 to 3 hours, pour off liquid remaining at the top. The resulting material is milk of magnesia substrate.
Physician may order use of other solutions or combinations.

Soft, bland diet is prescribed.

Dental care with a soft toothbrush (mild stomatitis) or cotton swabs (severe stomatitis) is important.

Analgesia: Xylocaine Viscous 15 ml every 3 to 4 hours may be prescribed. Drug is swished around in the mouth and may be swallowed if the pharynx is also sore. A topical local anesthetic spray may also be used.

6-22. SUPERINFECTION

Signs and symptoms: Black furry tongue; glossitis; ulcerations of the mouth; anogenital itching; vaginal itching and discharge; diarrhea; fever.

6-23. TARTRAZINE SENSITIVITY

Tartrazine is FD&C Yellow No. 5, a food dye and coloring. Products containing tartrazine may cause allergic-type reactions, including bronchial asthma, in susceptible individuals. Although the overall incidence of such reactions in the general population is low, it is most frequently seen in those who also have aspirin sensitivity. Not all yellow preparations contain tartrazine, and not all preparations labeled as containing tartrazine are yellow.

When a patient has a known sensitivity to aspirin, drugs containing tartrazine should be avoided, when possible. In some instances another brand of the drug can be used, because not all pharmaceutical firms producing a specific drug may include tartrazine in their product. If the drug containing tartrazine must be administered, the patient is closely observed for an allergic reaction and the physician is contacted immediately if bronchial asthma or other allergic symptoms occur.

6-24. THROMBOCYTOPENIA

Thrombocytopenia may occur with some antineoplastic agents as well as with other drugs such as cephalosporins, clindamycin, and aminoglycosides. This hematologic manifestation is usually more severe when antineoplastic agents are administered.

Nursing management: Observe patient closely for evidence of bleeding. Look for bruises, petechiae, bleeding gums, hematuria, bright red or tarry stools, epistaxis, prolonged bleeding from an injection site, heavy menstrual flow (if the patient is menstruating), coffee-ground or black emesis or the vomiting of bright red blood, and prolonged bleeding from cuts.

Monitor vital signs every 4 hours. A drop in blood pressure and rise in the pulse rate may indicate internal bleeding. The temperature should be taken orally (unless the physician directs otherwise) to avoid trauma to and possible bleeding of rectal tissue.

When possible, parenteral injections are avoided. If necessary, apply prolonged pressure at the injection site.

Apply prolonged pressure at venipuncture sites.

Instruct patient to avoid cuts, bruises, and falls; use an electric razor for shaving; and avoid blowing his nose to minimize possibility of epistaxis.

Report all bleeding episodes promptly.

A stool softener may be ordered if the patient is constipated.

A soft toothbrush or gentle rinsing of the mouth is employed for oral care.

Platelet transfusions may be necessary to control bleeding.

Appendix 7
Controlled Substances

The Controlled Substances Act of 1970 regulates the manufacturing, distribution, and dispensing of drugs that have potential for abuse. The Drug Enforcement Administration (DEA) within the U.S. Department of Justice is the leading federal agency responsible for enforcement of the act.

DEA SCHEDULES

Drugs under jurisdiction of the Controlled Substances Act are divided into five schedules based on their potentials for abuse and physical and psychological dependence. All controlled substances listed in this book are identified by schedule as follows:

Schedule I (C-I): High abuse potential and no accepted medical use (heroin, marijuana, LSD).

Schedule II (C-II): High abuse potential with severe dependence liability (narcotics, amphetamines, barbiturates).

Schedule III (C-III): Less abuse potential than schedule II drugs and moderate dependence liability (nonbarbiturate sedatives, nonamphetamine stimulants, limited amounts of certain narcotics).

Schedule IV (C-IV): Less abuse potential than schedule III drugs and limited dependence liability (some sedatives and antianxiety agents, nonnarcotic analgesics).

Schedule V (C-V): Limited abuse potential. Primarily small amounts of narcotics (codeine) used as antitussives or antidiarrheals. Under federal law, limited quantities of certain C-V drugs may be purchased without a prescription directly from a pharmacist. The purchaser must be at least 18 years of age and must furnish suitable identification. All such transactions must be recorded by the dispensing pharmacist.

Prescribing physicians and dispensing pharmacies must be registered with the DEA. Separate records must be maintained of all purchases and dispensations of controlled substances. A physical inventory of all controlled substances must be made every 2 years. Prescriptions for controlled substances must be written in ink and must include date issued; full name and address of the patient; and name, address, and DEA registration number of the physician. Oral prescriptions must be promptly committed to writing. Controlled substance prescriptions may not be dispensed or refilled more than 6 months after the date issued, nor may they be refilled more than five times. A written prescription order signed by the physician is required for schedule II drugs. In case of an emergency, oral prescriptions for schedule II substances may be filled; however, the physician must provide a signed prescription within 72 hours. Schedule II prescriptions cannot be refilled.

In many cases, state laws are more restrictive than federal laws and therefore impose additional requirements.

The following pharmacologic agents are controlled substances:

SCHEDULE II (C–II) DRUGS

Alphaprodine HCl
Amobarbital
Amobarbital sodium
Amphetamine combinations
Amphetamine complex
Amphetamine mixtures
Amphetamine sulfate
Cocaine
Codeine phosphate
Codeine sulfate
Dextroamphetamine sulfate
Fentanyl citrate and droperidol
Hydrochlorides of opium alkaloids (Pantopon)
Hydrocodone bitartrate
Hydromorphone HCl
Levorphanol tartrate
Meperidine HCl
Methadone HCl
Methamphetamine HCl
Methylphenidate HCl
Morphine HCl
Morphine sulfate
Opium tincture deodorized
Oxycodone HCl
Oxymorphone HCl
Pantopon (hydrochlorides of opium alkaloids)
Pentobarbital
Pentobarbital sodium
Phenmetrazine HCl
Secobarbital
Secobarbital sodium

SCHEDULE III (C–III) DRUGS

Aprobarbital
Benzphetamine HCl
Butabarbital sodium
Chlorphentermine HCl
Glutethimide
Mazindol
Metharbital

Methyprylon
Paregoric tincture
Pentobarbital sodium (suppositories)
Phendimetrazine tartrate
Secobarbital sodium (suppositories)
Talbutal
Thiamylal sodium
Thiopental sodium

SCHEDULE IV (C–IV) DRUGS

Alprazolam
Brown mixture
Chloral hydrate
Chlordiazepoxide
Clonazepam
Clorazepate dipotassium
Diazepam
Diethylpropion HCl
Ethchlorvynol
Ethinamate
Fenfluramine HCl
Flurazepam HCl
Mephobarbital
Meprobamate
Methohexital sodium
Paraldehyde
Pemoline
Pentazocine
Phenobarbital
Phenobarbital sodium (injection)
Propoxyphene HCl
Propoxyphene HCl and acetaminophen
Propoxyphene HCl and aspirin
Propoxyphene HCl and aspirin, phenacetin, caffeine
Propoxyphene napsylate
Propoxyphene napsylate and acetaminophen
Propoxyphene napsylate and aspirin
Temazepam
Triazolam

SCHEDULE V (C–V) DRUGS

Diphenoxylate w/atropine sulfate
Loperamide HCl

Appendix 8
Abbreviations

<	less than	FDA	Food and Drug Administration
>	greater than	Fe	iron
A.C.	before meals	Fl	fluoride
ADH	antidiuretic hormone	g	gram
ADL	activities of daily living	gal	gallon
AgNO$_3$	silver nitrate	GFR	glomerular filtration rate
ANC	acid-neutralizing capacity	GI	gastrointestinal
bid	twice daily	G6PD	glucose-6-phosphate dehydrogenase
C	Celsius (centigrade)	GU	genitourinary
Ca	calcium	h	hour
Ccr	creatinine clearance	HBr	hydrobromide
CDC	Centers for Disease Control	HCl	hydrochloride
CHF	congestive heart failure	HCO$_3$	bicarbonate
ci	curie	HDL	high-density lipoprotein
Cl	chloride	Hg	mercury
CNS	central nervous system	5-HIAA	5-hydroxyindoleacetic acid
COPD	chronic obstructive pulmonary disease	H.S.	at bedtime (hour of sleep)
		HSV	herpes simplex virus
CRNA	certified registered nurse anesthetist	I	iodine
CSF	cerebrospinal fluid	IM	intramuscular
CTZ	chemoreceptor trigger zone	IOP	intraocular pressure
cu	cubic	IPPB	intermittent positive pressure breathing
Cu	copper		
CVA	cerebrovascular accident	IU	international units
DIC	disseminated intravascular coagulation	IV	intravenous
		K	potassium
DKA	diabetic ketoacidosis	kcal	kilocalorie (calorie)
dl	deciliter	KCl	potassium chloride
ECT	electroconvulsive therapy (shock therapy)	kg	kilogram
		KVO	keep vein open
F	Fahrenheit	lb	pound
FBS	fasting blood sugar (glucose)	LDL	low-density lipoprotein

m	meter	PT	prothrombin time
m^2	square meter	PTT	partial thromboplastin time
MAO	monoamine oxidase	qh	every hour
MAOI	monoamine oxidase inhibitor	qid	four times daily
mcg	microgram	RDA	recommended dietary (daily) allowance
mCi	millicurie		
MDR	minimum daily requirement	REM	rapid eye movements
mEq	milliequivalent	ROM	range of motion (exercises)
mg	milligram	Rx	prescription only
Mg	magnesium	SIADH	syndrome of inappropriate ADH secretion
MI	myocardial infarction		
MIC	minimum inhibitory concentration	SGOT	serum glutamic-oxaloacetic transaminase
ml	milliliter		
mm	millimeter	SGPT	serum glutamic-pyruvic transaminase
mM	millimole	t½	half-life
Mn	manganese	tbsp	tablespoon
mU	milliunits	TCA	tricyclic antidepressant
Na	sodium	tid	three times daily
NaCl	sodium chloride	U	unit
NF	National Formulary	UD	unit dose package
ng	nanogram	USP	*United States Pharmacopeia*
otc	over-the-counter (nonprescription)	UTI	urinary tract infection
oz	ounce	VLDL	very low-density lipoproteins
P	phosphorus	VMA	vanillylmandelic acid
P.C.	after meals	w/	with
PID	pelvic inflammatory disease	WBCT	whole blood clotting time
PO	by mouth	WHO	World Health Organization
ppm	parts per million	w/o	without
prn	as needed	Zn	zinc
pt	pint		

Appendix 9
Glossary

Acetones   *see* Ketones

Acidosis   a disturbance in the acid–base balance of the body, with a shift toward the acid state

Additive effect   a response, following administration of two drugs (*e.g.,* barbiturates and alcohol), equal to the sum of the individual drug responses

Adrenergic   having an action similar to that of epinephrine

Adrenergic blocking agent   an agent inhibiting response to adrenergic nerve stimulation; an antiadrenergic drug

Adsorbent   an agent that binds chemicals to its surface (*e.g.,* activated charcoal)

Agonist   a narcotic capable of activating specific opiate receptors in the brain

Agranulocytosis   a decrease in the number of leukocytes

Akathisia   motor restlessness; urgent need for movement

Akinesia   complete or partial loss of muscle movement

Alkaloid   a naturally occurring substance from plants that reacts with an acid to form a salt

Alkalosis   a disturbance in the acid–base balance, with an accumulation of alkali

Alopecia   loss of hair

Amaurosis   complete loss of vision without evidence of a pathologic condition of the eye

Amebicide   an agent capable of destroying amebas

Amelioration   an improvement

Amenorrhea   absence of menstruation

Amine   an organic compound containing nitrogen

Anabolic   promoting anabolism

Anabolism   building up of body tissue; opposite of catabolism (*adj:* anabolic)

Analeptic   an agent used to stimulate the central nervous system, especially one that stimulates the respiratory center and wakefulness

Analogue   one of two or more drugs that have similar properties but different chemical structures

Anaphylactic shock   *see* Anaphylaxis

Anaphylactoid reaction   *see* Anaphylaxis

Anaphylaxis   an immediate and serious hypersensitive response to a drug or foreign protein characterized by severe hypotension, bronchospasm, dyspnea, cyanosis, and unconsciousness

Androgen   a male sex hormone; a substance producing and maintaining secondary male sex characteristics

Angioneurotic edema   a hypersensitive drug response characterized by large wheals or hives and swelling of submucous or subcutaneous tissues

Anhidrosis   diminishment or absence of sweat

Anosmia   loss of the sense of smell

Antagonism   an opposing effect; a reduced or abolished effect due to administration of a second drug

Anthelmintic   an agent used to treat parasitic worm infestations in the intestine

Antiadrenergic   an adrenergic blocking agent

Antibiotic an agent destroying or preventing the growth of microorganisms

Antibody a protein substance formed by the body in response to an antigen or foreign body

Anticholinergic an agent decreasing the activity of cholinergic nerve fibers; parasympatholytic

Anticoagulant an agent delaying coagulation of the blood

Anticonvulsant an agent used to control or prevent convulsive disorders

Antidepressant an agent used to treat depression

Antidote a drug or substance used to neutralize poisons or the actions or effects of another agent

Antiemetic an agent used to prevent or treat nausea and vomiting

Antigen a substance that induces the formation of antibodies

Antihistamine an agent that appears to compete with histamine receptor sites and is used in the treatment of allergies and motion sickness

Antikaliuretic an agent that reduces or prevents excretion of potassium in the urine

Antimetabolite an agent interfering with the use of metabolites necessary for cell growth

Antineoplastic an agent used in treatment of neoplastic diseases

Antipyretic an agent that reduces fever

Antiseptic an agent that prevents or slows the growth of microorganisms

Antitoxin a specific antibody produced by the body following exposure to a specific toxin

Antivenin a substance prepared from immunized animal sera used to neutralize venom from a poisonous animal or insect

Anuria suppression of urinary output

Aphakia absence of the crystalline lens of the eye

Aphasia inability to speak; inability to understand the meaning of written or spoken words

Aphthous characterized by ulcers

Argyria permanent discoloration of skin or conjunctiva due to use of silver compounds

Arrhythmia abnormal heart rhythm

Arthralgia joint pain

Asterixis involuntary, intermittent, jerking muscular movements caused by contraction of a group of muscles

Atopic 1. displaced; 2. allergic

Azotemia an excess of nitrogen-containing compounds in the blood

Bactericidal destructive to bacteria

Bacteriostatic inhibiting or retarding bacterial growth

Benign not malignant; not serious

Bioavailability the rate and extent to which a specific dose of a drug enters the bloodstream and reaches the site(s) of action; also, the rate of absorption and availability at the site of drug action of the active drug ingredient

Biotransformation a physiological process that changes the characteristics of a substance so that it can be metabolized and excreted

Borborygmus a rumbling or gurgling sound heard over the large intestine

Bradykinesia (*adj:* bradykinetic) slowness of movement

Bromhidrosis an offensive, fetid odor to sweat

Bronchodilator an agent that dilates the bronchi

Bulla a bleb filled with fluid or air

Cachexia a state of wasting or emaciation

Carcinogen an agent capable of causing cancer

Carcinogenesis the production of cancer

Carcinogenic causing cancer

Cardiotonic an agent that increases the force of myocardial contraction

Catabolism the breaking down of tissue; opposite of anabolism

Catecholamines organic compounds found in the sympathetic nervous system (*e.g.,* epinephrine, norepinephrine)

Cerumen waxy secretion in the outer ear canal

Cervicitis inflammation of the cervix

Cheilitis inflammation of the lips

Cheilosis fissures of the lips and at the corners of the mouth

Chloasma hyperpigmentation of the skin, usually due to pregnancy; may also be seen in liver disorders or during menstruation or menopause

Chloruretic effect promotion of excretion of chlorides in the urine

Cholinergic agents agents that mimic the actions of the parasympathetic nervous system; parasympathomimetics

Cholinergic blocking agents agents that inhibit the activity of the parasympathetic nervous system

Chronotropic effect an effect on the heart rate

Chvostek's sign spasm of the facial muscles produced by tapping in front of the ear over the facial nerve or its branches; a sign evoked in tetany

Clonic *see* Clonus

Clonus alternate spasm and relaxation of muscles (*adj:* clonic)

Corticoids same as corticosteroids

Corticosteroids agents with actions similar to those of hormones produced by the adrenal cortex

Cross-allergenicity *see* Cross-sensitivity

Cross-resistance resistance shared by two groups of drugs; an individual resistant to one group may also be resistant to the other group

Cross-sensitivity sensitivity (allergy) shared by two groups of drugs; an individual sensitive to one group may be sensitive to the other group

Cumulative effect   an increasing response to repeated doses of a drug occurring when the rate of administration exceeds the rate of drug excretion; usually seen in those with renal failure

Cycloplegia   paralysis of the ciliary muscle of the eye, resulting in difficulty in focusing

Cycloplegics   agents producing cycloplegia

Cytotoxic   an agent having a deleterious effect on cells; used in the treatment of malignant neoplasms

Decongestant   an agent that reduces congestion

Demulcent   an agent that soothes

Depressant   an agent that depresses nerve activity and some vital processes such as respiration or heartbeat

Detritus   waste material; disintegrated matter or debris

Diathesis   constitutional predisposition or susceptibility to a certain disease

Diluent   a liquid or solid that dilutes; a substance that increases the bulk of a drug or liquefies a solid

Diplopia   double vision

Disinfectant   a substance that kills bacteria

Diuresis   production and passage of abnormally large amounts of urine

Diuretic   an agent that promotes the excretion of water and electrolytes

Diurnal   pertaining to the daytime

Dysesthesia   sensation of pins and needles; a crawling sensation

Dysgeusia   impairment of taste

Dyskinesia   difficulty in movement

Dysmenorrhea   painful menstruation

Dysphagia   difficulty in swallowing

Dysphoria   malaise; restlessness; unrest without apparent cause

Dysplasia   abnormal development or overgrowth of tissue

Edentulous   without teeth

Elixir   a sweetened alcohol and water preparation

Endogenous   originating within the body

Enteric coating   a layer on the outer surface of a tablet or capsule preventing dissolution in the stomach

Enteric pathogens   pathogens in the intestinal tract

Envenomation   the introduction of venom by means of a bite

Enzyme   an organic catalyst produced by cells, capable of acting independently and inducing a chemical change in other substances without undergoing a change in itself

Eosinophilia   an increase in the number of eosinophils in the blood

Epilation   removal of hair

Epinephrine   a hormone produced by the adrenal medulla; also known as adrenalin

Erythema multiforme   a skin reaction involving the sudden appearance of lesions on the face, neck, extremities, and dorsal surface of the hands and feet; the severe form, which can be fatal, is called Stevens-Johnson syndrome

Erythrocyte   a red blood cell

Erythromelalgia   burning pain and redness of the extremities

Euthyroid   normal activity of the thyroid gland; a state of normal thyroid gland activity

Exanthema   an eruption or rash on the skin accompanied by inflammation

Exogenous   originating outside the body

Expectorant   an agent that facilitates removal of bronchopulmonary secretions

Extract   an active, concentrated drug principle obtained by a chemical process or by distillation

Extrasystole   premature contraction of the heart

Extravasation   the escape of fluid into surrounding tissue

Fluidextracts   extracts made from a vegetable drug and made into a fluid by addition of alcohol

Formication   a creeping or crawling sensation

Galactorrhea   excessive flow of milk from the mammary gland

Generic drug   a nonproprietary name of a drug; a drug marketed under various trade names

Globus hystericus   the (subjective) sensation of a lump in the throat in hysteria

Glossitis   inflammation of the tongue

Glucocorticoid   one of the hormones of the adrenal gland that affect carbohydrate and protein metabolism and protect the body in times of stress

Gravid   pregnant

Gynecomastia   enlargement of the male breast

Hematopoiesis   the production and development of blood and its constituents, which normally takes place in the bone marrow

Hematopoietic   an agent that stimulates the production of blood and its constituents

Hemeralopia   diminishing vision in bright light; day blindness

Hemostatic   an agent that promotes clot formation

Heterotopia   displacement; development in an abnormal position

Hirsutism   excessive or abnormal growth of hair

Hydrocholeretic   an agent that increases the output of bile of low specific gravity by the liver

Hydrophilic   an agent with water-absorbing qualities

Hyperacusis   abnormal acuteness of hearing

Hyperammonemia excess ammonia in the blood

Hyperchloremia excessive chlorides in the blood

Hypercholesterolemia excess cholesterol in the blood

Hyperglycemia an increase in blood glucose

Hyperhidrosis excessive sweating

Hyperkalemia excessive amount of potassium in the blood

Hyperkeratosis corneal hypertrophy; overgrowth of the corium of the skin

Hypermagnesemia excessive amount of magnesium in the blood

Hypernatremia excessive amount of sodium in the blood

Hypernoia excessive mental activity

Hypersensitivity (drug) a response greater than usual from a given dose of a drug

Hypertrophy increase in the size of an organ or structure without an increase in the number of cells

Hypervolemia an abnormal increase in the volume of circulating blood

Hyphemia blood in the anterior chamber of the eye

Hypochloremia a decrease in chlorides in the blood

Hypodermoclysis the introduction of fluid into subcutaneous tissue; may be used as a method of administering parenteral fluids

Hypogeusia a diminution in taste perception

Hypoglycemia a decrease in the blood glucose

Hypokalemia a decrease in the amount of potassium in the blood

Hypomagnesemia a decrease in the amount of magnesium in the blood

Hyponatremia a decrease in the amount of sodium in the blood

Hypovolemia an abnormal decrease in the volume of circulating blood

Idiosyncrasy an abnormal drug response; may be an exaggerated response or a diminished response

Immunity resistance to disease by means of a production of antibodies specific for that disease

Immunogenic producing immunity

Inotropic effect an increase in the force of contraction of the heart

Intraocular within the eye

Kaliuretic an agent that promotes excretion of potassium in the urine

Keratolytic an agent that promotes softening and then shedding of the skin

Ketonemia the presence of ketones in the blood

Ketones a group of compounds produced by the oxidation of fatty acids; also called acetones

Ketonuria the presence of ketones in the urine

Laxative an agent that promotes the evacuation of feces

Leukocyte a white blood cell

Lipids a group of fats or fatlike substances

Lipolysis decomposition of fat

Livido reticularis a reddish blue mottling of the skin of the extremities

Mastalgia pain in the breast

Mastodynia pain in the breast

Metabolite the product of metabolism

Miliaria cutaneous changes associated with sweat retention

Mineralocorticoids a group of hormones produced by the adrenal cortex having a marked effect on the retention and excretion of minerals, chiefly sodium and potassium

Miosis an abnormal contraction of the pupil of the eye

Miotic an agent causing miosis

Mitosis the process of cell division

Monocyte a mononuclear leukocyte

Morphologic pertaining to shape and structure

Mucolytic an agent that reduces the thickness of bronchopulmonary mucus

Mucositis inflammation of a mucous membrane

Muscarinic receptors receptors in effector cells stimulated by postganglionic neurons of the sympathetic nervous system; drugs with a muscarinic effect act directly on muscarinic-type fibers

Mutagenesis the induction of genetic mutation

Mutagenic an agent capable of inducing genetic mutation

Myasthenia muscle weakness

Mydriasis abnormal dilatation of the pupil

Mydriatic an agent that dilates the pupil

Myelocyte a bone-marrow cell that gives rise to granular leukocytes in the circulating blood

Myopia nearsightedness

Nadir the lowest point

Naris external nostril (*pl:* nares)

Natriuretic an agent enhancing the excretion of sodium in the urine

Nephrocalcinosis the deposit of calcium phosphate in renal tubules

Nidation implantation of a fertilized ovum in the lining of the uterus

Norepinephrine a hormone produced by the adrenal medulla as well as formed at certain nerve endings of sympathetic nerves

Normovolemia a normal blood volume

Nyctalopia inability to see well in dim or faint light or at night; night blindness

Ointments topical preparations containing medicinal substances with a base of lanolin, petrolatum, or other substances

Oligomenorrhea scanty or infrequent menstrual flow

Oligospermia abnormally low number of sperm

Oncogenic a substance capable of causing tumor formation

Oncolytic destructive to tumor cells

Opiate an opium derivative; a synthetic drug that produces pharmacologic effects similar to those of morphine

Orthostatic hypotension hypotension occurring when standing in an upright position for a period of time

Over-the-counter (otc) drug a drug that does not require a prescription

Oxytocic an agent that stimulates uterine contractions

Pancytopenia abnormal depression of all the formed elements of the blood

Parasympathomimetic an agent producing effects similar to those resulting from stimulation of parasympathetic nerve fibers

Pathogen a disease-producing microorganism or substance

Phlebosclerosis hardening of the walls of a vein

Photophobia an aversion or intolerance to light

Porcine resembling a pig or swine; of pork origin

Postural hypotension hypotension resulting from a change in posture, usually upon rising from a sitting or lying position

Proptosis a downward displacement

Prostaglandin a substance detected in almost every tissue of the body and body fluid, having widespread effects such as contraction of smooth muscle and dilation of vascular beds

Proteolytic enzyme an agent used to liquefy purulent and fibrinous exudates

Pruritus severe itching

Psychotropic an agent affecting the function of the mind

Pyrosis a burning sensation

Rhabdomyolysis disintegration of striated muscle fibers

Saluresis excretion of sodium and chloride in the urine

Saluretic an agent promoting the excretion of sodium and chloride in the urine

Scotoma a gap in the visual field (*pl:* scotomata)

Sialadenopathy enlargement of the salivary gland

Sialoadenitis inflammation of the salivary gland

Sialorrhea excessive salivation

Spasmolytic an agent that relieves spasms

Steroids *see* Corticosteroids

Stomatitis inflammation of the mouth

Suspension a combination of a fluid and a solid in which the particles are suspended, but not dissolved, in the fluid vehicle

Symblepharon adhesion between the eyelid conjunctiva and the eyeball

Sympathomimetic an agent producing effects similar to those resulting from stimulation of sympathetic nerve fibers

Synechiae adhesions, especially in the eye

Synergism an effect greater than the sum of the separate actions of two or more drugs

Syrup an aqueous sugar solution often used to disguise the taste and/or odor of a drug or solution

Tachyphylaxis **1.** rapid immunization by means of injecting small doses; **2.** rapid development of tolerance after only a few doses of a drug

Teratogens agents capable of causing malformation or deformity in the developing embryo

Tolerance (drug) decreased drug response after repeated administration; usually requires an increase in dose to elicit the desired effect

Tranquilizer an agent that reduces mental tension and anxiety

Trismus tonic contraction of the muscles used for chewing

Trousseau's sign elicitation of carpopedal spasm by compression of the upper arm

Uricosuric an agent increasing the excretion of uric acid

Vaccine a suspension of attenuated (weakened) or killed infectious microorganisms

Vasoconstrictor an agent causing constriction of blood vessels

Vasodilator an agent causing relaxation (dilatation) of blood vessels

Viscid *see* Viscous

Viscous thick, sticky, gelatinous

Xanthopsia a visual defect in which objects have a yellow appearance

Xerophthalmia dryness of the conjunctiva

Xerosis cutis dry skin

Xerostomia dry mouth

Appendix 10
Combination
Chemotherapeutic
Regimens

Combinations of antineoplastic agents are superior to single drug therapy in the management of many diseases, leading to higher response rates and increased duration of remissions. This improved response may be due to the different mechanisms by which the agents work. Neoplastic cells that acquire rapid resistance to a single agent by random mutation develop resistance less rapidly when treated with a combination of agents. Selection of agents for combination chemotherapeutic regimens is based on a number of factors, including mechanism of drug action, cell-cycle specificity of action, responsiveness to dosage schedules, and drug toxicity. Increased responsiveness to combination therapy may permit dosage reductions and therefore decrease toxicity. Some of the commonly used combination chemotherapeutic regimens are listed below.

ABVD

Use:	Hodgkin's disease, induction (resistant to MOPP)
Regimen:	doxorubicin 25 mg/m^2/day IV, days 1 and 14
	bleomycin 10 units/m^2/day IV, days 1 and 14
	vinblastine 6 mg/m^2/day IV, days 1 and 14
	dacarbazine 375 mg/m^2/day IV, days 1 and 14
	Repeat every 38 days for 6 cycles

ACe

Use:	breast cancer, metastatic or recurrent disease
Regimen:	cyclophosphamide 200 mg/m^2/day PO, days 3 through 6
	doxorubicin 40 mg/m^2 IV, day 1
	Repeat every 21 or 28 days

A-COPP

Use:	Hodgkin's disease, induction (children only)
Regimen:	doxorubicin 60 mg/m^2 IV, day 1
	cyclophosphamide 300 mg/m^2/day IV, days 14 and 20
	vincristine 1.5 mg/m^2/day IV, days 14 and 20 (max. dose 2 mg)
	procarbazine 100 mg/m^2/day PO, days 14 through 28
	prednisone 40 mg/m^2/day PO, days 1 through 27 (1st and 4th cycles only)
	prednisone 40 mg/m^2/day PO, days 14 through 27 (2nd, 3rd, 5th, and 6th cycles)

Repeat every 42 days for 6 cycles

Adria + BCNU

Use: multiple myeloma, multiple myeloma in relapse (alkylator resistant)

Regimen: doxorubicin 30 mg/m^2 IV, day 1
carmustine 30 mg/m^2 IV, day 1

Repeat every 21 or 28 days

Ara-C + ADR

Use: acute myelocytic leukemia, induction

Regimen: cytarabine 100 mg/m^2/day, continuous 24 hour IV infusion for 7 to 10 days
doxorubicin 30 mg/m^2/day IV for 3 days

Ara-C + DNR + PRED + MP

Use: acute myelocytic leukemia (children only)

Induction: daunorubicin 25 mg/m^2 IV for 1 day
cytarabine 80 mg/m^2/day IV for 3 days
prednisolone 40 mg/m^2 PO daily
mercaptopurine 100 mg/m^2 PO daily

Repeat weekly until remission

Maintenance: Repeat every month or 28 days

Ara-C + 6-TG

Use: acute myelocytic leukemia

Induction: cytarabine 100 mg/m^2 q12h IV for 10 days
thioguanine 100 mg/m^2 q12h PO for 10 days

Repeat both drugs every 30 days until remission marrow is obtained

Maintenance: cytarabine 100 mg/m^2 q12h IV for 5 days
thioguanine 100 mg/m^2 q12h PO for 5 days

Repeat every month

BCVPP

Use: Hodgkin's disease, induction

Regimen: carmustine 100 mg/m^2 IV, day 1
cyclophosphamide 600 mg/m^2 IV, day 1
vinblastine 5 mg/m^2 IV, day 1
procarbazine 100 mg/m^2/day PO, days 1 through 10
prednisone 60 mg/m^2/day PO, days 1 through 10

Repeat every 28 days for 6 cycles

CAF

Use: breast cancer, metastatic disease

Regimen: cyclophosphamide 100 mg/m^2/day PO, days 1 through 14
doxorubicin 30 mg/m^2/day IV, days 1 and 8
fluorouracil 500 mg/m^2/day IV, days 1 and 8

Repeat every 4 weeks until a total cumulative dose of 450 mg/m^2 of doxorubicin is given, then discontinue doxorubicin and substitute methotrexate 40 mg/m^2 IV and increase fluorouracil to 600 mg/m^2 IV

CAMP

Use: lung cancer, non–oat cell carcinomas

Regimen: cyclophosphamide 300 mg/m^2/day IV, days 1 and 8
doxorubicin 20 mg/m^2/day IV, days 1 and 8
methotrexate 15 mg/m^2/day IV, days 1 and 8
procarbazine 100 mg/m^2/day PO, days 1 through 10

Repeat every 28 days

CAV

Use:	Small cell lung cancer, induction
Regimen:	cyclophosphamide 750 mg/m^2 IV every 3 weeks doxorubicin 50 mg/m^2 IV every 3 weeks vincristine 2 mg IV every 3 weeks

CAVe

Use:	Hodgkin's disease, induction (resistant to MOPP)
Regimen:	lomustine 100 mg/m^2 PO, day 1 doxorubicin 60 mg/m^2 IV, day 1 vinblastine 5 mg/m^2 IV, day 1
	Repeat every 6 weeks for 9 cycles

CHL + PRED

Use:	chronic lymphocytic leukemia
Regimen:	chlorambucil 0.4 mg/kg/day PO for 1 day every other week prednisone 100 mg/day PO for 2 days every other week
	Adjust dosage according to blood counts every 2 weeks prior to therapy; increase initial dose of 0.4 mg/kg by 0.1 mg/kg every 2 weeks until toxicity or disease control occurs.

CHOP

Use:	non-Hodgkin's lymphoma, lymphomas with unfavorable histology
Regimen:	cyclophosphamide 750 mg/m^2 IV, day 1 doxorubicin 50 mg/m^2 IV, day 1 vincristine 1.4 mg/m^2 IV, day 1 (max. dose 2 mg) prednisone 60 mg/day PO, days 1 through 5
	Repeat every 21 to 28 days for 6 cycles

CHOR

Use:	lung cancer, small cell carcinoma
Regimen:	cyclophosphamide 750 mg/m^2/day IV, days 1 and 22 doxorubicin 50 mg/m^2/day IV, days 1 and 22 vincristine 1 mg IV, days 1, 8, 15, and 22
	Radiation total dose 3000 rad, 10 daily fractions over a 2-week period beginning with day 36

CISCA

Use:	urinary tract, metastatic disease
Regimen:	cyclophosphamide 650 mg/m^2 IV, day 1 doxorubicin 50 mg/m^2 IV, day 1 cisplastin 100 mg/m^2 IV infusion over 2 hours, day 2
	Repeat every 21 days; discontinue doxorubicin when it reaches a total cumulative dose of 450 mg/m^2, then increase cyclophosphamide to 1000 mg/m^2 IV

CMC-High dose

Use:	lung cancer, small cell carcinoma
Regimen:	cyclophosphamide 1000 mg/m^2/day IV, days 1 and 29 methotrexate 15 mg/m^2/day IV twice weekly for 6 weeks lomustine 100 mg/m^2 PO day 1
	If disease responds, proceed to maintenance therapy

CMF

Use:	breast cancer, metastatic or recurrent disease and adjuvant therapy (various regimens)
Regimen:	cyclophosphamide 100 mg/m^2/day PO, days 1

through 14
methotrexate 40 to 60 mg/
m²/day IV, days 1 and 8
fluorouracil 600 mg/m²/
day IV, days 1 and 8

Repeat every 28 days

CMFP

Use:	breast cancer, metastatic disease
Regimen:	cyclophosphamide 100 mg/m²/day PO, days 1 through 14 methotrexate 60 mg/m²/day IV, days 1 and 8 fluorouracil 700 mg/m²/day IV, days 1 and 8 prednisone 40 mg/m²/day PO, days 1 through 14

Repeat every 28 days

CMFVP   (Cooper's Regimen)

Use:	breast cancer, metastatic or recurrent disease
Regimen:	cyclophosphamide 2 mg/kg PO daily methotrexate 0.75 mg/kg IV weekly fluorouracil 12 mg/kg IV weekly vincristine 0.025 mg/kg IV weekly (max. dose 2 mg) prednisone 0.75 mg/kg PO, days 1 through 21, then taper

COP

Use:	non-Hodgkin's lymphoma, lymphomas with favorable histology
Regimen:	cyclophosphamide 800 to 1000 mg/m² IV, day 1 vincristine 1.4 mg/m² IV, day 1 (max. dose 2 mg) prednisone 60 mg/m²/day PO, days 1 through 5

Repeat every 21 days for 6 cycles

COPP OR "C" MOPP

Use:	non-Hodgkin's lymphoma, lymphomas with unfavor-

able histology, Hodgkin's disease

Regimen:	cyclophosphamide 650 mg/m²/day IV, days 1 and 8 vincristine 1.4 mg/m²/day IV, days 1 and 8 (max. dose 2 mg) procarbazine 100 mg/m²/day PO, days 1 through 14 prednisone 40 mg/m²/day PO, days 1 through 14

Repeat every 28 days for 6 cycles

CVP

Use:	non-Hodgkin's lymphoma, lymphomas with favorable histology
Regimen:	cyclophosphamide 400 mg/m²/day PO, days 2 through 6 vincristine 1.4 mg/m² IV, day 1 (max. dose 2 mg) prednisone 100 mg/m²/day PO, days 2 through 6

Repeat every 21 days for 6 cycles

CY-VA-DIC

Use:	soft-tissue sarcomas, adult sarcomas
Regimen:	cyclophosphamide 500 mg/m² IV, day 1 vincristine 1.4 mg/m²/day IV, days 1 and 5 (max. dose 2 mg) doxorubicin 50 mg/m² IV, day 1 dacarbazine 250 mg/m²/day IV, days 1 through 5

Repeat every 21 days

FAC

Use:	breast cancer, metastatic disease
Regimen:	fluorouracil 500 mg/m²/day IV, days 1 and 8 doxorubicin 50 mg/m² IV, day 1 cyclophosphamide 500 mg/m² IV, day 1

Repeat every 3 weeks

FAM

Use: lung cancer, non–oat cell carcinomas

Regimen: fluorouracil 600 mg/m^2/day IV, days 1, 8, 28, and 36
doxorubicin 30 mg/m^2/day IV, days 1 and 28
mitomycin 10 mg/m^2 IV, day 1

Repeat every 8 weeks

Use: gastric carcinoma, advanced disease

Regimen: fluorouracil 600 mg/m^2/day IV, days 1, 8, 29, and 36
doxorubicin 30 mg/m^2/day IV, days 1 and 29
mitomycin 10 mg/m^2 IV, day 1

Repeat every 8 weeks

Use: pancreatic carcinoma, advanced disease

Regimen: fluorouracil 600 mg/m^2/week IV, weeks 1, 2, 5, 6, and 9
doxorubicin 30 mg/m^2/week IV, weeks 1, 5, and 9
mitomycin 10 mg/m^2/week IV, weeks 1 and 9

M-2 Protocol

Use: multiple myeloma

Regimen: vincristine 0.03 mg/kg IV, day 1 (max. dose 2 mg)
carmustine 0.5 mg/kg IV, day 1
cyclophosphamide 10 mg/kg IV, day 1
melphalan 0.25 mg/kg/day PO, days 1 through 4
prednisone 1 mg/kg/day PO, days 1 through 7; then taper to day 21

Repeat every 35 days until progression of the disease

MACC

Use: lung cancer, non–oat cell carcinoma

Regimen: methotrexate 40 mg/m^2 IV, day 1
doxorubicin 40 mg/m^2 IV, day 1
cyclophosphamide 400 mg/m^2 IV, day 1
lomustine 30 mg/m^2 PO, day 1

Repeat every 21 days

MOPP

Use: Hodgkin's disease, induction

Regimen: mechlorethamine 6 mg/m^2/day IV, days 1 and 8
vincristine 2 mg/m^2/day IV, days 1 and 8 (max. dose 2 mg)
procarbazine 100 mg/m^2/day PO, days 1 through 14
prednisone 40 mg/m^2/day PO, days 1 through 14

Repeat every 28 days for 6 cycles

MOPP-LO BLEO

Use: Hodgkin's disease, induction

Regimen: mechlorethamine 6 mg/m^2/day IV, days 1 and 8
vincristine 1.5 mg/m^2/day IV, days 1 and 8 (max. dose 2 mg)
procarbazine 100 mg/m^2/day PO, days 2 through 7 and 9 through 12
prednisone 40 mg/m^2/day PO in divided doses, days 2 through 7 and 9 through 12
bleomycin 2 units/m^2/day IV, days 1 and 8

Repeat monthly for 6 cycles

MPL + PRED (MP)

Use: multiple myeloma

Regimen: melphalan 8 mg/m^2/day PO, days 1 through 14
prednisone 75 mg/m^2/day PO, days 1 through 7

Repeat every 28 days for 6 cycles

MTX + MP

Use: acute lymphocytic leuke-mia, maintenance therapy

Regimen: methotrexate 20 mg/m^2/ week IV

mercaptopurine 50 mg/m^2/ day PO

Continue both drugs until relapse of disease or after 3 years of remission

MTX + MP + CTX

Use: acute lymphocytic leuke-mia, maintenance therapy

Regimen: methotrexate 20 mg/m^2/ week IV

mercaptopurine 50 mg/m^2/ day PO

cyclophosphamide 200 mg/ m^2/week IV

Continue all 3 drugs until relapse of disease or after 3 years of remission

POCC

Use: lung cancer, small cell carcinoma

Regimen: procarbazine 100 mg/m^2/ day PO, days 1 through 14

vincristine 2 mg/day IV, days 1 and 8 (max. dose 2 mg)

cyclophosphamide 600 mg/ m^2/day IV, days 1 and 8

lomustine 60 mg/m^2 PO, day 1

Repeat every 28 days

T-2 Protocol

Use: Ewing's sarcoma

Regimen: **Cycle #1**

Month one

dactinomycin 0.45 mg/m^2/ day IV, days 1 through 5

doxorubicin 20 mg/m^2/day IV, days 20 through 22

radiation days 1 through 21, then 2 weeks rest period

Month two

doxorubicin 20 mg/m^2/day IV, days 8 through 10

vincristine 1.5 to 2 mg/m^2 IV, day 24 (max. dose 2 mg)

cyclophosphamide 1200 mg/m^2 IV, day 24

radiation days 8 through 28

Month three

vincristine 1.5 to 2 mg/m^2/ day IV, days 3, 9, and 15 (max. dose 2 mg)

cyclophosphamide 1200 mg/m^2 IV, day 9

Cycle #2: repeat Cycle #1 without radiation

Cycle #3

Month one

dactinomycin 0.45 mg/m^2/ day IV, days 1 through 5

doxorubicin 20 mg/m^2/day IV, days 20 through 22

Month two

vincristine 1.5 to 2 mg/m^2/ day IV, days 8, 22, and 28 (max. dose 2 mg)

cyclophosphamide 1200 mg/m^2/day IV, days 8 and 22

Month three: no drugs given for 28 days

Cycle #4: repeat Cycle #3

VAC Pulse

Use: soft-tissue sarcomas, rhab-domyosarcoma (pediatric)

Regimen: vincristine 2 mg/m^2/week IV, weeks 1 through 12 (max. dose 2 mg)

dactinomycin 0.015 mg/kg/ day IV for 5 days, weeks 1 and 13. Continue 5-day courses every 3 months for 5 to 6 courses (max. dose 0.5 mg/day)

cyclophosphamide 10 mg/ kg/day IV or PO for 7 days; continue every 6 weeks for 2 years

VAC Standard

Use:

soft-tissue sarcomas, rhab-domyosarcoma, and undif-ferentiated sarcoma

Regimen:

vincristine 2 mg/m^2/week IV, weeks 1 through 12 (max. dose 2 mg)

dactinomycin 0.015 mg/kg/day IV for 5 days, every 3 months for 5 to 6 courses (max. dose 0.5 mg/day)

cyclophosphamide 2.5 mg/kg/day PO; continue daily for 2 years

VBP

Use:

disseminated testicular cancer

Regimen:

vinblastine 0.2 mg/kg/day IV, days 1 and 2 (every 3 weeks for 5 courses)

cisplatin 20 mg/m^2/day IV infusion over 15 minutes, 6 hours after vinblastine, days 1 through 5. Repeat every 3 weeks for 3 courses.

bleomycin 30 units/week IV 6 hours after vinblastine on the second day of each week for 12 weeks to a total cumulative dose of 360 units

VP

Use:

acute lymphocytic leuke-mia, induction

Regimen:

vincristine 2 mg/m^2/week IV for 4 to 6 weeks (max. dose 2 mg)

prednisone 60 mg/m^2/day PO in divided doses for 4 weeks; taper dose weeks 5 through 7

VP-L-Asparaginase

Use:

acute lymphocytic leuke-mia, induction

Regimen:

vincristine 2 mg/m^2/week IV for 4 to 6 weeks (max. dose 2 mg)

prednisone 60 mg/m^2/day PO for 4 to 6 weeks; then taper

L-asparaginase 10,000 units/m^2/day IV for 14 days

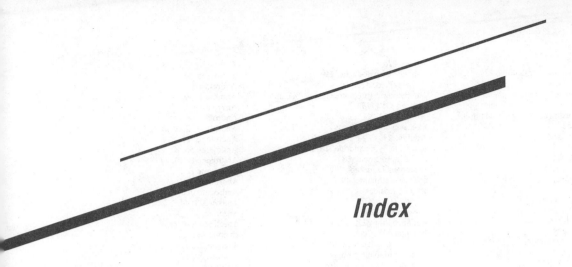

Index